CHILD NEUROLOGY

[There was] . . . a time when theses in medicine could still be beautifully literary, since ignorance about diseases and the human body still required that medicine be an art.
—Kurt Vonnegut, Jr.

Be kind to my mistakes, and live happy!
—Anonymous translator of *Robinson Crusoe* into Italian; cited by Walter De La Mare

CHILD NEUROLOGY

Sixth Edition

Edited by

John H. Menkes, M.D.
Departments of Neurology and Pediatrics
University of California, Los Angeles, UCLA School of Medicine
Department of Pediatric Neurology
Cedars-Sinai Medical Center
Los Angeles, California

and

Harvey B. Sarnat, M.D.
Departments of Pediatric Neurology and Neuropathology
University of Washington School of Medicine
Children's Hospital and Regional Medical Center
Seattle, Washington

with 16 contributing authors

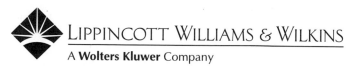

LIPPINCOTT WILLIAMS & WILKINS
A **Wolters Kluwer** Company
Philadelphia · Baltimore · New York · London
Buenos Aires · Hong Kong · Sydney · Tokyo

Acquisitions Editor: Charles W. Mitchell
Developmental Editor: Joyce A. Murphy
Supervising Editor: Mary Ann McLaughlin
Production Editor: Shannon Garza, Silverchair Science + Communications
Manufacturing Manager: Kevin Watt
Cover Designer: Mark Lerner
Compositor: Silverchair Science + Communications
Printer: Courier Westford

© 2000 by LIPPINCOTT WILLIAMS & WILKINS
530 Walnut Street
Philadelphia, PA 19106 USA
LWW.com

Printed in the USA

Library of Congress Cataloging-in-Publication Data
Child neurology / edited by John H. Menkes and Harvey B. Sarnat.-- 6th ed.
    p. ; cm.
  Includes bibliographical references and index.
  ISBN 0-7817-2385-X
  1. Pediatric neurology. I. Title: Child neurology. II. Menkes, John H., 1928- III. Sarnat, Harvey B. IV. Menkes, John H., 1928- Textbook of child neurology.
  [DNLM: 1. Child. 2. Nervous System Diseases--Infant. WS 340 M545 2000]
RJ486 .M45 2000
616.92'8--dc21
                                                                    99-046285

Care has been taken to confirm the accuracy of the information presented and to describe generally accepted practices. However, the authors, editors, and publisher are not responsible for errors or omissions or for any consequences from application of the information in this book and make no warranty, expressed or implied, with respect to the currency, completeness, or accuracy of the contents of the publication. Application of this information in a particular situation remains the professional responsibility of the practitioner.

The authors, editors, and publisher have exerted every effort to ensure that drug selection and dosage set forth in this text are in accordance with current recommendations and practice at the time of publication. However, in view of ongoing research, changes in government regulations, and the constant flow of information relating to drug therapy and drug reactions, the reader is urged to check the package insert for each drug for any change in indications and dosage and for added warnings and precautions. This is particularly important when the recommended agent is a new or infrequently employed drug.

Some drugs and medical devices presented in this publication have Food and Drug Administration (FDA) clearance for limited use in restricted research settings. It is the responsibility of health care providers to ascertain the FDA status of each drug or device planned for use in their clinical practice.

10 9 8 7 6 5 4 3 2 1

To Joan, my wife, for giving me the pleasure of her company
and
To my teachers:
B.G.B.
(1901–1988)
S.S.G.
A.S.N.
S.C.
D.B.C.
(1913–1992)

—J.H.M.

To my wife, Laura

—H.B.S

Contents

Contributing Authors

Richard G. Ellenbogen, M.D.
Associate Professor
Department of Neurological Surgery
University of Washington School of Medicine
Children's Hospital and Regional Medical Center
4800 Sand Point Way, NE
Seattle, Washington 98105

Rena E. Falk, M.D.
Professor
Department of Pediatrics
University of California, Los Angeles, UCLA
School of Medicine
Steven Spielberg Pediatric Research Center
Cedars-Sinai Medical Center
8700 Beverly Boulevard
Los Angeles, California 90048

Burton W. Fink, M.D.
Clinical Professor
Department of Pediatrics
University of California, Los Angeles, UCLA
School of Medicine
8700 Beverly Boulevard
Los Angeles, California 90048

William D. Graf, M.D.
Associate Professor
Departments of Pediatrics and Neurology
University of Washington School of Medicine
Children's Hospital and Regional Medical Center
4800 Sand Point Way, NE
Seattle, Washington 98105

Carole G. H. Hurvitz, M.D.
Clinical Professor
Department of Pediatrics
University of California, Los Angeles, Center
for the Health Sciences
Director
Department of Pediatric Hematology and
Oncology
Cedars-Sinai Medical Center
8700 Beverly Boulevard, Room 4310
Los Angeles, California 90048

Carol B. Hyman, M.D.
Associate Professor
Department of Pediatrics
University of Southern California School of
Medicine
Children's Hospital of Los Angeles
Cedars-Sinai Medical Center
8700 Beverly Boulevard, #4310
Los Angeles, California 90048

Victor Israele, M.D.
Department of Pediatrics
Fundación Centro de Estudios Infectiológicos
(FUNCEI)
Castex 3345
Piso 5B
Buenos Aires, Argentina 1425

Stanley C. Jordan, M.D.
Professor
Department of Pediatrics
University of California, Los Angeles,
UCLA School of Medicine
Director
Department of Pediatric Nephrology and
Transplant Immunology
Cedars-Sinai Medical Center
8700 Beverly Boulevard
Los Angeles, California 90048

Marcel Kinsbourne, M.D.
Professor
Department of Cognitive Studies
Tufts University
11 Miner Hall
Medford, Massachusetts 02155

Bernard L. Maria, M.D., M.B.A.
Professor
Department of Pediatrics
University of Florida College
of Medicine
1600 Archer Road
Gainesville, Florida 32610

John H. Menkes, M.D.
Professor Emeritus
Departments of Neurology and Pediatrics
University of California, Los Angeles,
  UCLA School of Medicine
Department of Pediatric Neurology
Cedars-Sinai Medical Center
8700 Beverly Boulevard
Los Angeles, California 90048

Franklin G. Moser, M.D.
Director
Department of Clinical and Interventional
  Neuroradiology
Cedars-Sinai Medical Center
8700 Beverly Boulevard
Los Angeles, California 90048

Robert Rust, M.A., M.D.
Professor
Department of Neurology
University of Virginia School of Medicine
Box 394
Charlottesville, Virginia 22908

Raman Sankar, M.D., Ph.D.
Associate Professor
Departments of Neurology and Pediatrics
University of California, Los Angeles, UCLA
  School of Medicine
Mattel Children's Hospital at UCLA
Los Angeles, California 90095

Harvey B. Sarnat, M.D., F.R.C.P.C.
Professor
Departments of Pediatric Neurology and Neu-
  ropathology
University of Washington School of Medicine
Children's Hospital and Regional Medical Center
4800 Sand Point Way, NE
Seattle, Washington 98105

Elaine Tuomanen, M.D.
Professor
Department of Pediatrics
University of Tennessee, Memphis, College of
  Medicine
Member and Chair
Department of Infectious Diseases
St. Jude Children's Research Hospital
332 N. Lauderdale Street
Memphis, Tennessee 38105

Frederick Watanabe, M.D.
Assistant Professor
Department of Pediatrics
University of California, Los Angeles,
  UCLA School of Medicine
Center for Liver Diseases and
  Transplantation
Cedars-Sinai Medical Center
8700 Beverly Boulevard
Los Angeles, California 90048

Marvin Lee Weil, M.D.
Professor Emeritus
Departments of Pediatrics and Neurology
University of California, Los Angeles,
  UCLA School of Medicine
Los Angeles, California 90048
and
Academic Visitor
Department of Biochemistry
University of Oxford
82 Thames Street
Oxford, England OX1 1SU

Preface to the Sixth Edition

A text such as this one, which strives to blend the neurosciences with clinical pediatric neurology, must be prepared to adapt itself to the continuous advances in both fields. It must be ready to render the increasing complexity of molecular biology, genetics, neurochemistry, neurophysiology, and neuropathology into terms that are readily apprehended by the clinician and lead him or her to understand how the innumerable developments in the various areas of research impact on the diagnosis, care, and treatment of patients.

My predecessors had an easier task. Frank R. Ford, under whose tutelage I had the good fortune to learn my basic neurology, wrote what for many years was the standard text of pediatric neurology, *Diseases of the Nervous System in Infancy, Childhood and Adolescence*. Even so, I recall that in 1954 he said to me on inscribing my text, "Doctor, there are many things in here I don't know much about." Thomas Farmer, Patrick Bray, and many others have been the sole authors of excellent textbooks of pediatric neurology, but these texts were also published decades ago, and now it is no longer possible for a single person to write a text that is both comprehensive and accurate. The one exception is Jean Aicardi's new text, *Diseases of the Nervous System in Childhood*, a tour de force that somehow defies the laws of gravity.

To obtain a broader point of view, I have therefore called on Harvey B. Sarnat and his expertise in neuroembryology, muscle diseases, and neonatal neurology to assist me as coeditor of this edition. The list of authors has also been enlarged, with contributors in infectious diseases, cytogenetics, neuroimaging, neuroimmunology, and neuro-oncology. As before, I have enlisted experts in pediatric cardiology, pediatric hematology and oncology, pediatric nephrology, and organ transplantation to help me with the chapter that deals with the neurologic manifestations of systemic disease. Marcel Kinsbourne and William D. Graf have rewritten the chapter that deals with disorders of mental development. Theirs was an unenviable task.

Errors of omission and commission are inevitable in a text of this breadth and size. What will also be inevitable is a failure to keep the text abreast of the latest developments: a lag period of at least 1 year between completion of scientific work and its citation in this text is the best we could do. At the same time, we have retained and sometimes even enlarged the number of classic citations. Too often, younger practitioners tend to forget the names and contributions of some of the pioneers in our field. We have taken care that these were not cast aside in the process of updating the text.

My thanks also go to William R. Wilcox and Andre Vanderhal of the Department of Pediatrics, Cedars-Sinai Medical Center, and the staff of Cedars-Sinai Medical Library for their assistance in preparing the new edition.

John H. Menkes, M.D.

Preface to the First Edition

Even in a textbook, prefaces are written not to be read but rather to blunt inevitable criticisms. One must therefore first ask, why, in view of the existence of several first-rate pediatric neurology texts, was this book ever written. The main excuse for becoming involved in such an undertaking, and for imposing another book upon an already overwhelmed medical audience, is the hope of being able to offer a new viewpoint of the field. More than any other branch of clinical neurology, pediatric neurology has felt the impact of the many recent advances in the neurosciences. Their magnitude becomes evident when the neurologic literature of the last century is read. At that time, clinical descriptions achieved a degree of clarity and conciseness, which has not been improved upon, and which at present is only rarely equaled. Yet the reader who finds the explanation of Tay-Sachs disease* offered during the last years of the nineteenth century must experience a sense of achievement at the great strides made during a relatively brief historical period. However, at the same time, one cannot but wonder how many of our "explanations" accepted and taught today, will make as little sense fifty years hence.

It is the aim of this text to incorporate some of the knowledge derived from the basic neurologic sciences into the clinical evaluation and management of the child with neurologic disease. Obviously, this can only be done to a limited extent. For some conditions the basic sciences have not yet offered any help, while for others, available experimental data only provide tangential information. Even when biochemical or physiologic information is pertinent to the conditions under discussion, their full presentation has been avoided, for to do so with any degree of completeness would require an extensive review of several scientific disciplines, which would go far beyond the intent of the text. The author and his colleagues have therefore chosen to review only aspects of the neurologic sciences with immediate clinical impact, and to refer the reader to the literature for some of the remaining information. They have also deemed it appropriate *not* to include a section on the neurologic examination of children. This subject is extremely well presented by R. S. Paine and T. E. Oppe, in *The Neurologic Examination of Children*,** a work everyone seriously interested in pediatric neurology should read.

In covering the field, extensive use of literature references has been made. These generally serve one or more of the following purposes:

(1) A classic or early description of the condition.
(2) Background information pertaining to the relevant neurologic sciences.
(3) A current review of the condition.
(4) In the case of some of the rarer clinical entities, the presentation of several key references was preferred to a brief and obviously inadequate summary.

It is hoped that this approach will serve to keep the text reasonably compact, yet allow it to be used as a guide for further reading.

John H. Menkes, M.D.
Los Angeles, California

---

*Namely, "an inherited weakness of the central nervous system, especially of the ganglion cells, and a premature degeneration due to exhaustion caused by this."
**London, Wm. Heinemann, 1966.

Regarding every disease now incurable we may entertain the hope—faint it may be with respect to some, stronger in the case of others—that our powerlessness may not be permanent, and that we, or those who come after us, may be able to speak in very different terms.
—W. R. Gowers, 1879

Introduction

Neurologic Examination of the Child and Infant

John H. Menkes, °Harvey B. Sarnat, and †Franklin G. Moser

Departments of Neurology and Pediatrics, University of California, Los Angeles, UCLA School of Medicine, and Department of Pediatric Neurology, Cedars-Sinai Medical Center, Los Angeles, California 90048; °Departments of Pediatric Neurology and Neuropathology, University of Washington School of Medicine, and Children's Hospital and Regional Medical Center, Seattle, Washington 98105; and †Department of Clinical and Interventional Neuroradiology, Cedars-Sinai Medical Center, Los Angeles, CA 90048

The ever-increasing sophistication and accuracy of neurodiagnostic procedures might cause younger physicians to view the neurologic examination of the pediatric patient as obsolete, and, like cardiac auscultation, a nostalgic ceremony engaged in by physicians trained before magnetic resonance imaging (MRI) and DNA hybridization (1). This is not how we view it. Excessive reliance on diagnostic procedures at the expense of an organized plan of approach, the "let's order a computed tomographic scan and an electroencephalogram and then take a look at the kid" attitude, not only has been responsible for the depersonalization of neurologic care, and the escalation of its costs, but also has made the analysis of neurologic problems unduly complex for the pediatrician or general practitioner. For these reasons, a presentation of some of the techniques of neurologic examination is still in order.

The pediatric neurologist who, through experience, has individualized the examination will find little new in this section, which was written with the pediatrician and general neurologist in mind. The pediatrician will find the section on the neurologic examination helpful; the general neurologist, who at times is called on to consult on an infant not much larger than the palm of the hand, may benefit from the section on the neurologic examination of the infant.

At its best, the neurologic evaluation is a challenge in logical deduction. It requires a clear plan at each step with the goal of answering the following questions:

1. Does the child have a neurologic disorder?
2. If so, where is the site of the lesion, or, as so often is the case in pediatric neurology, does it involve all parts of the brain to an equal degree?
3. What pathologic lesions are most likely to produce lesions at this site or sites? The course of the illness, be it acute, subacute, static, or remitting, may provide a clue to the nature of the disease process.

It is at this point, and only at this point, that the physician draws up a differential diagnosis and calls on neurodiagnostic procedures to help decide which of the suspected conditions is the most likely.

If this systematic approach is followed, useless diagnostic procedures are avoided. For instance, an assay for arylsulfatase to exclude metachromatic leukodystrophy is inappropriate in a neurologic disorder that is clearly static. Similarly, neither computed tomography (CT) scans nor MRI of the brain assist materially in the differential diagnosis of a lower motor neuron disease.

NEUROLOGIC HISTORY

An accurate history, obtained from one or more members of the family, is often the most vital part of the neurologic evaluation. Additionally, if properly questioned, a child older than 3 to 5 years might provide information that not only is valuable, but may be more reliable than that related by his or her parents. In taking a history from a youngster, the physician must learn not to ask leading questions, and not to phrase them to obtain yes or no answers. The physician also must be responsive to the youngster's mood, and cease taking a history as soon as fatigue or restlessness becomes evident. In a younger child, or one with a limited attention span, the salient points of the history are best secured at the onset of the evaluation. The history is followed by the neurologic examination, and, finally, by a second, more extensive review of the history.

In the assessment of a neurologic problem, an accurate review of the presenting illness is important. This is particularly the case in the youngster with headaches, seizures, or other types of recurrent disease, and for the youngster with a learning disability or an attention deficit disorder. In such patients, the history, particularly its social and environmental aspects, can be extensive enough to require more than one appointment.

A review of the developmental history necessitates a survey of antenatal, perinatal, and postnatal development. This includes questioning the mother about the length of the pregnancy, any complications, including intercurrent infections, and drug intake. The mother who is concerned about her youngster may already have reviewed her pregnancy many times and may well provide much irrelevant information. For instance, an accident occurring during the second trimester is hardly the explanation for a meningomyelocele. The physician might well interrupt the questioning to reassure the mother that this event was not responsible for the child's neurologic defect.

A review of the perinatal events is always in order. As a rule, the youngster who has had an uncomplicated neonatal period and was discharged with the mother will not have sustained perinatal asphyxia, even though the infant might have had low Apgar scores or passage of meconium. The physician should not forget to obtain some information about the feeding history.

Many children who later present with delayed development have had feeding problems, notably regurgitation, excessive *colic*, or frequent formula changes. A history of abnormal sleeping habits is also not unusual in the brain-damaged youngster.

The developmental milestones must always be recorded. Most mothers recall these and can compare one youngster with the siblings. Failure to remember any of the milestones is unusual, even in the lower socioeconomic classes; it suggests a postpartum depression.

A system review focuses on the major childhood illnesses, immunizations, and injuries. Recurrent injuries suggest hyperactivity, impaired coordination, or poor impulse control.

The family history is relevant in some of the neurologic disorders. The physician should remember that most neurodegenerative disorders are transmitted as a recessive gene, and that questions about the health of siblings and the presence of consanguinity are in order. On the other hand, some of the epilepsies or migraine headaches tend to be transmitted as dominant traits; in fact, in children experiencing migraine headaches, a history of migraine in a first-degree relative can almost always be elicited.

GENERAL PHYSICAL EXAMINATION

The child's height, weight, blood pressure, and head circumference must always be measured and recorded. The youngster should be undressed by the parents, with the physician absent.

The physician should note the general appearance of the child, in particular the facial configuration and the presence of any dysmorphic features. Cutaneous lesions such as café au lait spots, angiomas, or areas of depigmentation are clues to the presence of phakomatoses. The condition of the teeth provides information about antenatal defects or kernicterus. The location of the hair whorl and the appearance of the palmar creases should always be noted. Abnormalities of whorl patterns can indicate the presence of cerebral malformations (2). The quality of the scalp hair, eyebrows, and nails also should be taken into account. It is important to inspect the midline of the neck, back, and pilonidal area for any defects, particularly for small dimples that might indicate the presence of a dermoid sinus tract. Comparison of the size of the thumb nails and their convexity might disclose a growth disturbance, a frequent accompaniment to a hemiparesis. Examination of chest, heart, and abdomen and palpation of the femoral pulses should always be part of the general physical examination. Finally, the presence of an unusual body odor may offer a clue to a metabolic disorder.

NEUROLOGIC EXAMINATION OF THE CHILD

In addition to the standard instruments used in neurologic examination, the following have been found useful: a tennis ball; a few small toys, including a toy car that can be used to assess fine motor coordination; a bell; and some object that attracts the child's attention (e.g., a pinwheel). A flashlight with a rubber adapter for transillumination is still used; it is cheaper and quicker than a CT scan or an ultrasound and often provides the same information. Most pediatric neurologists do not wear white coats.

In most intellectually healthy school-aged children, the general physical and neurologic examinations can be performed in the same manner as for adults, except that their more uncomfortable aspects, such as funduscopic examination, corneal and gag reflexes, and sensory testing, should be postponed until the end.

In younger children, the neurologic examination is a catch-as-catch-can procedure, with a considerable amount of information revealed by the youngster's play activities, including the child's dominant handedness and the presence of cerebellar deficits, a hemiparesis, and perhaps even a visual field defect.

The toddler is more difficult to examine. The toddler is best approached by seating the child in the mother's or father's lap, and talking to the child. Because toddlers are fearful of strangers, the physician must first observe the youngster, and defer touching him or her until some degree of rapport has been established. Offering a small, interesting toy may bridge the gap. In any case, the physician must be patient and wait for the youngster to make the first approach. Once frightened, most toddlers are difficult to reassure and are lost for the remainder of the examination.

SKULL

The general appearance of the skull can suggest the presence of macrocephaly, microcephaly, or craniosynostosis. Prominence of the venous pattern might accompany increased intracranial pressure. Flattening of the occiput is seen in many developmentally delayed youngsters. Conversely, occipital prominence can indicate the Dandy-Walker syndrome. Biparietal enlargement suggests the presence of subdural hematomas and should raise the suspicion of child abuse. Palpation of the skull can disclose ridging of the sutures, as occurs in craniosynostosis. Biparietal foramina are usually benign and are often transmitted as a dominant trait (3). Prominence of the metopic suture is seen in some youngsters with developmental malformations. Percussion of the skull can reveal areas of tenderness resulting from localized osteomyelitis, an indication of an underlying brain abscess. Macewen (*cracked pot*) sign accompanies the separation of sutures and reflects increased intracranial pressure.

If accurately measured, serial head circumferences continue to be one of the most valuable parameters for assessing the presence of hydrocephalus or microcephaly. After multiple measurements are made with a good cloth or steel tape to ensure that the maximum circumference has been obtained, the value should be recorded on a head growth chart (Fig. I.1). Delayed head growth, particularly with evidence of arrest or slowing of head growth, reflects impaired brain growth from a variety of causes. Scalloping of the temporal fossae frequently accompanies microcephaly and suggests underdeveloped frontal and temporal lobes. Occasionally, one encounters a youngster, usually a girl, with a head circumference at or below the third percentile, whose somatic measurements are commensurate, and whose intellectual development is normal.

Palpation of the anterior fontanelle provides a simple way of estimating intracranial pressure. Normally, the fontanelle is slightly depressed and the pulsations are hardly felt. Auscultation

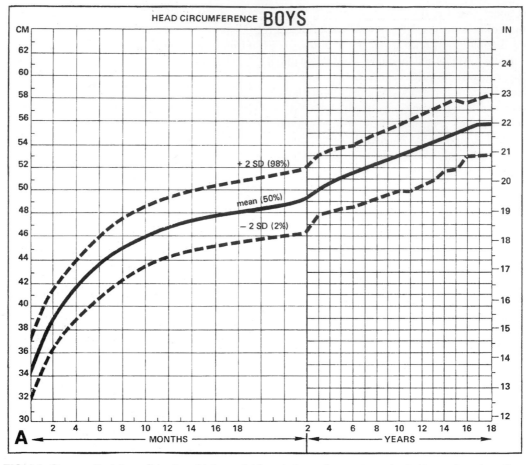

FIG. I.1. Composite international and interracial head circumference graph. **A:** Boys. *(continued)*

of the skull using a bell stethoscope with the child in the erect position is performed over six standard listening points: both globes, the temporal fossae, and the retroauricular or mastoid regions. In all cases, conduction of a cardiac murmur should be excluded. Spontaneous intracranial bruits are common in children. These are augmented by contralateral carotid compression. Wadia and Monckton (4) heard unilateral or bilateral bruits in 60% of 4- to 5-year-old children, 10% of 10-year-old children, and 45% of 15- to 16-year-old adolescents. Intracranial bruits are heard in more than 80% of patients with angiomas. Unlike benign bruits, they are accompanied by a thrill and are much louder and harsher. Intracranial bruits are heard

in a variety of other conditions characterized by increased cerebral blood flow. These include anemia, thyrotoxicosis, and meningitis. Bruits also accompany hydrocephalus and some (not necessarily vascular) intracranial tumors. The technique and the history of auscultation for intracranial bruits is reviewed by Mackenzie (5).

Cranial Nerves

Olfactory Nerve

The olfactory nerve is only rarely assessed. Loss of olfactory nerve function can follow a head injury with fracture of the cribriform plate. Nerve function also can be lost when a tumor

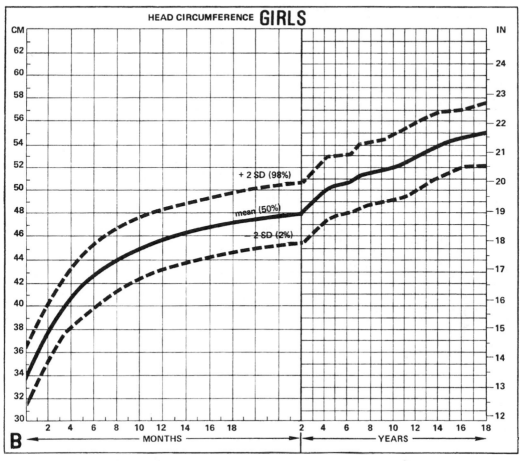

HEAD CIRCUMFERENCE GIRLS

FIG. I.1. *Continued.* **B:** Girls. SD, standard deviation. (Courtesy of Dr. G. Nellhaus, Napa V. A. Hospital, Napa, CA.)

involves the olfactory bulbs. Olfactory sensation as transmitted by the olfactory nerve is not functional in the newborn, but is present by 5 to 7 months of age. By contrast, newborns do respond to inhalation of irritants, such as ammonia or vinegar, as the reflex is transmitted by the trigeminal nerve; hence, this reflex is preserved in the infant with arhinencephaly (6).

Optic Nerve

Much can be learned from a funduscopic examination, and more time is often spent with this than with any other part of the neurologic examination. With assistance from the parent or nurse, it is possible to examine even the most uncooperative youngster. If necessary, a mydriatic such as 2.5% or 10.0% phenylephrine (Neo-Synephrine) or 1% cyclopentolate (Cyclogyl) is used. Particular attention is paid to the optic discs, maculae, and appearance of the retina. In infants, the optic disc is normally pale and gray, an appearance similar to optic atrophy in later life. Optic nerve hypoplasia can be diagnosed if the discs are less than one-half normal size. The macular light reflex is absent until approximately 4 months of age. Premature and newborn infants have incompletely developed uveal pigment, resulting in a pale appearance of the fundus and a clear view of the choroidal blood vessels. Obliteration of the disc margins and absent pulsations of the central veins are the earliest and most important indications for papilledema. The differential diagnosis of papilledema is reviewed in Chapter 10.

Retinal hemorrhages are seen in one-third of vaginally delivered newborns. They are usually small and multiple, and their presence does not necessarily indicate intracranial bleeding. Persistence of the hyaloid artery is common in premature infants and is seen in approximately 3% of full-term infants. Chorioretinitis suggests an intrauterine infection. Less extensive and grouped pigmentation resembling the footprints of an animal (*bear tracks*) represents a harmless and common anomaly. This condition must be distinguished from the more extensive pigmentation seen in retinitis pigmentosa.

Visual acuity can be tested in the older child by standard means. In the toddler, an approximation can be obtained by observing him or her at play or by offering objects of varying sizes. Optokinetic nystagmus can be elicited by rotating a striped drum or by drawing a strip of cloth with black and white squares in front of the child's eyes. The presence of optokinetic nystagmus confirms cortical vision; its absence, however, is inconclusive. Unilateral optokinetic nystagmus suggests the presence of hemianopia. The visual fields can be assessed in toddlers and in infants younger than 12 months of age. The baby is placed in the mother's lap, and the physician is seated in front of them, using a small toy to attract the baby's attention. An assistant standing in back of the infant brings another object into the field of vision, and the point at which the infant's eyes or head turns toward the object is noted.

The blink reflex, closure of the eyelids when an object is suddenly moved toward the eyes, is often used to determine the presence of functional vision in small infants. The reflex is absent in the newborn and does not appear until 3 or 4 months of age. It is present in approximately one-half of healthy 5-month-old infants and should be present in all infants by 1 year of age (7).

Oculomotor, Trochlear, and Abducens Nerves: Extraocular Movements

The physician notes the position of the eyes at rest. Noting the points of reflection of a flashlight assists in detecting a nonparallel alignment of the eyes. Paralysis of the oculomotor nerve results in lateral and slightly downward deviation of the affected eye. Paralysis of the abducens nerve produces a medial deviation of the affected eye, whereas paralysis of the trochlear nerve produces little change at rest. The *setting sun* sign, a forced downward deviation of the eyes at rest with paresis of upward gaze, is an indication of increased intracranial pressure, in particular pressure on the quadrigeminal plate causing impairment of the vertical gaze centers. This phenomenon also can be elicited in healthy infants younger than 4 weeks of age by suddenly changing the position of the head, and in infants up to 20, or even 40, weeks of age by removing a bright light that had been placed in front of their eyes (8). Downward deviation of the eyes, skew deviation, and intermittent opsoclonus (irregular, chaotic oscillations of the eyes in horizontal, vertical, or oblique directions) may be noted transiently in healthy newborns (9).

Ocular bobbing refers to abnormal spontaneous vertical eye movements. In its most typical appearance, it consists of intermittent, often conjugate, fast downward movement of the eyes followed by, after a brief tonic interval, a slower return to the primary position (10). It is generally seen with pontine pathology, but also can be encountered in encephalitis, and in some metabolic encephalopathies. It probably reflects residual eye movements of patients who have severe limitations of horizontal and vertical eye movements.

The doll's-eye phenomenon refers to the apparent turning of the eyes to the opposite direction in response to rotation of the head. It is seen in healthy newborns, in coma, and whenever optic fixation is impaired.

The size of the pupils, their reactivity to light, and accommodation and convergence are noted. In infants younger than 30 weeks' gestation, pupils are large and no response to light occurs. After 32 weeks' gestation, an absent light response is abnormal (11).

The association of meiosis, enophthalmos, ptosis, and lack of sweating on the ipsilateral side of the face was first described in 1869 and is known as Horner syndrome (12). The condition can

Rt. sup. rectus III

Lt. inf. oblique III

Rt. inf. oblique III

Lt. sup. rectus III

RIGHT LATERAL GAZE

LEFT LATERAL GAZE

Rt. ext. rectus VI

Lt. medial rectus III

Rt. medial rectus III

Lt. ext. rectus VI

RIGHT DOWNWARD GAZE

LEFT DOWNWARD GAZE

FIG. I.2. Extraocular muscles involved in the various eye movements. Ext., exterior; inf., inferior; Lt., left; Rt., right; sup., superior. (Adapted from Farmer TW. *Pediatric neurology*, 3rd ed, New York: Harper & Row, 1983. With permission.)

result from damage to the cervical sympathetic nerves when it accompanies brachial plexus injuries, or can be congenital, being transmitted as an autosomal dominant condition (13). A slight degree of anisocoria is not unusual, particularly in infants and small children. Anisocoria also has been noted to be transmitted as an autosomal dominant trait.

Eye movements are examined by having the child follow an object while the mother holds the child's head. If he or she permits it, the movement of each eye is examined separately while the other one is kept covered. The actions of the extraocular muscles are depicted in Figure I.2. At birth, doll's-eye movements are normally elicitable, but little or no conjugation occurs. Shortly after birth, the eyes become conjugated, and by 2 weeks of age, the infant moves the eyes toward light and fixates. Following movements are complete in all directions by approximately 4 months of age, and acoustically elicited eye movements appear at 5 months of age (14). Depth perception using solely binocular cues appears by 24 months of age along with stable binocular alignment and optokinetic nystagmus.

Strabismus owing to muscular imbalance can be differentiated from a paralytic strabismus. In the former, the ocular movements are concomitant and full. In the latter, the disassociation of the eyes increases when the eyes enter the field of action of the paralyzed muscle. In abducens nerve palsies, failure of abduction is readily demonstrable. The combination of defective adduction and elevation with outward and downward displacement of the eye suggests a third nerve palsy. Internuclear ophthalmoplegia (syndrome of the median longitudinal fasciculus) in its classical appearance consists of paralysis of adduction of the contralateral eye on lateral gaze, with nystagmus of the abducting eye and preservation of convergence. Ptosis and a large pupil with impaired constriction to light also can be present. Unilateral or bilateral congenital ptosis is relatively common, being transmitted as a dominant trait in some instances (15). In others, reflex elevation or closure of the ptotic lid occurs in response to swallowing or movements of the jaw. Elevation has been termed the *Marcus Gunn sign*, and closure, the *reverse Marcus Gunn sign*. In instances of trochlear nerve palsy, the eye fails to move down when adducted. This defect is often accompanied by a head tilt.

In describing the presence of nystagmus, the physician should note the position of the eyes that produces the greatest amplitude of the nystagmus, the direction of the fast movement, and the quality or speed of the nystagmus. When the nystagmus is of small amplitude, it might be noted only on funduscopic examination.

Trigeminal Nerve

The action of the temporalis and masseter muscles is noted. Unilateral lesions of the trigeminal nerve result in a deviation of the jaw to the paralytic side and atrophy of the temporalis muscle. The jaw jerk can be elicited by placing one's finger below the lower lip of the slightly open mouth and tapping downward. An absent jaw jerk is rarely significant; upper motor neuron lesions above the level of the pons exaggerate the reflex.

The corneal reflex tests the intactness of the ophthalmic branch of the trigeminal nerve. A defect should be suspected when spontaneous blinking on one side is slower and less complete. The frequency of blinking increases with maturation and decreases in toxic illnesses.

Facial Nerve

Impaired motor function is indicated by facial asymmetry. Involvement of the facial nucleus or the nerve produces a lower motor neuron weakness in which upper and lower parts of the face are paralyzed. Normal wrinkling of the forehead is impaired, and the eye either cannot be closed or can be opened readily by the examiner. Weakness of the face can be obvious at rest and is accentuated when the child laughs or cries. When facial weakness is caused by corticobulbar involvement (upper motor neuron facial weakness), the musculature of the upper part of the face is spared. Although this sparing was believed to reflect bilateral enervation of the upper facial motor neurons, it now appears that upper facial motor neurons receive little direct cortical input, whereas lower facial neurons do (16).

Weakness is accentuated with volitional movements, but disappears when the child laughs or cries. The converse, upper motor facial weakness associated with emotion and not evident on volitional movements, can be seen in thalamic lesions (17). The McCarthy reflex, ipsilateral blinking produced by tapping the supraorbital region, is diminished or absent in lower motor neuron facial weakness. Like the palpebral reflex, bilateral blinking induced by tapping the root of the nose, it can be exaggerated by upper motor neuron lesions.

An isolated weakness of the depressor of the corner of the mouth (depressor anguli oris) is relatively common in children. It results in a failure to pull the affected side of the mouth backward and downward when crying.

The sense of taste from the anterior two-thirds of the tongue is conveyed by the chorda tympani. Taste can be tested in children by applying solutions of sugar or salt to the previously dried and protruded tongue by cotton-tipped applicator sticks, making certain that the child does not withdraw the tongue into the mouth.

Cochlear and Vestibular Nerves

Hearing can be tested in the younger child by observing the child's response to a bell. Small infants become alert to sound; the ability to turn the eyes to the direction of the sound becomes evident by 7 to 8 weeks of age, and turning with eyes and head appears by approximately 3 to 4 months of age. Hearing is tested in older children by asking them to repeat a whispered word or number. For more accurate evaluation of hearing, audiometry or brainstem auditory-evoked potentials are necessary.

Vestibular function can be assessed easily in infants or small children by holding the youngster vertically and facing the examiner, then turning the child several times in a full circle. Clockwise and counterclockwise rotations are performed. The direction and amplitude of the quick and slow movements of the eye are noted. The healthy infant demonstrates full deviation of the eyes in the direction toward which the examiner is rotating, with the quick phase of the nystagmus backward. When rotation ceases, these directions are reversed. This test has been found to be valuable in a newborn suspected of perinatal asphyxia, with an abnormal response suggesting impaired brainstem function between the vestibular and the oculomotor nuclei.

Glossopharyngeal and Vagus Nerves

Asymmetry of the resting uvula and palate and failure to elevate the palate during phonation indicate impaired vagal motor function. When upper or lower motor neuron involvement of the vagus nerve exists, the uvula deviates toward the unaffected side, and with movement, the palate is drawn away from the affected side.

The gag reflex tests the afferent and efferent portions of the vagus. This reflex is absent in approximately one-third of healthy individuals (18). Testing taste over the posterior part of the tongue is extremely difficult and, in some opinions, generally not worth the effort.

Spinal Accessory Nerve

Testing the sternocleidomastoid muscle can be done readily by having the child rotate his or her head against resistance.

Hypoglossal Nerve

The position of the tongue at rest should be noted with the mouth open. The tongue deviates toward the paretic side. Fasciculations are seen as small depressions that appear and disappear quickly at irregular intervals. They are most readily distinguished on the underside of the tongue. Their presence cannot be determined with any reliability if the youngster is crying.

Motor System

The child's station (i.e., posture while standing) can usually be discerned before the start of the examination. Similarly, the walking and running gaits can be seen by playing with the youngster and asking him or her to retrieve a ball and run outside of the examining room. In the course of such an informal examination, sufficient information can be obtained so that the formal testing of muscle strength is only confirmatory.

Evaluation of the motor system in a school-aged child can be done in a formal manner.

Examination of selected proximal and distal muscles of the upper and lower extremities is usually sufficient. A book originally published by the Medical Research Council is invaluable for this purpose (19): Muscle strength is graded from 0 to 5. The following grading system has been suggested:

0. No muscle contraction
1. Flicker or trace of contraction
2. Active movement with gravity eliminated
3. Active movement against gravity
4. Active movement against gravity and resistance
5. Normal power

Muscle tone is examined by manipulating the major joints and determining the degree of resistance. In toddlers or infants, inequalities of tone to pronation and supination of the wrist, flexion and extension of the elbow, and dorsi and plantar flexion of the ankle have been found to provide more information than assessment of muscle strength or reflexes.

A sensitive test for hypotonia of the upper extremities is the pronator sign, in which the hand on the hypotonic side hyperpronates to palm outward as the arms are raised over the head. Additionally, the elbow may flex (Fig. I.3). In the lower extremities, weakness of the flexors of the knee can readily be tested by having the child lie prone and asking the child to maintain his or her legs in flexion at right angles at the knee (Barré sign).

Coordination

Coordination can be tested by applying specific tests for cerebellar function, such as having the youngster reach for and manipulate toys. One may be reluctant to use marbles for this purpose for fear that a small child might swallow them. Ataxia with tremor of the extremities can be demonstrated in the older child on finger-to-nose and heel-to-shin testing. Accentuation of the tremor as the extremity approaches the target is characteristic of cerebellar dysfunction (intention tremor). In the finger-to-nose test, the arm must be maintained abducted at the shoulder. The examiner can discover minor abnor-

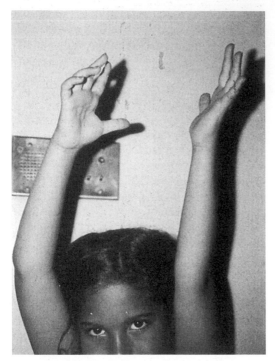

FIG. I.3. The pronator sign. Weakness of the right upper extremity in a girl with a Brown-Séquard syndrome after spinal cord trauma.

malities by moving the finger to a different place each time. The ability to perform rapidly alternating movements can be assessed by having the child repeatedly pat the examiner's hand, or by having the child perform rapid pronation and supination of the hands. In the lower extremities, rapid tapping of the foot serves a similar purpose. Pyramidal and extrapyramidal lesions slow rapid succession movements, but leave intact the execution of each stage of the movement so that no true dissociation occurs. The heel-to-shin test is not an easy task for many youngsters to comprehend, and performance must be interpreted with regard to the child's age and level of intelligence.

A variety of involuntary movements can be noted in the course of the examination. They may be seen when the child walks or is engaged in various purposeful acts.

Athetosis indicates an instability of posture, with slow swings of movement most marked in the distal portions of the limbs. The movements fluctuate between two extremes of posture in the hand, one of hyperextension of the fingers with pronation and flexion of the wrist and supination of the forearm, and the other of intense flexion and adduction of the fingers and wrist and pronation of the forearm.

Choreiform movements refer to more rapid and jerky movements similar in their range to the athetoid movements, but so fluid and continuous that the two extremes of posture are no longer evident (20). They commonly involve the muscles of the face, tongue, and proximal portions of the limbs. In children, athetosis and choreiform movements occur far more frequently as associated, rather than as isolated, phenomena.

Dystonia is characterized by fixation or relative fixation in one of the athetotic postures. When dystonia results from perinatal asphyxia, it is nearly always accompanied by other involuntary movements. The other manifestations of basal ganglia disorder (tremors and myoclonus) are usually less apparent. Tremors are rhythmic alterations in movement, whereas myoclonus is a relatively unpredictable contraction of one or more muscle groups. It can be precipitated by a variety of stimuli, particularly sudden changes in position, or by the start of voluntary movements. In addition to these movement disorders, children with dystonic cerebral palsy also exhibit sudden increases in muscle tone, often precipitated by attempts at voluntary movement (*tension*). These movements must be distinguished from seizures.

Small, choreiformlike movements are common in the healthy infant. They are transient; emerging at approximately 6 weeks of age, they become maximal between 9 and 12 weeks of age, and taper off between 14 and 20 weeks of age. According to Prechtl and coworkers, their absence is highly predictive of neurologic abnormalities (21).

Sensory Examination

A proper sensory examination is difficult at any age, and almost impossible in an infant or toddler. Sensory modalities can be tested in the older child using a pin or preferably a tracing wheel. In infants or toddlers, abnormalities in skin temperature or in the amount of perspiration indicate the level of sensory deficit. The ulnar surface of the hand has been found to be the most sensitive, and by moving the hand slowly up the child's body, one can verify changes that one marks on the skin, and rechecks on repeat testing.

Object discrimination can be determined in the healthy school-aged child by the use of coins, or small, well-known items, such as paper clips or rubber bands.

Reflexes

The younger the child, the less informative the deep tendon reflexes. Reflex inequalities are common and less reliable than inequalities of muscle tone in terms of ascertaining the presence of an upper motor neuron lesion. The segmental levels of the major deep tendon reflexes are presented in Table I.1.

Little doubt exists that the Babinski response is the best known sign of disturbed pyramidal tract function. To elicit it, the plantar surface of the foot is stimulated with a sharp object, such as the tip of a key, from the heel forward along the lateral border of the sole, crossing over the distal ends of the metatarsals toward the base of the great toe. Immediate dorsiflexion of the great toe and subsequent separation (fanning) of the other toes constitutes a positive response. Stimulation of the outer side of the foot is less objectionable and can be used in children who cannot tolerate the sensation of having their soles stimulated. The response is identical. An extensor plantar response must be distinguished from voluntary withdrawal, which, unlike the true Babinski response, is seen after a moment's delay. It also

TABLE I.1. *Segmental levels of major deep tendon reflexes*

Reflex	Segmental level
Jaw jerk	V-trigeminal nerve
Biceps	C5–6
Triceps	C6–8
Radial periosteal	C5–6
Patellar	L2–4
Ankle	S1–2
Hamstrings	L4–S2

must be distinguished from athetosis of the foot (*striatal toe*). According to Paine and Oppe, a positive response to Babinski sign is seen normally in the majority of 1-year-old children and in many up to 2½ years of age (22). In the sequential examination of infants conducted by Gingold and her group, the plantar response becomes consistently flexor between 4 and 6 months of age (22a).

Many eponyms, 20, according to Wartenberg (23), have been attached to the reflexes elicitable from the sole of the foot. Some, such as Rossolimo reflex, which is elicited by tapping the plantar surface of the toe and producing a stretching of the plantar flexors, are muscle stretch reflexes. Others, such as Oppenheim reflex (a firm stroke with finger and thumb down the anterior border of the tibia) or Gordon reflex (a hard squeeze of the calf muscle), are variants of Babinski response.

In the upper extremity, Hoffmann reflex is elicited by flicking the terminal phalanx of the patient's middle finger downward between the examiner's finger and thumb. In hyperreflexia, the thumb flexes and adducts, and the tips of the other fingers flex. Wartenberg sign is elicited by having the patient supinate the hand, slightly flexing the fingers. The examiner pronates his or her own hand and links his or her own flexed finger with the patient's. Both flex their fingers against each other's resistance. In pyramidal tract disease, the thumb adducts and flexes strongly, a reemergence of the forced grasp reflex.

Clonus is a regular repetitive movement of a joint elicited by a sudden stretching of the muscle and maintaining the stretch. It is most easily demonstrable at the ankle by dorsiflexion of the foot. Clonus represents increased reflex excitability. Several beats of ankle clonus can be demonstrated in some healthy newborns and in some tense older children. A sustained ankle clonus is abnormal at any age and suggests a lesion of the pyramidal tract.

Chvostek sign, a contraction of the facial muscles after percussion of the pes anserinus of the facial nerve (just anterior to the external auditory meatus), is evidence of increased irritability of the motor fibers to mechanical stimulation such as occurs in hypocalcemia (24).

Children with developmental disabilities, such as minimal brain dysfunction and attention deficit disorders, are often found to have *soft signs* on neurologic examination (see Chapter 16). These represent persistence of findings considered normal at a younger age. Of the various tests designed to elicit soft signs, tandem walking, hopping on one foot, and the ability of the child to suppress overflow movements when asked to repetitively touch the index finger to the thumb have been found to be the most useful. Forward tandem gait is performed successfully by 90% of 5-year-old children; 90% of 7-year-old children also can hop in one place, and synkinesis becomes progressively suppressed between 7 and 9 years of age (25).

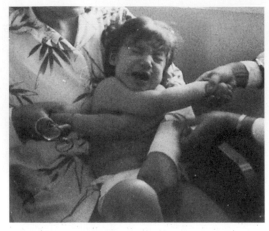

FIG. I.4. Scarf sign in an infant with upper extremity hypotonia on a cerebral basis.

Cognitive Function

Evaluation for the presence of cognitive limitations is an important part of the neurologic examination of developmentally delayed youngsters and of children with ostensibly normal intelligence who are referred because of school failure. Such an examination is extremely time consuming and might require a return visit. An outline of an evaluation of intelligence, speech, and disorders of cognitive function is presented in Chapter 16. Also provided are suggestions on how to interpret psychological data.

NEUROLOGIC EXAMINATION OF THE INFANT

The neurologic examination of an infant younger than 1 year of age can be divided into three parts: evaluation of posture and tone, evaluation of primitive reflexes, and examination of items that are relatively age invariable.

Posture and Muscle Tone

Evaluation of posture and muscle tone is a fundamental part of the neurologic examination of infants. It involves examination of the resting posture, passive tone, and active tone. Posture is appreciated by inspecting the undressed infant as the infant lies undisturbed. During the first few months of life, normal hypertonia of the

flexors of the elbows, hips, and knees occurs. The hypertonia decreases markedly during the third month of life, first in the upper extremities and later in the lower extremities. At the same time, tone in neck and trunk increases. Between 8 and 12 months of age, a further decrease occurs in the flexor tone of the extremities, together with increased extensor tone (26).

Evaluation of passive tone is accomplished by determining the resistance to passive movements of the various joints with the infant awake and not crying. Because limb tone is influenced by tonic neck reflexes, it is important to keep the child's head straight during this part of the examination. Passive flapping of the hands and the feet are simple means of ascertaining muscle tone. In the upper extremity, the scarf sign is a valuable maneuver. With the infant sustained in a semireclining position, the examiner takes the infant's hand and pulls the arm across the infant's chest toward the opposite shoulder (Fig. I.4). The position of the elbow in relationship to the midline is noted. Hypotonia is present if the elbow passes the midline. In the lower extremity, the fall-away response serves a similar purpose. The infant is suspended by the feet, upside down, and each lower extremity is released in turn. The rapidity with which the lower extremity drops when released is noted. Normally, the extremity maintains its position for a few

TABLE I.2. *Postural reactions*

Postural reflex	Stimulus	Origin of afferent impulses	Age reflex appears	Age reflex disappears
Local static reactions				
Stretch reflex	Gravitation	Muscles	Any age	
Positive supporting action			Well developed in 50% of newborns	Indistinguishable from normal standing
Placing reaction			37 weeks	Covered up by voluntary action
Segmental static reactions	Movement	Contralateral muscles		
Crossed extensor reflex			Newborn	7–12 mo
Crossed adductor reflex to quadriceps jerk			3 mo	8 mo
General static reactions	Position of head in space	Otolith Neck muscles Trunk muscles		
Tonic neck reflex			Never complete and obligatory	
Neck-righting reflex			4–8 mo	Covered up by voluntary action
Grasp reflex				
Palmar			28 weeks	4–5 mo
Plantar			Newborn	9–12 mo
Moro reflex			28–32 weeks	4–5 mo
Labyrinthine accelerating reactions	Change in rate of movement	Semicircular canals		
Linear acceleration			4–9 mo	Covered up by voluntary action
Parachute reaction				
Angular acceleration			Any age	
Postrotational nystagmus				

From Menkes JH. The neuromotor mechanism. In: Cooke RE, ed. *The biologic basis of pediatric practice.* New York: McGraw-Hill, 1968. With permission.

moments, then drops. In hypotonia, the drop occurs immediately; in hypertonia, the released lower extremity remains up.

The traction response is an excellent means of ascertaining active tone. The examiner, who should be sitting down and facing the child, places his or her thumbs in the infant's palms and fingers around the wrists, and gently pulls the infant from the supine position. In the healthy infant younger than 3 months of age, the palmar grasp reflex becomes operative, the elbows tend to flex, and the flexor muscles of the neck are stimulated to raise the head so that even in the full-term neonate the extensor and flexor tone are balanced, and the head is maintained briefly in the axis of the trunk. The test is abnormal if the head is pulled passively and drops forward, or if the head is maintained backward. In the former case, abnormal hypotonia of the neck and trunk muscles exists; in the latter case, abnormal hypertonia of the neck extensors exists. With abnormal hypertonia, one also might note the infant's head to be rotated laterally and extended when the infant is in the resting prone position.

Primitive Reflexes

The evaluation of various primitive reflexes is an integral part of the neurologic examination of the infant. Many of the reflexes exhibited by the newborn infant also are observed in a *spinal animal*, one in which the spinal cord has been permanently transected. With progressive maturation, some of these reflexes disappear (Tables I.2 and

TABLE I.3. *Percentage of healthy babies showing various infantile reflexes with increasing age*

	Signs that disappear with age			Signs that appear with age				
	Moro	Tonic neck reflex	Crossed adduction to knee jerk	Neck-righting reflex	Supporting reaction	Landau	Parachute	Hand grasp
Degree of sign tabulated	Extension even without flexor phase	Imposable even for 30 in. or inconstant	Strong or slight	Imposable but transient	Fair or good	Head above horizontal and back arched	Complete	Thumb to forefinger alone
Age (mo)								
1	93	67	?[a]	13	50	0	0	0
2	89	90	?[a]	23	43	0	0	0
3	70	50	41	25	52	0	0	0
4	59	34	41	26	40	0	0	0
5	22	31	41	38	61	29	0	0
6	0	11	21	40	66	42	3	0
7	0	0	12	43	74	42	29	16
8	0	0	15	54	81	44	40	53
9	0	0	6	67	96	97	76	63
10	0	0	3	100	100	100	79	84
11	0	0	3	100	100	100	90	95
12	0	0	2	100	100	100	100	100

[a]Divergence of experience and opinion between different examiners.
From Jampel RS, Quaglio ND. Eye movements in Tay-Sachs disease. *Neurology* 1964;14:1013–1019. With permission.

I.3). This disappearance should not be construed as meaning that they are actually lost, for a reflex once acquired in the course of development is retained permanently. Rather, these reflexes, which develop during intrauterine life, are gradually suppressed as the higher cortical centers become functional.

Segmental Medullary Reflexes

A number of segmental medullary reflexes become functional during the last trimester of gestation. They include (a) respiratory activity, (b) cardiovascular reflexes, (c) coughing reflex mediated by the vagus nerve, (d) sneezing reflex evoked by afferent fibers of the trigeminal nerve, (e) swallowing reflex mediated by the trigeminal and glossopharyngeal nerves, and (f) sucking reflex evoked by the afferent fibers of the trigeminal and glossopharyngeal nerves and executed by the efferent fibers of the facial, glossopharyngeal, and hypoglossal nerves.

Flexion Reflex

Another reflex demonstrable in the isolated spinal cord is the flexion reflex. This response is elicited by the unpleasant stimulation of the skin of the lower extremity, most consistently the dorsum of the foot, and consists of dorsiflexion of the great toe and flexion of the ankle, knee, and hip. This reflex has been elicited in immature fetuses and can persist as a fragment, the extensor plantar response, for the first 2 years of life. It is seen also in infants whose higher cortical centers have been profoundly damaged. Reflex stepping, which is at least partly a function of the flexion response, is present in the healthy newborn when the infant is supported in the standing position; it disappears in the fourth or fifth month of life.

Moro Reflex

The Moro reflex is best elicited by a sudden dropping of the baby's head in relation to its trunk. Moro, however, elicited this reflex by hitting the infant's pillow with both hands (27). The infant opens the hands, extends and abducts the

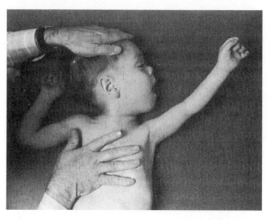

FIG. I.5. Obligatory tonic neck response in a 6-year-old boy with severe spastic quadriplegia and extrapyramidal symptoms secondary to perinatal asphyxia.

upper extremities, and then draws them together. The reflex first appears between 28 and 32 weeks' gestation and is present in all newborns. It fades out between 3 to 5 months of age (22a). Its persistence beyond 6 months of age, or its absence or diminution during the first few weeks of life, indicates neurologic dysfunction.

Tonic Neck Response

The tonic neck response is obtained by rotating the infant's head to the side while maintaining the chest in a flat position. A positive response is extension of the arm and leg on the side toward which the face is rotated, and flexion of the limbs on the opposite side (Fig. I.5). An asymmetric tonic neck response is abnormal, as is an obligatory and sustained pattern (i.e., one from which the infant is unable to extricate him- or herself). Inconstant tonic neck responses can be elicited for as long as 6 to 7 months of age and can even be momentarily present during sleep in the healthy 2- to 3-year-old child (22a).

Righting Reflex

With the infant in the supine position, the examiner turns the head to one side. The healthy infant rotates the shoulder in the same direction, followed by the trunk, and finally the pelvis. An obligate neck-righting reflex in which the shoulders, trunk, and pelvis rotate simultaneously, and in which the infant can be rolled over and over like a log, is always abnormal. Normally, the reflex can be imposed briefly in newborns, but the infant is soon able to break through it.

Palmar and Plantar Grasp Reflexes

The palmar and plantar grasp reflexes are elicited by pressure on the palm or sole. Generally, the plantar grasp reflex is weaker than the palmar reflex. The palmar grasp reflex appears at 28 weeks' gestation, is well established by 32 weeks, and becomes weak and inconsistent between 2 and 3 months of age, when it is covered up by voluntary activity. Absence of the reflex before 2 or 3 months of age, persistence beyond that age, or a consistent asymmetry is abnormal. The reappearance of the grasp reflex in frontal lobe lesions reflects the unopposed parietal lobe activity.

Vertical Suspension

The examiner suspends the child with his or her hand under its axillae and notes the position of the lower extremities. Marked extension or scissoring is an indication of spasticity (Fig. I.6).

Landau Reflex

To elicit the Landau response, the examiner lifts the infant with one hand under the trunk, face downward. Normally, a reflex extension of the vertebral column occurs, causing the newborn infant to lift the head to slightly below the horizontal, which results in a slightly convex upward curvature of the spine. With hypotonia, the infant's body tends to collapse into an inverted U shape.

Buttress Response

To elicit the buttress response, the examiner places the infant in the sitting position and displaces the center of gravity with a gentle push on one shoulder. The infant extends the contralateral arm and spreads the fingers. The reflex normally appears at approximately 5 months of age. Delay in its appearance and asymmetries are significant.

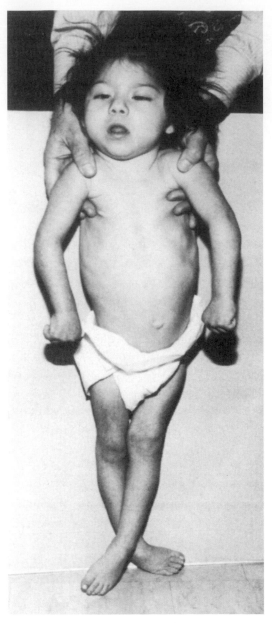

FIG. I.6. Infant with upper motor neuron lesion demonstrates scissoring of the lower extremities when held in vertical suspension. Spastic quadriparesis followed perinatal asphyxia.

Parachute Response

The parachute reflex is tested with the child suspended horizontally about the waist, face down. The infant is then suddenly projected toward the floor, with a consequent extension of the arms and

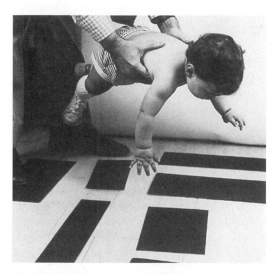

FIG. I.7. Infant demonstrating the parachute reaction. Note the extended arms and spreading of the fingers. The minimal asymmetry in the response may be the consequence of an antecedent meningitis.

spreading of the fingers. Between 4 and 9 months of age, this reflex depends on visual and vestibular sensory input and is proportional to the size of the optic stimulus pattern on the floor (28) (Fig. I.7).

Reflex Placing and Stepping Responses

Reflex placing and stepping responses are of lesser value. Reflex placing is elicited by stimulating the dorsum of the foot against the edge of the examining table. Reflex stepping, which is at least partly a function of the flexion response to noxious stimuli, is present in the healthy newborn when the newborn is supported in the standing position. The response disappears by 4 to 5 months of age.

Other Reflexes

A number of other primitive reflexes have been described. They include the curious bowing reflex first described by Gamper. This reflex, which occasionally can be demonstrated in healthy premature infants of 7 months' gestation, is invariably present in anencephalics. It can be elicited by placing the infant into the supine position and extending the thighs at the

hip joints. The head then lifts itself slowly, followed by the trunk, so that the infant ultimately achieves the sitting position.

Other primitive reflexes add little to the neurologic examination of the infant. The physician should gather experience in a few selected tests, rather than try and elicit the entire gamut of responses.

Age-Invariable Tests

The last part of the neurologic examination involves tests similar to those performed in older children or adults, such as the funduscopic examination and the deep tendon reflexes. These have been discussed already in the cranial nerves and reflexes sections. Though a variety of deep tendon reflexes can be elicited in the infant, they are of limited value except when they are clearly asymmetric. The triceps and brachioradialis reflexes are usually difficult to elicit during the period of neonatal flexion hypertonia. The patellar reflex is accompanied by adduction of the opposite thigh, the crossed adductor reflex. This reflex disappears by 9 to 12 months of age (22a). An unsustained ankle clonus is common in the healthy neonate.

The ready availability of head ultrasound has for most practitioners relegated transillumination of the infant's skull to the scrap heap of history. Nevertheless, when performed correctly, it remains a quick and useful test to detect the presence of hydrocephalus, subdural effusions, porencephalic cysts, and posterior fossa cysts (29).

It is not always possible to summarize the neurologic examination result of the infant as being normal or abnormal. Rather, an intermediate group of infants exists whose examination results are suspect. The examination should be recorded as such, with the ultimate decision being left to subsequent examinations. Only some 1% of these suspect infants turn out to have gross neurologic deficits (30).

NEURODIAGNOSTIC PROCEDURES

At the conclusion of history taking and physical examination, the physician sets up a differential diagnosis and calls on a variety of diagnostic procedures to ascertain the cause of the neuro-logic illness.

Some of the more commonly used proce-dures are commented on briefly to describe their applicability to various diagnostic problems and to direct the reader to more extensive sources.

Cerebrospinal Fluid

In most cases, a sample of the cerebrospinal fluid (CSF) is obtained by lumbar puncture, a proce-dure introduced in 1891 by Quincke as a means of reducing the increased intracranial pressure in children with hydrocephalus (31). To perform a spinal tap, the child is held in the lateral recum-bent position with the spine maintained maxi-mally flexed. In the newborn or small infant, the tap is best performed with the baby in the sitting position. A small pillow placed against the abdomen keeps the spine flexed, while an assis-tant maintains the head in a perfect anteroposte-rior alignment. After cleaning the back with an antibacterial solution, the tap is performed. One may omit local anesthesia because it entails twice as much struggling than a tap performed without it. A controlled clinical trial has come to a similar conclusion (32). In one medical center, eutectic mixture of local anesthetics (EMLA) cream, a topical anesthetic of mixture of 2.5% lidocaine and 2.5% prilocaine, applied as a thick layer over the puncture site approximately 1 hour before the tap has made the procedure eas-ier for the child and doctor. For a small child or toddler, a 22-gauge needle is preferable, whereas for the newborn, a 23-gauge needle without a stylet is optimal. The needle is inserted into the L3–4, or for a newborn, whose spinal cord ter-minates at a lower level than the older child's, into the L4–5 interspace, with the bevel being maintained parallel to the longitudinal dural fibers to decrease the size of the dural tear. The needle is then pushed forward as slowly as pos-sible. Entry into the subarachnoid space can be felt by a sudden pop. A bloody tap usually results from the needle's going too deep and penetrating the dorsal epidural venous plexus overlying the vertebral bodies. Less often it is caused by injury to the vessels along the cauda equina. The person who holds the child in a perfect position is more

important to the success of a lumbar puncture than the person who inserts the needle. Bonadio and coworkers have constructed a graph relating the depth to which the needle must go to obtain clear CSF with body surface area (33).

If an opening pressure is essential, the stylet is replaced with a manometer, taking care to lose as little spinal fluid as possible. Because examination of the CSF for cells is more impor-tant than a pressure reading in most cases, a few drops of CSF should be collected at this point. An accurate recording of CSF pressure requires total relaxation of the child, a difficult and at times impossible task. The cooperative child may be released and the legs extended, because falsely high pressures result when the knees are pressed against the abdomen. When the needle has been placed correctly, the fluid can be seen to move up and down the manometer with res-pirations. In older children, normal CSF pres-sure is less than 180 mm H_2O; usually it is between 110 and 150 mm H_2O. Pressure is approximately 100 mm H_2O in the newborn. Ellis and coworkers have proposed that CSF pressure can be estimated by counting the num-ber of drops that are collected through the nee-dle during a fixed period of time, ranging from 12 to 39 seconds, depending on the temperature of the child and the gauge and the length of the needle. Their paper presents the counting period for which the number of drops counted equals the CSF pressure in centimeters of water (34). This method is not useful in cases in which the CSF viscosity is significantly increased. Queck-enstedt test, compression of the jugular veins to determine the presence of a spinal subarachnoid block, has lost its usefulness. After the spinal tap is completed, the stylet, if such is used, is replaced, and the needle is given half a turn before being removed to prevent extensive spinal fluid leakage (35). This manipulation is believed to reduce the likelihood for a postlum-bar puncture headache (36).

The normal CSF is crystal clear. A cloudy fluid indicates the presence of cells. Fluid that contains more than 500 red blood cells per μL appears grossly bloody. If so, the possibility of a traumatic tap should be excluded by performing cell counts on three sequential samples of fluid.

In the presence of an intracranial hemorrhage, little difference exists in the counts obtained from the first and last specimens. Performing sequential cell counts is a more reliable method of demonstrating intracranial bleeding than observing the presence of a xanthochromic fluid or crenated red cells (37). Crenation of red cells in CSF occurs promptly, whereas xanthochromia can be noted whenever contamination by red cells is heavy. In the term neonate, the mean protein concentration is 90 mg/dL; in the premature neonate, it is 115 mg/dL (38). The presence of blood from any source raises the total protein by 1.5 mg/dL of fluid for every 1,000 fresh red blood cells per μL (39). The number of white cells in normal CSF is higher in infants than in children. In the study conducted by Ahmed and colleagues, the mean white cell count in normal, noninfected neonates was 7, with a range of 0 to 130 per μL (40).

In children older than 12 months of age, normal values range up to 3 cells per μL. Whereas polymorphonuclear cells can be present in the newborn, they are not found in CSF taken from healthy children older than 12 months of age (41). Blood-contaminated CSF complicates the determination of pleocytosis. Although it is frequently stated that the ratio of white blood cells to red blood cells does not differ from that present in peripheral blood (1:300), actual determinations by several groups of workers indicate that only approximately 20% of the predicted number of white blood cells are present in CSF; consequently, recalculation is necessary (42).

The normal IgG values for pediatric patients have been compiled by Rust and coworkers (43). In tuberculous meningitis, a cobweb can form at the bottom of the tube; staining of this material can reveal the presence of acid-fast organisms. It is appropriate to consider the complications of lumbar puncture performed under these and other circumstances.

The possibility of herniation in the presence of increased intracranial pressure must be considered not only in cases of brain tumor, but also in purulent meningitis. The incidence of this complication in both groups of patients is 12%, and it is likely that subjects who develop this adverse reaction already had formed tentorial or cerebellar pressure cones before the lumbar puncture (44).

The most common complication of lumbar puncture is headache. Its onset is between 15 minutes and 4 days after the tap, and it can persist for up to 2 weeks. It is most severe with the patient upright and subsides in the recumbent position. Nausea, vomiting, and, less often, vertigo can accompany the headache. It is generally accepted, although not proven conclusively, that the headache results from persistent leakage of CSF through a hole in the dura and arachnoid, with cerebral hypotension and a consequent stretching and displacement of pain-sensitive structures (45). The major factor in headache induction is the diameter of the hole made in the dura by the needle (46,47). Neither the amount of fluid removed nor the position of the patient during the puncture is important. Use of a small-gauge needle reduces the incidence of the complication, although if CSF pressures are to be measured, the physician should allow sufficient time for equilibration.

The best current treatment of postlumbar puncture headache is strict bed rest and the use of analgesics. Neither overhydration nor use of a variety of drugs (notably, caffeine and diphenhydramine) has proven effective (48). Backache as a result of the trauma of the lumbar puncture is relatively common, but in children is generally not sufficiently severe to represent a major problem.

Less common complications of lumbar puncture include diplopia caused by unilateral or bilateral abducens palsy. This usually clears within a few days or weeks.

Trauma to the arachnoid and to dural vessels at the base of the vertebrae is fairly common, particularly in small infants, but unless the patient is suffering from a bleeding disorder, it is asymptomatic. An epidural hematoma, and even less likely, a subdural hematoma, and a subarachnoid hemorrhage after a lumbar puncture are extremely unusual complications (49). Frequent lumbar punctures, particularly when performed for the introduction of intrathecal medications, may result in the implantation of an epidermal tumor. Other, rarer complications, together with 789 references on complications of lumbar puncture, can be found in a review by Fredericks (50).

Cytologic studies can be performed on CSF after centrifugation and can assist in determining whether tumors have spread to the meninges or to the spinal subarachnoid space, as may occur in a medulloblastoma (51). Occasionally, the CSF contains choroid plexus and ependymal cells. These are particularly prominent in hydrocephalic infants (52,53).

Electroencephalography

Electroencephalography (EEG) remains the central tool for the clinical investigation of seizures and other paroxysmal disorders, although the increasing importance of neuroimaging studies has circumscribed its usefulness.

EEG does not exclude the presence of epilepsy or organic disease, and its role in diagnosing the neuropsychiatric disorders is limited. A single normal tracing is of little value in excluding the diagnosis of epilepsy, and conversely, insignificant EEG abnormalities can accompany gross structural brain disease. Neither the technique of EEG nor the interpretation of normal and abnormal tracings are covered at this point. Rather, the reader is referred to a basic text such as that of Fisch (54), a more comprehensive one by Niedermeyer and Lopes da Silva (55), or one on EEG of neonates by Stockard-Pope, Werner, and Bickford (56). Specific EEG abnormalities and their interpretations are covered in Chapter 13.

EEG is indicated in transient alterations in cerebral function or behavior, central nervous system degenerative disorders (with photic stimulation), unexplained coma, prognosis after anoxic episodes and other acute cerebral problems, and the determination of brain death. It is of little help in developmental retardation, static encephalopathies unaccompanied by seizures, minimal brain dysfunction, attention deficit disorders, and neuropsychiatric disorders.

Quantitative methods for data analysis of brain electrical activity (BEAM) can be used to compare signals from the various electrodes and so construct multicolor contour maps of brain activity. BEAM has found relatively little applicability in pediatric neurology. Even though this technique facilitates the detection of asymmetries, it remains investigational in mild to moderate head injuries, learning disabilities, and the attention deficit disorders. At present, no clinical application exists for quantitative EEG analysis without analysis of an accompanying routine EEG, and quantitative EEG by itself has not been proven useful in either the diagnosis or treatment of children with learning or attention deficits (57–59).

Polysomnography

As interest in sleep disorders has increased, the polysomnogram has become more readily available, not only in university centers, but also in clinical sleep laboratories. The procedure consists of the simultaneous recording of multiple physiologic variables during sleep. These include an EEG, electromyogram, electrocardiogram, and electro-oculogram. Additionally, respiration is recorded. The procedure is invaluable in the evaluation of sleep apnea of infancy, and the diagnosis of suspected nocturnal seizures, narcolepsy, periodic movement disorders, and parasomnias (60,61) (see Chapter 13).

Electromyography

A concentric needle electrode inserted into muscle records the action potentials generated by muscle activity. These are amplified and displayed on a cathode ray oscilloscope. The amplified input also can be fed into a loud speaker.

Normal resting muscle is electrically silent, except for a small amount of electrical activity produced by insertion of the needle that rapidly dies away. This is termed the *insertion potential*. With slight voluntary activity, single action potentials become evident. With increasing volitional activity, motor unit discharges increase in number, and the frequency of discharge increases until an interference pattern of continuous motor activity is achieved.

The number or rate of motor unit discharge, as well as the amplitude or shape of the individual discharges, can be abnormal. In establishing the diagnosis of myopathy, the duration of the discharge is more important than the amplitude, inasmuch as the latter varies with age and with the muscle tested. Spontaneous discharges may be elicited from resting muscle or the insertion potential may be increased. After denervation of muscle, fibrillation potentials appear. They result from the periodic rhythmic twitching of single muscle fibers resulting from their hyper-excitability consequent to denervation. Fibrillation potentials appear on the average between 10 and 20 days after nerve section, and, as a rule, the greater the distance between the site of injury and the muscle, the longer it takes for the abnormality to develop. Spontaneous fibrillations also can be seen in hyperkalemic period paralysis, botulinus intoxication, muscular dystrophy, and some myopathies. They can be recorded in the proximal musculature of some term babies younger than 1 month of age, and in some preterm infants (62).

Electromyography (EMG) is an integral part of the investigation of the patient with lower motor neuron disease. It is nonspecifically abnormal in upper motor neuron disease and in extrapyramidal disorders, and, therefore, has only limited use in these entities. High spatial resolution EMG, a noninvasive surface EMG technique, has been proposed for the diagnosis of pediatric neuromuscular disorders. As used in various European centers its diagnostic validity appears to be similar to that of needle EMG (63). For a more extensive coverage of this procedure, the reader is referred to texts by Kimura (64) or Aminoff (65).

Nerve Conduction Studies

The conduction rates of motor nerves can be measured by stimulating the nerve at two points and recording the latency between each stimulus and the ensuing muscle contraction. The conduction rate depends on the patient's age and on the nerve tested. Normal values for pediatric patients have been presented by Gamstorp (66).

Nerve conduction velocities can be used to distinguish demyelination from axonal degeneration of the peripheral nerve and also from muscular disorders. In peripheral nerve demyelination, nerve conduction velocities are generally reduced, whereas they are normal in axonal degenerations and in muscular diseases (see also Chapters 2 and 14). The procedure also provides information about the distribution of peripheral nerve lesions.

Sensory nerve conduction velocity can be determined in infants and children, but is a more difficult procedure. It is useful in the study of the hereditary sensory and autonomic neuropathies and some of the heredodegenerative disorders.

Evoked Potentials

Evoked potentials are the brain's response to an external stimulus. Most evoked potentials, being of low amplitude (0.120 µV), cannot be seen on routine EEG, but must be extracted from background activity by computed signal averaging after repeated stimuli. The presence or absence of one or more evoked potential waves and their latencies (the time from stimulus to wave peaks) is used in clinical interpretations.

In pediatric neurology, visual-evoked responses (VERs), brainstem auditory-evoked responses (BAERs), and somatosensory-evoked potentials (SSEPs) are the most commonly used tests.

Visual-Evoked Responses

Flash and pattern shift VERs are in use. In one institution, pattern shift stimuli are preferred for older children in that they are more reliable and also can provide some information about visual acuity. Flash stimuli are used for infants and older but uncooperative youngsters. The amplitude and latencies of the VER as recorded from both occipital lobes are used for clinical purposes, with the former being less valuable in pediatrics because it is contingent on attention span and visual acuity.

VERs have found their place in the diagnosis of a variety of leukodystrophies, demyelinating diseases, and lipidoses. They can demonstrate clinically silent optic neuritis such as is present in spinocerebellar ataxia and various other system degenerations. VERs can be recorded reliably from neonates and have been used to measure visual acuity in infants and follow the development of the visual system (67,68).

Brainstem Auditory-Evoked Responses

A series of clicks delivered to one ear sequentially activates cranial nerve VIII, cochlear nucleus, superior olivary nucleus, nuclei of the lateral lemniscus, and inferior colliculus. In the neonate, the waves representing cranial nerve VIII (I), the superior olivary nucleus (III), and the inferior colliculus (V) are the most readily detectable. The BAER can be elicited in premature infants after 26 weeks' gestation, with amplitude increasing and latency decreasing as a function of increasing gestational age. Clinical interpretation of the BAER is based on the time interval between the waves and the interpeak latencies. These reflect the intactness of the brainstem auditory tract.

Diseases of the peripheral auditory nerve affect the latencies of all waves, but do not alter interpeak latencies. The BAER is abnormal in various leukodystrophies, with most patients having central abnormalities. Clinically inapparent abnormalities of the auditory nerve can be demonstrated by BAER in Friedreich ataxia and the various hereditary motor and sensory neuropathies. The BAER is also abnormal in brainstem disease, such as occurs in neonates as a consequence of perinatal asphyxia or hyperbilirubinemia. It is also abnormal in bacterial meningitis and in the various viral encephalitides.

Indicative of brainstem damage, the BAER has been used for prognostic purposes in patients who are comatose subsequent to head trauma, cardiorespiratory arrest, or increased intracranial pressure.

Somatosensory-Evoked Potentials

SSEPs are recorded after stimulation of peripheral sensory nerves. Like BAERs, the waveforms and the anatomy of the sensory tracts are closely correlated. The cell bodies of the large-fiber sensory system lie in the dorsal root ganglia; their central processes travel rostrally in the posterior columns of the spinal cord to synapse in the dorsal column nuclei at the cervicomedullary junction. Second-order fibers cross the midline to the thalamus, whence third-order fibers continue to the frontoparietal sensorimotor cortex. Painless electrical stimuli at 4 to 5 per second are delivered to the skin overlying the median nerve at the wrist, the tibial nerve at the ankle, or the common peroneal nerve at the knee. Their intensity is adjusted to excite the largest myelinated fibers in the peripheral nerve. Waveforms are recorded along the somatosensory pathway: above the clavicle overlying the brachial plexus, at the posterior midline at the C2 vertebra to record the dorsal column nuclei, and on the scalp overlying the sensory cortex contralateral to the stimulated limb. When the lower extremities are stimulated, a recording electrode is placed over L1–3.

Clinical interpretation is based on interpeak latency, with particular attention paid to differences between the two sides. SSEPs can provide information on the integrity of the brachial plexus, and on spinal cord lesions if these involve the posterior columns. SSEPs can be used to evaluate children with myelodysplasia and provide useful information in patients with Friedreich ataxia and in the hereditary motor and sensory neuropathies. The role of multimodality evoked potential recordings in the diagnosis of brain death is covered in Chapter 15.

The SSEP appears in the fetus at approximately 29 weeks of gestation, with a progressive decrease of response latency with increasing gestational age.

Electronystagmography

This procedure measures the rate and amplitude of eye movements at rest and after caloric or rotational stimulation. It is useful in the evaluation of children with vertigo and in the postconcussion syndrome (69,70).

NEUROIMAGING

Skull Radiography

Radiographs of the skull are hardly as valuable as they were before the advent of CT scan and MRI. Currently, they are used occasionally to detect and interpret localized lytic lesions, such as are seen in histiocytosis X, and to evaluate various congenital anomalies of the cranium, such as occur in achondroplasia, cleidocranial dysostosis, wormian bones, or hyperostosis. Plain skull radiography is clearly inferior to CT in the assessment of the child who has suffered a head injury, although, on occasion, radiography is better than CT in demonstrating a horizontal skull fracture.

In children, particularly in those between 4 and 8 years of age, prominence of convolutional markings is not a reliable indication of increased intracranial pressure. Separation of sutures is rare in children older than 10 years of age and is practically nonexistent beyond the age of 20 years.

Computed Tomography

The advent of CT and MRI revolutionized the diagnostic evaluation of the neurologic patients and eliminated the need for invasive studies such as pneumonencephalography and ventriculography.

The technique of CT was introduced by Hounsfield (71), who developed a scanning instrument based on theoretical work of Oldendorf (72). It permits visualization of even slight differences in the density of the intracranial contents without the need for and the complications of an invasive procedure. In essence, scattering of radiation is eliminated by the use of a thin x-ray beam so that the photon absorption by tissues can be calculated accurately using a sodium iodide crystal or solid state detector. The x-ray tube and the detector move across the head and obtain readings of photon transmission through the head. The exact matrix depends on the particular scanning instrument used. After completion of the scan, the unit is rotated one degree and the process is repeated. In this fashion, the tube and the detector are rotated 180 degrees around the head. The resulting readings are fed into a computer that calculates the x-ray absorption coefficients of each of the voxels. The most current machines make standard serial cuts of the head 5 mm thick, but when required for examination of the posterior fossa, the orbit, or the perisellar region, they can reduce the thickness to less than 1 mm. The total radiation dose for a complete scan is approximately 6 rads, somewhat less than that produced by a routine skull series.

Many of the developed scanners have the ability to acquire spiral or helical scans. With this technique, the gantry rotates continuously as the table moves. The helical data set is then reconstructed into artificial slices for viewing. This technique shortens the scan time considerably. The newest scanners can acquire multiple slices concurrently, further shortening the scan time.

The CT scanning procedure takes some 5 to 30 minutes, and because even a slight degree of motion results in an artifact, the normally active child younger than 5 years of age requires sedation to prevent movement of the head. Chloral hydrate, rectal sodium pentothal (40 mg/kg), and meperidine (Demerol; 2 mg/kg up to 50 mg) are reliable and safe agents for this purpose. Chloral hydrate is administered orally as an initial dose of 60 to 75 mg/kg, with a subsequent dose of 45 to 50 mg/kg for those children in whom the initial dose was ineffective.

Nonionic contrast media of the iodide type (e.g., iohexol) can be used to facilitate recognition of structure and vascularity. They have for the greater part replaced ionic contrast media because of their lower incidence of anaphylactoid reactions and other complications (73). Enhancement of tumors and surrounding abnormal tissue results from a breakdown of the blood–brain barrier.

A CT scan is the procedure of choice for the emergency evaluation of the child who has suffered head trauma or who is suspected of having a subarachnoid hemorrhage. The CT scan is also preferable to MRI for the detection of intracranial calcifications such as are seen in intrauterine infections, the phakomatoses, and brain tumors. It also can be used to localize and define a brain abscess and to follow its course under therapy.

Although catheter angiography is still the procedure of choice for the ultimate delineation of vascular lesions, these are readily detected by CT scans, MRI, and MR angiography. The latter procedures also provide information not obtainable by catheter angiography, such as the presence and extent of an associated hematoma, subarachnoid blood, or edema. CT angiography is a noninvasive technique that uses a rapid intravenous contrast bolus and thin spiral scans of a defined area of vascular anatomy. It is most useful in evaluat-

TABLE I.4. *Relative value of magnetic resonance imaging and computed tomographic scanning*

Disease	Magnetic resonance imaging	Computed tomographic scanning	Metrizamide-enhanced computed tomographic scanning
Tumors			
Low grade			
Supratentorial	+ + +	+ +	
Infratentorial	+ + + +	+ +	
High grade			
Supratentorial	+ + + +	+ + + +	
Infratentorial	+ + + +	+ +	
Metastases			
Supratentorial	+ + +	+ +	
Infratentorial	+ + +	+	
Demyelinating diseases	+ + + +	+ +	
Trauma			
Craniocerebral	+ +	+ + +	
Spinal	+ + +[a]	+ + +	+ + +
Vasculitis (systemic lupus erythematosus)	+ + +	±	
Cervicomedullary junction and cervical spinal cord			
Congenital anomalies	+ + + +	+	+ +
Tumors (intraaxial)			
Brainstem	+ + + +	+	+ +
Cerebellopontine angle	+ + +	+ +	+ + +
Cervical spine	+ + + +	±	+ +
Tumors (extraaxial)			
Brainstem	+ + + +	+	+ +
Cervical spine	+ + + +	±	+ + +

+ + + +, preferred initial approach; + + +, of definite value; + +, of value, but should not be considered as the initial diagnostic approach; +, of some value, but other procedures are superior; ±, of questionable value.

[a]Radiographic computed tomographic scanning is superior in visualizing bone abnormalities whereas magnetic resonance imaging may be superior in demonstrating blood and spinal cord injury.

Adapted from Council of Scientific Affairs, Report of the Panel on Magnetic Resonance Imaging. Magnetic resonance imaging of the central nervous system. *JAMA* 1988;259:1211. With permission.

ing complex circle of Willis aneurysms (73a). CT angiography can be performed as a dedicated study or can be done retrospectively by reconstructing data obtained from a conventional diagnostic spiral CT scan (73b).

A CT scan is inferior to ultrasonography for the diagnosis of many of the early intracranial complications of prematurity and for the evaluation of an infant with hydrocephalus. The CT scan is also inferior to MRI in the detection of minor central nervous system malformations, the evaluation of structural epileptogenic lesions, and demyelinating processes.

Magnetic Resonance Imaging

Magnetic resonance imaging is a versatile and noninvasive procedure, whose clinical use was first described in 1977 (74). It provides infor-mation on brain structure without exposure to ionizing radiation. For a discussion of the fundamental physical principles of MRI and an explanation of its terminology, subjects far beyond the scope of this text, and for a more extensive presentation of its application, the reader is referred to books such as those by Lee, Rao, and Zimmerman (75). This section reviews the applications of MRI of the brain and compares them with those for CT scanning. Table I.4 shows the relative efficacy of the two procedures. Generally, T1-weighted images provide a better view of structural anatomy, whereas T_2-weighted images are preferred for the detection of abnormalities.

In the evaluation of tumors, MRI is generally superior to CT scanning for the detection and characterization of posterior fossa lesions, particularly when these are isodense and thus require contrast infusion for their delineation. It is also superior for the detection and delineation of low-grade tumors and provides a more precise definition of associated features, such as mass effects, hemorrhage, and edema. In a brainstem glioma, for instance, sagittal scans demonstrate the rostrocaudal extent of tumor, and tumors involving the sella or the chiasmatic cistern are more readily delineated by MRI than CT scanning, because interference from surrounding bone limits the accuracy of CT scanning. The infusion of chelated gadolinium (i.e., gadopentetate dimeglumine) provides contrast enhancement for intracranial lesions with abnormal vascularity, such as the more malignant tumors, and detects lesions that disrupt the blood–brain barrier. These are best seen on T1-weighted images (76). Enhanced MRI facilitates the distinction between tumor and edema, and between viable tissue and necrotic tissue. It also delineates any leptomeningeal spread of metastases, and the spinal cord metastases so common in medulloblastomas. Gadolinium contrast infusions also have been used to delineate the cerebral lesions of neurofibromatosis and tuberous sclerosis. Gadolinium contrast has proven to be an exceedingly safe material, with a complication rate of less than 1 in 10,000. The use of neuroimaging in the diagnosis of central nervous system tumors is discussed more extensively in Chapter 10.

In spinal cord tumors, MRI is the procedure of choice. It is far superior in examination of inherent bone disease and in evaluation of the bone marrow.

In addition, MRI, by providing good gray-white differentiation, offers valuable information on the status of myelin in demyelinating diseases and during normal and abnormal development. When T2-weighted images are viewed, white matter appears lighter (higher signal intensity) than gray matter for the first 6 to 7 months of life. Between 8 and 12 months of age, the signal intensities from white and gray matter are approximately equal (Fig. I.8). Thereafter, the brain has the adult appearance with gray matter lighter than white matter (77,78). This progression is delayed frequently in developmentally retarded youngsters (see Fig. I.8). MRI

of the brain in preterm infants younger than 30 weeks' gestation demonstrates the presence of the germinal matrix at the margins of the lateral ventricles as small areas of high signal intensity on T1-weighted images and low signal intensity on T2-weighted images (79,80). The MRI also can be used to demonstrate the maturation of the cortical sulci (see Chapter 4).

For the evaluation of developmentally delayed children, particularly when anomalies of cortical architecture are suspected, MRI is far superior to CT scanning in that it can depict areas of micropolygyria, lissencephaly, or heterotopic gray matter. Additionally, the quality of images is superior to that offered by CT scans.

MRI is the procedure of choice for the evaluation of patients with refractory complex or simple partial seizures and is preferred to CT scanning in demonstrating abnormalities at the cervicomedullary junction and the cervical spinal cord. The procedure is, therefore, used as a follow-up study for the patient who has sustained cervical trauma or who is suspected of having an Arnold-Chiari malformation.

MRI has been used to map the distribution of brain iron (79). In the healthy brain, the concentration of iron is maximal in the globus pallidus, caudate nucleus, and putamen. It increases in the Hallervorden-Spatz syndrome, making MRI useful in its diagnosis.

Finally, in choosing between CT scanning and MRI, the physician should not forget that the critically ill patient with a variety of infusions and requiring respiratory support cannot be managed properly in many MRI units, and that the procedure costs 20% to 300% more than CT scans (80).

Diffusion-Weighted Magnetic Resonance Imaging

In images obtained with diffusion-weighted MRI, contrast depends on differences in the molecular motion of water. Acute strokes, such as occur in sickle cell disease, and hypoxic-ischemic changes in mature brain are detected earlier by this technique than by conventional MRI (81,82). The advantages of this technique in neonatal hypoxic-ischemic encephalopathy are

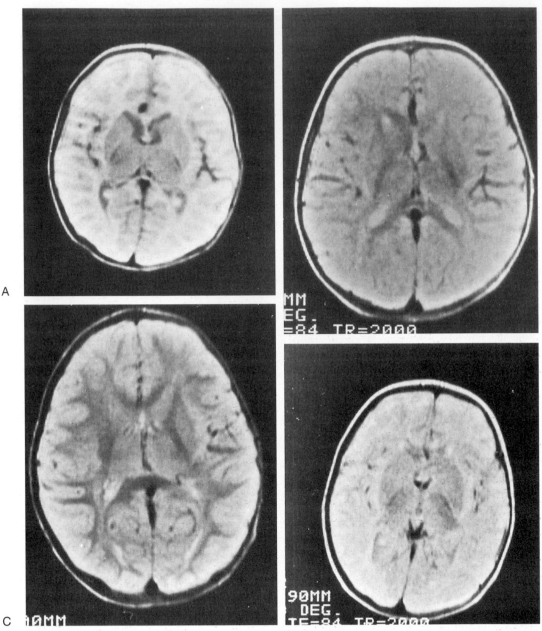

FIG. I.8. Magnetic resonance imaging studies in normal and abnormal development. **A:** Normal development, age 3 months. Axial spin-echo (SE) (2,000/84). White matter has higher signal intensity than adjacent gray matter. Myelin is already present in the region of the thalamus and the posterior limbs of the internal capsule. A small amount of myelin is present in the occipital white matter. **B:** Normal development, age 10 months. Axial SE (2,000/84). The gray and white matter are isointense. Myelin is now present also in the anterior limbs of the internal capsule. **C:** Normal development, age 18 months. Axial SE (2,000/84). The white matter is hypointense relative to the gray matter. The area of myelinated white matter has now extended peripherally. **D:** Delayed development, age 18 months. Axial SE (2,000/84). White matter is transitional between having higher signal intensity than the adjacent gray matter and being isointense with gray matter. Myelin is present in the thalamus and the posterior limbs of the internal capsule. This picture is consistent with a normal development of between 3 and 6 months of age. (Courtesy of Dr. Rosalind B. Dietrich.)

not as clear (83). Several methods, notably fluid-attenuated inversion recovery pulse sequences, have been used to reduce CSF signal and produce heavy T2-weighting and thus provide additional anatomic detail. These are discussed in detail by Oatridge and colleagues (84). In the authors' institution, a combination of fluid-attenuated inversion recovery and diffusion-weighted images are used to evaluate the patient with hyperacute infarction (within 3 hours of onset).

Magnetic Resonance Angiography

Magnetic resonance angiography (85) is a non-invasive technique that allows visualization of blood vessels. In the pediatric age group, who have a higher cerebral blood flow than adults, the large cerebral arteries and their major branches are routinely visualized. This procedure has replaced traditional angiography for most purposes and has proved helpful in evaluating dural sinuses, cerebral aneurysms, and in studying arterial and venous components of an arteriovenous malformation. In particular, it is a noninvasive diagnostic tool for the evaluation of children with vascular accidents. Some centers use gadolinium enhancement to visualize veins and arteries with slower blood flow (86,87) (see Chapter 12).

Magnetic Resonance Spectroscopy

Magnetic resonance spectroscopy (MRS) is performed using the same magnets and computers as conventional MRI. Proton MRS is used more widely than ^{31}P-MRS. Unlike MRI, MRS provides information on the cerebral metabolites and some neurotransmitters in one or more small regions of interest (voxels). The major metabolites that can be detected by proton MRS include *N*-acetyl compounds, primarily *N*-acetylaspartate (NAA); creatine (including phosphocreatine and its precursor, creatine); and choline-containing compounds, including free choline, phosphoryl, and glycerophosphoryl choline. NAA is a neuronal marker, whereas the choline compounds are released in the course of membrane disruption. Proton MRS also can be used to determine the concentration of lactate, which accumulates as a result of tissue damage and consequent anaerobic metabolism (88,89,89a). Neurotransmitters, such as gamma-aminobutyric acid and glutamate, also can be estimated using proton MRS. In neonates, the dominant peaks are the choline-containing compounds and *myo-inositol*. With maturation, NAA increases so that by 4 months of age, it becomes the major metabolic peak. As a consequence, the NAA/choline and NAA/creatine ratios increase rapidly with maturation, whereas the choline/creatine ratio decreases (88).

Concentrations of adenosine triphosphate, phosphocreatine, and some of the other high-energy phosphates involved in cellular energetics can be assessed using ^{31}P-MRS.

Spectra can be acquired within 1 hour, and changes in intracellular pH and metabolites can be followed. Proton and phosphorus MRS has been used in the evaluation of muscle diseases, localization of epileptic foci, evaluation of the extent of post-traumatic lesions, classification of brain tumors, and diagnosis of the various mitochondrial disorders, leukodystrophies, and other demyelinating disorders. These techniques also have been used to determine the extent, timing, and prognosis of perinatal asphyxia (89,90).

Ultrasonography

As is more extensively discussed in Chapter 5, ultrasonography is widely used for the recognition of intracranial hemorrhage in the newborn and for the detection of a variety of nonhemorrhagic lesions, notably intracranial tumors, hydrocephalus, periventricular leukomalacia, and polycystic encephalomalacia (91). Additionally, ultrasonography detects areas of calcification, such as those caused by cytomegalovirus or *Toxoplasma* infections. Because the procedure is performed through the open anterior fontanelle, its accuracy decreases with the decreasing size of the fontanelle.

Positron Emission Tomography

Positron emission tomography (PET) enables one to detect localized functional abnormalities of the brain. It is based on the emission by certain unstable isotopes of positrons (positively charged electrons), which, after brief passage through tissue, collide with negatively charged electrons and emit energy that can be localized by tomography. Isotopes of carbon, nitrogen, oxygen, and fluorine have been used for PET scanning. All have short half-lives and are generally prepared by an on-site or nearby cyclotron. ^{18}F-labeled 2-fluorodeoxyglucose is particularly useful for measuring transport and phosphorylation of glucose in that it is not metabolized beyond deoxyglucose-6-phosphate and, therefore, remains within the brain. ^{18}F-labeled 2-fluorodeoxyglucose allows accurate measurements of cerebral blood flow and of local oxygen and glucose metabolism. Because the hallmark of an epileptic focus is an interictal area of reduced cerebral glucose metabolism, the PET scan has become invaluable in the assessment of candidates for surgical therapy of epilepsy (92). The PET scan is being used also for the early diagnosis of Huntington disease, the differential diagnoses of dementias, and in the differentiation between radiation necrosis and tumor recurrence. Specific ligands have been used to investigate dopamine, opiate, and benzodiazepine receptor binding in various movement disorders. For the most part, these studies have not had any clinical applicability in pediatric cases. Finally, the PET scan has shown considerable promise in the study of the functional development of the normal and diseased human brain (93).

Single Photon Emission Computed Tomography

The so-called poor man's PET scan, single photon emission computed tomography (SPECT), depends on the gamma-ray emission of certain neutral lipophilic isotopes, notably ^{99}Tc, to measure regional cerebral blood flow. In the pediatric population, SPECT finds considerable use for the study of refractory epilepsies. In essence, the results with SPECT parallel those with PET scanning; generalized hyperperfusion is seen during a seizure in the generalized epilepsies, and regional hyperperfusion is seen for a few

minutes before and during a seizure in an area that corresponds to the epileptic focus in partial seizures (94). Ictal hyperperfusion extends for approximately 10 minutes into the postictal period with hyperperfused surround that often is extensive (95). Interictally, a large proportion of patients show areas of hypoperfusion corresponding to the epileptic focus. For the purpose of localizing an epileptic focus, interictal hypoperfusion is less reliable than the data obtained by a combination of SPECT and MRI (94).

The simplicity and economy of SPECT is its biggest advantage. However, several drawbacks to this technique exist. For one, SPECT tracers are not natural biological molecules, and their physiologic behavior is not fully understood. Spatial resolution of SPECT is poorer than resolution by PET, and SPECT gives no information with respect to brain metabolism, nor does it permit quantitation of blood flow. Because in most instances brain metabolism and cerebral blood flow are closely linked, and the isotopes used in SPECT do not require on-site production, this procedure has an important role in the evaluation of the difficult seizure patient (96). At present, no isotopes of carbon, oxygen, or nitrogen with usable half-lives and energies exist; this procedure has been therefore mainly limited to the study of cerebral perfusion (97). Newer pharmaceuticals, notably ^{99}mTc-methoxy-isobutylisonitrile, have been used to detect the metabolic activity of tumors (97a).

Functional Magnetic Resonance Imaging

In the authors' institution, the clinical applications of functional MRI are principally in the preoperative localization of the sensorimotor, visual, and language cortex in patients with intracranial tumors (98). Functional MRI allows the identification of cortical activation by examination of the oxygen level of the cortical veins. Oxygenated hemoglobin has different signal characteristics than hemoglobin. Blood flow to an actively functioning cortex provides more oxygen to neurons than is consumed by them, and as a result, the oxygen level in the corresponding veins increases.

Cerebral Arteriography

The visualization of cerebral blood vessels by the injection of radiopaque dyes was introduced by Moniz in 1927 (99). Currently, various techniques are used for arteriography in children, most commonly cannulation of the brachial or femoral arteries under direct visualization. The exact amount injected depends on the size of the child, but generally nonionic contrast medium is injected directly. With the small catheters that are now available, selective angiography of the cerebral vessels can be performed on even the smallest infant (99a). Lateral and anteroposterior views of the skull are taken simultaneously or with successive injections. The principal indication for the procedure is in the evaluation of vascular abnormalities, including arteriovenous malformations, aneurysms, and occlusive vascular disease (see Chapter 12). Tumors of the cerebral hemispheres are localized by the distortion of the normal vascular patterns of the carotid arterial or venous system, or by the presence of abnormal vasculature. Although CT and MRI provide first-line evidence of the size and location of a brain tumor, arteriography using digital subtraction techniques offers excellent confirmatory data in terms of blood supply to the mass lesion.

Current angiographic techniques have permitted the development of interventional neuroradiology. Percutaneous endovascular procedures have become the major mode of treatment for a wide array of vascular lesions, including malformations of the vein of Galen, arteriovenous malformations, fistulas, and intracerebral aneurysms (see Chapter 12).

Radiography of the Spine and Myelography

Spinal radiographs and CT are important in the management of the youngster who has been subjected to craniocerebral or spinal trauma. In interpreting spine films, the pediatric neurologist must consider a number of relatively common normal variations. These include the forward subluxation of C2 on C3, a variety of anomalies of the odontoid process, including the presence of an accessory ossicle, and the occipitalization of C1 (100).

MRI is the optimal study for the delineation of spinal cord tumors, diastematomyelia, the tethered cord, and various spinal cord anomalies that are reviewed in Chapter 4.

Pneumoencephalography and Ventriculography

Because these procedures are of purely historical interest, a brief review suffices. In 1918, Dandy introduced the technique of visualizing the cerebral ventricles and subarachnoid spaces by the injection of air into the lumbar spinal canal (101).

When this technique was used, localization of intracranial neoplasms relied on the presence of abnormalities in ventricular size and location. The morbidity of the procedure was considerable. When air was used as the contrast medium, its introduction into the ventricular system almost invariably resulted in headache and vomiting. Less often, hypotensive episodes and focal or generalized seizures and CSF pleocytosis occurred.

REFERENCES

1. Craige E. Should auscultation be rehabilitated? *N Engl J Med* 1988;318:1611–1613.
2. Tirosh E, Jaffe M, Dar H. The clinical significance of multiple hair whorls and their association with unusual dermatoglyphics and dysmorphic features in mentally retarded Israeli children. *Eur J Pediatr* 1987;146: 568–570.
3. Goldsmith WM. "The catlin mark": the inheritance of an unusual opening in the parietal bones. *J Hered* 1922;13:69–71.
4. Wadia NH, Monckton G. Intracranial bruits in health and disease. *Brain* 1957;80:492–509.
5. Mackenzie I. The intracranial bruit. *Brain* 1955;78: 350–367.
6. Peiper A. *Cerebral function in infancy and childhood.* New York: Consultants Bureau, 1963:49–53.
7. Kasahara M, Inamatsu S. Der Blinzelreflex im Säuglingsalter. *Arch Kinderhk* 1931;92:302.
8. Cernerud L. The setting-sun eye phenomenon in infancy. *Dev Med Child Neurol* 1975;17:447–455.
9. Hoyt CS, Mousel DK, Weber AA. Transient supranuclear disturbances of gaze in healthy neonates. *Am J Ophthalmol* 1980;89:708–713.
10. Mehler MF. The clinical spectrum of ocular bobbing and ocular dipping. *J Neurol Neurosurg Psychiatry* 1988;51:725–727.
11. Isenberg SJ. Clinical application of the pupil examination in neonates. *J Pediatr* 1991;118: 650–652.
12. Horner JF. Ueber eine Form von Ptosis. *Klin Mbl Augenheilk* 1869;7:193.
13. Hageman G, Ippel PF, te Nijenhuis FC. Autosomal dominant congenital Horner's syndrome in a Dutch family. *J Neurol Neurosurg Psychiatry* 1992; 55:28–30.

14. Jampel RS, Quaglio ND. Eye movements in Tay-Sachs disease. *Neurology* 1964;14:1013–1019.
15. Engle EC, et al. A gene for isolated congenital ptosis maps to a 3-cM region within 1p32-p34.1. *Am J Hum Genet* 1997;60:1150–1157.
16. Jenny AB, Saper CB. Organization of the facial nucleus and corticofacial projection in the monkey: a reconsideration of the upper motor neuron facial palsy. *Neurology* 1987;37:930–939.
17. Ross RT, Mathiesen R. Volitional and emotional supranuclear facial weakness. *N Engl J Med* 1998; 338:1515.
18. Davies AE, et al. Pharyngeal sensation and gag reflex in healthy subjects. *Lancet* 1995;345:487–488.
19. Medical Research Council. *Aids to the examination of peripheral nerve injuries.* London: Balliere Tindall, 1986.
20. Denny-Brown D. *The basal ganglia,* Oxford: Oxford University Press, 1962.
21. Prechtl HFR, et al. An early marker for neurological deficits after perinatal brain lesions. *Lancet* 1997; 349:1361–1363.
22. Paine RS, Oppe TE. *Neurological examination of children: clinics in developmental medicine,* Vol. 20/21. London: William Heinemann, 1966.
22a. Gingold MK, et al. The rise and fall of the plantar response in infancy. *J Pediatr* 1998;133:568–570.
23. Wartenberg R. *The examination of reflexes,* Chicago: Yearbook Publishers, 1945.
24. Chvostek F. Weitere Beiträge zur Tetanie. *Wiener Mediz Presse* 1879;20:1201,1233,1268,1301.
25. Denckla MB. Development of motor coordination in normal children. *Dev Med Child Neurol* 1974;16: 729–741.
26. Amiel-Tison C. A method for neurologic evaluation within the first year of life. *Curr Probl Pediatr* 1976;7:1.
27. Moro E. Das erste Trimenon. *Münchn Med Wchschr* 1918:1147.
28. Wenzel D. The development of the parachute reaction: a visuo-vestibular response. *Neuropädiatrie* 1978;9: 351–359.
29. Dodge PR, Porter P. Demonstration of intracranial pathology by transillumination. *Arch Neurol* 1961; 5:594–605.
30. Nelson KB, Ellenberg JH. Neonatal signs as predictors of cerebral palsy. *Pediatrics* 1979;64:225–232.
31. Quincke H. Die Lumbarpunktion des Hydrocephalus. *Klin Wochenschr* 1891;28:929–933,965–968.
32. Porter FL, et al. A controlled clinical trial of local anesthesia for lumbar punctures in newborns. *Pediatrics* 1991;88:663–669.
33. Bonadio WA, et al. Estimating lumbar puncture depth in children. *N Engl J Med* 1988;319:952–953.
34. Ellis RW, et al. A simple method of estimating cerebrospinal fluid pressure during lumbar puncture. *Pediatrics* 1992;89:895–897.
35. Nelson DA. Dangers of lumbar spinal needle placement. *Ann Neurol* 1989;25:310.
36. Strupp M, Brandt T. Should one reinsert the stylet during lumbar puncture? *N Engl J Med* 1997;336:1190.
37. McMenemy WH. The significance of subarachnoid bleeding. *Proc R Soc Med* 1954;47:701.
38. Volpe JJ. Neonatal intracranial hemorrhage. Pathophysiology, neuropathology, and clinical features. *Clin Perinatol* 1977;4:77–102.
39. Tourtellotte WW, et al. A study on traumatic lumbar punctures. *Neurology* 1958;8:129–134.
40. Ahmed A, et al. Cerebrospinal fluid values in the term neonate. *Pediatr Infec Dis J* 1996;15:298–303.
41. Portnoy JM, Olson LC. Normal cerebrospinal fluid values in children: another look. *Pediatrics* 1985;75: 484–487.
42. Rubenstein J, Yogev R. What represents pleocytosis in blood-contaminated ("traumatic tap") cerebrospinal fluid in children? *J Pediatr* 1985;107: 249–251.
43. Rust RS, Dodson WE, Trotter JL. Cerebrospinal fluid IgG in childhood: the establishment of reference values. *Ann Neurol* 1988;23:406–410.
44. Duffy GP. Lumbar puncture in the presence of raised intracranial pressure. *BMJ* 1969;1:407–409.
45. Tourtellotte WW, et al. *Postlumbar puncture headaches.* Springfield, IL: Charles C Thomas Publisher, 1964.
46. Tourtellotte WW, et al. A randomized, double-blind clinical trial comparing the 22 versus 26 gauge needle in the production of the postlumbar puncture syndrome in normal individuals. *Headache* 1972;12: 73–78.
47. Gernes RH. Posture and headache after lumbar puncture. *Lancet* 1980;2:33.
48. Raymond JR, Raymond PA. Postlumbar puncture headache: ideology and management. *West J Med* 1988;148:551–554.
49. Kirkpatrick D, Goodman SJ. Combined subarachnoid and subdural spinal hematoma following spinal puncture. *Surg Neurol* 1975;3:109–111.
50. Fredericks JAM. Spinal puncture complications: complications of diagnostic lumbar puncture, myelography, spinal anesthesia and intrathecal drug anesthesia. In: Vinken PJ, Bruyn GW, Klawans HL, Frankel HL, eds. *Handbook of clinical neurology Vol. 17(61): spinal cord trauma.* Amsterdam, New York: Elsevier Science, 1992:147–189.
51. Glass JP, et al. Malignant cells in cerebrospinal fluid (CSF): the meaning of a positive CSF cytology. *Neurology* 1979;29:1369–1375.
52. de Reuck J, Vanderdonckt P. Choroid plexus and ependymal cells in CSF cytology. *Clin Neurol Neurosurg* 1986;88:177–179.
53. Wilkins RH, Odom GL. Ependymal-choroid cells in cerebrospinal fluid. Increased incidence in hydrocephalic infants. *J Neurosurg* 1974;41:555–560.
54. Fisch BJ. *Spehlmann's EEG primer,* 2nd ed. Amsterdam, New York: Elsevier Science, 1991.
55. Niedermeyer E, Lopes da Silva FH. *Electroencephalography: basic principles, clinical applications, and related fields,* 4th ed. Baltimore: Williams & Wilkins, 1998.
56. Stockard-Pope JE, Werner SS, Bickford RG. *Atlas of neonatal electroencephalography,* 2nd ed. New York: Raven Press, 1992.
57. Binnie CD, Macgillivray BB. Brain mapping—a useful tool or a dangerous toy? *J Neurol Neurosurg Psychiatry* 1992;55:527–529.
58. Duffy FH, et al. Neurophysiological studies in dyslexia. *Res Publ Assoc Res Nerv Ment Dis* 1988;66:149–169.
59. Nuwer M. Assessment of digital EEG, quantitative EEG, and brain mapping: report of the American Academy of Neurology and the American Clinical Neurophysiology Society. *Neurology* 1997;49:277–292.
60. Guilleminault C. *Sleep and its disorders in children,* New York: Raven Press, 1987.
61. Ferber R, Kryger M, eds. *Principles and practice of sleep medicine in the child,* Philadelphia: WB Saunders, 1995.

62. Gamstorp I. *Pediatric neurology,* 2nd ed. London, Boston: Butterworth–Heinemann, 1985:45–47.
63. Huppertz HJ, et al. Diagnostic yield of noninvasive high spatial resolution electromyography in neuromuscular diseases. *Muscle Nerve* 1997;20: 1360–1370.
64. Kimura J. *Electrodiagnosis in diseases of nerve and muscle. Principles and practice.* Philadelphia: FA Davis Co, 1983.
65. Aminoff MJ. *Electromyography in clinical practice: clinical and electrodiagnostic aspects of neuromuscular disease,* 3rd ed. New York: Churchill Livingstone, 1997.
66. Gamstorp I. Normal conduction velocity of ulnar, median and peroneal nerves in infancy, childhood and adolescence. *Acta Paediatr Stockholm* 1963; 146[Suppl]:68–77.
67. Moskowitz A, Sokol S. Developmental changes in the human visual system as reflected by the latency of the pattern reversal VEP. *Electroencephalogr Clin Neurophysiol* 1983;56:115.
68. Kos-Pietro S, et al. Maturation of human visual evoked potentials: 27 weeks conceptional age to 2 years. *Neuropediatrics* 1997;28:318–323.
69. Taylor MJ, Boor R, Ekert PG. Preterm maturation of the somatosensory evoked potential. *Electroencephalogr Clin Neurophysiol* 1996;100:448–452.
70. Baloh RW, Halmagyi GM, eds. *Disorders of the vestibular system.* London: Oxford University Press, 1996.
71. Ambrose J, Hounsfield GN. Computerized transverse axial tomography. *Br J Radiol* 1973;46:148–149.
72. Oldendorf W. Isolated flying spot detection of radiodensity discontinuities displaying the internal structural pattern of a complex object: IRE Trans Biomed Electronics. *Biomed Mater Eng* 1961; 8:68–72.
73. Federle MP, Willis LL, Swanson DP. Ionic versus nonionic contrast media: a prospective study of the effect of rapid bolus injection on nausea and anaphylactoid reactions. *J Comput Assist Tomogr* 1998;22: 341–345.
73a. Vieco PT. CT angiography of the intracranial circulation. *Neuroimaging Clin N Am* 1998;8:577–592.
73b. Rankin SC. CT angiography. *Eur Radiol* 1999;9: 297–310.
74. Hinshaw WS, Bottomley PA, Holland GN. Radiographic thin-section image of the human wrist by nuclear magnetic resonance. *Nature* 1977;270: 722–723.
75. Lee SH, Rao KCVG, Zimmerman RA. *Cranial and spinal MRI and CT,* 4th ed. New York: McGraw–Hill, 1996.
76. Edelman RR, Warach S. Magnetic resonance imaging. *N Engl J Med* 1993;328:708–716.
77. Dietrich RB, et al. MR evaluation of early myelination patterns in normal and developmentally delayed infants. *Am J Neuroradiol* 1988;9:69–76.
78. Byrd SE, Darling CF, Wilczynski MA. White matter of the brain: maturation and myelination on magnetic resonance in infants and children. *Neuroimag Clin North Am* 1993;3:247–266.
79. Battin MR, et al. Magnetic resonance imaging of the brain in very preterm infants: visualization of the germinal matrix, early myelination and cortical folding. *Pediatrics* 1998;101:957–962.
80. van Wezel-Meijler G, et al. Magnetic resonance imaging of the brain in premature infants during the neonatal period: normal phenomena and reflection of mild ultrasound abnormalities. *Neuropediatrics* 1998;29:89–96.
81. Baird AE, Warach S. Magnetic resonance imaging of acute stroke. *J Cereb Blood* 1998;18:583–609.
82. Cowan FM, et al. Early detection of cerebral infarction and hypoxic ischemic encephalopathy in neonates using diffusion-weighted magnetic resonance imaging. *Neuropediatrics* 1994;25:172–175.
83. Tuor UI, et al. Diffusion- and T2-weighted increases in magnetic resonance images of immature brain during hypoxia-ischemia: transient reversal posthypoxia. *Exp Neurol* 1998;150:321–328.
84. Oatridge A, et al. MRI diffusion-weighted imaging of the brain: contributions to image contrast from CSF signal reduction, use of a long echo time and diffusion effects. *Clin Radiol* 1993;47:82–90.
85. Zimmerman RA, Bilaniuk LT. Pediatric brain, head and neck, and spine magnetic resonance angiography. *Magn Reson Q* 1992;8:264–290.
86. Zimmerman RA, Bogdan AR, Gusnard DA. Pediatric magnetic resonance angiography: assessment of stroke. *Cardiovasc Intervent Radiol* 1992;15: 60–64.
87. Brant-Zawadzki M, Heiserman JE. The roles of MR angiography, CT angiography and sonography in vascular imaging of the head and neck. *Am J Neuroradiol* 1997;18:1820–1825.
88. Holshouser BA, et al. Proton MR Spectroscopy after acute central nervous system injury: outcome prediction in neonates, infants and children. *Radiology* 1997;202:487–496.
89. Groenendaal F, et al. Cerebral lactate and *N*-acetylaspartate/choline ratios in asphyxiated full-term neonates demonstrated in vivo using proton magnetic resonance spectroscopy. *Pediatr Res* 1994;35: 148–151.
89a. Novotny E, Ashwal S, Shevell M. Proton magnetic resonance spectroscopy: an emerging technology in pediatric neurology research. *Pediatr Res* 1998; 44: 1–10.
90. Wang Z, Zimmerman RA, Sauter R. Proton MR spectroscopy of the brain: clinically useful information obtained in assessing CNS diseases in children. *Am J Radiol* 1996;167:191–199.
91. Teele RL, Share JC. Cranial ultrasonography. In: Teele RL, Share JC, eds. *Ultrasonography of infants and children.* Philadelphia: WB Saunders, 1991:156.
92. Duncan JS. Imaging and epilepsy. *Brain* 1997;120: 339–377.
93. Chugani HT. Functional brain imaging in pediatrics. *Pediatr Clin North Am* 1992;39:777–799.
94. Baumgartner C, et al. Preictal SPECT in temporal lobe epilepsy: regional cerebral blood flow is increased prior to electroencephalography-seizure onset. *J Nucl Med* 1998;39:978–982.
95. Uvebrant P, et al. Brain single photon emission computed tomography (SPECT) in neuropediatrics. *Neuropediatrics* 1991;22:3–9.
96. Schulder M, et al. Functional image-guided surgery of intracranial tumors located in or near the sensorimotor cortex. *J Neurosurg* 1998;89:412–418.
97. Prichard JW, Brass LM. New anatomical and functional imaging methods. *Ann Neurol* 1992;32: 395–400.
97a. O'Tuama LA, et al. Thallium-201 versus technician-99m-MIBI SPECT in evaluation of childhood brain tumors: a

within-subject comparison. *J Nucl Med* 1993;34:
1045–1051.

98. Turner R. Magnetic resonance imaging of brain function. *Ann Neurol* 1994;35:637–638.

99. Moniz E. L'encephalographie arterielle, son importance dans la localization des tumeurs cerebrales. *Rev Neurol (Paris)* 1927;2:72–90.

99a. Burrows PE, Robertson RI. Neonatal central nervous system vascular disorders. *Neurosurg Clin N Am* 1998; 9:155–180.

100. Cattel HS, Filtzer DL. Pseudosubluxation and other normal variations in the cervical spine in children. *J Bone Joint Surg* 1965;47A:1295–1309.

101. Dandy WE. Ventriculography following the injection of air into the cerebral ventricles. *Ann Surg* 1918; 68:5.

Chapter 1

Metabolic Diseases of the Nervous System

John H. Menkes

Departments of Neurology and Pediatrics, University of California, Los Angeles,
UCLA School of Medicine, and Department of Pediatric Neurology, Cedars-Sinai Medical Center, Los
Angeles, California 90048

The diseases considered in this chapter result from a single mutant gene that codes for an enzymatic protein that in most instances is involved in a catabolic pathway. The consequent homeostatic disturbances produce a neurologic or developmental abnormality. The separation between conditions considered in this chapter and those in Chapter 2 is admittedly arbitrary. Both chapters deal with single gene defects, except that for diseases covered in this chapter, the defective gene is normally expressed in one or more organs, not necessarily in the nervous system, and chemical analyses of tissues are frequently diagnostic. Conditions considered in Chapter 2 are also the result of a single defective gene, but one that is mainly or exclusively expressed in the nervous system. Consequently, these entities lack characteristic chemical abnormalities of tissues or body fluids.

Since 1975, almost all of the nearly 500 neurologic and neuromuscular diseases caused by known enzymatic or protein defects have been mapped to a specific chromosome region, and a large proportion of them have been cloned (1). In the course of these advances, a large amount of metabolic, molecular, and genetic detail has become available, whose full discussion is outside the domain of this text. Rather, the emphasis of this chapter is on the clinical presentation of the diseases, their diagnosis and treatment, and, when known, the mechanisms that induce the neurologic deficits. For a more extensive discussion of the genetic and molecular basis of the neurologic disorders, the reader is referred to a text by Rosenberg and coworkers (2).

Inborn errors of metabolism affect only approximately 1 in 5,000 live births and are therefore relatively uncommon in the practice of pediatric neurology. Their importance rests in part on the insight they offer into the relationship between a genetic mutation, the resultant disturbance in homeostasis, and a disorder of the nervous system.

The mechanisms by which inborn errors of metabolism produce brain dysfunction remain largely uncertain, although, for some conditions, a plausible theory of pathogenesis has been proposed. Not all enzyme defects lead to disease; a large number of harmless metabolic variants exist. These include pentosuria, one of the original four inborn errors of metabolism described by Garrod (3), cystathioninuria, hydroxyprolinemia (4), and sarcosinemia. Many of these variants were discovered when inmates of institutions for the mentally retarded were screened for metabolic defects.

An introduction to the fundamentals of molecular genetics is far beyond the scope of this text. The reader interested in this subject is referred to books by Lodish and colleagues (5) and Lewin (6).

For practical purposes, metabolic disorders are divided into the following groups:

Disorders of amino acid metabolism
Disorders of membrane transport
Disorders of carbohydrate metabolism
Organic acidurias
Lysosomal storage diseases
Disorders of lipid and lipoprotein metabolism
Peroxisomal disorders
Familial myoclonus epilepsies
Ceroid lipofuscinosis and other lipidoses
Disorders of metal metabolism
Disorders of purine and pyrimidine metabolism
Mitochondrial disorders

TABLE 1.1. *Clinical syndromes suspect for an underlying metabolic cause*

Neurologic disorder, including mental retardation replicated in sibling or close relative
Recurrent episodes of altered consciousness or unexplained vomiting in an infant
Recurrent unexplained ataxia or spasticity
Progressive central nervous system degeneration
Mental retardation without obvious cause

EVALUATION OF THE PATIENT SUSPECTED OF HAVING A METABOLIC DISORDER

The spectacular advances of molecular biology have facilitated the diagnosis and prevention of genetic diseases and have brought humanity to the threshold of gene therapy. The clinician must, therefore, strive for an early diagnosis of inborn errors of metabolism to offer treatment whenever possible, provide appropriate genetic counseling, and, in many instances, give parents an opportunity for an antenatal diagnosis on the occasion of a subsequent pregnancy (7,8).

Since the initial descriptions of phenylketonuria and maple syrup urine disease, the protean clinical picture of the various inborn metabolic errors has become apparent. As a consequence, these disorders must be included in the differential diagnosis of neurologic problems whenever other causes are not evident from the child medical history and physical examination.

Two questions should be considered: What type of patient is suspect for an inborn error of metabolism, and what laboratory tests should be included in the diagnostic evaluation? It is clear that the greater the suspicion of a metabolic disorder, the more intense the investigative process must be.

Table 1.1 lists some clinical syndromes arranged according to decreasing likelihood of an underlying metabolic cause.

Frequently, a carefully obtained history and a physical examination provide important clues to the presence of a metabolic disorder and its specific diagnosis (Table 1.2).

Metabolic investigations are less imperative for children who have focal neurologic disorders or who suffer from mental retardation in conjunction with major congenital anomalies. Dysmorphic features, however, have been found in some of the peroxisomal disorders, including Zellweger syndrome, in pyruvate dehydrogenase deficiency, glutaric acidemia type II, and Smith-Lemli-Opitz syndrome.

When embarking on a metabolic investigation, procedures are performed in ascending order of complexity and discomfort to patient and family.

Metabolic Screening

Routine screening of plasma and urine detects the overwhelming majority of disorders of amino acid metabolism and disorders manifested by an abnormality of organic acids, as well as the common disorders of carbohydrate metabolism. At our institution, metabolic screening usually includes plasma amino acids and urinary organic acids. The yield on these tests is low, and a high frequency of nonspecific or nondiagnostic abnormalities occurs. Urea cycle disorders are characterized by elevated concentrations of blood ammonia with the patient in the fasting state or on a high-protein intake (4 g/kg per day). A number of genetic disorders are characterized by hypoglycemia or intermittent acidosis. Elevated lactic and pyruvic acid levels in serum or cerebrospinal fluid (CSF) are found in a number of the mitochondrial disorders. Hence, determination of fasting blood sugar, serum pH, pCO_2, and lactic and pyruvic acids is indicated as part of a metabolic workup. Should the suspicion for a metabolic disorder be high, these determinations should be repeated with the child on a high-protein intake or after a high-carbohydrate meal. Other biochemical determinations required in the evaluation of a patient with a suspected metabolic defect include serum and urine uric acid, serum cholesterol, serum carnitine

TABLE 1.2. *Clinical clues to the diagnosis of metabolic diseases of the nervous system*

Clue	Diagnosis
Cutaneous abnormalities	
Increased pigmentation	Adrenoleukodystrophy
Telangiectases (conjunctiva, ears, popliteal areas)	Ataxia-telangiectasia
Perioral eruption	Multiple carboxylase deficiency
Absent adipose tissue	Cockayne syndrome
Angiokeratoma (red macules or maculopapules) of hips, buttocks, scrotum	Fabry disease, sialidosis, fucosidosis type II
Oculocutaneous albinism	Chédiak-Higashi syndrome
Xanthomas	Cerebrotendinous xanthomatosis
Subcutaneous nodules	Ceramidosis (Farber disease)
Ichthyosis	Sjögren-Larsson syndrome (spasticity, seizures)
	Refsum disease (neuropathy, ataxia, phylanic acid)
	Dorfman-Chanarin syndrome (lipid storage in muscle, granulocytes, and so forth)
Abnormal urinary or body odor	
Musty	Phenylketonuria
Maple syrup or caramel	Maple syrup urine disease
Sweaty feet or ripe cheese	Isovaleric acidemia
Sweaty feet	Glutaric acidemia type II
Cat urine	3-Methylcrotonyl-CoA carboxylase deficiency
Cat urine	Multiple carboxylase deficiency
Hair abnormalities	
Alopecia	Multiple carboxylase deficiency
Kinky hair	Kinky hair disease
	Argininosuccinic aciduria
	Multiple carboxylase deficiency
	Giant axonal neuropathy
	Trichothiodystrophy (Pollitt syndrome; mental retardation, seizures)
Unusual facies	Mucopolysaccharidoses (Hunter-Hurler syndrome)
Coarse	I-cell disease (mucolipidosis II)
	GM_1 gangliosidosis (infantile)
Slight coarsening (difficult to notice without comparing other family members)	Sanfilippo syndrome
	Mucolipidosis III (pseudo-Hurler dystrophy)
	Fucosidosis II
	Mannosidosis
	Sialidosis II
	Aspartylglucosaminuria
Ocular abnormalities	
Cataracts	Galactosemia
	Cerebrotendinous xanthomatosis
	Homocystinuria
	Cockayne syndrome
Corneal clouding	Hurler syndrome
	Hunter syndrome (late in severe cases)
	Morquio syndrome
	Maroteaux-Lamy syndrome
Cherry-red spot	Tay-Sachs, Sandhoff diseases (GM_2 gangliosidosis)
	GM_1 gangliosidosis (infantile)
	Niemann-Pick disease (types A and C)
	Infantile Gaucher disease (type II)
	Sialidosis

levels (including total, acyl, and free carnitine), immunoglobulins, T_4, T_3, serum copper, ceruloplasmin, and magnesium. Assay of the very-long-chain fatty acids diagnoses adrenoleukodystrophy and other peroxisomal disorders.

Radiography

Radiographic examination of the vertebrae and long bones can be used to diagnose most of the mucopolysaccharidoses, Gaucher diseases, Niemann-Pick diseases, and GM_1 gangliosidosis. Neuroimaging studies, including magnetic resonance imaging (MRI), have been less helpful in pointing to any inborn metabolic error. Abnormalities such as agenesis of the corpus callosum and a large operculum seen in a few of the conditions covered in this chapter are nonspecific. The yield is much higher when a child with mental retardation with or without seizures is subjected to MRI. As a rule, the more severe the mental retardation, the higher the yield. Thus, the computed tomographic (CT) scanning or MRI shows a significant abnormality in approximately 80% of patients presenting with profound mental retardation (8). As a rule, MRI provides more information than CT. As is noted in Chapter 2, in the Diseases with Degeneration Primarily Affecting White Matter section, MRI is useful also in the diagnosis of the various leukodystrophies.

Serum Lysosomal Enzyme Screen

A serum lysosomal enzyme screen should be performed. In particular, assays for β-galactosidase, arylsulfatase, and the hexosaminidases can be run accurately in a number of centers.

Structural and Biochemical Alterations

In a number of metabolic disorders, notably the lipidoses and white matter degenerations, diagnosis requires clinical evaluation and combined microscopic, ultrastructural, and biochemical studies on biopsied tissue. In the past, a brain biopsy was required for this purpose. It has become clear that, if adequately sought, structural and biochemical alterations can be detected outside the central nervous system (CNS) in almost every leukodystrophy or lipidosis. Table 1.3 shows what diseases (discussed in Chapters 1 and 2) are likely to be diagnosed by examination of various tissues.

TABLE 1.3. *Common diseases diagnosed by study of tissues*

Tissue studied	Disease
Peripheral nerve	Metachromatic leukodystrophy
	Globoid cell leukodystrophy
	Infantile neuroaxonal dystrophy
	Fabry disease
	Refsum disease
	Tangier disease
Skin, conjunctivae, lymphocytes	Most lipidoses, particularly late infantile and juvenile neuronal ceroid lipofuscinosis
	Lafora disease
	Neuroaxonal dystrophy[a]
	Mucolipidosis
	Sanfilippo syndromes
	Fabry disease
Muscle	Late infantile and juvenile neuronal ceroid lipofuscinosis
	Familial myoclonus epilepsy
	Mitochondrial disorders
Bone marrow	Niemann-Pick diseases
	Gaucher diseases
	GM_1 gangliosidosis
Brain	All lipidoses, and degenerative diseases of gray matter
	All white matter degenerations, with the possible exception of Pelizaeus-Merzbacher disease
	None of the movement disorders, except Huntington disease

[a]When storage is confined to nerve fibers (e.g., neuroaxonal dystrophy), conjunctival biopsy is not diagnostic.

At this time, rectal biopsy and biopsies of other tissues such as kidney or tonsils are indicated only rarely. A liver biopsy is occasionally required to verify the actual enzymatic defect and is used to measure copper content in the diagnosis of Wilson disease, Menkes disease, and their variants. When tissue biopsy suggests a specific metabolic disorder, highly sophisticated enzyme assays are required to confirm the diagnosis.

DISORDERS OF AMINO ACID METABOLISM

Phenylketonuria

Phenylketonuria (PKU) has long been the prototype for an inborn metabolic error that produces serious neurologic symptoms. Fölling, in 1934, first called attention to the condition in a report of 10 mentally defective patients who excreted large amounts of phenylpyruvic acid (9). The disease has since been found in all parts of the world, although it is rare in blacks and Ashkenazi Jews. Its incidence in the general population of the United States, as determined by screening programs, is approximately 1 in 14,000 (10).

Molecular Genetics and Biochemical Pathology

Phenylketonuria is an autosomal recessive disorder that results in an inability to hydroxylate phenylalanine to tyrosine. The complete hydroxylation system consists in part of phenylalanine hydroxylase (PAH), a PAH stabilizer, the tetrahydrobiopterin cofactor (BH_4), dihydropteridine reductase, which is required to recycle BH_4, and a BH_4 synthesizing system. This system involves guanosine triphosphate (GTP) cyclohydrolase, and 6-pyruvoyl tetrahydropteridine synthetase (Fig. 1.1) (11).

PAH is normally found in liver, kidney, and pancreas, but not in brain or skin fibroblasts. The enzyme is an iron-containing metalloprotein dimer of identical subunits with a molecular weight of approximately 100,000. The gene coding for the enzyme has been cloned and localized to the long arm of chromosome 12 (12q22-24). The gene is approximately 90 kilobase (kb) long and codes for a mature RNA of

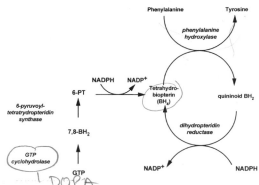

FIG. 1.1. Phenylalanine metabolism. Phenylalanine is converted to tyrosine by the holoenzyme, phenylalanine hydroxylase. Phenylalanine hydroxylase requires tetrahydrobiopterin (BH_4) as cofactor. BH_4 is recycled by dihydropteridine reductase. BH_4 is synthesized from guanosine triphosphate (GTP) by a series of reactions that involve GTP cyclohydrolase and 6-pyruvoyltetrahydropteridin (6-PT) synthase. Genetic defects in all these steps can result in hyperphenylalaninemia. A defect in GTP cyclohydrolase is seen also in dopa-responsive dystonia (see Chapter 2). [$NADP^+$, nicotinamide-adenine dinucleotide phosphate (oxidized form); NADPH, nicotinamide-adenine dinucleotide phosphate (reduced form).]

approximately 2,400 bases. Availability of this clone has facilitated the molecular genetic analysis of patients with PKU and has confirmed that PKU is the consequence of numerous mutant alleles arising in various ethnic groups. More than 200 mutations have been recorded, with the frequency of the mutations differing considerably between ethnic groups. Most patients with PKU are compound heterozygotes rather than homozygotes in the precise meaning of the term (12). Some mutations result in little or no PAH activity, whereas others produce a mutant PAH protein that has significant enzyme activity (13,13a). As a rule, the biochemical phenotype (i.e., the degree of phenylalanine elevation) correlates well with the activity of PAH as predicted from the genetic mutation. In the experience of Ramus and colleagues, however, no good correlation existed between PAH activity and intellectual function of untreated patients, and a good likelihood exists that various environmental factors and modifying gene may affect intellectual function in these subjects (13b).

Dihydropteridine reductase, a heat-stable enzyme involved in phenylalanine hydroxylation (see Fig. 1.1), is coded by a gene that has been localized to chromosome 4. It is present in normal amounts in classic PKU, but is absent or defective in one type of the non-PKU phenylalaninemias.

The infant with classic PKU is born with only slightly elevated phenylalanine blood levels, but because of the absence of PAH activity, the amino acid derived from food proteins and postnatal catabolism accumulates in serum and CSF and is excreted in large quantities. In lieu of the normal degradative pathway, phenylalanine is converted to phenylpyruvic acid, phenylacetic acid, and phenylacetylglutamine.

The transamination of phenylalanine to phenylpyruvic acid is sometimes deficient for the first few days of life, and the age at which phenylpyruvic acid can be first detected varies from 2 to 34 days. From the first week of life, o-hydroxyphenylacetic acid also is excreted in large amounts.

In addition to the disruption of phenylalanine metabolism, tryptophan and tyrosine are handled abnormally. Intestinal transport of L-tryptophan and tyrosine is impaired in PKU, and fecal content of tryptophan and tyrosine is increased. These abnormalities are reversed by dietary correction of the plasma phenylalanine levels (14). Miyamoto and Fitzpatrick suggested that a similar interference might occur in the oxidation of tyrosine to 3-(3,4-dihydroxyphenyl)alanine (dopa), a melanin precursor, and might be responsible for the deficiency of hair and skin pigment in phenylketonuric individuals (15). The biochemical pathology of PKU is reviewed to a greater extent by Scriver and colleagues (11).

Pathologic Anatomy

Alterations within the brain are nonspecific and diffuse. They involve gray and white matter, and they probably progress with age. Three types of alterations exist.

Interference with the Normal Maturation of the Brain

Brain growth is reduced, and microscopic examination shows impaired cortical layering, delayed outward migration of neuroblasts, and heterotopic gray matter (16). Additionally, the amount of Nissl granules is markedly deficient. This is particularly evident in those areas of the brain that are not fully developed at birth. Dendritic arborization and the number of synaptic spikes are reduced within the cortex (17). These changes point to a period of abnormal brain development extending from the last trimester of gestation into postnatal life (Fig. 1.2).

Defective Myelination

Defective myelination may be generalized or limited to areas where one would expect postnatal myelin deposition. Except for adult subjects with PKU with neurologic deterioration, products of myelin degeneration are unusual (18). Myelin is usually relatively pale, and a mild degree of gliosis (Fig. 1.3) and irregular areas of vacuolation (status spongiosus) can be present. Areas of vacuolation usually are seen in central white matter of the cerebral hemispheres and in the cerebellum.

Diminished or Absent Pigmentation of the Substantia Nigra and Locus Ceruleus

Because substantia nigra and locus ceruleus are normally pigmented in albinos, and tyrosinase activity cannot be demonstrated in normal neurons within the substantia nigra, diminished or absent pigmentation is not a result of tyrosinase inhibition by phenylalanine or its derivatives (19). Rather, neuromelanogenesis in the phenylketonuric patient must be interrupted at some other metabolic point, such as the metal-catalyzed pseudoperoxidation of dopamine derivatives probably responsible for the melanization of lipofuscin in the substantia nigra (19).

Clinical Manifestations

Phenylketonuric infants appear healthy at birth. In untreated infants, vomiting, which at times is projectile, and irritability are frequent during the first 2 months of life. By 49 months, delayed intellectual development becomes apparent (20). In the untreated classic case, mental retardation is severe, precluding speech and toilet training. Children in this category have an IQ

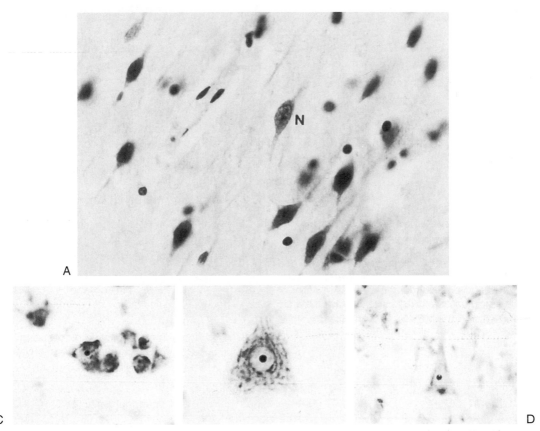

FIG. 1.2. Phenylketonuria. **A:** Cresyl-violet-stained section showing spindle-shaped immature neuron (N) (×350). (Courtesy of Dr. Nathan Malamud, Langley Porter Neuropsychiatric Institute, San Francisco, CA.) **B:** Photomicrograph of Nissl-stained giant Betz cell from a healthy 4-month-old child. **C:** Photomicrograph of Nissl-stained Betz cells from a healthy 14-year-old child. **D:** Photomicrograph of Nissl-stained Betz cell from a 19-year-old with untreated phenylketonuria. Patient's developmental level was 4.6 months at age 5 years and 10 months; he was microcephalic and had seizures commencing at 10 years of age. Note that the Betz cells are reduced in size, with a pale cytoplasm and few well-formed Nissl granules. These cytoarchitectural abnormalities are nonspecific. (**B**, **C**, and **D** from Bauman ML, Kemper TL. Morphologic and histoanatomic observations of the brain in untreated human phenylketonuria. *Acta Neuropathol* 1982;58:55–63. With permission.)

below 50. Seizures, common in the more severely retarded, usually start before 18 months of age and can cease spontaneously. During infancy, they often take the form of infantile spasms, later changing into tonic-clonic attacks.

The untreated phenylketonuric child is blond and blue-eyed, with normal and often pleasant features. The skin is rough and dry, sometimes with eczema. A peculiar musty odor, attributable to phenylacetic acid, can suggest the diagnosis. Significant neurologic abnormalities are rare, although hyperactivity and autistic features are not unusual. Microcephaly may be present, as well as a mild increase in muscle tone, particularly in the lower extremities. A fine, irregular tremor of the outstretched hands is seen in approximately 30% of the subjects. Parkinsonianlike extrapyramidal symptoms also have been encountered (21). The plantar response is often extensor.

A variety of electroencephalographic (EEG) abnormalities has been found, but hypsarrhythmic patterns, recorded even in the absence of seizures, and single and multiple foci of spike

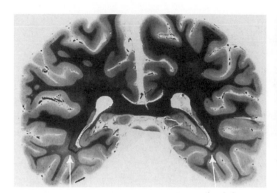

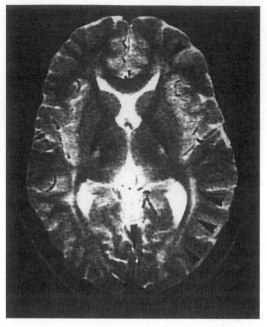

FIG. 1.3. Phenylketonuria. Cerebrum of a 35-year-old man stained for myelin by the Loyez method. The individual was never treated. He sat at 1 year and walked at 3 years. He was microcephalic, spastic, and never developed speech. Death was caused by pulmonary tuberculosis and dehydration. The visual radiations (*arrows*) stand out against the background of persisting pallor of the association tracts and nonspecific thalamic radiations. In a healthy brain of that age, the visual radiations are not distinguishable by tonality of staining from the completely myelinated white matter. (From Bauman ML, Kemper TL. Morphologic and histoanatomic observations of the brain in untreated human phenylketonuria. *Acta Neuropathol* 1982;58:55–63. With permission.)

FIG. 1.4. T2-weighted magnetic resonance imaging of a 16-year-old girl with phenylketonuria. The girl was treated from early infancy, and the diet was stopped at 12 years of age. At the time of the scan, her neurologic examination was normal, but her phenylalanine level was 27.0 mg/dL (1,639 μmol/L). The scan shows areas of high signal, particularly in the parieto-occipital areas, but also at the tips of the anterior horns of the lateral ventricles. (Courtesy of Dr. Alan J. Thompson, Neurorehabilitation Section, Institute of Neurology, University of London.)

and polyspike discharges are the most common (22). Neurologic examination of subjects who were treated before 2 months of age was abnormal in 40% in the experience of Thompson and colleagues (23). Abnormalities included hyperactive reflexes, tremors, and occasional seizures.

MRI is abnormal in almost every subject, regardless of when treatment was initiated. On T2-weighted imaging, one sees increased signal in the periventricular and subcortical white matter of the posterior hemispheres. Increased signal can extend to involve the deep white matter of the posterior hemispheres and the anterior hemispheres. No signal abnormalities are seen in brainstem, cerebellum, or cortex, although cortical atrophy can exist (Fig. 1.4) (24,25). The severity of the abnormality is unrelated to the subject's IQ, but is significantly associated with the phenylalanine level at the time of imaging. In adult patients with PKU who had come off their diets, resumption of dietary treatment can improve MRI abnormalities within a few weeks

or months, an observation that strongly suggests that at least some of the MRI changes are the result of edema (23,25).

Heterozygous mothers tend to have elevated plasma phenylalanine levels and somewhat reduced tyrosine values during the latter part of pregnancy and after delivery. Mothers suffering from PKU have a high incidence of spontaneous abortions. A sufficient number of offspring have been examined to indicate that when maternal blood phenylalanine levels are more than 20 mg/dL (1212 μmol/L), fetal brain damage is almost inevitable, with mental retardation encountered in 92% of offspring and microcephaly in 73%. Offspring have an unusual facies: upturned nose, underdeveloped philtrum, and a thin upper lip (26). Additionally, a significant incidence of congenital heart disease and prenatal and postnatal growth retardation occurs (27). MRI in these children shows hypoplasia or partial agenesis of the corpus callosum, and delayed myelination (28). These observations are best explained by a deleterious effect of elevated phenylalanine on the myelinating ability of oligodendrocytes.

Much, if not all, of the fetal damage appears preventable by placing phenylketonuric mothers on a phenylalanine-restricted diet before conception and maintaining blood phenylalanine levels below 6 mg/dL (360 μmol/L) throughout pregnancy (29). Birth weight and head circumference in infants of mothers so managed were normal, and no evidence existed for fetal nutritional deficiency. Offspring of mothers who experience mild PKU as defined by phenylalanine levels of less than 400 μmol/L (6.6 mg/dL) appear to be normal, and mothers do not require dietary intervention (30).

The pathogenesis of mental retardation in PKU is still unclear (31). At present, no evidence exists that phenylpyruvic acid or any of the other phenylalanine metabolites are neurotoxic at concentrations in which they are seen in PKU (32). Probably no single factor is responsible, rather impairment of amino acid transport across the blood–brain barrier; disruption of the brain amino acid pool; and consequent defective proteolipid protein synthesis, impaired myelination, and low levels of neurotransmitters, such as serotonin, are responsible to varying degrees (33,34).

Diagnosis

Phenotypically, the diagnosis of PKU can be suspected from the clinical features of the disease and from the examination of the patient's urine using a ferric chloride test. Currently, most patients with PKU are identified through a newborn screening program (35,36). As mentioned in the section on Molecular Genetic and Biochemical Pathology, plasma phenylalanine levels are elevated in the cord blood of phenylketonuric infants and increase rapidly within a few hours of birth. A screening program that involves spectrofluorometric or microbiological estimation of blood phenylalanine

is used commonly. Tandem mass spectrometric analysis of phenylalanine and other amino acids as well as of the acylcarnitines of the various organic acids also has been used in some laboratories (36a), and trials of this method for newborn screening are being instituted in several states, including California. Whatever the method, the screening test requires a drop of whole blood placed on a filter paper. If positive [a value greater than 2 to 4 mg/dL (120 to 240 μmol/L)], the diagnosis is confirmed by quantitative analysis of phenylalanine and tyrosine in blood. Although most infants whose blood phenylalanine levels are above the threshold value do not have PKU, such patients require prompt reevaluation by an appropriate laboratory to determine whether hyperphenylalaninemia is persistent and to determine whether it is caused by PAH deficiency.

Of considerably greater concern are the false-negative test results. It is now clear that routine screening tests, when correctly performed after 12 hours of life, detect all infants with classic PKU. In a group of such infants, the lowest phenylalanine value recorded at 24 hours was 5.6 mg/dL (339 μmol/L), at 48 hours, 7.5 mg/dL (454 μmol/L), and at 72 hours, 8.4 mg/dL (509 μmol/L). Thus, even at 24 hours, none of the infants with classic PKU would have escaped detection (37). As a rule, breast-fed PKU infants have higher phenylalanine levels than those who are formula-fed. In all cases, a second screening blood specimen should be obtained from all infants whose first blood specimen was drawn during the first 24 hours of life (38,39).

The widespread screening programs to detect newborns with blood phenylalanine concentrations higher than normal also have uncovered other conditions in which blood phenylalanine levels are increased in the neonatal period. Patients with moderate and mild PKU and mild hyperphenylalaninemia, as these entities are termed, have phenylalanine levels that tend to be lower than those seen in classic PKU and have a less severe mutation in the gene for PAH (13a). Some of these various phenotypes are the result of different phenotypic severity of the various mutations in the PAH gene, with most of the mild hyperphenylalaninemias representing compound heterozygotes for a mutation that abolishes catalytic activity of PAH, and one that reduces it (13a,40,41). With normal protein intakes, their phenylalanine levels range between 4 and 20 mg/dL (242 and 1,212 μmol/L), and the majority appear to have unimpaired intelligence, even when untreated.

In infants with mild hyperphenylalaninemia, the increase in blood phenylalanine is sufficiently slow to allow some to escape detection even when routine screening is performed at 72 hours. When follow-up phenylalanine determinations are run between ages 2 and 6 weeks, positive test results are found in some patients with the milder hyperphenylalaninemias and in patients with PKU whose initial screening test result was reported negative as a result of a laboratory error (42). An evaluation of patients with PKU who missed being diagnosed by screening during the neonatal period (approximately 1 for every 70 detected) indicates that laboratory errors are responsible for 58% of the missed cases and inadequate follow-up for 21% (43). Approximately one-third of these missed diagnoses result in legal action.

Genotypically, prenatal determination of the heterozygote or homozygote can be performed by gene mapping techniques using DNA restriction fragment polymorphisms derived from DNA extracted from lymphocytes. Radiolabeled nucleotides specific for the most common mutations have been prepared by the polymerase chain reaction technique using DNA isolated from lymphocytes of classic patients with PKU. This method exponentially amplifies specific DNA sequences *in vitro*, so that considerable quantities become available and can be used by hybridization studies to determine whether this specific pathologic sequence is present in the DNA of a given subject (Fig. 1.5) (44,45).

Other Conditions Characterized by Hyperphenylalaninemia

Three forms of phenylalaninemia, accounting for 13% of cases of elevated phenylalanine levels in white infants, and characterized by progressive brain degeneration and many neurologic deficits, are aptly termed *malignant phenylalaninemia*. Biochemically, these conditions are characterized by a defect in the production of tetrahydrobiopterin (BH$_4$), the cofactor in the hydroxylation of phenylalanine to tyrosine.

The first and most common of these conditions to be recognized is characterized by undetectable dihydropteridine reductase activity in liver, brain, and cultured fibroblasts, but normal hepatic PAH activity (46). Dihydropteridine reductase is responsible for the regeneration of tetrahydrobiopterin from quinoid dihydrobiopterin (see Fig. 1.1). BH$_4$ levels are low in blood, urine, CSF, and a number of tissues. Because BH$_4$ is an essential coenzyme for hydroxylation of not only phenylalanine, but also tyrosine and tryptophan, affected children show a defect in the synthesis of dopamine, norepinephrine, epinephrine, and serotonin.

The clinical picture of dihydropteridine reductase deficiency is one of developmental delay associated with the evolution of marked hypotonia, involuntary movements, oculogyric crises, and tonic-clonic and myoclonic seizures. None of these symptoms responds to restriction of phenylalanine intake (47,48). Progressive intracranial calcifications can be demonstrated by CT scanning. These might be the consequence of reduced intracranial tetrahydrofolate (49), because folate deficiency, whether it is caused by inadequate intake or defective absorption, can induce intracranial calcifications. MRI demonstrates white matter abnormalities and cystic loss of parenchyma (50).

Treatment for patients with dihydropteridine reductase deficiency requires restriction of phenylalanine intake and administration of catechol and serotonin precursors. The former is given as levodopa-carbidopa (Sinemet), and the latter as 5-hydroxytryptophan (8 to 10 mg/kg per day). Additionally, folinic acid (12.5 mg per day) is added to the diet (51). Treatment of the other variants is discussed by Kaufman (52).

Increased phenylalanine levels can result not only from decreased regeneration of BH$_4$ as a result of dihydropteridine reductase deficiency, but also from inadequate biopterin synthesis. Thus, in the second type of malignant hyperphenylalaninemia, the defect is localized to the synthetic pathway of BH$_4$ at the point of the formation of 6-pyruvoyl-tetrahydropterin (6-PT) (see Fig. 1.1). The enzyme deficiency can be complete, partial, or transient or might affect only nonneural tissue (47,52–54).

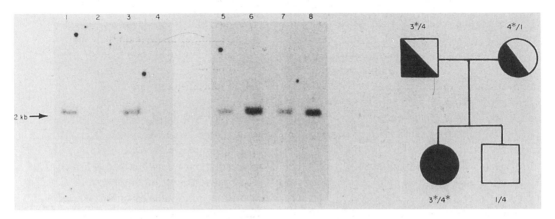

FIG. 1.5. Oligonucleotide hybridization analysis. Lanes 1 and 5, father; lanes 2 and 6, mother; lanes 3 and 7, child with phenylketonuria (PKU); lanes 4 and 8, unaffected child. A mutant splicing probe specific for the exon/intron 12 splice junction was used for lanes 1 to 4, and the normal splicing probe for the junction was used for lanes 5 to 8. DNA was isolated from leukocytes of family members, digested with the restriction enzyme Pvu II, and subjected to electrophoresis. The segregation of PKU alleles (*) and the restriction fraction polymorphism haplotypes for each family member are shown on the right. In this family, the father has a mutant haplotype 3 gene that hybridizes to the mutant splicing probe (lane 1), and a normal haplotype 4 gene that hybridizes to the normal splicing probe (lane 5). The mother has a mutant haplotype 4 gene and a normal haplotype 1 gene. The mutant splicing probe does not hybridize to her DNA (lane 2), whereas the normal splicing probe hybridizes strongly (lane 6). The data show that the PKU mutation associated with the mother's mutant haplotype 4 allele is not the same as that associated with the father's mutant haplotype 3 allele. The PKU child in this family inherited the mutant haplotype 3 gene from his father and the mutant haplotype 4 gene from his mother. DNA isolated from this child hybridized to both the mutant and the normal splicing probes (lanes 3 and 7). This PKU child, therefore, has two different mutant phenylalanine hydroxylase alleles, and, consequently, is a compound heterozygote. The unaffected sibling has inherited the normal haplotype 4 allele from his father and the normal haplotype 1 allele from his mother. He hybridizes strongly to the normal probe (lane 8), but not to the mutant probe (lane 4). A probe for the other mutant was not available. (From DiLella AG, Woo SL. Molecular basis of phenylketonuria and its clinical applications. *Mol Biol Med* 1987;4:183. With permission.)

The clinical picture of this entity is much like that of dihydropteridine reductase deficiency: progressive neurologic deterioration highlighted by hypotonia, involuntary movements, and seizures. Diagnosis of this variant depends on normal assays for PAH and dihydropteridine reductase and on determination of urinary pterins (55). MRI in this disorder is similar to that seen in classical PKU (56).

Another rare cause for persistent hyperphenylalaninemia is a defect of GTP-cyclohydrolase, needed for the first step of BH_4 biosynthesis (see Fig. 1.1) (57,58). Symptoms include hypotonia, seizures, and hyperthermia. Mutations in GTP-cyclohydrolase are also responsible for dopa-responsive dystonia, a condition covered in the section on Primary Dystonia. Symptoms in this condition differ considerably from those seen in

hyperphenylalaninemia. The best explanation for the phenotypic diversity is that the mutant enzyme has a dominant negative effect on the normal enzyme (58a).

Elevated blood phenylalanine levels also are observed in 25% of premature infants and occasionally in full-term newborns. In all of these patients, tyrosine levels are increased to a much greater extent than are phenylalanine levels.

Treatment

Treatment of PKU can be attempted on two levels: modification of the phenotypic expression of the defective gene and definitive treatment by correcting the gene defect. Only the first approach has been used in clinical practice.

On referral of an infant with a confirmed positive screening test result, the first step is quantitative determination of serum phenylalanine and tyrosine levels. All infants whose blood phenylalanine concentration is greater than 10 mg/dL (600 μmol/L) and whose tyrosine concentration is low or normal (1 to 4 mg/dL) should be started on a low-phenylalanine diet immediately. Infants whose blood phenylalanine concentrations remain in the range of 6.6 to 10.0 mg/dL (400 to 600 μmol/L) should be treated also.

The generally accepted therapy for classic PKU is restriction of the dietary intake of phenylalanine by placing the infant on one of several low-phenylalanine formulas. The diet should be managed by a team consisting of a nutritionist, a physician with expertise in metabolic disorders, and a person to ensure dietary compliance. To avoid symptoms of phenylalanine deficiency, milk is added to the diet in amounts sufficient to maintain blood levels of the amino acid between 2 and 6 mg/dL (120 and 360 μmol/L). Generally, patients tolerate this diet quite well, and within 1 to 2 weeks, the serum concentration of phenylalanine becomes normal. Serum phenylalanine determinations are essential to ensure adequate regulation of diet. These are performed twice weekly during the first 6 months of life, and twice monthly thereafter.

Strict dietary control should be maintained for as long as possible, and most centers strive to keep levels below 6.0 mg/dL (360 μmol/L), even in patients with moderate and mild PKU. Samples of low-phenylalanine menus are given by Buist and colleagues (59), and the nutritional problems inherent in prolonged use of a restricted diet are discussed by Acosta and colleagues (60). Dietary lapses frequently are accompanied by progressive white matter abnormalities on MRI. Some workers have suggested supplementation of the low-phenylalanine diet with tyrosine, but no statistical evidence exists that this regimen results in a better intellectual outcome. Failure to treat subjects with mild hyperphenylalaninemias does not appear to produce either intellectual deficits or MRI abnormalities.

Dietary therapy has for the greater part been effective in preventing mental retardation in patients with severe PKU. It has become apparent that the outcome depends on several factors. Most important is the age at which the diet was initiated. Smith and coworkers found that patients' IQ fell approximately four points for each month between birth and start of treatment (61). The average phenylalanine concentration while receiving treatment also affects outcome, with optimal average phenylalanine levels in the most recent cohorts being 5.0 to 6.6 mg/dL (300 to 400 μmol/L). Additionally, hypophenylalaninemia during the first 2 years of life [i.e., the length of time that phenylalanine concentration was below 2.0 mg/dL (120 μmol/L)], also affected outcome adversely. Even patients with normal IQ scores and with the most favorable diagnostic and treatment characteristics have lower IQs than other members of their families and suffer from cognitive deficits, educational difficulties, and behavioral problems, notably hyperactivity (61–63). Dietary supplementation with tyrosine, although used in several centers, does not appear to improve performance on neuropsychological tests (64). The most likely explanations for these deficits are inadequate dietary control or unavoidable prenatal damage by elevated phenylalanine on the developing brain with induction of minor structural malformations (see Fig. 1.2) (16).

When patients who already have developed symptoms caused by classic PKU are placed and maintained on a low-phenylalanine diet, their seizures disappear and their EEG results tend to revert to normal. Microcephaly, if present, can correct itself, and abnormally blond hair regains its natural color.

Considerable uncertainty exists about when, if ever, to terminate the diet (65). In the series of Waisbren and coworkers (66), one-third of youngsters whose diet was discontinued at 5 years of age had a reduction in IQ of 10 points or more during the ensuing 5 years. The blood phenylalanine level when the children were off the restrictive diet predicted the change in IQ. Of the children whose IQs dropped 20 or more points, 90% had blood phenylalanine levels of 18 mg/dL (1,090 μmol/L) or higher, and 40% of

TABLE 1.4. *Some neurogenetic diseases that may be treated by bone marrow transplantation*

Disease	Expression	Results of treatment
Chédiak-Higashi syndrome	Expression of genetic defect restricted to lymphoid and hematopoietic cells	Correctable by BMT
Gaucher disease (adult form)	Generalized genetic defect; symptoms restricted to lymphohematopoietic cells	Correctable by BMT
Adrenoleukodystrophy	Generalized genetic defect; generalized clinical symptoms with central nervous system involvement	May be correctable by BMT
Metachromatic leukodystrophy	—	Adult form may be stabilized
Globoid cell leukodystrophy	—	—
Mucopolysaccharidoses		
Hurler disease	—	Visceral symptoms improve, neurologic symptoms may stabilize
Hunter disease	—	Visceral symptoms improve, neurologic symptoms appear to progress
Sanfilippo disease	—	No effect on neurologic symptoms
Phenylketonuria	Lymphohematopoietic cells do not express normal gene product	Not correctable by BMT

BMT, bone marrow transplantation.
Adapted from Parkman R. The application of bone marrow transplantation to the treatment of genetic diseases. *Science* 1986;232:1373–1378.

those whose IQs rose 10 points or more had a phenylalanine level of less than 18 mg/dL (1,090 µmol/L). In young adult patients with PKU, discontinuation of the diet was accompanied by the evolution of spasticity and worsening of white matter abnormalities as observed on serial MRI (67). Reinstitution of diet results in clear clinical improvement and resolution of new MRI abnormalities. Reports such as these speak against early relaxation of the restrictions on phenylalanine intake and indicate that dietary therapy for patients with classical PKU should be lifelong (68,68a).

The inadequacies of dietary therapy underline the need for a more definitive approach to the treatment of PKU. Allogeneic or autologous bone marrow transplants are being used for the treatment of a variety of genetic diseases (Table 1.4). The likelihood that this procedure will cure or at least stabilize a genetic disease depends on the tissue-specific expression of the normal gene product, the patient's clinical symptoms, and the cellular transport of the normal gene product (69,70). In PKU, the defective enzyme is not normally expressed in bone marrow–derived cells, and bone marrow transplantation has no therapeutic value (see Table 1.4). To date, liver transplantation for the treatment of inborn errors

of metabolism affecting the nervous system has been limited to Wilson disease, glycogen storage disease, Crigler-Najjar disease, and tyrosinemia type I (71).

Another approach to treating the patient with PKU is the introduction of PAH gene into affected hepatic cells. Recombinant viruses containing human PAH have been introduced into mouse hepatoma cells, where they are able to continue expressing the human enzyme (72). The next step would be to find a virus that can infect human liver, maintain itself there without inducing damage to the organ, and allow the human gene to continue functioning in the new host. The use of implanted microencapsulated genetically engineered cells to remove phenylalanine is under investigation (73).

Treatment of phenylalaninemia caused by tetrahydrobiopterin deficiency involves administration of tetrahydrobiopterin or a synthetic pterin and replenishment of the neurotransmitters (levodopa, 5-hydroxy-tryptophan) because synthesis of these substances is impaired also.

Tyrosinosis and Tyrosinemia

Several clinically and biochemically distinct disorders are characterized by an elevation in

TABLE 1.5. *Clinical and genetic features of the tyrosinemias*

Condition	Clinical manifestations	Enzyme defect	Reference
Tyrosinemia type I	Acute episodes of weakness, pain, self-mutilation, porphyrialike axonopathic process; seizures and extensor hypertonia; hepatic necrosis, renal tubular damage; carrier rate 1 in 20 in French-Canadian isolates	Fumarylacetoacetase	106,107
Tyrosinemia type II	Mental retardation, herpetiform corneal ulcers, palmoplantar keratoses	Tyrosine transaminase soluble form	108,109
Tyrosinemia type III	Mild mental retardation	HPPA oxidase	110–112
Tyrosinosis	Only one reported case, asymptomatic	?	113
Tyrosinemia of prematurity	No clinical abnormalities, follow-up suggests impaired visual-perceptual function	Inactivation of HPPA oxidase by its substrate	114,115
Hawkinsinuria	Metabolic acidosis, failure to thrive, dominant inheritance, unusual, swimming pool odor	Excretion of a cysteine or glutathione-conjugated intermediate in conversion of HPPA to homogentisic acid (Hawkinsin[a])	116

HPPA, 4-hydroxyphenyl pyruvic acid.
[a]The name *Hawkinsin* is derived from the family in whom the disease was first described (117).

serum tyrosine and the excretion of large amounts of tyrosine and its metabolites (74). Their clinical and biochemical characteristics are outlined in Table 1.5.

Maple Syrup Urine Disease

Maple syrup urine disease (MSUD) is a familial cerebral degenerative disease caused by a defect in branched chain amino acid metabolism and characterized by the passage of urine that has a sweet, maple syrup–like odor. It was first described in 1954 by Menkes and coworkers (75). Since then, numerous other cases have been diagnosed throughout the world, and its incidence is estimated at 1 in 220,000 births (76). In some inbred populations, such as the Mennonites, the incidence, however, is as high as 1 in 176 births (77). The disease occurs in all races and is transmitted in an autosomal recessive manner.

Molecular Genetics and Biochemical Pathology

MSUD is characterized by the accumulation of three branched chain ketoacids: α-ketoisocaproic acid, α-ketoisovaleric acid, and α-keto-β-methylvaleric acid, the derivatives of leucine, valine, and isoleucine, respectively (78,79). Their accumulation is the consequence of a defect in oxidative decarboxylation of branched chain ketoacids (Fig. 1.6).

The branched chain α-ketoacid dehydrogenase complex is located within the mitochondrial inner membrane matrix compartment. It is a multienzyme complex comprising six proteins: $E_{1\alpha}$ and $E_{1\beta}$, which form the decarboxylase; E_2; E_3; and a branched chain–specific kinase and phosphatase. The last two enzymes regulate the activity of the complex by phosphorylating and dephosphorylating the dehydrogenase. E_1 is a thiamin pyrophosphate–dependent enzyme. The second enzyme (E_2), dihydrolipoyltransacylase, transfers the acyl group from the first enzyme to coenzyme A. The third enzyme (E_3), dihydrolipoyldehydrogenase, a flavoprotein, reoxidizes the disulfhydryl form of lipoamide. The same enzyme is common to other α-ketoacid dehydrogenases, such as pyruvate and α-ketoglutarate dehydrogenase (80). The complex removes carboxyl groups from all three branched chain ketoacids and converts those ketoacids to their respective coenzyme A derivatives (see Fig. 1.6, step 2).

With six genes involved in the function of the branched chain ketoacid dehydrogenase complex, considerable room for heterogeneity exists. Mutations in the genes for $E_{1\alpha}$, $E_{1\beta}$, E_2, and E_3 have been described, with many MSUD

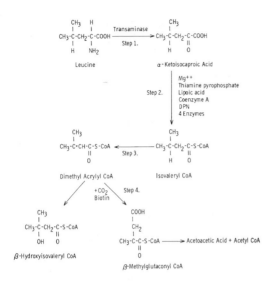

FIG. 1.6. Degradation of leucine in mammalian tissues. In maple syrup urine disease, the metabolic block is located at step 2. In isovaleric acidemia, the block is confined to step 3. A rare entity with a possible metabolic block at step 4 also has been reported.

patients being compound heterozygotes. These induce a continuum of disease severity that ranges from the severe, classic form of MSUD to mild and intermittent forms.

As a consequence of the enzymatic defect, the branched chain ketoacids accumulate in serum and CSF and are excreted in large quantities in urine (79). Plasma levels of the respective amino acids (e.g., leucine, isoleucine, and valine) are elevated secondary to the increase in ketoacid concentrations. Alloisoleucine, which is formed by transamination of α-keto-β-methylvaleric acid, also has been found in serum (81). In some cases, the branched chain hydroxyacids, most prominently α-hydroxyisovaleric acid (82), are excreted also. Sotolone, a derivative of α–ketabutyric acid, the decarboxylation of which is impaired by accumulation of α-keto-β-methylvaleric acid, is responsible for the characteristic odor of the patient's urine and perspiration (78a).

Pathologic Anatomy

Structural alterations in the nervous system in untreated infants with MSUD are similar to, but

more severe than, those seen in PKU. In infants dying during the acute phase of the disease, diffuse edema occurs (75). The cytoarchitecture of the cortex is generally immature, with fewer cortical layers and the persistence of ectopic foci of neuroblasts, an indication of disturbed neuronal migration. Dendritic development is abnormal, and the number of oligodendrocytes and the amount of myelin are less than would be seen in a healthy brain of comparable age (83). Marked astrocytic gliosis and generalized cystic degeneration occur (84). Little clinical or pathologic evidence exists for demyelination in subjects who are treated early (85,86). On chemical examination, the concentration of myelin lipids is markedly reduced, with cerebrosides, sulfatides, and proteolipid protein almost completely absent. These abnormalities are not found in infants dying of the disease within the first days of life, or in patients treated by restriction of branched chain amino acid intake (86).

Clinical Manifestations

Various mutations result in five fairly distinct clinical phenotypes of MSUD. Patients can be homozygotes for the same allele or compound heterozygotes for different alleles. The classic form of MSUD accounts for approximately 75% of patients (77). In the original four patients reported by Menkes and coworkers (75), as well as in subsequent cases, opisthotonos, intermittent increase in muscle tone, and respiratory irregularities appeared within the first week of life in babies apparently healthy at birth (87). Subsequently, rapid deterioration of the nervous system occurred, and all but one died within 1 month. In some patients, cerebral edema is marked and can be fatal (88). Other patients, spastic and intellectually retarded, have survived without treatment for several years. A fluctuating ophthalmoplegia correlates in intensity with serum leucine levels (89). Presentation with pseudotumor cerebri also has been reported. Approximately 50% of patients with the classic form of MSUD develop severe hypoglycemia; this is probably the consequence of a defective gluconeogenesis from amino acids, particularly alanine (90).

MRI during the acute stage of the disease before treatment is characteristic. It demonstrates edema that is maximal in cerebellar deep white matter, the posterior portion of the brainstem, and the posterior limb of the internal capsule. Edema also is seen in the cortical U fibers, the head of the caudate, and the putamen (91,92). These findings are consistent with the location of status spongiosus noted on pathologic examination. The cause of the acute cerebral edema and its unique localization are unknown. Because a reduced intake of branched chain amino acids prevents the evolution of the more severe neurologic symptoms, damage probably results from their accumulation or from accumulation of their ketoacid metabolites. As is the case in PKU, chronic brain damage is probably caused by interference with amino acid transport into the brain, a deranged amino acid environment, and, consequently, failure in biosynthesis of proteolipids, myelin, and neurotransmitters (93). In treated subjects, the MRI discloses symmetric bilateral periventricular high signal intensity on T2-weighted images. This picture is similar to that seen in PKU and suggests focal dysmyelination (85).

The intermittent form of MSUD results from a variety of mutations in the gene for E_2, and branched chain dehydrogenase activity is higher than in the classic form, usually 5% to 20% of normal (94). The clinical picture is that of intermittent periods of ataxia, drowsiness, behavior disturbances, and seizures that make their first appearance between ages 6 and 9 months. Attacks are generally triggered by infections, immunizations, or other forms of stress (95).

In the intermediate form, the clinical picture is one of mild to moderate mental retardation (96). Branched chain dehydrogenase activity ranges from 5% to 20% of normal, and the defect is usually in the gene coding for $E_{1\alpha}$ (80).

A thiamin-responsive variant represents an entity in which, in some cases at least, a mutant exists in the gene for E_2. The reason for the effectiveness of thiamin therapy in this variant is unclear; addition of thiamin increases the activity of the branched chain dehydrogenase complex *in vivo*, but not in cultured cells (97,98).

Mutants defective in the gene for E_3 present with hypotonia, rapid neurologic deterioration, and severe lactic acidosis. This entity is covered with the various other organic acidemias.

Diagnosis

Clinically, MSUD is diagnosed by the characteristic odor of the patient and by a positive 2,4-dinitrophenylhydrazine urine test. Plasma branched chain amino acids are elevated by the time the infant is 24 hours old, even in those infants who have not yet been given protein (99). Routine newborn screening for the condition using a bacterial inhibition assay analogous to that used for the neonatal diagnosis of PKU is performed in many states in the United States and in many countries abroad (100). Tandem mass spectroscopy also can be used and has the advantage of obtaining rapid quantitative measurements of all three branched chain amino acids (36a). The presence of the branched chain ketoacid decarboxylases in cultivated amniocytes and chorionic villi allows the antenatal diagnosis of the disease as early as 10 weeks' gestation (101).

Treatment

Treatment consists of restricting the dietary intake of the branched chain amino acids through the use of one of several commercially available formulas (102). For optimal results, infants should be placed on the diet during the first few days of life and should receive frequent measurements of serum amino acids. Prompt and vigorous treatment of even mild infections is mandatory; a number of children on this synthetic diet have died of septicemia (87).

Peritoneal dialysis or multiple exchange transfusions have been used to correct coma or other acute neurologic symptoms in the newly diagnosed infant (102). Another, simpler approach is to provide intravenously or by nasogastric tube an amino acid mixture devoid of the branched chain amino acids (103). Most of the children in whom long-term dietary therapy was initiated during the first 2 weeks of life, and whose dietary control was meticulously maintained, achieved normal or nearly normal IQs (104). In the experience of Hilliges and coworkers, the mean IQ of MSUD patients at 3 to 16 years of age was 74 ± 14, as compared with 101 ± 12 for early treated patients with PKU. The length of time after birth that plasma leucine concentrations remain elevated appears to affect the IQ, as does the amount, if any, of residual branched chain ketoacid dehydrogenase activity (105). The thiamin-responsive child is treated with 10 to 1,000 mg thiamin per day (102).

Nonketotic Hyperglycinemia (AR) *Hiccups)*

This relatively common family of diseases is marked by genetic and phenotypic heterogeneity, and considerable variation occurs in the severity of neurologic symptoms (118). In the infantile form, neurologic symptoms begin during the neonatal period. They are highlighted by profound hypotonia, intractable generalized or myoclonic seizures, apnea, and progressive obtundation with coma and respiratory arrest. The EEG demonstrates a burst-suppression pattern or, later, hypsarrhythmia (119). Nystagmus and a marked depression of the electroretinogram results (ERG) also are seen. The majority of affected infants die during the neonatal period; those who survive are profoundly retarded. A transient neonatal form has been recognized that initially is clinically indistinguishable from the permanent form of nonketotic hyperglycinemia. However, symptoms remit abruptly after a few days or months and youngsters are left unimpaired (120).

A less severe form becomes apparent during the latter part of the first year of life after several months of normal development. It is marked by progressive dementia leading to decerebrate rigidity. Extrapyramidal signs are not uncommon (121). A juvenile form with mild mental retardation, hyperactivity, and language deficits also has been reported, as has a neurodegenerative picture (119,122).

Pathologic examination of the brain in the infantile form of the disease discloses a reduction in white matter with an extensive spongy degeneration accompanied by marked gliosis (122). Partial or complete agenesis of the corpus callosum has been described, an indication of a significant intrauterine insult (119).

The marked increase in plasma and CSF glycine, and the markedly elevated ratio of CSF glycine to blood glycine are diagnostic of the condition (119). The MRI shows decreased or absent supratentorial white matter, with thinning of the corpus callosum and cortical atrophy (123).

The basic defect in this condition is localized to the mitochondrial glycine cleavage system, which converts glycine to serine and is expressed in liver and brain. This complex reaction requires four protein components and, to date, defects in one or another of three of these components have been documented (119). Some correlation exists between the clinical expression of the disease and the genetic lesion. The classic neonatal form of the disease usually is associated with virtual absence of the pyridoxal-containing decarboxylase (P protein), and the milder atypical forms with the tetrahydrofolate-requiring transfer protein (T protein) (119,124).

The pathophysiology of the neurologic abnormalities has not been established fully. Glycine is an inhibitory neurotransmitter that acts mainly at spinal cord and brainstem levels. It also acts as a coagonist for the N-methyl-D-aspartate glutamate receptor, modulating its activity and probably producing seizures by an excitotoxic mechanism (119). The inhibitory effects of glycine are blocked by strychnine, but its effectiveness on the basic course of the illness is questionable. Blockers of the N-methyl-D-aspartate receptor, such as dextromorphan or ketamine, may have beneficial effects in isolated cases, but the clinical variability of the condition precludes their accurate assessment (125,126).

Defects in Urea Cycle Metabolism

Six inborn errors in the urea cycle have been described. Five of these represent a lesion at each of the five steps in the conversion of ammonia to urea (Fig. 1.7). These include argininosuccinic aciduria, citrullinuria, hyperargininemia, and two conditions termed *hyperammonemia*, the more common one attributable to a defect of ornithine transcarbamylase (OTC), and the other the result of a defect in mitochondrial carbamyl

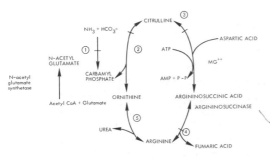

FIG. 1.7. Normal urea cycle. The cycle is completely reversible. In argininosuccinic aciduria, the cycle is blocked at step 4. In citrullinuria, the block occurs at step 3. In ornithine transcarbamylase deficiency, the block is at step 2. In carbamoylphosphate synthetase deficiency, the block is at step 1. A defect in N-acetylglutamate synthetase results in hyperammonemia by depriving step 1 of its activator, N-acetylglutamate. The enzyme is inhibited by a variety of organic thioesters, notably propionyl-CoA and isovaleryl-CoA. In hyperargininemia, the defect is one of arginase, step 5.

phosphate synthetase (CPS). The genes for all components of the urea cycle have been cloned. Additionally, a deficiency of N-acetylglutamate synthetase has been reported (127). This enzyme is responsible for the formation of N-acetylglutamate, a required activator for mitochondrial CPS. The biochemical aspects of the urea cycle have been reviewed by Batshaw (128).

Because most systemic and neurologic symptoms in these diseases are the consequences of hyperammonemia or the accumulation of urea cycle intermediates, clinical manifestations of the urea cycle defects are nonspecific and overlap considerably. In their classic presentation, which occurs in some 60% of cases (129), the conditions become apparent between 24 and 72 hours of life. Initial symptoms include vomiting, lethargy, and hypotonia. These progress rapidly to seizures and coma. The EEG often shows suppression bursts, and neuroimaging indicates the presence of cerebral edema.

When the enzyme deficiency is less severe, hyperammonemic episodes are delayed to late infancy or childhood. Subjects have recurrent episodes of lethargy, vomiting, and, less often, seizures. Hyperactivity, behavioral abnormalities, and moderate to severe mental retardation are

common, as is intolerance of protein-containing foods (130).

Argininosuccinic Aciduria

Argininosuccinic aciduria is one of the more common of the urea cycle disorders. The condition is characterized by mental retardation, poorly formed hair, and accumulation of argininosuccinic acid in body fluids. It was first described in 1958 by Allan and others (131).

Molecular Genetics and Biochemical Pathology

Argininosuccinic acid is a normal intermediary metabolite in the synthesis of urea (see Fig. 1.7). A deficiency in argininosuccinate lyase, an enzyme whose gene is on chromosome 7, has been demonstrated in liver and skin fibroblast cultures (132).

The synthesis of urea is only slightly depressed, but a large proportion of labeled ammonium lactate administered to affected individuals is converted to glutamine (133). The manner in which children synthesize urea is not clear. It appears likely that in argininosuccinic aciduria, as well as in the other defects of urea cycle, substrate accumulates to a concentration at which the decreased substrate-binding capacity of the mutant enzyme is overcome by the accumulation of precursor to levels greater than the Km for the mutated enzyme (134).

Pathologic Anatomy

The liver architecture is abnormal, with increased fat deposition. The brain in one patient who died at age 9 days was edematous, with poor demarcation of gray and white matter. The cortical layers were poorly developed, and myelination was defective with vacuolated myelin sheaths and cystic degeneration of white matter (135). An older patient had atypical astrocytes similar to the Alzheimer II cells seen in Wilson disease and in severe chronic liver disease (136).

Clinical Manifestations

As ascertained by newborn screening, the incidence of argininosuccinic aciduria in Massachusetts is 1 in 70,000, and 1 in 91,000 in Austria (137). Three distinct clinical forms have been recognized, each resulting from a different genetic mutation (138).

The most severe entity is the neonatal form. Infants feed poorly, become lethargic, develop seizures, and generally die within 2 weeks (135,139). In a second form, progression is less rapid, but similar symptoms appear in early infancy. In the majority of patients, including those described by Allan and coworkers (131), the presenting symptoms are mental retardation, recurrent generalized convulsions, poorly pigmented brittle hair (trichorrhexis nodosa), ataxia, and hepatomegaly (140). Some patients have been seizure free, however, and have presented with little more than learning difficulties, and others (approximately 20% of all affected children) have had normal intelligence without treatment (141).

Diagnosis

The presence of elevated blood ammonia should suggest a disorder in the urea cycle. Initial evaluation of such a child should include routine blood chemistries, plasma lactate levels, liver function tests, quantitative assay of plasma amino acids, and assay of urine for organic acids and orotic acid (128). The specific diagnosis of argininosuccinic aciduria can be made by a significant elevation of plasma citrulline, and the presence of large quantities of plasma, urinary, and CSF argininosuccinic acid. In some instances, fasting blood ammonia level can be normal or only slightly elevated, but marked elevations occur after protein loading. Increased excretion of orotic acid is seen in all urea cycle defects, with the exception of CPS deficiency (142).

Treatment

Hyperammonemic coma in the neonate caused by any of the urea cycle defects requires prompt intervention. In essence, treatment consists of detoxification and removal of the excess ammonia, and reduction in the formation of ammonia. Quantitative amino acid chromatography should be performed on an emergency basis, and the infant should be given a high dose of intravenous glucose with insulin to suppress protein catabolism. The elevated ammonia levels can be reduced by hemodialysis if available, or by peritoneal dialysis (143). Details of treatment are presented by Brusilow and Horwich (141) and Batshaw and colleagues (144). Treatment for increased intracranial pressure, which frequently accompanies neonatal hyperammonemia, is symptomatic.

The long-term management of an infant who suffers a urea cycle defect is directed toward lowering blood ammonia levels and maintaining them as close to normal as possible. This is accomplished by providing the infant with alternative pathways for waste nitrogen synthesis and excretion. Infants with argininosuccinic aciduria are placed on a protein-restricted diet (1.2 to 2.0 g/kg per day), which is supplemented with L-arginine (0.4 to 0.7 g/kg per day), which promotes the synthesis of citrulline and argininosuccinate as waste nitrogen products, and citrate, which improves weight gain and reduces hepatomegaly (141,144).

Episodes of hyperammonemia are generally triggered by intercurrent infections. Prevention of a rapid progression to death requires hospitalization and the use of intravenous therapy (141).

On this regimen, children with argininosuccinic aciduria do well. Reduction of blood ammonia levels is accompanied by improved growth, reduction in liver size, cessation of seizures, and, in some patients, normal hair. Intellectual function is significantly impaired, however. In the experience of Batshaw and coworkers, all infants with the severe, neonatal form of the disease survived, although those who have been followed the longest have shown a significant lowering of their IQs (144). Children with the late-onset variant fare much better, and with therapy, achieve normal development (140). As a rule, the individual's ultimate IQ is a function of the severity and duration of hyperammonemic coma, and children who have not recovered from coma within 5 days do poorly (145). Valproic acid cannot be used in the treatment of seizures associated with this and with the other urea cycle defects because it induces severe hyperammonemia at even low dosages (146).

Citrullinemia (Argininosuccinic Acid Synthetase Deficiency)

In 1963, McMurray and associates reported a mentally retarded infant who had a metabolic block in the conversion of citrulline to argininosuccinic acid (see Fig. 1.7, step 3) (147). Since then, it has become clear that this condition, like many of the other inborn metabolic errors, is heterogeneous. The gene coding for the enzyme catalyzing this step (argininosuccinic acid synthetase) has been cloned. It is carried on chromosome 9 (148). To date, at least 20 different genetic mutations have been recorded for infants with neonatal citrullinuria (149).

As a result of the enzymatic defect, the concentration of citrulline in urine, serum, and CSF is markedly increased, and administration of a protein meal results in a dramatic increase of blood ammonia and urinary orotic acid. Blood and urinary urea values are normal, indicating that urea production is not completely blocked.

Several forms of citrullinemia have been recognized. In Western countries, the most common of these presents in the newborn infant as a fulminant condition with lethargy, hypotonia, and seizures (150). In other instances, the disease is less severe, even though recurrent bouts of vomiting, ataxia, and seizures can start in infancy. A third form presents with mental retardation. Completely asymptomatic subjects also have been encountered (147,150). A late-onset variant with loss of enzymatic activity in liver, but not in kidney or fibroblasts, is seen predominantly in Japan, where it constitutes the most common form of citrullinemia (151). It presents with cyclical changes in behavior, dysarthria, and motor weakness.

Treatment for citrullinemia is similar to treatment for argininosuccinic aciduria, except that for long-term therapy, the low-protein diet is supplemented with arginine and sodium phenylbutyrate (141,144).

Citrullinuria in the absence of citrullinemia has been seen in patients with cystinuria. In this instance, citrulline is derived from arginine, which is poorly absorbed from the intestine (152).

Ornithine Transcarbamylase Deficiency

Ornithine transcarbamylase is an enzyme coded by an X-linked gene and located in the mitochondrial matrix. Deficiency of OTC in the male infant is characterized biochemically by a catastrophic elevation of blood ammonia. This is accompanied by an increased excretion of orotic acid and a generalized elevation of plasma and urine amino acids. The disease was first reported in 1962 by Russell and coworkers (153) and is the most common of the urea cycle defects. The gene coding for the enzyme has been cloned and localized to the short arm of the X chromosome (Xp21.1), close to the Duchenne muscular dystrophy locus. More than 140 mutations have been recorded, and most families have their own unique mutation (154). The enzyme defect can be complete or, as occurs in some 10% to 20% of hemizygous male subjects, it can be partial (155). As a consequence, blood ammonia levels are strikingly and consistently elevated (0.4 to 1.0 mg/dl or 230 to 580 µmol/L, contrasted with normal values of less than 0.1 mg/dL or 50 µmol/L), and CSF ammonia is at least 10 times normal. Additionally, an accumulation of glutamine, glutamate, and alanine; a striking reduction in plasma citrulline; and an increased excretion of orotic acid occur. This is the consequence of a diffusion of excess carbamyl phosphate from mitochondria into cytosol, where it is converted into orotic acid (156).

As is the case in argininosuccinic aciduria, the neuropathologic picture is highlighted by the presence of Alzheimer II astrocytes throughout the brain (157). Unlike hepatic encephalopathy, a striking degree of neuronal necrosis also exists. Electron microscopic examination of liver can reveal striking abnormalities of the mitochondria (158).

As a rule, the magnitude of the enzymatic defect correlates with the severity of clinical symptoms. In male subjects, the clinical picture is marked by severe hyperammonemia. When the condition presents during the neonatal period it is rapidly progressive, with a high incidence of mortality or profound neurologic residua. Symptoms usually are delayed until the second day of life and are highlighted by feeding difficulties, lethargy, and respiratory distress. The plasma ammonia level is at least five times normal, thus distinguishing the condition from sepsis (158a).

Less severe cases present with failure to thrive and with episodic attacks of headache and vomiting, followed by periods of lethargy and stupor. These attacks are often the consequence of protein ingestion and are accompanied by high blood ammonia levels (159). Although hyperammonemia is probably responsible for a considerable proportion of the neurologic symptoms, alterations in neurotransmitters, notably quinolinic acid, a known excitotoxin that accumulates as a result of increased tryptophan transport across the blood–brain barrier, also could be involved (128).

The disease is expressed more variably in the heterozygous female subject, with manifestations ranging from apparent normalcy to profound neurologic deficits (156). In symptomatic female subjects, behavioral abnormalities are almost invariable. In the series of Rowe and coworkers, irritability, temper tantrums, inconsolable crying, and hyperactivity were seen in every patient. Episodic vomiting and lethargy were also invariable. Ataxia was seen in 77% of female patients, reduced physical growth in 38%, and developmental delay in 35%. Seizures, generalized or focal, were seen in 23% (156). Blood ammonia and urinary orotic acid levels were elevated consistently when girls were symptomatic. Other girls are asymptomatic except for an aversion to protein-rich foods and possible subtle cognitive deficits (160). Valproate therapy can induce fatal hepatotoxicity in male subjects with OTC deficiency, and in heterozygous female subjects (161).

Treatment of OTC deficiency in the male or female subject is similar to treatment for argininosuccinic aciduria. It is directed at decreasing protein intake by means of a low-protein diet and increasing waste nitrogen excretion by the addition of sodium phenylbutyrate and arginine or citrulline to the diet (162). Prospective treatment of infants at risk for neonatal OTC deficiency has been attempted with some success in that such infants appear to have a better neurologic outcome than those who have to be rescued from hyperammonemic coma (163). Orthoptic liver transplantation presents another option, but is best postponed for a few years until a lower likelihood exists of surgical complications (164).

In some hemizygous male subjects, OTC deficiency is not complete, and the clinical course is not as severe. It can consist of several months of normal development followed by progressive cerebral degeneration or by the acute onset of cerebral and hepatic symptoms resembling those of Reye syndrome (165).

Ornithine transcarbamylase is expressed only in liver and in the small intestine; prenatal diagnosis therefore depends on linkage analysis. Because many cases represent new mutations, this technique is of limited use, except for offspring of obligate gene carriers (166,167). The availability of a cDNA probe for OTC enables the diagnosis of heterozygotes by linkage analysis with restriction fragment polymorphisms in or around the gene, but does not predict whether the female subject will be asymptomatic or severely affected (155).

Carbamyl Phosphate Synthetase Deficiency

Carbamyl phosphate synthetase deficiency is a disorder of the urea cycle manifested by a reduction in hepatic mitochondrial CPS activity (see Fig. 1.7, step 1). This condition was reported first by Freeman and associates (168).

Symptoms of CPS deficiency are the most severe of any of the urea cycle defects, and the neonatal form of the condition, which is associated with complete absence of the enzyme, is usually fatal. In partial CPS deficiency, symptoms appear in infancy and consist of recurrent episodes of vomiting and lethargy, convulsions, hypotonia or hypertonia, and irregular eye movements. Autopsy reveals ulegyria of cerebral and cerebellar cortex, and hypomyelination of the centrum semiovale and the central part of the brainstem. In contrast to argininosuccinic aciduria, no Alzheimer cells are seen, probably because these cells take some time to develop, and CPS deficiency is usually rapidly fatal (157,169).

Carbamyl phosphate synthetase deficiency is diagnosed by the presence of hyperammonemia in the absence of an elevation of plasma citrulline, argininosuccinic acids, or arginine. In contrast to OTC deficiency, orotic acid excretion is low or normal. Treatment for the neonatal and the less severe older-onset forms of CPS deficiency is similar to that for OTC deficiency (141,145).

Hyperargininemia

Hyperargininemia, the least common of urea cycle disorders, has a clinical picture that differs from that of the other urea cycle disorders. Seizures can begin during the neonatal period. In other instances, mental retardation, microcephaly, spastic diplegia, or quadriparesis becomes apparent during the first few months or years (170). The concentration of arginine in plasma and CSF is elevated, and excretion of arginine, cystine, and lysine is increased, a urinary amino acid pattern resembling that of cystinuria. Additionally, a marked orotic aciduria and an increased excretion of guanidine compounds that can act as excitatory neurotransmitters exist. Plasma ornithine levels are usually normal. A deficiency of arginase has been documented in red cells and liver (171). A second arginase, localized to mitochondria, is encoded by a different gene and is normal.

Patients are treated with a diet consisting of a mixture of essential amino acids, exclusive of arginine, and supplemented by a commercial formula that furnishes fats, carbohydrates, vitamins, and minerals (172). Replacement of arginase by means of periodic exchange transfusions has been suggested as a supplementary means of controlling blood and CSF arginine concentrations (173). The effectiveness of bone marrow transplants is still unknown.

N-*Acetylglutamate Deficiency*

N-Acetylglutamate deficiency results from a defect in *N*-acetylglutamate synthetase. In the absence of the enzyme, a deficiency of *N*-acetylglutamate exists, an activator of mitochondrial CPS (174). Clinical manifestations are similar to those of the urea cycle defects.

Other Genetic Causes of Hyperammonemia

Hyperammonemia is seen in several other genetic disorders.

Hyperammonemia, with increased excretion of orotic acid, is seen in periodic hyperlysinemia. For reasons as yet unknown, hyperammonemia can be induced by administration of large amounts of lysine, and the condition diagnosed by the excretion of large amounts of lysine. It is considered with the other defects of lysine metabolism.

Another cause for intermittent hyperammonemia is ornithinemia. This is a heterogeneous entity, clinically and biochemically. At least two conditions have been delineated.

A partial defect of ornithine decarboxylase [hyperammonemia, hyperornithinemia, homocitrullinuria (HHH syndrome)], in which, as the name indicates, elevated plasma ornithine levels are accompanied by hyperammonemia, homocitrullinuria, and a lowered activity of carbamoylphosphate synthetase. The clinical picture is of prolonged neonatal jaundice, mental retardation, infantile spasms, and intermittent ataxia (175). The basic defect appears to be localized to the transport of ornithine across the inner mitochondrial membrane, possibly because of an abnormality of the transport protein (176).

The other condition is ornithine-ketoacid aminotransferase deficiency. In this entity, ornithinemia is accompanied by gyrate atrophy of the choroid and retina, leading to night blindness. Intelligence is preserved, and no neurologic or muscular symptoms occur, although type 2 muscle fiber atrophy is seen on biopsy (177). Nearly 40 allelic variants have been described. In some of these, ornithinemia is corrected by treatment with pyridoxine. Ocular symptoms seem to be ameliorated by a low-arginine diet (178).

Transient hyperammonemia with consequent profound neurologic depression can be encountered in asphyxiated infants (179,180). This entity should be differentiated not only from the various urea cycle defects, but also from the various organic acidemias, notably methylmalonic acidemia and propionic acidemia, which can induce hyperammonemia (181). In these conditions, the accumulation of organic acids inhibits the formation of *N*-acetylglutamine, the activator of mitochondrial CPS, and the activities of all five enzymes of the urea cycle are depressed. On a clinical basis, the organic acidemias can be distinguished from urea cycle defects in that infants with a urea cycle defect are asymptomatic for the first 24 hours of life, and only rarely develop coma before 72 hours. Additionally, they demonstrate tachypnea rather than a respiratory distress syndrome. In contrast to the distressed neonates with hyperammonemia, infants with the various organic acidemias demonstrate ketonuria or ketonemia (182). Asymptomatic hyperammonemia is relatively common in low-birth-weight neonates, but its cause is still unclear (183).

Histidinemia

Histidinemia is a harmless metabolic variant that is caused by a defect in histidase, the enzyme that converts histidine to urocanic acid. An ensuing elevation of plasma histidine levels and an excretion of large amounts of the amino acid occur (184).

Two other rare defects of histidine metabolism, urocanic aciduria and formiminotransferase deficiency, are also thought to represent benign conditions (184).

Defects in the Metabolism of Sulfur Amino Acids

Homocystinuria

The increased excretion of homocystine is a manifestation of several inborn errors of methionine metabolism. The most common of these errors is marked by multiple thromboembolic episodes, ectopia lentis, and mental retardation. Although discovered as late as 1962 by Field and reported subsequently by Carson and associates (185), the prevalence of homocystinuria varies considerably from one country to another, ranging from 1 in 65,000 in Ireland to approximately 1 in 335,000 worldwide (186). The condition is transmitted by an autosomal recessive gene, localized to the long arm of chromosome 21 (21q22).

Molecular Genetics and Biochemical Pathology

In the most common genetic form of homocystinuria, the metabolic defect affects cystathionine synthase, the enzyme that catalyzes the formation of cystathionine from homocysteine and serine (Fig. 1.8) (187). The enzyme as purified from human liver has two identical subunits and contains bound pyridoxal phosphate (188). It also has been found in brain and skin fibroblasts (189). Considerable genetic hetero-

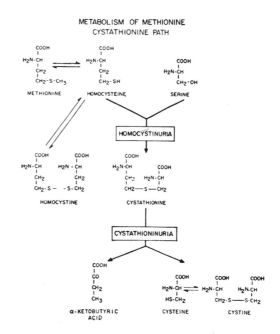

FIG. 1.8. Normal metabolism of sulfur amino acids. In the most common form of homocystinuria, the defect is in the conversion of homocysteine to cystathionine. In cystathioninuria, the block is located in the conversion of cystathionine to cysteine. A block in the conversion of homocysteine to methionine also produces homocystinuria, but serum methionine levels remain normal.

geneity exists among various cystathionine synthase–deficient families, but in the majority, the lesion resides in a structural gene for the enzyme (190). In most homocystinuric subjects, the mutation does not cause dysfunction of the catalytic domain of this enzyme, but rather interferes with its activation by pyridoxine (191). As a result, enzyme activity is either completely absent, or as is the case in a significant proportion of affected families (approximately 25% to 50% of patients with homocystinuria), residual activity occurs. In the latter group, addition of pyridoxine stimulates enzyme activity and partially or completely abolishes the excretion of homocystine, the oxidized derivative of homocysteine (189). Pyridoxine-responsive patients tend to have a milder phenotype of the disease.

As a result of the block, increased amounts of homocystine, the oxidized derivative of homocysteine and its precursor, methionine, are found in urine, plasma, and CSF. Administration of a methionine load to affected individuals produces a striking and prolonged increase in plasma methionine, but little alteration in the homocystine levels. In part, this reflects the low renal threshold for homocystine (192).

In the most common forms of homocystinuria, administration of oral pyridoxine, the coenzyme for cystathionine synthase, does not alter homocystine excretion. In the pyridoxine-responsive variant, large doses of the vitamin (500 mg/day or more) eliminate homocystine from plasma and urine (193).

Homocystinuria also can result from an impaired methylation of homocysteine to methionine (see Fig. 1.8). When the metabolic block is at this point, plasma methionine concentrations are normal rather than increased, as is the case in the more common form of homocystinuria owing to cystathionine synthase deficiency. Methylation uses N^5-methyltetrahydrofolate as a methyl donor and a vitamin B_{12} derivative (methylcobalamin) as a cofactor. Methylation can be impaired as a result of lack of cofactor or enzyme. When synthesis of the vitamin B_{12} cofactor is defective, the biochemical picture is characterized by increased excretion of methylmalonic acid and homocystine. Methylmalonic aciduria (MMA) is the result of a reduced activity of methylmalonyl-CoA mutase, a cobalamin-dependent enzyme. Several errors in cobalamin metabolism have been recognized; the clinical picture includes mental retardation, seizures, failure to thrive, hypotonia, ataxia, and megaloblastic anemia. Auditory- and visual-evoked potentials can be abnormal. Ectopia lentis or skeletal abnormalities are not found. These entities often respond to large doses of vitamin B_{12}. The conditions are covered in the section on Organic Acidurias, later in this chapter.

Another cause for homocystinuria is a defect in the methylation enzyme, methylene tetrahydrofolate reductase. The clinical picture in these patients is protean. Some are retarded or have been diagnosed as schizophrenic; others have recurrent episodes of vomiting and lethargy or muscular weakness and seizures. Vascular thromboses also have been encountered, but the

skeletal and ocular changes of homocystinuria are absent (194,195). Folic acid has reduced the biochemical abnormalities in some patients with this condition, but has been ineffectual in others.

Pathologic Anatomy

The primary structural alterations in homocystinuria are noted in blood vessels of all calibers (196). Most of these show intimal thickening and fibrosis; in the aorta and its major branches, fraying of elastic fibers might be observed. Arterial and venous thromboses are common in a number of organs. Within the brain are usually multiple infarcted areas of varying age. The existence of dural sinus thrombosis has been recorded.

How the metabolic defect induces a propensity to vascular thrombosis is still uncertain, but it probably occurs on several levels. This topic has been reviewed by Welch and Loscalzo (197). It also has become evident that an increased plasma homocysteine concentration is an independent risk factor for atherosclerotic vascular disease.

Clinical Manifestations

The pyridoxine-unresponsive form of homocystinuria is more severe in its manifestations than the pyridoxine-responsive form.

Homocystinuric infants appear healthy at birth, and their early development is unremarkable until seizures, developmental slowing, or cerebrovascular accidents occur between 5 and 9 months of age. Ectopia lentis is seen in more than 90% of affected individuals. Lenticular dislocation has been recognized as early as age 18 months, but it generally occurs between 3 and 10 years of age. The typical older homocystinuric child's hair is sparse, blond, and brittle, and multiple erythematous blotches are seen over the skin, particularly across the maxillary areas and cheeks. The gait is shuffling, the extremities and digits are long, and genu valgum is present in most instances. Secondary glaucoma and cataracts are common (198).

In approximately 50% of the patients reported, major thromboembolic episodes have occurred on one or more occasions. These include fatal thromboses of the pulmonary artery, coronary arteries, and renal artery and vein. Multiple major cerebrovascular accidents also result in hemiplegia, and ultimately in a picture that closely resembles pseudobulbar palsy. Thromboembolic events are particularly common after even minor surgical procedures. It is likely that minor and unrecognized cerebral thrombi are the cause of the mental retardation that occurs in 50% of the patients (199,200). Routine laboratory study results are normal, but in a high proportion of subjects, electromyography suggests myopathy (200).

Radiography reveals a biconcavity of the posterior aspects of the vertebrae (*codfish vertebrae*) (201). Additionally, scoliosis and osteoporosis become apparent in late childhood. Abnormalities of the hands and feet are noted also. These include metaphyseal spicules, enlargement of carpal bones, and selective retardation of the development of the lunate bone (202).

Diagnosis

The diagnosis of homocystinuria suggested by the appearance of the patient can be confirmed by the increased urinary excretion of homocystine, by elevated plasma methionine and homocystine, and by a positive urinary cyanide-nitroprusside reaction. Enzyme activity can be determined in cultured skin fibroblasts or in liver biopsy specimens.

Although ectopia lentis, arachnodactyly, and cardiovascular symptoms are seen also in Marfan syndrome, homocystinuria can be distinguished by its autosomal recessive transmission (in contrast to the dominant transmission of Marfan syndrome), the thromboembolic phenomena, the early appearance of osteoporosis, the biconcave vertebrae, and the peculiar facial appearance (203). The relatively long fingers seen in Marfan syndrome are present at birth, and the skeletal disproportion remains constant. In homocystinuria, the skeleton is normal for the first few years of life, but the limbs grow disproportionately long. Ectopia lentis is seen not only in homocystinuria, but also as an isolated congenital defect in the Weill-Marchesani syndrome and in sulfite oxidase deficiency. In the

latter condition, it occurs in conjunction with profound mental retardation, seizures commencing shortly after birth, acute hemiplegia, opisthotonos, and hyperacusis. Because the majority of cases are the result of a deficiency of the molybdenum cofactor rather than of the apoenzyme, this condition is covered more fully in the section dealing with disorders of metal metabolism.

Cystathionine synthase has been found in cultivated amniotic fluid cells, and the condition, therefore, can be diagnosed prenatally (204).

Treatment

Restriction of methionine intake lowers plasma methionine and eliminates the abnormally high urinary excretion of homocystine. Commercially available diets that are methionine free and are supplemented by carbohydrates, fats, and fat-soluble vitamins generally lower plasma methionine levels to the normal range (200). The diets are supplemented with cystine.

Other dietary measures include the addition of folic acid, based on the assumption that the mental defect is related to low serum folate levels (205). Wilcken and coworkers have recommended treatment with betaine hydrochloride in subjects who do not respond to pyridoxine (206).

In pyridoxine-responsive patients, large doses of the vitamin (250 to 1,200 mg/day) reduce or eliminate biochemical abnormalities. The effectiveness of antithrombotic agents, such as aspirin or dipyridamole, has not yet been proven.

Early therapy appears to improve the ultimate IQ and delays the onset of thromboembolic episodes and ectopia lentis in those who do not respond to pyridoxine (193). In pyridoxine-responsive homocystinuria, early therapy results in a normal IQ and delays the various complications of homocystinuria to a greater extent than in nonpyridoxine-responsive homocystinuria. In the series of Mudd and coworkers, pyridoxine-responsive patients treated from the neonatal period on had an IQ ranging from 82 to 110. Virtually all patients with IQs more than 90 were found to be responsive to pyridoxine (193).

Cystathioninuria

A grossly increased urinary excretion of the amino acid cystathionine has been observed in a few individuals, the result of a defect in cystathionase (see Fig. 1.8), a pyridoxal phosphate-dependent enzyme. This condition is a benign metabolic variant, and the association with neurologic symptoms reported in the past is fortuitous (207).

Hypermethioninemia

Several other conditions are marked by elevated plasma methionine levels. The most common of these is a transitory methioninemia, seen in 13-month-old infants, many of whom are premature and receiving a high-protein diet (at least 7 g/kg per day). It is likely that the biochemical abnormality is caused by delayed maturation of one or more of the enzymes of methionine metabolism.

Methioninemia, with or without tyrosinemia, accompanied by hepatorenal disease (tyrosinemia I) is considered in the section on Tyrosinosis and Tyrosinemia (see Table 1.5).

Persistent methioninemia associated with a deficiency of hepatic methionine adenosyltransferase is a benign metabolic variant unaccompanied by neurologic symptoms or impairment of cognition (208).

Neurologic symptoms are not commonly part of the clinical picture of early-onset or infantile nephropathic cystinosis. However, with the successful management of end-stage renal disease and longer survival of patients, neurologic complications are becoming apparent (209). Cystine accumulates in the form of cystine crystals in lysosomes of a variety of organs. In the brain, they are seen in the interstitial macrophages of choroid plexus (210). Two forms of neurologic disorder have been recognized. One form is marked by progressive cerebellar signs, spasticity, pseudobulbar palsy, and dementia. The second form presents with the sudden onset of changes in consciousness and hemiparesis (211). A myopathy caused by accumulation of cystine in and around muscle fibers, and oral motor dysfunction also has been recorded (212). CT scans have revealed progressive ventricular dilatation and calcifications in the periventricular white matter (213). A young man with a progressive parkinsonian movement disorder has been seen at our hospital. Treatment with cysteamine can be effective in some cases with encephalopathy (211).

Iminoacidurias

Several inborn metabolic errors are characterized by the increased excretion of proline and hydroxyproline, the two principal imino acids. Like so many other inborn errors of metabolism, these conditions were discovered by screening mentally retarded children, and a cause-and-effect relationship was assumed. It is now clear that these disorders are benign and that the initial association with mental retardation and photosensitive epilepsy was fortuitous.

Hyperlysinemias

Several inborn errors are marked by an elevation in blood lysine levels and by increased urinary excretion of the amino acid.

Hyperlysinemia and saccharopinuria were first observed in patients with mental retardation and seizures. These conditions also have been described in healthy infants and, as is the case for the iminoacidemias, the neurologic abnormalities have turned out to be fortuitous (214). Another benign metabolic variant is hyperdibasic aminoaciduria. This condition is marked by abnormally high excretion of the dibasic amino acids (lysine, arginine, and ornithine) in the presence of normal plasma levels and a normal cystine excretion (214).

Increased excretion of lysine and arginine accompanied by hyperammonemia also is seen in familial protein intolerance with dibasic aminoaciduria. Two forms have been recognized, which are probably not allelic. In type I, the presenting symptoms include mental retardation, recurrent vomiting, and diarrhea, but no hyperammonemia or protein intolerance (214,215). Type II is not uncommon in Finland, where its incidence has been estimated at between 1 in 60,000 to 80,000 (215). It manifests with protein intolerance, bouts of hyperammonemia, and mental retardation. The gene for this recessive disorder has been mapped to the long arm of chromosome 14 (14q11.2). The defective gene is believed to code for one of several permeases involved in renal and intestinal transport of basic amino acids (216,216a).

TABLE 1.6. *Some rarely encountered defects of amino acid metabolism associated with neurologic symptoms*

Disease (reference)	Enzymatic defect	Clinical features	Diagnosis
Hypervalinemia (221)	Valine transaminase	Vomiting, failure to thrive, nystagmus, mental retardation	Increased blood and urine valine; no increased excretion of ketoacid
Hyper-β-alaninemia (222)	β-Alanine-α-keto-glutarate transaminase	Seizures commencing at birth, somnolence	Plasma urine β-alanine and β-aminoisobutyric acid elevated; urinary γ-aminobutyric acid elevated
Carnosinemia (223)	Carnosinase	Grand mal and myoclonic seizures, progressive mental retardation	Increased serum and urine carnosine; increased CSF homocarnosine
α-Methylacetoacetic aciduria (224,225)	3-Ketothiolase	Recurrent severe acidosis	α-Methyl acetoacetate and α-methyl-β-hydroxy butyric acid in urine
Hypertryptophanemia (226,227)	Tryptophan transaminase	Ataxia, spasticity, mental retardation, pellagralike skin rash, cataracts	Elevated serum tryptophan, diminished or normal kynurenine, massive excretion of indole-acetic, -lactic, -pyruvic acids
Aspartylglycosaminuria (228,229)	Aspartylglucos-aminidase	Progressive mental retardation, coarse facial features, changes in tubular bones of hand, vacuolated lymphocytes, mitral valve insufficiency	Elevated urine aspartylglu-cosamine
Glutamyl ribose-5-phosphate storage disease (230)	Deficiency of ADP-ribose protein hydrolase	Mental deterioration, seizures, microcephaly, proteinuria, coarse facies	Accumulation of glutamyl ribose-5-phosphate in brain and kidney
Glutamyl cysteine synthetase deficiency (231)	γ-Glutamylcysteine synthetase	Hemolytic anemia, spino-cerebellar degeneration, peripheral neuropathy	Reduced erythrocyte glutathione, generalized aminoaciduria
Hyperoxaluria (232,233)	Type I: excessive oxalate synthesis; type II: defective hydroxypyruvate metabolism	Progressive renal insufficiency, dementia, peripheral neuropathy; type II milder than type I	Increased urinary oxalic acid with glycolic acid (type I) or L-glyceric acid

ADP, adenosine 5^1-diphosphate; CSF, cerebrospinal fluid.

Another disorder of lysine metabolism is pipecolatemia. This entity is identical with Zellweger cerebrohepatorenal syndrome and is discussed in the section on Peroxisomal Disorders, later in this chapter.

The diagnosis of the various hyperlysinemias rests on the increased serum levels of lysine. High urinary excretion of lysine, usually accompanied by increased cystine excretion but with normal blood levels of both amino acids, also is seen in some heterozygotes for cystinuria (217).

Two other defects of lysine metabolism involve the conversion of α-aminoadipic acid to glutaconyl CoA. In α-aminoadipic aciduria, first recognized in a mentally retarded youngster and his apparently healthy brother, the defect is in the conversion of α-aminoadipic acid to α-ketoadipic acid (218). In α-ketoadipic aciduria, first observed in a mentally retarded child, the defect is in the conversion of α-ketoadipic acid to glutaryl-CoA (219). As yet, it is not clear whether these conditions represent benign metabolic variants or truly have the potential of inducing neurologic symptoms. Increased excretion of α-aminoadipic acid has been seen in children receiving vigabatrin for their seizures (220).

Other Rare Metabolic Defects

A few other extremely rare defects of amino acid metabolism associated with neurologic symptoms are presented in Table 1.6. Past experience

TABLE 1.7. *Defects in amino acid transport*

Transport system	Condition	Biochemical features	Clinical features
Basic amino acids	Cystinuria (three types) (234)	Impaired renal clearance and defective intestinal transport of lysine, arginine, ornithine, and cystine	Renal stones, no neurologic disease; ? increased prevalence in subjects with mental disease
Generalized	Lowe syndrome	? Impaired intestinal transport of lysine and arginine; ? impaired tubular transport of lysine	Severe mental retardation, glaucoma, cataracts, myopathy; gender-linked transmission
Acidic amino acids	Dicarboxylic aminoaciduria (235)	Increased excretion of glutamic, aspartic acids	Harmless variant
Neutral amino acids	Hartnup disease	Defective intestinal and renal tubular transport of tryptophan and other neutral amino acids	Intermittent cerebellar ataxia; photosensitive rash
Proline, hydroxyproline, glycine	Iminoglycinuria (236,237)	Impaired tubular transport of proline, hydroxyproline, and glycine	Harmless variant; transient iminoglycinuria normal in early infancy
β-Amino acids	None known	Excretion of β-aminoisobutyric acid and taurine in β-alaninemia is increased owing to competition at the tubular level	—

with disorders such as the iminoacidemias, cystathioninuria, and histidinemia should caution the reader against accepting a causal relationship between metabolic and neurologic defects. A number of neurologic disorders that are accompanied by aminoaciduria are not included in Table 1.6. Most investigators have noted that when mentally retarded children are screened, a few exhibit pathologic aminoaciduria. Deficiency diseases, notably rickets, often caused by lack of sunlight, in combination with anticonvulsant therapy, can account for some of these; the remainder are unexplained.

DISORDERS OF AMINO ACID TRANSPORT

Renal amino acid transport is handled by five specific systems that have nonoverlapping substrate preferences. The disorders that result from genetic defects in each of these systems are listed in Table 1.7.

Hartnup Disease

Hartnup disease is a rare familial condition characterized by photosensitive dermatitis, intermittent cerebellar ataxia, mental disturbances, and renal aminoaciduria. The name is that of the family in which it was first detected (238). The chromosomal locus for the gene is as yet unknown.

Molecular Genetics and Biochemical Pathology

The symptoms are the result of an extensive disturbance in sodium-dependent transport of neutral amino acids across the membrane of the brush border of the small intestine and the proximal renal tubular epithelium. Four main biochemical abnormalities exist: a renal aminoaciduria, increased excretion of indican, an abnormally high output of nonhydroxylated indole metabolites, and increased fecal amino acids. These deficits are discussed in detail by Milne and colleagues (239) and Scriver (240).

Pathologic Anatomy

No pathologic studies have yet been reported in typical patients with Hartnup disease.

Clinical Manifestations

The incidence of the biochemical lesion responsible for Hartnup disease is 1 in 18,000 in Massachusetts, 1 in 70,000 in Vienna, and 1 in 33,000 in New South Wales, Australia (241). Clinical manifestations of Hartnup disease are the consequence of several factors. Polygenic inheritance is the major determinant for plasma amino acid levels, and symptoms are seen only in subjects with the lowest amino acid concentrations. Because protein malnutrition further lowers amino acid levels, the disease itself, as distinguished from its biochemical defect, is seen mainly in malnourished children. Whenever dietary intake is satisfactory, neither neurologic nor dermatologic signs appear (241). Also, no difference exists in rate of growth or IQ scores between groups with Hartnup disease and control groups. In the series of Scriver and coworkers, 90% of Hartnup subjects had normal development (242). However, low academic performance and impaired growth were seen in those patients with Hartnup disease who, for genetic reasons, tended to have the lowest plasma amino acid levels (242).

When present, symptoms are intermittent and variable, and tend to improve with increasing age. A characteristic red, scaly rash appears on the exposed areas of the face, neck, and extensor surfaces of the extremities. This rash resembles the dermatitis of pellagra and, like it, is aggravated by sunlight. Cerebral symptoms can precede the rash for several years. They include intermittent personality changes, psychoses, migrainelike headaches, photophobia, and bouts of cerebellar ataxia. Changes in hair texture also have been observed. The four children of the original Hartnup family underwent progressive mental retardation, but this is not invariable. Renal and intestinal transport is impaired in 80% of patients, renal transport alone in 20% (242). A patient with the clinical picture of Hartnup disease, impaired intestinal absorption of neutral amino acids, but no renal aminoaciduria has been observed. A somewhat similar case has been reported by Borrie and Lewis (243). The MRI is nonspecific; it demonstrates delayed myelination (244).

Diagnosis

Hartnup disease should be considered in patients with intermittent cerebral symptoms, even without skin involvement.

Numerous metabolic disorders with a partial enzymatic defect produce intermittent cerebellar ataxia. These include MSUD, lactic acidosis, pyruvate dehydrogenase deficiency, and some of the diseases caused by defects in the urea cycle. Additionally, in familial intermittent cerebellar ataxia, no metabolic lesion has been found (245). Another rare condition to be considered in the differential diagnosis of Hartnup disease is hypertryptophanemia (see Table 1.6) and a disorder in kynurenine hydroxylation (246). Chromatography of urine for amino acids and indolic substances in the presence of a normal serum pattern is diagnostic for Hartnup disease.

Treatment

The similarity of Hartnup disease to pellagra has prompted treatment with nicotinic acid (25 mg/day). Tryptophan ethylester also has been effective (247). However, the tendency for symptoms to remit spontaneously and for general improvement to occur with improved dietary intake and advancing age makes such therapy difficult to evaluate.

Lowe Syndrome (Oculocerebrorenal Syndrome)

Lowe syndrome is a gender-linked recessive disorder whose gene has been localized to the long arm of the X chromosome (Xq25-26) and is characterized by severe mental retardation, myopathy, and congenital glaucoma or cataract. Biochemically, it is marked by a generalized aminoaciduria of the Fanconi type, renal tubular acidosis, and hypophosphatemic rickets (248). The gene responsible for the disorder has been cloned (249). It encodes a protein that has considerable similarity to inositol polyphosphate-5-phosphatase, an enzyme that is involved in the conversion of extracellular signals into intracellular signals (250). It is not yet clear how the genetic lesion relates to the basic phenotypic defect, which is believed to be a defect in membrane transport (251).

Neuropathologic examination has disclosed rarefaction of the molecular layer of the cerebral cortex and parenchymal vacuolation or little more than ventricular dilatation (252,253). The urinary levels of lysine are more elevated than those of the other amino acids, and defective uptake of lysine and arginine by the intestinal mucosa has been demonstrated in two patients (251).

The clinical picture is that of a developmental delay or of progressive loss of acquired skills. This is accompanied by hypotonia, areflexia, and evidence of peripheral neuropathy with loss of myelinated fibers (254,255). CT scans reveal reduced density of periventricular white matter and marked scalloping of the calvarial bones, especially in the occipital region (256). T2-weighted MRI shows patchy, irregular areas of increased signal intensity (254,256). Additionally, multiple periventricular cystic lesions have been observed (257).

Heterozygous female subjects are neurologically healthy, with normal renal function, but have micropunctate cortical lens opacities (258).

DISORDERS OF CARBOHYDRATE METABOLISM

Galactosemia

Hepatomegaly, splenomegaly, and failure to thrive associated with the excretion of galactose were first pointed out by von Reuss in 1908 (259). Galactosemia is transmitted in an autosomal recessive manner. In the United States, it is seen with a frequency of 1 in 62,000; in Austria, it is 1 in 40,000 to 46,000; and in England, it is 1 in 72,000 (260).

Molecular Genetics and Biochemical Pathology

In 1917, Göppert demonstrated that galactosemic children excreted galactose after the ingestion of lactose (milk) and galactose (261). In 1956, Schwarz and associates found that administration of galactose to affected children gave rise to an accumulation of galactose-1-phosphate (262). This was confirmed by Kalckar and his group, who were able to demonstrate a deficiency in galactose-1-phosphate uridyltransferase (GALT), the enzyme that catalyzes the conversion of galactose-1-phosphate into galactose uridine diphosphate (UDP-galactose) (Fig. 1.9) (263). The gene for galactosemia has been mapped to

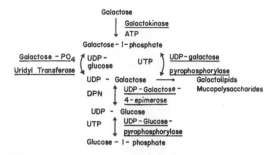

FIG. 1.9. Normal galactose metabolism. In galactosemia, galactose-1-phosphate uridyltransferase is defective. (ATP, adenosine triphosphate; DPN, disphosphopyridine nucleotide; UDP, uridine diphosphate; UTP, uridine triphosphate.)

the small arm of chromosome 9 (9p13). It has been cloned and sequenced, and more than 50 point mutations have been identified (264). The most common genetic lesion in classic galactosemia is a point mutation (Q188R) that has a prevalence of 60% to 70% in whites and results in a complete enzyme deficiency; the remainder have detectable amounts of enzyme activity (264). In black patients, the most common mutation (S135L) accounts for 45% of the mutant alleles. Patients homozygous for the S135L allele have residual red cell GALT activity and a milder clinical course (264). Homozygotes of two other mutant alleles, the Los Angeles and Duarte variants, are essentially asymptomatic.

In classic galactosemia, the metabolic block is essentially complete. Lactose of human or cow's milk is hydrolyzed to galactose and glucose, the latter being handled in a normal manner. The metabolism of galactose, however, stops after the sugar is phosphorylated to galactose-1-phosphate. This phosphate ester accumulates in erythrocytes, lens, liver, and kidney (265). Galactitol, the alcohol of galactose, also is found in the lens, brain, and urine of galactosemic individuals (266), and directly or indirectly can be a major factor in the development of mental retardation. Other factors responsible can include a deficiency of uridine diphosphate galactose; a reduction of glycolytic intermediates; a loss of adenosine triphosphate (ATP); and hyperosmolar dehydration (266,267).

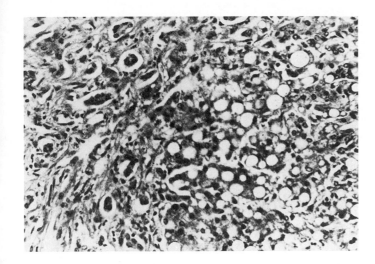

FIG. 1.10. Galactosemia. High-power view of liver shows periportal fibrosis, a marked disruption of hepatic architecture, and an increase in the number of bile ducts. Considerable numbers of cells are distended with large, pale vacuoles. (Courtesy of Dr. G. N. Donnell, Children's Hospital, Los Angeles, CA.)

Administration of galactose to affected infants results in marked hypoglycemia. This has been explained by an increased insulin release, prompted by the large amounts of circulating reducing substance, or by assuming interference by galactose-1-phosphate with normal glycogen breakdown. The peripheral hypoglycemia is enhanced by competition between glucose and galactose at the level of the hexose transport across the blood–brain barrier. As a consequence, the brain in galactosemic subjects is in a constant hypoglycemic environment.

Intolerance to galactose decreases with increasing age. In part, this intolerance might be a result of the decreasing importance of milk as a food item. In subjects with classic galactosemia who have been tested repeatedly, no increase in erythrocyte transferase activity has been found (268).

Pathologic Anatomy

The main pathologic lesions are found in the liver and brain. In the liver, several stages are recognized. Initially one sees a severe, diffuse, fatty metamorphosis. The hepatic cells are filled with large, pale, fat-containing vacuoles (Fig. 1.10) (269). If the disease remains untreated, the liver cell cords are transformed into pseudoglandular structures. The final stage is pseudolobular cirrhosis. Cerebral alterations are nonspecific. Edema, fibrous gliosis of white matter, and marked loss of cortical neurons and Purkinje cells are the most prominent findings (270).

Clinical Manifestations

Infants with galactosemia appear healthy at birth, although their cord blood can already contain abnormally high concentrations of galactose-1-phosphate, and a few already have cataracts and hepatic cirrhosis, probably as a consequence of intrauterine galactosemia (271). In severe cases, symptoms develop during the first week of life. These include vomiting, diarrhea, listlessness, and failure to gain weight. Increased intracranial pressure can be a presenting sign (272). Infants are jaundiced. This may represent a persistence of neonatal jaundice or can appear at age 3 to 5 days (273). On a normal diet, hypoglycemia is not common. By age 2 weeks, hepatosplenomegaly and lenticular opacifications are easily detectable. The cataracts can be cortical or nuclear and can be present at birth (266). The most frequently observed opacity is a central refractile ring (274). The infants are hypotonic and often have lost the Moro reflex. Pseudotumor cerebri as a result of cerebral edema is not uncommon (272). Sepsis caused by *Escherichia coli* occurs with high frequency and is responsible for the majority of deaths during the neonatal period (275). Other secondary effects of deranged galactose metabolism include ovarian failure or atrophy and testicular atrophy (276). On MRI, a high incidence of abnormalities is seen. Most commonly, multiple areas of increased signal are seen in white matter, predominantly in the periventricular region (277).

If galactosemia is untreated, growth failure becomes severe, and the infant develops the usual signs of progressive hepatic cirrhosis. In some infants, the disease can be less severe and does not manifest until age 3 to 6 months, at which time the presenting symptoms are delayed physical and mental development. By then, cataracts can be well established and the cirrhosis far advanced.

In another group of galactosemic individuals, the diagnosis is not made until patients are several years old, often on evaluation for mental retardation. They might not have cataracts or albuminuria. Intellectual retardation is not consistent in untreated galactosemic children. When present, it is moderate; IQs range between 50 and 70. Asymptomatic homozygotes also have been detected. Most of these have some residual transferase activity.

Diagnosis

The enzyme defect is best documented by measuring the erythrocyte GALT activity. Several methods are currently available and can be used for state and nationwide screening. They are reviewed by Beutler (278).

Galactosuria, usually in combination with glucosuria or fructosuria, is seen in severe hepatic disorders of the neonatal period (e.g., neonatal hepatitis, tyrosinosis, congenital atresia of the bile ducts). Families in which several members are mentally defective and have congenital cataracts without an abnormality in galactose metabolism have been described by Franceschetti and others (279).

The antenatal diagnosis of galactosemia can be made by assay of GALT activity on cultured amniocytes or chorionic villi (280).

Treatment

When milk is withdrawn and lactose-free products such as Nutramigen or Prosobee are substituted, gastrointestinal symptoms are rapidly relieved and normal growth is reinstituted. The progression of cirrhosis is arrested, and in 35% of patients, the cataracts disappear (273). Because infants have developed hypoglycemia when first placed on a galactose-free diet, it might be useful to add some glucose to the formula.

The propensity of galactosemic neonates for *E. coli* sepsis requires securing cultures of blood, urine, and CSF and treating against this organism until the test results are negative (275). In the larger series of Waggoner, sepsis was suspected in 30% of neonates and confirmed in 10% (281).

The composition of a low-galactose diet has been published by Cornblath and Schwartz (282). Maintenance of the galactose-free diet and avoidance of milk and milk products is recommended until at least after puberty. In several children who returned to a milk-containing diet before puberty, cataracts flared up. Even after that age, some continue to be sensitive to milk products and prefer to avoid them. Intermittent monitoring of erythrocyte galactose-1-phosphate levels has been suggested. Even children with well-controlled galactosemia have elevated galactose-1-phosphate levels. These usually range between 30 and 45 μg/mL, as contrasted with normal levels of 5 to 10 μg/mL (283). Endogenous formation of galactose-1-phosphate from glucose-1-phosphate by way of the epimerase reaction (see Fig. 1.9) is believed to be responsible.

The long-term outlook for galactosemic subjects is not as good as was initially believed, even when the diet is carefully monitored. A number of cases of progressive cerebellar ataxia and extrapyramidal movement disorders have been reported (284,285). In the series of Waggoner and colleagues, cerebellar deficits were seen in 18% (281); in the series of Kaufman and colleagues, the incidence was 27% (285). The cause for this syndrome is unclear, and MRI studies on patients with this syndrome do not differ from those without it (285). Rogers and Segal postulate that the syndrome results from an endogenous product of galactose-1-phosphate from UDP-glucose via the epimerase reaction (286). Another possibility is that a deficiency of UDP-galactose could limit the formation of cerebral glycoproteins and galactolipids. Administration of uridine, which has been suggested to prevent these complications, has not been effective (287).

Cognitive deficits are common. In 70% of galactosemic children treated from birth, the IQ was 90 or higher; however, approximately 50% of the youngsters had significant visual and perceptual deficits, and 33% had EEG abnormalities (288). Studies confirm that most subjects have cognitive deficits in one or more areas. Verbal dyspraxia occurs in some 62%. Patients are unable to program their speech musculature and also show frequent disturbances in speech rhythm. Receptive language is normal (285,289). In addition, there appears to be a progressive decline in IQ with age (281,285). Neither IQ scores nor the presence of the dyspractic speech disorder are highly related with the age at which therapy is initiated or quality of control (281). Rather, cognitive and language deficits are likely to result from the *in utero* formation of potentially neurotoxic galactose-1-phosphate and the continued generation of galactose from glucose via UDP-galactose-4-epimerase (see Fig. 1.9) (266,290).

By restricting the galactose intake during pregnancy of women who previously had borne galactosemic children, Donnell and associates were able to reduce the incidence of congenital galactosemic cataracts (291).

Two other defects of galactose metabolism have been recognized. A deficiency of galactokinase (see Fig. 1.9) has been discovered in patients with juvenile cataracts. Neither hepatomegaly nor neurologic deficits are present (292). Deficiency of epimerase, the enzyme that converts UDP-glucose to UDP-galactose (see Fig. 1.9), can result in galactosuria, failure to thrive, and mental retardation (293,294).

Fructose Intolerance

Fructose intolerance, as distinguished from benign fructosuria, was first described by Chambers and Pratt in 1956 (295). The condition is transmitted as an autosomal recessive trait and is the consequence of a deficiency in the principal hepatic aldolase, aldolase B (296). Aldolase A, normally found in muscle and renal medulla, and aldolase C, found in brain, are normal (297). The gene coding for aldolase B is located on the long arm of chromosome 9 (9q21.3 to 9q22.2), and more than 20 mutations have been documented (298).

Molecular Genetics and Biochemical Pathology

As a consequence of the metabolic defect, ingested fructose (or sucrose, which is split into fructose and glucose) is converted to fructose-1-phosphate, which accumulates in tissues and is responsible for renal and hepatic damage. Additionally, plasma lactate and urate levels increase (299). A glucagon-unresponsive hypoglycemia results from the blockage of glycogenolysis by fructose-1-phosphate at the point of phosphorylase and from the interruption of gluconeogenesis by the phosphate ester at the level of the mutant fructose-1,6-diphosphate aldolase (300).

Pathologic Anatomy

The main pathologic abnormality is hepatic cirrhosis similar to that seen in galactosemia. The brain shows retarded myelination and neuronal shrinkage attributable to hypoglycemia (301). An associated coagulation defect can induce intracerebral hemorrhage.

Clinical Manifestations

Hereditary fructose intolerance is relatively rare in the United States but far more common in Europe. In Switzerland, the gene frequency is 1 in 80, and in Great Britain, 1 in 250 (299). The condition manifests by intestinal disturbances, poor weight gain, and attacks of hypoglycemia after fructose ingestion. Transient icterus, hepatic enlargement, fructosuria, albuminuria, and aminoaciduria follow intake of large quantities of fructose. Mild mental deficiency is frequent, and there may be a flaccid quadriparesis (302). Heterozygotes are predisposed to gout (299).

Diagnosis

The diagnosis of hereditary fructose intolerance is based in part on the patient's clinical history,

on the presence of a urinary reducing substance, and on the results of an intravenous
fructose tolerance test (0.25 g/kg). An oral tolerance test is contraindicated in view of the
ensuing severe gastrointestinal and systemic
symptoms (303). In most cases, administration
of this amount of fructose produces gastrointestinal symptoms, hypoglycemia, and a
decrease in the level of serum phosphorus. In
the urine, tyrosine, phenylalanine, proline, and
phenolic acid excretion is increased. For confirmation, a jejunal or liver biopsy with determination of fructose-1-phosphate aldolase levels
is necessary (304). MR spectroscopy has been
used to confirm the diagnosis and to determine
heterozygosity (299).

Other causes of increased fructose excretion
include impaired liver function, and fructosuria,
which is an asymptomatic metabolic variant
caused by a deficiency of fructokinase.

Treatment

Treatment of hereditary fructose intolerance is
relatively simple but is needed lifelong. It
involves avoiding the intake of fruits and cane or
beet sugar (sucrose). The composition of fruc-
tose-free diets has been published (282).

Other Disorders of
Carbohydrate Metabolism

Fructose-1,6-diphosphatase deficiency is a rare
disorder that manifests during the neonatal
period with hyperventilation, hyperbilirubinemia, seizures, coma, and laboratory evidence of
ketosis, hypoglycemia, and lactic acidosis
(305). The diagnosis is difficult, and a variety of
other causes for intermittent neonatal hypoglycemia must be excluded. The enzyme defect
can be demonstrated by liver biopsy (306).

Of the various forms of mellituria seen in
infancy and childhood, the most common are
caused by the increased excretion of a single
sugar, predominantly glucose. Isolated lacto-
suria and fructosuria are encountered also. Lac-
tosuria usually is explained on the basis of
congenital lactose intolerance or secondary lactose intolerance associated with enteritis, celiac

disease, and cystic fibrosis. Essential pentosuria, one of the original inborn errors of metabolism described by Garrod, is a result of the
excretion of L-xylulose. Ribosuria occurs in
Duchenne muscular dystrophy, probably as the
result of tissue breakdown. Sucrosuria has been
reported in association with hiatus hernia and
other intestinal disturbances.

A mixed sugar excretion also can be seen in
acute infections, liver disease, and gastroenteritis.

ORGANIC ACIDURIAS

A number of disorders of intermediary metabolism are manifested by intermittent episodes
of vomiting, lethargy, acidosis, and the excretion of large amounts of organic acids. Even
though the enzymatic lesions responsible are
not related, they are grouped together because
they are detected by analysis of urinary
organic acids.

Propionic Acidemia
(Ketotic Hyperglycinemia)

Propionic acidemia, the first of the organic
acidurias to be described, is characterized by
intermittent episodes of vomiting, lethargy,
and ketosis. Hsia and coworkers demonstrated
a defect in propionyl-CoA carboxylase, a
biotin-dependent enzyme that converts propionyl-CoA to methylmalonyl-CoA (307). The
enzyme consists of two polypeptides, α and β,
coded by genes (PCCA and PCCB) that are
located on chromosomes 13 and 3, respectively. Considerable genetic heterogeneity
exists, with defects in each of the two structural genes encoding the two subunits of propionyl-CoA carboxylase (308). The clinical
presentation of the two forms appears to be
comparable; the original family had the PCCA
type of propionic acidemia.

As a consequence of the metabolic block, not
only is serum propionate elevated, but also several propionate derivatives accumulate (309).
Hyperammonemia is frequent, probably as a consequence of an inhibition by the accumulating
organic acids of N-acetylglutamate synthetase,
the enzyme that forms N-acetylglutamate, a stim-

ulator of carbamoyl-phosphate synthetase (see Fig. 1.7) (310). The severity of hyperammonemia appears to be proportional to the serum propionate levels (311). The mechanism for hyperglycinemia in this and in several of the other organic acidurias has not been fully elucidated. It appears likely, however, that propionate interferes with one of the components of the mitochondrial glycine cleavage system.

In the classic form of the disease, symptoms start shortly after birth (312). In other cases, they might not become apparent until late infancy or childhood and are precipitated by upper respiratory or gastrointestinal infections. Marked intellectual retardation and a neurologic picture of a mixed pyramidal and extrapyramidal lesion ultimately become apparent (313). Attacks are precipitated by ingestion of proteins and various amino acids, notably leucine. In addition to ketoacidosis, hyperammonemia, persistent neutropenia, and thrombocytopenia occur. Propionic acidemia is seen in all patients, and plasma and urinary glycine levels are increased (314). In some patients, MRI shows increased signal in the caudate nucleus and putamen on T2-weighted images (315).

Structural abnormalities in the brain are similar to those seen in PKU and other diseases of amino acid metabolism, namely retarded myelination and a spongy degeneration of white matter (316).

Treatment involves a diet low in valine, isoleucine, threonine, and methionine, with carnitine supplementation (60 to 200 mg/kg per day). A commercial formula is available.

Propionic acidemia is biochemically and clinically distinct from familial glycinuria, a condition in which serum glycine levels are normal and the nervous system is unaffected (317). It also should be distinguished from iminoglycinuria and from nonketotic hyperglycinemia. Isovaleric acidemia and α-ketothiolase deficiency also can present with episodes of ketoacidosis and hyperglycinemia.

Methylmalonic Aciduria

The classic presentation of MMA is one of acute neonatal ketoacidosis, with lethargy, vomiting, and profound hypotonia. Several genetic entities have been recognized. In all, the conversion of methylmalonyl-CoA to succinyl-CoA is impaired, a result either of a defect in the mitochondrial apoenzyme, methylmalonyl-CoA mutase, or in the biosynthesis, transport, or absorption of its adenosylcobalamin cofactor (318). The gene for methylmalonyl-CoA mutase has been cloned, and more than two dozen mutations have been recognized (319).

Approximately one-third of patients with MMA have the classic form of the disease (318). In this condition, the defect is localized to the apoenzyme methylmalonyl-CoA mutase. In the majority of patients, the enzyme is totally inactive, whereas in other patients with MMA, the apoenzyme defect is partial (320). In the remainder of patients with MMA, constituting approximately 50% of a series of 45 patients assembled by Matsui and her group (318), dramatic biochemical improvement occurs with the administration of adenosylcobalamin, the cofactor for the mutase. In most of the responders, synthesis of adenosylcobalamin is blocked at the formation of the cofactor from cobalamin (cobalamin adenosyltransferase) or at one of the mitochondrial cobalamin reductases. In a small proportion of patients, the defect appears to involve adenosylcobalamin and methylcobalamin. Because the latter serves as cofactor for the conversion of homocysteine to methionine, children with this particular defect demonstrate homocystinuria and MMA (321). The various disorders in cobalamin absorption, transport, and use are reviewed by Shevell and colleagues (322).

As ascertained by routine screening of newborns, a large proportion of infants with persistent MMA are asymptomatic and experience normal growth and mental development (323). These children may represent the mildest form of partial mutase deficiency.

Infants suffering from the classic form of the disease (absence of the apoenzyme methylmalonyl-CoA mutase) become symptomatic during the first week of life, usually after the onset of protein feedings. The clinical picture is highlighted by hypotonia, lethargy, recurrent vomiting, and profound metabolic acidosis (318). The prognosis for survival is poor, with death occurring in one of many episodes of metabolic acidosis and ketosis. Survivors have a poor outcome, with spastic quadriparesis, dystonia, and severe developmental delay. When the apoenzyme defect is partial, patients generally become symptomatic in late infancy or childhood and are not as severely affected (320). MRI studies of the brain resemble those obtained on subjects with propionic acidemia with delayed myelination and changes in the basal ganglia (324). Pathologic changes within the brain also involve the basal ganglia predominantly, with neuronal loss and gliosis, or spongy changes in the globus pallidus and putamen.

Abnormal laboratory findings in the classic form of MMA include ketoacidosis and an increased amount of methylmalonic acid in blood and urine. Hyperglycinemia is seen in 70% of classic cases, and hyperammonemia is seen in 75% (318). Hematologic abnormalities, notably leukopenia, anemia, and thrombocytopenia, are encountered in approximately 50% of the cases. These abnormalities result from the growth inhibition of marrow stem cells by methylmalonic acid (325).

Most children with the early onset form of apoenzyme deficiency die by 18 months of age. Almost all of the survivors have some degree of neurologic impairment. This is in part the consequence of diminished protein tolerance and frequent bouts of metabolic decompensation. Late-onset patients fare better, and some have relatively minor neuromotor and mental handicaps (326).

At least four disorders of cobalamin absorption and transport and seven disorders of cobalamin utilization exist. In two of the cobalamin utilization defects, the output of methylmalonic acid is increased (cblA, cblB); in three, MMA and homocystinuria occur (cblC, cblD, and cblF); and in two, there is an increased excretion of homocystine (cblE and cblG) (322).

The clinical course of children experiencing a cofactor deficiency is not as severe as that of children with an apoenzyme deficiency, and nearly 60% of patients with the most common cobalamin utilization defect, cobalamin reductase deficiency (cblC), do not become symptomatic until after age 1 month (318). The clinical picture is variable (327). The majority of children present in infancy or during the first year of life, with failure to thrive, developmental delay, and megaloblastic anemia. In others, the disease presents during adolescence, with dementia and a myelopathy (328,329). A progressive retinal degeneration has been observed (330). Pathologic findings in the cblC defect include a subacute combined degeneration of the spinal cord and a thrombotic microangiopathy (331).

The diagnosis of MMA can be suspected when urine treated with diazotized p-nitroaniline turns emerald green. MMA also is seen in pernicious anemia and vitamin B_{12} deficiency. Cultured fibroblasts are used for the further delineation of the various metabolic defects responsible for MMA.

Infants with MMA should first be tested for vitamin B_{12} responsiveness. In those who fail to respond, a low-protein diet (0.75 to 1.2 g protein/kg per day) with the addition of L-carnitine is required (332). Vitamin B_{12}-responsive patients are treated with intramuscular hydroxocobalamin (1 mg every 3 weeks), supplemented with L-carnitine (250 mg/kg per day) (332). In the child who does not respond to hydroxocobalamin, a trial of deoxyadenosylcobalamin is indicated (332). In children with the various cofactor deficiencies, the biochemical and clinical response to therapy is gratifying (327,332a). Even an occasional patient with the apoenzyme deficiency can improve with therapy.

Isovaleric Aciduria

A striking odor of urine, perspiration, and exhaled air, resembling stale perspiration, is characteristic of patients with isovaleric aciduria. The enzymatic lesion in this condition has been localized to isovaleryl-CoA dehydrogenase (see Fig. 1.6, step 3), a mitochondrial enzyme (333). The gene for this enzyme has been mapped to the long arm of chromosome 15 (15q12-15) and has been cloned (334). As a consequence of the enzymatic defect, serum isovaleric acid concentrations are several hundred times normal, and the administration of L-leucine produces a sustained increase in isovaleric acid levels.

In addition to abnormally elevated concentrations of isovaleric acid in blood and urine, moderate hyperammonemia occurs. This is particularly evident during the neonatal period. Large quantities of isovaleryl glycine are excreted during acute episodes of acidosis and while the patient is in remission. During attacks, 3-hydroxyisovaleric acid, 4-hydroxyisovaleric acid and its oxidation products (methylsuccinic acid and methaconic acids), and isovaleryl glucuronide are excreted also (335). The acidosis seen during an attack appears to result from an accumulation of ketone bodies rather than from the presence of isovaleric acid.

Two clinical phenotypes are seen: an acute and commonly fatal neonatal form in which infants develop recurrent acidosis and coma during the first week of life, and a chronic form with recurrent attacks of vomiting, lethargy, ataxia, and ketoacidosis (336). Acute and chronic forms can be present in the same family. No correlation exists between the amount of residual enzyme activity and the clinical form of the disease. Rather, the severity of the disease appears to be a function of the effectiveness with which isovaleryl-CoA is detoxified to its glycine derivative (337). Attacks are triggered by infections or excessive protein intake. Pancytopenia is not uncommon; it is caused by arrested maturation of hematopoietic precursors (338).

Treatment involves a low-protein diet (1.5 to 2 g/kg per day) with oral glycine supplementation (250 mg/kg per day). Additionally, L-carnitine (100 mg/kg per day) has been given. Glycine and carnitine aid in the mitochondrial detoxification of isovaleryl-CoA (337). For infants who survive the neonatal period, the outlook for normal intellectual development is fairly good, and four of nine subjects treated by Berry and coworkers at Children's Hospital of Philadelphia had IQs of more than 95 (337). A clinical picture resembling isovaleric aciduria develops after intoxication with achee, the fruit that induces Jamaican vomiting sickness and that contains hypoglycin, an inhibitor of several acyl-CoA dehydrogenases, including isovaleryl-CoA dehydrogenase (339).

Glutaric Acidurias

Several completely different genetic defects have been grouped under the term *glutaric aciduria*.

Glutaric aciduria I is a recessive disorder with an incidence of approximately 1 in 30,000 caused by a defect in the gene that codes for glutaryl-CoA dehydrogenase. Biochemically, the condition is marked by the excretion of large amounts of glutaric acid. The clinical picture is protean, and the disorder is frequently undiagnosed or misdiagnosed. In approximately 20% of patients, glutaric aciduria I takes the form of a neurodegenerative condition commencing during the latter part of the first year of life and characterized by hypotonia, dystonia, choreoathetosis, and seizures (340). In most of the remaining patients, development is normal for as long as 2 years of age, and then after what appears to be an infectious, an encephalitic, or a Reye syndrome–like illness, neurologic deterioration occurs (341,342). In yet other cases, the clinical picture resembles extrapyramidal cerebral palsy (343). Macrocephaly is noted in 70% of cases (344). Lack of appetite, sleeplessness, and profuse sweating also is noted, as is hypoglycemia (344,345). No molecular basis for the clinical variability exists (346).

Neuroimaging shows frontotemporal cortical atrophy giving what has been termed a *bat wing* appearance. This is often accompanied by increased signal in the basal ganglia on T2-weighted images and caudate atrophy. Bilateral subdural hematomas have also been described (Fig. 1.11). When these are accompanied by retinal hemorrhages, an erroneous diagnosis of child abuse frequently is made. Neuropathology shows temporal and frontal lobe hypoplasia, degeneration of the putamen and globus pallidus, mild status spongiosus of white matter, and heterotopic neurons in cerebellum (347). It is not clear why so much of the damage is localized to the basal ganglia. It has been postulated that this results from depletion of gamma-aminobutyric acid (GABA) as a consequence of glutaric acid and its derivative 3-hydroxyglutaric acid inhibiting glutamic acid decarboxylase, the enzyme responsible for the synthesis of GABA from glutamate. Other possibilities are that increased glutaminergic neurotransmission occurs by interference with glutamate reuptake or by activation of glutamatergic binding sites (346,348).

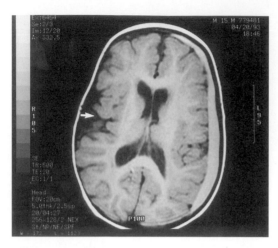

FIG. 1.11. Glutaric aciduria I. Magnetic resonance imaging study. This T1-weighted image demonstrates an enlarged operculum on the right (*arrow*), and an extensive left subdural hematoma.

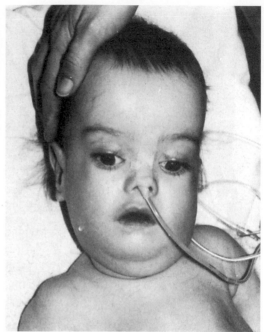

A

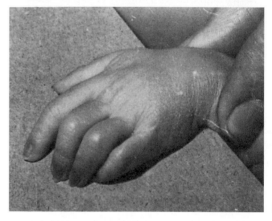

B

FIG. 1.12. Zellweger syndrome. **A:** Typical facies with high forehead and flat facies. Redundant skin of the neck is seen. (Courtesy of the late Dr. H. Zellweger, University of Iowa.) **B:** Hand, demonstrating camptodactyly of third, fourth, and fifth fingers. (Courtesy of Dr. J. M. Opitz, Shodair Children's Hospital, Helena, MT.)

A low-protein, high-caloric diet and carnitine supplementation have sometimes prevented further deterioration, but almost all patients are left with a severe dystonic-dyskinetic disorder (344).

In glutaric aciduria type II, a defect occurs in one of three genes involved in the mitochondrial β-oxidation of fatty acids: those coding for the α and β subunits of the electron transfer flavoprotein and that coding for the electron transfer flavoprotein dehydrogenase (349,350). As a result, the activities of all acyl-CoA dehydrogenases served by these enzymes are deficient. Therefore, increased excretion occurs, not only of glutaric acid, but also of other organic acids, including lactic, ethylmalonic, isobutyric, and isovaleric acids.

Glutaric aciduria II can present in the neonatal period with an overwhelming and generally fatal metabolic acidosis coupled with hypoglycemia, acidemia, and a cardiomyopathy. Affected infants can have an odor of sweaty feet. Dysmorphic features are prominent in approximately one-half of cases (351). They include macrocephaly, a large anterior fontanelle, a high forehead, flat nasal bridge, and malformed ears. This appearance is reminiscent of Zellweger syndrome (Fig. 1.12). Glutaric aciduria II also can develop later in life with episodic vomiting, acidosis, and hypoglycemia. Other cases present in early childhood with progressive spastic ataxia and high signal intensity on T2-weighted MRI in supratentorial white matter, a picture mimicking a leukodystrophy (352). The neuropathologic picture is marked by diffuse gliosis of cerebrum, brainstem, and cerebellum, with foci of leukomalacia and striatal degeneration (351,353).

Some infants with glutaric aciduria II respond dramatically to riboflavin (100 mg three times a day). This riboflavin-responsive multiple acyl-CoA dehydrogenase deficiency may be identical to ethylmalonic-adipic aciduria (352,354,355).

Disorders of Fatty Acid Oxidation

Up to 18 defects of hepatic fatty acid oxidation have been recognized (356,357). These include eight defects of the β-oxidation cycle. Affected subjects are unable to use fatty acids derived from adipose tissue or diet for energy production or hepatic ketone synthesis. Because fatty acids are the principal energy source during fasting, infants rapidly decompensate in the neonatal period or during a febrile illness. Taken collectively, these conditions are not rare, and their incidence in Great Britain has been estimated at 1 in 5,000 live births (358). In addition to the acute metabolic decompensation that results when infants are fasted, resulting in a rapid evolution of seizures and coma, the clinical presentation of most of these conditions is marked by episodes of a nonketotic or hypoketotic hypoglycemia. The esterified-to-free-carnitine ratio is increased, and generally hypocarnitinemia occurs. In the experience of Rinaldo and colleagues, mortality of the first such episode is

59% (359). Some infants have been diagnosed as having Reye syndrome; others have died from an episode that is similar to sudden infant death syndrome (SIDS). When the enzyme defect is limited to muscle, it can present with cardiomyopathy, muscle weakness, and myoglobinuria. These symptoms are features of defects in the transport of fatty acids into mitochondria and are covered in the section on Mitochondrial Diseases, later in this chapter.

Medium-Chain Acyl-CoA Dehydrogenase Deficiency

The most common of the disorders of fatty acid oxidation is a defect involving medium-chain acyl-CoA dehydrogenase (MCAD) deficiency (360). The incidence of this entity varies considerably. In whites, it has been estimated to be between 1 in 6,400 and 1 in 23,000 live births; thus, it appears to be as common as PKU (361–363).

Because MCAD is active over the range of C_4 to C_{12} carbons, its deficiency permits fatty acid oxidation to progress only up to the point at which the carbon chain has been reduced to 12 (357). A single-point mutation in the gene is responsible for the condition in more than 90% of white subjects. This mutation results in the substitution of glutamine for lysine in the MCAD precursor. This disrupts folding of the mature form and its assembly in mitochondria, with subsequent disappearance of the mutant MCAD. Clinical symptoms usually develop during the

TABLE 1.8. *Fatty acid oxidation disorders*

Disorder	Reference
Carnitine cycle	
Carnitine transport defect	Stanley et al. (377)
Carnitine palmitoyl transferase I	Haworth et al. (378)
Carnitine-acylcarnitine translocase	Stanley et al. (379)
Carnitine palmitoyl transferase II	Land et al. (380)
Mitochondrial β-oxidation	
Medium-chain CoA acyldehydrogenase deficiency	Iafolla et al. (362)
Long-chain CoA acyldehydrogenase deficiency	Treem et al. (381)
Short-chain CoA acyldehydrogenase deficiency	Bhala et al. (382)
Very-long-chain CoA acyldehydrogenase deficiency	Souri et al. (383), Andresen et al. (367a)
Long-chain 3-hydroxyacyl-CoA dehydrogenase deficiency	Tyni et al. (384), Tein et al. (384a)
Short-chain 3-hydroxyacyl-CoA dehydrogenase deficiency	Bennett et al. (385)
Electron transfer flavoprotein deficiency (glutaric aciduria II)	Loehr et al. (350)
Electron transfer flavoprotein dehydrogenase deficiency (glutaric aciduria II)	Wilson et al. (351)

TABLE 1.9. *Some of the organic acidurias of infancy and childhood*

Condition	Unique manifestations	Reference
Propionic aciduria	Mixed pyramidal and extrapyramidal deficits	Childs et al. (312)
Glutaric aciduria I	Spasticity, extrapyramidal dysfunction, macrocephaly	Hoffman et al. (344)
Glutaric aciduria II	Dysmorphic features, sweaty feet odor	Wilson et al. (351)
Isovaleric aciduria	Sweaty feet odor	Tanaka et al. (333)
2-Hydroxyglutaric aciduria	Mental deficiency, cerebellar dysfunction, brainstem and cerebellar atrophy, extrapyramidal tract signs, progressive macrocephaly	Chen et al. (386), Barbot et al. (387), van der Knaap et al. (387a)
Oxyprolinuria (glutathione synthetase deficiency)	Neonatal acidosis with or without neurologic damage	Spielberg et al. (388)
4-Hydroxybutyric aciduria (γ-hydroxybutyric aciduria)	Severe ataxia, hypotonia, mild mental retardation	Rating et al. (389), Gibson et al. (390), Chambliss et al. (391)
3-Hydroxyisobutyric aciduria	Intracerebral calcifications, lissencephaly, polymicrogyria	Ko et al. (392), Chitayat et al. (393)
3-Methylglutaconic aciduria (three types; also seen in Smith-Lemli-Opitz syndrome)	Delayed speech, mental retardation, choreoathetosis, optic atrophy, cardiomyopathy	Gibson et al. (394), Zeharia et al. (395)
Ethylmalonic aciduria (also seen in short-chain acyl-CoA dehydrogenase deficiency)	Developmental delay, central nervous system malformations, petechiae, acrocyanosis, chronic diarrhea; excretion of ethylmalonic and methyl succinic acid	Nowaczyk et al. (396)
3-Hydroxy-3-methylglutaric aciduria	Fasting hypoglycemic coma	Robinson et al. (397), Thompson et al. (398)

first year of life and are characterized by episodes of hypoketotic hypoglycemia triggered by fasting or infections. These episodes result in lethargy, vomiting, and altered consciousness. In the series of Iafolla and coworkers, 36% of subjects had sudden cardiorespiratory arrest (362). Although the last presentation resembles that of SIDS, Miller and colleagues were unable to find any homozygotes for the glutamine to lysine mutation leading to MCAD deficiency in 67 SIDS babies (364), and Boles and colleagues found an incidence of only 0.6% among cases diagnosed as SIDS (365). In the latter study, another 0.6% of SIDS cases were believed to have glutaric aciduria II (365).

The MCAD deficiency is treated by supplemental L-carnitine, a low-fat diet, and avoidance of fasting, which rapidly initiates a potentially fatal hypoglycemia. The efficacy of these mea-

sures is still unclear. On follow-up of patients, a significant proportion of survivors has global developmental delays, attention deficit disorder, and language deficits (362).

The other disorders of fatty acid β-oxidation are much less common. They are summarized in Table 1.8. In long-chain acyl-CoA deficiency, the defect is at the start of the fatty acid β-oxidation cycle. Subjects are unable to metabolize fatty acids with 12 to 18 carbons (366,367). Three forms have been recognized: a severe form with early onset and a high incidence of cardiomyopathy; a milder, childhood-onset form; and an adult form with rhabdomyolysis and myoglobinuria. The clinical picture appears to correlate with the amount of residual enzyme activity (367a).

Short-chain acyl-CoA dehydrogenase is active from four to six carbons, and infants excrete large amounts of butyrate, methylmalonate, and methylsuccinate (368,369). Whereas patients with MCAD and long-chain acyl-CoA deficiency tend to develop hypoketotic hypoglycemia, patients with short-chain acyl-CoA dehydrogenase deficiency may not have hypoglycemia. Most patients have hypotonia, hyperactivity, and developmental delay. The condition can be intermittent.

Defects in branched chain acyl-CoA dehydrogenation also have been recognized. They are listed in Table 1.9.

The diagnosis of these disorders depends on the presence of the various dicarboxylic acids in urine. Levels of free carnitine in blood are decreased, and the ratio of esterified to free carnitine is increased. According to Hale and Bennett, a total carnitine level in blood of 30 μmol/L or less should suggest a disorder in fatty acid oxidation (356). Because organic acids are not always present in the interval between acute episodes, Rinaldo and coworkers have suggested an assay for urinary hexanoylglycine and phenylpropionylglycine, both by-products of fatty acid oxidation, which is said to be highly specific for the MCAD defect (359). Others prefer to obtain a urine for organic acids when the child is acutely ill.

Disorders of Biotin Metabolism

Four biotin-dependent enzymes exist, all carboxylases: propionyl-CoA carboxylase, 3-methylcrontonyl-CoA carboxylase, pyruvate carboxylase, and acetyl-CoA carboxylase. The covalent binding of biotin to these enzymes is catalyzed by holocarboxylase synthetase. A significant proportion of infants with organic aciduria is found to have impaired function of these biotin-containing carboxylases (370). The clinical picture for the multiple carboxylase deficiencies is fairly specific. Two forms are recognized, neonatal and juvenile.

The neonatal form presents with metabolic acidosis, ketosis, and an erythematous rash. It is caused by a defect in biotin holocarboxylase synthetase (371). Symptoms are usually reversed by biotin.

A second, more common, form is characterized by the onset of symptoms after the neonatal period, usually between ages 2 and 3 months.

Although symptoms resulting from a deficiency of holocarboxylase synthetase can appear as late as 8 years of age (372), the late-onset form of multiple carboxylase deficiency is usually caused by a defect in biotinidase. Biotinidase hydrolyzes the bond between biotin and lysine, the bound form in which biotin exists in the diet, and thus recycles biotin in the body (373). The enzyme deficiency can be complete or partial, with patients who have a partial deficiency tending to be asymptomatic unless stressed by prolonged infections representing heterozygotes (374). Considerable heterogeneity exists in profound biotinidase deficiency, and numerous biochemical and immunologic phenotypes have been recognized (375). As ascertained by a screening program, the incidence of complete biotinidase deficiency in the United States is 1 in 166,000. The condition is rare in Asians (376).

Symptoms in complete biotinidase deficiency include lactic acidosis, alopecia, ataxia, spastic paraparesis, seizures, and an erythematous rash. Developmental delay soon becomes apparent. Hearing loss, acute vision loss, optic atrophy, and respiratory irregularities are seen in a significant proportion of cases (370). Plasma and urinary biotin levels are subnormal, and clinical and biochemical findings are reversed by the administration of oral biotin (5 to 10 mg/kg/day).

A unique familial syndrome of acute encephalopathy appearing between 1 and 14 years of age, and marked by confusion and lethargy progressing to coma, has been reported (376a). The condition is associated with dystonia, chorea, rigidity, and, at times, opisthotonus and external ophthalmoplegia. It is completely reversible by the administration of biotin (5 to 10 mg/kg per day). MRI shows increased signal on T2-weighted images within the central part of the caudate, and in parts, or all of the putamen. Its cause is unknown, and all enzyme assay results have been normal.

Some of the other, much rarer organic acidurias are summarized in Table 1.9, together with any distinguishing clinical features. In most conditions, however, symptoms are indistinguishable; they consist mainly of episodic vomiting, lethargy, convulsions, and coma. Laboratory features include acidosis, hypoglycemia, hyper-

TABLE 1.10. *Molecular lesions in the lysosomal storage diseases*

No immunologically detectable enzyme; includes conditions with grossly abnormal structural genes.
Immunologically detectable, but catalytically inactive polypeptide. Stability or transport of polypeptide abnormal.
Enzyme catalytically active, but not segregated into lysosomes.
Enzyme catalytically active, unstable in prelysosomal or lysosomal compartments.
Lysosomal enzyme synthesized normally and transported into lysosomes. Activator protein missing.
Lysosomal enzyme deficiency results from intoxication with inhibitor of lysosomal enzyme.[a]

[a]Not yet determined in humans, but inhibition of α-mannosidase by an alkaloid has been demonstrated.
Data from Kornfeld S. Trafficking of lysosomal enzymes in normal and disease states. *J Clin Invest* 1986;77:1–6. With permission.

ammonemia, and hyperglycinemia. The organic acidurias can be diagnosed during an acute episode by subjecting serum or, preferably, urine to organic acid chromatography. In addition, a marked reduction in plasma-free carnitine exists, and an increased esterified carnitine to free carnitine ratio exists. These assays should be performed on any child with neurologic symptoms who has an associated metabolic acidosis, or who is noted to have hyperglycinemia or hyperammonemia on routine biochemical analyses.

LYSOSOMAL STORAGE DISEASES

Lysosomes are subcellular organelles containing hydrolases with a low optimal pH (acid hydrolases) that catalyze the degradation of macromolecules. The lysosomal storage diseases, as first delineated by Hers (399), are characterized by an accumulation of undegraded macromolecules within lysosomes. The various groups are named according to the nature of the storage product. They include type II glycogenosis, the mucopolysaccharidoses, the mucolipidoses, the glycoproteinoses, the sphingolipidoses, and the acid lipase deficiency diseases. The combined prevalence of all lysosomal storage diseases is 1 in 6,600 to 1 in 7,700 live births (399a). The disease entities result from various single gene mutations, with each of the enzyme defects resulting from one of several different abnormalities on the

genomic level (Table 1.10). The heterogeneity of the disorders is overwhelmingly complex (400). The enzyme itself can be defective, the result of a variety of single-base mutations or deletions that produce immunologically responsive or unresponsive enzyme proteins. The defect can cause a defective glycosylation of the enzyme protein or cause a failure to generate a recognition marker that permits the enzyme to attach itself to the lysosomal membrane. Other mutations result in a lack of enzyme activator or substrate activator proteins, or a defective transport of the substrate across the lysosomal membrane.

Glycogen Storage Diseases (Glycogenoses)

Of the various glycogenoses, only type II (Pompe disease) is a lysosomal disorder. For convenience sake, however, all the other glycogenoses are considered here as well.

Neuromuscular symptoms are seen in all but one of the eight types of glycogenoses (Table 1.11). Hypoglycemia is seen in types I, II, III, and VI, and in the condition characterized by a defect in glycogen synthesis (type I0). In type Ia, hypoglycemia is frequently severe enough to induce convulsions.

Seizures also can be seen in type Ia glycogenosis without documented hypoglycemia, and focal neurologic signs, including hemiparesis, can sometimes be detected. Whether these are consequences of minor intracranial hemorrhages owing to an associated bleeding diathesis is unknown (401).

A myopathy presenting with muscular stiffness and easy fatigability has been recognized in type IIIa glycogenosis. Undoubtedly, it is related to the accumulation of glycogen within muscle (402).

Hypotonia has been seen in the various type I glycogenoses and also has been the presenting symptom in type IV glycogenosis (403). Types V and VII glycogenoses are discussed in Chapter 13.

Type II Glycogenosis (Pompe Disease)

Type II glycogenosis, first described by Pompe (404) in 1932, is a rare autosomal recessive disorder characterized by glycogen accumulation

TABLE 1.11. *Enzymatically defined glycogenoses*

Type	Defect	Structure of glycogen	Involvement	Neuromuscular symptoms
0	UDPG-glycogen transferase	Normal	Liver, muscle	Hypoglycemic seizures
Ia	Glucose-6-phosphatase complex (G6Pase)	Normal	Liver, kidney, intestinal mucosa	Hypoglycemic seizures, growth retardation, lactic acidemia
IaSP	Regulatory protein for glucose-6-phosphatase	Normal	Liver	Hypoglycemic seizures
Ib	Hepatic microsomal glucose-6-phosphate transport system	Normal	Liver	As Ia, but also impaired neutrophil function
Ic	Transporter of microsomal phosphate	Normal	Liver	Hypoglycemic seizures
Id	Defective microsomal glucose transport	Normal	Liver	As Ia
II	Lysosomal acid-α-1,4-glucosidase	Normal	Generalized	Progressive weakness
IIIa	Glycogen debrancher deficiency	Limit dextrinlike (short outer chains)	Muscle	Hypoglycemia, muscle weakness becomes more marked with age
IIIb	Glycogen debrancher deficiency	Limit dextrinlike	Liver	Hepatomegaly, hypoglycemia
IV	Brancher deficiency (Amylo-1, 4–1,6-transglucosylase)	Amylopectinlike (long outer chains)	Generalized	Hypotonia, failure to thrive
V	Muscle phosphorylase	Normal	Muscle	Muscular cramps, weakness, atrophy (see Chapter 14)
VI	Liver phosphorylase	Normal	Liver, leukocytes	Hypoglycemia
VII	Phosphofructokinase	Normal	Muscle, erythrocytes	Muscular cramps, weakness (see Chapter 14)
VIII	Phosphorylase kinase	Normal	Liver	None

UDPG, uridine diphosphoglucose.

in the lysosomes of skeletal muscles, heart, liver, and CNS.

Molecular Genetics and Biochemical Pathology

Two groups of enzymes are involved in the degradation of glycogen. Phosphorylase initiates one set of breakdown reactions, cleaving glycogen to limit dextrin, which then is acted on by a debrancher enzyme (oligo-1,4-glucanotransferase, and amyl-1,6-glucosidase) to yield a straight-chain polyglucosan, which is cleaved to the individual glucose units by phosphorylase. A second set of enzymes includes α-amylase, which cleaves glycogen to a series of oligosaccharides, and two α-1,4-glucosidases, which cleave the α-1,4 bonds of glycogen. Two of these terminal glucosidases exist. One, located in the microsomal fraction, has a neutral pH optimum (neutral maltase); the other, found in lysosomes, has its maximum activity at an acid pH (3.5) (acid α-glucosidase). The

gene for the latter enzyme has been mapped to the long arm of chromosome 17 (17q23) and has been cloned.

In type II glycogenosis, lysosomal acid α-glucosidase is deficient in liver, heart, and skeletal muscle; consequently, glycogen accumulates in these organelles as a result of tissue turnover (399). Like every other lysosomal protein, α-glucosidase is synthesized in a precursor form on membrane-bound polysomes and is sequestered in the lumen of the rough endoplasmic reticulum as a larger glycosylated precursor. Whereas the primary translational product of α-glucosidase mRNA is 100 kd, it becomes glycosylated to yield a 110-kd precursor, which in turn undergoes a posttranslational modification by phosphorylation to yield the mannose-6-phosphate recognition marker (405). Phosphorylation is an important step, as formation of the marker distinguishes the lysosomal enzymes from secretory proteins and allows the lysosomal enzymes to be channeled to the lysosomes to which they

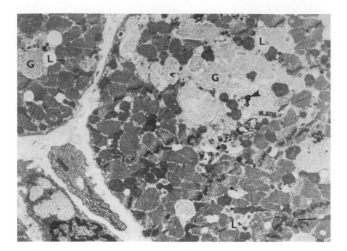

FIG. 1.13. Glycogen storage disease type II (Pompe disease). Electron micrograph of several myofibers of various sizes demonstrating varying degrees of glycogen accumulations in sarcoplasm (G). Also seen are irregular electron-dense accumulations suggestive of lysosomes or autophagosomes (*arrowhead*). Large lipid droplets (L) appear between myofibrils (uranyl acetate and lead citrate, original magnification ×9,600). (From Sarnat H. Lipid storage myopathy in infantile Pompe disease. *Arch Neurol* 1982;39:180. Copyright 1982, American Medical Association. With permission.)

become attached by a membrane-bound mannose-phosphate–specific receptor. Additionally, the 110-kd precursor undergoes proteolytic processing to yield the two 76-kd and one 70-kd mature lysosomal enzyme polypeptides. With such a complex processing system, it is not surprising to encounter extensive clinical heterogeneity in glycogenosis II. Considerable biochemical heterogeneity exists, and a variety of nonsense, frame shift, and missense mutations have been described. These result in partial or complete loss of enzyme activity. As a rule, good correlation exists between the amount of residual enzyme activity and the severity of the disease. Two relatively common mutations are responsible for a large proportion of the infantile form of Pompe disease. In whites, one of the more common mutations is a deletion of exon 18, which results in total loss of enzyme activity and the clinical manifestations of infantile glycogen storage disease (406).

Pathologic Anatomy

Glycogen can be deposited in virtually every tissue. The heart is globular, the enlargement being symmetric and primarily ventricular. In the infantile form, massive glycogen deposition occurs within the muscle fibers. In cross-section, these appear with a central, clear area, giving a *lacunate* appearance. Glycogen also is deposited in striated muscle (particularly the tongue), in smooth muscle, and in the Schwann cells of

peripheral nerves, kidney, and liver (Fig. 1.13). Ultrastructural studies of muscle show glycogen to be present in lysosomal sacs where it occurs in conjunction with cytoplasmic degradation products. Additionally, it occurs free in cytoplasm (407). In the CNS, glycogen accumulates within neurons and in the extracellular substance (408). The anterior horn cells are affected predominantly, although deposits are seen in all parts of the neuraxis, including the cerebral cortex (409). Chemical analysis indicates an excess of glycogen in cerebral cortex and white matter and a deficiency in total phospholipid, cholesterol, and cerebroside. No evidence exists for primary demyelination.

Clinical Manifestations

Pompe disease can take one of three forms. In the classic, infantile form, the first symptoms usually appear by the second month of life. They include difficulty in feeding, with dyspnea and exhaustion interfering with sucking. Gradually, muscular weakness and impaired cardiac function become apparent. Marked cardiac enlargement is present at an early age. The heart appears globular on radiographic examination; murmurs are usually absent, but the heart tones have a poor quality and a gallop rhythm is often audible. Affected infants have poor muscle tone and few spontaneous movements, although the deep tendon reflexes are often intact. Skeletal muscles are often enlarged and gradually acquire a peculiar rubbery consistency. Electromyography shows lower motor neuron degeneration (410). Convulsions, intellectual impairment, and coma also have been observed. The liver, although usually not enlarged, is abnormally firm and easily palpable. Splenomegaly is rare. Infants are prone to intercurrent infections, particularly pneumonia, and usually die of these or bulbar paralysis by 1 year of age. In most of the patients belonging to this clinical form, lysosomal α-glucosidase is catalytically inactive, although the protein is present in some families. The most common form of this variant, termed *Antopol disease*, is marked by severe cardiomyopathy, a mild myopathy, and mental retardation (411).

α-Glucosidase deficiency also has been seen in older children and adults (juvenile and adult forms, respectively) (412). In these patients, organomegaly is absent, and muscle weakness is often slowly progressive or nonprogressive with maximum involvement of the proximal musculature of the lower extremities (413). Pharyngeal muscles can be involved as a consequence of glycogen storage in brainstem neurons (414). In most of the slowly progressive cases, residual lysosomal α-glucosidase activity is more than 10%. In others, the enzyme activity is undetectable, but the 110-kd precursor is present. Other individuals appear to be compound heterozygotes for different mutant alleles (406).

Diagnosis

When cardiac symptoms predominate, a differentiation from other causes of cardiomegaly and congestive failure in the absence of significant murmurs is required. These other causes include endocardial fibroelastosis, acute interstitial myocarditis, and aberrant coronary artery. When muscular weakness predominates, infantile spinal muscular atrophy (Werdnig-Hoffmann disease), the muscular dystrophies, myasthenia gravis, and hypotonic cerebral palsy must be considered (see Chapter 14). Cardiac involvement is generally late in Werdnig-Hoffmann disease and in the muscular dystrophies. In contrast to glycogen storage disease, the intellectual deficit in hypotonic cerebral palsy is usually severe and begins early. A muscle biopsy is usually required to confirm the diagnosis. Blood chemistry, including fasting blood sugars and glucose tolerance tests, is normal. α-Glucosidase activity of muscle and leukocytes is markedly diminished, and this assay serves as an excellent diagnostic aid (415). α-Glucosidase activity also can be shown in fibroblasts grown from normal amniotic fluid cells. This method can be used for the antepartum diagnosis of Pompe disease and for the detection of heterozygotes.

Treatment

No effective treatment exists for Pompe disease. Several approaches to the treatment of glycogenosis II, as well as the other lysosomal defects, have been proposed. For enzyme replacement therapy to be successful, α-glucosidase must be taken up by the lysosomes of affected organs. Enzyme replacement therapy, using the recombinant human enzyme or an α-glucosidase precursor, with phosphorylated, *N*-linked, mannose-containing carbohydrate chains appears to be the most promising (416,417). The major problems inherent in this approach include the protection of the enzyme from immunologic and proteolytic attack, its delivery in sufficient amounts to the affected cell lysosomes, and its proper localization within them. Additionally, no evidence exists that sufficient amounts of the enzyme are able to cross the blood–brain barrier even when its permeability has been temporarily increased by one of the several measures available. Adenovirus-mediated gene transfer holds some promise in delivering α-glucosidase to muscle (418). The problems inherent in gene delivery to the brain are discussed by Kennedy (419).

Allogeneic bone marrow transplantation offers more promise for the treatment of lysosomal storage diseases. In glycogenosis II, however, no beneficial result has been reported, despite successful engraftment. Liver transplantation has been used with some effect in type IV glycogen storage disease (brancher deficiency) (420). After transplant, the cells of the host organs become mixed with cells of the donor genome that migrate from the allograft into the tissues of the recipient and serve as enzyme carriers. This observation explains why some

TABLE 1.12. *Classification of the mucopolysaccharidoses*

Type	Eponym	Clinical features				Urinary mucopolysaccharides					Enzyme defect
		Corneal clouding	Dwarfism	Neurologic signs	Cardiovascular involvement	Heparan sulfate	Dermatan sulfate	Keratan sulfate	Chondroitin-4-sulfate	Chondroitin-6-sulfate	
I H	Hurler	Severe	Marked	Marked	Marked	+	+	–	–	–	α-l-iduronidase
I S	Scheie	Severe	Mild	None	Late	+	+	–	–	–	α-l-iduronidase
I H/S	Hurler-Scheie	Severe	Mild	None or mild	Late	+	+	–	–	–	α-l-iduronidase
II A	Hunter (severe)	None	Marked	Mental retardation	Late	+	+	–	–	–	Iduronate sulfatase
II B	Hunter (mild)	None	Mild	Normal intellect, hearing deficits	Mild	+	+	–	–	–	Iduronate sulfatase
III A	Sanfilippo A	Absent	Moderate	Profound mental deterioration	Rare	+	–	–	–	–	Heparan-N-sulfatase
III B	Sanfilippo B	Absent	Moderate	Profound mental deterioration	Rare	+	–	–	–	–	α-N-acetylglucosaminidase
III C	Sanfilippo C	Absent	Moderate	Slow mental deterioration	Rare	+	–	–	–	–	Acetyl CoA: α-glucosaminide acetyltransferase
III D	Sanfilippo D	Absent	Moderate	Mild mental retardation	Rare	+	–	–	–	–	N-acetylglucosaminide 6-sulfate sulfatase
IV A	Morquio A	Late	Marked	None	Late	–	–	+	–	+	Galactose 6-sulfate sulfatase
IV B	Morquio B	Late	Marked	None	Late	–	–	+	–	–	β-Galactosidase
VI	Maroteaux-Lamy	Severe	Marked	None	Present	–	+	–	–	–	N-acetylgalactosamine 4-sulfate sulfatase
VII	Sly	Variable	Marked to severe	Variable: none	Present	±	±	–	+	+	β-Glucuronidase

patients with such lysosomal storage diseases as type 1 Gaucher disease, Niemann-Pick disease, and Wolman disease receive more benefit from liver transplants than simply improved hepatic functions.

Mucopolysaccharidoses

A syndrome consisting of mental and physical retardation, multiple skeletal deformities, hepatosplenomegaly, and clouding of the cornea was described by Hunter in 1917 (421), by Hurler in 1919 (422), and by Pfaundler in 1920 (423). To Ellis and associates in 1936, the "large head, inhuman facies, and deformed limbs" suggested the appearance of a gargoyle (424). The syndrome is now known to represent six major entities, some with two or more subgroups that are distinguishable by their clinical picture, genetic transmission, enzyme defect, and urinary mucopolysaccharide (MPS) pattern (Table 1.12).

Molecular Genetics and Biochemical Pathology

The principal biochemical disturbance in the various mucopolysaccharidoses involves the metabolism of MPS. The chemistry of the MPS, also known as *glycosaminoglycans*, has been reviewed by Alberts and colleagues (425) and more extensively by Kjellen and Lindahl (426). These substances occur as large polymers having a protein core and multiple carbohydrate branches. Chondroitin-4-sulfate is found in cornea, bone, and cartilage. It consists of alternating units of D-glucuronic acid and sulfated *N*-acetylgalactosamine (Fig. 1.14).

Dermatan sulfate is a normal minor constituent of connective tissue and a major component of skin. It differs structurally from chondroitin-4-sulfate in that the uronic acid is principally L-iduronic rather than glucuronic acid (see Fig. 1.14).

Heparan sulfate consists of alternating units of uronic acid and glucosamine. The former may be L-iduronic or D-glucuronic acid. Glucosamine can be acetylated on the amino nitrogen, as well as sulfated on the amino nitrogen and hydroxyl

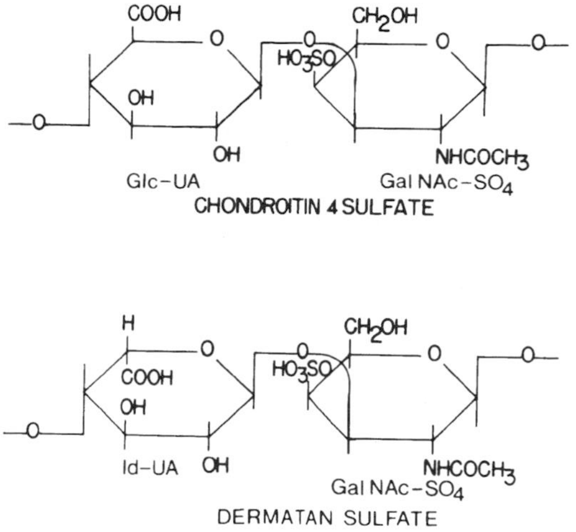

FIG. 1.14. Structure of chondroitin-4-sulfate and dermatan sulfate.

group (Fig. 1.15). Generally, the MPS chains are linked to the serine of the protein core by means of a xylose-galactose-galactose-glucuronic acid-*N*-acetylhexosamine bridge.

The pathways of MPS biosynthesis are well established. The first step is the formation of a protein acceptor. Hexosamine and uronic acid moieties are then attached to the protein, one sugar at a time, starting with xylose. Sulfation occurs after completion of polymerization. The sulfate groups are introduced through the intermediary of an active sulfate. This is a labile nucleotide, identified as adenosine-3'-phosphate-5'-sulfatophosphate.

In the mucopolysaccharidoses, degradation of MPS is impaired because of a defect in one of several lysosomal hydrolases. This results in the accumulation of incompletely degraded molecules within lysosomes and the excretion of MPS fragments. The initial steps of MPS degradation (cleavage from the protein core) are intact in the mucopolysaccharidoses. In tissue where amounts of MPS are pathologic, such as liver, spleen, and urine, the protein core is completely lacking or represented only by a few amino acids.

In all of these diseases, therefore, the metabolic defect is located along the further degradation of the MPS, and in all but one, it involves the breakdown of dermatan sulfate and heparan sul-

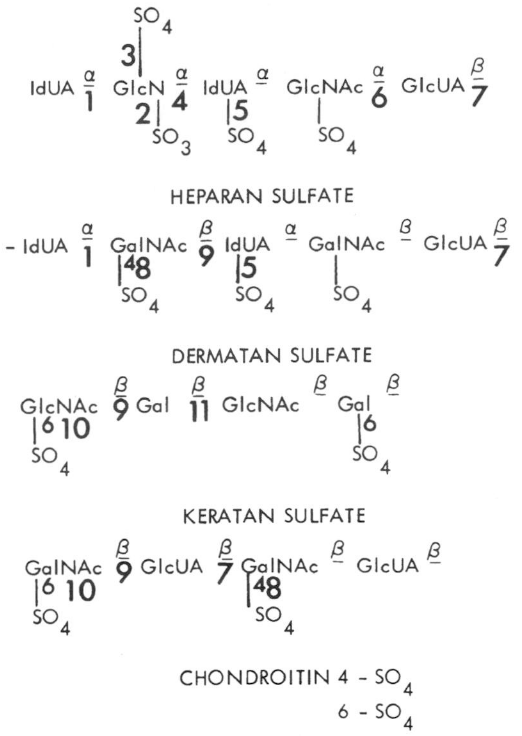

$$\text{IdUA} \overset{\alpha}{\underset{1}{-}} \overset{\overset{\displaystyle SO_4}{\displaystyle |}}{\underset{\underset{\displaystyle SO_3}{\displaystyle 2|}}{\text{GlcN}}} \overset{3}{\underset{4}{\alpha}} \overset{\alpha}{\underset{\underset{\displaystyle SO_4}{\displaystyle |5}}{=}} \text{IdUA} \; \text{GlcNAc} \overset{\alpha}{\underset{\underset{\displaystyle SO_4}{\displaystyle |}}{6}} \text{GlcUA} \overset{\beta}{\underset{7}{-}}$$

HEPARAN SULFATE

$$-\text{IdUA} \overset{\alpha}{\underset{1}{-}} \underset{\underset{\displaystyle SO_4}{\displaystyle |48}}{\text{GalNAc}} \overset{\beta}{\underset{9}{-}} \underset{\underset{\displaystyle SO_4}{\displaystyle |5}}{\text{IdUA}} \overset{\alpha}{=} \underset{\underset{\displaystyle SO_4}{\displaystyle |}}{\text{GalNAc}} \overset{\beta}{=} \text{GlcUA} \overset{\beta}{\underset{7}{-}}$$

DERMATAN SULFATE

$$\underset{\underset{\displaystyle SO_4}{\displaystyle |^6 10}}{\text{GlcNAc}} \overset{\beta}{\underset{9}{-}} \text{Gal} \overset{\beta}{\underset{11}{-}} \text{GlcNAc} \overset{\beta}{=} \text{Gal} \overset{\beta}{\underset{\underset{\displaystyle SO_4}{\displaystyle |6}}{=}}$$

KERATAN SULFATE

$$\underset{\underset{\displaystyle SO_4}{\displaystyle |^6 10}}{\text{GalNAc}} \overset{\beta}{\underset{9}{-}} \text{GlcUA} \overset{\beta}{\underset{7}{-}} \underset{\underset{\displaystyle SO_4}{\displaystyle |48}}{\text{GalNAc}} \overset{\beta}{=} \text{GlcUA} \overset{\beta}{=}$$

CHONDROITIN 4 - SO_4

6 - SO_4

FIG. 1.15. Pathway of degeneration of mucopolysaccharides stored in the various mucopolysaccharidoses. The defects in the various entities as indicated by numbers: (1) Hurler and Scheie syndromes; (2) Sanfilippo syndrome type A; (5) Hunter syndrome; (6) Sanfilippo syndrome type B; (7) β-glucuronidase deficiency (MPS VII); (8) Maroteaux-Lamy syndrome; (9) Tay-Sachs and Sandhoff diseases (GM_2 gangliosidoses); (10) Morquio syndrome; and (11) GM_1 gangliosidosis. Step (3) is blocked by Sanfilippo syndrome type D. In Sanfilippo syndrome type C, acetylation of the free amino group of glucosamine (4) is defective. (Gal, galactose; GalNAc, N-acetylgalactosamine; GlcN, glucosamine; GlcNAc, N-acetylglucosamine; GlcUA, glucuronic acid; IdUA, iduronic acid.) (Courtesy of Dr. R. Matalon, Research Institute, Miami Children's Hospital, Miami, FL.)

fate (see Figs. 1.14 and 1.15). As a result, large amounts (75 to 100 mg/24 hours) of fragmented chains of these MPSs are excreted by individuals afflicted with the two major genetic entities: the autosomally transmitted Hurler syndrome (MPS IH; see Table 1.12) and the rarer gender-linked Hunter syndrome (MPS II). These values com-

pare with a normal excretion of 5 to 25 mg per 24 hours for all MPSs. Normal MPS excretion is distributed between chondroitin-4-sulfate (31%), chondroitin-6-sulfate (34%), chondroitin (25%), and heparan sulfate (8%) (427).

The biochemical lesions in the various mucopolysaccharidoses have been reviewed by Neufeld and Muenzer (428).

In the Hurler syndromes (MPS I), the activity of α-L-iduronidase is deficient (see Fig. 1.15, step 1) (428). The iduronic acid moiety is found in dermatan and heparan sulfates (see Fig. 1.15); therefore, the metabolism of both MPSs is defective. The gene for α-L-iduronidase has been mapped to chromosome 4 and has been cloned. More than 50 mutations have been described, with the frequency of each mutation differing from one genetic stock to the next. As a consequence of the genetic variability, a wide range of clinical phenotypes exists, from the most severe form, Hurler syndrome (IH), through an intermediate form (I H/S) to the mildest form, Scheie syndrome or MPS IS (429). Among patients of European origin, two mutations account for more than 50% of alleles (429).

In Hunter syndrome (MPS II), iduronate sulfatase activity is lost (Fig. 1.15, step 5) (428). Like L-iduronidase, this enzyme also is involved in the metabolism of dermatan and heparan sulfates. The gene for the enzyme is located on the distal portion of the long arm of the X chromosome (Xq28) in close proximity to the fragile X site. It has been cloned and considerable genetic heterogeneity exists, and, in contrast to Hurler syndrome, there is a high incidence of gene deletions or rearrangements. In contrast to Hurler syndrome, only a few mutations are seen in more than one family (430). Several phenotypic forms of Hunter syndrome have been distinguished, and, as a rule, gene deletions result in a severe clinical picture. Hunter syndrome can occur in female subjects; in these circumstances, it results from X:autosome translocation or the unbalanced inactivation of the nonmutant maternal chromosome (431).

In the four types of Sanfilippo syndrome (MPS IIIA, B, C, and D), the basic defect involves the enzymes required for the specific degradation of heparan sulfate. In the A form of the disease, a lack of heparan-N-sulfatase (heparan sulfate sulfatase) occurs (Fig. 1.15, step 2), which is the enzyme that cleaves the nitrogen-bound sulfate moiety (428). In the B form, the defective enzyme is N-acetyl-α-D-glucosaminidase (Fig. 1.15, step 6) (428). In Sanfilippo syndrome, type C, the defect is localized to the transfer of an acetyl moiety from acetyl-CoA to the free amino group of glucosamine (Fig. 1.15, step 4) (428). In type D, the sulfatase for N-acetyl-glucosamine-6-sulfate is defective (Fig. 1.15, step 3) (428). The gene has been mapped to the long arm of chromosome 6 and has been cloned. Because all four of these enzymes are specific for the degradation of heparan sulfate, dermatan sulfate metabolism proceeds normally.

In Morquio syndrome (MPS IV) type A, the enzymatic lesion involves the metabolism of the structurally dissimilar keratan sulfate and chondroitin-6-sulfate. It is located at N-acetyl-galactosamine-6-sulfate sulfatase (Fig. 1.15, step 10) (428). Morquio syndrome type B, a clinically milder form, is characterized by a defect in β-galactosidase. The gene for this condition has been cloned. As a consequence of its defect, the removal of galactose residues from keratan sulfate is impaired. The defect is allelic with GM_1 gangliosidosis, a condition in which a deficiency of β-galactosidase interrupts the degeneration of keratan sulfate and GM_1 ganglioside (432). As a consequence of these defects, the urinary MPS in both forms of Morquio syndrome consists of approximately 50% keratan sulfate and lesser amounts of chondroitin-6-sulfate (see Table 1.12).

In Maroteaux-Lamy syndrome (MPS VI), the abnormality is an inability to hydrolyze the sulfate group from N-acetyl-galactosamine-4-sulfate (Fig. 1.15, step 8) (428). This reaction is involved in the metabolism of dermatan sulfate and chondroitin-4-sulfate (see Figs. 1.14 and 1.15). The gene has been mapped to the long arm of chromosome 5 and has been cloned. Numerous mutations have been documented, and the phenotype of the condition is quite variable.

In MPS VII (Sly syndrome), a lack of β-glucuronidase (Fig. 1.15, step 7) has been demonstrated in a variety of tissues (428). The gene for this enzyme has been mapped to the long arm of chromosome 7 (7q21.11) and has been cloned. Numerous mutations have been described. As is the case for the other MPS, these allelic forms have been postulated to explain differences in clinical manifestations in patients having the same enzymatic lesion.

Hurler Syndrome (Mucopolysaccharide I and IH)

Pathologic Anatomy

Visceral alterations in Hurler syndrome are widespread and involve almost every organ. Large vacuolated cells containing MPS can be seen in cartilage, tendons, periosteum, endocardium, and vascular walls, particularly the intima of the coronary arteries (433). Abnormalities occur in the cartilage of the bronchial tree, and the alveoli are filled with lipid-laden cells. The bone marrow is replaced in part by connective tissue that contains many vacuolated fibroblasts. The liver is unusually large, most parenchymal cells being at least double their normal size. On electron microscopy, MPSs are noted to accumulate in the lysosomes of most hepatic parenchymatous cells (434). The Kupffer cells are swollen and contain abnormal amounts of MPS. In the spleen, the reticulum cells are larger than normal and contain the same storage material.

Changes within the CNS are widespread. The leptomeninges are edematous and thickened. The Virchow-Robin spaces are filled with MPS, and the periadventitial space in white matter is dilated and filled with viscous fluid and mononuclear cells containing MPS-positive vacuoles. The meningeal alterations produce partial obstruction of the subarachnoid spaces, which, in association with a narrowed foramen magnum, is responsible for the hydrocephalus that is often observed. The neurons are swollen and vacuolated, and their nuclei are peripherally displaced. Neuronal distention is most conspicuous in the cerebral cortex, but cells in the thalamus, brainstem, and particularly in the anterior

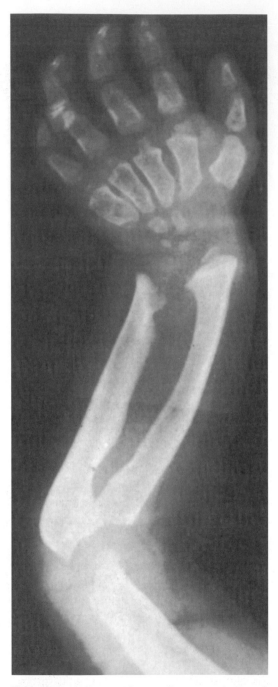

FIG. 1.16. Hurler syndrome. Roentgenogram of upper extremity. The ulna and radius are short and wide, and their epiphyseal ends are irregular. The metacarpal bones and phalanges are also thickened and irregular.

horns of the spinal cord are involved also. In the cerebellum, the Purkinje cells contain abnormal lipid material and demonstrate a fusiform swelling of their dendrites. On electron microscopy, the storage material is in the form of membranes, *zebra bodies*, and, least common, lipofuscin material (435). The relationship of the pathologic appearance of neurons to the neurologic defects has been studied extensively. Because it has been best delineated in GM_2 gangliosidosis, it is discussed under that section.

From a chemical viewpoint, the material stored in the brain is of two types. Within neurons are large amounts of two gangliosides: the GM_2 ganglioside, which also is stored in the various GM_2 gangliosidoses (Tay-Sachs disease), and the hexosamine-free hematocyte (GM_3 ganglioside). The greater proportion of the stored material is within mesenchymal tissue and is in the form of dermatan and heparan sulfates (435).

Clinical Manifestations

A detailed review of the clinical manifestations of the various mucopolysaccharidoses can be found in the book by Beighton and McKusick (436). Hurler syndrome is inherited as an autosomal recessive disorder with an estimated incidence of 1 in 144,000 births (437). Affected children usually appear healthy at birth and, except for repeated infections, otitis in particular, remain healthy for the greater part of their first year of life. Slowed development can be the first evidence of the disorder. Bony abnormalities of the upper extremities are observed by 12 years of age. These changes are much more marked there than in the lower extremities, with the most striking being swelling of the central portion of the humeral shaft and widening of the medial end of the clavicle (Fig. 1.16), alterations that result from a thickening of the cortex and dilatation of the medullary canal (438).

The typical patient is small with a large head and peculiar gross features (Fig. 1.17). The eyes are widely spaced. The bridge of the nose is flat and the lips are large. The mouth is open and an almost constant nasal obstruction or upper respiratory infection exists. Kyphosis is marked

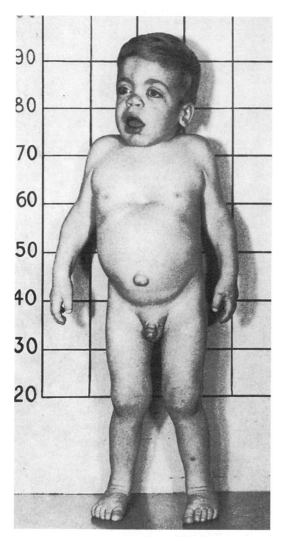

FIG. 1.17. Hurler syndrome in a 4-year-old boy. The patient demonstrates the unusual, coarse facies, depressed bridge of the nose, open mouth, and large tongue. The hands are spade-like, the abdomen protrudes, and an umbilical hernia is present. (Courtesy of Dr. V. A. McKusick, Johns Hopkins Hospital, Baltimore, MD.)

and appears early. The hands are wide and the fingers are short and stubby, with contractures that produce a claw-hand deformity. A carpal tunnel syndrome caused by entrapment of the median nerve is common, as is odontoid hypoplasia, which can lead to C1–2 vertebral displacement and quadriplegia. The abdomen protrudes, an umbilical hernia is often present,

and gross hepatosplenomegaly occurs. The hair is profuse and coarse. In older children, a unique skin lesion is observed occasionally (439). It consists of an aggregation of white, nontender papules of varying size, found symmetrically around the thorax and upper extremities. Corneal opacities are invariable. In most cases, progressive spasticity and mental deterioration occur. Blindness results from a combination of corneal clouding, retinal pigmentary degeneration, and optic atrophy. Optic atrophy is the consequence of prolonged increased intracranial pressure, meningeal infiltration constricting the optic nerve, and infiltration of the optic nerve itself. Cortical blindness caused by MPS storage in neurons of the optic system also has been observed. A mixed conductive and sensorineural deafness occurs (440).

Untreated, the disease worsens relentlessly, progressing more slowly in those children whose symptoms have a somewhat later onset. Many of the slower progressing patients suffer from the intermediate Hurler-Scheie syndrome (MPS I H/S). A curious and unique feature of this particular variant is the presence of arachnoid cysts. Spinal cord compression is not unusual; in Hurler syndrome, it generally results from dural thickening.

Radiographic abnormalities in Hurler syndrome are extensive and have been reviewed by Caffey (see Fig. 1.16) (438). They are the prototype for the other mucopolysaccharidoses. The CSF is normal. When blood smears are studied carefully, granulocytes can be seen to contain darkly azurophilic granules (Reilly granules). Some 20% to 40% of lymphocytes contain metachromatically staining cytoplasmic inclusions. These are also seen in Hunter and Sanfilippo syndromes, and in the GM_1 gangliosidoses. MRI not only in Hurler but also in Hunter and Sanfilippo diseases shows multiple cystic lesions of the corona radiata, periventricular white matter, corpus callosum, and less frequently, basal ganglia. These lesions have low signal intensity of T1-weighted images and high signal on T2-weighted images. They reflect MPS deposition in the perivascular spaces. In the more advanced cases, increased patchy or diffuse signal is seen in periventricular white matter on T2-weighted images. Ultimately, cerebral atrophy and communicating hydrocephalus occur. In the series of Lee and colleagues, a 57% incidence of associated posterior fossa cysts also occurred (441).

Death is usually a result of airway obstruction or bronchopneumonia secondary to the previously described pulmonary and bronchial alterations. Coronary artery disease and congestive heart failure caused by MPS infiltration of the heart valves also can prove fatal, even as early as 7 years of age (442).

Diagnosis

Although classic Hurler syndrome offers little in the way of diagnostic difficulty, in many children, particularly in infants, some of the cardinal signs, such as hepatosplenomegaly, mental deficiency, bony abnormalities, or a typical facial configuration, are minimal or completely lacking (Fig. 1.18) (443). A qualitative screening test for increased output of urinary MPS usually confirms the diagnosis, whereas quantitative determinations of the various MPSs indicate the specific disorder. False-negative and false-positive test results are encountered, with the latter being fairly common in newborns. A more definitive diagnosis requires an assay for α-L-iduronidase. If Hurler disease is suspected, the assay can be performed on serum or plasma. Enzyme assays for the other MPSs are best performed on lymphocytes or cultured fibroblasts (428). These assays also can serve for carrier detection or prenatal diagnosis (428).

In a number of conditions, the facial configuration seen in Hurler syndrome, the body abnormalities, and hepatosplenomegaly are unaccompanied by an abnormal MPS excretion. The first of these entities to have been defined was generalized GM_1 gangliosidosis, formerly known as *pseudo-Hurler syndrome*. This condition is characterized by hepatosplenomegaly, mental retardation, and bony abnormalities, but a normal MPS output. The basic defect is one of ganglioside degradation (see Sphingolipidoses, later in this chapter).

Patients presenting with dwarfism, early psychomotor retardation, unusual facies, but a clear or only faintly hazy cornea, and normal MPS

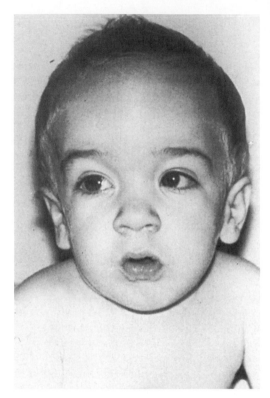

FIG. 1.18. Infant with Hurler disease showing mild coarse features, presence of metopic suture, mild corneal clouding, and chronic rhinorrhea. (From Matalon R, Kaul R, Michals K. The mucopolysaccharidoses and the mucolipidoses. In: Rosenberg RN, et al., (eds). *The molecular and genetic basis of neurological disease.* Stoneham, MA: Butterworth–Heinemann, 1993. With permission.)

excretion manifest the syndrome termed *mucolipidosis II*, or I-cell disease. This entity is discussed with the mucolipidoses.

Other conditions to be considered in the differential diagnosis are mucolipidoses III and IV and the various disorders of glycoprotein degradation: mannosidosis, fucosidosis, sialidosis, and aspartylglycosaminuria. Finally, cretinism must always be excluded in the youngster with small stature, developmental retardation, and unusual facies.

Treatment

Bone marrow transplantation has dramatically improved the course of Hurler disease and its prognosis. The beneficial effects result from the replacement of enzyme-deficient macrophages and microglia by marrow-derived macrophages that provide a continuous source of normal enzyme that can enter the brain and digest stored MPS. Several hundred patients with Hurler, Hunter, and Sanfilippo disease have undergone bone marrow transplantation with considerable improvement of their dysmorphic features, cardiac defects, hepatosplenomegaly, and hearing. Macrocephaly tends to resolve, as does odontoid hypoplasia (444). In the British series of Vellodi and colleagues, the intelligence of 60% of children improved or showed no further deterioration after bone marrow transplant (445). In the American series of Guffon and colleagues, 46% had normal intelligence, and 15% had borderline intelligence (446). Because little improvement occurs in mental function in children who are severely retarded, Vellodi and colleagues do not recommend bone marrow transplants for those older than 2 years of age (445). Guffon and colleagues consider an initial IQ of lower than 70 to be the main criterion for excluding a patient from consideration for transplant (446). As a rule, no improvement occurs in corneal clouding, and orthopedic problems, particularly the carpal tunnel syndrome, tend to persist. Complications and mortality of bone marrow transplant are still significant; they are considered in Chapter 15.

Other forms of therapy have less to offer. Enzyme replacement therapy has had only limited success and is still in the experimental stages (419).

Hunter Syndrome (Mucopolysaccharide II)

This condition is transmitted as an X-linked recessive disorder, with a variety of alleles believed responsible for differences in severity of clinical manifestations. Its frequency in British Columbia is 1 in 111,000 births (447).

Depending on whether mental deterioration is present, the syndrome is separated into mild and severe forms (II A and II B, respectively). In the mild form, the abnormal facial configuration is first noted during early childhood. Dwarfism, hepatosplenomegaly, umbilical hernia, and frequent respiratory infections are almost invari-

able. Cardiac disease, particularly with valvular abnormalities, was seen in more than 90% of patients in the series of Young and Harper and was the most common cause of death (448). Additionally, joints are involved widely, with a particular predilection for the hands. Neurologic symptoms in the mild form of Hunter syndrome are limited to progressive head growth (generally unaccompanied by ventricular enlargement or hydrocephalus), sensorineural deafness, and retinitis pigmentosa with impaired visual-evoked responses. The latter two symptoms are explained by the autopsy finding of vacuolated ganglion cells in the eighth nerve nucleus and retina (449). Papilledema is common; seen in the presence of normal CSF pressure and normal-sized ventricles, it probably results from local infiltrative processes around the retinal veins. It can be present for 8 years or longer without apparent loss of vision (450).

In the severe form of the disease, the clinical picture is highlighted by the insidious onset of mental retardation, first noted between ages 2 and 3 years. Seizures are seen in 62%, and a persistent, unexplained diarrhea in 65% of patients (451). Upper airway obstruction is common and difficult to correct because tracheostomy presents major anesthetic risks (450). Corneal clouding is unusual, but its presence does not speak against the diagnosis of Hunter syndrome (452). In the series of Young and Harper, death occurred at an average age of 12 years (451). Multiple nerve entrapments can occur in Hunter as well as in Hurler syndromes as the consequence of connective tissue thickening through MPS deposition (453).

Alterations within the brain are similar to those seen in Hurler syndrome. Considerable leptomeningeal MPS storage occurs, mainly in the form of dermatan and heparan sulfates. The neuronal cytoplasm is distended with lipid-staining material, probably of ganglioside nature (454). Electron microscopy reveals the presence of lamellar figures in cortical neurons (455). The storage process commences during early intrauterine development (456).

The enzyme deficiency can be ascertained in serum, lymphocytes, and fibroblasts. Prenatal diagnosis of Hunter syndrome can be performed by examining amniotic fluid cells and by assaying for idurono-sulfate-sulfatase in cell-free amniotic fluid (428). Approximately one-fourth of mothers are noncarriers (i.e., their affected male offspring represent a new mutation).

Sanfilippo Syndrome (Mucopolysaccharide III A, B, C, and D)

This heterogeneous syndrome, first described in 1963 by Sanfilippo and coworkers, is characterized by mental deterioration that commences during the first few years of life. It is accompanied by subtle somatic features of a mucopolysaccharidosis (457). With an incidence of at least 1 in 24,000, it is the most common of the mucopolysaccharidoses (428).

Four genetically and biochemically, but not clinically, distinct forms have been recognized. In all, delayed development is the usual presenting symptom. It is first noted between ages 2 and 5 years and is gradually superseded by evidence of neurologic regression. This is most rapid in type A. Abnormally coarse facial features are usually evident even earlier, but generally go unnoticed because they are never as prominent as in the other mucopolysaccharidoses (Fig. 1.19). No growth retardation, no corneal opacification, and only mild hepatosplenomegaly occur. Diarrhea is seen in more than 50% of patients (458). Loss of extension of the interphalangeal joints was present in all patients in the series of Danks and coworkers, whereas limitation of elbow extension was characteristic for the rare type D (458,459). In addition to mental deterioration, the neurologic examination can disclose ataxia, coarse tremor, progressive spasticity, and, as the illness advances, bulbar palsy. The changes seen on MRI are similar to those for Hurler and Hunter syndromes (441). Although hydrocephalus can be caused by meningeal thickening, it is more often the result of malformations of the foramen magnum or of an underdeveloped dens, with increased thickness of the ligaments surrounding it (460).

Other common radiographic features are widening of the anterior two-thirds of the ribs and elongation of the radius. Peripheral blood smears can reveal cytoplasmic inclusions in

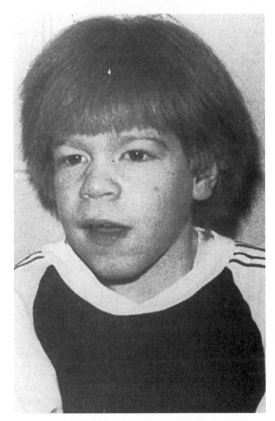

FIG. 1.19. Patient with Sanfilippo A syndrome, showing the relatively mild coarsening of facial features. (From Matalon R, Kaul R, Michals K. The mucopolysaccharidoses and the mucolipidoses. In: Rosenberg RN, et al., eds. *The molecular and genetic basis of neurological disease.* Stoneham, MA: Butterworth–Heinemann, 1993. With permission.)

lymphocytes or polymorphs, and bone marrow aspirates can be positive for storage material.

The disease is inexorably progressive, and most patients die before 20 years of age. Generally, the downhill course is most rapid in the type A variant (461).

Morphologic alterations within the CNS are similar to those seen in Hurler syndrome, but heparan sulfate is the major MPS stored in the leptomeninges and brain (435,454).

The clinical diagnosis of Sanfilippo syndrome is difficult to establish and also can be missed on random MPS screening. It must be considered in any mentally retarded child who has only minor physical stigmata (see Fig. 1.19). Examination of a 24-hour urine collection discloses the excretion of heparan sulfate (see Table 1.12). Enzyme assays on serum, skin fibroblasts, and lymphocytes confirm the diagnosis and identify the specific type. Treatment of type A disease with bone marrow transplantation does not appear to be of benefit (462).

Morquio Syndrome (Mucopolysaccharide IV A and B)

The clinical manifestations of Morquio syndrome involve the skeleton primarily and the nervous system only secondarily. Skeletal manifestations include growth retardation and deformities of the vertebral bodies and epiphyseal zones of the long bones. Generally, type A is more severe than type B. However, type A shows considerable clinical heterogeneity. Absence or severe hypoplasia of the odontoid process or atlantoaxial instability is invariable (463), and neurologic symptoms result from chronic or acute compression of the spinal cord. This compression can be the result of atlantoaxial subluxation, the presence of a gibbus, or dural thickening as a consequence of MPS deposition. These complications are best visualized by MRI. The mild form of Morquio syndrome (MPS IV B) presents with growth retardation, bony abnormalities (dysostosis multiplex), and corneal opacities. Mental functioning generally remains normal. Corneal opacities, sensorineural hearing loss, and mental retardation are encountered occasionally (464). Neuroimaging studies can show ventricular dilatation and progressive white matter disease.

It is not clear why the nervous system is generally spared in Morquio syndrome B, whereas an equally severe defect of β-galactosidase results in GM_1 gangliosidosis. The best explanation is that in Morquio syndrome type B, the mutation affects the activity of β-galactosidase for keratan sulfate, whereas in GM_1 gangliosidosis, the mutation affects the enzyme's ability to degrade ganglioside. β-Galactosidase deficiency also can be caused by a lack of a protective protein. This is the case in mucolipidosis I, in which a deficiency of β-galactosidase and sialidase occurs.

Pathologic examination of the brain reveals leptomeningeal thickening and neuronal storage. Neuronal storage tends to be localized; Koto and coworkers found it primarily within the thalamus and hippocampus. On ultrastructural examination, the material appears similar to that stored in Hurler syndrome (464).

The diagnosis of Morquio syndrome can be made by the presence of keratan sulfate in urine (see Table 1.12) and by assaying for *N*-acetyl-hexosamine-6-sulfatase activity.

Scheie Syndrome (Mucopolysaccharide IS)

In Scheie syndrome, the major manifestation is corneal clouding (465). Intelligence is unaffected until late in life, and until then, neurologic symptoms are limited to a high incidence of carpal tunnel syndrome (compression of the median nerve as it transverses the carpal tunnel of the wrist).

On autopsy, relatively little MPS storage is found within the leptomeninges, and the neurons appear normal (435).

Scheie syndrome is diagnosed in patients who have the biochemical and enzymatic defects of Hurler syndrome, but lack skeletal and severe neurologic involvement. Hurler-Scheie genetic compounds also have been reported (MPS I H/S). These disorders are characterized by hepatosplenomegaly, corneal clouding, slow mental deterioration, and, ultimately, the evolution of increased intracranial pressure resulting from obstruction at the basilar cisterns (436). Winters and associates described neuronal storage (466).

Maroteaux-Lamy Syndrome (Mucopolysaccharide VI)

In this condition, first described in 1963 by Maroteaux, Lamy, and colleagues (467), neurologic complications result from compression myelopathy and hydrocephalus (436,468). Several clinical variants with differing severity of expression have been recognized. The severe form resembles Hurler syndrome, except that the intellect remains normal. Skeletal and corneal involvement is generally severe in this form, and the facial appearance is characteristic for a mucopolysaccharidosis. The milder forms of the disease show some of the clinical manifestations, but in a less marked form.

The excretion of dermatan sulfate in the absence of urinary heparan sulfate is strongly suggestive of the diagnosis (see Table 1.12). The enzyme implicated in the disease (N-acetyl-galactosamine-4-sulfate sulfatase, or arylsulfatase B) is readily assayed in a variety of tissues, and antenatal diagnosis has been possible.

Sly Syndrome (Mucopolysaccharide VII)

The clinical appearance of patients with Sly syndrome varies considerably. Some have been of normal intelligence, or only mildly retarded, whereas others have presented with severe retardation and macrocephaly (468). Hepatomegaly is generally present, and the facial and skeletal abnormalities are characteristic for a mucopolysaccharidosis. The increased excretion of heparan sulfate and dermatan sulfate is shared with MPS I, II, and V, but a deficiency of β-glucuronidase (see Table 1.12) is readily detected in serum, leukocytes, and fibroblasts (469).

Mucolipidoses

Mucolipidoses have the clinical features of both the mucopolysaccharidoses and the lipidoses. At least four mucolipidoses have been distinguished, characterized by MPS storage despite normal excretion of MPS. All of them are rare.

The most likely to be encountered is mucolipidosis II [ML-II or inclusion cell (I-cell) disease]; its prevalence in the French-Canadian isolate is 1 in 6,000 (470). This condition is the consequence of a defect in UDP-N-acetylglucosamine: N-acetylglucosaminyl-1-phosphotransferase, the enzyme that is responsible for attaching a phosphate group to mannose and synthesizing mannose-6-phosphate, which acts as a recognition marker for lysosomal enzymes. In the absence of this recognition marker, lysosomal enzymes are prevented from reaching lysosomes and instead are routed into the extracellular space and excreted (471).

As in all other lysosomal disorders, considerable clinical and biochemical heterogeneity exists. The clinical and radiologic features of this autosomal recessive disorder are reminiscent of Hurler syndrome, although in distinction, I-cell disease is apparent at birth. Features seen in the affected newborn include hypotonia, coarse facial appearance, striking gingival hyperplasia, congenital dislocation of the hips, restricted joint mobility, and tight, thickened skin (471). Radiographic changes of dysostosis multiplex develop between 6 and 10 months of age. Subsequently, growth failure, microcephaly, and progressive mental deterioration become apparent. Hepatomegaly and corneal clouding are inconstant. Most patients die during childhood (471). Nonimmune hydrops fetalis can be seen in some pregnancies.

Cultured fibroblasts contain numerous inclusions. Visible by phase-contrast microscopy, these inclusions represent enlarged lysosomes filled with MPS and membranous material. The brain has no significant neuronal or glial storage, and the clinically evident mental deterioration cannot, as yet, be explained on a morphologic basis (472).

In ML-II and -III, a number of lysosomal enzymes (e.g., α-L-iduronidase, β-glucuronidase, and β-galactosidase) are elevated markedly in plasma and deficient in fibroblasts. Enzyme levels in liver and brain are normal (473).

ML-III is a milder form of ML-II. In this condition, the defect in the phosphorylation of mannose is also defective, although to a lesser degree than in ML-II. In this condition, as well as in ML-II, the activity of N-acetylglucosaminyl-1-phosphotransferase is considerably reduced.

Symptoms of ML-III do not become apparent until after age 2 years, and learning disabilities or mental retardation are mild. Restricted mobility of joints and growth retardation occur. Radio-graphic examination shows a pattern of dysostosis multiplex with severe pelvic and vertebral abnormalities. Fine corneal opacities and valvular heart disease are occasionally present (474). The disease can be diagnosed by the presence of elevated lysosomal enzymes in plasma.

ML-IV is a relatively common disease in Ashkenazi Jews (475). The symptoms are nonspecific, and probably many cases go undiagnosed. Developmental delay and impaired vision become apparent during the first year of life. Corneal opacities are almost invariable, as is strabismus and an ERG with markedly reduced amplitude. Photophobia was noted in 25% of the children in the Israeli series of Amir and coworkers (475). A striking hypotonia and extrapyramidal signs also have been encountered, and some patients have been evaluated for a congenital myopathy. Seizures are not part of the clinical picture. Skeletal deformities and visceromegaly are absent (475). Curiously, patients with ML IV are constitutionally achlorhydric (476). Although visual function deteriorates, Amir and coworkers found no intellectual deterioration. MRI consistently demonstrates a hypoplastic corpus callosum; additionally, there can be delayed myelination (477). MPS excretion is normal, but the urine contains large quantities of GM_3 gangliosides, phospholipids, and neutral glycolipids. The diagnosis is made by visualizing the polysaccharide and lipid-containing inclusion organelles using electron microscopy of a conjunctival or skin biopsy. In contrast to ML II, ML IV shows a variety of inclusions in neurons, glia, and the perivascular cells of brain (478). The metabolic defect underlying ML-IV has not been identified, and the responsible gene has not been mapped. A defect in the transport of lipids along the lysosomal pathway has been postulated (479).

Mucolipidosis I (sialidosis) is considered with the glycoproteinoses.

Glycoproteinoses

In four storage diseases, the primary enzymatic defect involves the degradation of glycoproteins. These substances, which in essence are peptides linked to oligosaccharides, are widely distributed within cells, the cell membrane, and outside the cells; they are particularly abundant in nervous tissue (480). Because some of the same oligosaccharide linkages also are found in glycolipids, a single enzymatic lesion affects the degradation of more than one macromolecule. For this reason, some of the sphingolipid storage diseases and the mucolipidoses have an impaired glycoprotein breakdown, and, con-

versely, the glycoproteinoses also can have a defective sphingolipid catabolism.

Fucosidosis

Although a severe and a mild form of this autosomal recessive disorder have been distinguished on clinical grounds, both forms have been identified within the same family and there appears to be a continuous clinical spectrum (481). A deficiency of α-L-fucosidase can be documented. Fucosidase is responsible for cleavage of the fucose moieties linked to *N*-acetylglucosamine (Fig. 1.20). The gene for the enzyme has been mapped to the distal portion of the short arm of chromosome 1 (1p34.1-1.p36.1). It has been cloned and sequenced. Considerable genetic heterozygosity exists, and numerous mutations have been recognized (482).

In approximately 60% of patients, the condition has a rapidly progressive course, with intel-

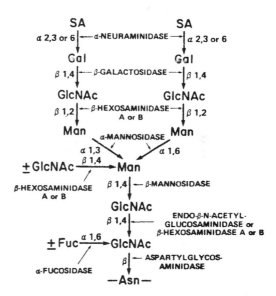

FIG. 1.20. Probable steps for degradation of a complex type oligosaccharide structure. (Asn, asparigine; Fuc, fucose; Gal, galactose; GlcNAc, *N*-acetylglucosamine; Man, mannose; SA, sialic acid.) (From Beaudet AL. Disorder of glycoprotein degradation: mannosidosis, fucosidoses, sialidosis and aspartylglycosaminuria. In: Stanbury JB, et al., eds. *The metabolic basis of inherited diseases*, 5th ed. New York: McGraw–Hill, 1983:788. With permission.)

lectual deterioration and spasticity commencing at approximately 1 year of age. The facial features are coarse, and skeletal abnormalities (dysostosis multiplex) are present. The chloride content of sweat is increased markedly. Seizures and growth retardation are common and the patient usually dies by age 35 years. When the condition is more protracted, the clinical picture is similar, except that angiokeratoma of the skin, particularly of the gingiva and genitalia, is invariable. These skin manifestations are indistinguishable from those seen in Fabry disease and sialidosis and are not seen when the disease progresses rapidly (483).

Pathologic examination discloses cytoplasmic vacuolization in most organs, notably in liver. Vacuolization also occurs in neurons and glial cells within brain and spinal cord (484).

Biochemical analysis reveals fucose-rich glycolipids in a variety of organs. In brain, the storage material is of two types: One is probably a MPS, and the other is a complex lipid. Structurally, the stored sphingolipid resembles the erythrocyte oligosaccharides responsible for H and Lewis blood group activity. As a consequence, Lewis activity in red cells and saliva is expressed to an unusually high degree.

α- and β-*Mannosidosis*

α-Mannosidosis, first described in 1967, is characterized by a Hurlerlike facial appearance, mental retardation, skeletal abnormalities, hearing loss, and hepatosplenomegaly (485). Considerable clinical heterogeneity exists, with a severe infantile form (type I) and a milder, juvenile-adult form (type II) having been distinguished (480).

Neuronal storage of mannose-rich oligosaccharides is widespread within the brain and spinal cord (486). The basic metabolic lesion is a deficiency of α-mannosidoses A and B in liver, brain, peripheral leukocytes, serum, and skin fibroblasts. Mannosidase normally hydrolyses the trisaccharide mannose-mannose-*N*-acetylglucosamine (see Fig. 1.20), which consequently is excreted in large amounts (487).

A defect in β-mannosidase also has been reported (488). It is marked by developmental regression and coarse facial features, and occasionally, a peripheral neuropathy, but neither organomegaly nor corneal clouding (488,489).

Sialidosis

Under the name *sialidosis* are grouped several conditions that share a defect in glycoprotein sialidase (neuraminidase), the lysosomal enzyme that catalyzes the hydrolysis of terminal sialic acid residues of glycoconjugates (see Fig. 1.20) (490). The gene that codes for sialidase has been mapped to the short arm of chromosome 6. It has been cloned and several mutations have been documented (491).

Two clinical forms are recognized. In type I sialidosis (cherry-red spot myoclonus syndrome), neurologic symptoms begin after age 10 years. Initially, these include diminished visual acuity (notably night blindness), a macular cherry-red spot, ataxia with gait abnormalities, nystagmus, and myoclonic seizures. Neuropathy and punctate lenticular opacities also can be present (492). Patients do not have dysmorphic features or deterioration of intelligence and have a normal life span.

In type II, the congenital form of primary neuraminidase deficiency with dysmorphic features is characterized by hepatosplenomegaly, corneal opacifications, dysostosis multiplex, hydrops fetalis, ascites, and a pericardial effusion. The condition is rapidly fatal. Pathologic examination of the brain discloses membrane-bound vacuoles in cortical neurons and Purkinje cells, and *zebra bodies* in spinal cord neurons. Vacuoles are also seen in the glomerulus and tubular epithelial cells of the kidney, and in hepatocytes, endothelial cells, and Kupffer cells of the liver (493).

In addition, there is a condition in which neuraminidase and β-galactosidase deficiencies are combined (galactosialidosis or Goldberg syndrome). One form has its onset early in life, with hydrops, coarse facies, and skeletal changes (494). The other has a juvenile onset, with coarse facies, dysostosis multiplex, conjunctival telangiectases, corneal clouding, a macular cherry-red spot, hearing loss, mental retardation, and seizures (494). Angiokeratoma is seen in galactosialidosis, which is particularly common among Japanese (495). The combined enzymatic deficiencies are the result of a lack of a lysosomal protective protein, which is required for activity of both sialidase and β-galactosidase (496).

Sialuria

Several clinical disorders of sialic acid metabolism are marked by lysosomal storage and an abnormally increased urinary excretion of sialic acid. The most common of these entities has been termed *Salla disease*, after a small town in northern Finland close to the Russian border, where this disease is particularly prevalent (497). It is characterized by growth retardation, coarse facies, early delay in mental development, and the evolution of ataxia, spasticity, and extrapyramidal movements. The disease is slowly progressive and is compatible with a normal life span. Free sialic acid is elevated in urine, blood, and fibroblasts. The combination of early-onset psychomotor retardation and a normal life span without any evidence for deterioration throughout childhood makes this entity unique among lysosomal storage diseases.

Similar entities that are more rapidly progressive but also are marked by an increased excretion of free sialic acid have been reported from France, Italy, and the United States (498). The clinical picture is highlighted by developmental delay, slightly coarse facies with a large tongue, hypotonia, and, occasionally, visceromegaly. The slowly and the rapidly progressive forms are linked to the long arm of chromosome 6 and are believed to represent allelic disorders (499).

The basic defect for the Finnish and the non-Finnish forms is believed to be located in the carrier-mediated system that transports sialic acid out of lysosomes (500). It thus resembles the defect for cystinosis. The sialurias are probably more common than has been appreciated up to now. The diagnosis can be suspected from the presence of cytoplasmic vacuoles in lymphocytes and from the presence of membrane-bound vacuoles in a conjunctival biopsy (501). Unfortunately, none of the screening tests for oligosaccharides can detect free sialic acid, and all lysosomal enzymes are normal.

Aspartylglycosaminuria

This condition is caused by a defect in the enzyme that cleaves the *N*-acetylglucosamine-asparagine bond (see Fig. 1.20, see Table 1.6). Like Salla disease, aspartylglycosaminuria is common in Finland. The clinical picture is one of mental deterioration commencing between ages 6 and 15 years, coarse facial features, lenticular opacities, bony changes (dysostosis multiplex), and mitral insufficiency. Vacuolated lymphocytes are noted in the majority of patients. The disease is identified by the excretion of a variety of glycoasparagines and, therefore, is detected by routine amino acid chromatography (228,229).

Sphingolipidoses

This group of disorders includes a number of hereditary diseases characterized by an abnormal sphingolipid metabolism, which in most instances leads to the intralysosomal deposition of lipid material within the CNS. Clinically, these conditions assume a progressive course that varies only in the rate of intellectual and visual deterioration.

With the rapid advances in the knowledge of the composition, structure, and metabolism of cerebral lipids, these disorders are best classified according to the chemical nature of the storage material or, if known, according to the underlying enzymatic block. Although such an arrangement is adhered to in this section, the chemistry and metabolism of sphingolipids often prove too complex for the clinician who is not continuously involved in this field. To make matters more difficult, diseases with a similar phenotypic expression can be caused by completely different enzymatic blocks; conversely, an apparently identical biochemical defect can produce completely different clinical pictures.

A more practical grouping of the lipid storage diseases, intended to assist in the bedside diagnosis of these disorders, is presented in Table 1.13.

TABLE 1.13. *Lipid storage diseases*

Condition	Storage material in brain	Enzymatic defect	Clinical characteristics
Without marked visceromegaly			
GM$_2$ gangliosidosis (Tay-Sachs disease)	GM$_2$ ganglioside Hexosaminidase A and B (Sandhoff disease) GM$_2$ activator deficiency	Hexosaminidase A	Cherry-red spot; onset first year of life; visceromegaly in Sandhoff disease
Niemann-Pick C disease	Cholesterol	Impaired intracellular cholesterol transport	Intellectual deterioration, usually starting in late infancy, early childhood; retinal cherry-red spot common; visceromegaly may be present
Juvenile Gaucher disease	Unknown	Glucocerebrosidase	Progressive dementia
With marked visceromegaly			
Generalized gangliosidosis GM$_1$	GM$_1$ ganglioside	β-Galactosidase	Infantile onset: Hurler appearance; bony abnormalities; retinal cherry-red spots
Gaucher disease: acute neuronopathic form (type 2)	Usually none	Glucocerebrosidase	Bulbar signs common early in disease; occasional cherry-red spot
Niemann-Pick disease Type A	Sphingomyelin	Sphingomyelinase	Intellectual deterioration, anemia, hepatosplenomegaly
Gaucher disease: subacute neuronopathic form (type 3)	Unknown	Glucocerebrosidase	Slow intellectual deterioration, myoclonus, ataxia, horizontal supranuclear gaze palsy

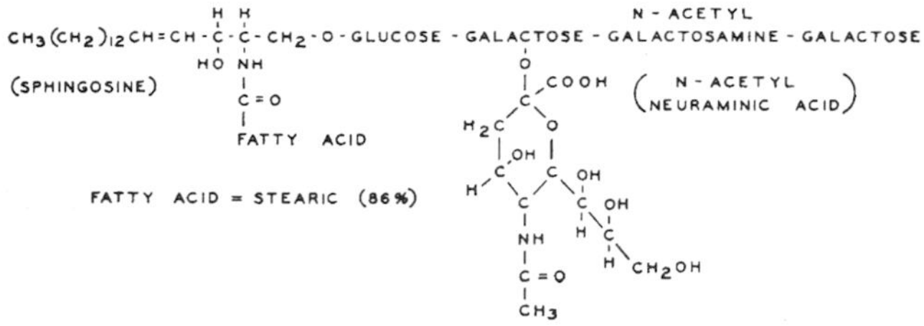

FIG. 1.21. Structure of a monosialoganglioside.

Gangliosides

In choosing the name *gangliosides*, Klenk emphasized the localization of these lipids within the ganglion cells of the neuraxis (502). His finding has since been amply confirmed by work indicating that gangliosides are found mainly in nuclear areas of gray matter and are present in myelin in only small amounts.

Gangliosides are components of the plasma membranes. They are composed of sphingosine, fatty acids, hexose, hexosamine, and neuraminic acid (Fig. 1.21). The sphingosine–fatty acid moiety (ceramide) is hydrophobic and acts as a membrane anchor, whereas the hexose, hexosamine, and neuraminic moieties are hydrophilic and extracellular. The pattern of gangliosides is cell-type specific and changes with growth and differentiation. Gangliosides interact at the cell surface with membrane-bound receptors and enzymes; they are involved in cellular adhesion processes and signal transduction events. In addition, they are believed to play a role in the binding of neurotransmitters and other extracellular molecules. They also have a neuronotropic function, which is discussed in the pathogenesis of neurologic deficits in some of the gangliosidoses. Gangliosides are degraded in the cellular lysosomal compartment. The plasma membranes containing gangliosides that are destined for degradation are endocytosed and are transported through the endosomal compartments to the lysosome. There, a series of hydrolytic enzymes cleave the sugar moieties sequentially to yield ceramide, which is further degraded to sphingosine and fatty acids.

At least 10 different gangliosides have been isolated from brain. Of these, four are major components and account for more than 90% of the total ganglioside fraction of brain.

As is depicted in Figure 1.21, the major gangliosides contain the skeleton ceramide-glucose-galactose-galactosamine-galactose. *N*-Acetylneuraminic acid (NANA) is attached to the proximal galactose in the monosialoganglioside, whereas in the two major disialospecies, an additional NANA unit is attached either to the terminal galactose or to the first NANA.

GM_2 Gangliosidoses (Tay-Sachs Disease)

Tay-Sachs disease, the prototype of this group of diseases, was first described by Tay, who noted the retinal changes in 1881 (503), and by Sachs in 1887 (504).

Molecular Genetics and Biochemical Pathology. On chemical analysis of brain tissue, the most striking abnormality is the accumulation of GM_2 ganglioside in cerebral gray matter and cerebellum 100 to 300 times the normal level. The structure of GM_2 ganglioside that accumulates in Tay-Sachs disease is depicted in Figure 1.22. It consists of ceramide to which 1 mol each of glucose, galactose, *N*-acetylgalactosamine, and *N*-acetylneuraminic acid has been attached. Cerebral white matter, liver, spleen, and serum also contain increased amounts of GM_2 ganglioside. The ganglioside content of viscera is not increased. Several other glycosphingolipids are found in lesser amounts.

In most instances, storage of GM_2 ganglioside is the result of a defect in hexosaminidase. Two isozymes of hexosaminidase have been recognized. Hexosaminidases A and B are the two major tissue isozymes; hexosaminidase A is composed of one α subunit and one β subunit, whereas hexosaminidase B is composed of two

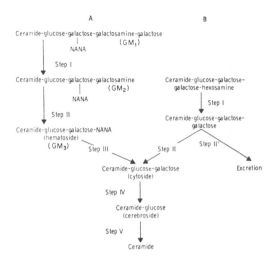

FIG. 1.22. Degradative pathways for sphingolipids. Metabolic defects are located at the following points: generalized gangliosidosis GM_1 at step A I; Tay-Sachs disease and variants of generalized gangliosidosis GM_2 at step A II; adult Gaucher disease at step A V; and Fabry disease at step B II. Enzymes for most of these reactions have been demonstrated in mammalian brain. (NANA, *N*-acetylneuraminic acid.)

slightly different β subunits. The gene locus for the α subunit has been mapped to chromosome 15 (15q23-q24); for the β subunit, it is on the long arm of chromosome 5 (5q11.2-13.3) (505).

In the classic form of Tay-Sachs disease, the disorder affects the α chain, and hexosaminidase A is inoperative (Fig. 1.22, step A II) in brain, blood, and viscera (506). Total hexosaminidase activity is usually normal, but the hexosaminidase B component in the CNS acting on its own is unable to hydrolyze GM_2 ganglioside *in vivo*. The genes coding for the α and β subunits have been coded. At least 78 mutations in the gene coding for the α subunit have been documented (507). These have been catalogued by Kolodny (505).

In the Jewish form of generalized GM_2 gangliosidoses, three molecular lesions have been found in what had once been considered a pure genetic entity, and a large proportion of patients are compound heterozygotes. The most common mutation, accounting for 73% of Ashkenazi Jews carrying the gene for Tay-Sachs disease in the series of Grebner and Tomczak (508), is a four-

base pair insertion in exon 11 (505). In 18%, there was a single base substitution in intron 12 resulting in defective splicing of the messenger RNA, whereas in 3.3% there was a point mutation on exon 7 (505). In French-Canadian patients, an ethnic group in whom the gene frequency for Tay-Sachs disease is equal to that in Ashkenazi Jews, a large deletion in the gene coding for the α chain has been recognized. The deletion involves part of intron 1, all of exon 1, and probably also the promoter region for the gene. As a consequence, neither mRNA nor immunoprecipitable hexosaminidase A protein is produced. Clinically, this variant is indistinguishable from the Jewish form of Tay-Sachs disease (509).

Mutations in the gene that codes for the gene for the β subunit result in a deficiency of hexosaminidase A and hexosaminidase B, a condition that is termed *Sandhoff disease*. The most common genetic defect producing this condition is a large deletion in the gene coding for the β subunit (505). Infants with this disorder are non-Jewish, have a mild visceromegaly, and accumulate much larger amounts of globoside (ceramide-glucose-galactose-galactose-galactosamine) in viscera than infants with Tay-Sachs disease (510). Sandhoff disease accounts for approximately 7% of the GM_2 gangliosidoses (511).

A defect at a third gene locus that codes for the GM_2 activator protein produces the AB variant. The action of the activator is to extract a single GM_2 molecule from its micelles to form a water-soluble protein-lipid complex that acts as the true substrate for hexosaminidase A (512). In this entity, accounting for less than 4% of the GM_2 gangliosidoses in the United Kingdom (511), both hexosaminidase components are present but are inactive with respect to hydrolyzing GM_2 gangliosides. The clinical picture of this condition resembles that of classical Tay-Sachs disease. Aside from the GM_2 activator, four other sphingolipid activator proteins have been recognized; their genetically inherited defects lead to lysosomal storage diseases (511a).

Some children who show the clinical picture of late infantile or juvenile amaurotic idiocy (see Generalized GM_1 Gangliosidosis, later in this chapter) have been found to have GM_2 gan-

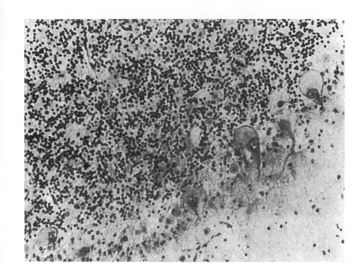

FIG. 1.23. Tay-Sachs disease. Purkinje cells, showing swollen cell bodies and an occasional *antlerlike* dendrite. In general, lipid storage in the cerebellum is less extensive than in the cerebral cortex (cresyl violet, ×150). (Courtesy of the late Dr. D. B. Clark, University of Kentucky, Lexington, KY.)

gliosidosis and a partial defect of hexosaminidase A (513). They account for approximately 25% of English patients with GM_2 gangliosidosis (511). Patients with the adult or chronic form of GM_2 gangliosidosis are compound heterozygotes between one of the infantile mutations and a point mutation at exon 7 in the gene for the α chain (505). The clinical picture is one of a child with learning disability, who, over the years, develops a gradually progressive muscular weakness. At times, this picture is complicated by ataxia, at other times by dystonia (514). Finally, there are asymptomatic individuals with little more than 10% residual hexosaminidase A activity (511a).

Pathologic Anatomy. The pathologic changes in Tay-Sachs disease are confined to the nervous system and represent the most fulminant of all the cerebroretinal degenerations. Almost every neuron in the cerebral cortex is distended markedly, its nucleus is displaced to the periphery, and the cytoplasm is filled with lipid-soluble material (Fig. 1.23). A similar substance is stored in the apical dendrites of the pyramidal cells. As the disease progresses, the number of cortical neurons diminishes, with only a few pyknotic cells remaining. The gliotic reaction is often extensive. In the white matter, myelination can be arrested, and in the terminal stages, demyelination, accumulation of lipid breakdown products, and widespread status

spongiosus are observed commonly. Similar alterations affect the cerebellar Purkinje cells, and to a somewhat lesser degree, the larger neurons of the brainstem and spinal cord. In the retina, the ganglion cells are distended with lipid. At the margin of the fovea, considerable reduction in the number of ganglion cells and an accumulation of large phagocytic cells occurs.

On electron microscopic examination of the involved neurons, the lipid is found in the membranous cytoplasmic bodies, which are round, oval, and 0.5 to 2.0 μm in diameter. They occupy a considerable portion of the ganglion cell cytoplasm (Fig. 1.24). The membranous bodies also can be located in axis cylinders, glial cells, and perivascular cells (515). Membranous cytoplasmic bodies consist of aggregates of lipids (90%) and protein (10%). The composition of lipids is approximately one-third to one-half gangliosides (mainly GM_2), approximately 20% phospholipids, and 40% cholesterol. *In vitro* experiments show membranous cytoplasmic bodies to be formed in neurons as a consequence of high ganglioside concentrations in the presence of phospholipids and cholesterol.

By means of Golgi stains and electron microscopy, massively expanded neuronal processes can be demonstrated even in the earliest stages of Tay-Sachs disease. These meganeurites are found specifically at the axon

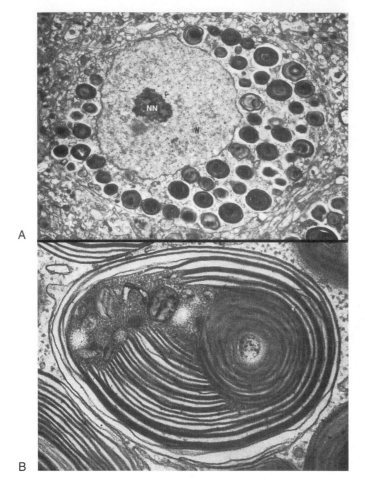

A

B

FIG. 1.24. Tay-Sachs disease, cortical biopsy. **A:** Neuron showing cytoplasmic granules. These are ganglioside in nature. Electron microscopic examination (×10,000). (NN, nucleolus; N, nucleus; C, cytoplasmic granule.) **B:** Cytoplasmic granule showing lamellar arrangement. Lamellae are approximately 25 Angstrom thick. Electron microscopic examination (×10,000). (From Terry RD, Weiss M. Studies in Tay-Sachs disease: ultrastructure of cerebrum. *J Neuropathol Exp Neurol* 1963;22:18–55. With permission.)

hillock of the cell and displace distally the initial segment of the axon. With progressive enlargement, they become interspersed between the neuronal soma and the axon. Growth of new neurites is increased, probably as a response to excessive amounts of gangliosides, and dendritic spines are lost (516). Abnormal synapses are formed. As a consequence, GABA-ergic connections are enhanced, and the cholinergic connections are altered. The synaptic alterations can be seen early in the disease, much before ganglioside storage has produced a mechanical disruption of cell cytoplasm and organelles (517). Their presence readily explains the neuronal dysfunction and the early onset of neurologic deficits. Similar but less prominent meganeurites have been observed in Hurler syndrome,

Sanfilippo syndrome, and in some of the other gangliosidoses.

Clinical Manifestations. Before the 1970s, the classic form of Tay-Sachs disease usually occurred in Jewish families, particularly those of Eastern European background. Now the condition is encountered in a variety of ethnic groups. It is transmitted as an autosomal recessive trait. In the United States, the gene frequency is 1 in 27 among Ashkenazi Jews and 1 in 380 among non-Jews.

Infants appear healthy at birth. Until 3 to 10 months of age, growth and development are essentially unremarkable. Listlessness and irritability are usually the first indications of the illness, as well as hyperacusis in approximately one-half of the infants. Soon thereafter, an arrest in intellectual development and a loss of acquired abilities are observed. Examination at this time shows a generalized hypotonia and what is termed a *cherry-red spot* in both macular areas. The cherry-red spot is characteristic of Tay-Sachs disease, although it is also seen in the other forms of GM_2 gangliosidosis and occasionally is observed in Niemann-Pick disease (types A and C), generalized GM_1 gangliosidosis, Farber lipogranulomatosis, infantile Gaucher disease, metachromatic leukodystrophy, and sialidosis (518). In Tay-Sachs disease, it is invariably present by the time neurologic symptoms have developed.

No significant enlargement of liver or spleen occurs. The neurologic symptoms progress rapidly to complete blindness and loss of all voluntary movements. Pupillary light reflexes remain intact, however. The hypotonia is replaced by spasticity and opisthotonus. Convulsions appear at this time and can be generalized, focal, myoclonic, or gelastic. In the final stages, a progressive enlargement of the head has been observed; it is invariably present if the disease has lasted more than 18 months (519). The condition terminates fatally by the second or third year of life.

The CSF is normal. In the early stages of the disease, neuroimaging shows low density on CT scans in caudate, thalamus and putamen, and cerebral white matter, with increased signal on T2-weighted MRI in these areas (520). The caudate nuclei appear swollen and protrude into the lateral ventricles.

The clinical pictures of Sandhoff disease and the AB form of GM_2 gangliosidosis are similar to that of classic Tay-Sachs disease. Juvenile variants of Sandhoff disease have been described. As a rule, these children have late infantile or juvenile progressive ataxia (521).

Other clinical variants of GM_2 gangliosidosis have been recognized in which the picture is highlighted by motor neuron disease (522) or by a movement disorder (523). As a rule, such patients have traces of hexosaminidase A activity.

Diagnosis. The diagnosis of Tay-Sachs disease is made easily on clinical grounds in an infant with a progressive degenerative disease of the nervous system, when the infant has the characteristic retinal cherry-red spot and lacks significant visceromegaly (see Table 1.13). Hexosaminidase assay of serum confirms the clinical impression and also can be used to detect the heterozygote. Prenatal diagnosis by assaying the hexosaminidase A content of amniotic fluid or of fibroblasts cultured from amniotic fluid is possible during the second trimester of gestation (524).

The serum hexosaminidase assay has been automated and used in mass screening surveys. It is accurate in genotype assignment in 96% of instances, and the chance of missing a Tay-Sachs carrier has been estimated as 1 in 30,000 (525). False-positive results are seen in some women who are on oral contraceptives. In these instances, assay of leukocyte hexosaminidase is required to verify the genotype. The apparent deficiency of the enzyme in clinically healthy individuals has already been discussed in this section on Molecular Genetics and Biochemical Pathology.

Treatment. No effective treatment is known for this condition. The process of GM_2 ganglioside accumulation, and subsequent degeneration of brain structure and function, is already well established by the second trimester of fetal development, so that postnatal enzyme replacement therapy and bone marrow transplantation cannot be expected to be effective. Prevention of lysosomal storage by administration of *N*-butyldeoxynojirimycin, an inhibitor of glycosphingolipid synthesis, has been found to prevent GM_2 storage in the brain of mice with Tay-Sachs disease. This approach might be of help in patients with some residual hexosaminidase activity (525a).

Generalized GM_1 Gangliosidosis (Familial Neurovisceral Lipidosis, Pseudo-Hurler Syndrome)

Although it is customary to classify GM_1 gangliosidosis into infantile, late infantile or juvenile, and adult forms according to the age of onset, a continuum of onset occurs, and this classification is merely one of convenience.

GM_1 gangliosidosis is not a rare condition, the infantile form being known as a variant of Tay-Sachs disease with visceral involvement or as pseudo-Hurler syndrome. It was delineated in

1964 by Landing and coworkers (526). The basic enzymatic lesion, a defect in lysosomal β-galactosidase and storage of a monosialoganglioside GM_1 (see Fig. 1.22, step A I), was discovered in 1965 by O'Brien and coworkers (527).

The clinical picture of the late infantile and juvenile forms of generalized GM_1 gangliosidosis resembles the Batten-Bielschowsky or Spielmeyer-Vogt types of late infantile and juvenile amaurotic idiocies, whereas the adult form of GM_1 gangliosidosis is a slowly progressive disease characterized by focal neurologic signs, such as ataxia and movement disorders.

Molecular Genetics and Biochemical Pathology. Total ganglioside content of brain and viscera is increased, and the stored GM_1 ganglioside constitutes up to 90% of total gray matter gangliosides. Additionally, the asialo derivative of GM_1 (GA_1) is present in large amounts. The ganglioside also is stored in liver and spleen. The ultrastructure of the stored material in the liver, however, is entirely different from the membranous cytoplasmic bodies found in neurons. This difference has been attributed to the accumulation of numerous mannose-containing oligosaccharides, which probably result from defective glycoprotein catabolism (528). It is the storage of these compounds that accounts for the hepatomegaly seen in generalized GM_1 gangliosidosis, but not in GM_2 gangliosidosis. A profound deficiency (less than 0.1% of normal) of β-galactosidase, the enzyme that catalyzes the cleavage of the terminal galactose of GM_1 (see Fig. 1.22, step A I), has been demonstrated in several tissues of all patients with GM_1 gangliosidoses regardless of their clinical course (529).

The β-galactosidase is synthesized in a precursor form, which is processed via an intermediate form to the mature enzyme that aggregates in lysosomes as a high-molecular-weight complex of β-galactosidase, a *protective protein*, and a lysosomal neuraminidase. The β-galactosidase precursor is encoded on the short arm of chromosome 3, and numerous mutations have been recognized, with most patients being compound heterozygotes, and the degree of residual β-galactosidase activity determining the clinical course of the disease. In type B Morquio disease, several other mutations of the β-galactosidase gene have been identified (530).

It is of note that the same mutation can result in type B Morquio disease and in GM_1 gangliosidosis with the phenotypic expression being dependent on the nature of the second allele with which it is paired (531). Type B Morquio disease is considered in the section on the mucopolysaccharidoses. A combined defect in β-galactosidase and neuraminidase produces a clinical picture of cherry-red spots and myoclonus. It is the consequence of a defective protective protein and considered in the section on sialidase deficiency.

Pathologic Anatomy. The pathologic picture shows neuronal storage resembling that of GM_2 gangliosidosis (Tay-Sachs disease). The neurons are distended with *p*-aminosalicylic acid (PAS)–positive lipid material; electron microscopy shows that they contain a large number of membranous cytoplasmic bodies similar to those seen in Tay-Sachs disease (532). Additionally, many unusual membrane-bound organelles appear to be derived from lysosomes. Abnormalities also are seen in the extraneural tissues. In the kidneys, a striking vacuolization of the glomerular epithelial cells and the cells of the proximal convoluted tubules occurs. In the liver, a marked histiocytosis is associated with vacuolization of the parenchymal cells. Visceral storage of GM_1 is less prominent in the slower progressive forms.

Clinical Manifestations. For clinical purposes, it is preferable to adhere to the traditional classification of the disease and to divide generalized gangliosidosis into three types. The infantile form of GM_1 is a severe cerebral degenerative disease that can be clinically evident at birth. The infant is hypotonic with a poor sucking reflex and poor psychomotor development. Characteristic facial abnormalities include frontal bossing, depressed nasal bridge, macroglossia, large low-set ears, and marked hirsutism. Hepatosplenomegaly usually is present after age 6 months. Approximately 50% of patients have cherry-red spots. The skeletal deformities (dysostosis multiplex) are similar to those seen in Hurler syndrome (438,533). Patients with hepatosplenomegaly and rapid neurologic deterioration that begins during the first few months of life, but without facial coarsening or many skeletal deformities, also have been recognized (534).

In the late infantile and juvenile forms of generalized GM$_1$ gangliosidosis, neurologic symptoms usually become manifest after 1 year of age. Hyperacusis can be striking, seizures occur in approximately 50% of the patients, and a slowly progressive mental deterioration develops. Bony abnormalities and hepatosplenomegaly are absent, and optic atrophy, when present, is usually unaccompanied by a cherry-red spot (535).

In the chronic adult form, progressive intellectual deterioration becomes apparent between 6 and 20 years of age. It is accompanied by ataxia, a variety of involuntary movements, and spasticity. In other cases, the condition is marked by progressive athetosis or dystonia, but no dementia (536). Pathologic studies reveal that in this, as well as in other sphingolipidoses, the storage material in the more chronically progressive disorders is localized predominantly to the basal ganglia, notably the caudate and lenticular nuclei (537). In this region, axonal and dendritic changes analogous to those seen in GM$_2$ gangliosidosis are maximal. The cause for the regional predilection is utterly obscure

Diagnosis. The diagnosis of GM$_1$ gangliosidosis is suggested by the early onset of clinical manifestations and rapid neurologic deterioration in a patient who has features and radiologic bone changes reminiscent of Hurler syndrome, and by the absence of β-galactosidase in conjunctiva, leukocytes, skin, urine, or viscera. Because so many phenotypic variants of this disorder exist, it is advisable to perform a conjunctival biopsy or to assay for β-galactosidase in any patient with an unexplained progressive neurologic disorder. Enzyme assays on fibroblasts cultured from amniotic fluid allow an antenatal diagnosis in offspring of affected families (538).

Treatment. No treatment is available at this time. GM$_1$ gangliosidosis has not been treated successfully by bone marrow transplantation.

Gaucher Disease

Under the name of Gaucher disease are grouped three fairly distinct clinical conditions (chronic, infantile, and juvenile Gaucher disease) that are characterized by storage of cerebrosides in the reticuloendothelial system. The entity was first described by Gaucher in 1882 (539).

The most common form is chronic non-neuronopathic (type 1) Gaucher disease, a slowly progressive condition with marked visceral involvement but no nervous system involvement, except in a few instances in which it develops late in life. Occasionally, this form can appear at birth or during early childhood.

The acute neuronopathic form (type 2) is a rare disorder, with a rapid downhill course and marked cerebral involvement. The subacute or juvenile neuronopathic form (type 3) is characterized by splenomegaly, anemia, and neurologic deterioration that develop in the first decade of life. A high incidence of this condition has been reported from the northern part of Sweden, and it therefore is also known as *Norbottnian Gaucher disease.*

Molecular Genetics and Biochemical Pathology

The enzymatic defect in the various forms of Gaucher disease is an inactivity of a lysosomal ceramide glucoside-cleaving enzyme, glycosyl ceramide β-glucosidase (glucocerebrosidase) (540). The gene for this enzyme is localized to the long arm of chromosome 1. It has been isolated and sequenced. Numerous mutations have been identified, with two point mutations accounting for some 80% of mutant alleles. As yet, poor correlation exists between the genetic mutation and the ensuing clinical picture, and an individual's genotype predicts neither the severity nor the course of the illness, although, as a rule, the clinical picture is similar in siblings (541).

As a consequence of the genetic lesion, glucocerebrosidase is defective, and glucocerebroside is the principal sphingolipid stored within the reticuloendothelial system in adult Gaucher disease (542). In affected subjects, the spleen contains greatly increased amounts of ceramide glucoside, ceramide dihexosides, and hematosides (ceramide-glucose-galactose-NANA) (543).

Pathologic Anatomy

The outstanding feature of all types of Gaucher disease is the widespread presence of large numbers of Gaucher cells in spleen, liver, lymph nodes, and bone marrow (Fig. 1.25). These are

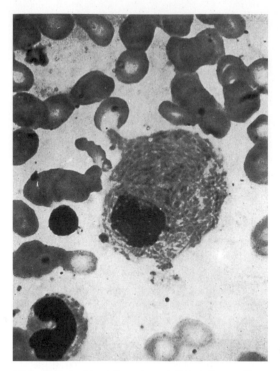

FIG. 1.25. Typical Gaucher cell together with a lymphocyte and a juvenile neutrophil from the sternal bone marrow in a patient with Gaucher disease. (From Wintrobe MM, et al. *Clinical hematology*, 8th ed. Philadelphia: Lea & Febiger, 1981. With permission.)

modified macrophages, appearing as spherical or oval cells between 20 and 50 μm in diameter with a lacy, striated cytoplasm that contrasts with the vacuolated foam cells of Niemann-Pick disease. Electron microscopy reveals irregular inclusion bodies containing tubular elements (544).

In the neuronopathic form (type 2) of Gaucher disease, the cerebral alterations are of five types. These are foci of acute cell loss with neuronophagia, microglial nodules, and chronic neuronal dropout accompanied by gliosis. Additionally, perivascular Gaucher cells can be seen in white matter, particularly in the subcortical area. They are derived from vascular adventitial histiocytes. Finally, a subtle neuronal cytoplasmic accumulation of a PAS-positive material occurs, which on electron microscopy appears as tubular and fibrillar inclusions, similar to the

tubules of isolated glucocerebrosides (545). These are detected principally in the large nerve cells outside the cerebral cortex. A marked degree of cytoplasmic storage is not characteristic of infantile Gaucher disease.

The interrelation between the lipid storage and neuronal cell death is not clear. Glucosylsphingosine and galactosylsphingosine (psychosine), which accumulate in the brain of the neuronopathic forms of Gaucher disease, may be responsible for neuronal damage. Psychosine is known to be cytotoxic and is, in addition, a powerful inhibitor of protein kinase C, which is prominently involved in signal transduction and cellular differentiation (546).

Clinical Manifestations

In the neuronopathic (type 2 infantile) form of Gaucher disease, the onset of symptoms is generally noted at age 4 or 5 months with anemia, apathy, and loss of intellectual achievements (547,547a). These are followed by a gradually progressive spasticity. Neck retraction and bulbar signs are observed frequently, and the infant can have considerable difficulty in swallowing. An acquired oculomotor apraxia also has been noted (548). Splenomegaly is usually quite marked, but liver and lymph nodes might not be enlarged. Pulmonary infiltration owing to aspiration or alveolar consolidation by Gaucher cells can be noted. Occasionally, retinal cherry-red spots are present. Radiographic examination reveals rarefaction at the lower ends of the femora. Laboratory studies show only anemia and thrombocytopenia. A neonatal form of Gaucher disease is associated with congenital ichthyosis, hepatosplenomegaly, hydrops fetalis, and a rapidly progressive downhill course (549).

The subacute neuronopathic form (type 3) becomes apparent during the first decade of life, manifesting by a slowly progressive hepatosplenomegaly, intellectual deterioration, cerebellar ataxia, myoclonic seizures, and spasticity (550). A horizontal supranuclear gaze palsy can develop early in the disease (551). A disproportionately large number of patients have been encountered in Norbotten in northern Sweden (552).

The chronic nonneuronopathic (type 1) form of Gaucher disease, which is much more common and which occasionally is clinically evident during infancy, rarely involves the CNS. Two patients with abducens nerve paralysis and one patient with pseudopapilledema, however, have been encountered by me.

The diagnosis of neuronopathic Gaucher disease must be considered in a child with anemia, splenomegaly, and intellectual deterioration. The presence of Gaucher cells in bone marrow aspirates supports the diagnosis, although Gaucher cells also can be seen in chronic myelocytic leukemia, or, occasionally, in thalassemia major. The main difficulty, from a clinical standpoint, is excluding Niemann-Pick disease type A. Assay of glucocerebrosidase in leukocytes and fibroblast cultures, using synthetic or labeled natural substrates, provides a definitive diagnosis and can be used to identify the heterozygote for intrauterine diagnosis of the disease (553).

The diagnosis of type 2 Gaucher disease can be made by finding Gaucher cells in a bone marrow aspirate. Neuroimaging studies are generally unremarkable (551).

Treatment

Three forms of therapy have been proposed for Gaucher disease: bone marrow transplantation, enzyme replacement, and genetic therapy.

Bone marrow transplantation has been attempted in the subacute form (type 3) of the disease with an encouraging response in some cases (554). Although extremely costly, enzyme replacement using macrophase-targeted glucocerebrosidase (Ceredase) has been used to treat types 1 and 3 Gaucher disease. As a rule, systemic manifestations are reversed, and patients show no significant neurologic deterioration (551,555). No evidence to date shows that type 2 patients benefit from enzyme replacement therapy. As is the case for the other lysosomal storage diseases, gene therapy using retroviral vectors to transfer the cDNA for the human glucocerebrosidase gene into hematopoietic stem cells is still in the experimental phase.

Fabry Disease

This rare metabolic disorder is characterized by the storage of ceramide trihexoside and dihexoside and is transmitted as a gender-linked condition with occasional penetrance into the heterozygous female subject (556).

Molecular Genetics and Biochemical Pathology

The basic defect involves α-galactosidase A, an enzyme that is specific for cleavage of the terminal galactose moiety of ceramide trihexoside, which has an α-configuration (see Fig. 1.22, step B II) (557). The gene for α-galactosidase A is localized to the long arm of the X chromosome (Xq21.33-q22). It has been completely sequenced and a large number of mutations have been documented with every family having their own private mutation, making phenotype difficult to predict from genotype (558). Examination of the synthesis and processing of the enzyme indicates that Fabry disease, like most other lysosomal storage diseases, represents a heterogeneous group of mutations affecting enzyme synthesis, processing, and stability. In some subjects, deficiency of α-galactosidase A is the result of a complete absence of the protein; in others, the α-galactosidase A polypeptides are synthesized but are rapidly degraded after their transport to lysosomes (559). Yet other patients, with a milder clinical form of the disease, have residual enzyme activity. As a consequence of the enzymatic defect, large amounts of trihexoside (ceramide-glucose-galactose-galactose), normally present in minute amounts in plasma and kidneys, have been isolated from affected tissues, and lesser quantities of a ceramide dihexoside (ceramide-galactose-galactose) are found in kidney (560).

Pathologic Anatomy

On pathologic examination, foam cells with vacuolated cytoplasm are found in smooth, striated, and heart musculature; bone marrow; reticuloendothelial system; and renal glomeruli.

In the CNS, lipid storage is highly selective and is primarily confined to the lysosomes of vascular endothelium, including that of the choroid plexus. The accumulation of the glyco-lipid leads to degenerative and proliferative changes and tissue ischemia and infarctions. In some cases, glycolipid also occurs in neurons of the autonomic nervous system, such as the inter-mediolateral cell columns of the thoracic cord, the dorsal autonomic nuclei of the vagus, hypo-thalamus, amygdala, and anterior nuclei of the thalamus (561). In these areas, the permeability of the blood–brain barrier can be sufficiently great to allow entrance of the glycolipid (562). On ultrastructural examination, the intraneuronal inclusions resemble those seen in Hurler syn-drome, in that zebra bodies are prominent (561).

Clinical Manifestations

Fabry disease was first described in 1898 on the basis of its dermatologic lesions (563). It is a rare condition with an incidence of approxi-mately 1 in 40,000 (556). Manifestations usu-ally begin in childhood, but can be delayed into the second or third decade of life. The clinical picture is believed to result from direct involve-ment of various tissues by lipid deposits or by vascular disease involving the small arteries and arterioles, predominantly in the posterior circu-lation (564). The disease is a systemic disorder. The punctate, angiectatic skin rash, which gave the condition its original name, *angiokeratoma corpus diffusum*, is commonly its earliest mani-festation, and usually, as in Fabry original case, appears in late childhood (565). It is most fre-quently seen about the hips and genitalia, but can sometimes assume a butterfly distribution over the face. Younger patients have episodes of sustained fever, weight loss, and pain in joints and abdomen. Corneal opacifications, best seen by slit-lamp examination, are common. They have been seen in infancy (566). A peripheral neuropathy affecting the small myelinated and unmyelinated fibers commonly develops as the disease progresses (567). In older patients, hypertension, recurrent cerebral infarction, and hemorrhage are the usual neurologic complica-tions. Neuroimaging studies can be used to delineate the cerebrovascular alterations (568). The illness is progressive; death is usually caused by renal failure or cardiac dysfunction.

Variants atypical through lack of cutaneous manifestations or isolated renal and corneal involvement (cornea verticillata) are fairly com-mon (569).

Heterozygous female subjects can be totally asymptomatic or can show corneal opacities, skin lesions, or intermittent pain in the extremities.

Diagnosis

Fabry disease should be considered in older boys who have intermittent burning pain in their feet, legs, and fingertips, aggravated by warm weather. In the early stages of the disease, angiomas must be sought with care. The scrotum is the most likely site (565). The diagnosis also can be made by finding lipidlike inclusions in the endothelium and smooth muscle of skin biopsies. Biopsy of the peripheral nerve can reveal swelling and disrup-tion of unmyelinated axons and zebra bodies in perineural fibroblasts (567). The diagnosis is con-firmed by finding a marked deficiency of α-galac-tosidase A in plasma or serum leukocytes or in cultured skin fibroblasts (570). Heterozygotes can be diagnosed using restriction fragment length polymorphisms in close proximity to the gene for α-galactosidase (571).

Treatment

Phenytoin, carbamazepine, or a combination of the two drugs can be of considerable benefit in relieving the intermittent pain. When phenytoin is used, plasma levels of only 4 µg/mL or above are adequate in providing relief (572). No specific treatment exists for the cerebrovascular complica-tions (564). Treatment of the enzyme defect with renal transplant appears to improve sensory symp-toms and arrest cerebrovascular complications (573). The graft functions normally for at least several years and does not show the microscopic changes of the Fabry kidney. Enzyme replace-ment therapy and gene therapy using retroviral vectors are still in their experimental phases.

Schindler Disease

Schindler disease, a rare disorder first recognized in 1988, is the consequence of a defect in lysosomal α-*N*-acetylgalactosaminidase (α-galactosidase B). The condition is marked by storage of glycopeptides and oligosaccharides with a termination α-*N*-acetylgalactosaminyl moieties. The neuropathologic picture resembles that of infantile neuroaxonal dystrophy (Seitelberger disease), a condition covered in Chapter 2, in that axonal spheroid are seen throughout the neocortex. The condition generally becomes apparent during the second year of life and manifests by developmental deterioration, myoclonic seizures, and cortical blindness. No organomegaly occurs and no vacuolization of peripheral lymphocytes or granulocytes. The diagnosis is made by analysis of plasma lysosomal enzymes, and oligosaccharides in nondesalted urine (574).

Niemann-Pick Diseases

The prototype of these conditions was first described in 1914 by Niemann (575). Their traditional nomenclature as proposed in 1958 by Crocker (576) implies that these conditions are biochemically and enzymatically related. Actually, this is not the case. Niemann-Pick disease types A (NPA) and B (NPB) are recessively inherited lysosomal storage diseases that feature a deficiency in sphingomyelinase activity and an accumulation of sphingomyelin in the reticuloendothelial system. They are allelic and result from mutations in the gene that codes for sphingomyelinase. Types C (NPC) and D (NPD) are characterized by an accumulation of cholesterol and sphingomyelin. They result from an abnormal intracellular translocation of cholesterol derived from low-density lipoproteins with NPD being an allelic variant of NPC. In 1989, Spence and Callahan (577) proposed a classification by which the various conditions are grouped into type I (formerly types A and B) and type II (formerly types C and D). From a clinical point of view, it is still preferable, however, to retain the older classification.

Niemann-Pick Disease Type A

Clinically, NPA is characterized by autosomal recessive transmission with a predilection for Ashkenazi Jewish families [approximately 30% of patients in the series of Crocker and Farber (576)]. Symptoms become apparent during the first year of life with hepatosplenomegaly, which can lead to massive abdominal distention, and with poor physical and mental development. Other systemic symptoms include persistent neonatal jaundice, diarrhea, generalized lymphadenopathy, and pulmonary infiltrates.

In approximately one-third of patients, neurologic symptoms predominate initially, and few children survive beyond infancy without apparent involvement of the nervous system. Seizures, particularly myoclonic jerks, are common, and marked spasticity can develop before death. Approximately one-half of the infants have hypotonia; with progression of the disease, the nerve conduction velocities slow. On biopsy of the peripheral nerves, the Schwann cells are filled with inclusion bodies (578). Retinal cherry-red spots are found in approximately 25% of patients and can antedate neurologic abnormalities (576). Corneal and lenticular opacifications are common (579). The progression of the disease is variable, but death usually occurs before age 5 years.

The pathologic hallmark of NPA is the presence of large, lipid-laden cells in the reticuloendothelial system, mostly in spleen, bone marrow, liver, lungs, and lymph nodes. In the brain, massive, generalized deposition of foam cells and ballooned ganglion cells occurs, primarily in the cerebellum, brainstem, and spinal cord (580). Lipid storage also occurs in the endothelium of cerebral blood vessels, in arachnoid cells, and in the connective tissue of the choroid plexus.

Biochemical examination documents the storage of sphingomyelin in affected organs. This compound was first described in 1884 by Thudichum, the father of neurochemistry (581), and was found to have the structure depicted in Figure 1.26.

Chemical and histochemical studies have shown sphingomyelin to be a major myelin constituent. It is also a normal component of spleen. Sphingomyelinase, which cleaves sphingomyelin into phosphatidylcholine and ceramide, is normally present in liver, kidney, spleen, and brain. Two forms of this enzyme have been distinguished.

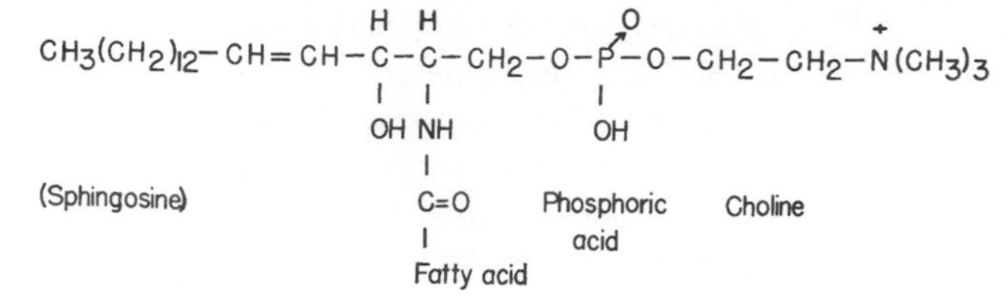

FIG. 1.26. Structure of a sphingomyelin.

The lysosomal form has an acidic pH optimum, which distinguishes it from the microsomal form, which has a basic pH optimum. In NPA, the lysosomal enzyme is defective. The gene for lysosomal (acid) sphingomyelinase has been localized to the short arm of chromosome 11. It has been cloned and sequenced, and a variety of different mutations have been described. Mutations in which no catalytically active sphingomyelinase exists result in NPA, whereas mutations that produce a defective enzyme with residual catalytic activity result in NPB (582). Two common mutations are responsible for more than 50% of Ashkenazi Jewish patients with NPA (583).

Niemann-Pick Disease Type B

The absence of any neurologic manifestations in NPB precludes its extensive discussion. Suffice it to say that the clinical picture is one of hepatosplenomegaly and interstitial pulmonary infiltrates. In some cases, sphingomyelin storage occurs in retinal neurons, peripheral nerves, and the endothelium of the cerebral vasculature (584).

Niemann-Pick Disease Type C

Niemann-Pick disease type C is as common as NPA and NPB combined and is seen in a variety of ethnic groups. It has been described under a variety of terms, notably Niemann-Pick types E and F, a condition in which vertical supranuclear ophthalmoplegia and sea-blue histiocytes were accompanied by hepatic cirrhosis, and juvenile dystonic lipidosis. As can be surmised from the variety of eponyms, the clinical picture is extremely heterogeneous, even within the same family, and a continuum of severity occurs, with the appearance of neurologic symptoms ranging from 3 months to 55 years (585). In its most severe form, the disease presents in infancy with prolonged neonatal jaundice, often associated with cholestasis and giant cell hepatitis, hepatosplenomegaly, and a rapid progression (586). Neurologic signs or symptoms may not be apparent (587). In the late infantile form, a more common entity, the disease makes its first appearance between ages 2 and 4 years. Neurologic symptoms predominate and are contingent on the age when the disease appears. Whereas in the infantile form hypotonia and developmental arrest predominate, in children under 5 years cerebellar ataxia is the presenting feature, and older children, who develop the juvenile form of the disease, present with dementia. Dystonia and other basal ganglia symptoms are common as are myoclonic or akinetic seizures, ataxia, and macular cherry-red spots. A supranuclear paralysis of vertical gaze is characteristic for this condition. Hepatosplenomegaly is found in some 90% of subjects, but is not as striking as in NPA and can become less marked as the illness progresses (588). Sea-blue histiocytes and foam cells are seen in the bone marrow in virtually every instance (589).

The gene whose mutation is responsible for most cases of NPC has been localized to chromosome 18. It has been cloned and encodes a protein that is believed to participate in the transfer of plasma membrane cholesterol to the endoplasmic reticulum and mitochondria and also to export lysosomal cholesterol to the plasma membrane (590,591). The protein may also be involved in glycolipid transport (591a). A number of mutations have been documented, and a second, phenotypically similar, but genetically distinct form of NPC (NPC2) has been described. NPC2 gene mutations are seen in approximately 5% of NPC patients (591b).

Niemann-Pick Disease Type D

The clinical presentation of NPD, now known to be allelic with NPC is indistinguishable from the slowly progressive form of NPC, except that patients are from southwestern Nova Scotia, a geographic isolate where the heterozygote frequency for this condition ranges between 1 in 4 and 1 in 10 (592,593).

Diagnosis

Hepatosplenomegaly, anemia, and failure to thrive in children who show intellectual deterioration can indicate one of the forms of Niemann-Pick disease with neurologic involvement. This diagnosis is best confirmed by bone marrow aspiration, peripheral nerve or lymph node biopsy (578), and, in NPA, a deficiency of sphingomyelinase in leukocytes and skin fibroblasts. Sphingomyelinase activity has been found in cultured amniotic fibroblasts, allowing an intrauterine diagnosis of NPA or NPB (584). The presence of sea-blue histiocytes in the bone marrow serves to diagnose NPC. More specific assays involve the demonstration of increased amounts of unesterified cholesterol in fibroblasts, or quantitation of impaired cholesterol ester synthesis in fibroblasts or lymphocytes (594).

Treatment

Liver or bone marrow transplantation has been unsuccessful in the treatment of NPA and NPC. Enzyme replacement therapy is also still in its experimental stages. No evidence indicates that dimethylsulfoxide or cholesterol-lowering agents improve neurologic symptoms in NPC.

Wolman Disease
(Acid Lipase Deficiency Disease)

This condition was first described by Wolman and his group in 1956 (595). The clinical manifestations resemble those of NPA and include failure in weight gain, a malabsorption syndrome, and adrenal insufficiency. Lipoproteins and plasma cholesterol are reduced, and acanthocytes are evident (596). A massive hepatosplenomegaly occurs, and radiographic examination reveals the adrenals to be calcified. Neurologic symptoms are usually limited to delayed intellectual development. Patho-

logic examination shows xanthomatosis of the viscera. Sudanophilic material is stored in the leptomeninges, retinal ganglion cells, and nerve cells of the myenteric plexus. Sudanophilic granules outline the cortical capillaries, and sudanophilic demyelination occurs (597).

A striking accumulation of cholesterol esters and triglycerides occurs in affected tissues. Lipid accumulation is greatest in tissues that synthesize the most cholesterol esters. These tissues include the adrenal cortex, liver, intestine, spleen, and lymph nodes. Relatively little lipid storage occurs in brain. The basic enzymatic defect is a deficiency in acid lipase, a lysosomal enzyme normally active against medium- and long-chain triglycerides, as well as cholesterol esters (598). The gene coding for this enzyme has been mapped to the long arm of chromosome 10 and has been cloned. Acid lipase deficiency has been demonstrated in fibroblasts, which lack the ability to hydrolyze cholesterol esters entering the cells bound to low-density lipoproteins. Because free low-density lipoproteins are not present in the cell, the suppression of 3-hydroxy-3-methylglutaryl-CoA reductase, which normally regulates endogenous cholesterol synthesis, also is impaired (599).

Wolman disease should be distinguished from cholesterol ester storage disease, a more benign entity that is allelic with Wolman disease and in which no lipid storage occurs within the CNS (600). In most but not all instances, patients with cholesterol ester storage disease have genetic mutations that result in residual acid lipase activity, whereas the mutations resulting in Wolman disease produce a nonfunctioning enzyme (601). Wolman disease also should be distinguished from triglyceride storage disease type I, in which only the hydrolysis of triglycerides is impaired, and in which infants are developmentally retarded (602).

A variant of Wolman disease characterized by tapetoretinal degeneration, deafness, progressive mental deterioration, and tubular nephropathy has been reported (603). The clinical picture of the patient resembled that of Alström syndrome, a condition for which an underlying enzymatic defect has not yet been delineated.

Ceramidosis (Lipogranulomatosis)

Ceramidosis, which is probably the rarest of the lysosomal storage diseases, was first described by Farber and associates (604). The clinical features are unique and manifest during the first few weeks of life. The infant becomes irritable, has a hoarse cry, and develops nodular erythematous swelling of the wrists. Over subsequent months, nodules develop in numerous sites, particularly in areas subject to trauma, such as joints and the subcutaneous tissue of the buttocks. Severe motor and mental retardation occur. Hepatosplenomegaly has been seen in approximately one-fourth of reported cases. In approximately two-thirds of cases, the disease progresses rapidly, and death usually occurs by 2 years of age. As a rule, the earlier the dermal nodules appear, the more malignant the ill!ness. Variants that resemble a malignant form of histocytosis X have been reported (605).

The basic pathologic lesion is a granuloma formed by the proliferation and ballooning of mesenchymal cells that ultimately become enmeshed in dense hyaline fibrous tissue. Within the CNS, neurons and glial cells are swollen and contain stored material (606).

The enzymatic defect responsible has been localized to lysosomal acid ceramidase, which is absent from brain, kidney, and skin fibroblasts (607). The gene coding for the enzyme has been cloned and molecular lesions have been defined (608). A consequence of the defect is a striking increase in ceramides in affected tissues. Gangliosides also are increased, particularly in the subcutaneous nodules, which have the ganglioside concentration of normal gray matter. Mildly affected patients in whom mental function is unimpaired also have been encountered (609). Bone marrow transplantation has been unsuccessful in correcting the neurologic deficits and, as yet, no treatment exists for this disorder (610).

DISORDERS OF LIPID METABOLISM

Globoid cell leukodystrophy and metachromatic leukodystrophy have been shown to result from a disorder in lipid metabolism. These conditions are discussed in Chapter 2 with the other leukodystrophies.

Cerebrotendinous Xanthomatosis

Although cerebrotendinous xanthomatosis, a rare but well-defined familial disease, was first described by van Bogaert and associates in 1937 (611), its unique chemical feature, deposition of cholestanol (dihydrocholesterol) within the nervous system, was uncovered only in 1968 by Menkes and associates (612). The disease is characterized by xanthomas of tendons and lungs, cataracts, slowly progressive cerebellar ataxia, spasticity, and dementia. It has a predilection for Sephardic Jews of Moroccan ancestry.

Although, as a rule, the disease is not apparent until late childhood, some 35% of patients in the series of Berginer and colleagues were symptomatic before age 10 years (613). Progression is generally slow, and in many instances, the illness does not interfere with a normal life span. The triad of progressive spinocerebellar ataxia, pyramidal signs, and mental retardation is seen in the large majority of patients with cerebrotendinous xanthomatosis, and mental retardation is seen in more than 90% (613). Cataracts are present in 76% and generally are seen as early as 56 years of age. Seizures are encountered in 40% to 50% and can be the presenting symptom (614). Intractable diarrhea can be a major manifestation during childhood (615). A sensory and motor neuropathy also has been documented (613). Tendon xanthomas can be apparent in childhood, most commonly over the Achilles and triceps tendons. Serum cholesterol levels are normal, but cholestanol concentrations in serum and erythrocytes are elevated (613). CT reveals the presence of hyperdense nodules in the cerebellum, and diffuse white matter hypodensity. MRI demonstrates atrophy of cerebrum and cerebellum, with occasional atrophy of the brainstem and corpus callosum. Also, cerebral white matter hypodensity is present, an indication of cholestanol infiltration and demyelination (616).

On pathologic examination, the brainstem and cerebellum are the two areas within the nervous system most affected. Myelin destruction, a variable degree of gliosis, and xanthoma cells are visible (617).

On chemical examination, large amounts of free and esterified cholestanol are found stored in the nervous system. The sterol is located not only in such affected areas as the cerebellum, but also in histologically normal myelin. The content of cholestanol in the tendon xanthomas is increased, but here the predominant sterol is cholesterol (612).

The defect in cerebrotendinous xanthomatosis has been localized to the mitochondrial sterol 27-hydroxylase (618). The gene has been cloned and numerous mutations have been documented (619). As a consequence of the enzymatic defect, cholic acid biosynthesis proceeds via the 25-hydroxylated intermediates. The deposition of cholestanol within the CNS has been explained by a disorder in the blood–brain barrier induced by the presence of large amounts of bile alcohol glucuronides (620).

Treatment with chenodeoxycholic acid (15 mg/kg per day) reverses the elevated CSF cholestanol levels and induces a 50% reduction of plasma cholestanol, an increase in IQ, and a reversal of neurologic symptoms (621). Additionally, improvement occurs in the EEG, somatosensory-evoked potentials, and the MRI (613,621).

Smith-Lemli-Opitz Syndrome

Smith-Lemli-Opitz syndrome, an autosomal recessive condition, is marked by the combination of mental retardation, hypotonia, midface hypoplasia, congenital or postnatal cataracts, and ptosis. Anomalies of the external male genitalia and the upper urinary tract are common (622). The prevalence of Smith-Lemli-Opitz syndrome has been estimated at 1 in 20,000, making it one of the more common metabolic causes for mental retardation (623,624). The basic biochemical defect involves the gene coding for sterol delta-7-reductase, the enzyme that converts 7-dehydrocholesterol to cholesterol, the last step of cholesterol biosynthesis. The gene has been mapped to the long arm of chromosome 11 and has been coded. A number of mutations have been documented that result in reduced expression of the enzyme (625,626). As a consequence of the enzymatic defect, the concentration of plasma 7-dehydrocholesterol is markedly increased, and plasma cholesterol is significantly reduced.

The clinical picture of Smith-Lemli-Opitz syndrome ranges in severity from little more than syndactyly of the toes to holoprosencephaly with profound mental retardation (626). As a rule, the lower the plasma cholesterol, the more severe the clinical picture. Although the disease has been divided into two types, with type II being more severe than type I, it is more likely that there is a continuum of clinical severity. A low plasma cholesterol level should suggest the diagnosis, which can be confirmed by finding an elevated 7-dehydrocholesterol level on gas-liquid chromatography/mass spectroscopy (627). In 10% of patients, plasma cholesterol levels are normal, and the diagnosis depends on quantitation of 7-dehydrocholesterol (627). Some patients excrete large amounts of 3-methylglutaconic acid, and this can be detected on screening of urinary organic acids (628).

Smith-Lemli-Opitz syndrome has been treated with dietary cholesterol supplementation. Initial results appear to be encouraging, although on theoretical grounds one would not expect dietary cholesterol to cross the blood–brain barrier (629).

Cholesterol Storage Diseases

Several conditions characterized by intracerebral cholesterol deposition have been described. The metabolic defect for any of them is not known.

Involvement of the CNS in histiocytosis X, although rare, has been well documented (630,631). Most frequently, the granulomatous lesion of the membranous bones of the skull extends into the tuber cinereum or about the cranial nerves at the base of the brain. Demyelination and perivascular lipid deposition are noted occasionally, particularly in the cerebellum. As a consequence, one can see visual field defects, hemiparesis or other signs of pyramidal tract involvement, or a cerebellar syndrome. Seizures and parietal lobe signs are less common (632). Feigin has recorded a case in which cholesterol-containing nodules were deposited within the cerebral gray matter (633).

PEROXISOMAL DISORDERS

Peroxisomes are ubiquitous organelles containing more than 50 enzymes involved in anabolic and catabolic reactions, including plasmalogen and bile acid biosynthesis, gluconeogenesis, the removal of excess peroxides, purine catabolism, and β-oxidation of very-long-chain fatty acids. Peroxisomes do not contain DNA, and peroxisomal matrix and membrane proteins, therefore, must be imported from the cytosol where they are synthesized. Peroxisomal structure and function and peroxisomal biogenesis have been reviewed by Wanders and coworkers (634), Moser (635), and Baumgartner and colleagues (635a). At least 20 disorders of peroxisomal function have been identified to date. They can be classified into three groups.

In group 1, a disorder of peroxisome biogenesis, the number of peroxisomes is reduced and the activities of many peroxisomal enzymes are deficient. Zellweger cerebrohepatorenal syndrome, neonatal adrenoleukodystrophy, and infantile Refsum disease belong to this group.

In group 2, peroxisomal structure and function are normal, and the defect is limited to a single peroxisomal enzyme. At least eight disorders exist in which a single peroxisomal enzyme is defective. X-linked adrenoleukodystrophy, in which peroxisomal fatty acid β-oxidation is defective, and adult Refsum disease in which phytanic acid α-oxidation is deficient, belong to this group. X-linked adrenoleukodystrophy is covered in Chapter 2 with the other leukodystrophies.

In group 3, peroxisomal structure and function are normal, but the activities of several peroxisomal enzymes are reduced. An entity termed *rhizomelic chondrodysplasia punctata* has been assigned to this group. The various disorders are outlined in Table 1.14.

Disorders of Peroxisomal Biogenesis

The basic defect in disorders of peroxisomal biogenesis involves the incorporation of the peroxisomal proteins into peroxisomes. The proteins of peroxisomal matrix and membranes are encoded by nuclear genes and are synthesized on cytoplasmic polyribosomes. They are then targeted to the peroxisomes. Protein targeting is

TABLE 1.14. *Peroxisomal disorders*

Condition	Clinical manifestations	Reference
Disorders of peroxisomal biogenesis		
Zellweger syndrome	Typical facies, weakness, hypotonia, renal cysts, hepatomegaly, cirrhosis, cataracts, chorioretinitis, optic atrophy	Moser (635)
Neonatal adrenoleukodystrophy	Seizures, hypotonia, marked developmental delay, dysmorphic features	Mobley (657), Powers (658)
Infantile Refsum disease	Mild dysmorphic features, retinitis pigmentosa, hypotonia, developmental regression	Budden (659), Powers (658)
Disorders of single peroxisomal enzyme		
X-Linked adrenoleukodystrophy	—	See Chapter 2
Mevalonate kinase deficiency	—	Hoffmann (653)
Adult Refsum disease	—	Watkins (650)
Bifunctional protein deficiency	Severe hypotonia at birth, neonatal seizures, disturbances of neuronal migration	Watkins (660)
Acyl-CoA oxidase deficiency	Less severe than bifunctional protein deficiency; moderate hypotonia at birth, seizures	Watkins (660)
Peroxisomal thiolase deficiency	Severe hypotonia at birth, dysmorphic features, enlarged liver	Schram (661)
Disorders of multiple peroxisomal enzymes		
Rhizomelic chondrodysplasia punctata	Shortening of limbs, flat facies, stippled epiphysitis, mental retardation	Moser (635)

achieved through the interaction of specific peroxisomal targeting signals on these proteins with their cognate cytoplasmic receptors. The major targeting signal is a C-terminal tripeptide (PTS1). Less commonly a 9-amino acid signal is used (PTS2). These receptors, bound to their cargo, interact with specific docking proteins in the peroxisomal membrane. Finally, by a process still not understood, the peroxisomal proteins enter the peroxisome (636). As ascertained from the results of complementation analyses, at least 12 different groups of defects affect peroxisomal biogenesis, implying that at least 12 genes are involved in the formation of normal peroxisomes and in the transport of peroxisomal enzymes (635). No correlation exists between the complementation group and the phenotypic features, and Zellweger syndrome is represented in each of the complementation groups (635).

As a consequence of the defect of peroxisomal membrane proteins, enzymes normally found within the peroxisomal matrix are absent or located in the cytosol, and cultured fibroblasts derived from patients with Zellweger syndrome contain empty membranous sacs, designated as *peroxisomal ghosts* (637).

Zellweger Syndrome

The differentiation of the disorders of peroxisomal biogenesis into Zellweger syndrome, neonatal adrenoleukodystrophy, and infantile Refsum disease is not based on a fundamental genetic difference, but on the severity of the disease, with Zellweger syndrome the most severe, and infantile Refsum disease the least severe. All three entities are autosomal recessive disorders, with the Zellweger form having a frequency of 1 in 100,000 births. Several genetic defects cause the disorders of peroxisomal biogenesis. Mutations in either one of two adenosinetriphosphatases (ATPases) (PEX1 and PEX6) are the most common causes of these disorders (638), but several other genetic mutations have been delineated.

In its classic form, Zellweger syndrome is marked by intrauterine growth retardation, hypotonia, profound developmental delay,

hepatomegaly, variable contractures in the limbs, and renal glomerular cysts. Impaired hearing and nystagmus are common, as are irregular calcifications of the patellae. Facies are unusual with a large fontanel, a high forehead with shallow supraorbital ridges, a low or broad nasal bridge, and a variety of eye and ear anomalies (639) (see Fig. 1.12). A number of migrational disorders of the brain have been documented, including macrogyria, polymicrogyria, and heterotopic gray matter (640,641). Muscle biopsy might disclose a mitochondrial myopathy (642). MRI discloses impaired myelination and diffusely abnormal gyral patterns with areas of pachygyria and micropolygyria. These abnormalities are most severe in the perisylvian and perirolandic regions (643).

The plasma fatty acid pattern in Zellweger syndrome is abnormal, with large amounts of very-long-chain fatty acids. Most subjects also have elevations in plasma or urinary pipecolic acid. Additionally, phytanic levels are elevated, and the urinary excretion of dicarboxylic acids is increased (644).

Neonatal Adrenoleukodystrophy and Infantile Refsum Disease

These two entities represent less severe expressions of disordered peroxisomal biogenesis. Neonatal adrenoleukodystrophy is an autosomal recessive disease, in contrast to the X-linked adrenoleukodystrophy of later onset, with symptoms becoming apparent during the first 3 months of life. It is marked by dysmorphic features, hearing deficit, hypotonia, hepatomegaly, seizures, and retinal degeneration (645).

The clinical features of infantile Refsum disease are similar. They include a sensorineural hearing loss, retinitis pigmentosa, and mental retardation. Facial dysmorphism and hypotonia are less marked, and neonatal seizures are less common (645). As in Zellweger syndrome, serum phytanic acid, pipecolic acid, and very-long-chain fatty acids are present in increased amounts in plasma, and urinary pipecolic acid is elevated (635,635a).

The diagnosis of these conditions is best made by assay of plasma very-long-chain fatty acids and can be confirmed by phytanic acid and pipecolic acid determinations in plasma or urine (635a). Morphologic examination of established fibroblast cultures or tissue obtained by liver biopsy is also of diagnostic assistance (635,635a).

Single Peroxisomal Enzyme Defects

Refsum Disease
(Heredopathia Atactica Polyneuritiformis)

Although Refsum disease has been known since 1944, when Refsum described two families with polyneuritis, muscular atrophy, ataxia, retinitis pigmentosa, diminution of hearing, and ichthyosis, an underlying disorder in lipid metabolism was uncovered only some 20 years later (646,647).

The disease usually makes its appearance between ages 4 and 7 years, most commonly with partial, intermittent peripheral neuropathy. This neuropathy can be accompanied by sensorineural deafness, ichthyosis, and cardiomyopathy. The CSF shows an albuminocytologic dissociation with a protein level between 100 and 600 mg/dL.

In brain, lipids are deposited in swollen nerve cells and in areas of demyelination with the formation of fatty macrophages (648). The characteristic alterations in peripheral nerve are hypertrophy, sometimes with *onion bulb* formation, and a loss of myelinated fibers. Electron microscopy reveals Schwann cells to contain paracrystalline inclusions. In all organs, including the brain, quantities of lipids are increased. The lipids contain, as one of their major fatty acids, a branched chain compound, 3,7,11,15-tetramethylhexadecanoic acid (phytanic acid). Blood levels of phytanic acid are increased. In contrast to normal levels of 0.2 mg/dL or less, they range between 10 and 50 mg/dL.

These changes result from a defect in the gene that codes for phytanoyl-coenzyme A hydroxylase. As a consequence, there is a block in the peroxisomal α-oxidation of phytanic to prostanoic acid (Fig. 1.27) (649). Phytanic acid is almost exclusively of exogenous origin and derived mainly from dietary phytol ingested in

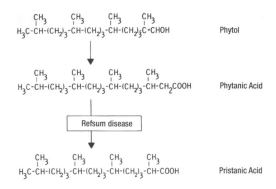

FIG. 1.27. Phytol metabolism. In Refsum disease, the metabolic block is located at the conversion of phytanic to pristanic acid.

the form of nuts, spinach, or coffee. When patients are placed on a phytol-free diet, blood phytanic acid levels decrease slowly, and within 1 year reach levels of approximately one-fourth of the original values (650). This change is accompanied by increased nerve conduction velocities, return of reflexes, and improvement in sensation and objective coordination. Periodic plasma exchanges have been used to reduce body stores of phytanic acid and appear to be particularly effective during the early phases of therapy (650).

The mechanism by which phytanic acid produces the variety of clinical manifestations is not clear. Steinberg proposes that its structural similarity to the farnesol and the geranyl-geranyl groups permits phytanic acid to interfere with the formation of cytosolic prenylated proteins, and prevents anchoring of cytosolic proteins to membranes (651).

The differential diagnosis of Refsum disease includes other causes of chronic and intermittent polyneuritis, such as α-lipoprotein deficiency (Tangier disease), which can be diagnosed by examination of the plasma lipoproteins and by the low serum cholesterol levels. Other similar clinical entities are relapsing infectious polyneuritis, the mitochondrial myopathies (*ophthalmoplegia plus*), acute intermittent porphyria, recurrent exposures to toxins, particularly alcohol or lead, and the various hereditary sensory motor neuropathies described in Chapter 2.

Mevalonic Aciduria

Mevalonic aciduria is an inborn error of cholesterol biosynthesis whose clinical picture is highlighted by neonatal acidosis, the evolution of cataracts, and seizures. Profound diarrhea and a malabsorption syndrome are common. Hepatomegaly, lymphadenopathy, and anemia can suggest a congenital infection. Affected infants have a triangular face with down-slanted eyes and large, posteriorly rotated, low-set ears. The diagnosis can be suspected by a markedly reduced blood cholesterol level and confirmed by analysis of urinary organic acids. The defect is localized to mevalonate kinase, a peroxisomal enzyme, which is virtually absent in fibroblasts. The pathogenesis of the clinical manifestations is still unknown, but could be related to the increased output of leukotriene E_4 (652,653). Mevalonate kinase is also deficient in livers of patients with Zellweger syndrome (654).

Some of the other defects of peroxisomal enzymes are summarized in Table 1.14.

Defects of Multiple Peroxisomal Enzymes

Rhizomelic Chondrodysplasia Punctata

Rhizomelic chondrodysplasia punctata, an autosomal recessive disorder, is marked by severe proximal shortening of humeri and femora and mental retardation with or without spasticity. Patients have flat facies and a low nasal bridge; cataracts are seen in 72% and ichthyosis in 28% (635). Radiography shows punctate epiphyseal and extraepiphyseal mineralization. Similar calcifications are seen in warfarin embryopathy and in Conradi-Hünermann syndrome, an autosomal dominant disorder in which intelligence is relatively preserved (655).

Neuropathologic examination in rhizomelic chondrodysplasia punctata shows little more than cortical atrophy; no abnormality in myelination or disorders of cortical migration occur. Three unrelated enzymes, acyl-CoA-dihydroxy-acetone phosphate acyl transferase, phytanoyl-

CoA hydroxylase, and 3-oxoacyl-CoA thiolase are affected in this condition. The basis for this disorder has been pinpointed to the gene that codes for the receptor for the sequence of the amino-terminal of 3-oxoacyl-CoA thiolase, the targeting sequence PTS2 (656).

CARBOHYDRATE-DEFICIENT GLYCOPROTEIN SYNDROMES

Carbohydrate-deficient glycoprotein syndromes (CDGS) were first described in 1987 by Jackon et al (656a). They represent a group of heterogeneous genetic neurologic disorders with multisystem involvement that results from the abnormal synthesis of *N*-linked oligosaccharides (656b). CDGS has been reported throughout the world; all entities are transmitted as autosomal recessive traits.

N-Linked oligosaccharides are a prominent structural feature of cell surfaces and are essential to the function of cell surface receptors, protein targeting and turnover, and cell-to-cell interaction. The characteristic biochemical abnormality in CDGS is the hypoglycosylation of glycoproteins. As a result, the carbohydrate side chain of glycoproteins is either truncated or completely absent. At this time, at least seven subtypes have been recognized (Table 1.15).

Type I is the most common form of CDGS. The typical presentation is that of a hypotonic and hyporeflexic infant with failure to thrive. Numerous dysmorphic features occur. Most frequently, inverted nipples and an abnormal distribution of fat in the suprapubic area and buttocks are seen. Facies are unusual with a high nasal bridge, prominent jaw, and large pinnae (662). Afebrile seizures and strokelike episodes, the latter possibly the consequence of a transient coagulopathy, also have been observed. MRI studies show cerebellar hypoplasia, brainstem atrophy, and occasionally Dandy-Walker malformation.

The condition tends to be nonprogressive. Older children develop ataxia, retinitis pigmentosa, and hypogonadism. Microcephaly can develop or can be present at birth. The diagnosis of all forms of CDGS is best made by the presence of abnormal transferrin and by its pattern, as demonstrated by isoelectric focusing of serum

TABLE 1.15. *Carbohydrate-deficient glycoprotein syndromes*

Type	Central nervous system symptoms	Systemic symptoms	Neuroimaging	Molecular defect	Reference
Ia	Most common: hypotonia, hyporeflexia, seizures, strokelike episodes, retinitis pigmentosa	Failure to thrive, dysmorphic facies, inverted nipples, fat pads in pubic and gluteal areas, pericardial effusion	Cerebellar hypoplasia, brainstem atrophy, Dandy-Walker malformation	Phosphomannomutase	Krasnewich and Gahl (662)
Ib	None	Protein-losing enteropathy, recurrent thrombotic events	—	Phosphomannose isomerase	Niehues et al. (663)
Ic	Less severe than in Ia	—	—	Defective biosynthesis of dolichol-linked oligosaccharides	Burda et al. (664)
II	Severe delay, hypotonia, hand-washing movements	Coarse facies, low-set ears	Cerebellar hypoplasia, generalized dysmyelination	N-acetylglucosaminyl transferase II	Ramaekers et al. (665)
III	Hypotonia progressing to spastic quadriparesis, infantile spasms, optic atrophy	—	Cortical atrophy, general dysmyelination, Dandy-Walker malformation	Unknown	Stibler et al. (666)
IV	Severe developmental delay, infantile spasms, evolving spastic quadriparesis, optic atrophy	Dysplastic ears, adducted thumbs	Cerebellar, cerebral atrophy	Unknown	Stibler et al. (667)
V	Same as Ia	Same as Ia	—	Dolichylglucosyl transferase	Korner et al. (668)

transferrin (656b,667). Isoelectric focusing with Western blotting of antithrombin, thyroxin-binding globulin, and α_1-antitrypsin is also abnormal (667). Plasma amino acids and urine organic acids are normal, as are the immune responses (662). The condition cannot be diagnosed prenatally until at least 36 weeks' gestation (669). Therapy with intravenous mannose has been suggested, but is probably not effective.

FAMILIAL MYOCLONUS EPILEPSIES

Five major conditions produce progressive myoclonus epilepsy: the sialidoses, myoclonus epilepsy with ragged red fibers, and the neuronal ceroid lipofuscinosis (670). These three conditions are considered in the sections Glycoproteinoses, Mitochondrial Diseases, and Neuronal Ceroid Lipofuscinoses, respectively. Lafora disease and Unverricht-Lundborg disease are covered in this section.

Lafora Disease

Lafora disease, first described by Lafora in 1911 (671), is marked by generalized, myoclonic, and focal occipital seizures, commencing between 11 and 18 years of age, and accompanied by a fairly rapidly progressive dementia. It is clinically and genetically distinct from Unverricht-Lundborg disease, first described by Unverricht in 1891 (672). The gene for Lafora disease has been localized to the long arm of chromosome 6 (6q23-25). It encodes a protein, named *laforin*, which functions as a tyrosine phosphatase. A variety of mutations in the gene have been described and co-segregate with Lafora disease (673). However, a small proportion of clinically typical patients do not show linkage to chromosome 6q23-25 (673a).

The pathologic picture of Lafora disease is unique. Many concentric amyloid (Lafora) bodies are found within the cytoplasm of ganglion cells throughout the neuraxis, particu-

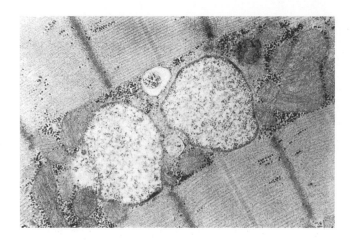

FIG. 1.28. Myoclonus epilepsy. Electron micrograph showing inclusion bodies in muscle. (Courtesy of Dr. M. Anthony Verity, Department of Pathology, University of California, Los Angeles, Los Angeles, CA.)

larly in the dentate nucleus, substantia nigra, reticular substance, and hippocampus (Fig. 1.28). Histochemically, these inclusions react as a protein-bound MPS. Similar amyloid material has been found in heart and liver (674). In the liver, the material causes cells to acquire a ground-glass appearance with eccentric nuclei and clear halos at their periphery. The cytoplasm contains PAS-positive basophilic material. Electron microscopy reveals short, branching filaments (675). Inclusions also are seen in eccrine sweat glands and muscle (676). Isolation and hydrolysis of organelles from the brain has shown them to consist of polyglucosan, a glucose polymer (linked in the 1:4 and 1:6 positions) chemically related to glycogen.

Lafora disease appears between ages 11 and 18 years with the onset of grand mal and myoclonic seizures. At first, the myoclonic seizures are triggered by photic stimulation or proprioceptive impulses and are much more frequent when formal tests of coordination are attempted, simulating the intention tremor of cerebellar ataxia. The EEG is usually abnormal, with generalized and focal and multifocal posterior epileptiform discharges (676). The interval between the bilateral sharp waves and the myoclonus is 15 ms in the upper extremities and 25 ms in the lower extremities, suggesting that cortical discharges and myoclonic seizures are secondary to a brainstem focus.

With progression of the disease, the major seizures become less frequent, myoclonus increases in intensity, and intellectual deterioration occurs. A terminal stage of dementia, spastic quadriparesis, and almost constant myoclonic seizures is reached within 4 to 10 years of the first symptoms.

The diagnosis of Lafora disease is confirmed by the characteristic polyglucosan storage material in muscle and in the sweat glands (obtained by skin biopsy). In liver, PAS-positive material is found in the extracellular spaces (677). Electron microscopy reveals a disrupted endoplasmic reticulum and large vacuoles containing electron-dense material (678). Storage material can be detected in liver before the appearance of neurologic symptoms (679).

No therapy has been found to arrest the progression of neurologic symptoms. The seizures are generally difficult if not impossible to control with anticonvulsants.

Unverricht-Lundborg Disease

Unverricht-Lundborg disease is an autosomal recessive disorder that tends to start somewhat earlier than Lafora disease. It manifests by myoclonic and generalized seizures and a slowly progressive intellectual deterioration. The condition is common in the Baltic region; in Finland, its incidence is 1 in 20,000 (676). The Baltic and Mediterranean forms of Unverricht-Lundborg disease are the consequence of a defect in the gene encoding cystatin B, one of several cysteine protein inhibitors whose function is to inactivate proteases that leak out of lysosomes. The gene has been localized to the long arm of chromosome 21 (21q22.3). In the majority of patients, the mutation is an unstable minisatellite repeat expansion in the promoter region of the cystatin B gene (680). A defect in another cysteine protein inhibitor, cystatin C, is responsible for hereditary cerebral amyloid angiopathy.

The pathologic picture of Unverricht-Lundborg disease is marked by neuronal loss and gliosis, particularly affecting the Purkinje cells the cerebellum, and cells in the medial thalamus and spinal cord.

The disorder becomes manifest between 6 and 16 years of age, with the mean age of onset 10 years of age. Stimulus-sensitive myoclonus initiates the disease in approximately one-half of the children, and tonic-clonic seizures initiates it in the remainder. Myoclonus is induced by maintenance of posture or initiation of movements. Myoclonus and seizures are difficult to control, and a slow and interfamily variable progression to ataxia and dementia occurs (670). The EEG shows progressive background slowing and 3- to 5-Hz spike wave or multiple spike wave activity. The temporal relationship between the electrical discharges and the myoclonus is variable. Marked photosensitivity and giant somatosensory-evoked potentials occur.

Treatment of myoclonus is difficult, and in many patients it is aggravated by phenytoin. The tonic-clonic seizures tend to respond to the usual anticonvulsant therapy, notably valproate, clonazepam, and lamotrigine. The use of *N*-acetylcysteine together with other antioxidants has been suggested by Hurd and colleagues. It may reduce the severity of the myoclonus and induce some normalization of the somatosensory-evoked potentials (681).

Myoclonic seizures also occur in idiopathic epilepsy and in a variety of degenerative diseases, most commonly the infantile and juvenile amaurotic idiocies. They also are found in the mitochondrial myopathies, sialidosis, and subacute sclerosing panencephalitis. Finally, dentatorubral atrophy (Ramsay Hunt syndrome) must be considered in the differential diagnosis of myoclonic seizures. As depicted by Hunt in 1921, the last is a progressive cerebellar ataxia accompanied by myoclonic seizures and atrophy of the dentate nucleus and superior cerebellar peduncles without the presence of amyloid bodies (see Chapter 2).

NEURONAL CEROID LIPOFUSCINOSES (BATTEN DISEASE)

Neuronal ceroid lipofuscinoses (NCL) are characterized by the accumulation of autofluorescent neuronal storage material within neuronal lysosomes, leading to neuronal death and cerebral atrophy. The various NCLs are differentiated according to the age at which neurologic symptoms first become evident, the ultrastructural morphology, and the genetic analysis. The major subtypes are the infantile form, first reported from Finland in 1973 by Santavuori and her associates (682), the late infantile form first described by Jansky in 1909 (683), and subsequently by Bielschowsky (684) and Batten (685), the juvenile form described by Spielmeyer (686), and the adult form first described by Kufs (687). All are transmitted in an autosomal recessive manner. Their relative frequencies in the clinical and pathologic series of Wisniewski and colleagues are as follows: infantile NCL, 11.3%; late infantile NCL (LINCL), 36.3%; juvenile NCL, 51.1%; and adult NCL, 1.3% (688). The molecular genetics of the various NCLs are outlined in Table 1.16.

Infantile Neuronal Ceroid Lipofuscinosis (Santavuori Disease, CLN1)

This condition was first reported in Finland in 1973 by Santavuori and associates (682). Its incidence in that country is 1 in 13,000, but the disease has been reported worldwide. The gene for infantile NCL has been localized to the short arm of chromosome 1 (1p32). It encodes a lysosomal enzyme, palmitoyl-protein thioesterase (689,689a).

The principal features of the illness include intellectual deterioration that becomes apparent between 9 and 19 months of age (later than the generalized GM_2 gangliosidoses), ataxia, myoclonic seizures, and visual failure, with a

TABLE 1.16. *Molecular genetics of the neuronal ceroid lipofuscinoses*

Clinical description	Ultrastructural characteristics	Location of gene	Gene defect	Reference
Infantile NCL (Santavuori)	Granular osmiophilic deposits	1p32	Palmitoyl-protein thioesterase (CLN1)	Das et al. (689)
Late infantile NCL (Jansky-Biel-schowsky)	Curvilinear bodies	11p15.5	Lysosomal pepstatin-insensitive carboxy peptidase (CLN2)	Sleat et al. (690)
Juvenile NCL (Spielmeyer-Vogt)	Fingerprint profiles, curvilinear bodies, granular osmiophilic deposits	16p12.1	Protein of unknown function (CLN3); also CNL1	Munroe et al. (691)
Adult NCL (Kufs)	Ceroid lipofuscin, curvilinear bodies	?	CLN4	International Batten Disease Consortium (693)
Finnish variant of late infantile NCL	Subunit c of mitochondrial adenosine triphosphate synthase	13q22	Transmembrane protein (CLN5)	Tyynela et al. (692) Savukoski (694)
Indian variant of late infantile NCL	Curvilinear bodies, finger print profiles	15q21-23	CLN6	Sharp et al. (695)

NCL, neuronal ceroid lipofuscinoses.

brownish pigmentation of the macula, hypopigmentation of the fundi, and optic atrophy (696). A retinal cherry-red spot is absent, but a pigmentary retinal degeneration is not unusual (697). Head growth ceases early, and in contrast to GM_2 gangliosidosis, most infants become microcephalic before age 24 months.

The EEG shows a progressive decrease in amplitude and an increased proportion of slow waves. Concurrently, a progressive loss of the ERG and the visual-evoked responses occur

(696,698). The MRI can be abnormal before the development of neurologic symptoms.

Pathologic examination shows the brain to be small with diffuse cortical atrophy. Microscopic examinations performed during the early stages of the illness show the neuronal cytoplasm to be slightly distended by granular, PAS-, and Sudan black–positive, autofluorescent material. On ultrastructural examination, this material consists of granular osmiophilic deposits (Fig. 1.29). It resembles ordinary lipofuscin, except

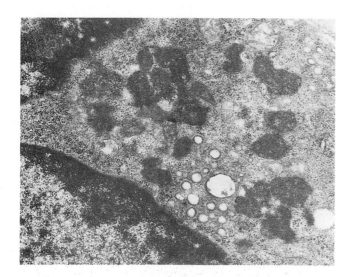

FIG. 1.29. Electron micrograph showing granular osmiophilic deposits in the cytoplasm of an eccrine clear cell. Biopsy of a 3-year-old child with blindness, dementia, and spastic quadriparesis, who began having seizures and myoclonus at age 15 months (×25,000). (Courtesy of Dr. Stirling Carpenter, Montreal Neurological Institute, Montreal, Canada.)

that the granules are far more uniform, and no associated lipid droplet component exists. Similar storage material can be found in approximately 20% of lymphocytes (699). Chemically, the storage material consists mainly of sphingosine activator proteins A and D. These are small lysosomal proteins that activate the various hydrolases required for the degradation of sphingolipids (511a). The relationship between the defect in the gene coding for palmitoyl-protein thioesterase and the accumulation of the sphingosine activator proteins is still unclear (692). As the disease progresses, a gradual and ultimately near total loss of cortical neurons occurs (696).

Late Infantile Neuronal Ceroid Lipofuscinosis (Late Infantile Amaurotic Idiocy, Jansky-Bielschowsky Disease, CLN2)

The onset of the clinical syndrome occurs later than that of the classic form of GM_2 gangliosidosis. The condition does not affect Jewish children predominantly, its progression is slower, and patients lack the usual retinal cherry-red spot. The gene for the condition has been mapped to the short arm of chromosome 11 (11p15.5). It encodes a lysosomal pepstatin-insensitive carboxypeptidase (690,700).

Late infantile NCL is characterized by normal mental and motor development for the first 24 years of life, although in many instances, slight clumsiness or a slowing in the acquisition of speech can be recalled retrospectively. The usual presenting manifestations are myoclonic or major motor seizures. Ataxia develops subsequently and is accompanied by a slowly progressive retinal degeneration, which is generally not obvious until the other neurologic symptoms have become well established. Visual acuity is decreased, and a florid degeneration occurs in the macular and perimacular areas. The macular light reflex is defective, and a fine brown pigment is deposited. The optic disc is pale. Photic stimulation at two or three flashes per second elicits high-amplitude polyphasic discharges at the time of the child's first seizure or within a few months thereafter (701). These abnormalities

have been noted even before the onset of neurologic symptoms.

The ERG is abnormal and is lost early in the course of the disease as a consequence of storage material in the rod and cone layer of the retina. This finding is in marked contrast to the preservation of the ERG in the GM_2 gangliosidoses in which retinal lipid storage is limited to the ganglion layer. The visual-evoked responses are also abnormal in that the early components are grossly enlarged (698). Marked spasticity, as well as a parkinsonian picture, can develop terminally. The condition progresses fairly slowly, and death does not occur until late childhood.

Laboratory studies have rarely shown an increase in CSF protein. CT scans and MRI show nonspecific changes with generalized atrophy most evident in the cerebellum (702). However, these studies distinguish the lipofuscinoses from the various leukodystrophies in which striking alterations of white matter occur.

Microscopic examination of the affected brain reveals generalized neuronal swelling of lesser amplitude than in generalized GM_2 gangliosidosis. The intraneuronal material stains with PAS and Sudan black, but, unlike the lipid stored in GM_2 gangliosidosis, it is nearly insoluble in lipid solvents and is invariably autofluorescent. The material is principally the hydrophobic mitochondrial ATP synthase subunit c, a normal component of the inner mitochondrial membrane (703). Sleat and coworkers have postulated this protein to be a substrate for the defective carboxypeptidase (690).

On ultrastructural examination, the storage material most commonly seen consists of curved stacks of lamellae with alternating dark and pale lines, the so-called curvilinear bodies (Fig. 1.30) (704). In a few cases, the storage material has a "fingerprint" configuration (Fig. 1.31), which is more typical of juvenile NCL. This designation is based on its appearance in groups of parallel lines, each pair separated by a thin lucent space. Some cases have only granular osmiophilic material (see Fig. 1.29). These different appearances of the storage material probably reflect differences in the genetic lesions in phenotypically similar patients, and mutations in CLNI gene have been documented in some of these cases (689a).

The stored material is distributed widely and is seen not only in neurons and astrocytes, but

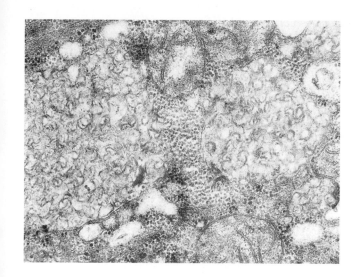

FIG. 1.30. Curvilinear body storage disease. Electron micrograph showing curvilinear bodies in an eccrine clear cell. Skin biopsy of a 4-year-old boy with seizures, myoclonus, and visual impairment, whose symptoms started at age 3 years (×50,000). (Courtesy of Dr. Stirling Carpenter, Montreal Neurological Institute, Montreal, Canada.)

also in Schwann cells, smooth and skeletal muscle, fibroblasts, and secretory cells in such organs as thyroid, pancreas, and eccrine sweat glands (704).

By electron microscopy, the material can be identified in biopsies of skin, skeletal muscle and conjunctivae, and peripheral lymphocytes, as well as in urinary sediment (705).

A variant of LINCL (CLN5) has been encountered in Finland, where it is a relatively common disease, with an incidence of 1 in 21,000 (706). The gene for this entity has been mapped to chromosome 13q22. It encodes a transmembrane protein of unknown function (696). The disease is marked by a somewhat later onset of symptoms (usually between 4 and

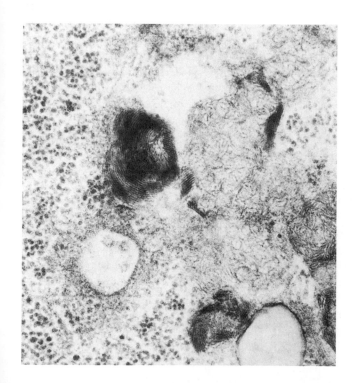

FIG. 1.31. "Fingerprint" profiles. Skin biopsy from a 5-year-old boy with a 6-month history of akinetic and myoclonic seizures and pigmentary retinal degeneration. Fingerprint profiles are present in sweat glands (×115,000). (Courtesy of Dr. Stirling Carpenter, Montreal Neurological Institute, Montreal, Canada.)

TABLE 1.17. *Clinical differentiation of the neuronal ceroid lipofuscinoses*

	Infantile (Santavuori) CLN1	Late infantile (Jansky-Bielschowsky) CLN2	Variant late infantile CLN5	Juvenile (Spielmeyer-Vogt) CLN3
Age at onset	9–19 mo	2–4 yr	5–7 yr	4–10 yr
Visual failure	Early	Late	Early	Early
Ataxia	Marked	Marked	Marked	Mild and late
Myoclonic seizures	Present	Present	Present	Occasional
Retinal pigment aggregation	Not seen	Rarely seen	Not seen	Invariable after 11–13 yr
Abnormal photic stimulation	Not seen	Positive early and persists	Develops late, disappears	Not seen
Visual-evoked potentials	Abolished early	Abnormal early and persists	Abnormal early, abolished later	Abolished early
Lymphocyte-electron microscopy	Granular amorphous inclusions	Inclusions with curvilinear bodies, fingerprint bodies	Negative	Vacuoles containing fingerprint bodies

Adapted from Santavuori P, et al. A variant of Jansky-Bielschowski disease. *Neuropediatrics* 1982;13:135–141. With permission.

7 years of age), early visual failure, a somewhat slower progression, and the presence of curvilinear and "fingerprint" storage material in all tissues but lymphocytes (Table 1.17).

Juvenile Neuronal Ceroid Lipofuscinosis (Juvenile Amaurotic Idiocy; Spielmeyer-Vogt Disease, CLN3)

Juvenile neuronal ceroid lipofuscinosis was first mentioned in 1893 by Freud (707), and subsequently by Spielmeyer (686) and Vogt (708). The gene for this condition has been localized to the long arm of chromosome 16 (16p12.1) (695). It encodes a membrane protein of as yet unknown function (689a,691). The most common genomic mutation involves a 1.02-kb deletion.

As described in the classic monographs, visual and intellectual deterioration first becomes apparent between 4 and 10 years of age. Funduscopic examination at that time reveals abnormal amounts of peripheral retinal pigmentation and early optic atrophy. In the majority of patients, seizures develop between the ages of 8 and 13 years (709). Loss of motor function becomes apparent subsequently. Ataxia and seizures are usually not seen; in the series of Järvelä and colleagues, extrapyramidal signs, notably parkinsonism, were seen during the second to third decade of life in approxi-

mately one-third of patients homozygous for the 1.02-kb deletion (709). Although many patients whose illness commences during the early school years follow this clinical pattern, variations do occur.

The EEG is generally abnormal in that it demonstrates large-amplitude slow wave and spike complexes, often without the photosensitivity noted in LINCL. The ERG is absent, even in the early stages of the illness, and the visual-evoked potentials lose their amplitude as the disease progresses. Large complexes such as are present in LINCL are not noted (700). The MRI shows mild to moderate atrophy (709).

Light microscopy reveals mild ballooning of cortical neurons, often with storage apparent in the initial segment of the axon. The cell is packed with PAS- and Sudan black–positive, autofluorescent material that is resistant to lipid solvents. Electron microscopy reveals inclusions consisting of prominent "fingerprint" formations (see Fig. 1.31). These also are seen in some cases of LINCL. They may be interspersed with poorly organized lamellar material, sometimes referred to as *rectilinear profiles*. These inclusions are thin stacks of lamellae with the same periodicity as curvilinear bodies, but more likely to be straight than curved (703). "Fingerprint" profiles also can be seen in a variety of other cell types throughout the body, but the extent of storage is considerably less than in LINCL, and much more variability is present from case to case and organ to organ. The "fingerprint" profiles are found regularly within eccrine sweat gland secretory cells and in some lymphocytes (710). In rare instances, clinically indistinguishable from the majority of juvenile NCL cases, the cytoplasmic inclusions are composed of granular osmiophilic material (see Fig. 1.29). Granular osmiophilic and fingerprint inclusions also have been seen in Kufs disease (CLN4), the adult form of NCL (711).

Biochemical studies on the storage material show the presence of the subunit c of the mitochondrial ATP synthase (692).

Several other NCLs have been described, and the heterogeneity of the various clinical entities has become fully apparent.

Diagnosis of the Ceroid Lipofuscinoses

The ceroid lipofuscinoses should be considered in the differential diagnosis of the infant or child who presents with seizures and loss of acquired milestones coupled with progressive visual impairment. The first step in the diagnostic process is an EEG, with emphasis on photic stimulation at 2-3 Hz. Curvilinear storage disease generally gives an exaggerated photic response. The visual-evoked potentials and ERGs also tend to be abnormal in these disorders. A lysosomal enzyme screen must be performed to exclude the majority of the lysosomal storage diseases. Imaging studies exclude the various white matter degenerations. The definitive diagnosis usually can be arrived at by a morphologic examination of readily available tissue, such as skin, conjunctiva, muscle, peripheral nerves, or lymphocytes. In all instances, electron microscopy and histochemical examinations are necessary for a diagnosis (see Table 1.17). On skin biopsy in children with LINCL, the curvilinear storage material is best seen in histiocytes and smooth muscle cells, but it can be found in virtually any cell type. In the other ceroid lipofuscinoses, examination of sweat glands is mandatory because other cell types are involved inconsistently (703); in the hands of some investigators, electron microscopic examination of muscle obtained on biopsy is equally reliable (712).

Rectal biopsy with its attendant discomfort is no longer indicated. When skin, conjunctiva, and muscle have failed to yield a diagnosis, a brain biopsy might have to be performed. This procedure has the advantage that histologic, histochemical, and ultrastructural studies can be combined with chemical analysis of the cerebral lipids. Generally, the presence of progressive intellectual deterioration can be considered sufficient incentive to suggest the procedure for prognostic and diagnostic purposes. Biopsies are usually taken from the frontal lobe. A single cube, at least 1.5 cm in dimension and including both gray and white matter, is removed and divided. One part is placed in 10% formalin-saline for histologic examination or is fixed in phosphate-buffered 5% glutaraldehyde for electron microscopy, whereas the other portion is frozen for chemical studies.

Human immunodeficiency virus encephalopathy is becoming an important cause for progressive intellectual deterioration. Although in most instances CNS involvement is preceded by bouts of systemic infection, this is not invariable. The condition is covered more fully in Chapter 6. Finally, despite its present rarity, juvenile paresis, caused by congenital syphilitic infection, which is often accompanied by retinal degeneration, must always be included in the differential diagnosis.

DISORDERS OF SERUM LIPOPROTEINS

Abetalipoproteinemia

Abetalipoproteinemia, an unusual disorder, was first described by Bassen and Kornzweig in 1950 (713). The main clinical manifestations include acanthocytosis (large numbers of burr-shaped erythrocytes) (Fig. 1.32), hypocholesterolemia, progressive combined posterior column degeneration, peripheral neuritis, mental retardation, retinitis pigmentosa, and steatorrhea. The disorder is transmitted in an autosomal recessive manner.

In the first year of life, infants develop a typical celiac syndrome with abdominal distention, diarrhea, foul-smelling stools, decreased fat absorption, and, occasionally, osteomalacia. The

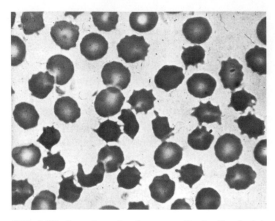

FIG. 1.32. Acanthocytes from a patient with abetalipoproteinemia. (From Wintrobe MM, et al. *Clinical hematology*, 8th ed. Philadelphia: Lea & Febiger, 1981. With permission.)

majority of affected infants are below the third percentile for height and weight. Neurologic symptoms are first noted between ages 2 and 17 years, and 33% of patients are symptom-atic before age 10 years. Commonly, the initial symptom is unsteadiness of gait. This is caused by a combination of ataxia, proprioceptive loss, and muscle weakness. Deep tendon reflexes are generally absent, and cutaneous sensory loss is often demonstrable (714). Extensor plantar responses are noted occasionally. Mental retardation has been seen in approximately 33% of patients (715). The retinal degeneration is accompanied by decreased visual acuity and night blindness. The ERG and the visual-evoked potentials are often abnormal even in the early stages of the disease. Somatosensory-evoked potentials were abnormal in some 40% of patients in the series of Brin and coworkers (716). Cardiac abnormalities, including irregularities of rhythm, are common.

Autopsy reveals extensive demyelination of the posterior columns and spinocerebellar tracts, and neuronal loss in the anterior horns, cerebellar molecular layer, and cerebral cortex (717). Ceroid and lipofuscin deposits are seen in muscle. They are similar to the inclusions in cystic fibrosis patients and probably reflect vitamin E deficiency (718).

Characteristic laboratory findings include low serum cholesterol (usually in the range of 20 to 50 mg/dL), low serum triglycerides (2 to 13 mg/dL), depressed total serum lipids (80 to 285 mg/dL), and vitamin E levels below 1.3 μg/mL, as contrasted with a normal range of 5 to 15 μg/mL (716,719).

As indicated by its name, the hallmark of the disease is the complete absence of serum β-lipoproteins. This in turn leads to an absence of all apolipoprotein β-containing lipoproteins (i.e., chylomicrons, very-low-density lipoproteins, and low-density lipoproteins).

In the majority of cases, the disease is caused by a defect in the gene that codes for the microsomal triglyceride transfer protein (720). This protein mediates the transfer of lipid molecules from their site of synthesis in the membranes of the endoplasmic reticulum to the nascent lipoprotein particles in the endoplasmic reticulum. In some cases, the lack of microsomal transfer protein could reflect its down-regulation in response to another more proximate defect, or could result from a defect in a factor that controls the concentration of microsomal transfer protein. The gene for apobetalipoprotein has been excluded as a cause for abetalipoproteinemia.

As a consequence of the absence of β-lipoproteins, fat absorption is deficient. Normally, ingestion of fat is followed by absorption of lipids by the mucosal cells, from which the lipids are released in the form of chylomicrons and discharged into the lymphatic system. In abetalipoproteinemia, no fat is detectable in the lymphatic spaces of the small bowel and no chylomicrons appear in the plasma after fat loading. This defect is consequent to a defect in lipid transport from the mucosal cells into the lymphatic system, β-lipoproteins apparently being necessary to form chylomicrons. Fat-soluble vitamins transported in chylomicrons are also poorly absorbed, resulting in the low serum levels of vitamins E and A.

Neurologic symptoms are probably the result of inadequate body stores of vitamin E, with resulting peroxidation of the unsaturated myelin phospholipids. In support of this hypothesis is the finding of a nearly identical neurologic picture when vitamin E deficiency results from chronic fat malabsorption, as is seen in cystic fibrosis and cholestatic liver disease (see Chapter 15).

Supplementation of the diet with vitamin E (100 mg/kg per day given orally) appears to prevent the development or progression of neurologic and retinal lesions. All children started on such high dosages of vitamin E before age 16 months have remained normal neurologically and developmentally up to at least 27 years of age (720,721). No evidence exists that intramuscular vitamin E is superior. In addition to vitamin E, current therapeutic regimens suggest administration of vitamin A (200 to 400 IU/kg per day) and vitamin K_1 (5 mg/day). Improvement of patients can best be followed by repeated somatosensory-evoked potentials (722).

The presence of low blood cholesterol should alert the clinician to abetalipoproteinemia. Low cholesterol also is seen in hypobetalipoproteinemia, malnutrition, and a variety of absorption defects.

The occurrence of acanthocytes in peripheral blood is not limited to abetalipoproteinemia. Acanthocytes are mature erythrocytes with many irregularly arranged spiny projections (see Fig. 1.32). They are best detected on a fresh blood smear using conventional light microscopy. A 1:1 saline dilution may reveal their presence when undiluted blood fails to show the cells. Acanthocytes occasionally have been seen in patients with anemia or advanced cirrhosis. It also has been present in patients with triglyceride hyperlipemia and in families with extrapyramidal movement disorders resembling Hallervorden-Spatz disease. Several other families have been reported in whom an extrapyramidal disorder (parkinsonism, chorea, vocal tics), motor neuron disease, areflexia, and mental retardation were associated with the presence of acanthocytes, but in whom serum lipids were normal (neuroacanthocytosis) (723,724). In most instances, the disease has its onset between 25 and 45 years of age. The gene for this autosomal recessive condition has been mapped to chromosome 9q2, but the molecular etiology is still unknown (725).

Several forms of hypobetalipoproteinemia have been recognized. In the majority of affected children or adolescents, neurologic symptoms are absent or are limited to a loss of deep tendon reflexes; in others, evidence exists for progressive demyelination, with ataxia, and mental deterioration (720). By contrast to abetalipoproteinemia, the defect in this condition has been localized to the gene coding for the apoprotein B. Treatment with vitamin E appears to arrest the progressive neurologic symptoms.

Tangier Disease (Hypoalphalipoproteinemia)

Tangier disease is a hereditary disorder of lipid metabolism distinguished by almost complete absence of high-density plasma lipoproteins, reduction of low-density plasma lipoproteins, cholesterol, and phospholipids, normal or elevated triglyceride levels, and storage of cholesterol esters in the reticuloendothelial system of the liver, spleen, lymph nodes, tonsils, and cornea. The name of the disease refers to an island in Chesapeake Bay, where the first two patients were found.

Symptoms usually are limited to enlargement of the affected organs, notably the tonsils. Retinitis pigmentosa and peripheral neuropathy have been observed (726). Peripheral neuropathy was noted in nearly 50% of the reported patients. Nerve biopsy reveals three different types of changes. One group had a multifocal demyelination with large amounts of neutral lipids within Schwann cells, particularly those associated with unmyelinated fibers. In another group (whose clinical manifestations include facial weakness, weakness of the small hand muscles, spontaneous pain and loss of pain and temperature sensations), no demyelination occurs, but lipid is deposited in Schwann cells. A third type is a distal sensory neuropathy (727). It is not clear whether lipid deposition follows fiber degeneration or represents a primary storage process of cholesterol esters. The nature of the metabolic disorder is under considerable investigation. Plasma contains reduced amounts of high-density lipoproteins that are similar but not identical to the normal lipoproteins. The two apoproteins of the high-density lipoproteins are also reduced. The gene has been mapped to chromosome 9q31, but the nature of the defect is still unknown (728). The most plausible explanation is a defect in the transfer of the high-density lipoproteins causing them to be diverted into the lysosomal compartment and degraded rather than being secreted (729).

DISORDERS OF METAL METABOLISM

Wilson Disease
(Hepatolenticular Degeneration)

Wilson disease is an autosomal recessive disorder of copper metabolism that is associated with cirrhosis of the liver and degenerative changes in the basal ganglia. The fact that, once diagnosed, Wilson disease is eminently treatable prompts a more extensive discussion than would otherwise be justified by the frequency of the disease.

During the second half of the nineteenth century, a condition termed *pseudosclerosis* was distinguished from multiple sclerosis by the lack of ocular signs. In 1902, Kayser observed green corneal pigmentation in one such patient (730); in 1903, Fleischer, who had also noted the green pigmentation of the cornea in 1903, commented on the association of the corneal rings with pseudosclerosis (731). In 1912, Wilson gave the classic description of the disease and its pathologic anatomy (732).

Because the derangement of copper metabolism is one of the important features of this condition, it is pertinent to review briefly the present knowledge of the field (733).

Copper homeostasis is an important biological process. By balancing intake and excretion, the body avoids copper toxicity on the one hand, and on the other hand ensures the availability of adequate amounts of the metal for a variety of vital enzymes, such as cytochrome oxidase and lysyl oxidase. The daily dietary intake of copper ranges between 1 and 5 mg. Healthy children consuming a free diet absorb 150 to 900 µg/day,

or approximately 40% of dietary copper (734). Cellular copper transport consists of three processes: copper uptake, intracellular distribution and use, and copper excretion.

The site of copper absorption is probably in the proximal portion of the gastrointestinal tract. The metallothioneines (MTs), a family of low-molecular-weight metal-binding proteins containing large amounts of reduced cysteine, are involved in regulating copper absorption at high copper intakes. In addition to playing a role in the intestinal transport of the metal, MTs are probably also involved in the initial hepatic uptake of copper. Two major isoforms of the protein exist, MT-I and MT-II. All MT genes have been mapped to the long arm of chromosome 16.

After its intestinal uptake, copper enters plasma, where it is bound to albumin in the form of cupric ion. Within 2 hours, the absorbed copper is incorporated into a liver protein. The concentration of the metal in normal liver ranges from 20 to 50 µg/g dry weight. In liver, copper is either excreted into bile, stored in liver lysosomes in what is probably a polymeric form of MT, or combined with apoceruloplasmin to form ceruloplasmin, which then enters the circulation. More than 95% of serum copper is in this form.

Ceruloplasmin is an α-globulin with a single continuous polypeptide chain and a molecular weight of 132 kd; it has six copper atoms per molecule. The protein has multiple functions. Although it is not involved in copper transport from the intestine, it is considered to be the major vehicle for the transport of the metal from the liver and to function as a copper donor in the formation of a variety of copper-containing enzymes. Ceruloplasmin controls the release of iron into plasma from cells, in which the metal is stored in the form of ferritin. It is also the most prominent serum antioxidant, and as such, it catalyses the oxidation of ferrous ion to ferric ion and prevents the oxidation of polyunsaturated fatty acids and similar substances. Finally, it modulates the inflammatory response and can regulate the concentration of various serum biogenic amines.

The concentration of ceruloplasmin in plasma is normally between 20 and 40 mg/dL. It is elevated in a variety of circumstances, including pregnancy or other conditions with high estrogen concentrations, infections, cirrhosis, malignancies, hyperthyroidism, and myocardial infarction. The concentration of ceruloplasmin is low in healthy infants up to approximately 2 months of age and in children experiencing a combined iron and copper deficiency anemia. In the nephrotic syndrome, low levels are caused by the vast renal losses of ceruloplasmin. Ceruloplasmin also is reduced in kinky hair disease (KHD; Menkes disease), a condition discussed in the subsequent section.

Several other copper-containing proteins have been isolated from mammalian tissues. Most prominently, these include the enzymes cytochrome c oxidase, dopamine β-hydroxylase, superoxide dismutase, and tyrosinase. None of these is altered in Wilson disease.

Molecular Genetics and Biochemical Pathology

Knowledge of disturbed copper metabolism in Wilson disease did not progress for more than three decades. In 1913, 1 year after Wilson report, Rumpel found unusually large amounts of copper in the liver of a patient with hepatolenticular degeneration (735). Although this finding was confirmed and an elevated copper concentration also was detected in the basal ganglia by Lüthy (736), the implication of these reports went unrecognized until 1945 when Glazebrook demonstrated abnormally high copper levels in serum, liver, and brain in a patient with Wilson disease (737). In 1952, 5 years after the discovery of ceruloplasmin, several groups of workers simultaneously found it to be low or absent in patients with Wilson disease. Although for many years it was believed that Wilson disease was caused by ceruloplasmin deficiency, it has become evident that absence of ceruloplasmin (aceruloplasminemia) results in a severe disorder of iron metabolism (738,739).

The gene for Wilson disease is located on the long arm of chromosome 13. It has been cloned and encodes a copper-transporting P-type ATPase that is expressed in liver and kidney (740). The ATPase is present in two forms: one is localized to the cellular trans-Golgi network where it is probably involved in the delivery of copper to apoceruloplasmin. The other form, probably representing a cleavage product, is found in mitochondria (741,741a). A large number of mutations have been characterized. Some are large deletions that completely destroy gene function and result in an early onset of symptoms; others that reduce but do not eliminate copper transport are consistent with a later onset of symptoms. Most patients are compound heterozygotes (742).

The genetic mutation induces extensive changes in copper homeostasis. Normally, the amount of copper in the body is kept constant through excretion of copper from the liver into bile. The two fundamental defects in Wilson disease are a reduced biliary transport and excretion of copper, and an impaired formation of plasma ceruloplasmin (743). Biliary excretion of copper is between 20% and 40% of normal, and fecal output of copper is reduced also (744). Because ceruloplasmin is present in the liver of patients with Wilson disease, a posttranslational defect appears to be responsible for the absence of ceruloplasmin from bile and serum.

Most important, copper accumulates within liver. At first, it is firmly bound to copper proteins, such as ceruloplasmin and superoxide dismutase, or is in the cupric form complexed with MT. When the copper load overwhelms the binding capacity of MT, cytotoxic cupric copper is released, causing damage to hepatocyte mitochondria and peroxisomes (745). Ultimately, copper leaks from liver into blood, where it is taken up by other tissues, including brain, which in turn are damaged by copper (746).

Several other abnormalities are consistently found in patients with Wilson disease, including low to low-normal levels of plasma iron-binding globulin. This abnormality occurs in the asymptomatic carrier and suggests that Wilson disease also may encompass a disorder of iron metabolism. This may result from the deficiency of hephaestin, a ceruloplasmin homologue, which has been implicated in intestinal iron transport and

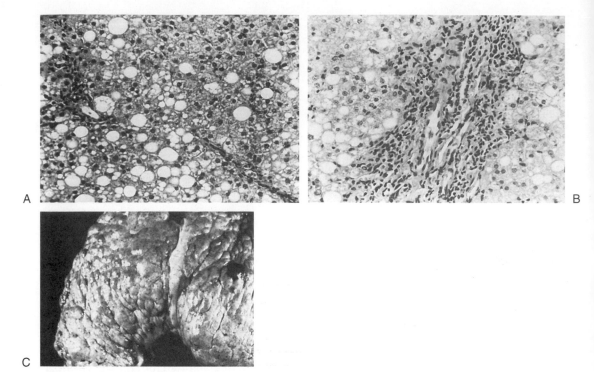

FIG. 1.33. Wilson disease. Morphologic alterations in liver. **A:** Needle biopsy specimen in a 6-year-old asymptomatic boy. Some of the earliest pathologic findings visible by light microscopy include hepatocytes of irregular appearance, with lipid droplets of varying sizes, prominent Kupffer cells, moderate cellular infiltrates, and a slender fibrous band. Liver copper: 1,158 µg/g dry weight (normal, 947 µg/g dry weight). **B:** More pronounced cellular infiltrate in another portion of the liver biopsy specimen in **A**. **C:** Liver showing nodular cirrhosis typical of the end stages of this condition. (From Scheinberg IH, Sternlieb I. *Wilson disease*. Philadelphia: Saunders, 1984. With permission.)

may be involved in the transfer of iron from tissue cells to plasma transferrin (746a).

Another abnormality consistently found in patients with Wilson disease is persistent aminoaciduria. This is most marked during the later stages but may be noted in some asymptomatic patients. The presence of other tubular defects (e.g., impaired phosphate resorption in patients without aminoaciduria) suggests that a toxic action of the metal on renal tubules causes the aminoaciduria.

Pathologic Anatomy

The abnormalities in copper metabolism result in a deposition of the metal in several tissues. In the brain, the largest proportion of copper is located in the subcellular soluble fraction, where it is bound not only to cerebrocuprein, but also to a number of other normal cerebral proteins. Anatomically, the liver shows a focal necrosis that leads to a coarsely nodular, postnecrotic cirrhosis. The nodules vary in size and are separated by bands of fibrous tissues of different widths (Fig. 1.33C). Some hepatic cells are enlarged and contain fat droplets, intranuclear glycogen, and clumped pigment granules; other cells are necrotic with regenerative changes in the surrounding parenchyma (see Fig. 1.32) (747).

Electron microscopic studies indicate that copper is initially spread diffusely within cytoplasm, probably as the monomeric MT complex.

Later in the course of the disease, the metal is sequestered within lysosomes, which become increasingly sensitive to rupture (Fig. 1.34) (746). Copper probably initiates and catalyses oxidation of the lysosomal membrane lipids, resulting in lipofuscin accumulation. Within the kidneys, the tubular epithelial cells can degenerate, and their cytoplasm can contain copper deposits.

In the brain, particularly in patients whose symptoms commenced before the onset of puberty, the basal ganglia show the most striking alterations. They have a brick-red pigmentation; spongy degeneration of the putamen frequently leads to the formation of small cavities (732). Microscopic studies reveal a loss of neurons, axonal degeneration, and large numbers of protoplasmic astrocytes, including giant forms termed *Alzheimer cells*. These cells are not specific for Wilson disease; they also can be seen in the brains of patients dying in hepatic coma or as a result of argininosuccinic aciduria or other disorders of the ammonia cycle. Opalski cells, also seen in Wilson disease, are generally found in gray matter. They are large cells with a rounded contour and finely granular cytoplasm. They probably represent degenerating astrocytes. In approximately 10% of patients, cortical gray matter and white matter are more affected than the basal ganglia. Here, too, extensive spongy degeneration and proliferation of astrocytes is seen (748). Copper is deposited in the pericapillary area and within astrocytes, but it is uniformly absent from neurons and ground substance.

Lesser degenerative changes are seen in the brainstem, dentate nucleus, substantia nigra, and convolutional white matter. Copper also is found throughout the cornea, particularly the substantia propria, where it is deposited in an alcohol-soluble, and probably chelated, form. In the periphery, the metal appears in granular clumps close to the endothelial surface of Descemet membrane. Here, the deposits are responsible for the appearance of the Kayser-Fleischer rings. The color of the Kayser-Fleischer ring varies from yellow to green to brown. Copper deposition in this area occurs in two or more layers, with particle size and distance

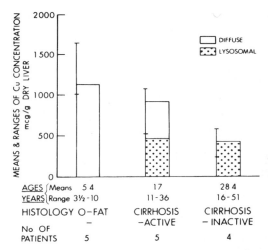

FIG. 1.34. Mean values and ranges of hepatic copper concentrations in patients with Wilson disease, grouped according to age and stage of disease (mean age, 5.4 years). Asymptomatic children with minimal histologic abnormalities (mean age, 17 years). Adolescents and young adults with active liver disease (mean age, 28.4 years). Adults with neurologic symptoms of Wilson disease and inactive cirrhosis. The height of the bar graph indicates the concentration of copper in each group. A striking decrease is seen with advancing age and progression of the disease, and the intracellular distribution of copper changes from its diffuse cytoplasmic distribution in the hepatocytes of children to its lysosomal concentration in the hepatocytes of patients with advanced disease. (From Scheinberg IH, Sternlieb I. *Wilson disease*. Philadelphia: Saunders, 1984. With permission.)

between layers influencing the ultimate appearance of the ring (749).

Clinical Manifestations

Wilson disease is a progressive condition with a tendency toward temporary clinical improvement and arrest (746). It is transmitted in an autosomal recessive manner with a high rate of consanguinity in parents of affected children. The condition occurs in all races, with a particularly high incidence in Eastern European Jews, in Italians from southern Italy and

Sicily, and in people from some of the smaller islands of Japan—groups with a high rate of inbreeding.

In a fair number of cases, primarily in young children, initial symptoms can be hepatic, such as jaundice or portal hypertension, and the disease can assume a rapidly fatal course without any detectable neurologic abnormalities (750,751). In many of these patients, an attack of what appears to be an acute viral hepatitis heralds the onset of the illness (752). The presentation of Wilson disease with hepatic symptoms is common among affected children in the United States. In the series of Werlin and associates, who surveyed patients in the Boston area, the primary mode of presentation was hepatic in 61% of patients younger than age 21 years (753). In approximately 10% of affected children in the United States, Wilson disease presents as an acute or intermittent, Coombs-test-negative, nonspherocytic anemia that is accompanied by leukopenia and thrombocytopenia (753).

When neurologic symptoms predominate, the appearance of the illness is delayed until 10 to 20 years of age, and the disease progresses at a slower rate than in the hepatic form. The youngest reported child with cerebral manifestations of Wilson disease was 4 years old. The first signs are usually bulbar; these can include indistinct speech and difficulty in swallowing. A rapidly progressive dystonic syndrome is not unusual when the disease presents in childhood. Such patients can present with acute dystonia, rigidity, and fever, with an occasional elevation of serum creatine phosphokinase (754).

In the experience of Arima and his group, 33% of children presented with hepatic symptoms, mainly jaundice or ascites (750). They were 4 to 12 years old at the time of medical attention. Cerebral symptoms, notably dystonia, drooling, or gait disturbances, were the presenting symptoms in 30% of children. These patients were 9 to 13 years of age. The remainder had a mixed hepatocerebral picture and were 6 to 12 years old at the time of medical attention. Minor intellectual impairment or emotional disturbances also can be observed, but seizures or mental deterioration are not prominent features of the disease.

Before long, the patient has a characteristic appearance. A fixed smile is a result of retraction of the upper lip; the mouth hangs open and drools. Speech is often severely impaired. Tremors are usually quite marked. Though they often are unilateral during the early stages of the disease, sooner or later they become generalized. The tremors are present at rest, but become exaggerated with movements and emotional disturbance. Initially fine, they gradually become coarse as the illness progresses until they assume a characteristic "wing-beating" appearance. Rigidity, contractures, and tonic spasms advance steadily and can involve the extremities. Dementia can be severe in some patients, whereas other patients are merely emotionally labile. A nearly pure parkinsonlike syndrome and progressive choreoathetosis or hemiplegia also have been described. In essence, Wilson disease is a disorder of motor function; despite often widespread cerebral atrophy, no sensory symptoms or reflex alterations occur.

Without treatment, death ensues within 1 to 3 years of the onset of neurologic symptoms and is usually a result of hepatic insufficiency.

The intracorneal, ring-shaped pigmentation, first noted by Kayser and Fleischer, might be evident to the naked eye or might appear only with slit-lamp examination. The ring can be complete or incomplete and is present in 75% of children who present with hepatic symptoms, and in all children who present with cerebral or a combination of cerebral and hepatic symptoms (750). The Kayser-Fleischer ring can antedate overt symptoms of the disease and has been detected even in the presence of normal liver functions. In the large clinical series of Arima, it was never present before 7 years of age (750). "Sunflower" cataracts are less commonly encountered.

CT scans usually reveal ventricular dilatation and diffuse atrophy of the cortex, cerebellum, and brainstem. Approximately one-half of the patients have hypodense areas in the thalamus and basal ganglia. Increased density owing to copper deposition is not observed. Generally, MRI correlates better with clinical symptoms than CT. It demonstrates abnormal signals (hypointense on T1-weighted images and hyperintense on T2-weighted images) most commonly in the putamen, thalami, and the head of the caudate nucleus. The midbrain is also abnormal, as is the pons and cerebellum. Cortical atrophy and focal lesions in cortical white matter also are noted. Correlation with clinical symptoms is not good in that patients with neurologic symptoms can have normal MRI results, and other subjects with no neurologic symptoms can have abnormal MRI results (755,756). PET demonstrates a widespread depression of glucose metabolism, with the greatest focal hypometabolism in the lenticular nucleus. This abnormality precedes any alteration seen on CT scan (757).

Diagnosis

When Wilson disease presents with neurologic manifestations, some of the diagnostic features are the progressive extrapyramidal symptoms commencing after the first decade of life, abnormal liver function, aminoaciduria, cupriuria, and absent or decreased ceruloplasmin. The presence of a Kayser-Fleischer ring is the single most important diagnostic feature; its absence in a child with neurologic symptoms rules out the diagnosis of Wilson disease. The ring is not seen in the majority of presymptomatic patients, nor is it seen in 15% of children in whom Wilson disease presents with hepatic symptoms (752).

An absent or low serum ceruloplasmin level is of lesser diagnostic importance; some 5% to 20% of patients with Wilson disease have normal levels of the copper protein. In affected families, the differential diagnosis between heterozygotes and presymptomatic homozygotes is of utmost importance, inasmuch as it is generally accepted that presymptomatic homozygotes should be treated preventively (758).

The presymptomatic child with Wilson disease can have a Kayser-Fleischer ring (seen in 33% of presymptomatic patients in Walshe series), an increased 24-hour urine copper level (greater than 100 µg/24 hours), hepatosplenomegaly (seen in 38%), and abnormal neuroimaging (seen in approximately one-fourth).

Approximately one-half of the patients with presymptomatic Wilson disease had no physical findings, and urinary copper excretion can be normal in children younger than the age of 15 years. Should the diagnosis in a child at risk still be in doubt, an assay of liver copper is indicated (758). Low ceruloplasmin levels in an asymptomatic family member only suggest the presymptomatic stage of the disease; some 10% of heterozygotes have ceruloplasmin levels below 15 mg/dL. Because gene carriers account for approximately 1% of the population, gene carriers with low ceruloplasmin values are seen 40 times more frequently than patients with Wilson disease and low ceruloplasmin values. Therefore, when low ceruloplasmin levels are found on routine screening and are unaccompanied by any abnormality of hepatic function or copper excretion, the subject is most likely a heterozygote for Wilson disease (746).

When a liver biopsy has been decided on, histologic studies with stains for copper and copper-associated proteins and chemical quantitation for copper are performed. In all confirmed cases of Wilson disease, hepatic copper is greater than 3.9 µmol/g dry weight (237.6 µg/g) as compared with a normal range of 0.2 to 0.6 µmol/g. Because of the large number of mutations causing the disease, a combination of mutation and linkage analysis is required for prenatal diagnosis. As a rule, this technique is not useful in the diagnosis of an individual patient. However, about one-third of North American Wilson disease patients have a point mutation (His 1069 Glu), and screening for this mutation can be performed readily (758a).

Wilson disease is one of a number of metabolic diseases that can present with extrapyramidal signs and symptoms. These conditions and the best means of diagnosing them are listed in Table 1.18.

Treatment

All patients with Wilson disease, whether symptomatic or asymptomatic, require treatment. The aims of treatment are initially to remove the toxic amounts of copper and secondarily to prevent tissue reaccumulation of the metal (759,760).

TABLE 1.18. *Genetic metabolic diseases presenting with basal ganglia signs*

Disease	Diagnostic tests
Dihydropteridine reductase deficiency	Blood phenylalanine
Dihydrobiopterine synthetase deficiency	Blood phenylalanine
Propionic acidemia	Urinary organic acids
Nonketotic hyperglycinemia	Blood amino acids
Glutaric aciduria type I	Urine organic acids
Mucolipidosis type IV	Conjunctival biopsy
Salla disease	Urinary sialic acid
GM_1 gangliosidosis, juvenile	Conjunctival biopsy
GM_2 gangliosidosis	Conjunctival biopsy
Niemann-Pick disease type C (juvenile dystonic lipidosis)	Bone marrow aspirate
Neuroacanthocytosis	Blood smear
Wilson disease	Ceruloplasmin, slit-lamp, urinary Cu
Wilson disease variant	Serum copper
Kinky hair disease variant	Serum copper
Lesch-Nyhan disease	Urinary uric acid
Creatine deficiency syndrome	Magnetic resonance spectroscopy of brain
Cystinosis	Bone marrow aspiration

Treatment can be divided into two phases: the initial phase, when toxic copper levels are brought under control, and maintenance therapy. No agreed on regimen exists for the treatment of the new patient with neurologic or psychiatric symptoms. In the past, most centers recommended starting patients on D-penicillamine (600 to 3,000 mg per day). Although this drug is effective in promoting urinary excretion of copper, adverse reactions during the initial and maintenance phases of treatment are seen in approximately 25% of patients. These include worsening of neurologic symptoms during the initial phases of treatment, which frequently is irreversible. Skin rashes, gastrointestinal discomfort, and hair loss are encountered also. During maintenance therapy, one may see polyneuropathy, polymyositis, and nephropathy. Some of these adverse effects can be prevented by giving pyridoxine (25 mg per day).

Because of these side effects, many institutions now advocate initial therapy with ammonium tetrathiomolybdate (60 to 300 mg per day, administered in six divided doses, three with meals and three between meals). Tetrathiomolybdate forms a complex with protein and copper and when given with food blocks the absorption of copper. The major drawback to using this drug is that it still has not been approved for general use in this country.

Triethylene tetramine dihydrochloride (trientine) (250 mg four times a day, given at least 1 hour before or 2 hours after meals) is also a chelator that increases urinary excretion of copper. Its effectiveness is less than that of penicillamine, but the incidence of toxicity and hypersensitivity reactions is lower.

Zinc acetate (50 mg of elemental zinc acetate three times a day) acts by inducing intestinal MT, which has a high affinity for copper and prevents its entrance into blood. Zinc is far less toxic than penicillamine but is much slower acting. Diet does not play an important role in the management of Wilson disease, although Brewer recommends restriction of liver and shellfish during the first year of treatment (760).

Zinc is the optimal drug for maintenance therapy and for the treatment of the presymptomatic patient. Trientine in combination with zinc acetate has been suggested for patients who present in hepatic failure. Liver transplantation can be helpful in the patient who presents in end-stage liver disease. The procedure appears to correct the metabolic defect and can reverse neurologic symptoms (763).

With these regimens, gradual improvement in neurologic symptoms occurs. As a rule, brainstem auditory-evoked potentials improve within 1 month of the onset of therapy, with the somatosensory-evoked responses being somewhat slower to return to normal (761). The Kayser-Fleischer ring begins to fade within 6 to 10 weeks of the onset of therapy and disappears completely in a couple of years (762). Improvement of neurologic symptoms starts 5 to 6 months after therapy has begun and is generally complete in 24 months. As shown by serial neuroimaging studies, a significant regression of lesions occurs within thalamus and basal ganglia (755). Successive biopsies show a reduction in the amount of hepatic copper. Total serum copper and ceruloplasmin levels decrease, and the aminoaciduria and phosphaturia diminish. Evoked potentials also have been used to assess the response to treatment.

As a rule, patients who are started on therapy before the evolution of symptoms remain healthy. Children who have had hepatic disease exclusively do well, and in 80%, hepatic functions return to normal. Approximately 40% of children who present with neurologic symptoms become completely asymptomatic and remain so for 10 or more years. Children with the mixed hepatocerebral picture do poorly. Less than 25% recover completely, and approximately 25% continue to deteriorate, often with the appearance of seizures. In all forms of the disease, the earlier the start of therapy, the better the outlook (750).

When symptom-free patients with Wilson disease discontinue chelation therapy, their hepatic function deteriorates in 9 months to 3 years, a rate that is far more rapid than deterioration after birth (764). Scheinberg and coworkers postulate that penicillamine not only removes copper from tissue but also detoxifies the metal by inducing MT synthesis (765).

Several variants of Wilson disease have been recognized. One type begins in adolescence and is marked by progressive tremor, dysarthria, disturbed eye movements, and dementia. It is characterized biochemically by low serum copper and ceruloplasmin. Kayser-Fleischer rings are absent, and liver copper concentrations are low. Metabolic studies using labeled copper suggest a failure in copper absorption from the lower gut (766).

In another type, the patient developed extrapyramidal movements, but no liver disease. Kayser-Fleischer rings were not present. Blood copper levels were low, but hepatic copper was markedly elevated, with the metal stored in cytoplasm (767).

In familial apoceruloplasm in deficiency, the clinical presentation is with dementia, retinal degeneration, and a variety of movement disorders (739). MRI and neuropathologic examinations demonstrate iron deposition in the basal ganglia. The clinical and pathologic findings confirm the essential role of ceruloplasmin in iron metabolism and in brain iron homeostasis. The relationship between this condition and Hallervorden-Spatz syndrome is unclear.

Kinky Hair Disease (Menkes Disease)

This focal degenerative disorder of gray matter was described in 1962 by Menkes and associates (768). It is transmitted as an X-linked disorder.

Molecular Genetics and Biochemical Pathology

The characteristic feature of KHD, as expressed in the human infant, is a maldistribution of body copper, so that it accumulates to abnormal levels in a form or location that renders it inaccessible for the synthesis of various copper enzymes (769). Most of the clinical manifestations can be explained by the low activities of the various copper-containing enzymes. Patients absorb little or no orally administered copper; when the metal is given intravenously, they experience a prompt increase in serum copper and ceruloplasmin (770). Copper levels are low in liver and brain, but are elevated in several other tissues, notably intestinal mucosa, muscle, spleen, and kidney. The copper content of cultured fibroblasts, myotubes, or lymphocytes derived from patients with KHD is several times greater than control cells; however, the kinetics of copper uptake are normal (771). Excess copper is bound to MT, which is present in increased amounts.

The gene for KHD has been mapped to Xq13.3 and codes for a P-type ATPase. This enzyme is expressed in most tissues, including brain, but not in liver. The ATPase is one of a family of membrane proteins that transports cations across plasma and endoplasmic reticulum membranes, and which in KHD is believed to be involved in the transport of copper out of cells (772). At basal copper levels the protein is located in the trans-Golgi network, the sorting station for proteins exiting from the Golgi apparatus where it is involved in copper uptake into its lumen. At increased intra- and extracellular copper concentrations the MNK protein shifts towards the plasma membrane, presumably to enhance removal of excess copper from the cell (772a). Numerous mutations have been recognized, and it appears as if almost every family has its own private mutation.

As a consequence of the defect in the transport protein, copper becomes inaccessible for the synthesis of ceruloplasmin, superoxide dismutase, and a variety of other copper-containing enzymes, notably ascorbic acid oxidase, cytochrome oxidase, dopamine β-hydroxylase, and lysyl oxidase.

Because of the defective activity of these metalloenzymes, a variety of pathologic changes are set into motion. Arteries are tortuous, with irregular lumens and a frayed and split intimal lining. These abnormalities reflect a failure in elastin and collagen cross-linking caused by dysfunction of the key enzyme for this process, copper-dependent lysyl oxidase.

Changes within the brain result from vascular lesions, copper deficiency, or a combination of the two. Extensive focal degeneration of gray matter occurs, with neuronal loss and gliosis and an associated axonal degeneration in white matter. Cellular loss is prominent in the cerebellum. Here, Purkinje cells are hard hit; many are lost, and others show abnormal dendritic arborization (*weeping willow*) and perisomatic processes. Focal axonal swellings (*torpedoes*) are observed also (768,773). Electron microscopy often shows a marked increase in the number of mitochondria in the perikaryon of Purkinje cells, and to a lesser degree in the neurons of cerebral cortex and the basal ganglia (774). Mitochondria are enlarged, and intramitochondrial electron-dense bodies are present. The pathogenesis of these changes is a matter of controversy, but they are believed to result from a reduction in the activity of the mitochondrial, copper-containing enzymes.

Clinical Manifestations

KHD is not a rare disorder; its frequency has been estimated at 1 in 114,000 to 1 in 250,000 live births (774). Baerlocher and Nadal have provided a comprehensive review of the clinical features (775). Symptoms appear during the neonatal period. Most commonly, hypothermia, poor feeding, and impaired weight gain are observed. Seizures soon become apparent. Marked hypotonia, poor head control, and progressive deterioration of all neurologic function are seen. The facies has a cherubic appearance with a depressed nasal bridge and reduced movements (776). The optic discs are pale, and microcysts of the pigment epithelium are seen (777). The most striking finding is the appearance of the scalp hair; it is colorless and friable. Examination under the microscope reveals a variety of abnormalities, most often pili torti (twisted hair) and trichorrhexis nodosa (fractures of the hair shaft at regular intervals) (768).

Radiography of long bones reveals metaphyseal spurring and a diaphyseal periosteal reaction, reminiscent of scurvy (778). On MR arteriography, the cerebral vessels are markedly elongated and tortuous. Similar changes are seen in the systemic vasculature (779). The urinary tract is not spared. Hydronephrosis, hydroureter, and bladder diverticula are common (780).

Neuroimaging discloses cerebral atrophy and cortical areas of encephalomalacia. A progressive tortuosity and enlargement of intracranial vessels also can be shown by MRI (781). Asymptomatic subdural hematomas are almost invariable. EEGs show multifocal paroxysmal discharges or hypsarrhythmia. Visual-evoked potentials are of low amplitude or completely absent (782).

The course is usually inexorably downhill, but the rate of neurologic deterioration varies, considerably. The author of this chapter has seen a patient in his 20s, and numerous patients have been reported, whose clinical manifestations are less severe than those seen in the classic form of KHD, and it appears likely that a continuum in disease severity exists. One of the most important variants is occipital horn syndrome. As originally described, this condition is characterized by occipital exostoses, which appear as bony horns on each side of the foramen magnum, cutis laxa, and bladder diverticula (783). Lysyl oxidase, a copper enzyme, is severely deficient. In some families, the clinical manifestations combine those of occipital horn syndrome and KHD (783).

Diagnosis

The clinical history and the appearance of the infant should suggest the diagnosis. Serum ceruloplasmin and copper levels are normally low in the neonatal period and do not reach adult levels until 1 month of age. Therefore, these determinations must be performed serially to demonstrate a failure of the expected increase. The diagnosis can best be confirmed by demonstrating the intracellular accumulation of copper and decreased efflux of Cu^{64} from cultured fibroblasts (784). The increased copper content of chorionic villi has been used for first-trimester diagnosis of the disease (784). These analyses require considerable expertise, and few centers can perform them reliably.

In heterozygotes, areas of pili torti constitute between 30% and 50% of the hair. Less commonly, skin depigmentation is present. Carrier detection by measuring the accumulation of radioactive copper in fibroblasts is possible, but is not very reliable (784). The full neurodegenerative disease, accompanied by chromosome X/2 translocation, has been encountered in girls (785).

Trichorrhexis nodosa also can be seen not only in argininosuccinic aciduria, but in a number of other conditions that result in a structural abnormality of the hair shaft. A condition characterized by short stature, ataxia, mental retardation, ichthyosis, and brittle hair and nails with low sulfur content has been termed *tricho-*

thiodystrophy (786). Approximately one-half of the patients have photosensitivity. Several genetically distinct entities are probably included in this group, with some having a defect in the nucleotide-excision repair gene (786). Other disorders in the hair shaft are reviewed in conjunction with photographs of their microscopic appearance in an article by Whiting (787).

Treatment

Copper supplementation, using daily injections of copper-histidine, appears to be the most promising treatment. Parenterally administered copper corrects the hepatic copper deficiency and restores serum copper and ceruloplasmin levels to normal. The effectiveness of treatment in arresting or reversing neurologic symptoms probably depends on whether some activity of the copper-transporting enzyme has been preserved, and whether copper supplementation has been initiated promptly (784,788). Therefore, it is advisable to commence copper therapy as soon as the diagnosis is established and to continue therapy until it becomes evident that cerebral degeneration cannot be arrested.

Molybdenum Cofactor Deficiency

Three enzymes require molybdenum for their function: sulfite oxidase, xanthine dehydrogenase, and aldehyde oxidase. An autosomal recessive disorder marked by intractable seizures, often starting in the neonatal period, severe developmental delay, and multiple cerebral infarcts results from a deficiency of the molybdenum cofactor (789). The gene for the disease has been mapped to the short arm of chromosome 6 (790). Molybdenum cofactor deficiency can be suspected by elevated serum lactate levels, low serum and urinary uric acid, and increased urinary sulfite. A dipstick test (Merckoguant, Merck, Darmstadt, Germany) applied to fresh urine detects the presence of sulfites (790a). Treatment with dietary restriction of methionine has been attempted (791). Isolated sulfite oxidase deficiency also results in a profound developmental delay, hypotonia, and seizures, which generally start in the neonatal period. Dislocated lenses are apparent in some cases (792,793).

DISORDERS OF PURINE AND PYRIMIDINE METABOLISM

Lesch-Nyhan Syndrome

The occurrence of hyperuricemia in association with spasticity and severe choreoathetosis was first reported by Catel and Schmidt in 1959 (794). Since then, the disease has been observed in all parts of the world. It is transmitted as an X-linked disorder, with the gene mapped to Xq26-q27.2 (795).

Molecular Genetics and Biochemical Pathology

The structure of the gene whose defect is responsible for Lesch-Nyhan syndrome has been elucidated. It codes for the enzyme hypoxanthine guanine phosphoribosyltransferase (HGPRT), which is defective in this condition. More than 100 mutations have been recorded to date; some 85% of these are point mutations or small deletions (796). The same mutation is encountered rarely in unrelated subjects (797). As a consequence of the genetic mutation, HGPRT activity is reduced to less than 0.5% of normal in a number of tissues, including erythrocytes and fibroblast cultures.

Because of HGPRT deficiency, hypoxanthine cannot be reused, and whatever hypoxanthine is formed is either excreted or catabolized to xanthine and uric acid. Additionally, phosphoribosylpyrophosphate, a known regulator of de novo purine synthesis, is increased. For these reasons, de novo uric acid production is increased markedly, and serum urine and CSF uric acid levels are elevated. The excretion of other purines, such as xanthine and hypoxanthine, is increased also (798).

The mechanism by which the neurologic disorder is induced is still unclear, although an abnormality in the dopaminergic system has been well documented. In basal ganglia, notably in the terminal-rich regions of the caudate, putamen, and nucleus accumbens septi, the dopamine concentration is reduced, as are the activities of dopa decarboxylase and tyrosine hydroxylase. Such findings point to a functional loss of a significant proportion of nigrostriatal and mesolimbic dopamine tracts. Using a ligand that binds to dopamine transporters, Wong and coworkers have shown a reduction in the density of dopamine-containing neurons (799). A reduced dopamine turnover also is indicated by abnormally low CSF homovanillic acid. A reduction in norepinephrine turnover and a diminution in the function of the striatal cholinergic neurons also have been documented. These alterations of the normal neurotransmitter balance within basal ganglia could account for the movement disorder characteristic of Lesch-Nyhan syndrome (800). Based on animal data, it has been postulated that the self-injurious behavior that is so characteristic of the condition is the consequence of destruction of dopaminergic fibers early in development, and subsequent exposure to dopamine agonists (796). Uric acid itself appears not to be directly involved in producing the neurologic disorder; more likely it is a toxic substance accumulating as a consequence of the enzymatic defect.

As would be expected from the Lyon hypothesis, the heterozygote female subject has two cell populations, one with full enzymatic activity and the other enzyme deficient. Heterozygotes can be ascertained by determining HGPRT activity in hair follicles.

Pathologic Anatomy

The morphologic alterations seen in the brain are sparse and can be explained by the uremia, which is often present terminally (801). The dopamine-producing cells in the substantia nigra appear grossly unaffected. Chemical analyses show marked reductions in dopamine and homovanillic acid content and tyrosine hydroxylase and dopa decarboxylase activity (796).

Clinical Manifestations

Affected children appear healthy at birth, and initial gross motor milestones are achieved appropriately. During the first year of life, psychomotor retardation becomes evident. Extrapyramidal movements appear between 8 and 24 months of age and persist until obliterated by progressive spasticity. Seizures occur in approximately 50% of the patients. A curious and unexplained feature of the disease is the invol-

TABLE 1.19. *Disorders of purine and pyrimidine metabolism with neurologic phenotypes*

Disorder	Biochemical abnormality	Clinical manifestations
Lesch-Nyhan (HGPTR deficiency)	Elevated urine uric acid	Extrapyramidal disorder, self-mutilation
Phosphoribosylpyrophosphate synthase superactivity	Elevated urine uric acid	Developmental delay, ataxia, sensori-neural deafness (807)
Adenosine monophosphate deaminase deficiency 1 (myoadenylate deaminase)	Decreased lactate formation on ischemic forearm test	Hypotonia, exertional myalgia, poor exercise tolerance or no symptoms (812,813)
Purine nucleotide phosphorylase deficiency	Elevated urine/plasma inosine, guanosine	T-cell immunodeficiency, cerebral vasculopathy, strokes (811)
Adenylosuccinate lyase (Adenyl Sucoinase) deficiency	Succinyl adenosine, succinyl-aminoimidazole carboxamide ribotide elevated in plasma, urine, CSF	Severe mental retardation, seizures, autistic features (808,814)
Uridine monophosphate syn-thase deficiency	Orotic acid elevation in urine	Mental retardation (815)
Dihydropyrimidine dehydrogenase deficiency	Increased excretion of uracil, thymine, 5-hydroxymethyluracil	Mental retardation, adverse reaction to 5-fluorouracil (809)
Dihydropyrimidinase deficiency	Increased excretion of uracil, thymine	Dysmorphic features, intractable seizures, severe developmental delay (810)

CSF, cerebrospinal fluid; HGPTR, hypoxanthine guanine phosphoribosyl transferase.

untary self-destructive biting of fingers, arms, and lips, which becomes apparent by 4 years of age. Children are disturbed by their compulsion to self-mutilation and are happier when maintained in restraints. Hematuria and renal calculi are seen in the majority of individuals, and ultimately renal failure develops. Gouty arthritis and urate tophi are also late complications. A megaloblastic anemia is common. Intellectual levels range from moderate mental retardation to low average (802). In later years, a large proportion of patients develop vocal tics, reminiscent of those seen in Tourette disease.

Numerous variants of the condition have been recognized. In one such variant, a partial enzyme deficiency leads to excessive uric acid production, gouty arthritis, and mild neurologic symptoms, most commonly a spinocerebellar syndrome (803). In another variant, partial HGPRT deficiency is accompanied by mild mental retardation, short stature, and spasticity (796,804).

Diagnosis

The features of the illness, in particular self-mutilation and extrapyramidal movements, make a diagnosis possible on clinical grounds. Although serum uric acid is usually elevated, diagnosis is best confirmed from the urinary uric acid content, a urinary uric acid to creatine ratio of 3 to 1 or higher being almost diagnostic (796). Enzymatic analyses of lysed erythrocytes, cultured skin fibroblasts, cultured amniotic fluid cells, or other tissue are easily carried out and confirm the diagnosis and can be used for antenatal diagnosis (796,805). Routine MRI studies reveal mild cerebral atrophy. Volumetric MRI shows a one-third reduction in caudate volume (806).

A variety of other disorders of purine and pyrimidine metabolism are summarized in Table 1.19.

An X-linked syndrome marked by developmental delay, ataxia, and sensorineural deafness in which hyperuricemia is caused by superactivity of phosphoribosyl pyrophosphate synthetase and excessive purine production has been reported (807). Another disorder of purine metabolism (Adonylsuccinate lyase deficiency) is manifested by the presence of large amounts of succinyladenosine and succinylaminoimidazolc carboxamide riboside in body fluids. The clinical picture is one of severe mental retardation, seizures, and autistic features. Curiously, the CSF protein has been abnormally low in the three reported patients (808,814). These disorders are best identified by identification of the purine metabolites in urine and plasma by high-performance liquid chromatography.

Treatment

Allopurinol (20 mg/kg per day), a xanthine oxidase inhibitor, which blocks the last steps of uric acid synthesis, has been used in treating the renal and arthritic manifestations of the disease. The decrease in uric acid excretion induced by this drug is accompanied by an increase of hypoxanthine and xanthine. A variety of drugs has been used in an attempt to suppress self-mutilation. The most effective appears to be L-5-hydroxytrophan given in conjunction with carbidopa and fluphenazine (796). Bone marrow transplantation and retroviruses have been suggested as a genetic vector for the delivery of the missing enzyme to bone marrow cells. The former has been unsuccessful in improving neurologic symptoms (796).

Disorders of Pyrimidine Metabolism

A condition, termed *thymine-uraciluria*, in which increased excretion of uracil, thymine, and 5-hydroxymethyluracil are accompanied by mental retardation has been reported. The defect is one of dihydropyrimidine dehydrogenase. Subjects develop severe reactions to 5-fluorouracil, with cerebellar ataxia and progressive obtundation (809).

CREATINE DEFICIENCY SYNDROME

Creatine deficiency syndrome, a newly discovered disorder of creatine biosynthesis, is caused by a deficiency in hepatic guanidinoacetate methyltransferase. The condition is marked by a progressive extrapyramidal movement disorder, seizures, and microcephaly. On MRI, delayed myelination is seen, and on MR spectroscopy, the creatine and creatine phosphate peaks are virtually absent. Treatment with oral creatine (400 to 500 mg/kg per day) results in gradual improvement in some of the symptoms (816).

PORPHYRIA

Of the various inherited disorders of the heme biosynthetic pathway that result in the accumulation of porphyrin or porphyrin precursors, only congenital erythropoietic porphyria is observed with any frequency during childhood. It results in cutaneous photosensitivity and hemolytic anemia, but it is not accompanied by neurologic symptoms.

Acute intermittent porphyria is transmitted as an autosomal dominant trait with variable, but generally low, penetrance. Symptoms usually begin at puberty or shortly thereafter, are most pronounced in young adults, and commonly are aggravated or precipitated by the ingestion of barbiturates. They consist of recurrent attacks of autonomic dysfunction, intermittent colicky abdominal pain, convulsions, and a polyneuritis, which usually predominantly affects the motor nerves. The upper limbs are generally more involved, and the paralysis progresses until it reaches its maximum within several weeks. Seizures are relatively rare. Mental disturbances, notably anxiety, insomnia, and confusion, are common, but no skin lesions develop (817,818). Attacks can be precipitated by a variety of drugs, notably anticonvulsants.

Decreased activity of porphobilinogen deaminase to 50% of normal has been demonstrated in several tissues, notably in erythrocytes, where the enzyme can be assayed most readily. The gene for the enzyme is located on the long arm of chromosome 11 (11q23-11qter), and more than 100 allelic variants have been documented (819). This heterogeneity is in part responsible for the variable expression of the disease. A presumed homozygous patient was noted to have porencephaly and severe mental retardation (819a).

The pathogenesis of the neurologic symptoms is poorly understood (820). The most likely explanation is that multiple factors, notably δ-aminolevulinic acid (ALA), act on the nervous system concomitantly or sequentially (820). Kappas and coworkers postulate that drugs, such as barbiturates, evoke acute intermittent porphyria by inducing hepatic ALA synthetase, with consequent overproduction of ALA (821). As hepatic heme synthesis

TABLE 1.20. *Neurologic symptoms in the hereditary porphyrias*

Disease	Neurologic signs and symptoms
Acute intermittent porphyria	Recurrent attacks of autonomic dysfunction, abdominal pain, seizures, motor polyneuropathy
δ-Aminolevulinic acid dehydratase deficiency	Motor polyneuropathy
Congenital erythropoietic porphyria	No neurologic symptoms, severe cutaneous photosensitivity
Porphyria cutanea tarda	No neurologic symptoms, cutaneous photosensitivity
Hereditary coproporphyria	As in acute intermittent porphyria, cutaneous photosensitivity
Variegate porphyria	Acute neurovisceral crises, photosensitive skin; rarely starts before third decade of life
Protoporphyria	Cutaneous photosensitivity, no neurologic symptoms except in end-stage liver disease

increases, porphobilinogen deaminase becomes rate limiting, and an increased production of ALA is required to provide more porphobilinogen to maintain heme formation (821).

The diagnosis is arrived at by demonstrating increased urinary porphobilinogen and urinary ALA during an attack. Between attacks, the excretion of both metabolites decreases, but is rarely normal. Clinically silent carriers do not excrete increased amounts of these metabolites (822).

The neurologic signs and symptoms of the various porphyrias are summarized in Table 1.20. Increased excretion of ALA without increased porphobilinogen excretion is seen in lead poisoning and hereditary tyrosinemia.

MITOCHONDRIAL DISEASES (MITOCHONDRIAL CYTOPATHIES)

More than 200 different defects of mitochondrial DNA (mtDNA) have been described. The majority of these are accompanied by neuromuscular deficits.

Molecular Genetics and Biochemical Pathology

Mitochondria have been termed "the power plant of the cell". One of the cell's largest organelles, they occupy as much as 25% of cytoplasmic volume and the number of mitochondria per cell ranges from hundreds to thousands. Mitochondria have their own DNA, distinct from nuclear DNA (nDNA). MtDNA is a predominantly double circular molecule that functions as an independent genetic unit, with each mitochondrion containing from 2 to 10 genomes (823). The mutation rate of mtDNA is high, probably 7 to 10 times greater than nDNA. MtDNA contains 37 genes. These encode subunits of four of the five enzyme complexes involved in the electron transport chain, two ribosomal RNAs, and 22 transfer RNAs (tRNA). Although mitochondria are sufficiently large to be seen under a light microscope, their structural details can be viewed only under an electron microscope. In essence, mitochondria generate the high-energy phosphate bond in ATP by phosphorylation of adenosine diphosphate (ADP). The considerable amount of energy required for this reaction is derived from the oxidation of the metabolic products of carbohydrates, fatty acids, and proteins. It is this process of energy generation, referred to collectively as *oxidative phosphorylation*, that is the primary function of mitochondria. Several biochemical domains have been distinguished, and defects in each have been documented (Fig. 1.35).

Oxidation of Pyruvate to Acetyl Coenzyme A by the Pyruvate Dehydrogenase Complex

Pyruvate dehydrogenase is one of the most complex enzymes known, with a molecular weight of more than 7 million. It contains multiple subunits of three catalytic enzymes (E_1, E_2, and E_3), two regulatory polypeptides, and five different coenzymes.

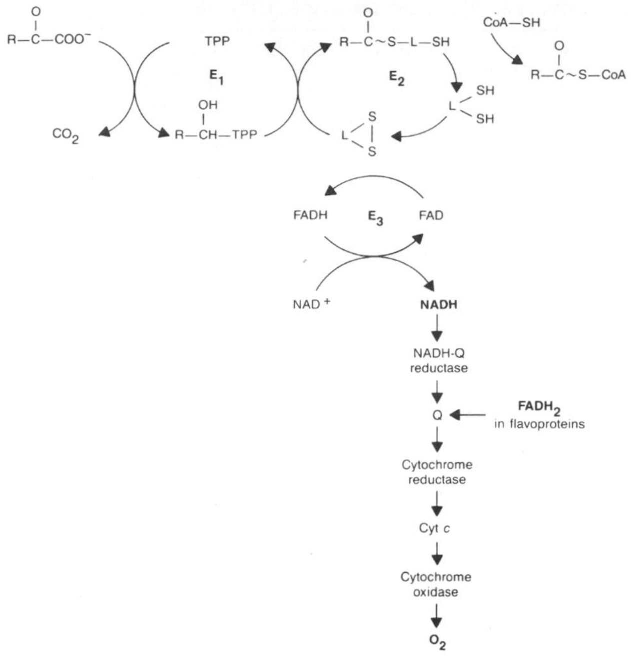

FIG. 1.35. The pyruvate dehydrogenase complex and its relationship to the electron carriers in the respiratory chain. Electrons are transferred from nicotinamide adenine dinucleotide (reduced form) (NADH) through a chain of three protein complexes: NADH dehydrogenase (ubiquinone) (NADHQ reductase), cytochrome reductase, and cytochrome oxidase. Q, coenzyme Q, the reduced form of ubiquinone, which also can accept electrons from $FADH_2$, which is formed in the citric acid cycle by the oxidation of succinate to fumarate. Cytochrome reductase contains cytochrome b and cytochrome c_1. Electrons are passed from cytochrome b, to cytochrome c_1, and then to cytochrome c. Cytochrome oxidase catalyses their transfer from cytochrome c to oxygen. (E_1, pyruvate dehydrogenase; E_2, dihydrolipoamide acetyltransferase; E_3, dihydrolipoamide dehydrogenase; TPP, thiamine pyrophosphate.)

Oxidation of Acetyl Coenzyme A to Carbon Dioxide, and Generation of the Reduced Electron Carriers

Oxidation of acetyl coenzyme A to carbon dioxide and generation of the reduced electron carriers, a set of nine reactions, are carried out within the mitochondrial matrix by the citric acid (Krebs) cycle.

Reoxidation of the Reduced Coenzymes by Molecular Oxygen

These reactions are carried out on the inner mitochondrial membrane by the electron transport chain, a set of electron carriers grouped into five multienzyme complexes. The free energy released during oxidation is stored in an electrochemical proton gradient across the inner mitochondrial membrane. The movement of protons back across the mitochondrial membrane is then coupled with the synthesis of ATP from ADP and phosphate. Seven subunits of nicotinamide-adenine dinucleotide (reduced form) (NADH) coenzyme Q reductase (complex I), the cytochrome b

subunit of $CoQH_2$-cytochrome c reductase (complex III), three of the subunits for cytochrome c oxidase (complex IV), and two subunits of ATPase (complex V) are encoded by mtDNA. All other subunits of the respiratory chain are coded by nDNA (823a). Because in the formation of the zygote, almost all mitochondria are contributed by the ovum, mtDNA is maternally inherited (824). Maternal inheritance appears to be operative in a small but significant proportion of inherited mitochondrial diseases; in the remainder transmission is as an autosomal recessive trait, or is sporadic or unpredictable (825).

Transport of Free Fatty Acids into Mitochondria by Carnitine

Within mitochondria, the fatty acids are uncoupled from carnitine, a carrier molecule, and react with CoA to form an acyl-CoA. By a series of four sequential reactions (β-oxidation), each molecule of acyl-CoA is oxidized to form one molecule of acetyl-CoA and an acyl-CoA shortened by two carbon atoms. Because most defects of β-oxidation present with organic aciduria, these conditions are considered in the section dealing with organic acidurias.

Oxidation of Amino Acids within Mitochondria

After transamination to their respective ketoacids, alanine, aspartic acid, and glutamic acid enter the citric acid cycle.

Clinical Manifestations

Mitochondrial diseases can result from mutations in mtDNA, mutations of nDNA coding for those subunits of the multienzyme complexes not encoded by mitochondria, defects in nuclear genes that regulate mtDNA replication and expression, and defects in which nuclear and mitochondrial genes are involved. Although some 200 mutations of mtDNA have been described, little is known with respect to mutations of nDNA involved in mitochondrial structure and function. The protein subunits encoded by nDNA are synthesized in the cytosol and then transported into the mitochondria across the impermeable inner membrane. The transport process is extremely complex and requires unfolding and refolding of the protein subunits and targeting of the protein to receptors on the mitochondrial membrane.

Mitochondrial mutations fall into two groups: rearrangements (i.e., deletions and duplications of the mitochondrial genome) and point mutations. The majority of rearrangements are sporadic and not transmitted. Point mutations of mtDNA are inherited maternally (826). In the Queen Square series of mitochondrial diseases reported by Petty and coworkers, similarly involved relatives were seen in some 20% of cases, but no consistent pattern of inheritance existed, although maternal transmission was nine times as frequent as paternal transmission (827).

Clinical presentations of the disorders of mitochondrial function are protean. They range from a mild muscle ache and weakness after prolonged exercise to a severe and fatal lactic acidosis developing within a few days of birth. To complicate matters, different mutations of mtDNA can produce the same symptoms and signs (phenocopies), and identical mtDNA mutations may not produce identical diseases (genocopies). The confusing clinical pictures are undoubtedly caused by the following factors: (a) the large number of nuclear and mitochondrial genes involved in electron transport and other mitochondrial functions; (b) the variability in the distribution of mutant mtDNA in the various organs; and (c) the variable presence of a population of mutant mitochondrial genomes (mutant homoplasmy) and mixed mutant and wild-type mitochondrial genomes (heteroplasmy). Random segregation of mitochondria during cell division results in an unequal distribution of mutant and wild type mtDNA in daughter cells. The clinical picture is related to the mutation load, and to the susceptibility of various tissues to the effects of mutant mtDNA.

A number of authorities have classified diseases of mitochondria, according to the nature of the biochemical defect, or as to whether they involve the mitochondrial genome, nuclear genome, or both genomes simultaneously. In this chapter, mitochondrial diseases are grouped according to their major clinical presentation. The molecular lesions and the clinical picture resulting from them are presented in Table 1.21.

Leber Disease (Hereditary Optic Atrophy)

This degenerative disorder, which primarily affects the optic nerves, was first described by Leber in 1871 and is characterized by an insidiously progressive loss of central vision with sparing of the peripheral fields (828).

Molecular Biology

Several point mutations have been recognized. The most common of these is located at base pair 11778. This mutation results in the substitution of histidine for arginine in mitochondrially derived NADH ubiquinone oxidoreductase (complex I) and results in deficient respiratory chain function. Less often mutations occur at base pair 3460 or at base pair 14484. These mutations also result in amino acid changes in complex I. Many other

TABLE 1.21. *Molecular lesions in mitochondrial diseases*

Disease	MtDNA lesion
Leber optic atrophy (at least three major mutations)	11778 ND 1 subunit of complex I (72% of cases)
	14459 ND 6 subunit of complex I
	3460 ND 1 subunit of complex I
	14484 ND 6 subunit of complex I
Leber optic atrophy with dystonia	14459 ND 6 subunit for complex I
Mitochondrial myopathy	3250 tRNA leucine
	3251 tRNA leucine
	3302 tRNA leucine
	Deletion COX III subunit of complex IV
Mitochondrial myopathy and cardiomyopathy	3260 tRNA leucine
Mitochondrial cardiomyopathy	3303 tRNA leucine
	4269 tRNA isoleucine
	9997 tRNA glycine
Leigh syndrome	9176 ATPase 6
	8993 ATPase 6
MERRF	8344 tRNA lysine
	8356 tRNA leucine
	3243 tRNA leucine
MELAS/MERRF	8356 tRNA leucine
	7512 tRNA serine
	3256 tRNA leucine
Sensorineural hearing loss plus ataxia	7512 tRNA serine
	7445 tRNA serine
MELAS	3243 tRNA leucine most common
	3252, 3271, 3291 tRNA leucine
	1642 tRNA valine
Progressive external ophthalmoplegia	Deletion affecting several genes
	Multiple deletions
	3243, 3256, 5703 tRNA leucine
	5692 tRNA aspartate
Kearns-Sayre syndrome	Deletion affecting several genes
Mitochondrial neurogastrointestinal encephalo-myopathy	Multiple deletions affecting several genes
Diabetes insipidus, diabetes mellitus, optic atrophy, deafness	Single deletion affecting several genes
	Multiple deletions affecting several genes
Hearing loss, ataxia, myoclonus	7472 tRNA serine
Chronic progressive external ophthalmoplegia and intestinal obstruction	10006 tRNA glutamic acid

MELAS, mitochondrial myopathy, encephalopathy, lactic acidosis, and strokelike episodes syndrome; MERRF, myoclonus epilepsy with ragged red fibers syndrome.

mitochondrial point mutations have been identified with a greater frequency in patients with Leber disease than in controls. Because normal mtDNA is highly polymorphic, the role of these other point mutations in causing or contributing to the manifestations of the disease is not clear. Individuals with Leber disease usually show nearly complete homoplasmy for mutant mtDNA, with only trace amounts of normal mtDNA. Although vision loss is more likely when the patient has homoplasmy for the mutant mtDNA, relatively poor correlation exists between disease severity and the degree of heteroplasmy in lymphocytes. The predominance of male subjects among patients with Leber disease is still unexplained (828). As a rule, men never pass the disease to their offspring, but nearly 100% of women carriers transmit the condition whether they are clinically affected or not.

Pathology

Pathologic examination reveals a loss of ganglion cells from the retinal fovea centralis, marked atrophy of the optic nerves, and demyelination of the papillomacular bundle, chiasm, and tracts. The geniculate bodies show a striking cell loss and gliosis. The visual cortex is normal (829). Examination of muscle by electron microscopy reveals aggregates of enlarged mitochondria in the subsarcolemmal region. The myofilaments are disrupted, and occasional nemaline rods are seen. These alterations point to a disorder of mitochondrial function even in the absence of clinically discernible muscle weakening (830). It is still not known what triggers the sudden deterioration of vision. Cyanide, which previously has been suggested as an exogenous factor, acts as an inhibitor for cytochrome c oxidase, rather than for complex I.

Clinical Manifestations

Relatively little difference in the clinical picture of Leber disease exists between patients containing the three major mutations (828). As a rule, the younger the onset of symptoms, the better the ultimate outcome, and some 80% of subjects with onset of vision loss before 20 years of age recovered sufficiently to be able to drive a car (828). The variability in the severity of clinical symptoms might be accounted for by the presence of additional exogenous or endogenous factors, notably the intragenic suppressor mutation on the mitochondrial gene coding for complex I (831).

The onset of symptoms is insidious, usually occurring between 18 and 25 years of age and without any obvious precipitating cause. vision loss progresses rapidly until it reaches a static phase. The initial complaint is a sudden blurring of central vision that progresses to dense central scotomas. In many patients, vision loss is at first unilateral. Examination of the fundi in the earliest stages of the illness can reveal a tortuosity of the arterioles most evident in the circumpapillary area (832). This tortuosity suggests that the vasculopathy is the primary retinal abnormality. Vascular tortuosity is limited to arteries, and in contrast to papilledema, veins are neither tortuous nor distended. In the late stages of the illness, temporal pallor of the optic discs can occur (833).

In the early stages of the illness, the visual-evoked potential is delayed and reduced in amplitude. With progression, it is extinguished completely (834). Abnormalities of the visual-evoked potentials are found in 50% of descendants from the female linkage, but also in one-third of descendants from the male linkage. MRI has shown bilateral sharply defined low-signal areas in the putamen (835). Associated neurologic symptoms occur in many families, including some who are homoplasmic for the arginine-histidine mutation. These include an extrapyramidal-pyramidal syndrome developing during childhood, seizures, cerebellar signs, spasticity, and mental retardation (828). The association of Leber disease and dystonia has been well described. It results from a mutation in the ND 6 gene for complex I (836). It is marked by the childhood onset of severe generalized dystonia associated with dementia, bulbar dysfunction, corticospinal tract dysfunction, and short stature. The MRI demonstrates bilateral symmetric abnormalities on T2-weighted images in putamen and caudate. Blood lactate is rarely elevated, and ragged red fibers are absent (836a).

Approximately one-half of patients recover some degree of vision. Recovery does not occur for many months or years after the initial vision loss, with the mutation at base pair 3460 having a better prognosis than other mutations (828).

Diagnosis

The uniqueness of Leber disease rests on the X-linked transmission and the rapid loss of central vision. The association of these symptoms with one of the three primary mutations of mtDNA virtually establishes the diagnosis. In the absence of such data and in the absence of similar symptoms in family members, the presence of an optic nerve tumor must be excluded by appropriate neuroimaging studies. Families in whom optic atrophy is associated with other neurologic symptoms are better considered as variants of the hereditary cerebellar degenerations and are covered in Chapter 2, as are various other forms of hereditary optic neuronatrophy (835).

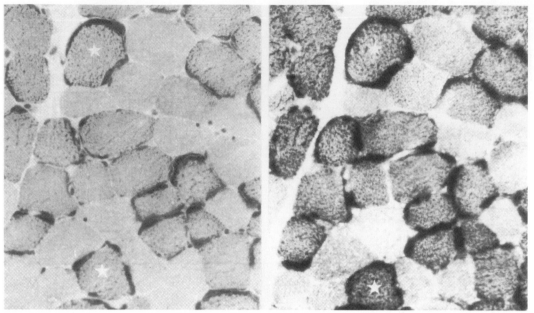

A   B

FIG. 1.36. Ragged red fibers seen in serial sections of human skeletal muscle. **A:** Modified Gomori trichrome stain. **B:** Succinate dehydrogenase enzyme activity is more sensitive. Stars denote ragged red fibers. (Courtesy of Dr. Eduardo Bonilla, Columbia University, New York, NY.)

Treatment

No treatment exists, but the patient or family can be assured that vision loss does not progress to complete blindness.

Impairment of Muscle Function

Two main clinical phenotypes have been encountered. The first is a progressive, but often fluctuating, weakness commencing at any time between birth and the seventh decade of life, with the majority of cases having their onset in the first two decades of life. Muscle weakness is mainly proximal, and the upper extremities tend to be more affected. The second clinical phenotype is a myopathy complicated by ptosis and a chronic progressive external ophthalmoplegia. In the series of Petty and coworkers, the latter clinical picture was seen in 73% of subjects. Because their patients were ascertained from muscle biopsy files, this incidence is undoubtedly too high (827). Some patients have a recurrent myoglobinuria, and cardiac muscle also can

be involved. Others have a pigmentary degeneration of the retina. In the Queen Square experience, pigmentary degeneration was seen in 36% of patients presenting with muscular involvement, and was most frequently of the "salt and pepper" type (827); a retinitis pigmentosa appearance was much less common (837).

Muscle biopsy discloses the presence of ragged red muscle fibers. Ragged red fibers are characterized by the accumulation of abnormal mitochondria under the sarcolemmal membrane. They are the morphologic hallmark of an abnormal mitochondrial proliferation. They are best visualized by means of the modified Gomori trichrome reaction or by succinate dehydrogenase stain. On electron microscopy, an increased number of bizarre and often enlarged mitochondria are seen, accompanied by crystalline and, in some instances, lipid inclusions (Fig. 1.36). As a rule, ragged red fibers are seen primarily in defects of oxidative phosphorylation because of impaired mitochondrial protein synthesis. Phosphorus MR spectroscopy of affected muscle shows an abnormal intracellular energy state as evidenced by increased inorganic phosphate and diminished phosphocreatine concentrations (838).

Patients with chronic progressive external ophthalmoplegia (CPOE) and myopathy generally harbor a mitochondrial deletion in muscle. In the Queen Square series of Holt and coworkers, 69% of subjects with CPOE and proximal myopathy harbored deletions of the mitochondrial genome. When retinopathy accompanied CPOE, the incidence of demonstrable mitochondrial deletions increased to 92%. By contrast, patients whose limb weakness was unaccompanied by CPOE did not show mitochondrial deletions (839). Rather they are likely to show various point mutations in the gene for the transfer RNA (tRNA) for leucine (see Table 1.21). A myopathy accompanied by cardiomyopathy is associated with several point mutations in the gene for the tRNA for leucine, whereas isolated cardiomyopathy is associated with mutations in the gene for the tRNA for isoleucine.

A severe and rapidly fatal myopathy that develops at birth or a few months thereafter and is accompanied by lactic acidosis and ragged red fibers has been associated with a marked depletion of muscle mitochondrial DNA (840). The condition is believed to be transmitted as a recessive trait and could be caused by a mutation in a nuclear gene that controls mitochondrial DNA levels in early development (841) (see Table 1.21).

PROGRESSIVE OR INTERMITTENTLY PROGRESSIVE DETERIORATION OF NEUROLOGIC FUNCTION

Neurologic deficits can be generalized or focal. Several clinical syndromes have been recognized; they overlap considerably.

Leigh Syndrome (Subacute Necrotizing Encephalomyelitis)

As originally described (842), the affected infant suffered from a rapidly progressive neurologic illness marked by somnolence, blindness, deafness, and spasticity. The clinical picture in subse-quently reported cases has been fairly characteristic. In the majority of cases, neurologic symptoms are first noted during the first year of life. Psychomotor delay and hypotonia are the most common initial signs. As the disease progresses, abnormalities in extraocular movements, optic atrophy, cerebellar dysfunction, and disturbances of respiration appear. A peripheral neuropathy also has been prominent, and cardiomyopathy can contribute to an early demise. In the New York series of Macaya and colleagues, movement disorders, notably dystonia or myoclonus, formed a prominent part of the neurologic picture in 86% of patients (843); in some, they were the presenting sign (844). A male predominance occurs; 66% of patients in the series of DiMauro and colleagues, were male (845).

Arterial or CSF lactate is almost invariably elevated. T2-weighted MRI studies are diagnostic of the condition. They show symmetric areas of increased signal in the putamen. Less often, additional lesions are seen in the caudate nuclei, globus pallidus, and substantia nigra (846). Pathologic findings are highlighted by a spongy degeneration of the neurophile, usually involving the spinal cord and the gray matter of the brainstem, basal ganglia, and thalamus. This degeneration is accompanied by an astrocytic reaction and an intense capillary proliferation (847), the latter probably the response to a chronic increase in brain lactate. Muscle biopsy is usually normal; specifically, it does not disclose a ragged red myopathy (848).

Several disorders of mitochondrial function have been implicated in Leigh syndrome. In the survey of United Kingdom patients by Morris and coworkers, the most common defect was cytochrome c oxidase deficiency (complex IV) seen in 23% of pedigrees. An isolated complex I deficiency was seen in 10% of pedigrees, and a pyruvate dehydrogenase complex deficiency was seen in 7% of pedigrees (849). Two mutations at base pair 8993 of the ATPase 6 gene (complex V) also have been described and are believed to account for a significant proportion of patients with the variant of Leigh syndrome that consists of neurogenic atrophy, ataxia, and retinitis pigmentosa as first described by Holt (850,851). Less often other mutations exist in the ATPase 6 gene (852), point mutations in mitochondrial tRNA genes, and a mutation in succinate dehydrogenase (853). In one isolated instance, a deficiency in fumarase, an enzyme involved in the citric acid cycle, has been demonstrated (854). In the Australian series of Rahman and colleagues, a defect in complex I was the most common cause for Leigh syndrome (853). In both series, the cause for nearly one-half of Leigh syndrome patients could not be defined (849,853). The cause of the cytochrome oxidase deficiency in Leigh syndrome is still unclear. Several groups have suggested that it is the result of a defect in assembling the active enzyme complex (855). SURF1, a "housekeeping" gene of unknown function, involved in the assembly of the complex is defective in the majority of subjects with cytochrome oxidase deficiency (856,856a).

When Leigh syndrome is the result of a pyruvate dehydrogenase deficiency, treatment with a ketogenic diet appears to be of benefit, with improvement of lactate and pyruvate levels, MRI abnormalities, and perhaps even prevention of irreversible brain damage (857,857a).

Kearns-Sayre Syndrome (Ophthalmoplegia Plus)

First described by Kearns and Sayre in 1958, this is the most likely mitochondrial CNS syndrome to be encountered. It is also the best studied from clinical and molecular aspects (858).

As defined by DiMauro and coworkers (859), the condition is characterized by its onset before age 15 years, the presence of CPOE, pigmentary degeneration of the retina, and one of the following: heart block, cerebellar deficits, or a CSF protein of more than 100 mg/dL. A myopathy affecting facial, cervical, and limb muscle is also common. The complete clinical picture of this condition is protean, and various incomplete forms have been described, such as one in which CPOE and a myopathy are associated with hearing loss, ataxia, and cardiac abnormalities (860). In almost all instances, growth retardation antedates the onset of neurologic symptoms, which generally appear after age 5 years. Ragged red fibers are generally

found by muscle biopsy. An associated peripheral neuropathy is not unusual, and abnormal mitochondria are demonstrable on sural nerve biopsy (861). Cataracts, nerve deafness, ichthyosis, a variety of endocrinopathies, cardiomyopathy, and proximal renal tubular acidosis also have been recorded (862,863).

Serum creatine kinase values are normal or moderately increased. Blood lactate and pyruvate levels are frequently increased, and, in many other instances, CSF lactate is elevated in the absence of an elevated blood lactate. Some 80% of patients suffering from Kearns-Sayre syndrome have a large deletion in their mitochondrial genome (839,864). Deletions range in size from 1.3 to 8 kb, and vary in location. One particular 4.9-kb deletion, seen in approximately one-third of patients, arises from what appears to be a hot spot and is flanked by direct repeats (865). Deletions are usually seen in all tissues, and no obvious correlation exists between the severity of neurologic symptoms and the size or location of the deletion (866). The cause of the various deletions is still uncertain. Because deletions are generally sporadic, they most likely result from a spontaneous mutation of mitochondrial DNA at a stage preceding organogenesis, or from homologous recombination of mitochondrial DNA (867). With progression of the disease, the fraction of mitochondrial DNA containing the deletion increases. This could reflect the fact that mitochondria containing deletions replicate preferentially and accumulate in the ragged red fibers (868,869). However, muscle fibers regenerating at the site of a muscle biopsy taken from a patient with Kearns-Sayre syndrome and a point mutation in the gene for a tRNA for leucine were essentially homoplasmic for the wild-type mtDNA (870). Deletions in all tissues also have been detected in Pearson syndrome, a condition marked by refractory anemia, exocrine pancreatic dysfunction, insulin-dependent diabetes mellitus, lactic acidosis, and 3-methylglutaconic aciduria. This disease is generally fatal during the first few years of life, but survivors can develop signs of Kearns-Sayre syndrome (871). As already mentioned in this section, deletions are seen in patients presenting with CPOE without the full clinical picture of Kearns-Sayre syndrome. In contrast to those seen in Kearns-Sayre syndrome, they tend to be localized to muscle (839,860). Deletions have not been found in patients suffering from the other mitochondrial myopathies, including mitochondrial myopathy, encephalopathy, lactic acidosis, and strokelike episodes (MELAS syndrome) and myoclonus epilepsy with ragged red fibers (MERRF syndrome) (864,872) (see Table 1.21).

The neuropathologic picture in Kearns-Sayre syndrome is marked by the presence of status spongiosus in gray and white matter. In cerebrum and cerebellum, white matter is affected principally, whereas in the brainstem, gray matter is primarily affected. Additionally, prominent neuronal loss occurs in brainstem and cerebellum, with demyelination paralleling the severity of spongy degeneration. Calcium deposits are seen in the globus pallidus and thalamus. In brain, mitochondrial structural abnormalities have not been documented consistently (873). As yet, it is not clear how the mitochondrial defects translate into neuropathologic abnormalities. The most plausible explanation is that failure in oxidative phosphorylation results in tissue anoxia in the presence of a continued supply of blood and glucose. With glycolysis being maintained, lactate levels increase, which in turn induce cellular damage (874).

Myoclonus Epilepsy with Ragged Red Fibers Syndrome

Myoclonus epilepsy with ragged red fibers syndrome (MERRF) was first described by Fukuhara and colleagues (875). As the name suggests, the syndrome is highlighted by myoclonic and generalized seizures. Additionally, progressive dementia, ataxia, weakness, spasticity, and a sensorineural hearing loss occur (876,877). Optic atrophy and cardiac involvement have been seen. In contrast to Kearns-Sayre syndrome, patients develop neither ophthalmoplegia nor retinal degeneration.

The most common molecular abnormality, seen in some 80% of cases, is a point mutation in the mitochondrial gene at 8344 coding for the lysine tRNA (866,878). Other mutations in the

genes for the tRNA for leucine also have been observed (see Table 1.21). As a consequence, there is a partial defect in one or more of the various respiratory complexes that require mitochondrially encoded subunits. As a rule, an imperfect relationship exists between the proportion of mutant mtDNA in tissue and the presence or absence of disease, which suggests that other factors, such as a second mutation in the tRNA gene, operate to determine phenotype (879). Maternal inheritance has been well demonstrated, but in most families, the maternal relatives have few if any symptoms (880).

Ragged red fibers are found on muscle biopsy, and mutant mitochondrial DNA can be demonstrated in blood (881). On pathologic examination of the brain, neuronal degeneration and gliosis is seen in the dentate nucleus, cerebellar cortex, midbrain, medulla, and spinal cord. The distribution and nature of the lesions differ markedly from those seen in Kearns-Sayre syndrome and MELAS. Sparaco postulates that the different regional expression of lesions reflects an uneven distribution of the wild-type and mutant mitochondria, a different threshold to metabolic damage in various areas of the CNS, or a selective vulnerability of cells to toxic factors such as lactate (873).

Mitochondrial Myopathy, Encephalopathy, Lactic Acidosis, and Strokelike Episodes Syndrome

MELAS syndrome was defined by Pavlakis and associates (882). It is characterized by strokelike episodes caused by focal brain lesions predominantly localized to the parieto-occipital lobes, and lactic acidosis, ragged red fibers, or both. Other signs include dementia, focal or generalized seizures, and deafness (866). In the extensive series of Ciafaloni and colleagues, the onset of symptoms was before 15 years of age in 62% of cases (883,884). Strokes were present in all patients; in none did they represent the initial symptom. Hemianopia or cortical blindness and seizures were seen in every patient. Recurrent headaches, vomiting, and dementia were also frequent symptoms. Although ophthalmoplegia or retinitis pigmentosa was seen occasionally, no patient in the series of Ciafaloni and colleagues had the complete triad of CPOE, retinitis pigmentosa, and cardiomyopathy.

The most common molecular pathology that underlies the MELAS syndrome is a heteroplasmic point mutation on the tRNA gene for leucine at 3243, which is seen in some 80% of patients. Several other point mutations in the gene coding for the tRNA for leucine have been reported, as well as mutations for the tRNA for other amino acids such as valine (866,883). As a consequence, deficiencies occur in one or more of the respiratory chain enzymes, most commonly in complex IV. In approximately 90% of pedigrees, family history is compatible with maternal transmission, and the point mutation can be demonstrated in blood or muscle in mildly symptomatic or asymptomatic relatives (884). Blood DNA can be used to diagnose the mitochondrial deletion. This technique is useful for children, in whom mutant mitochondrial levels in blood are high in relation to those in muscle (885). The correlation between genotype and phenotype is not good, and the 3243 point mutation also has been documented in families with maternally inherited progressive external ophthalmoplegia, isolated myopathy, or diabetes mellitus and deafness (866).

In addition to the presence of ragged red fibers in muscle, the characteristic pathologic lesion in MELAS syndrome is a focal necrosis involving the cerebral cortex, the subcortical white matter, basal ganglia, and thalamus. Calcium deposits are found in basal ganglia, particularly the globus pallidus, and are demonstrable by CT scans. The mechanism of the strokelike episodes in this condition is still unknown (886).

Alpers Syndrome

This condition, as first described by Alpers (887), manifests by progressive deterioration of mental function, seizures, hypotonia, and impaired vision and hearing. Many subjects with this clinical picture have an elevation of lactic and pyruvic acid levels in the CSF and blood or solely in the CSF. A variety of defects in cerebral mitochondrial function have been implicated. These include deficiencies in either

complex I or complex III (887a). Ragged red fibers are not seen in this condition (877). The nosology of Alpers syndrome is problematic, and many authors use this eponym to refer to a clinical entity in which progressive neuronal degeneration is associated with liver disease. This entity is considered in Chapter 2.

Congenital Lactic Acidosis

Congenital lactic acidosis is one of the most severe presentations of disordered mitochondrial function. Several biochemical defects are responsible. In 1962, Hartmann and associates described a 3-year-old girl with Down syndrome who since early infancy had suffered from chronic acidosis caused by an accumulation of blood lactate and pyruvate (888). Since then, a fairly large number of infants with this clinical picture have been encountered, with the most prominent feature being metabolic acidosis, usually commencing in the neonatal period, accompanied by tachypnea, lethargy, vomiting, and muscular hypotonia. Seizurelike episodes can be observed, as well as athetotic movements (889). Serum and CSF lactate levels are markedly elevated, the latter as much as fivefold over the normal. MRI can be normal or can show increased signal in the frontal lobes on T2-weighted images (889). When a positron emission tomography scan is performed before the onset of chronic brain damage, one observes a markedly increased rate of cerebral glucose metabolism. This is the consequence of the defect in oxidative phosphorylation and the increased need for glucose when the glycolytic pathway has to fulfill the energy needs of the brain (889).

Several enzyme deficiencies are responsible for congenital lactic acidosis. These have been localized to two distinct areas of intermediary metabolism: pyruvate dehydrogenation and gluconeogenesis.

Of the enzymes constituting the pyruvate dehydrogenation complex, a deficiency in pyruvate dehydrogenase (E_1) is the most frequently documented cause of lactic acidosis (890,891). The pyruvate dehydrogenase component is a tetramer of two different subunits, $\alpha_2\beta_2$, with the gene for the E_1 α subunit being localized to the X chromosome. Generally, there is no good correlation between the residual activity of the enzyme complex and the severity of the clinical picture, except that infants who die during the neonatal period tend to have less than 20% residual enzyme activity (892,893). For reasons as yet unexplained, several of the infants were found to have dysmorphic features reminiscent of fetal alcohol syndrome, and others had agenesis of the corpus callosum. Also encountered have been defects of the other enzymes of the pyruvate dehydrogenase complex: E_2 (dihydrolipoyltransacetylase) (894), E_3 (dihydrolipoyldehydrogenase) (895), and pyruvate dehydrogenase phosphatase (896). In dihydrolipoyldehydrogenase deficiency, pyruvate and α-ketoglutarate dehydrogenases are defective. Mitochondrial structure is normal in the various defects of the pyruvate dehydrogenase complex, and ragged red fibers are absent in muscle. The various forms of pyruvate carboxylase deficiency are covered with the organic acidurias. Other causes for lactic acidosis are presented in Table 1.22.

Whereas in some children the signs of a metabolic disturbance are obvious, others have intermittent ataxia and choreoathetosis, with attacks after nonspecific febrile illnesses that last several hours or as long as 1 week (897). One such patient had optic atrophy and mental retardation, whereas another had normal intelligence (898).

Treatment with dichloroacetate has been suggested by a number of workers (899,899a). The drug activates the pyruvate dehydrogenase system by inhibiting pyruvate decarboxylase kinase, thus locking up pyruvate decarboxylase in its unphosphorylated active form. Dichloroacetate appears to produce some clinical benefits in approximately one-third of patients. Patients with MELAS syndrome are most likely to show improvement.

Defects in Mitochondrial Energy Conservation and Transduction

In Luft disease, an extremely rare condition, hypermetabolism manifests by a lifelong history of heat intolerance, excessive sweating, low-grade

TABLE 1.22. *Conditions producing lactic acidosis in infancy and childhood*

Pyruvate dehydrogenase complex
  Pyruvate decarboxylase (E_1)
  Dihydrolipoamide acetyltransferase (E_2)
  Dihydrolipoamide dehydrogenase (E_3)
Pyruvate dehydrogenase phosphatase
  Pyruvate decarboxylase activator
Gluconeogenesis
  Glucose-6-phosphatase (glycogen storage
    disease type I)
  Fructose 1,6-diphosphatase
  Pyruvate carboxylase
Carboxylase defects
  Propionyl-CoA carboxylase
  3-Methylcrotonyl-CoA carboxylase
  Multiple carboxylase deficiency
Organic acidurias
  Glutaric aciduria I
  Glutaric aciduria II
  Phosphoenolpyruvate carboxykinase deficiency
Nongenetic causes
  Sepsis
  Circulatory failure, shock, hypoxia
  Short-bowel syndrome
  Urinary tract infection caused by *Enterobacter cloacae* (a lactic acid–producing organism) (366)
  Seizures
  Reye syndrome
  Salicylate poisoning
  Liver failure
  Administration of intravenous glucose in newborns
  Bacterial meningitis (cerebrospinal fluid lactic acid)

fever, and mild weakness (900). Chemical study on muscle biopsy shows complete uncoupling of oxidative phosphorylation (900,901). This condition probably represents a nuclear defect.

Structural Defects

Morphologically abnormal muscle mitochondria also are seen in a variety of other disorders. These include hypothyroid myopathy, KHD, zidovudine myopathy, and the lipid storage myopathies (902).

Diagnosis

Because of the wide spectrum of their clinical presentations, an organized diagnostic approach to the mitochondrial myopathies is necessary.

Whenever clinical evidence suggests a mitochondrial disorder, the initial laboratory test should be the determination of CSF and blood levels of lactate and pyruvate. Because venous lactate increases rapidly with the hyperventilation and struggling that attends venipuncture, arterial lactate and pyruvate or, preferably, the values obtained in CSF generally are more reliable. Additionally, in some mitochondrial defects, the blood lactate level is normal but CSF lactate is elevated (903). Normal values for CSF lactate are 1.3 ± 0.3 mmol/L or 11.7 ± 2.7 mg/dL (903a).

Lactate concentration in blood and CSF depends on the pyruvate concentration and on the relative amounts of reduced and oxidized cytosolic NAD. As the ratio of NAD to NADH decreases, as occurs in disorders of the citric acid cycle, the ratio of lactate to pyruvate increases.

Should CSF lactate be normal, a mitochondrial disorder is not likely, unless symptoms are confined to muscle. In such cases, even mild exercise can induce a lactic acidosis. If this occurs, a muscle biopsy with biochemical and structural examination is indicated.

Should CSF lactate be elevated, the physician must distinguish between a primary and a secondary elevation (see Table 1.22). Additionally, the ratio of lactate to pyruvate is of diagnostic assistance. A normal ratio (less than 25) points to a defect in gluconeogenesis or in the pyruvate dehydrogenase complex, whereas an elevated lactate to pyruvate ratio suggests a respiratory chain defect or a pyruvate carboxylase deficiency.

Evaluation of lactic acidosis also requires determination of blood ammonia and serum amino acids. Hyperammonemia has been noted in several disorders of mitochondrial function (904,905), and an elevated serum alanine is often encountered in some of the disorders of the pyruvate dehydrogenase complex (906).

The next step in the evaluation of lactic acidosis is the quantitation of total and esterified serum carnitine. An elevation of esterified carnitine is seen in a variety of organic acidurias and, therefore, should be pursued by chromatography of the urinary organic acids (907). Low serum levels of free carnitine suggest a systemic carnitine deficiency and should be followed up by a muscle biopsy. The biopsy specimen should be sent for electron microscopy, measurement of muscle carnitine, and appropriate enzymologic studies.

Should serum free and esterified carnitine levels be normal, the possibility of one of the various disorders of gluconeogenesis must be excluded (see Table 1.22). These entities are usually characterized by a fasting hypoglycemia without ketosis (908).

If lactic acidosis is not explainable by the previously mentioned studies in this section, a muscle biopsy must be performed (859). Should light microscopy suggest the presence of ragged red fibers, confirmed by electron microscopy, the defect is most likely to be a mitochondrial deletion or a defect in one of the genes coding for a tRNA. If the increased lipid content overshadows the mitochondrial abnormalities, the various lipid storage myopathies must be considered. These are covered in Chapter 14. Should the muscle biopsy result be normal, a defect of the pyruvate decarboxylase complex or of pyruvate carboxylase is likely. Pinpointing the biochemical defect requires assays of the various respiratory chain complexes in muscle or skin fibroblast cultures. Details of the techniques used are given by Robinson and colleagues (909).

Treatment

This careful diagnostic evaluation is not solely academic. It assists in genetic counseling and reveals the entities that appear to be at least partly amenable to treatment. Some patients with MELAS syndrome showed transient muscle strengthening, seizure control, and lowering of elevated serum lactate and pyruvate with corticosteroid therapy. Riboflavin (100 mg/day) has been suggested in the treatment of the myopathy caused by a deficiency of complex I (NADH-CoQ reductase). In patients with Kearns-Sayre syndrome owing to an impairment in complex I (NADH-CoQ reductase), prolonged treatment with coenzyme Q (120 mg/day orally) has improved exercise tolerance, reduced cerebellar deficits, and lowered serum lactate and pyruvate levels (910). Coenzyme Q also might improve neurologic symptoms in some of the other mitochondrial myopathies (910). Dichloroacetate, an activator of the pyruvate dehydrogenase complex, has been used to treat patients with lactic acidosis caused by a deficiency in the E_1 enzyme (899,899a,911). Finally, in some infants, cytochrome oxidase deficiency has been found to be spontaneously reversible (912). This probably reflects a gradual selection of muscle fibers containing a wild-type mitochondrial genome over those containing mainly mutant genomes (845).

REFERENCES

1. Harding AE, Rosenberg RN. A neurologic gene map. In: Rosenberg RN, et al., eds. *The molecular and genetic basis of neurological disease*, 2nd ed. Boston: Butterworth–Heinemann, 1997:23–28.
2. Rosenberg RN, et al., eds. *The molecular and genetic basis of neurological disease*, 2nd ed. Boston: Butterworth–Heinemann, 1997.
3. Garrod AE. The Croonian lectures on inborn errors of metabolism. Lecture IV. *Lancet* 1908;2:214–220.
4. Kim SZ, et al. Hydroxyprolinemia: comparison of a patient and her unaffected twin sister. *J Pediatr* 1997;130:437–441.
5. Lodish H, et al. eds. *Molecular cell biology*, 3rd ed. New York: Scientific American Books, 1995.
6. Lewin B. *Genes VI*. New York: Oxford University Press, 1997.
7. Burton BK. Inborn errors of metabolism. The clinical diagnosis in early infancy. *Pediatrics* 1987;79:359–369.
8. Curry CJ, et al. Evaluation of mental retardation: recommendations of a Consensus Conference. *Am J Med Genet* 1997;72:468–477.
9. Fölling A. Uber Ausscheidung von Phenylbrenztraubensäure in den Harn als Stoffwechselanomalie in Verbindung mit Imbezillität. *Ztschr Physiol Chem* 1934;227:169–176.
10. Berman JL, et al. Causes of high phenylalanine with normal tyrosine. *Am J Dis Child* 1969;117:654–656.
11. Scriver CR, et al. The hyperphenylalaninemias. In: Scriver CR, Beaudet AL, Sly WS, Valle D, eds. *The metabolic and molecular basis of inherited disease*, 7th ed. New York: McGraw-Hill, 1995:1015–1075.
12. Okano Y, et al. Molecular basis of phenotypic heterogeneity in phenylketonuria. *N Engl J Med* 1991;324:1232–1238.
13. Eisensmith RC, et al. Molecular basis of phenylketonuria and a correlation between genotype and phenotype in a heterogenous southeastern US population. *Pediatrics* 1996;97:512–516.
13a. Goldberg P, et al. A European multicenter study of phenylalanine hydroxylase deficiency: classification of 105 mutations and a general system for genotype-based prediction of metabolic phenotype. *Am J Hum Genet* 1998;63:71–79.
13b. Ramus SJ, et al. Genotype and intellectual phenotype in untreated phenylketonuria patients. *Pediatr Res* 1999;45:474–481.
14. Yarbro MT, Anderson JA. L-tryptophan metabolism in phenylketonuria. *J Pediatr* 1966;68:895–904.
15. Miyamoto M, Fitzpatrick TB. Competitive inhibition of mammalian tyrosinase by phenylalanine and its relationship to hair pigmentation in phenylketonuria. *Nature* 1957;179:199–200.
16. Malamud N. Neuropathy of phenylketonuria. *J Neuropathol Exp Neurol* 1966;25:254–268.
17. Bauman ML, Kemper TL. Morphologic and histoanatomic observations of the brain in untreated human phenylketonuria. *Acta Neuropathol* 1982;58:55–63.
18. Crome L. The association of phenylketonuria with leucodystrophy. *J Neurol Neurosurg Psychiatr* 1962;25:149–153.
19. Barden H. The histochemical relationship of neuromelanin and lipofuscin. *J Neuropathol Exp Neurol* 1969;28:419–441.
20. Partington MW. The early symptoms of phenylketonuria. *Pediatrics* 1961;27:465–473.
21. MacLeod MD, et al. Management of the extrapyramidal manifestations of phenylketonuria with L-dopa. *Arch Dis Child* 1983;58:457–458.
22. Gross PT, et al. EEG in phenylketonuria. Attempt to establish clinical importance of EEG changes. *Arch Neurol* 1981;38:122–126.
23. Thompson AJ, et al. Brain MRI changes in phenylketonuria: associations with dietary status. *Brain* 1993;116:811–824.
24. Pearson KD, et al. Phenylketonuria: MR imaging of the brain with clinical correlation. *Radiology* 1990;177:437–440.
25. Cleary MA, et al. Magnetic resonance imaging in phenylketonuria: reversal of cerebral white matter changes. *J Pediatr* 1995;127:251–255.
26. Kang E, Paine RS. Elevation of plasma phenylalanine levels during pregnancies of women heterozygous for phenylketonuria. *J Pediatr* 1963;63:282–289.
27. Lenke RR, Levy HL. Maternal phenylketonuria and hyperphenylalaninemia: an international survey of the outcome of treated and untreated pregnancies. *N Engl J Med* 1980;303:1202–1208.
28. Levy HL, et al. Maternal phenylketonuria: magnetic resonance imaging of the brain in offspring. *J Pediatr* 1996;128:770–775.
29. Koch R, et al. The North American Collaborative Study of maternal phenylketonuria (PKU). *Int Pediatr* 1993;8:89–96.
30. Levy HL, et al. Maternal mild hyperphenylalaninaemia: an international survey of offspring outcome. *Lancet* 1994;344:1589–1594.
31. Scriver CR, Clow CL. Phenylketonuria: epitome of human biochemical genetics. *N Engl J Med* 1980;303:1336–1342.
32. Kaufman S. An evaluation of the possible neurotoxicity of metabolites of phenylalanine. *J Pediatr* 1989;114:895–900.
33. Menkes JH, Koch R. Phenylketonuria. In: Vinken PJ, Bruyn GW, eds. *Handbook of clinical neurology*. Vol. 29. Amsterdam: North-Holland Publishing Co, 1977:29–51.
34. Hommes FA. On the mechanism of permanent brain dysfunction in hyperphenylalaninemia. *Biochem Med Metabol Biol* 1991;46:277–287.

35. Guthrie R, Susi A. A simple phenylalanine method for detecting phenylketonuria in large populations of newborn infants. *Pediatrics* 1963;32:338–343.

36. McCaman MW, Robins E. Fluorometric method for the determination of phenylalanine in serum. *J Lab Clin Med* 1962;59:885–890.

36a. Bartlett K, Eaton SJ, Pourfarzam M. New developments in neonatal screening. *Arch Dis Child Fetal Neonatal Ed* 1997;77:F151–F154.

37. Koch R, Friedman EG. Accuracy of newborn screening programs for phenylketonuria. *J Pediatr* 1981;98:267–269.

38. Doherty LB, Rohr FJ, Levy HL. Detection of phenylketonuria in the very early newborn population. *Pediatrics* 1991;87:240–244.

39. Sinai L, et al. Phenylketonuria screening: effect of early newborn discharge. *Pediatrics* 1995;96:605–608.

40. Economou-Petersen E, et al. Molecular basis for non-phenylketonuria hyperphenylalanemia. *Genomics* 1992;14:15.

41. Guttler F, et al. Correlation between polymorphic DNA haplotypes at phenylalanine hydroxylase locus and clinical phenotypes of phenylketonuria. *J Pediatr* 1987;110:68–71.

42. Sepe SJ, Levy HL, Mount FW. An evaluation of routine follow-up infants for phenylketonuria. *N Engl J Med* 1979;300:606–609.

43. Holtzman C, et al. Descriptive epidemiology of missed cases of phenylketonuria and congenital hypothyroidism. *Pediatrics* 1986;78:553–558.

44. DiLella AG, Huang WM, Woo SLC. Screening for phenylketonuria mutations by DNA amplifications with the polymerase chain reaction. *Lancet* 1988;1:497–499.

45. Ledley FD. Clinical application of genotypic diagnosis for phenylketonuria: theoretical considerations. *Eur J Pediatr* 1991;150:752–756.

46. Gröbe H, et al. Hyperphenylalaninemia due to dihydropteridine reductase deficiency. *Eur J Pediatr* 1978;129:93–98.

47. Dhondt JL. Tetrahydrobiopterin deficiencies: preliminary analysis from an international survey. *J Pediatr* 1984;104:501–508.

48. Smith I, et al. Neurological aspects of biopterin metabolism. *Arch Dis Child* 1986;61:130–137.

49. Woody RC, Brewster MA, Glasier C. Progressive intracranial calcification in dihydropteridine reductase deficiency prior to folinic acid therapy. *Neurology* 1989;39:673–675.

50. Sugita R, et al. Brain CT and MR findings in hyperphenylalaninemia due to dihydropteridine reductase deficiency (variant of phenylketonuria). *J Comput Assist Tomogr* 1990;14:699–703.

51. Irons M, et al. Folic acid therapy in treatment of dihydropteridine reductase deficiency. *J Pediatr* 1987;110:61–67.

52. Kaufman S. Unsolved problems in diagnosis and therapy of hyperphenylalaninemia caused by defects in tetrahydrobiopterin metabolism. *J Pediatr* 1986;109:572–578.

53. Dhondt JL, et al. Neonatal hyperphenylalaninaemia presumably caused by a new variant of biopterin synthetase deficiency. *Europ J Pediat* 1988;147:153–157.

54. Thony B, et al. Hyperphenylalaninemia due to defects in tetrahydrobiopterin metabolism: molecular characterization of mutations in 6-pyruvoyl-tetrahydropterin synthase. *Am J Hum Genet* 1994;54:782–792.

55. Hoganson G, et al. Biopterin synthesis defects: problems in diagnosis. *Pediatrics* 1984;74:1004–1011.

56. Brismar J, et al. Malignant hyperphenylalaninemia: CT and MR of the brain. *Am J Neuroradiol* 1990;11:135–138.

57. Niederwieser A, et al. GTP cyclohydrolase I deficiency, a new enzyme defect causing hyperphenylalaninemia with neopterin, biopterin, dopamine and serotonin deficiencies and muscular hypotonia. *Eur J Pediatr* 1984;141:208–214.

58. Blau N, et al. A missense mutation in a patient with guanosine triphosphate cyclohydrolase I deficiency missed in the newborn screening program. *J Pediatr* 1995;126:401–405.

58a. Hirano M, Yanagihara T, Ueno S. Dominant negative effect of GTP cyclohydrolase I mutations in dopa-responsive hereditary progressive dystonia. *Ann Neurol* 1998;44:365–371.

59. Buist NRM, et al. Towards improving the diet for hyperphenylalaninemia and other metabolic disorders. *Int Pediatr* 1993;8:80–88.

60. Acosta PB, et al. Nutrition studies in treated infants with phenylketonuria. *Int Pediatr* 1993;8:63–73.

61. Smith I, Beasley MG, Ades AE. Intelligence and quality of dietary treatment in phenylketonuria. *Arch Dis Child* 1990;65:472–478.

62. Brunner RL, Jordan MK, Berry HK. Early treated phenylketonuria: neuropsychologic consequences. *J Pediatr* 1983;102:831–835.

63. Smith I, et al. Behavior disturbance in 8-year-old children with early treated phenylketonuria. *J Pediatr* 1988;112:403–408.

64. Smith ML, et al. Randomised controlled trial of tyrosine supplementation on neuropsychological performance in phenylketonuria. *Arch Dis Child* 1998;78:116–121.

65. Holtzman NA, et al. Effect of age at loss of dietary control on intellectual performance and behavior of children with phenylketonuria. *N Engl J Med* 1986;314:593–598.

66. Weisbren SE, et al. Predictors of intelligence quotients and intelligence quotient change in persons treated for phenylketonuria early in life. *Pediatrics* 1987;79:351–355.

67. Thompson AJ, et al. Neurological deterioration in young adults with phenylketonuria. *Lancet* 1990;336:602–605.

68. Villasana D, et al. Neurological deterioration in adult phenylketonuria. *J Inherited Metab Dis* 1989;12:451–457.

68a. Endres W. Diet in phenylketonuria: how long? Policies under discussion. *Ann Nutr Metab* 1998;4:221–227.

69. Parkman R. The application of bone marrow transplantation to the treatment of genetic diseases. *Science* 1986;232:1373–1378.

70. Hoggerbrugge PM, Valerio D. Bone marrow transplantation and gene therapy for lysosomal storage diseases. *Bone Marrow Transplant* 1998;21[suppl 2]:S34–S36.

71. Whitington PF, Alonso EM, Piper J. Liver transplantation for inborn errors of metabolism. *Int Pediatr* 1993;8:30–39.

72. Peng H, et al. Retroviral mediated gene transfer and expression of human phenylalanine hydroxylase in primary mouse hepatocytes. *Proc Natl Acad Sci U S A* 1988;85:8146–8150.

73. Chang TM, Prakash S. Therapeutic uses of microencapsulated genetically engineered cells. *Mol Med Today* 1998;4:221–227.

74. Scriver CR, Larochelle J, Silverberg M. Hereditary tyrosinemia and tyrosyluria in a French-Canadian geographic isolate. *Am J Dis Child* 1967;113:41–46.

75. Menkes JH, Hurst PL, Craig JM. A new syndrome: progressive familial infantile cerebral dysfunction associated with unusual urinary substance. *Pediatrics* 1954;14: 462–467.

76. Roth KS. Newborn metabolic screening: a search for "nature's experiments." *South Med J* 1986;79:47–54.

77. Cox RP, Chuang JL, Chuang DT. Maple syrup urine disease: clinical and molecular genetic considerations. In: Rosenberg RN, et al., eds. *The molecular and genetic basis of neurological disease*, 2nd ed. Boston: Butterworth–Heinemann, 1997:1175–1193.

78. Menkes JH. Maple syrup disease: investigations into the metabolic defect. *Neurology* 1959;9:826–835.

78a. Podebrad F, et al. 4,5-dimethyl-3-hydroxy-2[5H]-furanone (sotolone)—the odor of maple syrup urine disease. *J Inherit Metabol Dis* 1999;22:107–114.

79. Menkes JH. Maple syrup disease: isolation and identification of organic acids in the urine. *Pediatrics* 1959;23:348–353.

80. Chuang DT. Maple syrup urine disease: it has come a long way. *J Pediatr* 1998;132:S17–S23.

81. Mamer OA, Reimer ML. On the mechanisms of the formation of L-alloisoleucine and the 2-hydroxy-3-methylvaleric acid stereoisomers from L-isoleucine in maple syrup urine disease patients and in normal humans. *J Biol Chem* 1992;267:22141–22147.

82. Lancaster G, Mamer OA, Scriver CR. Branched-chain α-keto acids isolated as oxime derivatives. Relationship to the corresponding hydroxy acids and amino acids in maple syrup urine disease. *Metabolism* 1974;23: 257–265.

83. Kamei A, et al. Abnormal dendritic development in maple syrup urine disease. *Pediatr Neurol* 1992;8: 145–147.

84. Martin JJ, Schlote W. Central nervous system lesions in disorders of amino-acid metabolism: a neuropathological study. *J Neurol Sci* 1972;15:49–76.

85. Müller K, Kahn T, Wendel U. Is demyelination a feature of maple syrup disease? *Pediatr Neurol* 1993;9: 375–382.

86. Menkes JH, Solcher H. Effect of dietary therapy on cerebral morphology and chemistry in maple syrup disease. *Arch Neurol* 1967;16:486–491.

87. Dickinson JP, et al. Maple syrup urine disease. Four years' experience with dietary treatment of a case. *Acta Paediat Scand* 1969;58:341–351.

88. Riviello JJ, et al. Cerebral edema causing death in children with maple syrup urine disease. *J Pediatr* 1991;119:42–45.

89. MacDonald JT, Sher PK. Ophthalmoplegia as a sign of metabolic disease in the newborn. *Neurology* 1977; 27:971–973.

90. Haymond MW, Ben-Galim E, Strobel KE. Glucose and alanine metabolism in children with maple syrup urine disease. *J Clin Invest* 1978;62:398–405.

91. Felber SR, et al. Maple syrup urine disease: metabolic decompensation monitored by proton magnetic resonance imaging and spectroscopy. *Ann Neurol* 1993;33: 396–401.

92. Brismar J, et al. Maple syrup urine disease: findings on CT and MRI scans of the brain in 10 infants. *Am J Neuroradiol* 1990;11:1219–1228.

93. Menkes JH. The pathogenesis of mental retardation in phenylketonuria and other inborn errors of amino-acid metabolism. *Pediatrics* 1967;39:297–308.

94. Tsuruta M, et al. Molecular basis of intermittent maple syrup urine disease: novel mutations in the E_2 gene of the branched-chain alpha-keto acid dehydrogenase complex. *J Hum Genet* 1998;43:91–100.

95. Goedde HW, Langenbeck U, Brackertz D. Clinical and biochemical-genetic aspects of intermittent branched-chain ketoaciduria. *Acta Paediatr Scand* 1970;59: 83–87.

96. Schulman JD, et al. A new variant of maple syrup urine disease (branched chain ketoaciduria): clinical and biochemical evaluation. *Am J Med* 1970;49: 118–124.

97. Ellerine NP, et al. Thiamin-responsive maple syrup urine disease in a patient antigenically missing dihydrolipoamide acyltransferase. *Biochem Med Metab Biol* 1993;49:363–374.

98. Scriver CR, Clow CL, George H. So-called thiamin-responsive maple syrup urine disease: 15-year follow-up of the original patient. *J Pediatr* 1985;107:763–765.

99. Wendel U, et al. Maple-syrup-urine disease. *N Engl J Med* 1983;308:1100–1101.

100. Naylo EW, Guthrie R. Newborn screening for maple syrup urine disease (branched-chain ketoaciduria). *Pediatrics* 1978;61:262–266.

101. Elsas LJ, et al. Maple syrup urine disease: coenzyme function and prenatal monitoring. *Metabolism* 1974; 23:569–579.

102. Chuang DT, Shih VE. Disorders of branched-chain amino acid and keto acid metabolism. In: Scriver CR, Beaudet AL, Sly WS, Valle D, eds. *The metabolic and molecular basis of inherited disease*, 7th ed. New York: McGraw-Hill, 1995:1239–1278.

103. Nyhan WL, et al. Treatment of the acute crisis in maple syrup urine disease. *Arch Pediatr Adolesc Med* 1998;152:593–598.

104. Clow CL, Reade TM, Scriver CR. Outcome of early and long-term management of classical maple syrup urine disease. *Pediatrics* 1981;68:856–862.

105. Hilliges C, Awiszus D, Wendel U. Intellectual performance of children with maple syrup urine disease. *Eur J Pediatr* 1993;152:144–147.

106. Mitchell G, et al. Neurologic crises in hereditary tyrosinemia. *N Engl J Med* 1990;322:432–437.

107. Laine J, et al. The nephropathy of Type I tyrosinemia after liver transplantation. *Pediatr Res* 1995;37:640–645.

108. Westphal EM, et al. The human tyrosine aminotransferase gene: characterization of restriction fragment length polymorphisms and haplotype analysis in a family with tyrosinemia type II. *Hum Genet* 1988; 79:260–264.

109. Andersson S, et al. Persistent tyrosinemia associated with low activity of tyrosine aminotransferase. *Pediatr Res* 1984;18:675–678.

110. Menkes JH, Jervis GA. Developmental retardation associated with an abnormality in tyrosine metabolism. *Pediatrics* 1961;28:399–409.

111. Endo F, et al. 4-Hydroxyphenylpyruvic acid oxidase deficiency with normal fumarylacetoacetase: a new variant form of hereditary hypertyrosinemia. *Pediatr Res* 1983;17:92–96.

112. Ruetschi U, Rymo L, Lindstedt S. Human 4-hydroxy-phenylpyruvate dioxygenase gene (HPD). *Genomics* 1997;44:292–299.

113. Medes G. A new error of tyrosine metabolism: tyrosinosis. The intermediary metabolism of tyrosine and phenylalanine. *Biochem J* 1932;26:917–940.

114. Menkes JH, et al. Relationship of elevated blood tyrosine to the ultimate intellectual performance of premature infants. *Pediatrics* 1972;49:218–224.

115. Mamunes P, et al. Intellectual deficits after transient tyrosinemia in the term neonate. *Pediatrics* 1976;57: 675–680.

116. Borden M, et al. Hawkinsinuria in two families. *Am J Med Genet* 1992;44:52–56.

117. Niederweiser A, et al. A new sulfur amino-acid, named hawkensin, identified in a baby with transient tyrosinemia and her mother. *Clin Chim Acta* 1977;76:345–356.

118. Tada K. Nonketotic hyperglycinemia: clinical metabolic aspects. *Enzyme* 1987;38:27–35.

119. Hamosh A, Johnston MV, Valle D. Nonketotic hyperglycinemia. In: Scriver CR, Beaudet AL, Sly WS, Valle D, eds. *The metabolic and molecular basis of inherited disease*, 7th ed. New York: McGraw-Hill, 1995: 1337–1348.

120. Luder AS, et al. Transient nonketotic hyperglycinemia in neonates. *J Pediatr* 1989;114:1013–1015.

121. Frazier DM, Summer GK, Chamberlin HR. Hyperglycinuria and hyperglycinemia in two siblings with mild developmental delays. *Am J Dis Child* 1978; 132:777–781.

122. Trauner DA, et al. Progressive neurodegenerative disorder in a patient with nonketotic hyperglycinemia. *J Pediatr* 1981;98:272–275.

123. Press GA, et al. Abnormalities of the brain in nonketotic hyperglycinemia: MR manifestations. *Am J Neuroradiol* 1989;10:315–321.

124. Tada K, et al. Genomic analysis of nonketotic hyperglycinemia: a partial deletion of P-protein gene. *J Inherit Metab Dis* 1990;13:766–770.

125. Schmitt B, et al. Nonketotic hyperglycinemia: clinical and electrophysiological effects of dextromorphan, an antagonist of the NMDA receptor. *Neurology* 1993; 43:421–423.

126. Deutsch SI, Rosse RB, Mastropaolo J. Current status of NMDA antagonist interventions in the treatment of nonketotic hyperglycinemia. *Clin Neuropharmacol* 1998;21:71–79.

127. Elpeleg ON, et al. Late-onset form of partial *N*-acetyl-glutamate synthetase deficiency. *Eur J Pediatr* 1990; 149:634–636.

128. Batshaw ML. Inborn errors of urea synthesis. *Ann Neurol* 1994;35:133–141.

129. Matsuda I, et al. Retrospective survey of urea cycle disorders: Part I. Clinical and laboratory observations of thirty-two Japanese male patients with ornithine transcarbamylase deficiency. *Am J Med Genet* 1991;38: 85–89.

130. Rowe PC, Newman SL, Brusilow SW. Natural history of symptomatic partial ornithine transcarbamylase deficiency. *N Engl J Med* 1986;314:541–547.

131. Allan JD, et al. A disease, probably hereditary, characterized by severe mental deficiency and a constant gross abnormality of amino acid metabolism. *Lancet* 1958;1:182–187.

132. O'Brien WE, Barr RH. Argininosuccinate lyase: purification and characterization from human liver. *Biochemistry* 1981;20:2056–2060.

133. Crane CW, Gay WMB, Jenner FA. Urea production from labeled ammonia in argininosuccinic aciduria. *Clin Chim Acta* 1969;24:445–448.

134. Kay JD, et al. Effect of partial ornithine carbamoyltransferase deficiency on urea synthesis and related biochemical events. *Clin Sci* 1987;72: 187–193.

135. Carton, D, et al. Argininosuccinic aciduria: neonatal variant with rapid fatal course. *Acta Paediatr Scand* 1969;58:528–534.

136. Lewis PD, Miller AL. Argininosuccinic aciduria: case report with neuropathological findings. *Brain* 1970;93: 413–422.

137. Levy HL, Coulombe JT, Shih VE. Newborn urine screening. In: Bickel H, et al. eds. *Neonatal screening for inborn errors of metabolism*. Berlin: Springer-Verlag, 1980:89.

138. Walker DC, et al. Molecular analysis of human argininosuccinate lyase: mutant characterization and alternative splicing of the coding region. *Proc Nat Acad Sci* 1990;87:9625–9629.

139. Glick NR, Snodgrass PJ, Schafer IA. Neonatal argininosuccinicaciduria with normal brain and kidney but absent liver argininosuccinate lyase activity. *Am J Hum Genet* 1976;28:22–30.

140. Widhalm K, et al. Long-term follow-up of 12 patients with the late-onset variant of argininosuccinic acid lyase deficiency: no impairment of intellectual and psychomotor development during therapy. *Pediatrics* 1992;87:1182–1184.

141. Brusilow SW, Horwich AL. Urea cycle enzymes. In: Scriver CR, Beaudet AL, Sly WS, Valle D, eds. *The metabolic and molecular basis of inherited disease*, 7th ed. New York: McGraw-Hill, 1995:1187–1232.

142. Bachmann C, Colombo JP. Diagnostic value of orotic acid excretion in heritable disorders of the urea cycle and in hyperammonemia due to organic acidurias. *Eur J Pediatr* 1980;134:109–113.

143. Rutledge SL, et al. Neonatal hemodialysis: effective therapy for the encephalopathy of inborn errors of metabolism. *J Pediatr* 1990;116:125–128.

144. Batshaw ML, et al. Treatment of inborn errors of urea synthesis. Activation of alternative pathways of waste nitrogen synthesis and excretion. *N Engl J Med* 1982; 306:1387–1392.

145. Msall M, et al. Neurologic outcome in children with inborn errors of urea synthesis: outcome of urea-cycle enzymopathies. *N Engl J Med* 1984;310:1500–1505.

146. Morgan HB, Swaiman KF, Johnson BD. Diagnosis of argininosuccinic aciduria after valproic acid-induced hyperammonemia. *Neurology* 1987;37:886–887.

147. McMurray WC, et al. Citrullinuria. *Pediatrics* 1963; 32: 347–357.

148. Beaudet AL, et al. The human argininosuccinate locus and citrullinemia. *Adv Hum Genet* 1986;15: 161–196.

149. Kobayashi K, et al. Heterogeneity of mutations in argininosuccinate synthetase causing human citrullinemia. *J Biol Chem* 1990;265:11361–11367.

150. Wick H, et al. Variants of citrullinaemia. *Arch Dis Child* 1973;48:63–64.

151. Oyanagi K, et al. Citrullinemia: quantitative deficiency of argininosuccinate synthetase in the liver. *Tohoku J Exp Med* 1986;148:385–391.

152. Milne MD, London DR, Asatoor AM. Citrullinuria in cases of cystinuria. *Lancet* 1962;2:49–50.

153. Russell A, et al. Hyperammonaemia: a new instance of an inborn enzymatic defect of the biosynthesis of urea. *Lancet* 1962;2:699–700.

154. Tuchman M, et al. The biochemical and molecular spectrum of ornithine transcarbamylase deficiency. *J Inherit Metab Dis* 1998;21[suppl 1]:40–58.

155. Wendel U, et al. DNA analysis of ornithine transcarbamylase deficiency. *Eur J Pediatr* 1988;147:368–371.

156. Rowe PC, Newman SL, Brusilow SW. Natural history of symptomatic partial ornithine transcarbamylase deficiency. *N Engl J Med* 1986;314:541–546.

157. Dolman CL, Clasen RA, Dorovini-Zis K. Severe cerebral damage in ornithine transcarbamylase deficiency. *Clin Neuropathol* 1988;7:10–15.

158. Shapiro JM, et al. Mitochondrial abnormalities of liver in primary ornithine transcarbamylase deficiency. *Pediatr Res* 1980;14:735–739.

158a. Maestri NE, Clissold D, Brusilow SW. Neonatal onset ornithine transcarbamylase deficiency: a retrospective analysis. *J Pediatr* 1999;134:268–272.

159. Bachmann C. Ornithine transcarbamoyl transferase deficiency: findings, models and problems. *J Inherit Metab Dis* 1992;15:578–591.

160. Batshaw ML, et al. Cerebral dysfunction in asymptomatic carriers of ornithine transcarbamylase deficiency. *N Engl J Med* 1980;302:482–485.

161. Hjelm M, et al. Evidence of inherited urea cycle defect in a case of fatal valproate toxicity. *BMJ* 1986;292:23–24.

162. Maestri NE, et al. Long-term treatment of girls with ornithine transcarbamylase deficiency. *N Engl J Med* 1996;335:855–859.

163. Maestri NE, et al. Prospective treatment of urea cycle disorders. *J Pediatr* 1991;119:923–928.

164. Todo S, et al. Orthoptic liver transplantation for urea cycle enzyme deficiency. *Hepatology* 1992;15:419–422.

165. Yudkoff M, et al. Ornithine transcarbamylase deficiency in a boy with normal development. *J Pediatr* 1980;96:441–443.

166. Tuchman M, et al. Identification of "private" mutations in patients with ornithine transcarbamylase deficiency. *J Inherit Metab Dis* 1997;20:525–527.

167. Svirklys LG, et al. Family studies in ornithine transcarbamylase deficiency. *Arch Dis Child* 1988;63:297–302.

168. Freeman JM, et al. Congenital hyperammonemia. *Arch Neurol* 1970;23:430–437.

169. Ebels EJ. Neuropathological observations in a patient with carbamylphosphate synthetase deficiency and in two sibs. *Arch Dis Child* 1972;47:47–51.

170. Terheggen HG, et al. Familial hyperargininaemia. *Arch Dis Child* 1975;50:57–62.

171. Cederbaum SD, Shaw KN, Valente M. Hyperargininemia. *J Pediatr* 1977;90:569–573.

172. Snyderman SE, et al. Argininemia treated from birth. *J Pediatr* 1979;95:61–63.

173. Mizutani N, et al. Enzyme replacement therapy in a patient with hyperargininemia. *Tohoku J Exp Med* 1987;151:301–307.

174. Bachmann C, et al. *N*-acetylglutamate synthetase deficiency: a disorder of ammonia detoxification [Letter]. *N Engl J Med* 1981;1:543.

175. Zammarchi E, et al. Neonatal onset of hyperornithemia-hyperammonemia-homocitrullinuria syndrome with favorable outcome. *J Pediatr* 1997;131:440–443.

176. Hommes FA, et al. Decreased transport of ornithine across the inner mitochondrial membrane as a cause of hyperornithinaemia. *J Inherit Metab Dis* 1982;5:41–47.

177. Valtonen M, et al. Skeletal muscle of patients with gyrate atrophy of the choroid and retina and hyperornithinaemia in ultra-low-field magnetic resonance imaging and computed tomography. *J Inherit Metab Dis* 1996;19:729–734.

178. McInnes RR, et al. Hyperornithinemia and gyrate atrophy of the retina: improvement of vision during treatment with a low arginine diet. *Lancet* 1981;1:513–516.

179. Van Geet C, et al. Possible platelet contribution to pathogenesis of transient neonatal hyperammonemia syndrome. *Lancet* 1991;337:73–75.

180. Ellison PH, Cowger ML. Transient hyperammonemia in the preterm infant: neurologic aspects. *Neurology* 1981;31:767–770.

181. Ogier de Baulny H, et al. Neonatal hyperammonemia caused by a defect of carnitine-acylcarnitine translocase. *J Pediatr* 1995;127:723–728.

182. Hudak ML, Jones MD, Brusilow SW. Differentiation of transient hyperammonemia of the newborn and urea cycle enzyme defects by clinical presentation. *J Pediatr* 1985;107:712–719.

183. Batshaw ML, Brusilow SW. Asymptomatic hyperammonemia in low-birth-weight infants. *Pediatr Res* 1978;12:221–224.

184. Levy HL, Taylor RG, McInnes RR. Disorders of histidine metabolism. In: Scriver CR, Beaudet AL, Sly WS, Valle D, eds. *The metabolic and molecular basis of inherited disease*, 7th ed. New York: McGraw-Hill, 1995:1107–1123.

185. Carson NAJ, Cusworth DC, Dent CE. Homocystinuria: a new inborn error of metabolism associated with mental deficiency. *Arch Dis Child* 1963;38:425–436.

186. Naughten ER, Yap S, Mayne PD. Newborn screening for homocystinuria: Irish and world experience. *Eur J Pediatr* 1998;157[suppl 2]:S84–S87.

187. Mudd SH, et al. Homocystinuria: an enzymatic defect. *Science* 1964;143:1443–1445.

188. Kraus J, et al. Purification and properties of cystathionine-β-synthase from human liver. *J Biol Chem* 1978;253:6523–6528.

189. Uhlendorf BW, Conerly EB, Mudd SH. Homocystinuria: studies in tissue culture. *Pediatr Res* 1973;7:645–658.

190. Fowler B, et al. Homocystinuria: evidence for three distinct classes of cystathionine-β-synthase mutants in cultured fibroblasts. *J Clin Invest* 1978;61:645–653.

191. Shan X, Kruger WD. Correction of disease-causing CBS mutations in yeast. *Nat Genet* 1998;19:91–93.

192. Brenton DP, Cusworth DC, Gaull GE. Homocystinuria: metabolic studies on 3 patients. *J Pediatr* 1965;67:58–68.

193. Mudd SH, et al. The natural history of homocystinuria due to cystathionine-β-synthase deficiency. *Am J Hum Genet* 1985;37:1–31.

194. Haworth JC, et al. Symptomatic and asymptomatic methylene tetrahydrofolate reductase deficiency in two adult brothers. *Am J Med Genet* 1993;45:572–576.

195. Freeman JM, Finkelstein JD, Mudd SH. Folate-responsive homocystinuria and "schizophrenia": A defect in methylation due to deficient 5, 10-methylene tetrahy-

drofolate reductase activity. *N Engl J Med* 1975;292: 491–496.

196. Gibson JB, Carson NA, Neill DW. Pathological findings in homocystinuria. *J Clin Pathol* 1964;17: 427–437.

197. Welch GN, Loscalzo J. Homocysteine and atherosclerosis. *N Engl J Med* 1998;338:1042–1050.

198. Presley GD, Sidbury JB. Homocystinuria and ocular defects. *Am J Ophthalmol* 1967;63:1723–1727.

199. Wilcken B, Turner G. Homocystinuria in New South Wales. *Arch Dis Child* 1978;53:242–245.

200. Mudd SH, Levy HL, Skovby F. Disorders of transsulfuration. In: Scriver CR, Beaudet AL, Sly WS, Valle D, eds. *The metabolic and molecular basis of inherited disease*, 7th ed. New York: McGraw-Hill, 1995:1279–1327.

201. Thomas PS, Carson NA. Homocystinuria: the evolution of skeletal changes in relation to treatment. *Ann Radiol* 1978;21:95–104.

202. Schedewie H, et al. Skeletal findings in homocystinuria: a collaborative study. *Pediatr Radiol* 1973;1:12–23.

203. Brenton DP, et al. Homocystinuria and Marfan's syndrome: a comparison. *J Bone Joint Surg* 1972;54B: 277–298.

204. Kurczynski TW, et al. Maternal homocystinuria: studies of an untreated mother and fetus. *Arch Dis Child* 1980;55:721–723.

205. Morrow G, Barness LA. Combined vitamin responsiveness in homocystinuria. *J Pediatr* 1972;81:946–954.

206. Wilcken DE, et al. Homocystinuria—the effects of betaine in the treatment of patients not responsive to pyridoxine. *N Engl J Med* 1983;309:448–453.

207. Lyon ICT, Procopis PG, Turner B. Cystathioninuria in a well-baby population. *Acta Paediatr Scand* 1971;60: 324–328.

208. Mudd SH, et al. Isolated persistent hypermethioninemia. *Am J Hum Genet* 1995;57:882–892.

209. Jonas AJ, et al. Nephropathic cystinosis with central nervous system involvement. *Am J Med* 1987;83: 966–970.

210. Levine S, Paparo G. Brain lesions in a case of cystinosis. *Acta Neuropathol* 1982;57:217–220.

211. Broyer M, et al. Clinical polymorphism of cystinosis encephalopathy. Results of treatment with cysteamine. *J Inherit Metab Dis* 1996;19:65–75.

212. Gahl WA, et al. Myopathy and cystine storage in muscles in a patient with nephropathic cystinosis. *N Engl J Med* 1988;319:1461–1464.

213. Cochat P, et al. Cerebral atrophy and nephropathic cystinosis. *Arch Dis Child* 1986;61:401–403.

214. Simell O. Lysinuric protein intolerance and other cationic aminoacidurias. In: Scriver CR, Beaudet AL, Sly WS, Valle D, eds. *The metabolic and molecular basis of inherited disease*, 7th ed. New York: McGraw-Hill, 1995:3603–3627.

215. Simell O, et al. Lysinuric protein intolerance. *Am J Med* 1975;59:229–240.

216. Lauteala T, et al. Lysinuric protein intolerance (LPI) gene maps to the long arm of chromosome 14. *Am J Hum Genet* 1997;60:1479–1486.

216a. Borsani G, et al. SLC7A7, encoding a putative permease-related protein, is mutated in patients with lysinuric protein intolerance. *Nature Genet* 1999;21:297–301.

217. Harris H, et al. Phenotypes and genotypes in cystinuria. *Ann Hum Genet* 1955;10:57–71.

218. Fisher MH, Gerritsen T, Opitz JM. α-Aminoadipic aciduria, a non-deleterious inborn metabolic defect. *Hum Genet* 1974;24:265–270.

219. Wilson RW, et al. α-Ketoadipic aciduria: a description of a new metabolic error in lysine-tryptophan degeneration. *Pediatr Res* 1975;9:522–526.

220. Vallat C, et al. Treatment with vigabatrin may mimic alpha-aminoadipic aciduria. *Epilepsia* 1996;37: 803–805.

221. Wada Y, Tada K, Minagawa A. Idiopathic hypervalinemia: probably a new entity of inborn error of valine metabolism. *Tohoku J Exp Med* 1963;81:46–55.

222. Higgins JJ, et al. Pyridoxine-responsive hyper-β-alaninemia associated with Cohen's syndrome. *Neurology* 1994;44:1728–1732.

223. Willi SM, et al. A deletion in the long arm of chromosome 18 in a child with serum carnosinase deficiency. *Pediatr Res* 1997;41:210–213.

224. Yamaguchi S, et al. Defect in biosynthesis of mitochondrial acetoacetyl-coenzyme A thiolase in cultured fibroblasts from a boy with 3-ketothiolase deficiency. *J Clin Invest* 1988;81:813–817.

225. Fukao T, et al. Identification of a novel exonic mutation at -13 from 5' splice site causing exon skipping in a girl with mitochondrial acetoacetyl-coenzyme A thiolase deficiency. *J Clin Invest* 1994;93:1035–1041.

226. Salih MAM, Bender DA, McCreanor GM. Lethal familial pellagra-like skin lesions associated with neurologic and developmental impairment and the development of cataracts. *Pediatrics* 1985;76:787–793.

227. Martin JR, Mellor CS, Fraser FC. Familial hypertryptophanemia in two siblings. *Clin Genet* 1995; 47:180–183.

228. Isenberg JN, Sharp HL. Aspartylglucosaminuria: psychomotor retardation masquerading as a mucopolysaccharidosis. *J Pediatr* 1975;86:713–717.

229. Tollersrud OK, et al. Aspartylglucosaminuria in northern Norway: a molecular and genealogical study. *J Med Genet* 1994;31:360–363.

230. Williams JC, et al. Progressive neurologic deterioration and renal failure due to storage of glutamyl ribose-5-phosphate. *N Engl J Med* 1984;311: 152–155.

231. Konrad PN, et al. γ-Glutamyl-cysteine synthetase deficiency. A cause of hereditary hemolytic anemia. *N Engl J Med* 1972;286:557–561.

232. Small KW, Letson R, Scheinman J. Ocular findings in primary hyperoxaluria. *Arch Ophthalmol* 1990;108:89–93.

233. Seargeant LE, et al. Primary oxaluria type 2 (L-glyceric aciduria): a rare cause of nephrolithiasis in children. *J Pediatr* 1991;118:912–914.

234. Scriver CR, et al. Cystinuria: increased prevalence in patients with mental disease. *N Engl J Med* 1970;283: 783–786.

235. Melancon SB, et al. Dicarboxylic aminoaciduria: an inborn error of amino acid conservation. *J Pediatr* 1977;91:422–427.

236. Scriver CR. Membrane transport in disorders of amino acid metabolism. *Am J Dis Child* 1967;113:170–174.

237. Procopis PG, Turner B. Iminoaciduria: a benign renal tubular defect. *J Pediatr* 1971;79:419–422.

238. Barton DN, et al. Hereditary pellagra-like skin rash with temporary cerebellar ataxia, constant renal aminoaciduria, and other bizarre biochemical features. *Lancet* 1956;2:421–426.

239. Milne MD, et al. The metabolic disorder in Hartnup disease. *Q J Med* 1960;29:407–421.

240. Scriver CR. Hartnup disease: a genetic modification of intestinal and renal transport of certain neutral α-amino acids. *N Engl J Med* 1965;273:530–532.

241. Wilcken B, Yu JS, Brown DA. Natural history of Hart-nup disease. *Arch Dis Child* 1977;52:38–40.

242. Scriver CR, et al. The Hartnup phenotype: mendelian transport disorder multifactorial disease. *Am J Hum Genet* 1987;40:401–412.

243. Borrie PF, Lewis CA. Hartnup disease. *Proc R Soc Med* 1962;55:231–232.

244. Erly W, et al. Hartnup disease: MR findings. *Am J Neuroradiol* 1991;12:1026–1027.

245. Hill W, Sherman H. Acute intermittent familial cerebellar ataxia. *Arch Neurol* 1968;18:350–357.

246. Clayton PT, et al. Pellagra with colitis due to a defect in tryptophan metabolism. *Eur J Pediatr* 1991;150: 498–502.

247. Jonas AJ, Butler IJ. Circumvention of defective neutral amino acid transport in Hartnup disease using tryptophan ethyl ester. *J Clin Invest* 1989;84: 200–204.

248. Lowe CU, Terry M, MacLachlan EA. Organic aciduria, decreased renal ammonia production, hydrophthalmos and mental retardation: a clinical entity. *Am J Dis Child* 1952;83:164–184.

249. Lin T, Orrison BM, Leahey AM, et al. Spectrum of mutations in the OCR1 gene in the Lowe oculocerebrorenal syndrome. *Am J Hum Genet* 1997;60: 1384–1388.

250. Attree O, et al. The Lowe's oculocerebrorenal syndrome gene encodes a protein highly homologous to inositol polyphosphate-5-phosphatase. *Nature* 1992; 358:239–242.

251. Bartsocas CS, et al. A defect in intestinal amino acid transport in Lowe's syndrome. *Am J Dis Child* 1969;117:93–95.

252. Richards W, et al. The oculo-cerebro-renal syndrome of Lowe. *Am J Dis Child* 1965;109:185–203.

253. Matin MA, Sylvester PE. Clinicopathological studies of oculocerebrorenal syndrome of Lowe, Terrey and MacLachlan. *J Ment Defic Res* 1980;24:1–17.

254. Charnas L, et al. MRI findings and peripheral neuropathy in Lowe's syndrome. *Neuropediatrics* 1988;19:7–9.

255. Charnas LR, Gahl WA. The oculocerebrorenal syndrome of Lowe. *Adv Pediatr* 1991;38:75–101.

256. O'Tuama LA, Laster DW. Oculocerebrorenal syndrome: case report with CT and MR correlates. *Am J Neuroradiol* 1987;8:555–557.

257. Demmer LA, Wippold FJ, Dowton SB. Periventricular white matter cystic lesions in Lowe (oculocerebrorenal) syndrome. A new MR finding. *Pediatr Radiol* 1992;22: 76–77.

258. Cibis CW, et al. Lenticular opacities in carriers of Lowe's syndrome. *Ophthalmology* 1986;93:1041–1045.

259. von Reuss A. Zuckerausscheidung im Säuglingsalter. *Wien Med Wochenschr* 1908;58:799–803.

260. Shih V, et al. Galactosemia screening of newborns in Massachusetts. *N Engl J Med* 1971;284:753–757.

261. Göppert F. Galaktosurie nach Milchzuckergabe bei angeborenem, familiärem chronischem Leberleiden. *Berl Klin Wochenschr* 1917;54:473–477.

262. Schwarz V, et al. Some disturbances of erythrocyte metabolism in galactosaemia. *Biochem J* 1956;62: 34–40.

263. Kalckar HM, Anderson EP, Isselbacher KJ. Galactosemia, a congenital defect in a nucleotide transferase. *Biochim Biophys Acta* 1956;62:262–268.

264. Wang BB, et al. Molecular and biochemical basis of galactosemia. *Mol Genet Med* 1998;63:263–269.

265. Schwarz V, Golberg L. Galactose-1-phosphate in galactose cataract. *Biochim Biophys Acta* 1955;18:310–311.

266. Holton JB. Galactosaemia: pathogenesis and treatment. *J Inherit Metab Dis* 1996;19:3–7.

267. Granett SE, et al. Studies on cerebral energy metabolism during the course of galactose neurotoxicity in chicks. *J Neurochem* 1972;19:1659–1970.

268. Segal S, Berry GT. Disorders of galactose metabolism. In: Scriver CR, Beaudet AL, Sly WS, Valle D, eds. *The metabolic and molecular basis of inherited disease*, 7th ed. New York: McGraw-Hill, 1995:967–1000.

269. Smetana HF, Olen E. Hereditary galactose disease. *Am J Clin Pathol* 1962;38:3–25.

270. Haberland C, et al. The neuropathology of galactosemia. *J Neuropathol Exp Neurol* 1971;30:431–447.

271. Allen JT, et al. Evidence of galactosemia in utero [Letter]. *Lancet* 1980;1:603.

272. Huttenlocher PR, Hillman RE, Hsia YE. Pseudotumor cerebri in galactosemia. *J Pediatr* 1970;76:902–905.

273. Hsia DY, Walker FA. Variability in the clinical manifestations of galactosemia. *J Pediatr* 1961;59:872–883.

274. Walsh FB, Hoyt WF. *Clinical Neuro-Ophthalmology*, 3rd ed. Baltimore: Williams & Wilkins, 1969:802.

275. Levy HL, et al. Sepsis due to Escherichia coli in neonates with galactosemia. *N Engl J Med* 1977;297: 823–825.

276. Kaufman FR, et al. Correlation of ovarian function with galactose-1-phosphate uridyl transferase levels in galactosemia. *J Pediatr* 1988;112:754–756.

277. Nelson MD, et al. Galactosemia: evaluation with MR imaging. *Radiology* 1992;184:255–261.

278. Beutler E. Disorders of galactose metabolism. In: Rosenberg RN, et al., eds. *The molecular and genetic basis of neurological disease*, 2nd ed. Boston: Butterworth–Heinemann 1997:1099–1108.

279. Franceschetti A, Marty F, Klein D. Un syndrome rare: heredoataxie avec cataracte congenitale et retard mental. *Confin Neurol* 1956;16:271–275.

280. Jakobs C, et al. Prenatal diagnosis of galactosemia. *Eur J Pediatr* 1995;154[suppl 2]:S33–S36.

281. Waggoner DD, Buist NRM, Donnell GN. Long-term prognosis in galactosemia: results of a survey of 350 cases. *J Inherit Metab Dis* 1990;13:802–818.

282. Cornblath M, Schwartz R. *Disorders of carbohydrate metabolism in infancy*, 3rd ed. Oxford: Blackwell Scientific Publications, 1991:Appendix II.

283. Komrower GM. Galactosaemia thirty years on: the experience of a generation. *J Inherit Metab Dis* 1982;5[suppl 2]:96–104.

284. Böhles H, Wenzel D, Shin YS. Progressive cerebellar and extrapyramidal motor disturbances in galactosemic twins. *Eur J Pediatr* 1986;145:413–417.

285. Kaufman FR, et al. Cognitive functioning, neurologic status and brain imaging in classical galactosemia. *Eur J Pediatr* 1995;154[suppl 2]:S2–S5.

286. Rogers S, Segal S. Modulation of rat tissue galactose-1-phosphate uridyltransferase by uridine and uridinetriphosphate. *Pediatr Res* 1991;30:222–226.

287. Manis FR, et al. A longitudinal study of cognitive functioning in patients with classical galactosemia, including a cohort treated with oral uridine. *J Inherit Metab Dis* 1997;20:535–549.

288. Fishler K, et al. Developmental aspects of galactosemia from infancy to childhood. *Clin Pediatr* 1980;19:38–44.

289. Nelson CD, et al. Verbal dyspraxia in treated galactosemia. *Pediatrics* 1991;88:346–350.

290. Gitzelmann R, Steinmann B. Galactosemia: how does

long-term treatment change the outcome? *Enzyme* 1984;32:37–46.

291. Donnell GN, Koch R, Bergren WR. Observations on results of management of galactosemic patients. In: Hsia DYY, ed. *Galactosemia*. Springfield: Charles C Thomas, 1969:247.

292. Gitzelmann R, Wells HJ, Segal S. Galactose metabolism in a patient with hereditary galactokinase deficiency. *Eur J Clin Invest* 1974;4:79–84.

293. Henderson MJ, Holton JB, MacFaul R. Further observations in a case of uridine diphosphate galactose-4-epimerase deficiency with a severe clinical presentation. *J Inherit Metab Dis* 1983;6:17–20.

294. Maceratesi P, et al., Human UDP-galactose 4′epimerase (GALE) gene and identification of five missense mutations in patients with epimerase-deficiency galactosemia. *Mol Genet Med* 1998;63:26–30.

295. Chambers RA, Pratt RTC. Idiosyncrasy to fructose. *Lancet* 1956;2:340.

296. Nikkila EA, et al. Hereditary fructose intolerance: an inborn deficiency of liver aldolase complex. *Metabolism* 1962;11:727–731.

297. Schapira F, Gregori C, Hatzfeld A. Isoelectrofocusing of aldolase B from normal human livers and from livers with hereditary fructose intolerance. *Clin Chim Acta* 1977;78:1–8.

298. Ali M, Rellos P, Cox TM. Hereditary fructose intolerance. *J Med Genet* 1998;35:353–365.

299. Oberhaensli RD, et al. Study of hereditary fructose intolerance by use of ³¹P magnetic resonance spectroscopy. *Lancet* 1987;2:931–934.

300. Van den Berghe G, Hue L, Hers HG. Effect of the administration of fructose on the glycogenolytic action of glucagon. An investigation on the pathogeny of hereditary fructose intolerance. *Biochem J* 1973;134:637–645.

301. Lindemann R, et al. Amino acid metabolism in hereditary fructosemia. *Acta Paediat Scand* 1970;59:141–147.

302. Rennert OM, Greer M. Hereditary fructosemia. *Neurology* 1970;20:421–425.

303. Bender SW, et al. Hereditäre Fructose Intoleranz. *Monatsschr Kinderheilk* 1982;130:21–26.

304. Gitzelmann R, Steinmann B, Van den Berghe G. Disorders of fructose metabolism. In: Scriver CR, Beaudet AL, Sly WS, Valle D, eds. *The metabolic and molecular basis of inherited disease*, 7th ed. New York: McGraw-Hill, 1995:905–934.

305. Moses SW, et al. Fructose-1, 6-diphosphatase deficiency in Israel. *Isr J Med Sci* 1991;27:1–4.

306. Buhrdel P, Bohme HJ, Didt L. Biochemical and clinical observations in four patients with fructose-1,6-diphosphatase deficiency. *Eur J Pediatr* 1990;149:574–576.

307. Hsia YE, Scully KL, Rosenberg LE. Inherited propionyl-CoA deficiency in "ketotic hyperglycinemia." *J Clin Invest* 1971;50:127–130.

308. Ohura T, et al. Genetic heterogeneity of propionic acidemia: analysis of 15 Japanese patients. *Hum Genet* 1991;87:41–44.

309. Menkes JH. Idiopathic hyperglycinemia: isolation and identification of three previously undescribed urinary ketones. *J Pediatr* 1966;69:413–421.

310. Coude FX, Sweetman L, Nyhan WL. Inhibition by propionyl CoA of *N*-acetylglutamate synthetase in rat liver mitochondria. *J Clin Invest* 1979;64:1544–1551.

311. Wolf B, et al. Correlation between serum propionate and blood ammonia concentration in propionic acidemia. *J Pediatr* 1978;93:471–473.

312. Childs B, et al. Idiopathic hyperglycinemia and hyperglycinuria. A new disorder of amino acid metabolism. *Pediatrics* 1961;27:522–538.

313. Surtees RAH, Matthews EE, Leonard JV. Neurologic outcome of propionic acidemia. *Pediatr Neurol* 1992;8:333–337.

314. Ando T, et al. Propionic acidemia in patients with ketotic hyperglycinemia. *J Pediatr* 1971;78:827–832.

315. Bergman AJIW, et al. Magnetic resonance imaging and spectroscopy of the brain in propionic acidemia: clinical and biochemical considerations. *Pediatr Res* 1996;40:404–409.

316. Shuman RM, Leech RW, Scott CR. The neuropathology of the non-ketotic and ketotic hyperglycinemias: three cases. *Neurology* 1978;28:139–146.

317. de Vries A, et al. Glycinuria: a hereditary disorder associated with nephrolithiasis. *Am J Med* 1957;23:408–415.

318. Matsui SM, Mahoney MJ, Rosenberg LE. The natural history of the inherited methylmalonic acidemias. *N Engl J Med* 1983;308:857–861.

319. Adjalla CE, et al. Seven novel mutations in mut methylmalonic aciduria. *Hum Mutat* 1998;11:270–274.

320. Shevell MI, et al. Varying neurologic phenotypes among mut0 and mut- patients with methylmalonylCoA mutase deficiency. *Am J Med Genet* 1993;45: 619–624.

321. Mitchell GA, et al. Clinical heterogeneity in cobalamin C variant of combined homocystinuria and methylmalonic aciduria. *J Pediatr* 1986;108:410–415.

322. Shevell MI, Cooper BA, Rosenblatt DS. Inherited disorders of cobalamin and folate transport and metabolism. In: Rosenberg RN, et al., eds. *The molecular and genetic basis of neurological disease*, 2nd ed. Boston: Butterworth–Heinemann, 1997:1301–1321.

323. Ledley FD, et al. Benign methylmalonic aciduria. *N Engl J Med* 1984;311:1015–1018.

324. Brismar J, Ozand PT. CT and MR of the brain in disorders of the propionate and methylmalonate metabolism. *Am J Neuroradiol* 1994;15:1459–1473.

325. Inoue S, et al. Inhibition of bone marrow stem cell growth in vitro by methylmalonic acid: a mechanism for pancytopenia in a patient with methylmalonic acidemia. *Pediatr Res* 1981;15:95–98.

326. Van der Meer SB, et al. Clinical outcome of long-term management of patients with vitamin B_{12}-unresponsive methylmalonic acidemia. *J Pediatr* 1994;125: 903–908.

327. Rosenblatt DS, et al. New disorder of vitamin B_{12} metabolism (Cobalamin F) presenting as methylmalonic aciduria. *Pediatrics* 1986;78:51–54.

328. Shinnar S, Singer HS. Cobalamin C mutation (methylmalonic aciduria and homocystinuria) in adolescence: a treatable cause of dementia and myelopathy. *N Engl J Med* 1984;311:451–454.

329. Mitchell GA, et al. Clinical heterogeneity in cobalamin C variant of combined homocystinuria and methylmalonic aciduria. *J Pediatr* 1986;108:410–415.

330. Robb RM, et al. Retinal degeneration in vitamin B_{12} disorder associated with methylmalonic aciduria and sulfur amino-acid abnormalities. *Am J Ophthalmol* 1981;97:691–696.

331. Russo P, et al. A congenital anomaly of vitamin B_{12} metabolism: a study of three cases. *Hum Pathol* 1992;23:504–512.

332. Fenton WA, Rosenberg LE. Disorders of propionate and methylmalonate metabolism. In: Scriver CR, Beaudet AL, Sly WS, Valle D, eds. *The metabolic and molecular basis of inherited disease*, 7th ed. New York: McGraw-Hill, 1995:1439.

332a. Chalmers RA, et al. Enzymological studies on patients with methylmalonic aciduria: basis for a clinical trial of deoxyadenosylcobalamin in a hydroxocobalamin-unresponsive patient. *Pediatr Res* 1991;30:560–563.

333. Tanaka K, et al. Isovaleric acidemia; new genetic defect of leucine metabolism. *Proc. Nat Acad Sci, U S A* 1966;56;236–242.

334. Mohsen AW, et al. Characterization of molecular defects in isovaleryl-CoA dehydrogenase in patients with isovaleric acidemia. *Biochemistry* 1998;37: 10325–10335.

335. Hine DG, Tanaka K. The identification and the excretion pattern of isovaleryl glucuronide in the urine of patients with isovaleric acidemia. *Pediatr Res* 1984;18:508–512.

336. Ando T, et al. Isovaleric acidemia: identification of isovalerate, isovalerylglycine, and 3-hydroxyisovalerate in urine of a patient previously reported as butyric and hexanoic acidemia. *J Pediatr* 1973;82:243–248.

337. Berry GT, Yudkoff M, Segal S. Isovaleric acidemia: medical and neurodevelopmental effects of long-term therapy. *J Pediatr* 1988;113:58–64.

338. Kelleher JF, et al. The pancytopenia of isovaleric acidemia. *Pediatrics* 1980;65:1023–1027.

339. Tanaka K, Isselbacher KT, Shih V. Isovaleric and methylbutyric acidemias induced by hypoglycin A: mechanism of Jamaican vomiting sickness. *Science* 1972;175:69–71.

340. Goodman SI, et al. Glutaric aciduria: a "new" disorder of amino acid metabolism. *Biochem Med* 1975;12: 12–21.

341. Haworth JC, et al. Phenotypic variability in glutaric aciduria type I: report of fourteen cases in five Canadian Indian kindreds. *J Pediatr* 1991;118:52–58.

342. Goodman SI, et al. Glutaric aciduria: biochemical and morphologic considerations. *J Pediatr* 1977;90: 746–750.

343. Hauser SE, Peters H. Glutaric aciduria type I: an underdiagnosed cause of encephalopathy and dystonia-dyskinesia syndrome in children. *J Paediatr Child Health* 1998;34:302–304.

344. Hoffmann GF, et al. Clinical course, early diagnosis, treatment, and prevention of disease in glutaryl-CoA dehydrogenase deficiency. *Neuropediatrics* 1996;27: 115–123.

345. Dunger DB, Snodgrass GJ. Glutaric aciduria type I presenting with hypoglycaemia. *J Inherit Metab Dis* 1984;7:122–124.

346. Anikster Y, et al. Glutaric aciduria type I in the Arab and Jewish communities in Israel. *Am J Hum Genet* 1996;59:1012–1018.

347. Kimura S, et al. Two cases of glutaric aciduria type 1: clinical and neuropathological findings. *J Neurol Sci* 1994;123:38–43.

348. Superti-Furga A, Hoffmann GF. Glutaric aciduria type 1 (glutaryl-CoA-dehydrogenase deficiency): advances and unanswered questions. Report from an international meeting. *Eur J Pediatr* 1997;156:821–828.

349. Amendt BA, Rhead WJ. The multiple acyl-coenzyme A dehydrogenation disorders, glutaric aciduria type II and ethylmalonic-adipic aciduria: mitochondrial fatty acid oxidation, acyl-coenzyme A dehydrogenase, and electron transfer flavoprotein activities in fibroblasts. *J Clin Invest* 1986;78:205–213.

350. Loehr JP, Goodman SI, Frerman FE. Glutaric acidemia Type II: heterogeneity of clinical and biochemical phenotypes. *Pediatr Res* 1990;27:311–315.

351. Wilson GN, et al. Glutaric aciduria Type II: review of the phenotype and report of an unusual glomerulopathy. *Am J Med Genet* 1989;32:395–401.

352. Uziel G, et al. Riboflavin-responsive glutaric aciduria type II presenting as a leukodystrophy. *Pediatr Neurol* 1995;13:333–335.

353. Chow CW, et al. Striatal degeneration in glutaric acidaemia type II. *Acta Neuropathol* 1989;77:554–556.

354. Gregersen N, et al. Riboflavin responsive multiple acyl-CoA dehydrogenation deficiency. Assessment of 3 years of riboflavin treatment. *Acta Paediatr Scand* 1986;75: 676–681.

355. Green A, et al. Riboflavin-responsive ethylmalonic-adipic aciduria. *J Inherit Metab Dis* 1985;8:67–70.

356. Hale DE, Bennett MJ. Fatty acid oxidation disorders: a new class of metabolic diseases. *J Pediatr* 1992;121: 1–11.

357. Eaton S, Bartlett K, Pourfarzam M. Mammalian mitochondrial β-oxidation. *Biochem J* 1996;320:345–357.

358. Bennett MJ, Worthy E, Pollitt RJ. The incidence and presentation of dicarboxylic aciduria. *J Inherit Metab Dis* 1987;10:322–323.

359. Rinaldo P, et al. Medium-chain acyl-CoA dehydrogenase deficiency: diagnosis by stable isotope dilution analysis of urinary n-hexanoylglycine and 3-phenylpropionylglycine. *N Engl J Med* 1988;319:1308–1313.

360. Duran M, Wadman SK. Chemical diagnosis of inherited defects of fatty acid metabolism and ketogenesis. *Enzyme* 1987;38:115–123.

361. Matsubara Y, et al. Prevalence of K329E mutation in medium-chain acyl-CoA dehydrogenase gene determined from Guthrie cards. *Lancet* 1991;338:552–553.

362. Iafolla AK, et al. Medium-chain acyl-coenzyme A dehydrogenase deficiency: clinical course in 120 affected children. *J Pediatr* 1994;124:409–415.

363. Tanaka K, et al. A survey of the newborn populations in Belgium, Germany, Poland, Czech Republic, Hungary, Bulgaria, Spain, Turkey, and Japan for the G985 variant allele with haplotype analysis at the medium-chain acyl-CoA dehydrogenase gene locus: clinical and evolutionary considerations. *Pediatr Res* 1997;41: 201–209.

364. Miller ME, et al. Frequency of medium-chain acyl-CoA dehydrogenase deficiency G-985 mutation in sudden infant death syndrome. *Pediatr Res* 1992;31: 305–307.

365. Boles RG, et al. Retrospective biochemical screening of fatty acid oxidation disorders in postmortem livers of 418 cases of sudden death in the first year of life. *J Pediatr* 1998;132:924–933.

366. Hale DE, et al. Long-chain acyl coenzyme A dehydrogenase deficiency: an inherited cause of nonketotic hypoglycemia. *Pediatr Res* 1985;19:666–671.

367. Amendt BA, et al. Long-chain acyl-Coenzyme A dehydrogenase deficiency. Biochemical studies in fibroblasts from three patients. *Pediatr Res* 1988;23: 603–605.

367a. Andresen BS, et al. Clear correlation of genotype with disease phenotype in very-long-chain acyl-CoA dehydrogenase deficiency. *Am J Hum Genet* 1999;64: 479–494.

368. Amendt BA, et al. Short-chain acyl-coenzyme A dehydrogenase deficiency. Clinical and biochemical studies in two patients. *J Clin Invest* 1987;79:1303–1309.

369. Bhala A, et al. Clinical and biochemical characterization of short-chain acyl-coenzyme A dehydrogenase deficiency. *J Pediatr* 1995;126:910–915.

370. Wolf B, Heard SG. Screening for biotinidase deficiency in newborns: worldwide experience. *Pediatrics* 1990;85:512–517.

371. Burri B, Sweetman L, Nyhan W. Mutant holocarboxylase synthetase: evidence for the enzyme defect in early infantile biotin-responsive multiple carboxylase deficiency. *J Clin Invest* 1981;68:1491–1495.

372. Suormala T, et al. Five patients with a biotin-responsive defect in holocarboxylase formation: evaluation of responsiveness to biotin therapy *in vivo* and comparative biochemical studies *in vitro*. *Pediatr Res* 1997;41: 666–673.

373. Wolf B, et al. Clinical findings in four children with biotinidase deficiency detected through a statewide neonatal screening program. *N Engl J Med* 1985;313: 16–19.

374. Pomponio RJ, et al. Mutations in the human biotinidase gene that cause profound biotinidase deficiency in symptomatic children: molecular, biochemical, and clinical analysis. *Pediatr Res* 1997;42:840–848.

375. Hart PS, Hymes J, Wolf B. Biochemical and immunological characterization of serum biotinidase in profound biotinidase deficiency. *Am J Hum Genet* 1992;50: 126–136.

376. Wolf B. Disorders of biotin metabolism: treatable neurologic syndromes. In: Rosenberg RN, et al., eds. *The molecular and genetic basis of neurological disease*, 2nd ed. Boston: Butterworth–Heinemann, 1997: 1323–1339.

376a. Ozand PT, et al. Biotin-responsive basal ganglia disease: a novel entity. *Brain* 1998;121:1267–1279.

377. Stanley CA, et al. Chronic cardiomyopathy and weakness or acute coma in children with a defect in carnitine uptake. *Ann Neurol* 1991;30:709–716.

378. Haworth JC, et al. Atypical features of the hepatic form of carnitine palmitoyltransferase deficiency in a Hutterite family. *J Pediatr* 1992;121:553–557.

379. Stanley CA, et al. Brief report: a deficiency of carnitine-acylcarnitine translocase in the inner mitochon-drial membrane. *N Engl J Med* 1992;327:19–23.

380. Land JM, et al. Neonatal carnitine palmitoyltransferase-2-deficiency: a case presenting with myopathy. *Neuromusc Disord* 1995;5:129–137.

381. Treem WR, et al. Hypoglycemia, hypotonia, and cardiomyopathy: the evolving clinical picture of long-chain acyl-CoA dehydrogenase deficiency. *Pediatrics* 1991;87:328–333.

382. Bhala A, et al. Clinical and biochemical characterization of short-chain acyl-coenzyme A dehydrogenase deficiency. *J Pediatr* 1995;126:910–915.

383. Souri M, et al. Mutation analysis of very-long-chain acyl-coenzyme A dehydrogenase (VLCAD) deficiency: identification and characterization of mutant VLCADF cDNAs from four patients. *Am J Hum Genet* 1996;58:97–106.

384. Tyni T, et al. Long-chain 3-hydroxyacyl-coenzyme A dehydrogenase deficiency with the G1528C mutation: clinical presentation of thirteen patients. *J Pediatr* 1997;130:67–76.

384a. Tein I, et al. Long-chain L-3-hydroxyacyl-coenzyme A dehydrogenase deficiency neuropathy: response to cod liver oil. *Neurology* 1999;52:640–643.

385. Bennett MJ, et al. Mitochondrial short-chain L-3-hydroxyacyl coenzyme A dehydrogenase deficiency: a new defect of fatty acid oxidation. *Pediatr Res* 1996;39:185–188.

386. Chen E, et al. L-2-hydroxyglutaric aciduria: neuropathological correlations and first report of severe neurodegenerative disease and neonatal death. *J Inherit Metab Dis* 1996;19:335–343.

387. Barbot C, et al. L-2-hydroxyglutaric aciduria: clinical, biochemical and magnetic resonance imaging in six Portuguese pediatric patients. *Brain Dev* 1997;19: 268–272.

387a. van der Knaap MS, et al. D-2-hydroxyglutaric aciduria: biochemical marker or clinical disease entity? *Ann Neurol* 1999;45:111–119.

388. Spielberg SP, et al. 5-Oxoprolinuria: biochemical observations and case report. *J Pediatr* 1977;91:237–241.

389. Rating D, et al. 4-Hydroxybutyric aciduria: a new inborn error of metabolism. I. Clinical review. *J Inherit Metab Dis* 1984;1[suppl 1]:90–92.

390. Gibson KM, et al. The clinical phenotype of succinic semialdehyde dehydrogenase deficiency (4-hydroxybutyric aciduria): case reports of 23 new patients. *Pediatrics* 1997;99:567–574.

391. Chambliss KL, et al. Two exon-skipping mutations as the molecular basis of succinic semialdehyde dehydrogenase deficiency (4-hydroxybutyric aciduria). *Am J Hum Genet* 1998;63:399–408.

392. Ko FJ, et al. 3-Hydroxyisobutyric aciduria: an inborn error of valine metabolism. *Pediatr Res* 1991;30: 322–326.

393. Chitayat D, et al. Brain dysgenesis and congenital intracerebral calcification associated with 3-hydroxyisobutyric aciduria. *J Pediatr* 1992;121:86–89.

394. Gibson KM, et al. Multiple syndromes of 3-methylglutaconic aciduria. *Pediatr Neurol* 1993;9:120–123.

395. Zeharia A, et al. 3-Methylglutaconic aciduria: a new variant. *Pediatrics* 1992;89:1080–1082.

396. Nowaczyk MJ, et al. Ethylmalonic and methylsuccinic aciduria in ethylmalonic encephalopathy arise from abnormal isoleucine metabolism. *Metabolism* 1998; 47:836–839.

397. Robinson BH, et al. Hydroxymethylglutaryl CoA lyase deficiency: features resembling Reye syndrome. *Neurology* 1980;30:714–718.

398. Thompson GN, et al. Fasting hypoketotic coma in a child with deficiency of mitochondrial 3-hydroxy-3-methylglutaryl-CoA synthase. *N Engl J Med* 1997; 337:1203–1207.

399. Hers HG. Inborn lysosomal diseases. *Gastroenterology* 1965;48:625–633.

399a. Meikle PJ, et al. Prevalence of leposomal storage disorders. *J Am Med Assoc* 1999;281:249–254.

400. Kornfeld S. Trafficking of lysosomal enzymes in normal and disease states. *J Clin Invest* 1986;77:1–6.

401. Fine RN, Podosin R, Donnell GN. Acute hemiplegia in glycogen storage disease, type I. *Acta Paediatr Scand* 1969;58:621–624.

402. Murase T, et al. Myopathy associated with Type III glycogenosis. *J Neurol Sci* 1973;20:287–295.

403. Zellweger H, et al. Glycogenosis IV, a new cause of infantile hypotonia. *J Pediatr* 1972;80:842–844.

404. Pompe JC. Over idiopathische hypertrophie van het hart. *Ned Tijdschr Geneeskd* 1932;76:304–307.

405. Kross MA, et al. Two extremes of the clinical spectrum of glycogen storage disease type II in one family: a matter of genotype. *Hum Mutat* 1997;9:17–22.

406. Kleijer WJ, et al. Prenatal diagnosis of glycogen storage disease type II. Enzyme assay or mutation analysis? *Pediatr Res* 1995;38:103–106.

407. Engel AG, Hirschhorn R. Acid maltase deficiency. In: Engel AG, Franzini-Armstrong C, eds. *Myology. Basic and clinical*, 2nd ed. New York: McGraw–Hill 1994;2:1533–1553.

408. Gambetti T, DiMauro S, Baker L. Nervous system in Pompe's disease: ultrastructure and biochemistry. *J Neuropath Exp Neurol* 1971;30:412–430.

409. Martin JJ, et al. Pompe's disease: an inborn lysosomal disorder with storage of glycogen. *Acta Neuropathol* 1973;23:229–244.

410. Lenard HG, et al. Electromyography in Type II glycogenosis. *Neuropädiatrie* 1974;5:410–424.

411. Verloes A, et al. Nosology of lysosomal glycogen storage diseases without in vitro maltase deficiency. Delineation of a neonatal form. *Am J Med Genet* 1997;72:135–142.

412. Engel AG, et al. The spectrum and diagnosis of acid maltase deficiency. *Neurology* 1973;23:95–106.

413. Swaiman KF, Kennedy WR, Sauls HS. Late infantile acid maltase deficiency. *Arch Neurol* 1968;18: 642–648.

414. Matsuishi T, et al. Childhood acid maltase deficiency: a clinical, biochemical, and morphologic study of three patients. *Arch Neurol* 1984;41:47–52.

415. Broadhead DM, Butterworth J. α-Glucosidase in Pompe's disease. *J Inherit Metab Dis* 1978;1:153–154.

416. Kikuchi T, et al. Clinical and metabolic correction of Pompe disease by enzyme therapy in acid maltase-deficient quail. *J Clin Invest* 1998;101:827–833.

417. Yang HW, et al. Recombinant human acid α-glucosidase corrects acid α-glucosidase-deficient human fibroblasts quail fibroblasts and quail myoblasts. *Pediatr Res* 1998;43:374–380.

418. Nicolino MP, et al. Adenovirus-mediated transfer of the acid alpha-glucosidase gene into fibroblasts, myoblasts and myotubes from patients with glycogen storage disease type II leads to high level expression of enzyme and corrects glycogen accumulation. *Hum Mol Genet* 1998;7:1695–1702.

419. Kennedy PG. Potential use of herpes simplex virus (HSV) vectors for gene therapy of neurological disorders. *Brain* 1997;120:1245–1259.

420. Sterzl TE, et al. Chimerism after liver transplantation for type IV glycogen storage disease and type 1 Gaucher disease. *N Engl J Med* 1993;328:745–749.

421. Hunter C. A rare disease in two brothers. *Proc R Soc Med* 1917;10:104–116.

422. Hurler G. Uber einen Typ multipler Abartungen, vorwiegend am Skelett-system. *Z Kinderheilk* 1919;24: 220–234.

423. von Pfaundler M. Demonstrationen über einen Typus kindlicher Dysostose. *Jahrb f Kinderh* 1920;92: 420–421.

424. Ellis RWB, Sheldon W, Capon NB. Gargoylism (chondro-osteo-dystrophy, corneal opacities hepatosplenomegaly, and mental deficiency). *Q J Med* 1936;5: 119–139.

425. Alberts B, et al. The extracellular matrix of animals. In: Alberts B, et al., eds. *The molecular biology of the cell*, 3rd ed. New York: Garland Publishing, 1994:973–977.

426. Kjellen L, Lindahl V. The proteoglycans structures and functions. *Ann Rev Biochem* 1991;60:443–475.

427. Varadi DP, Cifonelli JA, Dorfman A. The acid mucopolysaccharides in normal urine. *Biochem Biophys Acta* 1967;141:103–117.

428. Neufeld EF, Muenzer J. The mucopolysaccharidoses. In: Scriver CR, Beaudet AL, Sly WS, Valle D, eds. *The metabolic and molecular basis of inherited disease*, 7th ed. New York: McGraw-Hill, 1995:2465–2494.

429. Scott HS, et al. Molecular genetics of mucopolysaccharidosis type I: diagnostic, clinical and biological implications. *Hum Mutat* 1995;6:288–302.

430. Froissant R, et al. Identification of iduronate sulfatase gene alterations in 70 unrelated Hunter patients. *Clin Genet* 1998;53:362–368.

431. Clarke JT, et al. Hunter disease (Mucopolysaccharidosis type II) associated with unbalanced inactivation of the X-chromosomes in a karyotypically normal girl. *Am J Hum Genet* 1991;49:289–297.

432. Groebe H, et al. Morquio syndrome (mucopolysaccharidosis IV B) associated with β-galactosidase deficiency: report of two cases. *Am J Hum Genet* 1980;32: 258–272.

433. Renteria VG, Ferrans VJ, Roberts WC. The heart in Hurler syndrome: gross histologic and ultrastructural observations in five necropsy cases. *Am J Cardiol* 1976;38:487–501.

434. Van Hoof F, Hers HG. L'ultrastructure des cellules hepatiques dans la maladie de Hurler (gargoylisme). *C R Acad Sci Paris* 1964;259:1281–1283.

435. Dekaban AS, Constantopoulos G. Mucopolysaccharidosis types I, II, III A and V. Pathological and biochemical abnormalities in the neural and mes- enchymal elements of the brain. *Acta Neuropathol* 1977;39:17.

436. Beighton P, McKusick VA. *Heritable disorders of connective tissue*, 5th ed. St. Louis: Mosby, 1993.

437. Lowry RB, et al. An update on the frequency of mucopolysaccharide syndromes in British Columbia. *Hum Genet* 1990;85:389–390.

438. Caffey J. Gargoylism (Hunter-Hurler disease, dysostosis multiplex, lipochondrodystrophy): prenatal and postnatal bone lesions and their early postnatal evolution. *AJR Am J Roentgenol* 1952;67:715–731.

439. Levin S. A specific skin lesion in gargoylism. *Am J Dis Child* 1960;99:444–450.

440. Friedmann I, et al. Histopathological studies of the temporal bones in Hurler's disease [Mucopolysaccharidosis (MPS) IH]. *J Laryngol Otol* 1985;99:29–41.

441. Lee C, et al. The mucopolysaccharidoses: characterization by cranial MR imaging. *Am J Neuroradiol* 1993;14:1285–1292.

442. Gross DM, et al. Echocardiographic abnormalities in the mucopolysaccharide storage diseases. *Am J Cardiol* 1988;61:170–176.

443. Roubicek M, Gehler J, Spranger J. The clinical spectrum of α-L-iduronidase deficiency. *Am J Med Genet* 1985;20:471–481.

444. Peters C, Shapiro EG, Krivit W. Hurler syndrome: past, present, and future. *J Pediatr* 1998;133:7–9.

445. Vellodi A, et al. Bone marrow transplantation for mucopolysaccharidosis type I: experience of two British centres. *Arch Dis Child* 1997;76:92–99.

446. Guffon N, et al. Follow-up on nine patients with Hurler syndrome after bone marrow transplantation. *J Pediatr* 1998;133:119–125.

447. Lowry RB, et al. An update on the frequence of mucopolysaccharide syndromes in British Columbia. *Hum Genet* 1990;85:389–390.

448. Young IS, Harper PS. Mild form of Hunter's syndrome: clinical delineation based on 31 cases. *Arch Dis Child* 1982;57:828–836.

449. Topping TM, et al. Ultrastructural ocular pathology of Hunter's syndrome. Systemic mucopolysaccharidosis type II. *Arch Ophthalmol* 1971;86:164–177.

450. Young ID, Harper PS. Long-term complications in Hunter's syndrome. *Clin Genet* 1979;16:125–132.

451. Young ID, Harper PS. The natural history of the severe form of Hunter's syndrome: a study based on 52 cases. *Dev Med Child Neurol* 1983;25:481–489.

452. Spranger J, et al. Mucopolysaccharidosis II (Hunter disease) with corneal opacities: report of two patients at the extremes of a wide clinical spectrum. *Eur J Pediatr* 1978;129:11–16.

453. Karpati G, et al. Multiple peripheral nerve entrapments: an unusual phenotypic variant of the Hunter syndrome (Mucopolysaccharidosis II) in a family. *Arch Neurol* 1974;31:418–422.

454. Constantopoulos G, McComb RD, Dekaban AS. Neurochemistry of the mucopolysaccharidoses: brain glycosaminoglycans in normals and four types of mucopolysaccharidoses. *J Neurochem* 1976;26:901–908.

455. Murphy JV, et al. Hunter's syndrome: ultrastructural features in young children. *Arch Pathol Lab Med* 1983;107:495–499.

456. Meier C, et al. Morphological observations in the nervous system of prenatal mucopolysaccharidosis II (M. Hunter). *Acta Neuropathol* 1979;48:139–143.

457. Sanfilippo SJ, et al. Mental retardation associated with acid mucopolysacchariduria (heparitin sulfate type). *J Pediatr* 1963;63:837–838.

458. Danks DM, et al. The Sanfilippo syndrome: clinical, biochemical, radiological, haematological and pathological features of nine cases. *Austr Paediat J* 1972;8:174–186.

459. Kaplan P, Wolfe LS. Sanfilippo syndrome type D. *J Pediatr* 1987;110:267–271.

460. Federico A, et al. Sanfilippo B syndrome (MPS III B): case report with analysis of CSF mucopolysaccharides and conjunctival biopsy. *J Neurol* 1981;225:77–83.

461. van de Kamp JJP, et al. Genetic heterogeneity and clinical variability in the Sanfilippo syndrome (types A, B, and C). *Clin Genet* 1981;20:152–160.

462. Shapiro EG, et al. Neuropsychological outcomes of several storage diseases with and without bone marrow transplantation. *J Inherit Metab Dis* 1995;18:413–429.

463. Nelson J, Thomas PS. Clinical findings in 12 patients with MPS IV A (Morquio's disease). Further evidence for heterogeneity. Part III: odontoid dysplasia. *Clin Genet* 1988;33:126–130.

464. Koto A, et al. The Morquio syndrome: neuropathology and biochemistry. *Ann Neurol* 1978;4:26–36.

465. Scheie HG, Hambrick GW, Barness LA Jr. A newly recognized forme fruste of Hurler's disease (gargoylism). *Am J Ophthalmol* 1962;53:753–769.

466. Winters PR, et al. α-L-iduronidase deficiency and possible Hurler-Scheie genetic compound. Clinical, pathologic, and biochemical findings. *Neurology* 1976;26:1003–1007.

467. Maroteaux P, et al. Une nouvelle dysostose avec elimination urinaire de chondroitine-sulfate B. *Presse Med* 1963;71:1849–1852.

468. Peterson DI, et al. Myelopathy associated with Maroteaux-Lamy syndrome. *Arch Neurol* 1975;32:127–129.

469. Beaudet AL, et al. Variation in the phenotypic expression of β-glucuronidase deficiency. *J Pediatr* 1978;86:388–394.

470. De Braekeleer M. Hereditary disorders in Saguenay-Lac-St. Jean (Quebec, Canada). *Hum Hered* 1991;41:141–146.

471. Beck M, et al. Inter- and intrafamilial variability in mucolipidosis II (I-cell disease). *Clin Genet* 1995;47:191–199.

472. Martin JJ, et al. I-cell disease (mucolipidosis II). A report on its pathology. *Acta Neuropathol* 1975;33:285–305.

473. Leroy LG, et al. I-cell disease; biochemical studies. *Pediatr Res* 1972;6:752–757.

474. Kelly TE, et al. Mucolipidosis III (Pseudo-Hurler polydystrophy). Clinical and laboratory studies in a series of 12 patients. *Johns Hopkins Med J* 1975;137:156–175.

475. Amir N, Zlotogora J, Bach G. Mucolipidosis type IV: clinical spectrum and natural history. *Pediatrics* 1987;79:953–959.

476. Schiffman R, et al. Constitutive achlorhydria in mucolipidosis type IV. *Proc Natl Acad Sci U S A* 1998;95:1207–1212.

477. Frei KP, et al. Mucolipidosis type IV. Characteristic MRI findings. *Neurology* 1998;51:565–569.

478. Tellez-Nagel I, et al. Mucolipidosis IV. *Arch Neurol* 1976;33:828–835.

479. Chen CS, Bach G, Pagano RE. Abnormal transport along the lysosomal pathway in mucolipidosis type IV disease. *Proc Natl Acad Sci U S A* 1998;95:6373–6378.

480. Johnson WG. Disorders of glycoprotein degradation: sialidosis, fucosidosis, alpha-mannosidosis, beta-mannosidosis, and aspartylglycosaminuria. In: Rosenberg RN, et al., eds. *The molecular and genetic basis of neurological disease*, 2nd ed. Boston: Butterworth–Heinemann, 1997:355–369.

481. Willems PJ, et al. Fucosidosis revisited: a review of 77 patients. *Am J Med Genet* 1991;38:111–131.

482. Cragg H, et al. Fucosidosis: genetic and biochemical analysis of eight cases. *J Med Genet* 1997;34:105–110.

483. Troost J, et al. Fucosidosis I. Clinical and enzymological studies. *Neuropaediatrie* 1977;8:155–162.

484. Larbrisseau A, Brochu P, Jasmin G. Fucosidose de type 1 Etude anatomique. *Arch Franc Pediatr* 1979;36:1013–1023.

485. Kistler JP, et al. Mannosidosis. New clinical presentation, enzyme studies and carbohydrate analysis. *Arch Neurol* 1977;34:45–51.

486. Sung JH, Hayano M, Desnick RJ. Mannosidosis: pathology of the nervous system. *J Neuropathol Exp Neurol* 1977;36:807–820.

487. Norden NE, et al. Characterization of two mannose-containing oligosaccharides from the urine of patients with mannosidosis. *Biochemistry* 1974;13:871–874.

488. Wenger DA, et al. Human β-mannosidase deficiency. *N Engl J Med* 1986;315:1201–1205.

489. Kleijer WJ, et al. β-Mannosidase deficiency: heterogenous manifestation in the first female patient and her brother. *J Inherit Metab Dis* 1990;13:867–872.

490. Young ID, et al. Neuraminidase deficiency: case report and review of the phenotype. *J Med Genet* 1987;24:283–290.

491. Pshezhetsky AV, et al. Cloning, expression and chromosomal mapping of human lysosomal sialidase and characterization of mutations in sialidosis. *Nat Genet* 1997;15:316–320.

492. Steinman L, et al. Peripheral neuropathy in the cherry-red spot-myoclonus syndrome (Sialidosis type I). *Ann Neurol* 1980;7:450–456.

493. Yamano T, et al. Pathological study on a severe sialidosis (α-neuraminidase deficiency). *Acta Neuropath* 1986;71:278–284.

494. Kleijer WJ, et al. Cathepsin A deficiency in galactosialidosis: studies of patients and carriers in 16 families. *Pediatr Res* 1996;39:1067–1071.

495. Okada S, et al. A case of neuraminidase deficiency associated with a partial β-galactosidase defect. *Eur J Pediatr* 1979;130:239–249.

496. Galjart NJ, et al. Expression of cDNA encoding the human "protective protein" associated with lysosomal β-galactosidase and neuraminidase. *Cell* 1988;54:755–764.

497. Renlund M, et al. Salla disease: a new lysosomal storage disorder with disturbed sialic acid metabolism. *Neurology* 1983;33:57–66.

498. Berra B, et al. Infantile sialic acid storage disease: biochemical studies. *Am J Med Genet* 1995;58:24–31.

499. Schleutker J, et al. Lysosomal free sialic acid storage disorders with different phenotypic presentations—infantile-form sialic acid storage disease and Salla disease—represent allelic disorders on 6q14-15. *Am J Hum Genet* 1995;57:893–901.

500. Mancini GMS, et al. Sialic acid storage diseases: a multiple lysosomal transport defect for acidic monosaccharides. *J Clin Invest* 1991;87:1329–1335.

501. Robinson RO, Fensom AH, Lake BD. Salla disease—rare or underdiagnosed. *Dev Med Child Neurol* 1997;39:153–157.

502. Klenk E. Beiträge zur Chemie der Lipoidosen: Niemann-Picksche Krankheit und amaurotische Idiotie. *Zschr Physiol Chem* 1939;262:128–143.

503. Tay W. Symmetrical changes in the region of the yellow spot in each eye of an infant. *Trans Ophthalmol Soc UK* 1880–1881;1:55–57.

504. Sachs B. On arrested cerebral development, with special reference to its cortical pathology. *J Nerv Ment Dis* 1887;14:541–553.

505. Kolodny EH. The GM2 gangliosidoses. In: Rosenberg RN, et al., eds. *The molecular and genetic basis of neurological disease*, 2nd ed. Boston: Butterworth–Heinemann 1997:473–490.

506. Mahuran DJ. The biochemistry of HEXA and HEXB gene mutations causing GM_2 gangliosidosis. *Biochim Biophys Acta* 1991;1096:87–94.

507. Myerowitz R. Tay-Sachs disease-causing mutations and neutral polymorphisms in the Hex A gene. *Hum Mutat* 1997;9:195–208.

508. Grebner EE, Tomczak J. Distribution of three α-chain β-hexosaminidase A mutations among Tay-Sachs carriers. *Am J Hum Genet* 1991;48:604–607.

509. Myerowitz R, Hogikyan ND. A deletion involving Alu sequences in the β-hexosaminidase α-chain gene of French Canadians with Tay-Sachs disease. *J Biol Chem* 1987;263:15396–15397.

510. Sandhoff K, Andreae U, Jatzkewitz H. Deficient hexosaminidase activity in an exceptional case of Tay-Sachs disease with additional storage of kidney globoside in visceral organs. *Life Sci* 1968;7:283–288.

511. Ellis RB, et al. Prenatal diagnosis of Tay-Sachs disease [Letter]. *Lancet* 1973;2:1144–1145.

511a. Sandhoff K, Kolter T. Biochemistry of glycosphingolipid degradation. *Clin Chim Acta* 1997;266:51–61.

512. Hama Y, Li YT, Li SC. Interaction of G_{M2} activator protein with glycosphingolipids. *J Biol Chem* 1997;272:2828–2833.

513. Menkes JH, et al. Juvenile GM_2 gangliosidosis. Biochemical and ultrastructural studies on a new variant of Tay-Sachs diseases. *Arch Neurol* 1971;25:14–22.

514. Navon R, et al. Ashkenazi-Jewish and non-Jewish adult G_{M2} gangliosidosis patients share a common genetic defect. *Am J Hum Genet* 1990;46:817–821.

515. Terry RD, Weiss M. Studies in Tay-Sachs disease: ultrastructure of cerebrum. *J Neuropathol Exp Neurol* 1963;22:18–55.

516. Walkley SU, et al. GM2 ganglioside as a regulator of pyramidal neuron dendritogenesis. *Ann NY Acad Sci* 1998;845:188–199.

517. Walkley SU. Pathobiology of neuronal storage disease. *Int Rev Neurobiol* 1988;29:191–244.

518. Kivlin JD, Sanborn GE, Myers GG. The cherry-red spot in Tay-Sachs and other storage diseases. *Ann Neurol* 1985;17:356–360.

519. Aronson SM, et al. The megaloencephalic phase of infantile amaurotic familial idiocy: cephalometric and pneumoencephalographic studies. *Arch Neurol Psychiatr* 1958;79:151–163.

520. Yoshikawa H, Yamada K, Sakuragawa N. MRI in the early stage of Tay-Sachs disease. *Neuroradiology* 1992;34:394–395.

521. Johnson WG. Genetic heterogeneity of hexosaminidase-deficiency diseases. *Res Publ Assoc Res Nerv Ment Dis* 1983;60:215–237.

522. Cashman NR, et al. N-acetyl-β-hexosaminidase β locus defect and juvenile motor neuron disease: a case study. *Ann Neurol* 1986;19:568–572.

523. Oates CE, Bosch EP, Hart EN. Movement disorders associated with chronic GM_2 gangliosidoses. *Europ Neurol* 1986;25:154–159.

524. O'Brien JS. Pitfalls in the prenatal diagnosis of Tay-Sachs disease. In: Kaback M, Rimoin D, eds. Tay-Sachs disease: screening and prevention. New York: Alan R. Liss, 1977:283.

525. Kaback M, et al. Tay-Sachs disease—carrier screening, prenatal diagnosis, and the molecular era. An international perspective, 1970–1993. The International TSD Data Collection Network. *JAMA* 1993;270:2307–2315.

525a. Platt FM, et al. Prevention of lysosomal storage in Tay-Sachs mice treated with N-butyldeoxynojirimycin. *Science* 1997;276:428–431.

526. Landing BH, et al. Familial neurovisceral lipidosis. An analysis of eight cases of a syndrome previously reported as "Hurler-variant," "pseudo-Hurler disease" and "Tay-Sachs disease" with visceral involvement. *Am J Dis Child* 1964;108:503–522.

527. O'Brien JS, et al. Generalized gangliosidosis: another inborn error of ganglioside metabolism? *Am J Dis Child* 1965;109:338–346.

528. Wolfe LS, et al. The structures of oligosaccharides accumulating in the liver of GM_1-gangliosidosis, Type I. *J Biol Chem* 1974;249:1828–1838.

529. Okada S, O'Brien JS. Generalized gangliosidosis: β-galactosidase deficiency. *Science* 1968;160:1002–1004.

530. Oshima A, et al. Human β-galactosidase gene mutations in Morquio B disease. *Am J Hum Genet* 1991;49:1091–1093.

531. Ishii N, et al. Clinical and molecular analysis of a Japanese boy with Morquio B disease. *Clin Genet* 1995;48:103–108.

532. Suzuki K, Suzuki K, Chen GC. Morphological, histochemical and biochemical studies on a case of systemic late infantile lipidosis (generalized gangliosidosis). *J Neuropathol Exp Neurol* 1968;27:15–38.

533. O'Brien JS. Generalized gangliosidosis. *J Pediatr* 1969;75:167–186.

534. Farrell DF, MacMartin MP. GM$_1$-gangliosidosis: enzymatic variation in a single family. *Ann Neurol* 1981;9:232–236.

535. Wolfe LS, et al. GM$_1$-gangliosidosis without chondrodystrophy or visceromegaly. *Neurology* 1970;20:23–44.

536. Guazzi GC, et al. Type 3 (chronic) GM$_1$ gangliosidosis presenting as infanto-choreo-athetotic dementia, without epilepsy, in three sisters. *Neurology* 1988;38:1124–1127.

537. Goldman JE, et al. Chronic GM$_1$-gangliosidosis presenting as dystonia. I. Clinical and pathologic features. *Ann Neurol* 1981;9:465–475.

538. Lowden JA, et al. Prenatal diagnosis of GM$_1$-gangliosidosis. *N Engl J Med* 1973;288:225–228.

539. Gaucher PCE. De l'épithélioma primitif de la rate. Thèse [thesis] de Paris 1882.

540. Brady RO, et al. Demonstration of a deficiency of glucocerebroside-cleaving enzyme in Gaucher's disease. *J Clin Invest* 1966;45:1112–1115.

541. Masuno M, et al. Non-existence of a tight association between a 444-leucine to proline mutation and phenotypes of Gaucher disease: high frequency of a NciI polymorphism in the non-neuronopathic form. *Hum Genet* 1990;84:203–206.

542. Lieb H. Cerebrosidspeicherung bei Splenomegalie Typus-Gaucher. *Ztschr Physiol Chem* 1924;140:305–315.

543. Philippart M, Rosenstein B, Menkes JH. Isolation and characterization of the main splenic glycolipids in the normal organ and in Gaucher's disease: evidence for the site of metabolic block. *J Neuropathol Exp Neurol* 1965;24:290–303.

544. Lee RE. The fine structure of the cerebroside occurring in Gaucher's disease. *Proc Natl Acad Sci U S A* 1968;61:484–489.

545. Grafe M, et al. Infantile Gaucher's disease: a case with neuronal storage. *Ann Neurol* 1988;23:300–303.

546. Hannun YA, Bell RM. Lysosphingolipids inhibit protein kinase C: implications for the sphingolipidoses. *Science* 1987;235:670–674.

547. Rodgers CL, Jackson SH. Acute infantile Gaucher's disease: case report. *Pediatrics* 1951;7:53–59.

547a. Sidransky E. New perspectives in type 2 Gaucher disease. *Adv Pediatr* 1997;44:73–107.

548. Tsuji S, et al. A mutation in the human glucocerebrosidase gene in neuronopathic Gaucher's disease. *N Engl J Med* 1987;316:570–575.

549. Sidransky E, Sherer D, Ginns EI. Gaucher disease in the neonate: a distinct Gaucher phenotype is analogous to a mouse model created by targeted disruption of the glucocerebrosidase gene. *Pediatr Res* 1992;32:494–498.

550. Nishimura RN, Barranger JA. Neurologic complications of Gaucher's disease, Type 3. *Arch Neurol* 1980;37:92–93.

551. Schiffman R, et al. Prospective study of neurological responses to treatment with macrophage-targeted glucocerebrosidase in patients with type 3 Gaucher's disease. *Ann Neurol* 1997;42:613–621.

552. Dreborg S, Erikson A, Hagberg B. Gaucher disease—Norrbottnian type I. General clinical description. *Eur J Pediatr* 1980;133:107–118.

553. Svennerholm L, Hakansson G, Dreborg S. Assay of the β-glucosidase activity with natural labeled and artificial substrates in leukocytes from homozygotes and heterozygotes with the Norrbottnian type (Type 3) of Gaucher disease. *Clin Chim Acta* 1980;106:183–193.

554. Erikson A, et al. Clinical and biochemical outcome of bone marrow transplantation for Gaucher disease of the Norrbottnian type. *Acta Paediatr Scand* 1990;79:680–685.

555. Erikson A, Åström M, Månssour JE. Enzyme infusion therapy of the Norrbottnian (type 3) Gaucher disease. *Neuropediatrics* 1995;26:203–207.

556. Desnick RJ, Eng CM. Fabry disease: α-galactosidase A deficiency. In: Rosenberg RN, et al., eds. *The molecular and genetic basis of neurological disease*, 2nd ed. Boston: Butterworth–Heinemann 1997:443–452.

557. Schram AW, et al. Enzymological properties and immunological characterization of α-galactosidase isoenzymes from normal and Fabry human liver. *Biochim Biophys Acta* 1977;482:125–137.

558. Eng CM, et al. Fabry disease: thirty-five mutations in the alpha-galactosidase A gene in patients with classic and variant phenotypes. *Mol Med* 1997;3:174–182.

559. Lemansky P, et al. Synthesis and processing of α-galactosidase A in human fibroblasts. Evidence for different mutations in Fabry disease. *J Biol Chem* 1987;262:2062–2065.

560. Sweeley CC, Klionsky B. Fabry's disease: classification as a sphingolipidosis and partial characterization of a novel glycolipid. *J Biol Chem* 1963;238:3148–3150.

561. Grunnet ML, Spilsbury PR. The central nervous system in Fabry's disease. *Arch Neurol* 1973;28:231–234.

562. Kaye EM, et al. Nervous system involvement in Fabry's disease: clinicopathological and biochemical correlation. *Ann Neurol* 1988;23:505–509.

563. Fabry J. Ein Beitrag zur Kenntnis der Purpura haemorrhagica nodularis (Purpura papulosa hemorrhagica Hebrae). *Arch Dermatol Syph* 1898;43:187–200.

564. Mitsias P, Levine SR. Cerebrovascular complications of Fabry's disease. *Ann Neurol* 1996;40:8–17.

565. deGroot WP. Fabry's disease in children. *Br J Dermatol* 1970;82:329–332.

566. Sher NA, Letson RD, Desnick RJ. The ocular manifestations of Fabry's disease. *Arch Ophthalmol* 1979;97:671–676.

567. Cable WJL, et al. Fabry disease: significance of ultrastructural localization of lipid inclusions in dermal nerves. *Neurology* 1982;32:347–353.

568. Crutchfield KE, et al. Quantitative analysis of cerebral vasculopathy in patients with Fabry disease. *Neurology* 1998;50:1746–1749.

569. Franceschetti AT, Philippart M, Franceschetti A. A study of Fabry's disease: I. Clinical examination of a family

with cornea verticillata. *Dermatologica* 1969;138: 209–221.

570. Desnick RJ, et al. Fabry's disease: enzymatic diagnosis of hemizygotes and heterozygotes: α-galactosidase activities in plasma, serum, urine, and leukocytes. *J Lab Clin Med* 1973;81:157–171.

571. Desnick RJ, et al. Fabry disease: molecular diagnosis of hemizygotes and heterozygotes. *Enzyme* 1987;38: 54–64.

572. Lockman LA, et al. Relief of the pain of Fabry's disease by diphenylhydantoin. *Neurology* 1973;23:871–875.

573. Donati D, Novario R, Gastaldi L. Natural history and treatment of uremia secondary to Fabry's disease: a European experience. *Nephron* 1987;46:353–359.

574. De Jong J, et al. Alpha-*N*-acetylgalactosaminidase deficiency with mild clinical manifestations and difficult biochemical diagnosis. *J Pediatr* 1994;125: 385–391.

575. Niemann A. Ein unbekanntes Krankheitsbild. *Jahrb Kinderheilk* 1914;79:1–10.

576. Crocker AC, Farber S. Niemann-Pick disease: a review of 18 patients. *Medicine* 1958;37:1–95.

577. Spence MW, Callahan JW. Sphingomyelin-cholesterol lipidoses: the Niemann-Pick group of disease. In: Scriver CR, et al., eds. *The metabolic basis of inherited disease*, 6th ed. New York: McGraw-Hill, 1989: 1655–1676.

578. Gumbinas M, Larsen M, Liu HM. Peripheral neuropathy in classic Niemann-Pick disease: ultrastructure of nerves and skeletal muscles. *Neurology* 1975;25: 107–113.

579. Walton DS, Robb RM, Crocker AC. Ocular manifestations of Group A Niemann-Pick disease. *Am J Ophthalmol* 1978;85:174–180.

580. Ivemark BI, et al. Niemann-Pick disease in infancy: report of two siblings with clinical, histologic, and chemical studies. *Acta Paediatr* 1963;52:391–401.

581. Thudichum JLW. *A treatise on the chemical constitution of the brain, based throughout upon original researches*. London: Bailliere, Tindall and Cox, 1884.

582. Takahashi T, et al. Identification and expression of five mutations in the human acid sphingomyelinase gene causing types A and B Niemann-Pick disease. Molecular evidence for genetic heterogeneity in the neuronopathic and non-neuronopathic forms. *J Biol Chem* 1992;267:12552–12558.

583. Levran O, Desnick RJ, Schuchman EH. Identification and expression of a common missense mutation (L302P) in the acid sphingomyelinase gene of Ashkenazi Jewish type A Niemann-Pick disease patients. *Blood* 1992;80:2081–2087.

584. Wenger DA, et al. Niemann-Pick disease type B: prenatal diagnosis and enzymatic and chemical studies on fetal brain and liver. *Am J Hum Genet* 1981;33:337–344.

585. Brady RO, Carstea ED, Pentchev PG. The Niemann-Pick diseases group. In: Rosenberg RN, et al., eds. *The molecular and genetic basis of neurological disease*, 2nd ed. Boston: Butterworth–Heinemann 1997: 387–403.

586. Guibaud P, et al. Forme infantile précoce, cholestatique, rapidement mortelle, de la sphingomyélinose type C. *Pediatrie* 1979;34:103–114.

587. Kelly, DA, et al. Niemann-Pick disease type C. Diagnosis and outcome in children, with particular reference to liver disease. *J Pediatr* 1993;123:242–247.

588. Philippart M, et al. Niemann-Pick disease: morphologic and biochemical studies in the visceral form with late central nervous system involvement (Crocker's group C). *Arch Neurol* 1969;20:227–238.

589. Vanier MT, et al. Niemann-Pick disease group C: clinical variability and diagnosis based on defective cholesterol esterification. A collaborative study on 70 patients. *Clin Genet* 1988;33:331–348.

590. Carstea ED, et al. Niemann-Pick C1 disease gene: homology to mediators of cholesterol homeostasis. *Science* 1997;277:228–231.

591. Lange Y, Ye J, Stock TL. Circulation of cholesterol between lysosomes and the plasma membrane. *J Biol Chem* 1998;273:18915–18922.

591a. Vanier MT. Lipid changes in Niemann-Pick disease type C brain: personal experience and review of the literature. *Neurochem Res* 1999;24;481–489.

591b. Millat G, et al. Niemann-Pick Cl disease: The 11061T substitution is a frequent mutant allele in patients of Western European descent and correlates with a classic juvenile phenotype. *Am J Hum Genet* 1999;65: 1321–1329.

592. Jan MM, Camfield PR. Nova Scotia Niemann-Pick disease (type D): clinical study of 20 cases. *J Child Neurol* 1998;13:75–78.

593. Greer WL, et al. The Nova Scotia (type D) form of Niemann-Pick disease is caused by a G3097→T transversion in NPC1. *Am J Hum Genet* 1998;63:52–54.

594. Argoff CE, et al. Type C Niemann-Pick disease: documentation of abnormal LDL processing in lymphocytes. *Biochem Biophys Res Commun* 1990;171:38–45.

595. Abramov A, Schorr S, Wolman M. Generalized xanthomatosis with calcified adrenals. *Am J Dis Child* 1956;91:282–286.

596. Eto Y, Kitagawa T. Wolman's disease with hypolipoproteinemia and acanthocytosis: clinical and biochemical observations. *J Pediatr* 1970;77:862–867.

597. Wolman M. Involvement of nervous tissue in primary familial xanthomatosis with adrenal calcification. *Pathol Eur* 1968;3:259–265.

598. Patrick AD, Lake BD. Deficiency of an acid lipase in Wolman's disease. *Nature* 1969;222:1067–1068.

599. Brown MS, et al. Restoration of a regulatory response to low density lipoprotein in acid lipase-deficient human fibroblasts. *J Biol Chem* 1976;251: 3277–3286.

600. Yatsu FM, Alam R. Wolman disease. In: Rosenberg RN, et al., eds. *The molecular and genetic basis of neurological disease*, 2nd ed. Boston: Butterworth–Heinemann, 1997:371–378.

601. Pagani F, et al. New lysosomal acid lipase gene mutants explain the phenotype of Wolman disease and cholesteryl ester storage disease. *J Lipid Res* 1998;39: 1382–1388.

602. Galton DJ, et al. Triglyceride storage disease. *QJM* 1974;43:63–71.

603. Philippart M, Durand P, Borrone C. Neutral lipid storage with acid lipase deficiency: a new variant of Wolman's disease with features of the Senior syndrome. *Pediatr Res* 1982;16:954–959.

604. Farber S, Cohen J, Uzman LL. Lipogranulomatosis: a new lipoglycoprotein storage disease. *J Mount Sinai Hosp N Y* 1957;24:816–837.

605. Antonarakis SE, et al. Phenotypic variability in siblings with Farber disease. *J Pediatr* 1984;104: 406–409.

606. Burck U, et al. A case of lipogranulomatosis Farber: some clinical and ultrastructural aspects. *Eur J Pediatr* 1985;143:203–208.
607. Chen WW, Moser AB, Moser HW. Role of lysosomal acid ceramidase in the metabolism of ceramide in human skin fibroblasts. *Arch Biochem* 1981;208: 444–455.
608. Koch J, et al. Molecular cloning and characterization of a full-length complementary DNA encoding human acid ceramidase. Identification of the first molecular lesion causing Farber disease. *J Biol Chem* 1996;271: 33110–33115.
609. Barriere H, Gillot F. La lipogranulomatose de Farber. *Nouv Presse Med* 1973;2:767–770.
610. Moser HW. Ceramidase deficiency: farber lipogranulomatosis. In: Rosenberg RN, et al., eds. *The molecular and genetic basis of neurological disease*, 2nd ed. Boston: Butterworth–Heinemann, 1997:379–386.
611. van Bogaert L, Scherer HJ, Epstein E. *Une forme cérébrale de la cholestérinose généralisée.* Paris: Masson & Cie, 1937.
612. Menkes JH, Schimschock JR, Swanson PD. Cerebrotendinous xanthomatosis: the storage of cholestanol within the nervous system. *Arch Neurol* 1968;19:47–53.
613. Berginer VM, Salen G, Shefer S. Cerebrotendinous xanthomatosis. In: Rosenberg RN, et al., eds. *The molecular and genetic basis of neurological disease*, 2nd ed. Boston: Butterworth–Heinemann, 1997:1051–1060.
614. Arlazaroff A, et al. Epileptic seizures as a presenting symptom of cerebrotendinous xanthomatosis. *Epilepsia* 1991;32:657–661.
615. Kuriyama M, et al. Cerebrotendinous xanthomatosis: clinical and biochemical evaluation of eight patients and review of the literature. *J Neurol Sci* 1991;102:225–232.
616. Berginer VM, et al. Magnetic resonance imaging in cerebrotendinous xanthomatosis: a prospective clinical and neuroradiological study. *J Neurol Sci* 1994; 122:102–108.
617. Schimschock JR, Alvord EC, Swanson PD. Cerebrotendinous xanthomatosis: clinical and pathological studies. *Arch Neurol* 1968;18:688–698.
618. Cali JJ, Russell DW. Characterization of human sterol 27-hydroxylase: a mitochondrial cytochrome P-450 that catalyzes multiple oxidation reactions in bile acid biosynthesis. *J Biol Chem* 1991;266:7774–7778.
619. Chen W, et al. Genetic analysis enables definite and rapid diagnosis of cerebrotendinous xanthomatosis. *Neurology* 1998;51:865–867.
620. Batta AK, et al. Increased plasma bile alcohol glucuronides in patients with cerebrotendinous xanthomatosis: effect of chenodeoxycholic acid. *J Lipid Res* 1987;28:1006–1012.
621. Van Heijst AF, et al. Treatment and follow-up of children with cerebrotendinous xanthomatosis. *Eur J Pediatr* 1998;157:313–316.
622. Johnson VP. Smith-Lemli-Opitz syndrome: review and report of two affected siblings. *Z Kinderheilk* 1975;119:221–234.
623. Smith DW, Lemli L, Opitz JM. A newly recognized syndrome of multiple congenital anomalies. *J Pediatr* 1964;64:210–217.
624. Tint GS, et al. Defective cholesterol biosynthesis associated with the Smith-Lemli-Opitz syndrome. *N Engl J Med* 1994;330:107–113.
625. Wassif CA, et al. Mutations in the human sterol delta7-reductase gene at 11q12-13 cause Smith-Lemli-Opitz syndrome. *Am J Hum Genet* 1998;63:55–62.
626. Fitzky BU, et al. Mutations in the delta7-sterol reductase gene in patients with the Smith-Lemli-Opitz syndrome. *Proc Natl Acad Sci U S A* 1998;95: 8181–8186.
627. Cunniff C, et al. Clinical and biochemical spectrum of patients with RSH/Smith-Lemli-Opitz syndrome and abnormal cholesterol metabolism. *Am J Med Genet* 1997;68:263–269.
628. Kelley RI, Kratz L. 3-Methylglutaconic acidemia in Smith-Lemli-Opitz syndrome. *Pediatr Res* 1995;37: 671–674.
629. Irons M, et al. Treatment of Smith-Lemli-Opitz syndrome: results of a multicenter trial. *Am J Med Genet* 1997;68:311–314.
630. Berry DH, Becton DL. Natural history of histiocytosis X. *Hematol Oncol Clin N Am* 1987;1:23–34.
631. Fabiani A, et al. Histiocytosis X: a reappraisal of a nosological concept with some remarks about brain pathology. *Zbl Neurochirurgie* 1981;42:221–234.
632. Burn DJ, et al. Langerhans' cell histiocytosis and the nervous system. *J Neurol* 1992;2390:345–350.
633. Feigin I. Xanthomatosis of nervous system. *J Neuropathol Exp Neurol* 1956;15:400–416.
634. Wanders RJA, Schutgens RBH, Barth PG. Peroxisomal disorders: a review. *J Neuropath Exp Neurol* 1995;54:726–739.
635. Moser HW. Peroxisomal disorders. In: Rosenberg RN, et al., eds. *The molecular and genetic basis of neurological disease*, 2nd ed. Boston: Butterworth–Heinemann 1997:273–314.
635a. Baumgartner MR, et al. Clinical approach to inherited peroxisomal disorders: a series of 27 patients. *Ann Neurol* 1998;44:720–730.
636. Subramani S. Components involved in peroxisome import, biogenesis, proliferation, turnover and movement. *Physiol Rev* 1998;78:171–188.
637. Santos MJ, et al. Peroxisomal membrane ghosts in Zellweger syndrome—aberrant organelle assembly. *Science* 1988;239:1536–1538.
638. Geisbrecht BV, et al. Disruption of a PEX1-PEX6 interaction is the most common cause of the neurologic disorders Zellweger syndrome, neonatal adrenoleukodystrophy, and infantile Refsum disease. *Proc Natl Acad Sci U S A* 1998;95:8630–8635.
639. Opitz JM, et al. The Zellweger syndrome (cerebrohepatorenal syndrome). *Birth Defects: Original Article Series.* 1969;5:144–160.
640. Kamei A, et al. Peroxisomal disorders in children: immunohistochemistry and neuropathology. *J Pediatr* 1993;122:573–579.
641. Volpe JJ, Adams RD. Cerebrohepatorenal syndrome of Zellweger: an inherited disorder of neuronal migration. *Acta Neuropath* 1972;20:175–198.
642. Sarnat HB, et al. Mitochondrial myopathy of cerebrohepatorenal (Zellweger) syndrome. *Can J Neurol Sci* 1983;10:170–177.
643. Barkovich AJ, Peck WW. MR of Zellweger syndrome. *Am J Neuroradiol* 1997;18:1163–1170.
644. Rocchiccioli F, Aubourg P, Bougnères PF. Medium-and long-chain dicarboxylic aciduria in patients with Zellweger syndrome and neonatal adrenoleukodystrophy. *Pediatr Res* 1986;20:62–66.

645. Moser AB, et al. Phenotype of patients with peroxisomal disorders subdivided into sixteen complementation groups. *J Pediatr* 1995;127:13–22.
646. Refsum S. Heredopathia atactica polyneuritiformis. *Acta Psychiatr Scand* 1946;38[suppl]:93–103.
647. Richterich R, Van Mechelen P, Rossi E. Refsum's disease (heredopathia atactica polyneuritiformis): an inborn error of lipid metabolism with storage of 3, 7, 11, 15-tetramethyl hexadecanoic acid. *Am J Med* 1965;39:230–236.
648. Cammermeyer J. Neuropathologic changes in hereditary neuropathies: manifestation of the syndrome heredopathia atactica polyneuritiformis in the presence of interstitial hypertrophic polyneuropathy. *J Neuropathol Exp Neurol* 1956;15:340–361.
649. Jansen GA, et al. Phytanoyl-Coenzyme A hydroxylase deficiency—the enzyme defect in Refsum's disease. *N Engl J Med* 1997;337:133–134.
650. Watkins PA, Mihalik SJ. Refsum disease. In: Rosenberg RN, et al., eds. *The molecular and genetic basis of neurological disease*, 2nd ed. Boston: Butterworth–Heinemann 1997:315–330.
651. Steinberg D. Refsum disease. In: Scriver CR, Beaudet AL, Sly WS, Valle D, eds. *The metabolic and molecular basis of inherited disease*, 7th ed. McGraw-Hill, New York, 1995:2351–2369.
652. Mayatepek E, Hoffmann GF, Bremer HJ. Enhanced urinary excretion of leukotriene E4 in patients with mevalonate kinase deficiency. *J Pediatr* 1993;123:96–98.
653. Hoffmann GF, et al. Clinical and biochemical phenotype in 11 patients with mevalonic aciduria. *Pediatrics* 1993;91:915–921.
654. Wanders RJ, Romeijn GJ. Differential deficiency of mevalonate kinase and phosphomevalonate kinase in patients with distinct defects in peroxisome biogenesis: evidence for a major role of peroxisomes in cholesterol biosynthesis. *Biochem Biophys Res Commun* 1998;247:663–667.
655. Happle R. X-linked chondrodysplasia punctata. Review of literature and report of a case. *Hum Genet* 1979;53:65–73.
656. Slavecki ML, et al. Identification of three distinct peroxisomal protein import defects in patients with peroxisomal biogenesis disorders. *J Cell Sci* 1995;108:1817–1829.
656a. Jacken J, Eggermont E, Stibler H. An apparent homozygous X-linked disorder with carbohydrate-deficient serum glycoproteins. *Lancet* 1987;2:1398.
656b. Freeze HH. Disorders of protein glycosylation and potential therapy: tip of an iceberg? *J Pediatr* 1998;133:593–600.
657. Mobley WC, et al. Neonatal adrenoleukodystrophy. *Ann Neurol* 1982;12:204–205.
658. Powers JM, Moser HW. Peroxisomal disorders: genotype, phenotype, major neuropathologic lesions and pathogenesis. *Brain Pathol* 1998;8:101–120.
659. Budden SS, et al. Dysmorphic syndrome with phytanic acid oxidase deficiency, abnormal very-long-chain fatty acids and pipecolic acidemia: studies in 4 children. *J Pediatr* 1986;108:33 39.
660. Watkins PA, et al. Distinction between peroxisomal bifunctional enzyme and acetyl CoA oxidase deficiencies. *Ann Neurol* 1995;38:472–477.
661. Schram AW, et al. Human peroxisomal 3-oxoacylcoenzyme A thiolase deficiency. *Proc Natl Acad Sci U S A* 1987;84:2494–2496.

662. Krasnewich D, Gahl WA. Carbohydrate-deficient glycoprotein syndrome. *Adv Pediatr* 1997;44:109–140.
663. Niehues R, et al. Carbohydrate-deficient glycoprotein syndrome type Ib. Phosphomannose isomerase deficiency and mannose therapy. *J Clin Invest* 1998;101:1414–1420.
664. Burda P, et al. A novel carbohydrate-deficient glycoprotein syndrome characterized by a deficiency in glucosylation of the dolichol-linked oligosaccharide. *J Clin Invest* 1998;102:647–652.
665. Ramaekers VT, et al. A new variant of the carbohydrate-deficient glycoproteins syndrome. *J Inherit Metab Dis* 1991;14:385–388.
666. Stibler H, et al. Carbohydrate-deficient glycoprotein (CDG) syndrome—a new variant, type III. *Neuropediatrics* 1993;24:51–52.
667. Stibler H, Stephani U, Kutsch U. Carbohydrate-deficient glycoprotein syndrome—a fourth subtype. *Neuropediatrics* 1995;26:235–237.
668. Korner C, et al. Carbohydrate-deficient glycoprotein syndrome type V: deficiency of dolichyl-P-Glc:Man9GlcNAc2-PP-dolichyl glucosyltransferase. *Proc Natl Acad Sci U S A* 1998;95:13200–13205.
669. Stibler H, Skovby F. Failure to diagnose carbohydrate-deficient glycoprotein syndrome prenatally. *Pediatr Neurol* 1994;11:71.
670. Berkovic SF, So NK, Andermann F. Progressive myoclonus epilepsies: clinical and neurophysiological diagnosis. *J Clin Neurophysiol* 1991;8:261–274.
671. Lafora GR. Über das Vorkommen amyloider Körperchen in Innern der Ganglienzell. *Virchows Arch Pathol Anat* 1911;205:295–303.
672. Unverricht H. *Die Myoklonie*. Leipzig: Franz Deuticke, 1891.
673. Minassian BA, et al. Mutations in a gene encoding a novel protein tyrosine phosphatase cause progressive myoclonus epilepsy. *Nature Genet* 1998;20:171–174.
673a. Minassian BA, et al. Genetic locus heterogeneity in Lafora's progressive myoclonus epilepsy. *Ann Neurol* 1999;5:262–265.
674. Harriman DGF, Millar JHD. Progressive familial myoclonic epilepsy in three families: its clinical features and pathological basis. *Brain* 1955;78:325–349.
675. Nishimura RN, et al. Lafora disease: diagnosis by liver biopsy. *Ann Neurol* 1980;8:409–415.
676. Berkovic SF, et al. Progressive myoclonus epilepsies: specific causes and diagnosis. *N Engl J Med* 1986;315:296–304.
677. Janeway R, et al. Progressive myoclonus epilepsy with Lafora inclusion bodies. I. Clinical, genetic, histopathologic and biochemical aspects. *Arch Neurol* 1967;16:565–582.
678. Odor DL, et al. Progressive myoclonus epilepsy with Lafora inclusion bodies. II. Studies of ultrastructure. *Arch Neurol* 1967;16:583–594.
679. Baumann RJ, Kocoshis SA, Wilson D. Lafora disease: liver histopathology in presymptomatic children. *Ann Neurol* 1983;14:86–89.
680. Virtaneva K, et al. Unstable minisatellite expansion causing recessively inherited myoclonus epilepsy, EPM1. *Nature Genet* 1997;15:393–396.
681. Hurd RW, et al. Treatment of four siblings with progressive myoclonus epilepsy of the Unverricht-Lundborg type with *N*-acetylcysteine. *Neurology* 1996;47:1264–1268.

682. Santavuori P, et al. Infantile type of so-called neu-
     ronal ceroid lipofuscinosis. Part I. A clinical study of
     15 patients. *J Neurol Sci* 1973;18:257–267.
683. Jansky J. Über einen noch nicht beschriebenen Fall
     der familiären amaurotischen Idiotie mit Hypoplasie
     des Kleinhirns. *Z Erforsch Behandl Jugendlich
     Schwachsinns* 1909;3:86–88.
684. Bielschowsky M. Über spätinfantile familiäre amau-
     rotische Idiotie mit Kleinhirn symptomen. *Deutsch Z
     Nervenheilk* 1914;50:7–29.
685. Batten FE. Family cerebral degeneration with macu-
     lar change (so-called juvenile form of family amau-
     rotic idiocy). *QJM* 1914;7:444–454.
686. Spielmeyer W. Weitere Mitteilung ueber eine besondere
     Form von familiaerer amaurotischer Idiotie. *Neurol Zbl*
     1905;24:1131–1132.
687. Kufs M. Über eine Spätform der amaurotischen Idiotie
     und ihre heredofamiliären Grundlagen. *Z Ges Neurol
     Psychiat* 1925;95:169–188.
688. Wisniewski KE, et al. Variability in the clinical and
     pathological findings in the neuronal ceroid lipofusci-
     noses: review of data and observations. *Am J Med Genet*
     1992;42:525–532.
689. Das AK, et al. Molecular genetics of palmitoyl-protein
     thioesterase deficiency in the U.S. *J Clin Invest*
     1998;102:361–370.
689a. Mole S, Gardener M. Molecular genetics of the neu-
     ronal ceroid lipofuscinoses. *Epilepsia* 1999;40
     [suppl3]:29–32.
690. Sleat DE, et al. Association of mutations in a lysoso-
     mal protein with classical late-infantile neuronal
     ceroid lipofuscinosis. *Science* 1997;277:1802–1805.
691. Munroe PB, et al. Spectrum of mutations in the Batten
     disease gene, CLN3. *Am J Hum Gent* 1997;61:
     310–316.
692. Tyynela J, et al. Sphingolipid activator proteins (SAP's)
     in neuronal ceroid lipofuscinosis. *Neuropediatrics*
     1997;28:49–52.
693. International Batten Disease Consortium. Isolation of a
     novel gene underlying Batten disease (CLN3). *Cell*
     1995;82:949–957.
694. Savukoski M, et al. CLN5, a novel gene encoding a
     putative transmembrane protein mutated in Finnish vari-
     ant late infantile neuronal ceroid lipofuscinosis. *Nature
     Genet* 1998;19:286–288.
695. Sharp JD, et al. Loci for classical and a variant late
     infantile neuronal ceroid lipofuscinosis map to chro-
     mosomes 11p15 and 15q21-23. *Hum Mol Genet*
     1997;6:591–595.
696. Santavuori P, Haltia M, Rapola J. Infantile type of so-
     called neuronal ceroid-lipofuscinosis. *Dev Med Child
     Neurol* 1974;16:644–653.
697. Bateman JB, Philippart M. Ocular features of the
     Hagberg-Santavuori syndrome. *Am J Ophthalmol*
     1986;102:262–271.
698. Harden A, Pampiglione G, Picton-Robinson N. Elec-
     troretinogram and visual evoked response in a form
     of "neuronal lipidosis" with diagnostic EEG fea-
     tures. *J Neurol Neurosurg Psychiatry* 1973;36:
     61–67.
699. Baumann RJ, Markesbery WR. Santavuori disease:
     diagnosis by leukocyte ultrastructure. *Neurology*
     1982;32:1277–1281.
700. Zhong N, et al. Two common mutations in the CLN2
     gene underlie late infantile neuronal ceroid lipofusci-
     nosis. *Clin Genet* 1998;54:234–238.

701. Pampiglione G, Harden A. So-called neuronal ceroid
     lipofuscinosis: neurophysiological studies in 60 chil-
     dren. *J Neurol Neurosurg Psychiat* 1977;40:323–330.
702. Seitz D, et al. MR imaging and localized proton MR
     spectroscopy in late infantile neuronal ceroid lipofus-
     cinosis. *Am J Neuroradiol* 1998;19:1373–1377.
703. Palmer DN, et al. Different patterns of hydrophobic pro-
     tein storage in different forms of neuronal ceroid lipo-
     fuscinosis (NCL, Batten disease). *Neuropediatrics*
     1997;28:45–48.
704. Carpenter S, et al. The ultrastructural characteristics
     of the abnormal cytosomes in Batten-Kufs' disease.
     Brain 1977;100:137–156.
705. Farrell DF, Sumi SM. Skin punch biopsy in the diagno-
     sis of juvenile neuronal ceroid-lipofuscinosis. *Arch Neu-
     rol* 1977;34:39–44.
706. Santavuori P, et al. A variant of Jansky-Bielschowski
     disease. *Neuropediatrics* 1982;13:135–141.
707. Freud S. Ueber familiaere Formen von cerebralen
     Diplegien. *Neurol Zentralbl* 1893;12:512–515,
     542–547.
708. Vogt H. Ueber familiaere amaurotische Idiotie und ver-
     wandte Krankheitsbilder. *Monatsschr Psychiat Neu-
     rol* 1905;18:161–171, 310–357.
709. Järvelä I, et al. Clinical and magnetic resonance imag-
     ing findings in Batten disease: analysis of the major
     mutation (1.02-kb deletion). *Ann Neurol* 1997;
     42:799–802.
710. Ikeda K, Goebel HH. Ultrastructural pathology of
     human lymphocytes in lysosomal disorders: a contri-
     bution to their morphological diagnosis. *Eur J Pediat*
     1982;138:179–185.
711. Kornfeld M. Generalized lipofuscinosis (generalized
     Kufs' disease). *J Neuropathol Exp Neurol* 1972;31:
     668–682.
712. Goebel HH, Zeman W, Pilz H. Significance of mus-
     cle biopsies in neuronal ceroid-lipofuscinoses. *J Neu-
     rol Neurosurg Psychiatry* 1975;38:985–993.
713. Bassen FA, Kornzweig AL. Malformation of erythro-
     cytes in cases of atypical retinitis pigmentosa. *Blood*
     1950;5:381–387.
714. Schwarz JF, et al. Bassen-Kornzweig syndrome: defi-
     ciency of serum β-lipoprotein. *Arch Neurol* 1963;8:
     438–454.
715. Kane JP, Havel RJ. Disorders in the biogenesis and
     secretion of lipoproteins containing the B apolipopro-
     teins. In: Scriver CR, Beaudet AL, Sly WS, Valle D, eds.
     The metabolic and molecular basis of inherited disease,
     7th ed. McGraw-Hill, New York, 1995: 1853–1885.
716. Brin MF, et al. Electrophysiologic features of abeta-
     lipoproteinemia: functional consequences of vitamin
     E deficiency. *Neurology* 1986;36:669–673.
717. Sobrevilla LA, Goodman ML, Kane CA. Demyelinat-
     ing central nervous system disease, macular atrophy,
     and acanthocytosis (Bassen-Kornzweig syndrome).
     Am J Med 1964;37:821–832.
718. Lazaro RP, et al. Muscle pathology in Bassen-
     Kornzweig syndrome and vitamin E deficiency. *Am J
     Clin Pathol* 1986;86:378–387.
719. Blum CB, et al. Role of apolipoprotein E-containing
     lipoproteins in abetalipoproteinemia. *J Clin Invest*
     1982;70:1157–1169.
720. Malloy MJ, Kane JP. Disorders of lipoproteins. In:
     Rosenberg RN, et al., eds. *The molecular and genetic
     basis of neurological disease*, 2nd ed. Boston: Butter-
     worth–Heinemann 1997:1003–1018.

721. Muller DPR, Lloyd JK. Effect of large oral doses of vitamin E on the neurologic sequelae of patients with abeta-lipoproteinemia. *Ann N Y Acad Sci* 1982;393: 133–144.

722. Fagan ER, Taylor MJ. Longitudinal multimodal evoked potential studies in abetalipoproteinemia. *Can J Neurol Sci* 1987;14:617–621.

723. Hardie RJ, et al. Neuroacanthocytosis: a clinical, haematological and pathological study of 19 cases. *Brain* 1991;114:13–49.

724. Bird TD, et al. Familial degeneration of the basal ganglia with acanthocytosis: a clinical, neuropathological, and neurochemical study. *Ann Neurol* 1978;3: 253–258.

725. Rubio JP, et al. Chorea-acanthocytosis: genetic linkage to chromosome 9q21. *Am J Hum Genet* 1997;61: 899–908.

726. Engel WK, et al. Neuropathy in Tangier disease. α-Lipoprotein deficiency manifesting as familial recurrent neuropathy and intestinal lipid storage. *Arch Neurol* 1967;17:19.

727. Thomas PK. Inherited neuropathies related to disorders of lipid metabolism. *Adv Neurol* 1988;48:133–144.

728. Rust S, et al. Assignment of Tangier disease to chromosome 9q31 by a graphical linkage exclusion strategy. *Nature Genet* 1998;20:96–98.

729. Schmitz G, et al. Tangier disease: a disorder of intracellular membrane traffic. *Proc Natl Acad Sci U S A* 1985;82:6305–6309.

730. Kayser B. Ueber einen Fall von angeborener grünlicher Verfärbung der Cornea. *Klin Monatsbl Augenheilkd* 1902;40:22–25.

731. Fleischer B. Über einer der "Pseudosklerose" nahestehende bisher unbekannte Krankheit (gekennzeichnet durch Tremor psychische Störungen, bräunliche Pigmentierung bestimmter Gewebe, insbesondere auch der Hornhautperipherie, Lebercirrhose). *Deutsch Z Nervenheilk* 1912;44:179–201.

732. Wilson SAK. Progressive lenticular degeneration: a familial nervous disease associated with cirrhosis of the liver. *Brain* 1912;34:295–509.

733. Menkes JH. Disorders of copper metabolism. In: Rosenberg RN, et al. eds. *The molecular and genetic basis of neurological disease*, 2nd ed. Boston: Butterworth–Heinemann 1997:1273–1281.

734. Vulpe CD, Packman S. Cellular copper transport. *Ann Rev Nutr* 1995;15:293–322.

735. Rumpel A. Über das Wesen und die Bedeutung der Leberveränderungen und der Pigmentierungen bei den damit verbundenen Fällen von Pseudosklerose, zugleich ein Beitrag zur Lehre der Pseudosklerose (Westphal-Strümpell). *Deutsch Z Nervenheilk* 1913;49: 54–73.

736. Lüthy F. Über die hepato-lentikuläre Degeneration (Wilson-Westphal-Strümpell). *Deutsch Z Nervenheilk* 1931;123:101–181.

737. Glazebrook AJ. Wilson's disease. *Edinburgh Med J* 1945;52:83–87.

738. Mukhopadhyay CK, Attieh ZK, Fox PL. Role of ceruloplasmin in cellular iron uptake. *Science* 1998;279: 714–716.

739. Gitlin JD. Aceruloplasminemia. *Pediatr Res* 1998;44: 271–276.

740. Tanzi RE, et al. The Wilson's disease gene is a copper-transporting ATPase with homology to the Menkes disease gene. *Nature Genet* 1993;5:344–350.

741. Lutsenko S, Cooper MJ. Localization of the Wilson's disease protein product to mitochondria. *Proc Natl Acad Sci U S A* 1998;95:6004–6009.

741a. Schaefer M, et al. Hepatocyte-specific localization and copper-dependant trafficking of the Wilson's disease protein in the liver. *Am J Phipiol* 1999;276:G639–646.

742. Thomas GR, et al. The Wilson disease gene: spectrum of mutations and their consequence. *Nature Genet* 1995;9:210–217.

743. Davis W, Chowrimootoo GF, Seymour CA. Defective biliary copper excretion in Wilson's disease: the role of caeruloplasmin. *Eur J Clin Invest* 1996;26:893–901.

744. Frommer DJ. Defective biliary excretion of copper in Wilson's disease. *Gut* 1974;15:125–129.

745. Iyengar V, et al. Studies of cholecystokinin-stimulated biliary secretions reveal a high molecular weight copper-binding substance in normal subjects that is absent in patients with Wilson's disease. *J Lab Clin Med* 1988;111:267–274.

746. Scheinberg IH, Sternlieb I. *Wilson's disease*, 2nd ed. Philadelphia: W.B. Saunders, 1999.

746a. Vulpe CD, et al. Hephaestin, a ceruloplasmin homologue implicated in intestinal iron transport, is defective in the sla mouse. *Nature Genet* 1999;21:195–199.

747. Strohmeyer FW, Ishak, KG. Histology of the liver in Wilson's disease: a study of 34 cases. *Am J Clin Pathol* 1980;73:12–24.

748. Richter R. The pallial component in hepatolenticular degeneration. *J Neuropathol Exp Neurol* 1948;7:1–18.

749. Uzman LL, Jakus MA. The Kayser-Fleischer ring: a histochemical and electron microscope study. *Neurology* 1957;7:341–355.

750. Arima M, et al. Prognosis of Wilson's disease in childhood. *Eur J Pediatr* 1977;126:147–154.

751. Slovis TL, et al. The varied manifestations of Wilson's disease. *J Pediatr* 1971;78:570–504.

752. Scott J, et al. Wilson's disease, presenting as chronic active hepatitis. *Gastroenterology* 1978;74:645–651.

753. Werlin SL, et al. Diagnostic dilemmas of Wilson's disease: diagnosis and treatment. *Pediatrics* 1978;62:47–51.

754. Kontaxakis V, et al. Neuroleptic malignant syndrome in a patient with Wilson's disease [Letter]. *J Neurol Neurosurg Psychiatr* 1988;51:1001–1002.

755. Prayer L, et al. Cranial MRI in Wilson's disease. *Neuroradiology* 1990;32:211–214.

756. King AD, et al. Cranial MR imaging in Wilson's disease. *Am J Roentgenol* 1996;167:1579–1584.

757. Hawkins RA, Mazziotta JC, Phelps ME. Wilson's disease studied with FDG and positron emission tomography. *Neurology* 1987;37:1707–1711.

758. Walshe JM. Diagnosis and treatment of presymptomatic Wilson's disease. *Lancet* 1988;2:435–437.

758a. Shah AB, et al. Identification and analysis of mutation in the Wilson disease gene (ATP7B): population frequencies, genotype-phenotype correlation, and functional analyses. *Am J Hum Genet* 1997;61:317–328.

759. Brewer GJ, Yuzbasiyan-Gurkan V. Wilson's disease. *Am J Med* 1992;71:139–164.

760. Brewer GJ. Practical recommendations and new therapies for Wilson's disease. *Drugs* 1995;50:240–249.

761. Grimm G, et al. Evoked potentials in assessment and follow-up of patients with Wilson's disease. *Lancet* 1990;336:963–964.

762. Mitchell AM, Heller GL. Changes in Kayser-Fleischer ring during treatment of hepatolenticular degeneration. *Arch Ophthalmol* 1968;80:622–631.

763. Bax RT, et al. Cerebral manifestation of Wilson's disease successfully treated with liver transplantation. *Neurology* 1998;51:863–865.

764. Walshe JM, Dixon AK. Dangers of non-compliance in Wilson's disease. *Lancet* 1986;1:845–847.

765. Scheinberg IH, et al. Penicillamine may detoxify copper in Wilson's disease. *Lancet* 1987;2:95.

766. Godwin-Austin RB, et al. An unusual neurological disorder of copper metabolism clinically resembling Wilson's disease but biochemically a distinct entity. *J Neurol Sci* 1978;39:85–98.

767. Heckmann J, Saffer D. Abnormal copper metabolism: another "non-Wilson's" case. *Neurology* 1988;38:1493–1495.

768. Menkes JH, et al. A sex-linked recessive disorder with growth retardation, peculiar hair, and focal cerebral and cerebellar degeneration. *Pediatrics* 1962;29: 764–779.

769. Danks DM, et al. Menkes' kinky hair syndrome: an inherited defect in copper absorption with widespread effects. *Pediatrics* 1972;50:188–201.

770. Bucknall WE, Haslam RH, Holtzman NA. Kinky hair syndrome: response to copper therapy. *Pediatrics* 1973;52:653–657.

771. van den Berg GJ, et al. Muscle cell cultures in Menkes' disease: copper accumulation in myotubes. *J Inherit Metab Dis* 1990;13:207–211.

772. Vulpe C, et al. Isolation of a candidate gene for Menkes disease and evidence that it encodes a coppertransporting ATPase. *Nature Genet* 1993;3:7–13.

772a. Goodyer ID, et al. Characterization of the Menkes protein copper-binding domains and their role in copper-induced protein relocalization. *Hum Molec Genet* 1999;8:1473–1478.

773. Hirano A, et al. Fine structure of the cerebellar cortex in Menkes Kinky-Hair disease. *Arch Neurol* 1977;34: 52–56.

774. Tønnesen T, Kleijer WJ, Horn N. Incidence of Menkes disease. *Hum Genet* 1991;86:408–410.

775. Baerlocher K, Nadal D. Das Menkes-Syndrom. *Ergeb Inn Mediz* 1988;57:79–144.

776. Grover WD, Johnson WC, Henkin RI. Clinical and biochemical aspects of trichopoliodystrophy. *Ann Neurol* 1979;5:65–71.

777. Seelenfreund MH, Gartner S, Vinger PE. The ocular pathology of Menkes' disease. *Arch Ophthalmol* 1968;80:718–720.

778. Wesenberg RL, Gwinn JL, Barnes GR. Radiologic findings in the kinky hair syndrome. *Radiology* 1968;92: 500–506.

779. Kim OH, Suh JH. Intracranial and extracranial MR angiography in Menkes disease. *Pediatr Radiol* 1997;27:782–784.

780. Wheeler EM, Roberts PF. Menke's steely hair syndrome. *Arch Dis Child* 1976;51:269–274.

781. Faerber EN, et al. Cerebral MR of Menkes' kinky-hair disease. *Am J Neuroradiol* 1989;10:190–192.

782. Ferreira RC, et al. Menkes disease. New ocular and electroretinographic findings. *Ophthalmology* 1998;105: 1076–1078.

783. Proud VK, et al. Distinctive Menkes disease variant with occipital horns: delineation of natural history and clinical phenotypes. *Am J Med Genet* 1996; 65:44–51.

784. Tümer Z, Horn N. Menkes disease: recent advance and new aspects. *J Med Genet* 1997;34:265–274.

785. Kapur S, et al. Menkes' syndrome in a girl with X-auto-some translocation. *Am J Hum Genet* 1987;26: 503–510.

786. Stefanini M, et al. A new nucleotide-excision-repair gene associated with the disorder trichothiodystrophy. *Am J Hum Genet* 1993;53:817–821.

787. Whiting DA. Structural abnormalities of the hair shaft. *J Am Acad Dermatol* 1987;16:1–25.

788. Kaler SG, et al. Early copper therapy in classic Menkes disease patients with a novel splicing mutation. *Ann Neurol* 1995;38:921–929.

789. Slot HMJ, et al. Molybdenum-cofactor deficiency: an easily missed cause of neonatal convulsions. *Neuropediatrics* 1993;139–142.

790. Shalata A, et al. Localization of a gene for molybdenum cofactor deficiency, on the short arm of chromosome 6, by homozygosity mapping. *Am J Hum Genet* 1998;63:148–154.

790a. Koch H. Dipsticks and convulsions. *Lancet* 1998;352: 1824.

791. Boles RG, et al. Short-term response to dietary therapy in molybdenum cofactor deficiency. *Ann Neurol* 1993;34:742–744.

792. Rupar CA, et al. Isolated sulfite oxidase deficiency. *Neuropediatrics* 1996;27:299–304.

793. Garrett RM, et al. Human sulfite oxidase R160Q; identification of the mutation in a sulfite oxidase-deficient patient and expression and characterization of the mutant enzyme. *Proc Natl Acad Sci U S A* 1998;95: 6394–6398.

794. Catel W, Schmidt J. Über familiäre gichtische Diathese in Verbindung mit zerebralen und renalen Symptomen bei einem Kleinkind. *Dtsch Med Wochenschr* 1959;84: 2145–2147.

795. Lesch M, Nyhan WL. A familial disorder of uric acid metabolism and central nervous system function. *Am J Med* 1964;36:561–570.

796. Sege-Peterson K, Nyhan WL. Lesch-Nyhan disease and hypoxanthine-guanine phosphoribosyltransferase deficiency. In: Rosenberg RN, et al., eds. *The molecular and genetic basis of neurological disease*, 2nd ed. Boston: Butterworth–Heinemann 1997:1233–1252.

797. Stout JT, Caskey CT. HPRT: gene structure, expression, and mutation. *Ann Rev Genet* 1985;19:127–148.

798. Seegmiller JE. Contributions of Lesch-Nyhan syndrome to the understanding of purine metabolism. *J Inherit Metab Dis* 1989;12:184–196.

799. Wong DF, et al. Dopamine transporters are markedly reduced in Lesch-Nyhan disease in vivo. *Proc Natl Acad Sci U S A* 1996;93:5539–5543.

800. Jankovic J, et al. Lesch-Nyhan syndrome: a study of motor behavior and cerebrospinal fluid neurotransmitters. *Ann Neurol* 1988;23:466–469.

801. Watts RW, et al. Clinical, postmortem, biochemical and therapeutic observations on the Lesch-Nyhan syndrome with particular reference to the neurological manifestations. *QJM* 1982;201:43–78.

802. Matthews WS, Solan A, Barabas G. Cognitive functioning in Lesch-Nyhan syndrome. *Dev Med Child Neurol* 1995;37:715–722.

803. Kelley WN, et al. Hypoxanthine-guanine phosphoribosyl transferase deficiency in gout. *Ann Intern Med* 1969;70:155–206.

804. Page T, Nyhan WL, Morena de Vega V. Syndrome of mild mental retardation, spastic gait, and skeletal

malformations in a family with partial deficiency of hypoxanthine-guanine phosphoribosyl transferase. *Pediatrics* 1987;79:713–717.

805. Page T, et al. Use of selective media for distinguishing variant forms of hypoxanthine phosphoribosyl transferase. *Clin Chim Acta* 1986;154:195–201.

806. Harris JC, et al. Craniocerebral magnetic resonance imaging measurement and findings in Lesch-Nyhan syndrome. *Arch Neurol* 1998;55:547–553.

807. Becker MA, et al. Inherited superactivity of phosphoribosylpyrophosphate synthetase: association of uric acid overproduction and sensorineural deafness. *Am J Med* 1988;85:383–390.

808. Jaeken J, et al. Adenylsuccinase deficiency: an inborn error of purine nucleotide synthesis. *Eur J Pediatr* 1988;148:126–131.

809. Diasio RB, Beavers TL, Carpenter JT. Familial deficiency of dihydropyrimidine dehydrogenase: biochemical basis for familial pyrimidinemia and severe 5-fluorouracil–induced toxicity. *J Clin Invest* 1988;81: 47–51.

810. Putman CWM, et al. Dihydropyriminidase deficiency: a progressive neurological disorder? *Neuropediatrics* 1997;28:106–110.

811. Tam DA, Leshner RT. Stroke in purine nucleoside phosphorylase deficiency. *Pediatr Neurol* 1995;12: 146–148.

812. Sinkeler SP, et al. Myoadenylate deaminase deficiency: a clinical, genetic, and biochemical study in nine families. *Muscle Nerve* 1988;11:312–317.

813. Shumate JB, et al. Adenylate deaminase deficiency in a hypotonic infant. *J Pediatr* 1980;96:885–887.

814. Sebesta I, et al. Adenylsuccinase deficiency: clinical and biochemical findings in 5 Czech patients. *J Inherit Metab Dis* 1997;20:343–344.

815. Suchi M, et al. Molecular cloning of the human UP synthase gene and characterization of point mutations in two hereditary orotic aciduria families. *Am J Hum Genet* 1997;60:525–539.

816. Schulze A, et al. Creatine deficiency syndrome caused by guanidinoacetate methyltransferase deficiency: diagnostic tools for a new inborn error of metabolism. *J Pediatr* 1997;131:626–631.

817. Barclay N. Acute intermittent porphyria in childhood. A neglected diagnosis? *Arch Dis Child* 1974;49: 404–406.

818. Becker DM, Kramer S. The neurological manifestations of porphyria: a review. *Medicine* 1975;56:411–423.

819. McDonagh AF, Bissell DM. Porphyria and porphyrinology—the past fifteen years. *Semin Liver Dis* 1998;18:3–15.

819a. Beukeveld GJ, et al. A retrospective study of a patient with homozygous form of acute intermittent porphyria. *J Inherit Metab Dis* 1990;13:673–683.

820. Meyer UA, Schuurmans MM, Lindberg RLP. Acute porphyrias: pathogenesis of neurological manifestations. *Semin Liver Dis* 1998;18:43–52.

821. Kappas A, et al. The porphyrias. In: Scriver CR, Beaudet AL, Sly WS, Valle D, eds *The metabolic and molecular basis of inherited disease*, 7th ed. McGraw-Hill, New York, 1995:2103–2159.

822. Kushner JP. Laboratory diagnosis of the porphyrias. *N Engl J Med* 1991;324:1432–1434.

823. Wallace DC. Diseases of the mitochondrial DNA. *Annu Rev Biochem* 1992;61:1175–1212.

823a. Smeitink JAM, et al. Nuclear genes of human complex I of the mitochondrial electron transport chain: state of the art. *Hum Molec Genet* 1998;7:1573–1579.

824. Chinnery PF, Turnbull DM. Mitochondrial medicine. *Q J Med* 1997;90:657–667.

825. Poulton J, Macaulay V, Marchington DR. Mitochondrial genetics '98. Is the bottleneck cracked? *Am J Hum Genet* 1998;62:752–757.

826. Chinnery PF, et al. MELAS and MERRF. The relationship between maternal mutation load and the frequency of affected offspring. *Brain* 1998;121: 1889–1894.

827. Petty RKH, Harding AE, Morgan-Hughes JA. The clinical features of mitochondrial myopathy. *Brain* 1986;109:915–938.

828. Riordan-Eva P, Harding AE. Leber's hereditary optic neuropathy: the clinical relevance of different mitochondrial DNA mutations. *J Med Genet* 1995;32:81–87.

829. Adams JH, Blackwood W, Wilson J. Further clinical and pathological observations on Leber's optic atrophy. *Brain* 1966;89:15–26.

830. Uemura A, et al. Leber's hereditary optic neuropathy: mitochondrial and biochemical studies on muscle biopsies. *Br J Ophthalmol* 1987;71:531–536.

831. Howell N, et al. Leber hereditary optic neuropathy: involvement of the mitochondrial ND1 gene and evidence for an intragenic suppressor mutation. *Am J Hum Genet* 1991;48:935–942.

832. Nikoskelainen E, et al. Fundus findings in Leber's hereditary optic neuroretinopathy. III. Fluorescein angiographic studies. *Arch Ophthalmol* 1984;102: 981–989.

833. Nikoskelainen E, et al. The early phase in Leber hereditary optic atrophy. *Arch Ophthalmol* 1977;95:969–978.

834. Nikoskelainen E, et al. Leber's hereditary optic neuroretinopathy, a maternally inherited disease. *Arch Ophthalmol* 1987;105:665–671.

835. Smith VC, Pokorny J, Ernest JT. Primary hereditary optic atrophies. In: Krill AE, ed. *Hereditary retinal and choroidal diseases*. Vol 2. New York: Harper & Row, 1977:1109–1135.

836. Jun AS, Brown MD, Wallace DC. A mitochondrial DNA mutation at nucleotide pair 14459 of the NADH dehydrogenase subunit 6 gene associated with maternally inherited Leber hereditary optic neuropathy and dystonia. *Proc Natl Acad Sci U S A* 1994;91:6206–6210.

836a. Shoffner JM, et al. Leber's hereditary optic neuropathy plus dystonia is caused by a mitochondrial DNA point mutation. *Ann Neurol* 1995;38:163–169.

837. DiMauro S, et al. Mitochondrial myopathies. *J Inherit Metab Dis* 1987;10[suppl 1]:113–128.

838. Matthews PM, et al. In vivo muscle magnetic resonance spectroscopy in the clinical investigation of mitochondrial disease. *Neurology* 1991;41:114–120.

839. Holt IJ, et al. Mitochondrial myopathies: clinical and biochemical features of 30 patients with major deletions of muscle mitochondrial DNA. *Ann Neurol* 1989;26:699–708.

840. Ricci E, et al. Disorders associated with depletion of mitochondrial DNA. *Brain Pathol* 1992;2:141–147.

841. Tritschler HJ, et al. Mitochondrial myopathy of childhood associated with depletion of mitochondrial DNA. *Neurology* 1992;42:209–217.

842. Leigh D. Subacute necrotizing encephalomyelopathy in an infant. *J Neurol Neurosurg Psych* 1951;14:216–222.

843. Macaya A, et al. Disorders of movement in Leigh syndrome. *Neuropediatrics* 1993;24:60–67.

844. Campistol J, et al. Dystonia as a presenting sign of subacute necrotizing encephalomyelopathy in infancy. *Eur J Pediatr* 1986;144:589–591.

845. DiMauro S, et al. Cytochrome c oxidase deficiency. *Pediatr Res* 1990;28:536–541.

846. Barkovich AJ, et al. Mitochondrial disorders: analysis of their clinical and imaging characteristics. *Am J Neuroradiol* 1993;14:1119–1137.

847. Egger J, et al. Cortical subacute necrotizing encephalitis. A study of two patients with mitochondrial dysfunction. *Neuropediatrics* 1984;15:150–158.

848. van Erven PMM, et al. Disturbed oxidative metabolism in subacute necrotizing encephalomyelopathy (Leigh syndrome). *Neuropediatrics* 1986;17:28–32.

849. Morris AAM, et al. Deficiency of respiratory chain complex I is a common cause of Leigh disease. *Ann Neurol* 1996;40:25–30.

850. Santorelli FM, et al. A T-C mutation at nt 8993 of mitochondrial DNA in a child with Leigh syndrome. *Neurology* 1994;44:972–974.

851. Holt LJ, et al. A new mitochondrial disease, associated with mitochondrial heteroplasmy. *Am J Hum Genet* 1990;46:428–433.

852. Thyagarajan D, et al. A novel mitochondrial ATPase 6 point mutation in familial bilateral striatal necrosis. *Ann Neurol* 1995;38:468–472.

853. Rahman S, et al. Leigh syndrome: clinical features and biochemical and DNA abnormalities. *Ann Neurol* 1996;39:343–351.

854. Zinn AB, Kerr DS, Hoppel CL. Fumarase deficiency: a new cause of mitochondrial encephalomyopathy. *N Engl J Med* 1986;315:469–475.

855. Adams PL, Lightowlers RN, Turnbull DM. Molecular analysis of cytochrome c oxidase deficiency in Leigh's syndrome. *Ann Neurol* 1997;41:268–270.

856. Zhu Z, et al. SURF1, encoding a factor involved in the biogenesis of cytochrome c oxidase, is mutated in Leigh syndrome. *Nature Genet* 1998;20:337–343.

856a. Tiranti V, et al. Loss-of-function mutations of SURF-1 are specifically associated with Leigh syndrome with cytochrome c oxidase deficiency. *Ann Neurol* 1999; 46:161–166.

857. Wijburg FA, et al. Leigh syndrome associated with a deficiency of the pyruvate dehydrogenase complex: results of treatment with a ketogenic diet. *Neuropediatrics* 1992;23:147–152.

857a. Wexler ID, et al. Outcome of pyruvate dehydrogenase deficiency treated with ketogenic diets. Studies in patients with identical mutations. *Neurology* 1997;49: 1655–1661.

858. Kearns TP, Sayre GP. Retinitis pigmentosa, external ophthalmoplegia and complete heart block: unusual syndrome with histologic study in one of two cases. *Arch Ophthalmol* 1958;60:280–289.

859. DiMauro S, et al. Mitochondrial myopathies. *Ann Neurol* 1985;17:521–538.

860. Yamamoto M, Clemens PR, Engel AG. Mitochondrial DNA deletions in mitochondrial cytopathies: observations in 19 cases. *Neurology* 1991;41:1822–1828.

861. Yiannikas C, et al. Peripheral neuropathy associated with mitochondrial myopathy. *Ann Neurol* 1986;20: 249–257.

862. Danta G, Hilton RC, Lynch PG. Chronic progressive external ophthalmoplegia. *Brain* 1975;98:473–492.

863. Karpati G, et al. The Kearns-Shy syndrome. A multisystem disease with mitochondrial abnormality demonstrated in skeletal muscle and skin. *J Neurol Sci* 1973;19:133–151.

864. Moraes CT, et al. Mitochondrial DNA deletions in progressive external ophthalmoplegia and Kearns-Sayre syndrome. *N Engl J Med* 1989;320:1293–1299.

865. Schon EA, et al. A direct repeat is a hotspot for large-scale deletion of human mitochondrial DNA. *Science* 1989;244:346–349.

866. Zeviani M, Tiranti V, Piantadosi C. Mitochondrial disorders. *Medicine* 1998;77:59–72.

867. Zeviani M, et al. Tissue distribution and transmission of mitochondrial DNA deletions in mitochondrial myopathies. *Ann Neurol* 1990;28:94–97.

868. Shoubridge EA, Karpati G, Hastings KEM. Deletion mutants are functionally dominant over wild-type mitochondrial genomes in skeletal muscle fiber segments in mitochondrial diseases. *Cell* 1990;62:43–49.

869. Larsson N, et al. Progressive increase of the mutated mitochondrial DNA fraction in Kearns-Sayre syndrome. *Pediatr Res* 1990;28:131–136.

870. Shoubridge EA, Johns T, Karpati G. Complete restoration of a wild-type mtDNA genotype in regenerating muscle fibres in a patient with a tRNA point mutation and mitochondrial encephalomyopathy. *Hum Mol Genet* 1997;6:2239–2242.

871. McShane MA, et al. Pearson syndrome and mitochondrial encephalopathy in a patient with a deletion of mtDNA. *Am J Hum Genet* 1991;48:39–42.

872. Holt IJ, Harding AE, Morgan-Hughes JA. Deletions of muscle mitochondrial DNA in patients with mitochondrial myopathies. *Nature* 1988;331:717–719.

873. Sparaco M, et al. Neuropathology of mitochondrial encephalomyopathies due to mitochondrial DNA defects. *J Neuropathol Exp Neurol* 1993;52:1–10.

874. Rehncrona S, Rosen I, Siesjö BK. Excessive cellular acidosis: an important mechanism of neuronal damage in the brain? *Acta Physiol Scand* 1980;110:435–437.

875. Fukuhara N, et al. Myoclonus epilepsy associated with ragged-red fibers (mitochondrial abnormalities): disease entity or syndrome? Light and electron-microscopic studies of two cases and review of the literature. *J Neurol Sci* 1980;47:117–133.

876. Hopkins LC, Rosing HS. Myoclonus and mitochondrial myopathy. *Adv Neurol* 1986;43:105–117.

877. Tulinius MH, et al. Mitochondrial encephalomyopathies in childhood. II. Clinical manifestations and syndromes. *J Pediatr* 1991;199:251–259.

878. Shoffner JM, et al. Myoclonic epilepsy and ragged red fiber disease (MERRF) is associated with a mitochondrial tRNALys mutation. *Cell* 1990;61:931–937.

879. Hammans SR, et al. The mitochondrial DNA transfer RNALeu(UUR) A→G (3243) mutation. A clinical and genetic study. *Brain* 1995;118:721–734.

880. Rosing HS, et al. Maternally inherited mitochondrial myopathy and myoclonic epilepsy. *Ann Neurol* 1985;17:228–237.

881. Larsson N, et al. Segregation and manifestations of the mtDNA tRNAlys A>G(8344) mutation of myoclonus epilepsy and ragged red fibres (MERRF) syndrome. *Am J Hum Genet* 1993;51:1201–1212.

882. Pavlakis SG, et al. Mitochondrial myopathy, encephalopathy, lactic acidosis and strokelike episodes (MELAS): a distinctive clinical syndrome. *Ann Neurol* 1984;16:481–488.

883. Taylor RW, et al. MELAS associated with a mutation in the valine transfer RNA gene of mitochondrial DNA. *Ann Neurol* 1996;40:459–462.

884. Ciafaloni E, et al. MELAS: clinical features, biochemistry, and molecular genetics. *Ann Neurol* 1992;31: 391–398.

885. Poulton J, Morten K. Noninvasive diagnosis of the MELAS syndrome from blood DNA. *Ann Neurol* 1993;34:1–16.

886. Ooiwa Y, et al. Cerebral blood flow in mitochondrial myopathy, encephalopathy, lactic acidosis and strokelike episodes. *Stroke* 1993;24:304–309.

887. Alpers BJ. Diffuse progressive degeneration of the gray matter of the cerebrum. *Arch Neurol Psychiatr* 1931;25:469–505.

887a. Schuelke M, et al. Mutant NDUFV1 subunit of mitochondrial complex I causes leukodystrophy and myoclonic epilepsy. *Nature Genet* 1999;21:260–261.

888. Hartmann AF Sr, et al. Lactate metabolism: studies of a child with a serious congenital deviation. *J Pediatr* 1962;61:165–180.

889. Duncan DB, et al. Positron emission tomography and magnetic resonance spectroscopy of cerebral glycolysis in children with congenital lactic acidosis. *Ann Neurol* 1995;37:351–358.

890. Robinson BH, Taylor J, Sherwood WG. The genetic heterogeneity of lactic acidosis: occurrence of recognizable inborn errors of metabolism in a pediatric population with lactic acidosis. *Pediatr Res* 1980;14: 956–962.

891. Kerr DS, et al. Systemic deficiency of the first component of the pyruvate dehydrogenase complex. *Pediatr Res* 1987;22:312–318.

892. Old SE, DeVivo DC. Pyruvate dehydrogenase complex deficiency: biochemical and immunoblot analysis of cultured skin fibroblasts. *Ann Neurol* 1989;26:746–751.

893. Robinson BH, et al. Variable clinical presentation in patients with defective E$_1$ component of pyruvate dehydrogenase complex. *J Pediatr* 1987;111:525–533.

894. Cederbaum SD, et al. Sensitivity to carbohydrate in a patient with familial intermittent lactic acidosis and pyruvate dehydrogenase deficiency. *Pediatr Res* 1976;10:713–720.

895. Robinson BH, Taylor J, Sherwood WG. Deficiency of dihydrolipoyl dehydrogenase (a component of the pyruvate and α–ketoglutarate dehydrogenase complexes): a cause of congenital lactic acidosis in infancy. *Pediatr Res* 1977;11:1198–1202.

896. Robinson BH, Sherwood WG. Pyruvate dehydrogenase phosphatase deficiency: a cause of congenital chronic lactic acidosis in infancy. *Pediatr Res* 1975;9:935–939.

897. Blass JP, Avigan J, Uhlendorf BW. A defect in pyruvate decarboxylase in a child with an intermittent movement disorder. *J Clin Invest* 1970;49:423–432.

898. Taylor J, Robinson BH, Sherwood WG. A defect in branched-chain amino acid metabolism in a patient with congenital lactic acidosis due to dihydrolipoyl dehydrogenase deficiency. *Pediatr Res* 1978;12: 60–62.

899. Stacpoole PW, et al. Treatment of congenital lactic acidosis with dichloroacetate. *Arch Dis Child* 1997;77:535–541.

899a. Morten KJ, Caky M, Matthew PM. Stabilization of the pyruvate dehydrogenase E1α subunit by dichloroacetate. *Neurology* 1998;51:1331–1335.

900. Luft R, et al. A case of severe hypermetabolism of non-thyroid origin with a defect in the maintenance of mitochondrial respiratory control. *J Clin Invest* 1962;41:1776–1804.

901. DiMauro S, et al. Luft's disease: further biochemical and ultrastructural studies of skeletal muscle in the second case. *J Neurol Sci* 1976;27:217–232.

902. Sengers RCA, Stadhouders AM. Secondary mitochondrial pathology. *J Inherit Metab Dis* 1987;10[suppl 1]: 98–104.

903. Brown GK, et al. "Cerebral" lactic acidosis: defects in pyruvate metabolism with profound brain damage and minimal systemic acidosis. *Eur J Pediatr* 1988;147: 10–14.

903a. Stacpoole PW, et al. The importance of cerebrospinal fluid lactate in the evaluation of congenital lactic acidosis. *J Pediatr* 1999;134:99–102.

904. Matsuo M, et al. Fatal case of pyruvate dehydrogenase deficiency. *Acta Paediatr Scand* 1985;74:140–142.

905. DiMauro S, Trevisan C, Hays A. Disorders of lipid metabolism in muscle. *Muscle Nerve* 1980;3: 369–388.

906. Stansbie D, Wallace SJ, Marsac C. Disorders of the pyruvate dehydrogenase complex. *J Inherit Metab Dis* 1986;9:105–119.

907. Turnbull DM, et al. Short-chain acyl CoA dehydrogenase deficiency associated with a lipid-storage myopathy and secondary carnitine deficiency. *N Engl J Med* 1984;311:1232–1236.

908. Chalmers RA. Organic acids in urine of patients with congenital lactic acidoses: an aid to differential diagnosis. *J Inherit Metab Dis* 1984;7[suppl 1];79–89.

909. Robinson BH, et al. The use of skin fibroblast cultures in the detection of respiratory chain defects in patients with lactic acidemia. *Pediatr Res* 1990;28: 549–555.

910. Bresolin N, et al. Clinical and biochemical correlations in mitochondrial myopathies treated with coenzyme Q10. *Neurology* 1988;38:892–899.

911. Toth PP, et al. Transient improvement of congenital lactic acidosis in a male infant with pyruvate decarboxylase deficiency treated with dichloroacetate. *J Pediatr* 1993;123:427–430.

912. DiMauro S, et al. Benign infantile mitochondrial myopathy due to reversible cytochrome c oxidase deficiency. *Ann Neurol* 1983;14:226–234.

In my conception of scientific work, history and research are so indivisibly linked that I cannot even conceive of one without the other.
—*T. Billroth,* Über das Lehren und Lernen der Medizinischen Wissenschaften

Chapter 2

Heredodegenerative Diseases

John H. Menkes

Departments of Neurology and Pediatrics, University of California, Los Angeles, UCLA School of Medicine, and Department of Pediatric Neurology, Cedars-Sinai Medical Center, Los Angeles, California 90048

Advances in molecular biology have pointed to a basic similarity between diseases of metabolic origin (Chapter 1) and heredodegenerative diseases. Nevertheless, essential differences remain. In metabolic disorders, the biochemical derangement of tissue or body fluids has led, in enzymopathies such as phenylketonuria or maple syrup urine disease, to the identification of the basic biochemical defect. Subsequent purification of the normal protein has permitted isolation of the gene that codes for it and has led to the determination of the molecular abnormality or abnormalities in the gene in patients with the disease. This process has been termed *functional cloning*.

Most of the conditions covered in this chapter as yet have no biochemical explanation. This lack has prompted the application of positional cloning (*reverse genetics,* i.e., a process in which the gene responsible for the disorder is isolated without its protein product being known). Theoretically, the process is simple; the approximate map position of the gene is established by linkage studies on extended families experiencing the disease. In many instances, cytogenetics and the use of a large number of polymorphic markers allow assignment of the gene to a specific chromosome with a resolution of roughly several million base pairs. This first step has been accomplished for quite a few of the conditions covered in this chapter. The second step involves a more exact localization of the gene site and

subsequent isolation and cloning of the gene. Although this has been a complicated and labor-intensive process, it has been achieved for a significant proportion of the heredodegenerative diseases covered in this chapter.

A shortcut to this process, which is also applicable to the rarer diseases, has been the use of *candidate genes.* A number of genes coding for proteins and enzymes vital to brain function have been mapped, cloned, and sequenced. When a new disease locus is assigned to a chromosomal region using linkage analysis, candidate genes from the same region are surveyed, and features of these candidate genes are compared with the features of the particular disease. Conversely, when a new gene is assigned to a chromosomal region, candidate diseases are analyzed by an analogous process. This approach has led to the observation that abnormalities in the gene for myelin proteolipid protein (PLP) are responsible for Pelizaeus-Merzbacher disease (PMD), with the gene for both PLP and the disease localized to the q22 segment of the X chromosome. One of the genes for Charcot-Marie-Tooth (CMT) disease [hereditary motor sensory neuropathy (HMSN) type IA] was isolated by this combined approach.

The interested reader is referred to reviews of this constantly evolving field by Lupski and Zoghbi (1) and Collins (2).

For the clinician, it is still best that the heredodegenerative diseases are grouped according to their clinical presentation and according to the site in the brain that incurs the major anatomic or functional insult. The various categories are (a) heredodegenerative diseases of the basal ganglia, (b) heredodegenerative diseases of the cerebellum, brainstem, and spinal cord, (c) heredodegenerative diseases of the peripheral and cranial nerves, and (d) diffuse cerebral degenerative diseases. A variety of intermediate forms have been well documented.

HEREDODEGENERATIVE DISEASES OF THE BASAL GANGLIA

Huntington Disease

Huntington disease (HD) is a chronic progressive degenerative disease characterized by involuntary movements, mental deterioration, and an autosomal dominant transmission. Although its essential features were first described by Waters (3) in 1841, Huntington provided its most accurate and graphic description in residents of East Hampton, Long Island (4).

The prevalence of HD in the general population has been estimated at between 5 and 10 per 100,000 (5). Although all patients early in United States' history were descendants of two English brothers, the disease has since been found in all races and nationalities.

Abnormalities are limited to the brain. Grossly, patients have gyral atrophy affecting primarily the frontal lobes, and generalized and symmetric dilatation of the lateral ventricles. The striatum (caudate nucleus and putamen) is markedly shrunken (Fig. 2.1). Light microscopic examination demonstrates three processes: neuronal loss, which is associated with the presence of brain macrophages and neuronal satellitosis; lipopigment deposition in neurons and astroglia in excess of that expected for the subject's age; and a relative astrocytic proliferation (6).

Electron microscopy of frontal lobe biopsies reveals a generalized, nonspecific derangement of all membrane structures, a consequence of cell death.

In adults, the main morphologic changes, namely neuronal loss and astrogliosis, are found in the caudate nucleus, putamen, and, to a lesser

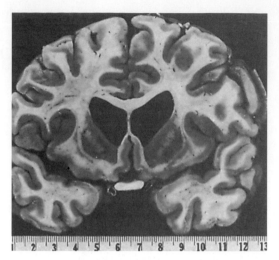

FIG. 2.1. Huntington disease. Gross atrophy of the caudate nucleus gives the lateral ventricles a butterfly appearance. (Courtesy of Dr. J. A. N. Corsellis, The Maudsley Hospital, London.)

extent, in the cortex, notably the frontal lobes (7). The ventrolateral thalamic nucleus, subthalamic nucleus, and, in some cases, spinal cord also may be involved. As a rule, the caudate nucleus, particularly its paraventricular portion, is more affected than the putamen, whereas the nucleus accumbens generally is spared until late in the disease process. The pathology of juvenile HD is somewhat similar. Children presenting with the rigid form of the disease appear to have a marked destruction of the putamen (8,9). Severe astrogliosis of the globus pallidus may occur without neuronal loss, and hyperpigmentation of the substantia nigra has been noted in some of the juvenile patients (10).

Cell death within the striatum does not affect all neurons equally. The medium-sized GABA-ergic spiny projection neurons, which make up approximately 95% of human striatal neurons and contain a variety of neuropeptides, notably enkephalins and substance P, are the first to be affected (11). They are the source of the striatal output projections to the external globus pallidus and to the substantia nigra pars reticulata. By contrast, medium-sized aspiny interneurons containing somatostatin and staining with the histochemical marker NADPH–diaphorase are relatively spared, as are the large aspiny, cholinergic neurons, and neurons immunoreactive for neuropeptide Y.

The mechanisms for this selective vulnerability are still unclear. Calabresi and colleagues have proposed that one factor involved is a selective sensitivity to ionotropic glutaminergic agonists. Differences in intracellular calcium handling, the expression of calcium-binding proteins, and differences in energy demands also may determine cellular sensitivity (12). This selective cellular vulnerability is unique to HD and is not seen in any other neurodegenerative condition (13). Selective cell loss also is observed in the cortex where a depletion of the large pyramidal neurons in cortical layers III, V, and VI and sparing of the GABA-ergic local circuit neurons occur (14). During the initial phases of the disease, cell loss is at least partially compensated by augmentation of the dendritic trees of the surviving pyramidal cells. This observation could explain the normal cortical metabolic activity that is observed in the early phase of the illness (15).

Pathogenesis and Molecular Genetics

The gene for HD has been mapped to the telomere (tip) of the short arm of chromosome 4 (16). This work represented the first successful linkage analysis in humans using polymorphic DNA markers. The gene whose mutation causes HD is widely expressed in all regions of normal and HD brain and in various other organs. It encodes a large cytoplasmic protein, named *huntingtin* (17). The function of huntingtin is still unclear. It is believed to be essential to normal embryonic development and neurogenesis (18), and its amino acid sequence differs from any other protein sequenced to date. HD results from an expansion of a trinucleotide repeat in the coding region of the gene (19). Trinucleotide repeats are repeated units of three nucleotides in genomic DNA. In the case of HD, it is the trinucleotide (triplet) cytosine-adenine-guanine (CAG) that is repeated. Whereas, in the normal population this trinucleotide repeat ranges from 9 to 34 copies, the length of this repeat is expanded in HD to a mean of 42 to 46 copies. This long run of CAGs in the HD gene encodes

TABLE 2.1. *Triplet repeat diseases*

Triplet repeat expansion in untranslated regions
Fragile X syndromes A and E: CGG expansions
Myotonic dystrophy: CTG expansion
SCA8 spinocerebellar ataxia
Intronic expansion
Friedreich ataxia (spinocerebellar degeneration): GAA expansion
CAG expansion in translated regions
Spinobulbar muscular atrophy (X-linked)
Spinocerebellar ataxia I (SCA1)
Spinocerebellar ataxia II (SCA2)
Machado-Joseph disease (SCA3)
Spinocerebellar ataxia 6 (SCA6)
Huntington disease
Dentatorubral-pallidoluysian atrophy (DRPLA)
CAG expansion in ? translated regions
Hereditary spastic paraplegia (SPG4)
?Triplet repeat expansion
Familial essential tremor (FET1)

a polyglutamine unit near the amino terminus of huntingtin. In HD the length of the repeat is highly unstable. Whereas during maternal transmission it changes by only a few repeats, and on rare occasions has been shown to contract, in paternal transmission the length of the repeat increases dramatically in approximately one-third of cases. Of patients with repeats of 55 or more, 90% have an onset of the disease by age 30, and a good negative correlation exists between the length of the repeat and the age of onset of neurologic symptoms with the longest repeats resulting in juvenile HD (20). When HD appears sporadically, it is often the result of an expansion from an already large repeat. Such an expansion is more likely to occur on the paternally derived allele and has been correlated with advanced paternal age (21). The basic processes responsible for the instability of some repeat trinucleotide DNA sequences, a process termed *dynamic mutation*, are still unclear (22).

A similar expansion of genes with triplet repeats is seen in a number of neurologic conditions (Table 2.1). It would now appear that whenever a dominantly transmitted heredodegenerative disease manifests genetic anticipation (i.e., whenever a progressively earlier onset of neurologic symptoms occurs in successive generations), a repeat expansion of trinucleotide repeats is suspect (23) (see Fig. 3.5). However,

Fraser has stressed that ascertainment bias, that is to say, that the younger generation has not yet reached the age when the disease becomes manifest, and truncation bias, meaning that parents with an early onset of disease do not have offspring, also should be considered as a cause for anticipation in neurologic conditions (24). Also, a high incidence of repeat expansions occurs in the normal population and between 30% and 35% of humans have CAG repeat lengths in their genomes that exceed 40 repeats, an indication that trinucleotide expansion is not invariably associated with a disease process.

As yet it is unclear how the expanded triplet repeat on the Huntington gene causes the disease. Currently, the most popular theory is that HD is the consequence of a gain of function mutation, in which the mutated protein would have a new property or be expressed inappropriately (18). Two factors are believed to be important in the pathogenesis of HD. The first is that the expanded polyglutamine tract alters the physical properties of huntingtin in a manner as to induce neuronal death. Several investigators have observed neuronal intranuclear inclusions immunoreactive for huntingtin epitopes in HD brain (25). Of note is the presence of ubiquitin in these inclusions. Ubiquitin is a small protein that is crucial for the degradation of many cytosolic nuclear and endoplasmic reticulum proteins (25a). Because binding of ubiquitin to proteins marks them for subsequent degradation, this finding suggests that mutant huntingtin has been targeted for proteolysis but that the degradation was somehow incomplete. How mutant huntingtin induces a selective cell death is the subject of much research. More than a dozen proteins interact with the amino terminal of huntingtin. Some are involved in intracellular signaling, and the function of others is still poorly characterized (26). Experimental work suggests that polyglutamine-expanded huntingtin acts within the nucleus to induce apoptotic cell death (27). Antiapoptotic compounds protect neurons against the mutant huntingtin, as does blocking nuclear localization of mutant huntingtin (27a). Death may be a cell-specific event, possibly a function of the sensitivity of certain cells to endogenous excitotoxins such as glutamate or quinolinate.

Quinolinate, an excitotoxin, induces neuronal cell death and has been postulated to cause the selective cell loss in HD by mechanisms that might involve the preferential loss of cells with a high density of N-methyl-D-aspartate receptors (28,29). In support of this hypothesis is the marked reduction in N-methyl-D-aspartate receptor binding in the putamen of brains in patients with HD as compared with normal brains (30).

A second factor is mitochondrial dysfunction. Respiratory complex II/III is deficient in putamen derived from patients with HD, but is normal in their cerebral cortex, cerebellum, or cultured fibroblasts. This observation suggests that mitochondrial dysfunction parallels the severity of neuronal loss and could be secondary to cell damage induced by excitotoxicity, and the ensuing generation of free radicals and superoxide (30a).

Clinical Manifestations

Although symptoms usually begin between ages 35 and 40 years, approximately 5% of patients are younger than 14 years (31). In general, the age when symptoms have their onset decreases as the number of affected male ancestors increases. This finding is most striking when both the affected parent and grandparent are male. In a large series of patients with juvenile HD (patients whose symptoms become apparent before 20 years of age), Myers and coworkers found that 83% inherited the disease from their fathers (31). The onset of neurologic symptoms in siblings of patients with juvenile HD is approximately 27 years. This timing is significantly earlier than in the general population of patients with HD (32). At present, the best explanation for the phenomenon of paternal inheritance of juvenile HD is that an expansion of the triplet repeat occurs during spermatogenesis.

The clinical picture of HD as it presents in children differs from that of affected adults (Table 2.2).

As surveyed by Cotton and colleagues (33), the initial stages of the illness are marked by mental deterioration or behavioral abnormalities (20 of 40 patients), gait disturbances, usually the consequence of rigidity (18 of 40 cases), cerebellar

TABLE 2.2. *Clinical features of Huntington disease of childhood (28 cases)*

Features	Number of patients
Age of onset	
Younger than 5 years of age	7
5 to 10 years of age	21
Hyperkinesia or choreoathetosis	13
Rigidity	19
Seizures	13
Mental deterioration	22
Cerebellar symptoms	5

Data from Jervis GA. Huntington's chorea in childhood. *Arch Neurol* 1963;9:244–257; and Markham CH, Knox JW. Observations in Huntington's chorea. *J Pediatr* 1965;67:46–57. With permission.

signs (15 of 40 cases), and, less commonly, seizures. In the Dutch series of Siesling and coworkers, behavioral disorders were the first feature of juvenile HD in 70%, and chorea was seen in 48% (34). Some 70% of children in this series who presented with chorea developed rigidity in the course of the disease. Mental deterioration can commence before 2 years of age (35). It is not clear whether the intellectual decline results from striatal or cortical dysfunction.

The clinical onset of rigid cases is earlier than in patients who have chorea as the predominant movement disorder (34). Additionally, in almost 90% of rigid juvenile HD cases, the disease is paternally inherited. This contrasts with approximately 70% for juvenile HD with chorea (34,36).

When present, choreoathetosis resembles that seen in Sydenham chorea, but the movements have a greater affinity for the trunk and proximal musculature, and, unlike those in Sydenham chorea, are rarely asymmetric. They are increased by voluntary physical activity and excitement and cease during sleep. Seizures are rare in adults with HD but affect approximately 50% of children. In some cases, they are the most prominent symptom and herald the onset of neurologic deterioration. Grand mal attacks are the most common; minor motor and myoclonic seizures and action myoclonus also have been observed (35). Spasticity, although rare in adults, can be prominent in juvenile HD (37). Cerebellar signs occasionally can be a major feature. Although optic nerve atrophy is not seen, impairment of ocular motility is an early sign and resembles oculomotor apraxia (9). In such

instances, requesting the patient to look from side to side elicits closure of the eyelids or a rapid, jerking movement of the head with an attendant delay in the movement of the eyeballs. Unlike in oculomotor apraxia, random and vertical eye movements also are affected.

The disease progresses more rapidly in children than in adults, with an average duration of illness in the reported juvenile cases of 8 years, as contrasted with a range of 10 to 25 years for adults (38). Rate of progression of the disease has been shown to be directly proportional to the number of CAG repeats.

Homozygotes for HD have been identified in a large Venezuelan kindred (39). Their neurologic picture and the age when symptoms became apparent did not differ from those of the heterozygotes, an indication that the HD gene is phenotypically completely penetrant in the heterozygous state.

Laboratory studies are normal, although the electroencephalogram result is often abnormal, and the cerebrospinal fluid (CSF) protein concentration is sometimes elevated. Computed tomography (CT) scanning and magnetic resonance imaging (MRI) are equally reliable in demonstrating caudate atrophy, but can show normal results even when there are significant neurologic symptoms. The appearance of images on these scans is not specific, however, and can be seen in various other neurodegenerative processes (40). A more sensitive and more specific study involves positron emission tomography (PET) scanning after the infusion of radiolabeled fluorodeoxyglucose. A marked reduction in caudate glucose metabolism is observed in all symptomatic patients, regardless of whether atrophy is evident on CT or MRI scans, and in approximately one-third of presymptomatic subjects at risk for the disease (41). A reduced glucose metabolism is accompanied by a reduction in dopamine D_1 and D_2 receptor binding in caudate and putamen. A good correlation exists between intellectual deterioration and the reduction in D_2 receptor binding (42).

Diagnosis

The capacity to monitor the size of the trinucleotide repeat in individuals at risk for HD has revolutionized preclinical and prenatal testing for the disorder. The following diagnostic guidelines have been established: (a) Allele sizes of 26 or less CAG repeats have never been associated with the HD phenotype, or with mutations to longer repeats; (b) Allele sizes of 27 to 35 repeats have not been associated with the HD phenotype, but have been associated with mutability when transmitted by a male subject. It is likely that some patients with sporadic HD represent the occasional expansion of high normal paternal alleles into the affected range; (c) Allele sizes of 36 to 39 have been associated with HD phenotype but also have been seen in apparently unaffected individuals; (d) Allele sizes of 40 or more CAG repeats have always been accompanied by HD pathology (43). In the experience of Kremer and colleagues, who obtained molecular data from 1,007 subjects, 1.2% of individuals with a clinical diagnosis of HD possessed repeats that fell into the normal range (44). It is not known whether these patients have a phenocopy of HD or whether they were misdiagnosed. Until effective treatment becomes available, the World Federation of Neurology does not advise that patients under 18 be tested for the disease (45). The author of this chapter believes this is a complex issue and that the decision to administer or not to administer the test to children must be evaluated on a case-by-case basis.

The clinical diagnosis of HD rests on the neurologic examination, a positive family history, and neuroimaging studies. HD should be differentiated from the various conditions in which a movement disorder arises during childhood or adolescence. These include idiopathic torsion dystonia (dystonia musculorum deformans), Hallervorden-Spatz syndrome, Wilson disease, and juvenile Parkinson's disease. When intellectual deterioration is the chief feature, the various lipidoses should be considered. Since 1980 there has been a resurgence of Sydenham chorea in the United States. Even though an antecedent streptococcal infection usually cannot be elicited, the distribution of the involuntary movements assists in the diagnosis, as does immune evidence of a streptococcal infection. Benign nonprogressive familial chorea is a rare

but clinically distinct entity (46). PET scans in patients with this condition also demonstrate caudate hypometabolism.

Several conditions are now recognized in which an extrapyramidal disorder is accompanied by the presence of acanthocytes. These are red blood cells with an irregular body and spicules of variable length that are irregularly distributed over the surface of the cell (see Fig. 1.32). The differentiation between acanthocytes and red cells with rounded projections (echinocytes) and their visualization is discussed by Feinberg and coworkers (47). Acanthocytes are seen in more than 50% of all red cells derived from patients with abetalipoproteinemia, but also have been observed in an occasional patient with Hallervorden-Spatz disease; in hypobetalipoproteinemia, acanthocytosis, retinitis pigmentosa, and pallidal degeneration (HARP) syndrome; and in a condition termed *chorea-acanthocytosis*.

Symptoms of HARP syndrome generally appear during the first decade of life and are marked by dystonia, dysarthria, and impaired gait (48).

Typically, chorea-acanthocytosis is characterized by chorea, orofacial dyskinesia with dysarthria, and depressed or absent reflexes. Seizures, dementia, and self-mutilation also have been observed. The age of onset is usually during the second decade or later (49). This condition is not rare in the south of Japan and can be transmitted in both a recessive and a dominant manner (50). The diagnosis of neuroacanthocytosis rests on the demonstration of acanthocytes in a dried blood smear or in saline-diluted wet preparations. Serum lipoprotein electrophoresis and vitamin E levels are normal. Neuroimaging demonstrates caudate atrophy, and MRI reveals increased signal in the caudate and lentiform nuclei. PET scans indicate a severe loss of striatal dopamine D_2-receptor binding sites, and a marked reduction in the $[^{18}F]$dopa uptake in the posterior putamen. These point to a selective degeneration of dopaminergic projections from the substantia nigra compacta to the posterior putamen (51). Further discussion of the various neurologic syndromes associated with peripheral acanthocytosis is found in Chapter 1.

Progressive choreoathetosis also can be observed in a variety of other genetic diseases. These are summarized in Table 1.18.

Treatment

So far, no treatment has been effective in reversing or arresting the progressive dementia. Choline, reserpine, or various phenothiazines, however, can alleviate the choreiform movements, and levodopa, bromocriptine, or amantadine can provide some benefit in the rigid form of the disease.

Primary Dystonia (Dystonia Musculorum Deformans, Torsion Dystonia)

Primary dystonia (dystonia musculorum deformans, torsion dystonia) is characterized by sustained muscle contraction frequently causing twisting and repetitive movements, or abnormal postures. It was first described by Schwalbe in 1908 as a variant of hysteria (52), and more definitively by Oppenheim in 1911 (53). It is now evident that dystonia musculorum deformans represents one or more distinct, genetically transmitted entities, distinguishable from the various acquired dystonias that result from perinatal asphyxia, trauma, toxins, or vascular disease.

Pathogenesis and Molecular Genetics

Several genes have been implicated in the various hereditary dystonias. The disorders are summarized in Table 2.3. The clinical entity that most commonly manifests during childhood has been termed *early onset dystonia* (DYT1). The gene for this condition has been mapped to chromosome 9q34. It codes for a protein termed *torsin A*, an adenosine triphosphate (ATP) binding protein, which is structurally similar to the heat shock proteins. A single mutation, a three-base pair deletion, in the coding sequence of the gene is found in almost all cases seen in Ashkenazi Jewish families (54). Identical gene mutations also have been documented in patients with completely different

TABLE 2.3. *Hereditary dystonias*

Disease	Gene locus	Inheritance	Ethnic predilection	Symptoms	Reference
DYT 1	9q34	AD	Ashkenazi Jewish	Childhood limb onset dystonia, becoming generalized	Ozelius et al. (54)
DYT 2	?	AR	Gypsy	Early onset of dystonia in extremities	Gimenez-Roldan et al. (55)
DYT 3	Xq13.1	X-linked recessive	Filipino	Adult onset; blepharospasm, torticollis, generalized dystonia, parkinsonism	Lee et al. (56)
DYT 4	?	?	?	Dysphonia	Ahmad et al. (57)
DYT 5a	14q 22.1 GTP cyclohydrolase I	AD	Japan	Childhood onset, generalized dystonia, diurnal fluctuations, dramatic response to DOPA	Nygaard et al. (58)
DYT 5b	11p11.5 tyrosine hydroxylase	AR	None	Childhood onset, generalized dystonia, diurnal fluctuations, dramatic response to DOPA	Knappskog et al. (59)
DYT 6	8	AD	Mennonite	Adult onset, cranial cervical dystonia	Almasy et al. (60)
DYT 7	18p	AD	None	Onset in sixth decade of life, torticollis, tremor, dysphonia	Leube et al. (61)
Dystonia, deafness	Xq22	X-linked recessive	None	Early-onset deafness and dystonia	Hayes et al. (62)
Infantile dystonia	?	AD	None	Delayed development, onset of generalized dystonia first year of life; normal intellect	Mostofsky et al. (63)

AD, autosomal dominant; AR, autosomal recessive; DYT, dystonia.

ethnicities. This suggests that DYT1 is an example of a recurrent mutation causing a dominantly inherited condition (59a, 59b).

The pathophysiology of primary dystonia (dystonia musculorum deformans) is unknown. Clinical and electrophysiologic observations indicate that dystonic movements and postures result from a functional disturbance of the basal ganglia. In particular, the striatal control of the globus pallidus and the substantia nigra pas reticulata is impaired. Microelectrode recording conducted in the course of pallidotomy shows a decreased discharge rate from both the internal and external segments of the globus pallidus, probably as a consequence of an increased inhibitory output from the striatum. In addition, the pattern of spontaneous neuronal activity is highly irregular (59c). As a result, there is an alteration of thalamic control of cortical motor planning and execution of movements, reducing the brainstem and spinal cord inhibitory mechanisms (64,65). As a consequence, prolonged abnormal co-contractions of agonist and antagonist muscles occur, with abnormal recruitment (overflow) to the more distant musculature. Marsden has postulated that a defect in the presynaptic inhibitory mechanisms in the spinal cord causes the failure in reciprocal inhibition (66).

Even though primary dystonia is believed to be a functional disorder of the basal ganglia, no consistent anatomic abnormalities are seen in this region. Neuropathologic examination of patients with dystonia musculorum deformans has been negative or has revealed nonspecific changes (67). When discrete lesions result in a secondary focal or hemidystonia, these lesions are localized to the thalamus, caudate nucleus, putamen, or globus pallidus (66).

Although manganese intoxication can induce dystonic symptoms (68), no evidence exists that this heavy metal or any other metal is implicated in primary dystonia.

Clinical Manifestations

Dystonia has been classified according to the body distribution of the abnormal movements. Generalized dystonia (dystonia musculorum deformans) is the most common form seen in children. In this condition, one or both legs and some other region of the body are affected (69). Focal dystonia refers to involvement of a single region. It includes the eyelids (blepharospasm), mouth (oromandibular dystonia), larynx (spastic dysphonia), neck (torticollis), and hand (writer's cramp). In segmental dystonia, two or more contiguous regions are involved. Focal and segmental dystonias are seen rarely during the first two decades of life. Torticollis, when seen in infants and children, is a relatively common condition but is unrelated to primary dystonia. It is considered in Chapter 5.

Generalized dystonia is transmitted as an autosomal dominant condition with a low penetrance, probably between 30% and 40% (70). The factors that control penetrance, be they genetic or environmental, are unknown (71). The degree of penetrance is not dependent on the gender of the transmitting parent.

Primary dystonia caused by a defect in the DYT1 gene is the most common type of childhood dystonia. It has a relatively high incidence among Ashkenazi Jews. This entity begins between the ages of 4 and 16 and is characterized by an initially rapid deterioration.

The first symptoms in both the childhood and late-onset forms of hereditary dystonia are involuntary movements or posturing of one portion of the body (72). Most commonly, the initial movement consists of a plantar, flexion-inversion movement of the foot that can first appear when walking (Fig. 2.2). Initially, symptoms are intermittent, and, being more severe under stress, they frequently are misdiagnosed as representing a hysterical reaction. In due time, however, they become constant. As the disease progresses, involuntary flexion or extension appears at the wrist, and finally, torsion spasms of the neck and trunk become evident. These movements can be triggered by motion of any other part of the body, or ultimately they can appear spontaneously. Eventually, the affected limbs assume a fixed, continuously maintained, abnormal attitude on which athetotic fluctuations in time are superimposed. On examination, the muscles resist passive movements and after forcible deflection, tend to return to their original position.

In some cases, the involuntary movements affect the face and interfere with speech and swallowing. Dystonia of the visceral musculature, particularly paroxysmal dyspnea, has been described. As a rule, all movements cease during sleep. The

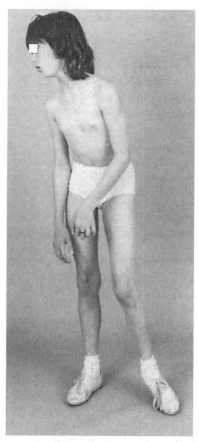

FIG. 2.2. Dystonia musculorum deformans. Dystonic posturing of left arm and left lower extremity. Flexion at the knee and equinovarus positioning of the foot are typical for this condition. Additionally, this 11½-year-old girl has torticollis. Symptoms started at age 9 years with a change in voice, followed by torsion of the distal portion of her left lower extremity at age 10 years.

intellect remains normal in all instances. The childhood-onset form of the disease tends to progress relentlessly, and, in general, the earlier the onset of symptoms, the more rapid their advance. In the experience of Marsden and Harrison (73), 79% of children whose involuntary movements appeared before 11 years of age progressed to generalized dystonia. Individuals whose sole symptom is a mixed resting and intention tremor, writer's cramp, or torticollis frequently are seen in affected families and probably represent a partial expression of the disease (72,74).

Neuroimaging in primary dystonia is usually unremarkable. In the secondary (sympto-

matic) dystonias, it is not uncommon to see abnormalities on either CT or on T2-weighted MRI in the basal ganglia, notably the thalamus, or in the putamen (67). On PET scan of a movement-free patient, a significant increase is seen in the cerebral glucose metabolism in the caudate and lentiform nuclei, cerebellum, and those areas of the frontal lobes that receive projections from the mediodorsal thalamic nucleus (65,75).

In contrast to the generalized forms of hereditary dystonia, segmental and focal forms are rarely encountered in children. The most common of these conditions is spasmodic torticollis, which can appear in isolation or as part of a segmental dystonia, with muscle spasms also affecting the upper extremity. Focal dystonias also include writer's cramp, blepharospasm, spasmodic dysphonia, and oromandibular dystonia. Although these entities tend to remain restricted, they progress in some instances to generalized dystonia (76). In most instances these forms represent a partial expression of primary dystonia (DYT1) (74).

A hereditary progressive form of dystonia with marked diurnal fluctuations and a striking response to low doses of dopaminergic drugs has been seen in Japan and accounts for approximately 5% to 10% of all dystonias seen in the West (58,77). Both autosomal dominant and autosomal recessive forms have been described (see Table 2.3). The autosomal dominant form is the result of a defect in the gene that codes for guanosine triphosphate (GTP) cyclohydrolase I; the recessive form is caused by a defect in the gene for tyrosine hydroxylase (58,59). GTP cyclohydrolase I deficiency also is seen in hyperphenylalaninemia (see Chapter 1). The clinical picture for both forms is similar to early-onset generalized dystonia, with onset during the first decade of life. In approximately one-fourth of children, the diurnal fluctuations are not apparent (58). The various other types of primary dystonia do not usually become apparent during childhood or adolescence (see Table 2.3). Patients with generalized dystonia and severe developmental delay and failure to achieve normal motor milestones also have been described. These patients are compound heterozygotes for mutations in the gene coding for GTP cyclohydrolase, but unlike patients with autosomal recessive GTP cyclohydrolase I deficiency, these subjects do not demonstrate a marked elevation of plasma phenylalanine. These individuals respond dramatically to therapy with a combination of levodopa and BH_4 (77a).

Myoclonic dystonia, a dominantly transmitted form in which torsion dystonia is accompanied by myoclonic jerks, can develop during childhood. Both myoclonus and dystonia improve dramatically with ingestion of alcohol, or with a combination of trihexyphenidyl hydrochloride and valproic acid (78).

The various paroxysmal dystonias are covered in Chapter 13.

Diagnosis

Primary dystonia (dystonia musculorum deformans) must be differentiated from dystonia arising as a consequence of a known central nervous system (CNS) insult (symptomatic or secondary dystonia), or because of other hereditary neurologic disorders. In children, dystonic symptoms are most often the result of perinatal asphyxia (see Chapter 5). Under such circumstances, the movement disorder generally appears before the third year of life, although, exceptionally, the involuntary movements do not begin until 5 to 15 years of age, or even later, with the child having exhibited minimal or no neurologic abnormalities before that time (79,80). In a number of these subjects, dystonic symptoms are not static, but continue to progress throughout life.

Dystonic movements also can develop after acute viral encephalitis, carbon monoxide poisoning, and the ingestion of various drugs, notably phenytoin, carbamazepine, phenothiazines, butyrophenones, benzamides (e.g., Tigan), tricyclic antidepressants, chloroquine, antihistamines (e.g., Benadryl), ketamine, and lithium (81). Many children who develop drug-induced dystonia suffered from preexisting brain damage. Dystonia also can follow craniocerebral trauma. Under these circumstances, it is typically unilateral (hemidystonia). Typical dystonia also can follow peripheral trauma, with the traumatized limb being the one initially affected by the movement disorder

(82,83). It is unclear what role trauma plays in the clinical expression that otherwise would have been asymptomatic for the DYT1 gene.

Dystonic movements also are seen in Leigh syndrome and Wilson disease. In Wilson disease, Kayser-Fleischer rings are invariable, the serum ceruloplasmin is generally depressed, and speech or the facial musculature is often preferentially affected. Other heredodegenerative diseases in which dystonia can be a prominent clinical feature include various lipidoses (GM_1 and GM_2 gangliosidosis, juvenile neuronal ceroid lipofuscinosis, and Niemann-Pick disease type C), metachromatic leukodystrophy (MLD), and glutaric acidemia type I.

Treatment

Two modes of treatment, pharmacologic agents and neurosurgery, have been used to alleviate the symptoms of dystonia. The effectiveness of drug treatment is unpredictable and inconsistent, but approximately one-half of the patients experience significant improvement. Trihexyphenidyl (Artane) is probably best used for DYT1 patients with this disease, whereas levo-dopa, given alone or with a decarboxylase inhibitor (Sinemet), appears to be most beneficial in patients with late-onset dystonia. Trihexyphenidyl is administered to children in extremely large dosages (60 to 80 mg/day or even more). Dosages begin at 2-4 mg/day, and the drug is gradually increased until maximum benefit or intolerable side effects are encountered (84). Tetrabenazine, a dopamine-depleting drug, can be given in dosages of 50 to 200 mg/day. Its effect is potentiated by combining it with lithium (approximately 900 mg/day) (85). In some patients, a combination of trihexyphenidyl, dextroamphetamine, and tetrabenazine appears to be fairly effective, as is the *cocktail* of trihexyphenidyl, pimozide, and tetrabenazine used in the United Kingdom (86). The concomitant administration of baclofen (40 to 120 mg/day) can enhance the effectiveness of drug therapy (87). Other drugs that can be beneficial to an occasional patient include carbamazepine (Tegretol), bromocriptine, and diazepam (Valium). Botulinum toxin (Botox) has been effective in the treatment of blepharospasm and other craniocervical dystonias, but it is used only rarely in generalized dystonia because of the number of large muscles affected.

Unilateral or bilateral pallidotomy is currently the surgical procedure of choice for severe primary dystonia. The experience of Ondo and colleagues and that of other neurosurgeons suggests that this procedure brings on a marked but gradual improvement over the course of several months (88). Cryothalamectomy, also has been used in several centers. This procedure can induce clinical remissions in a large proportion of patients with hemidystonia. Patients with spasmodic torticollis, whether isolated or part of a segmental dystonia, also can benefit from this treatment (89). The effectiveness of the procedure in children with generalized dystonia has not been nearly as good. The relapse rate is high and, in the experience of Andrew and coworkers, 56% of patients undergoing bilateral operations develop dysarthria. This complication is particularly likely if speech disturbances were present before surgery (89). Other complications include a mild hemiparesis, ataxia, and epilepsy. Implantation of a subcutaneous dorsal column stimulator in the high cervical region of the spinal cord is ineffectual. Unilateral or bilateral pallidal stimulation has been used with some success in adults with dystonia. Its effectiveness for the pediatric population has been determined (89a).

In general, it appears that patients with the early onset form of hereditary dystonia (DYT1) respond more favorably to drugs, whereas patients with focal or segmental dystonia are likely to be more amenable to surgery.

Tardive Dyskinesia

Tardive dyskinesia is encountered in the pediatric population in association with the use of neuroleptic medications, notably phenothiazines, butyrophenones, or diphenylbutylpiperidine (Pimozide) (90). The condition is not one entity, but a number of different syndromes. Its incidence is not known. Studies on an inpatient population of psychotic children and adolescents receiving neuroleptics suggest that extrapyramidal movement disorders are seen during drug therapy or on drug withdrawal in as many as 50% (91). In most instances, the movement disorder is transient. It is more common in children who have had prenatal and perinatal complications or those who have received high dosages of the medication for months or years or after an increase in the dosage (92). However, low dosages given over brief periods also have induced the movement disorder.

The severity of movements varies considerably. Characteristically, they consist of orofacial dyskinesias, notably stereotyped involuntary protrusion of the tongue, lip smacking, and chewing. A variety of other involuntary movements also can be present. After the medication is discontinued, these can improve in the course of several months or they can persist. Withdrawal dyskinesias generally disappear after a few weeks or months. Persistent dystonia has been associated with the use of neuroleptics. The clinical appearance of this movement disorder differs from tardive dyskinesia by the absence of orofacial dyskinesias.

Tardive dyskinesia is believed to result from a hypersensitivity of the dopamine receptors induced by the neuroleptic medications. A full review of the pathophysiology of this disorder is beyond the scope of this text.

Why this condition appears in some patients and not in others is unclear. Neither the concomitant administration of anticholinergic drugs predisposes to the appearance of tardive dyskinesia, nor do drug holidays prevent it. In the experience of this chapter's author, several patients with tardive dyskinesia have had a family history of a movement disorder (such as writer's cramp or tremor), suggesting a genetic predisposition.

In making the diagnosis of tardive dyskinesia, one should bear in mind that a number of movement disorders, notably HD or Wilson disease, are preceded by behavior problems, personality changes, or psychoses that could require the use of neuroleptic agents. It is also necessary to differentiate tardive dyskinesia from the choreiform movements of hyperkinetic children, the peculiar movements of institutionalized retarded youngsters, and the choreoathetosis of children with cerebral palsy that can be suppressed by neuroleptics.

A variety of drugs have been used for the treatment of persistent tardive dyskinesia. Jankovic and his group favor tetrabenazine given solely or in combination with lithium (85). In their series, which mainly comprised adults, a persistent excellent response was seen in 85% of subjects. A variety of other drugs (reserpine, clonidine, and clozapine) also have been used. In many instances, however, if the movement disorder has established itself and has failed to subside with withdrawal of the responsible neuroleptic, the outlook for remission is not good.

The neuroleptic malignant syndrome is another neurologic disorder believed to result from the administration of dopamine receptor–blocking neuroleptics. The principal clinical features of this condition are hyperthermia, muscular rigidity, tremors, rhabdomyolysis, and disorientation. Tachycardia and hypertension also can develop (93). The condition can be life-threatening, and prompt treatment is required. This involves the use of up to 1.5 mg/kg of dantrolene, a drug that has been effective in malignant hyperthermia, and a dopamine D_2 receptor agonist, bromocriptine (94).

Hallervorden-Spatz Disease

In 1922, Hallervorden and Spatz described Hallervorden-Spatz disease, a rare familial disorder that began before age 10 years and was characterized by clubfoot deformity, gradually increasing stiffness of all limbs, impaired speech, and dementia (95). Some neurologists distinguish Hallervorden-Spatz syndrome, a clinical entity, from Hallervorden-Spatz disease, which is a postmortem diagnosis.

Pathology

Three pathologic abnormalities occur in Hallervorden-Spatz disease. These are (a) intracellular and extracellular iron deposition in the globus pallidus, substantia nigra, and less often, cerebral cortex; (b) a variable degree of neuronal loss and gliosis in the globus pallidus and the pars reticularis of the substantia nigra; and

(c) widely disseminated rounded structures, identified as axonal spheroids and seen with particular frequency in the basal ganglia (96).

Microscopically, the pigment is located within neurons and glial cells and in the neuropil, particularly around large blood vessels of affected areas. Histochemical and chemical analyses indicate that it contains iron and is related to neuromelanin. The cytoplasm of the renal tubules contains a brown granular pigment, similar in composition to that deposited in nerve tissues (97). It is not clear whether the disorder represents a lipofuscin storage disease with an iron-catalyzed pseudoperoxidation of lipofuscin to neuromelanin, or whether it is the result of an abnormality in axonal metabolism (98). If the latter is true, Hallervorden-Spatz disease is a specific form of primary axonal dystrophy with a predilection for the substantia nigra and locus ceruleus; the excess pigmentation results from lipid deposition. The condition would, therefore, be related to other types of primary axonal dystrophies, such as occur in cystic fibrosis, vitamin E deficiency, infantile neuroaxonal dystrophy, and poisoning with organic cyanides (99).

The gene for Hallervorden-Spatz disease has been mapped to chromosome 20p12.3-13 (100), but up to now, the biochemical defect was still unclear. No systemic abnormality of iron metabolism has been demonstrated, and most genes implicated in iron metabolism and transport have been excluded (100). The finding of Perry and coworkers that an accumulation of cysteine and cystine and reduced activity of cysteine dioxygenase in the globus pallidus occurs has not been confirmed (101). Cysteine dioxygenase converts cysteine to L-cysteinesulfinic acid, the major catabolic product of cysteine. This observation of cysteine accumulation becomes particularly pertinent when one considers the parkinsonian symptoms of long-surviving patients with cystinosis.

Clinical Manifestations

Considerable variability occurs in time of onset of symptoms and in the major manifestations of Hallervorden-Spatz disease (102). In the classic form of the disease, symptoms become apparent during the latter part of the first decade or the second decade. These include a progressive impairment of gait caused by equinovarus pes deformity of the feet and rigidity of the legs, slowing and diminution of all voluntary movements, dysarthria, and mental deterioration (103). Approximately 50% of patients, however, have exhibited a choreiform and athetotic movement disorder. Spasticity has been evident in some cases and atrophy of distal musculature or seizures in others. Retinitis pigmentosa was seen in 20% of patients compiled by Dooling and colleagues (102). This feature is often accompanied by optic atrophy and is seen in patients whose disease has an earlier onset and more rapid progression (104).

Neuroimaging studies are of considerable assistance in the diagnosis of the disease. The CT scan shows bilateral high-density lesions within the globus pallidus (105). The presence of iron within the basal ganglia is best detected by MRI using a T2-weighted spin-echo pulse sequence at high field strength (1.5 Tesla). Marked hypointensity of the globus pallidus is seen, and the low-signal area surrounds a circumscribed region of high signal, the *eye-of-the-tiger sign* (106).

No treatment exists for the condition. In my experience, iron chelation has been ineffective. Movement disorders, notably dystonia, have been controlled by bilateral thalamotomy. Pallidotomy has not been effective at our institution.

Several variants of Hallervorden-Spatz disease have been encountered (96). In one of these, an associated acanthocytosis occurs (96,107). In some instances, this entity has been accompanied by retinitis pigmentosa and hypoprebetalipoproteinemia (see Chapter 1) (108). In another variant, the bone marrow contains sea-blue histiocytes (109). This phenomenon indicates the presence of complex lipids in histiocyte liposomes and is seen in a variety of other neurologic disorders, including GM_1 gangliosidosis, Fabry disease, Niemann-Pick disease C, Tangier disease, and Wolman disease (see Chapter 1). These cells also are found in chronic myelogenous leukemia, idiopathic thrombocytopenic purpura, and hyperlipoproteinemia type I.

Familial Calcification of Basal Ganglia (Fahr Disease)

Fahr disease is not a single entity, but several genetically and clinically distinct disorders that share the characteristic of calcific deposits within the basal ganglia (Fig. 2.3). A brain that demonstrated calcification within the basal ganglia was first described by Bamberger in 1856 (110). In 1930, Fahr reported a case of idiopathic calcification of the cerebral blood vessels in an adult with progressive neurologic symptoms (111). Since then, several genetic disorders subsumed under the term *Fahr disease* have been delineated (112).

One form of familial calcification of the basal ganglia is best exemplified by two sets of siblings reported by Melchior and coworkers (113). In these children, the disease was marked by mental deterioration, which became apparent

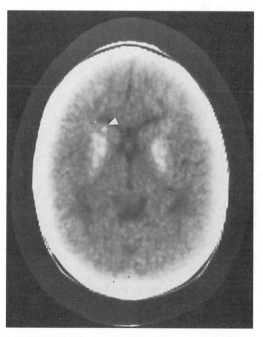

FIG. 2.3. Calcified basal ganglia in a 10-year-old girl. Computed tomographic scan without contrast. The calcification is principally in the putamen and globus pallidus. Additionally, a focus of calcification in the caudate nucleus appears on the left (*arrowhead*). (Courtesy of Drs. Hervey Segall, the late Robert Sedgwick, and the late Lawrence S. Fishman, Children's Hospital, Los Angeles, CA.)

within the first 2 years of life, and a choreo-athetotic movement disorder. Microcephaly and seizures also can be present, and in one patient, calcification could be seen on ophthalmoscopic examination of the fundi. An autosomal recessive transmission is likely.

Another group has been designated as Aicardi-Goutiéres disease. It is an autosomal recessive progressive encephalopathy, with its onset in infancy, first described in 1984 (114). Initial symptoms include feeding difficulties and irritability. In some patients, previously acquired skills are lost, and spasticity develops. Microcephaly is common (114a). The diagnostic features include basal ganglia calcifications, a mild but persistent CSF lymphocytosis, a protein elevation, and a high level of interferon-α in CSF and serum (114a). MRI studies show increased signal in central white matter (115).

An autosomal dominant type of calcification of the basal ganglia is represented by the family reported by Boller and coworkers (116). Affected members developed chorea and dementia in the third or fourth decade. The family reported by Moskowitz and coworkers was clinically similar, and its members excreted greater than normal amounts of 3',5'-AMP in response to administration of purified parathormone (117). In another family, calcification of the basal ganglia that was transmitted as an autosomal dominant trait was entirely asymptomatic (118).

On pathologic examination, calcium deposits are found within capillaries and the media of the larger vessels. Free calcium also is seen within brain tissue in the basal ganglia, cortex, and dentate nucleus of the cerebellum. There might be an accompanying demyelination (119).

Calcification of the basal ganglia also can be seen secondary to a number of well-delineated conditions. Most often, the picture is encountered in disorders of calcium metabolism, including hypoparathyroidism, pseudohypoparathyroidism, and hyperparathyroidism. Additionally, calcification of the basal ganglia, accompanied by deposition of the mineral in other parts of the brain, is seen in tuberous sclerosis, toxoplasmosis, cytomegalic inclusion disease, Cockayne syndrome, and Down syndrome (120). Calcification of the basal ganglia has variously been reported as a consequence of perinatal asphyxia, but in my experience, this situation is extremely unusual. A differential diagnosis of basal ganglia calcification as detected by CT scans was presented by Harrington and coworkers (121).

Hereditary (Familial) Tremor

Hereditary (familial) tremor represents the most common movement disorder seen in childhood. Symptoms usually become evident around puberty, although patients aged 5 years or younger have been observed.

The tremor is rhythmic, with the frequency of oscillation usually being between 4 and 8 Hz (122). The tremor increases with movement, becoming accentuated as the limb approaches its target, and, except in the most severe cases, is absent when the limb is at rest. It disappears with sleep. The tremor initially affects one or both of the upper extremities, but usually does not interfere with fine coordination. With tremor progression, the patient can develop head nodding. The lower extremities are affected less often, and intelligence, gait, and strength remain normal (123,124). Speech and eyelids are rarely affected during childhood. Brief episodes of shuddering or stiffening of the body, usually associated with excitement, might be observed in infancy or early childhood. They are believed to represent an antecedent to familial tremor (125). In approximately 10% of patients, essential tremor is associated with dystonia, and there is also an increased prevalence of Parkinson's disease (123).

Although the disease is progressive during its early stages, it arrests during much of adult life and interferes little with the patient's daily activity. In later life, however, the condition can suddenly become aggravated, and senile tremor can be a late manifestation of essential tremor.

An autosomal dominant transmission appears to be likely, and up to the present, two genes have been mapped. One was obtained by linkage analysis from a large American family and is on chromosome 2p22-p25 (FET2) (126). The other, obtained from an Icelandic family, is on chromosome 3q13 (FET1) (127). Evidence suggests that an expanded CAG trinucleotide sequence will turn out to be responsible for the disease in some families. Without doubt, other gene loci will be found in the course of the next few years.

The pathophysiology of familial tremor is still in dispute. Autopsy has shown no significant disorder. Marsden distinguished two forms. The first he termed an exaggerated physiologic essential tremor with a frequency of 8 to 12 Hz, which depends on a peripheral reflex. The second form represents a pathologic essential tremor, which has a frequency of 4 to 7 Hz and is largely dependent on an interaction between an overactive central generator, associated with the rubro-olivocerebellorubral loop, and the peripheral system, in particular the stretch reflex (122,128). On PET, overactivity of this loop is confirmed by the observed hypermetabolism of the medulla, presumably reflecting inferior olivary activity, and abnormal bilateral cerebellar blood flow during tremor and at rest (129).

The diagnosis of essential tremor rests on the exclusion of other disorders of the basal ganglia. Tremors can accompany dystonia musculorum deformans (123), spasmodic torticollis, and writer's cramp. They probably represent a partial expression of primary dystonia. Tremors also are seen in Wilson disease and HD. A family history of the disorder and examination of the parents and other family members are helpful.

Treatment

In most cases of familial tremor, the tremor is not a severe enough handicap to require treatment during childhood and adolescence. Propranolol, a nonselective β-adrenoreceptor antagonist, relieves familial tremor. It also has been used to treat shuddering attacks (130). For adults, dosages range from 120 to 240 mg/day, given in three doses because the half-life of the drug is 23 hours (128). No correlation exists between plasma levels of propranolol and tremorolytic action (131). Small dosages of primidone (50 mg/day) are equally or even more effective (132). Stereotactic thalamotomy, which reduces the amplitude of the tremor, has been used for severely affected adult patients (133).

Restless Legs Syndrome

Restless legs syndrome is a common disorder. It affects between 2% and 5% of the population. It is characterized by a creeping-crawling or aching sense of discomfort in both legs that creates the need to move them. Symptoms are most common at night before going to sleep. In addition, brief involuntary flexion of the lower extremities can be noted during sleep. Occasionally, the movements also affect the upper extremities. In approximately one-third of patients, there is a family history exists, propose an autosomal dominant transmission. The cause for the movements is not clear. Trenkwalder and colleagues suggest the presence of brainstem disinhibition that activates a spinal generator for the involuntary limb movements (134). In the experience of Walters and colleagues, approximately 20% of adult patients with restless legs syndrome had an age of onset before 10 years. Diagnosis was usually not made at that time; rather, the condition was considered as growing pains or attention deficit/hyperactivity disorder (135). The diagnosis is best made by polysomnography or videotaping, which discloses the periodic limb movements during sleep. Treatment with clonazepam or levodopa has been quite effective.

Juvenile Parkinson's Disease

As is commonly defined, juvenile Parkinson's disease refers to a condition in which symptoms of Parkinson's disease make their appearance before age 20 years. This is in distinction to early-onset Parkinson's disease, a condition that becomes apparent between the ages of 20 and 40 years. Our concepts of juvenile Parkinson's disease have undergone marked changes. Although it had been known for many years that when Parkinson's disease develops during the first two decades of life, the familial occurrence can be as high as 40%, but the genetic transmission had not been clarified until recently.

The initial report of juvenile Parkinson's disease by Hunt in 1917 probably described four unrelated adolescent patients with dopa-responsive dystonia (136). Since then, genetic analysis has confirmed the clinical impression that juvenile Parkinson's disease is a heterogeneous condition, and an autosomal dominant and an autosomal recessive form have been delineated. One of the genes for the autosomal dominant form has been mapped to chromosome 4q21-23

(137). This gene encodes α-synuclein, a neuron-specific presynaptic membrane protein, which is a component of Lewy bodies, the fibrous cytoplasmic inclusions seen in dopaminergic neurons of the substantia nigra in adult-onset Parkinson's disease (138). To date, two mutations in the gene for synuclein have been described (139). In addition, a second locus for autosomal dominant early-onset Parkinson's disease has been mapped to chromosome 2p13 (139a). The gene for the autosomal recessive form of juvenile Parkinson's disease has been mapped to chromosome 6q15.2-27 and has been cloned (140). It encodes a protein, named *parkin*, which is abundant in all parts of the brain, including the substantia nigra (141). A variety of mutations in the gene lead to a clinical picture of juvenile Parkinson's disease (141a). Kitada and coworkers have proposed that the defect in the expression of parkin interferes with the ubiquitin-mediated proteolytic pathway (141). The protein is related to the ubiquitin family of proteinases, which are a component of the filaments seen in Alzheimer disease, the Lewy bodies of adult Parkinson's disease, and the neuronal intranuclear inclusions seen in Huntington disease (25,141). Kitada and coworkers have proposed that the defect in the expression of parkin interferes with the ubiquitin-mediated proteolytic pathway (141). A variety of mutations in the gene, including deletions and point mutations, can lead to clinical picture of juvenile Parkinson's disease (141a,141b).

The clinical picture of both forms of juvenile Parkinson's disease is similar. However, the autosomal recessive form is encountered frequently in Japan (142). Symptoms appear as early as the second half of the first decade of life. Initial signs are a gait disturbance with retropulsion, a fine tremor, hyperreflexia, and dystonic posturing of the foot. Parkinsonian symptoms improve with sleep. Good response occurs with levodopa, although dopa-induced dyskinesia can appear within a few months of starting the medication. No intellectual deterioration occurs. MRI study results are normal (142). Neuropathologic studies show neuronal loss and gliosis in the pars compacta of the substantia nigra. In the median portion of the sub-

stantia nigra and in the locus ceruleus, neuronal loss and poor melanization of the nigral neurons occur. No Lewy bodies are detectable in either the autosomal recessive or the autosomal dominant forms (143,144).

Juvenile Parkinson's disease should be distinguished from Wilson disease, dopa-responsive dystonia, and olivopontocerebellar atrophy or other system degenerations presenting with parkinsonian symptoms. We have encountered identical twins with a clinical picture of the dystonic, dopa-responsive form of juvenile Parkinson's disease who were found to have neuronal intranuclear inclusion disease (145). Another condition to be considered is rapid-onset dystonia-parkinsonism, which can have its onset as early as the second decade of life (146).

Gilles de la Tourette Syndrome

Gilles de la Tourette syndrome, which straddles the fields of neurology and psychiatry, was first described in 1885 by Georges Gilles de la Tourette (147). It is characterized by multiple, uncontrollable muscular and vocal tics and in the classic cases, obscene utterances. Although, in the past, the condition was considered to be rare and caused by emotional and psychiatric factors, it is now clear that it represents a continuum of mild and transient tics at one end and the complete Tourette syndrome (TS) at the other.

Pathogenesis and Pathology

The pathogenesis of TS is still unknown. Although the current working hypothesis proposes an autosomal dominant transmission of the disease, no genetic linkage has been found. Specifically, no confirmed linkage exists to the various dopamine receptor genes or to the dopamine transporter gene. Failure to confirm the linkage could reflect diagnostic uncertainties, including an unclear definition of TS, the variable clinical expression of the disorder, and genetic heterogeneity. Walkup and coworkers have suggested that the susceptibility for TS is inherited by a major locus in combination with a multifactorial background (148). Because cases of secondary TS, such as after carbon monoxide poisoning, have shown lesions in the basal ganglia (149), a disorder in the circuitry of the basal ganglia has been postulated. Neuropathologic studies, however, have failed to find any consistent structural alterations in this region. The observation that children with TS have significantly increased anti-neuronal antibodies against human putamen points to an autoimmune mechanism. A number of studies have suggested a relationship between a prior streptococcal infection and various movement disorders aside from Sydenham chorea, but such a link has not yet been proven for TS (149a). This topic is covered more fully in Chapter 7 in the section on PANDAS.

The going hypothesis is that TS represents a supersensitivity of central dopamine receptors. However, observations of a disorder of the dopamine receptor system have neither been confirmed nor rejected by PET or functional imaging techniques (150). Abnormalities in neurotransmitter metabolism, a reduction in cyclic AMP, or a reduction in dynorphinlike immunoreactivity throughout the brain still requires confirmation (151,152). Volumetric MRI suggests that the left-sided predominance of the putamen visualized in healthy right-handed boys is absent in TS, and that a tendency to right-sided predominance exists (153).

Clinical Manifestations

A variety of estimates have been presented for the prevalence of TS in the United States. These range from 5 in 10,000, as determined in North Dakota children (154), to 2.5%. Boys are affected more frequently than girls by a ratio of between 3:1 and 5:1. The syndrome is rare in blacks; in Cleveland, 97% of TS patients were white (155). In approximately 33%, the condition is familial, and relatives can have multiple tics, an obsessive-compulsive disorder, or the complete TS (156,157).

Symptoms generally appear between ages 5 and 10 years. Although periods of remission occur, the condition usually persists for life. The initial clinical picture is usually one of multifocal tics affecting the face and head. These progress to vocal tics, such as grunting, coughing, sneezing, and barking, and, in the most severe cases, to coprolalia or compulsive echolalia. Tics can be voluntarily suppressed for variable periods, but an accompanying increase in internal tension ultimately results in a symptomatic discharge. Compulsive self-mutilation has been noted in a significant number. In patients in the Cleveland series, an attention deficit disorder was documented in 35%, learning disabilities in another 22%, and serious psychiatric disorders in 9% (155). Coprolalia was encountered in only 8%, an indication that even mild cases of the syndrome are currently coming to physicians' attention. As observed in the genetic studies, obsessive-compulsive traits also are characteristic; they tend to occur more frequently in girls (157).

Clinical findings suggest that brain function is abnormal in a high proportion of these children. On neurologic examination, a large number of patients exhibit "soft" signs. Approximately 15% of cases are precipitated by stimulant medications, such as methylphenidate hydrochloride (Ritalin), pemoline (Cylert), and dextroamphetamine sulfate (Dexedrine) (158).

The electroencephalogram results have been reported to be abnormal in as many as 55% of affected patients, sometimes even revealing frank paroxysmal discharges. Sleep is disturbed. The amount of stages 3 and 4 sleep is increased, the number of awakenings is increased, and the amount of rapid eye movement sleep is decreased. Sleep electroencephalography (EEG) show high-voltage slow waves with awakening and immature arousal pattern (159).

Dopamine receptor antagonists are generally the most reliable drugs for the treatment of TS. Most clinicians favor haloperidol or pimozide. Haloperidol (1.5 to 2.0 mg/day) improves symptoms in up to 80% of affected children, although side effects prevent the drug from being used for long-term therapy in more than one-third (160). Pimozide appears to be at least as effective as haloperidol, producing significant improvement in 70% of patients with fewer side effects (161). As recommended by Shapiro and coworkers, the starting dose for children is 1 mg, given at bedtime, with the dosage being increased 1 mg every 5 to 7 days until at least a 70% reduction of symptoms occurs, or until adverse side effects appear (161). Regeur and coworkers have used a dosage range of 0.5 to 9.0 mg/day (162). Other drugs that have been useful in the treatment of TS include tetrabenazine (85), clonidine, and fluphenazine.

Side effects are similar for all drugs but are least common with pimozide. Acute dystonia is seen in some 5% to 9% of patients receiving pimozide; akathisia is seen in some 25%, but usually disappears within the first 3 months of therapy. Tardive dyskinesia is seen with haloperidol and pimozide; it is more common with haloperidol (163). Other side effects include weight gain and gynecomastia, and, rarely, nonspecific alterations of the electrocardiogram results. Although several authorities have recommended clonidine hydrochloride, an α_2-adrenergic agonist, in dosages ranging from 0.05 to 0.9 mg/day (160), Goetz and coworkers found the drug to be ineffective in dosages ranging from 7.5 to 15.0 µg/kg per day (164). Leckman, however, has found that clonidine might not become effective until it has been given for some 3 months. He also noted that even after brief discontinuation, its reinstitution does not result in an improvement until after 2 weeks to 4 months (165).

TS lasts lifelong but tends to become less severe after adolescence. Although in one-fourth of patients symptoms can remit for as long as several years, only 8% of children have complete and permanent remission (161).

The treatment of the youngster with TS accompanied by an attention deficit disorder is difficult. Psychostimulant drugs increase the frequency of tics in 20% to 50% of children with TS, whereas haloperidol and pimozide can aggravate the attention deficit disorder (155).

PAROXYSMAL DYSKINESIAS

The first entity of this rare set of disorders which straddle the boundary between seizures and basal ganglia diseases was described by Mount and Reback in 1940 (166). In its classic form, it is characterized by paroxysmal attacks of choreiform, athetoid, dystonic, or tonic movements lasting from a few seconds to several minutes. Consciousness remains unimpaired. Goodenough and coworkers (167) classified the reported cases into familial and acquired (sporadic), with the majority falling into the latter group (168).

Lance distinguished two types of familial dyskinesias (169). In one group, termed *kinesigenic paroxysmal dyskinesias*, attacks are regularly precipitated by movement, especially movement occurring after prolonged immobility. Paroxysms begin almost always in childhood, usually between ages 6 and 16 years. The movements most often resemble dystonia, although some patients can exhibit a choreiform or even a ballistic component (170). Only rarely does significant family history of similar attacks exist (170). Attacks usually last less than 5 minutes. In the familial cases, the condition appears to be transmitted as an autosomal dominant trait. Attacks respond promptly to anticonvulsants, notably carbamazepine or phenytoin (170). Curiously, blood levels required to control attacks (4 to 5 µg/mL) are well below the range considered to be therapeutic for seizure disorders (171).

In the nonkinesigenic cases, attacks arise spontaneously or are triggered by fatigue. They first appear before 5 years of age, and most often take the form of dystonia, although a mixed movement disorder also can be seen (170). The family history is consistent with an autosomal dominant transmission, and the gene has been mapped to chromosome 2q34 (172). In the experience of Demirkiran and Jankovic, attacks usually last longer than 5 minutes in 65% of instances, but the duration of attacks cannot be used to classify the various paroxysmal dyskinesias (170). The response to anticonvulsants is not as good as in the kinesigenic cases. Between attacks, the child is usually in excellent health, although some children have shown mild choreiform movements or a seizure disorder (173,174). Another autosomal dominant nonkinesigenic dyskinesia has been mapped to the short arm of chromosome 1 (175). In this condition, a spastic paraplegia occurs during and between episodes of dyskinesia. Less often one encounters exertion-induced dyskinesias or sleep-induced dyskinesias (170).

Acquired paroxysmal dyskinesias are often seen in children who had previously experienced perinatal asphyxia or other static encephalopathies, as well as in patients with reflex epilepsy and metabolic disorders, notably idiopathic hyperparathyroidism. The condition also is seen in multiple sclerosis. In some cases of acquired paroxysmal dyskinesia, attacks have responded to diphenhydramine (174). Other patients respond to clonazepam or acetazolamide. Bressman and coworkers distinguish a psychogenic form of paroxysmal dystonia. Patients belonging to this group respond to placebo, hypnotherapy, or faith healing (168).

A transient form of dystonia arising during infancy is marked by periods of opisthotonos and dystonic posturing of the upper limbs, occurring during the waking state and generally lasting no more than a few minutes. The attacks resolve within a few months. No family history exists, and this entity is distinct from Sandifer syndrome, which accompanies hiatus hernia (see Chapter 5), and from paroxysmal torticollis, a precursor to migraine (176).

The essence of the paroxysmal dyskinesias is unknown. Stevens (177) and Homan and associates (171) postulated that they represent a convulsive disorder akin to the reflex epilepsies. During an attack, however, the EEG does not disclose any paroxysmal features and differs little from the interictal tracing. Most likely, in analogy with paroxysmal ataxia, a condition covered in the subsequent section, the paroxysmal dyskinesias will turn out to represent different types of channelopathies.

Familial startle disease or hyperexplexia is characterized by transient, generalized rigidity in response to unexpected loud noises or sudden tactile stimulation. A large number of subjects exhibit severe muscle stiffness at birth (*stiff baby syndrome*) (178). This is diagnosed frequently as spastic quadriparesis. Attacks of hypertonicity may result in apnea. Muscle tone returns to normal in early childhood, but patients continue to have sudden falls in response to startle, and they can suppress the startle reaction if they are able to anticipate the stimuli (179). The "Jumping Frenchmen of Maine" probably represent an extensive family with such a condition (180). The EEG and electromyography (EMG) results are generally normal. It has been suggested that the condition is related to cortical and reticular reflex

myoclonus (181). The condition can appear sporadically, or is transmitted as an autosomal dominant disorder with the gene localized to the long arm of chromosome 5 (5q33-q35) (182). As a consequence of a variety of mutations, there is a defect in the α-1 subunit of the inhibitory glycine receptor (183). Recessive cases differing in their mutations of the α-1 subunit of the glycine receptor and compound heterozygotes have also been described (183a). Symptoms improve markedly with administration of clonazepam or valproate.

Another rare entity that borders between seizures and movement disorders is one of hereditary chin trembling, which can be associated with nocturnal myoclonus (184). The condition responds to administration of botulinum toxin (185).

HEREDODEGENERATIVE DISEASES OF THE CEREBELLUM, BRAINSTEM, AND SPINAL CORD

Heredodegenerative diseases of the cerebellum, brainstem, and spinal cord involve a slow, progressive deterioration of one or more of the functions subserved by the cerebellum, brainstem, or spinal cord. This deterioration is caused by neuronal atrophy within the affected tract or tracts, commencing at the axonal periphery and advancing in a centripetal manner. Familial distribution is the usual pattern. In the past, classification of these disorders being based on clinical and pathologic data called forth numerous debates, which are now being resolved with the increasing availability of genetic data. Two groups can be distinguished: the autosomal recessive ataxias and the autosomal dominant ataxias. In this chapter, emphasis is placed on those conditions that are more prevalent during childhood and adolescence.

Friedreich Ataxia

Friedreich ataxia (FRDA) was first distinguished from syphilitic locomotor ataxia by Friedreich in 1863, who reported all the essential clinical and pathologic features of the condition (186). Characterized by ataxia, nystagmus, kyphoscoliosis, and pes cavus, it occurs throughout the world as an autosomal recessive trait.

Molecular Genetics, Pathology, and Pathogenesis

The gene for FRDA has been mapped to chromosome 9q13. It has been cloned and codes for a protein termed *frataxin* (187). Some 94% of FRDA patients are homozygous for an expanded GAA repeat in an intron of the gene. The remaining subjects, some 4%, are compound heterozygotes with an expanded repeat on one allele and a point mutation or deletion on the other (187). Compound heterozygotes have a somewhat earlier onset of symptoms and are more likely to show optic atrophy (187a). The number of GAA repeats ranges from 6 to 29 in healthy individuals and from 120 to 1,700 in FRDA patients, with the size of the expanded repeat correlating with age of onset and disease severity (188,189). The expression of frataxin is markedly reduced in FRDA, and the pattern of frataxin expression in normal tissues approximates the sites of pathologic changes in the disease (187). How reduced frataxin expression results in the disease process is still not quite clear. Frataxin is localized to mitochondria, and its reduced expression results in reduced activity of complexes I, II, and III of the mitochondrial respiratory chain (190). Impaired mitochondrial function is probably the result of iron overload in mitochondria and tissue damage from free radical toxicity (191,191a). Thus, FRDA is one of many mitochondrial diseases resulting from a mutation of the nuclear genome. How the GAA triplet-repeat expansion results in a reduced expression of frataxin in mitochondria is not clear. The most likely possibility is that the unusual DNA structure interferes with transcription (192). Interestingly, the previously reported abnormalities in the pyruvate dehydrogenase complex and in the activity of the mitochondrial malic enzyme can now be explained (193).

The essential pathologic process in FRDA, as well as in the other cerebellar degenerations, is a dying back of neurons in certain systems from the periphery to the center with eventual disappearance of the cell body (194). The principal lesions are found in the long ascending and descending tracts of the spinal cord (Fig. 2.4). The peripheral nerves also can be affected, as

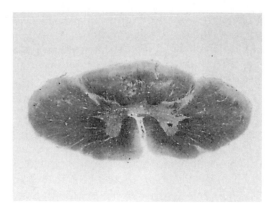

FIG. 2.4. Friedreich ataxia. Section of spinal cord stained for myelin. The area of myelination involves the posterior columns and the lateral and ventral spinocerebellar tracts. The corticospinal tracts are relatively spared, although demyelination is more extensive than would be expected from the clinical picture at the time of demise. (Courtesy of Dr. K. E. Earle, Armed Forces Institute of Pathology, Washington, DC.)

well as can the brainstem and, less often, the cerebellum. All these areas show axonal degeneration, demyelination, and a compensatory gliosis. Degenerative cellular changes are most striking in Clarke column and the dentate nucleus. They occur to a lesser extent in a variety of other nuclei of the lower brainstem and in the Purkinje cells. Cell loss and gliosis also are seen in the vestibular and auditory systems (195). Other areas of gray matter are usually unaffected. A reduction in glycolytic enzymes and an increase in oxidative and hydrolytic enzymes have been found on histochemical examination of the posterior columns of the spinal cord. Aside from the expected loss of proteolipid that accompanies demyelination, no lipid abnormalities have been documented in affected tracts (196).

Abnormalities of the viscera are limited to the heart. These are cardiomegaly, with myocytic hypertrophy and chronic interstitial fibrosis, and an inflammatory infiltrate (197).

Clinical Manifestations

Friedreich ataxia is not a common condition. The prevalence in Great Britain is approxi-

TABLE 2.4. *Frequency of neurologic symptoms in 72 patients with Friedreich ataxia*

Symptom	Percent incidence
Truncal ataxia	100
Dysarthria	82
Nystagmus	33
Dysmetria of upper extremities	89
Decreased vibration sense in lower extremities	72
Areflexia of lower extremities	100
Weakness of lower extremities	69
Atrophy of lower extremities	46
Extensor plantar reflex	83
Pes cavus	83
Scoliosis	78
Diabetes	15
Abnormal electrocardiographic results	79

Data from Klockgether T, Evert B. Genes involved in hereditary ataxias. *Trends Neurosci* 1998;21: 413–418. With permission.

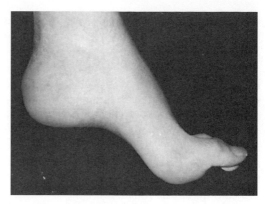

FIG. 2.5. Typical pes cavus foot deformity seen in Friedreich ataxia. The patient is a 12-year-old girl.

mately 1 in 48,000 (197). In western Norway, it is 1 in 100,000. Although considerable variability occurs in age of onset, in most families the disease begins at the same period of time in each affected individual. The first symptoms can be seen as early as age 2 years, and the mean age of onset is 10 years of age (198). The clinical manifestations are outlined in Table 2.4 (199). Children can be slow in learning to walk or can begin to stumble frequently. Less commonly, abnormal speech or incoordination of hand movements is the initial complaint.

Neurologic symptoms advance relentlessly. Although the disease evolves rapidly in a few children, progression is slow in the vast majority, and, occasionally, long static periods occur. Intercurrent infections frequently aggravate existing symptoms and bring new ones to light. The patient with fully developed FRDA has an immature, dysmorphic appearance with a number of skeletal deformities, some of which can exist from birth. In approximately three-fourths of the patients, the feet have a high arch (pes cavus), hammer toes, and wasting of the small muscles of the sole (Fig. 2.5). This abnormality, present at birth, might for many years represent the only sign of FRDA. Kyphoscoliosis is present in 75% to 90% of subjects (197,199).

The most prominent sign, however, is ataxia. As might be expected from the pathologic lesions, ataxia is caused by a combination of cerebellar asynergia and loss of posterior column sensation. Ataxia is usually more marked in the legs than in the arms and is most evident when the child's gait or station is examined. Speech is invariably involved and acquires a staccato or explosive character, which is the result of an incoordination of respiration and phonation. Nystagmus is seen in 20% to 40% of cases (197–199). It is usually bilateral and is present only on lateral movements of the eyes. Additionally, one frequently observes broken up, jerky pursuit movements. Nystagmus on upward gaze is rare as is optic atrophy (194). Optic atrophy can be congenital or can have its onset during early infancy, progressing rapidly after its inception.

Carroll found color vision to be impaired in 40% of patients and abnormalities in the visual-evoked potentials were seen in two-thirds of the patients (200). The two principal abnormalities were a generalized reduction in amplitude of the potentials and a prolongation in their latency. The reduction in amplitude is probably the consequence of a loss of functional fibers in the visual pathway. Electroretinogram results are usually normal. Vestibular involvement, including loss of caloric reactions and attacks of vertigo, was already described by Friedreich (186). Attacks of vertigo often appear early and ultimately are seen in approximately 50% of the patients. Deafness is also common, caused by degeneration of the cochlear neurons (195,201).

Weakness of the distal musculature of the lower limbs and wasting of the small muscles of the hands and feet are common and are out of proportion to the degree of disuse. A loss of vibratory and proprioceptive sensation occurs, and in the advanced cases, the other sensory modalities also are likely to be affected, notably in the distal portions of the extremities (194,197). Pains, cramps, and paresthesias are common.

In the experience of Harding, deep tendon reflexes were absent in 74% of patients, with the patellar reflex being lost in 99%. An extensor plantar response could be elicited in 89% (197,198).

MRI studies can show enlargement of the fourth ventricle and atrophy of the superior vermis, brainstem, and spinal cord (199). The somatosensory-evoked potentials recorded over the clavicles are abnormal even in the earliest stages of the disease (202). They are unaccompanied, however, by a delay in peripheral nerve conduction. Sphincter disturbance is rare except for occasional urgency of micturition (197). Neither mental retardation nor dementia was encountered in Harding large series (197,198). Electrocardiographic and echocardiographic evidence of myocarditis has been found in 80% to 90% of patients (199). T-wave abnormalities and congenital heart block are particularly common (203). Echocardiographic abnormalities are seen early; most commonly interventricular septal hypertrophy is seen (197). An unusually high incidence of diabetes and abnormal glucose tolerance has been recorded (198,199).

The patient with an advanced case of FRDA is bedridden with dysphagia and other bulbar signs. Death is caused by inanition, or, more commonly, by myocarditis with intractable congestive failure.

Heterozygotes for FRDA are neurologically normal. According to Harding, they demonstrate neither pes cavus nor scoliosis (197).

When patients with clinically typical FRDA are examined for GAA trinucleotide expansion, a small proportion with a typical phenotype does not show an expanded allele. It is possible that these subjects have point mutations or deletions in the gene for FRDA on both chromosomes (204), or have a genetically different disease with an FRDA phenotype. Conversely, triplet expansions have been seen in a number of subjects with atypical ataxia and in patients presenting with generalized chorea (205).

Diagnosis

In the typical patient, the clinical diagnosis is suggested by the presence of childhood-onset progressive ataxia, skeletal deformities, an abnormal visual-evoked potential, and an abnormal echocardiogram result. The diagnosis is established by determination of the size of GAA repeats, which can now be performed commercially. Ataxia-telangiectasia (see Chapter 11) is the second most common cause of childhood-onset progressive ataxia. It is distinguished clinically by cutaneous telangiectases, a history of frequent serious respiratory infections, absent or marked reduction of IgA globulins, an elevated α-fetoprotein, and a lack of skeletal deformities and sensory signs.

Harding described an autosomal recessive form of cerebellar ataxia in which deep tendon reflexes are preserved and in which optic atrophy, diabetes, and cardiac abnormalities cannot be demonstrated (197). Symptoms appear between 18 months and 20 years of age, and the progression of the illness is slower than in the classic form of FRDA. Approximately one-half of patients with this clinical picture harbor the GAA repeat expansion (206).

An infantile-onset spinocerebellar ataxia (SCA) is seen not infrequently in Finland and is probably identical with an entity termed *Behr disease*. Symptoms develop during the second year of life and are highlighted by cerebellar ataxia, a peripheral sensory neuropathy, deafness, optic atrophy, athetosis, and seizures. Hypogonadism can be documented in female patients (207,208). The gene for this condition, now termed *SCA 8*, has been mapped to chromosome 10q24 (208a). An untranslated CTG expansion appears to be responsible for the disease (208b) (Table 2.5).

An adult-onset SCA caused by a mutation of the α-tocopherol transfer protein has a clinical picture that resembles FRDA (209). Several other conditions are even rarer. These include an entity characterized by cerebellar ataxia, mental deficiency, congenital cataracts, impaired physical growth, and various skeletal anomalies. It was first described by Marinesco and Sjögren, Garland, and others (210,211). The brain shows marked cerebellar atrophy, especially affecting the vermis, with almost complete loss of Purkinje and granule cells and with gliosis of the dentate nucleus. The presence of a myopathy is suggested by EMG, and by the presence of fiber-type disproportion, fibrosis, and lipid deposition on biopsy (211). Electron microscopic studies on sural nerve biopsies demonstrate numerous abnormally enlarged lysosomes. Lysosomal enzyme study results, however, have been normal.

Several recessively inherited ataxias have been described in isolated enclaves, such as the Amish communities in the United States and the French Canadian community of Quebec (Troyer syndrome, Charlevoix-Saguenay syndrome) (212,213). These probably represent complicated forms of hereditary spastic paraplegia (197). A childhood-onset, recessive condition, marked by posterior column ataxia and retinitis pigmentosa has been mapped to the long arm of chromosome 1 (1q31-q32) (197a). Subjects have no clinical or neuroimaging evidence of cerebellar involvement; rather they show increased signals in the dorsal aspect of the spinal cord (197b).

Treatment

Children with SCA should remain active for as long as possible and participate in physical therapy and programmed remedial exercises. These should focus on balance training and muscle strengthening. In my experience, the cardiomyopathy has not interfered with such an exercise program. Orthopedic surgery for skeletal deformities, particularly progressive scoliosis, which is a major cause for morbidity, might be necessary if bracing does not arrest the progression of the scoliosis (214). No drug therapy has yet been found to be effective. However, in the experience of the University of California Los Angeles Ataxia Clinic, patients feel better when their carbohydrate intake is restricted. Children with FRDA should be seen by cardiologists and orthopedic surgeons at regular intervals (once or twice a year). With good supportive care, patients can expect to live into their 40s or 50s.

Spinocerebellar Ataxias (Olivopontocerebellar Atrophies)

The SCAs represent several genetically distinct autosomal dominant conditions, some of which were in the past designated as olivopontocerebellar atrophies and whose prototypes were first described by Menzel in 1890, by Déjérine and Thomas in 1900, and by Holmes in 1907 (215–217). Clinically, they manifest by progressive cerebellar ataxia, tremor, speech impairment, and, in some instances, marked extrapyramidal signs, cranial nerve palsies, and peripheral neuropathy. On the basis of molecular genetics, these conditions have been divided into

TABLE 2.5. *Molecular genetics of the autosomal dominant ataxias*

Disease	Chromosome	Mutation	Gene product	Reference
SCA1	6p	CAG repeat	Ataxin 1	Orr et al. (219)
SCA2	12q	CAG repeat	Ataxin 2	Pulst et al. (220)
SCA3	14q	CAG repeat	Ataxin 3	Kawaguchi et al. (221)
SCA4	16q	?	?	Flanigan et al. (222)
SCA5	11cen	?	?	Ranum et al. (223)
SCA6	19p	CAG repeat	α_{1A} Voltage-dependent calcium channel subunit	Zhuchenko et al. (224)
SCA7	3p12-13	CAG repeat	Ataxin 7	Benton et al. (225)
SCA8[a]	13q21	CTG expansion in untranslated region	—	Koob et al. (208b)
SCA9[b]	—	—	—	
SCA10	22q	—	—	Grewal et al. (232), Zu et al. (232a)

CAG, ctyosine-adenosine-guanine; CTG, cytosine-thymine-guanine; SCA, spinocerebellar ataxia.
[a]In the past, the designation of SCA8 had been reserved for an autosomal recessive disorder whose gene is on 10q24 (207). This disorder has now been reclassified as infantile onset spinocerebellar ataxia.
[b]This designation has been reserved.

10 types (191,218) (see Table 2.5). Approximately one-third of cases do not correspond to any of the mapped conditions, so that, over time, further genetic subtypes will undoubtedly be delineated.

SCA1, SCA2, SCA3, SCA6, and SCA7 are caused by the inheritance of an expansion of CAG repeats coding for an extended polyglutamine tract. Although the mean age of onset of these disorders is during the fourth decade of life, the conditions have been encountered in children. The length of the expanded repeat tends to increase from generation to generation, and an inverse correlation exists between the size of the repeat and the age when symptoms become apparent. As a result, a progressively earlier onset of symptoms occurs in successive generations, a phenomenon termed *anticipation* (218).

In the series of Benton and colleagues, some 6% of families with autosomal SCA have a defect in SCA1 (225). SCA1 codes for a protein, termed *ataxin 1*. It is found ubiquitously and is a nuclear protein in all cells with the exception of the cerebellar Purkinje cells where it is cytoplasmic as well as nuclear. As is the case for HD, the extended polyglutamine tract is believed to induce neuronal degeneration in an as yet undefined manner. In the series of Pandolfo and Montermini, 16% of SCA1 subjects developed symptoms before 15 years of age (218). Expanded repeats tend to increase in length more with paternal than with maternal transmission; as a consequence, the majority of patients with juvenile onset are offspring of affected male subjects. Characteristic symptoms include ataxia, ophthalmoplegia, and pyramidal and extrapyramidal signs. Neuropathologically, patients with SCA1 show gross atrophy of the cerebellum, cerebellar peduncles, and basis ponti. The Purkinje cells appear most affected. A marked reduction in the number of granule cells and neuronal loss in the dentate nucleus are seen. Pathologic changes can involve the basal ganglia, spinal cord, retina, and peripheral nervous system.

SCA2 is a phenotypically similar disease. The gene for the disease has been identified. It codes for a highly basic protein, ataxin 2, having no similarity with any other proteins. Ataxin 2 is found in all parts of the brain, but an ataxin 2–binding protein is predominantly expressed in the cerebellum

(224a). In the series of Benton and colleagues, SCA2 was encountered in 21% of families with autosomal dominant cerebellar ataxia (225). The onset of neurologic symptoms is before 10 years of age in some 3% of patients. In these children, the disease is nearly always paternally transmitted.

SCA3, also known as Machado-Joseph disease, is also phenotypically similar. In the series of Pandolfo and Montermini, the onset of neurologic symptoms was before 15 years of age in 7% of subjects (218). In Germany, this condition is the most common of the autosomal dominant cerebellar ataxias, being found in 42% of the families with autosomal dominant ataxia (226). In the series of Benton and colleagues, this condition was seen in only 8% of families (225).

SCA6 was seen in 11% of the families compiled by Benton and colleagues (225). It differs from the other autosomal dominant cerebellar ataxias in that the mutation affects a gene with a known function, the α_{1A} voltage-dependent calcium channel subunit CACNA1A, which has its strongest expression in Purkinje cells (191). Two other neurologic disorders are caused by mutations in the same gene: hereditary paroxysmal (episodic) ataxia (EA2), considered in another part of this section, and familial hemiplegic migraine, considered in Chapter 13. SCA6 is a slowly progressive disorder and does not develop during childhood (227). MRI shows little more than cerebellar and brainstem atrophy.

SCA7 is clinically distinct in that ataxia is almost always associated with early retinal degeneration (225,228). The condition can manifest as early as the first year of life, usually with ataxia and progressive vision loss (225,229). SCA7 appears to be phenotypically similar but genetically distinct from hereditary dentatorubral-pallidoluysian atrophy (Haw River syndrome). The latter entity has a predilection to Japanese families and results from a CAG trinucleotide expansion on chromosome 12p 13.1-p12.3 (230). The clinical picture of dentatorubral-pallidoluysian atrophy varies even within the same family. It may present with learning disabilities, followed by progressive cerebellar signs, choreoathetosis, myoclonus, and dementia. As implied by the name, degenerative changes are seen in the globus pallidus, dentate and red nuclei, and Purkinje cells (231).

Several families with autosomal dominant cerebellar ataxia cannot be documented to have any of the known SCA mutations (232). These made up 43% of families in the series of Benton and colleagues (225).

The diagnosis of autosomal dominant cerebellar ataxia is based on the underlying genetic mutation. Molecular genetic analyses for SCA1, SCA2, SCA3, and SCA6 can now be performed commercially.

Rare forms of familial cerebellar degenerations starting in infancy or childhood were described by Norman (233) Frontali (233a), and Jervis (234). In these entities, cerebellar ataxia, hypotonia, nystagmus, and mental deficiency were evident during infancy. These entities probably represent SCA7.

In the child who presents with progressive ataxia, the differential diagnosis depends on the rapidity with which the symptoms have appeared. When they are of short duration, ataxia is most likely to be neoplastic, toxic, or infectious. If the ataxia is slowly progressive, posterior fossa tumors must be excluded. Structural anomalies of the upper cervical spine and foramen magnum (e.g., platybasia) can present with ataxia, as does hydrocephalus caused by partial obstruction at the aqueduct of Sylvius (see Chapter 4). The lipidoses, particularly the group of late infantile amaurotic idiocies, also can present a primarily cerebellar picture (see Chapter 1).

Of the familial cerebellar degenerations presenting during childhood, ataxia-telangiectasia and FRDA are the most common. Several conditions, collectively termed *Ramsay Hunt syndrome*, present with progressive cerebellar ataxia, myoclonus, and seizures. Refsum disease is characterized by cerebellar ataxia, deafness, retinitis pigmentosa, and polyneuritis. It is produced by a defect in the oxidation of branched chain fatty acids (see Chapter 1). Sporadic cerebellar degenerations of childhood also can be caused by toxins such as lead or organic mercury compounds (see Chapter 9).

Familial Episodic (Paroxysmal) Ataxia

Two distinct forms of familial episodic (paroxysmal) ataxia have been recognized. Episodic ataxia 1 is characterized by brief bouts of ataxia or dysarthria lasting seconds to minutes, with interictal myokymia, usually involving the muscles about the eyes and the hands. Attacks are usually triggered by startle or exercise (235). In some families, acetazolamide is of marked benefit, in others anticonvulsants are helpful. Other findings are joint contractures and paroxysmal choreoathetosis. No progressive cerebellar degeneration occurs. This condition is linked to chromosome 12p and is the consequence of a mutation in the gene that codes for a brain potassium channel (KCNA1) (236).

A second form of episodic ataxia (episodic ataxia 2) is marked by attacks that last for up to several days. Attacks are triggered by emotional upset or physical exertion. The condition can have its onset as early as 3 years of age (237). In some patients, migrainelike headaches, vertigo, and nausea accompany the attacks, a clinical picture that suggests a diagnosis of basilar migraine (see Chapter 13). Interictal downbeat and rebound nystagmus is common. Progressive cerebellar ataxia can be present in some. The gene for episodic ataxia 2 has been mapped to chromosome 19p, and, like SCA6, codes for the α_{1A} voltage-dependent calcium channel subunit CACNA1A (238). The same gene also is affected in familial hemiplegic migraine. (See Chapter 13.)

Ramsay Hunt Syndrome (Dentatorubral Atrophy)

Ramsay Hunt syndrome (dentatorubral atrophy), a rare disorder, was first described by J. Ramsay Hunt in 1921 in a family with myoclonus epilepsy and cerebellar ataxia (239). Autopsy showed well-marked degeneration of the spinocerebellar tracts, atrophy of the dentate nucleus, and pallor of the superior cerebellar peduncle, including the dentatorubral tract.

As it has been redefined, Ramsay Hunt syndrome represents a recessively inherited degenerative disease marked by tonic-clonic or clonic seizures, intention myoclonus, myoclonic jerks, and cerebellar dysfunction. Onset is during the first or second decade of life. Mental deterioration is absent or minimal. The waking EEG result is normal or has a slightly slowed background with brief bursts of fast generalized spike-wave discharges (240,241). Because many families with this condition originate from countries around the Mediterranean Sea, Genton and coworkers have proposed the name *Mediterranean myoclonus* (240). Ramsay Hunt syndrome is distinct from Unverricht disease, also termed *Baltic myoclonus*, and Lafora disease, two conditions marked by myoclonic seizures and mental deterioration (see Chapter 1). Myoclonic seizures, ataxia, and mental deterioration also are seen in mitochondrial encephalopathy, sialidosis, the lipidoses, particularly in the late infantile neuronal ceroid lipofuscinoses, the juvenile form of HD, and cerebral anoxia resulting from transient cardiac arrest.

Although no treatment completely reverses the neurologic symptoms, I, as well as Genton and coworkers, have found valproic acid or clonazepam to be of considerable benefit.

Familial Spastic Paraplegia

Characterized by progressive spastic paraplegia, and first described by Seeligmüller in 1876 (242), familial spastic paraplegia (FSP) appears to be the most common system degeneration of childhood, with CMT disease and FRDA being far less common (243). The condition exhibits a variable mode of inheritance: In some families it is transmitted in a dominant manner; less often,

it is transmitted in an X-linked or in an autosomal recessive manner. In addition, Harding has further subdivided this condition into *pure* and *complicated* forms (197). Several gene loci responsible for pure FSP have been found. These are outlined in Table 2.6. Linkage to chromosome 2p is the most common of these (250a).

Pathology

The major changes occur in the spinal cord. Axonal degeneration of the pyramidal tracts is always present and is maximal in the terminal portions. In affected tracts, the myelin sheath is lost and the axis cylinder disappears. Ascending tracts also can be involved, in particular the posterior columns, spinocerebellar fibers, and cells of the dorsal root ganglion, which can degenerate and show satellitosis (251,252). No signs of primary demyelination are seen. It is of note that in the autosomal recessive form linked to chromosome 16q24.3 (see Table 2.6), the gene defect involves a protein (paraplegin), a nuclear-encoded mitochondrial metalloprotease, and that muscle biopsy discloses ragged red fibers (249a).

Clinical Manifestations

The Hereditary Spastic Paraplegia Working Group found that families in which the disease is transmitted by an autosomal dominant gene far outnumber those in whom an autosomal recessive gene has been implicated (253). In nearly one-half of families, the gene has not been mapped. The clinical picture of the various genetic forms of FSP

TABLE 2.6. *Molecular genetics of the familial spastic paraplegias*

Disease	Chromosome	Mutation	Gene product	Reference
SPG1 (X-linked)	Xq28	—	L1 cell adhesion molecule	Jouet et al. (244)
SPG2 (X-linked)	Xq22	—	Myelin proteolipid gene	Saugier-Veber et al. (245)
SPG3 (dominant)	14q11.2-q24.3	—	—	Huang et al. (246)
SPG4 (dominant)	2p21-p24	CAG repeat expansion	—	Dürr et al. (247), Benson et al. (248)
SPG5A (recessive)	8p12-q13	—	—	Hentati et al. (249)
SPG5B (recessive)	16q24.3	Deletion	Paraplegin	Casari et al. (249a)
SPG6 (SPG4A) (dominant)	15q11.1	—	—	Dübe et al. (250)
Dominant	8q23-24	—	—	Hedera et al. (250a)
Recessive	2q24-25	—	—	McHale et al. (250b)

CAG, cytosine-adenine-guanine; SPG, spastic paraplegia.

appears to be unrelated to the gene defect. In all forms, a marked intrafamilial variability in age of onset exists, and even in genetically homogenous kindred, the distinction between early and late-onset FSP proposed by Harding (254) does not hold true (247). In the recessive variants of FSP, the average age at onset of symptoms is 11.5 years; in the dominant forms, it is 20 years (254). However, 40% of patients develop symptoms before 5 years of age (197,254). Children can be slow in learning to walk, and once they do walk, their gait is stiff and awkward, and the legs are scissored. Muscle tone is increased, the deep tendon reflexes are hyperactive, and the plantar responses are extensor. No muscular atrophy occurs, and, despite the pathologic involvement of the posterior columns, usually no impairment of position or vibratory sensation occurs. Bladder and bowel control is retained during the early stages of the illness. As a rule, the rate of progress of the illness is extremely slow; it is faster in children affected with the recessive forms. When children suffer from one or other of the dominant forms, the condition often remains static until they are in their 30s, and in the experience of Harding, only one patient became unable to walk before 50 years of age (197). The upper extremities often remain virtually unaffected until the terminal stage of the disease.

At least two forms of X-linked spastic paraplegia have been recognized. Like the dominant types of FSP, these have been divided into pure and complicated forms. One of the genes for the pure form has been localized to Xq28 (SPG1) (244) (see Table 2.6). The other gene is on Xq21 and codes for the PLP, which is defective in PMD. A point mutation in the PLP protein results in X-linked FSP (SPG2, (see Table 2.6), whereas a deletion in the gene results in PMD. This indicates that these two conditions are allelic disorders (245).

Harding distinguished the pure form of FSP from the complicated type, which is marked by a variety of associated neurologic features (197,254). The range of additional clinical features is enormous, and overlap exists between the various groups. Grouped together, the complicated forms of FSPs are at least as common than the *pure* form. Harding subdivided them into five groups (197). The most commonly encountered complicated forms comprise a combination of mild paraparesis with moderate to severe amyotrophy of the small hand muscles and the distal portion of the lower extremities. In other families, spastic paraplegia is associated with dementia, seizures, optic neuritis, movement disorders, cardiac abnormalities, and hypopigmentation of the skin. In several families, ataxia, nystagmus, and dysarthria accompany spastic paraplegia. This mixed picture has been termed *spastic ataxia.* These syndromes have been seen in Amish families (Troyer syndrome) and in French Canadian isolates (Charlevoix-Saguenay syndrome). Most of the cases are dominantly inherited, but autosomal recessive, and X-linked complicated FSP have been reported. To date, none of the genes for complicated FSP has been mapped (255).

Diagnosis

In the absence of a family history, the diagnosis of FSP is determined by exclusion. Motor and sensory nerve conduction times are normal, but somatosensory-evoked potentials are absent or reduced, not only in affected subjects but also in clinically healthy family members at risk for the disease. Progression of symptoms speaks against spastic diplegia of perinatal origin (see Chapter 5). Sensory deficits and sphincter disturbances, which usually accompany spinal cord tumors, are rarely seen in the early stages of FSP (254). Nevertheless, in the absence of a convincing family history, MRI studies of the spinal cord are required to exclude a spinal cord neoplasm. In rare instances, arginase deficiency can present as progressive spastic paraparesis (see Chapter 1).

Treatment

In view of the slow progression of symptoms, an active physiotherapy program should be designed. Orthopedic surgery, unless essential to relieve contractures, should be discouraged.

Fazio-Londe Disease

Fazio-Londe disease, a rare condition, also termed *progressive bulbar paralysis of childhood*, is probably heterogeneous and distinct from spinal muscular atrophy (Werdnig-Hoffmann disease) (see Chapter 14) and from amyotrophic lateral sclerosis, which is a sporadic degeneration of the anterior horn cells and pyramidal fibers occurring in adult life.

The clinical picture reflects a progressive deterioration of the anterior horn cells, particularly those of the bulbar musculature and pyramidal tracts. Symptoms begin at a variable age. In a family the author of this chapter has encountered, symptoms began during early childhood. They progress fairly rapidly and lead to death in approximately one decade (256).

McShane and colleagues distinguished two forms of progressive bulbar palsy presenting in the first two decades (257). In bulbar hereditary motor neuropathy I, bilateral nerve deafness is prominent and accompanies involvement of the motor components of the cranial nerves. This condition is inherited as an autosomal recessive disorder. Bulbar hereditary motor neuropathy II is usually recessive. In some patients, the degree of pyramidal tract involvement is minimal and can be limited to extensor plantar responses; the clinical picture is, therefore, essentially that of the late-onset form of Werdnig-Hoffmann disease. In other families, clinical or pathologic evidence of posterior column deficit relates this particular form of heredodegenerative disease to the spinocerebellar group (258). When anterior horn cell involvement is exclusively distal and is accompanied by significant spasticity and slow progression, the condition can be related to the complicated form of FSP (197). This variant can be transmitted rarely as a dominant trait.

In a few families, progressive degeneration of the anterior horn cells and pyramidal tracts appears after age 20 years. Those families include a large series of cases among the Chamorro tribe of Guam, in whom anterior horn cell degeneration is associated frequently with parkinsonism and dementia. This condition has been linked to a plant-excitant neurotoxin (see Chapter 9).

The diagnosis rests on the presence of a pure motor neuronopathy, with or without the presence of long tract signs. Tumors of the brainstem must be excluded. When pyramidal tract signs are not striking, myasthenia gravis or an ocular muscle dystrophy should be excluded.

Treatment

No treatment is available.

HEREDODEGENERATIVE DISEASES OF THE PERIPHERAL AND CRANIAL NERVES

In the past, heredodegenerative diseases of the peripheral and cranial nerves were grouped according to their clinical presentation and the histopathology and electrophysiology of the peripheral nerves. Advances in molecular biology have permitted a classification to be made in terms of genetic characteristics (259). The frequencies of the various hereditary peripheral neuropathies in a pediatric population are depicted in Table 2.6 (260) and their clinical characteristics in Table 2.7. An excellent monograph on this subject is provided by Ouvrier, McLeod, and Pollard (261).

TABLE 2.7. *Specific diagnostic entities in 103 children with peripheral neuropathies*

Conditions	Number of patients
HMSN	63
CMT 1 (HMSN 1)	31
Autosomal dominant (CMT 1A, B, C)	21
Sporadic or recessive (CMT 4A, B)	10
CMT 2 (HMSN 2)	32
Autosomal dominant (CMT 2A, B)	27
Parents unknown	4
Sporadic or recessive (CMT 2D)	1
Hereditary sensory neuropathies	3
Heredodegenerative CNS disorders with peripheral neuropathies	37
Spastic paraplegias	9
Heredoataxias	6
Friedreich ataxia	3
Abetalipoproteinemia	2
Lysosomal disorders	9
Globoid cell leukodystrophy (Krabbe disease)	5
Other neurometabolic disorders	7
Unknown or undiagnosed	6

CMT, Charcot-Marie-Tooth disease; CNS, central nervous system; HMSN, hereditary motor and sensory neuropathies.

Adapted from Hagberg B, Westerberg B. The nosology of genetic peripheral neuropathies in Swedish children. *Dev Med Child Neurol* 1983;25:3–18. With permission.

Charcot-Marie-Tooth Disease (Peroneal Muscular Atrophy, Hereditary Motor Sensory Neuropathy Type I)

Charcot-Marie-Tooth disease, also called peroneal muscular atrophy or HMSN type I and CMT 1, was described by Virchow in 1855 (262), by Charcot and Marie in France in 1886 (263), and by Tooth in England in 1886 (264), who considered it as a peroneal type of familial progressive muscular atrophy. Two major subdivisions of CMT disease, CMT 1 and CMT 2, are used. CMT 1 is characterized pathologically by extensive segmental demyelination and remyelination and by a consequential thickening of peripheral nerves to the point at which they become palpably enlarged (259). By contrast, in CMT 2, which is a far less common entity, no pathologic evidence exists for demyelination, rather axonal degeneration occurs. The pathologic features of demyelination and remyelination are shared by an entity formerly termed *Lévy-Roussy syndrome* (hereditary areflexic dystasia) and by most cases of Déjérine-Sottas syndrome (HMSN III).

CMT 1 is a relatively common condition and constitutes 51% of pooled pediatric cases of hereditary peripheral neuropathies (265). The prevalence of all forms of CMT 1 is 3.8 per 10,000 population, and they are transmitted as autosomal dominant disorders with a high degree of penetrance (266).

Pathology, Pathogenesis, and Molecular Genetics

Because only a few complete postmortem examinations are available, the changes within the CNS have not been well documented. Most commonly, the patient has degeneration of the posterior columns, loss of anterior horn cells, and degeneration of the spinocerebellar tracts and the anterior and posterior nerve roots (267). Biopsy of the peripheral nerves reveals a diminution in fascicle size and a reduction in the number of myelinated fibers, with the greatest loss among those of large diameter. Unmyelinated fibers appear normal (259). As a consequence of repeated demyelination and remyelination, greater than normal variation exists in the distance between nodes.

Depending on the duration and severity of the disease, gross enlargement of the proximal portions of the peripheral nerves, plexi, and roots are seen, with lesser involvement of the distal peripheral nerves and cranial nerves. Microscopic examination shows increased thickness of the myelin sheath and endoneurium and an increase in collagen around the individual fibers. Because of their appearance on transverse section, the concentric lamellae surrounding the nerve fibers were first termed *onion bulbs* by Déjérine and Sottas (268) (Fig. 2.6). Electron microscopy shows these to contain only Schwann cells and their processes, and they probably reflect a nonspecific regenerative Schwann cell response to injury (269,270). The lamellae can be seen in even the youngest patients (271). Some demyelination occurs, particularly in younger patients (272). Degenerative changes in the skeletal muscles are secondary to damage of the peripheral nerves.

CMT 1 is genetically heterogeneous (272a). In the most common form, type 1A, the genetic defect is a large (1.5 Mb) submicroscopic duplication of the proximal portion of the short arm of chromosome 17 (17p11.212), a region that contains the gene for the peripheral myelin protein (PMP) 22 (273). This duplication arises as a spontaneous mutation in some 10% to 20% of subjects, and nearly 90% of sporadic cases of CMT demonstrate this abnormality. It has been conjectured, but it is still unproven, that PMP-22 is an important structural component of peripheral myelin. How overexpression of PMP-22 results in the clinical manifestations of CMT 1A has not been fully clarified. In animals, overexpression of PMP-22 interferes with the growth and differentiation of Schwann cells. This, however, does not appear to be the case in patients with CMT 1A (273). Approximately 30% of patients with CMT 1A show a point mutation in the gene for PMP-22 (274). Patients who have only one copy of the gene for PMP-22 develop the condition known as hereditary neuropathy with liability to pressure palsies, whereas patients with four copies of the gene have the clinical picture of Déjérine-Sottas disease. These entities are covered in the Déjérine-Sottas disease section later in this chapter.

The gene for the less common entity, CMT 1B, has been localized to the long arm of chromosome

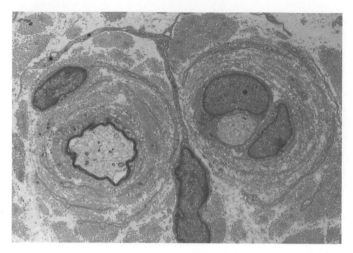

FIG. 2.6. Sural nerve biopsy in 2-year-old girl. Electron micrograph, hereditary motor sensory neuropathy type III (Déjérine-Sottas disease). Large *onion bulbs* are seen containing small fibers with absent or thin myelin sheaths. Symptoms of proximal weakness became apparent younger than 1 year of age, and the girl did not walk until 2½ years of age. Ataxia was seen, and the peripheral nerves were enlarged on clinical examination. Pupils were normal, and no cranial nerve deficits were seen. (Courtesy of Dr. Robert Ouvrier, The Children's Hospital, Camperdown, Sydney, Australia.)

1 (1q22-23). The major structural protein of peripheral myelin, P_0, a glycoprotein involved in the compaction of the multilamellar myelin sheaths, has been localized to this site, and both deletions and point mutations in this gene can cause CMT 1B (275).

At least three X-linked forms of CMT 1 also have been described (Table 2.8). Collectively these account for approximately 10% of all CMT cases (276). The gene for one form is on the short arm of the chromosome (Xp22.2); for the other, the gene is on the long arm (Xq13.1), and codes for connexin 32. At least 100 mutations in the gene sequence of connexin have been documented (277). Connexins are membrane-spanning proteins that are localized adjacent to the nodes of Ranvier and in the Schmidt-Lantermann incisures of peripheral nerve. They assemble to form gap junctions, channels that facilitate the transfer of ions and small molecules between cells (278).

In addition to these X-linked conditions, at least one other form of CMT 1 exists, designated CMT 1C, an autosomal dominant condition whose gene is located on an as yet undetermined autosome (see Table 2.8).

Clinical Manifestations

The various genetic subtypes of CMT 1 can manifest at any age, but in general, a bimodal distribution can be distinguished, with onset in the first two decades or after the fifth decade of life. Only the patients with the earlier onset are discussed here.

Symptoms can become apparent before 1 year of age (271). As a rule, the phenotype for CMT 1B is more severe than for CMT 1A, with somewhat earlier onset of symptoms (275). Patients with point mutations in the gene for PMP-22 tend to have a more severe expression of the disease than those who have a duplication, and onion bulbs can be detected in abundance on nerve biopsies at an early age (272). In general, the peroneal muscles are involved first, and delay in walking or a slapping storklike gait might motivate the parents to bring the child to the physician. In the upper extremities, weakness and atrophy are at first lim-

TABLE 2.8. *Heredodegenerative diseases of the peripheral nerves*

Name	Site	Transmission	Gene product	Clinical picture	Pathology	Reference
CMT 1A	17p11.2	AD	PMP-22	Weakness, wasting of lower then upper limbs, sensory loss, delayed NCV, pes cavus, scoliosis, tremor, onset first decade of life	Segmental demyelination, onion bulbs, hypertrophy	Hanemann and Müller (273)
CMT 1B	1q22	AD	P_0			
CMT 1C	?	AD	?			
CMT 2A	1p36-p35	AD	?	Similar to CMT 1, but onset in second decade of life, slower progress, normal NCV	Axonal degeneration	Suter and Snipes (278)
CMT 2B	3q13-q22	AD	?			
CMT 2C	?	AD	?	Similar to CMT 1, but with paresis of diaphragm and vocal cord	Axonal degeneration	Dyck et al. (287)
CMT 2D	7p14	AD	?	Clinically similar to CMT 2A, 2B, but upper extremities more involved than lower extremities	Axonal degeneration	Ionasescu et al. (286)
CMT X1	Xq13	X-linked	Connexin 32	Similar to CMT 1		Ionasescu et al. (296)
CMT X2	Xp22.2	X-linked				
CMT X3	Xq25	X-linked				
Déjérine-Sottas (CMT 3)	Various	AD + AR	PMP-22, P_0	Early hypotonia, mental retardation, slowed NCV	Hypomyelination, demyelination, onion bulb formation	Tyson et al. (289)
CMT 4A	8q13-q21.1	AR	?	Decreased NCV	Loss of large myelinated fibers, hypomyelination, onion bulb formation	Ben Othmane et al. (294)
CMT 4B	11q23	AR	?		Focally folded myelin	Bolino et al. (295)
HMSN V	5q23-q33	AR	?	Sensory-motor neuropathy starting in childhood or adolescence, pes cavus, scoliosis frequent Peripheral neuropathy and spastic paraplegia	Thin myelin sheaths, onion bulb formation	LeGuern et al. (285) Harding and Thomas (291)
HMSN VI				Peripheral neuropathy and optic atrophy		Macdermot and Walker (292), Ippel et al. (292a)
HMSN VII				Peroneal muscular atrophy and retinitis pigmentosa		Massion-Verniory et al. (293)
	3p14.1-q13	AD	?	Muscle cramps, proximal weakness > distal weakness, sensory loss, adult onset	Decreased number of large and small myelinated fibers	Takashima et al. (293a)
HSAN I	9q22.1-q22.3	AD	? ninjurin	Onset in second to fourth decade of life, sensory loss over feet, pain > touch, ulcers on feet, NCV normal	Loss of unmyelinated fibers, reduced small myelinated fibers, large myelinated fibers preserved	Chadwick et al. (297)

Continued

TABLE 2.8. *Continued.*

Name	Site	Transmission	Gene product	Clinical picture	Pathology	Reference
HSAN II		AR	?	Congenital, light touch, pain affected most, limbs more than trunk, unrecognized injuries	Total loss of myelinated fibers, reduced unmyelinated fibers	Davar et al. (298)
HSAN III (familial dysauto-nomia)	9q31-q33	AR	?	See Table 2.9	Decreased numbers of neurons in autonomic, spinal ganglia, absence of gamma-motor neurons	Eng et al. (299)
HSAN IV		AR	?	Bouts of high fever, anhidrosis, normal sensory nerve action potentials	Absence of unmyelinated fibers	Edwards-Lee et al. (300)
HSAN V	?	AR	?	Similar to HSAN IV	Selective loss of small myelinated fibers	Donaghy et al. (301)

AD, autosomal dominant; AR, autosomal recessive; CMT, Charcot-Marie-Tooth disease; HMSN, hereditary motor sensory neuropathy; HSAN, hereditary sensory and autonomic neuropathy; NCV, nerve conduction velocity.

ited to the small muscles of the hand, but later spread to the forearm. The face, trunk, and proximal muscles usually are spared, although nystagmus or facial weakness is not uncommon.

In the fully developed condition, examination reveals a pes cavus deformity (271,279), scoliosis, and contractures of the wrist and fingers that have produced a claw hand. The patient has striking atrophy and weakness of the distal musculature, which contrasts with the preservation of the bulk and strength of the proximal parts. Sensation, particularly vibratory and position sense, is reduced over the distal portions of the extremities. Vasomotor signs are common and include flushing and cyanosis or marbling of the skin. The ankle reflexes are generally lost; other deep tendon reflexes are preserved. The plantar responses can be difficult to elicit.

Progression of the disease is slow, and spontaneous arrests are common. The CSF protein level is elevated in one-half of the cases, but no other abnormalities exist. Median nerve sensory action potentials are generally absent, and motor nerve conduction velocities along the peroneal nerve are slowed. Slowed nerve conduction velocities are characteristic for the various forms of CMT 1 and can be recorded before any clinical manifestations or in cranial nerves that remain uninvolved (280). This feature distinguishes the various forms of CMT 1 from the forms of CMT 2 in which nerve conduction velocities are normal or only slightly decreased. Sensory neural deafness with or without mental retardation has accompanied CMT 1 in several families (281,282).

Diagnosis

CMT disease 1 is diagnosed on the basis of its dominant transmission, the characteristic distal distribution of the slowly progressive muscular wasting and weakness, and the presence of sensory deficits. In approximately 10% to 20% of subjects, the duplication of the PMP-22 gene is de novo and is usually of paternal origin. Sensory deficits distinguish the various forms of CMT 1 from the slowly progressive distal myopathies. Nerve conduction velocities are reduced markedly and, as a rule, also are abnormal in one of the parents (265,271,280). Conduction of

visual-evoked potentials is slowed in approximately one-half of the patients, including those who deny visual symptoms. Although histologic abnormalities are noted on biopsy of the peripheral nerves, they are not pathognomonic.

A dominantly inherited syndrome, considered to be an intermediate between peroneal muscular atrophy and FRDA, was described by Roussy and Lévy and by Symonds and Shaw in 1926 (283). This condition is now considered to be CMT 1 (197).

Treatment

Aside from orthopedic measures designed to prevent the disabling deformities and intensive physical therapy, no specific therapy is available. Prenatal diagnosis for CMT 1A is now available.

Charcot-Marie-Tooth Disease (Peroneal Muscular Atrophy), Axonal Type

CMT disease (peroneal muscular atrophy), axonal type, also genetically heterogeneous, is characterized by axonal degeneration of the peripheral nerves (see Table 2.8). The clinical picture is similar to that of CMT 1, except that the progression of the disability is slower. Because a significant proportion of axons is spared, nerve conduction velocities are often normal or near normal. EMG reveals denervation. Patients satisfying clinical and pathologic criteria for CMT 2 made up 5% of the pooled pediatric series of hereditary peripheral neuropathies compiled by Hagberg and Lyon (265). The various forms of CMT 2 are transmitted as a dominant trait (see Table 2.8), and one parent can show abnormalities on EMG (284).

Déjérine-Sottas Disease (Hypertrophic Interstitial Neuropathy of Infancy, Hereditary Motor Sensory Neuropathy Type III)

The prototype of a severe form of hereditary demyelinating neuropathy was described by Déjérine and Sottas (268). Déjérine-Sottas disease (hypertrophic interstitial neuropathy of infancy, hereditary motor sensory neuropathy type III) has been shown to consist of several genetically distinct entities, all of them marked by onset of symptoms in infancy or childhood, and progressing to severe disability. In the pooled series of Hagberg and Lyon, published in 1981, patients corresponding to HMSN III accounted for 12% of children with hereditary peripheral neuropathies (265). Several autosomal dominant and autosomal recessive conditions result in this clinical picture. They include mutations in the gene for PMP-22, mutations in the gene for P_0, and tandem duplications of the gene for P_0. In the majority, a de novo mutation or autosomal dominant transmission exists (288), whereas in other cases, there appears to be an autosomal recessive condition (289).

The pathologic picture of Déjérine-Sottas disease is highlighted by hypomyelination of the peripheral nerves, with hypertrophic changes and the presence of onion bulbs (289). In some patients with the clinical picture of Déjérine-Sottas disease, a unique pathologic picture of focally folded myelin sheaths is seen (289).

Clinical Manifestations

As first described in two siblings by Déjérine and Sottas in 1893 (268), the clinical picture is marked by hypotonia, muscular atrophy, and weakness, accompanied by ataxia and sensory disturbances. Facial weakness and an unusual thick-lipped, pouting (*tapir mouth*) appearance are characteristic. The disease begins early in life, prior to 1 year of age in the majority of patients (271). The rate of progression varies considerably, even within the same family (269). In approximately 10% of patients, the neuropathy is evident at birth (265).

Initial symptoms also include a delay in motor milestones, or in children with later onset of the illness, a disturbance of gait or weakness of the hands. Nerve conduction times are extremely slow, usually less than 10 per second. As the disease progresses, distal weakness and atrophy become evident. Distal sensory impairment is usual and tends particularly to affect vibration sense. In contrast to the initially reported cases, pupillary abnormalities are seen rarely. Kyphoscoliosis or pes cavus is common (occurring in two-thirds of cases in the series of Ouvrier and coworkers) (271). Intelligence remains unaffected.

Laboratory findings include an elevated CSF protein content (seen in 75% of patients) and abnormal sensory and motor nerve conduction velocities (290). EMG shows widespread evidence of peripheral denervation with frequent fibrillation potentials at rest.

Diagnosis

The diagnosis of Déjérine-Sottas disease (HMSN III) should be considered in any chronic progressive peripheral neuropathy of childhood. Clinical enlargement of the nerves was seen in all children in the series of Ouvrier and coworkers (271). This finding, however, was only seen in a small percentage of cases examined by Tyson and colleagues (289). Even when present, it is not specific for HMSN III, as it is also encountered in some one-fourth of patients with CMT 1 (HMSN I). Clinical enlargement also should be distinguished from nerves made easily visible by muscular atrophy.

Other conditions that produce a chronic demyelinating polyneuropathy with its onset in infancy include MLD, Niemann-Pick disease type C, and chronic polyneuropathy secondary to nonspecific infections.

Treatment

Aside from orthopedic measures and consistent, active physiotherapy, no specific treatment exists. Corticosteroids have been ineffective.

Several other entities have been designated as hereditary motor sensory neuropathies. These include Refsum disease (HMSN IV), which is considered in Chapter 1, HMSN V, which is associated with spastic paraplegia (291), HMSN VI, associated with optic atrophy (292,292a), and HMSN VII, associated with retinitis pigmentosa (293).

Hereditary Neuropathy with Liability to Pressure Palsies (Tomaculous Neuropathy)

Hereditary neuropathy with liability to pressure palsies (HNPP) is a dominantly transmitted condition characterized by recurrent peripheral nerve palsies, often precipitated by only slight trauma (302). Distal nerves are affected more commonly, and both patients and asymptomatic carriers show slowed motor and sensory conduction velocities even in childhood. Psychomotor development is unaffected. On nerve biopsy one almost always sees focal myelin thickenings, termed *tomacula*, which result from redundant loop formation within the myelin sheaths (303,304). HNPP can be accompanied by nerve deafness or scoliosis (305). In approximately 70% of subjects, HNPP results from a 1.5 mb deletion on chromosome 17 p11.2, the site that spans the gene for PMP-22 (302) with a consequent underexpression of PMP-22 (306).

The relationship between HNPP and Smith-Magenis syndrome is still unclear. The latter condition is a contiguous gene deletion syndrome of chromosome 17 p11.2. Smith-Magenis syndrome is characterized by brachycephaly, midface hypoplasia, and a moderate degree of mental retardation. In approximately one-half of subjects, deep tendon reflexes are decreased or absent, but no susceptibility exists to pressure palsies, and nerve conduction velocities are normal (307).

Hereditary Brachial Plexus Neuropathy

A dominantly transmitted form of brachial plexus neuropathy has been known for nearly 100 years. This condition is characterized by recurrent attacks of pain affecting the neck and shoulders, followed within hours or days by a weakness of muscles enervated by the brachial plexus. Attacks tend to be precipitated by infection or mild trauma. In addition to muscles enervated by the brachial plexus, the lower extremities are affected in approximately 20% of cases. Cranial nerves, notably X, VII, and VIII, also can be involved, resulting in hoarseness owing to paralysis of the vocal cords, impaired swallowing, facial weakness, and sensorineural deafness. Functional recovery takes place within a few months, but atrophy and weakness can persist. Associated anomalies are not unusual. Affected children have closely spaced eyes or other dysmorphic features (308,309). Although the condition usu-

ally presents during the second to third decade of life, it also can affect neonates, producing what appears to be a traumatic brachial plexus injury.

Nerve conduction velocities are normal during both the attack and the recovery period, but EMG can reveal evidence of denervation. Biopsy of the peripheral nerves reveals regions of tomaculous (sausagelike) thickening of the myelin sheath. Corticosteroid therapy has been suggested, but does not appear to affect the course of the attacks. The gene for this condition has been mapped to chromosome 17 q24-q25 (310).

Hereditary brachial plexus neuropathy can be distinguished on clinical grounds from HNPP. In the latter condition, attacks are not preceded by pain, and generally affect the distal nerves. Nerve biopsy is characteristic. Hereditary brachial plexus neuropathy also should be distinguished from acute brachial plexus neuropathy. This condition mainly affects adults, is bilateral in 25% to 33% of cases, and is triggered by infections and immunizations, notably by tetanus toxoid. Epidemics or clusters of brachial plexus neuropathy have been observed (311).

Hereditary Sensory and Autonomic Neuropathies

At least five clinical entities exist under hereditary sensory and autonomic neuropathies, all characterized by a progressive loss of function that predominantly affects the peripheral sensory nerves (312). These conditions are less common than the hereditary motor sensory neuropathies, and their incidence has been estimated at 1 in 25,000, approximately one-tenth that of CMT 1 (313), and collectively, these conditions accounted for 3% of the hereditary peripheral neuropathies of infants and children pooled by Hagberg and Lyon (265).

The clinical presentation depends on the population of affected neurons or axons. When degeneration of the large diameter afferent fibers occurs, such as occurs in FRDA, position sense is involved primarily. When the small afferent and autonomic fibers are affected, an increased threshold to nociception and thermal discrimination occurs, accompanied by autonomic and trophic changes.

Type I (Hereditary Sensory Radicular Neuropathy)

Hereditary sensory radicular neuropathy is the most common of the hereditary sensory and autonomic neuropathies. It is transmitted as an autosomal dominant trait and is characterized by a sensory deficit in the distal portion of the lower extremities, chronic perforating ulcerations of the feet, and progressive destruction of the underlying bones. It is identical to familial lumbosacral syringomyelia. Pathologic examination discloses degeneration of the dorsal root ganglia and of the dorsal roots of the spinal cord segments supplying the lower limbs (314).

Symptoms appear in late childhood or early adolescence. Initially, patients have episodes of cellulitis of the feet accompanied by a progressive loss of sensation in the lower extremities, which is associated with painless lacerations and trophic ulcers (Fig. 2.7). On examination, perception of pain is affected more than touch or deep pressure perception. Sweating is impaired. The distal portions of the upper extremities also can be affected. Sharp, brief pains can occur in the legs and resemble the lightning pains of tabes dorsalis. Many of the cases have had accompanying nerve deafness and atrophy of the peroneal muscles (314).

The gene for this disorder has been mapped to 9 q22.1-q22.3 (313). Ninjurin, a candidate gene, has been localized to this region (297). This is an adhesion protein that is upregulated in dorsal root ganglion neurons and Schwann cells after nerve injury and promotes neurite outgrowth. Histopathologic examination shows a marked reduction in the number of unmyelinated fibers. Small myelinated fibers are decreased to a lesser degree, and large myelinated fibers are affected least (312). Motor nerve conduction velocities are normal, but the sensory nerve action potentials are absent.

Type II (Congenital Sensory Neuropathy)

Congenital sensory neuropathy is characterized by its autosomal recessive inheritance and by an onset of symptoms in early infancy or childhood. The upper and lower extremities are affected with chronic ulcerations and multiple injuries to fingers and feet. Pain sensation is involved most, with

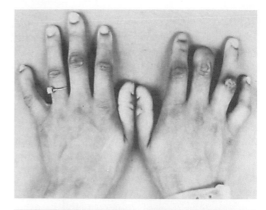

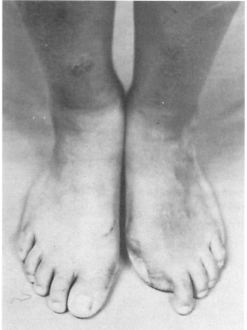

FIG. 2.7. Hereditary sensory radicular neuropathy. Trophic changes in digits of upper and lower extremities. (Courtesy of Dr. K. E. Astrom, Massachusetts General Hospital, Boston, MA.)

temperature and touch sensations affected to a lesser extent. Deep pain is impaired and the deep tendon reflexes are reduced (315). Autoamputation of the distal phalanges is common, as is a neuropathic joint degeneration (298). The condition progresses slowly, if at all (316). Sensory nerve action potentials are reduced or absent. Nerve biopsy shows a total loss of myelinated fibers and reduced numbers of unmyelinated fibers.

Type III (Familial Dysautonomia, Riley-Day Syndrome)

Although the name *familial dysautonomia* suggests that the disease is exclusively a disorder of the autonomic nervous system, peripheral sensory neurons, peripheral motor neurons, and other neuronal populations also are affected.

In the first description of the disease in 1949, Riley and coworkers pointed out excessive sweating, poor temperature control, skin blotching, defective lacrimation, indifference to pain, absent deep tendon reflexes, and motor incoordination (317). The condition is transmitted as an autosomal recessive trait and is confined to Jews of Eastern European descent. In the United States, the frequency of the carrier state in this ethnic group is 1 in 50 (318). The gene for dysautonomia has been localized to the distal region of the long arm of chromosome 9 (9q31). Two actin-like genes have been cloned from this region (318a). Mapping of the gene has permitted prenatal diagnosis and carrier detection in families with at least one affected child (299).

Pathology

No consistent structural abnormality has been found within the CNS. The sympathetic ganglia are hypoplastic, and the number of neurons in the spinal ganglia is reduced, with hypoplasia of the dorsal root entry zones and Lissauer tract (319). Substance P immune reactivity in the substantia gelatinosa of the spinal cord and the medulla is depleted, a finding consistent with a supposition that this undecapeptide is involved in the transmission of pain impulses (320).

Some patients have shown degenerative changes in the reticular substance of the pons and medulla with focal lack of myelination and neuronal depletion (321). Additionally, fibers are lost from the lateral and ventral spinothalamic tracts, the posterior columns, and the spinocerebellar tracts, and myelin sheaths are lacking in the mesencephalic roots of the trigeminal nerve. These changes are slowly progressive without neuronophagia or evidence of myelin breakdown.

In peripheral nerves, the number of myelinated and nonmyelinated axons is reduced, and the transverse fascicular area is diminished. Most important, the catecholamine endings appear to be absent (322). The primary genetic and biochemical lesions are still unknown, and no consistent abnormality in blood levels, urinary excretion, or tissue concentration of catecholamines or their metabolites has been found. Plasma norepinephrine levels are normal, but when patients assume the upright position, the expected increase in norepinephrine does not occur. Plasma dopamine β-hydroxylase activity is lower than normal, and sympathetic nerve stimulation fails to induce a significant increase (323). Most clinical and pathologic alterations can best be explained by a deficit of a trophic factor essential to antenatal development, which also continues to have a minor postnatal sustaining function.

Clinical Manifestations

Familial dysautonomia is characterized by symptoms referable to the sensory and autonomic nervous system. No single feature, but rather the association of several, points to the diagnosis.

Nervous system dysfunction is usually evident from birth as a poor or absent suck reflex, hypotonia, and hypothermia. Nursing difficulties result in frequent regurgitation (324). A high incidence of breech presentation (31%) is unrelated to the birth weight, but reflects intrauterine hypotonia. Retarded physical development, poor temperature control, and motor incoordination become prominent during early childhood, and subsequently other clinical features are detected (Table 2.9) (325). These include inability to produce overflow tears with the usual stimuli, absent or hypoactive deep tendon reflexes, absent corneal reflexes, postural hypotension, relative indifference to pain, and absence of the fungiform papillae on the tongue in association with a marked diminution in taste sensation (Fig. 2.8) (326). Many patients have serious feeding difficulties, including cyclic vomiting and recurrent pneumonia. In part, these problems can be attributed to absent or decreased lower esophageal peristalsis, a dilated esophagus, and impaired gastric motility (327). Taste and smell is significantly impaired (328). Scoliosis is frequent and becomes more marked with age. Intelligence remains normal. Many patients die from the disease during infancy or childhood. In some 40%, death is a consequence of cardiorespiratory arrest, usually during sleep or precipitated

TABLE 2.9. *Clinical features of familial dysautonomia*

Disturbances of autonomic nervous system	
Reduced or absent tears	+++
Peripheral vascular disturbances	
Hypertension with excitement	++
Postural hypotension	+++
Skin blotching with excitement or with eating	++
Cold hands and feet	+++
Excessive perspiration	+++
Erratic temperature control	++
Disturbed swallowing reflex	+++
Drooling beyond usual age	++
Cyclic vomiting	++
Disturbances of voluntary neuromuscular system	
Absent or hypoactive deep tendon reflexes	+++
Poor motor coordination	+++
Dysarthria	+++
Convulsions	+
Abnormal electroencephalographic results	++
Sensory disturbances	
Relative indifference to pain	+++
Corneal anesthesia	++
Psychological disturbances	
Apparent mental retardation	++
Breath-holding spells in infancy	++
Emotional lability	+++
Other disturbances	
Absence of fungiform papillae	+++
Corneal ulcerations	++
Frequent bronchopneumonia	++
Retardation of body growth	++
Scoliosis	++

+, common; ++, occurs frequently but not required for the diagnosis; +++, probably present in all cases.

by hypotension. A prolongation of the QT interval seen in approximately one-third of patients could predispose them to sudden death from ventricular arrhythmia (329). Aspiration or infectious pneumonia is another common cause for demise. Still, approximately one-third of living patients are 20 years of age or older (330). Some symptoms, notably cyclic vomiting, become less marked with age; others, in particular the sensory loss, are slowly progressive (331).

The brainstem auditory-evoked potentials are abnormally prolonged in most patients (332). Neuroimaging studies have been unremarkable.

Other clinical aspects of this systemic disease, including ophthalmologic abnormalities, anesthetic hazards, and various emotional problems, are discussed by Goldberg and associates (333) and Axelrod and Maayan (334).

Diagnosis

The diagnosis of dysautonomia rests on the patient's history, genetic background, and clinical features of the condition, in particular the absence of fungiform papillae, absent corneal reflexes, decreased or absent deep tendon reflexes, and decreased response to pain. Of the various tests designed to elicit autonomic dysfunction, I have found the intradermal histamine test to be the most reliable. In healthy subjects,

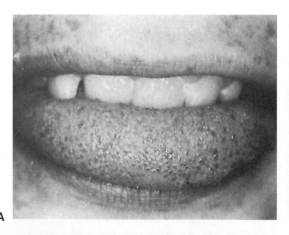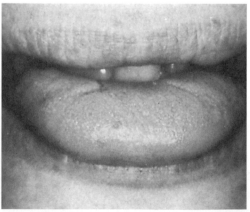

FIG. 2.8. Familial dysautonomia. **A:** Tip of the tongue of a healthy child. The dark spots are blood cells seen through the clear epithelium of the fungiform papillae. **B:** In familial dysautonomia, no fungiform papillae exist, and the tongue appears smooth. (Courtesy of Dr. Felicia Axelrod, Department of Pediatrics, New York University, New York, NY.)

intradermal injection of histamine phosphate (0.03 to 0.05 mL of a 1:1000 solution) produces a local wheal and a red erythematous flare extending 1 to 3 cm beyond the wheal. In dysautonomic patients beyond the newborn period, the flare response is absent. A similar lack of response can be seen in atopic dermatitis and in some disorders of the spinal cord or peripheral nerves (e.g., other progressive sensory neuropathies). Forms of congenital dysautonomia, other than Riley-Day syndrome, have been reported in families that are not of Ashkenazi Jewish extraction (335).

Treatment

Treatment is symptomatic (334). Impaired swallowing is best managed by experimenting with nipples of different sizes and with thickened feedings. If these methods fail, gavage feedings are necessary. When gastroesophageal reflux results in intractable pulmonary problems, gastrostomy feeding and fundal plication are required (336). Vomiting is managed by correcting the dehydration, which generally is isotonic. Gastric distention is relieved by using bethanechol chloride. Oral dosages range from 1 to 2 mg/kg per day, given in several divided doses, although the amount required varies from one child to the next. Cessation of vomiting is promoted by the use of diazepam (0.1 to 0.2 mg/kg per dose) given intravenously. Diazepam is also the most effective treatment for hypertension and is given intramuscularly in doses of 0.5 to 1.0 mg/kg. Crises are best handled with diazepam, or with the combination of diazepam and chlorpromazine (0.5 to 1.0 mg/kg given intramuscularly) (334). Aspiration pneumonia is prevented by maintaining the head in an elevated position. Feeding and swallowing difficulties in the infant might necessitate gavage. Hypertensive crises are treated with sedation and chlorpromazine.

Type IV (Congenital Insensitivity to Pain and Anhidrosis)

Congenital insensitivity to pain and anhidrosis is a recessive condition that becomes apparent in early life. Affected infants, usually boys, present with episodes of high fever often related to the environmental temperature, anhidrosis, and insensitivity to pain. Palmar skin is thickened, and Charcot joints (sensory arthropathy) are commonly present. Children respond to tactile stimulation, and deep tendon reflexes are preserved. Peripheral nerve biopsy shows the small unmyelinated fibers to be almost totally absent (337). Axonal microtubules are reduced, and the mitochondria are abnormally enlarged. Muscle biopsy discloses an accumulation of lipid droplets and reduced cytochrome C oxidase (300). In contrast to the other sensory neuropathies, motor and sensory nerve action potentials are normal. An autosomal recessive neuropathy seen in Navajo children is similar pathologically. Clinically, the Navajo children do not experience bouts of hyperpyrexia and are developmentally normal (338). A different and apparently unique motor sensory neuropathy also has been described in Navajo children. It is marked by corneal insensitivity and scarring, self-mutilation, and an associated encephalomyelopathy (339).

Type V (Hereditary Sensory and Autonomic Neuropathy)

Hereditary sensory and autonomic neuropathy also manifests with congenital insensitivity to pain and anhidrosis. It is distinct from congenital insensitivity to pain and anhidrosis by a selective absence of the small myelinated fibers (315). This condition, in association with neurotrophic keratitis, has been seen in Kashmir (301).

Other Hereditary Sensory Neuropathies

Several other, probably distinct, forms of hereditary sensory neuropathies have been reported. In addition, an entity exists termed *asymbolia to pain*, or congenital indifference to pain, in which pain sensation is appreciated, but its unpleasant quality is lost. It is an autosomal recessive disorder that is often accompanied by auditory imperception (340).

Giant Axonal Neuropathy

Giant axonal neuropathy, which is probably an autosomal recessive disorder, was described in

1972 by Berg and colleagues (341). It is characterized clinically by a chronically progressive,
peripherally mixed neuropathy having its onset in
early childhood. Most of those affected have pale
or slightly reddish hair, which is unusually tight
and curly. Ataxia and nystagmus are not unusual.
Biopsy of the motor and sensory nerves reveals
decreased numbers of myelinated and unmyelinated fibers, and the presence of focal axonal
enlargements that are more common distally, and
adjacent to a node of Ranvier. Ultrastructurally,
these swellings are replete with aggregates of
neurofilaments (342). Swollen axons also have
been found within the CNS (343).

The gene for this condition has been mapped
to chromosome 16 q24 (344). Its pathogenesis is
unknown, and to date no candidate genes have
been mapped to the region. The condition probably represents a generalized disorder of cytoplasmic microfilament formation (345). Similar
axonal enlargements have been seen in neuroaxonal dystrophy and in glue-sniffing neuropathy.

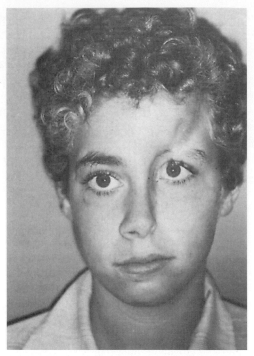

FIG. 2.9. Progressive facial hemiatrophy in a 16-
year-old boy. The scarlike coup de sabre is characteristic for this condition, but also may be seen
in scleroderma. (Courtesy of Dr. Creighton G.
Bellinger, Glendale, CA.)

Progressive Facial Hemiatrophy (Parry-Romberg Syndrome)

Progressive facial hemiatrophy (Parry-Romberg
syndrome) is characterized by progressive wasting of the face, including the subcutaneous tissue, fat, cartilage, and bone.

The disease makes its appearance in early
childhood and occasionally is present at birth.
Approximately 75% of patients with progressive facial hemiatrophy are affected before 20
years of age. In approximately 25%, local
trauma appears to predispose to the condition.
Initially, shrinkage of the subcutaneous tissue
occurs over the maxilla or at the upper corner of
the nasolabial fold. As the disease progresses
slowly over the course of several years, the
remainder of the facial half becomes involved
(Fig. 2.9). Patients experience no muscular
weakness, loss of trigeminal nerve function, or
atrophy of the skin. The hair, including the eye-
lashes and eyebrows, is affected commonly, and
alopecia and blanching, particularly along the
paramedian area, can precede all other manifestations of the condition.

Cerebral symptoms include seizures that
can be generalized or focal (particularly sensory focal) and minimal pyramidal tract signs
(347,348). No definite pathologic changes
have been found in the few brains examined,
although some have shown nonspecific
inflammatory processes (346,347). The CT
scan can be normal or show intracerebral calcifications or atrophy. The calcification is
generally ipsilateral to the facial hemiatrophy
(348). MRI demonstrates areas of ipsilateral
cortical dysgenesis or increased signal in the
ipsilateral white matter on T2-weighted
images (349).

Although the appearance of the patient with
progressive hemiatrophy is characteristic,
lipodystrophy and scleroderma should be considered in the differential diagnosis. In lipodystrophy, the involvement is bilateral and spares
cartilage and bone; in scleroderma, the skin
becomes cold, waxy, and inelastic and adheres

TABLE 2.10. *Neurologic disorders accompanying retinitis pigmentosa*

Errors in lipid metabolism
    3-Hydroxydicarboxylic aciduria (Poll-The, 372)
    Abetalipoproteinemia
    Refsum disease
Neuronal ceroid lipofuscinoses
    Infantile form
    Late infantile form
    Juvenile form
Errors in mucopolysaccharide metabolism
    Hurler disease (MPS IH)
    Hunter disease (MPS II)
    Scheie disease (MPS IS)
Peroxisomal disorders
    Zellweger disease
    Neonatal adrenoleukodystrophy
    Infantile Refsum's disease
Mitochondrial disorders
    Kearns-Sayre syndrome
Heredodegenerative diseases
    Friedreich ataxia
    Spinocerebellar ataxias
    Familial spastic paraplegias
    Hallervorden-Spatz disease
    Cockayne syndromes
    Chédiak-Higashi syndrome
    Hallgren syndrome (Hallgren, 373)
Other hereditary disorders
    Gyrate atrophy caused by ornithine aminotrans-
      ferase deficiency
    Sjögren-Larsson syndrome (Sjögren, 374)
    Laurence-Moon syndrome
    Allström syndrome (Allström, 375)
    Usher syndromes

MPS, mucopolysaccharides.

to the subcutaneous tissue. In familial hemiatrophy, the skin usually remains normal.

Aside from cosmetic surgery, no appropriate therapy for this condition is available. The atrophy progresses for several years but never becomes complete.

Progressive Hereditary Nerve Deafness

Various heredodegenerative diseases of the CNS are accompanied by a progressive sensory neural hearing loss. These include such heredodegenerations as CMT disease, FRDA, and the hereditary sensory neuropathies. Progressive nerve deafness also is seen in association with retinitis pigmentosa (Usher syndromes), recessive conditions with a variable degree of penetrance. In Refsum disease, nerve deafness

accompanies retinitis pigmentosa, ataxia, and polyneuropathy.

A number of syndromes in which progressive nerve deafness accompanies lesions of the visual system have been summarized by Fischel-Ghodsian and Falk (350) and by Fraser (351). In all of these, deafness begins insidiously and progresses slowly; the ability to hear high tones is usually lost first. A differential diagnosis of profound hearing loss in childhood is presented in Chapter 4 (see Table 4.15). Ménière disease, a condition characterized by progressive deafness, tinnitus, and paroxysms of vertigo, is essentially a disorder of middle life.

Retinitis Pigmentosa

Retinitis pigmentosa represents a common cause of hereditary visual impairment. The condition can be subdivided into a group in which the disease process is confined to the eye, and a group in which retinitis pigmentosa accompanies a systemic or heredodegenerative disorder. The latter disorders are listed in Table 2.10. A list of the various mapped or cloned human genes that cause retinal degenerations is provided by Heckenlively and Daiger (351a).

DIFFUSE CEREBRAL DEGENERATIVE DISEASES

Various hereditary diseases that affect the CNS in a nonselective manner are included in diffuse cerebral degenerative diseases. Although, in some, the evidence points to a defect in cerebral metabolism, the relationship between the enzymatic defect and the neurologic abnormalities has not yet been defined completely.

Diseases with Degeneration Primarily Affecting White Matter

Hereditary widespread demyelination of the cerebral white matter can be grouped by the histochemical characteristics of the myelin breakdown products. The following major entities have been distinguished: adrenoleukodystrophy (ALD), PMD, spongy degeneration of white matter (Canavan disease), Alexander disease, MLD, and Krabbe disease (globoid cell leukodystrophy).

Adrenoleukodystrophy

Adrenoleukodystrophy is the most common and clearly defined form of sudanophilic cerebral sclerosis, with an incidence of 1 in 10,000 male subjects. It is also the most common inherited peroxisomal disorder. The condition is characterized by visual and intellectual impairment, seizures, spasticity, and a more or less rapid progression to death. ALD is an X-linked condition in which CNS degeneration is often accompanied by adrenocortical insufficiency. The gene whose mutation causes the disease has been mapped to chromosome X q28.

Pathology, Molecular Genetics, and Pathogenesis

Pathologic features include widespread demyelination and gliosis of cerebral white matter. The demyelination generally spares subcortical fibers, and exhibits a rostrocaudal progression with the earliest abnormalities evident in the occipital and posterior parietal lobes. Inflammatory cells are common and are seen in a perivascular distribution. Macrophages are filled with material that has positive results for periodic acid–Schiff and oil red O. In the zona fasciculata and reticularis of the adrenal gland, ballooned cells are evident. Many of these have striated cytoplasm and vacuolations. Similar lipid inclusions are found in Schwann cells of the peripheral nerves and in testes (352). The structure of peroxisomes is normal.

Chemical analysis demonstrates the accumulation of very-long-chain fatty acids (VLCFA) with carbon chain lengths of 22 to 30 (C_{22} to C_{30}), notably C_{26}, in white matter cholesterol esters, cerebrosides, and gangliosides. VLCFA, particularly C_{26}, also are increased in cultured fibroblasts and serum (353,354). These VLCFA are partly of exogenous origin and their β-oxidation normally occurs within peroxisomes (355). The biochemical defect, however, does not directly involve the oxidation of VLCFA, as was originally surmised. Rather, it has been localized to the gene that codes for an ATP transporter. This is a member of the family of ATP-binding-cassette transport systems (called *cassette* because the ATP fits into the molecule like a cassette into a tape player). These proteins couple the hydrolysis of ATP to the translocation of a variety of substances, including VLCFA–coenzyme A (CoA) synthetase, across a biological membrane (356). As a result of the transporter defect, the first step in the β-oxidation of the VLCFA, namely the synthesis of VLCFA-CoA, is inoperative. The biological functions of the transporters have been reviewed by Schneider and Hunke (357). A large number of different mutations in the gene that codes for the VLCFA-CoA transporter, including deletions and point mutations, have been documented in patients with all different phenotypes of ALD, and no correlation exists between genotype and phenotype (358).

The pathogenesis of the CNS lesion in ALD is poorly understood (358a). The presence of the slowly progressive adult form and the severe childhood form of ALD in the same nuclear family, the observation of different phenotypes in identical twins (359), and the rapid progression of the disease after years of dormancy all suggest that nongenetic factors, modifier genes, or both are important in the expression of the disease. The increased expression of proinflammatory cytokines, such as tumor necrosis factor-α and interleukin-1_β in astrocytes and microglia in demyelinating lesions of patients with the childhood form of ALD, suggests an important role of cytokines in the pathogenesis of the disease (360). Moser postulates that a modifier gene acts by modulating the severity of the inflammatory response mounted by the brain (358).

Clinical Manifestations

Three phenotypes have been distinguished. The cerebral form of ALD is the most common; it represented 48% of the collected patients in Moser group (361). In the Australian series of Kirk and colleagues, it comprised 54% (362). Adrenomyeloneuropathy was found in 25% of ALD hemizygotes, and Addison disease without neurologic involvement in 10% of Moser cases (361), and in 25% and 16%, respectively, in the series of Kirk and colleagues (362). The various phenotypes frequently occur within the same family, and the manifestations of the disease can differ significantly in closely related family members (362a). In some individuals, progression is fairly rapid, whereas in others the course can be relapsing and remitting (363).

Onset of the cerebral form of ALD is usually between ages 5 and 8 years, with a gradual disturbance in gait and slight intellectual impairment. Abnormal pigmentation or classic adrenal insufficiency sometimes precedes neurologic abnormalities by several years. In other cases, adrenocortical atrophy is asymptomatic throughout life (352). Early seizures of several types are common, as are attacks of crying and screaming. Visual complaints are initially rare, whereas swallowing is disturbed in approximately one-third of the children. Spastic contractures of the lower extremities appear, and frequently the child becomes ataxic. Extrapyramidal symptoms also can be observed. Cutaneous melanosis or evidence of Addison disease can often be detected.

The CSF protein content can be elevated, and a mild lymphocytosis can develop. MRI is more sensitive than the CT scan in terms of showing the extent of abnormal white matter. Abnormalities that are seen as high signal on T2-weighted sequences are first seen in the periventricular posterior parietal and occipital regions, and extend anteriorly with progression of the disease. Demyelination can be accompanied by a contrast-enhancing area that probably represents an inflammatory reaction. Calcification is not unusual (364,365). The MRI and MR spectroscopy also are abnormal in the preclinical stage of the disease (358,366). Because patients may remain asymptomatic in the face of an abnormal MRI until as long as their seventh decade of life, there is little predictive significance to these neuroimaging abnormalities. Evoked potentials are normal when neurologic symptoms first make their appearance; they become abnormal as the demyelinating lesions extend into the brainstem and parieto-occipital lobes. The auditory-evoked potential, one of the most sensitive indices of brainstem demyelination, is abnormal in obligatory carriers (367). The urinary excretion of adrenal androgens and corticosteroids is decreased, and adrenocorticotropic hormone stimulation fails to produce an increase in the 17-hydroxycorticoid excretion.

Adrenomyeloneuropathy generally has its onset in adult life, with only 8% of cases developing before 21 years of age (361,368). The condition is characterized by spastic paraparesis, distal neuropathy, adrenal insufficiency, and hypogonadism. MRI of the brain is abnormal in approximately one-half of patients, and cognitive function is reduced in approximately 40% (361).

Between 15% and 20% of female carriers develop a spastic paraparesis or a mild peripheral neuropathy. The MRI is abnormal in 16% (361).

Diagnosis

The diagnosis is based on demonstrating abnormally high levels of plasma VLCFA, in particular a significantly elevated level of C_{26} saturated fatty acid, and abnormally high ratios of C_{26} to C_{22} and C_{24} to C_{22} fatty acids (353,358). Some 85% of obligatory heterozygotes also can be diagnosed by their increased VLCFA levels in plasma and cultured fibroblasts (358). Plasma VLCFA levels are unaffected by the usual food intake or by storage at room temperature for up to 2 weeks. Elevated levels of VLCFA also are seen in some of the other peroxisomal disorders (see Chapter 1).

Treatment

Two forms of therapy can be considered: dietary therapy and bone marrow transplantation. Although the VLCFAs are, in part, of dietary origin, restriction of their intake does not affect the progressive worsening of the condition (358). However, a diet containing 20% erucic acid, a monounsaturated 22 carbon fatty acid (22:1), in addition to 80% oleic acid normalizes the levels of plasma C_{26} within a month. This diet, which goes under the name *Lorenzo oil*, has been tested in various centers, but in view of the variability of the clinical course of ALD it is difficult to evaluate its effectiveness. In the experience of Kaplan and coworkers, dietary therapy with Lorenzo oil failed to improve the abnormal visual-evoked responses (369). However, some suggestion exists that dietary therapy is effective when started in presymptomatic boys (358). It is the opinion of Gartner and colleagues that no scientific evidence exists to recommend this diet for patients with neurologic symptoms (364). Thrombocytopenia is a fairly common complication of treatment with Lorenzo oil (370). Bone marrow transplantation has been used in several mildly affected patients and the results appear to be encouraging (358,364). The mortality of this procedure is high; 10% when the donor is related, 20% to 30% when the donor is unrelated. Immunosuppressants have had no beneficial effects (364). Other therapeutic approaches include the use of lovastatin, which normalizes plasma VLCFAs, and 4-phenylbutyrate, which normalizes brain VLCFAs in mice by enhancing an alternative pathway for VLCFA oxidation (370a).

In addition to the adrenoleukodystrophies, two other forms of sudanophilic diffuse sclerosis have been documented. The sporadic form is probably related to multiple sclerosis and is considered in Chapter 7. The other form is a sudanophilic diffuse sclerosis occurring as an autosomal recessive disorder, which in some families is accompanied by meningeal angiomatosis (371). It is not well substantiated as a discrete entity, and the white matter lesions are now believed to be hypoxic in nature.

Pelizaeus-Merzbacher Disease

Pelizaeus-Merzbacher disease is a rare, slowly progressive disorder of myelin formation first described by Pelizaeus (376) in 1885 and Merzbacher in 1910 (377). The classic form of the condition has its onset in infancy and is transmitted in a gender-linked manner with the gene localized to the long arm of the X chromosome (Xq21.2-Xq22). The families described by Pelizaeus and Merzbacher fall into this category, as do the cases reported by Seitelberger (378) and Boulloche and Aicardi (379).

Pathology, Pathogenesis, and Molecular Genetics

The pathologic picture demonstrates widespread lack of myelin, although islands of myelination, particularly around small blood vessels, are preserved. Little sudanophilic material is present, and chemical examination of the brain reveals the white matter lipids to be normal or reduced. As expected from the absence of sudanophilic material, and in contrast to ALD, no increase in cholesterol esters is seen (380). The axons in demyelinated areas are covered by their lipid sleeves, which give histochemical reactions for sphingolipids. Oligodendrocytes contain spherical lamellated cytoplasmic inclusions and numerous myelin balls at their periphery (380). This pathologic picture suggested that the basic defect is an impairment in myelin formation, a situation reminiscent of that observed in *jimpy* mice. In this animal model a defect in PLP exists, one of the two major myelin membrane proteins. Indeed, the gene that encodes PLP, the PLP gene, has been found to be defective in PMD. In addition to PLP, the PLP gene also encodes another myelin protein, DM20. PLP and DM20 are two isoforms. They are hydrophobic membrane proteins that account for approximately one-half of the protein content of adult brain. The mRNAs that encode them are synthesized by alternative splicing of the primary transcript of the PLP gene. A large number of missense mutations in this gene have been described in patients with PMD. These include point mutations, interstitial deletions and insertions, and an apparent complete deletion of the gene (381). These missense mutations account for some 10% to 25% of families with PMD. In a large proportion of the remaining families, duplications of the PLP gene occur (382). These can be detected by Fluoresance *in situ* hybridization, using a PLP probe (383). The phenotype for the various mutations and duplications appears to be fairly comparable (382). PMD is allelic with SPG2, one of the X-linked forms of hereditary spastic paraplegia (245) (see Table 2.6).

Clinical Manifestations

The clinical course differs from the other leukodystrophies only by the presence, before 3 months of age, of arrhythmically trembling and roving eye movements. Head control is poor, and cerebellar ataxia, including intention tremor and scanning speech, is frequent. Over the years, optic atrophy, involuntary movements, and spasticity become apparent, whereas the nystagmus can disappear. The disease progresses slowly, with many plateaus. The CSF is normal, as are other laboratory studies (384). Abnormalities of myelin are disclosed by MRI. Nezu and colleagues distinguish three patterns: diffuse alterations in hemispheric white matter and the corticospinal tracts, diffuse alterations in hemispheric white matter with a normal corticospinal tract, and least often, patchy changes in the white matter of the cerebral hemispheres (385). Little correlation exists between the type of MRI abnormality and the gene defect, and these changes do not appear to progress (385).

A connatal form of PMD that has an early, possibly prenatal onset, and progresses rapidly also has been reported. It appears to be allelic with the classic form of PMD (386).

Diagnosis

In the absence of other affected members of the family, the diagnosis cannot be made with certainty solely on clinical grounds or by neuroimaging. However, ocular and cerebellar symptoms of extremely slow progression and the gender-linked recessive transmission tend to differentiate PMD from other degenerative conditions. The absence of remissions and early onset distinguish it from multiple sclerosis. Restriction enzyme analysis of genomic DNA with the appropriate probes provides a diagnosis and seems to be valuable in prenatal ascertainment of the disease (387). Considerable doubt exists whether MRI can be used for carrier detection. An X-linked disease has been reported that clinically resembles PMD in which there were capillary calcifications in the basal ganglia and dentate nucleus and in which the gene locus was on the long arm of the X chromosome but outside the region for the PLP gene (388).

Treatment

No known effective treatment is available.

Spongy Degeneration of the Cerebral White Matter (Canavan Disease)

Spongy degeneration of the cerebral white matter (Canavan disease) is a rare familial degenerative disease of cerebral white matter first described by Canavan in 1931 (389). The condition is inherited as an autosomal recessive trait, with the gene having been mapped and cloned. It codes for an enzyme, aspartoacylase, which hydrolyzes *N*-acetylaspartic acid to L-aspartic acid. A point mutation in the gene for aspartoacylase is a common finding in Canavan disease. In the series of Kaul and coworkers, 12 of 17 patients with this condition had this abnormality, the remainder were compound heterozygotes with one allele having the point mutation (390).

The condition is fairly rare worldwide, but its incidence appears to be as high as 1 in 5,000 live births in the Ashkenazi Jewish population, with one point mutation being extremely common (391). In the most common clinical variant, symptoms appear between the second and fourth month of life and include failure of intellectual development, optic atrophy, and hypotonia. Subsequently, seizures appear, and a progressive increase occurs in muscular tone. Choreoathetotic movements are noted occasionally. A relative or absolute macrocephaly is often evident by age 6 months. It was seen in all Arab cases reported by Gascon and colleagues (392) and was seen in 92% of children in the series of Traeger and Rapin (392a). In almost all, it could be documented by 1 year of age. The visual-evoked responses are frequently absent or delayed; they were normal in only one of eight children reported by Gascon and colleagues (392). Nystagmus was seen in 88% of children, and seizures in 63% (392a). Death usually ensues before 5 years of age (393), although survival into the second or third decade of life is not uncommon (392a).

Variants in which the onset of neurologic symptoms occur within the first few days of

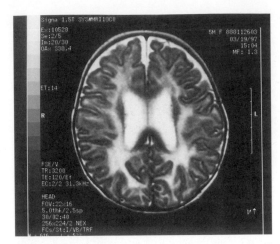

FIG. 2.10. Spongy degeneration of cerebral white matter (Canavan disease). Magnetic resonance imaging study. T2-weighted axial views show a marked increase in signal in the white matter that is most evident in the posterior portions of the hemispheres. (Courtesy of Dr. Franklin G. Moser, Division of Neuroradiology, Cedars-Sinai Medical Center, Los Angeles.)

life or after age 15 years also have been recognized (393).

The main pathologic findings are in white matter, particularly that of the convolutional areas, which is replaced by a fine network of fluid-containing cystic spaces that give the characteristic spongy appearance. The central portions and the internal capsule remain relatively spared. Edema fluid collects in the cytoplasm of astrocytes and intramyelinic vacuoles that result from splitting of the myelin sheath at the intraperiod lines (393,394). Products of myelin degradation cannot be found (395). Also, axonal degeneration of the peripheral nerves is present, with clumping and granular disintegration of axonal material (396).

The most striking finding in patients with Canavan disease is the increased amount of *N*-acetylaspartic acid in plasma and urine (391), the consequence of aspartoacylase deficiency. In brain, *N*-acetylaspartate is localized within neurons. Its function is not known; presumably it serves as a source of acetyl groups for the synthesis of myelin lipids (397).

The clinical diagnosis of Canavan disease rests on the progressive neurologic deterioration in a child with megalocephaly, optic atrophy, and seizures. It is confirmed by assay of urine for *N*-acetylaspartic acid. CT or ultrasonography demonstrates the cystic appearance of white matter (367). On MRI, diffuse white matter degeneration is seen, with abnormally high signal throughout cerebral white matter on T2-weighted images (398) (Fig. 2.10). As the disease progresses, cerebral atrophy becomes marked. On nuclear magnetic resonance spectroscopy, the ratio of *N*-acetylaspartic acid to creatine and choline is strikingly increased; the actual concentration of *N*-acetylaspartate is not increased (399).

In many cases the course of the disease is slowly progressive. The author of this chapter has seen children who were relatively intact neurologically even in the face of striking MRI abnormal results.

Alexander Disease

First described by Alexander in 1949 (400), this condition begins within the first year of life with intellectual deterioration, macrocephaly, spasticity, and seizures. Juvenile and adult forms also have been recognized. Bulbar signs are almost invariable additional symptoms in the juvenile form (401). The vast majority of cases of infantile and juvenile Alexander disease are isolated, and some doubt exists whether this is a genetically transmitted condition.

Microscopic examination of the brain reveals diffuse demyelination. The distinctive feature is the presence of innumerable Rosenthal fibers that are particularly dense around blood vessels. Rosenthal fibers are rounded, oval, or club-shaped densely osmiophilic bodies in the cytoplasm of enlarged astrocytes. It is believed that their formation is initiated by oxidative stress (402). The cells contain stress proteins, such as α-B-crystallin and HSP27. Crystallins are enormously large proteins normally secreted in the lens of the eye and in normal astrocytes. In Alexander disease, they form insoluble astrocytic aggregates (403). To date, no abnormality has been found in the gene coding for α-B-crystallin. Rosenthal fibers occur in smaller numbers in a variety of conditions associated with reactive or neoplastic astrocytes (404).

Diagnosis usually depends on microscopic examination of the brain. MRI results show increased periventricular signal. The location of the abnormal signal correlates with areas where an accumulation of Rosenthal fibers occurs (405). Although the appearance of neuroimaging studies has been claimed to be diagnostic for one or another of the leukodystrophies, their appearance is rarely specific. Rather, they show an evolution in the course of the disease from a normally appearing brain to one in which white matter is diffusely abnormal, to an ultimate picture of generalized gray and white matter atrophy. Because, as a rule, the lesions are more extensive when visualized by MRI than by CT scans, MRI is the imaging study of choice in an infant or child with suspected leukodystrophy (406).

Metachromatic Leukodystrophy

Metachromatic leukodystrophy is a lysosomal storage disease marked by the accumulation of cerebroside sulfate (sulfatide) within the nervous system and other tissue. Although first described in 1910 by Alzheimer (407), the condition was not fully delineated until 1933 when Greenfield noted it to be a form of diffuse sclerosis in which oligodendroglial degeneration was characteristic (408).

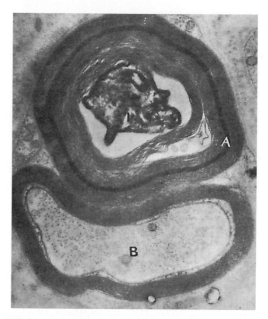

FIG. 2.11. Metachromatic leukodystrophy. Electron microscopic examination. Sural nerve biopsy (×18,400). Within the myelin loop is a circular band of increased density (A). Large cytoplasmic inclusions (I) corresponding in size and distribution to metachromatic material observed in frozen sections of the same nerve can be seen. The adjacent axon and myelin are normal (B). (Courtesy of Dr. H. De F. Webster, National Institutes of Health, Bethesda, MD.)

Pathology and Molecular Genetics

Diffuse demyelination and accumulation of metachromatically staining granules are the outstanding pathologic features. (Metachromatic staining implies that the tissue-dye complex has an absorption spectrum sufficiently different from the original dye to produce an obvious contrast in color. The spectral shift is caused by the polymerization of the dye, which is induced by negative charges such as RSO_3 present in close proximity to one another within the tissue.) Metachromatically staining granules are either free in the tissues or stored within glial cells and macrophages. Metachromatic material is almost always found in neuronal cytoplasm, distending the cell body as in GM_2 gangliosidosis, but to a lesser extent. Electron microscopy demonstrates cytoplasmic inclusions and alteration in the lamellar structure of myelin (Fig. 2.11). Demyelination is diffuse, but especially affects those tracts that myelinate during the latter part of infancy. All the involved areas have loss of oligodendroglia. Metachromatic granules also are found in the renal tubules, bile duct epithelium, gallbladder, islet cell and ductal epithelium of pancreas, reticular zone of adrenal cortex, and liver.

In 1959, Austin showed the metachromatic material to be a sulfatide (i.e., a sulfuric acid ester of cerebroside) and a major constituent of myelin glycolipids (409). Subsequently, Austin and associates (410) and Jatzkewitz and Mehl (411) found the basic enzymatic defect in late infantile MLD to be an inactivity of a heat-labile cerebroside sulfatase (arylsulfatase-A). This defect results in the blocked hydrolysis of sulfatides to cerebrosides (Fig. 2.12). A marked reduction but not complete absence of arylsulfatase-A activity has been found in gray and white matter, kidney, liver, urine, leukocytes, and cultured skin fibroblasts (412). The gene coding for

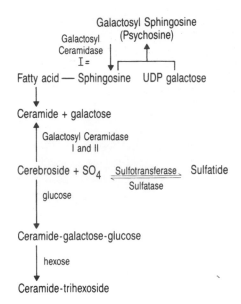

FIG. 2.12. Glycolipid metabolism in brain. In metachromatic leukodystrophy, sulfatase is defective. In globoid cell leukodystrophy, galactosylceramidase I is deficient. As a consequence, galactosyl sphingosine (psychosine) accumulates. Also, a secondary increase exists in ceramide dihexoside and trihexoside. (UDP, uridine diphosphate.)

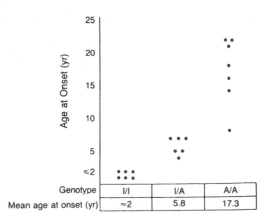

FIG. 2.13. Arylsulfatase-A genotype and age at onset of symptoms for metachromatic leukodystrophy. The arylsulfatase-A genotype was plotted against the age at onset of clinical symptoms in 19 patients for whom such data were available. (From Polten A, et al. Molecular basis of different forms of metachromatic leukodystrophy. *N Engl J Med* 1991;324:1822. With permission.)

arylsulfatase-A has been mapped to chromosome 22 q13.31-q ter. It has been cloned and characterized, and more than 50 mutations have been identified to date (413). Two mutations are particularly common in whites. In one [termed *allele I* by Polten and colleagues (414)], a G to A transition eliminates the splice donor site at the start of intron 2, with the resultant total loss of enzyme activity. Another common mutation (termed *allele A*), is characterized by a C to T transition that results in the substitution of leucine for proline at amino acid 426. This produces an enzyme with 3% residual activity. In the experience of Barth and colleagues, who studied mainly families from the United Kingdom, these two mutations accounted for 59% of the genetic lesions causing MLD (415). Numerous other, less common mutations in the gene have been demonstrated. These include both point mutations and gene deletions (413).

As a rule, the phenotype of each mutation can be inferred from their clinical expression in combination with other MLD mutations. In the series of Polten and colleagues, 21% of patients with the late infantile form of MLD were homozygous for the I/I genotype, another 48% had an I haplotype. Compound heterozygosity I/A was seen in 27% of juvenile cases (414) (Fig. 2.13). Homozygosity for allele A was seen in 45% of patients with the adult form of MLD, and another 27% had the A haplotype. A significant proportion of individuals with the A/A haplotype demonstrated the juvenile form of MLD. Thus, a considerable degree of phenotypic variation exists among patients with identical A/A genotypes, suggesting that nonallelic or environmental factors affect the age when neurologic symptoms make their appearance.

A reduction in arylsulfatase-A activity to 5% to 10% of control values is seen in up to 20% of the healthy population. This nonpathogenic reduction in enzyme activity is caused by homozygosity for a pseudodeficiency allele (416). Individuals who are homozygous for this allele are asymptomatic, although in some, MRI shows lesions of white matter (417).

Less commonly, MLD is caused by a deficient cerebroside sulfatase activator protein, saposin B. The saposins are small glycoproteins that are required for sphingolipid hydrolysis by lysosomal hydrolases. Four saposins arise through hydrolytic cleavage from one gene product, prosaposin; other saposins arise from different genes. To date, at least four different mutations in the gene for saposin B have been recognized (418). Patients with cerebroside activator protein deficiency present as the late infantile or juvenile form of MLD (413). The role of saposins in the various lysosomal storage diseases is reviewed by O'Brien and Kishimoto (419).

The mechanism by which sulfatide accumulation results in brain damage is not totally clear. Sulfatides are stored in oligodendrocytes and Schwann cells, and isolated myelin contains excess amounts of sulfatides. These are believed to result in an unstable molecular structure of myelin and myelin's consequent breakdown. Additionally, sulfatide accumulation might be responsible for the destruction of oligodendroglia and possibly for damage to neurons as well (420).

Clinical Manifestations

The incidence of the several forms of MLD is approximately 1 in 40,000 births. Symptoms can appear at any age. In the late infantile variant, a gait disorder, caused by either poor balance or a gradual stiffening, and strabismus occur by age 2 years. Impairment of speech, spasticity, and intellectual deterioration appear gradually, and, occasionally, coarse tremors or athetoid movements of the extremities develop. Deep tendon reflexes in the legs are reduced or even absent. Unexplained bouts of fever or severe abdominal pain can develop as the disease advances. Optic atrophy becomes apparent. Seizures are never prominent, although they can appear as the disease progresses (421). Progression is inexorable, with death occurring within 6 months to 4 years after the onset of symptoms. The CSF protein is elevated, the conduction velocity in the peripheral nerves is decreased, and the electroretinograms in contrast to the various juvenile amaurotic idiocies is normal. Auditory-evoked potentials can be abnormal even in presymptomatic patients (422). On MRI, the areas of demyelination are marked by high signal intensity on T2-weighted images. These are first seen in the periventricular regions and the centrum semiovale. The splenium and the

genu of the corpus callosum also are affected (423), as are the internal capsule and the pyramidal tracts. Characteristically, the subcortical white matter, including the arcuate fibers, tends to be spared until late in the disease (423).

The juvenile form of MLD is somewhat rarer. It was first described by Scholz (424) and subsequently by others (425). Neurologic symptoms become evident at between 5 years of age and adulthood and progress slowly. Older patients develop an organic mental syndrome and progressive corticospinal, corticobulbar, cerebellar, or, rarely, extrapyramidal signs (426). The adult form of MLD, which has been seen as early as 15 years of age, generally begins with a change in personality and psychiatric problems (427). Rarely, the disease begins as a peripheral neuropathy.

The variant forms with arylsulfatase-activator deficiency present a clinical picture of late infantile or juvenile MLD (413).

Multiple sulfatase deficiency (mucosulfatidosis) is characterized by mental deterioration, coarse facial features, hepatosplenomegaly, skeletal anomalies, and ichthyosis. The condition results from a defect in a posttranslational modification of sulfatases, by which a cystine residue is replaced with formylglycine to produce catalytically active sulfatases (428). At least 13 different sulfatases are defective. Patients accumulate sulfatides, acid mucopolysaccharides (heparan sulfate), and cholesterol sulfate in brain, liver, and kidney. Urinary excretion of mucopolysaccharides, notably heparan sulfate, is increased (429). The CSF protein content is elevated, and nerve conduction is slowed.

Diagnosis

The time of onset of neurologic symptoms, the presence of ataxia, spasticity, and particularly depressed deep tendon reflexes with elevated CSF protein content should suggest the diagnosis, which is confirmed by a marked reduction in urinary or leukocyte arylsulfatase-A activity. Other abnormal laboratory test results include slowed motor nerve conduction velocities, a reduced auditory-evoked brainstem response, and a nonfunctioning gallbladder. Brown metachromatic bodies can be found on biopsy of various

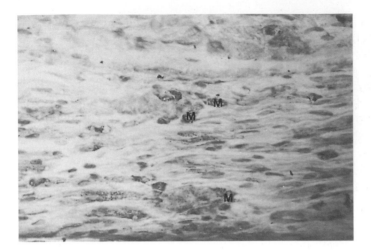

FIG. 2.14. Metachromatic leukodystrophy. Peripheral nerve biopsy, longitudinal section, stained with acetic cresyl violet (acid pH). Innumerable coarse and fine clumps of golden brown crystalline granules (M). The 5-year-old girl had onset of intellectual deterioration at 3½ years of age. This was accompanied by seizures and impaired coordination. Nerve conduction times were markedly prolonged, and cerebrospinal fluid protein was elevated.

peripheral nerves as early as 15 months after the onset of symptoms (Fig. 2.14). Segmental demyelination of peripheral nerves is encountered in other leukodystrophies, including globoid cell leukodystrophy, Canavan disease (396), and, rarely, GM_2 gangliosidosis and Spielmeyer-Vogt disease (430).

The assay of fibroblast arylsulfatase-A activity can be used for the biochemical identification of heterozygotes for MLD and for multiple sulfatase deficiency. Cultured amniotic fluid cells can serve for the antenatal diagnosis of the disorder. Asymptomatic individuals with pseudodeficiency of arylsulfatase are distinguished from presymptomatic individuals with MLD by the presence of normal levels of urinary sulfatides and normal nerve conduction velocities.

Treatment

As is the case for several of the other lysosomal disorders, bone marrow transplantation is being used to treat the late infantile and the juvenile forms of MLD. Long-term results in patients with the juvenile form of MLD have been particularly encouraging in that engraftment exists with normalization of leukocyte arylsulfatase-A activity, and a decrease in the sulfatide content of peripheral nerves, with consequent arrest of neurologic deterioration (413,431). Retroviral or adenovirus-mediated gene transfer has been suc-

cessful under experimental conditions, but as yet these techniques have not been applied to the patient population.

Globoid Cell Leukodystrophy (Krabbe Disease)

Globoid cell leukodystrophy (Krabbe disease) was first described in 1908 by Beneke (432) and more definitively in 1916 by Krabbe (433), who noted characteristic globoid cells in affected white matter.

Pathology

The white matter of the cerebrum, cerebellum, spinal cord, and cortical projection fibers is extensively demyelinated, with only minimal sparing of the subcortical arcuate fibers (434). Additionally, an almost total loss of oligodendroglia occurs. In areas of recent demyelination, mononuclear epithelioid cells and large (20 to 50 μm) multinucleated globoid cells are seen around the smaller blood vessels (Fig. 2.15). The globoid cells are believed to arise from vascular adventitia. Histochemical reactions and chemical analyses on globoid cell-rich fractions prepared by differential centrifugation show that a protein-bound cerebroside is stored within them. The appearance of globoid cells is believed to be stimulated by the release of cerebrosides from myelin, because a similar cellular

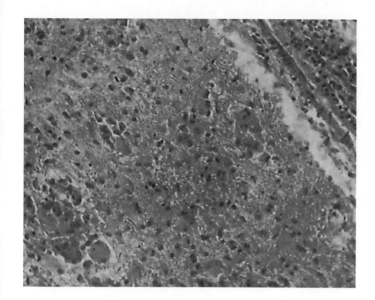

FIG. 2.15. Globoid cell leuko-dystrophy. Cerebral white matter. Aggregates of globoid cells are seen in the vicinity of a blood vessel in the lower left corner. A considerable increase in cellularity occurs in the demyelinated area (hematoxylin and eosin, ×280).

response can be produced in experimental animals through intercerebral injection of natural and synthetic cerebrosides (435).

Small clusters of globoid cells occur in a number of degenerative diseases of myelin, and the distinguishing feature of Krabbe disease is not the mere presence of these cellular elements, but rather their vast number. Ultrastructural examination reveals intracellular and extracellular crystalline inclusions, most commonly seen within the globoid cells, which correspond to the periodic acid–Schiff positive material (436). The peripheral nerves show segmental demyelination and marked endoneurial fibrosis. Electron microscopy reveals curved or straight tubular structures in the cytoplasm of Schwann cells, around small blood vessels, or in the proliferated endoneurial collagenous tissue (437). Globoid cells also have been noted in lungs, spleen, and lymph nodes (438).

Biochemical Pathology and Molecular Genetics

The basic biochemical defect in this condition is a deficiency of a galactosylceramidase (galacto-cerebroside β-galactosidase) (see Fig. 2.12). Galactosylceramidase activity is reduced in a number of tissues, including leukocytes, brain, liver, spleen, and cultured skin fibroblasts (439). Because galactosylsphingosine (psychosine) is broken down only by galactosylceramidase, the substance accumulates in brain, peripheral nerve, liver, and kidney. Galactosylsphingosine has profound cytotoxic effects, inhibiting mitochondrial functions and inducing a globoid cell response and the destruction of oligodendrocytes (440). With the disappearance of oligodendrocytes, cerebroside biosynthesis ceases and the formation of myelin is arrested.

The gene coding for galactocerebrosidase has been mapped to chromosome 14q23.3-q32. The gene has been cloned and more than 40 mutations have been documented. These include deletions of varying sizes and numerous point mutations. In general terms, a fair inverse correlation exists between the amount of residual galactocerebrosidase activity and the severity of the clinical manifestations. However, as is the case for ALD, and some of the disorders of lysosomal function, intrafamilial variability of clinical manifestations has been described (441), including symptomatic and asymptomatic siblings harboring the same genetic mutation (442). The factors responsible for this variability are still unknown.

Clinical Manifestations

Three clinical forms of Krabbe disease have been distinguished: the classic infantile form, the late infantile or juvenile form, and the adult form. In the infantile form, the disease begins acutely at 46 months of age with restlessness, irritability, and progressive stiffness. Convulsions can develop later. Frequently, these are tonic spasms induced by light, noise, or touch. Infants show increased muscular tone, with few spontaneous movements. Optic atrophy and hyperacusis are seen often. The deep tendon reflexes are characteristically difficult to elicit and can be absent in the legs. Terminally, infants are flaccid and develop bulbar signs (440).

A small proportion of patients has a later onset and slower evolution of their illness. Their neurologic symptoms include most commonly a slowly evolving spastic paraparesis. Less often the predominant symptoms include a motor and sensory neuropathy, hemiparesis, cerebellar ataxia, or cortical blindness (442).

Laboratory studies in the infantile form reveal a consistent elevation of CSF protein content. Conduction velocity of motor nerves is reduced. In the late-onset forms, both CSF protein and nerve conduction time can be normal (443). The MRI shows increased signal on T2-weighted images in the affected white matter, notably in the parietal lobes (418,419). In the late-onset Krabbe disease, the white matter lesions are more restricted and mainly affect the periventricular region, corpus callosum, or occipital lobes (442).

Diagnosis

The salient clinical diagnostic feature for the infantile form of globoid cell leukodystrophy is peripheral nerve involvement: depressed deep tendon reflexes, elevated CSF protein, and delayed nerve conduction in a deteriorating infant. Various other degenerative conditions present a clinical picture akin to Krabbe disease. In general, GM_2 gangliosidosis (Tay-Sachs disease) can be distinguished by the characteristic retinal changes. Juvenile amaurotic idiocy and MLD have a somewhat later onset. In the rare progressive degenerations of the gray matter, seizures tend to appear earlier and more frequently. The marked white matter involvement as seen on MRI and the near absence of serum, leukocyte, or skin fibroblast galactosylceramidase are probably the most defin-

itive tests. An antenatal diagnosis can be made by means of this enzymatic assay (440).

Treatment

Allogeneic bone marrow transplantation has arrested the anticipated evolution of neurologic signs in a number of patients with Krabbe disease. Nerve conduction studies improved, and the CSF protein levels decreased after hematopoietic stem cell transplantation (444). Entrance of donor-derived mononuclear cells into the CNS occurs over the course of several months to years. As a consequence, the procedure is much less effective in the rapidly progressive infantile form than in the more slowly developing late-onset forms (444). *In utero* bone marrow transplantation also has been attempted (445).

Other Hereditary Demyelinating Conditions

Several entities in which demyelination is part of the pathologic picture are mentioned here.

Cockayne Syndrome

Cockayne syndrome is one of several known disorders of DNA repair (446). This rare condition, transmitted as an autosomal recessive trait, was first described by Cockayne in 1936 (447). It is a progressive disorder, characterized by an unusual progeroid facies (large ears and sunken eyes), failure of growth first manifested after the second year of life, slowly progressive intellectual deterioration, lack of subcutaneous fat, pigmentary retinal degeneration, nerve deafness, and hypersensitivity of skin to sunlight (448,449). In the Turkish patients of Özdirim and colleagues, ocular abnormalities including cataracts, retinitis pigmentosa, optic atrophy, and miosis unresponsive to mydriatics was recorded in 88% of children (448). A peripheral neuropathy also has been demonstrated, and nerve conduction and brainstem auditory-evoked responses are abnormal (448,450). Radiographic examinations reveal thickening of the skull bones and kyphoscoliosis. Calcifications, particularly involving the basal ganglia are common. MRI reveals loss of white matter and white matter hyperintensity on T2-weighted images (448,450).

On pathologic examination, generally patchy demyelination and atrophy of white matter and cerebellum are seen. The brain can undergo perivascular calcification in the basal ganglia and cerebellum, changes termed a *calcifying vasopathy* (451).

The basic disorder in Cockayne syndrome has been localized to the nucleotide excision repair pathway, a process that is responsible for the removal from DNA of a variety of lesions, including those induced by ultraviolet light. Nucleotide excision repair is a six-step process requiring a large number of gene products. It recognizes and removes lesions from DNA by a dual incision around the lesion in the damaged strand along with flanking nucleotides. Excision is followed by repair synthesis using the undamaged strand as template and by ligation. As determined by hybridization in culture using cell fusion agents, seven excision-deficient complementation groups have been identified to date, of which at least two have the clinical picture of Cockayne syndrome (452). Skin fibroblasts derived from patients with Cockayne syndrome show marked sensitivity to ultraviolet light. This is the consequence of a specific defect in the repair of lesions in strands of actively transcribed genes (453). The precise nature of the defect in this process has not yet been established. The presence of the two complementation groups (Cockayne syndrome A and B) points to the existence of genetic defects at more than one step in the repair pathway. A mutation in CSB protein, which functions as an RNA polymerase elongation factor, has also been found (453a). It

is not clear why the nervous system is singled out for defects in conditions in which impaired DNA repair exists. This extremely complex area is covered in a review by Wood (454).

Except in the classic case, diagnosis of Cockayne syndrome is difficult. Not all patients have a photosensitive dermatitis, intracranial calcifications are seen only in some 40% to 50% of subjects, and optic atrophy is seen in approximately one-half. Even fibroblast ultraviolet sensitivity is not present invariably (455).

Cockayne syndrome is one of three neurologic disorders in which an abnormality in DNA repair has been documented. Ataxia-telangiectasia is considered in Chapter 11. Xeroderma pigmentosum is also a markedly heterogeneous condition, with several complementation groups. In this condition, there is also a defect in the nucleotide excision pathway (453). Xeroderma pigmentosum is characterized by a variety of cutaneous abnormalities in the areas of skin exposed to sunlight. Additionally, neurologic symptoms develop in 20% of subjects (456). These include progressive mental deterioration, microcephaly, ataxia, choreoathetosis, a sensorineural hearing loss, and a peripheral neuropathy (457,458). Some patients with xeroderma pigmentosum can present with physical and mental retardation, optic atrophy, retinitis pigmentosa, premature senility, and other clinical features of Cockayne syndrome (453).

Other Diseases of Cerebral White Matter

The widespread use of MRI in the evaluation of children with neurologic disorders, particularly

TABLE 2.11. *Newer forms of leukoencephalopathy*

Clinical picture	Magnetic resonance imaging result	Reference
High incidence in Asian Indians, megalencephaly, slowly progressive course	Extensive white matter changes out of proportion to clinical picture	van der Knaap et al. (460), Singhal et al. (461)
Normal early development, onset 1.5 to 5.0 years of age, episodic deterioration triggered by minor infections, head trauma, accompanied by coma	White matter signal indistinguishable from cerebrospinal fluid, massive cavitating leukodystrophy	van der Knaap et al. (462)
Autosomal dominant, macrocephaly, nonprogressive, nystagmus, spasticity	Obstructive hydrocephalus caused by cerebellar enlargement, abnormal cerebellar white matter, progressing to atrophy	Gripp et al. (463)
Delayed initial development, spasticity, normal head circumference or microcephaly	Cystic lesions in anterior temporal lobes, periventricular demyelination	Olivier et al. (463a)

those with intellectual deterioration, has resulted in the description of at least four groups of patients who demonstrate white matter changes compatible with a leukodystrophy, but whose clinical picture does not fall into any of the previously described categories (Table 2.11). These conditions are not rare. In the series of Kristjáns-dóttir and colleagues of 78 patients with MRI abnormalities that primarily involved white matter, only 32 could be given a specific diagnosis. In the remaining 46 children, the cause of the white matter abnormalities could not be ascertained. Of these children, 17 (37%) had a clearly progressive course, and 13 (28%) were stationary over the course of at least 3 years (459).

Chédiak-Higashi Syndrome

Chédiak-Higashi syndrome, first described by Chédiak in 1952 (464), is characterized by partial albinism with decreased pigmentation of hair and eyes, photophobia, nystagmus, hepatosplenomegaly, lymphadenopathy, and the presence of giant, peroxidase-positive granules in polymorphonuclear leukocytes. Abnormalities in platelet and leukocyte function result in recurrent and ultimately lethal pyogenic infections. A variety of neurologic symptoms can be found. These include cranial and peripheral neuropathies, a progressive spinocerebellar degeneration, and mental retardation (465,466). Intracytoplasmic inclusions within the neurons and perivascular infiltrations are found throughout the nervous system, most prominently in the pons and cerebellum. Similar infiltrations are seen in peripheral nerves (467). The gene for the condition has been mapped to chromosome 1 q42.1-42.2, and a number of mutations have been documented. The cause of the neurologic symptoms is still obscure. Allogenic bone marrow transplantation from an HLA-identical donor has resulted in long-term improvement in the susceptibility to bacterial infections. The effects on neurologic symptoms have not yet been documented (468).

Neuroaxonal Dystrophies (Seitelberger Disease)

Neuroaxonal dystrophies (Seitelberger disease), are rare degenerative disorders of the nervous system, which share a pathologic picture of focal axonal swelling in myelinated and non-myelinated central and peripheral nervous system axons. Several entities have been described, the most likely of which to be encountered is the late infantile form. As first documented by Seitelberger (469), it has its onset between 1 and 2 years of age. The clinical picture is marked by mixed upper and lower motor neuron signs; the pathologic picture is one of axonal swelling throughout the neuraxis (470).

Affected subjects develop neurologic abnormalities within the first 2 years of life. These include progressive weakness, hypotonia, and muscular atrophy accompanied by evidence of corticospinal tract involvement and anterior horn cell disease. Tendon reflexes are usually hyperactive, and urinary retention is common, as are disturbances of ocular mobility and optic atrophy (470). Convulsions are rare. The most characteristic finding on neuroimaging is a diffuse and prominent hyperintensity of the cerebellar cortex seen on T2-weighted MRI (471). This is accompanied by diffuse cerebellar atrophy. The diagnosis can best be made by biopsy of the peripheral nerves, which demonstrates globular swellings (neuroaxonal spheroids) along the course of the axons, particularly at the neuromuscular junction. Similar changes are seen in the peripheral nerve endings of conjunctivae and on skin biopsy (472). These are best seen by electron microscopy. In some cases, biopsy results of peripheral tissue were negative, and the diagnosis rested on brain biopsy (473).

The presence of neuroaxonal spheroids is, however, nonspecific. They also are seen in a juvenile form of neuroaxonal dystrophy that becomes symptomatic between 9 and 17 years of age (474).

Axonal swelling also is encountered in numerous other conditions. These include vitamin E deficiency, Hallervorden-Spatz disease, the olivopontocerebellar atrophies, FRDA, human T-cell lymphotropic virus 1 tropic myeloneuropathy, GM_1 and GM_2 gangliosidoses, α-N-acetylgalactosaminidase deficiency (Schindler disease), and the amyotrophic lateral sclerosis-Parkinson's-dementia complex seen on Guam. Additionally, Begeer and coworkers have observed that the clinical and pathologic pictures of neuroaxonal dystrophy and giant axonal neuropathy might overlap, in that peripheral nervous system involvement can be seen in some patients with neuroaxonal dystrophy, and CNS involvement can occur in some patients with giant axonal neuropathy (475).

Rett Syndrome

Rett syndrome is a unique and relatively common condition with an incidence of 1 in 10,000 to 1 in 15,000 girls, which places it second as a cause for mental retardation in females. Inasmuch as progressive dementia is one of its main features, it is considered in this chapter.

A syndrome of cerebral atrophy and hyperammonemia occurring exclusively in girls was first described by Rett in 1966 (476). Since then, it has become evident that hyperammonemia is present only rarely in these children, and that in fact characteristic laboratory abnormalities are absent.

Approximately 99.5% of cases of Rett syndrome are sporadic (477). However, the incidence of familial cases is higher than is expected by chance. Four sets of monozygotic twins have been recorded, all concordant for the disease, whereas of three sets of dizygotic twins reported, only one set was affected (478). The disease affects females almost exclusively. The gene for Rett syndrome has been localized to Xq28 (478a). Amir and coworkers have shown that in about one-quarter of sporadic patients there were mutations in the gene that encodes X-linked methyl-CpG-binding protein 2 (MeCP2) (479). This protein is one of three known proteins which selectively bind methylated DNA and mediate transcriptional repression (480,481). MeCP2 is widely expressed and is abundant in brain. Amir et al. propose that loss of function of this protein leads to overexpression of some genes which could be detrimental during the later stages of cerebral maturation (479).

Pathologic examination of the brain discloses diffuse cerebral atrophy with increased amounts of neuronal lipofuscin, and an underpigmentation of the substantia nigra. Neuronal size is reduced and cell-packing density is increased throughout the brain. These changes are most evident in the medial temporal lobe (482). Decreased length and complexity of dendritic branching in premotor front, motor, and limbic cortex is seen (483). Abnormalities also are seen in the cerebellum with reduced numbers of Purkinje cells (482). These pathologic changes are most consistent with a curtailment of brain maturation early in development, perhaps before birth (482). Immunochemical studies of microtubule-associated proteins, which are expressed during dendritic formation in embryonic mammalian brain, also suggest a disturbance in the early stages of neocortical maturation (477). Neurochemical studies and evaluation of patients with PET point to abnormalities in the cholinergic and the dopaminergic pathways (477). It is not known whether these changes are primary or secondary to abnormalities in neurotrophins.

The clinical picture is fairly characteristic and suggests the diagnosis (477,484). Although hypotonia is often noted, girls develop normally until 6 to 12 months of age. Thereafter, a deceleration in head growth and a clear developmental regression occur. Microcephaly develops, as do pyramidal tract signs, and an autisticlike behavior. One-third of children experience seizures, and almost all have abnormal EEG results. Purposive hand use is lost between 6 and 30 months; it is replaced by hand wringing or hand-to-mouth (handwashing) movements (Fig. 2.16) (485). Gait apraxia and truncal ataxia develop subsequently. Intermittent hyperventilation with a disorganized breathing pattern during the waking state is characteristic and is seen as early as 2 years of age (486). Neuroimaging shows little more than progressive cortical atrophy and hypoplasia of the corpus callosum, the latter probably secondary to neuronal reduction (487).

Rett syndrome allows prolonged survival. By the second decade of life, patients become stable. Seizures may subside, children may regain their ability to walk, their hand use improves, and they often have improved social interaction (477). Supportive care and active physical therapy have been fairly effective in preventing contractures. In our experience, treatment with carbamazepine, even in the absence of overt seizures, appears to improve alertness.

In the differential diagnosis of Rett syndrome, other conditions that induce a developmental regression coupled with seizures, cerebellar

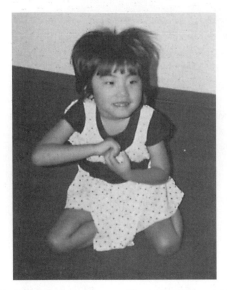

FIG. 2.16. Rett syndrome. The girl demonstrates the typical handwashing posture of the upper extremities.

signs, or autistic behavior have to be considered. These include some of the lipofuscinoses, Angelman syndrome, and the spinocerebellar degenerations. The characteristic loss of hand use, and the negative imaging studies and the negative biopsy results of conjunctivae and nerve assist in arriving at the diagnosis.

Diseases with Degeneration Primarily Affecting Gray Matter

Degenerative conditions that primarily affect cerebral gray matter are less common than those affecting white matter. Although clearly these entities do not represent a single genetic condition, they have in the past been referred to as *Alper syndrome* (488). The nature of the entities such as those described by Alpers in 1931 and by Ford and coworkers in 1951 (489) cannot be determined at the present time, but in retrospect one suspects that many were instances of metabolic defects, such as the mitochondrial encephalopathies.

In several forms of gray matter degeneration, the pathologic picture is unique. One of these conditions, which has aroused some interest, is intranuclear hyaline inclusion disease. This disor-

der is marked by slowly progressive pyramidal or extrapyramidal signs and mental deterioration. First symptoms appear between the ages of 3 and 12 years. Brainstem signs such as blepharospasm or cranial nerve palsies are common, as are oculogyric crises. Eosinophilic neuronal intranuclear inclusions are seen in neurons of the central and autonomic nervous system (145,490). Goutières and coworkers suggest rectal biopsy as a means of making a diagnosis during the patient's lifetime (491).

An autosomal recessive progressive neuronal degeneration with liver disease presents during the first year of life with developmental delay and failure to thrive. Seizures are prominent, and clinical and pathologic evidence of liver failure occurs (492,493). One such patient had a marked depletion of mitochondria in skeletal muscle, and no detectable activity of liver and muscle mitochondrial DNA polymerase γ (494). Because many children suffering from this condition have been placed on valproate for control of their seizures, this degenerative disease can mimic valproate-induced hepatic encephalopathy.

REFERENCES

1. Lupski JR, Zoghbi HY. Molecular genetics and neurologic disease: an introduction. In: Rosenberg RN, et al. *The molecular and genetic basis of neurological disease*. 2nd ed. Boston: Butterworth–Heinemann, 1997:3–22.
2. Collins FS. Positional cloning moves from perditional to traditional. *Nat Gen* 1995;9:347–350.
3. Bruyn GW. Huntington's chorea—historical, clinical and laboratory synopsis. In: Vinken PJ, Bruyn GW, eds. *Handbook of neurology: diseases of the basal ganglia.* Amsterdam: North-Holland Publishing Co., 1968.
4. Huntington G. On chorea. *Med Surg Rep* 1872;26: 317–321.
5. Conneally PM. Huntington's disease: genetics and epidemiology. *Am J Hum Genet* 1984;36:506–526.
6. Tellez-Nagel I, Johnson AB, Terry RB. Studies on brain biopsies of patients with Huntington's chorea. *J Neuropathol Exp Neurol* 1974;33:308–332.
7. Bruyn GW, Bots GTAM, Dom R. Huntington's chorea: current neuropathological status. *Adv Neurol* 1979;23:83–93.
8. Jervis GA. Huntington's chorea in childhood. *Arch Neurol* 1963;9:244–257.
9. Markham CH, Knox JW. Observations in Huntington's chorea. *J Pediatr* 1965;67:46–57.
10. Carlier G, et al. Etude anatomoclinique d'une forme infantile de la maladie de Huntington. *Acta Neurol Belg* 1974;74:36–63.

11. Richfield EK, et al. Preferential loss of pre-proenkephalin versus preprotachykinin neurons from the striatum of Huntington's disease patients. *Ann Neurol* 1995;38: 852–861.

12. Calabresi P, et al. Striatal spiny neurons and cholinergic interneurons express differential ionotropic glutamatergic responses and vulnerability: implications for ischemia and Huntington's disease. *Ann Neurol* 1998;43:586–597.

13. Albin RL. Selective neurodegeneration in Huntington's disease. *Ann Neurol* 1995;38:4835–4836.

14. Storey E, et al. The cortical lesion of Huntington's disease: further neurochemical characterization and reproduction of some of the histological and neurochemical features by *N*-methyl-D-aspartate lesions of rat cortex. *Ann Neurol* 1992;32: 526–534.

15. Sotrell A, et al. Evidence for neuronal degeneration and dendritic plasticity in cortical pyramidal neurons of Huntington's disease: a quantitative Golgi study. *Neurology* 1993;43:2088–2096.

16. Gusella JF, et al. A polymorphic DNA marker genetically linked to Huntington's disease. *Nature* 1983;306: 234–238.

17. Sapp E, et al. Huntington localization in brains of normal and Huntington's disease patients. *Ann Neurol* 1997;42:604–612.

18. Duyao MP, et al. Inactivation of the mouse Huntington's disease gene homologue Hdh. *Science* 1995;269: 407–410.

19. The Huntington's Disease Collaborative Research Group. A novel gene containing a trinucleotide repeat that is expanded and unstable on Huntington's disease chromosomes. *Cell* 1993;72:971–983.

20. Duyao MP, et al. Trinucleotide repeat length instability and age of onset in Huntington's disease. *Nat Genet* 1993;4:387–392.

21. Myers RH, et al. De novo expansion of a $(CAG)_n$ repeat in sporadic Huntington's disease. *Nat Genet* 1993;5:168–173.

22. Richards RI, Sutherland GR. Simple repeat DNA is not replicated simply. *Nat Genet* 1994;6:114–116.

23. La Spada AR, et al. Trinucleotide repeat expansion in neurological disease. *Ann Neurol* 1994;36:814–822.

24. Fraser FC. Trinucleotide repeats not the only cause of anticipation. *Lancet* 1997;350:459–460.

25. Gourfinkel-An I, et al. Differential distribution of the normal and mutated forms of Huntington in the human brain. *Ann Neurol* 1997;42:712–719.

25a. Alves-Rodrigues A, Gregori L, Figueiredo-Pereira ME. Ubiquitin, cellular inclusions and their role in neurodegeneration. *Trends Neurosci* 1998;21:516–520.

26. Faber PW, et al. Huntington interacts with a family of WW domain proteins. *Hum Mol Genet* 1998;7: 1463–1474.

27. Lin YF. Expression of polyglutamine-expanded Huntington activates the SEK1-JNK pathway and induces apoptosis in a hippocampal neuronal line. *J Biol Chem* 1998;273:28873–28877.

27a. Saudou F, et al. Huntingtin acts in the nucleus to induce apoptosis but death does not correlate with the formation of intranuclear inclusions *Cell* 1998; 95:55–66.

28. Beal MF, et al. Replication of the neurochemical characteristics of Huntington's disease by quinolinic acid. *Nature* 1986;321:168–171.

29. Choi DW. Ionic dependence of glutamate neurotoxicity. *J Neurosci* 1987;7:369–379.

30. Young AB, et al. NMDA receptor losses in putamen from patients with Huntington's disease. *Science* 1988;241:981–983.

30a. Tabrizi SJ, et al. Biochemical abnormalities and excitotoxicity in Huntington's disease brain. *Ann Neurol* 1999;45:25–32.

31. Myers RH, et al. Maternal factors in onset of Huntington's disease. *Am J Hum Genet* 1985;37:511–523.

32. Hayden MR, Soles JA, Ward RH. Age of onset in siblings of persons with juvenile Huntington's disease. *Clin Genet* 1985;28:100–105.

33. Cotton JB, et al. La maladie de Huntington chez l'enfant: a propos d'une observation anatomoclinique. *Pediatrie* 1975;30:609–619.

34. Siesling S, Vegter-van der Vlis M, Roos RA. Juvenile Huntington's disease in the Netherlands. *Pediatr Neurol* 1997;17:37–43.

35. Haslam RHA, Curry B, Johns R. Infantile Huntington's disease. *Can J Neurol Sci* 1983;10:200–203.

36. van Dijk JB, et al. Juvenile Huntington's disease. *Hum Genet* 1986;73:235–239.

37. Katafuchi Y, et al. A childhood form of Huntington's disease associated with marked pyramidal signs. *Eur Neurol* 1984;23:296–299.

38. Myers RH, et al. Clinical and neuropathologic assessment of severity in Huntington's disease. *Neurology* 1988;38:341–347.

39. Young AB, et al. Huntington's disease in Venezuela: neurologic features and functional decline. *Neurology* 1986;36:244–249.

40. Simmons JT, et al. Magnetic resonance imaging in Huntington's disease. *Am J Neuroradiol* 1986;7:25–28.

41. Mazziotta JC, et al. Reduced cerebral glucose metabolism in asymptomatic subjects at risk for Huntington's disease. *N Engl J Med* 1987;316:357–362.

42. Laurence AD, et al. The relationship between striatal dopamine receptor binding and cognitive performance in Huntington's disease. *Brain* 1998; 121:1343–1355.

43. ACMG/ASHG Statement. Laboratory guidelines for Huntington disease genetic testing. *The American College of Medical Genetics/American Society of Human Genetics Huntington Disease Genetic Testing Working Group* 1998;62:1243–1247.

44. Kremer B, et al. A worldwide study of the Huntington's disease mutation. The sensitivity and specificity of measuring CAG repeats. *N Engl J Med* 1994; 330: 1401–1406.

45. World Federation of Neurology—Committee of the International Huntington's Association and the World Federation of Neurology. Ethical issues policy statement on Huntington's disease molecular genetics predictive test. *J Med Genet* 1990;27:34–38.

46. Stapert JLRH, et al. Benign (nonparoxysmal) familial chorea of early onset: an electroneurophysiological examination of two families. *Brain Dev* 1985;7: 38–42.

47. Feinberg TE, et al. Diagnostic tests for choreoacanthocytosis. *Neurology* 1991;41:100–106.

48. Orrell RW, et al. Acanthocytosis, retinitis pigmentosa, and pallidal degeneration: a report of three patients, including the second reported case with hypoprebetalipoproteinemia (HARP syndrome). *Neurology* 1995; 45:487–492.

49. Hardie RJ, et al. Neuroacanthocytosis: a clinical, haematological and pathological study of 19 cases. *Brain* 1991;114:13–49.
50. Shibasaki H, et al. Involuntary movements in chorea-acanthocytosis: a comparison with Huntington's chorea. *Ann Neurol* 1982;12:311–314.
51. Brooks DJ, et al. Presynaptic and postsynaptic striatal dopaminergic function in neuroacanthocytosis: a positron emission tomographic study. *Ann Neurol* 1991;30:166–171.
52. Schwalbe MW. *Eine eigentuehmliche, tonische Krampfform mit hysterischen Symptomen,* Inaug Dissert Berlin: G. Schade, 1908.
53. Oppenheim H. Ueber eine eigenartige Krampfkrankheit des kindlichen und jugentlichen Alters (dysbasia lordotica progressiva, dystonia musculorum deformans). *Neurol Centralbl* 1911; 30:1090–1107.
54. Ozelius LJ, et al. The early-onset torsion dystonia gene (DYT1) encodes an ATP-binding protein. *Nat Genet* 1997;17:40–48.
55. Gimenez-Roldan S, et al. Hereditary torsion dystonia in gypsies. *Adv Neurol* 1988;50:73–91.
56. Lee LV, et al. The phenotype of the X-linked dystonia-parkinsonism syndrome: an assessment of 42 cases in the Philippines. *Medicine* 1991;70: 179–187.
57. Ahmad F, et al. Evidence for locus heterogeneity in autosomal dominant torsion dystonia. *Genomics* 1993;15:9–12.
58. Nygaard TG, Marsden CD, Fahn S. Dopa-responsive dystonia: long-term treatment response and prognosis. *Neurology* 1991;41:174–181.
59. Knappskog PM, et al. Recessively inherited L-DOPA-responsive dystonia caused by a point mutation (Q381K) in the tyrosine hydroxylase gene. *Hum Mol Genet* 1995;4:1209–1212.
59a. Klein C, et al. De novo mutations (GAG deletion) in the DYT1 gene in two non-Jewish patients with early-onset dystonia. *Hum Mol Genet* 1998;7:1133–1136.
59b. Lebre AS, et al. DYT1 mutation in French families with idiopathic torsion dystonia. *Brain* 1999;122:41–45.
59c. Vitek JL, et al. Neuronal activity in the basal ganglia in patients with generalized dystonia and hemiballismus. *Ann Neurol* 1999;46:22–35.
60. Almasy L, et al. Idiopathic torsion dystonia linked to chromosome 8 in two Mennonite families. *Ann Neurol* 1997;42:670–673.
61. Leube B, et al. Idiopathic torsion dystonia: assignment of a gene to chromosome 18p in a German family with adult onset, autosomal dominant inheritance and purely focal distribution. *Hum Mol Genet* 1996;5: 1673–1677.
62. Hayes MW, et al. X-linked dystonia-deafness syndrome. *Mov Disord* 1998;13:303–308.
63. Mostofsky SH, et al. Autosomal dominant torsion dystonia with onset in infancy. *Pediatr Neurol* 1996;15: 245–248.
64. Berardelli A, et al. The pathophysiology of primary dystonia. *Brain* 1998;121:1195–1212.
65. Eidelberg D, et al. Functional brain networks in DYT1 dystonia. *Ann Neurol* 1998;44:303–312.
66. Marsden CD, et al. The anatomical basis of symptomatic hemidystonia. *Brain* 1985;108:463–483.
67. Zeman W. Dystonia: an overview. *Adv Neurol* 1976;14:91–103.
68. Cook DG, Fahn S, Brait KA. Chronic manganese intoxication. *Arch Neurol* 1974;30:59–64.
69. Fahn S. Concept and classification of dystonia. *Adv Neurol* 1988;50:1–8.
70. Gasser T, Fahn S, Breakefield XO. The autosomal dominant dystonias. *Brain Pathol* 1992;2:297–308.
71. Bird TD. Penetrating observations of dystonia. *Ann Neurol* 1998;44:299–300.
72. Marsden CD, Harrison MJG, Bundey S. Natural history of idiopathic torsion dystonia. *Adv Neurol* 1976;14:177–187.
73. Marsden CD, Harrison MJG. Idiopathic torsion dystonia: a review of 42 patients. *Brain* 1974;97: 793–810.
74. Bressman SB, et al. Clinical-genetic spectrum of primary dystonia. *Adv Neurol* 1998;78:79–91.
75. Karbe H, et al. Positron emission tomography demonstrates frontal cortex and basal ganglia hypometabolism in dystonia. *Neurology* 1992;42:1540–1544.
76. Sheehy MP, Marsden CD. Writer's cramp–a focal dystonia. *Brain* 1982;105:461–480.
77. Segawa M, et al. Hereditary progressive dystonia with marked diurnal fluctuation. *Adv Neurol* 1976;14: 215–233.
77a. Furukawa Y, et al. Dystonia with motor delay in compound heterozygotes for GTP-cyclohydrolase I gene mutations. *Ann Neurol* 1998;44:10–16.
78. Pueschel SM, Friedman JH, Shetty T. Myoclonic dystonia. *Childs Nerv Syst* 1992;8:61–66.
79. Hansen RA, Berenberg W, Byers RK. Changing motor patterns in cerebral palsy. *Dev Med Child Neurol* 1970;12:309–314.
80. Burke RE, Fahn S, Gold AP. Delayed onset dystonia in patients with "static" encephalopathy. *J Neurol Neurosurg Psychiatry* 1980;43:789–797.
81. Goetting MG. Acute lithium poisoning in a child with dystonia. *Pediatrics* 1985;76:978–980.
82. Schott GD. Induction of involuntary movements by peripheral trauma: an analogy with causalgia. *Lancet* 1986;2:712–716.
83. Trauma and dystonia [Editorial]. *Lancet* 1989;1: 759–760.
84. Burke RE, Fahn S, Marsden CD. Torsion dystonia: a double-blind, prospective trial of high-dosage trihexyphenidyl. *Neurology* 1986;36:160–164.
85. Jankovic J, Beach J. Long-term effects of tetrabenazine in hyperkinetic movement disorders. *Neurology* 1997;48:358–362.
86. Marsden CD, Marion MH, Quinn N. The treatment of severe dystonia in children and adults. *J Neurol Neurosurg Psychiatry* 1984;47:1166–1173.
87. Greene PE, Fahn S. Baclofen in the treatment of idiopathic dystonia in children. *Mov Disord* 1992;7:48–52.
88. Ondo WG, et al. Pallidotomy for generalized dystonia. *Mov Disord* 1998;13:693–698.
89. Andrew J, Fowler CJ, Harrison MJG. Stereotaxic thalamotomy in 55 cases of dystonia. *Brain* 1983;106: 981–1000.
89a. Krauss JK, et al. Bilateral stimulation of globus pallidus internus for treatment of cervical dystonia. *Lancet* 1999;354:837–838.
90. Singer HS. Tardive dyskinesia: a concern for the pediatrician. *Pediatrics* 1986;77:553–556.
91. Kumra S, et al. Case series: spectrum of neuroleptic-induced movement disorders and extrapyramidal side

effects in childhood-onset schizophrenia. *J Am Acad Child Adolesc Psychiatry* 1998;37:221–227.

92. Campbell M, et al. Neuroleptic-related dyskinesias in autistic children: a prospective, longitudinal study. *J Am Acad Child Adolesc Psychiatry* 1997;36: 835–843.

93. Joshi PT, Capozzoli JA, Coyle JT. Neuroleptic malignant syndrome: life-threatening complication of neuroleptic treatment in adolescents with affective disorders. *Pediatrics* 1991;87:235–239.

94. Goulon M, et al. Beneficial effects of dantrolene in the treatment of neuroleptic malignant syndrome. *Neurology* 1988;33:516–518.

95. Hallervorden J, Spatz H. Erkrankung im System mit besonderer Beteilung des Globus Pallidus und der Substantia Nigra. *Z Ges Neurol Psychiat* 1922;79: 254–302.

96. Halliday W. The nosology of Hallervorden-Spatz disease. *J Neurol Sci* 1995;134[Suppl]:84–91.

97. Nakai H, Landing BH, Schubert WK. Seitelberger's spastic amaurotic axonal idiocy: report of a case in a 9 year old boy with comment on visceral manifestations. *Pediatrics* 1960;25:441–449.

98. Park BE, Netsky MG, Betsill WL. Pathogenesis of pigment and spheroid formation in Hallervorden-Spatz syndrome and related disorders. *Neurology* 1975;25:1172–1178.

99. Vakili S, et al. Hallervorden-Spatz syndrome. *Arch Neurol* 1977;34:729–738.

100. Taylor TD, et al. Homozygosity mapping of Hallervorden-Spatz syndrome to chromosome 20p12.3-p13. *Nat Genet* 1996;14:479–481.

101. Perry TL, et al. Hallervorden–Spatz disease: cysteine accumulation and cysteine dioxygenase deficiency in the globus pallidus. *Ann Neurol* 1985;18: 482–489.

102. Dooling EC, Schoene WC, Richardson EP, Jr. Hallervorden-Spatz syndrome. *Arch Neurol* 1974;30:70–83.

103. Swaiman KF. Hallervorden-Spatz syndrome and brain iron metabolism. *Arch Neurol* 1991;48: 1285–1293.

104. Newell FW, Johnson RO, Huttenlocher PR. Pigmentary degeneration of the retina in Hallervorden-Spatz syndrome. *Am J Ophthalmol* 1979;88:467–471.

105. Savoiardo M, et al. Hallervorden-Spatz disease: MR and pathologic findings. *Am J Neuroradiol* 1993;14:155–162.

106. Sehti KD, et al. Hallervorden-Spatz syndrome: clinical and magnetic resonance imaging correlations. *Ann Neurol* 1988;24:692–694.

107. Swisher CN, et al. Coexistence of Hallervorden-Spatz disease with acanthocytosis. *Trans Am Neurol Assoc* 1972;97:212.

108. Higgins JJ, et al. Hypoprebetalipoproteinemia, acanthocytosis, retinitis pigmentosa, and pallidal degeneration (HARP syndrome). *Neurology* 1992;42:194–198.

109. Swaiman KF, et al. Sea-blue histiocytes, lymphocytic cytosomes, movement disorder and ^{59}Fe-uptake in basal ganglia: Hallervorden-Spatz disease or ceroid storage disease with abnormal isotope scan? *Neurology* 1983;33:301–305.

110. Bamberger H. Beobachtungen und Bemerkungen über Hirnkrankheiten. *Verh Phys Med Ges (Würzburg)*1885; 6:325–328.

111. Fahr T. Idiopatische Verkalkung der Hirngefässe. *Zentralbl Allg Pathol Pathol Anat* 1930;50:129–133.

112. Billard C, et al. Encephalopathy with calcifications of the basal ganglia in children: a reappraisal of Fahr's syndrome with respect to 14 new cases. *Neuropediatrics* 1989;20:12–19.

113. Melchior JC, Benda CE, Yakovlev PI. Familial idiopathic cerebral calcifications in childhood. *Am J Dis Child* 1960;99:787–803.

114. Aicardi J, Goutières F. A progressive encephalopathy in infancy with calcifications of the basal ganglia and chronic cerebrospinal fluid lymphocytosis. *Ann Neurol* 1984;15:49–54.

114a. Goutières F, et al. Aicardi-Goutières syndrome: an update and results of interferon-α studies. *Ann Neurol* 1998;44:900–907.

115. McEntagart M, et al. Aicardi-Goutières syndrome: an expanding phenotype. *Neuropediatrics* 1998;29: 163–167.

116. Boller F, Boller M, Gilbert J. Familial idiopathic cerebral calcifications. *J Neurol Neurosurg Psychiatry* 1977;40:280–285.

117. Moskowitz MA, Winickoff RN, Heinz ER. Familial calcification of the basal ganglions: a metabolic and genetic study. *N Engl J Med* 1971;285:72–77.

118. Okada J, et al. Familial basal ganglia calcifications visualized by computerized tomography. *Acta Neurol Scand* 1981;64:273–279.

119. Jervis GA. Microcephaly with extensive calcium deposits and demyelination. *J Neuropath Exp Neurol* 1954;13:318–329.

120. Marasco JA, Feczko WA. Basal ganglia calcification in Down's syndrome. *Comp Tomogr* 1979;3:111–113.

121. Harrington MG, et al. The significance of the incidental finding of basal ganglia calcification on computed tomography. *J Neurol Neurosurg Psychiatry* 1981;44: 1168–1170.

122. Marsden CD, Obeso J, Rothwell JC. Benign essential tremor is not a single entity. In: Yahr MD, ed. *Current Concepts in Parkinson's Disease*. Amsterdam: Excerpta Medica, 1983:31–46.

123. Koller WC, et al. The relationship of essential tremor to other movement disorders: report on 678 patients. *Ann Neurol* 1994;35:717–723.

124. Critchley M. Observation on essential (heredofamilial) tremor. *Brain* 1949;72:113–139.

125. Vanasse M, Bedard P, Andermann F. Shuddering attacks in children: an early clinical manifestation of essential tremor. *Neurology* 1976;26: 1027–1030.

126. Higgins JJ, Pho LT, Nee LE. A gene (ETM) for essential tremor maps to chromosome 2p22-p25. *Mov Disord* 1997;12:859–864.

127. Gulcher JR, et al. Mapping of a familial essential tremor gene, FET1, to chromosome 3q13. *Nat Genet* 1997;17:84–87.

128. Findlay LJ, Koller WC. Essential tremor: a review. *Neurology* 1987;37:1194–1197.

129. Jenkins IH, et al. A positron emission tomography study of essential tremor: evidence for overactivity of cerebellar connections. *Ann Neurol* 1993;34:82–90.

130. Barron TF, Younkin DP. Propanolol therapy for shuddering attacks. *Neurology* 1992;42:258–259.

131. Calzetti S, et al. Controlled study of metopronol and propanolol during prolonged administration in patients with essential tremor. *J Neurol Neurosurg Psychiatry* 1983;45:893–897.

132. Koller WC, Royse VL. Efficacy of primidone in essential tremor. *Neurology* 1986;36:121–124.

133. Lakie M, et al. Effect of stereotactic thalamic lesion on essential tremor. *Lancet* 1992;340:206–207.

134. Trenkwalder C, Bucher SF, Oertel WH. Electrophysiological pattern of involuntary limb movements in the restless legs syndrome. *Muscle Nerve* 1996;19:155–162.

135. Walters AS, et al. Restless legs syndrome in childhood and adolescence. *Pediatr Neurol* 1994;11:241–245.

136. Hunt JR. Progressive atrophy of the globus pallidus. (Primary atrophy of the pallidal system.) A system disease of the paralysis agitans type, characterized by atrophy of the motor cells of the corpus striatum: a contribution to the functions of the corpus striatum. *Brain* 1917;40:58–148.

137. Polymeropoulos MH, et al. Mapping of a gene for Parkinson's disease to chromosome 4q21-q23. *Science* 1996;274:1197–1199.

138. Nussbaum RL, Polymeropoulos MH. Genetics of Parkinson's disease. *Hum Mol Genet* 1997;6: 1687–1691.

139. Conway KA, Harper JD, Lansbury PT. Accelerated in vitro fibril formation by a mutant alpha-synuclein linked to early-onset Parkinson's disease. *Nat Med* 1998;4:1318–1320.

139a. Gasser T, et al. A susceptibility locus for Parkinson's disease maps to chromosome 2p13. *Nat Genet* 1998;18:262–265.

140. Jones AC, et al. Autosomal recessive juvenile parkinsonism maps to 6q25.2-q27 in four ethnic groups: detailed genetic mapping of the linked region. *Am J Hum Genet* 1998;63:80–87.

141. Kitada T, et al. Mutations in the Parkin gene cause autosomal recessive juvenile parkinsonism. *Nature* 1998;392:605–608.

141a. Hattori N, et al. Molecular genetic analysis of a novel Parkin gene in Japanese families with autosomal recessive juvenile parkinsonism: evidence for variable homozygous deletions in the Parkin gene in affected individuals. *Ann Neurol* 1998;44:935–941.

141b. Abbas N, et al. A wide variety of mutations in the Parkin gene are responsible for autosomal recessive parkinsonism in Europe. *Hum Mol Genet* 1999;8: 567–574.

142. Ishikawa A, Tsuji S. Clinical analysis of 17 patients in 12 Japanese families with autosomal-recessive type juvenile parkinsonism. *Neurology* 1996;47: 160–166.

143. Takahashi H, et al. Familial juvenile parkinsonism: clinical and pathologic study in a family. *Neurology* 1994;44:437–441.

144. Dwork AJ, et al. Dominantly inherited, early-onset parkinsonism: neuropathology of a new form. *Neurology* 1993;43:69–74.

145. Haltia M, et al. Neuronal intranuclear inclusion disease in identical twins. *Ann Neurol* 1984;15:316–321.

146. Dobyns WB, et al. Rapid-onset dystonia-parkinsonism. *Neurology* 1993;43:2596–2602.

147. de la Tourette G. Etude sur une affection nerveuse, characterisée par de l'incoordination motrice, accompagnée d'echolalie et de coprolalie. *Arch Neurol (Paris)* 1885;9:158–200.

148. Walkup JT, et al. Family study and segregation analysis of Tourette's syndrome: evidence for a mixed model of inheritance. *Am J Hum Genet* 1996;59:684–693.

149. Pulst S, Walshe TM, Romero JA. Carbon monoxide poisoning with features of Gilles de la Tourette's syndrome. *Arch Neurol* 1983;40:443–444.

149a. Singer HS, et al. Antibodies against human putamen in children with Tourette's syndrome. *Neurology* 1998; 50:1618–1624.

150. Wong DF, et al. D2-like dopamine receptor density in Tourette's syndrome measured by PET. *J Nucl Med* 1997;38:1243–1247.

151. Haber SN, et al. Gilles de la Tourette's syndrome: a postmortem neuropathological and immunohistochemical study. *J Neurol Sci* 1986;75:225–241.

152. Singer HS, et al. Tourette's syndrome: a neurochemical analysis of postmortem cortical brain tissue. *Ann Neurol* 1990;27:443–446.

153. Singer HS, et al. Volumetric MRI changes in basal ganglia of children with Tourette's syndrome. *Neurology* 1993;43:950–956.

154. Burd L, et al. A prevalence study of Gilles de la Tourette's syndrome in North Dakota school-age children. *J Am Acad Child Adolesc Psychiatry* 1980; 25: 552–553.

155. Ehrenberg G, Cruse RP, Rothner AD. Tourette's syndrome: an analysis of 200 pediatric and adolescent cases. *Clev Clin Q* 1986;53:127–131.

156. Golden GS. Tics and Tourette's: a continuum of symptoms? *Ann Neurol* 1978;4:145–148.

157. Chase TN, Friedhoff AJ, Cohen DJ, eds. Tourette syndrome: genetics, neurobiology, and treatment. *Adv Neurol* 1992;58.

158. Lowe TL, et al. Stimulant medications precipitate Tourette's syndrome. *JAMA* 1982;247:1729–1731.

159. Glaze DG, Frost JD, Jankovic J. Sleep in Gilles de la Tourette's syndrome: disorder of arousal. *Neurology* 1983;33:586–592.

160. Leckman JF, et al. Short-and long-term treatment of Tourette's syndrome with clonidine: a clinical perspective. *Neurology* 1985;35:343–351.

161. Shapiro AK, Shapiro E, Fulop G. Pimozide treatment of tic and Tourette disorders. *Pediatrics* 1987;79:1032–1039.

162. Regeur L, et al. Clinical features and long-term treatment with pimozide in 65 patients with Gilles de la Tourette's syndrome. *J Neurol Neurosurg Psychiatry* 1986;49:791–795.

163. Sallee FR, et al. Relative efficacy of haloperidol and pimozide in children and adolescents with Tourette's disorder. *Am J Psychiatr* 1997;154:1057–1062.

164. Goetz CG, et al. Clonidine and Gilles de la Tourette's syndrome: double-blind study using objective rating methods. *Ann Neurol* 1987;21:307–310.

165. Leckman JF, et al. Rebound phenomenon in Tourette's syndrome after abrupt withdrawal of clonidine. *Arch Gen Psychiatry* 1986;43:1168–1176.

166. Mount LA, Reback S. Familial paroxysmal choreoathetosis. *Arch Neurol Psychiatr* 1940;44:841–847.

167. Goodenough DJ, et al. Familial and acquired paroxysmal dyskinesias. *Arch Neurol* 1978;35:827–831.

168. Bressman SB, Fahn S, Burke RE. Paroxysmal nonkinesigenic dystonia. *Adv Neurol* 1988;50:403–413.

169. Lance JW. Familial paroxysmal dystonic choreoathetosis and its differentiation from related syndromes. *Ann Neurol* 1977;2:285–293.

170. Demirkiran M, Jankovic J. Paroxysmal dyskinesias: clinical features and classification. *Ann Neurol* 1995;38:571–579.

171. Homan RW, Vasko MR, Blaw M. Phenytoin concentrations in paroxysmal kinesigenic choreoathetosis. *Neurology* 1980;30:673–676.

172. Raskind WH, et al. Further localization of a gene for paroxysmal dystonic choreoathetosis to a 5-cM region on chromosome 2q34. *Hum Genet* 1998;102:93–97.

173. Pryles CV, Livingston S, Ford FR. Familial paroxysmal choreoathetosis of Mount and Reback: study of a second family in which this condition is found in association with epilepsy. *Pediatrics* 1952;9: 44–47.

174. Rosen JA. Paroxysmal choreoathetosis. *Arch Neurol* 1964;11:385–387.

175. Auburger G, et al. A gene for autosomal dominant paroxysmal choreoathetosis/spasticity (CSE) maps to the vicinity of a potassium channel gene cluster on chromosome 1p, probably within 2 cm between D1S443 and D1S197. *Genomics* 1996;31:90–94.

176. Angelini L, et al. Transient paroxysmal dystonia in infancy. *Neuropediatrics* 1988;19:171–174.

177. Stevens H. Paroxysmal choreoathetosis. *Arch Neurol* 1966;14:415–420.

178. Lingam S, Wilson J, Hart EW. Hereditary stiff-baby syndrome. *Ann Neurol* 1980;8:195–197.

179. Andermann F, et al. Startle disease or hyperekplexia: further delineation of the syndrome. *Brain* 1980;103: 985–997.

180. Stevens H. Jumping Frenchmen of Maine. *Arch Neurol* 1965;12:311–314.

181. Wilkins DE, Hallet M, Wess MM. Audiogenic startle reflex of man and its relationship to startle syndromes. *Brain* 1986;109:561–573.

182. Ryan SG, et al. Startle disease or hyperexplexia: response to clonazepam and assignment of the gene (STHE) to chromosome 5q by linkage analysis. *Ann Neurol* 1992;31:663–668.

183. Shiang R, et al. Mutations in the α1 subunit of the inhibitory glycine receptor cause the dominant neurologic disorder, hyperexplexia. *Nat Genet* 1993;5: 351–357.

183a. Vergouwe MN, et al. Hyperekplexia phenotype due to compound heterozygosity for GLRA1 gene mutations. *Ann Neurol* 1999;46:634–638.

184. Johnson LF, Kinsbourne M, Renuart AW. Hereditary chin-trembling with nocturnal myoclonus and tongue-biting in dizygous twins. *Dev Med Child Neurol* 1971;13:726–729.

185. Gordon K, Cadera W, Hinton G. Successful treatment of hereditary trembling chin with botulinum toxin. *J Child Neurol* 1993;8:154–156.

186. Friedreich N. Ueber degenerative Atrophie der spinalen Hinterstränge. *Virchows Arch Path Anat* 1863;26: 391–419.

187. Campuzano V, et al. Friedreich's ataxia: autosomal recessive disease caused by an intronic GAA triplet repeat expansion. *Science* 1996;271:1423–1427.

187a. Cossée M, et al. Friedreich's ataxia: point mutations and clinical presentation of compound heterozygotes. *Ann Neurol* 1999;45:200–206.

188. Dürr A, et al. Clinical and genetic abnormalities in patients with Friedreich's ataxia. *N Engl J Med* 1996;335:1169–1175.

189. Montermini L, et al. Phenotypic variability in Friedreich's ataxia: role of the associated GAA triplet repeat expansion. *Ann Neurol* 1997;41:675–682.

190. Rotig A, et al. Aconitase and mitochondrial iron-sulphur protein deficiency in Friedreich's ataxia. *Nat Genet* 1997;17:215–217.

191. Klockgether T, Evert B. Genes involved in hereditary ataxias. *Trends Neurosci* 1998;21:413–418.

191a. Pandolfo M. Molecular pathogenesis of Friedreich Ataxia. *Arch Neurol* 1999;56:1201–1208.

192. Bidchandani SI, Ashikawa T, Patel PI. The GAA triplet-repeat expansion Friedreich's ataxia interferes with transcription and may be associated with an unusual DNA structure. *Am J Hum Genet* 1998;62: 111–121.

193. Blass JP, Kark RAP, Menon NK. Low activities of the pyruvate and oxoglutarate dehydrogenase complexes in five patients with Friedreich's ataxia. *N Engl J Med* 1976;295:62–67.

194. Greenfield JG. *The spino-cerebellar degenerations*, Oxford: Blackwell, 1954.

195. Oppenheimer DR. Brain lesions in Friedreich's ataxia. *Can J Neurol Sci* 1979;6:173–176.

196. Robinson N. Chemical changes in the spinal cord in Friedreich's ataxia and motor neuron disease. *J Neurol Neurosurg Psychiatry* 1968;31:330–333.

197. Harding AE. *The hereditary ataxias and related disorders,* Edinburgh: Churchill Livingstone, 1984.

197a. Higgins JJ, Morton H, Loveless JM. Posterior column ataxia with retinitis pigmentosa (AXPC1) maps to chromosome 1q31-q32. *Neurology* 1999;52:146–150.

197b. Higgins JJ, et al. An autosomal recessive disorder with posterior column ataxia and retinitis pigmentosa. *Neurology* 1997;49:1717–1729.

198. Harding AE. Friedreich's ataxia: a clinical and genetic study of 90 families with an analysis of early diagnostic criteria and intrafamilial clustering of clinical features. *Brain* 1981;104:589–620.

199. De Michele G, et al. Childhood onset of Friedreich's ataxia: a clinical and genetic study of 36 cases. *Neuropediatrics* 1996;27:3–7.

200. Carroll WM, et al. The incidence and nature of visual pathway involvement in Friedreich's ataxia. *Brain* 1980;103:413–434.

201. van Bogaert L, Martin L. Optic cochleovestibular degeneration in the hereditary ataxias. I. Clinico-pathological and genetic aspects. *Brain* 1974;97: 15–40.

202. Jones SJ, Baraitser M, Halliday AM. Peripheral and central somatosensory nerve conduction defects in Friedreich's ataxia. *J Neurol Neurosurg Psychiatry* 1980;43:495–503.

203. Boyer SH, Chisholm AW, McKusick VA. Cardiac aspects of Friedreich's ataxia. *Circulation* 1962;25: 493–505.

204. Schols L, et al. Friedreich's ataxia: revision of the phenotype according to molecular genetics. *Brain* 1997;120: 2131–2140.

205. Hanna HG, et al. Generalized chorea in two patients harboring the Friedreich's ataxia gene trinucleotide repeat expansion. *Mov Disord* 1998;13:339–340.

206. Geschwind DH, et al. Friedreich's ataxia GAA repeat expansion in patients with recessive or sporadic ataxia. *Neurology* 1997;49:1004–1009.

207. Koskinen TP, et al. Infantile onset spinocerebellar ataxia with sensory neuropathy—a new inherited disease. *J Neurol Sci* 1994;121:50–56.

208. Koskinen TP, Pihko H, Voutilainen R. Primary hypogonadism in females with infantile onset spinocerebellar ataxia. *Neuropediatrics* 1995;26:263–266.

208a. Nikali K, et al. Toward cloning of a novel ataxia gene: refined assignment and physical map of the IOSCA locus (SCA8) on 10q 24. *Genomics* 1997;39:185–191.

208b. Koob MD, et al. An untranslated CTG expansion causes a novel form of spinocerebellar ataxia (SCA8). *Nat Genet* 1999;21:379–384.

209. Yokota T, et al. Friedreich-like ataxia with retinitis pigmentosa caused by the His[101] Gln mutation of the α-tocopherol transfer protein gene. *Ann Neurol* 1997;41:826–832.

210. Garland H, Moorhouse D. An extremely rare recessive hereditary syndrome including cerebellar ataxia, oligophrenia, cataract, and other features. *J Neurol Neurosurg Psychiatry* 1953;16:110–116.

211. McLaughlin JF, et al. Marinesco-Sjögren syndrome: clinical and magnetic resonance imaging features in three children. *Dev Med Child Neurol* 1996;38: 356–370.

212. Bouchard JP, et al. Autosomal recessive spastic ataxia of Charlevoix-Saguenay. *Can J Neurol Sci* 1978;5:61–69.

213. Cross HE, McKusick VA. The Troyer syndrome: a recessive form of spastic paraplegia with distal muscle wasting. *Arch Neurol* 1967;16:473-485.

214. Shapiro F, Bresnan MJ. Orthopedic management of childhood neuromuscular disease. II. Peripheral neuropathy, Friedreich's ataxia, and arthrogryposis multiplex congenita. *J Bone Joint Surg Am* 1982;64:949–953.

215. Menzel P. Beitrag zur Kentniss der hereditären Ataxie und Kleinhirnatrophie. *Arch Psychiatr Nervenkr* 1890;22:160–190.

216. Dejerine J, André-Thomas A. L'atrophie olivopontocérébelleuse. *Nouv Iconog Salpètr* 1900;13:330–370.

217. Holmes GM. A form of familial degeneration of the cerebellum. *Brain* 1907;30:466–489.

218. Pandolfo M, Montermini L. Molecular genetics of the hereditary ataxias. *Adv Genet* 1998;38:31–68.

219. Orr HT, et al. Expansion of an unstable trinucleotide CAG repeat in spinocerebellar ataxia type 1. *Nat Genet* 1993;4:221–226.

220. Pulst SM, et al. Moderate expansion of a normally biallelic trinucleotide repeat in spinocerebellar ataxia type 2. *Nat Genet* 1996;14:269–276.

221. Kawaguchi Y, et al. CAG expansions in a novel gene for Machado-Joseph disease at chromosome 14q32.1. *Nat Genet* 1994;8:221–226.

222. Flanigan K, et al. Autosomal dominant spinocerebellar ataxia with sensory axonal neuropathy (SCA4): clinical description and genetic localization to chromosome 16q22.1. *Am J Hum Genet* 1996;59:392–399.

223. Ranum LP, et al. Spinocerebellar ataxia type 5 in a family descended from the grandparents of President Lincoln: maps to chromosome 11. *Nat Genet* 1994;8:280–284.

224. Zhuchenko O, et al. Autosomal dominant cerebellar ataxia (SCA6) associated with small polyglutamine expansions in the alpha 1A-voltage-dependent calcium channel. *Nat Genet* 1997;15:62–69.

224a. Huynh DP, et al. Expression of ataxin-2 in brains from normal individuals and patients with Alzheimer's diease and spinocerebellar ataxia 2. *Ann Neurol* 1999;45:232–241.

225. Benton CS, et al. Molecular and clinical studies in SCA-7 define a broad clinical spectrum and the infantile phenotype. *Neurology* 1998;51:1081–1086.

226. Schöls L, et al. Autosomal dominant cerebellar ataxia: phenotypic differences in genetically defined subtypes? *Ann Neurol* 1997;42:924–932.

227. Ikeuchi T, et al. Spinocerebellar ataxia type 6: CAG repeat expansion in α$_{1a}$voltage-dependent calcium channel gene and clinical variations in Japanese populations. *Ann Neurol* 1997;42:879–884.

228. Gouw LG, et al. Autosomal dominant cerebellar ataxia with retinal degeneration: clinical, neuropathologic, and genetic analysis of a large kindred. *Neurology* 1994;44:1441–1447.

229. Van Leeuwen MA, van Bogaert L. Hereditary ataxia with optic atrophy of the retrobulbar neuritis type, and latent pallido-Luysian degeneration. *Brain* 1949;72:340–363.

230. Warner TT, et al. A clinical and molecular genetic study of dentatorubral-pallidoluysian atrophy in four European families. *Ann Neurol* 1995;37:452–459.

231. Takahashi H, et al. Hereditary dentatorubral-pallidoluysian atrophy: clinical and pathological variants in a family. *Neurology* 1988;38:1065–1070.

232. Grewal RP, et al. Clinical and genetic analysis of a distinct autosomal dominant spinocerebellar ataxia. *Neurology* 1998;51:1423–1426.

232a. Zu L, et al. Mapping of a new autosomal dominant spinocerebellar ataxia to chromosome 22. *Am J Hum Genet* 1999;64:594–599.

233. Norman RM. Primary degeneration of the granular layer of the cerebellum: An unusual form of familial cerebellar atrophy occurring in eary life. *Brain* 1940;63:365–379.

233a. Frontali M, et al. Autosomal dominant pure cerebellar ataxia: neurological and genetic study. *Brain* 1992; 115:1647–1654.

234. Jervis GA. Early familial cerebellar degeneration (report of 3 cases in one family). *J Nerv Ment Dis* 1950;111:398–407.

235. Brunt ER, can Weerden TW. Familial paroxysmal kinesigenic ataxia and continuous myokymia. *Brain* 1990;113:1361–1382.

236. Browne DL, et al. Episodic ataxia/myokymia syndrome is associated with point mutations in the human potassium channel gene KCNA1. *Nat Genet* 1994;8:136–140.

237. Baloh RW, et al. Familial episodic ataxia: clinical heterogeneity in four families linked to chromosome 19p. *Ann Neurol* 1997;41:8–16.

238. Ophoff RA, et al. Familial hemiplegic migraine and episodic ataxia type-2 are caused by mutations in the Ca^{2+} channel gene CACNL1A4. *Cell* 1996;87: 543–552.

239. Hunt JR. Dyssynergia cerebellaris myoclonica—primary atrophy of the dentate system. *Brain* 1921;44:490–538.

240. Genton P, et al. The Ramsay Hunt syndrome revisited: Mediterranean myoclonus versus mitochondrial encephalopathy with ragged-red fibers and Baltic myoclonus. *Acta Neurol Scand* 1990;81:8–15.

241. Marsden CD, et al. Progressive myoclonic ataxia (the Ramsay Hunt syndrome). *Arch Neurol* 1990;47: 1121–1125.

242. Seeligmüller A. Sklerose der Seitenstränge des Rückenmarks bei 4 Kindern derselben Familie. *Dtsch Med Wochenschr* 1876;2:185–186.

243. Dyken P, Krawiecki N. Neurodegenerative diseases of infancy and childhood. *Ann Neurol* 1983;13:351–364.

244. Jouet M, et al. X-linked spastic paraplegia (SPG1), MASA syndrome and X-linked hydrocephalus result from mutations in the L1 gene. *Nat Genet* 1994;7:402–406.

245. Saugier-Veber P, et al. X-linked spastic paraplegia and Pelizaeus-Merzbacher disease are allelic disorders at the proteolipid protein locus. *Nat Genet* 1994;6: 257–262.

246. Huang S, et al. Another pedigree with pure autosomal dominant spastic paraplegia (AD-FSP) from Tibet mapping to 14q11.2-q24.3. *Hum Genet* 1997;100: 620–623.

247. Dürr A, et al. Phenotype of autosomal dominant spastic paraplegia linked to chromosome 2. *Brain* 1996;119:1487–1496.

248. Benson KF, et al. CAG repeat expansion in autosomal dominant familial spastic paraparesis: novel expansion in a subset of patients. *Hum Mol Genet* 1998;7: 1779–1786.

249. Hentati A, et al. Linkage of "pure" autosomal recessive familial spastic paraplegia to chromosome 8 markers and evidence of genetic locus heterogeneity. *Hum Mol Genet* 1994;3:1263–1267.

249a. Casari G, et al. Spastic paraplegia and OXPHOS impairment caused by mutations in paraplegin, a nuclear-encoded mitochondrial metalloprotease. *Cell* 1998;93:973–983.

250. Dubé M-P, et al. Hereditary spastic paraplegia: LOD-score considerations for confirmation of linkage in a heterogeneous trait. *Am J Hum Genet* 1997;60: 625–629.

250a. Hedera P, et al. Novel locus for autosomal dominant hereditary spastic paraplegia, on chromosome 8q. *Am J Hum Genet* 1999;64:563–569.

250b. McHale DP, et al. A gene for autosomal recessive symmetrical spastic cerebral palsy maps to chromosome 2q24-25. *Am J Hum Genet* 1999;64: 526–532.

251. Behan WMH, Maia M. Strumpell's familial paraplegia: genetics and neuropathology. *J Neurol Neurosurg Psychiatry* 1974;37:8–20.

252. Schwarz GA, Liu C. Hereditary spastic paraplegia. *Arch Neurol Psychiatr* 1956;75:144–162.

253. Fink JK, et al. Hereditary spastic paraplegia: advances in genetic research. *Neurology* 1996;46: 1507–1514.

254. Harding AE. Hereditary "pure" spastic paraplegia: a clinical and genetic study of 22 families. *J Neurol Neurosurg Psychiatry* 1981;44:871–883.

255. Meierkord H, et al. "Complicated" autosomal dominant familial spastic paraplegia is genetically distinct from "pure" forms. *Arch Neurol* 1997;54:379–384.

256. Markand ON, Daly DD. Juvenile type of slowly progressive bulbar palsy: report of a case. *Neurology* 1971;21:753–758.

257. McShane MA, et al. Progressive bulbar paralysis of childhood: a reappraisal of Fazio-Londe disease. *Brain* 1992;115:1889–1900.

258. Engel WK, Kurland LT, Klatzo I. An inherited disease similar to amyotrophic lateral sclerosis with a pattern of posterior column involvement: an intermediate form? *Brain* 1959;82:203–220.

259. Dyck PJ, et al. Hereditary motor and sensory neuropathies. In: Dyck PJ, et al., eds. *Peripheral Neuropathy*. 3rd ed. Philadelphia: WB Saunders, 1993:1094–1136.

260. Hagberg B, Westerberg B. The nosology of genetic peripheral neuropathies in Swedish children. *Dev Med Child Neurol* 1983;25:3–18.

261. Ouvrier RA, McLeod JG, Pollard JD. *Peripheral neuropathy in childhood*, New York: Raven Press, 1990.

262. Virchow R. Ein Fall von progressiver Muskelatrophie. *Virchows Arch Path Anat* 1855;8:537–540.

263. Charcot JM, Marie P. Sur une forme particulière d'atrophie musculaire progressive, souvent familiales débutant par les pieds et les jambes, et atteignant plus tard les mains. *Rev Med (Paris)* 1885;6:97–138.

264. Tooth HH. *The peroneal type of progressive muscular atrophy*, Cambridge University Thesis. London: H.K. Lewis, 1886.

265. Hagberg B, Lyon G. Pooled European series of hereditary peripheral neuropathies in infancy and childhood. *Neuropaediatrie* 1981;12:9–17.

266. Dyck PJ, Lambert EH. Lower motor and primary sensory neuron diseases with peroneal muscular atrophy. II. Neurologic, genetic, and electrophysiologic findings in various neuronal degenerations. *Arch Neurol* 1968;18:619–625.

267. de Recondo J. Hereditary neurogenic muscular atrophies. In: Vinken PJ, Bruyn GW, eds. *Handbook of clinical neurology: system disorders and atrophies*, Part I, Vol 21. New York: Elsevier North Holland, 1975:271–317.

268. Dejerine J, Sottas J. Sur la nevrite interstitielle hypertrophique et progressive de l'enfance. *Compt Rend Soc Biol (Paris)* 1893;45:63–96.

269. Webster H deF, et al. The role of Schwann cells in formation of "onion bulbs" found in chronic neuropathies. *J Neuropathol Exp Neurol* 1967;26:276–299.

270. Behse F, Buchthal F. Peroneal muscular atrophy (PMA) and related disorders. II. Histological findings in sural nerves. *Brain* 1977;100:67–85.

271. Ouvrier RA, McLeod JG, Conchin TE. The hypertrophic forms of hereditary motor and sensory neuropathy. *Brain* 1987;110:121–148.

272. Gabreels-Festen AA, et al. Charcot-Marie-Tooth disease type 1A: morphological phenotype of the 17p duplication versus PMP point mutations. *Acta Neuropathol* 1995;90:645–649.

272a. Lupski JR. Charcot-Marie-Tooth polyneuropathy: duplication, gene dosage, and genetic heterogeneity. *Pediatr Res* 1999;45:159–165.

273. Hanemann CO, Muller HW. Pathogenesis of Charcot-Marie-Tooth 1A (CMT 1A) neuropathy. *Trends Neurosci* 1998;21:282–286.

274. Roa BB, et al. Charcot-Marie-Tooth disease type 1A: association with a spontaneous point mutation in the PMP22 gene. *N Engl J Med* 1993;329:96–101.

275. Bird TD, et al. Clinical and pathological phenotype of the original family with Charcot-Marie-Tooth type 1B: a 20-year study. *Ann Neurol* 1997;41:4663–4669.

276. Ionasescu VV, et al. Heterogeneity in X-linked recessive Charcot–Marie-Tooth neuropathy. *Am J Hum Genet* 1991;48:1075–1083.

277. Nicholson GA, Yeung L, Corbett A. Efficient neurophysiologic selection of X-linked Charcot-Marie-Tooth families: ten novel mutations. *Neurology* 1998;51: 1412–1416.

278. Suter U, Snipes GJ. Biology and genetics of hereditary motor and sensory neuropathies. *Annu Rev Neurosci* 1995;18:45–75.

279. Tyrer JH, Sutherland JM. The primary spinocerebellar atrophies and their associated defects, with a study of the foot deformity. *Brain* 1961;84:289–300.

280. Nicholson GA. Penetrance of the hereditary motor and sensory neuropathy Ia mutation: assessment by nerve conduction studies. *Neurology* 1991;41:547–552.

281. Hamiel OP, et al. Hereditary motorsensory neuropathy (Charcot-Marie-Tooth disease) with nerve deafness: a new variant. *J Pediatr* 1993;123:431–434.

282. Sabatelli M, et al. Hereditary motor and sensory neuropathy with deafness, mental retardation, and absence of sensory large myelinated fibers: confirmation of a new entity. *Am J Med Genet* 1998;23:75:309–313.

283. Roussy G, Lévy G. Sept cas d'une maladie familiale particuliere: troubles de la marche, pieds bots, et areflexie tendineuse generalisee, avec, accessoirement, legere maladresse des mains. *Rev Neurol (Paris)* 1926;1:427–450.

284. Hagberg B, et al. Peripheral neuropathies in childhood: Gothenburg 1973–78. *Neuropaediatrie* 1979; 10[Suppl]:426.

285. LeGuern E, et al. Homozygosity mapping of an autosomal recessive form of demyelination Charcot-Marie-Tooth disease to chromosome 5q23-q33. *Hum Mol Genet* 1996;5:1685–1688.

286. Ionasescu V, et al. Autosomal dominant Charcot-Marie-Tooth axonal neuropathy mapped on chromosome 7p (CMT2D). *Hum Mol Genet* 1996;5: 1373–1375.

287. Dyck PJ, et al. Hereditary motor and sensory neuropathy with diaphragm and vocal cord paresis. *Ann Neurol* 1994;35:608–615.

288. Lynch DR, et al. Autosomal dominant transmission of Dejerine-Sottas disease (HMSN III). *Neurology* 1997;49:601–603.

289. Tyson J, et al. Hereditary demyelinating neuropathy of infancy: a genetically complex syndrome. *Brain* 1997;120:47–63.

290. Bradley WG, Aguayo A. Hereditary chronic polyneuropathy: electrophysiologic and pathologic studies in affected family. *J Neurol Sci* 1969;9:131–154.

291. Harding AE, Thomas PK. Peroneal muscular atrophy with pyramidal features. *J Neurol Neurosurg Psychiatry* 1984;47:168–172.

292. MacDermot KD, Walker RWH. Autosomal recessive hereditary motor and sensory neuropathy with mental retardation, optic atrophy and pyramidal tract signs. *J Neurol Neurosurg Psychiatry* 1987;50:1342–1347.

292a. Ippel EF, et al. Genetic herogeneity of hereditary motor and sensory neuropathy type VI. *Child Neurol* 1995;10:459–463.

293. Massion-Verniory L, Dumont D, Potvin AM. Rétinite pigmentaire familiale compliqueé d'une amyotrophie neurale. *Rev Neurol (Paris)* 1946;78:561–571.

293a. Takashima H, et al. A new type of hereditary motor and sensory neuropathy linked to chromosome 3. *Ann Neurol* 1997;41:771–780.

294. Ben Othmane K, et al. Linkage of a locus (CMT4A) for autosomal recessive Charcot-Marie-Tooth disease to chromosome 8q. *Hum Mol Genet* 1993;2: 1625–1628.

295. Bolino A, et al. Localization of a gene responsible for autosomal recessive demyelinating neuropathy with focally folded myelin sheaths to chromosome 11q23 by homozygosity mapping and haplotype sharing. *Hum Mol Genet* 1996;5:1051–1054.

296. Ionasescu VV, et al. X-linked recessive Charcot-Marie-Tooth neuropathy: clinical and genetic study. *Muscle Nerve* 1992;15:368–373.

297. Chadwick BP, et al. The human homologue of the ninjurin gene maps to the candidate region of hereditary sensory neuropathy type I (HSNI). *Genomics* 1998;47:58–63.

298. Davar G, et al. Exclusion of p75NGFR and other candidate genes in a family with hereditary sensory neuropathy type II. *Pain* 1996;67:135–139.

299. Eng CM, et al. Prenatal diagnosis of familial dysautonomia by analysis of linked CA-repeat polymorphisms on chromosome 9q31-q33. *Am J Med Genet* 1995;59:349–355.

300. Edwards-Lee TA, Cornford ME, Yu KT. Congenital insensitivity to pain and anhidrosis with mitochondrial and axonal abnormalities. *Pediatr Neurol* 1997;17: 356–361.

301. Donaghy M, et al. Hereditary sensory neuropathy with neurotrophic keratitis. *Brain* 1987;110:561–583.

302. Mariman ECM, et al. Prevalence of the 1.5-Mb 17p deletion in families with hereditary neuropathy with liability to pressure palsies. *Ann Neurol* 1994;36: 650–655.

303. Behse F, et al. Hereditary neuropathy with liability to pressure palsies: electrophysiological and histopathological aspects. *Brain* 1972;95:777–794.

304. Sellman MS, Mayer RF. Conduction block in hereditary neuropathy with susceptibility to pressure palsies. *Muscle Nerve* 1987;10:621–625.

305. Gabreels-Festen AAWM, et al. Hereditary neuropathy with liability to pressure palsies in childhood. *Neuropediatrics* 1992;23:138–143.

306. Nicholson GA, et al. A frame shift mutation in the PMP22 gene in hereditary neuropathy with liability to pressure palsies. *Nat Genet* 1994;6:263–266.

307. Greenberg F, et al. Multi-disciplinary clinical study of Smith-Magenis syndrome. *Am J Med Genet* 1996; 62:247–254.

308. Thomas PK, Ormerod IE. Hereditary neuralgic amyotrophy associated with a relapsing multifocal sensory neuropathy. *J Neurol Neurosurg Psychiatry* 1993;56: 107–109.

309. Airaksinen EM, et al. Hereditary recurrent brachial plexus neuropathy with dysmorphic features. *Acta Neurol Scand* 1985;71:309–316.

310. Stogbauer P, et al. Refinement of the hereditary neuralgic amyotrophy (HNA) locus to chromosome 17 q24-q25. *Hum Genet* 1997;99:685–687.

311. Zeharia A, et al. Benign plexus neuropathy in children. *J Pediatr* 1990;116:276–278.

312. Dyck PJ. Neuronal atrophy and degeneration predominantly affecting peripheral sensory and autonomic neurons. In: Dyck PJ, et al., eds. *Peripheral neuropathy*. 3rd ed. Philadelphia: WB Saunders, 1993: 1065–1093.

313. Nicholson GA, et al. The gene for hereditary sensory neuropathy type I (HSN-I) maps to chromosome 9q22.1-q22.3 *Nat Genet* 1996;13:101–104.

314. Denny-Brown D. Hereditary sensory radicular neuropathy. *J Neurol Neurosurg Psychiatry* 1951;14: 237–252.

315. Dyck PJ, et al. Not "indifference to pain" but varieties of hereditary sensory and autonomic neuropathy. *Brain* 1983;106:373–390.

316. Verity CM, Dunn HG, Berry K. Children with reduced sensitivity to pain: assessment of hereditary sensory neuropathy types II and IV. *Dev Med Child Neurol* 1982;24:785–797.

317. Riley CM, et al. Central autonomic dysfunction with defective lacrimation. I. Report of five cases. *Pediatrics* 1949;3:468–478.

318. Mahloudji M, Brunt PW, McKusick VA. Clinical neurological aspects of familial dysautonomia. *J Neurol Sci* 1970;11:383–395.

318a. Chadwick BP, et al. Cloning, mapping, and expression of two novel actin genes, actin-like-7A (ACTL7A) and actin-like-7B (ACTL7B), from the familial dysautonomia candidate region on 9 q 31. *Genomics* 1999; 58:302–309.

319. Pearson J. Familial dysautonomia (a brief review). *J Auton Nerv Syst* 1979;1:119–126.

320. Pearson J, Brandeis L, Cuello AC. Depletion of substance-P-containing axons in substantia gelatinosa of patients with diminished pain sensitivity. *Nature* 1982;295:61–63.

321. Brown WJ, Beauchemin JA, Linde LM. A neuropathological study of familial dysautonomia (Riley-Day syndrome) in siblings. *J Neurol Neurosurg Psychiatry* 1964;27:131–139.

322. Pearson J, et al. The sural nerve in familial dysautonomia. *J Neuropathol Exp Neurol* 1975;34:413–424.

323. Ziegler MG, Lake CR, Kopin IJ. Deficient sympathetic nervous response in familial dysautonomia. *N Engl J Med* 1976;294:630–633.

324. Axelrod FB, Porges RF, Sein ME. Neonatal recognition of familial dysautonomia. *J Pediatr* 1987;110: 946–948.

325. Yatsu F, Zussman W. Familial dysautonomia (Riley-Day syndrome): case report with postmortem findings of a patient at age thirty-one. *Arch Neurol* 1964;10: 459–463.

326. Axelrod FB, Pearson J. Familial dysautonomia. In: Gomez MR, ed. *Neurocutaneous diseases: a practical approach.* Boston: Butterworth–Heinemann, 1987: 200–208.

327. Linde LM, Westover JL. Esophageal and gastric abnormalities in dysautonomia. *Pediatrics* 1962;29: 303–306.

328. Gadoth N, et al. Taste and smell in familial dysautonomia. *Dev Med Child Neurol* 1997;39:393–397.

329. Glickstein JS, et al. Abnormalities of the corrected QT interval in familial dysautonomia: an indicator of autonomic dysfunction. *J Pediatr* 1993;122: 925–928.

330. Axelrod FB, Abularrage JJ. Familial dysautonomia: a prospective study of survival. *J Pediatr* 1982;101: 234–236.

331. Axelrod FB, et al. Progressive sensory loss in familial dysautonomia. *Pediatrics* 1981;67:517–522.

332. Lahat E, et al. Brainstem auditory evoked potentials in familial dysautonomia. *Dev Med Child Neurol* 1992;34:690–693.

333. Goldberg MF, Payne JW, Brunt PW. Ophthalmologic studies of familial dysautonomia: the Riley-Day syndrome. *Arch Ophthalmol* 1968;80:732–743.

334. Axelrod FB, Maayan C. Familial dysautonomia. In: Burg FD, Ingelfinger JR, Wald ER, Polin RA, eds. *Gellis & Kagan's current pediatric therapy*,Vol 16. Philadelphia: WB Saunders Company, 1998: 466–469.

335. Alvarez E, et al. Evaluation of congenital dysautonomia other than Riley-Day syndrome. *Neuropediatrics* 1996;27:26–31.

336. Udassin R, et al. Nissen fundoplication in the treatment of children with familial dysautonomia. *Am J Surg* 1992;164:332–336.

337. Goebel HH, Veit S, Dyck PJ. Confirmation of virtual unmyelinated fiber absence in hereditary sensory neuropathy type IV. *J Neuropathol Exp Neurol* 1980;39:670–674.

338. Johnsen SD, Johnson PC, Stein SR. Familial sensory autonomic neuropathy with arthropathy in Navajo children. *Neurology* 1993;43:1120–1125.

339. Singleton R, et al. Neuropathy in Navajo children: clinical and epidemiological features. *Neurology* 1990;40:363–367.

340. Osuntokun BO, Odeku EL, Luzzato L. Congenital pain asymbolia and auditory imperception. *J Neurol Neurosurg Psychiatry* 1968;31:291–296.

341. Berg BO, Rosenberg SH, Asbury AK. Giant axonal neuropathy. *Pediatrics* 1972;49:894–899.

342. Maia M, Pires MM, Guimaraes A. Giant axonal disease: report of three cases and review of the literature. *Neuropediatrics* 1988;19:10–15.

343. Carpenter S, et al. Giant axonal neuropathy: a clinically and morphologically distinct neurological disease. *Arch Neurol* 1974;31:312–316.

344. Flanigan KM, et al. Localization of the giant axonal neuropathy gene to chromosome 16q24. *Ann Neurol* 1998;43:143–148.

345. Pena SD. Giant axonal neuropathy: an inborn error of organization of intermediate filaments. *Muscle Nerve* 1982;5:166–172.

346. Wartenberg R. Progressive facial hemiatrophy. *Arch Neurol Psychiatr* 1945;54:75–97.

347. Wolf SM, Verity MA. Neurological complications of progressive facial hemiatrophy. *J Neurol Neurosurg Psychiatry* 1974;37:997–1004.

348. Asher SW, Berg BO. Progressive hemifacial atrophy. *Arch Neurol* 1982;39:44–46.

349. Dupont S, et al. Progressive facial hemiatrophy and epilepsy: a common underlying dysgenetic mechanism. *Neurology* 1997;48:1013–1018.

350. Fischel-Ghodsian N, Falk RE. Deafness. In: Rimoin DL, Connor JM, Pyeritz RE, eds. *Principles and practice of medical genetics.* 3rd ed. New York: Churchill Livingstone, 1996:1149–1170.

351. Fraser GR. The causes of profound deafness in childhood. In: Wolstenholme GEW, Knight J, eds. *Sensorineural hearing loss.* London: J and A Churchill, 1970:5–40.

351a. Heckenlively JR, Daiger SP. Hereditary retinal and choroidal degenerations. In: Rimoin DL, Connor JM, Pyeritz RE, eds. *Principles and practice of medical genetics.* 3rd ed. New York: Churchill Livingstone 1996:2555–2576.

352. Schaumburg HH, et al. Adrenoleukodystrophy: a clinical and pathological study of 17 cases. *Arch Neurol* 1975;33:577–591.

353. Moser HW, et al. Adrenoleukodystrophy: increased plasma content of saturated very-long-chain fatty acids. *Neurology* 1981;31:1241–1249.

354. Menkes JH, Corbo LM. Adrenoleukodystrophy: accumulation of cholesterol esters with very-long-chain fatty acids. *Neurology* 1977;27:928–932.

355. Kishimoto Y, et al. Adrenoleukodystrophy: evidence that abnormal very-long-chain fatty acids of brain cholesterol tests are of exogenous origin. *Biochem Biophys Res Comm* 1980;96:69–76.

356. Mosser J, et al. The gene responsible for adrenoleukodystrophy encodes a peroxisomal membrane protein. *Hum Mol Genet* 1994;3:265–171.

357. Schneider E, Hunke S. ATP-binding-cassette (ABC) transport systems: functional and structural aspects of the ATP hydrolyzing subunits/domains. *FEMS Microbiol Res* 1998;22:1–20.
358. Moser H. Peroxisomal disorders. In: Rosenberg RN, et al. *The molecular and genetic basis of neurological disease.* 2nd ed. Boston: Butterworth–Heinemann, 1997;290–300.
358a. Dubois-Dalcq M, Feigenbaum V, Aubourg P. The neurobiology of X-linked adrenoleukodystrophy: a demyelinating peroxisomal disorder. *Trends Neurosci* 1999;22:4–12.
359. Korenke GC, et al. Cerebral adrenoleukodystrophy (ALD) in only one of monozygotic twins with an identical ALD genotype. *Ann Neurol* 1996;40:254–257.
360. Pahan K, Khan M, Singh I. Therapy for X-adrenoleukodystrophy: normalization of very-long-chain fatty acids and inhibition of induction of cytokines by cAMP. *J Lipid Res* 1998;39:1091–1100.
361. Moser HW, et al. Adrenoleukodystrophy: phenotypic variability and implications for therapy. *J Inherit Metab Dis* 1992;15:645–664.
362. Kirk EP, et al. X-linked adrenoleukodystrophy: the Australasian experience. *Am J Med Genet* 1998;76:420–423.
362a. Wichers M, et al. X-linked adrenomyeloneuropathy associated with 14 novel ALD-gene mutations: no correlation between type of mutation and age of onset. *Hum Genet* 1999;105:116–119.
363. Walsh PJ. Adrenoleukodystrophy: report of two cases with relapsing and remitting courses. *Arch Neurol* 1980;37:448–450.
364. Gartner J, et al. Clinical and genetic aspects of X-linked adrenoleukodystrophy. *Neuropediatrics* 1998;29:3–13.
365. Kumar AJ, et al. Adrenoleukodystrophy: correlating MR imaging with CT. *Radiology* 1987;165:497–504.
366. Rajanayagam V, et al. Proton MR spectroscopy and neuropsychological testing in adrenoleukodystrophy. *Am J Neuroradiol* 1997;18:1909–1914.
367. Moloney JBM, Masterson JG. Detection of adrenoleukodystrophy carriers by means of evoked potentials. *Lancet* 1982;2:852–853.
368. O'Neill BP, Marmion LC, Feringa ER. The adrenoleukomyeloneuropathy complex: expression in four generations. *Neurology* 1981;31:151–156.
369. Kaplan PW, et al. Visual evoked potentials in adrenoleukodystrophy: a trial with glycerol trioleate and Lorenzo Oil. *Ann Neurol* 1993;34:169–174.
370. Zinkham WH, et al. Lorenzo's Oil and thrombocytopenia in patients with adrenoleukodystrophy. *N Engl J Med* 1993;328:1126–1127.
370a. Kemp S, et al. Gene redundancy and pharmacological gene therapy: implications for X-linked adrenoleukodystrophy. *Nat Med* 1998;4:1261–1268.
371. Hooft DG, van Bogaert L, Guazzi GC. Sudanophilic leukodystrophy with meningeal angiomatosis in two brothers: infantile form of diffuse sclerosis with meningeal angiomatosis. *J Neurol Sci* 1965;2:30–51.
372.Poll-The BT, et al. Metabolic pigmentary retinopathies: diagnosis and therapeutic attempts. *Eur J Pediatr* 1992;151:2–11.
373.Hallgren B. Retinitis pigmentosa combined with congenital deafness with vestibular-cerebellar ataxia and mental abnormality in a proportion of cases: a clinical and geneticostatistical study. *Acta Psychiatr Scand* 1959[Suppl]:138:1–101.
374. Sjögren T, Larsson T. Oligophrenia in combination with congenital ichthyosis and spastic disorders: a clinical and genetic study. *Acta Psychiatr Scand* 1957;32[Suppl 113]:1–112.
375. Allstrom CH, et al. Retinal degeneration combined with obesity, diabetes mellitus and neurogenous deafness: a specific syndrome (not hitherto described) distinct from the Laurence-Moon-Bardet-Biedl syndrome. *Acta Psychiatr Neurol Scand* 1959;34[Suppl 129]:135.
376. Pelizaeus F. Ueber eine eigentümliche Form spastischer Lähmung mit Cerebralerscheinungen auf hereditärer Grundlage. *Arch Psychiatr Nervenkr* 1885;16:698–710.
377. Merzbacher L. Eine eigenartige familiär-hereditäre Erkrankungsform. *Z Ges Neurol Psychiatry* 1910;3:1–138.
378. Seitelberger F. Pelizaeus-Merzbacher disease. In: Vinken PJ, Bruyn GW, eds. *Handbook of clinical neurology,* Vol 10. New York: Elsevier North Holland, 1970:150–202.
379. Boulloche J, Aicardi J. Pelizaeus-Merzbacher disease: clinical and nosological study. *J Child Neurol* 1986;1:233–239.
380. Watanabe I, et al. Early lesion of Pelizaeus-Merzbacher Disease: electron microscopic and biochemical study. *J Neuropathol Exp Neurol* 1973;32:313–333.
381. Raskind WH, et al. Complete deletion of the proteolipid protein gene (PLP) in a family with X-linked Pelizaeus-Merzbacher disease. *Am J Hum Genet* 1991;49:1355–1360.
382. Sistermans EA, et al. Duplication of the proteolipid protein gene is the major cause of Pelizaeus-Merzbacher disease. *Neurology* 1998;50:1749–1754.
383. Woodward K, et al. Pelizaeus-Merzbacher disease: identification of Xq22 proteolipid-protein duplications and characterization of breakpoints by interphase FISH. *Am J Hum Genet* 1998;63:207–217.
384. Tyler HR. Pelizaeus-Merzbacher disease: a clinical study. *Arch Neurol Psychiatry* 1958;80:162–169.
385. Nezu A, et al. An MRI and MRS study of Pelizaeus-Merzbacher disease. *Pediatr Neurol* 1998;18:334–337.
386. Iwaki A, et al. A missense mutation in the proteolipid protein gene responsible for Pelizaeus-Merzbacher disease in a Japanese family. *Hum Mol Genet* 1993;2:19–22.
387. Bridge PJ, MacLeod PM, Lillicrap DP. Carrier detection and prenatal diagnosis of Pelizaeus-Merzbacher disease using a combination of anonymous DNA polymorphisms and the proteolipid protein (PLP) gene cDNA. *Am J Med Genet* 1991;38:616–621.
388. Lazzarini A, et al. Pelizaeus-Merzbacher-like disease: exclusion of the proteolipid protein locus and documentation of a new locus on Xq. *Neurology* 1997;49:824–832.
389. Canavan MM. Schilder's encephalitis periaxialis diffusa. *Arch Neurol Psychiatry* 1931;25:299–308.
390. Kaul R, et al. Cloning of the human aspartoacylase cDNA and a common missense mutation in Canavan's disease. *Nat Genet* 1993;5:118–123.
391. Matalon R, Kaul R, Michals K. Canavan disease. In: Rosenberg RN, et al. *The molecular and genetic basis of neurological disease,* 2nd ed. Boston: Butterworth–Heinemann, 1997:493–502.
392. Gascon GG, et al. Infantile CNS spongy degeneration—14 cases: clinical update. *Neurology* 1990;40:1876–1882.

392a. Traeger EC, Rapin I. The clinical course of Canavan disease. *Pediatr Neurol* 1998;18:207–212.

393. Adachi M, et al. Spongy degeneration of the central nervous system (van Bogaert and Bertrand type; Canavan's disease): a review. *Hum Pathol* 1973;4:331–447.

394. Gambetti P, Mellman WJ, Gonatas NK. Familial spongy degeneration of the central nervous system (van Bogaert-Bertrand Disease). *Acta Neuropathol* 1969;12:103–115.

395. Banker BQ, Robertson JT, Victor M. Spongy degenerations of the central nervous system in infancy. *Neurology* 1964;14:981–1001.

396. Suzuki K. Peripheral nerve lesion in spongy degeneration of the central nervous system. *Acta Neuropathol* 1968;10:95–98.

397. Birken DL, et al. *N*-acetyl-*L*-aspartic acid: a literature review of a compound prominent in 1HNMR spectroscopic studies of brain. *Neurosci Biobehav Rev* 1989;13:23–31.

398. Patel PJ, et al. Sonographic and computed tomographic findings in Canavan's disease. *Br J Radiol* 1986;59:1226–1228.

399. Barker PB, et al. Proton NMR spectroscopy of Canavan's disease. *Neuropediatrics* 1992;23:263–267.

400. Alexander WS. Progressive fibrinoid degeneration of fibrillary astrocytes associated with mental retardation in hydrocephalic infant. *Brain* 1949;72:373–381.

401. Pridmore CL, et al. Alexander's disease: clues to diagnosis. *J Child Neurol* 1993;8:134–144.

402. Castellani RJ, et al. Advanced lipid peroxidation endproducts in Alexander's disease. *Brain Res* 1998; 787:15–18.

403. Iwaki T, et al. α B-crystallin expressed in non-lenticular tissues and accumulates in Alexander's disease brains. *Cell* 1989;57:71–78.

404. Neal JW, et al. Alexander's disease in infancy and childhood: a report of two cases. *Acta Neuropathol* 1992;84:322–327.

405. Shah M, Ross JS. Infantile Alexander disease: MR appearance of a biopsy-proven case. *Am J Neuroradiol* 1990;11:1105–1106.

406. Mirowitz SA, et al. Neurodegenerative diseases of childhood: MR and CT evaluation. *J Comput Assist Tomogr* 1991;15:210–222.

407. Alzheimer A. Beiträge zur Kenntnis der pathologischen Neuroglia und ihrer Beziehungen zu den Abbauvorgängen im Nervengewebe: Histologische und histopathologische Arbeiten über die Grosshirnrinde 1910;3:401–562.

408. Greenfield JG. A form of progressive cerebral sclerosis in infants associated with primary degeneration of the interfascicular glia. *J Neurol Psychopathol* 1933;13:289–302.

409. Austin J. Metachromatic sulfatides in cerebral white matter and kidney. *Proc Soc Exp Biol Med* 1959;100: 361–364.

410. Austin JH, et al. A controlled study of enzymatic activities in three human disorders of glycolipid metabolism. *J Neurochem* 1963;10:805–816.

411. Jatzkewitz H, Mehl EL. Cerebrosidesulphatase and arylsulphatase: a deficiency in metachromatic leukodystrophy (ML). *J Neurochem* 1969;16:19–28.

412. Austin JH. Studies in metachromatic leukodystrophy. *Arch Neurol* 1973;28:258–264.

413. Kolodny EH. Metachromatic leukodystrophy and multiple sulfatase deficiency: sulfatide lipidosis. In: Rosenberg RN, et al. *The molecular and genetic basis of neurological disease*, 2nd ed. Boston: Butterworth–Heinemann, 1997:433–442.

414. Polten A, et al. Molecular basis of different forms of metachromatic leukodystrophy. *N Engl J Med* 1991;324:18–22.

415. Barth ML, Fensom A, Harris A. Prevalence of common mutations in the arylsulphatase: a gene in metachromatic leukodystrophy patients diagnosed in Britain. *Hum Genet* 1993;91:73–77.

416. Harvey JS, Carey WF, Morris CP. Importance of the glycosylation and polyadenylation variants in metachromatic leukodystrophy pseudodeficiency phenotype. *Hum Mol Genet* 1998;7:1215–1219.

417. Penzien JM, et al. Compound heterozygosity for metachromatic leukodystrophy and arylsulfatase: a pseudodeficiency allele is not associated with progressive neurological disease. *Am J Hum Genet* 1993; 52:557–564.

418. Zhang XL, et al. The mechanism for a 33 nucleotide insertion in mRNA causing sphingolipid activator protein (SAP1) deficient metachromatic leukodystrophy. *Hum Genet* 1991;87:211–215.

419. O'Brien JS, Kishimoto Y. Saposin proteins: structure, function, and role in human lysosomal storage disorders. *FASEB J* 1991;5:301–308.

420. Morrell P, Wiesmann U. A correlative synopsis of the leukodystrophies. *Neuropediatrics* 1984;15[Suppl]: 62–65.

421. McFaul R. Metachromatic leucodystrophy: review of 38 cases. *Arch Dis Child* 1982;57:168–175.

422. Brown FR, et al. Auditory evoked brain stem response and high-performance liquid chromatography sulfatide assay as early indices of metachromatic leukodystrophy. *Neurology* 1981;31:980–985.

423. Kim TS, et al. MR of childhood metachromatic leukodystrophy. *Am J Neuroradiol* 1997;18:733–738.

424. Scholz W. Klinische, pathologische anatomische und erbiologische Untersuchungen bei familiärer diffuser Hirnsklerose im Kindesalter. *Z Ges Neurol Psychiat* 1925;99:651–717.

425. Menkes JH. Chemical studies of two cerebral biopsies in juvenile metachromatic leukodystrophy: the molecular composition of cerebroside and sulfatides. *J Pediatr* 1966;69:422–431.

426. Austin JH, et al. Metachromatic leukodystrophy (MLD): VIII. MLD in adults: diagnosis and pathogenesis. *Arch Neurol* 1968;18:225–240.

427. Alves D, et al. Four cases of late onset metachromatic leucodystrophy in a family: clinical, biochemical and neuropathological studies. *J Neurol Neurosurg Psychiatry* 1986;49:1417–1422.

428. Dierks T, Schmidt B, von Figura K. Conversion of cysteine to formylglycine: a protein modification in the endoplasmic reticulum. *Proc Natl Acad Sci* USA 1997;94:11963–11968.

429. Eto Y, et al. Various sulfatase activities in leukocytes and cultured skin fibroblasts from heterozygotes for the multiple sulfatase deficiency (Mukosulfatidosis). *Pediatr Res* 1983;17:97–100.

430. Hagberg B, Sourander P, Thoren L. Peripheral nerve changes in the diagnosis of metachromatic leucodystrophy. *Acta Paediatr Scand* 1962;51[Suppl 13S]: 63–71.

431. Kidd D, et al. Long-term stabilization after bone marrow transplantation in juvenile metachromatic leukodystrophy. *Arch Neurol* 1998;55:98–99.

432. Beneke R. Ein Fall hochgradigster ausgedehnter Sklerose des Zentralnervensystem. *Arch Kinderheilk* 1908;47:420–422.
433. Krabbe K. A new familial infantile form of diffuse brain sclerosis. *Brain* 1996;39:74–114.
434. Norman RM, Oppenheimer DR, Tingey AH. Histological and chemical findings in Krabbe's leucodystrophy. *J Neurol Neurosurg Psychiatry* 1961;24:223–232.
435. Austin JH, Lehfeldt D. Studies in globoid (Krabbe) leukodystrophy: III. Significance of experimentally produced globoidlike elements in rat white matter and spleen. *J Neuropathol Exp Neurol* 1965;24:265–289.
436. Andrews JH, et al. Globoid cell leukodystrophy (Krabbe's disease): morphological and biochemical studies. *Neurology* 1971;21:337–352.
437. Martin JJ, et al. Leucodystrophie à cellules globoïdes (maladie de Krabbe) lésions nerveuses périphériques. *Acta Neurol Belg* 1974;74:356–375.
438. Hager H, Oehlert W. Ist die diffuse Hirnsklerose des Typ Krabbe eine entzündliche Allgemeinerkrankung? *Z Kinderheilk* 1957;80:82–96.
439. Kobayashi T, et al. Globoid cell leukodystrophy is a generalized galactosylsphingosine (psychosine) storage disease. *Biochem Biophys Res* 1987;144:41–46.
440. Suzuki K, Suzuki Y, Suzuki K. Galactosylceramide lipidosis: globoid cell leukodystrophy (Krabbe's disease). In: Scriver CR, Beaudet AL, Sly WS, Valle D, eds. *The metabolic basis of inherited disease*. 7th ed. New York: McGraw-Hill, 1995:2671–2692.
441. De Gasperi R, et al. Molecular heterogeneity of late-onset forms of globoid cell leukodystrophy. *Am J Hum Genet* 1996;59:1233–1242.
442. Satoh JI, et al. Adult-onset Krabbe disease with homozygous T1853C mutation in the galactocerebrosidase gene: unusual MRI findings of corticospinal tract demyelination. *Neurology* 1997;49:1392–1399.
443. Loonen MCB, et al. Late-onset of globoid cell leucodystrophy (Krabbe's disease): clinical and genetic delineation of two forms and their relation to the early-infantile form. *Neuropediatrics* 1985;16:137–142.
444. Krivit W, et al. Hematopoietic stem-cell transplantation in globoid-cell leukodystrophy. *N Engl J Med* 1998;338:1119–1126.
445. Bambach BJ, et al. Engraftment following in utero bone marrow transplantation for globoid cell leukodystrophy. *Bone Marrow Transplant* 1997;19:399–402.
446. Woods CG. DNA repair disorders. *Arch Dis Child* 1998;78:178–184.
447. Cockayne EA. Dwarfism with retinal atrophy and deafness. *Arch Dis Child* 1936;11:1–8.
448. Ozdirim E, et al. Cockayne syndrome: review of 25 cases. *Pediatr Neurol* 1996;15:312–316.
449. Nance MA, Berry SA. Cockayne syndrome: review of 140 cases. *Am J Med Genet* 1992;42:68–84.
450. Sugita K, et al. Comparison of MRI white matter changes with neuropsychologic impairment in Cockayne syndrome. *Pediatr Neurol* 1992;8:295–298.
451. Moossy J. The neuropathology of Cockayne's syndrome. *J Neuropathol Exp Neurol* 1967;26:654–660.
452. Citterio E, et al. Biochemical and biological characterization of wild-type and ATPase-deficient Cockayne syndrome B repair protein. *J Biol Chem* 1998; 273:11844–11851.
453. Vermeulen W, et al. Xeroderma pigmentosum complementation group G associated with Cockayne syndrome. *Am J Hum Genet* 1993;53:185–192.
453a. Conaway JW, Conaway RC. Transcriptional elongation and human disease. *Annu Rev Biochem* 1999; 68:301–319.
454. Wood RD. DNA repair in eukaryotes. *Annu Rev Biochem* 1996;65:135–167.
455. Sugita K, et al. Cockayne syndrome with delayed recovery of RNA synthesis after ultraviolet irradiation but normal ultraviolet survival. *Pediatr Res* 1987; 21:34–37.
456. Butler IJ. Xeroderma pigmentosum. In: Rosenberg RN, et al. *The molecular and genetic basis of neurological disease*, 2nd ed. Boston: Butterworth–Heinemann, 1997: 959–967.
457. Kanda T, et al. Peripheral neuropathy in xeroderma pigmentosum. *Brain* 1990;113:1025–1044.
458. Mimaki T, et al. Neurological manifestations in xeroderma pigmentosum. *Ann Neurol* 1986;20:70–75.
459. Kristjansdottir R, et al. Disorders of the cerebral white matter in children: the spectrum of lesions. *Neuropediatrics* 1996;27:295–298.
460. van der Knaap MS, et al. Leukoencephalopathy with swelling and a discrepantly mild clinical course in eight children. *Ann Neurol* 1995;37:324–334.
461. Singhal BS, et al. Megalencephalic leukodystrophy in an Asian Indian ethnic group. *Pediatr Neurol* 1996;14:291–296.
462. van der Knaap MS, et al. A new leukoencephalopathy with vanishing white matter. *Neurology* 1997;48: 845–855.
463. Gripp KW, et al. Imaging studies in a unique familial dysmyelinating disorder. *Am J Neuroradiol* 1998;19: 1368–1372.
463a. Olivier M, et al. A new leukoencephalopathy with bilateral anterior temporal lobe cysts. *Neuropediatrics* 1998;29:225–228.
464. Chediak M. Nouvelle anomalie leucocytaire de caractere constitutionnel et familial. *Rev Hemat* 1952;7: 362–367.
465. Donohue WL, Bain HW. Chédiak-Higashi syndrome. A lethal familial disease with anomalous inclusions in the leukocytes and constitutional stigmata: report of a case with neuropathology. *Pediatrics* 1957;20: 416–430.
466. Sheramata W, Kott S, Cyr DP. The Chédiak-Higashi-Steinbrinck syndrome. *Arch Neurol* 1971;25:289–294.
467. Sung JH, et al. Neuropathological changes in Chédiak-Higashi disease. *J Neuropathol Exp Neurol* 1969; 28:86.
468. Haddad E, et al. Treatment of Chédiak-Higashi syndrome by allogenic bone marrow transplantation: report of 10 cases. *Blood* 1998;85:3328–3333.
469. Seitelberger F, Gross H. Ueber eine spätinfantile form der Hallervorden-Spatzschen krankheit. II. histochemische befunde, erörterung der nosologie. *Dtsch Z Nervenheilk* 1957;176:104–125.
470. Aicardi J, Castelein P. Infantile neuroaxonal dystrophy. *Brain* 1979;102:727–748.
471. Tanabe Y, et al. The use of magnetic resonance imaging in diagnosing infantile neuroaxonal dystrophy. *Neurology* 1993;43:110–113.
472. Ferreira RC, Mierau GW, Bateman JB. Conjunctival biopsy in infantile neuroaxonal dystrophy. *Am J Ophthalmol* 1997;123:264–266.

473. Ramaekers VT, et al. Diagnostic difficulties in infantile neuroaxonal dystrophy. *Neuropediatrics* 1987; 18:170–175.

474. Williamson K, et al. Neuroaxonal dystrophy in young adults: a clinicopathological study of two unrelated cases. *Ann Neurol* 1982;11:335–343.

475. Begeer JH, et al. Infantile neuroaxonal dystrophy and giant axonal neuropathy: are they related? *Ann Neurol* 1979;6:540–548.

476. Rett A. Ueber ein eigenartiges hirnatrophisches Syndrom bei Hyperammonamie im Kindesalter. *Wien Med Wochenschr* 1966;116:723–726.

477. Naidu S. Rett syndrome: a disorder affecting early brain growth. *Ann Neurol* 1997;42:3–10.

478. Wahlstrom J. Practical and theoretical considerations concerning the genetics of the Rett syndrome. *Brain Dev* 1987;9:466–468

478a. Sirianni N, et al. Rett syndrome: confirmation of X-linked dominant inheritance and localization of the gene to Xq28. *Am J Hum Genet* 1998;63:1552–1558.

479. Amir RE, et al. Rett syndrome is caused by mutations in X-linked NECP2, encoding methyl-CpG-binding protein 2. *Nat Genet* 1999;23:185–188.

480. Nan X, et al. Transcriptional repression by the methyl-CpG-binding protein MeCP2 involves a histone deacetylase complex. *Nature* 1998;393: 386–389.

481. Hendrich B, Bird A. Identification and characterization of a family of methyl-pG-binding proteins. *Mol Cell Biol* 1998;18:6538–6547.

482. Baumann ML, Kemper TL, Arin DM. Pervasive neuroanatomic abnormalities of the brain in three cases of Rett syndrome. *Neurology* 1995;45: 1581–1586.

483. Armstrong DD, Dunn K, Antalffy B. Decreased dendritic branching in frontal, motor and limbic cortex in Rett syndrome compared with trisomy 21. *J Neuropathol Exp Neurol* 1998;57:1013–1017.

484. The Rett Syndrome Diagnostic Criteria Work Group. Diagnostic criteria for Rett syndrome. *Ann Neurol* 1988;23:425–428.

485. Hagberg B, et al. A progressive syndrome of autism, dementia, ataxia, and loss of purposeful hand use in girls: Rett's syndrome—report of 35 cases. *Ann Neurol* 1983;14:471–479.

486. Glaze DG, et al. Rett's syndrome: characterization of respiratory patterns and sleep. *Ann Neurol* 1987;21: 377–382.

487. Nihei K, Naitoh H. Cranial computed tomographic and magnetic resonance imaging studies on the Rett syndrome. *Brain Dev* 1990;12:101–105.

488. Alpers BJ. Diffuse progressive degeneration of the cerebral gray matter. *Arch Neurol Psychiatry* 1931;25: 469–505.

489. Ford FR, Livingston S, Pryles CV. Familial degeneration of the cerebral gray matter in childhood, with convulsions, myoclonus, spasticity, cerebellar ataxia, choreoathetosis, dementia, and death in status epilepticus: differentiation of infantile and juvenile types. *J Pediatr* 1951;39:33–43.

490. Sung JH, et al. An unusual degenerative disorder of neurons associated with a novel intranuclear hyaline inclusion (neuronal intranuclear hyaline inclusion disease). *J Neuropathol Exp Neurol* 1980;39:107–130.

491. Goutières F, Mikol J, Aicardi J. Neuronal intranuclear inclusion disease in a child: diagnosis by rectal biopsy. *Ann Neurol* 1990;27:103–106.

492. Wilson DC, et al. Progressive neuronal degeneration of childhood (Alpers syndrome) with hepatic cirrhosis. *Eur J Pediatr* 1993;152:260–262.

493. Harding BN. Progressive neuronal degeneration of childhood with liver disease (Alpers-Huttenlocher syndrome): a personal review. *J Child Neurol* 1990;5:273–287.

494. Naviaux RK. Mitochondrial DNA polymerase α-deficiency and mtDNA depletion in a child with Alpers' syndrome. *Ann Neurol* 1999;45:54–58.

Chapter 3

Chromosomal Anomalies
and Contiguous Gene Syndromes

John H. Menkes and *Rena E. Falk

*Departments of Neurology and Pediatrics, University of California, Los Angeles, UCLA School of Medicine, and Department of Pediatric Neurology, Cedars-Sinai Medical Center, Los Angeles, California 90048; and *Department of Pediatrics, University of California, Los Angeles, UCLA School of Medicine, and Steven Spielberg Pediatric Research Center, Cedars-Sinai Medical Center, Los Angeles, California 90048*

This chapter considers conditions that develop as a result of chromosomal abnormalities. Abnormalities of chromosomes are either constitutional or acquired. Acquired chromosomal abnormalities develop postnatally, affect only one clone of cells, and are implicated in the evolution of neoplasia. Constitutional abnormalities on the other hand develop during gametogenesis or early embryogenesis and affect all or a major portion of the subject's cells. Until recently, detection of constitutional abnormalities was limited to disorders that resulted in gains or losses of an entire chromosome or large portions thereof—abnormalities readily visible by routine cytogenetics. The introduction of chromosomal banding techniques with increasing degrees of resolution, the widespread use of fluorescent in situ hybridization (FISH), and supplemental molecular analyses have refined cytogenetic analysis and have permitted detection of uniparental disomies and innumerable subtle, often submicroscopic (cryptogenic), deletions, duplications, or translocations—disorders that generally induce defects in multiple, contiguous genes (1). Because in humans more than 30,000 genes are expressed in brain, it comes as no surprise that impaired brain function is the most common symptom of chromosomal anomalies.

In considering the significance of some of the subtle chromosomal abnormalities, one must keep in mind that many of the abnormal chromosomal constitutions have been ascertained by searching the genome of mentally or neurologically handicapped individuals with multiple congenital abnormalities, thus introducing an obvious sampling bias. To complicate matters, chromosomal abnormalities are seen in only a fraction of handicapped individuals, whereas a sizable proportion of healthy adults have been found to have chromosomal variants. These include variations in Y chromosomal length, variations in satellite size or location, and variations in size of secondary constrictions, as well as some forms of mosaicism, balanced translocations, and differences in the intensity and appearance of bands revealed by staining techniques. Small supernumerary chromosomes (*marker chromosomes*) may serve as a case in point. This abnormality is seen in 0.3 to 1.2 of 1,000 newborns and in 0.7 to 1.5 of 1,000 fetuses on amniocentesis. Even though the origin of the marker chromosome may be ascertained by FISH, for the purpose of genetic counseling the prognosis of the marker is still uncertain in many cases (2).

An evaluation of the relationship of chromosomal abnormalities to neurologic deficits can be achieved by controlled, blind-coded cytogenetic surveys in groups of unclassifiable mentally retarded and control subjects. One such study using routine cytogenetics detected chromosomal abnormalities in 6.2% of mentally retarded patients and 0.7% of controls (3). Routine cytogenetic analyses have uncovered chromosomal anomalies in 40% of subjects with severe mental retardation [intelligence quotient (IQ) less than 55], and 10% to 20% in subjects with mild mental retardation (4). However, the cost of a systematic surveillance of the newborn population using both high-resolution chromosomal banding and DNA polymorphisms, as are being performed by Flint and colleagues, would be prohibitive (4).

Using banding techniques, Jacobs and colleagues found a 0.92% prevalence of structural chromosomal abnormalities in unselected newborns (5). The limitations of prenatal and neonatal surveillance programs are discussed more fully by Hook and colleagues (6). Studies in other species, as well as in humans, have shown that major duplications or deficiencies in autosomes tend to be lethal (7), with death occurring either *in utero* or in the immediate postnatal period (8). Few of the autosomal trisomies are compatible with survival. Thus, the most common trisomy, chromosome 16, accounts for 7.5% of all spontaneous abortions, but is not compatible with live birth, and only 2.8% of trisomy 13, 5.4% of trisomy 18, and 23.8% of trisomy 21 cases are live born (6).

This chapter confines itself to the neurologic sequels of chromosomal abnormalities. For the basic principles of cytogenetics, consult one of several excellent monographs (9). Schinzel (10), Jones (11), and de Grouchy and Turleau (12) present useful summaries of the phenotypic expressions of the various chromosomal deficits. A continuously updated catalogue of chromosomal variations has been published by Borgaonkar (13) and is available on line, http://www.wiley.co.uk/products/subject/life/borgaonkar.

AUTOSOMAL ABNORMALITIES

Down Syndrome (Trisomy 21)

Down syndrome (trisomy 21), the most common autosomal anomaly in live births and the most common single cause of mental retardation, was first differentiated from other forms of mental retardation in 1866 by Down (14) and Seguin

(15). Demographic factors, notably the higher proportion of older women bearing children, have caused an increase in the incidence of this condition. However, prenatal diagnosis programs also have affected the incidence. The most recent figures in the United States (1992) indicate an incidence of 1.04 per 1,000 newborns, and 34.1% occur in births to women aged 35 years and older (16). This is significantly less than the incidence of 1 in 500 recorded in 1950 (16a).

Etiology and Pathogenesis

Down syndrome is associated with either an extra chromosome 21 or an effective trisomy for chromosome 21 by its translocation to another chromosome, usually chromosome 14, or, less often another acrocentric chromosome, especially chromosome 21 or 22 (17).

A few terms require definition. In the general population one couple in more than 500 carries a reciprocal translocation. *Reciprocal translocation* is a structural alteration of chromosomes that usually results from breakage of two chromosomes with the subsequent exchange of the resultant chromosomal segments. In general, this event occurs during cell division, most frequently at prophase of the first meiotic division. The segments exchanged are nearly always from nonhomologous chromosomes and are usually not the same size. Such a rearrangement is said to be *balanced* when none of the chromosomal material appears to be duplicated or deleted on standard or high-resolution analysis.

Robertsonian translocation results from centromeric fusion of two acrocentric chromosomes. A larger chromosome is formed, with the resultant loss of the short arm regions of the participating chromosomes, resulting in a complement of 45 chromosomes in the *balanced carrier*. On a clinical basis, it is impossible to distinguish between patients with Down syndrome caused by regular trisomy 21 and those caused by translocation. The frequency of trisomy 21 increases with maternal age and reaches an incidence of 1 in 54 births in mothers aged 45 years or older (18). In contrast to ordinary trisomy, the incidence of translocation Down syndrome is independent of maternal age. Most translocations producing Down syndrome arise de novo in the affected child and are not associated with familial Down syndrome. Data obtained between 1989 and 1993 on prenatal and postnatal diagnoses of 1,811 Down syndrome subjects born to mothers aged 29 years or younger show trisomy 21 in 90.8% (17). Of a group of 235 translocation Down syndrome subjects, 42% involved a translocation between chromosome 21 and chromosome 14, whereas 38% showed a translocation involving two 21 chromosomes. In translocation, patients for whom cytogenetic results were available from both parents, 21;21 translocations were almost invariably de novo, whereas 37% of 14;21 translocations were inherited from the mother, and 4% derived from the father (17). Of 51 cases of 21;21 translocation investigated, 50 were de novo and one was of maternal origin (17).

Approximately 1% of couples experience the recurrence of Down syndrome as a result of regular trisomy 21. In most instances, this is caused by previously unrecognized mosaicism in one parent (19). In families in whom Down syndrome results from a translocation, the risk for subsequent affected children is significantly higher; it is 15% if the mother is the carrier, but less than 5% of the father is the translocation carrier (20).

By the use of polymorphic DNA markers, several studies have concluded that in more than 90% of instances the extra chromosome is maternally derived and mainly is the consequence of errors in the first meiotic division. The mean maternal age associated with errors in meiosis is approximately 33 years, significantly higher than the mean reproductive age in the United States. In 4.3%, there were errors in paternal meiosis. In these cases, and in the remainder, caused by errors in mitosis, maternal age is not increased (21). Several hypotheses have been put forth to account for the maternal age effect; the most likely is that with increasing age a decreasing number of chiasmata occurs, that is to say sites of crossovers, where recombination occurs because of breakage and reunion between homologous chromosomes (22).

To understand the molecular pathogenesis of Down syndrome, two questions must be answered: (a) What portion of chromosome 21 is responsible for the phenotypic expression of Down syndrome, and (b) how does the presence of a small acrocentric chromosome in triplicate produce the anatomic and functional abnormalities of the Down syndrome phenotype?

Studies on individuals with partial trisomy 21 have suggested that overexpression and subsequent interactions of genes on chromosome 21q22 contribute significantly to the phenotype of Down syndrome (23). It is of potential significance that the gene for a Down syndrome cell adhesion molecule has been mapped to chromosome 21q22.2-22.3. This gene is expressed in the developing nervous system, and like other cell adhesion molecules is critical for cellular migration, axon guidance, and the formation of neural connections (see Chapter 4) (22). However, duplication of regions distinct from 21q22 suffice to produce many of the typical Down syndrome features (23).

It also is not known how the presence of extra copies of genes and their regulatory sequences produces the Down syndrome phenotype. Although, on a theoretical basis, one would expect gene product levels 1.5 times normal, this is not always the case. Thus, amyloid precursor protein (APP), whose gene is located just outside the duplicated area critical to the Down syndrome phenotype, is expressed approximately four times normal in the brains of patients with Down syndrome (24).

Pathology

Malformations affect principally the heart and the great vessels. Approximately 20% to 60% of Down syndrome subjects have congenital heart disease. Defects in the atrioventricular septum were the most common abnormalities encountered by Rowe and Uchida in 36% of their patients, most of whom were younger than 2 years of age (25). A ventricular septal defect was present in 33%, and a patent ductus arteriosus was present in 10% of patients. Among the other malformations, gastrointestinal anomalies are the most common. These include duodenal stenosis or atresia, anal atresia, and megacolon. Hirschsprung disease is seen in approximately 6% of subjects (26). Malformations of the spine, particularly of the upper cervical region, can occasionally produce neurologic symptoms (27).

Grossly, the brain is small and spherical, and the frontal lobes, brainstem, and cerebellum are

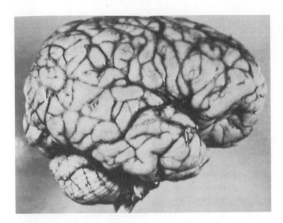

FIG. 3.1. Lateral view of the brain of a 10-year-old boy with Down syndrome showing the typical small superior temporal gyrus and the large operculum. (From Lemire RJ, et al. *Normal and abnormal development of the human nervous system.* Hagerstown, MD: Harper & Row, 1975. With permission.)

smaller than normal. The number of secondary sulci is generally reduced, the tuber flocculi persist, and the superior temporal gyrus is poorly developed (Fig. 3.1). A number of microscopic abnormalities also have been described (28,29). In essence, these involve reduction of neuronal density in various areas of the cortex, a loss of cortical interneurons, an accumulation of undifferentiated fetal cells in the cerebellum, and a reduction in the number of spines along the apical dendrites of pyramidal neurons (30). The reduction has been interpreted as indicating a reduction in the number of synaptic contacts. Interestingly, the dendritic tree is greater than normal in early infancy, but the excessive early outgrowth is followed by atrophy (31). Becker and colleagues have explained these observations as an abortive attempt by neurons to compensate for the decreased number of spines and synapses on their receptive surfaces (31).

Abnormalities of the basal nucleus have received particular attention, because an early and significant loss of neurons in this area is a feature of Down syndrome and Alzheimer disease. In Down syndrome the cell count is one-third normal, even before the onset of dementia, and it decreases progressively with age (32). In

a few patients, particularly those dying in infancy, demyelinated patches are observed in the periventricular white matter, where they are accompanied by fat-filled granular cells.

The relation of these pathologic findings to the clinical picture remains to be determined. A significant proportion of subjects with Down syndrome die of congenital heart disease or sepsis, processes that could result in some of the microscopic alterations. These findings, however, are not commonly noted in children without Down syndrome who die of complications resulting from sepsis or congenital heart disease. The most likely conclusion is that failure in gyral development and aplasia of the brainstem and cerebellum represent structural anomalies that are the direct result of the chromosomal disorder.

The most intriguing neuropathologic observation is the premature development of senile changes within the brain, compatible with a morphologic diagnosis of Alzheimer disease. The pattern of involvement of the brain by senile plaques and tangles follows that seen in Alzheimer disease. The amygdala, hippocampus, and the association areas of the frontal, temporal, and parietal cortex are particularly vulnerable to these changes (33). They are found in 7.5% of subjects aged 10 to 19 years, in 15.5% of subjects aged 20 to 29 years, and in 80% of subjects who die aged 30 to 39 years (34–36). Microscopic alterations include pigmentary degeneration of neurons, senile plaques, and calcium deposits within the hippocampus, basal ganglia, and cerebellar folia. The calcium deposits in the cerebellar folia can be extensive enough to be seen on neuroimaging studies. As in Alzheimer disease, the brains of subjects with Down syndrome have reduced choline acetyltransferase activity, not only in areas that contain plaques, but also in those that appear microscopically normal (37). Price and coworkers have postulated a selective degeneration of the cells in the nucleus basalis of Meynert, analogous to that encountered in the senile dementia of Alzheimer disease (38).

Underlying the evolution of Alzheimer disease in children with Down syndrome is an excessive buildup of amyloid β-protein. Amyloid β-protein aggregates to form both senile plaques and amyloid deposits in cerebral blood vessels. Soluble forms of amyloid β-protein as generated from the amyloid β-protein precursor most commonly end at C-terminal residue 40 (Aβ40), but a longer form, Aβ42, also is produced. Aβ42 precedes Aβ40 in amyloid deposition in Down syndrome (39), and Aβ42 is present in the brain of fetuses affected with Down syndrome as early as 21 weeks' gestation (40). The gene for APP has been mapped to the Down syndrome critical region of chromosome 21, suggesting that overexpression of APP suffices to lead to an increased amount of Aβ42 in brain, which in turn initiates the formation of senile plaques. Indeed, plasma concentrations of Aβ40 and Aβ42 are increased approximately threefold and twofold, respectively (41). Why the appearance of plaques and amyloid deposits is delayed for decades after the appearance of Aβ42 remains unclear.

Clinical Manifestations

The clinical picture of Down syndrome is protean and consists of an unusual combination of anomalies, rather than a combination of unusual anomalies (20). The condition is seen more frequently in male subjects, with one study showing a male to female ratio of 1:23, but with a female bias in mosaic subjects (17).

The birth weight of Down syndrome infants is less than normal, and 20% weigh 2.5 kg or less (42). Neonatal complications are more common than normal, a consequence of fetal hypotonia and a high incidence of breech presentations. Physical growth is consistently delayed, and the adult Down syndrome subject is significantly short statured (43). The mental age that is ultimately achieved varies considerably. It is related in part to environmental factors, including the age at institutionalization for non–home-reared individuals, the degree of intellectual stimulation, and the evolution of presenile dementia even before puberty. As a rule, the developmental quotient (DQ) is higher than the IQ and decreases with age (Table 3.1) (44). Most of the older patients with Down syndrome have IQs between 25 and 49, with the average approximately 43. The social adjustment tends to be approximately

TABLE 3.1. *Intellectual functioning of children with Down syndrome*

Age (yr)		Mean	Standard deviation	Range
0–1	Developmental quotient	65	±15	27–100
1–2	Developmental quotient	51	±11	23–73
2–3	Developmental quotient	46	±8	32–55
3–4	Intelligence quotient	43	±16	10–55
4–9	Intelligence quotient	43	±7	10–61

Modified from Smith GF, Berg JM. *Down's Anomaly.* 2nd ed. Edinburgh: Churchill Livingstone, 1976. With permission.

3 years ahead of that expected for the mental age (44). The decline in full-scale IQ with age is faster in those subjects who carry the E4 allele, an important risk factor for both sporadic and familial late-onset Alzheimer disease (44a).

Mosaicism can be found in approximately 2% to 3% of patients with Down syndrome. In these instances, the subject exhibits a mixture of trisomic and normal cell lines. These individuals tend to achieve somewhat higher intellectual development than nonmosaic subjects, and, in particular, they possess better verbal and visual-perceptual skills (45).

Aside from mental retardation, specific neurologic signs are rare and are limited to generalized muscular hypotonia and hyperextensibility of the joints. This is particularly evident during infancy and occurs to a significant degree in 44% of subjects younger than 9 years of age (46).

Whereas major motor seizures are seen no more frequently in Down syndrome infants than in the general population, the association between infantile spasms and Down syndrome is greater than chance (47). Attacks can occur spontaneously or, less often, follow insults such as perinatal hypoxia. The electroencephalogram (EEG) demonstrates hypsarrhythmia or modified hypsarrhythmia (48). The prognosis for seizure control is relatively good. In the experience of Stafstrom and Konkol, only 3 of 16 patients with Down syndrome with infantile spasms had persistent seizures, and the degree of cognitive impairment did not exceed that

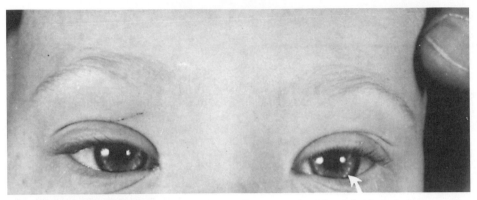

FIG. 3.2. Five-year-old child with Down syndrome demonstrating Brushfield spots (*arrow*). (Courtesy of the late Dr. H. Zellweger, Department of Pediatrics, University of Iowa.)

expected for the general Down syndrome population (48). A progressive disorganization of the EEG accompanies the evolution of Alzheimer dementia (49). Neuroimaging characteristically reveals large opercula, an indication of the underdeveloped superior temporal gyrus. In older subjects, evidence exists of premature aging (50). Symmetric calcifications in basal ganglia are common, particularly in adults (51).

Numerous case reports and series have associated atlantoaxial instability and dislocation with Down syndrome. The instability, seen in some 15% to 40% of patients, results from laxity of the transverse ligaments that hold the odontoid process close to the anterior arch of the atlas (52). The instability is usually asymptomatic, but neck pain, hyperreflexia, progressive impairment of gait, and urinary retention have been encountered (53). Other patients have experienced an acute traumatic dislocation. In view of this catastrophic complication, children with Down syndrome should undergo a complete neurologic examination, including neuroimaging of the cervical spine, if they plan to participate in competitive sports (e.g., Special Olympics) or in sports that could result in trauma to the head or neck. Children who have this abnormality should be excluded from these activities. Children with atlantoaxial instability who develop neurologic signs require surgical stabilization of the joint (54). Children with Down syndrome who do not participate in ath-

letics may be screened with lateral radiography of the cervical spine taken with the head in flexion and extension.

In addition to these neurologic abnormalities, patients with Down syndrome exhibit a number of stigmata. None of these is present invariably, nor are any consistently absent in the healthy population, but their conjunction contributes to the characteristic appearance of the subject.

The eyes show numerous abnormalities, almost all of which have been encountered in other chromosomal anomalies (55). The palpebral fissures are oblique (upslanting) and narrow laterally. Patients have a persistence of a complete median epicanthal fold, a fetal characteristic rarely present in healthy children older than age 10 years but observed in 47% of trisomy 21 patients aged 5 to 10 years and in 30% of older subjects (56). Brushfield spots are an accumulation of fibrous tissue in the superficial layer of the iris. They appear as slightly elevated light spots encircling the periphery of the iris (Fig. 3.2). According to Donaldson, Brushfield spots are present in 85% of Down syndrome subjects, as compared with 24% of controls (56,57). Blepharitis and conjunctivitis are common, as are lenticular opacifications and keratoconus, particularly in older subjects. Many children with Down syndrome benefit from spectacles to correct refractive errors and astigmatism.

Anomalies of the external ear are also frequent. The ear is small, low set, and often C

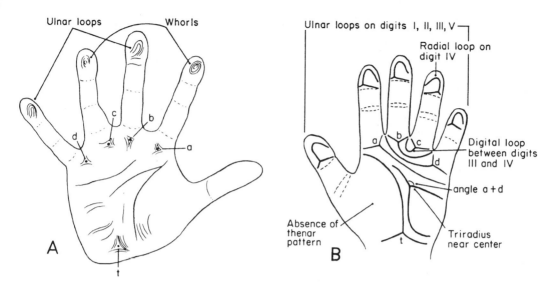

FIG. 3.3. Outlines of the digital, palmar, and plantar configurations. **A:** Healthy child. The triradii are a, b, c, d, and t—the meeting point of sets of parallel ridges; t is located near the base of the fourth metacarpal bone at some point on its axis. **B:** Child with Down syndrome. A transverse palmar crease occurs, fingers tend to have a loop pattern, and the triradius subtends an angle of approximately 80 degrees with points a and d instead of the normal 45 degrees. (Modified from Penrose LS. Fingerprints, palms and chromosomes. *Nature* 1963;197:933.)

shaped, with a simple helix and hypoplastic tragus. The cartilage is often deficient. Additionally, the diameter of the external auditory meatus is abnormally narrow, which precludes good visualization of the tympanic membrane.

Structural anomalies of the middle and inner ear might contribute significantly to the language delay commonly encountered in children with Down syndrome. Congenital malformations of the bones of the middle ear, permanent fixation of the stapes, and shortening of the cochlear spiral are encountered frequently (58). Additionally, children, particularly infants, are prone to acute and chronic otitis, middle ear effusions, and endolymphatic hydrops with subsequent conductive and neurosensory hearing loss.

According to Balkany and colleagues (59), 64% of patients with Down syndrome have binaural hearing loss. In 83%, the hearing loss is conductive, and in the remainder, sensorineural. Brainstem auditory-evoked potentials can be used to determine the type and severity of hearing loss in young or uncooperative children (60). Because of the frequency of impaired

hearing, a comprehensive hearing evaluation is indicated during the first 6 to 12 months of life.

The lips of the patient with Down syndrome have radial furrows, and, as a consequence of the generalized hypotonia, the tongue, often fissured, tends to protrude because the maxilla is too small and the palate is too narrow to accommodate it. A typical finding, particularly evident in infants, is a roll of fat and redundant skin in the nape of the neck, which combined with the short neck and low hairline, gives the impression of webbing.

The extremities are short. The fifth digit is curved in, and the middle phalanx is hypoplastic (clinodactyly). As a consequence, its distal interphalangeal crease is usually proximal to the proximal interphalangeal crease of the ring finger. Additionally, the distal and proximal interphalangeal creases are closely spaced, and there might be a single flexion crease on the fifth digits. The simian line, a single transverse palmar crease, is present bilaterally in 45% of patients (Fig. 3.3). In the feet, a diastasis between the first and second toes (sandal gap) is the most characteristic anatomic abnormality. A juvenile rheumatoid arthritislike progressive polyarthritis has been seen with some frequency. A number of other autoimmune disorders also have a greater than chance association with Down syndrome (61).

The dermatoglyphic pattern of the patient with Down syndrome shows several abnormalities. Of these, a distally displaced triradius, the palmar meeting point of three differently aligned fine creases, is seen in 88%, but in only 10% of controls (44). Dermatoglyphic abnormalities of the fingerprint patterns are equally characteristic (see Fig. 3.3) (44,62).

Abnormalities of the skin are common. Xeroderma and localized chronic hyperkeratotic lichenification are seen in 90% and 75% of subjects, respectively. Vitamin A levels are reduced in 15% to 20% of subjects.

Down syndrome is associated with several autoimmune conditions, notably diabetes mellitus type I, and with a variety of endocrine abnormalities (63). An elevation of antithyroid antibody is common, and nearly 50% of trisomy 21 subjects, mostly male, have reduced thyroid function in later life (64). Congenital hypothyroidism and primary gonadal deficiency are fairly common, but hypothyroidism can appear at any age. Gonadal deficiency progresses from birth to adolescence and becomes manifest in adult life with resultant infertility in virtually all nonmosaic male subjects (65).

Currently, 44% and 14% of Down subjects survive to 60 and 68 years of age, respectively (66). Several factors contribute to the reduced life expectancy. The most important of these is the high incidence of major cardiovascular malformations; these account for some 80% of deaths. In one study, 92.2% of Down syndrome subjects without congenital heart disease survived to age 24 years, as contrasted with 74.6% of subjects with congenital heart disease (67). As expected, mortality in those with congenital heart disease is the greatest during the first year of life (68). Of less significance in terms of influencing life expectancy is a 10- to 20-fold increase in lymphoid leukemia (69). As a rule, acute myeloid leukemia predominates in children with Down syndrome under age 4 years, whereas acute lymphoid leukemia predominates in older children (69). Also shortening the life expectancy of children with Down syndrome is a still unexplained high susceptibility to infectious illnesses, and the early appearance of Alzheimer disease, which results in a marked decrease in survival after 35 years of age (70). The clinical picture of Alzheimer disease in patients with Down syndrome corresponds to that in patients without Down syndrome. Deterioration of speech and gait are early findings. Epileptic seizures and myoclonus are common and were seen in 78% and 8% of patients in the Dutch series of Evenhuis (71). Loss of cognitive function, including memory loss, generally remains unrecognized until the later stages of the disease.

Diagnosis

The diagnosis of Down syndrome is made by the presence of the characteristic physical anomalies and is confirmed by cytogenetic analysis. Karyotyping of all cases of Down syndrome is indicated to identify those that result from chromosomal translocation. When translocation is present, the karyotype of both parents must be ascertained to determine whether one of them carries a balanced translocation.

Antenatal screening is indicated for mothers ages 35 or older at term, as well as in the young mother who has had a previous child with Down syndrome. Screening procedures for low-risk pregnancies can be conducted during the second trimester. Low maternal serum α-fetoprotein, reduction of unconjugated estriol, and elevated chorionic gonadotropins are independent predictors of Down syndrome. Using a combination of these markers, approximately two-thirds of Down syndrome fetuses can be detected (72). Inhibin, a glycoprotein of placental origin, is elevated in maternal serum in women with Down syndrome fetuses and has been suggested as another useful screening marker (73), as has pregnancy-associated protein A (73a). A positive result should prompt a follow-up ultrasound study and amniocentesis (72). Trials of first trimester screening are currently in progress.

Women with abnormal screening tests are offered ultrasound and amniocentesis. Cytogenetic studies of amniotic fluid or chorionic villi can be used for the antenatal diagnosis of Down syndrome as early as the third month of gestation. Current techniques of cell culture and karyotyping have been refined to the point that more than 99% of Down syndrome cases studied antenatally are diagnosed correctly. Even the diagnosis of a mosaic Down syndrome does not present any diagnostic difficulty except when the frequency of the abnormal karyotype is low (74). However, accurate prediction of the phenotype in mosaic cases can be problematic. Eventually, routine screening of all mothers for Down syndrome will be possible. One approach is the implementation of a polymerase chain reaction–based technique that uses chromosome 21 markers to detect abnormal gene copy numbers in fetal cells (75).

Treatment

Despite the number of vigorously and fervently advocated regimens, none has proved successful in improving the mental deficit of the child with Down syndrome. Medical intervention is directed toward treatment and prophylaxis of infections, treatment of hearing and visual deficits, early recognition and treatment of hypothyroidism, and if possible, correction of the congenital heart disease or any other significant malformation. Although not proven statistically, early intervention appears to be of benefit in enhancing communication and self-help skills.

The early administration of 5-hydroxytryptophan, a serotonin precursor, appears to reverse the muscular hypotonia characteristically present in the infant with Down syndrome (76), and in some instances can accelerate motor milestones. Unfortunately, this has no effect on the ultimate level of intelligence (77).

The treatment of the mentally retarded child with Down syndrome is similar to that of children retarded from any cause and having the same potential of intellectual and social function. The topic, particularly the role of early

intervention and total communication programs, is discussed in Chapter 16.

Other Abnormalities of Autosomes

Trisomies involving the other, larger chromosomes are associated with multiple severe malformations of the brain and viscera, and affected children usually do not survive infancy. The two entities most commonly encountered are trisomies of chromosomes 13 and 18. The incidence of these and other chromosomal abnormalities are presented in Table 3.2 (78).

Trisomy Chromosome 13 (Patau Syndrome)

Trisomy chromosome 13 (Patau syndrome) occurs in fewer than 1 of 5,000 births. Approximately one-half of cases are diagnosed prenatally through a combination of routine ultrasound and serum screening (79). The clinical picture is char-

TABLE 3.2. *Incidence of chromosomal anomalies among 3,658 newborns in a Danish population between 1980 and 1982*

Chromosomal anomalies	Total	Rate per 1,000
Autosomal chromosomes		
+ 13	0	
+ 18	1	0.27
+ 21	5	1.37
+ 8	1	0.27
+ ring	2	0.55
13/14 translocation	2	0.55
14/21 translocation	1	0.27
Reciprocal translocations	7	1.91
Inversion chromosome 2 and 6	2	0.55
Inversion chromosome 9[a]	35	9.57
Duplications	2	0.55
Others	1	0.27
Total autosomal anomalies	59	16.13
Sex chromosome anomalies		
47,XXY	3	1.60
47,XYY	2	1.07
47,XXX	3	1.68
45,XO (including mosaics)	4	2.24
Others	3	1.63
Total sex chromosome anomalies	15	4.10
Total chromosome anomalies	74	20.23

[a]No physical abnormalities accompany balanced translocations or inversion of chromosome 9.

Data from Nielsen J, et al. Incidence of chromosome abnormalities in newborn children. Comparison between incidences in 1969–1974 and 1980–1982 in the same area. *Hum Genet* 1982;61:98–101. With permission.

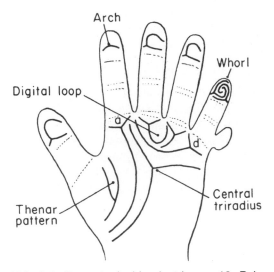

FIG. 3.4. Dermatoglyphics in trisomy 13. Polydactyly is present. The angle subtended by points a, d, and the central triradius is almost 90 degrees. Unlike in Down syndrome, both arches and whorls can be present. (Modified from Penrose LS. Fingerprints, palms and chromosomes. *Nature* 1963;197:933.)

acterized by feeding difficulties, apneic spells during early infancy, and striking developmental retardation (12,80–82). Subjects have varying degrees of median facial anomalies, including cleft lip or palate, and micrognathia. The ears are low set and malformed, and many infants are deaf. Polydactyly, flexion deformities of the fingers, and a horizontal palmar crease are common. The dermatoglyphics are abnormal (Fig. 3.4). Cardiovascular anomalies are present in 80% of patients, most commonly in the form of a patent ductus arteriosus or a ventricular septal defect. Approximately 33% of patients have polycystic kidneys. Also, an increased frequency of omphalocele and neural tube defects exists. Microcephaly is present in 83% and microphthalmus in 74% (81).

The major neuropathologic abnormality is holoprosencephaly (arrhinencephaly), a complex group of malformations that have in common absence of the olfactory bulbs and tracts and other cerebral anomalies, notably only one ventricle and absence of the interhemispheric fissure (see Chapter 4). On autopsy, a number of micro-

scopic malformations are observed, including heterotopic nerve cells in the cerebellum and in the subcortical white matter (83–85).

Absence of the olfactory apparatus is not specific for trisomy 13. In the series of Gullotta and coworkers (86), this malformation was encountered at autopsy in some 40% of trisomy 13 subjects. It also occurs with deletion of the short arm of chromosome 18 (18p), in the trisomy 18 syndrome, and with deletion of the long arm of chromosome 13 (13q). A condition termed *pseudotrisomy 13 syndrome* is fairly common. This entity is characterized by alobar holoprosencephaly and polydactyly, accompanied by apparently normal cytogenetics (87). Cardiac, pulmonary, genital, or other skeletal malformations also can be present (88).

The prognosis for children with chromosome 13 trisomy is poor. Approximately 50% die during the first month of life, and only 20% survive into the second year.

Trisomy Chromosome 18
(Edwards Syndrome)

Trisomy chromosome 18 (Edwards syndrome) was first discovered in 1960 by Edwards (89). Its incidence appears to be on the increase; it occurs in 1 of 555 conceptuses, with the most recently recorded frequencies in live-born infants in Dublin and Leicester being in the range of approximately 1 in 3,000 (90). The anomaly is seen four times more frequently in female subjects, suggesting that a high proportion of affected male fetuses succumb during gestation. Like other autosomal trisomies, trisomy 18 results from an error in maternal meiosis, with the additional chromosome demonstrating maternal origin in 96% of cases (91).

The clinical picture is highlighted by a long narrow skull with prominent occiput, characteristic facies, low-set malformed ears, a mildly webbed neck, and marked physical and mental retardation (81,86). A typical picture of camptodactyly (flexion contractures of the fingers) and abnormal palmar flexion creases occurs. The second and fourth fingers characteristically overlie the third, and the fifth finger overlies the fourth. Distally implanted, retroflexible thumbs are encountered frequently. As in chromosome 13 trisomy, omphalocele, polycystic kidneys, and congenital heart disease are common. A striking dermatoglyphic pattern, relatively less common in other autosomal anomalies, is the presence of simple arches on all fingers.

No consistent central nervous system malformation is associated with the trisomy 18 syndrome. The most common anomaly is agenesis of the corpus callosum, occasionally associated with nerve cell heterotopias of the cerebellum or white matter (84–86). In more than 50% of subjects, the brain is small, but normal on gross and routine microscopic examination (86). The prognosis for children with trisomy 18 is poor, and 90% die by 1 year of age. The mean survival time is 10 months for girls, and 23 months for boys (91). The natural history of trisomy 18 and trisomy 13 in long-term survivors has been well-characterized (91a,91b).

Other trisomies are much less common (see Table 3.2) but have been found with relatively high frequency in spontaneous human abortions (7). Mosaic trisomy syndromes have been recognized for chromosomes 8, 9, 16, and 20. Their clinical appearance is reviewed by de Grouchy and Turleau (12) and Tolmie (20).

STRUCTURAL AUTOSOMAL ANOMALIES

The best described of the numerous classical deletion syndromes are the 5p- (cri du chat), and the 4p- (Wolf-Hirschhorn) syndromes.

Cri du Chat Syndrome

A number of structural anomalies of the autosomal chromosomes have been reported and have been accompanied by neurologic defects, notably mental retardation and microcephaly. The most common of these entities is a deletion of the short arm of chromosome 5 (5p), which causes the cri du chat syndrome (92). Through the combined phenotypic and molecular analysis of affected individuals the genes responsible for this condition have been mapped to 5p15.2 and 5p15.3. Deletion of a critical region in 5p15.2 results in the characteristic facial features and the severe mental retardation, whereas deletion of 5p15.3 is associated only with the meowing cry (93).

Cri du chat syndrome is seen with a frequency of 1 in 20,000 to 50,000 births (20,92). A low birth weight and failure in physical growth are associated with a characteristic cry likened to that of a meowing kitten. Infants have microcephaly, large corneas, moon-shaped facies, ocular hypertelorism, epicanthal folds, transverse palmar (simian) creases, and generalized muscular hypotonia. The brain, although small, is grossly and microscopically normal, representing a rare example of true microcephaly (94).

Wolf-Hirschhorn Syndrome

The Wolf-Hirschhorn syndrome is caused by partial monosomy of the short arm of chromosome 4, with the region critical for the development of this disorder being 4p16.3 (95,96). The syndrome is characterized by a facies that has been likened to that of a Greek helmet. Frontal bossing, a high frontal hairline, a broad, beaked nose, prominent glabella, and ocular hypertelorism are seen. Major malformations occur commonly, especially cleft lip and palate, and mental retardation is usually severe. Deletions in the region responsible for Wolf-Hirschhorn syndrome overlap those seen in Pitt-Rogers-Danks syndrome. This entity has a somewhat different phenotype. It is marked by prenatal and postnatal growth retardation, microcephaly, prominent eyes, a large mouth, and maxillary hypoplasia. Mental retardation is somewhat less severe than is seen in the Wolf-Hirschhorn syndrome. As yet, no explanation exists for the phenotypes, and imprinting has been excluded (97).

Other structural autosomal anomalies associated with neurologic symptoms are summarized in Table 3.3. The various chromosomal anomalies have been tabulated by Borgaonkar (13).

Partial deletions and partial trisomies have been described for almost every chromosome, but few of these entities are sufficiently characteristic to allow the practitioner to suspect the diagnosis without cytogenetic analysis. In par-

TABLE 3.3. *Some structural autosomal anomalies associated with neurologic symptoms*

Chromosomal anomaly[a]	Clinical picture[b]	Reference
Trisomy short arm of 4	Microcephaly, growth retardation, prominent glabella, rounded nose, low-set ears	Rethore et al. (98)
Deletion short arm of 4	Microcephaly, hypotonia, hypertelorism, broad base of nose, ptosis, carplike mouth	Miller et al. (99), Hirschhorn et al. (100)
Deletion short arm of 5	Microcephaly, kitten cry during infancy	Lejeune et al. (92), Breg et al. (101)
Trisomy long arm of 7	Low birth weight, fuzzy hair, small palpebral fissures, micrognathia, abnormal low-set ears	Vogel et al. (102)
Trisomy of 8 (mosaic)	Long slender trunk, restricted articular function of large and small joints, thickened skin with deep furrows, absent patella	Riccardi (103)
Trisomy of 9 (mosaic)	Upward slanted eyes, small palpebral fissures, broad base and prominent tip of nose	Quazi et al. (104)
Trisomy short arm of 9	Microcephaly, enophthalmos, antimongoloid slant, bulbous nose with inverted nostrils, protruding ears	Centerwall and Beatty-DeSana (105)
Trisomy short arm of 10	Microcephaly, wide forehead, arched and widely spaced eyebrows, small palpebral fissures, carp mouth, microphthalmia	Klep-dePater et al. (106)
Trisomy short arm 11 (partial)	Short nose, long philtrum, micrognathia, retracted lower lip, micropenis	Pihko et al. (107)
Deletion 11q2 (Jacobsen syndrome)	Trigonocephaly, growth retardation, ptosis, congenital heart disease, pancytopenia	Wardinsky et al. (107a)
Deletion long arm 12, (partial)	Hypertonia, mental retardation, congenital anomalies	Tengstrom (108)
Trisomy distal portion short arm of 13	Microcephaly, narrow temples, long in-curved eyelashes, abnormal dentition, low-set or malformed ears	Schinzel et al. (109)
Ring 14	Mixed major and minor motor seizures; no major congenital anomalies and few facial stigmata	Lippe and Sparkes (110)
Deletion short arm of 18	Holoprosencephaly, congenital ptosis, microcephaly, hypertension, epicanthal folds	Nitowsky et al. (111)
Deletion long arm or 18	Hypoplasia first metacarpals, hypoplasia nasomaxillary region, microcephaly, carp mouth	Wertelecki et al. (112)
Deletion long arm of 21	Microcephaly, downward slant of palpebral fissures, low-set ears, high-arched or cleft palate	Mikkelsen and Vestermark (113)
Trisomy of 22	Microcephaly, large deep-set eyes, growth retardation, micrognathia, low-set malformed ears, preauricular skin tags, fingerlike thumbs, small penis, undescended testis	Hsu and Hirschhorn (114)
Trisomy long arm of 22	Coloboma of iris (cat's-eye syndrome), microcephaly, micrognathia, low-set ears	Hirschhorn et al. (115)

[a]p denotes short arm and q denotes long arm of the chromosome.
[b]Mental retardation is common to all of these chromosomes.

ticular, the phenotypic expressions of ring chromosomes overlap those of partial deletions, showing so much variability that one cannot arrive at any conclusions with respect to their clinical pictures (116). Furthermore, certain features are common to many of the chromosomal anomalies, and they also are encountered in the absence of any discernible chromosomal defect. Therefore, only those anomalies that occur with sufficient frequency to establish a fairly definite clinical picture are discussed here. The most complete review of the various neurologic deficits seen in chromosomal disorders is that by Kunze (117).

SEX CHROMOSOME ABNORMALITIES

Sex chromosome abnormalities consist of various aneuploidies involving the sex chromosomes. As determined by most surveys of the newborn population (118) or of cells obtained at amniocentesis (119), the incidence of sex chromosome abnormalities is approximately 2.5 in 1,000 phenotypic male subjects and 1.4 in 1,000 phenotypic female subjects (118). Although considerable geographic variation occurs, the two most common abnormalities in phenotypic male subjects are the XYY and the XXY (Klinefelter) syndromes (118). A significantly lower incidence of sex chromosome abnormalities is found in newborns than is found at amniocentesis, and in a large proportion of subjects with sex chromosome abnormalities, particularly phenotypic male subjects, the condition remains undiagnosed throughout life (119,120). The great majority of the abnormalities in female subjects (75%) involve the XXX syndrome, with less than 25% being X monosomy (Turner syndrome) or variants thereof (121).

Klinefelter Syndrome

Klinefelter syndrome was first described by Klinefelter in 1942 in male patients who suffered from increased development of breasts, lack of spermatogenesis, and increased excretion of follicle-stimulating hormone. The chromosome constitution of XXY, present in most subjects, was elucidated in 1959 (122).

The condition occurs in 1 in 600 male subjects (123). Although affected persons are relatively tall with an enunichoid habitus, the diagnosis is usually not made until adult life, and hormone assays are normal before the onset of puberty (124). Neurologic examination shows decreased muscle tone and some dysmetria or tremor; the major deficits encountered in unselected subjects are cognitive disorders. In the Denver series, IQs were some 10 points lower than controls (125), whereas in the Edinburgh series of Ratcliffe, the mean IQ of XXY patients was 96, as contrasted with a mean IQ of 105 for controls (126). A high incidence of impaired auditory sequential memory occurs, which results in delayed language development and a variety of learning disorders, notably dyslexia (127). An increase in the incidence of behavioral abnormalities also has been observed (126). EEG abnormalities, including spike and spike-wave discharges, are said to be common (128). A greater than chance association

exists between Klinefelter syndrome and midline suprasellar or pineal germinomas (129).

XYY Karyotype

The XYY karyotype is another common chromosomal anomaly encountered in the phenotypic male, with a frequency as high as 4 in 1,000 male newborns (130).

In the past, the XYY karyotype has been thought to be associated with unusually tall stature and dull normal intelligence. Controlled studies, however, have indeed shown a small, statistically significant deficit in the Webster Intelligence Test for Children Verbal and Full Scale IQs, but none in the Performance scores (131). Additionally, these boys can exhibit minor neurologic abnormalities, including intention tremor, mild motor incoordination, and limitation of motion at the elbows secondary to radioulnar synostoses (132,133). The last defect is also seen in Klinefelter syndrome.

The initial impression that a high proportion of XYY subjects exhibits antisocial behavior aroused much controversy. In some surveys, subjects had been ascertained by screening of psychiatric wards, prisons, and maximum security hospitals (134). However, careful behavioral studies have confirmed that XYY patients tend to have a high incidence of temper tantrums and to exhibit other forms of overt impulsive behavior, poor long-term planning, and an inability to handle aggression in a socially acceptable manner (131,135,136).

Other Sex Chromosonal Polysomies

In a phenotypically male subject, the greater the number of X chromosomes, the more severe the mental retardation. XYYY subjects, such as the one reported by Townes and associates, are only mildly retarded (137), whereas all of the 12 XXXYY male subjects reviewed by Schlegel had major intellectual deficit, with IQs varying from 35 to 74 (138). Subjects with the XXXY syndrome have severe mental retardation, small testes, microcephaly, and a variety of minor deformities (139). The XXXXY chromosomal anomaly is characterized by mental retardation, hypotonia, and a facial appearance reminiscent of

Down syndrome. The palpebral fissures are upslanted, and the individual has epicanthal folds, excess posterior cervical skin, and widely separated eyes. The fifth digits are usually shorter and curved inward (140).

In the phenotypic female subject, the presence of more than two X chromosomes also is associated with mental retardation. The most common of these disorders is the XXX syndrome, which is seen in 1 in 200 newborn female subjects (123). Although no specific clinical pattern exists for female subjects with the XXX sex chromosome complement and considerable variability exists in their cognitive abilities, the majority have an IQ less than that of their siblings and are at risk for language problems, learning disabilities, and impaired social adaptation (125). Additionally, the girls are clumsy and poorly coordinated, with hypotonia of their musculature. Tetrasomy and pentasomy X female subjects are usually mentally retarded, with the observed degree of retardation increasing with the number of supernumerary X chromosomes (141).

Turner Syndrome
(Ullrich-Turner Syndrome)

In 1938, Turner described a syndrome of sexual infantilism, cubitus valgus, and webbed neck in women of short stature (142). Ford, in 1959, found this condition to be generally associated with the 45,X chromosomal complement (143). In actuality, when cytogenetic techniques are combined with DNA analysis, the large majority, probably more than 75% of live-born individuals, are 45,X mosaics who have a normal XX cell line, another abnormal cell line, or both. In the experience of Kocova and colleagues, 40% of subjects whose karyotype was 45,X had some Y chromosome material (144). Other Turner subjects could have mosaicisms that are present in low frequencies (micromosaicism), which cannot be detected by the relatively insensitive techniques of conventional cytogenetics (145,146).

Turner syndrome is seen in approximately 0.2 per 1,000 female subjects (147). The clinical and endocrinologic picture of Turner syndrome is complex; this discussion is confined to the neurologic symptoms (148). As a rule, the apparent absence of the X chromosome is not associated with a gross intellectual deficit (149). However, severe mental retardation and a variety of gross congenital malformations are seen in some Turner syndrome patients with a tiny ring X chromosome (150). In these subjects, the XIST locus on their ring X chromosome is not present or is not expressed, resulting in defective X inactivation (151,152). The role of XIST in X chromosome inactivation is discussed by Kuroda and Meller (153).

Although the incidence of Turner syndrome is no greater in the institutionalized retarded than in the newborn (154), the majority of patients have a right-left disorientation and a defect in perceptual organization (*space-form blindness*) (155–157). This is particularly true for those subjects who have an apparent 45,X karyotype and is less marked in children with obvious mosaicism (158). Subjects in whom the X chromosome is paternally derived have better verbal skills and social adjustment than those in whom the X chromosome is maternally derived (159). The defects in perceptual organization correlate with magnetic resonance imaging evidence of reduced volume of cerebral hemisphere and parieto-occipital brain matter, including hippocampus, lenticular, and thalamic nuclei, being more marked on the right (160). Treatment with growth hormone has only a limited effect; but may be useful with or without concomitant anabolic corticosteroids (160a). It is not known whether early treatment improves cognitive deficits (161).

A syndrome that is phenotypically similar to Turner syndrome but occurs in karyotypically normal female and male subjects (Noonan syndrome) is associated commonly with short stature, congenital heart disease, hypertelorism, hypotonia, auditory nerve deafness, and mild mental retardation (162,163). Some patients have cortical dysplasia (164). As in Turner syndrome, lymphedema is a frequent occurrence; it results from dysplasia of the lymphatic vessels (165). The condition is transmitted as an autosomal dominant trait with the gene localized to the long arm of chromosome 12. The association of Noonan syndrome with neurofibromatosis has been reported by several authors. Evidence now exists for a second Noonan syndrome locus on 17q, and the concurrence of Noonan syndrome with neurofibromatosis type 1 may represent either a contiguous gene syndrome or the coincidental segregation of two autosomal dominant conditions (166).

Fragile X Syndrome

Even though the diagnosis of fragile X syndrome is now made by DNA analysis rather than cytogenetic analysis, this condition is best considered at this point.

The fact that a preponderance of patients in institutions for the mentally retarded are male has long been recognized, and various pedigrees corresponding to a sex-linked inheritance of mental retardation were recorded by Martin and Bell (167) and Renpenning and colleagues (168), among many others. No cytogenetic abnormality could be found consistently in these subjects until 1977, when Harvey and associates (169) and Sutherland (170) demonstrated a fragile site within the terminal region of the long arm of the X chromosome (Xq27) when cells were cultured in folic acid–deficient media.

Etiology, Pathogenesis, and Molecular Genetics

The progressive unraveling of the nontraditional inheritance pattern of the fragile X syndrome has been chronicled by Tarleton and Saul (171). The fragile X gene (*FMR-1*) has been isolated, cloned, and characterized. It contains a trinucleotide sequence (CGG), which in the normal genome is repeated from 6 to 55 times (172). In persons with the fragile X syndrome, this repeat is expanded (amplified) to several hundred copies (full mutation), whereas asymptomatic carriers for fragile X carry between 50 and 230 copies (premutation) (Fig. 3.5). The premutation tends to remain stable during spermatogenesis, but frequently expands to a full mutation during oogenesis. All male subjects with a full mutation, but only 53% of female subjects with a full mutation, are mentally impaired (173). The marked expansion of the CGG repeat sequence is accompanied by inacti-

vation through methylation of a sequence (CpG island) adjacent to, but outside of, the *FMR-1* gene, believed to initiate gene transcription. As a consequence, the *FMR-1* gene is not expressed in the majority of fragile X patients and its gene product, the fragile X mental retardation protein, a ribosome-associated RNA binding protein of uncertain function, is reduced or completely absent. Good correlation exists between the degree of methylation at the FMR-1 locus and phenotypic expression (174). It is becoming apparent that any mutation in the *FMR-1* gene, including deletions or point mutations such as the one described by Hammond and colleagues, which result in the failure to form the *FMR-1* gene product can give rise to the fragile X phenotype (175) although these are not detected by the standard tests described in the following sections.

Normally, the *FMR-1* gene is expressed in many tissues, including brain. There it is expressed in high levels in the neuronal perikarya where it is concentrated in ribosome-rich regions. The protein also has been localized to large- and small-caliber dendrites. The rapid production of fragile X mental retardation protein in response to stimulation of the glutamate receptor suggests that it is involved with dendritic function and normal maturation of synaptic connections (176,177).

Pathology

To date, no specific neuropathology has been recognized. On gross examination, the posterior vermis is reduced in size, with a compensatory increase in the size of the fourth ventricle. Magnetic resonance imaging studies have confirmed that the volume of the posterior vermis and the volume of the superior temporal gyrus are significantly reduced, whereas the volume of the hippocampus is increased (178,179). Ultramicroscopy shows abnormal synapses, suggesting defective neuronal maturation or arborization (180).

Clinical Manifestations

The condition is relatively common, second only to Down syndrome as a genetic cause for

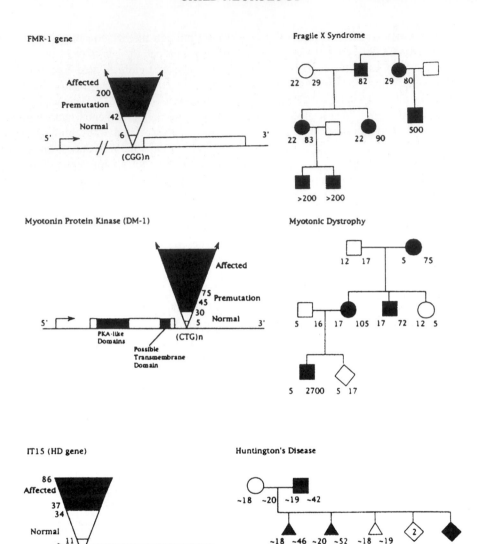

FIG. 3.5. Diseases caused by expansion of trinucleotide repeats. On the left, a schematic diagram of each gene, with the repeat region depicted as an inverted pyramid and the numbers of repeats beside it. Open regions represent the normal variation of repeat numbers. A representative pedigree for each disorder is depicted on the right, with the number of repeats in each allele displayed below the symbols. Open symbols represent unaffected individuals. Circles represent female subjects, squares represent male subjects, diamonds or triangles represent individuals whose sex is not identified, with a number inside to indicate more than one person. (Adapted from Ross CA, et al. Genes with triplet repeats: candidate mediators of neuropsychiatric disorders. *Trends Neurosci* 1993;16:254. With permission of Dr. C. A. Ross, Laboratory of Molecular Neurobiology, Departments of Psychiatry and Neuroscience, Johns Hopkins University School of Medicine, Baltimore, MD.)

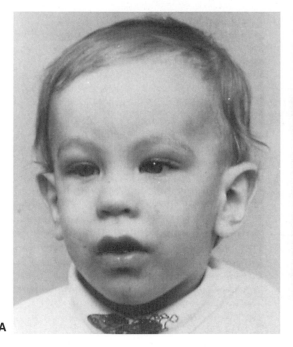 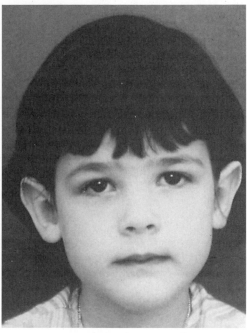

A   B

FIG. 3.6. A: Fragile X syndrome in a 2.5-year-old boy. Note long hypotonic face, high forehead, epicanthal folds, and prominent ears. **B:** Five-year-old fragile X–positive girl, referred because of behavior problems. Note prominent ears. (From Chudley AE, Hagerman RJ. Fragile X syndrome. *J Pediatr* 1987;110:821–831. With permission.)

mental retardation. It was seen with a frequency of 0.92 in 1,000 male subjects in British Columbia (181). In Coventry, England, the prevalence was 1 in 1,370 male subjects and 1 in 2,083 female subjects (182). Some 9% of male subjects with IQs between 35 and 60 and no neurologic signs have the fragile X syndrome (183). On screening using DNA analysis, 0.4% of unselected women have been found to carry premutations of 55 to 101 repeats (184).

Fragile X is a clinically subtle dysmorphic syndrome. The male has a long face, prominent brow, somewhat square chin, large, floppy ears, and macro-orchidism without any obvious evidence of endocrine dysfunction (Fig. 3.6A) (185). Although macro-orchidism can be present at birth (185), it is difficult to recognize in the prepubertal boy, as are most of the other physical features (186). Approximately 10% of subjects have a head circumference greater than the 97th percentile, and the fragile X syndrome may mimic the features of cerebral gigantism

(187,188). A number of clinical features reflect connective tissue dysplasia (186). These include hyperextensible finger joints, flat feet, aortic root dilatation, and mitral valve prolapse.

The neurologic picture is highlighted by retarded language development and hyperactivity. Delayed motor development is seen in some 20% of male subjects, and seizures have been experienced by 25% to 40% of male subjects. These are major motor or partial complex seizures and as a rule they respond well to anticonvulsant therapy (187). They do not correlate with the severity of the mental retardation. Gross neurologic deficits are the exception, although some subjects have been considered to be hypotonic (187). The severity of mental retardation varies considerably. Most male subjects are in the moderately to severely retarded range; in the experience of Hagerman and her group, 13% of boys have an IQ of 70 or higher, but experience significant learning disabilities (189). The majority of male subjects who carry a premuta-

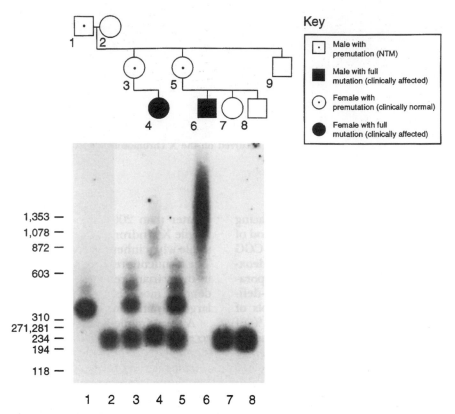

FIG. 3.7. Pedigree and polymerase chain reaction blot of fragile X family. Lane 1: Male subject with premutation (phenotypically normal transmitting male subject). The polymerase chain reaction blot shows only one band with a slightly greater molecular weight than normal. Lanes 2 and 7: Healthy female subjects. On polymerase chain reaction a single band occurs, with approximately 234 base pairs. Lanes 3 and 5: Female subjects with premutation. Their polymerase chain reaction blots show two groups of bands, one single band representing the normal X chromosome, and the other, a series of bands with amplification up to approximately 700 base pairs. Lane 4: Phenotypically affected female subject with full mutation. The polymerase chain reaction blot shows a band representing the normal X chromosome, and a smear of bands demonstrating the expansion. Lane 6: Male subject with full mutation. His polymerase chain reaction blot shows a smear of bands, which extends to over several thousand base pairs. Lane 8: Healthy male subject. (Courtesy of Genica Pharmaceuticals Corporation, Worcester, MA.)

tion are clinically unaffected, but some have significant learning disabilities (190).

The prevalence of autism among male subjects with the fragile X syndrome is considerable. Between 5% and 15% of autistic subjects have the fragile X syndrome, and, conversely, in the experience of Hagerman and coworkers, 16% of male subjects with the fragile X syndrome experience infantile autism (191). A large proportion of the remainder were found to have some autistic features, including poor eye con-

tact, fascination with spinning objects, and impaired relatedness. However, Einfeld and Hall could not detect any difference in the incidence of autistic behavior between subjects with fragile X and matched retarded controls (192). As many as 50% of fragile X male subjects with autistic symptoms have mosaicism (171).

In the affected female subject, clinical features are extremely variable. Typical physical features are generally absent or are relatively unremarkable (Fig. 3.6B). In the experience of

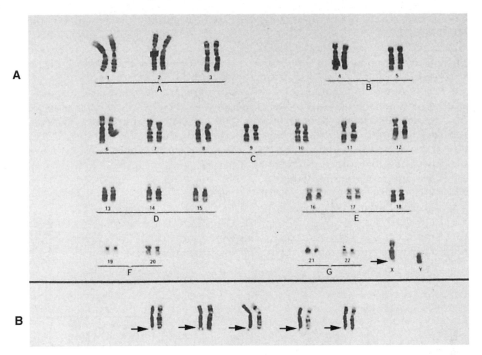

FIG. 3.8. X-linked mental retardation associated with the fragile X chromosome. **A:** Representative Giemsa (GTG) banded karyotype of a 12-year-old mentally retarded boy with relative macrocephaly, prominent brows, deep-set eyes, large ears, and megalotestes. The fragile site (*arrow*) was demonstrated in 28% of cells cultured in folic acid–deficient media. **B:** Fragile X chromosomes from same patient. Each pair represents the single X chromosome from a cell that was first analyzed unbanded (left), for easier recognition of the fragile site (*arrows*), then banded (right) to confirm that the fragile site occurred on the X chromosome. (Courtesy of Dr. Rena Falk, Cedars-Sinai Medical Center, Los Angeles, CA.)

Hagerman and her coworkers, 25% of girls had an IQ below 70, and another 28% had IQs between 70 and 84 (193). Of those girls who had a normal IQ, approximately one-half had learning difficulties. Conversely, in the experience of Turner and coworkers, approximately 5% of mildly retarded school girls had the marker X chromosome (194). No evidence exists for any deterioration in intelligence in female subjects, although the IQ of most boys with the full expansion decreases over time (190).

Diagnosis

Diagnosis of the fragile X syndrome in affected individuals and carriers can be made readily by means of molecular DNA techniques (Fig. 3.7). In the view of most experts in the field, this procedure has replaced cytogenetic fragile X testing as the diagnostic method of choice because the latter technique can result in false-negative results (195) (Fig. 3.8). Sutherland and Mulley argue that all patients with mental retardation should first be assessed by conventional cytogenetic techniques to detect the numerous other chromosomal abnormalities responsible for mental retardation in addition to fragile X (172).

Four other fragile sites have been found cytogenetically on the long arm of chromosome X. *FRAXE*, located on band Xq28, is often associated with a mild form of mental retardation. In this disorder, a GCC repeat occurs on Xq28 (196,197). Healthy individuals have up to 25 copies of the repeat; the mentally retarded have greater than 200 copies. In contrast to the fragile X syndrome (*FRAXA*), the repeat is equally unstable when

TABLE 3.4. Contiguous gene syndromes

Condition	Clinical manifestations	Chromosomal defect	References
Langer-Giedion	Mild to severe mental retardation, bulbous nose, redundant folds of skin over neck, multiple exostoses	8q24	Langer et al. (246), Ludecke et al. (247)
Beckwith-Wiedemann	Muscular hypertrophy, macroglossia, hypoglycemia, gigantism, omphalocele; increased risk for malignancies, notably Wilm tumor; some have paternal uniparental disomy	11p15.5	Hatada et al. (248), Koufos et al. (249), Pettenati et al. (250)
DiGeorge	Hypoparathyroidism, cellular immune deficiency, mental retardation	22q11.2	Driscoll et al. (251)
Aniridia, Wilm tumor	Aniridia, Wilm tumor, mental retardation, genitourinary anomalies, hemihypertrophy	11p13	Narahara et al. (252)
Smith-Magenis	Broad, flat midface, brachydactyly, hoarse, deep voice, mental retardation, peripheral neuropathy, characteristic self-hugging habit	17p11.2	

From Greenberg, F, et al. Multi-disciplinary clinical study of Smith-Magenis syndrome (deletion 17p11.2). *Am J Med Genet* 1996;62:247–254 and Elsea SH, et al. Gene for topoisomerase III maps within the Smith-Magenis syndrome critical region: analysis of cell-cycle distribution and radiation sensitivity. *Am J Med Genet* 1998;75:104–108.

inherited from father or mother. The frequent presence of normal intelligence in this variant reflects a relatively high incidence of mosaicism, with coexistent small and large amplifications (198).

FRAXF and *FRAXD* are less common. Subjects with *FRAXF* are mentally retarded with seizures (199), whereas *FRAXD*, located on band Xq27.2, is a common fragile site inducible in most healthy people and of no clinical significance (172).

The fragile X syndrome accounts for one-third to one-half of X-linked mental retardation. Additionally, more than 90 X-linked disorders exist, more than 40 of which have been mapped, in which mental retardation is a prominent clinical feature (172). One common entity, exemplified by the family originally reported by Renpenning and associates (168), is characterized by fairly severe mental retardation, microcephaly, short stature, and a normal karyotype (200). Patients belonging to the family reported by Martin and Bell (167) have subsequently been found to have the fragile X syndrome (172). The total estimated frequency of X-linked mental retardation is 1.8 in 1,000 male subjects, thus exceeding the incidence of Down syndrome (201).

Treatment

No specific treatment exists for youngsters with the fragile X syndrome. Rather, management involves a multidisciplinary approach with early speech and language therapy and behavior modification (186).

CHROMOSOMAL ANOMALIES IN VARIOUS DYSMORPHIC SYNDROMES (CONTIGUOUS GENE SYNDROMES, SEGMENTAL ANEUSOMY SYNDROMES)

In addition to deletions that are readily detected cytogenetically, combined molecular and cytogenetic analysis has led to the identification of small deletions in a number of clinically well-defined syndromes. These are outlined in Table 3.4. The term *contiguous gene syndrome*, coined by Schmickel (202), refers to the patterns of phenotypic expression resulting from the inactivation or overexpression as a result of deletion, duplication, or other means, of a set of adjacent genes in a specific chromosome region.

These conditions are distinct from the various syndromes that result from gross chromosomal deletion or duplication readily demonstrable by classic cytogenetic techniques (see Table 3.3) (203). The use of improved techniques for the examination of chromosomal structure has revealed that chromosomal anomalies are encountered in some syndromes with a far greater frequency than can be explained by chance. The number of recognizable syndromes has continued to multiply over the last decade or two, and their diagnosis has become increasingly difficult. Books by Jones (11) and Buyse (204) are invaluable assistants for that task, but even with their aid, diagnosis is often in dispute. An on-line database for the diagnosis of genetic and dysmorphic syndromes (OMIM) has been prepared by McKusick and his group and is continuously updated by the National Center for Biotechnology Information. It can be accessed at http://www.ncbi.nlm.nih.gov.

Two clinical disorders with a marked difference in clinical expression are associated with interstitial deletions of chromosome 15q11-q13, Prader-Willi and Angelman syndromes.

The observation that the clinical picture of deletion 15q11-q13 depended on whether the deleted chromosome is derived from mother or father, provided the first clear example of genomic imprinting in the human. Certain regions of the human genome normally exhibit gene expression from only the maternally or the paternally inherited allele. The term *genomic imprinting* refers to the differential expression of genetic material depending on whether it is inherited from the male or female parent. The absence of biparental contributions to the genome, which cannot be detected by routine cytogenetic examination, may be responsible for a large proportion of syndromes for which no chromosomal anomaly has as yet been demonstrated. Hall also has suggested that the phenotypic differences in any given chromosomal syndrome may reflect the parental origin of the affected chromosome (205). Some children with a cytogenetically normal karyotype have uniparental disomy (UPD) rather than biparental inheritance of a specific chromosome pair. UPD may exert a profound effect on the phenotype for several reasons. In some cases (isodisomy), it results in homozygosity for one or more deleterious genes. When imprinted regions are involved, UPD may result in loss of expression or overexpression of a critical imprinted gene or genes. In addition, Lalande suggests that genomic imprinting perturbs the timing of normal chromosomal replication (206). A more

extensive discussion of imprinting in Prader-Willi and Angelman syndromes is provided by Nicholls and colleagues (206a).

Prader-Willi Syndrome

Prader-Willi syndrome, marked by obesity, small stature, hyperphagia, and mental retardation, was first described by Prader and coworkers (207). It is not an unusual condition, and its prevalence has been estimated at 1 in 10,000 to 25,000 births (208).

When chromosomes are examined by FISH analysis, approximately 70% of patients with Prader-Willi syndrome demonstrate a deletion of the proximal part of the long arm of chromosome 15 (15q11-q13) (209). These deletions, which are occasionally visible by high-resolution banding techniques, occur exclusively on the paternally derived chromosome. Some of the remaining subjects with Prader-Willi syndrome have other abnormalities in the same region of chromosome 15, including molecular deletions, translocation, duplication, or inverted, repeated DNA elements (210). Other patients appear to have a normal karyotype, but restriction fragment length polymorphism analyses show the presence of two maternally derived chromosomes 15, and no paternal chromosome 15 (UPD) (211). Thus, in at least 95% of patients, partial or complete absence of the paternal chromosome 15 occurs. In the remainder of the patients, the disease results from mutations in the imprinting center (203,212,212a). Although monozygotic twins concordant for Prader-Willi syndrome have been reported and familial cases are known (213), the vast majority of cases occurs sporadically.

The clinical picture is fairly uniform (214). Breech presentation is common. Symptoms of hypothermia, hypotonia, and feeding difficulties become evident in infancy. Hypotonia is occasionally so striking that infants are evaluated for muscle disorders (214a). Small hands and feet are noted in early childhood. Over the years, hyperphagia and excessive weight gain develop. Hypotonia tends to improve, but short stature, hypogonadism, and mild to moderately severe mental retardation become evident (11,213,214).

Characteristically, the face is long, the forehead narrow, and the eyes almond shaped. Several endocrine abnormalities have been documented, but many of these reflect the severe obesity rather than an underlying disorder (208,214). Most patients have hypersomnolence; daytime hypoventilation also has been observed (215). Approximately one-half of Prader-Willi subjects are hypopigmented, a finding that is associated frequently with cytogenetic deletions and may be related to deletion of the *P* gene, which maps to the Prader-Willi syndrome region and which is associated with one form of oculocutaneous albinism (216). Many patients have strabismus, and, curiously, as is the case in albinos, visual-evoked potentials have demonstrated that optic fibers from the temporal retina cross at the chiasm, rather than projecting to the ipsilateral occipital lobe (217).

Anatomic examinations of the brain and of muscle biopsies have not been helpful in providing insight into the cause of the mental retardation and hypotonia. Electron microscopy of skin biopsies has revealed a reduction in the number of melanin-containing cells.

The diagnosis of Prader-Willi syndrome is prompted by historic and clinical features and is confirmed by high-resolution chromosome banding, FISH, or both with probes from the 15q11-q13 region to disclose deletions and other cytogenetically detectable anomalies. UPD can be diagnosed by analysis of the 15q11-q13 methylation status. Whereas healthy subjects have biparental and always different patterns, subjects with Prader-Willi or Angelman syndromes caused by either deletions or UPD show a uniform methylation pattern. This procedure is available commercially, and is less costly than microsatellite polymorphism typing, a procedure that requires parental DNA samples (Fig. 3.9) (218). Wevrick and Francke have proposed a polymerase chain reaction test for the expression of the gene for small nuclear ribonucleoprotein polypeptide N in blood leukocytes. This gene is not expressed in any of the Prader-Willi patients regardless of the underlying cytogenetic or molecular causes (219). One report suggests that disruption or failure of small nuclear ribonucleoprotein polypeptide N

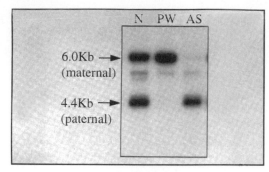

FIG. 3.9. Southern blot analysis exhibiting maternal 6.0-kb fragment and paternal 4.4-kb fragment in healthy person (lane N). In the patient with Prader-Willi syndrome (lane PW), the 4.4-kb fragment is lacking because of either deletion on paternal chromosome 15 or maternal uniparental disomy. In the patient with Angelman syndrome (lane AS), lack of the maternal 6.0-kb fragment indicates either deletion on maternal chromosome 15 or paternal uniparental disomy. (From Schad CR, Jalal SM, Thibodeau SN. Genetic testing for Prader-Willi and Angelman syndromes. *Mayo Clin Proc* 1995;70:1195–1196. With permission.)

expression is the cause of Prader-Willi syndrome (219a). The reliability and ease of the test for small nuclear ribonucleoprotein polypeptide N still need to be confirmed.

Angelman Syndrome

A submicroscopic deletion of the maternally derived chromosome 15q11-q13 is seen in approximately 70% of children with the Angelman "happy puppet" syndrome. Some 2% of patients with this condition have paternal UPD, and 2% to 3% have a defect in the imprinting center. The remaining 25% result from a defect in a gene involved in the ubiquitin-mediated protein degradation pathway (*UBE3A*) (203,220).

The incidence of Angelman syndrome is less than 1 in 10,000. The clinical picture is marked by severe mental retardation, microcephaly, and puppetlike, jerky, but not truly ataxic, movements. Frequent paroxysms of unprovoked laughter lend the syndrome its name. Several authors have noted that the lack of expressive speech in these children is disproportionate to the degree of retardation. Seizures are common and include almost every seizure type (221), most commonly atypical absences and myoclonic seizures (221a). The interictal EEG is said to be characteristic. It shows bifrontally dominant rhythmic runs of notched slow waves, or slow and sharp waves, especially during sleep when they can become continuous. At times, patients exhibit a rhythmic myoclonus involving hands and face that is accompanied by rhythmic 5- to 10-Hz EEG activity (222). With maturation, prolonged runs of 23-Hz high-amplitude (200 to 500 μV) spike and wave discharges make their appearance. This EEG result abnormality can be seen in the absence of seizures, and no correlation exists with electrical paroxysms and outbursts of laughter (223). As a rule, the seizure disorder is more severe in subjects with a chromosome 15q11-13 deletion than in those with UPD or mutations of the *UBE3A* gene (221a). The seizure disorder is probably the consequence of the deletion of one of the three $GABA_A$ receptors, such as GABRB3. Although a number of familial cases of Angelman syndrome have been reported, the recurrence risk for the condition is low except for those cases in which neither a deletion nor paternal UPD can be demonstrated. The latter cases may represent an autosomal recessive disorder caused by mutation in the *UBE3A* gene.

Examination of the brain shows mild cerebral atrophy, but normal gyral development. Marked cerebellar atrophy is seen, with loss of Purkinje and granule cells, and a marked decrease in dendritic arborizations (224).

Diagnosis may be made by FISH analysis in the case of deletions of 15q, but methylation studies detect a higher proportion of cases. Mutation analysis for *UBE3A* is not yet available commercially.

Miller-Dieker Syndrome

Miller-Dieker syndrome is characterized by lissencephaly, microcephaly, severe to profound mental retardation, and an unusual facies marked by a high forehead, vertical soft tissue furrowing, and a small, anteverted nose (11,225). More than 90% of subjects with this condition have visible or submicroscopic deletions of 17p13.3 (203). The chromosomal abnormality results in a deletion of one copy of *LIS-1*, a gene in this region. This gene encodes a protein that is a subunit of a brain platelet-activating factor acetylhydrolase. During early development, this protein is localized predominantly to the Cajal-Retzius cells, bipolar neurons of the preneuronal migration stage, and developing ventricular neuroepithelium (226).

The Miller-Dieker syndrome is a relatively rare cause of lissencephaly. This condition, which is discussed more extensively in Chapter 4, results from the arrest of migrating neurons in the formation of the cortical plate. In Gastaut series of 15 such cases, reported in 1987, only one was found to have an anomaly of chromosome 17 (227). However, subsequent studies using FISH have revealed that one-third of patients with isolated lissencephaly have deletions in 17p13.3. In other cases, molecular analysis may reveal point mutations in the *LIS-1* gene (228). For a more extensive discussion of lissencephaly, see Chapter 4.

Rubinstein-Taybi Syndrome

Rubinstein-Taybi syndrome was first described by Rubinstein and Taybi (229). It is marked by the presence of broad thumbs and great toes, a hypoplastic maxilla with a narrow palate, a prominent, beaked nose, and a moderate degree of mental retardation. Postnatal growth retardation occurs, and other facial abnormalities are common. These include downward-slanting palpebral fissures, low-set ears, heavy, highly arched eyebrows, and long eye-lashes (230). Although familial cases have been reported, the recurrence risk is on the order of 0.1%.

Many patients with the Rubinstein-Taybi syndrome have breakpoints or deletions of chromosome 16p13.3, and a gene for a nuclear protein that is involved in cyclic-AMP-regulated gene expression appears to be responsible for the clinical manifestations of the syndrome (203,231,232).

Cornelia de Lange Syndrome (Brachmann–de Lange Syndrome)

Cornelia de Lange syndrome (Brachmann–de Lange syndrome) is characterized by marked growth retardation, severe mental retardation, a

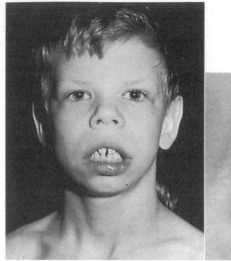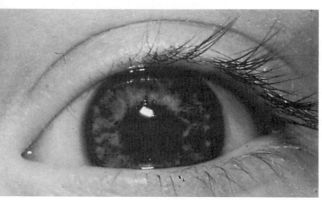

A   B

FIG. 3.10. A: Williams syndrome. The facial appearance in subjects is remarkably uniform. This boy's eyebrows flare medially, his nasal bridge is depressed, the epicanthal folds are prominent, and the nares are anteverted. Note prominent lips and full cheeks. (Courtesy of Professor K. Kruse, Medizinische Universität zu Lübeck, Germany, and Dr. R. Pankau, Universitäts Kinderklinik, Kiel, Germany.) B: Williams syndrome. A stellate pattern exists in the iris. (Courtesy Dr. G. Holmström, Department of Ophthalmology, Hospital for Sick Children, Great Ormond Street, London.)

low-pitched, growling cry, bushy eyebrows, hirsutism, and various malformations of the hands and feet (11,233). Although this condition is usually sporadic, it has a low recurrence rate. A number of patients have been found to have a partial duplication of the long arm of chromosome 3. They differ clinically from the classic form of the syndrome in that they usually do not demonstrate intrauterine growth retardation, they lack major limb abnormalities, and their facies are somewhat different from the typical de Lange patient (234). A homeobox gene that encodes one of the various transcription regulators controlling a variety of cell lines has been suggested as a candidate gene for the condition (235).

Williams Syndrome

Williams syndrome is a disorder marked by an unusual, elfinlike facies (Fig. 3.10A), supravalvular aortic stenosis, hypercalcemia, and significant physical and mental retardation. The

incidence of the condition has been estimated at 1 in 10,000 (203). Deletions at chromosome 7q11.23, inducing hemizygosity of *ELN*, the gene that encodes elastin, and a number of adjacent genes have been found in both maternally and paternally derived chromosomes. The other genes that are deleted commonly include *LIMK1*, which encodes a protein tyrosine kinase, *STX1A*, which encodes a component of the synaptic apparatus, and *FZD3*, which also is expressed in brain (235a,235c). Deletion of *LIMK1* is believed to be responsible for the defects in visuospatial construction seen in patients (235c,235d).

Mental retardation is usually not severe, and language ability may be quite good, with some children having an extraordinary talent for music. This contrasts with severe deficits in a number of nonverbal tasks, notably spatial cognition, planning, and problem solving (235b). An aortic systolic murmur, most commonly caused by supravalvular aortic stenosis is present in a large proportion of children. In addition, diffuse

TABLE 3.5. *Some of the rare malformation syndromes affecting the nervous system*

Condition	Manifestations	Reference
Bird-headed dwarf (Seckel)	Low birth weight, microcephaly, craniosynostosis, dislocation of joints, numerous bony defects, unusual facies, autosomal recessive inheritance	McKusick et al. (255), Seckel (256), Shanske et al. (257)
Börjeson syndrome	Seizures, hypogonadism, obesity, swelling of subcutaneous tissue of face, narrow palpebral fissures, large ears	Börjeson et al. (258), Gedeon et al. (259)
Cockayne syndromes	Impaired hearing, retinal degeneration, aged appearance, cataracts, intracranial calcifications, peripheral neuropathy	Chapter 2
Coffin-Siris syndrome	Mental retardation, coarse facial appearance, short fifth finger with absence of nail, Dandy-Walker deformity	Tunneson et al. (260), McPherson et al. (261)
De Sanctis-Cacchione syndrome (probably related to Cockayne syndromes)	Xeroderma pigmentosum, microcephaly; autosomal recessive transmission, defect in DNA repair	Reed et al. (262), Greenhaw et al. (263)
Hallermann-Streiff syndrome	Microphthalmia, hypotrichosis, malar hypoplasia, small nose, microcephaly	Hoefnagel and Bernirschke (264), Cohen (265)
Laurence-Moon syndrome	Obesity, mental retardation, polydactyly, retinitis pigmentosa, hypogonadism	Chapter 15
Leprechaunism	Large nares, low-set ears, sunken eyes, absent subcutaneous adipose tissue, short limbs, insulin resistance	Frindik et al (266), Kosztolanyi (267), Nakae et al (268)
Lowe syndrome	Cataracts, glaucoma, hypotonia, aminoaciduria, organic aciduria, choreoathetosis, X-linked transmission	Chapter 1
Schwartz-Jampel syndrome	Congenital blepharophimosis, continuous muscle contractions	Chapter 14
Sjögren-Larsson syndrome	Slowly progressive oligophrenia, spasticity, ichthyosis, deficiency of fatty alcohol:nicotinamide-adenine dinucleotide oxidoreductase	Hernell et al. (269), De Laurenzi et al. (270)
Sotos syndrome	Large-for-gestational-age infant, large hands and feet, macrocephaly, advanced bone age, wide range in IQ	Chapter 15
Zellweger syndrome (cerebrohepatorenal)	Hypotonia, high forehead with flat facies, poor suck, seizures, absent deep tendon reflexes, camptodactyly, peroxisomal disorder	Chapter 1

or segmental stenoses of a variety of arteries occur, including the carotid, which can result in cerebrovascular accidents (236,237). Early feeding difficulties, a hoarse cry, and small widely spaced teeth are other frequent manifestations. Hypertension is fairly common. More than one-half of children have a stellate pattern in their irises, which is uncommon in control subjects (Fig. 3.10B). The abnormality is believed to result from hypoplasia of the stroma of the iris (238). Magnetic resonance imaging shows cerebral hypoplasia and alterations in the relative size of paleocerebellar to neocerebellar portions of the vermis. Patients can die from azotemia or can become normocalcemic spontaneously. The cardiac murmur, characteristic facies, and mental retardation or borderline intellectual functioning persists into adult life (239). On pathologic examination, the brain is microcephalic, with paucity of gray matter neurons, foci of ectopic gray matter, and a variety of cytoarchitectural abnormalities (240).

Hypercalcemia is relatively infrequent and is not commonly documented by the time the diagnosis is made, although normocalcemic children can still have difficulty handling an intravenous load of calcium (241). No significant disturbance in vitamin D metabolism occurs, and the cause for the tendency to hypercalcemia still remains unexplained (242).

Velocardiofacial Syndrome

Velocardiofacial syndrome is a relatively common condition with an incidence that is comparable with or greater than that of Prader-Willi syndrome. It is characterized by a cleft palate, velopharyngeal insufficiency resulting in a distinctive hypernasal speech, cardiac malformations, a face marked by a prominent, bulbous nose, a squared nasal root, and micrognathia. The majority of children have learning disabilities or suffer from mild mental retardation (243). Approximately 25% of subjects develop a variety of psychiatric disorders in late adolescence or adult life, and there appears to be an increased susceptibility to schizophrenia (244). Hypocalcemia has been documented in approximately 20% of patients (243).

Cytogenetic analysis using FISH probes has shown deletions within 22q11. Some patients with velocardiofacial syndrome present with partial or typical DiGeorge syndrome associated with the 22q11 microdeletion (245). DiGeorge syndrome is phenotypically related to velocardiofacial syndrome. In addition to its clinical findings, thymic hypoplasia or aplasia and severe hypocalcemia also occur.

Other malformation syndromes are encountered frequently in the practice of child neurology. Most are characterized by mental retardation and small stature. Some of these conditions are outlined in Table 3.5. In due time and with a better understanding of molecular pathogenesis many of these entities will undoubtedly be found to represent contiguous gene syndromes or single gene defects.

ROLE OF CYTOGENETICS IN NEUROLOGIC DIAGNOSIS

Because chromosomal anomalies are seen in approximately 10% of moderately to profoundly retarded subjects, cytogenetic examination is an essential part of the evaluation of any youngster with a substantial mental handicap for which no obvious cause has been uncovered.

In most laboratories, phytohemagglutinin-stimulated lymphocytes serve for the analysis. However, in at least one entity, the Pallister-Kil-

TABLE 3.6. *Microdeletion syndromes for which fluorescent* in situ *hybridization probes are commercially available*

Condition	Chromosomal location
Angelman syndrome	15q11-13
Cri du chat syndrome	5p15.2
DiGeorge syndrome	22q11.2
Miller-Dieker syndrome	17p13.3
Prader-Willi syndrome	15q11-13
Smith-Magenis syndrome	17p11.2
Velocardiofacial syndrome	22q11.2
Wolf-Hirschhorn syndrome	4p16
Williams syndrome	7q11.23

Adapted from Jackson-Cook C, Pandya A. Strategies and logistical requirements for efficient testing in genetic disease. *Clinics Labor Med* 1995;15:839–857. With permission.

lian syndrome, a condition marked by profound mental retardation, streaks of hypopigmentation and hyperpigmentation, and facial dysmorphism, tetrasomy 12p has been detected in fibroblasts but not in lymphocytes (271). Some children with hypomelanosis of Ito have chromosomal mosaicism that may be demonstrated in skin and blood or only in fibroblast cultures. This condition is considered in Chapter 11.

Chromosomal banding is always indicated, and, at present, chromosomal analysis using only a conventional solid stain no longer has any role in pediatric neurology. The most popular banding technique in North America is Giemsa-trypsin banding (G banding). Quinacrine fluorescent banding (Q banding) and reverse banding (R banding) are additional techniques that are useful adjuncts in some cases. When an anomaly is identified, more than one banding technique might be needed to delineate its location and the size of any deletion or extra chromosomal fragment. When the location for the abnormality is suspected (e.g., chromosome 15q for Prader-Willi syndrome), molecular cytogenetic analyses using FISH techniques or high-resolution studies focusing on that site are indicated. FISH probes are now available for a number of microdeletion syndromes (Table 3.6) (272).

DNA studies are routine in the evaluation of the fragile X syndrome in the assessment of nonspecific mental retardation in both male and female subjects. When these study results are negative, and the phenotype is highly suggestive of the fragile X syndrome, cytogenetic analysis for fragile X should be performed also. An abnormal result would be an indication for *FMR-1* molecular analysis. Detection of the fragile X chromosome requires special culture conditions. Even so, only a relatively small proportion of cells (20% to 40%) show this marker (see Fig. 3.8). Additionally, the expression of fragile X can decrease with age, which complicates genetic analysis of families. Minor chromosomal deletions or other anomalies are best detected by examining cells in late prophase or early metaphase using high-resolution analysis, a technique much more laborious and expensive than standard analysis.

Unstable DNA sequences, as are seen in fragile X syndrome, myotonic dystrophy, and in several of the heredodegenerative conditions, can be detected by a repeat expansion detection technique. Such procedures are now available for clinical problems (273).

Because applying all the currently available cytogenetic techniques to the diagnosis of every mentally retarded child is not feasible, subjects with the greatest likelihood of chromosomal anomalies should be selected.

1. Chromosomal analysis is indicated in several circumstances: in the presence of clinically suspected autosomal syndromes (e.g., Down syndrome, cri du chat syndrome). In Down syndrome and in other trisomies, chromosomal analysis distinguishes nondisjunction trisomy from clinically identical translocation syndromes and mosaics.
2. In the presence of clinically suspected sex chromosome syndromes (e.g., Klinefelter syndrome, Turner syndrome).
3. Whenever mental retardation is accompanied by two or more major congenital anomalies, particularly when these involve the mesodermal or endodermal germ layers.
4. Whenever mental retardation is accompanied by minor congenital anomalies, particularly when these involve the face, hands, feet, or ears. In this respect, the frequency of minor anomalies of the face, mouth, ears, and extremities in a healthy population must

TABLE 3.7. *Incidence of stigmata in 74 healthy children*

Anomaly	Percentage
High palate	16.7
Head circumference >1 standard deviation outside normal range	15.3
Adherent ear lobes	14.0
Gap between first and second toe	11.7
Stubbed fifth finger	8.1
Curved fifth finger	7.7
Hypertelorism	6.8
Low-seated ears	4.5
Epicanthal folds	3.2
Syndactyly toes	2.7

From Walker HA. Incidence of minor physical anomalies in autistic patients. In: Coleman M, ed. *Autistic Syndrome*. New York: Elsevier Science, 1976:95–115. With permission.

be kept in mind. In a survey of 74 healthy children, Walker demonstrated between two and three such stigmata per subject (274). Their incidence in the healthy pediatric population is depicted in Table 3.7.

5. Whenever mental retardation is accompanied by small stature, physical underdevelopment, or dysmorphic features, including abnormalities of palmar creases (Fig. 3.11) or dermal ridge patterns (dermatoglyphics), or by abnormalities in the scalp hair whorl pattern (275,276). Because skin creases form at 11 to 12 weeks' gestation, these abnormalities point to an insult in early intrauterine life (276,277). Facial abnormalities are a particularly sensitive indicator of developmental anomalies of the brain. The explanation for this rests on the fact that facial development is dependent on prosencephalic and rhombencephalic organizing centers. Thus, any major defect in forebrain development can be reflected in the development of the face (278).
6. In the absence of a history of perinatal trauma, we obtain a cytogenetic survey in children who have microcephaly or the syndrome of muscular hypotonia with brisk deep tendon reflexes (atonic cerebral palsy). In addition, methylation studies or FISH for del (15q11.2) should be considered in the latter situation.

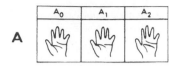

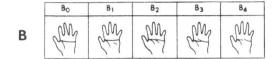

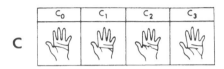

FIG. 3.11. Palmar crease variants. **A:** Normal palmar creases. AO is found in 94% of healthy children. **B:** Simian crease and its variants. **C:** Sydney line and its variants (274). The Sydney line is a proximal transverse crease that extends from beyond the hypothenar eminence to the ulnar margin of the palm. In contrast to the simian crease, a distal palmar crease also occurs (see Fig. 3.3) (276). **D:** Other unusual palmar creases. (Adapted from Dar H, Schmidt R, Nitowsky HM. Palmar crease variants and their clinical significance: a study of newborns at risk. *Pediatr Res* 1977;11:103–108. With permission. Further subvariants are depicted in the original publication.)

7. Whenever a family history exists of frequent unexplained stillbirths, neonatal deaths, or mental retardation.
8. In the presence of any new dominantly inherited syndrome (e.g., retinoblastoma) in addition to mental retardation.

Present cytogenetic techniques are so sensitive that they have uncovered minor chromosomal anomalies in unselected newborn populations (see Table 3.2). It is still unclear how many of the rarer chromosomal variations are consistently responsible for neurologic symptoms, and how

many are the consequences of the same environmental event (e.g., exposure to virus, drugs, irradiation) that induced the abnormal offspring. The coming availability of multicolor FISH to screen children with nonspecific mental retardation for cryptic subtelomeric deletions could well result in detection of abnormalities in a further 6% of mentally retarded children (4).

REFERENCES

1. Ledbetter DH Cryptic translocation and telomere integrity. *Am J Hum Genet* 1992;51:451–456.
2. Blennow E, et al. Fifty probands with extra structurally abnormal chromosomes characterized by fluor-escence in situ hybridization. *Am J Med Genet* 1995;55:85–94.
3. Tharapel AT, Summit RL. A cytogenetic survey of 200 unclassifiable mentally retarded children with congenital anomalies and 200 normal subjects. *Hum Genet* 1977;37:329–338.
4. Flint J, et al. The detection of subtelomeric chromosomal rearrangements in idiopathic mental retardation. *Nat Genet* 1995;9:132–140.
5. Jacobs PA, et al. Estimates of the frequency of chromosome abnormalities detectable in unselected newborns using moderate levels of banding. *J Med Genet* 1992;29:103–108.
6. Hook EB, Healy N, Willey A. How much difference does chromosome banding make? *Ann Hum Genet* 1989;54:237–242.
7. Griffin DK. The incidence, origin and etiology of aneu-ploidy. *Int Rev Cytol* 1996;167:263–296.
8. Kuleshov NP. Chromosome anomalies of infants dying during the perinatal period and premature newborn. *Hum Genet* 1976;31:151–160.
9. Ferguson-Smith M, Andrews T. Cytogenetic analysis. In: Rimoin DL, Connor JM, Pyeritz RE, eds. *Principles and practice of medical genetics*, 3rd ed. New York: Churchill Livingstone, 1996:253–276.
10. Schinzel A. *Catalogue of unbalanced chromosome aberrations in man.* Berlin/New York: Walter de Gruyter, 1984.
11. Jones KL. *Smith's recognizable patterns of human malformation.* 5th ed. Philadelphia: WB Saunders, 1997.
12. de Grouchy J, Turleau C, *Clinical atlas of human chromosomes.* 2nd ed. New York: John Wiley and Sons, 1984.
13. Borgaonkar DS. *Chromosomal variation in man: a catalog of chromosomal variants and anomalies.* 8th ed. New York: Wiley-Liss, 1997.
14. Down JLH. Observation on an ethnic classification of idiots. *Clin Lect Rep London Hospital* 1866;3: 259–262.
15. Seguin E. *Idiocy: Its treatment by the physiological method.* New York: William Wood, 1866.
16. Olsen CL, et al. The effects of prenatal diagnosis, population ageing, and changing fertility rates on the live birth prevalence of Down syndrome in New York State, 1983-1992. *Prenat Diagn* 1996;16: 991–1002.
16a. Böök JA, Reed SC. Empiric risk figures in mongolism. *J Am Med Assoc.* 1950;143:730–732.

17. Mutton D, Alberman E, Hook EB. Cytogenetic and epidemiological findings in Down syndrome, England and Wales 1989 to 1993. *J Med Genet* 1996;33: 387–394.

18. Pueschel M, ed. New *Perspectives on Down syndrome.* Baltimore: Paul Brookes, 1987.

19. Sachs ES, et al. Trisomy 21 mosaicism in gonads with unexpectedly high recurrence risks. *Am J Med Genet* 1990;[Suppl 7]:186–188.

20. Tolmie JL. Down syndrome and other autosomal trisomies. In: Rimoin DL, Connor JM, Pyeritz RE, eds. *Principles and Practice of Medical Genetics.* New York: Churchill Livingstone, 3rd ed, 1996:925–971.

21. Antonarakis SE. Human chromosome 21: Genome mapping and exploration, circa 1993. *Trends Genet* 1993;9:142–148.

22. Yamakawa K, et al. DSCAM: a novel member of the immunoglobulin superfamily maps in a Down syndrome region and is involved in the development of the nervous system. *Hum Molec Genet* 1998;7:227–237.

23. Korenberg JR, et al. Down syndrome phenotypes: The consequences of chromosomal imbalance. *Proc Natl Acad Sci U S A* 1994;91:4997–5001.

24. Neve RL, Finch EA, Dawes LP. Expression of the Alzheimer amyloid precursor gene transcripts in human brain. *Neuron* 1988;1:669–677.

25. Rowe DR, Uchida IA. Cardiac malformation in mongolism. A prospective study of 184 mongoloid children. *Am J Med* 1961;31:726–735.

26. Garver KL, Law JC. Garver B. Hirschsprung disease: a genetic study. *Clin Genet* 1985;28:503–508.

27. Finerman GA, Sakai D, Weingarten S. Atlantoaxial dislocation with spinal cord compression in the mongoloid child. A case report. *J Bone Joint Surg (Am)* 1976;58:408–409.

28. Ross MH, Galaburda AM, Kemper TL. Down's syndrome: Is there a decreased population of neurons? *Neurology* 1984;34:909–916.

29. Wisniewski KE, et al. Neuronal density and synaptogenesis in the postnatal stage of brain maturation in Down syndrome. In: Epstein CJ, ed. *Neurobiology of Down Syndrome.* New York: Raven Press, 1986: 29–44.

30. Suetsugu M, Mehraein P. Spine distribution along the apical dendrites of the pyramidal neurons in Down's syndrome. *Acta Neuropathol* 1980;50:207–210.

31. Becker LE, Armstrong DL, Chan F. Dendritic atrophy in children with Down's syndrome. *Ann Neurol* 1986;20:520–526.

32. Casanova MF, et al. Abnormalities of the nucleus basalis in Down's syndrome. *Ann Neurol* 1985;18: 310–313.

33. Hyman BT, et al. Neuropathological changes in Down's syndrome hippocampal formation. Effect of age and apolipoprotein E genotype. *Arch Neurol* 1995; 52:373–378.

34. Mann DMA. Alzheimer's disease and Down's syndrome. *Histopathology* 1988;13:125–137.

35. Wisniewski KE, Wisniewski HM, Wen GY. Occurrence of neuropathological changes and dementia of Alzheimer's disease in Down's syndrome. *Ann Neurol* 1985;17:278–282.

36. Olson MI, Shaw CM. Presenile dementia and Alzheimer's disease in mongolism. *Brain* 1969;92: 146–156.

37. Yates CM, et al. Alzheimer-like cholinergic deficiency in Down syndrome [Letter]. *Lancet* 1980;2:979.

38. Price DL, et al. Alzheimer's disease and Down's syndrome. *Ann NY Acad Sci* 1982;396:145–164.

39. Iwatsubo T, et al. Amyloid β protein (Aβ) deposition: Aβ42(43) precedes Aβ40 in Down syndrome. *Ann Neurol* 1995;37:294–299.

40. Teller JK, et al. Presence of soluble amyloid β peptide precedes amyloid plaque formation in Down's syndrome. *Nature Med* 1996;2:93–95.

41. Tokuda T, et al. Plasma levels of amyloid β proteins Aβ1-40 and Aβ1-42(43) are elevated in Down's syndrome. *Ann Neurol* 1997;41:271–273.

42. Levinson A, Friedman A, Stamps F. Variability of mongolism. *Pediatrics* 1955;16:43–54.

43. Cowie VA. *A Study of the early development of mongols.* Oxford: Pergamon Press, 1970.

44. Smith GF, Berg JM. *Down's Anomaly.* 2nd ed. Edinburgh: Churchill Livingstone, 1976.

44a. Del Bo R, et al. The apolipoprotein E epsilon4 allele causes a faster decline of cognitive performances in Down's syndrome subjects. *J Neurol Sci* 1997;14 5:87–91.

45. Fishler K, Koch R, Donnell GN. Comparison of mental development in individuals with mosaic and trisomy 21 Down's syndrome. *Pediatrics* 1976;58: 744–748.

46. Loesch-Mdzewska D. Some aspects of the neurology of Down's syndrome. *J Ment Defic Res* 1968;12: 237–246.

47. Pollack MA, et al. Infantile spasms in Down's syndrome. A report of 5 cases and review of the literature. *Ann Neurol* 1978;3:406–408.

48. Stafstrom CE, Konkol RJ. Infantile spasms in children with Down syndrome. *Dev Med Child Neurol* 1994;36:576–585.

49. Crapper DR, et al. Alzheimer degeneration in Down's syndrome. Electrophysiologic alterations and histopathologic findings. *Arch Neurol* 1975;32:618–623.

50. Roth GM, et al. Premature aging in persons with Down syndrome: MR findings. *Am J Neuroradiol* 1996;17:1283–1289.

51. Wisniewski KE, et al. Basal ganglia calcification (BGC) in Down's syndrome (DS)—Another manifestation of premature aging. *Ann N Y Acad Sci* 1982; 396:179–189.

52. Pueschel SM, Scola FH. Atlantoaxial instability in individuals with Down syndrome: Epidemiologic, radiographic, and clinical studies. *Pediatrics* 1987;80: 555–560.

53. Davidson RG. Atlantoaxial instability in individuals with Down syndrome: A fresh look at the evidence. *Pediatrics* 1988;81:857–865.

54. Lowry DW, et al. Upper cervical spine fusion in the pediatric population. *J Neurosurg* 1997;87: 671–676.

55. Ginsberg J, Bofinger MK, Roush JR. Pathologic features of the eye in Down's syndrome with relationship to other chromosomal anomalies. *Am J Ophthalmol* 1977;83:874–880.

56. Eissler R, Longenecker LP. The common eye findings in mongolism. *Am J Ophthalmol* 1962;54:398–406.

57. Donaldson DD. The significance of spotting of the iris in mongoloids: Bruschfield's spots. *Arch Ophthalmol* 1961;65:26–31.

58. Balkany TJ, et al. Ossicular abnormalities in Down's syndrome. *Otolaryngol Head Neck Surg* 1979;87: 372–384.

59. Balkany TJ, et al. Hearing loss in Down's syndrome: A treatable handicap more common than generally recognized. *Clin Pediatr* 1979;18:116–118.

60. Roizen NJ, et al. Hearing loss in children with Down syndrome. *J Pediatr* 1993;123:S9–S12.
61. Olson JC, et al. Arthropathy of Down syndrome. *Pediatrics* 1990;86:931–936.
62. Reed TE, et al. Dermatoglyphic nomogram for the diagnosis of Down's syndrome. *J Pediatr* 1970;77: 1024–1032.
63. Carlsson A, et al. Prevalence of IgA-antigliadin antibodies and IgA-antiendomysium antibodies related to celiac disease in children with Down syndrome. Pediatrics 1998;101:272–275.
64. Loudon MM, Day RE, Duke EM. Thyroid dysfunction in Down's syndrome. *Arch Dis Child* 1985;60: 1149–1151.
65. Hsiang YH, et al. Gonadal function in patients with Down syndrome. *Am J Med Genet* 1987;27: 449–458.
66. Baird PA, Sadovnick AD. Life expectancy in Down syndrome adults. *Lancet* 1988;2:1354–1356.
67. Hijii T, et al. Life expectancy and social adaptation in individuals with Down syndrome with and without surgery for congenital heart disease. *Clin Pediatr* 1997;36:327–332.
68. Hayes C, et al. Ten-year survival of Down syndrome births. *Int J Epidemiol* 1997;26:822–829.
69. Lange BJ, et al. Distinctive demography, biology, and outcome of acute myeloid leukemia and myelodysplastic syndrome in children with Down syndrome: Children's Cancer Group Studies 2861 and 2891. *Blood* 1998;91:608–615.
70. Strauss D, Eyman RK. Mortality of people with mental retardation in California with and without Down syndrome, 1986-1991. *Am J Ment Retard* 1996;100: 643–653.
71. Evenhuis HM. The natural history of dementia in Down's syndrome. *Arch Neurol* 1990;47: 263–267.
72. Haddow JE, et al. Prenatal screening for Down's syndrome with use of maternal serum markers. *N Engl J Med* 1992;327:588–593.
73. Aitken DA, et al. Dimeric inhibin as a marker for Down's syndrome in early pregnancy. *N Engl J Med* 1996;334:1231–1236.
73a. Brambati B, et al. Serum PAPP-A and free β-HCG are first trimester screening markers for Down syndrome. *Prenat Diagn* 1994;14:1043–1047.
74. Kardon NB, et al. Pitfalls in prenatal diagnosis resulting from chromosomal mosaicism. *J Pediatr* 1972;80:297–299.
75. Mansfield ES. Diagnosis of Down syndrome and other aneuploidies using quantitative polymerase chain reaction and small tandem repeat polymorphisms. *Hum Mol Genet* 1993;2:43–50.
76. Bazelon M, et al. Reversal of hypotonia in infants with Down's syndrome by administration of 5-hydroxytryptophan. *Lancet* 1967;1:1130–1133.
77. Weise P, et al. The use of 5-HTP in the treatment of Down's syndrome. *Pediatrics* 1974;54:165–168.
78. Nielsen J, et al. Incidence of chromosome abnormalities in newborn children. Comparison between incidences in 1969–1974 and 1980–1982 in the same area. *Hum Genet* 1982;61:98–101.
79. Abramsky L, Chapple J. Room for improvement? Detecting autosomal trisomies without serum screening. *Publ Health* 1993;107:349–354.
80. Patau K, et al. Multiple congenital anomaly caused by an extra autosome. *Lancet* 1960;1:790–793.
81. Taylor AI. Autosomal trisomy syndromes: A detailed study of 27 cases of Edwards' syndrome and 27 cases of Patau's syndrome. *J Med Genet* 1968;5:227–252.
82. Zoll B, et al. Trisomy 13 (Patau syndrome) with an 11-year survival. *Clin Genet* 1993;43:46–50.
83. Norman RM. Neuropathological findings in trisomies 13-15 and 17-18 with special reference to the cerebellum. *Dev Med Child Neurol* 1966;8:170–177.
84. Inagaki M, et al. Comparison of brain imaging and neuropathology in cases of trisomy 18 and 13. *Neuroradiology* 1987;29:474–479.
85. Moerman P, et al. The pathology of trisomy 13 syndrome. A study of 12 cases. *Hum Genet* 1988;80: 349–356.
86. Gullotta F, Rehder H, Gropp A. Descriptive neuropathology of chromosomal disorders in man. *Hum Genet* 1981;57:337–344.
87. Boles RG, et al. Pseudo-trisomy 13 syndrome with upper limb shortness and radial hypoplasia. *Am J Med Genet* 1992;44:638–640.
88. Cohen MM, Gorlin RJ. Pseudo-trisomy 13 syndrome. *Am J Med Genet* 1991;39:332–335.
89. Edwards JH, et al. A new trisomic syndrome. *Lancet* 1960;1:787–789.
90. Bergin A, et al. Trisomy 18: A nine year review. *Ir J Med Sci* 1988;157:57.
91. Fisher JM, et al. Molecular studies of trisomy 18. *Am J Hum Genet* 1993;52:1139–1140.
91a. Baty BJ, et al. Natural history of trisomy 18 and trisomy 13: I. Growth, physical assessment, medical histories, survival, and recurrence risk. *Am J Med Genet* 1994;49:175–188.
91b. Baty BJ, et al. Natural history of trisomy 18 and trisomy 13: II. Psychomotor development. *Am J Med Genet* 1994;49:189–194.
92. Lejeune J, et al. Three cases of partial deletion of the short arm of chromosome 5. *C R Acad Sci (Paris)* 1964;257:3098–3102.
93. Gersh M, et al. Development of diagnostic tools for the analysis of 5p deletions using interphase FISH. *Cytogenet Cell Genet* 1997;77:246–251.
94. Solitare GB. The cri-du-chat syndrome: Neuropathologic observations. *J Ment Defic Res* 1967;11: 267–277.
95. Fang YY, et al. High resolution characterization of an interstitial deletion of less than 1.9 Mb at 4p16.3 associated with Wolf-Hirschhorn syndrome. *Am J Med Genet* 1997;71:453–457.
96. Gandelman KY, et al. Molecular definition of the smallest region of deletion in the Wolf-Hirschhorn syndrome. *Am J Hum Genet* 1992;51:571–578.
97. Kant SG, et al. Pitt-Rogers-Danks syndrome and Wolf-Hirschhorn syndrome are caused by a deletion in the same region on chromosome 4p16.3. *J Med Genet* 1997;34:569–572.
98. Rethore MO, et al. La trisomie 4p. *Ann Genet* 1974;17:125–128.
99. Miller OJ, et al. Partial deletion of the short arm of chromosome no. 4 (4p-): Clinical studies in five unrelated patients. *J Pediatr* 1970;77:792–801.
100. Hirschhorn K, Cooper HL, Firschein I. Deletion of short arms of chromosome 4-5 in a child with defects of midline fusion. *Humangenetik* 1965;1:479–482.

101. Breg WR, et al. The cri-du-chat syndrome in adolescents and adults: Clinical findings in 13 older patients with partial deletion of the short arm of chromosome No. 5 (5p-). *J Pediatr* 1970;77:782–791.

102. Vogel W, Siebers JW, Reinwein H. Partial trisomy 7q. *Ann Genet* 1973;16:227–280.

103. Riccardi VM. Trisomy 8: An international study of 70 patients. *Birth Defects* 1977;13:171–184.

104. Quazi QH, et al. Trisomy 9 syndrome. *Clin Genet* 1977;12:221–226.

105. Centerwall WR, Beatty-DeSana, J.W. The trisomy 9p syndrome. *Pediatrics* 1975;56:748–755.

106. Klep-dePater JM, et al. Partial trisomy 10q: A recognizable syndrome. *Hum Genet* 1979;46:29–40.

107. Pihko H, Therman E, Uchida IA. Partial 11q trisomy syndrome. *Hum Genet* 1981;58:129–134.

107a. Wardinskym TD, et al. Partial deletion of the long arm of chromosome 11 [del(11)q23.3-qter)] with abnormal white matter. *Am J Med Genet* 1990;35:60–63.

108. Tengstrom C, et al. Partial trisomy 12q: Clinical and cytogenetic observations. *Clin Genet* 1985;28:112–117.

109. Schinzel A, Schmid W, Mursett G. Different forms of incomplete trisomy 13: Mosaicism and partial trisomy for the proximal and distal long arm. *Humangenetik* 1974;22:287–298.

110. Lippe BM, Sparkes RS. Ring 14 chromosome: association with seizures. *Am J Med Genet* 1981;9:301–305.

111. Nitowsky, HM, et al. Partial 18 monosomy in the cyclops malformation. *Pediatrics* 1966;37:260–269.

112. Wertelecki W, Gerald PS. Clinical and chromosomal studies of the 18q- syndrome. *J Pediatr* 1971; 78:44–52.

113. Mikkelsen M, Vestermark S. Karyotype 45, XX,-21/46, XX, 21q- in an infant with symptoms of the G-deletion syndrome. *J Med Genet* 1974;11:389–393.

114. Hsu LY, Hirschhorn K. The trisomy 22 syndrome and the cat eye syndrome. In: Yunis JJ, ed. *New Chromosomal Syndromes*. New York: Academic, 1977:339.

115. Hirschhorn K, Lucas M, Wallace I. Precise identification of various chromosome abnormalities. *Ann Hum Genet* 1973;36:375–379.

116. Hecht F, Vlietinck RF. Autosomal rings and variable phenotypes. *Hum Genet* 1973;18:99–100.

117. Kunze J. Neurological disorders in patients with chromosomal anomalies. *Neuropädiatrie* 1980;11:203–249.

118. Hamerton JL, et al. Cytogenetic survey of 14,069 newborn infants: I. Incidence of chromosome abnormalities. *Clin Genet* 1975;8:223–243.

119. Ferguson-Smith MA, Yates JRW. Maternal age specific rates for chromosome aberration and factors influencing them: Report of a collaborative study on 52,965 amniocenteses. *Prenat Diagn* 1984;4:5–44.

120. Abramsky L, Chapple J. 47,XXY (Klinefelter syndrome) and 47,XYY: estimated rates of and indication for postnatal diagnosis with implications for prenatal counselling. *Prenat Diagn* 1997;17:363–368.

121. Lubs HA, Ruddle FH. Application of quantitative karyotyping to chromosome variation in 4400 consecutive newborns. In: Jacobs PA, Price WH, Law P, eds. *Human population cytogenetics*. Baltimore: Williams & Wilkins. 1970.

122. Jacobs PA, Strong JA. A case of human intersexuality having a possible XXY sex-determining mechanism. *Nature* 1959;183:302–303.

123. Robinson A, de la Chapelle A. Sex chromosome abnormalities. In: Rimoin DL, Connor JM, Pyeritz RE. eds. *Principles and practice of medical genetics*. 3rd ed., New York: Churchill Livingstone, 1996: 973–997.

124. Salbenblatt JA, et al. Pituitary-gonadal function in Klinefelter syndrome before and during puberty. *Pediatr Res* 1985;19:82–86.

125. Robinson A, et al. Sex chromosome aneuploidy: The Denver prospective study. *Birth Defects* 1991;26:59–115.

126. Ratcliffe SG, et al. Klinefelter's syndrome in adolescence. *Arch Dis Child* 1982;57:612.

127. Bender B, et al. Speech and language development in 41 children with sex chromosome anomalies. *Pediatrics* 1983;71:262–267.

128. Dumermuth G. EEG Untersuchungen beim jugendlichen Klinefelter-syndrom. *Helv Paediatr Acta* 1961;16: 702–710.

129. Hashimoto M, et al. Medulla oblongata germinoma in association with Klinefelter syndrome. *Surg Neurol* 1992;37:384–387.

130. Sergovich F, et al. Chromosome aberrations in 2159 consecutive newborn babies. *N Engl J Med* 1969;280:851–855.

131. Radcliffe SG, Butler GE, Jones M. Edinburgh study of growth and development of children with sex chromosome abnormalities. IV. *Birth Defects* 1991;26:144.

132. Daly DF. Neurological abnormalities in XYY males. *Nature* 1969; 221:472–473.

133. Cleveland WW, Arias D, Smith GF. Radio-ulnar syno-stosis, behavioral disturbance and XYY chromosomes. *J Pediatr* 1969;74:103–106.

134. Jacobs PA, et al. Chromosome studies on men in a maximum security hospital. *Ann Hum Genet* 1968;31:339–358.

135. Noel B, et al. The XYY syndrome: Reality or myth. *Clin Genet* 1974;5:387–394.

136. Money J, et al. Cytogenetics, hormones and behavior disability: Comparison of XYY and XXY syndromes. *Clin Genet* 1974;6:370–382.

137. Townes PL, Ziegler NA, Lenhard LW. A patient with 48 chromosomes (XYYY). *Lancet* 1965;1:1041–1043.

138. Schlegel RJ, et al. Studies on a boy with XXYY chromosome constitution. Pediatrics 1965;36:113–119.

139. Zollinger H. XXXY Syndrome: Two new observations at early age and review of literature. *Helv Paediatr Acta* 1969;24:589–599.

140. Zaleski WA, et al. The XXXXY chromosome anomaly: Report of three new cases and review of 30 cases from the literature. *Can Med Assoc J* 1966;94: 1143–1154.

141. Brody J, Fitzgerald MG, Spiers ASD. A female child with five X chromosomes. *J Pediatr* 1967;70:105–109.

142. Turner HH. A syndrome of infantilism, congenital webbed neck and cubitus valgus. *Endocrinology* 1938;23:566–574.

143. Ford CE, et al. A sex chromosome anomaly in case of gonadal dysgenesis (Turner's syndrome). *Lancet* 1959;1:711–713.

144. Kocova M, et al. Detection of Y chromosome sequences in Turner's syndrome by Southern blot analysis of amplified DNA. *Lancet* 1993;342: 140–143.

145. Held KR, et al. Mosaicism in 45,X Turner syndrome: Does survival in early pregnancy depend on the presence of two sex chromosomes? *Hum Genet* 1992;88:288–294.

146. Henn W, Zang KD. Mosaicism in Turner's syndrome. *Nature* 1997;390:569.
147. Gravholt CH, et al. Morbidity in Turner syndrome. *J Clin Epidemiol* 1998;51:147–158.
148. Saenger P. Turner's syndrome. *N Engl J Med* 1996;335:1749–1754.
149. Money J. Two cytogenetic syndromes: Psychologic comparisons. I. Intelligence and specific factor quotients. *J Psychiatr Res* 1964;2:223–231.
150. Van Dyke DL, et al. Ullrich-Turner syndrome with a small ring X chromosome and presence of mental retardation. *Am J Med Genet* 1992;43:996–1005.
151. Migeon BR, et al. The severe phenotype of females with tiny ring X chromosomes is associated with inability of these chromosomes to undergo X inactivation. *Am J Hum Genet* 1994;55:497–504.
152. Herzing LBK, et al. Xist has properties of the X-chromosome inactivation centre. *Nature* 1997;386:272–275.
153. Kuroda MI, Meller VH. Transient Xist-ence. *Cell* 1997;91:9–11.
154. Miller OJ. The sex chromosome anomalies. *Am J Obstet Gynecol* 1964;90:1078–1139.
155. Alexander D, Walker HT, Money J. Studies in direction sense. I. Turner's syndrome. *Arch Gen Psychiatry (Chicago)* 1964;10:337–339.
156. Waber DP. Neuropsychological aspects of Turner's syndrome. *Dev Med Child Neurol* 1979;21:58–70.
157. Bender B, et al. Cognitive development of unselected girls with complete and partial X monosomy. *Pediatrics* 1984;73:175–182.
158. Temple CM, Carney RA. Intellectual functioning of children with Turner syndrome: A comparison of behavioural phenotypes. *Dev Med Child Neurol* 1993;35:691–698.
159. Skuse DH, et al. Evidence from Turner's syndrome of an imprinted X-linked locus affecting cognitive function. *Nature* 1997;387:705–708.
160. Murphy DGM, et al. X-chromosome effects on female brain: A magnetic resonance imaging study of Turner's syndrome. *Lancet* 1993; 342:1197–2000.
160a. Saenger P. Turner's syndrome. *N Engl J Med* 1996;335:1749–1754.
161. Buchanan CF, Law CM, Milner RD. Growth hormone in short, slowly growing children and those with Turner's syndrome. *Arch Dis Child* 1987;62:912–916.
162. Noonan JA. Hypertelorism with Turner's phenotype: New syndrome with associated congenital heart disease. *Am J Dis Child* 1968;116:373–380.
163. Sharland M. et al. A clinical study of Noonan syndrome. *Arch Dis Child* 1992;67:178–183.
164. Saito Y, et al. A case of Noonan syndrome with cortical dysplasia. *Pediatr Neurol* 1997;17:266–269.
165. Witt DR, et al. Lymphedema in Noonan syndrome: Clues to pathogenesis and prenatal diagnosis and review of the literature. *Am J Med Genet* 1987;27:841–856.
166. Bahuau M, et al. Novel recurrent nonsense mutation causing neurofibromatosis type 1 (NF1) in a family segregating both NF1 and Noonan syndrome. *Am J Med Genet* 1998;75:265–272.
167. Martin JP, Bell J. Pedigree of mental defect showing sex-linkage. *J Neurol Psychiatry* 1943;6:154–157.
168. Renpenning H, et al. Familial sex-linked mental retardation. *Can Med Assoc J* 1967;87:954–956.
169. Harvey J, Judge C, Wiener S. Familial X-linked retardation with an X chromosome abnormality. *J Med Genet* 1977;14:46–50.
170. Sutherland GR. Heritable fragile sites on human chromosomes. Demonstration of their dependence on the type of tissue culture medium. *Science* 1977;197:265.
171. Tarleton JC, Saul RA. Molecular genetic advances in fragile X syndrome. *J Pediatr* 1993;122:169–185.
172. Sutherland GR, Mulley JC. Fragile X syndrome and other causes of X-linked mental handicap. In: Rimoin DL, Connor JM, Pyeritz RE. eds. *Principles and practice of medical genetics*, 3rd ed. New York: Churchill Livingstone, 1996:1745–1766.
173. Rousseau F, et al. Direct diagnosis by DNA analysis of the fragile X syndrome of mental retardation. *N Engl J Med* 1991;325:1673–1681.
174. McConkie-Rosell A, et al. Evidence that methylation of the FMR-1 locus is responsible for variable phenotypic expression of the fragile X syndrome. *Am J Hum Genet* 1993;53:800–809.
175. Hammond LS, et al. Fragile X syndrome and deletions in FMR1: new case and review of the literature. *Am J Med Genet* 1997;72:430–434.
176. Feng Y, et al. Fragile X mental retardation protein: nucleocytoplasmic shuttling and association with somatodendritic ribosomes. *J Neurosci* 1997;17:1539–1547.
177. Weiler IJ, et al. Fragile X mental retardation protein is translated near synapses in response to neurotransmitter activation. *Proc Nat Acad Sci USA* 1997;94:5395–5400.
178. Reiss AL. Lee J, Freund L. Neuroanatomy of fragile X syndrome: the temporal lobe. *Neurology* 1994;44:1317–1324.
179. Mostofsky SH, et al. Decreased cerebellar posterior vermis size in fragile X syndrome: correlation with neurocognitive performance. *Neurology* 1998;50: 121–130.
180. Rudelli RD, et al. Adult fragile X syndrome. Clinico-neuropathologic findings. *Acta Neuropathol* 1985;67:289–295.
181. Herbst DS. Non-specific X-linked mental retardation. I. A review with information from 24 new families. *Am J Med Genet* 1980;7:443–460.
182. Webb TP, et al. Population incidence and segregation ratios in the Martin-Bell syndrome. *Am J Med Genet* 1986;23:573–580.
183. Webb TP, et al. The frequency of the fragile X chromosome among school children in Coventry. *J Med Genet* 1987;29:711–719.
184. Rousseau F, et al. Prevalence of carriers of premutation-size alleles of the FMR1 gene and implications for the population genetics of the fragile X syndrome. *Am J Hum Genet* 1993;57:1006–1018.
185. De Arce MA, Kearns A. The fragile X syndrome: The patients and their chromosomes. *J Med Genet* 1984;21:84–91.
186. Chudley AE, Hagerman RJ. Fragile X syndrome. *J Pediatr* 1987;110:821–831.
187. Wisniewski KE, et al. Fragile X syndrome: Associated neurological abnormalities and developmental disabilities. *Ann Neurol* 1985;18:665–669.
188. Beemer FA, Veenema H, de Pater JM. Cerebral gigantism (Sotos syndrome) in two patients with Fra (X) chromosomes. *Am J Med Genet* 1986;23:221–226.
189. Hagerman RJ, et al. High functioning fragile X males: demonstration of an unmethylated, fully

expanded FMR1 mutation associated with protein expression. *Am J Med Genet* 1994;51:298–308.

190. Hagerman RJ. et al. Learning-disabled males with a fragile X CGG expansion in the upper premutation size range. *Pediatrics* 1996;97:122–126.

191. Hagerman RJ, et al. An analysis of autism in 50 males with the fragile X syndrome. *Am J Med Genet* 1986;23:359–374.

192. Einfeld S, Hall W. Behavior phenotype of the fragile X syndrome. *Am J Med Genet* 1992;43:56–60.

193. Hagerman RJ, et al. Girls with fragile X syndrome: Physical and neurocognitive status and outcome. *Pediatrics* 1992;89:395–400.

194. Turner G, et al. Heterozygous expression of X-linked mental retardation and X-chromosome marker fra(X) q27. *N Engl J Med* 1980;303:662–664.

195. Gringras P, Barnicoat A. Retesting for fragile X syndrome in cytogenetically normal males. *Dev Med Child Neurol* 1998;40:62–64.

196. Gu Y, et al. Identification of FMR2, a novel gene associated with the FRAXE CCG repeat and CpG island. *Nat Genet* 1996;13:109–113.

197. Barnicoat AJ, et al. Clinical, cytogenetic, and molecular analysis of three families with FRAXE. *J Med Genet* 1997;34:13–17.

198. Knight SJ, et al. Trinucleotide repeat amplification and hypermethylation of a CpG island in FRAXE mental retardation. *Cell* 1993;74:127–134.

199. Hirst MC, et al. The identification of a third fragile site, FRAXF, in Xq27-q28 distal to both FRAXA and FRAXE. *Hum Molec Genet* 1993;2:197–200.

200. Fox P, Fox D, Gerrard JW. X-linked mental retardation: Renpenning revisited. *Am J Med Genet* 1980;7:491–495.

201. Schwartz CE. X-linked mental retardation. *Am J Hum Genet* 1993;52:1025–1031.

202. Schmickel RD. Contiguous gene syndromes. A component of recognizable syndromes. *J Pediatr* 1986;109:231–241.

203. Budarf ML, Emanuel BS. Progress in the autosomal segmental aneusomy syndromes (SASs): single or multi-locus disorders. *Human Molec Genet* 1997;6:1657–1665.

204. Buyse ML. *Birth defects encyclopedia*. Cambridge, MA: Blackwell Science, 1990.

205. Hall JG. Genomic imprinting: Review and relevance to human disease. *Am J Hum Genet* 1990;46:857–873.

206. Lalande M. Parental imprinting and human disease. *Ann Rev Genet* 1996;30:173–195.

206a. Nicholls RD, Saitoh S. Horsthemke B. Imprinting in Prader-Willi and Angelman syndromes. *Trends Genet* 1998;14:194–200.

207. Prader A, Labhart A, Willi H. Ein Syndrom von adipositas, Kleinwuchs, Kryptorchismus, und Oligophrenie nach myotonieartigen Zustand im Neugeborenenalter. *Schweiz Med Wschr* 1956;86: 1260–1261.

208. Bray GA, et al. The Prader-Willi syndrome: A study of 40 patients and a review of the literature. *Medicine* 1983;62:59–80.

209. Mascari MJ, et al. The frequency of uniparental disomy in Prader-Willi syndrome: Implications for molecular diagnosis. *N Engl J Med* 1992;326: 1599–1607.

210. Donlon TA, et al. Isolation of molecular probes associated with the chromosome 15 instability in the Prader-Willi syndrome. *Proc Natl Acad Sci U S A* 1986; 83:4408–4412.

211. Nicholls RD, et al. Genetic imprinting suggested by maternal heterodisomy in non-deletion Prader-Willi syndrome. *Nature* 1989;342:281–285.

212. Glenn CC, et al. Genomic imprinting: potential function and mechanisms revealed by the Prader-Willi and Angelman syndromes. *Molec Human Reprod* 1997;3:321–332.

212a. Ohta T, et al. Imprinting-mutation mechanisms in Prader-Willi syndrome. *Am J Hum Genet* 1999;64:397–413.

213. Hall BD, Smith DW. Prader-Willi syndrome. A resume of 32 cases including an instance of affected first cousins, one of whom is of normal stature and intelligence. *J Pediatr* 1972;81:286–293.

214. Holm VA, et al. Prader-Willi syndrome: Consensus diagnostic criteria. *Pediatrics* 1993;91:398–402.

214a. Miller SP, Riley P, Shevell MI. The neonatal presentation of Prader-Willi syndrome revisited. *J Pediatr* 1999;134:226–228.

215. Kaplan J, et al. Sleep and breathing in patients with the Prader-Willi syndrome. *Mayo Clin Proc* 1991;66: 1124–1126.

216. Spritz RA, et al. Hypopigmentation in the Prader-Willi syndrome correlates with P gene deletion but not with haplotype of the hemizygous P allele. *Am J Med Genet* 1997;71:57–62.

217. Creel DJ, et al. Abnormalities of the central visual pathways in Prader-Willi syndrome associated with hypopigmentation. *N Engl J Med* 1986; 314:1606–1609.

218. Schad CR, Jalal SM, Thibodeau SN. Genetic testing for Prader-Willi and Angelman syndromes. *Mayo Clin Proc* 1995;70:1195–1196.

219. Wevrick R, Francke U. Diagnostic test for the Prader-Willi syndrome by SNRPN expression in blood. *Lancet* 1996;348:1068–1069.

219a. Kuslich CD, et al. Prader-Willi syndrome is caused by disruption of the SNRPN gene. *Am J Hum Genet* 1999;64:70–76.

220. Kishino T, Lalande M, Wagstaff J. UBE3A/E6-AP mutations cause Angelman syndrome. *Nat Genet* 1997;15:70–73.

221. Matsumoto A, et al. Epilepsy in Angelman syndrome associated with chromosome 15q deletion. *Epilepsia* 1992;33:1083–1090.

221a. Minassian BA, et al. Angelman syndrome: Correlations between epilepsy phenotypes and genotypes. *Ann Neurol* 1998;43:485–493.

222. Guerrini R, et al. Cortical myoclonus in Angelman syndrome. *Ann Neurol* 1996;40:39–48.

223. Boyd SG, Harden A, Patton MA. The EEG in early diagnosis of the Angelman (happy puppet) syndrome. *Eur J Pediatr* 1988;147:508–513.

224. Jay V, et al. Puppet-like syndrome of Angelman: A pathologic and neurochemical study. *Neurology* 1991;41:416–422.

225. Jones KL, et al. The Miller-Dieker syndrome. *Pediatrics* 1980;66:277–281.

226. Clark GD, et al. Predominant localization of the LIS family of gene products to Cajal-Retzius cells and ventricular neuroepithelium in the developing human cortex. *J Neuropath Exp Neurol* 1997;56:1044–1052.

227. Gastaut H, et al. Lissencephaly (Agyria-pachygyria). Clinical findings and serial EEG studies. *Dev Med Child Neurol* 1987;29:167–180.

228. Lo Nigro C, et al. Point mutations and an intragenic deletion in LIS1, the lissencephaly causative gene in

isolated lissencephaly sequence and Miller-Dieker syndrome. *Hum Mol Genet* 1997;6:157–164.

229. Rubinstein JH, Taybi H. Broad thumbs and toes and facial abnormalities. *Am J Dis Child* 1963;105: 588–608.

230. Hennekens RCM, Stevens CA, Van de Kamp JJP. Etiology and recurrence risk in Rubinstein-Taybi syndrome. *Am J Med Genet* 1990;[Suppl 6]:17–29.

231. Petrij F, et al. Rubinstein-Taybi syndrome caused by mutations in the transcriptional co-activator CBP. *Nature* 1995;376:348–351.

232. Tanaka Y, et al. Abnormal skeletal patterning in embryos lacking a single Cbp allele: A partial similarity with Rubenstein-Taybi syndrome. *Proc Natl Acad Sci U S A* 1997;94:10251–10220.

233. Ptacek LJ, et al. The Cornelia de Lange syndrome. *J Pediatr* 1963;63:1000–1020.

234. Beck B, Mikkelsen M. Chromosomes in the Cornelia de Lange syndrome. *Hum Genet* 1981;59:271–276.

235. Semina EV, Reiter, RS, Murray JC. A new human homeobox gene OGI2X is a member of the most conserved homeobox gene family and is expressed during heart development in mouse. *Hum Mol Genet* 1998;7:415–422.

235a. Rossen ML, Sarnat HB. Why should neurologists be interested in Williams syndrome? *Neurology* 1998; 51:8–9.

235b. Karmiloff-Smith A, et al. Language and Williams syndrome: how intact is "intact"? *Child Dev* 1997;68: 246–262.

235c. Tassabehji M, et al. Williams syndrome: use of chromosomal microdeletions as a tool to dissect cognitive and physical phenotypes. *Am J Hum Genet* 1999;64: 118–125.

235d. Meng X, et al. Complete physical map of the common deletion region in Williams syndrome and identification and characterization of three novel genes. *Hum Genet* 1998;103:590–599.

236. Wollack JB, et al. Stroke in Williams syndrome. *Stroke* 1996;27:143–146.

237. Sadler LS, Gingell R, Martin DJ. Carotid ultrasound examination in Williams syndrome. *J Pediatr* 1998;132:354–356.

238. Holmström G, et al. The iris in Williams syndrome. *Arch Dis Child* 1990;65:987–989.

239. Morris CA. et al. Natural history of Williams syndrome: Physical characteristics. *J Pediatr* 1988;113: 318–326.

240. Crome L, Sylvester P.E. A case of severe hypercalcaemia of infancy with an account of the neuropathological findings. *Arch Dis Child* 1960;35:620–625.

241. Jones KL, Smith DW. The Williams elfin facies syndrome. *J Pediatr* 1975;86:718–723.

242. Kruse K, et al. Calcium metabolism in Williams-Beuren syndrome. *J Pediatr* 1992;121:902–907.

243. Goldberg R, et al. Velo-Cardio-Facial Syndrome: A review of 120 patients. *Am J Med Genet* 1993;45: 313–319.

244. Karayiorgou M. et al. Schizophrenia susceptibility associated with interstitial deletions of chromosome 22q11. *Proc Natl Acad Sci USA* 1995;92:7612–7616.

245. Driscoll DA, Emanuel BS. DiGeorge and velocardiofacial syndromes: The 22q11 deletion syndrome. *Mental Retard Dev Disabil Res Rev* 1996;2:130–138.

246. Langer LO, et al. the tricho-rhino-phalangeal syndrome with exostoses (Langer-Giedion syndrome):

four additional patients without mental retardation and review of the literature. *Am J Med* 1984;19:81–111.

247. Ludecke HJ, et al. Molecular dissection of a contiguous gene syndrome: localization of the genes involved in the Langer-Giedion syndrome. *Hum Mol Genet* 1995;4:31–36.

248. Hatada I, et al. New p57KIP2 mutations in Beckwith-Wiedemann syndrome. *Hum Genet* 1997;100: 681–683.

249. Koufos A, et al. Loss of heterozygosity in three embryonal tumours suggests a common pathogenetic mechanism. *Nature* 1985;316:330–334.

250. Pettenati MJ, et al. Wiedemann-Beckwith syndrome: presentation of clinical and cytogenetic data on 22 new cases and review of the literature. *Hum Genet* 1986;74:143–154.

251. Driscoll DA, et al. Prevalence of 22q11 microdeletions in DiGeorge and velo-cardio-facial syndromes: implications for genetic counselling and prenatal diagnosis. *J Med Genet* 1993;30:813–817.

252. Narahara K, et al. Regional mapping of catalase and Wilms tumor—aniridia, genitourinary abnormalities, and mental retardation triad loci to the chromosomal segment 11 p1305–p1306. *Hum Genet* 1984;66: 181–185.

253. Greenberg, F, et al. Multi-disciplinary clinical study of Smith-Magenis syndrome (deletion 17p11.2). *Am J Med Genet* 1996;62:247–254.

254. Elsea SH, et al. Gene for topoisomerase III maps within the Smith-Magenis syndrome critical region: analysis of cell-cycle distribution and radiation sensitivity. *Am J Med Genet* 1998;75:104–108.

255. McKusick VA, et al. Seckel's birdheaded dwarfism. *N Engl J Med* 1967;277:279–286.

256. Seckel HP. *Bird-headed dwarfs.* Springfield: Charles C Thomas Publisher, 1960.

257. Shanske A, et al. Central nervous system anomalies in Seckel syndrome: report of a new family and review of the literature. *Am J Med Genet* 1997;70: 155–158.

258. Borjeson M, Forssman H, Lehmann O. An X-linked, recessively inherited syndrome characterized by grave mental deficiency, epilepsy, and endocrine disorder. *Acta Med Scand* 1962;171:13–21.

259. Gedeon AK et al. Refinement of the background genetic map of Xq26-q27 and gene localisation for Borjeson-Forssman-Lehmann syndrome. *Am J Med Genet* 1996;64:63–68.

260. Tunneson WW, McMillan JA, Levin MA. The Coffin-Siris syndrome. *Am J Dis Child* 1978;132:393–395.

261. McPherson EW, et al. Apparently balance t(1;7) (q21.3;q34) in an infant with Coffin-Siris syndrome. *Am J Med Genet* 1997;71:430–433.

262. Reed W, May SB, Nickel WR. Xeroderma pigmentosum with neurological complications: The de Sanctis-Cacchione syndrome. *Arch Dermatol (Chicago)* 1965;91:224–226.

263. Greenhaw GA, et al. Xeroderma pigmentosum and Cockayne syndrome: Overlapping clinical and biochemical phenotypes. *Am J Hum Genet* 1992;50: 677–689.

264. Hoefnagel D, Bernirschke K. Dyscephalia and mandibulo-oculo-cephalis (Hallermann-Streiff syndrome). *Arch Dis Child* 1965;40:57–61.

265. Cohen MM, Hallermann-Streiff syndrome. A review. *Am J Med Genet* 1991;41:488–499.

266. Frindik JP, et al. Phenotypic expression in Donohue syndrome (leprechaunism): a role for epidermal growth factor. *J Pediatr* 1985;107:428–430.

267. Kosztolanyi G. Leprechaunism/Donohue syndrome/ insulin receptor gene mutations: a syndrome delineation story from clinicopathological description to molecular understanding. *Eur J Pediatr* 1997;156: 253–255.

268. Nakae J, et al. Long-term effect of recombinant human insulin-like growth factor I on metabolic and growth control in a patient with leprechaunism. *J Clin Endocrin Metab* 1998;8:542–549.

269. Hernell O, et al. Suspected faulty essential fatty acid metabolism in Sjögren–Larsson syndrome. *Pediatr Res* 1982;16:45–49.

270. De Laurenzi V, et al. Sjögren-Larsson syndrome is caused by mutations in the fatty aldehyde dehydrogenase gene. *Nat Genet* 1996;12:54-57.

271. Schubert R, et al. Report of two new cases of Pallister-Killian syndrome confirmed by FISH: tissue-specific mosaicism and loss of i(12p) by in vitro selection. *Am J Med Genet* 1997;72:106–110.

272. Jackson-Cook C, Pandya A. Strategies and logistical requirements for efficient testing in genetic disease. *Clinics Labor Med* 1995;15:839–857.

273. Schalling M, et al. Direct detection of novel expanded trinucleotide repeats in the human genome. *Nat Genet* 1993;4:135–139.

274. Walker HA. Incidence of minor physical anomalies in autistic patients. In: Coleman M, ed. *Autistic Syndrome*. New York: Elsevier Science, 1976:95–115.

275. Smith DW, Gong BT. Scalp hair patterning as a clue to early fetal development. *J Pediatr* 1973;83: 374–380.

276. Purvis-Smith SG. The Sydney line: A significant sign in Down's syndrome. *Aust Paediatr J* 1972;8: 198–200.

277. Shioni H, et al. The Sydney line and the simian line: The incidence in Down's syndrome patients with mental retardation and Japanese controls. *J Ment Defic Res* 1982;26:3–10.

278. Winter RM. What's in a face? *Nat Genet* 1996;12: 124–129.

279. Dar H, Schmidt R, Nitowsky HM. Palmar crease variants and their clinical significance: A study of newborns at risk. *Pediatr Res* 1977;11:103–108.

Chapter 4

Neuroembryology, Genetic Programming, and Malformations of the Nervous System

Part 1: The New Neuroembryology

Harvey B. Sarnat and *John H. Menkes

*Departments of Pediatric Neurology and Neuropathology, University of Washington School of Medicine, and Children's Hospital and Regional Medical Center, Seattle, Washington 98105; and *Departments of Neurology and Pediatrics, University of California, Los Angeles, UCLA School of Medicine, and Department of Pediatric Neurology, Cedars-Sinai Medical Center, Los Angeles, California 90048*

Preformation is represented by DNA, not by . . . a tiny adult in every sperm.

—*Antonio García-Bellido, 1998* (1)

Classic embryology is descriptive morphogenesis: detailed observations of gross and microscopic changes in organs and tissues in the developing embryo and fetus. The new neuroembryology is an integration of classic embryology with the insight of molecular genetic programs that direct cellular and regional differentiation to provide an explanation for the precise spatial and temporal sequences of these anatomic changes.

By means of molecular genetics, the focus of the concepts of normal and abnormal development of the nervous system has shifted from traditional categories of structural change, such as neuronogenesis, cell migration, axonal projection, and synapto-genesis, to an understanding of preprogrammed mechanisms that allow these overlapping processes to proceed. Inter-

actions of genes or their transcription products specify differentiation; developmental genes may be expressed only transiently in the embryo or continuously throughout life. After development appears complete, they conserve the identity of individual cellular types even in the adult and perhaps provide clues to degenerative processes that begin after the nervous system is mature.

The relevance of the new neuroembryology to clinical pediatric neurology, apart from new insights, is in its promise of new approaches for the prevention, and perhaps even potential treatment, of malformations of the nervous system. As a result of these new concepts, one must consider an entirely new and still largely unfamiliar classification of cerebral malformations. Such a classification is to be based on the defective expression or coexpression of transcription products of various developmental genes that determine and coordinate every aspect of neuroembryonic development, from gastrulation and the creation of a neuroepithelium to the last detail of postnatal synaptogenesis and myelination.

GASTRULATION

It is not birth, marriage, or death, but gastrulation which is truly the most important time in your life.

—Lewis Wolpert, 1978 (2)

Gastrulation is the birth of the nervous system. In simple chordates, such as amphioxus and amphibians, gastrulation is the invagination of a spherical blastula. In birds and mammals, the blastula is collapsed as a flattened, bilayered disc, and gastrulation appears not as an invagination but as a groove between two ridges on one surface of this disc, the primitive streak on the epiblast. The primitive streak establishes, in each embryo, the basic body plan of all vertebrates: a midline axis, bilateral symmetry, rostral and caudal ends, and dorsal and ventral surfaces.

As the primitive streak extends forward, an aggregate of cells at one end is designated the primitive node or Hensen node. Hensen node defines rostral. Cells of the epiblast on either side move toward the primitive streak, stream through it, and emerge beneath it to pass into the narrow cavity between the two sheets of cells, the epiblast above and the hypoblast below. These migratory cells give rise to the mesoderm and endoderm internally, and some then replace the hypoblast (2).

After extending approximately halfway across the blastoderm (epiblast), the primitive streak with Hensen node reverses the direction of its growth to retreat, moving posteriorly as the head fold and neural plate form anterior to Henson node. As the node regresses, a notochordal process develops in the area rostral to it and somites begin to form on either side of the notochord, the more caudal somites differentiating first and successive ones anterior to somites already formed. The notochord induces epiblast cells to form neuroectoderm (see the following Induction section).

INDUCTION

Experimental studies of the formation of the neural plate have yielded extraordinarily interesting information as the way one part of a developing embryo may influence the differentiation of other parts.

—B. M. Patten, 1951 (3)

Induction is a term denoting the influence of one embryonic tissue on another, so that both the inducer and the induced differentiate as different mature tissues. In the case of the nervous system, the creation and subsequent development of the neural tube may be defined in terms of gradients of inductive influences.

Induction usually occurs between germ layers, as with the notochord (mesoderm) inducing the floor plate of the neural tube (ectoderm). Induction also may occur within a single germ layer, however. An example is the optic cup (neuroectoderm) inducing the formation of a lens and cornea from the overlying epithelium (surface ectoderm) that otherwise would have simply differentiated as more epidermis. Neural induction is the differentiation or maturation of structures of the nervous system from undifferentiated ectodermal cells because of the influence of surrounding embryonic tissues.

Induction was discovered in 1924 by Hans Spemann and Hilde Mangold, who demonstrated that the dorsal lip of the newt gastrula was capable of inducing the formation of an ectopic second nervous system when transplanted to another site in a host embryo, another individual of the same species, or in a ventral site of the same embryo (4). This dorsal lip of the amphibian gastrula (also known as the *Spemann organizer*) is homologous with Hensen node of embryonic birds and mammals. The transplantation of the primitive node in a similar manner as in the Spemann and Mangold experiments in amphibians yields similar results.

The first gene isolated from the Spemann organizer was goosecoid (*gsc*), a homeodomain protein (for definition, see Patterning of the Neural Tube: Organizer Genes and Regulator Genes section) able to recapitulate the transplantation of the dorsal lip tissue. When injected into an ectopic site, *gsc* also normally induces the prechordal mesoderm and contributes to prosencephalic differentiation (5–7). Another gene also expressed in Hensen node and even before the primitive streak is fully formed, *Wnt-8C*, also is essential for the regulation of axis formation and later for hindbrain patterning in the region of the future rhombomere 4 (see Segmentation section) (8). The regulatory gene *Cnot*, with major domains in the primitive node, notochord, and prenodal and postnodal neural plate, is another important molecular genetic factor responsible for the induction of prechordal mesoderm and for the formation of the notochord in particular (9). The gene (transcription factor) gooseberry (*gox*) is unique in being the only identified gene to be expressed in the primitive streak that loses expression at the onset of notochord formation. The *gox* gene probably regulates the primitive streak either positively, by promoting its elongation, or negatively, by suppressing formation of the notochordal process. Another possible function is to promote a mesodermal lineage of epiblast cells as they ingress through the primitive streak. Several other genes essential in creating the fundamental architecture of the embryo and its nervous system are already expressed in the primitive node (7), and many reappear later to influence more advanced stages of ontogenesis.

The specificity of induction is not the inductive molecule, but rather the receptor in the induced cell. This distinction is important because foreign molecules similar in structure to the natural inductor molecule may at times be recognized erroneously by the receptor as identical; such foreign molecules thus can behave as teratogens if the embryo is exposed to such a toxin. Induction occurs during a precise temporal window; the time of responsiveness of the induced cell is designated its competence, and it is incapable of responding either before that precise time or thereafter (10).

Induction receptors are not necessarily in or on the plasma membrane of the cell, but also can be in the cytoplasm or in the nucleoplasm. Retinoic acid (see Retinoic Acid section) is an example of a nuclear inducer. In some cases, the stimulus acts exclusively at the plasma membrane of target cells and does not require actual

penetration of the cell (10,11). The receptors that represent the specificity of induction also are genetically programmed: a gene known as *Notch* is particularly important in regulating the competence of a cell to respond to inductive cues from within the neural tube and in surrounding embryonic tissues (12). Some mesodermal tissues, such as smooth muscle of the fetal gut, can act as mitogens on the neuroepithelium by increasing the rate of cellular proliferation (13,14), but this phenomenon is not true neural induction because the proliferating cells do not differentiate or mature. Some organizer and regulatory genes of the nervous system, such as *Wnt-1*, also exhibit mitogenic effects (15), and both insulinlike and basic fibroblast growth factors (bFGF) act as mitogens as well (16–18).

The early formation of the neural plate is not accomplished exclusively by mitotic proliferation of neuroepithelial cells, but also by a conversion of surrounding cells to a neural fate. In amphibians, a gene known as *achaete-scute* (*XASH-3*) is expressed early in the dorsal part of the embryo from the time of gastrulation and acts as a molecular switch to change the fate of undifferentiated cells to become neuroepithelium rather than surface ectodermal or mesodermal tissues (19). Some cells differentiate as specific types because they are actively inhibited from differentiating as other cell types. All ectodermal cells are preprogrammed to form neuroepithelium, and neuroepithelial cells are preprogrammed to become neurons if not inhibited by genes that direct their differentiation along a different lineage, such as epidermal, glial, or ependymal (20–22).

SEGMENTATION

The primitive segmentation of the vertebrate brain is a problem which has probably attracted as much of the attention of morphologists as any one of the great, unsettled questions of the day, and many views have been advanced.

—*C. F. W. McClure, 1890 (23)*

Over a century ago, the concept of segmentation was already an issue actively debated by biolo-

TABLE 4.1. *Segmentation of the neural tube*

Neuromere*	Derived structures in mature central nervous system
Rhombomere 8	Entire spinal cord; caudal medulla oblongata; cranial nerves XI, XII
Rhombomere 7	Medulla oblongata; cranial nerves IX, X; neural crest
Rhombomere 6	Medulla oblongata; cranial nerves VIII, IX
Rhombomere 5	Medulla oblongata; cranial nerves VI, VII; no neural crest
Rhombomere 4	Medulla oblongata; cranial nerves VI, VII; neural crest
Rhombomere 3	Caudal pons; cranial nerve V; no neural crest
Rhombomere 2	Caudal pons; cranial nerves IV, V; cerebellar nuclei
Rhombomere 1	Rostral pons; cerebellar cortex
Mesencephalic neuromere	Midbrain; cranial nerve III; neural crest
Diencephalic prosomere 2	Dorsal diencephalon
Diencephalic prosomere 1	Ventral diencephalon
Prosencephalic prosomere 2	Telencephalic nuclei; olfactory bulb
Prosencephalic prosomere 1	Cerebral cortex; hippocampus; corpus callosum

*Rhombomere 3 is associated with the first branchial arch; rhombomeres 4 and 5 are associated with the second branchial arch; rhombomere 7 is associated with the third branchial arch.

gists who were intrigued by the repeating units along the rostrocaudal axis of many worms and insects as well as by the somites of embryonic vertebrates. Segmentation of the neural tube creates intrinsic compartments that restrict the movement of cells by physical and chemical boundaries between adjacent compartments. These embryonic compartments are known as *neuromeres*.

The spinal cord has the appearance of a highly segmented structure, but is not intrinsically segmented in the embryo, fetus, or adult. It rather corresponds in its entirety to the caudalmost of the eight neuromeres that create the hindbrain. The apparent segmentation of the spinal cord is caused by clustering of nerve roots imposed by true segmentation of surrounding tissues derived from mesoderm, tissues that form the neural arches of the vertebrae, the somites, and associated structures. Neuromeres of the hindbrain are designated rhombomeres (24–27). The entire cerebellar cortex, vermis, floculonodular lobe, and lateral hemispheres, develops from rhombomere 1, but the dentate and other deep cerebellar nuclei are formed in rhombomere 2 (28,29). The rostral end of the neural tube forms a mesencephalic neuromere and probably six forebrain neuromeres, as two diencephalic and two or four telencephalic prosomeres, although these may possibly be subdivided further (30–32). The segmentation of the human embryonic brain into neuromeres is summarized in Table 4.1.

The segments of the embryonic neural tube are distinguished by physical barriers formed by processes of early specializing cells that resemble the radial glial cells that appear later in development (33,34) and also by chemical barriers from secreted molecules that repel migratory cells. Cell adhesion is increased in the boundary zones between rhombomeres, which also contributes to the creation of barriers against cellular migration in the longitudinal axis (34). Limited mitotic proliferation of the neuroepithelium occurs in the boundary zones between rhombomeres. Although cells still divide in this zone, their nuclei remain near the ventricle during the mitotic cycle and do not move as far centrifugally within the elongated cell cytoplasm during the interkinetic gap phases as they do in general (34). The rhombomeres of the brainstem also may be visualized as a series of transverse ridges and grooves on the dorsal surface, the future floor of the fourth ventricle; these ridges are gross morphologic markers of the hindbrain compartments (23,27).

The first evidence of segmentation is a boundary that separates the future mesencephalic neuromere from rhombomere 1 of the hindbrain. More genes play a role in this initial segmentation of the neural tube than in the subsequent formation of other boundaries that develop to separate other neuromeres. Furthermore, the mesencephalic-metencephalic region

TABLE 4.2. *Programs of developmental genes*

Organizer genes
  1. Cell proliferation
  2. Identity of organs or tissues (e.g., neural, renal)
  3. Axes of polarity and growth
    a. Ventrodorsal
    b. Dorsoventral
    c. Rostrocaudal
    d. Mesiolateral
  4. Segmentation
  5. Left-right symmetry or asymmetry
Regulator genes
  1. Differentiation of structures and specialization within organ
  2. Cell lineage: differentiation and specialization of individual cells
  3. Inhibition of other genetic programs in order to change a cell lineage

appears to develop early as a single independent unit or *organizer* for other neuromeres rostral and caudal to that zone (35,36). The organizer genes recognized at the mesencephalic-metencephalic boundary for this earliest segmentation of the neural tube include *Pax-2*, *Wnt-1*, *En-1*, *En-2*, *Pax-5*, *Pax-8*, *Otx-1*, *Otx-2*, *Gbx-2*, *Nkx-2.2*, and *FGF-8*.

The earliest known gene with regional expression in the mouse is *Pax-2*, expressing itself even before the neural plate forms. It is the earliest gene recognized in the presumptive region of the midbrain-hindbrain boundary (37,38). In invertebrates, *Pax-2* is important for the activation of Wingless (*Wg*) genes; this relationship is relevant because the first gene definitely associated with an identified midbrain-hindbrain boundary in vertebrates is *Wnt-1*, a homologue of *Wg*. The regulation of *Wnt-1* may be divided into two phases: in the early phase (one to two somites), the mesencephalon broadly expresses the gene throughout. In the later phase (15 to 20 somites), expression is restricted to dorsal regions, the roof plate of the caudal diencephalon, mesencephalon and myelencephalon, and spinal cord. It also is expressed in a ring that extends ventrally just rostral to the midbrain-hindbrain boundary and in the ventral midline of the caudal diencephalon and mesencephalon (39–41). *Wnt-1* is essential in activating and preserving the function of the Engrailed genes *En-1* and *En-2*. *En-*

1 is coexpressed with *Wnt-1* at the one-somite stage, in a domain only slightly caudal to *Wnt-1*, which includes the midbrain and rhombomere 1, the rostral half of the pons, and the cerebellar cortex, but excludes the diencephalon (42). The activation of *En-2* begins at the four-somite stage, and its function in mesencephalic and rhombomere 1 development is similar, with differences in some details, particularly their roles in cerebellar development (43,44). Finally, the homeobox gene *Otx-2* appears early in the initial boundary zone of the midbrain-hindbrain and, as with *Wnt-1*, it appears to be essential for the later expression of *En-1* and *En-2* and also of *Wnt-1* (45,46).

The creation of neuromeres allows the development of structures within regions of the brain without the neuroblasts that form these nuclei wandering to other parts of the neuraxis where they would not be able to later establish their required synaptic relations. The interaction of genes with one another is a complexity that makes analysis of single gene expression more difficult in interpreting programmed malformations of the brain.

PATTERNING OF THE NEURAL TUBE: ORGANIZER GENES AND REGULATOR GENES

Basic characteristics of the body plan are called *patterning* (24). They are the anatomic expression of the genetic code within the nuclear DNA of every cell, but they also may result from signals from neighboring cells, carried by molecules that are secretory translation products of various families of organizer genes, each in a highly precise and predictable temporal and spatial distribution.

The early development of the central nervous system (CNS) of all vertebrates, even before the closure of the neural placode or plate to form the neural tube, requires the establishment of a fundamental body plan of bilateral symmetry, cephalization or the identity of head and tail ends, and dorsal and ventral surfaces. These axes of the body itself, and of the CNS, require the expression of genes that impose gradients of differentiation and growth. The genes that determine the polarity and gradients of the anatomic axes are called *organizer genes*. Many express themselves not only in the CNS but in other organs and tissues as well (2,41). The bilateral symmetry of many organs and programmed asymmetries, probably including such neural structures as the different targets of the left and right vagal nerves and left-right asymmetries in the cerebral cortex, is determined in large part by *Pitx-2*, a gene expressed as early as in the primitive node (47).

The RNA that represents a transcript of the DNA translates a peptide, a glycoprotein, or some other molecule that acts to induce or at times to serve as a growth factor. Some genes also function to stimulate or inhibit the expression of others, or an antagonism or equilibrium exists between certain families of genes, exemplified by those that exert a dorsoventral gradient and those that cause a ventrodorsal gradient.

The difference between an organizer gene and a regulator gene is really its function, and often the same gene subserves both roles at different stages of development. The definitions and programs of these two groups are summarized in Tables 4.2 and 4.3.

Evolutionary Conservation of Genes

The sequences of nucleotides of DNA are so primordial to animal life that identical or nearly identical base pairs exist not only in all vertebrates, but in all invertebrates as well, from the simplest worms to the most complex primates (48). The evolutionary biologists of the nineteenth century, such as Charles Darwin and Thomas Huxley, were constantly searching for "the missing links" between mammals and other vertebrates, between humans and other primates and, most of all, between invertebrates and vertebrates, because comparative anatomy did not provide a sufficiently satisfactory answer. They never found the missing link because the technology of their day could not elucidate this fundamental and profound question. The missing link sought by the nineteenth-century evolutionary biologists is the identical sequence of nucleic acids residues that forms the same organizer genes in all animals, from the simplest worms to humans.

Despite evolutionary conservation of genes, there may be some variability between species in the compartmental site within the embryonic neural tube of structures programmed by these genes. For example, the abducens motor nucleus forms in rhombomere 6 in elasmobranchs (sharks) but in rhombomere 5 in mammals; the trigeminal/facial boundary shifts from rhombomere 4 in lampreys to rhombomere 3 in birds and mammals.

Transcription Factors and Homeoboxes

The genes that program the development of the nervous system are specific series of DNA base pairs linked to small proteins called *transcription factors*. These transcription factors are essential for the functional expression of these genes. A frequent transcription factor is the basic helix-loop-helix structure. It is so fundamental to the evolution of life that it appears for the first time in certain bacteria, even before a cell nucleus exists to concentrate the DNA evolved (48).

The zinc finger is another DNA-binding, gene-specific transcription factor. It consists of 28 amino acid repeats with pairs of cysteine and histidine residues, each sequence folded around a zinc ion (49). *Krox-20* (this gene name is applied to the mouse; in the human it is redesignated *EGR2*) is a zinc finger gene expressed in alternating rhombomeres, especially rhombomere 3 and rhombomere 5; neural crest tissue does not differentiate from those two rhombomeres, although it does in adjacent segments including rhombomere 4 (50). *Krox-20* also serves an additional function in the peripheral nervous system where it regulates myelination by Schwann cells (51). Finally, *Krox-20* regulates the expression of some other genes, most notably those of the *Hox* family (50,52–55). Examples of other zinc fingers include *Zic*, *TFIIIA*, *cSnR* (snail-related), and *PLZF* (human promyelocytic leukemia zinc finger) (56).

Complexes of retinoic acid with its intranuclear receptor form still another transcription factor important in nervous system development, both normal and abnormal (see Retinoic Acid section). A unique transcription factor

TABLE 4.3. *Organizer and regulator genes of the embryonic and fetal nervous system*[a]

Gene	Regions	Functions	References
Achaete-scute	Epiblast	Changes the fate of undifferentiated cells to form neuroepithelium	19
BMP4 (bone morpho-genic protein)	Hensen node; neural plate	Inhibits cells from forming neural tissue; dorsalizing to neural tube; of transforming growth factor β family	21,22
Cart1	Head mesenchyme	Organizes head mesoderm before neural crest arrival	47a
Cnot	Hensen node	Induces the primitive node to form notochordal process; induces neural placode	9
Delta	—	Antagonizes Notch; inhibits neural differentiation	—
Dab1 (disabled 1)	Laminated cortices	Acts downstream of rein for terminal neuroblast migration and cortical lamination	—
Dix1, Dix2 (distal-less)	Prosomeres; ventral thalamus; anterior hypothal-amus; corpus striatum	Subcortical neuroblast migration; interneuron migration from basal forebrain to neocortex	47b
Dorsalin1	Neural tube	Dorsalizing; of transforming growth factor β family	193
Doublecortin	Telencephalon	Neuroblast migration; Xq22.3-q23 locus; defective in subcortical laminar heterotopia (band hetero-topia; double cortex syndrome)	201,202
EMX2	Telencephalon	Neuroblast migration; defective in schizencephaly	52a
En1, En2 (engrailed)	Mesencephalon, r1	Formation of mesencephalon and metencephalon, including entire cerebellar cortex	28,29,35,39, 41–44, 79,81,99
Filamin 1	Telencephalon	Neuroblast migration; defective in X-linked domi-nant periventricular heterotopia	60a,204
Gbx2 (unplugged)	r1–r3	Specification of anterior hindbrain; contributes to formation of the cerebellum, motor trigeminal nerve	36
gox (Gooseberry)	Primitive streak	Regulates elongation of primitive streak; disappears at onset of notochord formation; related to Otx homeobox; promotes epiblast cells to become mesoderm	—
gsc (Goosecoid)	Hensen node, neural plate	Induces prechordal mesoderm and prosencephalon; ectopically duplicates neural tube	5–7
Hex3	Prosencephalon	Folate-dependent gene; defective in septo-optic dysplasia	—
HNF3 β (winged helix)	Notochord	Regulates floor plate development; suppresses dorsalizing influence of Pax3	65a
Hox 1.5	r3; r5	Segmentation; formation of parathyroid, thymus (ref. Hox family)	—
Hox 1.6 (Hoxa 1)	r4–r7	Rostrocaudal gradient and segmentation	25–27,73, 74,76–78
Hox 2.1	r8	Rostrocaudal gradient of spinal cord	—
Hox 2.6	Border r6/7–r8	Rostrocaudal gradient and segmentation	—
Hox 2.8	Border r2/3–r8	Rostrocaudal gradient and segmentation; regu-lates axonal projections from r3	—
Hox 2.9 (Hoxb1)	r4	Formation of neural crest	54,74
HNF (forkhead)	Neural plate	Patterning of the midline of the neural tube	—
Islet1	Ventral neural tube	Motor neuroblast differentiation	136
Islet3	Neural plate	Floor plate differentiation; suppresses Pax3	88,102
Krox20 (EGR2)	r3; r5	Zinc finger; regulates expression of Hox genes; regulates myelination of Schwann cells	50–55
L1CAM	Mesencephalon; telencephalon	Formation of aqueduct; cerebral neuroblast migra-tion defective in X-linked hydrocephalus with aqueductal stenosis and also reported in hemimegalencephaly	190,205
Lhx2	Prosomeres	LIM family homeobox; development of hippocampus and cellular proliferation for neocortex; devel-opment of eye before formation of optic cup	89

Continued

TABLE 4.3. *Continued*

Gene	Regions	Functions	References
LIM	Neural plate; pre-chordal mesen-chyme	Organizer of cephalic mesenchyme before migration of neural crest; organizer of neural placode	88,102,134
LIS1	Cortical plate	Neuroblast migration; 17p13.3 locus; defective in lissencephaly type I	176,198–200
Math1	r1, cerebellum	Differentiation of cerebellar granule cells	130
Math5	Optic cup	Retinal differentiation	70a
MNR	Motor neuroblasts	Motor neuron identity	70b
NeuroD	Ectodermal cells	Neuronal differentiation; three subtypes on human chromosomes 2, 5, 17; related to gene regulating transcription of insulin; retinal development	75a,b,80a,b, 91a,b, 94a,b
Neurogenin (ngn)	Ectodermal cells	Neuronal differentiation in CNS and peripheral nervous system; expressed earlier than neuroD; interacts with Delta and Notch; family of subtypes	100a,b,c
Nkx2.1	Prosomeres	Differentiation of hypothalamus; induced by *Shh*	97
Nkx2.2	All neuromeres	Specifies diencephalic neuromeric boundaries; interacts with Dix1 and transcription factor TTF1 for prosencephalic differentiation	96,97
Nkx6.1	Diencephalon-r8; motor neurons	Induced by *Shh* and repressed by BMP7; coex-pressed with Islet1 in motor neurons	97
Nkx6.2	Diencephalon-r8	Same as gtx; glial cell differentiation	97
Noggin	Hensen node	Inhibits BMP4 to allow neural plate differentiation	21,22,111a,
Notch	Neural plate; neuro-epithelium	Regulates the competence of cells to respond to inductive signals; differentiation of neural pla-code; asymmetric distribution in cytoplasm during mitotic cycle	115a,150
Null	Neuroepithelium	Inhibits differentiation of neural identity; asymmetric distribution in cytoplasm of during mitotic cycle	—
Numb	Neural plate; fetal neuroepithelium	Antagonizes Notch by preventing neural differentiation	115a,149
Otx1 (orthodenticle)	Mesencephalon/r1 boundary; telen-cephalon; sen-sory nerves	Onset of neuromere formation; corticogenesis; sense organ development	—
Otx2 (orthodenticle)	Prestreak blastomere; neural plate	Gastrulation; specification and maintenance of anterior neural plate	45,46
Pit1 (pituitary-specific)	Adenohypophysis	Differentiation of anterior pituitary	—
ptc (patched)	Cerebellar cortex	Regulates granule cell proliferation; tumor-suppressor gene	106–109, 123a
Pax2 (paired)	Primitive streak; r2–r8; prosomeres	Dorsalizing polarity gradient; segmentation regu-lated by notochord and floor plate; formation of ventral half of optic cup, retina, and optic nerve; overlaps and partially redundant with Pax5	35,37–39, 71,101
Pax3 (paired)	r1; r8	Identity of Bergmann glia; active spinal cord dorsalizing gradient	71
Pax5 (paired)	r1	Partially redundant with Pax2 for differentiation of cerebellar cortex; dorsalizing gradient	71,101
Pax6 (paired)	r1; r8; prosomeres	Identity of cerebellar granule cells; active in spinal cord as dorsalizing gradient; neuroblast migration to cerebral cortex and deep telencephalic nuclei	70,71
Pitx	Primitive streak	Determines right-left asymmetries of internal organs	47
Rein (reelin)	Laminar cortices	Extracellular matrix glycoprotein product secreted by Cajal-Retzius neurons and cerebellar granule cells, essential for terminal neuroblast migration and laminar architecture	174,175, 193,222
RhoB	Dorsal neural tube	Delamination of neural crest cells; BMP gene	137a
Shh (Sonic hedgehog)	Notochord; floor plate; prechordal mesoderm	Induces floor plate; ventralizing influence of neural tube; ventral midline of prosencephalon; induction of motor neurons; mitogen to cere-bellar granule cells	61–65,68, 69,108, 123a,131

Continued

TABLE 4.3. *Continued*

Gene	Regions	Functions	References
Slug	Neural crest	Neural crest differentiation; homologue of Snail in invertebrates	140
SMN (survival motor neuron)	Motor neuroblasts	Arrests apoptosis of motor neuroblasts	166,167
TSC1, TSC2	Neuraxis	Encodes proteins hamartin and tuberin; TSC1 at 9q34 locus; TSC2 at 16p13.3 locus; both defective in tuberous sclerosis	242–247
Twist	Hensen node	Organizer of cephalic mesenchyme before migration of neural crest; cranial neural tube morphogenesis	138a
TOAD64 (unc33)	Growth cones	Promotes axonal outgrowth	219
Wnt1 (wingless)	r1; r3–r8	Formation of mesencephalic-metencephalic boundary; formation of mesencephalon, rostral pons, and cerebellum; essential for expression of En1; weak dorsal polarizing influence in r3–r8; mitogen	28,35,39, 42,72,80, 132,133
Wnt3 (wingless)	mes; r1; r3–r8	Overlaps and redundant with Wnt1 in mesencephalic neuromere and r1; strong dorsal polarizing influence in r3–r8 including spinal cord; differentiation of brainstem nuclei; identity of Purkinje cells	72,103
Wnt7 (wingless)	Prosomeres	Differentiation of structures of diencephalon and telencephalon	32
Wnt8 (wingless)	Epiblast; primitive streak; r1–r8	Primitive streak formation; segmentation	8
Zic1	Cerebellum	Zinc finger; differentiation of granule cells	128,129

[a]An *organizer gene* is defined as one that programs the differentiation of the neural placode, neural axes, and gradients and segmentation of the neural plate and neural tube; a *regulator gene* is defined as one that programs the differentiation of specific structures and cellular types in the developing nervous system and conserves their identity and mediates developmental processes such as neuroblast migration or synaptogenesis. The genes are listed alphabetically rather than by function because many of the same genes serve various functions at different stages, as organizer genes in early ontogenesis and as regulator genes at later periods. This is a partial list of some of the most important in the nervous system, of the more than 80,000 genes that have already been identified in the human genome. Developmental genes recognized in invertebrates such as *Drosophila*, but for which the vertebrate homologue has not yet been identified, are excluded.

r1, rhombomere 1; r2, rhombomere 2, and so forth.

with coactivation domain requirements, *pit*, programs anterior pituitary differentiation (57,58).

Growth factors, which also are molecules created by DNA sequences, are other influences on the establishment of the plan of the neural tube. Biologically, they act as transcription factors: bFGF behaves as an auxiliary inductor of the longitudinal axis with a rostrocaudal gradient during the formation of the neural tube (59).

Some transcription factors include homeoboxes. These are restricted DNA sequences of 183 base pairs of nucleotides that encode a class of proteins sharing a common or similar 60–amino acid motif, termed the *homeodomain* (24). Homeodomains contain sequence-specific DNA-binding activities and are integral parts of

the larger regulatory proteins, the transcription factors. Homeoboxes or homeotic genes are classified into various families with common molecular structure and similar general expression in ontogenesis. Homeoboxes are associated especially with genes that program segmentation and rostrocaudal gradients of the neural tube. Some of the important families of homeobox genes in the development of the vertebrate nervous system are *gsc*, *Hox*, *En*, *Wnt*, *Shh*, *Nkx*, *LIM*, and *Otx*.

Families of Developmental Genes of the Central Nervous System

The genes that program the axes and gradients of the neural tube may be classified as families by their similar nucleic acid sequences and also by their similar general functions, although important differences occur within a family in the site or neuromere where each gene is expressed and in the anatomic structures they form. A dorsalizing gene not only has a dorsal territory of expression, but also causes the ventral parts of the neural tube to differentiate as dorsal structures if influences from ventralizing genes do not antagonize them with sufficient strength, and vice versa. A good example is the development of the somite. The sclerotome, which forms cartilage and bone of the vertebral body, normally is situated ventral to the myotome, which forms muscle cells, and the dermatome. Ectopic cells of the floor plate or of the notochord implanted next to the somite of the chick embryo cause a ventralization of the somite, so that excess cartilage and bone are formed and a deficiency of muscle and dermis occurs (60,61). The floor plate or notochord, in this instance, is the ventralizing inductor of the mesodermal somite, and it is now known that the genetic factor responsible is the transcription product of the gene *Sonic hedgehog* (*Shh*), which also serves as a strong ventralizing gradient force in the neural tube (22,62–65). If a section of notochord is implanted ectopically dorsal or lateral to the neural tube, a second floor plate forms opposite the notochord and motor neurons differentiate on either side of it, despite the presence of a normal floor plate and motor neurons in the normal position (66). *Shh*, a strong gene of the ventrodorsal gradient that becomes expressed as early as in the primitive node, has induced the ventralization of a dorsal region of the neural tube or duplicates the neural tube. Such an influence in the human fetus, the so-called split notochord, could be an explanation of the rare cases of diplomyelia or diastematomyelia (67). Excessive *Shh*, particularly its N-terminus cleavage product, upregulates floor plate differentiation at the expense of motor neuron formation (63) and might even induce duplication of the neuraxis. Furthermore, *Shh* also exerts a strong influence in the differentiation of ventral and medial structures of the prosencephalon (68), and the defective expression because the mutation of this gene is thought to be the molecular basis of the human malformation holoprosencephaly (69).

To establish an equilibrium with genes with a ventralizing influence, other families of genes exercise a dorsalizing influence, causing the differentiation of dorsal structures of the neural tube; the *Pax* family is an example (70,71). The *Wnt* family also is dorsalizing in the hindbrain; *in situ* hybridization shows its transcription products expressed diffusely only in the early neuroepithelium and restricted to dorsal regions as the neural tube develops (72). The zinc finger gene *Zic2* has a dorsalizing gradient in the forebrain. The rostrocaudal axis of the neural tube and segmentation, or the formation of neuromeres, are directed in large part by a family of 38 genes, divided into four groups, that are called *Hox* genes (25,26,73–77). Each of 13 *Hox* genes is expressed in certain rhombomeres and not in others (see Table 4.3). In addition to their functions in establishing the compartments or rhombomeres of the brainstem and effecting the differentiation of certain anatomic structures, *Hox* genes also serve as guides of growth cones that are forming the long descending and ascending pathways between the brain and spinal cord (78).

Genes that direct the specific differentiation of structures are called *regulatory genes*, and frequently are the same genes that served as organizer genes in an earlier period. The most important families for the development of the brainstem and midbrain are *Engrailed* (*En*), *Wingless* (*Wnt*), *Hox*, *Krox*, and *Paired* (*Pax*). Table 4.3 summarizes the sites of expression and functions of the most important organizer and regulator genes. Genes have peculiar names that do not correspond to their function. At times the same gene is given a slightly different name in vertebrates and invertebrates, despite an identical nucleotide sequence. For example, *Sonic hedgehog* in vertebrates is simply *hedgehog* in invertebrates. Other hedgehog genes in vertebrates are *Desert hedgehog* and *Indian hedgehog*, but these do not appear to be involved in the ontogenesis of the neural tube.

Many genes exert influences on the expression of others and some serve redundant functions with others. The gene *En-1* has a strong domain in the mesencephalic neuromere and also in rhombomere 1, the rhombomere that forms the rostral half of the pons and the cerebellar cortex. This same territory corresponds to the neuromeric expressions of *Wnt-1* and *Wnt-3*. One of the *Wnt* genes is necessary to augment the expression of *En-1*; if a loss of *Wnt-1* or *Wnt-3* occurs by mutation, the other *Wnt* gene is able to compensate alone and no malformation of the brain is observed in homozygotes. The overlapping and redundant expression of these two *Wnt* genes provides a kind of plasticity at the molecular level for the developing nervous system. If *Wnt-1* expression is lost, however, the expression of *Wnt-3* is insufficient to compensate in the rostral regions of the future brainstem, and the result is a defective midbrain and pons and cerebellar hypoplasia (35,42,79,80). The genes *En-1* and *En-2* have similar functions with differences in some details and are demonstrated in the human fetus as well as in the mouse (81).

Another complexity in gene interrelationships is that many regulatory genes change their territories of expression in different stages of development, increasing to include more rhombomeres or broader expression early in development and more restricted domains later. At times, the expression of a gene in the wrong neuromere, called *ectopic expression*, interferes with normal development.

Retinoic Acid

Retinoic acid, the alcohol of which is vitamin A, is a hydrophobic molecule secreted by the notochord and by ependymal floor plate cells (82). Retinoid-binding proteins and receptors are already strongly expressed in mesenchymal cells of the primitive streak and in the preotic region of the early developing hindbrain (83). Ependymal cells other than those of the floor plate and neuroepithelial cells have retinoic acid receptors, but do not secrete this compound.

Retinoic acid diffuses across the plasma membrane without requiring active transport and binds to intracellular receptors. It enters the cell nucleus where it binds to a specific nuclear receptor protein and changes the structural configuration of that protein, enabling it to attach to a specific receptor on a target gene, where the complexes formed by retinoic acid and its receptor then function as a transcription factor for neural induction (84,85). Other transcription factors of developmental genes already mentioned are the basic helix-loop-helix and zinc fingers.

Retinoic acid functions as a polarity molecule for determining the anterior and posterior surfaces of limb buds and, in the nervous system, is important in segmentation polarity and is a strong rostrocaudal polarity gradient (2,86,87). Excessive retinoic acid acts on the neural tube of amphibian tadpoles to transform anterior neural tissue to a posterior morphogenesis, resulting in extreme microcephaly and suppression of optic cup formation (85). Failure of optic cup formation may be caused by retinoic acid suppression by genes of the *LIM* family, such as *Islet-3* and *Lim-1* (88,89). Retinoic acid upregulates homeobox genes, those of the *Hox* family and *Krox-20* in particular, and causes ectopic expression of these genes in rhombomeres where normally they are not expressed (54,90). An excess of retinoic acid, whether endogenous or exogenous as in mothers who take an excess of vitamin A during early gestation, results in severe malformations of the hindbrain and spinal cord. A single dose of retinoic acid administered intraperitoneally to maternal hamsters on embryonic day 9.5 results in the Chiari type II malformation and often meningomyelocele in the fetuses (91–93). In cell cultures of cloned CNS stem cells from the mouse, retinoic acid enhances neuronal proliferation and also astroglial differentiation (94).

SUMMARIZED PRINCIPLES OF GENETIC PROGRAMMING

The molecular genetic regulation of neural tube development may be summarized as a series of principles of genetic programming.

Principle 1: *Developmental genes are reused repeatedly.* Nature recognizes useful genes and uses them over and over again during embryonic development, but developmental genes play different roles at different stages. An organizer gene of the neural axis or of segmentation may later serve as a regulator gene for the differentiation and maintenance of specific cells of the CNS. Genes of growth factors also are reused at different stages; the fibroblast growth factor gene *EGF8* is active during gastrulation, but later contributes to cardiac, craniofacial, midbrain, cerebellar, and forebrain development (95). The classification of a gene as an *organizer* or *regulator*, therefore, depends on the specific embryonic stage and its function at that stage of development.

Principle 2: *Domains of organizer genes change in successive stages*. The domains, or territories of expression, of organizer genes generally are diffuse initially and become more localized or confined to certain neuromeres as the neural tube develops.

Principle 3: *Relative gene domains may differ in various neuromeres*. The domain of one gene may be dorsal to another in rostral neuromeres, and ventral to it in caudal neuromeres, at any given stage of development. An example is *Nkx2.2* and *Nkx6.1*, both of which are coexpressed throughout most of the length of the neural tube. The domain of *Nkx2.2* is dorsal to that of *Nkx6.1* in the diencephalic and mesencephalic neuromeres, but shifts to a position ventral to that of *Nkx6.1* in the hindbrain and spinal cord (96,97).

Principle 4: *Some genes activate, regulate, or suppress the expression of others*. Some organizer genes act sequentially, so that one already expressed gene initiates the expression of another that follows or that becomes coexpressed. A failure of the first gene thus may result in a lack of expression of others, producing a more extensive developmental defect than might be anticipated from the loss of the first gene alone. An example is the normal cascade of *Pax-2* activating *Wnt-1* at the mesencephalic-metencephalic boundary at the beginning of neuromere formation; *Wnt-1* then activates *En-1* and *En-2*. Another example is the activation by *Shh* of *Nkx-2.1* in the rostral neural plate and *Nkx-6.1* in the caudal neural plate (97).

Some genes act by inhibiting or antagonizing the genetic programs of others. *Notch* and *Achaete-scute* change the fate of undifferentiated cells to form neuroepithelium and signal the formation of the neural plate; *Numb* and *Delta* antagonize these genes and inhibit neural differentiation. *Bone morphogenic protein 4 (BMP4)*, expressed in Hensen node, inhibits ectodermal germ cells from forming neural tissue and promotes epidermal differentiation, but *Noggin* inhibits *BMP4*, thus allowing neural plate formation to proceed (21,22). The formation of dorsal structures including the neural plate in the early embryo depends on the absence of BMP4 expression. *Wnt-1* and *Wnt-3* cause neural crest cells to form melanocytes instead of proceeding with neuronal fates (98).

All neuroepithelial cells are preprogrammed to form neurons; glial and ependymal cells can form only when this program is inhibited (21,99,100).

Principle 5: *Defective homeoboxes usually have reduced domains*. A defective homeobox gene, especially one of segmentation, usually is expressed in fewer neuromeres than normal, a reduction in its domain; it may even lose all of its expression. These changes occur in the homozygous and not the heterozygous state of genetic animal models.

Principle 6: *Some genes may compensate for the loss of others if their domains overlap: redundancy and synergy*. Some genes coexpressed in the same neuromeres may compensate, in part or in full, for the loss of expression of one of the pair, so that anatomic development, maturation, and function of the nervous system all proceed normally. An example is the coexpression of *Wnt-1* and *Wnt-3* in the myelencephalic rhombomeres. If *Wnt-1* is defective in rhombomere 4 to 9 of the mouse, but *Wnt-3* continues to be normally expressed, the hindbrain develops normally. This principle is known as *redundancy*. In the continued expression in adult life of some regulator genes to conserve cell identity, oculomotor, trochlear, and abducens neurons, but not hypoglossal or spinal motor neurons, are conserved by *Wnt-1* and *LIM* family genes. These genes can compensate for loss of expression of other genes expressed in all motor neurons to preserve normal extraocular muscle innervation in spinal muscular atrophy.

A variation of the principle of redundancy is synergy, a cooperation of two or more genes to produce effects that none is capable of achieving alone. An example is the synergy between *Pax-2* and *Pax-5* in midbrain and cerebellar development (101). If one of this pair is lost, partial but not total compensation may occur.

Principle 7: An organizer gene may be upregulated to be expressed in ectopic domains. Certain molecules may act as teratogens in the developing nervous system, if the embryo is exposed to an excess, whether the excess is exogenous or endogenous in origin. The inductive mechanism is the upregulation of organizer genes, to become expressed in ectopic domains such as in neuromeres where they do not normally play a role in development. An example is retinoic acid that induces ectopic expression of *Hox* genes.

Upregulation of some genes may suppress the expression of others, also contributing to dysgenesis. The overexpression of *LIM* proteins containing only *Islet-3* homeodomains in the zebrafish causes an early termination of expression of *Wnt-1*, *En-2,* and *Pax-2* in the midbrain neuromere and rhombomere 1. This results in severe mesencephalic and metencephalic defects and prevents the formation of optic vesicles. These defects can be rescued by the simultaneous overexpression of *Islet-3* (102).

Principle 8: Developmental genes regulate cell proliferation to conserve constant ratios of synaptically related neurons. An example of this principle is the constant, fixed ratio maintained between Purkinje cells and granule cells in the cerebellar cortex (103). This ratio is lower in less complex mammals than in humans. The ratio is 1:778 in the mouse and 1:2,991 in the human in one study (104) and 1:449 in the rat and 1:3,300 in the human in another (105). To regulate granule cell proliferation, *Shh* and its receptor *patched* (*ptc*) are important genes. *Ptc* protein is localized to granule cells and *Shh* to Purkinje cells, thus providing a molecular substrate for signaling between these synaptically related neurons to establish the needed amount of granule cell production (106,107). *Shh* in Purkinje cells acts as a mitogen on external granule cells (108). To make the system even more complex, *ptc* also interacts through activation of another gene, *smoothened*. A hemizygous deletion of *ptc* in mice results in uncontrolled, excessive prolif-

eration of granule cells and often also leads to neoplastic transformation to medulloblastoma (106). Mutations in the human *ptc* gene are associated with sporadic basal cell carcinomas of the skin and also primitive neuroectodermal tumors of the cerebellum, so that this gene is involved in at least a subset of human medulloblastomas (109). Theoretically, the focal loss of *ptc* expression also might be a basis for dysplastic gangliocytoma of the cerebellum, also known as Lhermitte-Duclos disease, a focal hamartoma, rather than a neoplasm (67).

NEURULATION

The bending of the neural placode to form the neural tube requires both extrinsic and intrinsic mechanical forces, in addition to the dorsalizing and ventralizing genetic effects in the Patterning of the Neural Tube section (Table 4.4).

These forces arise in part from the growth of the surrounding mesodermal tissues on either side of the neural tube, the future somites (110). After surgical removal of mesoderm and endoderm from one side of the neuroepithelium in the experimental animal, the neural tube still closes, but is rotated and becomes asymmetric (111). The mesoderm appears to be important for orientation, but not for closure, of the neural tube. The expansion of the surface epithelium of the embryo is the principal extrinsic force for

TABLE 4.4. *Factors involved in closure of neuroepithelium to form the neural tube*

I. Extrinsic mechanical forces
   A. Surrounding mesodermal tissues
   B. Surface epithelium
II. Intrinsic mechanical forces
   A. Wedge shape of floor plate cells
   B. Differential growth in dorsal and ventral zones
   C. Adhesion molecules
   D. Orientation of mitotic spindles of neuroepithelium
   E. Large fetal central canal
III. Molecular genetic programming
   A. Induction of floor plate by *Sonic hedgehog*
   B. Ventralizing gene transcription products
   C. Dorsalizing gene transcription products
   D. Genetic transcription products that regulate axonal guidance, both attraction and repulsion, across midline and in longitudinal axis
IV. Separation of neural crest

the folding of the neuroepithelium to form the neural tube (112). Cells of the neural placode are mobile and migrate beneath the surface ectoderm, raising the lateral margins of the placode toward the dorsal midline. The growth of the whole embryo itself does not appear to be an important factor because neurulation proceeds equally well in anamniotes (e.g., amphibians) that do not grow during this period and in amniotes (e.g., mammals) that grow rapidly at this time (113).

Among the intrinsic forces of the neuroepithelium, the cells of the floor plate have a wedge shape, narrow at the apex and broad at the base, that facilitates bending (114). Although the width of the floor plate is small, its site in the ventral midline is crucial and sufficient to allow a significant influence. It represents yet another aspect of floor plate induction by the notochord, apart from its influence on the differentiation of neural cells (115). Ependymal cells that form the floor plate are the first neural cells to differentiate, and they induce a growth of the parenchyma of the ventral zone more than in the dorsal regions (67,116); this mechanical effect also may facilitate the curving of the neural placode. The direction of proliferation of new cells in the mitotic cycle, determined in part by the orientation of the mitotic spindle, becomes another mechanical force shaping the neural tube (113,114). Adhesion molecules are probably yet another important mechanical factor for neurulation. In later stages, the ependymal-lined central canal, which is much larger in the fetus than in the newborn, may have a role in exerting a centrifugal force for the tubular shape. In early spinal cord development the central canal is a tall, narrow, midline slit, and only later in fetal life does it assume a rounded contour as seen in transverse sections (67).

Neuroepithelial cells of the neural placode or plate downregulate the polarity of their plasma membrane, so that apical and basilar surfaces are not as distinct, before neural tube closure; cell differentiation in general involves such changes in cell polarity (117). Finally, the rostrocaudal orientation of the majority of mitotic spindles of the neuroepithelium and the direc-

tion in which they push by the mass of daughter cells they form also influences the shape of the neural tube (118).

The neural tube closes in the dorsal midline first in the cervical region, with the closure then extending rostrally and caudally, so that the anterior neuropore of the human embryo closes at 24 days and the posterior neuropore closes at 28 days, the distances from the cervical region being unequal. This traditional view of a continuous zipperlike closure is an oversimplification. In the mouse embryo, the neural tube closes in the cranial region at four distinct sites, with the closure proceeding bidirectionally or unidirectionally and in general synchrony with somite formation (119,120). An intermittent pattern of anterior neural tube closure involving multiple sites also has been described in human embryos (121). In this closure, the principal rostral neuropore closes bidirectionally (122) to form the lamina terminalis, an essential primordium of the forebrain (67).

The bending of the neural plate to form the neural tube is primary neurulation. The term *secondary neurulation* refers only to the most caudal part of the spinal cord (i.e., conus medullaris) that develops from the neuroepithelium caudal to the site of posterior neuropore closure. This part of the spinal cord forms not as a tube, but rather as a solid cord of neural cells in which ependymal cells differentiate in its core and *canalize* the cord, often giving rise to minor aberrations (123). It was previously believed that this is the manner in which the entire spinal cord of fishes is formed, but dorsal folding of the neural plate actually occurs as in other vertebrates (124).

A rare anomaly of a human tail may occur. A true vestigial tail is the most distal remnant of the embryonic tail and contains adipose and connective tissue, central bundles of striated muscle, blood vessels, nerves and is covered by skin, but bone, cartilage, and spinal cord are lacking. Pseudotails are usually an anomalous elongation of the coccygeal vertebrae. In many instances, they contain lipomas, gliomas, teratomas, or even a thin, elongated parasitic fetus (125). Pseudotails often cause tethering of the spinal cord or may even be associated with spinal dysraphism (126,127).

EXPRESSION OF REGULATOR GENES AFTER THE FETAL PERIOD: CONSERVATION OF CELL IDENTITY

Many developmental genes continue to be expressed after the period of ontogenesis and into adult life. In particular, those that direct the differentiation of particular types of cells also may preserve the unique identity of these distinct cells in the mature state. In the cerebellar cortex, *Wnt-3* preserves the identity of Purkinje cells (103); *Pax-3* is responsible for the preservation of Bergmann glia (71); granule cells are supported by several genes, the most important being *Pax-6*, *Zic-1*, and *Math-1* (71,128–130). If one of these genes fails to be expressed, there may be compensation because of the principle of redundancy, but if this phenomenon is incomplete or fails to occur, the motor neurons may never differentiate or may later die by apoptosis and disappear. Theoretically, although not yet proved, such a mechanism might explain human cases of granuloprival cerebellar hypoplasia in which a sparse number or total absence of granule cells are seen in the presence of a normal complement of Purkinje cells and other cellular elements of the cerebellar cortex (67). On the other hand, the preservation of *Wnt-3* expression in Purkinje cells also depends in part on its relations with granule cells (103), so that synaptic contacts probably also impart genetic information between mature neurons.

Another example of genetic expression to preserve cell identity is in motor neurons. The earliest stimulus of motor neuron differentiation is *Shh*, induced by the notochord and floor plate (62,63,65,131). Despite the similar morphologic appearance and function of ocular and spinal motor neurons, differences exist in the genes that program their development and maintenance. *Wnt-1* knockout mice fail to develop oculomotor and trochlear nuclei and their extraocular muscles are altered or deficient, but spinal and hypoglossal motor neurons are not altered (60,132,133). Even among the three pairs of motor nuclei subserving the various extraocular muscles, abducens motor neurons may be selectively involved or spared in relation to motor neurons of the trochlear and oculomotor nuclei (132). Genes of the large *LIM* family, particularly *Lim-1*, *Lim-2*, *Islet-1*, and *Islet-2*, also are expressed in motor neurons and each individual gene in this family defines a subclass of motor neurons for the topographic projection of axonal projections (134–136). Insulinlike growth factor also has been identified as a regulator of apoptosis of developing motor neurons and may express a differential effect (137). These differences in genetic programming of motor neurons in various neuromeres perhaps explain oculomotor sparing with progressive degeneration of spinal and hypoglossal motor neurons in spinal muscular atrophy (Werdnig-Hoffmann disease).

ANATOMIC AND PHYSIOLOGIC PROCESSES OF CENTRAL NERVOUS SYSTEM DEVELOPMENT

Traditional embryology recognizes a series of developmental processes that are not entirely sequential because of a great deal of temporal overlap as the various processes proceed simultaneously.

Redundancy

One of the most important general principles of neuroembryology is that of redundancy. The redundancy of some genes with overlapping domains and their ability to compensate for lack of expression of the other has already been mentioned in the Patterning of the Neural Tube section. Another redundancy is the production of neuroblasts. An overproduction by 30% to 50% of neuroblasts occurs in all regions of the nervous system, depending on the number of symmetric mitotic cycles, followed by apoptosis of the surplus cells that are not needed to be matched to targets. Immature axonal projections are redundant because many collaterals form diffuse projections, followed during maturation by retraction of many to leave fewer but more specific connections. Synapses also are overly produced, followed by synaptic pruning to provide greater precision.

Embryologic Zones of the Neural Tube

After neurulation, the closed neural tube has an architecture of two concentric rings as viewed in transverse section: The inner ring is the ventricular zone, consisting of the proliferative, pseudostratified columnar neuroepithelium; the outer ring is the marginal zone, a cell-sparse region of fibers and extracellular matrix proteins (67). Details of the mitotic patterns in the ventricular zone are discussed later (see Neuronogenesis section).

With further development, four concentric zones appear. A subventricular zone outside the proliferative ventricular zone is composed of postmitotic, premigratory neuroblasts and glioblasts, and radial glial cells. After radial migration of neuroblasts begins, an intermediate zone is formed by the radial glial processes and the migratory neuroblasts adherent to them; this intermediate zone eventually becomes the deep subcortical white matter of the cerebral hemispheres. In the cerebrum, migratory neuroblasts destined to form the cerebral cortex begin to form an unlaminated cortical plate within the marginal zone. This event divides that zone into an outermost, cell-sparse region, thereafter known as the *molecular layer* (eventually layer 1 of the mature cerebral cortex), and the innermost portion of the marginal zone isolated by the intervening cortical plate, known as the *subplate zone*. This region contains many neurons that form transitory pioneer axons to establish the corticospinal and other long projection pathways, but eventually the subplate zone becomes incorporated into layer 6 of the maturing cortex and disappears as a distinct anatomic region.

The two and later four concentric zones clearly identified in the cerebrum are similar, although in modified form in the brainstem and spinal cord. They become even further altered in the cerebellum with an apparent inversion, the granule cells migrating from the surface inward rather than from the periventricular region outward. An ependymal epithelium eventually forms at the ventricular surface of the ventricular zone, creating an additional, innermost zone not present in the embryo except for the floor plate in the ventral midline (see Role of the Fetal Ependyma section).

Separation and Migration of the Neural Crest

Neural crest cells arise from the dorsal midline of the neural tube at the time of closure or shortly thereafter and migrate extensively along prescribed routes through the embryo to differentiate as the peripheral nervous system. This includes dorsal root and sympathetic ganglia, chromaffin cells such as those of the adrenal medulla and carotid body, melanocytes or pigment cells, and a few other cell types of both ectodermal and mesodermal origin. The facial skeleton including the orbits, connective tissue of the eye, ciliary ganglion, part of the trigeminal ganglia, and Schwann cells of nerves also are formed by the neural crest (138,139). The vertebrate gene *Slug*, a homologue of the *Snail* gene of insects, is expressed in early neural crest before its migration begins and probably is important in its differentiation (140).

The most rostral origin of neural crest cells from the neural tube is from the midbrain neuromere; these cells migrate as a uniform sheet, whereas those migrating from hindbrain and spinal cord rhombomeres do so segmentally (141,142). Rhombomeres 3 and 5 do not appear to generate neural crest cells; alternative hypotheses are that these cells undergo accelerated apoptosis or deviate rostrally and caudally to migrate with cells of adjacent rhombomeres (141,142). Migratory pathways of neural crest cells outside the neural tube are created in large part by attractant and repulsive molecules secreted by surrounding tissues, such as the otic capsule, somites, and vertebral neural arches (143). In addition, neural crest cells possess integrin receptors for interacting with extracellular matrix molecules (141,142). Changes in the distribution of extracellular matrix components impose migratory guidance limits as well (143).

The precise origin of neural crest cells is still incompletely understood, because they represent diverse mature populations that include elements of mesodermal as well as ectodermal primitive germ layers. Why neural crest precursors are so heterogeneous, why neural crest stem cells with multiple potentials exist, and even whether stem cells arising from the neural tube are joined by surrounding cells from the mesoderm are questions that are not as well understood as the pathways the precursors follow within the body of the embryo (144). As with other parts of the neural tube, neural crest tissue follows a rostrocaudal gradient of differentiation. The fate of neural crest cells is influenced by whether they migrate early or late, and by neurotrophic factors [e.g., neurotropin-3 is essential for survival of sympathetic neuroblasts and the innervation of specific organs (145)].

Neuroepithelial Cell Proliferation

Early cleavages in the fertilized ovum to form the blastula and the blastomere (gastrula) involve a simple proliferation of cells cycling between the mitotic (M-phase) and resting (S-phase) states, a process similar to DNA replication in bacteria. As the neuroectoderm forms in the epiblast at postovulatory week 3 in the human embryo, it becomes organized as a pseudostratified columnar epithelium, a sheet of bipolar cells all oriented so that one cytoplasmic process extends to the dorsal (future ventricular) surface and the other process extends to the ventral (future pial) surface. The nucleus of each of these spindle-shaped cells moves to and fro within its own cytoplasmic extensions. M-phase occurs at or near to the ventricular surface and S-phase occurs at the other end. Transitional periods between these two states are known as gap phases: G1 when the nucleus moves distally toward the pial surface and G2 when the nucleus approaches the ventricular surface (146). The introduction of gap phases in the mitotic cycle allows for adjustments to be made in the replication of DNA during G1, and the sequence ensures that G2 cells do not undergo an extra round of S-phase, which might lead to a change in ploidy as the chromosomes segregate in the dividing cell (147). In this way, errors may be corrected before the next mitosis, thus allowing for more plasticity than the all-or-none principle of simple cell division.

Mitoses continue to occur at the ventricular surface as the neural plate folds and becomes a neural tube. The differentiation of an ependyma

TABLE 4.5. *Generation of motor neurons in the lumbar spinal cord of the chick embryo*

Progenitor stem cells	60
Motor neuroblasts generated	24,000
Mature motor neurons required	12,000
Motor neurons generated in seven symmetric mitotic cycles	7,680
Motor neurons generated in eight symmetric mitotic cycles	15,360

From Burek MJ, Oppenheim RW. Programmed cell death in the developing nervous system. *Brain Pathol* 1996;6:427–446. With permission.

at the ventricular surface signals the termination of mitotic activity and indeed of the ventricular zone, as the remaining cells in the periventricular region all are postmitotic premigratory neuroblasts and glioblasts, hence of the subventricular zone (67,116).

Because mitoses increase cell populations exponentially, a finite number of mitotic cycles are needed to produce the requisite number of neurons needed in a given part of the nervous system. In the cerebrum of the rat, 10 mitotic cycles in the ventricular zone generate all the neurons of the cerebral cortex; in the human, 33 mitotic cycles generate a much larger number of neurons than simply three times the number in the rat cortex (148). Eight symmetric mitotic cycles are required to produce the minimum essential number of motor neuroblasts in the spinal cord of the chick (Table 4.5) (149).

The orientation of the mitotic spindle at the ventricular surface is important in the fate of the daughter cells after each mitosis, because certain gene products are distributed asymmetrically within the mother cell, and because with some orientations both daughter cells do not retain their attachments to the ventricular wall (150–152). *Notch*, *numb*, and *null* are genes with antagonistic functions, situated at opposite poles of the neuroepithelial cell. If the cleavage plane of the mitotic spindle is perpendicular to the ventricular surface, the daughter cells each retain an attachment to that surface and inherit equal amounts of *notch*, *numb*, and *null*. This situation is called *symmetric cleavage* and both daughter cells reenter the mitotic cycle in the same manner as their common precursor cell. If, however, the mitotic spindle is parallel to the ventricular surface, the two daughter cells are unequal because only one can retain an attachment to the ventricle, and one inherits most of the *notch* and *numb* whereas the other inherits most of the *null* gene product. This situation is asymmetric cleavage. Only one of the cells, the one at the ventricular surface, reenters the mitotic cycle, and the other, more distal cell, has completed its final mitosis and rapidly moves away from its sister to begin differentiation as a neuroblast and prepare for radial migration from the subventricular zone.

Neuronal polarity, establishing from which side of the cell the axon will sprout and from which cell surfaces the dendrites will form, is determined at least in part at the time of the final mitosis. Microtubule arrays are the most fundamental components of the mitotic spindle, forming during prophase as the centrosome replicates; the *minus* ends of the microtubules remain associated with the centrosome, whereas the *plus* ends emanate outward, with the duplicated centrosomes driven to opposite poles of the cell as a direct result of microtubule organization. The mitotic spindle consists of regions in which microtubules are uniformly oriented in tandem and in parallel and other regions where the microtubules are more haphazardly oriented; the former becomes the axonal end of the cell and the latter, the opposite pole or the dendritic end (153).

In the postnatal human infant, mitotic activity of neuronal precursors continues to be seen, although sparse, in the outer half of the external granule cell layer of the cerebellum; external granule cells do not complete their migration until after 1 year of age; hence the potential for regeneration after prenatal and even postnatal loss of some of these cells still exists. Another well-documented region of continued neuronal turnover in the human nervous system is the primary olfactory neurons (154).

A few neuroblasts appear to undergo division even during migration, which are exceptions to the general rule (155). A population of quiescent neuroepithelial stem cells in the subventricular zone of the mammalian forebrain retains a proliferative potential even in the adult (156). Great interest has been shown in this inconspicuous and sparse cell population because of its potential in neuronal regeneration and repair of the damaged brain and spinal cord.

Apoptosis

In every region of the nervous system, an overgeneration of neuroblasts occurs, more than are required at maturity by 30% to 70%. Surplus cells survive for a period of days or weeks and then spontaneously undergo a cascade of degenerative changes and disappear without inflammatory responses to cell death or the proliferation of glial scars. This physiologic process of programmed cell death, or apoptosis, was discovered in 1949 by Hamburger and Levi-Montalcini, who demonstrated its occurrence in the spinal dorsal root ganglion of the chick embryo (157). The phenomenon subsequently has been confirmed by numerous other independent investigators, and indeed it is a general principle of development in all animals, from the simplest worms to humans, and involves all organ systems, not just the nervous system (158–161). Examples of apoptosis that continues throughout life are found in any tissue that has a constant turnover of cells, such as the 120-day half-life of erythrocytes and the continuous replacement of intestinal mucosal epithelial cells (of mesodermal origin) and of epidermal cells of the skin (of ectodermal origin).

Apoptosis differs from cell death by necrosis (e.g., from ischemia, hypoxia, toxins, infections) in several important morphologic details, in addition to the absence of tissue reaction to the loss, except for the removal of the cellular debris by phagocytic microglial cells (i.e., modified macrophages). In neural cell apoptosis, the sequence begins with shrinkage of the nucleus, condensation of chromatin, and increased electron opacity of the cell. These events are followed by disappearance of the Golgi apparatus, loss of endoplasmic reticulum, and disaggregation of polyribosomes; final steps are the formation of ribosomal crystals and the breakdown of the nuclear membrane (157). Mitochondria are preserved until late stages of apoptosis, whereas they swell and disintegrate early in cellular necrosis.

Apoptosis is genetically patterned as with other events in nervous system development. The process is programmed into every cell, but its expression is blocked by the inhibitory influence of certain genes, such as *bcl-2* and the immediate early proto-oncogene c-*fos*, and this genetic regulation also is modulated by trophic factors of other cells in the vicinity that preserve metabolic integrity. For example, nerve growth factor and bFGF block cell death and preserve the identity of various cell lineages in the nervous system (162–164). The apoptotic process also may be accelerated or retarded by metabolic factors, such as plasma concentrations of thyroid hormone, serum ammonia, local neurotoxins including excitatory amino acids such as aspartate (165), lactic acidosis, and imbalances of calcium and electrolytes.

Synaptic relations are another *environmental factor* within the brain that affects apoptosis: An inverse relationship exists between the rate of apoptosis of spinal motor neurons and synaptogenesis. On the afferent side, neurons degenerate if they fail to be innervated or if they lose their entire afferent supply because of the loss of presynaptic neurons. This phenomenon is called *transsynaptic degeneration* and is exemplified in the lateral genicular body after optic nerve lesions and in the inferior olivary nucleus after destruction of the central tegmental tract. On the efferent side, motor neurons degenerate if they fail to match with target muscle fibers or if their muscle targets are removed, as after amputation of a limb bud of an embryo or even the amputation of an extremity in the adult.

Proteins programmed from exons 7 and 8 of the *survival motor neuron (SMN)* gene at the 5q11-q13 locus are defective in spinal muscular atrophy (Werdnig-Hoffmann and Kugelberg-Welander diseases); this is an example of a gene that normally arrests apoptosis in spinal motor neurons after all muscular targets are matched (166,167) (see Chapter 14). This degenerative disease thus occurs because a physiologic process in the early fetus becomes pathologic in late fetal life and the postnatal period because of its failure to stop, with continued progressive death of motor neurons.

Apoptosis occurs in two phases. The first is the programmed death of incompletely differentiated cells and represents the numerically most important phase of this process; even completely undifferentiated neuroepithelial cells undergo apoptosis, but the factors that select these short life cycles are poorly understood (168). The second phase is the cell death of mature, well-differentiated neurons. This process continues in the early postnatal period in the rat cervical spinal cord (169).

Transitory Neurons of the Fetal Brain

The process of apoptosis at times involves an entire population of neurons of the fetal brain that serve an important function in development but are not required after maturity. An example is the Cajal-Retzius neuron of the molecular layer of the fetal cerebral cortex. This cell already is present and mature in the marginal layer of the telencephalon before the first wave of radial migration from the subventricular zone as a part of the plexus that exists before formation of the cortical plate (67,170–173). The cells probably migrate rostrally from the midbrain neuromere at the time of neural tube formation. They are bipolar neurons that form axons and dendritic trunks running parallel to the pial surface of the brain. With formation of the cortical plate, axonal collaterals of Cajal-Retzius neurons plunge into the cortical plate to create the first intrinsic cortical synaptic circuits by forming synapses on neurons of layer 6 from the earliest waves of radial migration.

Cajal-Retzius neurons also appear to play an important role in radial neuroblast migration and in the developing laminar architecture of the cerebral cortex. The gene-associated antigen *reelin*, in the reeler mouse model, is expressed strongly in Cajal-Retzius neurons and is crucial to the laminar organization of cortical neurons (174,175). This gene programs an extracellular glycoprotein of the same name that is secreted by Cajal-Retzius cells in the cerebrum and by external granule cells in the cerebellum, and without which the laminar architecture of the cortex is disrupted severely. Cajal-Retzius cells also strongly express the *LIS* family of genes that have been shown to be defective in lissencephaly type I (Miller-Dieker syndrome)

(176). Cajal-Retzius neurons synthesize γ-aminobutyric acid as their principal neurotransmitter, and probably acetylcholine as well; immunocytochemical reactivity to calcium-binding proteins suggests that they represent a heterogeneous population (177). Cajal-Retzius cells persist until late fetal life in the molecular zone; they begin to disappear at approximately 32 weeks' gestation by a process of apoptosis and few remain at the time of birth, even these disappearing in early postnatal life (178). Subplate neurons of the deep layer of the marginal zone, isolated by the formation of the cortical plate, are another population of transitory neurons that produce pioneer axons and later disappear after permanent axonal projections from layer 5 pyramidal neurons are established.

The radial glial cell that provides the principal means of neuroblast migration is another cell of the fetal nervous system that is no longer recognized after maturity. Unlike the Cajal-Retzius neurons, radial glial cells do not disappear because of cell death but rather become transformed into mature fibrillary astrocytes of the white matter.

Role of the Fetal Ependyma

The ependyma of the mature brain is little more than a decorative lining of the ventricular system, serving minor functions in the transport of ions and small molecules between the ventricles and the cerebral parenchyma and perhaps having a small immunoprotective role. The fetal ependyma, by contrast, is an essential and dynamic structure that contributes to a number of developmental processes (67,116).

The floor plate is the first region of the neuroepithelium to differentiate as specific cells. It forms the ventral midline of the ependyma in the spinal cord and brainstem as far rostrally as the midbrain, but a floor plate is not recognized in the prosencephalon, perhaps not in diencephalic neuromeres because of the infundibulum in the ventral midline, or in the telencephalon. The floor plate has an active expression of *Shh* and contributes to the differentiation of motor neurons and of other parts of the ependyma. It also secretes retinoic acid,

unlike other ependymal cells that merely have retinoid receptors.

The ependyma develops in a precise temporal and spatial pattern. The last surfaces of the ventricular system to be completely covered by ependyma are in the lateral ventricles at 22 weeks' gestation. In some parts of the neuraxis, it is advantageous for ependymal differentiation to be delayed as long as possible to permit the requisite numbers of neuroblasts to be produced in the ventricular zone, because once the ependyma forms in a particular region, all mitotic activity ceases at the ventricular surface (116,179). One function of the fetal ependyma, therefore, is to regulate the arrest of mitotic proliferation of neuroepithelial cells.

The fetal ependyma is structurally different from the adult. Rather than a simple cuboidal epithelium as in the adult, it is a pseudostratified columnar epithelium, each cell having at least a slender cytoplasmic process contacting the ventricular surface even though its nucleus may be at some distance. This arrangement is needed so that ependymal cells do not divide after differentiation, and a provision is required for enough cells to cover the entire ventricular surface. With growth of the fetus, the extra layers of ependymal cells become thinned as the ependyma spreads to cover the expanding ventricular surface. At the basal surface of fetal ependymal cells is a process that radiates into the parenchyma. This process may reach the pial surface of the spinal cord and brainstem, but never spans the entire cerebral hemisphere and only extends into the subventricular zone (i.e., germinal matrix) and into the deeper portions of the intermediate zone. The fetal ependyma also differs from the adult in expressing certain intermediate filament proteins, such as vimentin and glial fibrillary acidic protein and some other molecules such as S-100β protein (180). As in the adult, the fetal ependyma is ciliated at its apical (i.e., ventricular) surface.

Ependymal cells are important elements in guiding the intermediate trajectories of axonal growth cones (181,182). In some places, the basal processes of fetal ependymal cells actually form mechanical tunnels to guide axonal growth in developing long tracts. Ependymal cells and their processes also secrete molecules that attract or repel axons and may be specific for some and not for other axons. Floor plate ependymal cells synthesize netrin, a diffusible neurotrophic factor, permitting the passage of commissural axons but repelling fibers of longitudinal tracts (183–185). Netrin may be bifunctional, acting as attractants of decussating axons at some sites, such as the floor plate in the spinal cord, but as repellants in other sites, such as trochlear axons (184). In the developing dorsal columns of the spinal cord, the dorsal median raphé formed by ependymal cells of the roof plate prevents the wandering to the wrong side of the spinal cord of rostrally growing axons, by secreting a proteoglycan, keratan sulfate, that strongly repels axonal growth cones (181). Ependymal processes do not guide migratory neuroblasts, despite their appearance resembling radial glial fibers.

The loss of S-100β protein from ependymal cells of the lateral ventricles appears to coincide with the end of cell migration from the subventricular zone and the beginning conversion of radial glial cells into mature astrocytes (116). Whether the ependyma is inducing this conversion is uncertain, but circumstantial evidence suggests such a function.

Neuroblast Migration

Almost no neurons occupy sites in the mature human brain that are the sites where these cells underwent their terminal mitosis and began differentiation. In some simple vertebrates, such as the salamander, mature neurons often are situated in the periventricular zone where they originated (186), but in humans, such periventricular maturation is regarded as heterotopic and pathologic. Neuroblasts thus migrate to sites often distant from their birthplace, to establish the needed synaptic relations with both similar and different types of neurons and to send axonal projections grouped with similar fibers to form tracts or fascicles to distant sites along the neuraxis. The synaptic architecture of the cerebral or cerebellar cortices would not be possible without such neuroblast migration.

Several mechanisms subserve neuroblast migration. The most important from the stand-point of transporting the majority of neuroblasts, whether into cortical or nuclear structures, is the use of radial glial fiber guides. In the cerebrum, glial cells of the subventricular zone develop a long, slender process that spans the entire cerebral mantle to terminate as an end-foot on the pial membrane at the surface of the brain (67,187). These specialized radial glial cells are transitory and, after all migration is complete, they retract their radial process and mature to become fibrillary astrocytes of the subcortical white matter. The radial glial process of these cells serves a unique function during fetal life of guiding migratory cells, both neuroblasts and glioblasts, from the subventricular zone or germinal matrix to their destination in the cerebral cortex or in other forebrain structures. They perform this function as a *monorail*, with migratory cells actually gliding along their surface. Fetal ependymal cells also have basal processes that extend into the germinal matrix, but they do not reach as far as the cortex or even into the deep white matter, differ morphologically, and serve entirely different functions that do not include the guidance of migratory cells (67,116). In the cerebellum, the specialized Bergmann glial cells, which occupy the Purkinje cell layer and have radiating processes that extend to the surface of the cerebellar cortex, provide a similar function for the migration inward of granule cells from the fetal external granular layer to the mature internal site within the folia (67). Bergmann cells and their processes persist into adult life, unlike the change that occurs before birth in the radial glial cells of the cerebrum.

The transport of migratory neuroepithelial cells along the radial glial fiber requires a number of adhesion molecules to prevent the cell from detaching too early. Adhesion molecules also lubricate their path of travel and perhaps provide nutrition to the cells as they move and continuously change their position in relation to capillaries within the white matter parenchyma (188). These molecules are secreted either by (a) the migratory neuroblast itself, (b) the radial glial cell, or (c) others already present in the extracellular matrix. Astrotactin is an example of a protein molecule produced by the neuroblast during migration that helps adhere the cell to the radial glial fiber and is essential in the establishment of the laminar architecture of the neocortex, hippocampus, olfactory bulb, and cerebellar cortex (189). The gene that encodes astrotactin is related also to the synthesis of epidermal growth factor and fibronectin (189). Examples of molecules synthesized by the radial glial cell for purposes of neuroblast adhesion are S-100β protein (116) and *L1-neural cell adhesion molecule* (*L1-NCAM*) (190); the defective expression of the gene that regulates the *L1-NCAM* protein results in polymicrogyria, pachygyria, and X-linked recessive fetal hydrocephalus (190). Other molecules synthesized by the radial glial cell also have been identified (191).

Finally, some molecules contributing to cell adhesion, such as fibronectin, laminins, and collagen type IV, needed for the formation of extracellular basement membranes, are found in the extracellular matrix (192). In addition to providing a substrate for normal neuroblast and glioblast migration, the motility and infiltration of brain parenchyma by neoplastic cells of neural origin depends largely on extracellular matrix proteins.

Reelin (*reln*) is a gene and glycoprotein transcription product secreted by Cajal-Retzius neurons in the cerebrum and by external granule cells in the cerebellum that is essential to terminal migration and the laminal architecture of cortices. The reeler mouse is a model that lacks expression of the *reln* gene and exhibits severe disruption of laminated structures of the brain (174,175). Another gene and its protein, *Disabled-1* (*dab-1*), acts downstream of *reln* in a signaling pathway of laminar organization, functioning in phosphorylation-dependent intracellular signal transduction (193).

Not all cells migrating within the developing brain use radial glial fibers. Some migrations proceed along the axons of earlier and now established cells in the brainstem, olfactory bulb, and cerebellum, using the axon in the same manner as a radial glial fiber. Tangential migrations perpendicular to the radial glial fibers also occur in the cerebral cortex and contribute to a mixture of clones in any given region so that all neurons are not from the same neu-

roepithelial stem cells originating in the same zone of the germinal matrix (194–197). The site of origin of these cells migrating tangentially is not well documented, but they begin their tangential course outside the proliferative ventricular zone (196). They might even represent the persistent stem cells that have in the 1990s been recognized in the adult brain and are of great interest because of their potential value in regeneration of the damaged nervous system if they can be stimulated and mobilized. How these tangential migrations occur, skipping from one radial glial fiber to another or traveling between radial glia, is incompletely resolved.

At the surface of the cerebrum, the migratory neuroblasts reverse direction so that the earlier migrations are displaced into deeper layers of the cortical plate by the more recent arrivals. Layer 6 therefore represents the earliest wave of radial neuroblast migration from the subventricular zone, and layer 2 consists of the last neurons to migrate.

The Cajal-Retzius cells of the molecular zone, which were in place before the first radial migrations occurred (171–173), are important to the architectural integrity of the developing cortex and appear to influence cell placement within the cortical plate, even before distinct lamination occurs. The pial membrane and the subpial granular layer of Brun (which in the human fetal cerebrum is a transitory layer of glial cells, unlike the cerebellar cortex in which the external granule cell layer is neuroblasts) are important in reversing the direction of migration as cells arrive at the surface. Deficiency of these components in certain malformations, such as holoprosencephaly, results in extensive overmigration with neuronal ectopia in the leptomeninges (67).

Several genes are now recognized to be defective in disorders of neuroblast migration in humans, although the precise mechanisms by which these genes mediate migration in the healthy fetus are incompletely understood. The *LIS1* gene at the 17p13.3 locus is responsible for lissencephaly type I in Miller-Dieker syndrome and also in isolated lissencephaly (198–200). *Doublecortin* is a gene (also denotes the gene product or signaling protein) that is defective or unexpressed in X-linked dominant subcortical laminar heterotopia, also known as band heterotopia or double cortex (201,202). Bilateral periventricular heterotopia, another X-linked dominant trait, is associated with deficiency of expression of *filamen-1* (203,204). The neural cell adhesion molecule *L1-CAM* is implicated in hemimegalencephaly (193) and also in X-linked recessive hydrocephalus with pachygyria and often with aqueductal stenosis (205).

Axonal Pathfinding

The outgrowth of a single axon precedes the formation of the multiple dendrites and is one of the first morphologic events marking the maturation of a neuroblast in becoming a neuron. It occurs at times even during the course of migration before the cell has arrived at its final destination and, in some cases, such as the external granule cells of the cerebellum, even occurs before migration starts. The tip of the growing axon, termed the *growth cone* by Ramón y Cajal (206), is neither pointed nor blunt, but rather is a constantly changing complex of cytoplasmic fingers or extension, the *filopodia*, enclosed by a membrane that extends between filopodia to form veils or webs. The cytoplasm of the filopodia is filled with microtubules, filaments, and mitochondria. Filopodia extend and retract with amoeboid movements.

To develop polarity, by which an axon emerges at one site and not at others, neuroblasts share membrane protein–sorting mechanisms with epithelial cells, the other important polarized type of cell. The axonal cell surface is analogous to the apical plasma membrane of epithelial cells, such as ependymal cells or intestinal mucosal cells, and the somatodendritic plasma membrane is analogous to the basolateral epithelial surface (207–209). A complex interaction of sorting signals from glycolipid proteins within the plasma membrane and soluble attachment protein receptors that promote the docking of vesicles with target membranes results in intracellular membrane fusions that differ in various parts of the neuroblast plasma membrane and are required for membrane assembly during axonal growth (208).

Three fundamental mechanisms guide axons to their destination, which may be at a great distance from the cell body (210,211). A fourth mechanism, proposed a century ago, has been resurrected as plausible. (a) *Cell-cell interactions*: Molecular signals generated by the target cell induce the growth cone to form a synapse. This mechanism is effective only as the axon approaches within 1 to 2 mm of the target. (b) *Cell-substrate interactions*: Molecules known as integrins bind the cell to an extracellular protein matrix, such as fibronectin or laminin. Such substrates serve as adhesive surfaces for growth cones, allowing them to pull themselves along, but also might provide directional cues as attractants or repellants. (c) *Chemotactic interactions*: Secretory molecules may release powerful attractants or repellants to keep the axon aligned along an intended course in its intermediate trajectory; growth cones are exquisitely sensitive to certain chemicals and grow toward or away from these molecules. (d) It was once thought that electrical or electromagnetic fields were important influences in orienting the growing axon; this discarded theory is being reconsidered in a more modern context, although its importance is still poorly substantiated. Local electrical fields might change the course of growing axons by altering receptive properties of their membrane to neurotransmitters and attractant and repellent molecules (212).

The glycosaminoglycans and proteoglycan molecules are important examples of growth cone repellants in the developing CNS. An example is keratan sulfate (unrelated biochemically to the epidermal protein keratin). This compound is secreted in many tissues of the fetal body at sites where nerves are not needed or desired: the epiphyseal plates of growing bones; the epidermis (to prevent nerves from growing through the skin); the notochordal sheath; and the developing neural arches of the vertebrae (to segment and guide nerve roots from the spinal cord between rather than through the somites) (211). The highly segmented somites are important early guides of neural crest cellular migration as well as of axonal projections peripherally (213). Within the CNS, fetal ependymal cells synthesize keratan sulfate, in part to prevent axons from growing into the ventricles of the brain, and in part to prevent aberrant decussation of developing long tracts and the wandering of axons toward wrong targets (116,181). The dorsal median raphe that separates the dorsal columns of the two sides of the spinal cord in the dorsal midline, probably programmed by dorsalizing genes such as those of the *Pax* family, is composed of ependymal roof plate processes that secrete keratan sulfate at the time when the axons of the dorsal columns are growing rostrally. The raphé serves to repel growth cones that might otherwise decussate prematurely, before reaching the gracile and cuneate nuclei of the medulla oblongata (181,182). The effects of such repellent molecules are selective, however. Keratan sulfate secreted by the floor plate and the dorsal median septum of the midbrain collicular plate does not prevent the passage of commissural fibers at those sites, although the substance repulses axons of descending and ascending long tracts. Perhaps the passage of commissural fibers is mediated by attractants of such fibers, such as netrin, that overcome a negative influence of keratan sulfate. The floor plate also repulses axons of developing motor neurons, so that they extend into the spinal roots only on the side of their soma (214). Another family of proteins, the semaphorins/collapsins, acts mainly as growth cone repellants both in neural tissue, including the floor plate, and throughout the body in nonneural tissues (215). Thus, the midline septa composed of floor and roof plate basal processes act as chemical barriers to some axons, but are not physical barriers despite their appearance in histologic stained sections, because commissural axons easily pass through them. Other examples of growth cone attractants are nerve growth factor and S-100 protein.

The cytoskeleton plays a central role in axonal guidance. The internal organization of actin filaments and microtubules changes rapidly within the growth cone before large-scale changes in growth cone shape are seen. These changes are evoked by local environmental molecules that stabilize local changes of cytoskeletal polymers in the growth cone (216). Although microtubule assembly in the growing axon is required for the axon to extend along its pathway, drugs that disrupt microtubule assembly do not impede the assembly and growth at the axonal tip (217). Growth cone collapse is a part of the normal process of axonal growth and may become pathologic if excessive; it is induced by a platelet-activation factor (218).

Finally, or perhaps first of all, homeobox-containing genes are involved in the regulation of axonal growth. A gene expressed early in neuronal differentiation, *TOAD-64* ("turned on after division"; with an identical nucleotide sequence to *unc-33* in nematodes) is strongly expressed by its protein transcription product in growth cones and is downregulated after axonal projection is complete. Mutations in this gene result in aberrations in axonal outgrowth in the mouse (219). The overexpression of *Hox-2* reverses axonal pathways from rhombomere 3 (78). Boundary regions between adjacent domains of regulatory gene expression influence where the first axons extend (209). Initial tract formation is associated with the selective expression of certain cell adhesion molecules and their regulatory gene transcripts (220).

Some long tracts are preceded by pioneer axons formed by transitory neurons that appear to serve as guides for the growth cones of permanent axons, and without which the permanent axons detour to heterotopic sites. An example is the pioneer axons from subplate neurons as the cortical plate is beginning to form; these pioneer axons establish the internal capsule and precede the passage of axons from pyramidal cells of the future layers 5 and 6 of the cortex. After the pyramidal cell axons are guided into the internal capsule, the pioneer axons and their cells of origin disappear, probably by apoptosis. An epidermal growth factor is expressed by pioneer neurons and by Cajal-Retzius cells in the reeler mouse, a model of migrational disorders and cortical dysgenesis (221,222).

Dendritic Proliferation and Synaptogenesis

Dendrites sprout only after the axon begins its projection from the same neuron. The branching pattern of dendrites and the formation of spines on these dendritic arborizations, on which synapses form, are varied and characteristic for each type of neuron. In the cerebral cortex, synaptogenesis occurs after migration of the neuron to its mature site is complete. In the cerebellar cortex, external granule cells project bipolar axons as parallel fibers in the molecular zone and form synapses with Purkinje cell dendrites before migrating to their mature site in the interior of the folium.

An excessive number of synapses generally forms, and many are later deleted with the retraction of redundant collateral axons (223). In addition, transitory neurons, such as the Cajal-Retzius neurons of the fetal cerebral cortex, form temporary synapses. As with other aspects of neural development, a critical period of synapse elimination occurs (224). Class 1 major histocompatibility complex glycoproteins may be involved in synaptic remodeling during fetal development and infancy. In the optic system, considerable amounts of these surface-expressed proteins are demonstrated on neurons of the lateral geniculate body in the late fetal and early postnatal periods, a period when synaptogenesis and especially synaptic retraction are most active (225).

Most of the dendritic arborization and synapatogenesis in the cerebral cortex occur during late gestation and early infancy, a circumstance that renders this developmental process particularly vulnerable to toxic, hypoxic, ischemic, and metabolic insults in the postnatal period, especially in neonates born prematurely.

When an axonal terminal reaches a dendritic spine and cell-cell contact is achieved, a chemical synapse usually forms rapidly. Some *promiscuous* neurons may even secrete transmitter before contacting their targets, inducing an overabundance of synapses that then undergo additional electrical activity–dependent refinement (226). Dendritic spines determine the dynamics of intracellular second-messenger ions, such as calcium, and probably provide for synaptic plasticity by establishing compartmentalization of afferent input based on biochemical rather than electrical signals (227).

Neurotropins play an important role in the modulation of synaptogenesis as selective retrograde messengers (228). Transsynaptic signaling by neurotropins and neurotransmitters also may influence neuronal architecture such as neurite sprouting and dendritic pruning (229,230). The effects of neurotrophic factors may be lamina-specific within the cortex and have opposite effects in different layers. Brain-derived neurotrophic factor stimulates dendritic growth in layer 4 neurons, whereas neurotropin-3 inhibits this growth; brain-derived neurotrophic factor is inhibitory and neurotropin-3 is stimulatory, by contrast, for neuroblasts in layer 6 (231).

Prostaglandins and their inducible synthetase enzymes (e.g., cyclo-oxygenase 2) are expressed by excitatory neurons at postsynaptic sites in the cerebral cortex and hippocampus. They modulate N-methyl-D-aspartate–dependent responses, such as long-term potentiation, and show a spatial and temporal sequence of expression that may be demonstrated in the fetal brain by immunocytochemistry. This expression is highly localized to dendritic spines and reflects functional rather than structural features of synapse formation (232–235). Prostaglandin signaling of cortical development, and synaptogenesis in particular, thus are mediated through dendrites, and the same is likely for neurotropin signaling (236).

Glial cells are important in promoting dendritic development (208,237). In addition to the axodendritic and axosomatic synapses, a few specialized sites in the developing brain show dendrodendritic contacts. An example is the spines of olfactory granule cells (220).

The electroencephalogram (EEG) is the most reliable and accessible noninvasive clinical measure of functional synaptogenesis in the cerebral cortex of the preterm infant. The maturation of EEG patterns involves a precise and predictable temporal progression of changes with conceptional age, including the development of sleep–wake cycles.

Neuronal and Glial Cell Maturation

Neuronal and epithelial cells are the most polarized cells of the body: Epithelial cells must have apical and basal surfaces, and neurons must form an axon at one end and dendrites at other cell surfaces (208,209,238,239). The development of cell polarity is one of the first events in neuronogenesis. The structural and molecular differences that distinguish axonal and dendritic domains play an integral role in every aspect of neuronal function (239). Neuronal polarity begins with the final mitosis of the neuroepithelial cell and is determined by the orientation of microtubules in the mitotic spindle (153).

Two other combined features distinguish neurons from all other cells in the body: an electrically polarizing and excitable plasma membrane and secretory function. Muscle cells have excitable membranes but do not secrete; endocrine and exocrine cells are secretory but do not have polarized membranes. Only neurons have both.

The development of electrical polarity of the cell membrane is an important maturational feature that denotes when a neuroblast becomes a neuron. This process depends on the development of ion channels as well as a means of delivering continuous energy production necessary to maintain a resting membrane potential. This membrane potential is mediated by voltage-gated ion channels and does not require another energy-generating mechanism such as the adenosine triphosphatase pumps mediated by Na^+/K^+, Ca^{2+}, or Mg^{2+}. The importance of glial cells for ion transport in this regard may be greater than once believed, and astrocytes play an important role in regulating the cerebral microenvironment, in addition to their nutritive functions and their contribution to the blood–brain barrier (237).

The onset of synthesis of neurotransmitter substances, their transport down the axon, and the formation of terminal axonal storage vesicles for these compounds are other features that denote the transition from neuroblast to neuron. Transmitter biosynthesis may begin before neuroblast migration is completed, although the secretion of these substances is delayed until synapses are formed with target cells. Some substances that later serve as neurotransmitters, including most of the neuropeptides, acetylcholine, and γ-aminobutyric acid, may be synthesized early in embryonic or fetal life before they could possibly function as transmitters and may serve a neurotrophic function.

A number of proteins are produced by mature neurons and not by immature nerve cells. Antibodies against such proteins may be used to demonstrate the maturation of neuroblasts in the human fetal brain (at autopsy) by immunocytochemistry. One such example is neuronal nuclear antigen (NeuN) (240). By coupling such studies with immunocytochemical markers of axonal maturation, such as the use of antibodies against synaptic vesicle proteins, it is possible to demonstrate the temporal relation of terminal axonal maturation and the maturation of their target neuron (241). This sequence may be altered in some cerebral malformations and may explain why some infants with severe malformations such as holoprosencephaly have intractable epilepsy whereas others with similar anatomic lesions, by imaging and even by histopathologic examination, have few or no seizures.

Some genes appear to be essential for the regulation of trophic factors or differentiation and growth of the individual neural cell. *TSC1* and *TSC2* are genes that produce products, respectively termed *hamartin and tuberin*, that are defective in tissues, both neural and nonneural, in patients with tuberous sclerosis (242–247) (see Chapter 11). *TSC1* is localized on chromosome 9q34 (244). It accounts for only the minority of patients with this autosomal dominant disease (245). TSC2 has its locus at 16p13.3.

Myelination

As with other aspects of nervous system development, myelination cycles (i.e., the time between onset and termination of myelination in a given pathway) are specific for each tract and precisely time linked. Some pathways myelinate in a rostrocaudal progression. The human corticospinal tract at birth is myelinated in the corona radiata, internal capsule, middle third of the cerebral peduncle, upper pons; very lightly myelinated in the pyramids; and unmyelinated in the spinal cord. Other pathways myelinate in their proximal and distal portions at the same time. Some pathways myelinate early and others late, but no axons myelinate during the growth of the axonal

TABLE 4.6. *Myelination cycles in the human central nervous system based on myelin tissue stains*[a]

Pathway	Begins	Completed
Spinal motor roots	16 wk	42 wk
Spinal sensory roots	20 wk	5 mo
Cranial motor nerves III, IV, V, VI	20 wk	28 wk
Ventral commissure, spinal cord	24 wk	4 mo
Dorsal columns, spinal cord	28 wk	36 wk
Medial longitudinal fasciculus	24 wk	28 wk
Habenulopeduncular tract	28 wk	34 wk
Acoustic nerve	24 wk	36 wk
Trapezoid body and lateral lemniscus	25 wk	36 wk
Acoustic radiations (thalamocortical)	40 wk	3 yr
Inferior cerebellar peduncle (inner part)	26 wk	36 wk
Inferior cerebellar peduncle (outer parts)	32 wk	4 mo
Middle cerebellar peduncle (pontocerebellar)	42 wk	3 yr
Superior cerebellar peduncle	28 wk	6 mo
Medial lemniscus	32 wk	12 mo
Optic nerve	38 wk	6 mo
Optic radiations (geniculocalcarine)	40 wk	6 mo
Ansa reticularis	28 wk	8 mo
Fornix	2 mo	2 yr
Mammillothalamic tract	8 mo	6 yr
Thalamocortical radiations	2 mo	7 yr
Corticospinal (pyramidal) tract	38 wk	2 yr
Corpus callosum	2 mo	14 yr
Ipsilateral intracortical association fibers, frontotemporal and frontoparietal	3 mo	32 yr

[a]Myelination determined by light microscopy using luxol fast blue and other myelin stains; composite from various authors. Gestational age stated in weeks; postnatal age stated in months and years.

From Sarnat HB. *Cerebral dysgenesis: embryology and clinical expression.* New York: Oxford University Press, 1992. With permission.

growth cone, before it reaches its target. The medial longitudinal fasciculus acquires myelin at 24 weeks' gestation and is fully myelinated within 2 weeks. The corticospinal tract begins myelinating at approximately 38 weeks and is not complete until 2 years of age. The corpus callosum begins mye-lination at approximately 4 months postnatally and is not complete until late adolescence. The last tract to complete myelination is the ipsilateral association bundle that interconnects the anterior frontal and the temporal lobes, which is not complete until 32 years of age (248). Myelination cycles as determined by special myelin stains of sections of fetal and postnatal CNS tissue at autopsy are summarized in Table 4.6. The traditional stain is luxol fast blue, but newer methods using gallocyanin stains (e.g. Lapham stain) and immunocytochemical demonstration of myelin basic protein provide earlier detection of myelin formation at the light microscopic level; electron microscopy remains the most sensitive morphologic method to document the onset of myelination in brain tissue. The sequences of proteins and lipids incorporated into myelin also may be studied biochemically at autopsy in immature brains.

Myelination also may be determined in living patients by magnetic resonance imaging (MRI). T1-weighted images are more sensitive than T2 sequences early, and T2 is more sensitive as myelination advances with maturation, but the present generation of imaging does not show the earliest onset of myelination that can be demonstrated histologically. This difference in sensitivity accounts for somewhat different tables of myelination used by neuroradiologists and neuropathologists (Table 4.7).

Myelination depends on the normal differentiation and integrity of oligodendrocytes in the CNS and Schwann cells in the peripheral nervous system (249–251). As with other developmental processes in the nervous system, the program-

TABLE 4.7. *First appearance of myelination in the human brain based on magnetic resonance imaging*

Anatomic region	T1-weighted	T2-weighted
Middle cerebellar peduncle	Birth	Birth to 2 mo
Cerebral white matter	Birth to 4 mo	3–5 mo
Internal capsule, posterior limb		
Anterior portion	Birth	4–7 mo
Posterior portion	Birth	Birth to 2 mo
Internal capsule, anterior limb	2–3 mo	7–11 mo
Corpus callosum, genu	4–6 mo	5–8 mo
Corpus callosum, splenium	3–4 mo	4–6 mo
Occipital white matter		
Central	3–5 mo	9–14 mo
Peripheral	4–7 mo	11–15 mo
Frontal white matter		
Central	3–6 mo	11–16 mo
Peripheral	7–11 mo	14–18 mo
Centrum semiovale	2–6 mo	7–11 mo

From Barkovich AJ. *Pediatric neuroimaging*, 2nd ed. New York: Raven, 1995. With permission.

ming of differentiation of these myelin-producing cells and of myelin formation is under genetic regulation (252,253). The *Krox-20* mouse gene (*EGR2* in humans), previously discussed as a zinc finger homeobox gene expressed in rhombomeres 3 and 5, also plays an important role in myelination by Schwann cells (51). It is a paradox that *Krox-20/EGR2* is expressed only in rhombomere 3 and rhombomere 5, rhombomeres that do not form neural crest tissue although adjacent and intervening rhombomeres do (56,57),

and Schwann cells are derived from neural crest. The *PMP-22* gene, which is defective in several hereditary motor sensory neuropathies, programs proteolipid protein by encoding an axonally regulated Schwann cell protein incorporated into peripheral myelin (253), but whether it serves a function in the CNS is uncertain.

In addition to their role in generating myelin sheaths around some axons, oligodendrocytes express nerve growth factor and may secrete other molecules that stimulate the growth of axons (254). Insulinlike growth factor also may play a role in central myelination and conserving axonal integrity (255). Gangliosides are complex lipids that form part of the myelinating membranes of oligodendrocytes and Schwann cells, and their composition is important in the development of myelin (256).

Oligodendrocytes may ensheath several axons in the CNS, but in the peripheral nervous system each Schwann cell myelinates only a single axon, though some Schwann cells may enclose one to four unmyelinated axons. At midgestation, a single Schwann cell may enclose as many as 25 axons, but this ratio becomes smaller with progressive maturation (257).

Myelination is an important parameter of the maturation of the brain in a clinically measurable index. Delayed myelination occurs in many metabolic diseases involving the nervous system, in fetal and postnatal malnutrition if the lipids and proteins are not available to be incorporated, and at times as a nonspecific feature of global developmental delay (67).

Part 2: Malformations of the Central Nervous System

John H. Menkes and °Harvey B. Sarnat

*Departments of Neurology and Pediatrics, University of California, Los Angeles, UCLA School of
Medicine, and Department of Pediatric Neurology, Cedars-Sinai Medical Center, Los Angeles,
California 90048; and °Departments of Pediatric Neurology and Neuropathology, University of Washington
School of Medicine, and Children's Hospital and Regional Medical Center, Seattle, Washington 98105*

Malformations of the brain and spinal cord may be genetically determined or acquired. The great majority of dysgeneses that occurs early in gestation have a genetic basis, whereas those that begin late in gestation are more likely to be secondary to destructive lesions such as infarcts that interfere with development of particular structures. The distinction between atrophy, the shrinkage of a previously well-formed structure, and hypoplasia, the deficient development of a structure that never achieves normal size, is not always clear in degenerative processes or in those acquired lesions of fetal life in which an insult is imposed on a structure that is not yet fully formed. Examples are ischemic lesions in fetal brain associated with congenital cytomegalovirus infections, and fetal degenerative diseases such as pontocerebellar hypoplasia, and polymicrogyria, which develop in zones of relative ischemia that surround porencephalic cysts resulting from an occlusion of the middle cerebral artery incurred in fetal life. White matter infarcts in the cerebrum may destroy radial glial fibers and prevent normal migration of neuroblasts and glioblasts from the subventricular zone or germinal matrix (see Chapter 5).

Regardless of their cause, malformations are traditionally classified as disturbances in developmental processes. These are outlined in Table 4.8.

Whereas this type of classification retains a validity for understanding the type of developmental process most disturbed, such as cellular proliferation or neuroblast migration, the new understanding of developmental genes and their role in the ontogenesis of the nervous system provides a new, complementary molecular genetic classification of early neurogenesis that recognizes the genetic regulation of development. An example of an attempt to use these new data to organize the thinking about developmental malformations of the brain is proposed in Table 4.9, a table that will undoubtedly undergo considerable revision in the coming years as more data become available.

Because the nervous system develops in a precise temporal as well as spatial sequence, it is often possible to assign a precise timing of a malformation, or at least to date the earliest time when the insult was first expressed. In most cases, an insult, whether caused by overexpression or underexpression of a developmental gene, or caused by an ongoing acquired process such as a congenital viral infection or repeated episodes of ischemia, affects nervous system development over an extended period of time. Thereby, the insult involves processes that occur at various stages of development, not just at a single precise moment. As discussed in the Patterning of the Neural Tube section, developmental genes may serve as organizer genes early in ontogenesis and as regulator genes later on, thus involving various processes. Defective expression of *Shh*, for example, may result in holoprosencephaly because of its early effects on midline ventralization in the prosencephalon, but may affect granule cell proliferation in the cerebellum as well; the timing of these two events is quite different.

The accounts that follow are traditional descriptions of major malformations of the human nervous system, but the new perspective of molecular genetic programming will forever be an integral part of the understanding of these disorders of development. Finally, it must

TABLE 4.8. *Traditional classification of central nervous system malformations as disorders of . . .*

1. Neurulation
2. Cell proliferation: neurogenesis and gliogenesis
3. Apoptosis
4. Migration of neuroblasts and glioblasts
5. Axonal projection and pathfinding
6. Dendritic sprouting and synaptogenesis
7. Myelination

always be recognized that just as no two adults, even monozygotic twins, are identical, no two fetuses are identical and no two cerebral malformations are identical. Individual biological variations occur in abnormal as well as in normal development and allowance must be made for

TABLE 4.9. *Proposed molecular genetic classification of malformations of early central nervous system development*

I. Disorders of the primitive streak and node
   A. Overexpression of genes
   B. Underexpression of genes
II. Disorders of ventralization of the neural tube
   A. Overexpression of the ventrodorsal gradient
      1. Duplication of spinal central canal
      2. Duplication of ventral horns of spinal cord
      3. Diplomyelia (and diastematomyelia?)
      4. Duplication of entire neuraxis
      5. Ventralizing induction of somite
         a. Segmental amyoplasia
   B. Underexpression of ventrodorsal gradient
      1. Fusion of ventral horns of spinal cord
      2. Sacral (thoracolumbosacral) agenesis
      3. Arhinencephaly
      4. Holoprosencephaly
III. Disorders of dorsalization of the neural tube
   A. Overexpression of dorsoventral gradient
      1. Duplication of dorsal horns of spinal cord
      2. Duplication of dorsal brainstem structures
   B. Underexpression of dorsalization of the neural tube
      1. Fusion of dorsal horns of spinal cord
      2. Septo-optic dysplasia (?)
IV. Disorder of the rostrocaudal gradient, segmentation, or both
   A. Decreased domains of homeoboxes
      1. Agenesis of mesencephalon and metencephalon
      2. Global cerebellar aplasia or hypoplasia
      3. Aplasia of basal telencephalic nuclei
   B. Increased domains of homeoboxes or ectopic expression
      1. Chiari II malformation

small differences while recognizing the principal patterns that denote pathogenesis.

The importance of disordered nervous system maturation in causing chronic abnormalities of brain function only recently has become fully apparent. Estimates suggest that 3% of neonates have major CNS or multisystem malformations (258), and 75% of fetal deaths and 40% of deaths within the first year of life are secondary to CNS malformations (259). Furthermore, 5% to 15% of pediatric neurology hospital admissions appear to be primarily related to cerebrospinal anomalies (260). Genetic and nongenetic interactions are responsible for 20% of CNS malformations; monogenic malformations, whether autosomal or X-linked, account for 7.5% of malformations; chromosomal factors account for 6%; and well-delineated environmental factors, including maternal infections, maternal diabetes, irradiation, and drugs (e.g., thalidomide, methylmercury) account for at least another 3.5%. In the remainder, more than 60%, the cause of the CNS malformation is unknown (261). As more associations with specific genes and their defective expression become known, this number will undoubtedly become smaller.

EMBRYOGENIC INDUCTION DISORDERS (0 TO 4 WEEKS' GESTATION)

Embryogenic induction disorders represent a failure in the mutual induction of mesoderm and neuroectoderm. The primary defect is a failure of the neural folds to fuse and form the neural tube (ectoderm), with secondary maldevelopment of skeletal structures enclosing the CNS (mesoderm). The defects range from anencephaly to sacral meningomyelocele in the cephalic to caudal direction of the neural tube, and from holoprosencephaly to craniospinal rachischisis (midline posterior splitting of skull and vertebral column) in the anterior to posterior direction. For convenience, they are divided into dorsal (posterior) and ventral (anterior) midline defects. The former is named *dysraphism* to indicate the persistent continuity between posterior neuroectoderm and cutaneous ectoderm. The latter are called *faciotelencephalopathy* to connote the fusion failure of anterior neural tube, cephalic mesoderm, and adjacent foregut entoderm, the anlagen for facial structures (259).

Dorsal Midline Central Nervous System–Axial Skeletal Defects: Dysraphism

A large number of midline anomalies occur, and the chance of several midline defects occurring conjointly is greater than the product of their individual occurrence (262).

Anencephaly

Anencephaly is the paradigm of the various dysraphic disorders. Although affected infants rarely survive early infancy, insight into the mechanics of neural ontogenesis provided by this disorder is enormous.

Pathogenesis and Pathology

Both genetic predisposition and environmental insults are responsible for the condition (263). The defect is time specific in that the insult probably occurs after the onset of neural fold development (16 days), but before closure of the anterior neuropore (24 to 26 days). The stimulus is nonspecific because a variety of insults have been implicated. These include drugs (264), infections (265), chemical disorders such as maternal diabetes or folic acid deficiency (266), and irradiation (267). Whatever the actual teratogenic stimulus might be, it induces three basic defects. A defective notochord causes a failure of the cephalic neural folds to fuse into a neural tube. This failure, in turn, leads to exposure of the well-differentiated brain to amniotic fluid, with subsequent degeneration of all forebrain germinal cells. Finally, mesoderm fails to differentiate into somites and hence into sclerotomes, the latter being the anlagen for the cranial base and the calvarium of the skull and the vertebrae. Thus, mutual induction between the three germ layers fails at time-specific stages, resulting in deformities of both nervous tissue and supporting axial bone (268).

Studies on human embryos have suggested that the splitting of an already closed neural tube

might account for anencephaly and other dysraphic conditions (269). Gardner and Brever have argued not only that dysraphic states are a consequence of neural tube rupture after closure, but also that a number of associated nonneural anomalies, including asplenia, renal agenesis, and tracheoesophageal fistula, result from the damage of anlagen for other organs by the overdistended neural tube (270). Osaka and coworkers discount these theories on the basis that in human embryos dysraphism can be observed before completion of neural tube closure (271,272). Muscle differentiates normally in anencephaly despite disruption of motor innervation, suggesting that motor innervation occurs after muscle development, and, therefore, after embryogenesis and neural tube closure (273).

Examination of the nervous system shows the spinal cord, brainstem, and cerebellum to be small. Descending tracts within the spinal cord are absent. Above this level, nothing save a few tangles of glial and vascular tissue and remnants of midbrain exists. The pituitary is absent with secondary adrenal hypoplasia. The optic nerves are absent, but the eyes are normal, indicating that the anterior cephalic end of the neural tube, from whence the optic vesicles spring, closed and diverticulated properly.

In addition to the primary defect of development, anencephaly involves an important encephaloclastic component. Because neural tissue is directly exposed to amniotic fluid, which is caustic, a progressive destruction of neural tissue and a compensatory proliferation of small blood vessels occurs to create the area cerebrovasculosa in the nubbin of tissue representing the residual prosencephalon. A poorly organized network of thin-walled vascular channels of variable size that are not mature capillaries, arterioles, or venules are enmeshed with glial processes and scattered (haphazardly oriented neurons and neuroblasts, lacking recognizable architecture as either nuclei or laminated cortex). Anencephaly is therefore difficult to analyze histopathologically because of the simultaneous presence of both primary dysplastic and secondary destructive processes.

The calvarium fails to develop, and the frontal, occipital, and parietal bones are partially absent. Malformations of the foramen magnum and cervical vertebrae are frequent. Some authors use the term *aprosencephaly* for cases in which the calvarium is intact, in distinction from atelencephaly in which the cranium is open (274,275). In exencephaly, a rare condition, the intramembranous bones of the vault are absent, and the preserved, but disorganized, brain is covered by vascular epithelium (276). The deformed forehead and relatively large ears and eyes lend a rather odd appearance to the face; however, all facial structures are normally developed, except for an occasional lateral cleft lip or palate. The condition is believed to be a stage in the development of anencephaly, with more complete destruction of the exposed brain being a matter of time (277).

Clinical Manifestations

Anencephaly is the most common major CNS malformation in the West (278). The incidence of this malformation differs in various parts of the world. It is high in Ireland, Scotland, and Wales and low in Japan. Other areas of high incidence include Egypt, the Arabian subcontinent, and New Zealand. As a rule, the incidence increases with increasing maternal age and decreasing socioeconomic status.

The rate of anencephaly, as well as that of the other neural tube defects, has declined. In the 1960s, the incidence ranged from 0.65 per 1,000 births in Japan to more than 3 in 1,000 in the British Isles, with a maximum incidence of 8 in 1,000 occurring in Ireland in 1960. Prior peaks in incidence had been recorded during the years of 1929 through 1932 and 1938 through 1941. Since then, there has been a steady decline in both the United States and the United Kingdom. Between 1971 and 1989, the annual rate of various forms of spina bifida has fallen from 2 in 1,000 to 0.6 in 1,000 (279), with a relative increase in the proportion of spina bifida to anencephaly (280). In part, this decline reflects the widespread use of antenatal screening, but other factors, notably the correction of maternal vitamin deficiency, also might be responsible (279,281).

Anencephaly is seen 37 times more frequently in female than in male newborns (282).

The recurrence rate in families with an affected child is 35%, although almost 10% of all siblings of anencephalics have major anomalies of neural tube closure anencephaly, spina bifida cystica, and encephalocele (283). The transmission appears to be matrilineal. No relationship to consanguinity is evident, nor to concordance in monozygotic twins, and the recurrence rate for a maternal half-sibling is the same as for a full sibling. These factors weigh against a simple polygenetic inheritance pattern and are more consistent with the interaction of genetic and environmental factors (284).

Anencephalic subjects do not survive infancy. During their few weeks of life, they exhibit slow, stereotyped movements and frequent decerebrate posturing. Head, facial, and limb movements can be spontaneous or pain induced. The Moro reflex and some brainstem functions and automatisms, such as sucking, rooting, and righting responses, are present and are more readily and more reproducibly elicited than in healthy infants. The *bowing reflex*, which occasionally can be demonstrated in healthy premature infants of 7 months' gestation, is invariably present in anencephalics (285) (see Introduction chapter). Seizures have been observed in anencephalic infants, an indication that some types of neonatal seizures originate in the deeper structures of the brain (286).

The presence of anencephaly and other open neural tube defects can be predicted by measuring α-fetoprotein (AFP) in amniotic fluid or maternal serum. AFP is the major serum protein in early embryonic life, representing 90% of total serum globulin. It is a fetus-specific α_1-globulin that is probably involved in preventing fetal immune rejection; it is produced first by the yolk sac and later by the fetal liver and gastrointestinal tract. It normally passes from fetal serum into fetal urine and then into amniotic fluid. Because of a substantial leak of fetal blood components directly into amniotic fluid, AFP concentrations in amniotic fluid and maternal serum AFP levels are elevated in anencephaly and in open spina bifida or cranium bifidum (287).

Normal AFP in adult serum is less than 10 ng/mL. In normal maternal serum and amniotic fluid, it ranges from 15 to 500 ng/mL. At 15 to 20 weeks' gestation, an AFP concentration of 1,000 ng/mL or more strongly suggests an open neural tube defect, and the current screening of serum detects 79% of cases of open spina bifida at 16 to 18 weeks (288). Determining gestational age is critical, however, because normal AFP concentration varies considerably with fetal age, peaking between 12 and 15 weeks' gestation. Amniotic fluid AFP screening is more reliable, detecting 98% of open spina bifida cases (289). The amniotic fluid must be assessed for contamination by fetal hemoglobin, which complicates amniocentesis, because a 200:1 AFP gradient exists between fetal serum and amniotic fluid. The reliability of ultrasonography depends on the experience of the operators; in good hands, the procedure is more than 99% specific (288). False-positive results are obtained in a variety of unrelated conditions, principally in the presence of multiple pregnancies, threatened abortion or fetal death, or when an error is made in dating the pregnancy. Amniotic fluid AFP obtained between 15 and 20 weeks' gestation is most specific (289); however, closed neural tube defects such as skin-covered lipomyelomeningoceles, encephaloceles, and meningoceles go undetected. These lesions constitute between 5% and 10% of total neural tube defects (290,291).

Mothers who have borne one or more children with neural tube defects, spinal dysraphism, or multiple vertebral anomalies; who have a family history of any of these disorders; or who, themselves, are surviving patients with spina bifida–risk bearing children with neural tube defects and should undergo screening.

Supplementation of the maternal diet with folic acid or with a multivitamin preparation that contains folic acid even before conception has been proposed to prevent neural tube defects. An extensive, controlled British study indicates that the recurrence rate of neural tube defects can be reduced sharply by folic acid supplementation (292). A multivitamin cocktail including folic acid, ascorbic acid, and riboflavin, given from at least 28 days before conception up to the second missed menstrual period, reduced the recurrence rates for neural tube defects from 4.2% to 0.5% in mothers with a previous neural tube defect

pregnancy, and from 9.6% to 2.3% in mothers who had given birth to two or more offspring with neural tube defects (293,294). These findings have been duplicated in an American study, which showed that a vitamin supplement including 0.8 mg of folic acid, started 1 month before conception, reduced significantly the incidence of neural tube defects (295). The reason for the apparent effect of folic acid is unclear, and the significance of these findings must be evaluated in the light of the declining incidence of neural tube defects in areas where no vitamin supplementation is used (281,296,297).

Spina Bifida and Cranium Bifidum

As the names imply, spina bifida and cranium bifidum share a failure of bone fusion in the posterior midline of the skull (cranium bifidum) or the vertebral column (spina bifida). The result is a bony cleft through which the meninges and varying quantities of brain or spinal cord tissue protrude. In cranium bifidum, the neural herniation is termed *encephalocele* and can consist of brain parenchyma and meninges, or only of meninges. These form the wall of a saclike cyst filled with cerebrospinal fluid (CSF). In spina bifida, the herniation is called *meningocele* or *myelomeningocele*, depending on whether the meninges herniate alone or in concert with spinal cord parenchyma and nerve roots.

Spina bifida occulta represents a fusion failure of the posterior vertebral arches unaccompanied by herniation of meninges or neural tissue. Spina bifida cystica collectively designates meningocele, myelomeningocele, and other cystic lesions (Fig. 4.1). Similarly, in the head, cranium bifidum comprises meningocele, a herniation of meninges containing only CSF, and the more commonly occurring encephalocele, in which the sac contains neural and glial tissue. *Rachischisis* refers to a severe condition with an extensive defect of the craniovertebral bone with exposure of the brain, spinal cord, and meninges.

Pathogenesis

Spina bifida and cranium bifidum are not only disorders of induction; they also are associated

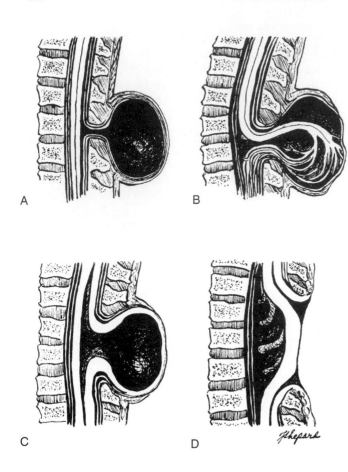

A

B

C

D

FIG. 4.1. Drawings of various forms of spinal dysraphic lesions (spina bifida cystica). **A:** Meningocele. Through the bony defect (spina bifida), the meninges herniate and form a cystic sac filled with spinal fluid. The spinal cord does not participate in the herniation and might or might not be abnormal. **B:** Myelomeningocele. The spinal cord is herniated into the sac and ends there or can continue in an abnormal way further downward. **C:** Myelocystocele or syringomyelocele. The spinal cord shows hydromyelia; the posterior wall of the spinal cord is attached to the ectoderm and is undifferentiated. **D:** Myelocele. The spinal cord is araphic; a cystic cavity is in front of the anterior wall of the spinal cord. (From Benda CE. *Developmental disorders of mentation and cerebral palsies.* New York: Grune & Stratton, 1952. With permission.)

with major abnormalities of cellular migration and secondary mechanical deformities of the nervous system. The continuity between neural and cutaneous ectodermal derivates is regarded as evidence that the primary defect is in the neural tube closure (298,299). Based on studies with embryos of mutant mice with genetically abnormal neurulation and a sacral neural tube defect, McLone and Naiditch (300) have proposed a unified theory for the development of the associated anomalies that incorporates some of the prior observations of Padget (269).

According to these authors, the initial event is a failure of the neural folds to close completely, leaving a dorsal myeloschisis. This is followed by a failure of the normal, transient occlusion of the central cavity of the spinal cord. These two events result in the escape of CSF into the amniotic cavity, and a collapse of the primitive ventricular system. The failure of the primitive cranial ventricular system to distend results in a posterior fossa that is too small to accommodate the growing cerebellum and leads to upward and downward herniation of the structures within the posterior fossa. Additionally, the failure of the normal distention of the ventricular system leads to inadequate support for the normal outward migration of neuroblasts, and a failure to maintain the normal pattern of ossification in the calvarium.

Marín-Padilla proposes that the primary defect is a limited injury to the primitive streak and primitive node, which impairs local growth of skeletal elements, which in turn interferes with closure of the neural tube (301). Although the specific genes involved have not yet been identified, this hypothesis may be expanded to invoke a mechanism of failed expression of one or more

TABLE 4.10. *Timetable of human central nervous system ontogenesis*

Days of gestation	Event	Effect of toxic stimulus
0–18	Three germ layers elaborate and early neural plate forms	No effect or death
18	Neural plate and groove develop	Anterior midline defects (18–23 days)
22–23	Optic vesicles appear	Induction hydrocephalus (18–60 days)
24–26	Anterior neuropore closed	Anencephaly (after 23 days to ?)
26–28	Posterior neuropore closed, ventral horns form	Cranium bifidum, spina bifida cystica, spina bifida occulta (after 26 days to ?)
28–32	Anterior and posterior nerve roots form	—
32	Cerebellar primordium, vascular circulation	Microcephaly (30–130 days), cellular proliferation syndromes (30–175 days), migration anomalies (30 days to complete development of each brain subdivision)
33–35	Prosencephalon cleaves to form paired telencephalon. Five cerebral vesicles, choroid plexi, dorsal root ganglion develop.	Holoprosencephaly
41	Region of olfactory bulb appears in forebrain	Arhinencephaly
56	Differentiation of cerebral cortex, meningitis, ventricular foramina, CSF circulation	Dandy-Walker malformation
70–100	Corpus callosum	Agenesis of corpus callosum
70–150	Primary fissures of cerebral cortex, spinal cord ends at L3 level	Lissencephaly, pachygyria
140–175	Neuronal proliferation in cerebral cortex ends	Defects of cellular architectonics, myelin defects (175 days to 4 years postnatally)
7–9 mo	Secondary and tertiary sulci	Destructive pathologic changes first noted
175 days to 4 yr postnatally	Neuron blast migration, glial cell production, myelin formation, axosomatic and axodendritic synaptic connections, spinal cord ends L1–2 level	—

organizer genes during the primitive streak and neural placode stages of early ontogenesis.

These defects are time specific, which is why the most common sites for the lesion in surviving children are either lumbosacral or occipital, these being the last levels at which neural tube closure normally occurs. The initiation of a defect at an earlier stage leads to a more extensive defect, which is incompatible with survival. In the same way, a simple meningocele results when the insult occurs after the spinal cord has formed, whereas a myelomeningocele arises from an earlier insult, which must occur before closure of the posterior neuropore (i.e., before 26 to 28 days' gestation) (Table 4.10) (302).

The cause of these anomalies is unknown. As is the case for anencephaly, it is likely that genetic defects, probably at more than one locus, interact with environmental factors to produce the varying dysraphic conditions. Spinal dysraphic lesions are one of the most common anomalies of the nervous system. As with anencephaly, the incidence is highest in Ireland and lowest in Japan and also is influenced by season, socioeconomic status, gender, ethnicity, and such maternal factors as parity, age, prior offspring with neural tube defects, and maternal heat exposure (303). Recurrence rates for mothers who have previously given birth to a child with an open neural tube defect are 1.5% to 2.0%, and for mothers with two affected children, the recurrence rate is 6% (304). The recurrence risk is also higher than normal if close relatives are affected. Less is known about the epidemiology of cranium bifidum, the incidence of which is approximately one-tenth that of spina bifida cystica (277,305).

TABLE 4.11. *Site of lesion of spina bifida cystica*

Level[a]	Number of patients
Cervical	51
Thoracic	103
Thoracolumbar	137
Lumbar	583
Lumbosacral	382
Sacral	119
Anterior	6
Thoracic	3
Pelvic	3
Undesignated	9
Total	1,396

[a]Level of the meningeal sac in 1,396 consecutive patients treated for spina bifida cystica in the Boston Children's Medical Center.

From Matson DD. *Neurosurgery of infancy and childhood*, 2nd ed. Springfield, IL: Charles C Thomas, 1969. With permission.

Pathology

Spina Bifida Cystica. Of the defects collectively termed *spina bifida cystica*, 95% are myelomeningoceles, and 5% are meningoceles. Locations of the defect in live-born infants are depicted in Table 4.11. A lumbar or lumbosacral defect is most common; it corresponds to the site of the posterior neuropore closure. Cervical lesions are the least frequent posterior defects. Anterior midline defects of the vertebral arches are uncommon and constituted less than 0.5% of cases in the experience of Matson (305). Approximately 100 anterior sacral meningoceles have been reported, the majority in female subjects (306). These conditions should be differentiated from spinal meningeal malformations, which can occur in isolation or in association with systemic malformations (307). Spinal meningeal malformations are relatively common in patients with the various mucopolysaccharidoses and in neurofibromatosis.

Cervical and thoracic meningoceles have narrow bases and are usually not associated with hydrocephalus. By contrast, 90% or more of lumbosacral myelomeningoceles are accompanied by Chiari type II malformations and hydrocephalus. As originally described by Chiari, type I malformations consist of ectopically, downwardly displaced cerebellar tonsils in the absence of space-occupying lesions other than hydrocephalus. Type III malformations consist of cervical spina bifida accompanied by a cerebellar encephalocele. Type IV is a heterogeneous

TABLE 4.12. *Central nervous system anomalies associated with meningomyelocele, hydrocephalus, and Arnold-Chiari malformation[a]*

	Percent of cases
Spinal cord malformation	88
Hydromyelia	68
Syringomyelia	36
Diplomyelia (complete duplication over several segments)	36
Diastematomyelia (splitting without duplication)	8
Brainstem malformation	76
Hypolasia of cranial nerve nuclei	20
Hypoplasia/aplasia of olivae	20
Hypoplasia/aplasia of basal pontile nuclei	16
Malformations of ventricular system	92
Aqueductal stenosis	52
Aqueductal forking	48
Aqueductal atresia	8
Cerebellar malformations	72
Heterotaxias (disordered combination of mature neurons and germinal cells)	48
Heterotopias	40
Cerebral malformations	92
Heterotopias	44
Polymicrogyria	40
Disordered lamination	24
Polymicrogyria	12
Agenesis of the corpus callosum	12

[a]Data are based on 25 autopsied patients with meningomyelocele and hydrocephalus.

Modified from Gilbert JN, et al. Central nervous system anomalies associated with meningomyelocele, hydrocephalus, and the Arnold-Chiari malformation: reappraisal of theories regarding the pathogenesis of posterior neural tube closure defects. *Neurosurgery* 1986;18:559–564. With permission.

variant in which the cerebellum and brainstem remained in their entirety within the posterior fossa, but in which cerebellar hypoplasia existed (308,309). Type IV is now an obsolete term of historical interest and is redesignated *cerebellar hypoplasia*.

In 88% of children with lumbar or lumbosacral meningomyeloceles, the spinal cord demonstrates abnormalities in the cervical region (Table 4.12) (298). The majority of instances involves hydrosyringomyelia; less often, diplomyelia, or winged and dorsally slit cords are present (310,311). In more than 70%, the medulla overrides the cervical cord dorsally, in association with type II Chiari malformation (Figs. 4.2 and 4.3). Of patients with spina bifida cystica, 70% show defects in the posterior arch of the atlas, which is bridged by a firm fibrous band, suggest-

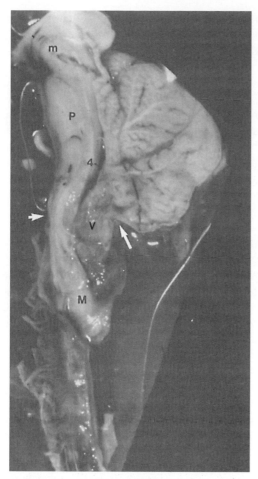

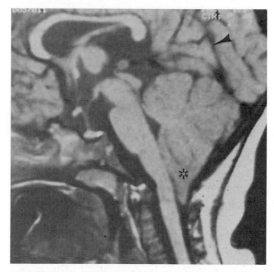

FIG. 4.3. Chiari type II malformation. Magnetic resonance imaging study. The fourth ventricle and aqueduct are stretched only slightly. Cerebellar ectopia includes both the inferior vermis and tonsil (*asterisk*). The tentorial opening is wide, and vertical orientation is seen at line of attachment along the straight sinus (*black arrowhead*). (Courtesy of Dr. Taher El Gammal, Department of Radiology, Medical College of Georgia, Augusta, Georgia, and the American Society of Neuroradiology.)

FIG. 4.2. Chiari type II malformation. Sagittal section through the cerebellum and brainstem in a newborn boy. Anterior is to the reader's left. Arrows mark the location of the foramen magnum. The medulla (M) protrudes below the foramen magnum into the cervical spinal cord canal to overlap the cervical spinal cord. The medulla buckles dorsally to form a kink. The cerebellar vermis (V) is indented by the posterior lip of the foramen magnum. The fourth ventricle (4) is elongated, and the midbrain (m) is beaked. The pons (P) is demonstrated also. (From Naidich TP, Mc Lone DG, Fulling KH. The Chiari II malformation: part IV. The hind-brain deformity. *Neuroradiology* 1983;25:179–197. With permission.)

ing that congenital atlantoaxial dislocation is a mild expression of an induction disorder (312). Examination of the parenchyma of the spinal cord reveals atrophic or poorly developed anterior horn cells, absent or abnormal corticospinal and sensory tracts, incomplete posterior horns, and exceedingly small and deranged anterior and posterior root fibers. These changes result in muscle denervation during fetal life and ultimately produce limb deformities and joint contractures.

Defects of cellular migration in the cerebral hemispheres are extremely common (see Table 4.12). These include gray matter heterotopia, schizencephaly, gyral anomalies, agenesis of the corpus callosum, and mesodermal heterotopia (298,313,314).

A number of mesodermal lesions accompany these ectodermal defects. In addition to the spinal canal being widened and the posterior arches being malformed, the vertebral bodies can be misshapen with resulting kyphosis or scoliosis. Rib anomalies are common. Mesodermal dysplasia of the skull produces defects in the membranous bones of the calvarium, a condition termed *craniolacunia* (*Lückenschadel*). This peculiar, honey-combed appearance of the skull is seen in some 85% of patients with the Chiari type II malformation. The skull changes are transient and disappear in the first few months after birth. They are probably the result of a defect in membranous bone formation and are not secondary to *in utero* intracranial hypertension, as is often stated (300).

Deformities of the lower extremities are common and are of two types. In the first type, the various clubfoot and rocker-bottom foot deformities result from the unopposed action of the intrinsic foot muscles or the muscles at the ankle joint. In the second type, the deformities are positional; they result from intrauterine pressure on the paralytic limbs.

Other anomalies accompany myelodysplasia with a greater than normal incidence. These include intestinal malformations (e.g., duodenal atresia, pyloric stenosis, anal stenosis), renal anomalies, notably renal agenesis, urogenital defects, cardiac malformations, and tracheoesophageal fistulas.

Spina Bifida Occulta. In spina bifida occulta, no herniation of the meninges is present and the skin of the back is completely epithelialized, although always showing some abnormality such as a nevus, dermal sinus and dimple (35%), an underlying lipoma (29%), or a hirsute area (304). Radiography reveals a variety of deformities, the most common of which are widening of the spinal canal, fusion of the vertebral bodies, fused and malformed laminae, spina bifida, and, sometimes, a midline bone mass within the spinal canal. These skin and bone abnormalities are indications that the cord and nerve roots are malformed also. There may be a localized doubling of the cord (diplomyelia), a sagittal splitting of the cord (diastematomyelia), absent or adherent nerve roots, or an intradural lipoma attached to the cord. Abnormalities of the filum terminale, notably a shortening, which gives the appearance of a lengthening of the cord but that actually results from a failure of the cord to dedifferentiate during early embryonic life, were seen in 24% of patients in Anderson series (315). Duplication of the spinal cord or portions of it, such as the central canal, is associated, as discussed in the Families of Developmental Genes section, with upregulation of an early ventralizing influence of a gene such as *Sonic hedgehog.*

These lesions must be recognized because they can cause progressive loss of neural func-

tioning during the childhood growth spurt. In many cases, operative intervention to free the cord or nerves is indicated to prevent further damage or prophylactically to avoid such damage. One distinction of occult dysraphism is that it never seems to coexist with the Chiari II malformation. However, its genetic origins are the same as those of spina bifida cystica, so that both types of spina bifida can occur in the same family. The chances that parents of a child with spina bifida occulta could have another offspring with spina bifida cystica are the same as when the proband has spina bifida cystica (316).

Cranium Bifidum. Several types of simple midline or paired paramedian skull defects are grouped under the term *cranium bifidum occultum.*

These include the persistence of wide fontanelles and parietal foramina (317). Persistently large foramina are seen in families, and the condition is sometimes transmitted as an autosomal dominant trait with the gene probably being located on the short arm of chromosome 11 (318). The condition has been termed *Caitlin marks,* named after the family in which it was described. Parietal foramina are generally asymptomatic, although they have been reported to be accompanied by a seizure disorder. The radiographic changes in the various congenital anomalies of the skull are reviewed by Kaplan and colleagues (319). Persistence of the fontanelle is sometimes accompanied by cleidocranial dysostosis, Marden-Walker syndrome, Schinzel-Giedion syndrome, and several other malformation syndromes (320).

Cranium bifidum (cephalocele, encephalocele) is a much more serious condition. Like anencephaly, it has been postulated to represent a defect in the closure of the anterior neuropore. Hoving and coworkers, however, have proposed that the underlying defect is a disturbance in the separation of neural and surface ectoderm (321). Marin-Padilla suggests that it results from a deficiency in local growth of the basicranium, with the timing of the insult and the amount of damage to mesodermal cells determining whether the result is anencephaly, Chiari II malformation, or cranium bifidum (301).

The incidence of cranium bifidum is approximately one-tenth that of spina bifida cystica. In the

Western world, approximately 85% of these lesions are dorsal defects involving the occipital bone. Parietal, frontal, or nasal encephaloceles are far less common. In Asia, the majority of encephaloceles is anterior and involves the frontal, nasal, and orbital bones (305,322,323). The lesions of cranium bifidum, regardless of whether they are a meningocele or contain neural tissue, and consequently are an encephalomeningocele, are usually classified together as encephaloceles. As with myelomeningoceles, the sac can be covered by partially transparent abnormal meninges, but in most lesions, the herniation is fully epithelialized with either dysplastic or normal skin. Cutaneous abnormalities are frequent and consist of port wine stains, abnormal patterning of hair in the posterior lumbosacral region, and, occasionally, excessive amounts of subcutaneous lipomatous tissue.

In the series of Simpson and coworkers, 34% of occipital meningoencephaloceles contained only cerebral tissue, 21% had cerebral and cerebellar tissue, and 37% had nodules of glial cells and dysplastic neural tissue (324). In 5% the sac contained cerebellar tissue only. Some of these infants would represent the Chiari III malformation. MRI is invaluable in determining the contents of the encephalocele (277).

Lorber and Schofield reported 147 cases of posteriorly located encephaloceles (323). Of this group, one-fifth were cranial meningoceles, and the remainder were encephalomeningoceles. Of those patients who survived into childhood, 25% of those who harbored a meningocele and 75% of those with an encephalomeningocele were retarded. All patients with microcephaly had neural tissue within the sac, and all were retarded. The presence of neural tissue in the sac usually was associated with malformations of the hindbrain or, less often, with holoprosencephaly or agenesis of the corpus callosum (325). In the series of Lorber and Schofield, 16% of patients with encephaloceles had other anomalies, including myelomeningocele, cleft palate, congenital malformations of the heart, and Klippel-Feil syndrome (323). Hydrocephalus was present in more than 59% of patients and was more common in those with encephalomeningoceles. In a small proportion of subjects with encephaloceles, the condition is part of a known syndrome. These

have been listed by Cohen and Lemire (326). Meckel-Gruber syndrome is probably the most common of these. It is an autosomal recessive condition with its gene mapped to chromosome 17q21-q24. It is characterized by an occipital encephalocele, holoprosencephaly, the Dandy-Walker syndrome, orofacial clefts, microphthalmia, polydactyly, polycystic kidneys, and cardiac anomalies (327).

In Western countries, only a small fraction of encephaloceles is located anteriorly. Most of these patients are otherwise completely healthy neurologically, and hydrocephalus is rare. The only associated CNS malformations are agenesis or lipomas of the corpus callosum (328). Anterior encephaloceles located at the cranial base often cause no external physical abnormalities, or they might be accompanied by such midline defects as hypertelorism, cleft lip, and cleft palate. An encephalocele presenting a mass that obstructs the nares can be mistaken for a nasal polyp. Its removal can result in a persistent CSF leak and meningitis.

On examination, the encephalocele is usually fully epithelialized, although the skin can be dysplastic. Its size ranges from the insignificant to a sac that can rival the calvarium in size. Pedunculate lesions are less likely to contain neural tissue than sessile lesions. Transillumination can provide an indication of neural tissue in the sac; however, neuroimaging studies are definitive and detect associated CNS abnormalities.

Meningocele. A meningocele, by definition, represents the herniation of only the meninges through the defective posterior arches; the sac does not contain neural elements. Meningoceles account for less than 5% of patients with spina bifida cystica (329). Myelomeningocele must be differentiated from meningocele because the prognoses are vastly different. An infant with a meningocele has little or no associated CNS malformation, rarely develops hydrocephalus, and usually has a normal neurologic examination. The anatomic distribution of meningoceles is the same as for myelomeningoceles. In general, meningoceles are fully epithelialized and tend to be more pedunculated than sessile lesions. Occasionally, a myelomeningocele is differentiated from a meningocele only at the time of operative repair. Some meningoceles contain a significant component of adipose tissue and are designated lipomeningoceles. These have a poorer long-term prognosis because the lipomatous portion often envelops nerve roots of the cauda equina and is not easily dissected from the roots at the time of surgery without sacrificing roots and creating a major neurologic deficit in the lower limbs and some visceral organs such as the urinary bladder.

Clinical Manifestations

Spina Bifida Cystica. At birth, spina bifida cystica can assume a variety of appearances. These range from complete exposure of neural tissue to a partially epithelialized membrane. Most often, a saclike structure is located at any point along the spinal column. Usually, the sac is covered by a thin membrane that is prone to tears, through which the CSF leaks. Of defects, 95% are myelomeningoceles and produce neurologic dysfunction corresponding to their anatomic level (330).

The lumbosacral region is the site of 80% of myelomeningoceles (see Table 4.11). These produce a variety of conus, epiconus, and cauda equina syndromes (Table 4.13). When the lesion is below L2, the cauda equina bears the brunt of the damage. Children exhibit varying degrees of

TABLE 4.13. *Neurologic syndromes with myelomeningoceles*

Lesion level	Spinal-related disability
Above L3	Complete paraplegia and dermatomal para-anesthesia Bladder and rectal incontinence Nonambulatory
L4 and below	Same as for above L3 except preservation of hip flexors, hip adductors, knee extensors Ambulatory with aids, bracing, orthopedic surgery
S1 and below	Same as for L4 and below except preservation of feet dorsiflexors, and partial preservation of hip extensors and knee flexors Ambulatory with minimal aids
S3 and below	Normal lower extremity motor function Saddle anesthesia Variable bladder-rectal incontinence

flaccid, areflexic paraparesis, and sensory deficits distal from the dermatome of L3 or L4. The sphincter and detrusor functions of the bladder are compromised and dribbling incontinence occurs. An absent or unilateral anal skin reflex and poor tone of the rectal sphincter are often apparent and can result in rectal prolapse. If the lesion is located at the thoracolumbar level or higher, the anal tone is often normal, and the bladder is hypertonic. Lesions below S3 cause no motor impairment, but can result in bladder and anal sphincter paralysis, and saddle anesthesia involving the dermatomes of S3 through S5. Electromyographic studies and nerve conduction velocities obtained in the lower extremities of affected newborns suggest that the paralysis is the outcome of a combined upper and lower motor neuron lesion (331). Upper motor neuron lesions that result from involvement of the corticospinal tracts, however, usually are obscured by the more severe involvement of the nerve roots, cauda equina, and anterior horn cells.

Cauda equina lesions produce muscular denervation *in utero*, resulting in joint deformities of the lower limbs. These are most commonly flexion or extension contractures, valgus or varus contractures, hip dislocations, and lumbosacral scoliosis. The expression of the contracture depends on the extent and severity of dermatome involvement.

Hydrocephalus associated with type II Chiari malformation complicates more than 90% of lumbosacral myelomeningoceles (332). It is manifest at birth in 50% to 75% of cases. In approximately 25% of infants with this condition, the head circumference is below the fifth percentile (300). In these infants and in the group whose head circumference is normal at birth, the ventricles are dilated at birth. This finding suggests that hydrocephalus almost always precedes operative closure of the myelomeningocele sac (333). Hammock and coworkers have proposed that some of the infants with large ventricles but normal head circumference have normal pressure hydrocephalus, and that these subjects, like adults with this syndrome, might benefit from shunting procedures (334).

Clinical signs of progressive hydrocephalus accompanying a myelomeningocele include an abnormal increase in head circumference, full fontanelle, spreading of sutures, hyperresonant calvarial percussion note, dilated scalp veins, deviation of the eyes below the horizontal (*setting sun sign*), strabismus, and irritability. MRI studies have become the definitive diagnostic procedure for the evaluation of spina bifida cystica and the various other dysraphic conditions (313). They reveal the downward displacement of the stretched brainstem, with a kink between the medulla and the cervical spinal cord, and herniation of the cerebellar vermis. These findings are best seen on sagittal views. As a consequence of these malformations, CSF circulation is blocked at the level of the foramen magnum. Additionally, a significant incidence of hydromyelia of the cervical or thoracic spinal cord occurs (335). MRI and cine-MRI also can be used to display the patency of the aqueduct (336). Using MRI, el Gammal and coworkers found aqueductal stenosis in 40% of patients with myelomeningocele (335).

Other cerebral anomalies also have been described (298). These include microgyria and other types of cortical dysgenesis. These are frequently visualized by MRI studies, but may be difficult to see if a deficit in cortical lamination is at the microscopic level, below the limit of resolution of imaging.

In the first few weeks or months of life, a small percentage of infants develop lower cranial nerve palsies and impaired brainstem function. This dysfunction is characterized by vocal cord paralysis with inspiratory stridor, retrocollis, apneic episodes, difficulty with feeding, and inability to handle secretions (337,338). Additionally, progressive spasticity of the upper extremities can develop (337). The reason for this progressive neurologic deficit is unclear. It might relate to compression of the cranial nerves and brainstem in the shallow posterior fossa. Downward pressure from inadequately controlled hydrocephalus has been suggested as an explanation for infants whose symptoms resolve with surgery. In others, brainstem hemorrhage, brainstem ischemia, or an underlying neuronal agenesis is present (337,339). Anterior

sacral meningoceles are characterized by unremitting and unexplained constipation and a smooth pelvic mass. Their presence can be diagnosed by MRI studies.

Radiography of the spine reveals the extent of the nonfused vertebrae. The relationship between the cord segment and the vertebral bodies is abnormal. Although at birth the terminal segments of the normal cord lie between the vertebral bodies of T11 and L1, in infants with myelomeningocele the cord can extend as far down as L5 or even lower. The position of the spinal cord segments remains normal in the lower cervical and upper thoracic levels (340).

A dysraphic lesion that straddles the categories of occult and cystic spina bifida is the subcutaneous lipoma extending intradurally through a posterior vertebral arch defect to end within the substance of a low-lying conus medullaris. A more extreme example of this type of lesion is the lipomyelomeningocele (Fig. 4.4A and B). This lesion can be included in either the cystic or the occult dysraphic category, because a huge mass is evident with some lesions, whereas others are but a minimal deformity of the back. The mass is invariably located in the lumbosacral region. It can be midline or eccentric, is fully epithelialized, and frequently is associated with a cutaneous angioma, a hair patch, one or more dimples, or a sinus tract. In addition to the fatty tissue, the mass can be cystic or occasionally it can contain cartilage. These lesions are usually not associated with the Chiari malformations, hydrocephalus, or other CNS anomalies.

Although some infants with lumbosacral lipoma have no neurologic deficit, it is more common to find the lower lumbar or sacral segments affected, with resultant motor or sensory loss in the feet and bladder and bowel dysfunction. The quantity of subcutaneous lipomatous material varies. It extends through the defective posterior arches to become intimate with the low-lying and tethered conus medullaris. The dura is dysplastic and blends into the fatty tissue or forms cystic cavities filled with CSF.

Surgical intervention is advised at approximately age 3 months, not simply for cosmetic reasons, but, more importantly, to decompress and

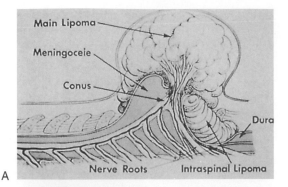

A

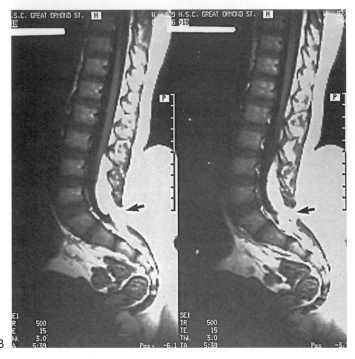

B

FIG. 4.4. A: Diagrammatic sagittal view of a lumbosacral lipomyelomeningocele. The subcutaneous lipoma extends through the defect in the posterior arches to end in the low-lying conus medullaris. The skin over the lesion is fully epithelialized and it had been covered by a large tuft of hair. (From Milhorat TH. *Pediatric neurosurgery*. Philadelphia: Davis, 1978. With permission.) **B:** Lipomyelomeningocele. T1-weighted magnetic resonance imaging shows the subcutaneous lipoma extending through the defect in the posterior arches (*arrow*) into the low-lying conus. (Courtesy of Dr. Brian Kendall, Institute of Neurology, London, UK.)

untether as far as possible the spinal cord, thus preventing progressive neurologic dysfunction. These patients require full orthopedic and urologic evaluation. A considerable proportion present with urologic symptoms, notably incontinence, soiling, and recurrent urinary tract infections (341).

Occasionally, a sacrococcygeal teratoma is mistaken for spina bifida cystica. Sacrococcygeal teratomas are only approximately one-fortieth as frequent as spina bifida cystica, with a marked female preponderance. As the name implies, a sacrococcygeal teratoma is located in the sacrococcygeal region, whereas the lesion of spina bifida cystica is above the coccyx. Other than the

breakdown of skin owing to tumor necrosis, no cutaneous abnormalities are seen. Deformities of the lower extremities and neurologic deficits are unusual, and radiography of the vertebral column is normal. Calcium deposits within the teratoma are seen in approximately one-third of patients. Imaging studies of the region confirm the diagnosis. A sacrococcygeal teratoma must be surgically removed in the first few days of life because the incidence of malignancy increases from 10% at birth to more than 50% by 2 months of age (342).

Malformations and infections of the genitourinary tract occur in up to 90% of newborns with spina bifida cystica, and renal disease is the most common cause of morbidity and mortality after age 3 years (343). Most commonly, a disturbance in bladder function is evident. One group, representing 33% of patients, shows more or less constant dribbling, and the bladder content is easily expressed manually. Direct cystometry reveals absent detrusor activity (344). In another, larger group of patients, detrusor contractions are weak, but bladder emptying is inefficient, and outlet obstruction at the level of the external sphincter occurs. This obstruction is believed to result from impaired coordination between the detrusor and sphincter functions and reflects a lesion of the spinal cord between the pontine-mesencephalic center regulating the vesicourethral unit and the sacral area. Bladder sensation is intact in some children. This latter type of upper motor neuron defect results in a high incidence of bladder trabeculation, an elevated resting bladder pressure, and dilatation of the upper urinary tract, often reaching enormous proportions (345). Continence appears to depend more on preservation of detrusor activity than of sphincter function. Serial neurologic evaluations indicate that these abnormalities are not static, but tend to change, particularly during the first year of life. Some children with complete or nearly complete denervation of the external sphincter improve, whereas others deteriorate (346). When deterioration occurs in childhood, it most likely occurs in patients with dyssynergia with a small, trabeculated, noncompliant bladder (347).

Persistent bacteriuria is seen in 50% of 2-year-old children, with hydronephrosis being found in 25% (348).

The three fundamental urologic problems are infection, incontinence, and retrograde high pressure on the upper urinary tract, producing hydronephrosis and hydroureter. Therefore, early and constant monitoring of the urinary tract with intravenous pyelograms, cultures with colony counts, and voiding cystography are an essential part of any therapeutic program (349). To assess the efficacy of clean intermittent catheterization and to time appropriate surgical intervention for the prevention or arrest of upper urinary tract damage, more complex urodynamic studies are available.

Spina Bifida Occulta. Spina bifida occulta, referring as it does to a simple bony anomaly in which there has not been complete fusion of the laminae in the midline, is extremely common. It is found in 25% of children hospitalized for any reason and in 10% of the general pediatric population. It generally involves the posterior arches of L5 and S1. Although it is usually asymptomatic and is found incidentally on radiographic examination, the skin of the low midback region can manifest a hairy tuft, dimple, dermal sinus, or mass caused by a subcutaneous lipoma or teratoma. In the child who has a neurogenic bladder, foot deformities, particularly a broad, shortened, or an elevated arch of the foot, or a variety of neurologic deficits of the lower limbs, spina bifida occulta can suggest an underlying malformation of the spinal cord (315,322). In these patients, neurologic deficits, even in the absence of urinary tract or cutaneous abnormalities, are an indication for neuroimaging studies.

Cranium Bifidum. The degree of neurologic and developmental damage in this condition depends on the quantity of herniated tissue, the degree of hydrocephalus, and the extent of hindbrain lesions or cerebral hemisphere dysplasias that result from the associated disorder of cellular migration and organization (277,314).

Often, no functional impairment is noted until childhood, by which time mild mental retardation, spastic diplegia, and impaired cognitive function or seizures can be evident. In the newborn, the mass must be distinguished from cephalhematoma, inclusion cysts of the scalp, cystic hygromas, caput succedaneum, and, in the case of anterior defects, nasal polyps. Its location along the midline, with pulsations synchronous with the heart rate, and absence of periosteal new bone formation distinguish cranium bifidum from these other conditions. Skull radiography reveals the bony defect, and neuroimaging studies define the ventricular system and quantity of neural tissue within the sac.

Treatment

Spina Bifida Cystica. The management of spina bifida cystica was given new energy by English orthopedic surgeons in the early 1960s (350,351). Their studies suggested that skin closure within 24 hours of birth reduces mortality and morbidity from meningitis and ventriculitis.

They argued that early closure not only prevents local infection and trauma to the exposed neural tissue, but also avoids stretching additional nerve roots, which is likely to occur as the cystic sac expands during the first 24 hours. As a consequence, further deterioration of lower limb function and sphincter control is prevented, and motor power of the legs is maintained (352).

In 1971, Lorber (353) proposed the principle of selective surgery and suggested four adverse criteria: a high level of paraplegia, clinically evident hydrocephalus present at birth, congenital lumbar kyphosis, and other major malformations. Other workers, however, have obtained a relatively good outcome in approximately one-half of infants who would have fared badly according to Lorber criteria (354). A further hindrance to the prediction of the future neurologic status of an infant with myelomeningocele is the subsequent progressive cavitation of the cervical and thoracic spinal cord that produces increasing weakness and spasticity of the upper extremities and causes progressive scoliosis (355).

The questions as to whether and when to operate on neonates with spina bifida cystica have perhaps generated more concern and anxiety than any others in pediatric neurosurgery. Many clinicians have refrained from operating on children who had one or more of Lorber adverse criteria. In a paper, published in 1974, these selected infants were found to have a 2-year survival rate of 0% to 4% (356).

The reluctance of many American clinicians to follow Lorber criteria in carefully selecting children to treat surgically has been justified by the observation that two or more of the contraindications to operation are commonly compatible with survival and with a quality of life more acceptable than had been expected. Also, with modern methods of management the purported selection criteria advocated in the past have been shown to have little prognostic value, and in terms of mortality, the ultimate outcome for patients in unselected series compares favorably with that of patients managed according to selection criteria. The effect of early treatment on disability is far less, however. As a rule, the higher the sensory level, the lower the survival rate, the lower the IQ, and the less the likelihood

of employability (357). For a review of the present position, see papers by McLone (358) and Hobbins (359). A survey, published in 1990, found that in an unselected adult population of myelomeningocele patients, some 50% of survivors were ambulatory and 25% were continent. Of the survivors, 50% were able to live without supervision in adapted accommodations and 70% were employable, 25% being able to manage competitive employment (357). McLone and coworkers conclude that "nearly all children born with a meningomyelocele should have the lesion repaired surgically within 24 hours of birth and should have hydrocephalus treated by shunt diversion . . . and other appropriate management" (360).

Almost all workers agree that when a patient has been selected for surgical treatment, the procedure should be undertaken within 24 hours of birth, and no later than 1 week of age. The claim that delivery by cesarean section before the onset of labor results in better motor function still requires confirmation (361), as do the benefits of an *in utero* repair of the myelomeningocele (362). Early surgery undoubtedly prevents further loss of functioning neural tissue as a result of trauma and infection. Additionally, prompt closure results in shorter hospitalization, easier care of the infant, and psychological benefit to the family and nursing staff. It is important to emphasize to the family that closing the defect does not reverse the neurologic impairment already present, and that often much additional treatment will be necessary. It is our view that if major malformations of other organ systems are present, or if MRI demonstrates major abnormalities of cortical architecture, parents should be advised of these malformations and of the likelihood of a poor intellectual and functional outcome. As a rule, intelligence is related to the thickness of the cortex at the time of shunt insertion and to the sensory level present at birth, with infants who had a lesion in the thoracic region faring worse than those who had a lumbar or sacral lesion (363,364). Children who required a shunt because of hydrocephalus did not perform as well intellectually as those who did not. In particular, those children whose shunt required one or more revisions showed a significant reduction in their cognitive score (364). Bier and colleagues also stress the importance of socioeconomic factors in the ultimate outcome, particularly in the verbal scores of affected children (364).

If the neonate is to be treated, as is usually the case, the sac is kept clean and moist before surgery by an undercover of gauze sponges wet with a povidone-iodine solution. To prevent colonization of the gastrointestinal tract and to keep the meconium sterile, the infant is not fed. Systemic broad-spectrum antibiotics, especially against *Staphylococcus* and coliform organisms, are started when the infant arrives at the hospital and are continued for several days after closure of the sac. Postoperatively, the infant is kept prone for the first week to diminish the risk of urine or feces contaminating the wound. If fluid is present beneath the skin at the repair site, it can be aspirated and a pressure dressing can be applied. Persistent fluid buildup indicates an accumulation of CSF at this location and requires the insertion of a ventriculoperitoneal shunt, even though the ventricles can still be only mildly dilated. Preventing the accumulation of CSF at the repair site allows the wound to heal completely and rarely is any additional surgery needed at this site. Bladder emptying is assured either with Credé maneuver or with intermittent catheterization. If Credé maneuver is used, occasionally catheterizing the infant is advisable to confirm that the residuals are low.

In the course of follow-up examinations, the head circumference and the appearance of the fontanelle are monitored, and imaging is used whenever the findings suggest increased intracranial pressure. As judged by imaging studies, more than 90% of infants with spina bifida cystica ultimately develop progressive hydrocephalus. Of these, 80% do so within the first 6 months of life and require a shunting procedure (365,366). Approximately 20% of children with myelomeningocele develop symptoms of hindbrain, cranial nerve, or spinal cord compression (367,368). In the majority of cases, manifestations develop before the age of 3 months (339). If the infant develops progressive lower cranial nerve palsies and brainstem signs,

it often becomes necessary to decompress the posterior fossa and upper cervical spine, assuming that the hydrocephalus is under good control (368).

Contracture deformities of the lower limbs require physical therapy, leg braces, and stabilization of dislocated hips. Muscle or tendon transplants and joint arthrodeses might be necessary in the ambulating child. Postoperatively, neuropathic fractures resulting from paralysis and prolonged immobility are common. They are best prevented by early active and passive range-of-motion exercises (369).

Kyphosis is an occasional serious and sometimes life-threatening development as the child assumes the sitting posture. It occurs in the more severe cases of extensive lumbosacral myelomeningocele as a result of the paralysis of trunk muscles and from the bone deformity associated with the primary lesion. The spinal deformity poses a threat to respiratory function, to the health of the skin overlying the repaired lesion, and sometimes to the function of surviving cord and nerves. An early decision with respect to reducing the deformity must be made in these circumstances. The deformity is best reduced by the difficult procedure of excision of the vertebral bodies at the level of the kyphosis. In some severe cases, it is possible to perform bony excision at the time of the primary operation. Not providing such treatment can cause a marked reduction in life expectancy.

Spinal cord tethering, of the type found in spina bifida occulta, is present in a small proportion of patients with myelomeningocele. This tethering occurs in addition to the obvious union of the neural elements with the superficial tissues, which is the essential feature of a myelomeningocele. Thus, diastematomyelia, other forms of tethering, and hydromyelia can be present. These additional lesions can be detected by MRI. In the series of Caldarelli and colleagues, routine MRI screening disclosed cavitation of the spinal cord in 22.5% of spina bifida patients. Approximately one-half of the lesions were clinically asymptomatic (370). Deciding whether and when to intervene surgically when such a lesion is found is difficult and requires considerable neurosurgical judgment.

Disorders of the excretory system are the most common cause of morbidity and mortality in patients who survive longer than 2 years. Fernandez and colleagues have outlined five points that are invaluable in the management of the child with neurogenic bladder. These are (a) achieving urinary continence, (b) good bladder emptying, (c) lowering intravesical pressure, (d) prevention of urinary tract infections, and (e) treatment of vesicoureteral reflux (371).

In lumbosacral spina bifida cystica, few children attain urinary continence, although McLone and his group believe that bladder and bowel control can be achieved by school age in almost 90% of surviving children (360). The mechanism for urinary incontinence cannot be predicted by the neurologic examination; rather it requires urodynamic testing, including cystometrography, uroflometry, and electromyography of the urinary sphincter (372). When these studies show the bladder to be atonic but with adequate urethral resistance, treatment is by intermittent catheterization, often in conjunction with cholinergic agents such as bethanechol, which can reduce the residual volume of the bladder. When the bladder is atonic and urethral resistance is inadequate, treatment should be directed to increasing outlet resistance. One way this can be accomplished is by creating an artificial urinary sphincter. Ephedrine, an α-adrenergic agent that acts on the bladder neck, or imipramine, can improve continence in the denervated bladder by increasing muscle tone, thereby increasing resistance to bladder outflow. Conversely, this resistance can be diminished by phenoxybenzamine or diazepam.

When incontinence results from a spastic bladder and decreased bladder capacity, and urethral resistance is adequate, the high intravesical pressure is managed with anticholinergic drugs. For this purpose, Fernandez and colleagues recommend oxybutynin chloride (0.2 mg/kg per day given in two divided doses), which inhibits the muscarinic action of acetylcholine on smooth muscle (371). Other drugs that have been suggested include propantheline bromide and imipramine hydrochloride. Serial cystometrograms are indicated to monitor drug response. When intermittent catheterization and anticholinergic drugs are insufficient, urinary diversion or bladder augmentation should be considered, with the latter procedure being used more frequently in children (371).

When incontinence is of mixed origin, a combination of medication, intermittent catheterization, and implantation of an artificial urinary sphincter should be tried. In all instances, however, an associated malformation of the urinary tract, such as double ureter or single kidney, must be kept in mind and must be diagnosed to provide comprehensive care.

In the absence of vesicoureteral reflux and in the presence of normal upper tracts, urine cultures taken every 6 months and urograms or imaging studies done every 13 years should suffice. Acute urinary tract infection demands prompt and appropriate antibiotics because infection inevitably leads to persistent vesicoureteral reflux. Such reflux, together with residual urine, produces trigonal hypertrophy and results in retrograde high pressure and eventual hydronephrosis.

Vesicoureteral reflux should be monitored by isotope cystography and requires long-term treatment with low dosages of antibiotics, such as nitrofurantoin or trimethoprim sulfa. Urinary acidification can be useful in inhibiting calculus formation.

Bowel incontinence owing to a flaccid external sphincter, although not as serious a medical problem as bladder incontinence, poses a much greater social disability. Constipation and impaction of stool are major problems after the first few years of life. Routine enemas or suppositories and biofeedback training have been used with some degree of success, especially when anorectal manometric data demonstrate some rectal sensation and when the patient is able to effect some contraction of skeletal muscle (373,374). Another approach to alleviating the fecal incontinence can be achieved in carefully selected and motivated children, who have failed to respond to the other approach, and who wish to avoid a colostomy. By means of an appendicostomy, a relatively simple operation, the appendix is inserted into the anterior aspect of the cecum, and retrograde colonic enemas can be performed. The slow washing out of the colonic contents by injection of water through the appendicostomy may be needed only every 24 to 48 hours, leaving the child free to take part in normal activities for the remainder of the time. The procedure can be carried out by itself or in combination with surgery for urinary incontinence (375).

The long-term care of the patient with spina bifida cystica requires a multidisciplinary effort. In addition to continuing neurologic and neurosurgical evaluations, the infant also should be seen at regular intervals by orthopedic surgeons, urologists, physiotherapists, and by the nursing and social services. Details of ongoing care are covered more extensively in a multiauthored book edited by Rekate (376).

Spina Bifida Occulta. The availability of neuroimaging has allowed a more complete diagnosis of occult dysraphism. Diagnosis is particularly important because the lesions are frequently multiple, and surgical intervention at more than one level is indicated.

Clear indications for surgery include the finding of progressive neurologic defects, the presence of an associated tumor or a dermal sinus that carries the risk of meningitis or deep abscess, or a history of meningitis. Considerable debate exists about the need to operate when a malformation has been discovered in the absence of a progressive neural loss. It is our opinion that a child with a lower limb malformation (a small and deformed foot is the most common manifestation) or with a skin stigmata should have plain radiography of the entire spine or MRI studies whenever these are available. When vertebral column malformation is disclosed on the radiographic films, follow-up imaging studies are necessary. Should these reveal an abnormal attachment of the cord or nerve roots, operative intervention to remove that attachment is required as a prophylactic measure, even when no history of progressive damage exists.

Meningocele. If the meningocele is fully epithelialized and not draining CSF, and if the skin over the sac is not ulcerated, immediate repair is not needed, and surgery can be deferred for several months. As is the case with spina bifida cystica, the possibility of an additional dysraphic anomaly such as a tethered cord or diastematomyelia requires complete imaging studies. Lesions that protrude minimally do not necessarily require surgical intervention. Imaging studies of the brain are suggested to assess ventricular size and to detect those few infants who develop hydrocephalus. A small proportion of meningoceles present ventrally as a pelvic mass, or even more uncommonly, as a posterior mediastinal mass. These lesions are usually not detected in the newborn period.

Cranium Bifidum Cysticum. Cranium bifidum cysticum requires immediate repair if CSF is leaking or if the defect is not covered by skin. If the defect is completely epithelialized, it should be closed before the infant's discharge from the hospital; if the lesion is small and less unsightly, closure can be postponed until later in the first year of life. When the lesion is tender and a source of distress to the infant, early surgical repair is indicated. Posterior encephaloceles are often associated with posterior fossa malformations leading to hydrocephalus. MRI should be done before surgical operation in all cases. Anterior encephaloceles should be repaired by a neurosurgeon working with a cosmetic surgeon.

Prognosis

Follow-up studies have been performed to compare the survival and quality of life among patients treated without surgery, patients who were operated on selectively (i.e., if they lacked the adverse criteria), and patients who received routine early operation (377). Some 45% of infants with myelomeningoceles who are not treated surgically die within the first year of life, most often as a consequence of hydrocephalus or CNS infections (378). Of the survivors, approximately 50% are minimally handicapped (379). The rest are severely handicapped. With operation, approximately 90% survive into their teens, but less than 33% of these are minimally handicapped (380).

Nonselective surgical intervention results in a large number of survivors with major disabilities. By adolescence, 66% of this group are wheelchair dependent, because many will have given up assisted walking as they gained weight. Furthermore, 40% have IQs below 80; 66% have no continence of bladder and bowel; 66% have visual defects, including strabismus, corneal scarring, and blindness; 25% have a seizure disorder; and 25% develop precocious puberty.

Approximately 90% experience pressure sores, burns, and fractures (381). Incontinence becomes the dominant issue in the surviving adolescent; some undergo urinary diversion, and others respond to intermittent catheterization. In most cases, incontinence adversely affects their academic and social life, and more than 90% can be expected to have some degree of personal, social, and economic dependence (382). Long-term studies on patients who had selective surgical intervention have not yet been completed.

When death occurs after early childhood, it is usually the result of urinary tract infection with sepsis and renal failure. Less often, it is the consequence of increased intracranial pressure resulting from poorly treated or intractable hydrocephalus. In some cases, death is the consequence of pulmonary disease caused by progressive kyphoscoliosis.

Even though surgical and medical advances have improved the prognosis for children with spina bifida cystica, the essence of treatment is prevention of the condition by correction of any maternal nutritional deficiency and prenatal screening programs not only of the high-risk population but also of the general population (383).

Chiari Malformations

The third major expression of dysraphism was first observed by Cleland in 1883 (384), but was more definitively described by Chiari in 1891 and 1896 (308,309). Chiari malformations are characterized by cerebellar elongation and protrusion through the foramen magnum into the cervical spinal cord. Primary anomalies of the hindbrain and skeletal structures with consequent mechanical deformities produce four different positions of the cerebellum and brainstem relative to the foramen magnum and upper cervical canal (385).

Pathogenesis

Traditional theories of the pathogenesis of the Chiari malformations have been mechanical in nature:

1. The traction theory suggests tethering of the spinal cord pulls the caudal medulla oblongata and posterior cerebellum through the foramen magnum as the spinal column grows faster than the spinal cord.

2. The pulsion theory suggests fetal hydrocephalus causes pressure and displacement downward of the brainstem and cerebellum during development.

3. The crowding theory suggests the posterior fossa itself is too small and the confined neural structures within it are forced through the foramen magnum as they grow. None of these theories fully accounts for all of the manifestations of Chiari malformations, such as the primary intramedullary dysplasia that usually is found in the brainstem and cerebellum, the accompanying aqueductal stenosis and hydromyelia in many cases, and inconstant forebrain anomalies in some, such as absence of the corpus callosum. The crowding theory of Marín-Padilla may play a role, however, as the posterior fossa is indeed pathologically reduced in volume, but it cannot explain the entire malformation.

4. The birth trauma theory is wholly without merit, and cases are well documented, both in the literature and in the neuropathologic experience of the present authors, of fetuses of less than 20 weeks' gestation with well-formed Chiari malformations.

5. The hypothesis that appears to have the greatest consistency with all aspects of Chiari malformations, particularly types II and III, is a molecular genetic hypothesis that the malformation is caused by ectopic expression of homeobox genes of rhombomere segmentation. Experimentally, Chiari II malformations and often meningomyeloceles may be created in fetal rodents by administering a single dose of retinoic acid (vitamin A) to the maternal animal on embryonic day 9.5 (386). Retinoic acid is known to cause ectopic expression of genes of the Hox and Krox families in mice, resulting in brainstem and cerebellar malformations.

Types

Type I. In type I malformation, clinically the least severe, the medulla is displaced caudally into the spinal canal, and the inferior pole of the cerebellar hemispheres is herniated through the foramen magnum in the form of two parallel, tonguelike processes. This herniation can extend as far down as the third cervical vertebra. Malformations at the base of the skull and the upper cervical spine are sometimes present. These include platybasia, basilar impression, atlas assimilation, atlantoaxial dislocation, asymmetric small foramen magnum, and Klippel-Feil syndrome. Hydromyelia, syringomyelia, syringobulbia, and diastematomyelia are frequently present (385). It should be noted that the terms *platybasia* and *basilar impression* frequently are used interchangeably. Platybasia refers to a malformation in which the angle formed by a line connecting the nasion, tuberculum sellae, and anterior margin of the foramen magnum is greater than 143 degrees. Platybasia is actually more of an anthropomorphic term than a strictly medical one, which anthropologists use, for example, to help distinguish *Homo neanderthalis* from *Homo sapiens*, and all healthy human infants have transitory platybasia to a degree in postnatal life. Basilar impression refers to an upward displacement of the occipital bone and cervical spine with protrusion of the odontoid process into the foramen magnum.

The Chiari malformation type I is generally asymptomatic in childhood, becoming clinically apparent only in adolescence or adult life. The ready availability of MRI studies that demonstrate the malformation has led to a more complete understanding of the clinical spectrum of this condition (387). Symptoms result from direct medullary compression, compromise of the vasculature supplying the medulla, or, less frequently, from hydrocephalus that develops from aqueductal stenosis or obstruction of the fourth ventricle at its outlet foramina or at the foramen magnum. With obstruction at the foramen magnum, torticollis, opisthotonus, and signs of cervical cord compression are evident. Headache, vertigo, laryngeal paralysis, and progressive cerebellar signs can be accompanied by lower cranial nerve deficits that are often asymmetric (388). Other symptoms of this condition include recurrent apneic attacks, and pain in the neck and the occipital region

that is exacerbated by laughing or straining. In the series of 43 patients reported by Nohria and Oakes, the mean age at presentation was 17.5 years (389). Hydrosyringomyelia was seen in 65% and scoliosis in 30%. Hydrocephalus was only seen in 12%.

Type II. In type II, the most common of the Chiari malformations to be diagnosed in childhood, any combination of features of type I malformation can be associated with noncommunicating hydrocephalus and lumbosacral spina bifida. Additionally, the medulla and cerebellum, together with part or all of the fourth ventricle, are displaced into the spinal canal (304,338). The medulla and pons are ventrally linked and juxtaposed (see Figs. 4.2 and 4.3). The pons and cranial nerves are elongated, and the cervical roots are compressed and forced to course upward, rather than downward, to exit through their respective foramina. Cervicothoracic hydromyelia and syringomyelia also can be present, and both the foramina of Luschka and Magendie and the basal cisterns are occluded as a result of impaction of the foramen magnum or atresia of the foramina outlets (390).

These anatomic features can be demonstrated readily by MRI studies. Additionally, one can observe that the posterior fossa is smaller than normal, and that the tentorium has a low attachment to the occipital bone (338). In 75% of patients, the underdeveloped tentorium allows inferior displacement of the medial posterior cerebrum (375).

In addition to these gross abnormalities, developmental arrests of the cerebellar and brainstem structures also occur, and heterotopias of cerebral gray matter, polygyria, and microgyria. Microgyria point to an additional defect in cerebral cellular migration (298,391).

In more than 90% of patients, type II Chiari malformation is seen in conjunction with spina bifida cystica, hydrocephalus, and any combination of the assorted defects already cited for type I (392). Conversely, all subjects with spina bifida cystica and hydrocephalus exhibit the type II defect. The clinical presentation of this condition was first noted in 1941 by Adams and colleagues, who demonstrated the lesion by intraspinal injection of lipiodol (393). In the

more recent experience of Vandertop and colleagues, 21% of patients develop signs of Chiari
II malformation despite good control of their
hydrocephalus (368). Symptoms usually develop
in infants. They include swallowing difficulties
seen in 71% of the series of Vandertop and
coworkers, stridor seen in 59%, arm weakness
in 53%, apneic spells in 29%, and aspiration in
12%. Surgical decompression and sectioning a
tight and dense fibrotic band that is often present
at the C1 level produces significant improvement
in the majority of infants.

Type III. Type III variant can have any of the
features of types I or II. Additionally, the entire
cerebellum is herniated through the foramen
magnum with a cervical spina bifida cystica.
Hydrocephalus is seen regularly and is the result
of differing degrees of atresia of the fourth ventricle foramina, aqueductal stenosis, or impaction
at the foramen magnum. Rhombencephalosynapsis can rarely be part of type III (394).

Type IV. Type IV, designated by Chiari, is
cerebellar hypoplasia and is covered with
other malformations of the posterior fossa. It
bears no relation to the other Chiari malformations.

Management

The clinical condition and therapeutic regimen
for the various Chiari syndromes are described
in other sections (see Spina Bifida Cystica, Cranium Bifidum, and Hydrocephalus).

Other Spinal Cord Dysraphic States

The vast majority of other dysraphic states are
confined to the spinal cord and its vertebral and
cutaneous environment. Like anencephaly and
spina bifida, they result from a combination of
environmental and genetic components (395).
They are of subtle expression and usually are
associated with spina bifida occulta, along with
a tethered cord, a mass lesion, or both (396). A
tethered conus medullaris is diagnosed by its
position below L2 and by a filum terminale that
is wider than 2 mm and is located in the posterior portion of the spinal cord. Tethering results
in traction and damage to neural tissue. If a

mass lesion is present (e.g., lipoma, syrinx),
compression of neural tissue occurs (396).

Neurologic dysfunction can be present
already in the neonate with an occult dysraphic
lesion. If so, it most frequently involves the lower
lumbar and sacral segments and produces motor
and sensory loss or sphincter impairment. Musculoskeletal deformities primarily involve the
foot, but scoliosis can develop. With somatic
growth, the neurologic deficit can worsen or can
become apparent, if not already present. The progression and development of neurologic symptoms is believed to result from the differential
growth between the spinal column and the spinal
cord, compression of neural elements, or damage
from repeated local trauma (328). Normally, the
conus medullaris ascends from the lower lumbar
to the upper lumbar level during growth. If tethered by a lipomatous mass, a hypertrophic filum
terminale, or by a bony spur such as is associated
with diastematomyelia, spinal cord ascent is
impaired, causing neural damage.

Dysraphisms are often heralded by cutaneous
or subcutaneous lesions, such as a hairy tuft,
hemangioma, lipoma, sinus, or dimple. We
advise imaging studies of the spine and the
spinal cord in any neonate with these cutaneous
abnormalities. If a patient has neurologic abnormalities and a bony defect in addition to the
cutaneous lesions, imaging and surgical exploration are indicated.

Diplomyelia and Diastematomyelia

The extensive use of neuroimaging has resulted
in a redefinition of diplomyelia and diastematomyelia. Pang and coworkers recommend the
term *split cord malformation* (SCM) for both
entities and distinguish two types (397). In type
I SCM, two hemicords are each contained within
their own dural tubes and separated by a rigid
osseocartilaginous median septum. This condition generally corresponds to diastematomyelia.
In type II SCM, a condition that generally corresponds to diplomyelia, the two hemicords are
housed in a single dural tube and are separated
by a nonrigid fibrous median septum. The state
of the dural tube and the nature of the median
septum can be demonstrated by imaging studies

(397). For this purpose, high-resolution, thin cut, axial computed tomographic (CT) myelography using bone algorithms is more sensitive than MRI (398).

According to Pang and colleagues, both types of SCM result from adhesions between ectoderm and endoderm, which lead to an accessory neuroenteric canal around which an endomesenchymal tract condenses, which bisects the developing notochord and causes the formation of two hemineural plates (397). Other workers consider diplomyelia to result from a split notochord, whereas diastematomyelia results from a single spinal cord that becomes separated into two parts with sequestered mesodermal tissue growing into the intervening space.

According to the old terminology *diplomyelia* represents a duplication of the spinal cord, usually in the lumbar region (79% in the series of Pang), and occasionally extending for 10 segments or more (398). Because it is a true duplication, each affected spinal segment has four dorsal roots and four anterior horns. The lesion can be associated with extensive spina bifida cystica or with tumors of the spinal cord, or it can occur in the absence of other neurologic deficits (399).

The term *diastematomyelia* is derived from the Greek *diastema*, meaning cleft. The condition is marked by a cleft in the spinal cord, which becomes divided longitudinally by a septum of bone and cartilage emanating from the posterior vertebral arch and extending anteriorly. Each half of the cord has its own dural covering. The cord or cauda equina becomes impaled by the bony spur, and differential growth between vertebral column and spinal cord results in stretching of the cord above its point of fixation. An alternative, pathogenetic hypothesis postulates that progressive cord or cauda equina damage results from minor trauma and traction at the spur during head and neck flexion in the growing child. In the majority of subjects, diastematomyelia is confined to the low thoracolumbar region, usually extending for one to two segments, rarely for as many as 10 segments (400). Finally, another hypothesis, which is supported by experimental genetic animal models, proposes that a strong ventralizing

gene such as *Sonic hedgehog* is upregulated during neural induction by the notochord, or that an even earlier gene expressed during gastrulation and primitive streak formation, such as *Wnt-8C*, is upregulated and causes duplication of the neuraxis.

Some 80% to 95% of patients with diastematomyelia are female (401). A variety of skin lesions mark the site of the defect. Most commonly [56% of cases in the series of Pang (398)], these are tufts of hair or dimples, but subcutaneous lipomas, vascular malformations, or dermal sinuses also can be present. Additionally, anomalies of the craniobasal bones may occur, as well as syringomyelia and hydromyelia (see Fig. 4.1C). A neurenteric cyst can be located in the cleft portions of the spinal cord (402).

Progressive sensorimotor deficits represent the most common clinical manifestation for both diplomyelia and diastematomyelia (398,403). They were seen in 87% of symptomatic children, and are commonly asymmetric. Pain was seen in 37% of children. Sensorimotor deficits may take two forms. The first is a predominantly unilateral, nonprogressive hypotonia and weakness. The second syndrome is seen in approximately two-thirds of cases. In this entity, the subject experiences weakness and spasticity of the lower extremities with awkward gait, incontinence of bladder and rectum, and, less commonly, posterior root pain. Symptoms either appear *de novo* or are superimposed on the first syndrome. A combination of upper and lower motor neuron signs in the lower extremities is associated with atrophy of the leg muscles and skeletal deformities of the feet (404). The difference in shape and dimensions of the lower limbs is often quite striking and is believed to result from a combination of prenatal and postnatal asymmetry of growth stimulus secondary to differences in nerve supply. Spinothalamic and posterior column sensory deficits correspond with the level of the lesion. With suspicion aroused by cutaneous anomalies and neurologic dysfunction of the lower limbs and sphincters, diagnosis can best be made by means of MRI of the spinal cord. Because sagittal images may be difficult to interpret in patients with severe scoliosis, coronal images should always be obtained.

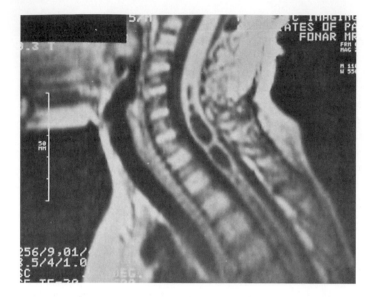

FIG. 4.5. Cervical syringomyelia. Magnetic resonance imaging study. The syrinx was essentially asymptomatic in this 4-year-old boy. It was discovered when imaging studies were done as part of an evaluation for a hemiplegia, which was found to be caused by a parietal porencephaly.

Surgery for SCM type I cases (diastematomyelia) has a higher risk of morbidity than is seen for SCM type II cases (diplomyelia), particularly when one hemicord is markedly smaller and, therefore, more delicate (398). Surgical removal of the bony spur allows the cord to become freely movable. Although this does not alter the nonprogressive hypoplastic syndrome, it prevents the onset or arrests and even improves the progressive *de novo* syndrome (402,405). The more recent the neurologic deficit, the more likely it is to be reversible; hence, prophylactic surgery for the infant or young child without neurologic deficit is indicated. Periodic postoperative follow-up is necessary because regrowth of bone spurs has been reported (406).

Syringomyelia and Hydromyelia

Syringomyelia and hydromyelia are traditionally believed to represent different expressions of the same pathologic process. As originally defined, syringomyelia is a condition of tubular cavitation within the spinal cord. When the cystic lesion extends into the medulla and pons, the condition is termed *syringobulbia*. When the condition is associated with Chiari type I or II malformation, as it often is, it is accompanied by tonsillar herni-

ation and an apparent occlusion of the outlet foramina of the fourth ventricle. The diameter of the cervical spinal canal is enlarged, and extensive scoliosis or kyphoscoliosis can be present. Some cases are post-traumatic, a condition more fully covered in Chapter 8 (Fig. 4.5). Others, nearly 20%, are associated with a spinal cord tumor (407). Rarely, spinal cord gray and white matter is disorganized, a microscopic picture analogous to schizencephaly of the cerebral cortex. In the majority of cases, however, the cause of syringomyelia remains essentially unknown despite numerous theories and many clinical and experimental studies intended to explain the condition (408). The most current theory, as proposed by Oldfield and colleagues, is based on their observations, supported by MRI and cine-MRI, that in subjects with syringomyelia associated with the Chiari I malformation the subarachnoid space is partially occluded at the level of the foramen magnum by the displaced brainstem and cerebellar tonsils (409). This displacement impedes the rapid upward and downward movement of CSF during the cardiac cycle and produces a systolic pressure wave in the spinal CSF that forces CSF into the spinal cord through the perivascular and interstitial spaces.

Hydromyelia is a dilated central canal without extension into the spinal cord parenchyma and resembles the healthy fetal condition at midgestation, although often in a more extreme form. At 6 to 12 weeks' gestation, the central canal is a tall, vertical slit extending almost the entire vertical axis of the neural tube. It is initially lined by undifferentiated neuroepithelium with mitotic activity at the surface of the central canal; a pseudostratified columnar ependymal epithelium then develops and stops all mitotic activity, first at the basal plate and later at the alar plate. The slit becomes round in transverse sectional views, and progressively narrows as the fetus and infant mature. In early adult life the canal ceases to exist altogether, and its site is identified by clusters and rosettes of residual ependymal cells, but the lumen is obliterated. Hydromyelia of the cervical and often of the thoracic and lumbosacral spinal cord usually accompanies Chiari II malformations, and the ependyma lining it overexpresses vimentin as a persistent fetal feature that normally disappears by 34 weeks' gestation. Vimentin expression continues into adult life in subjects with Chiari malformations, but does so only in the regions of dysgenesis of the ventricles, not in the normal lateral or third ventricles or in normal segments of the spinal cord (H. B. Sarnat, unpublished data).

Although sometimes recognized during childhood, syringomyelia usually does not become symptomatic until adult life (410). The vast majority of lesions involves the cervical cord and, therefore, the upper extremities are preferentially involved. However, a syrinx is sometimes encountered in spinal dysraphism of the lower spine, when it is usually associated with other malformations in this region. Because the cavities tend to be more central than eccentric, they damage fibers crossing through the central white matter of the cord and thus compromise temperature and pain sensation, sparing sensory modalities mediated by the posterior columns. This disassociated anesthesia is responsible for cutaneous trophic, sudomotor, and vasomotor disorders, including painless ulcerations, coldness, cyanosis, and hyperhidrosis. It also causes the painless arthropathies, the Charcot joints similar to those seen in tabes dorsalis, but involving joints of the upper rather than the lower extremities.

As the syrinx enlarges, involvement of anterior horn cells, pyramidal tracts, and posterior columns in the cervical region leads to segmental asymmetric lower motor neuron signs in the upper and lower extremities. Spasticity, hyperreflexia, and loss of position and vibratory sense occur. In children, the first sign can be a rapidly progressive scoliosis (411). In syringobulbia, asymmetric lower cranial nerve palsies occur, and the condition is almost always associated with anomalies of the craniobasal bones. Brainstem tumors are occasionally present. Syrinxes in the child or adult can impinge on dorsal motor nuclei of the vagus nerve, producing episodic stridor with laryngospasm, or they can compromise the nucleus ambiguous, causing chronic stridor and vocal cord paralysis (412).

Diagnosis is best made by MRI studies. Sagittal views provide excellent visualization of the cystic cavity and of the anatomy at the level of the foramen magnum. Gadolinium enhancement can be used to verify the presence of an adjoining tumor (413). Considerable dispute exists about the best means of managing the lesion (407,414). Posterior fossa and upper cervical decompression currently is the recommended treatment for the most common form of syringomyelia seen in the pediatric population (i.e., that associated with Chiari type II malformation and downward displacement of the cerebellar tonsils and outlet obstruction of the fourth ventricle) (407,415). In patients in whom such decompression fails to stabilize the neurologic deterioration and in whom persistence of a dilated cyst can be demonstrated, shunting of the CSF from the cystic cavity into the neighboring subarachnoid space is recommended (407,413). The value of occluding the opening from the fourth ventricle into the syringomyelic cavity has come under question, but is still recommended when syringomyelia is associated with the Dandy-Walker syndrome (407,416). Follow-up examinations by MRI are required.

Sacral Agenesis

Sacral agenesis is marked by total absence of the coccyx and the lower two or three sacral vertebrae, and hypoplasia of the vertebrae just above the aplastic segments. An associated anomalous development of the lumbosacral cord and other major or minor dysraphisms occur. Lipoma of the conus medullaris and filum terminale often accompany the defect (417). Sacral agenesis is associated in animals and humans with underexpression of *Sonic hedgehog* at the caudal end of the neural tube. The same molecular defect when expressed only at the rostral end of the neural tube is associated with holoprosencephaly. The gene for sacral agenesis has been mapped to chromosome 7q36, the same region that contains a gene for holoprosencephaly (418). Sacral agenesis, therefore, represents a genetic disorder of neural induction and of failure in induction of the sclerotome in the ventral half of the paired somites. In severe cases, the entire somite may fail to develop at the sacral and lumbar levels, hence the myotome is affected as well and fails to generate myocytes, resulting in segmental amyoplasia. Sensory innervation from the dorsal horns and dorsal roots remains well preserved, by contrast, and autonomic neural structure and function are variably involved (419).

Neurologic signs are those of a flaccid neurogenic bladder with dribbling incontinence, motor deficits, to a lesser extent sensory deficits of the lower extremities, lower extremity muscle hypoplasia, and skeletal arthrogryposis (419). Recurrent urinary tract infection and hydronephrosis, aggravated by delay in diagnosing the primary process, are major sources of morbidity (420). The defect has been associated with imperforate anus, malrotation of the bowel, and genital anomalies. All malformations can be dated to the first 7 weeks of gestation (421). Sacral agenesis is seen in approximately 1% of offspring of diabetic mothers, and Passarge and Lenz have postulated that insulin interferes with the differentiation of caudal chordamesoderm (422).

Neurodermal Sinus

The majority of dermal sinuses (e.g., the pilonidal sinus) does not connect with the CNS and are therefore of limited neurologic importance.

Neurodermal sinuses are relatively frequent among cases of occult spinal dysraphism (315).

They represent a communication lined by stratified squamous epithelium between skin and any portion of the neuraxis. Most commonly, the defects are in the lumbosacral region and the occiput, defects in the lumbosacral region occurring approximately nine times as frequently as those in the occiput. These two levels are at the terminal closure sites of the neural tube.

The sinus is often surrounded by a small mound of skin, the dimple, or other cutaneous lesions such as tufts of hair or angiomas. It often overlies a spina bifida occulta. It can expand into an epidermoid or dermoid cyst at its proximal end, causing segmental neurologic deficits, either through mass effect or by traction on the neuraxis. Cerebellar and brainstem signs or, on occasion, hydrocephalus can be produced by a neurodermal sinus in the occipital region. The presence of an open sinus tract can provide a portal of entry for bacterial infections, and a neurodermal sinus is an important cause for recurrent meningitis. In other cases, the dermoid cyst enlarges rapidly through infection of its contents, becoming an intraspinal abscess. When the lesion is in the lumbosacral region, coliform bacteria and staphylococci are the most common invaders; a sinus tract in the occiput is more likely to produce recurrent staphylococcal meningitis. Such defects must be scrupulously sought in any case of CNS infection (423). Any dermal sinus ending that is above the level of the lower sacrum should be traced with neuroimaging studies.

These lesions require surgical exploration and complete excision of the sinus before the development of symptoms. An occipital sinus is treated by primary excision of the entire sinus tract, and of the proximal cyst if it is present. In Matson's experience, surgical results were poorer when performed after the development of infection, with death resulting from chronic meningitis or hydrocephalus (305).

Congenital Scalp Defect

A congenital defect of the scalp, also known as *aplasia cutis congenita*, is a relatively rare anomaly seen in either sex. It can occur in isolation or in combination with a wide variety of other cerebral or extracranial anomalies (424). Rarely, congenital scalp defects are associated with similar cutaneous lesions elsewhere on the body. In 80% of instances the defect is sporadic, in the remainder it is inherited as autosomal dominant or autosomal recessive traits (277). The defect can vary from one that is small to one that includes most of the calvarial surface. Although in two-thirds of cases the underlying skull is intact, other cases involve underlying defects of periosteum, skull, and dura that often close spontaneously during the first few months after birth. The defect is generally at the vertex, although some lesions occur off the midline. The brain is usually normal, but imaging is justified to verify this assumption. Posterior midline scalp defects can be accompanied by mental retardation, congenital deafness, and hypothyroidism, the Johanson-Blizzard syndrome, and are seen in infants with deletion of the short arm of chromosome 4 (425). A small skin defect can be closed, but if it is large, grafting might be required. It is important to keep the lesion clean and moist before surgical repair.

Congenital Defects of the Cranial Bones

Congenital defects of the skull bones without loss of overlying skin or underlying dura result from a failure of ossification that usually occurs at the vertex either as enlarged persistent biparietal foramina or as an absence of the sphenoid wing. The latter can result in a pulsating exophthalmos that can damage the globe or optic nerve. In approximately 50% of the cases, this defect is associated with neurofibromatosis. Diagnosis is made by radiography or CT.

DEVELOPMENTAL ANOMALIES OF THE CEREBELLUM

In the Chiari malformation, the cerebellar hemispheres that remain in the posterior fossa are frequently hypoplastic. On microscopic examination, the cerebellum often shows disorganization of the normal lamination with the Purkinje cells being heterotopic or focally absent.

Complete cerebellar aplasia is a rare condition. It is believed to result from destruction of

the cerebellum, rather than representing a true aplasia (426). However, molecular genetic manipulations in mice demonstrate that global cerebellar hypoplasia results from homozygous deletion of the *Wnt-1*, *En-1*, or both genes, and *En-2* defective expression results in cerebellar hypoplasia with differentiation of a small amount of cerebellar cortex. Whether these same mechanisms are operative in humans remains speculative, but it seems likely that they account for at least some cases, perhaps the majority, of isolated cerebellar hypoplasias and aplasias, and especially if cerebellar aplasia is associated with agenesis of other structures derived from rhombomere 1, the midbrain and upper pons (metencephalon).

Cerebellar Hypoplasias

Under *cerebellar hypoplasias* are grouped several entities in which the cerebellum does not achieve its full developmental potential. Cerebellar hypoplasia can be categorized as global or as selective for the vermis or the lateral hemispheres.

Global hypoplasia of the cerebellum can be caused by a variety of endogenous or exogenous factors. It is seen as an autosomal recessive trait, in a variety of chromosomal disorders, and as a result of intrauterine exposure to drugs or irradiation. Patients with the autosomal recessive condition demonstrate a small cerebellum with an atrophic cerebellar cortex. Granule cells are markedly reduced or absent. Purkinje cells can be normal or can demonstrate a variety of abnormalities. Clinically, children present with delayed development, generalized muscular hypotonia, fixation nystagmus, esotropia, and in the more severe cases, microcephaly and a seizure disorder (427). Ataxia and intention tremor were seen in all such patients reported by Sarnat and Alcalá (428). Migrational disorders of the cerebral cortex frequently accompany this condition (429). Two syndromes of an autosomal recessive form of pontocerebellar hypoplasia have been reported. One type is accompanied by anterior horn cell degeneration similar to that seen in infantile spinal muscular atrophy, the other is marked by progressive microcephaly and extrapyramidal movements appearing during the first year of life (430).

Aplasia of the Vermis

Selective aplasia of the vermis results from a variety of teratogens acting on the brain during the seventh to eighth week of gestation, a time when the neural folds of the developing cerebellum meet in the midline to enclose the fourth ventricle and form the vermis (431). Hypoplasia of the cerebellar vermis occurs sporadically, as an autosomal dominant trait (432), or as Joubert syndrome, an autosomal recessive condition. Since its first description in 1969 by Joubert and coworkers (433), this disorder has been reported from all parts of the world. Patients usually present in infancy with respiratory irregularities, notably hyperpnea alternating with apnea. These were seen in 44% of subjects in the series of Kendall and colleagues (434). Abnormal eye movements, notably nystagmus and impaired supranuclear control, were seen in 67%. Reduced visual acuity or retinal dystrophy were seen in 44%. Cyclic conjugate lateral deviation of the eyes accompanied by head turning also has been described (435). Hypotonia and mental retardation are common, as are polycystic kidneys and congenital anomalies of the extremities.

Selective aplasia of the vermis may leave a CSF-filled extension of the subarachnoid space that separates the medial borders of the preserved lateral hemispheres, as in Joubert syndrome, or may be associated with fusion of the medial wall of the hemispheres and of the dentate nuclei that obliterates this space and also causes the fourth ventricle to be shallow and distorted. This latter condition is termed *rhombencephalosynapsis* and is most often a cerebellar component of the forebrain malformation septo-optic-pituitary dysplasia, but not of holoprosencephaly. The condition occasionally is associated with the Chiari III malformation (394). Children present with cerebellar deficits and mental retardation of variable severity (426,429).

Partial or complete absence of the vermis can be visualized by neuroimaging or on pathologic examination. In some cases the cerebellar folia

are normal, in others the hemispheres are hypoplastic with hypomyelination of cerebellar white matter. The brainstem is often hypoplastic with absence of the pyramidal decussations, and a variety of abnormalities at the cervicomedullary junction (434). Commonly, an associated atrophy of the cerebral hemispheres occurs. Diagnosis of the condition is best made by MRI. In some cases the secondary enlargement of the cisterna magna bears some resemblance to the Dandy-Walker syndrome (436).

A rare, sporadic malformation in which hypoplasia of the vermis is associated with an occipital encephalocele and ventrolateral dislocation of the hypoplastic cerebellar hemispheres has been termed *inverse cerebellum* or *tecto-cerebellar dysraphia*. Hydrocephalus, microcephaly, agyria, and dysplasia of the corpus callosum are associated findings (437).

The Dandy-Walker syndrome, which, in part, is characterized by complete or partial agenesis of the vermis, is covered in another section of this chapter.

Aplasia of the Cerebellar Hemispheres

Selective agenesis of the cerebellar hemispheres with preservation of the vermis is associated with secondary degeneration of cerebellofugal and cerebellipetal tracts, abnormalities in the basal ganglia, microcephaly, and mental retardation (437). Generalized disorganization of the cerebellar cortex usually is accompanied by such major cerebral malformations as holoprosencephaly. Because migration of the external granular layer of the cerebellum continues into the second year of postnatal life, focal dysplasias of the cerebellum can result from either prenatal or perinatal insults. When the dysplasias are prenatal, they are marked by heterotopias of undifferentiated neuroepithelial cells and hypertrophy and proliferation of the cells of the cerebellar cortex.

The condition known as *cerebellar hypertrophy, dysplastic gangliocytoma of the cerebellum,* or *Lhermitte-Duclos syndrome* manifests as a cerebellar tumor. It is covered in Chapter 10, although it is really a malformation and not a true neoplasm.

DEVELOPMENTAL ANOMALIES OF THE BASE OF THE SKULL AND UPPER CERVICAL VERTEBRAE

Platybasia

Platybasia is a term sometimes applied to a familial disorder characterized by a deformity of the osseous structures at the base of the skull that produces an upward displacement of the floor of the posterior fossa and a narrowing of the foramen magnum. The condition is transmitted as an autosomal dominant trait with occasional lack of penetrance (438). In the Chiari Malformations section, the diagnosis of platybasia in young infants should be made cautiously, as it also represents a normal transitory developmental stage.

As a rule, neurologic symptoms do not appear until the second or third decade of life. When they do, they are progressive and are caused by compression of the cervical spinal cord. Commonly, they include progressive spasticity, incoordination, and nystagmus with lower cranial nerve palsies. Platybasia can be associated with other malformations of the CNS, including the Chiari malformations and aqueductal stenosis.

The diagnosis is suggested by a short neck and a low hair line. It is confirmed by radiography of the skull and upper cervical spine. These reveal an odontoid process that extends above a line drawn from the dorsal lip of the foramen magnum to the dorsal margin of the hard palate.

Treatment is by surgical decompression of the posterior fossa and upper cervical cord (439).

Klippel-Feil Syndrome

Klippel-Feil syndrome, first described in 1912 by Klippel and Feil (440), is characterized by a fusion or reduction in the number of cervical vertebrae. The embryonic defect is a failure of segmentation of the chordamesoderm and its derivative sclerotomes that ultimately go on to form the cervical vertebrae. In most cases the syndrome appears sporadically; in isolated families an autosomal dominant transmission has been recorded.

On examination, affected children have a short neck and a low hairline. Passive and active movements of the neck are limited. Neurologic symptoms are variable. Progressive paraplegia owing to compression of the cervical cord can appear early in life. Some children are retarded or show learning deficits. An association with mirror movements has been reported. It could reflect the *soft signs* seen in children with mild intellectual

TABLE 4.14. *Unusual congenital defects of the cranial nerves and related structures*

Condition	Effects	Reference
Marcus Gunn syndrome	Eyelid lifts when jaw is opened and closes when jaw is closed, or vice versa	Falls et al. (788)
Duane syndrome	Fibrosis of one or both lateral rectus muscles results in retraction of the globe on adduction of the eye	Duane (789)
Congenital optic nerve hypoplasia	Congenitally small and atrophic disks; poor vision, diminished pupillary light response; occasionally accompanied by hypopituitarism	Margalith et al. (790), Skarf and Hoyt (791)
Congenital nystagmus	Rapid and fine nystagmus, often pendular; head often turned so that eyes are in the position of least nystagmus, may be dominant or sex-linked recessive trait	
Congenital anomaly of facial nerve	Weakness associated with deformities of ipsilateral ear	Dickinson et al. (792)
Congenital hypoplasia of depressor of anguli oris	Asymmetric face when crying; may have associated congenital heart disease, genitourinary or skeletal anomalies	Nelson and Eng (793)
CHARGE syndrome	Congenital anomaly of facial nerve, arhinencephaly, coupled with coloboma of iris, congenital heart disease, choanal atresia, mental retardation, genital hypoplasia, ear anomalies	Pagon et al. (794)

TABLE 4.15. *Common causes for profound hearing loss in childhood*

Condition	Associated anomalies	Incidence (% of total deaf children)	Reference
Genetically determined			
Clinically undifferentiated			
Autosomal recessive	None	25.4	Fraser (784)
Autosomal dominant	None	12.2	
Sex-linked	None	1.7	Parker (785)
Autosomal recessive syndromes			
Pendred syndrome	Sporadic goiter	5.6	
Usher syndrome	Retinitis pigmentosa, impaired vestibular function, ataxia	1.2	Konigsmark (774)
Surdocardiac syndrome	Syncopal attacks, impaired cardiac conduction	0.7	Jervell and Lange-Nielson (786)
Autosomal dominant syndromes			
Waardenburg syndrome	Widely spaced median canthi, flat nasal root, white forelock, heterochromia iridis	<1	Waardenburg (778)
Wildervanck syndrome	Klippel-Feil anomalies, osseous malformations of labyrinth, cleft palate, abducens palsy, female/male ratio 10:1	<1	Wildervanck (787)
Malformations			
Malformations of middle ear	Defective embryogenesis of first and second branchial arches, conductive and sensorineural hearing loss	1.8	
	Ear pits, preaurical tubercle, malformed ears; conductive and sensorineural hearing loss		
Prenatally acquired			
Rubella	Cataracts, congenital heart disease, microcephaly	8.0	
Syphilis		Rare	
Toxoplasmosis			
Drug ingestion (streptomycin, quinine)			
Perinatally acquired	Associated cerebral palsy, rarely associated kernicterus	16.0	
Postnatally acquired			
Head injury	Variable	22.9	
Meningitis	Variable		
"Mild" virus infections	Often unilateral		

Adapted from Fraser GR. The causes of profound deafness in childhood. In: Worstenholme GE, Knight J, eds. *Sensorineural hearing loss. A CIBA Foundation Symposium.* London: J. & A. Churchill, 1970:5–40. With permission.

deficits, or result from an inadequate decussation of the pyramidal tracts or dorsal closure of the cord (441). Associated malformations are common and include spina bifida, syringomyelia, and fibrosis of the lateral rectus muscle of the eye (Duane syndrome) (Table 4.14). The constellation of Klippel-Feil syndrome, congenital sensorineural hearing loss, and abducens palsy is known as the Wildervanck syndrome (Table 4.15). Wildervanck syndrome is limited to female subjects, suggesting that the condition is lethal in the hemizygous male subject. Klippel-Feil syndrome also can be accompanied by congenital heart disease (442,443).

The diagnosis of Klippel-Feil syndrome rests on radiographic demonstration of fused cervical or cervicothoracic vertebrae, hemivertebrae, or atlanto-occipital fusion. MRI can demonstrate compression of the cervical cord, syringomyelia, or other CNS anomalies.

With clinical evidence for compression of the cervical cord, laminectomy is indicated.

Cleidocranial Dysostosis

Cleidocranial dysostosis is transmitted as an autosomal dominant trait and is characterized by rudimentary clavicles, a broad head, delayed or defective closure of the anterior fontanelle, mental deficiency, and a variety of cerebral malformations (444). Other skeletal malformations are common. These include spina bifida, short and wide fingers, and delayed ossification of the pelvis.

ANTERIOR MIDLINE DEFECTS (FACIOTELENCEPHALOPATHY)

Holoprosencephaly

Just as anencephaly is the most catastrophic dysraphism, so holoprosencephaly is the most devastating of the anterior anomalies. Holoprosencephaly is a defect of ventralizing induction of the forebrain or prosencephalon by the prechordal mesoderm, and a defective expression of the transcription product of the gene *Sonic hedgehog* (*Shh*) has been shown to be the responsible molecular event, both in animal models and in humans (445,446). As a consequence, the formation of a median fissure and the development of paired telencephalic hemispheres from the prosencephalon fail (447). The defect in cleavage continues to influence subsequent cerebral development. This accounts for the associated defect in the formation of the corpus callosum, and the various migrational abnormalities. Like anencephaly, the dysplasia is time specific and stimulus nonspecific. Normally, cleavage of the hemispheres occurs at 33 days' gestation. Thus, of the major induction malformations, holoprosencephaly has the shortest vulnerable period.

Holoprosencephaly may result from multiple genetic defects. *Shh* expression can be altered in inborn metabolic diseases of cholesterol synthesis, notably, in the Smith-Lemli-Opitz syndrome in which the conversion of the cholesterol precursor, 7-dehydrocholesterol, to cholesterol is defective. In this condition, which is frequently accompanied by holoprosencephaly, the *Shh* protein product undergoes autoproteolysis to form a cholesterol-modified active product (448) (see Chapter 1). In other cases of holoprosencephaly, a mutation of the zinc-finger gene *Zic2* occurs. Because this genetic defect is associated with 13q deletions, it may be the cause of holoprosencephaly in infants with 13 trisomy (449).

Holoprosencephaly generally is sporadic. In Japan, the incidence is 0.4% of aborted fetuses and 6 in 10,000 live-born babies (450). A variety of chromosomal abnormalities are linked with holoprosencephaly. Aside from trisomy of chromosome 13, these include a partial deletion of the long arm of chromosome 13, ring chromosome 13, trisomy of chromosome 18, partial deletion of the short arm of chromosome 18, ring chromosome 18, and partial trisomy of chromosome 7 (451,452) (see Chapter 3). The malformation also is associated with such maternal disorders as diabetes mellitus, syphilis, cytomegalic inclusion disease, and toxoplasmosis (453). The risk of recurrence in siblings of affected patients is 6%. If a chromosomal anomaly is identified, the risk for recurrence is 2%, but is higher should the mother be older than 35 years of age (454). Second to chromosomal disorders, maternal diabetes mellitus, including gestational diabetes, is the most common condition associated with holoprosencephaly.

An autosomal dominant form of holoprosencephaly has been well described. The gene for this disorder has been localized to the telomeric region of the long arm of chromosome 7 (7q36.2) and has been shown to be associated with defective expression of *Shh* (418,455). In several reported families with this disorder, penetrance has been 88%, with mental retardation representing a mild expression of the defect (456). In rare instances, holoprosencephaly has been transmitted as an autosomal recessive condition (457).

Holoprosencephaly has been recognized in various degrees of severity (458,459). In its most complete expression (alobar holoprosencephaly), the brain is characterized by a single midline ventricular cavity encompassed within an undivided prosencephalic vesicle (Fig. 4.6). The thalamus

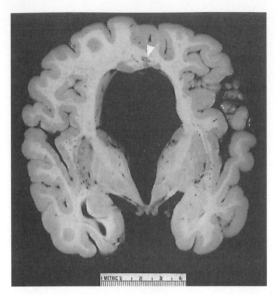

FIG. 4.6. Holoprosencephaly. In this coronal section, note the common lateral and third ventricles. Midline fusion of the frontal lobes is seen in the absence of the interhemispheric fissure. Note the subependymal heterotopias at the usual location of the corpus callosum (*arrowhead*). These may give rise to seizure foci. (Courtesy of Dr. Hideo H. Itabashi, Department of Pathology, Los Angeles County Harbor Medical Center.)

remains undivided, the inferior frontal and temporal regions are often absent, and the remainder of the isocortex is rudimentary, with only the primary motor and sensory cortex present. The olfactory diverticula and rhinencephalon are absent, but the brainstem and cerebellum are present and fully differentiated. Minor focal dysplasias of the cerebellar cortex may be present, however. Gray matter heterotopia and agenesis of the septum pellucidum result from abnormal cellular migration (460). The lamination and general architecture of the cortex is abnormal, and extensive sites of overmigration occur beyond the limits of the pia mater into the leptomeninges. Some of these overmigrated nodules become isolated from the brain as ectopia, and others remain attached to the cerebral surface or connected by a stalk. These nodules are sometimes known by the ignoble term *brain warts*. In holoprosencephaly, absence or severe deficiency occurs of the external granular layer of Brun, a transient layer of glial cells at the cerebral

cortical surface during the stage of radial migrations. Its absence could account for the failure to limit overmigration (461).

The clinical picture of this condition is highlighted by midline facial abnormalities, which are seen in the large majority of children with alobar holoprosencephaly and in many cases with milder forms of holoprosencephaly (462). The clinical and imaging classification of holoprosencephaly into alobar, semilobar, and lobar forms probably reflects the degree of genetic deficiency and how far caudally in the neural tube the underexpression extends, rather than fundamental differences in pathogenesis. In alobar holoprosencephaly, the neurologic picture is characterized by severe to profound mental retardation, seizures, rigidity, apnea, and temperature imbalance. Hydrocephalus can develop as a consequence of aqueductal obstruction, and associated hypothalamic or pituitary malformation can induce endocrine disorders. Diagnostic studies should include facial radiography to show deformed anterior craniobasal bones, cytogenetics, and MRI for definitive evaluation of the CNS abnormalities. The EEG, visual-evoked potentials, and auditory-evoked potentials are generally abnormal. When the patient has many extracephalic abnormalities, a chromosomal anomaly is likely, whereas in their absence the karyotype is usually normal.

Other Faciotelencephalopathies

Numerous other forms of partial fusion of the cerebral hemispheres have been described. In semilobar holoprosencephaly, an incomplete hemispheric fissure is seen posteriorly, and the occipital lobes and the occipital horns of the lateral ventricles are fairly normal. In lobar holoprosencephaly partial fusion of the hemispheres occurs frontally, with complete separation occipitally. The clinical hallmarks of this group of anomalies are a median cleft in the frontonasal portion of the face, and the absence or hypoplasia of the intermaxillary segment. These result in a spectrum of facies, ranging from cyclopia through ethmocephaly and cebocephaly to its mildest expression, orbital hypotelorism with a midline cleft lip, a hypoplastic intermaxillary region, or both (463). Skeletal changes include anomalous development of the orbital, nasal, maxillary, and ethmoid bones. A single central incisor has been observed in approximately 25% of the autosomal dominant form of holoprosencephaly (456). As a rule, the severity of facial anomalies reflects the severity of the cerebral malformations (i.e., the face predicts the brain) (464).

In cyclopia, the face is marked by a single median orbital fossa and eye with a protruding, noselike appendage above the orbit. Other dysplastic features include polydactyly and cardiac and digestive tract anomalies. Hypotelorism, a median cleft lip, and a nose that lacks its bridge, columella, or septum almost always denote some degree of holoprosencephaly, even if not associated with any of the aforementioned major anomalies (451,463). The diagnosis of hypotelorism should be based on formal measurements of the interpupillary, interorbital, and intercanthal distances (465).

In cebocephaly the nose is laid down on its side and orbital hypotelorism is seen (466). Many patients have a fairly normal neocortex and often survive with little or no neurologic dysfunction. Some, however, have a fully developed holoprosencephaly with severe neurologic impairment, and they often exhibit abnormal karyotypes.

The term *arhinencephaly* has been used to describe a variety malformations ranging from isolated absence or hypoplasia of the olfactory bulbs and tracts, to the association of this anomaly with the various forms of holoprosencephaly (451,459). Arhinencephaly can be unilateral and associated with hemifacial microsomia and oculoauriculovertebral dysplasia (Goldenhar syndrome) (467). It also can be accompanied by hypogonadotropic hypogonadism (Kallmann syndrome) (468).

Septo-Optic-Pituitary Dysplasia

Septo-optic-pituitary dysplasia, first described in 1956 by DeMorsier (469), may represent a form of holoprosencephaly. It is also possible that it is the result of a defect in dorsalizing genetic influence on the rostral end of the neural tube from genes such as *Pax-2* and *Pax-5*, rather than a defect in the ventralizing *Sonic hedgehog*. Septo-optic-pituitary dysplasia includes agenesis of the septum pellucidum, hypoplasia of the optic nerves and chiasm with resultant blindness or severe visual impairment, hypoplasia of the infundibulum with growth hormone deficiency and short stature, and in approximately one-third of children, diabetes insipidus (470,471). Although growth hormone deficiency is the most common isolated posterior pituitary insufficiency in septo-optic-pituitary dysplasia, some patients have panhypopituitarism. Endocrine function, therefore, should be evaluated in all children in whom the diagnosis is confirmed by imaging. Psychomotor function can be preserved (472). Optic nerve hypoplasia can occur in the absence of any other developmental anomaly, and as such it is a relatively common congenital anomaly (473). The condition is reviewed by Zeki and Dutton (474). The insult responsible for septo-optic-pituitary dysplasia probably begins at approximately 37 days' gestation, though underexpression of an organizer gene would begin even earlier. A variety of causes have been recorded, including maternal diabetes, maternal anticonvulsant intake, and cytomegalic inclusion disease (475). Additionally, optic nerve hypoplasia is seen in conjunction with the Klippel-Trenaunay-Weber syndrome, chondrodysplasia punctata, and Kallmann syndrome (hypogonadotropic hypogonadism) (475,476).

Noncleft Median Face Syndrome

Noncleft median face syndrome includes several syndromes familiar to pediatricians, such as Treacher Collins syndrome, Crouzon disease, and Apert syndrome. It also embraces the chromosomal trisomies 18 and 21. The facial deformities are mild but stereotyped, characterized by mongoloid and antimongoloid slants, and abnormally spaced eyes (hypertelorism or hypotelorism). In a significant proportion of cases, pathologic examination or neuroimaging studies of the brain reveal maldevelopment of the neocortex with frequent migration anomalies causing defective cortical lamination, and occasional failure of inductive diverticulation.

DISORDERS OF CELLULAR MIGRATION AND PROLIFERATION (1 TO 7 MONTHS' GESTATION)

Although disorders of organ induction are known to produce secondary histogenic migration or proliferation anomalies, this section confines itself to those disorders of cellular migration that are unassociated with defects of embryogenesis. Over the last few years, MRI has permitted diagnosis of these conditions during the lifetime of the affected child, and it is becoming apparent that their incidence is much greater than had previously been estimated. Barth and Barkovich and coworkers have published reviews of these various disorders (477,478).

The various conditions associated with migration defects are listed in Table 4.16. They include the phakomatoses; a variety of metabolic, genetic, and chromosomal syndromes; and maternal and environmental causes.

Migratory disorders develop when neuroblasts of the subventricular zone (i.e., the germinal matrix), which forms the wall of the lateral ventricles, fail to reach their intended destination in the cerebral cortex. This results in focal or generalized structural deformities of the cerebral hemispheres. These are discussed in sequence of their ontogenetic chronology.

Schizencephaly

Schizencephaly is characterized by clefts placed symmetrically within the cerebral hemispheres and extending from the cortical surface to the underlying ventricular cavity (Figs. 4.7 and 4.8) (314,479). The walls of the cleft may be in apposition or separated. The cerebral cortex that surrounds the cleft may be normal or show areas of polymicrogyria. This suggests that in many instances schizencephaly results from pathogenetic processes similar to those that cause polymicrogyria, but are more extensive and involve the entire thickness of the developing cerebral hemispheres (480).

A mutation of the homeobox gene *EMX-2* has been identified in schizencephaly (481,482). This mutation does not account for all cases, however, and some are not really primary devel-

TABLE 4.16. *Conditions associated with neuronal migration disorders[a]*

Metabolic diseases
Zellweger disease
Neonatal adrenoleukodystrophy
Glutaric aciduria, type II
Kinky hair disease
GM_2 gangliosidosis
Chromosomal anomalies
Trisomy 13
Trisomy 18
Trisomy 21
Deletion 4p
Deletion 17p13 (Miller-Dieker syndrome)
Neuromuscular disease
Walker-Warburg syndrome
Fukuyama muscular dystrophy
Myotonic dystrophy
Anterior horn arthrogryposis
Neurocutaneous syndromes
Incontinentia pigmenti
Neurofibromatosis
Hypermelanosis of Ito
Encephalocraniocutanous lipomatosis (499)
Tuberous sclerosis
Epidermal nevus syndrome (500)
Multiple congenital anomalies syndromes
Smith-Lemli-Opitz syndrome
Potter syndrome (501)
Cornelia de Lange syndrome
Meckel-Gruber syndrome
Orofacial-digital syndrome
Coffin-Siris syndrome
Other syndromes
Thanatophoric dysplasia (502)
Pachygyria and congenital nephrosis (503)
Aicardi syndrome
Joubert syndrome
Hemimegalencephaly
Maternal and environmental causes
Infection
Cytomegalovirus
Intoxication
Carbon monoxide
Isoretinoic acid (504)
Fetal alcohol syndrome
Methylmercury
Ionizing radiation

[a]Reference citations are given for syndromes not covered in this textbook.

Adapted from Barth P. Disorders of neuronal migration. *Can J Neurol Sci* 1987;14:1–16. With permission.

opmental malformations at all, but occur secondary to porencephaly or other encephaloclastic lesions acquired during midfetal life (461).

Schizencephaly should be distinguished from a porencephalic cyst caused by a variety of vascular or infectious insults to the brain during late fetal or early infantile life (314). A poren-

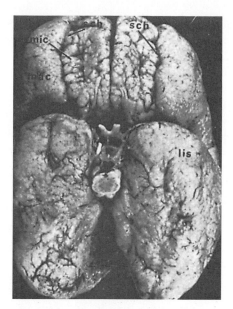

FIG. 4.7. Schizencephaly (sch). Ventral view of the brain in a severely retarded 10-year-old boy. In addition to the symmetric clefts in the orbital walls of the frontal lobes, the brain also shows failure of sulcation (lissencephaly, lis) and microgyria (mic) of the frontal lobes. (From Yakovlev PI, Wadsworth RC. Schizencephalies. A study of the congenital clefts in the cerebral mantle. *J Neuropathol Exp Neurol* 1946;5:116, 169. With permission.)

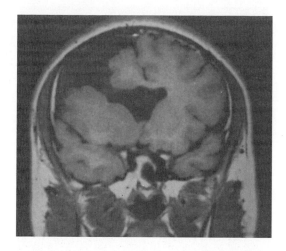

FIG. 4.8. Schizencephaly. T1-weighted magnetic resonance imaging study of a 17-year-old subject with seizures and mild developmental delay. Coronal images reveal a large unilateral cleft, lined with cortex. (Courtesy of Dr. A. J. Barkovich, Department of Radiology, University of California, San Francisco.)

cephalic cyst results from the dissolution of necrotic regions of brain, with cavitation and cyst formation within the parenchyma of the cerebral hemispheres. Porencephalic cysts might or might not communicate with the ventricular system or with the cerebral cortical surface. Occasionally, they act as a space-occupying lesion, causing symptoms of increased intracranial pressure (483). Most important, they are asymmetric, not aligned with the primary fissures, and unassociated with major cerebral migration defects.

The clinical picture of schizencephaly is characterized by a wide range of neurologic and developmental defects. Epilepsy may be the most serious complication and seizures often are the presenting symptom. Hypotonia, hemiparesis, or spastic quadriparesis can be accompanied by a seizure disorder and microcephaly. Imaging studies usually show bilateral, symmet-

ric, or asymmetric clefts (484,485). On clinical grounds porencephaly differs from schizencephaly in that the patient frequently has a well-documented history of a destructive insult to the brain, and neurologic deficits are often focal, asymmetric, or silent and compatible with relatively normal development. Unlike schizencephaly, a porencephalic cyst can occur as a one-way ball valve-type communication with the ventricular system. It can enlarge progressively and behave like an expanding lesion impinging on the ventricular system to produce hydrocephalus (305).

Lissencephaly (Agyria-Pachygyria, Macrogyria)

Lissencephaly, a term coined by Owen in 1868, literally means *smooth brain*. The term is used synonymously with agyria. In pachygyria (macrogyria), the pathology is less severe than that in lissencephaly and areas of normal laminar organization are seen. Lissencephaly and pachygyria may occur together in the same

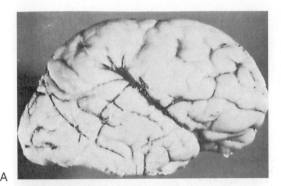

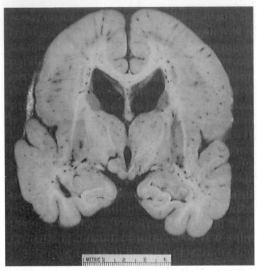

FIG. 4.9. Lissencephaly (agyria). **A:** External view of the brain. Note the severe degree of diffuse pachygyria with a large area of frontoparietal agyria from a 6½-year-old with marked hypotonia, profound retardation, and minor motor seizures. Microscopic examination of the brain showed an abnormally laminated cortex in the temporoparietal and occipital regions, abnormally formed neurons, almost complete loss of Purkinje cells, and loss of granule cells in cerebellum. (From Druckman R, et al. A case of atonic cerebral diplegia with lissencephaly. *Neurology* 1959;9:806. With permission.) **B:** Coronal section of another brain showing the typical deep cortical mantle and sparse central white matter. The mediotemporal areas show a cortical ribbon of normal appearance. The deep nuclei are grossly intact. (Courtesy Dr. Hideo H. Itabashi, Department of Pathology, Los Angeles County Harbor Medical Center.)

brain and are not mutually exclusive, but represent degrees of the same fundamental disorder in cell migration and cortical organization.

In lissencephaly the cerebral hemispheres approximate the smooth 24-month fetal cerebral cortex, with the absence of secondary sulci. The condition results from a migratory defect believed to occur between 12 and 16 weeks' gestation. The insult, whatever it may have been, prevents succeeding waves of migrating neurons from reaching their destined positions in the cerebral cortex. Thus, gray matter heterotopia, macrogyria, polymicrogyria, and schizencephaly, together with defective cortical lamination, often accompany this condition (Fig. 4.9) (486).

Two major types of lissencephaly have been defined by pathologic examination of the brain, and by MRI (477,487). In the Miller-Dieker syndrome, classical or type I lissencephaly (Figs. 4.10A and B), a point mutation and microdeletion of the *LIS1* gene occurs at the 17p13.3 locus (488–490). The *LIS1* gene is strongly expressed in Cajal-Retzius neurons and periventricular neuroepithelium and is essential for the normal course of radial migration (491). Intracellular levels of the *LIS1* protein correlate well with clinical and imaging findings (492). The precise genetic defect in lissencephaly type II has not yet been identified.

Pathologic examination of the brain in lissencephaly type I reveals that the cortex is four layered. Layer 1 corresponds to the molecular layer; layer 2 contains neurons of the normal layers III, V, and VI; layer 3 is cell sparse, possibly representing persistence of the fetal subplate zone; and layer 4 is thick and extends almost to the ependyma from which it is separated by a band of white matter (493). This layer contains heterotopic, incompletely migrated neurons (486).

Lissencephaly type II is characterized by an almost complete absence of cortical layering. Instead, vascular bundles and fibroglia tissue are seen perpendicular to the surface. These penetrate the brain from the thickened meninges and separate the cortex into glomeruluslike nests of neurons. Hydrocephalus often accompanies lissencephaly type II. It results from meningeal

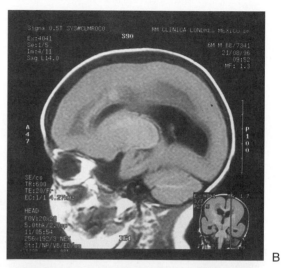

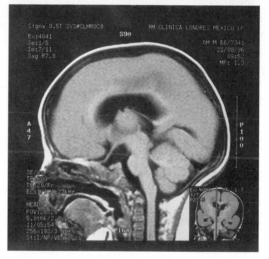

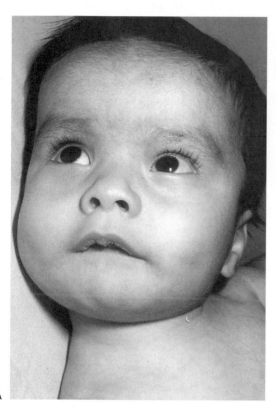

FIG. 4.10. A 7-month-old boy with Miller-Dieker syndrome. **A:** The face shows characteristic features of a high forehead, long philtrum of the upper lip and upturned nares; **B:** midsagittal; and **C:** parasagittal T1-weighted magnetic resonance imaging showing lissencephaly with grossly well-formed brainstem and cerebellum. The corpus callosum is thin. Lateral ventricles are mildly dilated and the subarachnoid spaces over the cerebral hemispheres and brainstem cisternae are wide. (Courtesy of Dr. Laura Flores Dinorin, Instituto Nacional de Pediatría, Mexico City, Mexico.)

thickening that obliterates the subarachnoid space around the brainstem and at the base of the brain (436).

Although the lissencephalies were previously considered to be rare, they are now more readily diagnosable with MRI studies (Fig. 4.11). Lissencephaly type I is the most common and accounted for 43% of the lissencephalies in the series of Aicardi. Pachygyria was seen in 26%, and lissencephaly type II in 14% of all lissencephalies (493). The clinical picture of complete lissencephaly type I is homogenous. All patients have profound mental retardation, marked hypotonia (hypotonic cerebral palsy), and seizures. These may include massive myoclonus and tonic seizures, which often are

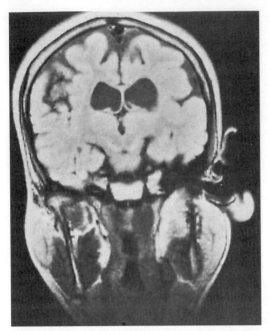

FIG. 4.11. Lissencephaly. T1-weighted magnetic resonance imaging study shows a number of anomalies. These include areas of total absence of gyri (lissencephaly), areas of large, broad gyri (pachygyria), and abnormal sulcation of the right parietal operculum. The left parietal operculum is also abnormal in that the sylvian fissure is enlarged. This 19-year-old man has had a long-standing seizure disorder, characterized by grand mal and atonic seizures, resistant to anti-convulsant therapy. He is functioning in the borderline range.

tion, by which time the primary sulci have already become elaborated. Thus, secondary sulcation is abortive and tertiary sulcation is prevented. Other migrational anomalies are associated, and the clinical picture is similar to that seen in lissencephaly type I, but less severe. Because the anomalies tend to be more asymmetric, the neurologic deficits are often lateralized (see Chapter 5). Areas of focal cortical dysplasia frequently act as an epileptic focus giving rise to focal clonic seizures or focal myoclonus. These architectonic abnormalities can now be visualized by MRI (Fig. 4.13) (497).

Lissencephaly type II is seen in the Walker-Warburg syndrome, an autosomal recessive disorder characterized by the additional features of hydrocephalus, retinal, or other ocular malformations, and the occasional presence of an occipital encephalocele. Most patients with this condition die before 2 years of age. The underlying cause of this type of lissencephaly is still a matter of dispute. Genetic or inflammatory processes are believed to be operative. Other syndromes associated with lissencephaly type II include muscle-eye-brain disease of Santavuori, most common in Finland, and the Fukuyama type of muscular dystrophy, almost exclusively limited to the Japanese population.

Although lissencephaly is seen in the Miller-Dieker syndrome (495) (see Chapter 3), only 5% of infants demonstrated this chromosomal anomaly in Aicardi series (493). The malformation also can be seen after cytomegalovirus infection and in a variety of other, rarer syndromes. These are listed in Table 4.16 and in a review by Dobyns and coworkers (498).

preceded by infantile spasms. In 76% of cases, the EEG shows high-amplitude (300 μv) 10- to 16-Hz rhythms (493). Microcephaly was present in approximately one-half of subjects in the series of Gastaut and coworkers (494). The high frequency of seizures, particularly infantile spasms, was also noted by Alvarez and his group (495).

In pachygyria, the MRI study shows an abnormally thick cortex, with white matter not penetrating into the convolutions. The whole hemisphere can be involved, the pachygyric areas can be unilateral, as in hemimegalencephaly (496), or restricted to the opercular area (Fig. 4.12). The toxic stimuli that induce macrogyria can occur up to the fifth month of gesta-

Polymicrogyria

Polymicrogyria results from an insult to the nervous system sustained before the fifth month of gestation. The affected brain resembles a chestnut kernel and is characterized by an excess of secondary and tertiary sulci, resulting in gyri that are too small and too numerous (Fig. 4.14). In addition to the gyral anomalies, polymicrogyria is characterized by other migrational defects, gray matter heterotopia, defective cortical cell polarization, and abnormal cellular lam-

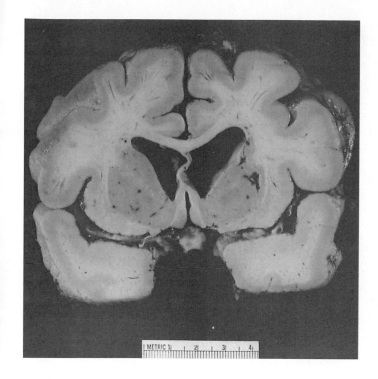

FIG. 4.12. Pachygyria (macrogyria). This developmental disturbance of the convolutional pattern has thickened and irregular convolutions. Note the scarcity of sulci, especially in the temporal lobes. This patient survived for many years. (Courtesy of Dr. Hideo H. Itabashi, Department of Pathology, Los Angeles County Harbor Medical Center.)

ination. Microscopically, the brain resembles that of a 4- to 6-month-old fetus. Layering abnormalities are generally present and tend to be of two types. In one type, four cellular layers of cerebral cortex occur, compared with the normal six, and the layering is irregular and more columnar than laminar. The reduced number of migrating cells results in a decreased amount of white matter and in hypoplastic pyramidal tracts. In the other form, no layers can be discerned (477). The anomaly can be generalized or affect only focal areas of the cerebral cortex. The cerebellum also shows deformities, with a failure in the development of a normal folial pattern. Gray matter heterotopia occurs along the brainstem and cerebellar axis. The abnormal cellular architecture serves to distinguish this anomaly from microgyria seen as a consequence of perinatal destructive lesions.

The mechanism causing polymicrogyria is still under dispute (477). Barth suggests that early fetal accidents, possibly ischemic cortical damage, at 13 to 16 weeks' gestation cause the unlayered form of polymicrogyria, whereas late

fetal accidents occurring between 20 and 24 weeks cause four-layered polymicrogyria. Other cases clearly are primary malformations.

The clinical picture in polymicrogyria is generally one of mental retardation and spasticity, or hypotonia with active deep tendon reflexes (hypotonic cerebral palsy; see Chapter 5). The important role of focal polymicrogyria in producing an intractable seizure disorder has become evident by neuroimaging studies. In particular, a syndrome of opercular polymicrogyria has been delineated. In addition to seizures, patients present with mental retardation, dysarthria, abnormal tongue movements, and dysphagia (505). Polymicrogyria is seen in the insular and opercular region, and at times the malformation extends to involve the parietal and the superior temporal region. Guerrini and colleagues have described a syndrome of symmetric parasagittal parieto-occipital polymicrogyria. The condition manifests by seizures and mild developmental delay. The lesion is located in the watershed vascular territory between the anterior cerebral artery and the posterior cere-

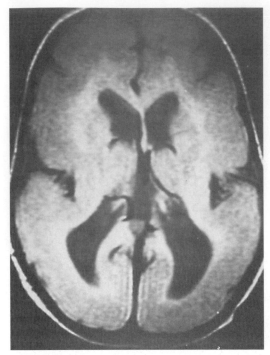

FIG. 4.13. Pachygyria. T1-weighted magnetic resonance imaging study of a 4-month-old infant presenting with seizures. Axial image demonstrates thickening of gray matter and thinning of white matter in this patient with lissencephaly. Pachygyria is present in the frontal lobes with agyria in the temporoparieto-occipital region. The distribution of the more severely affected regions posteriorly and the less severely affected anteriorly suggests a vascular component to this anomaly. (Courtesy of Dr. A. J. Barkovich, Department of Radiology, University of California, San Francisco.)

bral artery, and the authors have suggested that it is the consequence of perfusion failure occurring between the 20th and 24th weeks' of gestation (506). The predisposition of the opercular region to polymicrogyria has been confirmed by other groups and by our clinical experience (507,508).

MRI sometimes diagnoses polymicrogyria during the patient's lifetime (Fig. 4.15) (509), but in other cases the abnormal pattern of gyration is difficult to detect by MRI and nearly impossible by CT scan. In some cases, the abnormality can be detected by demonstrating a focal area of delayed maturation of subcortical

white matter (510). The distinction between polymicrogyria and macrogyria cannot always be made by MRI. In both conditions one can see a thickened cortex with absence of detectable gyri, and the irregularities on the surface of what is believed to be a macrogyric cortex actually represent polymicrogyria. Approximately 25% of patients with polymicrogyria have abnormally prolonged T2 relaxation of the underlying white matter (509).

Subcortical Laminar Heterotopia (Band Heterotopia, Double Cortex)

Subcortical laminar heterotopia is a rare genetic disorder that is transmitted as an X-linked dominant trait, so that nearly all patients are female (511). A few male subjects have survived spontaneous fetal loss and been born live; these boys have a particularly severe form of the disorder with lissencephaly in addition (512). The defective gene and its transcription product, called *doublecortin*, have been identified (513–515).

On pathologic examination, arrested radial neuroblast migration in the cerebrum is seen, so that a layer of gray matter heterotopia forms beneath the normal surface cortex and the periventricular zone, separated from both the cortex and the subependymal region by white matter (Fig. 4.16A and B). Because of the distinctive appearance by MRI, the condition has sometimes been termed the *double cortex syndrome*, but the internal architecture of the subcortical heterotopia is not laminar as in normal cortex, although the overlying cerebral cortex has normal structure. Synaptic connections between the disorganized subcortical heterotopia and the overlying cortex probably account for the severe seizure disorder. Positron emission tomography demonstrates that the subcortical heterotopia has the same degree of glucose metabolism as the overlying true cortex (516).

Bilateral Periventricular Nodular Heterotopia

Bilateral periventricular nodular heterotopia is another X-linked dominant trait that occurs almost exclusively in girls and is expressed clinically with epilepsy and mental retardation

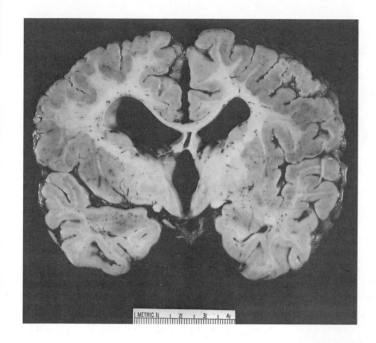

FIG. 4.14. Polymicrogyria. Coronal section of frontal lobe. Excessive secondary and tertiary sulci are present, resulting in gyri that are too small and too numerous. (Courtesy of Dr. Hideo H. Itabashi, Department of Pathology, Los Angeles County Harbor Medical Center.)

(517–521). Some, but not all, families exhibit dysmorphic facies and anomalies in the urinary tract and rectal polyps (520). Postmitotic premigratory neuroblasts of the germinal matrix fail to migrate altogether and mature in situ in the subependymal region, where they form nodules of gray matter that often protrude into the lateral ventricle and form internal connections but cannot establish the synaptic relations with cortical neurons at the surface of the brain. The surface cortex also has abnormal architecture, however, which probably accounts for the severe epilepsy (521). The diagnosis is established by MRI or by neuropathologic examination. It should not be confused with subependymal glial nodules that occur as a reactive change to periventricular leukomalacia, infantile hydrocephalus, ventriculitis, congenital infections, or acquired complications of prematurity.

Agenesis of the Corpus Callosum

The corpus callosum is the largest interhemispheric commissure. Agenesis of the corpus callosum is a relatively common condition in the developmentally disabled population, with an incidence as detected by CT of 2.3% (522) (Fig. 4-17). Sarnat postulates that agenesis of the cor-

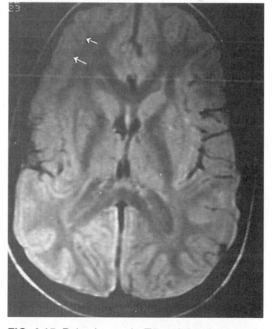

FIG. 4.15. Polymicrogyria. T2-weighted magnetic resonance imaging study of an 8-year-old child presenting with developmental delay. Axial images reveal thickening of right posterior frontal cortex (*arrows*). This region has no gyri; instead, paradoxically smooth cortex is seen, as in all cases of polymicrogyria. The normal fingerlike projections of white matter are absent. (Courtesy of Dr. A. J. Barkovich, Department of Radiology, University of California, San Francisco.)

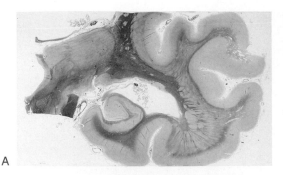

A

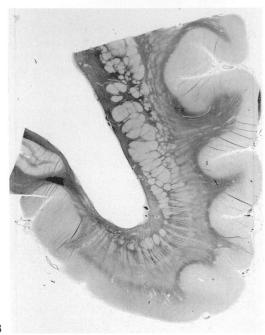

B

FIG. 4.16. Subcortical laminar heterotopia in a young adult woman with intractable epilepsy who died in status epilepticus. This is an X-linked dominant trait. Islands of nonlaminated and disorganized gray matter are found in the subcortical white matter of the **(A)** temporal and **(B)** occipital lobes, forming a *double cortex* as a second layer of gray matter beneath the "normal" cortex at the surface and separated from it and from the ventricular wall by white matter (Luxol fast blue/periodic acid–Schiff reaction). (Courtesy of Dr. Ellsworth C. Alvord, Jr., University of Washington, Seattle.)

pus callosum results from the failure of the programmed cell death, in this instance glial cells of the lamina terminalis that form the initial septum do not degenerate in time to permit the passage of callosal axons (67). Experimental evidence of

this mechanism is demonstrated in a murine model (523). The normally formed callosal fibers, being unable to cross the midline, are diverted to follow a path of least resistance, forming the bundle of Probst in the dorsomedial wall of the ipsilateral hemisphere, from which some fibers eventually make aberrant decussations. The anterior commissure is usually enlarged by some of these heterotopic axons. The bundle of Probst is interposed between the medial hemispheric wall and the lateral ventricle, splaying the lateral ventricles apart and giving a characteristic appearance in imaging studies.

The presence of heterotopic callosal axons that cannot cross the midline distinguishes agenesis of the corpus callosum with formation of the bundle of Probst from agenesis of the corpus callosum such as is seen in holoprosencephaly, in which callosal axons do not form. Most callosal axons in normal brains arise from the pyramidal cells of layer 3 of the cerebral cortex, unlike the corticospinal axons that originate mainly from pyramidal cells of layers 5 and 6.

Agenesis of the corpus callosum takes one of two forms. In one type, partial or complete agenesis of the corpus callosum, is accompanied solely by defects of contiguous and phylogenetically related structures. Abnormalities include a disturbance in the convolutional pattern of the medial wall of the hemisphere, which assumes a radiate arrangement. A complete or partial absence of the cingulate gyrus and of the septum pellucidum also can be observed. The most striking feature in these brains is the presence of the bundle of Probst. In this type of agenesis of the corpus callosum, significant neurologic abnormalities can be absent. If present and nonspecific, they can include seizures or mild to moderate mental retardation and impaired visual, motor, and bimanual coordination (see Fig. 4.1) (524,525).

As the corpus callosum forms from anterior to posterior, partial agenesis generally manifests by the presence of the anterior portions, the genu and body, and absence of the posterior portions, the splenium and rostrum (526). Myelination starts in the posterior portion of the corpus callosum, which begins to show increased signal on T1-weighted images at 3 to 4 months of age; the genu shows increased signal at 6 months of age (527).

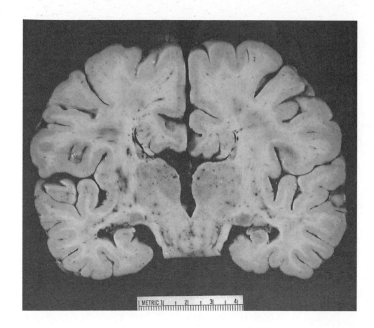

FIG. 4.17. Agenesis of corpus callosum. Coronal section of brain. In this instance, the anomaly was not accompanied by abnormalities of cellular proliferation. (Courtesy of Dr. Hideo H. Itabashi, Department of Pathology, Los Angeles County Harbor Medical Center.)

In the second form, agenesis of the corpus callosum is accompanied by numerous abnormalities of cellular proliferation, including polymicrogyria and heterotopias of gray matter. In these patients, and in families in which the trait is transmitted by one of at least two X-linked genes, severe intellectual retardation and seizures are present (528–530). The cortical anomalies are demonstrable by MRI or by positron emission tomography (529).

Agenesis of the corpus callosum accompanies a variety of chromosomal defects and the Dandy-Walker syndrome. It also was seen in 17% of patients with inherited metabolic disorders in the series of Bamforth and coworkers (531). These conditions include nonketotic hyperglycinemia, Zellweger syndrome, neonatal adrenoleukodystrophy, Menkes disease, glutaric aciduria type II, and pyruvate dehydrogenase deficiency, especially when the $E_1\alpha$ subunit is affected (532). Thus, the possibility of an inborn metabolic error should be considered in patients with agenesis of the corpus callosum.

A diminished width (hypoplasia) of the corpus callosum can be secondary to a reduced number of cortical neurons that give rise to callosal axons. This is not a developmental malformation. It may result from a variety of acquired insults and is a common consequence of supratentorial atrophy (533).

Agenesis of the corpus callosum is an integral part of Aicardi syndrome. This condition, which up to now has been described in female subjects only, is characterized by severe mental retardation, generalized tonic-clonic and myoclonic seizures that have their onset between birth and age 4 months, and chorioretinal lacunae. Hemivertebrae and costovertebral anomalies are common. In most instances, no other siblings are affected, and the syndrome is believed to result from an intrauterine insult between 4 and 12 weeks' gestation (534,535). The question as to whether an increased lethality of male fetuses occurs and the role of nonrandom inactivation of the X chromosome in the phenotypic expression of this condition remain unclarified.

Agenesis of the corpus callosum is also seen in the FG syndrome (FG stands for the initials of one of the families in which the syndrome was described). This syndrome is transmitted as an X-linked condition and is marked by the additional presence of constipation, imperforate anus, and a facial configuration highlighted by epicanthal folds and a fish-shaped (inverted V) mouth (530,536).

Colpocephaly

In colpocephaly the occipital horns of the lateral ventricles are disproportionately enlarged.

Colpocephaly can occur in association with agenesis of the posterior fibers of the corpus callosum, as a primary developmental malformation, or as an acquired lesion, a consequence of severe periventricular leukomalacia, or intrauterine infections. This acquired form is probably the most common cause of colpocephaly. The clinical picture is nonspecific. As a rule, mental retardation of variable severity and seizures occur (537). Hypertelorism can be present. The diagnosis is made by neuroimaging studies, although the condition should be distinguished from generalized ventriculomegaly in which the occipital horns are somewhat more dilated than the other portions of the ventricular system.

Cavum Septi Pellucidi

The development of the cavum septi pellucidi depends on and follows the evolution of the corpus callosum (538). The cavum is present in healthy fetal brain, in 97% of preterm infants, and in 56% of term infants (539). Its incidence diminishes further with increasing age. Persistence of its posterior extension, the cavum vergae, is less common; it is seen in only 7% of term neonates. The presence of a cavum septi pellucidi or both the cavi septi pellucidi and the cavum vergae generally represents incidental findings in healthy subjects. Less commonly, these defects occur in association with induction or migration disorders (540). A large cavum septi pellucidi more frequently occurs in brains with other dysgeneses, with generalized atrophy, or in metabolic encephalopathies, hence it should alert the clinician to investigate further (541,542). Neuroimaging studies establish the diagnosis and also may reveal associated defects of cellular proliferation and migration. Although in agenesis of the corpus callosum the cavum appears to be absent by neuroimaging, careful neuropathologic studies disclose that the leaves of the septum pellucidum are actually displaced laterally and adhere to the widely separated medial walls of the lateral ventricles.

MICROCEPHALY

Microcephaly has in the past been defined by a head circumference, as measured around the fore- head and the occipital protuberance, that is more than two standard deviations below the mean for age, sex, and race (see Fig. I.1) (543). This definition has been challenged, because 1.9% of healthy school children were found to have a head circumference less than 2 standard deviations below the mean (544), and because in some families with normal intelligence, microcephaly and short stature are inherited as dominant or recessive traits (545,546). When children with a head circumference less than two standard deviations but greater than three standard deviations below the mean are examined, 10.5% had an IQ below 70, 28.1% had a borderline IQ (71 to 80), and 14.0% had an IQ above 100. Of children with both height and head circumference less than two standard deviations below the mean, 13.3% had an IQ below 70. When children with a head circumference of less than three standard deviations below the mean were tested at 7 years of age, 51.2% had an IQ below 70 and 17.1% were borderline. None had an IQ above 100 (547).

Except in cases of premature closure of the sutures (craniosynostosis), the small size of the skull reflects a small brain, but it is not the size of the brain that determines the presence of mental retardation, rather it is the underlying structural pathology of the brain. An abnormally small brain results either from anomalous development during the first 7 months of gestation (primary microcephaly) or from an insult incurred during the last 2 months of gestation or during the perinatal period (secondary microcephaly).

Primary Microcephaly

Primary microcephaly results from a variety of genetic and environmental insults that cause anomalies of induction and migration.

Genetic Defects

Primary microcephaly can be transmitted as an autosomal recessive or as an autosomal dominant disorder (485,548,549). The brain can weigh as little as 500 g and resemble that of a 3–5-month-old fetus (550). Numerous migration anomalies are seen, including schizencephaly, lissencephaly, pachygyria, polymicrogyria, and

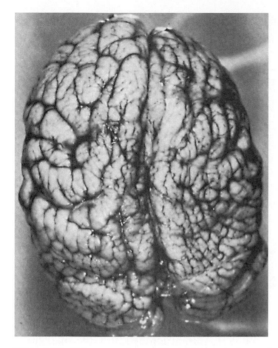

FIG. 4.18. Primary microcephaly. Dorsal view of the brain of a 9-year-old boy with severe microcephaly (brain weight was 700 g) and polymicrogyria. Note the regional differences, with the parieto-occipital regions being more severely involved, and a gradation to a more normal pattern frontally, especially in the larger hemisphere. Other malformations are not unusual. (From Lemire RJ, et al. *Normal and abnormal development of the human nervous system.* Hagerstown, MD: Harper & Row, 1975. With permission.)

In the other, more frequently encountered form, microcephaly was complicated by spasticity and seizures. Patients with this genetically transmitted microcephaly exhibited a receding forehead, and profound retardation was seen (551). Eye abnormalities, including chorioretinopathy and cataracts also have accompanied primary microcephaly (552,553). We have seen two siblings, brother and sister, with associated insulin-dependent diabetes mellitus (see Chapter 14).

In some patients, microcephaly results from an arrest in neuronogenesis before the requisite number of mitotic cycles are completed in the telencephalic neuroepithelium. One factor known to arrest mitotic activity is precocious differentiation of the ependyma, perhaps induced by fetal exposure to some toxin or virus that acts as a teratogen by imitating an inductive gene or molecule that normally initiates ependymal differentiation in a preprogrammed temporal sequence (461).

The recurrence of microcephaly after one affected child is relatively high, the exact frequency in each of the reported series depending on the incidence of autosomal recessive microcephaly. It was 19% in the series of Tolmie and colleagues (551). Prenatal diagnosis by ultrasound has been attempted by serial biparietal diameter measurements. This procedure discriminates poorly between affected and unaffected fetuses until the third trimester of gestation (551).

Disorders of Karyotype

Numerous chromosomal disorders, including trisomies, deletions, and translocation syndromes, are associated with primary microcephaly (see Table 3.3). Also, at least 20 well-defined dysmorphic syndromes with normal karyotypes, inherited or not inherited (e.g., Cornelia de Lange, Hallermann-Streiff, and Seckel syndromes) are associated with microcephaly (see Table 3.5).

Irradiation

Microcephaly can result from exposure to ionizing radiation during the first two trimesters, par-

agenesis of the corpus callosum (Figs. 4.18 and 4.19). Gray matter heterotopias occur, and neurons are reduced in number and abnormal in configuration (Figs. 4.19 and 4.20). Cortical lamination is defective, with grouping of cortical neurons in columnar blocks.

Numerous families with primary microcephaly have been recorded. In at least one, the gene has been mapped to the short arm of chromosome 8 (8pter-8p22). Tolmie and colleagues have distinguished two forms of autosomal recessive microcephaly, all of them characterized by a head circumference at birth that was more than five standard deviations below the mean. In one form, affected subjects were in the mildly retarded range with a normal facial appearance.

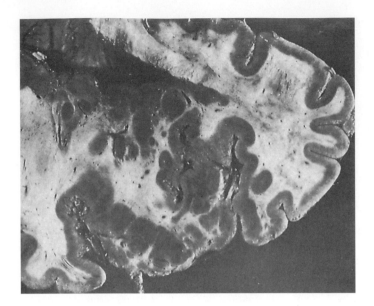

FIG. 4.19. Heterotopia of gray matter. Disruption of the cortex is present, with islands of heterotopic gray matter extending between the ependyma of the lateral ventricle and the surface. (From Layton DD. Heterotopic cerebral gray matter as an epileptogenic focus. *J Neuropathol Exp Neurol* 1962;21: 244. With permission.)

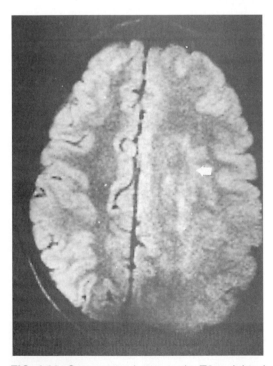

FIG. 4.20. Gray matter heterotopia. T2-weighted magnetic resonance imaging study of a 7-year-old child presenting with seizures reveals foci that are isointense with gray matter lying within the centrum semiovale (*arrow*). (Courtesy of Dr. A. J. Barkovich, Department of Radiology, University of California, San Francisco.)

ticularly between 4 and 20 weeks' gestation (554,555). The earlier the insult, the smaller the brain and the more disabling the resulting neurologic abnormalities. Maternal exposure within 1,500 m of the epicenter of the Hiroshima atomic bomb resulted in microcephaly when the gestational age at the time of exposure was 15 weeks or less (556). During the first 4 months of gestation, diagnostic irradiation of 1 cGy or less appears to pose little or no risk (557).

Infections In Utero

A variety of infectious agents, notably cytomegalovirus, *Toxoplasma*, and the rubella virus, are responsible for microcephaly. These disorders are discussed in Chapter 6.

Chemical Agents

In experimental animals, a wide variety of chemical agents have been found to produce microcephaly associated with induction and migration anomalies. Drugs implicated include cortisone, sulfhydryl enzyme inhibitors, aminopterin, triethylenemelamine, and nitrogen mustard. Additionally, mothers who suffer from untreated phenylketonuria have a high risk of bearing microcephalic offspring. This problem is considered in Chapter 1.

All causes of primary microcephaly, genetic, irradiation, chromosomal, infectious, or chemical, are time specific in that the toxic stimulus must occur during the period of induction and major cellular migration.

Secondary Microcephaly

A variety of insults, infectious, traumatic, metabolic, and anoxic, occurring during the last part of the third trimester, the perinatal period, and early infancy, cause destruction of brain with multiple areas of cystic degeneration, encephalomalacia, and porencephaly, accompanied by inflammatory gliotic scarring and shrinkage. As a consequence, little postnatal growth occurs and sutures close early. In secondary microcephaly, brain anomalies such as those in primary microcephaly are absent except for instances of cerebellar gray matter heterotopia and hypoplasia.

Clinical Manifestations

It is clear that both primary and secondary microcephaly display a broad spectrum of neurologic disorders. These disorders range from decerebration to a mild impairment of fine motor coordination, from complete nonresponsiveness to educable mental retardation, and from severe autistic behavior to mild hyperkinesis.

Diagnosis

In the diagnostic evaluation of the microcephalic child, various possible causes must be considered. Serologic studies for intrauterine infections, cytogenetics, amino acid screening, and CT for intracranial calcifications should be considered. MRI demonstrates abnormalities in cortical architecture (558). Craniosynostosis can be distinguished from microcephaly by an abnormally shaped skull and by the presence at birth of bony union between sutures. In the experience of Matson, in no patient with craniosynostosis was the affected suture open at birth (305).

The prognosis for relative microcephaly (i.e., a head circumference within the normal range, above the tenth percentile for gestational age, but proportionately small compared with length or weight) was examined by Brennan and coworkers, who used data collected as part of the Collaborative Perinatal Project. In their series, such infants do not show any developmental delay when tested at 7 years of age (559). It is otherwise for infants whose head circumference at birth is below the tenth percentile for gestational age. Both term infants and those small for gestational age having small head circumferences fare poorly, and according to Lipper and coworkers, head circumference at birth appears to be the most important variable for future neurodevelopmental outcome (560).

Microcephaly on rare occasions can be reversed with treatment of the underlying cause. This has been reported for phenylketonuria, chronic hypoglycemia, and diet-induced hypochloremic metabolic alkalosis (see Chapter 15).

CRANIOSYNOSTOSIS

Craniosynostosis was first described by Homer in the person of Thersites, "whose skull went up to a point . . . fluent orator though . . . the ugliest man who came beneath Ilion." Virchow, in 1851, provided a more complete clinical characterization (561).

Craniosynostosis is defined as the premature closure at birth of one or more cranial sutures. It is termed *simple* when only one suture is fused and *compound* when two or more sutures are affected. Primary craniosynostosis results from an abnormality of the mesenchymal matrix and is not the consequence of impaired brain growth. Secondary craniosynostosis is the consequence of one of various mechanical, metabolic, or hematologic disorders. Craniosynostosis can be an isolated phenomenon or can form part of a generalized dysmorphologic, chromosomal, or genetic syndrome (562).

In the healthy newborn, all sutures are separated by several millimeters, except the metopic suture, which closes antenatally. Metopic craniosynostosis, which manifests itself by a midfrontal ridge, is relatively common in small infants, but is of little or no clinical significance. No known neurologic consequences exist, and surgery is contraindicated.

TABLE 4.17. *Distribution of suture involvements in 136 patients with craniosynostosis*

Suture affected	Term	Male	Female	Total	Percent
Sagittal	Scaphocephaly (dolichocephaly)	45	10	55	40
Both coronals	Acrocephaly	12	16	28	20.5
One coronal	Plagiocephaly	10	12	22	16
All in vault	Oxycephaly	7	5	12	9
Sagittal and coronal	—	4	8	12	9
Metopic	Trigonocephaly	4	2	6	4.5
Sagittal and lambdoid	—	1	0	1	1
Total		83	53	136	100

From Till K. *Paediatric neurosurgery.* Oxford: Blackwell Scientific Publications, 1975. With permission.

By age 3 months, the posterior fontanelle is closed. By age 6 months, fibrous union of suture lines occurs and serrated edges interlock. By age 20 months, the anterior fontanelle is closed. At age 8 years, ossification of craniobasal bones is complete. By age 12 years, the sutures cannot be separated by raised intracranial pressure; they continue to be visible on radiography till age 20 years. Solid bony union of all sutures is complete by the eighth decade of life.

Etiology

No histologic abnormality of the prematurely fused sutures exists, and the pathogenesis is heterogeneous, with more than 100 syndromes of developmental defects having been described. These syndromes, which taken together constitute approximately 10% of craniosynostoses, are listed in monographs by David and coworkers (562) and Cohen (563). It appears likely therefore that calvarial involvement represents but one expression of a more widespread fundamental germ layer disturbance (564). To date, the molecular basis of several craniosynostosis syndromes has been identified. Dominant mutations in three fibroblast growth factor receptor genes have been shown to be responsible for Crouzon, Jackson-Weiss, Pfeiffer, and Apert syndromes (565,566). Doubtless other genetic mutations will be uncovered. Although animal experiments have shown that immobilization of a suture can lead to its fusion, the importance of intrauterine constraint in producing craniosynostosis has been questioned (567,568).

Secondary synostosis can be caused by a variety of metabolic disorders, including hyperthyroidism (569), Hurler syndrome, Conradi syndrome (570), and various forms of rickets, notably vitamin D deficiency, hypophosphatemia, hypophosphatasia, and azotemic osteodystrophy (571). It also is associated with such hematologic disorders as thalassemia and sickle cell anemia (572). In microcephaly and after reduction of increased intracranial pressure (as occurs with surgical treatment of hydrocephalus), a secondary premature fusion of the sutures occurs. In general, the deformities produced by secondary synostosis are much less pronounced than those with the primary form and rarely, if ever, appear to impair brain growth. Hence, corrective surgery for secondary synostosis is not indicated.

Clinical Manifestations

Craniosynostosis occurs in less than 5 in 10,000 births. The anatomic classification of craniosynostosis depends on the description of head contour or on the suture or sutures involved. The final skull shape depends on which sutures close, the duration and order of the closure process, and the success or failure of other sutures to compensate by expansion. As a rule, skull growth is inhibited in a direction at right angles to the closed sutures. The frequency of the various types of craniosynostosis is depicted in Table 4.17 (573).

Premature closure of the sagittal suture, the most common form of craniosynostosis, results in elongation of the skull in the anteroposterior direction. Associated anomalies are seen in 26% of patients, and between 5% and 40% of affected children are retarded (574,575). When the coronal suture fuses prematurely, the brain expands in a lateral direction. In this condition, the incidence of associated anomalies is higher: 33% with involvement of one coronal suture and 59% with involvement of both coronal sutures (305). Approximately 50% of affected children with synostosis of both coronal sutures are mentally retarded (574).

Of all types of craniosynostosis, oxycephaly can produce the most severe CNS involvement. Increased intracranial pressure, divergent strabismus, optic atrophy, anosmia, and bilateral pyramidal tract signs can either occur as associated CNS anomalies or because nonfused sutures are not sufficient to allow for expansion of the brain.

Psychomotor retardation can result from prolonged increased intracranial pressure, but more often it is caused by associated cerebral malformations or concurrent hydrocephalus (574,576). Retardation is noticeably absent in the majority of children with sagittal craniosynostosis, however, so that the need to treat is at times debatable.

In Crouzon syndrome (craniofacial dysostosis), premature closure of multiple sutures is associated with an abnormally high forehead, hypertelorism, shallow orbits with resultant exophthalmos, micrognathia, choanal atresia, prognathism, beaked nose, and high arched palate, but is usually associated with normal intellect. Chronic tonsillar herniation accompanies Crouzon syndrome and was seen in 73% of subjects studied by Cinalli and coworkers (577). Hydrocephalus develops in a large proportion of patients. It is believed to result from intracranial venous hypertension (578) or from the early closure of the lambdoid sutures (577). Crouzon syndrome tends to be hereditary or familial, and its gene has been mapped to the long arm of chromosome 10 (10q26). It codes for fibroblast growth factor receptor 2. Numerous mutations of fibroblast growth factor receptor 2 have been described and have been found to cause various craniosynostotic syndromes aside from Crouzon syndrome (565,579,580).

In Apert syndrome (acrocephalosyndactyly), the head and facial configuration are similar to that seen in Crouzon syndrome, but syndactyly or polydactyly is present as well. Most cases are sporadic. In the majority, the condition results from one of two mutations in the gene for fibroblast growth factor receptor 2 (581). Nonprogressive ventriculomegaly, hydrocephalus, and megalencephaly are often demonstrated (577). When measured, intracranial pressure is increased in some 80% of patients. The most likely cause of this phenomenon is impaired flow of CSF through the basilar cisterns. Only a small proportion of patients with Apert syndrome have normal intelligence, and malformations of the imbic structures, corpus callosum, and gyral abnormalities are common (582,582a).

A variety of other genetic or sporadically occurring constitutional dysplastic features are associated with craniosynostosis (562,563,583).

Diagnosis

In the small infant, the diagnosis can be suspected in the presence of an abnormally shaped head or face. CT is usually definitive. It reveals the extent of premature fusion and frequently shows an increased density of the fused suture. The early radiologic change is a loss of the pattern of interdigitations of the bone, until the suture becomes a simple line of separation of the bones. Bridging of this gap then begins, followed by a thickening of the bone along the line of the former suture. If the sagittal suture is involved, the anterior fontanelle is obliterated. With increased intracranial pressure, imaging studies performed after age 6 months can show demineralization and thinning of bone with increased digital impressions. MRI is necessary if hydrocephalus or abnormalities of cortical architecture are suspected.

One important differential diagnosis is that of microcephaly. Oxycephaly in particular, characterized by deformity of skull contour, closure of sutures at birth or during the neonatal period, and increased intracranial pressure, can mimic primary microcephaly. The differentiation of infants with unilambdoid synostosis (plagiocephaly) from those with positional flattening (deformational occipital plagiocephaly) can be difficult. In the experience of Menard and David, only 1% of children with unilateral occipital plagiocephaly were found to have true lambdoid synostosis (583).

The shape of the skull of a newborn who has been in the breech position *in utero* can suggest sagittal synostosis. In the breech baby, however, the biparietal diameter is normal, and no ridging is present at the sagittal suture, which appears normal on radiography. With time, the misshapen head can be expected to improve spontaneously (584).

Treatment

Craniosynostosis is treated surgically in children with multiple suture closure to prevent any brain damage that could result from chronic increased intracranial pressure, and in children with synostosis by only one suture to affect a good cosmetic result.

A consensus exists regarding the need for a surgical procedure in the presence of increased intracranial pressure (585). There has been considerable debate, however, regarding the need for surgery in children with synostosis of only one suture, particularly in plagiocephaly and scaphocephaly (premature closure to the sagittal suture). Some clinicians believe that scaphocephaly is rarely complicated by intellectual or neurologic dysfunction and that skull surgery is not justified for cosmetic reasons alone (574). Considerable debate exists concerning the optimal management of plagiocephaly. Rekate has reviewed the literature and found no prospective randomized controlled trials. Currently, the various recommended treatment options include observation only, mechanical correction of the deformity by wrapping of the head, and various types of surgical interventions. At present, it is not known whether children whose plagiocephaly has gone uncorrected have suffered from failure in intervention (586).

We believe that surgery for craniosynostosis should be viewed as a corrective rather than a cosmetic procedure and that a child with uncorrected synostosis and a significant skull deformity is fated to a lifetime of being considered and treated as abnormal.

It is fortunate that scaphocephaly is the disorder in most of the patients with synostosis; the technical procedure to correct this condition is easy, and if properly performed, it produces uniformly excellent results. The most common method of treating sagittal synostosis is to remove the midline strip of bone several centimeters in width from anterior to the coronal suture, to posterior to the lambdoidal sutures. Interpositional material is placed on the bony edges to prevent early refusion. Removal of a much wider strip of bone without interpositional material can serve the same purpose. The application of a fixative solution, such as Zenker, to the dura mater for this or any form of synostosis, with the intent to retard reossification, is definitely not recommended because the solution can penetrate the dura and injure the brain (587), or it can destroy the ossifying potential of the dura, necessitating subsequent cranioplasty (588).

Several techniques are currently advocated for the correction of the other synostoses (589). These are necessarily complex in most cases, particularly if surgical treatment has been delayed until later in childhood, and particularly when multiple sutures are involved, as in Crouzon disease. Surgery during the first 6 months of life is far more successful, having the advantage of using brain growth to assist in achieving a more normal skull shape, as well as removing any impediment to brain development.

Morbidity consists of local hematoma, wound infection, or rarely, the development of a leptomeningeal cyst. The more complex procedures should be performed only at centers with frequent experience with them, where the operative mortality is virtually nil, and prolonged morbidity is less than 1% (590).

MACROCEPHALY

Macrocephaly is defined as a head circumference that is more than two standard deviations more than the mean for age, sex, race, and gestation (see Fig. I.1). It is not a disease, but a syndrome of diverse causes. Table 4.18 outlines the most important diagnostic considerations appropriate for each age group. We should stress that evaluation of a child is necessary whenever a single head circumference measurement is outside the range of normal, or when graphing of serial measurements documents a progressive,

TABLE 4.18. *Common causes of macrocephaly and time of clinical presentation*

Early infantile (Birth to 6 mo of age)	Hydrocephalus (progressive or "arrested") Induction disorders	Spina bifida cystica, cranium bifi- dum, Chiari malformations (types I, II, and III), aqueductal stenosis, holoprosencephaly
	Mass lesions	Neoplasms, atrioventricular malfor- mations, congenital cysts
	Intrauterine infections	Toxoplasmosis, cytomegalic inclu- sion disease, syphilis, rubella
	Perinatal or postnatal infections	Bacterial, granulomatous, parasitic
	Perinatal or postnatal hemorrhage	Hypoxia, vascular malformation, trauma
	Hydranencephaly Subdural effusion Hemorrhagic, infectious, cystic hygroma Normal variant (often familial)	

Late infantile
(6 mo to 2 yr of age)
	Hydrocephalus (progressive or "arrested")
	  Space-occupying lesions
	  Postbacterial or granulomatous meningitis
	  Posthemorrhagic
	Dandy-Walker syndrome
	Subdural effusion
	Increased intracranial pressure syndrome
	  Pseudotumor cerebri
		Tumors, cysts, abscess
		
		Trauma or vascular malformation
		
		Lead, tetracycline, hypoparathy-
		roidism, corticosteroids, excess
		or deficiency of vitamin A, cya-
		notic congenital heart disease

	Primary skeletal cranial dysplasias (thick-
	ened or enlarged skull)
	  Osteogenesis imperfecta, hyperphos-
	  phatemia, osteopetrosis, rickets
	Megalencephaly (increase in brain substance)
	  Metabolic CNS diseases
		
		Leukodystrophies (e.g., Canavan,
		Alexander), lipidoses (Tay-
		Sachs), histiocytosis,
		mucopolysaccharidoses

	Proliferative neurocutaneous syndromes	von Recklinghausen tuberous scle- rosis, hemangiomatosis, Sturge- Weber
	Cerebral gigantism Achondroplasia Primary megalencephaly	Sotos syndrome May be familial and unassociated with abnormalities of cellular architecture, or associated with abnormalities or cellular archi- tecture

Early to late childhood
(Older than 2 yr of age)
	Hydrocephalus (progressive or "arrested")
	  Space-occupying lesions
	  Preexisting induction disorder
	  Postinfectious
	  Hemorrhagic
	  Chiari type I malformation
	Megalencephaly
	  Proliferative neurocutaneous syndromes
	  Familial
	Pseudotumor cerebri
	Normal variant
		
		Aqueductal stenosis

relative enlargement of the head as evidenced by the crossing of one or more percentile lines.

The differential diagnosis of macrocephaly takes into account the various conditions most likely for the age of the patient. The history must answer three important questions: Was the patient abnormal from birth or was there a period of normal growth and development before deterioration set in? Is there a family history of neurologic or cutaneous abnormalities? Is there a history of CNS trauma or infection?

The patient and family should be examined for cutaneous lesions such as angiomas, café-au-lait spots, vitiligo, shagreen patches, telangiectasia, and subcutaneous nodules. Measurements of the head circumference of both parents provides valuable information. We should stress that we have seen children with proven hydrocephalus with parents who have exceptionally large heads. The fundi must be evaluated for papilledema, macular degeneration such as is seen in lipidoses, for chorioretinitis and cataracts produced by intrauterine infections, and for optic nerve tumors caused by phakomatoses. The fontanelle, if open, is palpated for increased intracranial pressure, and its size is measured. The ranges of normal size have been recorded by Popich and Smith (591).

In 90% of healthy infants, the anterior fontanelle closes between 7 and 19 months of age, and in the remainder, by 26 months. The average time of closure is 16.3 months for boys and 18.8 months for girls (592). Persistent enlargement of the fontanelle is seen not only in hydrocephalus, but also in athyrotic hypothyroidism, achondroplasia, cleidocranial dysostosis, Down syndrome, trisomies 13 and 18, osteogenesis imperfecta, and the rubella syndrome. In addition to examination of the fontanelle, the skull should be auscultated for intracranial bruits.

Should ultrasonography demonstrate ventricular enlargement, the next question to be answered is whether ventriculomegaly is atrophic or caused by obstruction and increased intracranial pressure. Routine MRI, or cine-MRI, is useful to ascertain the presence of CSF flow through the foramen of Monro, aqueduct of Sylvius, and foramen of Magendie. MRI pro-

vides evidence for a mass lesion such as a neoplasm, a vascular malformation, subdural fluid collections, or porencephalic cysts. CT scans are essential to assess the presence of intracranial calcifications produced by prenatal infections, hypoparathyroidism, or parasitic cysts. Long bone radiographs can be used to determine the presence of spinal dysraphism. Increased cortical thickness of long bones suggests primary skeletal disturbances; fractures in different stages of healing suggest the diagnosis of a battered infant and a subdural hematoma.

Additional studies depend on diagnostic expectations for each age group (see Table 4.18).

Megalencephaly

Megalencephaly results from excessive amounts of normal brain constituents, cellular proliferation, or storage of metabolites. This condition is reviewed in a monograph by Gooskens (593).

In true megalencephaly, the increase in all neural elements is usually accompanied by overgrowth, abnormal migration, abnormal organization of some or all cellular and fiber elements of gray and white matter, giant neurons, gray matter heterotopias, and defective cortical lamination. The brain, which normally weighs 350 g at term (1,250 to 1,400 g at maturity), can be twice as heavy as expected for the age. True megalencephaly is primarily a proliferation disorder of embryonic origin, hamartomatous in nature with occasional malignant transformation, and, therefore, related to such phakomatoses as tuberous sclerosis and neurofibromatosis.

The classical clinical picture of true megalencephaly is one of mental retardation, seizures, hypotonia or mild pyramidal tract, and cerebellar deficits. These symptoms are occasionally progressive. The skull bones are thin, the anterior fontanelle is large, and sutures are slow in closing. The head reveals neither frontal bossing suggestive of hydrocephalus, nor lateral bulging seen so often with infantile subdural fluid collections. Multiple minor congenital anomalies are frequently present, including hypertelorism, abnormal dermatoglyphics, and high arched palate. These stigmata also are seen in cerebral gigantism

(Sotos syndrome) (see Chapter 15). Megalencephaly accompanies cutaneous and subcutaneous abnormalities in a variety of syndromes, notably disseminated hemangiomatosis, neurofibromatosis, multiple hemangiomas and pseudopapilledema, angiomatosis and lipomatosis, Bannayan syndrome (594), Beckwith-Wiedemann syndrome (see Chapter 14), and Klippel-Trenaunay-Weber syndrome (see Chapter 12). A dominantly inherited syndrome of megalencephaly, hypotonia, proximal muscle weakness, and increased intercellular muscle lipids has been described (595). A number of patients also have café-au-lait lesions and pigmented lesions of the penis, thus this condition may be identical to the Ruvalcaba-Myhre-Smith and Bannayan syndromes (596).

Although the prevalence of megalencephaly is increased in children with learning disabilities (597), the majority of children with this condition have normal to superior intelligence, and a large brain has been seen in many geniuses (598). In the large series of Lorber and Priestley, 88% of children with megalencephaly had normal to superior intelligence and 5% were in the borderline range (599). Sandler and coworkers found that when children with macrocephaly were compared with unaffected siblings, the former group had delayed motor milestones, speech and articulation problems, and difficulties with visuomotor integration (600). In the series of Lorber and Priestley, the male-to-female ratio was 4:1, height and weight were within the normal range in 90% and 91%, respectively, and at least 39% had a family history of an enlarged head, most commonly in the child's father (599). In such families, transmission of the condition is most likely to be as an autosomal dominant trait.

Hydrocephalus

Hydrocephalus is commonly defined as a pathologic increase in the cerebral ventricular volume. Although this increase can occur from a reduction in the volume of cerebral tissue resulting from either malformation or atrophy (hydrocephalus ex vacuo), the type of hydrocephalus considered here is that which results from an imbalance between the formation of CSF and its absorption. With the single possible exception of choroid plexus papilloma, in which CSF overproduction has been postulated to occur, hydrocephalus results from impaired absorption. An impairment to the normal flow or to the return of CSF into the blood leads to an increase in ventricular pressure because no mechanism exists for homeostasis and reduction of CSF formation. The increased pressure and the ventricular enlargement that follows account for the clinical findings. The timing, site of the obstruction, and cause of hydrocephalus, particularly the presence or absence of associated cerebral malformations, determine the type of hydrocephalus, the extent of any brain damage, and the outcome.

Physiology of the Cerebrospinal Fluid

Excellent books reviewing the embryology, anatomy, and physiology of the CSF dynamics and of the ventricular and subarachnoid spaces are those by Fishman, who also discusses the alterations of CSF in various disease processes (601), and by Davson and colleagues (602). Noted in Table 4.10, closure of the neural tube and primordial cephalization occur by 28 days' gestation. In humans, the cerebral vesicles with a central lumen develop from the cephalic end of the neural tube. These represent the major brain subdivisions and the tentatively defined ventricles, both of which become further elaborated as certain regions constrict and others expand to form the basic pattern of the ventricular system.

During the second month of gestation, choroid plexi primordia develop, first as a mesenchymal invagination of the roof of the fourth ventricle, then by a similar invagination of the lateral and third ventricles (603). By the third month, the plexi fill 75% of the lateral ventricle and then begin to decrease in relative size. During the third trimester, the plexi become cellular and glycogen rich. After birth, glycogen is lost as the cells begin aerobic oxidation (604).

As the plexi develop in the second month, the fetal ventricles are large relative to the thickness of the cortical wall, and this relative dilatation disappears with further development of white and gray matter. By the second to third trimester, the ventricles normally undergo restricted ependymal loss without subependymal gliosis (605). It is not clear when CSF secretion is initiated, but complete circulation from ventricle to the subarachnoid spaces does not occur until after 2 months' gestation (605).

At this time, the fourth ventricle exit foramina develop. These are the foramina of Luschka, two lateral apical roof apertures leading to the pontine cistern, and the foramen of Magendie, a single median posterior roof aperture leading to the cisterna magna (606). Initially, the outlets from the fourth ventricle are covered with a membrane, which does not impair CSF outflow, because drainage occurs via intercellular pores in the membrane. The membrane develops progressively larger pores and becomes progressively thinner until it no longer is present (606). The fully developed choroid plexi are outpouchings into the ventricular cavity of ependyma-lined blood vessels of the pia mater. Most of the CSF is produced within the ventricular system by the choroid plexi; however, a sizable proportion, some 10% to 20%, evidently is formed by the parenchyma of cerebrum and spinal cord (607).

The currently accepted view is that CSF bulk flow occurs from the site of its production in the ventricles to its absorption in the arachnoid (pacchionian) granulations. In the adult human, CSF is secreted at a rate of 500 mL per 24 hours or between 0.2% and 0.5% of the total volume per minute (601,608). The rate of CSF formation ranges from 0.3 to 0.4 mL/min in children (609) and adults (602). Total CSF volume in the newborn is 50 mL and increases with age to an adult volume of 150 mL. At CSF pressures below 200 mm H_2O, production of CSF is independent of pressure (610); however, a prolonged and marked increase in intraventricular pressure owing to hydrocephalus can slightly reduce the rate of CSF formation (610).

The mechanisms responsible for the formation of CSF are primarily active and specific transport, simple diffusion, and carrier-mediated diffusion. The choroid plexus has the morphologic characteristics associated with secretory function. It has been compared with the proximal renal tubules in that it can both secrete and absorb a number of substances (602). Unlike parenchymal capillaries, in which the tight junctions between endothelial cells constitute the blood–brain barrier, the capillaries of the choroid plexus are fenestrated and devoid of tight junctions. Tight junctions are found on the astrocytic side of the choroid epithelium, however, and these constitute the blood–CSF barrier (611).

CSF is not quite an ultrafiltrate of plasma. Its concentrations of potassium, calcium, bicarbonate, and glucose are lower than in an ultrafiltrate, whereas those of sodium, chloride, and magnesium are higher. These small differences are important because they affect the excitability of neurons.

CSF appears to be formed in a two-step process. The first step is the formation by hydrostatic pressure of a plasma ultrafiltrate through the nontight-junctioned choroidal capillary endothelium into the connective tissue stroma beneath the epithelium of the villus. The passage is driven by hydrostatic pressure. The ultrafiltrate is transformed subsequently into a secretion by an active metabolic process within the choroidal epithelium. Although the exact mechanism for this process is unknown, one model suggests that sodium and potassium–activated adenosine triphosphatase pumps sodium into the basal side of the cell with water passively following the osmotic gradient thus created.

Carbonic anhydrase catalyzes the formation of bicarbonate inside the cell, with the hydrogen ion being fed back to the sodium pump as a counter-ion to potassium (601). In a manner analogous to that on the basal side of the epithelium, sodium-potassium adenosine triphosphatase located in the microvilli on the astrocytic surface extrudes sodium into the ventricle, followed by osmotically drawn water. Because the cells do not swell or shrink, the sum of the two processes must be in balance.

The absorption of CSF depends in the main on bulk flow. Pulsatile movements of the CSF, as generated by the systolic expansion of the vasculature of the cerebral and basilar arterial systems, can be demonstrated by cine-MRI. No evidence exists, however, that they contribute significantly to the circulation of the CSF. Based on his data obtained by radiocisternography and gated MRI, Greitz argues that CSF flow is primarily pulsatile, and that no significant bulk flow occurs except within the ventricles, notably in the aqueduct (612). He suggests that CSF absorption is not limited to the arachnoid granulations, but can occur anywhere in the CNS via the brain extracellular space, which communicates with the subarachnoid space.

Whatever the actual forces involved in CSF absorption, 80% enters directly into the cisternal system with subsequent drainage from the cerebral subarachnoid space into the cortical venous system; 20% circulates into the subarachnoid space of the spinal cord, but eventually is drained to a great extent from cerebral subarachnoid space, with lesser drainage from the spinal subarachnoid space into the spinal venous system. Spinal descent of CSF, however, might prove to be an important alternative pathway in pathologic conditions.

CSF drainage occurs in part by way of the arachnoidal villi and granulations. These are essentially microtubular envaginations of the subarachnoid space into the lumen of large dural and venous sinuses (613). The distinction between arachnoid villi and granulations is one of size, and arachnoid granulations probably develop from villi with increasing age. Arachnoid villi are present in the fetus and newborn infant, arachnoid granulations become evident by 18 months of age and are visible to the naked eye by 3 years of age (614). They are located principally in the parieto-occipital region of the superior sagittal sinus, in the lateral sinuses of the posterior fossa, and at dural reflections over cranial nerves.

Three factors control CSF drainage: CSF pressure, pressure within the dural sinuses and the cortical venous system, and resistance of the arachnoidal villi to CSF flow (615). Changes in any of these variables significantly affect CSF flow. Normally, pressure is greater in the subarachnoid CSF than in the sagittal sinus, whether the body is recumbent or erect. The normal lumbar CSF pressure is 150 mm H_2O in the laterally recumbent adult and up to 180 mm H_2O in the child, substantially greater than the mean pressure of 90 mm H_2O in the superior sagittal sinus. The capacity for drainage is two to four times the normal rate of CSF production (609).

The labyrinth of small tubules in the villi can behave as one-way valves, in that they are closed by high pressure in the venous sinus and opened by high CSF pressure (613). The factors that control CSF drainage in the human are still uncertain, and the only proven force is that of a hydrostatic gradient. Increased CSF pressure does not facilitate the flow of macromolecules through the villi from the CSF, which suggests that the *valves* do not enlarge in response to increased pressure (616). Furthermore, it appears that drainage does not depend on the colloid osmotic pressure difference between CSF and sinus blood because the tubules are permeable to protein (613). To date, ultrastructural analysis of human specimens has failed to demonstrate the one-way valves of the villi seen in animals (617).

Experimental work with animals, including primates, suggests that a significant amount, perhaps as much as one-half of the CSF, drains through the lymphatics (618,619). To what extent this process exists in humans is still unknown, but support for the concept comes from the clinical observation that children with an obstructed CSF-diverting shunt occasionally develop nasal congestion and periorbital or facial swelling. The lymphatic drainage of CSF might play a role in the pathophysiology of hydrocephalus, either as an alternative pathway for drainage, or, in cases of impaired access to the lymphatic system, as a cause of hydrocephalus.

The question of whether CSF can be absorbed by the brain is still unresolved. The penetration of substances into the periventricular region of hydrocephalic animals has been well documented (620). CT scans demonstrate periventricular hypodensity in the presence of hydrocephalus, the result of CSF migrating into the area surrounding the ventricles in the presence of increased intraventricular pressure (621). This hypodensity is confirmed by MRI studies that show increased signal intensity in the periventricular regions. The presence of CSF in brain parenchyma, however, does not necessarily equate with absorption of CSF, and experimental evidence supports the contention that the brain, rather than absorbing CSF, acts as a conduit for fluid to move from the ventricles into the subarachnoid spaces or into the prelymphatic channels of the blood vessels (622).

CSF also can drain from the subarachnoid spaces surrounding the cranial and spinal nerve root sleeves, with entry into the lymphatic system. Studies by Nabeshima and colleagues (623) have shown that an outer arachnoid layer between the subarachnoid spaces and the dura functions as the blood–CSF barrier at this location. At higher than normal intraventricular pressures, this barrier can be disrupted with resultant penetration of macromolecules into the extracellular space of the dura mater and the dural lymphatic channels. It is possible that at high pressures, disruption of this arachnoid barrier permits significant absorption of CSF.

Pathogenesis

Any block in the CSF pathway from the site of formation to that of absorption results in increased CSF pressure. By convention, hydrocephalus is divided into noncommunicating and communicating forms. In noncommunicating hydrocephalus, the subarachnoid space is usually compressed; in communicating hydrocephalus it is enlarged. With one possible exception (discussed subsequently), all hydrocephalic conditions are obstructive.

In noncommunicating hydrocephalus, the obstructive site is within the ventricular system, including the outlet foramina of the fourth ventricle. In communicating hydrocephalus, the obstruction occurs distal to the fourth ventricle foramina, in the cisterns or cerebral subarachnoid space itself.

A condition termed *external hydrocephalus* has been identified with increasing frequency by means of neuroimaging studies. It is seen in infants with enlarged heads or rapid head growth. In all instances, subarachnoid spaces are widened bilaterally in the frontal and sometimes in the frontoparietal regions. The ventricles are of normal size or only slightly enlarged. The condition gradually resolves during the second year of life, and the large majority of infants, 89% in the series of Alvarez and coworkers (624) and 100% in the series of Andersson and coworkers (625), were developmentally normal. External hydrocephalus is more common in premature infants, and in 88% of cases a family history of enlarged head exists (624). It probably results from a developmental delay in arachnoidal function.

CSF formation in hydrocephalus is normal or nearly normal (626). In compensated hydrocephalus, the rate of absorption equals the rate of formation, whereas in uncompensated hydrocephalus only a small fraction of the total amount formed is not absorbed. As CSF formation is relatively constant, CSF pressure depends on the change in resistance to flow or absorption, and on the resistance to ventricular enlargement by brain elasticity, and by the meninges, skull, and scalp. Thus, the intracranial pressure in an infant with hydrocephalus whose head can enlarge fairly easily can be just a little above normal, whereas the same impairment of flow in an older child or adult with more rigid sutures causes a greater and more rapid increase in pressure.

Impaired CSF absorption in communicating hydrocephalus can occur at some or all of the following sites: the arachnoid villi, lymphatic channels associated with the cranial and spinal nerves, lymphatic channels in the adventitia of the cerebral vessels, and arachnoid membrane. If CSF outflow from the ventricles is blocked, as occurs in noncommunicating hydrocephalus, absorption could still occur through the adventitia of the blood vessels, through the stroma of the choroid plexus, and by passage of CSF through the extracellular space of the cortical mantle to reach the brain surface. Additional ways for CSF to exit the ventricles would be through the dilated spinal cord central canal (627) or through a fistulous opening created by a rupture of the ventricular system into the subarachnoid space at the lamina terminalis or the suprapineal recess (340).

The rate of ventricular enlargement depends on the degree to which the resistance to absorption has increased and on the distensibility of the ventricular system.

Regardless of the site of obstruction, it is the arterial pulse thrust, not only of the choroid plexus, but also of the cerebral arteries, that is believed to be responsible for compressing the ventricular wall, enlarging the ventricular cavity (628), and producing parenchymal disruption (629). This pulse thrust increases with increasing mean CSF pressure and splits the ventricular ependymal lining, as demonstrated in the experimental animal (629,630). Splitting of the ependymal lining, in turn, produces transependymal flow of CSF into white matter, resulting in spongy and edematous white matter, dissolution of nerve fibers, and a significant degree of neuronal and astrocytic swelling in the deep areas of gray matter (631). This transependymal flow, if it continues for long, is a likely cause of the loss of neural and glial tissue (cerebral atrophy), contributing to the thinning of the cerebral mantle. The more immediate cause of cerebral thinning, however, is the loss of extracellular water absorbed into the blood. A reversal of this process allows the remarkably rapid reduction in ventricular size that can be observed when the ventricular pressure is relieved by drainage or shunting.

Additionally, the cilia that normally cover the ependymal surfaces of the ventricular walls disappear (632). The impact of their loss on CSF dynamics and metabolism is still unknown. Also unclear is the extent to which normally nonfunctioning drainage routes, including the choroid plexi and the periventricular capillaries, become operative with increased CSF pressure and contribute to equalizing the rates of CSF formation and absorption in the human hydrocephalic patient. However, in both hydrocephalic animals (633,634) and humans (635), stabilization of ventricular pressure and the cessation of growth of the ventricular cavity appear to result from the availability of these other drainage pathways. In hydrocephalic children, ventricular pressure varies greatly with respiration, cardiovascular changes, and activity (636). Because ventricular pressure is increased by sucking and crying, normal pressure and high-pressure hydrocephalus might be the same phenomenon, differing only in time and rate of development, degree of obstruction, and parenchymal integrity (625).

Additionally, the combination of ventriculomegaly and increased intracranial pressure can produce brain damage by reducing cerebral blood flow, in particular through the anterior cerebral arteries, and thus lead to ischemic injury of the cerebral cortex adjacent to the interhemispheric fissure and the basal forebrain (637).

Pathology

The three general causes of hydrocephalus are excess secretion caused by choroid plexus papilloma, obstruction within the ventricular cavity (noncommunicating hydrocephalus), and absorptive block within the subarachnoid space (communicating hydrocephalus).

Excess Secretion Caused by Choroid Plexus Papilloma

The papilloma is a large aggregate of choroidal fronds that are microscopically similar to normal choroid plexi and produce great quantities of CSF. Accounting for 1% to 4% of childhood intracranial tumors, they usually occur after infancy and are associated with signs of increased intracranial pressure, although some of the more than 400 reported cases were found incidentally at postmortem examination. Whereas, in a number of instances the mass effect of the tumor or the presence of proteinaceous and xanthochromic CSF, most likely the result of bleeding stemming from the neoplasm, has suggested that obstruction of CSF flow is responsible for hydrocephalus, preoperative and postoperative studies of CSF production have substantiated earlier suggestions that, in at least some cases, the tumor produces hydrocephalus by CSF oversecretion (638,639).

Obstruction within the Ventricular Cavity

Any obstruction from the foramina of Monro or to the foramina of Magendie and Luschka produces noncommunicating hydrocephalus. Space-occupying lesions in the cerebral hemispheres tend to compress the ventricular system, whereas tumors in the posterior fossa or arteriovenous malformations involving the vein of Galen can produce kinking or obstruction of the aqueduct or obstruction at the fourth ventricular outflow. These conditions are discussed in Chapter 10. The other, more complex causes of aqueductal obstruction are discussed here.

Aqueductal Stenosis. Aqueductal stenosis is responsible for 20% of cases of hydrocephalus. Its incidence ranges from 0.5 to 1.0 in 1,000 births, with a recurrence risk in siblings of 1.0% to 4.5% (640). Normally, the aqueduct, lined by ependyma, is 3 mm in length at birth and its mean cross-section is 0.5 mm^2 (641), with the cross-sectional area ranging from 0.2 to 1.8 mm^2 (642). The cross-section is somewhat larger in the fetus, but after birth does not change significantly with age. In aqueductal stenosis, the aqueduct is smaller but remains histologically normal. In particular, no gliosis is present. Constrictions of the aqueduct to less than 0.14 mm^2 can occur at two points: the first is beneath the midline of the superior quadrigeminal bodies, and the second is at the intercollicular sulcus (643).

The onset of symptoms is usually insidious and can occur at any time from birth to adulthood. In many instances, aqueductal stenosis is accompanied by aqueductal forking, or marked branching of the channels. Associated malformations in neighboring structures are common. These include fusion of the quadrigeminal bodies, fusion of the third nerve nuclei, and more caudal defects of neural tube closure such as spina bifida cystica or occulta. These associated anomalies raise the possibility that aqueductal stenosis itself probably represents a mild expression of a neural tube defect (644).

A small percentage of the anomalies (approximately 2%) are caused by one or more sex-linked recessive genes (645). This entity, more correctly known as X-linked hydrocephalus because not all cases actually have aqueductal stenosis as the only basis, has been shown to be caused by a mutation in the *L1* gene, a member of the superfamily of cell adhesion molecules (646). Numerous such mutations have been documented (647). Yamasaki and colleagues have divided them into three groups. Mutations that disrupt only the cytoplasmic domain of *L1* result in the mildest phenotype. Point mutations and truncations of the *L1* extracellular domain produce a more severe phenotype with pronounced

hydrocephalus and profound mental retardation (647). This disorder also results in pachygyria and polymicrogyria, and the acronym of CRASH syndrome has been proposed to account for the major features of the disorders: corpus callosum hypoplasia, retardation, adducted thumbs, spastic paraplegia, and hydrocephalus (647). The presence of these malformations helps explain the intellectual, cognitive, and motor handicaps even after the hydrocephalus is compensated by shunting (648).

In at least some instances, noninflammatory aqueductal stenosis is the consequence of inapparent viral infections (see Chapter 6).

Aqueductal Gliosis. Aqueductal gliosis, a postinfectious noninflammatory process, is usually secondary to a perinatal infection or hemorrhage (643). With the increasing survival of newborns affected with bacterial meningitis or intracranial hemorrhage, this condition has assumed greater importance. The ependymal lining is permanently destroyed because it is highly vulnerable to insult and cannot regenerate (649). Marked fibrillary gliosis of adjacent tissue is evident, and granular ependymitis is seen below the obstruction. The occlusion is progressive, and like aqueductal stenosis, its onset is insidious. No foreign inflammatory cells are found in the region of the cerebral aqueduct either during the period of active fetal infection or afterward.

Aqueductal gliosis occasionally accompanies neurofibromatosis. A variant, also postinflammatory, appears as a septal obstruction at the caudal end of the aqueduct. This obstruction is the result of a membrane of neuroglial overgrowth associated with a granular ependymitis (643). Aqueductal stenosis and gliosis have been produced in experimental animals by intrauterine viral infections, and a patient has been reported with aqueductal stenosis after mumps encephalitis (see Chapter 6).

Descending from the ventricular system, the next major area of obstruction is at the fourth ventricle. This is the site of obstruction in approximately one-half of hydrocephalic children.

Chiari Malformations. Chiari malformations, congenital malformations involving the fourth ventricle, which alone or combined with

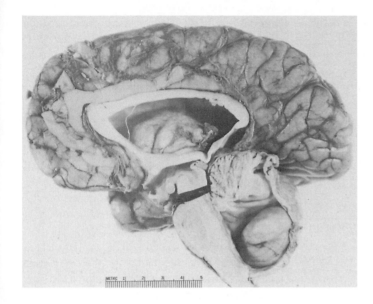

FIG. 4.21. Dandy-Walker syndrome with obstruction of the foramina of Magendie and Luschka. Midsagittal section showing absence of posterior cerebellar tissue. A dilatation of the fourth ventricle and a huge cyst within the posterior fossa confluent with the fourth ventricle are seen. The tentorium is displaced upward, and the lateral ventricle is markedly enlarged. (Courtesy of Dr. Hideo H. Itabashi, Department of Pathology, Los Angeles County Harbor Medical Center.)

other anomalies account for 40% of all hydrocephalic children, are discussed in the Chiari Malformation section.

Dandy-Walker Syndrome. Dandy-Walker syndrome, described in 1914 by Dandy and Blackfan (650), is characterized by a triad of complete or partial agenesis of the cerebellar vermis, cystic dilatation of the fourth ventricle, and an enlarged posterior fossa with upward displacement of the transverse sinuses, tentorium, and torcular (429). The basic embryonic failure in this malformation is still controversial. It is unrelated to occlusion of the foramina of Luschka and Magendie for three reasons. First, the foramina are open in as many as 80% of subjects. Second, the associated malformations of vermis and fourth ventricle occur before development of the foramina, which is after the fourth month of gestation in the case of the foramen of Magendie, and even later for the foramina of Luschka (67). Third, the lack of massive hydrocephalus at birth in most infants suggests that CSF circulation is present at that time. Currently, the best explanation is that of Benda and others who consider the Dandy-Walker syndrome to be a defect of neural tube closure at the cerebellar level occurring at approximately 4 weeks' gestation (485,651). Of uncertain relevance to humans is a phylogenetic

perspective that many birds normally have an expanded posterior membrane of the fourth ventricle without apertures, resembling a Dandy-Walker malformation, and the large membrane permits sufficient transudate of fluid between the fourth ventricle and subarachnoid space to provide adequate CSF flow.

The most striking abnormality is the presence of a hugely dilated fourth ventricle that acts as a cyst and is roofed by a neuroglial-vascular membrane lined with ependyma. This *cyst* herniates caudally and separates the cerebellar hemispheres posteriorly, displacing them anteriorly and laterally (Fig. 4.21). The vermis and choroid plexi are rudimentary. The foramina of the fourth ventricle are often occluded by membranes or are atretic. Hart and coworkers, however, were able to demonstrate patency of the foramen of Magendie in 7% of their cases (651).

Other associated neural and systemic anomalies include agenesis of the corpus callosum, aqueductal stenosis, occipital encephalocele, polymicrogyria, syringomyelia, heterotopias, facial angiomas, midline cleft palate, cardiovascular malformations, and polycystic kidneys (652,653).

A variant, in which cystic dilatation of the fourth ventricle and hypoplasia of the cerebellar

TABLE 4.19. *Clinical features in 40 cases of Dandy-Walker syndrome*

Disorder	Number of cases
Macrocrania	29
Hypotonia	10
Headache and vomiting	6
Downwardly displaced eyeballs	6
Spasticity	3
Hemiparesis	1
Seizures	6
Enlarged posterior fossa	6
Seventh nerve palsy	1
Cerebellar syndrome	1
Associated anomalies	
Agenesis of corpus callosum	3
Occipital encephalocele	7
Hemispheric malformation	1
Facial angiomas	4
Malformed fingers	2
Onset of hydrocephalus	
At birth	6
By 1 year of age	31

Adapted from Hirsh JF, et al. The Dandy-Walker malformation: a review of 40 cases. *J Neurosurg* 1984;61:515–522. With permission.

vermis exists without enlargement of the posterior fossa is more common than the classic Dandy-Walker malformation and accounts for one-third of posterior fossa malformations. A number of supratentorial malformations accompany this condition (426).

The Dandy-Walker syndrome also must be distinguished from retrocerebellar arachnoidal cysts (mega cisterna magna), and posterior fossa arachnoid cysts (654). In mega cisterna magna the vermis is intact, the cisterna magna is markedly enlarged, and the posterior fossa is enlarged. Mental retardation caused by associated supratentorial anomalies is common. In posterior fossa arachnoid cysts, symptoms arise from hydrocephalus, which occasionally is accompanied by cerebellar deficits (426).

The incidence of Dandy-Walker syndrome is 1 per 25,000 to 30,000 births, with the condition having a slight predilection for female subjects (653). Hydrocephalus is not present at birth; it appears by 3 months of age in some 75% of infants, and the diagnosis is established by 1 year of age in 80%. In some instances, hydrocephalus fails to develop and the condition remains asymptomatic throughout life (652). In addition to the clinical features outlined in Table 4.19,

infants can have a large occiput, with an inion that is higher than normal. They can experience recurrent attacks of pallor, ataxia, and abnormal respirations. In the series of Tal and coworkers, 7 of 10 infants died of sudden respiratory arrest (652). Because in 5 of those 7 infants previously placed ventricular shunts were patent, pressure of the cyst on the pontine respiratory center appears likely. Mental retardation is common and is probably the consequence of cortical malformations. In the series of Maria and coworkers 47% of children had normal intelligence, another 26% had learning disabilities, and the remainder had moderate or severe delay (655). The syndrome also is associated with a number of other conditions, including the Klippel-Feil syndrome, Cornelia de Lange syndrome, Rubinstein-Taybi syndrome, and hypertelorism.

Correction of hydrocephalus involves cystoperitoneal, ventriculoperitoneal, or both kinds of shunts (652,653). Cystoperitoneal shunting, because it avoids the risk of an entrapped fourth ventricle, is at present considered by many to be the best procedure for this condition (653). Fewer shunt malfunctions occur in part because the cyst does not collapse (656). Curless and coworkers suggest that cine-MRI be used to determine the presence of aqueductal flow, and that if normal flow is present, a single posterior ventricular shunt can safely be placed (657). McLaurin and Crone state that the incidence of aqueductal stenosis is sufficiently high to warrant Y shunting of the cyst and the lateral ventricles, or shunting of the cyst (656).

Other conditions that frequently obstruct fourth ventricular outflow are space-occupying lesions, particularly those involving the posterior fossa. Less often, a retrocerebellar subdural hematoma or bacterial or granulomatous meningitis occludes the foramina of Magendie and Luschka (658).

Absorptive Block
within the Subarachnoid Space

Of all childhood hydrocephalus, 30% are communicating. After the CSF passes through the exit foramina of the fourth ventricle, it normally traverses the basal cisterns around the brainstem and midbrain on the way to the cortical sub-arachnoid compartment and is absorbed through the arachnoid villi. Meningeal scarring can result from subarachnoid hemorrhage or bacterial meningitis. When this scarring occludes the exits from the cisterns or involves the arachnoid villi, the CSF circulation is impeded. The resulting increase in intracranial pressure then enlarges not only the four ventricles but also the subarachnoid compartment over the cerebral hemispheres.

Intraventricular hemorrhage is common in premature infants, particularly in babies weighing less than 1,500 g. Subarachnoid hemorrhage is usually seen in both premature and full-term infants. The pathogenesis and pathology of these conditions are discussed in Chapter 5. The fibrosis of the pacchionian granulations is so slow that decompensation and hydrocephalus often do not present clinically until 6 to 12 months after the perinatal hemorrhagic event.

Meningitis can produce communicating hydrocephalus in the acute phase by the clumping of purulent fluid in the drainage channels, and in the chronic phase by the organizing of exudate and blood, resulting in fibrosis of the subarachnoid spaces (see Chapter 6). As a rule, bacterial meningitis tends to produce cerebral cortical arachnoiditis, whereas granulomatous or parasitic meningitis produces cisternal obstruction. Rarely, viral meningitis can result in obstruction at either point. Intrauterine infections are discussed in Chapter 6.

Two causes of communicating hydrocephalus, although uncommon, deserve mention. The first is a diffuse meningeal malignant tumor caused by lymphoma or leukemia. This condition is discussed in Chapter 15. The second is an extra-axial arachnoid cyst that can be located in the basal cistern, over the cerebral cortex, or in the paramesencephalic region (659). This condition is considered later in this chapter.

Finally, chronic obstruction of the vein of Galen or the major sinuses has been held responsible for communicating hydrocephalus. Rosman and Shands postulate that increased intracranial venous pressure produces hydrocephalus if the patient is under 18 months of age. If increased venous pressure develops in a child older than 3 years of age, pseudotumor cerebri is more likely to result. The difference in response to venous obstruction might relate to an expansile calvarium and softer, less myelinated periventricular parenchyma in the infant, which permit greater ventricular dilatation under high pressure (660). Little experimental evidence supports this clinical impression (661). Occasionally, however, large space-occupying lesions within the posterior fossa can cause hydrocephalus without impinging on the fourth ventricle, perhaps as the result of venous obstruction.

Other Types of Hydrocephalus

Normal-Pressure Hydrocephalus (Hakim Syndrome) and Arrested (Compensated) Hydrocephalus

With advancing diagnostic and surgical technology, these conditions, which can be seen with any of the various types of hydrocephalus, have assumed increased importance (662). Normal-pressure hydrocephalus, conceptually and clinically defined primarily by Hakim, is an instance of indolently progressive hydrocephalus in which CSF pressure is within the physiologic range, but in which a marked increase in CSF pulse pressure results in slow ventricular expansion and progressive white matter damage (663). The cause and pathophysiology of the condition remain poorly understood, and the condition may represent a primary disorder in the cerebral parenchyma rather than a compromise of CSF compensatory pressure mechanisms (664). The pathogenesis of normal-pressure hydrocephalus, as it is seen in the elderly, undoubtedly differs from that in infants and children in whom the most common cause is communicating hydrocephalus with incomplete arachnoidal obstruction to CSF drainage. Primary events include neonatal intraventricular hemorrhage, spontaneous subarachnoid hemorrhage, intracranial trauma, infections, and surgery (664,665). The clinical presentation in childhood resembles that seen in adult life. In the series of Bret and Chazal, psychomotor retardation, psychoticlike behavior, gait abnormalities, and sphincter disturbances were seen in a large proportion of children (665).

Arrested hydrocephalus occurs when CSF formation and absorption are in balance and no more CSF accumulates. Milhorat (666) defines arrested hydrocephalus as the surgical or spontaneous termination of a hydrocephalic condition, with subsequent return to normal of the pressure gradient across the cerebral mantle. Others regard this condition as hydrocephalus that has been treated or resolved rather than arrested, and they are skeptical about whether hydrocephalus can ever be truly arrested. Indeed, in some patients, hydrocephalus can progress so slowly that the advancing neurologic dysfunction becomes evident only over the course of several years. In other cases, hydrocephalus becomes reactivated after a seemingly insignificant head trauma or viral illness. Even if no further net accumulation of CSF occurs, the increased resistance to CSF absorption establishes a new equilibrium at an increased intracranial pressure.

As a consequence, the head circumference is usually near or above the 97th percentile, and if above the 97th percentile, it generally parallels it. On neuroimaging studies, the ventricles are moderately to markedly dilated. The larger the ventricles, the less likely that ventricular size will further increase. On clinical evaluation, these children tend to be clumsy and uncoordinated, with a verbal IQ better than the performance IQ. Tone and deep tendon reflexes are often increased, and optic atrophy, papilledema, and visual field defects can be present.

Fetal Hydrocephalus

The advent and refinement of high-resolution ultrasonography has allowed the prenatal diagnosis of much fetal pathology. In particular, the diagnosis of hydrocephalus has made it possible to consider intrauterine shunting of ventricular fluid into the amniotic sac (667,668). The majority of fetuses that have undergone such shunting have had aqueductal stenosis or communicating hydrocephalus. Treatment at present must be regarded as experimental in view of the inability to be sure that intraventricular pressure is high

relative to the intrauterine pressure, together with our imperfect knowledge of the natural history of fetal hydrocephalus. A number of factors need to be considered before surgery is selected. These include the presence of other CNS malformations such as spina bifida cystica and the Chiari deformity. It is usually considered wrong to attempt amelioration of hydrocephalus in such cases. Karyotyping and screening of the family for X-linked hydrocephalus are also necessary. Renier and coworkers have stressed that antenatal ventriculomegaly is not synonymous with hydrocephalus, and a significant proportion of infants with ventriculomegaly are found to have normal CSF pressures after birth (669). It is also difficult to determine from ultrasonography alone whether hydrocephalus is so severe that treatment is contraindicated, or whether it is sufficiently mild to allow the pregnancy to go to term (670).

In approximately one-half of the cases collected by Glick and coworkers, hydrocephalus was accompanied by other major anomalies, which precluded treatment (670). Even when treatment is selected, the outlook is poor. In Renier series of 106 infants with hydrocephalus at birth, 62% survived to 10 years of age. Of the survivors, 28% had IQs over 80, and 50% had IQs below 50 (669). Although grim, this prognosis is still better than that for infants who develop hydrocephalus secondary to a perinatal intraventricular hemorrhage.

If intrauterine surgery is elected, the shunt should be inserted before 32 weeks' gestation. If at ventriculostomy the pressure is less than 60 mm H_2O, the insertion of a shunting tube might not be justified. The current mortality for this procedure is 15% to 20%. Follow-up ultrasonographic studies may document an arrest of progressive ventricular enlargement or decompression. At birth, the shunt is converted to a ventriculoperitoneal bypass.

Clinical Manifestations

Four major factors influence the clinical course in hydrocephalus: the time of onset, duration of increased intracranial pressure, rate at which intracranial pressure increases, and any preexisting structural lesions. The time when hydrocephalus develops in relation to closure of the cranial sutures determines whether enlargement of the head is the presenting sign. Before 2 years of age, progressive enlargement of the head is almost invariably a presenting complaint. When hydrocephalus develops after 2 years of age, any changes in head circumference are overshadowed by other neurologic manifestations. In older infants and children, the space-occupying lesions responsible for hydrocephalus often produce focal neurologic signs before causing CSF obstruction.

Neonatal Period through Infancy (0 to 2 Years)

Hydrocephalus causing an abnormally large head or abnormally accelerating head growth during this time is usually caused by a major defect in embryogenesis. Chiari malformations with or without spina bifida cystica, aqueductal stenosis, and aqueductal gliosis account for 80% of all hydrocephalus in this period and represent 60% of all hydrocephalus regardless of age (671). The remainder of cases are a consequence of intrauterine infection, anoxic or traumatic perinatal hemorrhage, and neonatal bacterial or viral meningoencephalitis. Rare causes include congenital midline tumor, choroid plexus papilloma, and arteriovenous malformation of the vein of Galen or straight sinus. Apart from the features unique to each disease, they all produce a stereotyped clinical picture.

The etiology, presenting signs, management, and sequels of perinatal intracranial hemorrhage are described in Chapter 5.

The head grows at an abnormal rate and is macrocephalic within 12 months, if not at birth. The forehead is disproportionately large, giving an inverted triangular appearance to the head. The skull is thin, hair can be sparse, and the sutures are excessively separated. This results in an accentuated *cracked pot* sound on percussion of the skull. The anterior fontanelle is tense and the scalp veins are dilated, strikingly so when the infant cries. A divergent strabismus with the eyeballs rotated downward is often noted. This *setting-sun sign* is caused by pressure of the third ventricle's suprapineal recess on the mes-

encephalic tectum, causing impairment of the vertical gaze centers. The sign, however, also can be elicited in healthy infants (see Introduction chapter). Other ocular disturbances include unilateral or bilateral abducens nerve paresis, nystagmus, ptosis, and a diminished pupillary light response. Optic atrophy caused by compression of the chiasm and optic nerves by a dilated anterior portion of the third ventricle can occur. Papilledema is rare, perhaps because of the presence of open sutures.

Early infantile automatisms persist, indicating a failure in the development of normal cortical inhibition. Responses such as the parachute reflex, which is expected to appear later in infancy, fail to develop. Opisthotonus can be striking. A common finding is spasticity of the lower extremities, resulting from proportionately more stretching and distortion of myelinated paracentral corticospinal fibers arising from the leg area of the motor cortex. These fibers have a longer distance to travel around the dilated ventricle than do the corticospinal and corticobulbar fibers supplying the upper extremities and face. Mild spasticity and weakness, however, occur in the upper limbs. Clinical signs are caused more by myelin disruption than by cellular loss (672).

Of great importance is the development of deranged lower brainstem function caused by bilateral corticobulbar disruption, a condition termed *pseudobulbar palsy*. This is manifested by difficulty in sucking, feeding, and phonation, and results in regurgitation, drooling, and aspiration. Laryngeal stridor, although not common, is distressing. Some of these symptoms also can be the consequence of an associated Chiari II malformation, causing vagal nerve traction or perhaps infarction of the vagal nuclei in the medulla. Corticobulbar deficits together with a change in acoustic properties of brain and calvarium are believed to account for the characteristic shrill, brief, and high-pitched cry.

Other features of early infantile hydrocephalus relate more to specific causes. The clinical picture of Dandy-Walker syndrome is fairly characteristic and is covered in another section of this chapter (see Dandy-Walker Syndrome section, previously).

The Chiari malformation type II is almost always associated with spina bifida cystica and, occasionally, with short, malformed necks that result from basilar impression or the Klippel-Feil anomaly.

If hydrocephalus is rapidly progressive, as in acute bacterial meningitis or diffuse cortical thrombophlebitis, then emesis, somnolence, irritability, seizures, and cardiopulmonary embarrassment occur despite open sutures. Neonates with severe hydrocephalus associated with congenital anomalies usually do not survive the neonatal period.

Early to Late Childhood (2 to 10 Years)

In this age group, neurologic symptoms caused by increased intracranial pressure or by focal deficits referable to the primary lesion tend to appear before any significant changes in head size.

The most common causes for hydrocephalus during this period of life are posterior fossa neoplasms and obstructions at the aqueduct. The Chiari type I malformation, with abnormalities of the craniobasal bones and cervical vertebrae, also can be encountered in this age group.

The clinical picture of the various space-occupying lesions is discussed in Chapter 10. A unique hydrocephalic syndrome (the bobble-head doll syndrome) is characterized by two to four head oscillations per second, psychomotor retardation, and obstructive lesions in or around the third ventricle or aqueduct (673). It is important to recognize that head bobbing can be a sign of obstructive hydrocephalus in which, it is postulated, a dilated third ventricle impinges on the medial aspect of the dorsomedial nucleus of the thalamus.

Between 2 and 10 years of age, the infections most likely to cause hydrocephalus are tuberculosis and fungal or parasitic infections. Hydrocephalus resulting from any one of these agents has its special features; however, in almost all instances, increased intracranial pressure produces papilledema, strabismus, and headache on awakening in the morning that improves after emesis or upright posture. The cracked pot sound is prominent on skull percussion. Pyramidal tract signs are more marked in the lower limbs for reasons noted previously.

Additional features seen in this late onset group are encountered also in the early onset group in whom hydrocephalus has become arrested or marginally compensated, either spontaneously or because of surgical intervention. These features include endocrine changes resulting in small stature with growth hormone deficiency (674), obesity, gigantism, delayed or precocious puberty, primary amenorrhea or menstrual irregularities, absent secondary sexual characteristics, hypothyroidism, and diabetes insipidus (675,676). They are probably caused by abnormal hypothalamic-pituitary axis function, which is a consequence of compression of this axis by an enlarged third ventricle, a particular risk in aqueductal stenosis. Spastic diplegia is prominent, and both upper limbs exhibit mild pyramidal tract signs resulting in fine motor incoordination. Perceptual motor deficits and visual-spatial disorganization ensue as a consequence of stretched corticospinal fibers of parietal and occipital cortex owing to dilated posterior horns of the lateral ventricles. Performance intelligence is considerably worse than verbal intelligence, and learning problems are common (677). Children are sociable and conversationally bright, and they exhibit relatively good memory, but they are often hyperkinetic, emotionally labile, and unable to conceptualize (678).

Diagnosis

In infants, the initial diagnosis of hydrocephalus is based on a head circumference that, regardless of absolute size, crosses one or more grid lines (1 cm on the chart) (see Figs. I.1 and 4.22). Such infants require prompt diagnostic evaluation, even when overt neurologic signs are absent.

An evaluation of a premature infant for possible hydrocephalus must take into account its normal postnatal head growth (679). In preterm infants whose weight is appropriate for gestational age, head growth velocity increases progressively after birth, with maximum velocity occurring between 30 and 40 days (680). The less mature the infant, the smaller the initial increments of head growth, and the later the

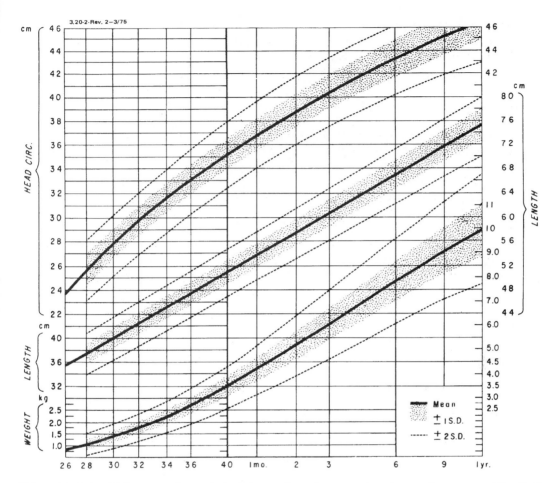

FIG. 4.22. A fetal-infant growth graph for infants of varying gestational ages. (Courtesy of Dr. S. G. Babson, Department of Pediatrics, University of Oregon School of Medicine, Portland, Oregon.)

time of maximal growth. The initial delay of head growth and probably of brain growth is related, in part, to the presence of respiratory distress and possibly also to exposure to oxygen (681). It does not correlate with caloric intake. A special head circumference chart applicable to preterm infants has been compiled by Babson and Benda (Fig. 4.22) (682).

Because acceleration of skull growth occurs later than increase in ventricular size, skull circumference measurements poorly reflect the increase in ventricular size. This is particularly the case for children older than age 18 months, in whom head circumference might not be abnormally large in the presence of hydrocephalus.

Various diagnostic studies of different complexities are used for the diagnosis of hydrocephalus and increased ventricular size. Transillumination of the skull is the least complex diagnostic study; nowadays, unfortunately, it is only rarely used (683).

Ultrasonography has proven invaluable in monitoring the ventricular system in infants with hydrocephalus (Fig. 4.23). Because the technique does not delineate intracranial anatomy as well as CT scans or MRI, its value lies not so much in establishing the diagnosis of hydrocephalus as in permitting sequential assessment of the adequacy of medical and surgical therapy (684,685). Fetal ultrasonography

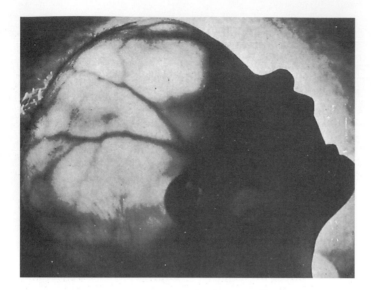

FIG. 4.23. Hydrocephalus in a neonate. Coronal ultrasonographic scan of hydrocephalus in a 2-day-old child with lumbosacral myelomeningocele. Marked dilatation of the bodies of the lateral ventricles (*LV*) and their temporal horns (*LV,t*) is present. The third ventricle (*V3*) is enlarged also, but to a lesser degree. (From Babcock DS, Han BK. The accuracy of high-resolution, real-time, ultrasonography of the head in infancy. *Radiology* 1981;139:665. With permission.)

also has been useful in the diagnosis of hydrocephalus and Dandy-Walker syndrome (686).

Although in the past CT scans have proven of value in the diagnostic evaluation of the infant or child with hydrocephalus, we believe that MRI is the preferred procedure. It demonstrates not only the size and position of the ventricles, but also the width of the subarachnoid spaces at the base of the brain and over its convexity. It is also the preferred means to measure changes in ventricular size after a shunting procedure.

MRI is also the optimal method to determine the cause of the hydrocephalus. The Dandy-Walker syndrome can be diagnosed by observing an enlarged fourth ventricle and a large posterior fossa cyst on sagittal views. Communicating hydrocephalus manifests by dilatation of the entire ventricular system and the subarachnoid spaces at the base of the brain and over the lower portion of the convexity. Aqueductal stenosis can be demonstrated by the dilatation of the lateral and third ventricles, the presence of a normal sized or small fourth ventricle, and absence of the normal flow-related signal void in the aqueduct (687,688).

It is sometimes difficult to distinguish between ventricular enlargement secondary to hydrocephalus and that resulting from white matter atrophy. Some findings that point to

hydrocephalus include dilatation of the temporal horns commensurate with dilatation of the lateral ventricles, enlargement of the anterior and posterior recesses of the third ventricle, and effacement of the cortical sulci (689).

A high-resolution axial technique can be used to quantitate CSF flow through the aqueduct and is a useful adjunct to MRI (690). Additionally, MRI can delineate a variety of cerebral anomalies and readily excludes the presence of tumors or larger arteriovenous malformations. Differentiation of normal and increased pressure hydrocephalus by MRI studies is under investigation (691,692). Cine-MRI also holds great promise in the evaluation of CSF dynamics in obstructive and communicative hydrocephalus (693,694).

Angiography for the diagnostic evaluation of hydrocephalus has largely been replaced by CT or MRI.

Information concerning CSF clearance, particularly in subjects with normal-pressure hydrocephalus, is provided by radioisotope cisternography. This procedure consists of the injection into the lumbar sac or cisterna of ^{131}I-labeled serum albumin, technetium, or indium (695). Emission of gamma radiation is measured by an external scanner. In communicating hydrocephalus, the radioisotope collects entirely within the ventricular system and persists there for 24 to 48 hours (696). In noncommunicating hydrocephalus and in healthy subjects, no retrograde filling is present. In the healthy subject, all the supratentorial cisterns are well visualized within 4 hours. By 12 to 24 hours, the radioisotope concentrates over the cerebral convexities toward the parasagittal area. By 48 hours, the CSF is clear.

When hydrocephalus develops after infancy, children show symptoms and signs of increased intracranial pressure. Their diagnostic evaluation is similar to that suggested for tumor suspects (see Chapter 10).

Treatment

The general principles of treatment are surgical correction of CSF obstruction, reduction of CSF production by drugs or surgical therapy, ventricular bypass into a normal intracranial channel in noncommunicating hydrocephalus, and ventricular bypass into an extracranial compartment in either noncommunicating or communicating hydrocephalus.

In the child with rapidly progressive hydrocephalus of whatever cause, the need for therapy is obvious. However, the patient in whom hydrocephalus progresses slowly or who is suspected of having an arrested process presents a difficult therapeutic problem (697). Ultimately, clinical findings and serial imaging studies will determine whether treatment is indicated. At present, we believe that the diagnosis of arrested hydrocephalus cannot be made in a patient with macrocephaly, despite a normal head growth curve and normal CSF pressures, unless ventricular size stabilizes as ascertained by imaging studies (662,666). We concur with the suggestion of McLone and Aronyk that children older than 3 years of age with stable ventricular size be monitored if their intellectual performance is within the normal range and appears stable (697). Children younger than 3 years of age with large ventricles should be shunted, not because we know what the likely outcome of nontreatment is, but because we do not.

Ventriculomegaly after meningitis or in conjunction with spina bifida cystica does not require a shunting procedure, unless serial imaging studies demonstrate it to be progressive. Once progression has become evident, needless procrastination or failure to treat can result in further compromise of both cognitive function and fine and gross motor coordination. Although the underlying cause of hydrocephalus and serial developmental examinations can provide clues to the ultimate prognosis, they cannot be used as the basis for a decision on whether to perform surgery.

Medical Treatment

As a rule, medical management of hydrocephalus has failed because in most cases hydrocephalus is the result of impaired CSF absorption, and the pharmacologic agents currently available have little or no effect on this process. Most agents known to decrease CSF formation under experimental conditions cannot be tolerated by human subjects when given in sufficiently high doses to diminish CSF production. Notable exceptions are acetazolamide and furosemide. These agents, given singly or in conjunction (e.g., 100 mg/kg per day of acetazolamide and 1 mg/kg per day of furosemide), decrease CSF production, acetazolamide by inhibiting choroid plexus carbonic anhydrase and furosemide probably by inhibiting chloride transport. Each agent reduces CSF formation by approximately 50%, but the combined effect of the two drugs appears to be greater than the additive effect. Reduction of normal CSF production by one-third reduces intracranial pressure by only 1.5 cm H_2O. This differential explains the clinical limitations of agents that reduce CSF formation (698,699). Currently, these drugs are used as a temporizing measure or are used preoperatively in patients with acute hydrocephalus in whom immediate surgery is not possible. Nephrocalcinosis is a potentially serious complication.

Surgical Treatment

Several methods of surgical treatment have been used.

Direct Attack. The best treatment for hydrocephalus is to remove the obstruction. This is possible only in the small proportion of patients in whom a tumor or cyst within or beyond the ventricular system can be resected. Surgical attempts to eliminate the obstruction in aqueductal stenosis, Dandy-Walker malformation, and Chiari malformation type II associated with myelodysplasia have been abandoned because the failure rate has been high, and the associated morbidity and mortality are considerable.

Indirect Attack. Two techniques of indirect attack are of great historical interest: endoscopic choroid plexus extirpation (plexectomy or electric coagulation) and third or fourth ventriculostomy. Choroid plexus extirpation had been used successfully in communicating hydrocephalus, with an arrest rate of 65% (700). Although complicated by intracerebral hemorrhage and, potentially, by cystic dilatations of the endoscopic tracts, as well as an operative mortality of 10%, the elimination of the choroid plexus pulse effect, one of the reasons for ventricular dilatation, provided a pathophysiologic rationale for this approach.

Ventricular Bypass. Therapeutically, the distinction between communicating (extraventricular) and noncommunicating (intraventricular) hydrocephalus has been rendered less important by modern shunt technology. In both types, the lateral ventricle is used as the drained reservoir. The CSF is bypassed from the ventricle, the site of its production, around the obstruction, and into a freely draining compartment of the body.

Surgical fenestration of the third ventricle into the basal cisterns and placement of a tube between a lateral ventricle and the cervical subarachnoid space (ventriculocisternostomy or Torkildsen procedure) are ways of bypassing the obstruction in noncommunicating hydrocephalus. Use of these methods depends on the patency of the basal cisterns and subarachnoid spaces, a condition that is not always present and must be verified before surgery. In general, these shunts are restricted to older children with noncommunicating hydrocephalus or to children with hydrocephalus caused by posterior fossa mass lesions obstructing outflow (694). In the experience of Cinalli and colleagues, when this procedure is performed using endoscopic guidance, good results were obtained in some 70% of infants or children with

primary aqueductal stenosis, and they consider this procedure preferable to shunt placement (701).

Extracranial Shunts

Ventriculoperitoneal Shunts. The modern era of extracranial shunts began in 1949 when Matson introduced diversion of CSF into the ureter (702). Subsequent development of pressure-regulated one-way flow valves made this procedure unnecessary and avoided the sacrifice of a kidney. Additionally, ureteral shunts were associated with such major complications as gram-negative ventriculitis and life-threatening electrolyte imbalances (590). Steady improvement in shunting hardware and a progressive decline in shunt-related complications have made extracranial shunting the procedure of choice whenever the direct surgical removal of the obstruction is not possible.

Extracranial shunts currently used include the ventriculoperitoneal, ventriculoatrial, ventriculopleural, and lumboperitoneal varieties. Although the ventriculoatrial shunt was the first to enjoy widespread success, it has largely been supplanted by the ventriculoperitoneal shunt because the latter is technically easier to insert and is associated with less severe complications. Ventriculoperitoneal shunts were not widely used until the last three decades because the peritoneal end frequently became obstructed. The development of newer silicone elastomers and the insertion of sufficient tubing to allow the abdominal end to move freely about the peritoneal cavity have largely eliminated this problem.

Several types of valves are used. The Holter valve consists of two stainless steel check valves connected by silicone tubing. The Pudenz-Heyer-Schulte valve is a plastic bubble pump placed under the scalp with its distal end connected to the slit valve. Both apparatuses can be pumped. The Holter valve can be attached to many types of reservoirs placed in the burr hole to measure ventricular pressure and to instill antibiotics. Other, increasingly sophisticated devices are used currently. Of note are the programmable valves (i.e., valves whose flow characteristics can be altered by application of a magnetic field external to the head) and the Delta Valve. The Delta Valve incorporates an antisiphon device and adjusts the flow automatically to maintain intraventricular pressure within a narrow range in the face of the significant changes in CSF pressure that result from changes in posture or altered intracranial conditions. Many shunt valves can be preset to open at high or low CSF pressures, depending on the individual needs of the patient, such as the size of the lateral ventricles and thickness of the cerebral mantle. The various shunting devices currently available are discussed by Post (703).

Ventriculovascular Shunts. The ventriculo-vascular shunt was the preferred pathway before improvement of the peritoneal shunt, and it still is preferred in some adult patients. A medium- or high-pressure valve is required. The slit one-way valve opens at a predetermined intraventricular pressure and closes once the pressure decreases below that level, thus preventing retrograde flow of venous blood into the ventricular cavity.

Lumboperitoneal and Other Shunts. Lumboperitoneal and other shunts are used infrequently in the pediatric age group because they are limited to the treatment of communicating hydrocephalus and pseudotumor cerebri. In pseudotumor cerebri, the narrower ventricles can make the insertion of a ventricular catheter technically difficult. Insertion of a lumboperitoneal shunt and its subsequent revision require a greater amount of operative manipulation than with other shunts and can be associated with scoliosis and nerve root irritation. Although the CSF can be diverted into the pleural cavity, frequent and progressive pleural effusions that require subsequent removal of the shunt in infants and small children restrict use of this type of a procedure to the older child or adult.

Complications of Shunts. The best way to avoid shunt complications is not to insert a shunt. Shunt complications can be divided into those that are common to all types of shunts and those that are unique to one particular type (704). All shunts are subject to obstruction, disconnection, and infection, and revisions are often required periodically with somatic growth. The frequency and location of obstruction and

disconnection depend to a degree on the shunting hardware. In general, the most frequent malfunction is that of occlusion of the ventricular catheter by choroid plexus or glial tissue that actually grows into the lumen of the catheter. Disconnection can occur at any point within the system, but most commonly it occurs where the various components are joined. Pressure-regulated valves in the shunting system can cause obstruction, drain CSF at higher or lower pressures than intended, and, rarely, allow retrograde flow. The last is of concern only in ventriculovascular shunts.

Use of a shunt valve that opens at too low a CSF pressure in an infant with a thin cerebral mantle and greatly enlarged lateral ventricle might result in collapse of the brain and massive subdural hematoma formation.

Although considerable apprehension has been expressed that an elevated CSF protein content can obstruct the valves, this has never been confirmed (705). We have noted, however, that increased CSF protein is commonly associated with a higher incidence of ventricular catheter obstruction. We advocate the use of radiopaque material to visualize the entire length of the shunt and thus determine the continuity of the shunting system on plain radiography. We also recommend that a reservoir be placed in the system to allow access to the CSF. By tapping the reservoir, pressures can be measured, functioning of the system can be ascertained, and CSF can be obtained for examination as necessary.

Imaging techniques that use contrast agents or radioisotopes can be used to determine the patency of the shunt. Each type of shunting system has its own peculiarities that determine how best to ascertain the adequacy of its function. That most shunting systems contain a pumping mechanism, in either the valve or the reservoir, that is designed to test whether the shunt is functioning properly is unfortunate, because the correlation between the response to pumping and functioning of the shunt is poor. Many functioning shunts do not pump normally, whereas other shunts that pump well are malfunctioning. We therefore strongly advocate that the response to pumping of the shunt not be used to establish its adequacy. In a shunt-dependent child, malfunction results in a progressive increase in intracranial pressure, which can be acute or chronic, depending on the rate at which intracranial pressure becomes elevated. The symptoms differ little from those seen before the insertion of the shunt.

The implantation of foreign material, even when it is completely tissue compatible, carries the risk of infection in the neighboring areas (706). Prevention of infection, clearly of primary importance, can be achieved only by meticulous attention to aseptic technique during insertion, revision, or tapping. The value of antibiotic prophylaxis in preventing shunt infections has been established (707). In our hospitals, coverage for gram-positive organisms is given preoperatively and for the first 24 hours after operation, using first-generation cephalosporins, such as cephalothin or cefazolin. To prevent emergence of vancomycin-resistant organisms, vancomycin is not used for bacterial prophylaxis. Reduction of operating time and the use of experienced neurosurgeons also has a beneficial effect on the occurrence of infection, which now occurs in 1% to 5% of procedures in many pediatric neurosurgical centers. Superficial sepsis in the area of the wound usually responds to antibiotic treatment, whereas deeper infection is uncommon when proper operative technique has been used.

More frequent is the development of infection secondary to colonization of the valve or catheters, which leads to peritonitis with a ventriculoperitoneal shunt or bacteremia with a ventriculoatrial shunt. Although insidious in onset and sometimes difficult to diagnose, infection secondary to colonization usually develops within 6 months of shunt insertion. In the experience of Meirovitch and his group, reporting from Israel on patients collected between 1972 and 1984, 44% of infections developed during the first postoperative week, and over one-half developed during the first postoperative month (708). As a rule, the infection rate is higher in neonates and small infants (709). In the experience of one center, the incidence is 15.7% when shunts are performed in infants younger than 6 months of age, as contrasted to 5.6% when patients older than 6 months are shunted. As a rule, the incidence of infection is inversely proportional to the experience of the neurosurgeon. Some centers propose the use of prophylactic antibiotics to reduce the incidence of infections.

The most common organisms encountered are coagulase-positive or coagulase-negative staphylococci (710,711). These accounted for 67% of infections in the 1992 series of Pople and colleagues (709). The remainder represents a variety of pathogens. Nearly all the organisms that have been responsible for shunt infections are normal skin commensals, and intensive typing procedures have shown that the invading organism is usually indistinguishable from the patient's own skin flora. Most infections occur within 4 months of the placement of an initial shunt and within 2 months of the placement of a revised shunt (711). Shunt infection can manifest by fever, shunt malfunction, irritability, vomiting, meningism, and swelling or redness over a portion or all of the shunting tract (708,711). Less commonly, one sees generalized symptoms such as meningitis or peritonitis with a ventriculoperitoneal shunt, or septicemia with a ventriculoatrial shunt. Peripheral leukocytosis is seen in approximately one-half of instances. In the case of a ventriculoperitoneal shunt, obstruction owing to infection usually occurs at the distal end.

Infections also can occur as a result of breakdown of the skin over the hardware. In some instances, the infection is confined to the ventricular system and the shunt, without any external evidence of infection. Initial and recurrent infection rates are similar in all types of shunts (708).

The most reliable way to confirm a shunt infection is to identify organisms on a Gram-stained smear, or to obtain multiple CSF cultures from the shunting system (710). A less time-consuming test is to measure serum C-reactive protein, supplemented by coagulase-negative staphylococcus antibody testing in the CSF (706). Increased CSF eosinophilia is seen in approximately 28% of shunt infections. In approximately 80% of these it is accompanied by blood eosinophilia. The distribution of infectious agents in shunt infections with eosinophilia is no different than in those without it (712).

The management of shunt infections remains a matter of debate. All authorities advocate the use of appropriate intraventricular and systemic antibiotics, combined with one of four approaches: removal of the infected shunt and placement of an external ventricular drainage system; removal of the infected shunt without replacement until a short course of antibiotics is completed, with the hydrocephalus being controlled by an external ventricular drain or repeated CSF aspirations; removal of the infected shunt with immediate insertion of a new shunt; or clearing of the infection without replacement of the shunting system (706,708,710,711). We advocate complete removal of the entire infected shunt, placement of a ventricular drain, and replacement of the shunt at a subsequent time. In the experience of Ronan and colleagues, this approach had a better outcome, with a relapse rate of only 4.5% (711). The appropriate antibiotic, chosen, if possible, according to the sensitivity of the organisms, is injected into the ventricles; at the same time, a broad-spectrum antibiotic is given systemically. The infection is usually overcome in 4 days, and on the seventh day the shunt can be reinserted.

Complications unique to peritoneal shunts include ascites, pseudocyst formation, perforation of a viscus or of the abdominal wall, and intestinal obstruction (713). The use of a coiled spring inside the peritoneal catheter to prevent its kinking (Raimondi catheter) is responsible for the majority of abdominal complications (714). The length of the tube in the peritoneal cavity does not appear to be a factor in subsequent complications (714).

The older the shunted patient is and the bigger the ventricles are at the time of surgery, the greater the likelihood of a significant subdural fluid collection. Fluid collection can occur spontaneously or after seemingly minor head trauma. Its incidence can be reduced by the use of a higher pressure valve. If it is asymptomatic, treatment is not indicated, but if it is accompanied by clinical symptoms, the fluid should be drained, usually by insertion of a subdural peritoneal shunt.

The incidence of seizures in patients with shunted hydrocephalus is higher than in unshunted patients (704,715). That the shunting procedure contributes to a seizure disorder is substantiated by EEG abnormalities localized to the site of shunt insertion (716). We do not believe that anticonvulsants should be given prophylactically.

Another, rarer complication of the shunting procedure is the slit ventricle syndrome. This condition refers to symptoms and signs of intermittent intracranial hypertension in a child who has been treated for hydrocephalus by the insertion of a shunt, and whose ventricular system is found to be much smaller than normal. The patient, whose condition has usually been stable for months or years after the initial shunt placement, develops headache, vomiting, or impaired consciousness. A large proportion of subjects, 27% in the series of Baskin and colleagues, develop Parinaud syndrome (716a). The cause for this potentially fatal syndrome has not been satisfactorily explained; it might represent several different entities (717). Rekate has suggested that chronic monitoring of intracranial pressure will uncover the cause of the syndrome (718). In a significant proportion of patients with small ventricles, intracranial pressure monitoring has revealed paroxysms of high pressure, even though the shunt appears to function normally. This may be the result of intermittent occlusion of the ventricular catheter in a shunt-dependent patient. In others, intracranial pressure is extremely low. This could result from an acquired rigidity of the periventricular tissue. In either case, the failure for ventriculomegaly to develop remains unexplained. Epstein has suggested that the diminished CSF volume is insufficient to buffer the normally occurring fluctuations in intracranial blood pressure and blood volume (717). Small ventricles revealed by neuroimaging studies, however, are often seen in patients who are clinically asymptomatic.

Regular monitoring by neuroimaging studies to monitor ventricle size should prevent the development of slit ventricle syndrome. Additionally, the appearance of a seizure disorder or the deterioration of the EEG should suggest this condition (719).

Treatment of the established condition is difficult and often ineffective. Baskin and colleagues suggest that patients undergo fiberoptic intracranial pressure monitoring after removal or externalization of their shunts. They found that a significant number of patients tolerated removal of their shunts. Those who demonstrated a need for CSF drainage underwent endoscopic third ventriculostomy with improvement or resolution of complaints in 73% (716a). No attempt should be made to insert a new ventricular catheter, because its failure and consequent hemorrhage are likely. Another approach would be to insert a valve that opens at a moderately higher pressure than the one already present, or to use an antisiphoning device (718). The newer, self-adjustable or externally adjustable valves might also prove to be capable of avoiding the syndrome.

Prognosis

Based on studies of the natural course of untreated (720) and spontaneously arrested hydrocephalus (678,721), it is clear that surgery reduces mortality and limits morbidity. Untreated, hydrocephalus has a 50% mortality. In one study, 50% of the survivors were mentally retarded in the illiterate range or worse, and fewer than 10% were intellectually normal. Over two-thirds of survivors had major physical handicaps (720). Other studies of spontaneously arrested hydrocephalus revealed an IQ over 90 in one-third of survivors, and disabling neurologic defects in two-thirds (678). These defects included ataxia, spastic diplegia, compromised fine motor coordination, and perceptual deficits.

In surgically treated hydrocephalus, survival rate is at least 90%, and the IQ is normal or nearly normal in approximately two-thirds of patients. As a rule, verbal IQ is higher than performance IQ, and the classic *cocktail chatter* of a hydrocephalic child is a common occurrence (722). Neither site of obstruction nor number of shunt revisions or infections have an adverse effect on IQ. No evidence exists that prompt shunting enhances the ultimate IQ. Rather IQ is a function of the etiology of the hydrocephalus, in particular, the presence or absence of concurrent cerebral malformations (723). Posterior fossa malformations do not affect IQ (722). In general,

the narrower the cortical mantle and the smaller the brain mass, the worse the eventual outcome. The outcome for normal cognitive function in preterm infants with shunted posthemorrhagic hydrocephalus is poor. This topic is covered in greater detail in Chapter 5.

The question whether a shunt, once placed, can ever be removed has been considered by Hemmer and Böhm (724). In their series, only 9% of shunts could be removed in children with communicating hydrocephalus or hydrocephalus associated with myelomeningoceles. We believe that no asymptomatic shunting device should ever be removed because, in many instances, it is impossible to establish beyond doubt whether the shunt is totally nonfunctional (725,726). In this respect, it is reassuring to remember that a nonfunctioning shunt rarely, if ever, becomes infected.

Hydranencephaly

Pathology

In hydranencephaly, the greater portions of both the cerebral hemispheres and the corpus striatum are reduced to membranous sacs composed of glial tissue covered by intact meninges and encompassing a cavity filled with clear CSF. Occasionally, the CSF is opaque and protein rich. Basal portions of frontal, temporal, and occipital lobe are preserved, together with scattered islands of cortex elsewhere. The diencephalon, midbrain, and brainstem are usually normal except for rudimentary descending corticobulbar and corticospinal tracts. The cerebellum can be normal, hypoplastic, or damaged (727,728). In some cases, the ependyma lining the covering membrane is intact, the choroid plexus is preserved, and the aqueduct is stenotic. Other patients have large bilateral schizencephalic clefts in which pia and ependyma are joined, and they demonstrate other migration anomalies of fetal morphogenesis. In still other brains, bilateral porencephalic cysts replace the parenchyma normally perfused by the middle and anterior cerebral arteries. The latter instances show pathologic evidence of a destructive lesion.

Pathogenesis

The pathology suggests at least four different pathogenetic mechanisms. Some authorities, citing the presence of preserved ependyma and aqueductal stenosis in some cases, have argued that hydranencephaly is a type of hydrocephalus that has run its course *in utero*. In other instances, hydranencephaly can be the consequence of intrauterine infections or other gestational insults (728,729). In other cases, the condition can represent a genetically determined defect in vascular ontogenesis or can be the outcome of vascular occlusion of both internal carotid arteries or their main branches (727,730). A proliferative vasculopathy with an autosomal recessive inheritance also has been described (731). A few cases appear to be caused by defects in embryogenesis and subsequent cellular migration, resulting in schizencephaly and cortical agenesis (314).

Clinical Manifestations

Infants appear healthy at birth or have a somewhat large head that enlarges progressively. Spontaneous and reflex activity is often normal. However, failure in the development of cerebrocortical inhibition results in the persistence and exaggeration of reflexes, which becomes apparent by the second or third postnatal week. Over the subsequent weeks, hyperreflexia, hypertonia, quadriparesis, and decerebration develop, together with irritability, infantile spasms, and dysconjugate extraocular movements. Generalized or minor motor seizures also become apparent. EEG can be normal at first, but later becomes abnormal, varying from a diffusely slow to an isoelectric pattern. The visual-evoked responses are absent, but brainstem auditory-evoked responses are preserved (732). Environmentally related behavioral automatisms can occur in those surviving early infancy (733).

Diagnosis

In an infant with an enlarged head or abnormally accelerating head growth, ultrasonography is mandatory to exclude severe hydrocephalus and expanding bilateral porencephalic cysts under increased pressure. Neuroimaging studies exclude massive bilateral subdural effusions that can mimic hydranencephaly on ultrasonography. Most infants with hydranencephaly do not survive beyond 23 months of life; they succumb to intercurrent infections or to an unexplained deficit of vital function. Survival for several years has been reported, however (733).

Treatment

No treatment is available for hydranencephaly.

Arachnoidal Cysts

Arachnoidal cysts are fluid-filled cavities situated within the arachnoid membrane and lined with collagen and cells arising from the arachnoid. They are believed to result from an anomalous splitting of the arachnoid membrane and to date from the sixth to the eighth fetal week. Some communicate freely with the subarachnoid space; in other patients contrast material introduced into the subarachnoid space does not enter the cyst or only does so slowly. Approximately one half of the cysts are located in the middle cranial fossa (734), one-third are in the posterior fossa, and 10% are found in the suprasellar region (Fig. 4.24). Approximately one-fourth of the middle cranial fossa cysts are bilateral and some are accompanied by hypogenesis or compression of the temporal lobe (735). Additionally, they can cause a diffuse expansion and thinning of the bones of the vault, and an elevation of the lesser wing of the sphenoid (573).

Although in many instances a small cyst is clinically silent, larger cysts or cysts located in the posterior fossa can produce signs and symptoms of increased intracranial pressure. The cyst has the potential of producing hydrocephalus by increasing the resistance to CSF flow in the subarachnoid space. As the cyst enlarges, it eventually produces extrinsic compression of the ventricular system or of the subarachnoid channels. Symptoms can begin at any time during life. Aside from hydrocephalus, they include headaches and seizures. The relationship

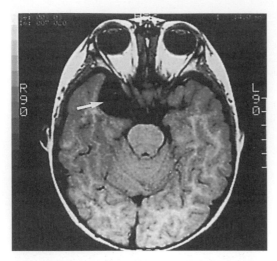

FIG. 4.24. Arachnoid cyst. The T1-weighted (466/16/1) axial magnetic resonance imaging demonstrates the presence of a discrete low-intensity structure (*arrow*) in the right middle fossa that displaces the anterior temporal lobe laterally. The lesion had high intensity on T2-weighted images, consistent with CSF signal characteristics. The patient was a 3.5-year-old boy who presented with headaches and whose neurologic examination was benign. No evidence exists of a pressure effect on the imaging study.

between headaches or seizures and the presence of an arachnoid cyst is often difficult to establish. Hemorrhage into an arachnoid cyst can cause the sudden onset of focal neurologic signs. A subdural hematoma has been reported to originate from a preexisting arachnoid cyst (736). Spinal cord arachnoid cysts can be intradural or less frequently extradural. They may present as space-occupying lesions with radicular pain, progressive weakness and spasticity, scoliosis, recurrent urinary tract infections, and constipation (737). An accompanying neural tube defect is common (738).

With the increased use of imaging studies, many cysts are discovered accidentally, particularly in the course of evaluating a seizure patient. Gandy and Heier believe that removal of the cyst does not improve seizure control (659). In other instances, removal of the cyst has been associated with complete or improved seizure control (739). Because the large major-

ity of cysts remain constant in size, and only large cysts tend to expand, we suggest only those cysts that present as space-occupying lesions should require surgical removal.

Achondroplasia

Achondroplasia is an abnormality of endochondral bone development transmitted as an autosomal dominant trait. It occurs in approximately 1 in 25,000 births, and 80% occur sporadically as new mutations. The gene for achondroplasia has been mapped to the tip of the short arm of chromosome 4 (4p16.3) in close proximity to the gene for Huntington disease (740). The gene (*FGFR3*) codes for a tyrosine kinase transmembrane receptor for fibroblast growth factor (740). *FGRFs* are members of a superfamily that bind fibroblast growth factors and initiate an intracellular signaling cascade. Remarkable genetic homogeneity exists, and almost all achondroplastic subjects have the same point mutation.

Clinically, a decrease in the rate of endochondral bone formation is seen with normal membranous bone formation. The condition is characterized by dwarfism and a variety of skeletal abnormalities. Neurologic symptoms are the result of macrocephaly, which might or might not be accompanied by hydrocephalus, and cervicomedullary compression.

Because the cranial base is the only portion of the skull that is preformed in cartilage, its growth is selectively impaired, and a compensatory growth of the calvaria and an increase in the vertical diameter of the skull occur. The skull base is narrowed and the petrous pyramids tower. This results in an abnormal orientation of inner and middle ear structures (741). These growth changes produce a characteristic brachycephalic configuration and narrowing of all foramina that pass through the base of the skull.

As Dandy (742) demonstrated in 1921 using pneumoencephalography, the ventricular system is enlarged in approximately 50% of achondroplastic individuals (743). The cause for ventricular dilatation is still under debate. Some authorities have suggested that it results from a mechanical block to the flow of CSF in the area of the foramen magnum, which is abnormally small in almost all patients with achondroplasia. This is confirmed by invasive monitoring, which has demonstrated an elevation of intracranial pressure (743). In addition, venography of the jugular veins demonstrates stenosis at the level of the jugular foramen and a pressure gradient across the foramen. Flodmark suggests that this phenomenon is responsible for venous hypertension and impaired CSF absorption (736). Yamada and colleagues have confirmed the presence of both causes for hydrocephalus (744). Venous decompression at the jugular foramen, and construction of a venous bypass from the transverse sinus to the jugular vein, have reduced ventriculomegaly, as has venous decompression at the jugular foramen (744,745).

Cervicomedullary compression resulting from stenosis of the foramen magnum is a serious complication, presenting at any time from infancy to adult life. In the series of Ryken and Menezes, 3.2% of subjects with achondroplasia demonstrated symptoms or signs of progressive compression of neural structures at the level of the foramen magnum (746). These included a variety of respiratory complications that are frequent in achondroplasia, notably apnea and respiratory irregularities. In the series of Nelson and coworkers, the incidence of apnea was 28% (747). Other signs include ataxia and spastic quadriparesis. In some instances brainstem compression can be insidious and can lead to syringobulbia, tetraplegia, and sudden infant death syndrome (748). Rarely, other neurologic signs are seen, including weak cry, failure to thrive, hypersomnia, and persistent papilledema (748,749). Paraplegia can develop as a result of compression of the spinal cord in the thoracic area (750). Mental retardation and seizures are not common features of achondroplasia (751). Although sensorineural hearing loss is common and subtle cognitive deficits have been uniformly demonstrated, general intelligence is within normal limits in most patients.

Considerable controversy exists as to who and when to perform suboccipital decompressive surgery (748,752,753). On the one hand, surgery is not without risk, and almost all achondroplastic infants who present with spasticity ultimately attain normal motor develop-

ment if left alone (752). In addition, because the foramen magnum grows faster than the spinal cord, the impingement of the posterior rim of the foramen magnum on the cord decreases with maturation. On the other hand, MRI and pathologic evidence suggest deformational and traumatic changes to the spinal cord as a result of foramen magnum stenosis (753). We believe MRI evidence of notching or indentation of the spinal cord at the level of the foramen magnum has little clinical significance, and that unless evidence exists of spasticity or increased signal within the spinal cord on T2-weighted images, decompressive surgery can be deferred.

Osteopetrosis

The osteopetroses are a rare and heterogeneous group of disorders characterized by generalized bone sclerosis with thickening and increased fragility of cortical and spongy bone. Both autosomal dominant and autosomal recessive forms have been encountered, with the former being more common. As a result of a defect in osteoclast function bone resorption is reduced, and the skull base is thickened and the foramina are narrowed. The autosomal dominant form has a benign prognosis, and subjects may remain asymptomatic. The recessive form is characterized by delayed psychomotor development, optic atrophy, conductive hearing loss, and facial nerve palsy (754,755). Other neurologic complications include hydrocephalus and intracranial hemorrhage (755). The earlier the onset of symptoms, the more malignant the course.

Cerebral atrophy with secondary ventricular dilatation is frequently evident. A combination of calvarial thickening and hydrocephalus explains the degree of macrocephaly only in part. The process involves all skeletal bone and results in hematologic and bleeding disorders and in frequent fractures.

Computed tomographic scans are diagnostic. MRI often reveals delayed myelination and cerebral atrophy. Calcifications can be seen in the periventricular area and the falx (756). The only curative treatment is early allogeneic bone marrow transplantation. Surgical decompression can stabilize cranial nerve deficits, especially optic nerve entrapments. Visual-evoked potentials and electroretinography can be used to show the first indications of visual impairment (757).

A syndrome of osteopetrosis, renal tubular acidosis, and cerebral calcification is inherited as an autosomal recessive trait. Mental retardation is common, and patients have unusual facies. The primary defect in this entity appears to be one of carbonic anhydrase II, one of two enzymes catalyzing the association of water and carbon dioxide to form bicarbonate (758,759). Osteopetrosis also has been associated with infantile neuroaxonal dystrophy (760).

CONGENITAL DEFECTS OF CRANIAL NERVES AND RELATED STRUCTURES

Möbius Syndrome

Möbius syndrome, first described by Harlan in 1880 (761), by Chisholm in 1882 (762), and more extensively by Möbius in 1888 and 1892 (763,764), is characterized by congenital paralysis of the facial muscles and impairment of lateral gaze.

Möbius syndrome results from diverse causes. Pathologic lesions include complete or partial absence of the facial nuclei, dysplasia of the facial musculature, and hypoplasia of the facial nerve. The entity also has been seen in a variety of conditions involving progressive disease of muscle, anterior horn cells, or peripheral neurons. In some instances, absence, faulty attachment, or fibrosis of the extraocular muscles is present, whereas in other cases, the brainstem nuclei showed multiple areas of calcification and necrosis, suggesting a prenatal vascular etiology (765–767). The symmetric calcified lesions with chronic gliosis, including gemistocytes, are in the tegmentum of the pons and medulla oblongata, a watershed zone of the brainstem between the territories of the paramedian penetrating arteries and the long circumferential arteries, both branches of the basilar artery. The vascular anatomy and the histopathologic findings at birth indicate a period of systemic hypotension in fetal life at least 4 to 6 weeks before birth (768). In a few cases, the electromyogra-

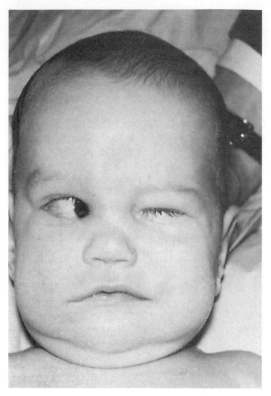

FIG. 4.25. Möbius syndrome. As the infant cries, she demonstrates the bilateral weakness of the lower facial musculature and the marked weakness of the right upper facial muscles. Additionally, a palsy of both external recti, tongue, and palatal musculature occurred, requiring gastrostomy feeding.

phy points to the presence of a supranuclear lesion (769,770).

Most patients with Möbius syndrome have a variable degree of unilateral, asymmetric, or symmetric bilateral facial paralysis, with an inability to abduct the eyes beyond the midline (771). Occasionally, the weakness is restricted to portions or quadrants of the face (Fig. 4.25). Atrophy of the tongue, paralysis of the soft palate or masseters, congenital clubfoot, deafness, or a mild spastic diplegia also can be present. Because of bulbar deficits, the language and communication disorder is far greater than general intelligence would predict (772). Möbius syndrome is nonprogressive. In some instances, however, myotonic dystrophy or muscular dystrophy can accompany Möbius syndrome (773).

Congenital Sensorineural Deafness

Congenital deafness resulting from a lesion of the acoustic nerve can occur in isolation or in combination with a variety of anomalies. The conditions can appear sporadically or be transmitted in a dominant, recessive, or sex-linked manner (774,775). In the experience of Das, a family history of deafness was elicited in 23% of children assessed for bilateral sensorineural hearing loss. Perinatal asphyxia was believed responsible for 13%, congenital infections for 8.2%, bacterial meningitis for 6.5%, chromosomal anomalies for 5.3%, and a variety of syndromes, notably Waardenburg syndrome, for 5.3%. In 34%, the cause was unknown (776). Mutations in the *connexin 26* gene are the single most common cause of genetic hearing loss (777). Other causes for profound hearing loss occurring in childhood are outlined in Table 4.15.

In a significant proportion of patients, dermatologic manifestations accompany the hearing loss. Waardenburg syndrome, probably the most common entity of this group, is characterized by widely spaced medial canthi, a flat nasal root, a white forelock, and heterochromia iridis. It is transmitted as a dominant trait (778). The gene defective in Waardenburg syndrome (*PAX3*) is located on the long arm of chromosome 2 (2q35-2q37), and normally codes for a protein termed HuP2. HuP2 protein binds DNA and the gene that codes for it is suspected to be one of a family of genes, the homeobox genes, which regulate mammalian development; in animals, mutations in these genes result in major developmental abnormalities (779,780).

In another group of syndromes, congenital sensorineural deafness is associated with visual symptoms. In Usher syndrome, a condition transmitted in an autosomal recessive manner, congenital neural hearing loss is seen in conjunction with progressive visual impairment and retinitis pigmentosa (774,781). Usher syndrome is the most common of a number of conditions in which retinitis pigmentosa is combined with deafness. These are reviewed by Mills and Calver (781). When a sensorineural hearing loss accompanies a neurologic disorder, it is usually in the framework of a peripheral neuropathy, and the hearing loss is progressive rather than congenital (774).

A distinct syndrome of congenital weakness of the musculature of the face, tongue, and palate unassociated with atrophy has been termed *congenital suprabulbar paresis* by Worster-Drought (782). This condition is related to the perisylvian syndrome, in which facio-lingual-masticatory diplegia results from bilaterally anterior opercular infarctions. In the congenital form of this condition, marked feeding difficulties are accompanied by dysarthria, restricted tongue movements, and an absent gag reflex. Intellect is relatively preserved. In the series of Kuzniecky and coworkers, seizures were documented in 87% (783). These tend to have their onset after the age of 5 years, and most commonly are atonic and tonic drop attacks. Neuroimaging studies frequently disclose polymicrogyria, which has a predilection for the opercular areas. Associated malformations, notably arthrogryposis, clubfeet, and spastic quadriparesis are not uncommon (782,783).

Other congenital disorders of the cranial nerves and the musculature innervated by them are presented in Table 4.14.

REFERENCES

1. García-Bellido A. The development of concepts on development: a dialogue with Antonio García-Bellido (Interview by Enrique Cerda-Olmedo). *Int J Dev Biol* 1998;42:233–236.
2. Wolpert L, Beddington R, Brocken J, et al. *Principles of development*, Oxford and NY: Oxford University Press, 1998.
3. Patten BM. *Early embryology of the chick*, 4th ed. New York: McGraw-Hill, 1951.
4. Spemann H, Mangold H. Über Induktion von Embryonalanlagen durch Implantation vonfremder Organisatorcn. *Wilhelm Roux Arch Entwick* 1924;100: 599–638.
5. Cho KWY, Blumberg B, Steinbeisser H, De Robertis EM. Molecular nature of Spemann's organizer: the role of the Xenopus homeobox gene goosecoid. *Cell* 1991;67:1111–1120.
6. Wakamiya M, Rivera-Pérez JA, Baldini A, Behringer RR. Goosecoid and goosecoid-related genes in mouse embryogenesis. *Cold Springs Harbor Symp Quant Biol* 1997;62:145–149.
7. De Robertis EM, Kim S, Leyns L, et al. Patterning by genes expressed in Spemann's organizer. *Cold Springs Harbor Symp Quant Biol* 1997;62:169–175.

8. Hume CR, Dodd J. Cwnt-8C: a novel Wnt gene with a potential role in primitive streak formation and hindbrain organization. *Development* 1993;119:1147–1160.

9. Stein S, Kessel M. A homeobox gene involved in node, notochord and neural plate formation of chick embryos. *Mech Dev* 1995;49:37–48.

10. Duprat AM, Gualandris L, Kan P, et al. Review: neural induction. *Arch d'Anat Microsc Morphol Exp* 1987;75:211–227.

11. Tiedemann H. The molecular mechanism of neural induction: neural differentiation of Triturus ectoderm exposed to Hepes buffer. *Roux's Arch Dev Biol* 1986;195:399–402.

12. Fortini ME, Artavanis-Tsakonas S. Notch: neurogenesis is only part of the picture. *Cell* 1993;75:1245–1247.

13. Fontaine-Pérus JC, Chanconie M, Le Douarin NM, et al. Mitogenic effect of muscle on the neuroepithelium of the developing spinal cord. *Development* 1989;107:413–422.

14. Fontain-Pérus J. Migration of crest-derived cells from gut: gut influences on spinal cord development. *Brain Res Bull* 1993;30:251–255.

15. Dickson ME, Krumlauf R, McMahon AP. Evidence for a mitogenic effect of Wnt-1 in the developing mammalian central nervous system. *Development* 1994;120:1453–1471.

16. DiCicco-Bloom E, Black IB. Insulin growth factors regulate the mitotic cycle in cultured rat sympathetic neuroblasts. *Proc Natl Acad Sci USA* 1988;85:4066–4070.

17. Tao Y, Black LB, DiCicco-Bloom E. Neurogenesis in neonatal rat brain is regulated by peripheral injection of basic fibroblast growth factor (bFGF). *J Comp Neurol* 1996;376:653–663.

18. Tao Y, Black IB, DiCicco-Bloom E. In vivo neurogenesis is inhibited by neutralizing antibody to basic fibroblast growth factor. *J Neurobiol* 1997;33:289–296.

19. Turner DL. Weintraub H. Expression of achaete-scute homolog 3 in Xenopus embryos converts ectodermal cells to a neural fate. *Genes Dev* 1994;8:1434–1447.

20. Anderson DJ. A molecular switch for the neuron-glia developmental decision. *Neuron* 1995;15:1219–1222.

21. Hemmati-Brivantou A, Melton D. Vertebrate embryonic cells will become nerve cells unless told otherwise. *Cell* 1997;88:13–17.

22. Tanabe Y, Jessell TM. Diversity and pattern in the developing spinal cord. *Science* 1996;274:1115–11123.

23. McClure, CFW. The segmentation of the primitive vertebrate brain. *J Morphol* 1890;4:35–56.

24. Keynes R, Lumsden A. Segmentation and the origin of regional diversity in the vertebrate central nervous system. *Neuron* 1990;2:1–9.

25. McGinnis W, Krumlauf R. Homeobox genes and axial patterning. *Cell* 1992;68:283–302.

26. Keynes R, Krumlauf R. Hox genes and regionalization of the nervous system. *Annu Rev Neurosci* 1994;17:109–132.

27. Guthrie S. Patterning the hindbrain. *Curr Opin Neurobiol* 1996;6:41–48.

28. Wassef M, Joyner AL. Early mesencephalon/metencephalon patterning and development of the cerebellum. *Perspect Dev Neurobiol* 1997;5:3–16.

29. Goldowitz D, Hamre K. The cells and molecules that make a cerebellum. *Trends Neurosci* 1998;21:375–382.

30. Figdor MC, Stem CD. Segmental organization of embryonic diencephalon. *Nature* 1993;363:630–634.

31. Rubenstein JLR, Shimamura K, Martínez S. Regionalization of the prosencephalic neural plate. *Ann Rev Neurosci* 1998;21:445–477.

32. Rubenstein JLR, Beachy PA. Patterning of the embryonic forebrain. *Curr Opin Neurobiol* 1998;8:18–26.

33. Mai JK, Andrressen C, Ashwell KWS. Demarcation of prosencephalic regions by CD15-positive radial glia. *Eur J Neurosci* 1998;10:746–751.

34. Guthrie S, Butcher M, Lumsden A. Patterns of cell division and interkinetic nuclear migration in the chick embryo hindbrain. *J Neurobiol* 1991;22:742–754.

35. Joyner AL. Engrailed Wnt and Pax genes regulate midbrain-hindbrain development. *Trends Genet* 1996;12:15–20.

36. Wassarman KM, Lewandoski M, Campbell K., et al. Specification of the anterior hindbrain organizer is dependent on Gbx2 gene function. *Development* 1997;124:2923–2934.

37. Nomes HO, Dressler GR, Knapik EW, et al. Spatially and temporally restricted expression of Pax-2 during neurogenesis. *Development* 1990;109:797–809.

38. Puschel AW, Westerfeld M, Dressler G. Comparative analysis of Pax-2 protein distributions during neurulation in mice and zebrafish. *Mech Dev* 1992;38:197–208.

39. Rowitch DH, McMahon AP. Pax-2 expression in the murine neural plate precedes and encompasses the expression domains of Wnt-1 and En-1. *Mech Dev* 1995;52:3–8.

40. Rowitch DH, Danielian PS, Lee SMK, et al. Cell interactions in patterning the mammalian midbrain. *Cold Springs Harbor Symp Quant Biol* 1997;62:535–544.

41. Wurst W, Auerback AB, Joyner AL. Multiple developmental defects in Engrailed-1 mutant mice: an early mid-hindbrain deletion and patterning defects in forelimbs and sternum. *Development* 1994;120:2065–2075.

42. McMahon AP, Joyner AL, Bradley A, et al. The midbrain-hindbrain phenotype of Wnt-1-/Wnt-1- mice results from stepwise deletion of engrailed-expressing cells by 9.5 days postcoitum. *Cell* 1992;69:581–595.

43. Millen KJ, Hui C-C, Joyner AL. A role for En-2 and other murine homologues of Drosophila segment polarity genes in regulating position information in the developing cerebellum. *Development* 1995;121:3935–3945.

44. Kuemerle B, Zanjani H, Joyner A, Herrup K. Pattern deformities and cell loss in Engrailed-2 mutant mice suggest two separate patterning events during cerebellar development. *J Neurosci* 1997;17:7881–7889.

45. Rhinn M, Dierich A, Shawlot W, et al. Sequential roles for Otx2 in visceral endoderm and neuroectoderm for forebrain and midbrain induction and specification. *Development* 1989;125:845–856.

46. Acampora D, Simeone A. Understanding the roles of Otx1 and Otx2 in the control of brain mophogenesis. *Trends Neurosci* 1999;22:116–122.

47. Ryan AK, Blumberg B, Rodríguez-Estaban C, et al. Pitx2 determines left-right asymmetry of internal organs in vertebrates. *Nature* 1998;394:545–551.

47a. Zhao Q, Behringer RR, de Crombrugghe B. Prenatal folic acid treatment suppresses acrania and meroanencephaly in mice mutant for the Cart1 homeobox gene. *Nat Genet* 1996;13:275–283.

47b. Anderson SA, Eisenstat DD, Shi L, Rubenstein JLR. Interneuron migration from basal forebrain to neocortex: dependence on Dix genes. *Science* 1997;278:474–476.

48. De Pomerai D. *From gene to animal: an introduction of the molecular biology of animal development*, 2nd ed. Cambridge, U.K: Cambridge University Press, 1990.

49. El-Baradi T, Pieler T. Zinc finger proteins: what we know and what we would like to know. *Mech Devel* 1991;35:155–169.

50. Schneider-Maunoury S, Topilko P, Seitanidou T, et al. Disruption of Krox-20 results in alteration of rhombomeres 3 and 5 in the developing hindbrain. *Cell* 1993;75:1199–1214.

51. Topilko P, Schneider-Maunoury S, Levi G, et al. Krox-20 controls myelination in the peripheral nervous system. *Nature* 1994;371:796–799.

52. Nieto MA, Sechrist J, Wilkinson DG, Bronner-Fraser M. Relationship between spatially restricted Krox-20 gene expression in branchial neural crest and segmentation in the chick embryo hindbrain. *EMBO J* 1995;14:1697–1710.

52a. Faina GT, Cardini FA, D'Incerti L, et al. Familial schizencephaly associated with EMX2 mutation. *Neurology* 1997;48:1403–1406.

53. Wilkinson DG, Krumlauf R. Molecular approaches to the segmentation of the hindbrain. *Trends Neurosci* 1990;13:335–339.

54. Morriss-Kay GM, Murphy P, Hill RE, Davidson DR. Effects of retinoic acid excess on expression of Hox-2.9 and Krox-20 and on morphological segmentation in the hindbrain of mouse embryos. *EMBO J* 1991;10:2985–2995.

55. Nonchev S, Maconochie M, Vesque C, et al. The conserved role of Krox-20 in directing Hox gene expression during vertebrate hindbrain segmentation. *Proc Natl Acad Sci U S A* 1996;93:9339–9345.

56. Cook M, Gould A, Brand N, et al. Expression of the zinc-finger gene PLZF at rhombomere boundaries in the vertebrate hindbrain. *Proc Natl Acad Sci U S A* 1995;92:2249–2253.

57. Ingraham HA, Chen PRP, Mangalan HJ, et al. A tissue-specific transcription factor containing a homeodomain specifies a pituitary phenotype. *Cell* 1988;55:519–529.

58. Xu L, Lavinsky RM, Dasen JS. Signal-specific coactivator domain requirements for Pit-1 activation. *Nature* 1998;395:301–306.

59. Doniach T. Basic FGF as an inducer of anteroposterior neural pattern. *Cell* 1995;83:1067–1070.

60. Brand-Saberi B, Ebensperger C, Wilting J, et al. The ventralizing effect of the notochord on somite differentiation in chick embryos. *Anat Embryol* 1993;188:239–245.

60a. Fox JW, Lamperti ED, Eksioglu YZ, et al. Mutations in filamin 1 prevent migration of cerebral cortical neurons in human periventricular heterotopia. *Neuron* 1998;21:1315–1325.

61. Pourquié O, Coltey M, Teillet M-A, et al. Control of dorsoventral patterning of somite derivatives by notochord and floor plate. *Proc Natl Acad Sci U S A* 1993;90:5242–5246.

62. Martí E, Bumcrot DA, Takada R, McMahon AP. Requirement of 19K form of Sonic hedgehog for induction of distinct ventral cell types in CNS explants. *Nature* 1995;375:322–325.

63. Roelink H, Porter JA, Chiang C, et al. Floor plate and motor neuron induction by different concentrations of the amino-terminal cleavage product of Sonic hedgehog autoproteolysis. *Cell* 1995;81:445–455.

64. Tabin CJ, McMahon AP. Recent advances in hedgehog signalling. *Trends Cell Biol* 1997;7:442–446.

65. Goulding M. Specifying motor neurons and their connections. *Neuron* 1998;21:943–946.

65a. Sasaki H, Hogan BLM. HNF-3β as a regulator of floor plate development. *Cell* 1994;76:103–115.

66. van Straaten HWM, Hekking JWM, Wiertz-Hoessels EJLM, et al. Effect of the notochord on the differentiation of the floor plate area in the neural tube of the chick embryo. *Anat Embryol* 1988;177:317–324.

67. Sarnat HB. *Cerebral dysgenesis: embryology and clinical expression*, New York: Oxford University Press, 1992.

68. Ericson J, Muhr J, Placzek M, et al. Sonic hedgehog induces the differentiation of ventral forebrain neurons: a common signal for ventral patterning within the neural tube. *Cell* 1995;81:747–756.

69. Roessler E, Belloni E, Gaudenz K, et al. Mutations in the human Sonic hedgehog gene cause holoprosencephaly. *Nature Genet* 1996;14:357–360.

70. Callaerts P, Halder G, Gehring WJ. Pax-6 in development and evolution. *Annu Rev Neurosci* 1997;20: 483–532.

70a. Brown NL, Kanekar S, Vetter ML, et al. Math5 encodes a murine basic helix-loop-helix transcription factor expressed during early stages of retinal neurogenesis. *Development* 1998;125:4621–4633.

70b. Tanabe Y, William C, Jessell TM. Specification of motor neuron identity by the MNR2 homeodomain protein. *Cell* 1998;95:67–80.

71. Stoykova A, Gruss P. Roles for Pax genes in developing and adult brain as suggested by expression patterns. *J Neurosci* 1994;14:1395–1412.

72. Saint-Jeannet J-P, He X, Varmus HE, Dawid IB. Regulation of dorsal fate in the neuraxis by Wnt-1 and Wnt-3a. *Proc Natl Acad Sci U S A* 1997;94:13713–13718.

73. Keynes R, Krumlauf R. Hox genes and regionalization of the nervous system. *Annu Rev Neurosci* 1994; 17:109–132.

74. Murphy P, Hill RE. Expression of the mouse labial-like homebox-containing genes, Hox-2.9 and Hox-1.6, during segmentation of the hindbrain. *Development* 1991; 111:61–74.

75. Boncinelli E, Somma R, Acampora D, et al. Organization of human homeobox genes. *Hum Reprod* 1988;3:880–886.

75a. Lee JE, Hollenberg SM, Snider I, et al. Conversion of Xenopus ectoderm into neurons by NeuroD: a basic helix-loop-helix protein. *Science* 1995;268:836–844.

75b. Yokoyama M, Nishi Y, Miyamoto Y, et al. Molecular cloning of a human neuroD from a neuroblastoma cell line specifically expressed in the fetal brain and adult cerebellum. *Brain Res Mol Brain Res* 1996;42: 135–139.

76. Capecchi MR. Hox genes and mammalian development. *Cold Springs Harbor Symp Quant Biol* 1997;62: 273–281.

77. Stern CD, Foley AC. Molecular dissection of Hox gene induction and maintenance in the hindbrain. *Cell* 1998;94:143–145.

78. Kessel M. Reversal of axonal pathways from rhombomere 3 correlates with extra Hox expression domains. *Neuron* 1993;10:379–393.

79. Millen KJ, Wurst W, Herrup K, Joyner AL. Abnormal embryonic cerebellar development and patterning of postnatal foliation in two mouse Engrailed-2 mutants. *Development* 1994;120:695–706.

80. Mastick GS, Fan C-M, Tessier-Lavigne M, et al. Early deletion of neuromeres in Wnt-1-/- mutant mice: evalu-

ation by morphological and molecular markers. *J Comp Neurol* 1996;374:246–258.

80a. Lee JE. NeuroD and neurogenesis. *Dev Neurosci* 1997;19:27–32.

80b. Katayama M, Mizuta I, Sakayama Y, et al. Differential expression of neuroD in primary cultures of cerebral cortical neurons. *Exp Cell Res* 1997;236:412–417.

81. Zec N, Rowitch DH, Bitgood MJ, Kinney HC. Expression of the homeobox-containing genes EN1 and EN2 in human fetal midgestational medulla and cerebellum. *J Neuropathol Exp Neurol* 1997;56:236–242.

82. Wagner M, Thaller C, Jessell T, et al. Polarizing activity and retinoid synthesis in the floor plate of the neural tube. *Nature* 1990;345:819–822.

83. Ruberte E, Dolle P, Chambon P, et al. Retinoid acid receptors and cellular retinoid binding proteins. II. Their differential pattern of transcription during early morphogenesis in mouse. *Development* 1991;111:45–60.

84. Summerbell D, Maden M. Retinoic acid, a developmental signalling molecule. *Trends Neurosci* 1990;13:142–147.

85. Momoi M, Yamagata T, Ichihashi K, et al. Expression of cellular retinoic-acid binding protein in the developing nervous system of mouse embryos. *Dev Brain Res* 1990;54:161–167.

86. Thaller C, Eichele G. Isolation of 3,4-didehydroretinoic acid: a novel morphogenetic signal in the chick wing bud. *Nature* 1990;345:815–819.

87. Brockes J. Reading the retinoid signals. *Nature* 1990;345:766–768.

88. Kikuchi Y, Segawa H, Tokumoto M, et al. Ocular and cerebellar defects in zebrafish induced by overexpression of the LIM domains of the Islet-3 LIM/homeodomain protein. *Neuron* 1997;18:369–382.

89. Porter FD, Drago J, Xu Y, et al. Lhx2, a LIM homeobox gene, is required for eye, forebrain, and definitive erythrocyte development. *Development* 1997;124:2935–2944.

90. Durston AJ, Timmermans JPM, Hage WJ, et al. Retinoic acid causes an anteroposterior transformation in the developing central nervous system. *Nature* 1989;340:140–144.

91. Marín-Padilla M, Marin-Padilla MT. Mophogenesis of experimentally induced Arnold-Chiari malformation. *J Neurol Sci* 1981;50:29–55.

91a. Morrow EM, Furukawa T, Lee JE, Cepko CL. NeuroD regulates multiple functions in the developing neural retina in rodent. *Development* 1998;126:23–36.

91b. Yan RT, Wang SZ. NeuroD induces photoreceptor cell overproduction in vivo and de novo generation in vitro. *J Neurobiol* 1998;15:485–496.

92. Marín-Padilla M. Embryology and pathology of the axial skeleton and neural dysraphic disorders. *Can J Neurol Sci* 1991;18:153–169.

93. Alles AJ, Sulik KK. Retinoic acid-induced spina bifida: evidence for a pathogenetic mechanism. *Development* 1990;108:73–81.

94. Wohl CA, Weiss S. Retinoic acid enhances neuronal proliferation and astroglial differentiation in cultures of CNS stem cell-derived precursors. *J Neurobiol* 1998;37:281–290.

94a. Tamimi R, Steingrimsson E, Copeland NG, et al. The NEUROD gene maps to human chromosome 2q32 and mouse chromosome 2. *Genomics* 1996;34:418–421.

94b. Yamimi RM, Steingrimsson E, Montgomery-Dyer K, et al. NEUROD2 and NEUROD3 genes map to human

chromosomes 17q12 and 5q23-q31 and mouse chromosomes 11 and 13, respectively. *Genomics* 1997;40:355–357.

95. Meyers EN, Lewandoski M, Martin GR. An Fgf8 mutant allelic series generated by Cre- and Flp-mediated recombination. *Nature Genet* 1998;18:136–141.

96. Price M, Lazzaro D, Pohl T, et al. Regional expression of the homeobox gene Nkx-2.2 in the developing mammalian forebrain. *Neuron* 1992;8:241–255.

97. Qiu M, Shimamuira K, Sussel L, et al. Control of anteroposterior and dorsoventral domains of Nkx-6.1 gene expression relative to other Nkx genes during vertebrate CNS development. *Mech Dev* 1998;72:77–88.

98. Dorsky RI, Moon RT, Raible DW. Control of neural crest cell fate by the Wnt signaling pathway. *Nature* 1998;396:370–373.

99. Condron BG, Patel NH, Zinn K. Engrailed controls glial/neuronal cell fate decisions at the midline of the central nervous system. *Neuron* 1994;13:541–554.

100. Shah NM, Marchionni MA, Isaacs I, et al. Glial growth factor restricts mammalian neural crest stem cells to a glial fate. *Cell* 1994;77:349–360.

100a. Ma Q, Kinter C, Anderson DJ. Identification of neurogenin—a vertebrate neuronal determination gene. *Cell* 1996;87:43–52.

100b. Sommer I, Ma Q, Anderson DJ. Neurogenins: a novel family of atonal-related bHLH transcription factors are putative mammalian neuronal determination genes that reveal progenitor cell heterogeneity in the developing CNS and PNS. *Mol Cell Neurosci* 1996;8:221–241.

100c. Ma Q, Chen Z, del Barco Barrantes I, et al. Neurogenin1 is essential for the determination of neuronal precursors for proximal cranial sensory ganglia. *Neuron* 1998;20:469–482.

101. Urbnek P, Fetka I, Meisler MH, Busslinger M. Cooperation of Pax2 and Pax5 in midbrain and cerebellum development. *Proc Natl Acad Sci USA* 1997;94:5703–5708.

102. Kikuchi Y, Segawa H, Tokumoto M, et al. Ocular and cerebellar defects in zebrafish induced by overexpression of the LIM domains of the Islet-3 LIM/homeodomain protein. *Neuron* 1997;18:369–382.

103. Salinas PC, Fletcher C, Copeland NG, et al. Maintenance of Wnt-3 expression in Purkinje cells of the mouse cerebellum depends on interaction with granule cells. *Development* 1994;120:1277–1286.

104. Lange W. Regional differences in the cytoarchitecture of the cerebellar cortex. In: Palay SL, Chan-Palay V, eds. *The cerebellum: new vistas.* Berlin: Springer-Verlag, 1982:93–107.

105. Korbo L, Andersen BB, Ladefoged O, Moller A. Total numbers of various cell types in rat cerebellar cortex using an unbiased stereological method. *Brain Res* 1993;609:262–268.

106. Goodrich LV, Mienkovi L, Higgins KM, Scott MP. Altered neural cell fates and medulloblastoma in mouse patched mutants. *Science* 1997;277:1109–1113.

107. Traiffort E, Charaytoniuk DA, Faure H, Ruat M. Regional distribution of Sonic hedgehog, Patched and Smoothened mRNA in the adult rat brain. *J Neurochem* 1998;70:1327–1330.

108. Wechsler-Reya, Scott MP. Control of neuronal precursor proliferation in the cerebellum by Sonic hedgehog. *Neuron* 1999;22:103–114.

109. Walter M, Reifenberger J, Summer C, et al. Mutations in the human homologue of the Drosophila segment polarity gene patched (PTCH) in sporadic basal cell carcinomas of the skin and primitive neuroectodermal tumors of the central nervous system. *Cancer Res* 1997;57:2581–2585.
110. Smith JL, Schoenwolf GC. Neurulation: coming to closure. *Trends Neurosci* 1997;20:510–517.
111. Schoenwolf GC, Smith JL. Mechanisms of neurulation: traditional viewpoint and recent advances. *Development* 1990;109:243–270.
111a. McMahon JA, Takada S, Zimmerman LB, et al. Noggin-mediated antagonism of BMP signaling is required for growth and patterning of the neural tube and somite. *Genes Dev* 1998;12:1438–1452.
112. Alvarez I, Schoenwolf GC. Expansion of surface epithelium provides the major extrinsic force for bending of the neural plate. *J Exp Zool* 1992;261:340–348.
113. Jacobson AG. Experimental analysis of the shaping of the neural plate and tube. *Am Zool* 1991;31:628–643.
114. Schoenwolf GC, Franks MV. Quantitative analyses of changes in cell shapes during bending of the avial neural plate. *Dev Biol* 1984;105:257–272.
115. Smith J, Schoenwolf GC. Notochordal induction of cell wedging in the chick neural plate and its role in neural tube formation. *J Exp Zool* 1989;25:49–62.
115a. Zhong W, Jiang M-M, Weinmaster G, et al. Differential expression of mammalian Numb, Numblike and Notch1 suggests distinct roles during mouse cortical neurogenesis. *Development* 1997;124:1887–1897.
116. Sarnat HB. Role of the human fetal ependyma. *Pediatr Neurol* 1992;8:163–178.
117. Aaku-Saraste E, Oback B, Hellwig A, Huttner WB. Neuro-epithelial cells downregulate their plasma membrane polarity prior to neural tube closure and neurogenesis. *Mech Dev* 1997;69:71–81.
118. Sausedo RA, Smith JL, Schoenwolf GC. Role of randomly oriented cell division in shaping and bending of the neural plate. *J Comp Neurol* 1997;381:473–488.
119. Juriloff DM, Harris JM, Tom C, et al. Normal mouse strains differ in the site of initiation of closure of the cranial neural tube. *Teratology* 1991;44:225–233.
120. Golden JA, Chernoff GF. Intermittent pattern of neural tube closure in two strains of mice. *Teratology* 1993;47:73–80.
121. Busam KJ, Roberts DJ, Golden JA. Clinical teratology counseling and consultation. Case report: two distinct anterior neural tube defects in a human fetus: evidence for an intermittent pattern of neural tube closure. *Teratology* 1993;48:399–403.
122. O'Rahilly R, Müller F. Bidirectional closure of the rostal neuropore in the human embryo. *Am J Anat* 1989;184:259–268.
123. Lemire RJ. Variations in development of the caudal neural tube in human embryos (Horizons XIV-XXI). *Teratology* 1969;2:361–370.
123a. Goodrich LV, Scott MP. Hedgehog and Patched in neural development. *Neuron* 1998;21:1243–1257.
124. Papan C, Campos-Ortega JA. On the formation of the neural keel and neural tube in the zebrafish Danio (Brachydanio) rerio. *Roux's Arch Dev Biol* 1994;203:178–186.
125. Dao AH, Netsky MG. Human tails and pseudotails. *Hum Pathol* 1984;15:449–453.
126. Lu FL, Wang P-J, Teng R-J, Yau K-IT. The human tail. *Pediatr Neurol* 1998;19:230–233.
127. James HE, Canty TG. Human tail and associated spinal anomalies. *Clin Pediatr* 1995;34:386–388.
128. Aruga J, Yokota N, Hashimoto M, et al. A novel zinc finger protein, Zic, is involved in neuronogenesis, especially in the cell lineage of cerebellar granule cells. *J Neurochem* 1994;63:1880–1890.
129. Aruga J, Minowa O, Yaginuma H, et al. Mouse Zic1 is involved in cerebellar development. *J Neurosci* 1998;18:284–293.
130. Ben-Arie N, Bellen HJ, Armstrong DL, et al. Math1 is essential for genesis of cerebellar granule neurons. *Nature* 1997;390:169–172.
131. Ericson J, Briscoe J, Rashbass P, et al. Graded Sonic hedgehog signaling and the specification of cell fate in the ventral neural tube. *Cold Springs Harbor Symp Quant Biol* 1997;62:451–466.
132. Fritzsch B, Nichols DH, Echelard Y, McMahon AP. Development of midbrain and anterior hindbrain ocular motoneurons in normal and Wnt-1 knockout mice. *J Neurobiol* 1995;27:457–469.
133. Porter JD, Baker RS. Absence of oculomotor and trochlear motorneurons leads to altered extraocular muscle development in the Wnt-1 null mutant mouse. *Dev Brain Res* 1997;100:121–126.
134. Tsuchida T, Ensini M, Morton SB, et al. Topographic organization of embryonic motor neurons defined by expression of LIM homeobox genes. *Cell* 1994;79:957–970.
135. Appel B, Korzh V, Glasgow E, et al. Motoneuron fate specification revealed by patterned LIM homeobox gene expression in embryonic zebrafish. *Development* 1995;121:4117–4125.
136. Pfaff SL, Mendelsohn M, Stewart CL, et al. Requirement of LIM homeobox gene Is/1 in motor neuron generation reveals a motor neuron-dependent step in interneuron differentiation. *Cell* 1996;84:309–320.
137. D'Costa AP, Prevette DM, Houenou LJ, et al. Mechanisms of insulin-like growth factor regulation of programmed cell death of developing avian motoneurons. *J Neurobiol* 1998;36:379–394.
137a. Jeh-Ping L, Jessell TM. A role for rhoB in the delamination of neural crest cells from the dorsal neural tube. *Development* 1998;125:5055–5067.
138. Le Douarin N. *The Neural Crest*, Cambridge, UK: Cambridge University Press, 1982.
138a. Chen Z-F, Behringer RR. Twist is required in head mesenchyme for cranial neural tube morphogenesis. *Genes Dev* 1995;9:686–699.
139. Tan SS, Morriss-Kay GM. The development and distribution of the cranial neural crest in the rat embryo. *Cell Tissue Res* 1985;240:403–416.
140. Gerhart J, Kirschner M. *Cells, embryos and evolution*, Malden: Blackwell Science, 1997.
141. Bronner-Fraser M. Neural crest formation and migration in the developing embryo. *FASEB J* 1994;8:699–706.
142. Bronner-Fraser M. Origins and developmental potential of the neural crest. *Exp Cell Res* 1995;218:405–417.
143. Sadaghiani B, Crawford BJ, Vielkind JR. Changes in the distribution of extracellular matrix components during neural crest development in Xiphophorus spp. Embryos. *Can J Zool* 1994;72:1340–1353.
144. Selleck MAJ, Scherson TY, Bronner-Fraser M. Origins of neural crest diversity. *Dev Biol* 1993;159:1–11.

145. ElShamy WM, Linnarsson S, Lee K-F, et al. Prenatal and postnatal requirements of NT-3 for sympathetic neuroblast survival and innnervation of specific targets. *Development* 1996;122:491–500.

146. Sauer FC. Mitosis in the neural tube. *J Comp Neurol* 1935;62:377–405.

147. Nurse P. Ordering S-phase and M-phase in the cell cycle. *Cell* 1994;79:547–550.

148. Caviness VS Jr, Pinto-Lord MC, Evrard P. The development of laminated patterns in the mammalian neocortex. In: Connelly TG, ed. *Morphogenesis and pattern formation*. New York: Raven Press, 1981:103–126.

149. Burek MJ, Oppenheim RW. Programmed cell death in the developing nervous system. *Brain Pathol* 1996;6:427–446.

150. Chenn A, McConnell SK. Cleavage orientation and the asymmetric inheritance of Notch1 immunoreactivity in mammalian neurogenesis. *Cell* 1995;82:631–641.

151. Zhong W, Feder JN, Jiang M-M, et al. Asymmetrical localization of a mammalian numb homolog during mouse cortical neuronogenesis. *Neuron* 1996;17:43–53.

152. Mione MC, Cavanaugh JFR, Harris B, Parnavelas JG. Cell fate specification and symmetrical/asymmetrical divisions in the developing cerebral cortex. *J Neurosci* 1997;17:2018–2029.

153. Bass PW. Microtubules and neuronal polarity: lessons from mitosis. *Neuron* 1999;22:23–31.

154. Crews L, Hunter D. Neurogenesis in the olfactory epithelium. *Perspect Dev Neurobiol* 1994;2:151–161.

155. Menezes JRL, Smith CM, Nelson KC, Luskin MB. The division of neuronal progenitor cells during migration in the neonatal mammalian forebrain. *Mol Cell Neurosci* 1995;6:496–508.

156. Kendler A, Golden JA. Progenitor cell proliferation outside the ventricular and subventricular zones during human brain development. *J Neuropathol Exp Neurol* 1996;55:1253–1258.

157. Hamburger V, Levi-Montalcini R. Proliferation, differentiation and degeneration in the spinal ganglia of the chick embryo under normal and experimental conditions. *J Exp Zool* 1949;111:457–502.

158. O'Connor TM, Wyttenback CR. Cell death in the embryonic chick spinal cord. *J Cell Biol* 1974;60:448–459.

159. Okado N, Oppenheim RW. Cell death of motorneurons in the chick embryo spinal cord. *J Neurosci* 1984;4:1639–1652.

160. Harris AJ, McCaig CD. Motorneuron death and motor unit size during embryonic development of the rat. *J Neurosci* 1984;4:13–24.

161. Ferrer I, Serrano T, Soriano E. Naturally occurring cell death in the subicular complex and hippocampus in the rat during development. *Neurosci Res* 1990;8:60–66.

162. Diener PS, Bregman BS. Neurotrophic factors prevent the death of CNS neurons after spinal cord lesions in newborn rats. *NeuroReport* 1994;5:1913–1917.

163. Pittman RN, Wang S, DiBenedetto AJ, et al. A system for characterizing cellular and molecular events in programmed neuronal cell death. *J Neurosci* 1993;13:3669–3680.

164. Gómez-Pinilla F, Lee JW-K, Cotman CW. Distribution of brain fibroblast growth factor in the developing brain. *Neuroscience* 1994;61:911–923.

165. Page KJ, Saha A, Everitt BJ. Differential activation and survival of basal forebrain neurons following infusions of excitatory amino acids: studies with the intermediate early gene c-*fos*. *Exp Brain Res* 1993;93:412–422.

166. Lefebvre S, Burglen L, Reboullet S, et al. Identification and characterization of a spinal muscular atrophy determining gene. *Cell* 1995;80:155–165.

167. Roy N, Mahadevan MS, McLean M, et al. The gene for neuronal apoptosis inhibitor protein is partially deleted in individuals with spinal muscular atrophy. *Cell* 1995;80:167–178.

168. Homma S, Yaginuma H, Oppenheim RW. Programmed cell death during the earliest stages of spinal cord development in the chick embryo: a possible means of early phenotypic selection. *J Comp Neurol* 1994;345:377–395.

169. Nurcombe V, McGrath PA, Bennett MR. Postnatal death of motor neurons during the development of the brachial spinal cord of the rat. *Neurosci Lett* 1981;27:249–254.

170. Duckett S, Pearse AGE. The cells of Cajal-Retzius in the developing human brain. *J Anat* 1968;102:183–187.

171. Marín-Padilla M. Dual origin of the mammalian neocortex and evolution of the cortical plate. *Anat Embryol* 1978;152:109–126.

172. Bayer SA, Altman J. Development of layer 1 and the subplate in the rat neocortex. *Exp Neurol* 1990;107:48–62.

173. Marín-Padilla M. Cajal-Retzius cells and the development of the neocortex. *Trends Neurosci* 1998;21:64–71.

174. Ogawa M, Miyata T, Nakajima K, et al. The reeler gene-associated antigen on Cajal-Retzius neurons is a crucial molecule for laminar organization of cortical neurons. *Neuron* 1995;14:899–912.

175. Curran T, D'Arcangelo G. Role of reelin in the control of brain development. *Brain Res Rev* 1998;26:285–294.

176. Clark DC, Mizuguchi M, Antalffy B, et al. Predominant localization of the LIS family of gene products to Cajal-Retzius cells and ventricular neuroepithelium in the developing human cortex. *J Neuropathol Exp Neurol* 1997;56:1044–1052.

177. Huntley GW, Jones EG. Cajal-Retzius neurons in developing monkey neocortex show immunoreactivity to calcium binding proteins. *J Neurocytol* 1990;19:200–219.

178. Derer P, Derer M. Cajal-Retzius cell ontogenesis and death in mouse brain visualized with horseradish peroxidase and electron microscopy. *Neuroscience* 1990;32:707–717.

179. Smart IHM. Proliferative characteristics of the ependymal layer during the early development of the spinal cord in the mouse. *J Anat* 1972;111:365–380.

180. Sarnat HB. Regional differentiation of the human fetal ependyma: immunocytochemical markers. *J Neuropathol Exp Neurol* 1992;51:58–75.

181. Snow DM, Steindler DA, Silver J. Molecular and cellular characterization of the glial roof plate of the spinal cord and optic tectum: a possible role for a proteoglycan in the development of an axon barrier. *Dev Biol* 1990;138:359–376.

182. Bovolentá P, Dodd J. Guidance of commissural growth cones at the floor plate in embryonic rat spinal cord. *Development* 1990;109:435–447.

183. Kennedy TE, Serafini T, de la Torre J, et al. Netrins are diffusible chemotropic factors for commissural axons in the embryonic spinal cord. *Cell* 1994;78:425–435.

184. Colamarino SA, Tessier-Lavigne M. The axonal chemoattractant netrin-1 is also a chemorepellant for trochlear motor neurons. *Cell* 1995;81:621–629.

185. Keynes R, Cook GMW. Axonal guidance molecules. *Cell* 1995;83:161–169.
186. Sarnat HB, Netsky MG. *Evolution of the nervous system*, 2nd ed. New York: Oxford University Press, 1981.
187. Roessmann U, Gambetti P. Astrocytes in the developing human brain: an immunohistochemical study. *Acta Neuropathol* 1986;70:308–313.
188. Anton ES, Cameron RS, Rakic P. Role of neuron-glial junctional domain proteins in the maintenance and termination of neuronal migration across the embryonic cerebral wall. *J Neurosci* 1996;16:1193–2283.
189. Zheng C, Heintz N, Hatten ME. CNS gene encoding astrotactin which supports neuronal migration along glial fibers. *Science* 1996;272:417–419.
190. Jouet M, Kenwrick S. Gene analysis of L1 neural cell adhesion molecule in prenatal diagnosis of hydrocephalus. *Lancet* 1995;345:161–162.
191. Herman J-P, Victor JC, Sanes JR. Developmentally regulated and spatially restricted antigens of radial glial cells. *Dev Dynamics* 1993;197:307–318.
192. Thomas LB, Gates MA, Steindler DA. Young neurons from the adult subependymal zone proliferate and migrate along an astrocyte, extracellular matrix-rich pathway. *Glia* 1996;17:1–14.
193. Rice DS, Sheldon M, D'Arcangelo G, et al. Disabled-1 acts downstream of Reelin in a signaling pathway that controls laminar organization in the mammalian brain. *Development* 1998;125:3719–3729.
194. O'Rourke NA, Dailey ME, Smith SJ, McConnell SK. Diverse migratory pathways in the developing cerebral cortex. *Science* 1992;258:299–302.
195. Rakic P. Radial versus tangential migration of neuronal clones in the developoing cerebral cortex. *Proc Natl Acad Sci U S A* 1995;92:11323–11327.
196. O'Rourke NA, Sullivan DP, Kaznowski CE, et al. Tangential migration of neurons in the developing cerebral cortex. *Development* 1995;121:2165–2176.
197. Wichterle H, García-Verdugo JM, Alvarez-Buylla A. Direct evidence for homotypic glia-independent neuronal migration. *Neuron* 1997;18:779–791.
198. Dobyns WB, Reiner O, Carrozzo R, Ledbetter DH. Lissencephaly: a human brain malformation associated with deletion of the LIS1 gene located at chromosome 17p13. *JAMA* 1993;270:2838–2842.
199. Lo Nigro C, Chong SS, Smith ACM, et al. Point mutations and an intragenic deletion in LIS1: the lissencephaly causitive gene in isolated lissencephaly sequence and Miller-Dieker syndrome. *Hum Mol Genet* 1997;6:157–164.
200. Chong SS, Pack SD, Roschke AV, et al. A revision of the lissencephaly and Miller-Dieker syndrome critical regions in chromosome 17p13.3. *Hum Mol Genet* 1997,6.147–155.
201. Gleeson JG, Allen KM, Fox JW, et al. Doublecortin, a brain-specific gene mutated in human X-linked lissencephaly and double cortex syndrome, encodes a putative signaling protein. *Cell* 1998;92:63–72.
202. des Portes V, Pinard JM, Billuart P, et al. A novel CNS gene required for neuronal migration and involved in X-linked subcortical laminar heterotopia and lissencephaly syndrome. *Cell* 1998;92:51–61.
203. Eksioglu YZ, Scheffer IE, Cardena P, et al. Periventricular heterotopia: an X-linked dominant epilepsy locus causing aberrant cerebral cortical development. *Neuron* 1996;16:77–87.

204. Fox JW, Lamperti ED, Eksioglu YZ, et al. Mutations in filamin 1 prevent migration of cerebral cortical neurons in human periventricular heterotopia. *Neuron* 1998;21:1315–1325.
205. Tsuru A, Mizuguchi M, Uyemura K, et al. Immunohistochemical expression of cell adhesion molecule L1 in hemimegalencephaly. *Pediatr Neurol* 1997;16:45–49.
206. Ramón y Cajal, S de. *Histologie du systéme nerveux central de l'homme et des vértébrés*, Paris: Maloine, 1909–1911.
207. Dotti CG, Simons K. Polarizing sorting of viral glycoproteins to at the axon and dendrites of hippocampal neurons in culture. *Cell* 1990;62:63–72.
208. Higgins D, Burack M, Lein P, Banker G. Mechanisms of neuronal polarity. *Curr Opin Neurobiol* 1997;7: 599–604.
209. Bredt DS. Sorting out genes that regulate epithelial and neuronal polarity. *Cell* 1998;94:691–694.
210. Tessier-Lavigne M, Placzek M, Lumsden AGS, et al. Chemotropic guidance of developing axons in the mammalian central nervous system. *Nature* 1988; 336:775 778.
211. Oakley RA, Tosney KW. Contact-mediated mechanisms of motor axon segmentation. *J Neurosci* 1993;13:3773–3792.
212. Erskine L, McCaig CD. Growth cone neurotransmitter receptor activation modulates electric field-guided nerve growth. *Dev Biol* 1995;171:330–339.
213. Tosney KW. Somites and axon guidance. *Scan Electron Microsc* 1988;2:427–442.
214. Guthrie S, Pini A. Chemopulsion of developing motor axons by the floor plate. *Neuron* 1995;14:1117–1130.
215. Dodd J, Schuchardt A. Axon guidance: a compelling case for repelling growth cones. *Cell* 1995;81:471–474.
216. Tanaka E, Sabry J. Making the connection: cytoskeletal rearrangements during growth cone guidance. *Cell* 1995;83:171–176.
217. Yu W, Baas PW. The growth of the axon is not dependent upon net microtubule assembly at its distal tip. *J Neurosci* 1995;15:6827–6833.
218. Clark GD, McNeil RS, Bix GL, Swann JW. Platelet-activating factor produces neuronal growth cone collapse. *NeuroReport* 1995;6:2569–2575.
219. Minturn JE, Fryer HJL, Geschwing DH, et al. TOAD-64P: a gene expressed early in neuronal differentiation in the rat is related to unc-33, a *C. elegans* gene involved in axon outgrowth. *J Neurosci* 1995;15:6757–6766.
220. Wilson SW, Placzek M, Furley AJ. Border disputes: do boundaries play a role in growth-cone guidance? *Trends Neurosci* 1993;16:316–323.
221. Chédodtal A, Pourquié O, Sotelo C. Initial tract formation in the brain of the chick embryo: selective expression of the BEN/SCI/DM-GRASP cell adhesion molecule. *Eur J Neurosci* 1995;7.193–212.
222. Hirotsune S, Takahara T, Sasaki N, et al. The reeler gene encodes a protein with an EGF-like motif expressed by pioneer neurons. *Nat Genet* 1995; 10:77–83.
223. Purves D, Lichtman JW. Elimination of synapses in the developing nervous system. *Science* 1980;210: 153–157.
224. Van Huizen F, Romijn HJ, Corner MA. Indications for a critical period for synapse elimination in developing rat cerebral cortex cultures. *Dev Brain Res* 1987;31:1–6.

225. Corriveau RA, Huh GS, Shatz CJ. Regulation of Class I MHC gene expression in the developing and mature CNS by neural activity. *Neuron* 1998;21:506–520.

226. Haydon PG, Drapeau P. From contact to connection: early events during synaptogenesis. *Trends Neurosci* 1995;18:196–201.

227. Koch C, Zador A. The function of dendritic spines: devices subserving biochemical rather than electrical compartmentalization. *J Neurosci* 1993;13:413–422.

228. Thoenen H. Neurotrophins and neuronal plasticity. *Science* 1995;270:593–598.

229. Greenough WT. Structural correlates of information storage in the mammalian brain: a review and hypothesis. *Trends Neurosci* 1984;7:229–233.

230. Lipton SA, Kater SB. Neurotransmitter regulation of neuronal outgrowth, plasticity and survival. *Trends Neurosci* 1989;12:265–270.

231. McAllister AK, Katz LC, Lo DC. Opposing roles for endogenous BDNF and NT-3 in regulating cortical dendritic growth. *Neuron* 1997;18:767–778.

232. Breder CD, Dewitt D, Kraig RP. Characterizatin of inducible cyclooxygenase in rat brain. *J Comp Neurol* 1995;355:296–315.

233. Kaufmann WE, Worley PF, Pegg J, et al. Cox-2: a synapatically induced enzyme is expressed by excitatory neurons at postsynaptic sites in rat cerebral cortex. *Proc Natl Acad Sci U S A* 1996;93:2317–2321.

234. Lerea LS, McNamara JO. Ionotropic glutamate receptor subtypes activate c-*fos* transcription by distinct calcium-requiring intracellular signaling pathways. *Neuron* 1993;10:31–41.

235. Williams JH, Errington ML, Lynch MA, et al. Arachidonic acid induces a long-term activity-dependent enhancement of synaptic transmission in the hippocampus. *Nature* 1989;341:739–742.

236. Shepherd GM, Greer CA. The dendritic spine: adaptations of structure and function for different types of synaptic integrations. In: Lesek R, Black M, eds. *Intrinsic determinants of neuronal form and function.* New York: AR Liss, 1989:245–314.

237. Walz W. Role of glial cells in the regulation of the brain microenvironment. *Progr Neurobiol* 1989;33:309–333.

238. Prochianz A. Neuronal polarity: giving neurons heads and tails. *Neuron* 1995;15:743–746.

239. Craig AM, Banker G. Neuronal polarity. *Annu Rev Neurosci* 1994;17:267–310.

240. Sarnat HB, Nochlin D, Born DE. Neuronal nuclear antigen (NeuN): a marker of neuronal maturation in the early human fetal nervous system. *Brain Dev* 1998;20:88–94.

241. Sarnat HB, Born DE. Synaptophysin immunocytochemistry with thermal intensification: a marker of terminal axonal maturation in the human fetal nervous system. *Brain Dev* 1999;21:41–50.

242. Menchine M, Emeline JK, Mischel PS, et al. Tissue and cell-type specific expression of the tuberous sclerosis gene, TSC2, in human tissues. *Modern Pathol* 1996;9:1071–1080.

243. Wienecke R, Maize JC Jr, Reed JA, et al. Expression of the TSC2 product tuberin and its target Rap1 in normal human tissues. *Am J Pathol* 1997;150:43–50.

244. van Slegtenhorst M, de Hoogt R, Hermans C, et al. Identification of the tuberous sclerosis gene TSC1 on chromosome 9q34. *Science* 1997;277:805–808.

245. Ali JB, Sepp T, Ward S, et al. Mutations in the TSC1 gene account for a minority of patients with tuberous sclerosis. *J Med Genet* 1998;35:969–972.

246. Au KS, Rodriguez JA, Finch JL, et al. Germ-line mutational analysis of the TSC2 gene in 90 tuberous sclerosis patients. *Am J Hum Genet* 1998;62:286–294.

247. Kwiatkowska J, Jozwiak S, Hall F, et al. Comprehensive mutational analysis of the TSC1 gene: observations on frequency of mutation, associated features, and nonpenetrance. *Ann Hum Genet* 1998;18:9365–9375.

248. Yakovlev PI, Lecours A-R. The myelination cycles of regional maturation of the brain. In: Minkowsky A, ed. *Regional development of the brain in early life.* Philadelphia: FA Davis Co, 1967:3–70.

249. Hasegawa M, Houdou S, Mito T, et al. Development of myelination in the human fetal and infant cerebrum: a myelin basic protein immunohistochemical study. *Brain Dev* 1992;14:1–6.

250. Colello RJ, Pott U. Signals that initiate myelination in the developing mammalian nervous system. *Mol Neurobiol* 1997;15:83–100.

251. Compston A, Zajicek J, Sussman J, et al. Glial lineages and myelination in the central nervous system. *J Anat* 1997;190:161–200.

252. Yu W-P, Collarini EJ, Pringle NP, et al. Embryonic expression of myelin genes: evidence for a focal source of oligodendrocyte precursors in the ventricular zone of the neural tube. *Neuron* 1994;12:1353–1362.

253. Lemke G. The molecular genetics of myelination: an update. *Glia* 1993;7:263–271.

254. Byravan S, Foster LM, Phan T, et al. Murine oligodendroglial cells express nerve growth factor. *Proc Natl Acad Sci USA* 1994;91:8812–8816.

255. Zumkeller W. The effect of insulin-like growth factors on brain myelination and their potential therapeutic application in myelination disorders. *Eur J Paediatr Neurol* 1997;4:91–101.

256. Ogawa-Goto K, Abe T. Gangliosides and glycosphingolipids of peripheral nervous system myelins: a minireview. *Neurochem Res* 1998;23:305–310.

257. Hasan SU, Sarnat HB, Auer RN. Vagal nerve maturation in the fetal lamb: an ultrastructural and morphometric study. *Anat Rec* 1993;237:527–537.

258. Kalter H, Warkany, J. Medical progress. Congenital malformations: etiologic factors and their role in prevention. (First of 2 parts). *N Engl J Med* 1983;308:424–431.

259. Adams RD, Sidman RL. *Introduction to neuropathology,* New York: McGraw-Hill, 1968.

260. Bird TD, Hall JG. Clinical neurogenetics: a survey of the relationship of medical genetics to clinical neurology. *Neurology* 1977;27:1057–1060.

261. Carter CO. Genetics of common single malformations. *Br Med Bull* 1976;32:21–26.

262. Opitz JM, Gilbert EF. CNS anomalies and the midline as a "developmental field." *Am J Med Genet* 1982;12:443–455.

263. Nance WE. Anencephaly and spina bifida: an etiologic hypothesis. *Birth Defects Original Article Series* 1971;7:97–102.

264. Robert E, Guibaud P. Maternal valproic acid and congenital tube defects. *Lancet* 1982;2:937.

265. Johnson RT. Effects of viral infection on the developing nervous system. *N Engl J Med* 1972;287:599–604.

266. Navarrete VN, et al. Subsequent diabetes in mothers delivered of a malformed infant. *Lancet* 1970;2:993–994.

267. Giroud A. Causes and morphogenesis of anencephaly. In: Wolstenholme GE, O'Connor CM, eds. *CIBA Foundation Symposium on Congenital Malformations*. London: Churchill Livingstone, 1960.
268. Müller F, O'Rahilly R. Development of anencephaly and its variants. *Am J Anat* 1991;190:193–218.
269. Padget DH. Development of so-called dysraphism with embryologic evidence of clinical Arnold-Chiari and Dandy-Walker malformations. *Johns Hopkins Med J* 1972;130:127–165.
270. Gardner WJ, Breuer AC. Anomalies of heart, spleen, kidneys, gut and limbs may result from an overdistended neural tube: a hypothesis. *Pediatrics* 1980; 65:508–514.
271. Osaka K, et al. Myeloschisis in early human embryos. *Child's Brain* 1978;4:347–359.
272. Osaka K, et al. Myelomeningocele before birth. *J Neurosurg* 1978;49:711–724.
273. Toop J, Webb JN, Emery AE. Muscle differentiation in anencephaly. *Dev Med Child Neurol* 1973;15:164–170.
274. Garcia CA, Duncan C. Atelencephalic microcephaly. *Dev Med Child Neurol* 1977;19:227–232.
275. Iivanainen M, Haltia M, Lydecken K. Atelencephaly. *Dev Med Child Neurol* 1977;19:663–668.
276. Hendricks SK, et al. Exencephaly: clinical and ultrasonic correlation to anencephaly. *Obstetr Gynecol* 1988;72:898–900.
277. Naidich TP, et al. Cephaloceles and related malformations. *Am J Neuroradiol* 1992;13:655–690.
278. Naggan L, Macmahon B. Ethnic differences in the prevalence of anencephaly and spina bifida in Boston, Massachusetts. *N Engl J Med* 1967;277:1119–1123.
279. Stone DH. The declining prevalence of anencephalus and spina bifida: its nature, causes and implications. *Dev Med Child Neurol* 1987;29:541–546.
280. Yen IH, et al. The changing epidemiology of neural tube defects: United States 1968–1989. *Amer J Dis Child* 1992;146:857–861.
281. Carstairs V, Cole S. Spina bifida and anencephaly in Scotland. *BMJ* 1984;289:1182–1184.
282. Nakano KK. Anencephaly: a review. *Dev Med Child Neurol* 1973;15:383–400.
283. Fedrick J. Anencephalus in the Oxford record linkage study area. *Dev Med Child Neurol* 1976;18:643–656.
284. James WH. The sex ratios of anencephalics born to anencephalic-prone women. *Dev Med Child Neurol* 1980;22:618–622.
285. Peiper A, Hempel HC, Wunscher W. Der gampersche verbeugungsreflex. *Mschr Kinderhk* 1959;107:393–622.
286. Danner R, Shewman A, Sherman MP. Seizures in an atelencephalic infant: is the cortex essential for neonatal seizures? *Arch Neurol* 1985;42:1014–1016.
287. Brock DJ. Biochemical and cytological methods in the diagnosis of neural tube defects. *Prog Med Genet* 1977;2:1–37.
288. Nicolaides KH, et al. Ultrasound screening for spina bifida: cranial and cerebellar signs. *Lancet* 1986;2:72–74.
289. Brock DJ. α-fetoprotein and the prenatal diagnosis of central nervous system disorders: a review. *Child's Brain* 1976;2:1–23.
290. Laurence KM. Fetal malformations and abnormalities. *Lancet* 1974;2:939–942.
291. Milunsky A. Prenatal detection of neural tube defects: false positive and negative results. *Pediatrics* 1977;59:782–783.
292. MRC Vitamin Study Research Group. Prevention of neural tube defects: result of the Medical Research Council Vitamin Study. *Lancet* 1991;338:131–137.
293. Smithells RW, et al. Further experience of vitamin supplementation for prevention of neural tube defect recurrences. *Lancet* 1983;1:1027–1031.
294. Rhoads GG, Mills JL. Can vitamin supplements prevent neural-tube defects? Current evidence and ongoing investigations. *Clin Obstet Gynecol* 1986;29:569–1986.
295. Czeizel AE, Dudas I. Prevention of the first occurrence of neural-tube defects by preconceptional vitamin supplementation. *N Engl J Med* 1992;327:1832–1835.
296. Lemire RJ. Neural tube defects. *JAMA* 1988;259:558–562.
297. Morrison K, et al. Susceptibility to spina bifida: an association study of five candidate genes. *Ann Hum Genet* 1998;62:379–396.
298. Gilbert JN, et al. Central nervous system anomalies associated with meningomyelocele, hydrocephalus, and the Arnold-Chiari malformation: reappraisal of theories regarding the pathogenesis of posterior neural tube closure defects. *Neurosurgery* 1986;18:559–564.
299. Dekaban AS. Anencephaly in early human embryos. *J Neuropathol Exp Neurol* 1963;22:533–548.
300. McLone DG, Naidich TP. Developmental morphology of the subarachnoid space, brain vasculature, and contiguous structures, and the cause of the Chiari II malformation. *Am J Neuroradiol* 1992;13:463–482.
301. Marin-Padilla M. Embryology and pathology of axial skeletal and neural dysraphic disorders. *Can J Neurol Sci* 1991;18:153–169.
302. Dryden R. The fine structure of spina bifida in an untreated three-day chick embryo. *Dev Med Child Neurol* 1971;25[Suppl]:116–124.
303. Milunsky A, et al. Maternal heat exposure and neural tube defects. *JAMA* 1992;268:882–885.
304. Milunsky A. Prenatal detection of neural tube defects. VI. Experience with 20,000 pregnancies. *JAMA* 1980;244:2731–2735.
305. Matson DD. *Neurosurgery of infancy and childhood*, 2nd ed. Springfield, IL: Charles C Thomas, 1969.
306. Anderson FM, Burke BL. Anterior sacral meningocele. *JAMA* 1977;237:39–42.
307. Richaud J. Spinal meningeal malformations in children (without meningoceles or meningomyeloceles). *Childs Nerv Syst* 1988;4:79–87.
308. Chiari H. Ueber Veränderungen des Kleinhirns infolge von Hydrocephalie des Grosshirns. *Dtsch Med Wochenschr* 1891;17:1172–1175.
309. Chiari H. Über die Veränderungen des Kleinhirns, des Pons und der Medulla Oblongata in Folge von congenitaler Hydrocephalie des Grosshirns. *Denkschrift Akad Wissenschaften in Wien* 1895;63:71–116.
310. Mackenzie NG, Emery JL. Deformities of the cervical cord in children with neurospinal dysraphism. *Dev Med Child Neurol* 1971;25[Suppl]:58–67.
311. Emery JL, Lendon RG. Clinical implications of cord lesions in neurospinal dysraphism. *Dev Med Child Neurol* 1972;27[Suppl]:45–51.
312. Blaauw G. Defect in posterior arch of atlas in myelomeningocele. *Dev Med Child Neurol* 1971; 25[Suppl]:113–115.
313. Brunberg JA, et al. Magnetic resonance imaging of spinal dysraphism. *Radiol Clin North Am* 1988;26:181–205.

314. Yakovlev PI, Wadsworth RC. Schizencephalies: a study of the congenital clefts in the cerebral mantle. *J Neuropathol Exp Neurol* 1946;5:116–130, 169–206.

315. Anderson FM. Occult spinal dysraphism: a series of 73 cases. *Pediatrics* 1975;55:826–834.

316. Carter CO, Evans KA, Till K. Spinal dysraphism: genetic relation to neural tube malformations. *J Med Genet* 1976;13:343–350.

317. Little BB, et al. Hereditary cranial bifidum and symmetric parietal foramina are the same entity. *Am J Med Genet* 1990;35:453–458.

318. Bartsch O, et al. Delineation of a contiguous gene syndrome with multiple exostoses, enlarged parietal foramina, craniofacial dysostosis, and mental retardation caused by deletions in the short arm of chromosome 11. *Am J Hum Genet* 1996;58:734–742.

319. Kaplan SB, Kemp SS, Oh KS. Radiographic manifestations of congenital anomalies of the skull. *Radiol Clin North Am* 1991;29:195–218.

320. Jones KL. *Smith's recognizable patterns of human malformation*, 5th ed. Philadelphia: WB Saunders, 1997:778–779.

321. Hoving EW, Vermeij-Keers C, Mommaas-Kienhuis AM, Separation of neural and surface ectoderm after closure of the rostral neuropore. *Anat Embryol* 1990;182:455–463.

322. Suwanwela C, Suwanwela N. A morphological classification of sincipital encephalomeningoceles. *J Neurosurg* 1972;36:201–211.

323. Lorber J, Schofield JK. The prognosis of occipital encephalocele. *Z Kinderchir* 1979;28:347–351.

324. Simpson DA, David DJ, White J. Cephaloceles: treatment, outcome and antenatal diagnosis. *Neurosurgery* 1984;15:14–21.

325. Smith MT, Huntington HW. Inverse cerebellum and occipital encephalocele: a dorsal fusion uniting the Arnold-Chiari and Dandy-Walker spectrum. *Neurology* 1977;27:246–251.

326. Cohen MM, Lemire RM. Syndromes with cephaloceles. *Teratology* 1982;25:161–172.

327. Summers MC, Donnenfeld AE. Dandy-Walker malformation in the Meckel syndrome. *Am J Med Genet* 1995;55:57–61.

328. Zee CS, et al. Lipomas of the corpus callosum associated with frontal dysraphism. *J Comput Assist Tomogr* 1981;5:201–205.

329. French BN. Midline fusion defects and defects of formation. In: Youmans JR, ed. *Neurological surgery*. 3rd ed. Philadelphia: WB Saunders, 1990:1081–1235.

330. Stark GD. Neonatal assessment of the child with a meningomyelocele. *Arch Dis Child* 1971;46:539–548.

331. Mortier W, von Bernuth H. The neural influence on muscle development in myelomeningocele: histochemical and electrodiagnostic studies. *Dev Med Child Neurol* 1971;25[Suppl]:82–89.

332. Laurence KM. The natural history of spina bifida cystica: detailed analysis of 407 cases. *Arch Dis Child* 1964;39:41–57.

333. Lorber J. Ventriculo-cardiac shunts in the first week of life. *Dev Med Child Neurol* 1969;20[Suppl]:13–22.

334. Hammock MK, Milhorat TH, Baron IS. Normal pressure hydrocephalus in patients with myelomeningocele. *Dev Med Child Neurol* 1976; 37[Suppl]:55–68.

335. el Gammal T, Mark EK, Brooks BS. MR imaging of Chiari II malformation. *AJR Am J Roentgenol* 1988;150:163–170.

336. Quencer RM. Intracranial CSF flow in pediatric hydrocephalus: evaluation with cine MR imaging. *Am J Neuroradiol* 1992;13:601–608.

337. Charney EB, et al. Management of Chiari II complications in infants with myelomeningocele. *J Pediatr* 1987;111:364–371.

338. Venes JL, Black KL, Latack JT. Preoperative evaluation and surgical management of the Arnold-Chiari II malformation. *J Neurosurg* 1986;64:363–370.

339. Bell WO, et al. Symptomatic Arnold-Chiari malformation: review of experience with 22 cases. *J Neurosurg* 1987;66:812–816.

340. Naik DR, Emery JL. The position of the spinal cord segments related to the vertebral bodies in children with meningomyelocele and hydrocephalus. *Dev Med Child Neurol* 1968;16[Suppl]:62–88.

341. Kaplan WE, McLone DG, Richards I. The urological manifestations of the tethered spinal cord. *Z Kinderchir* 1987;42[Suppl 1]:27–31.

342. Altman RP, Randolph JG, Lilly JR. Sacrococcygeal teratoma: American Academy of Pediatrics, Surgical Section Survey-1973. *J Pediatr Surg* 1974;9:389–398.

343. Smith ED. *Spina bifida and the total care of spinal meningomyelocele*, Springfield, IL: Charles C Thomas, 1965.

344. Stark G. Prediction of urinary continence in myelomeningocele. *Dev Med Child Neurol* 1971;13:388–389.

345. Stark G. The pathophysiology of the bladder in myelomeningocele and its correlation with the neurological picture. *Dev Med Child Neurol* 1968; 16[Suppl]:76–86.

346. Spindel MR, et al. The changing neurourologic lesion in myelodysplasia. *JAMA* 1987;258:1630–1633.

347. Brem AS, et al. Long-term renal risk factors in children with meningomyelocele. *J Pediatr* 1987;110:51–55.

348. Thomas M, Hopkins JM. A study of the renal tract from birth in children with myelomeningocele. *Dev Med Child Neurol* 1971;25[Suppl]:96–100.

349. Guthkelch AN. Aspects of the surgical management of myelomeningocele: a review. *Dev Med Child Neurol* 1986;28:525–532.

350. Sharrard WJ, Zachary RB, Lorber J. Survival and paralysis in open myelomeningocele with special reference to the time of repair of the spinal lesion. *Dev Med Child Neurol* 1967;11[Suppl]:35–50.

351. Sharrard WJ, et al. A controlled trial of immediate and delayed closure of spina bifida cystica. *Arch Dis Child* 1963;38:18–22.

352. Brocklehurst G. *Spina bifida for the clinician*, London: William Heinemann Med Books, 1976.

353. Lorber J. Spina bifida cystica: results of treatment of 270 consecutive cases with criteria for selection for the future. *Arch Dis Child* 1972;47:8548–8573.

354. Soare PL, Raimondi AJ. Intellectual and perceptual motor characteristics of treated myelomeningocele children. *Am J Dis Child* 1977;131:199–204.

355. Park TS, et al. Progressive spasticity and scoliosis in children with myelomeningocele. *J Neurosurg* 1985;62:367–375.

356. Lorber J. Selective treatment of myelomeningocele: to treat or not to treat? *Pediatrics* 1974;53:307–308.

357. Hunt GM. Open spina bifida: outcome for a complete cohort treated unselectively and followed into adulthood. *Dev Med Child Neurol* 1990;32:108–118.

358. McLone DG. Care of the neonate with a myelomeningocele. *Neurosurg Clin N Am* 1998;9:111–120.

359. Hobbins JC. Diagnosis and management of neural-tube defects today. *N Engl J Med* 1991;324:690–691.

360. McLone DG. Continuing concepts in the management of spina bifida. *Pediatr Neurosurg* 1992;18:254–256.

361. Luthy DA, et al. Cesarean section before the onset of labor and subsequent motor function in infants with meningomyelocele diagnosed antenatally. *N Engl J Med* 1991;324:662–666.

362. Tulipan N, Bruner JP. Myelomeningocele repair in utero: a report of three cases. *Pediatr Neurosurg* 1998; 28:177–180.

363. Hunt GM, Holmes AE. Some factors relating to intelligence in treated children with spina bifida cystica. *Am J Dis Child* 1976;130:823–827.

364. Bier JB, et al. Medical and social factors associated with cognitive outcome in individuals with myelomeningocele. *Dev Med Child Neurol* 1997;39:263–266.

365. Carmel PW. Management of the Chiari malformation in childhood. *Clin Neurosurg* 1983;30:385–406.

366. Laurence KM, Tew BJ. Follow-up of 65 survivors from 425 cases of spina bifida born in South Wales between 1956 and 1962. *Dev Med Child Neurol* 1967; 11[Suppl]:13.

367. Paul KS, et al. Arnold-Chiari malformation: review of 71 cases. *J Neurosurg* 1983;58:183–187.

368. Vandertop WP, et al. Surgical decompression for symptomatic Chiari II malformation in neonates with myelomeningocele. *J Neurosurg* 1992;77:541–544.

369. Drummond DS, et al. Postoperative neuropathic fractures in patients with myelomeningocele. *Dev Med Child Neurol* 1981;23:147–150.

370. Caldaerelli M, Di Rocco C, La Marca F. Treatment of hydromyelia in spina bifida. *Surg Neurol* 1998;50: 411–420.

371. Fernandez ET, et al. Neurogenic bladder dysfunction in children: review of pathophysiology and current management. *J Pediatr* 1994;124:1–7.

372. Gonzalez R. Urinary incontinence. In: Kelalis PK, et al, eds. *Clinical pediatric urology*. Philadelphia: WB Saunders, 1992:384–398.

373. Whitehead WE, et al. Biofeedback treatment of fecal incontinence in patients with meningomyelocele. *Dev Med Child Neurol* 1981;23:313–320.

374. Wald A. Use of biofeedback in treatment of fecal incontinence in patients with meningomyelocele. *Pediatrics* 1981;68:45–49.

375. Malone PS, Ransley PG, Kiely EM. Preliminary report: the antegrade continence enema. *Lancet* 1990;336:1217–1218.

376. Rekate HL. *Comprehensive management of spina bifida*, Boca Raton, FL: CRC Press, 1991.

377. Laurence KM. Effect of early surgery for spina bifida cystica on survival and quality of life. *Lancet* 1974;1:301–304.

378. Menzies RG, Parkin JM, Hey EN. Prognosis for babies with meningomyelocele and higher lumbar paraplegia at birth. *Lancet* 1985;2:993–997.

379. Hide DW, Williams HP, Ellis HL. The outlook for the child with a myelomeningocele for whom early surgery was considered inadvisable. *Dev Med Child Neurol* 1972;14:304–307.

380. McLaughlin JF, et al. Influence of prognosis on decisions regarding the care of newborns with myelodysplasia. *N Engl J Med* 1985;312:1589–1594.

381. Hunt GM. Spina bifida: implications for 100 children at school. *Dev Med Child Neurol* 1981;23:160–172.

382. Gilbertson M, et al. ASBAH-independence. *Z Kinderchir Grenzgeb* 1979;28:425–432.

383. Leonard CO, Freeman JM. Spina bifida: a new disease. *Pediatrics* 1981;68:136–137.

384. Cleland J. Contribution to the study of spina bifida, encephalocele, and anencephalus. *J Anat Physiol* 1883; 17:257–292.

385. Harding B, Copp AJ. Malformations. In: Graham DI, Lantos PL, eds. *Greenfield's neuropathology*. 6th ed. New York: Oxford University Press, 1997:417–422.

386. Marin-Padilla M, Marin-Padilla MT. Morphogenesis of experimentally induced Arnold-Chiari malformation. *J Neurol Sci* 1981;50:29–55.

387. Elster AD, Chen MY. Chiari I malformations: clinical and radiological reappraisal. *Radiology* 1992;183: 347–353.

388. Pascual J, et al. Headache in type I Chiari malformation. *Neurology* 1992;42:1519–1521.

389. Nohria V, Oakes WJ. Chiari I malformation: a review of 43 patients. *Pediatr Neurosurg* 1990–1991;16: 222–227.

390. Gardner WJ. Anatomic features common to the Arnold-Chiari and the Dandy-Walker malformations suggests a common origin. *Cleve Clin Q* 1959;26: 206–222.

391. Peach B. Arnold-Chiari malformation: anatomic features of 20 cases. *Arch Neurol* 1965;12:613–621.

392. Emery JL, MacKenzie NG. Medullocervical dislocation deformity (Chiari II deformity) related to neurospinal dysraphism (meningomeylocele). *Brain* 1973;96:155–162.

393. Adams RD, Schatzki R, Scoville WB. The Arnold-Chiari malformation diagnosis: demonstration by intraspinal lipiodol and successful surgical treatment. *N Engl J Med* 1941;225:125–131.

394. Schachenmayr W, Friede RL. Rhombencephalosynapsis: a Viennese malformation? *Dev Med Child Neurol* 1982;24:178–182.

395. Carter CO, et al. Spinal dysraphism: genetic relation to neural tube malformations. *J Med Genet* 1976;13: 343–350.

396. James CC, Lassman LP. *Spinal dysraphism: spina bifida occulta*, London: Butterworth, 1972.

397. Pang D, Dias MS, Ahab-Barmada M. Split cord malformation: Part I: a unified theory of embryogenesis for double spinal cord malformations. *Neurosurgery* 1992;31:451–480.

398. Pang D. Split cord malformation: Part II: clinical syndrome. *Neurosurgery* 1992;31:481–500.

399. Yamada S, Zinke DE, Sanders D. Pathophysiology of "the tethered cord syndrome." *J Neurosurg* 1981;54: 494–503.

400. Dryden RJ. Duplication of the spinal cord: a discussion of the possible embryogenesis of diplomyelia. *Dev Med Child Neurol* 1980;22:234–243.

401. Naidich TP, et al. Congenital anomalies of the spine and spinal cord. In: Atlas SW, ed. *Magnetic Resonance Imaging of the brain and spine*. New York: Raven Press, 1991:902–907.

402. Bremer JL. Dorsal intestinal fistula; accessory neurenteric canal; diastematomyelia. *Arch Pathol Lab Med* 1952;54:132–138.

403. Guthkelch AN. Diastematomyelia with median septum. *Brain* 1974;97:729–742.

404. Sheptak PE, Susen AF. Diastematomyelia. *Am J Dis Child* 1967;113:210–213.

405. Hendrick EB. On diastematomyelia. *Prog Neurol Surg* 1971;4:277–288.
406. Pang D, Parrish RG. Regrowth of diastematomyelic bone spur after extradural resection: case report. *J Neurosurg* 1983;59:887–890.
407. Batzdorf U. *Syringomyelia: concepts in diagnosis and treatment*, Baltimore: Williams & Wilkins, 1990.
408. Williams B. Pathogenesis of syringomyelia. In: Batzdorf U, ed. *Syringomyelia: current concepts in diagnosis and treatment*. Baltimore: Williams & Wilkins, 1991:59–90.
409. Oldfield EH, et al. Pathophysiology of syringomyelia associated with Chiari I malformation of the cerebellar tonsils: implications for diagnosis and treatment. *J Neurosurg* 1994;80:3–15.
410. Williams B. Syringomyelia. *Neurosurg Clin N Am* 1990;1:653–685.
411. Hall PV, et al. Myelodysplasia and developmental scoliosis: a manifestation of syringomyelia. *Spine* 1976;1:48–56.
412. Alcalá H, Dodson WE. Syringobulbia as a cause of laryngeal stridor in childhood. *Neurology* 1975;25:875–878.
413. Powell M. Syringomyelia: how MRI aids diagnosis and management. *Acta Neurochir* 1988;43[Suppl]:17–21.
414. Wisoff JH. Hydromyelia: a critical review. *Child Nerv Syst* 1988;4:1–8.
415. Filizzolo F, et al. Foramen magnum decompression versus terminal ventriculostomy for the treatment of syringomyelia. *Acta Neurochir* 1988;96:96–99.
416. Logue V, Edwards MR. Syringomyelia and its surgical treatment—an analysis of 75 patients. *J Neurol Neurosurg Psychiatry* 1981;44:273–284.
417. Towfighi J, Housman C. Spinal cord abnormalities in caudal regression syndrome. *Acta Neuropathol* 1991;81:458–466.
418. Lynch SA, Bond PM, Copp AJ, et al. A gene for autosomal dominant sacral agenesis maps to the holoprosencephaly region at 7q36. *Nat Genet* 1995;11:93–95.
419. Sarnat HB, Case ME, Graviss R. Sacral agenesis: neurologic and neuropathologic features. *Neurology* 1976;26:1124–1129.
420. Thompson IM, Kirk RM, Dale M. Sacral agenesis. *Pediatrics* 1974;54:236–238.
421. Mills JL, Baker L, Goldman AS. Malformations in infants of diabetic mothers occur before the seventh gestational week: implications for treatment. *Diabetes* 1979;28:292–293.
422. Passarge E, Lenz W. Syndrome of caudal regression in infants of diabetic mothers: observation of further cases. *Pediatrics* 1966;37:672–675.
423. Matson DD, Jerva MJ. Recurrent meningitis associated with congenital lumbo-sacral dermal sinus tract. *J Neurosurg* 1966;25:288–297.
424. Frieden IJ. Aplasia cutis congenita: a clinical review and proposal for classification. *J Am Acad Dermatol* 1986;14:646–660.
425. Hurst JA, Baraitser M. Johanson-Blizzard syndrome. *J Med Genet* 1989;26:45–48.
426. Altman NR, Naidich TP, Braffman BH. Posterior fossa malformations. *Am J Neuroradiol* 1992;13:691–724.
427. Pascual-Castroviejo I, et al. Primary degeneration of the granular layer of the cerebellum: a study of 14 patients and review of the literature. *Neuropediatrics* 1994;25:183–190.
428. Sarnat HB, Alcala H. Human cerebellar hypoplasia: a syndrome of diverse causes. *Arch Neurol* 1980;37:300–305.
429. Friede RL. *Developmental neuropathology*, 2nd ed. Berlin: Springer Verlag, 1989:361–371.
430. Barth PG, et al. The syndrome of autosomal recessive pontocerebellar hypoplasia, microcephaly, and extrapyramidal dyskinesia (pontocerebellar hypoplasia type 2): compiled data from 10 pedigrees. *Neurology* 1995;45:311–317.
431. Isaac M, Best P. Two cases of agenesis of the vermis of the cerebellum with fusion of the dentate nuclei and cerebellar hemispheres. *Acta Neuropathol* 1987;74:278–280.
432. Tomiwa K, Baraitser M, Wilson J. Dominantly inherited congenital ataxia with atrophy of the vermis. *Pediatr Neurol* 1987;3:360–362.
433. Joubert M, et al. Familial agenesis of the cerebellar vermis. *Neurology* 1969;19:813–825.
434. Kendall B, et al. Joubert syndrome: a clinico-radiological study. *Neuroradiology* 1990;31:502–506.
435. Legge RH, et al. Periodic alternating gaze deviation in infancy. *Neurology* 1992;42:1740–1743.
436. Bordarier C, Aicardi J, Goutières F. Congenital hydrocephalus and eye abnormalities with severe developmental brain defects: Warburg's syndrome. *Ann Neurol* 1984;16:60–65.
437. Robain O, Dulac O, Lejeune J. Cerebellar hemispheric agenesis. *Acta Neuropathol* 1987;60:137–141.
438. Bull JS, Nixon WLP, Pratt RTC. Radiological criteria and familial occurrence of primary basilar impression. *Brain* 1955;78:229–247.
439. DeLong WB, Schneider RC. Surgical management of congenital spinal lesions associated with abnormalities of the cranio-spinal junction. *J Neurol Neurosurg Psychiatry* 1966;29:319–322.
440. Klippel M, Feil A. Anomalie de la colonne vertebrale par d'absence des vertèbres cervicales. *Bull et Mém Soc Anat Paris* 1912;87:185–188.
441. Gunderson CH, Solitare GB. Mirror movements in patients with Klippel-Feil syndrome. *Arch Neurol* 1968;18:675–679.
442. Morrison SG, Perry LW, Scott LP. Congenital brevicollis (Klippel-Feil syndrome) and cardiovascular anomalies. *Am J Dis Child* 1968;115:614–620.
443. Foster JB, Hudgson P, Pearce GW. The association of syringomyelia and congenital cervico-medullary anomalies: pathological evidence. *Brain* 1969;92:25–34.
444. Bach C, et al. La dysostose cléido-cranienne étude de six observations: association à des manifestations neurologiques. *Ann Pediatr (Paris)* 1966;13:67–77.
445. Belloni E, et al. Identification of *Sonic hedgehog* as a candidate gene responsible for holoprosencephaly. *Nat Genet* 1996;14:353–356.
446. Roessler E, et al. Mutations in the human *Sonic hedgehog* gene cause holoprosencephaly. *Nat Genet* 1996;14:357–360.
447. Müller F, O'Rahilly R. Mediobasal prosencephalic defects, including holoprosencephaly and cyclopia, in relation to the development of the human forebrain. *Am J Anat* 1989;185:391–414.
448. Kelley RL, et al. Holoprosencephaly in RSH/Smith-Lemli-Opitz syndrome: does abnormal cholesterol metabolism affect the function of *Sonic hedgehog*? *Am J Med Genet* 1996;66:78–84.
449. Brown SA, et al. Holoprosencephaly due to mutations in *ZIC2*, a homologue of Drosophila odd-paired. *Nat Genet* 1998;20:180–183.

450. Matsunaga E, Shiota K. Holoprosencephaly in human embryos: epidemiologic study of 150 cases. *Teratology* 1977;16:261–272.
451. Kobori JA, Herrick MK, Urich H. Arhinencephaly: the spectrum of associated malformations. *Brain* 1987;110:237–260.
452. Ming PL, Goodner DM, Park TS. Cytogenetic variants in holoprosencephaly. Report of a case and review of the literature. *Am J Dis Child* 1976;130:864–867.
453. Barr M, Hanson JW, Currey K. Holoprosencephaly in infants of diabetic mothers. *J Pediatr* 1983;102:565–568.
454. Burck U. Genetic counselling in holoprosencephaly. *Helv Paediatr Acta* 1982;37:231–237.
455. Gurrieri F, et al. Physical mapping of the holoprosencephaly critical region on chromosome 7q36. *Nat Genet* 1993;3:247–251.
456. Ardinger HH, Bartley JA. Microcephaly in familial holoprosencephaly. *J Craniofac Genet Dev Biol* 1988;8:53–61.
457. McKusick VA. Holoprosencephaly. In: *Mendelian inheritance in man. Catalogs of autosomal dominant, autosomal recessive, and X-linked phenotypes.* 10th ed. Baltimore: Johns Hopkins University Press, 1992: 1443–1444.
458. De Meyer W. The median cleft face syndrome. *Neurology* 1967;17:961–972.
459. De Meyer W. Classification of cerebral malformations. *Birth Defects Original Article Series* 1971;7:78–93.
460. Dekaban AS. Arhinencephaly. *Am J Ment Defic* 1948;63:428–432.
461. Sarnat HB. Role of human fetal ependyma. *Pediatr Neurol* 1992 ;8:163–178.
462. Jellinger K, et al. Holoprosencephaly and agenesis of the corpus callosum: frequency of associated malformations. *Acta Neuropathol* 1981;55:1–10.
463. De Meyer W. Median facial malformations and their implications for brain malformations. *Birth Defects Original Articles Series* 1975;7:155–181.
464. Winter RM. What's in a face? *Nature Genet* 1996;12:124–129.
465. De Meyer W. Orbital hypertelorism. In: Vinken PJ, Bruyn GW, eds. *Handbook of clinical neurology. Vol. 30. Congenital malformations of the brain and skull. Part I.* New York: Elsevier North Holland, 1977:235–255.
466. De Meyer W, Zeman W, Palmer CG. Familial alobar holoprosencephaly (arhinencephaly) with median cleft lip and palate. *Neurology* 1963;13:913–918.
467. Aleksic S, et al. Unilateral arhinencephaly in Goldenhar Gorlin syndrome. *Dev Med Child Neurol* 1975; 17:498–504.
468. Merriam GR, Beitins IZ, Bode HH. Father-to-son transmission of hypogonadism with anosmia. *Am J Dis Child* 1977;131:1216–1219.
469. DeMorsier G. Études sur les dysgraphies cranioencéphaliques. II. Agénesie du septum lucidum avec malformation du tractus optique. La dysplasie septo-optique. *Schweiz Arch Neurol Psychiat* 1956;77:267–292.
470. Roessmann U, et al. Neuropathology of "septo-optic dysplasia" (de Morsier's syndrome) with immunohistochemical studies of the hypothalamus and pituitary gland. *J Neuropath Exp Neurol* 1987;46:597–608.
471. Masera N, et al. Diabetes insipidus with impaired osmotic regulation in septo-optic dysplasia and agenesis of the corpus callosum. *Arch Dis Child* 1994;70:51–53.
472. Michaud J, Mizrahi EM, Urich H. Agenesis of the vermis with fusion of the cerebellar hemispheres, septo-optic dysplasia and associated anomalies. *Acta Neuropathol* 1982;56:161–166.
473. Fielder AR, Levene MI, Trounce JQ. Optic nerve hypoplasia in infancy. *J Roy Soc Med* 1986;79:25–29.
474. Zeki SM, Dutton GN. Optic nerve hypoplasia in children. *Br J Ophthalmol* 1990;74:300–304.
475. Nelson M, Lessell S, Sadun AA. Optic nerve hypoplasia and maternal diabetes mellitus. *Arch Neurol* 1986;43:20–25.
476. Parr JH. Midline cerebral defect and Kallmann's syndrome. *J Roy Soc Med* 1988;81:355–356.
477. Barth P. Disorders of neuronal migration. *Can J Neurol Sci* 1987;14:1–16.
478. Barkovich AJ, Gressens P, Evrard P. Formation, maturation, and disorders of brain neocortex. *Am J Neuroradiol* 1992;13:423–446.
479. Dekaban A. Large defects in cerebral hemispheres associated with cortical dysgenesis. *J Neuropathol Exp Neurol* 1965;24:512–530.
480. Barkovich AJ, Kjos B. Schizencephaly: correlation of clinical findings with MR characteristics. *Am J Neuroradiol* 1992;13:85–94.
481. Faina GT, et al. Familial schizencephaly associated with EMX2 mutation. *Neurology* 1997;48:1403–1406.
482. Granata T, et al. Familial schizencephaly associated with EMX2 mutation. *Neurology* 1997;48:1403–1406.
483. Tardieu M, Evrard P, Lyon G. Progressive expanding congenital porencephalies: a treatable cause of progressive encephalopathy. *Pediatrics* 1981; 68:198–202.
484. Miller GM, et al. Schizencephaly: a clinical and CT study. *Neurology* 1984;34:997–1001.
485. Benda CE. *Developmental disorders of mentation and cerebral palsies*, New York: Grune & Stratton, 1952.
486. Steward RM, Richman DP, Caviness VS. Lissencephaly and pachygyria: an architectonic and topographical analysis. *Acta Neuropathol* 1975;31:1–12.
487. Barkovich AJ, Koch TK, Carrol CL. The spectrum of lissencephaly: report of 10 patients analyzed by magnetic resonance imaging. *Ann Neurol* 1991;30:139–146.
488. Dobyns WB, et al. Lissencephaly: a human brain malformation associated with deletion of the LIS1 gene located at chromosome 17p13. *JAMA* 1993;270:2838–2842.
489. Lo Nigro C, et al. Point mutations and an intragenic deletion in LIS1: the lissencephaly causative gene in isolated lissencephaly sequence and Miller-Dieker syndrome. *Hum Mol Genet* 1997;6:157–164.
490. Chong SS, et al. A revision of the lissencephaly and Miller-Dieker syndrome critical regions in chromosome 17p13.3. *Hum Mol Genet* 1997;6:147–155.
491. Clark DC, et al. Predominant localization of the LIS family of gene products to Cajal-Retzius cells and ventricular neuroepithelium in the developing human cortex. *J Neuropathol Exp Neurol* 1997;56:1044–1052.
492. Fogli A, et al. Intracellular levels of the LIS1 protein correlate with clinical and neuroradiological findings in patients with classical lissencephaly. *Ann Neurol* 1999;45:154–161.
493. Aicardi J. The agyria-pachygyria complex: a spectrum of cortical malformations. *Brain Develop* 1991;13: 1–8.
494. Gastaut H, et al. Lissencephaly (Agyria-pachygyria): clinical findings and serial EEG studies. *Dev Med Child Neurol* 1987;29:167–180.
495. Alvarez LA, et al. Miller-Dieker syndrome: a disorder affecting specific pathways of neuronal migration. *Neurology* 1986;36:489–493.

496. Robain O, et al. Hemimegalencephaly: a clinico-pathological study of four cases. *Neuropathol Appl Neurobiol* 1988;14:125–135.
497. Kuzniecky R, Berkovic S, Andermann F. Focal cortical myoclonus and rolandic cortical dysplasia: clarification by magnetic resonance imaging. *Ann Neurol* 1988;23:317–325.
498. Dobyns WB, Stratton RF, Greenberg F. Syndromes with lissencephaly. Miller-Dieker and Norman-Roberts syndrome and isolated lissencephaly. *Am J Med Genet* 1984;18:509–526.
499. Haberland C, Perou M. Encephalocraniocutaneous lipomatosis. *Arch Neurol* 1970;22:144–155.
500. Choi BH, Kudo M. Abnormal neuronal migration and gliomatosis cerebri in epidermal nevus syndrome. *Acta Neuropathol* 1981;53:319–325.
501. Grunnet ML, Bale JF. Brain abnormalities in infants with Potter syndrome (oligohydramnios tetrad). *Neurology* 1981;31:1571–1574.
502. Shigematsu H, et al. Neuropathological and Golgi study on a case of thanatophoric dysplasia. *Brain Develop* 1985;17:628–632.
503. Robain O, Deonna T. Pachygyria and congenital nephrosis: disorder of migration and neuronal orientation. *Acta Neuropathol* 1983;60:137–141.
504. Hansen LA, Pearl GS. Isoretinoin teratogenicity: case report with neuropathological findings. *Acta Neuropathol* 1985;65:335–337.
505. Kuzniecky R, et al. Congenital bilateral perisylvian syndrome: study of 31 patients. *Lancet* 1993;341:608–612.
506. Guerrini R, et al. Bilateral parasagittal parietooccipital polymicrogyria and epilepsy. *Ann Neurol* 1997;41:65–73.
507. Gropman AL, et al. Pediatric congenital bilateral perisylvian syndrome: clinical and MRI features in 12 patients. *Neuropediatrics* 1997;28:198–203.
508. Becker PS, Dixon AM, Troncoso JC. Bilateral opercular polymicrogyria. *Ann Neurol* 1989;25:90–92.
509. Palmini A, et al. Focal neuronal migration disorders and intractible partial epilepsy: a study of 30 patients. *Ann Neurol* 1991;30:741–749.
510. Sankar R, et al. Microscopic cortical dysplasia in infantile spasms: evolution of white matter abnormalities. *Am J Neuroradiol* 1995;16:1265–1272.
511. Palmini A, et al. Diffuse cortical dysplasia or the "double cortex" syndrome. *Neurology* 1991;41:1656–1662.
512. Pinard J-M, et al. Subcortical laminar heterotopia and lissencephaly in two families: a single X-linked dominant gene. *J Neurol Neurosurg Psychiatry* 1994;57:914–920.
513. Gleeson JG, Allen KM, Fox JW. *Doublecortin*, a brain-specific gene mutated in human X-linked lissencephaly and double cortex syndrome, encodes a putative signaling protein. *Cell* 1998;92:63–72.
514. Gleeson JG, et al. Characterization of mutations in the gene *doublecortin* in patients with double cortex syndrome. *Ann Neurol* 1999;45:146–153.
515. des Portes V, et al. A novel CNS gene required for neuronal migration and involved in X-linked subcortical laminar heterotopia and lissencephaly syndrome. *Cell* 1998;92:51–61.
516. Miura K, Watanabe K, Maeda N, et al. Magnetic resonance imaging and positron emission tomography of band heterotopia. *Brain Dev* 1993;15:288–290.
517. Huttenlocher PR, Taravath S, Mojtahedi S. Periventricular heterotopia and epilepsy. *Neurology* 1994;44:51–55.
518. Dubeau F, Tampieri D, Lee N. Periventricular and subcortical nodular heterotopia: a study of 33 patients. *Brain* 1995;118:1273–1287.
519. Li LM, et al. Periventricular nodular heterotopia and intractable temporal lobe epilepsy: poor outcome after temporal lobe resection. *Ann Neurol* 1997;41:662–668.
520. Musumeci SA, et al. A new family with periventricular nodular heterotopia and peculiar dysmorphic features. *Arch Neurol* 1997;54:61–64.
521. Eksioglu YZ, et al. Periventricular heterotopia: an X-linked dominant epilepsy locus causing aberrant cerebral cortical development. *Neuron* 1996;16:77–87.
522. Jeret JS, et al. Frequency of agenesis of the corpus callosum in the developmentally disabled population as determined by computerized tomography. *Pediatr Neurosci* 1986;12:101–103.
523. Zaki W. Le processus dégénératif au cours du développement du corps colleux. *Arch Anat Micr Morphol Expér* 1985;74:133–149.
524. Ettlinger G, et al. Agenesis of the corpus callosum: a behavioral investigation. *Brain* 1972;95:327–346.
525. Serur D, Jeret JS, Wisniewski K. Agenesis of the corpus callosum: clinical, neuroradiological and cytogenetic studies. *Neuropediatrics* 1988;19:87–91.
526. Barkovich AJ, Lyon G, Evrard P. Formation, maturation, and disorders of white matter. *Am J Neuroradiol* 1992;13:447–461.
527. Barkovich AJ, Kjos B. Normal postnatal development of the corpus callosum as demonstrated by MR imaging. *Am J Neuroradiol* 1988;9:487–491.
528. Menkes JH, Philippart M, Clark DB. Hereditary partial agenesis of the corpus callosum. *Arch Neurol* 1964;11:198–208.
529. Khanna S, et al. Corpus callosum agenesis and epilepsy: PET findings. *Pediatr Neurol* 1994;10:221–227.
530. Graham JM, et al. FG syndrome: report of three new families with linkage to Xq12-q22.1. *Am J Med Genet* 1998;80:145–156.
531. Bamforth F, et al. Abnormalities of corpus callosum in patients with inherited metabolic diseases. *Lancet* 1988;2:451.
532. Dobyns WB. Agenesis of the corpus callosum and gyral malformations are frequent manifestations of nonketotic hyperglycinemia. *Neurology* 1989;39:817–820.
533. Njiokiktjien C, Valk J, Ramaekers G. Malformation or damage of the corpus callosum? A clinical and MRI study. *Brain Develop* 1988;10:92–99.
534. deJong JG, et al. Agenesis of the corpus callosum, infantile spasms, ocular anomalies (Aicardi's syndrome). *Neurology* 1976;26:1152–1158.
535. Bertoni JM, von Loh S, Allen RJ. The Aicardi syndrome: report of 4 cases and review of the literature. *Ann Neurol* 1979;5:475–482.
536. Burn J, Martin N. Two retarded male cousins with odd facies, hypotonia, and severe constipation: possible examples of the X-linked FG syndrome. *J Med Genet* 1983;20:97–99.
537. Landman J, et al. Radiological colpocephaly: a congenital malformation or the result of intrauterine and perinatal brain damage. *Brain Develop* 1989;11:313–316.
538. Rakic P, Yakovlev P. Development of the corpus callosum and cavum septi in man. *J Comp Neurol* 1968;132:45–72.

539. Nakajima Y, et al. Ultrasonographic evaluation of cavum septi pellucidi and cavum vergae. *Brain Develop* 1986;8:505–508.

540. Miller ME, Kido D, Horner F. Cavum vergae: association with neurologic abnormality and diagnosis by magnetic resonance imaging. *Arch Neurol* 1986;43:821–823.

541. Bodensteiner JB. The saga of the septum pellucidum: a tale of unfunded clinical investigations. *J Child Neurol* 1995;10:227–231.

542. Pauling KJ, et al. Does selection bias determine the prevalence of the cavum septi pellucidi? *Pediatr Neurol* 1998;19:195–198.

543. Nellhaus G. Head circumference from birth to 18 years. *Pediatrics* 1968;41:106–114.

544. Sells CJ. Microcephaly in a normal school population. *Pediatrics* 1977;59:262–265.

545. Burton BK. Dominant inheritance of microcephaly with short stature. *Clin Genet* 1981;20:25–27.

546. Dorman C. Microcephaly and intelligence. *Dev Med Child Neurol* 1991;33:267–269.

547. Dolk H. The predictive value of microcephaly during the first year of life for mental retardation at 7 years. *Dev Med Child Neurol* 1991;33:974–983.

548. Book JA, Schut JW, Reed AC. A clinical and genetical study of microcephaly. *Am J Ment Defic* 1953;57: 637–660.

549. Merlob P, Steier D, Reisner SH. Autosomal dominant isolated ("uncomplicated") microcephaly. *J Med Genet* 1988;25:750–753.

550. Connolly CJ. The fissural pattern of primate brain. *Am J Phys Anthropol* 1936;21:301–422.

551. Tolmie JL, et al. Microcephaly: genetic counselling and antenatal diagnosis after the birth of an affected child. *Am J Med Genet* 1987;27:583–594.

552. McKusick VA, et al. Chorioretinopathy with hereditary microcephaly. *Arch Ophthalmol* 1966;75:597–600.

553. Scott-Emuakpor A, et al. A syndrome of microcephaly and cataracts in four siblings: a new genetic syndrome? *Am J Dis Child* 1977;131:167–169.

554. Miller RW, Blot WJ. Small head after in utero exposure to atomic radiation. *Lancet* 1972;2:784–787.

555. Dekaban A. Abnormalities in children exposed to x-radiation during various stages of gestation: tentative timetable of radiation injury to the human fetus, Part I. *J Nucl Med* 1968;9:471–477.

556. Wood JW, Johnson KG, Omori Y. In utero exposure to the Hiroshima atomic bomb: an evaluation of head size and mental retardation 20 years later. *Pediatrics* 1967;39:385–392.

557. Amatuzzi R. Hazards to the human fetus from ionizing radiation at diagnostic dose levels: review of the literature. *Perinatol Neonatal* 1980;4:23–30.

558. Steinlin M, et al. Contribution of magnetic resonance imaging on the evaluation of microcephaly. *Neuropediatrics* 1991;22:184–189.

559. Brennan TL, Funk SG, Frothinghom TE. Disporportionate intrauterine head growth and developmental outcome. *Dev Med Child Neurol* 1985;27:746–750.

560. Lipper E, et al. Determinants of neurobehavioral outcome in low-birth-weight infants. *Pediatrics* 1981;67:502–505.

561. Virchow R. Ueber den Cretinismus, namentlich in Franken, and über pathologische Schädelformen. *Verh Phys Med Ges (Würzburg)* 1851;2:230–271.

562. David JD, Poswillo D, Simpson D. *The craniosynostoses*, Berlin: Springer-Verlag, 1982.

563. Cohen MM Jr. Craniosynostosis update 1987. *Am J Med Genet* 1988;4[Suppl]:99–148.

564. Park EA, Powers GF. Acrocephaly and scaphocephaly with symmetrically distributed malformations of the extremities: A study of the so-called acrocephalosyndactylism. *Am J Dis Child* 1920;20:235–315.

565. Moloney DM, et al. Prevalence of Pro250Arg mutation of fibroblast growth factor receptor 3 in coronal craniosynostosis. *Lancet* 1997;349:1059–1062.

566. Passos-Bueno MR, et al. Description of a new mutation and characterization of FGFR1, FGFR2, and FGFR3 mutations among Brazilian patients with syndromic craniosynostoses. *Am J Med Genet* 1998;78:237–241.

567. Graham JM, Badura RJ, Smith DW. Coronal craniostenosis: fetal head constraint as one possible cause. *Pediatrics* 1980;65:995–999.

568. Babler WJ, et al. Skull growth after coronal suturectomy, periostectomy, and dural transection. *J Neurosurg* 1982;56:529–535.

569. Menking M, et al. Premature craniosynostosis associated with hyperthyroidism in 4 children with reference to 5 further cases in the literature. *Mschr Kinderheilk* 1972;120:106–110.

570. Comings DE, Papazian C, Schoene HR. Conradi's disease: Chondrodystrophia calcificans congenita, congenital stippled epiphyses. *J Pediatr* 1968;72:63–69.

571. Reilly BJ, Leeming JM, Fraser D. Craniosynostosis in the rachitic spectrum. *J Pediatr* 1964;64:396–405.

572. Cohen MM Jr. Perspectives on craniosynostosis. *West J Med* 1980;132:507–513.

573. Till K. *Paediatric neurosurgery*, Oxford: Blackwell Scientific Publications, 1975.

574. Freeman JM, Borkowf S. Craniostenosis: review of the literature and report of 34 cases. *Pediatrics* 1962; 30:57–70.

575. Müke R. Neue gesichtspunkte zur pathogenese und therapie der kraniosynostose. *Acta Neurochir* 1972; 26:191–250, 293–326.

576. Fishman MA, et al. The concurrence of hydrocephalus and craniosynostosis. *J Neurosurg* 1971;34:621–629.

577. Cinalli G, et al. Chronic tonsillar herniation in Crouzon's and Apert's syndromes: the role of premature synostosis of the lambdoid suture. *J Neurosurg* 1995;83:575–582.

578. Francis PM, et al. Chronic tonsillar herniation and Crouzon's syndrome. *Pediatr Neurosurg* 1992;18:202–206.

579. Steinberger D, et al. The mutations of FGFR2-associated craniosynostoses are clustered in five structural elements of immunoglobulin-like domain III of the receptor. *Hum Genet* 1998;102:145–150.

580. Schaefer F, et al. Novel mutation in the FGFR2 gene at the same codon as the Crouzon syndrome mutations in a severe Pfeiffer syndrome type 2 case. *Am J Med Genet* 1998;75:252–255.

581. Park WJ, et al. Analysis of phenotypic features and FGFR2 mutations in Apert syndrome. *Am J Hum Genet* 1995;57:321–328.

582. Cohen MM, Kreiborg S. The central nervous system in the Apert syndrome. *Am J Med Genet* 1990;35:36–45.

582a. Ladda RL, et al. Craniosynostosis associated with limb reduction malformations and cleft lip/palate: a distinct syndrome. *Pediatrics* 1978;61:12–15.

583. Menard RM, David DJ. Unilateral lambdoid synostosis: morphological characteristics. *J Craniofac Surg* 1998;9:240–246.

584. Lee FA, McComb JG. The breech head. (Personal communication.)
585. Dohn DF. Surgical treatment of unilateral coronal craniosynostosis (plagiocephaly): report of three cases. *Clev Clin Quart* 1963;30:47–54.
586. Rekate HL. Occipital plagiocephaly: a critical review of the literature. *J Neurosurg* 1998;89:24–30.
587. McComb JG, Withers GJ, Davis RL. Cortical damage from Zenker's solution applied to the dura mater. *Neurosurgery* 1981;6:68–71.
588. Anderson FM. Treatment of coronal and metopic synostosis: 107 cases. *Neurosurgery* 1981;8:143–149.
589. Marsh JL, Schwartz HG. The surgical correction of coronal and metopic craniosynostoses. *J Neurosurg* 1983;59:245–251.
590. Shillito J, Matson DD. Craniosynostosis: a review of 519 surgical patients. *Pediatrics* 1968;41:829–853.
591. Popich GA, Smith DW. Fontanels: range of normal size. *J Pediatr* 1972;80:749–752.
592. Aisenson MR. Closing of the anterior fontanelle. *Pediatrics* 1950;6:223–226.
593. Gooskens RHJM. *Megalencephaly: a subtype of macrocephaly*, Wijk bij Duurstede: Drukwerkverzorging ADDIX, 1987.
594. Saul RA, et al. Mental retardation in the Bannayan syndrome. *Pediatrics* 1982;69:642–644.
595. Powell BR, Budden SS, Buist NRM. Dominantly inherited megalencephaly, muscle weakness, and myoliposis: a carnitine-deficient myopathy within the spectrum of the Ruvalcaba-Myhre-Smith syndrome. *J Pediatr* 1993;123:70–75.
596. Cohen MM. Bannayan-Riley-Ruvalcaba syndrome: renaming three formerly recognized syndromes as one etiologic entity. *Am J Med Genet* 1990;35:291.
597. Smith RD. Abnormal head circumference in learning-disabled children. *Dev Med Child Neurol* 1981;23:626–632.
598. Wilson SAK. Megalencephaly. *J Neurol Psychopathol* 1934;14:173–186.
599. Lorber J, Priestley BL. Children with large heads: a practical approach to diagnosis in 557 children with special reference to 109 children with megalencephaly. *Dev Med Child Neurol* 1981;23:494–504.
600. Sandler AD, et al. Neurodevelopmental dysfunction among nonreferred children with idiopathic megalencephaly. *J Pediatr* 1997;31:320–324.
601. Fishman RA. *Cerebrospinal fluid in diseases of the nervous system*, 2nd ed. Philadelphia: WB Saunders, 1992.
602. Davson H, Welch K, Segal MB. *Physiology and pathophysiology of the cerebrospinal fluid*. Edinburgh/New York: Churchill Livingstone, 1987.
603. Müller F, O'Rahilly R. The human brain at stages 18-20, including the choroid plexuses and the amygdaloid and septal nuclei. *Anat Embryol* 1990;182:285–306.
604. Shuangshoti S, Netsky MG. Histogenesis of choroid plexus in man. *Am J Anat* 1966;118:283–316.
605. Dooling EC, Chi Je G, Gilles FH. Ependymal changes in the human fetal brain. *Ann Neurol* 1977;1:535–541.
606. McComb JG. Cerebrospinal fluid physiology of the developing fetus. *Am J Neuroradiol* 1992;13:595–599.
607. Rottenberg DA, Howieson J, Deck MDF. The rate of CSF formation in man: preliminary observations on metrizamide washout as a measure of CSF bulk flow. *Ann Neurol* 1977;2:503–510.
608. Masserman JH. Cerebrospinal hydrodynamics. IV. Clinical experimental studies. *Arch Neurol Psychiatr* 1934;32:523–553.
609. Cutler RWP, et al. Formation and absorption of cerebrospinal fluid in man. *Brain* 1968;91:707–720.
610. Lorenzo AV, Page LK, Watters GV. Relationship between cerebrospinal fluid formation, absorption and pressure in human hydrocephalus. *Brain* 1970;93:679–692.
611. Rubin LL, Staddon JM. The cell biology of the blood-brain barrier. *Annu Rev Neurosci* 1999;22:11–28.
612. Greitz D. Cerebrospinal fluid circulation and associated intracranial dynamics: a radiologic investigation using MR imaging and radionuclide cisternography. *Acta Radiol* 1993;34[Suppl 386]:1–23.
613. Welch K, Friedman V. The cerebrospinal fluid valves. *Brain* 1960;83:454–469.
614. Upton ML, Weller RO. The morphology of cerebrospinal fluid drainage pathways in human arachnoid granulations. *J Neurosurg* 1985;63:867–875.
615. Mann JD, et al. Regulation of intracranial pressure in rat, dog, and man. *Ann Neurol* 1978;3:156–165.
616. James AE, et al. The effect of cerebrospinal fluid pressure on the size of the drainage pathways. *Neurology* 1976;26:659–663.
617. Shabo AL, Maxwell DS. The morphology of the arachnoid villi: a light and electronmicroscopic study in the monkey. *J Neurosurg* 1968;29:451–463.
618. McComb JG, et al. Cerebrospinal fluid drainage as influenced by ventricular pressure in the rabbit. *J Neurosurg* 1982;56:790–797.
619. McComb JG. Recent research into the nature of cerebrospinal fluid formation and absorption. *J Neurosurg* 1983;59:369–383.
620. James AE Jr, et al. An alternative pathway of cerebrospinal fluid absorption in communicating hydrocephalus: transependymal movement. *Radiology* 1974;111:143–146.
621. Hiratsuka H, et al. Evaluation of periventricular hypodensity in experimental hydrocephalus by metrizamide CT ventriculography. *J Neurosurg* 1982;56:235–240.
622. Zervas NT, et al. Cerebrospinal fluid may nourish cerebral vessels through pathways in the adventitia that may be analogous to systemic vasa vasorum. *J Neurosurg* 1982;56:475–481.
623. Nabeshima S, et al. Junctions in the meninges and marginal glia. *J Comp Neurol* 1975;164:127–170.
624. Alvarez LA, Maytal J, Shinnar S. Idiopathic external hydrocephalus: natural history and relationship to benign familial macrocephaly. *Pediatrics* 1986;77:901–907.
625. Andersson H, Elfverson J, Svendson P. External hydrocephalus in infants. *Childs Brain* 1984;11:398–402.
626. Lorenzo AV, Bresnan MJ, Barlow CF. Cerebrospinal fluid absorption deficit in normal pressure hydrocephalus. *Arch Neurol* 1974;30:387–393.
627. Murthy VS, Deshpande DH. The central canal of the filum terminale in communicating hydrocephalus. *J Neurosurg* 1980;53:528–532.
628. Bering EA. Circulation of the cerebrospinal fluid: demonstration of the choroid plexuses as the generator of the force of flow of fluid and ventricular enlargement. *J Neurosurg* 1962;19:405–413.
629. Weller RO, Wisniewski H. Histological and ultrastructural changes with experimental hydrocephalus in adult rabbits. *Brain* 1969;92:819–828.

630. Milhorat TH, et al. Structural, ultrastructural and permeability changes in the ependyma and surrounding brain favoring equilibrium in progressive hydrocephalus. *Arch Neurol* 1970;22:397–407.

631. Weller RO, Shulman K. Infantile hydrocephalus: clinical, histological, and ultrastructural study of brain damage. *J Neurosurg* 1972;36:255–267.

632. Bannister CM, Chapman SA. Ventricular ependyma of normal and hydrocephalic subjects: a scanning electronmicroscopic study. *Dev Med Child Neurol* 1980; 22:725–735.

633. Levin VA, et al. Physiological studies on the development of obstructive hydrocephalus in the monkey. *Neurology* 1971;21:238–246.

634. Hochwald GM, et al. Experimental hydrocephalus: changes in cerebrospinal fluid dynamics as a function of time. *Arch Neurol* 1972;26:120–129.

635. Shulman K, Marmarou A. Pressure-volume considerations in infantile hydrocephalus. *Dev Med Child Neurol* 1971;25[Suppl]:90–95.

636. Hayden PW, Shurtleff DB, Foltz EL. Ventricular fluid pressure recordings in hydrocephalic patients. *Arch Neurol* 1970;23:147–154.

637. Hill A, Volpe JJ. Decrease in pulsatile flow in the anterior cerebral arteries in infantile hydrocephalus. *Pediatrics* 1982;69:4–7.

638. Milhorat TH, et al. Choroid plexus papilloma. I. Proof of cerebral spinal fluid overproduction. *Child's Brain* 1976;2:273–289.

639. Eisenberg HM, McComb JG, Lorenzo AV. Cerebrospinal fluid overproduction and hydrocephalus associated with choroid plexus papilloma. *J Neurosurg* 1974;40:381–385.

640. Adams C, Johnston WP, Nevin NC. Family study of congenital hydrocephalus. *Dev Med Child Neurol* 1982;24:493–498.

641. Emery JL, Staschak MC. The size and form of the cerebral aqueduct in children. *Brain* 1972;95:591–598.

642. Woollam DHM, Millen JW. Anatomical considerations in the pathology of stenosis of the cerebral aqueduct. *Brain* 1953;76:104–112.

643. Russell DS. Observations on the pathology of hydrocephalus. *Medical Research Council Special Report Series. No. 265.* London: His Majesty's Stationery Office, 1949:138.

644. McMillan JJ, Williams B. Aqueduct stenosis: case review and discussion. *J Neurol Neurosurg Psychiatry* 1977;40:521–532.

645. Edwards JH, Norman RM, Roberts JM. Sex-linked hydrocephalus: report of a family with 15 affected members. *Arch Dis Child* 1961;36:481–485.

646. Jouet M, Kenwrick S. Gene analysis of L1 neural cell adhesion molecule in prenatal diagnosis of hydrocephalus. *Lancet* 1995;345:161–162.

647. Yamasaki M, Thompson P, Lemmon V. CRASH syndrome: Mutations in L1CAM correlate with severity of the disease. *Neuropediatrics* 1997;28:175–178.

648. Graf WD, Born DE, Sarnat HB. The pachygyria-polymicrogyria spectrum of cortical dysplasia in X-linked hydrocephalus. *Eur J Pediatr Surg* 1999 (in press).

649. Sarnat HB. Ependymal reactions to injury: a review. *J Neuropathol Exp Neurol* 1995;54:1–15.

650. Dandy WE, Blackfan KD. Internal hydrocephalus: an experimental, clinical and pathological study. *Am J Dis Child* 1914;8:406–482.

651. Hart NM, Malamud N, Ellis WG. The Dandy-Walker syndrome: a clinicopathological study based on 28 cases. *Neurology* 1972;22:771–780.

652. Tal Y, et al. Dandy-Walker syndrome: analysis of 21 cases. *Dev Med Child Neurol* 1980;22:189–201.

653. Hirsh JF, et al. The Dandy-Walker malformation: a review of 40 cases. *J Neurosurg* 1984;61:515–522.

654. Cartwright MJ, Eisenberg MB, Page LK. Posterior fossa arachnoid cyst presenting with an isolated twelfth nerve paresis: case report and review of the literature. *Clin Neurol Neurosurg* 1991;93:69–72.

655. Maria BL, et al. Dandy-Walker syndrome revisited. *Pedatr Neurosci* 1987;13:45–51.

656. McLaurin RL, Crone KR. Dandy-Walker malformation. In: Wilkins RH, Rengachary SS, eds. *Neurosurgery*, 2nd ed. New York: McGraw-Hill, 1996:3669–3672.

657. Curless RG, et al. Magnetic resonance demonstration of intracranial CSF flow in children. *Neurology* 1992;42:377–381.

658. Gilles FH, Shillito J. Infantile hydrocephalus: retrocerebellar subdural hematoma. *J Pediatr* 1970;76: 529–537.

659. Gandy SE, Heier LA. Clinical and magnetic resonance features of primary intracranial arachnoid cysts. *Ann Neurol* 1987;21:342–348.

660. Rosman NP, Shands KN. Hydrocephalus caused by increased intracranial venous pressure: a clinicopathological study. *Ann Neurol* 1978;3:445–450.

661. Beck DJK, Russell DS. Experiments on thrombosis of the superior longitudinal sinus. *J Neurosurg* 1946;3:337–347.

662. Gordon N. Normal pressure hydrocephalus and arrested hydrocephalus. *Dev Med Child Neurol* 1977; 19:540–543.

663. Hakim S, et al. The physics of the cranial cavity, hydrocephalus and normal pressure hydrocephalus: mechanical interpretation and mathematical model. *Surg Neurol* 1976;5:187–210.

664. Mori K, Mima T. To what extent has the pathophysiology of normal pressure hydrocephalus been clarified? *Crit Rev Neurosurg* 1998;8:232–243.

665. Bret P, Chazal J. Chronic ("normal pressure") hydrocephalus in childhoodand adolescence: a review of 16 cases and reappraisal of the syndrome. *Childs Nerv Syst* 1995;11:687–691.

666. Milhorat TH. Hydrocephalus and the cerebrospinal fluid. Baltimore: Williams & Wilkins, 1972:137, 170.

667. Rogers M, Kaplan AM, Ben-Ora A. Fetal hydrocephalus. Use of ultrasound in diagnosis and management. *Perinatol Neonatol* 1980;4(6):31–34.

668. Johnson ML, et al. Fetal hydrocephalus: diagnosis and management. *Semin Perinatol* 1983;7:83–89.

669. Renier D, et al. Prenatal hydrocephalus: outcome and prognosis. *Child's Nerv Syst* 1988;4:213–222.

670. Glick PL, et al. Management of ventriculomegaly in the fetus. *J Pediatr* 1984;105:97–105.

671. Laurence KM. The pathology of hydrocephalus. *Ann Roy Coll Surg Engl* 1959;24:388–401.

672. Rubin RC. The effect of the severe hydrocephalus on size and number of brain cells. *Dev Med Child Neurol* 1972;27[Suppl]:117–120.

673. Tomasovic JA, Nellhaus G, Moe PG. The Bobble-head doll syndrome: an early sign of hydrocephalus. Two new cases and review of the literature. *Dev Med Child Neurol* 1975;17:777–783.

674. Hier DB, Wiehl AC. Chronic hydrocephalus associated with short stature and growth hormone deficiency: case report. Ann Neurol 1977;2:246–248.

675. Kim CS, Bennett DR, Roberts TS. Primary amenorrhea secondary to noncommunicating hydrocephalus. Neurology 1969;19:533–535.

676. Fiedler R, Krieger DT. Endocrine disturbances in patients with congenital aqueductal stenosis. Acta Endocrinol 1975;80:1–13.

677. Miller E, Sethi L. The effect of hydrocephalus on perception. Dev Med Child Neurol 1971;25[Suppl]:77–81.

678. Hagberg B, Sjörgen I. The chronic brain syndrome of infantile hydrocephalus: a follow-up study of 63 spontaneously arrested cases. Am J Dis Child 1966;112:189–196.

679. Sher PK, Brown SB. A longitudinal study of head growth in preterm infants. I. Normal rates of head growth. Dev Med Child Neurol 1975;17:705–710.

680. Fujimura M, Seryu J. Velocity of head growth during the perinatal period. Arch Dis Child 1977;52:105–112.

681. Fujimura M. Factors which influence the timing of maximum growth rate of the head in low birthweight infants. Arch Dis Child 1977;52:113–117.

682. Babson SG, Benda GI. Growth graphs for the clinical assessment of infants of varying gestational age. J Pediatr 1976;89:814–820.

683. Dodge PR, Porter P. Demonstration of intracranial pathology by transillumination. Arch Neurol 1961;5:594–605.

684. Horbar JD, et al. Ultrasound detection of changing ventricular size in posthemorrhagic hydrocephalus. Pediatrics 1980;66:674–678.

685. Afschrift M, et al. Ventricular taps in the neonate under ultrasonic guidance: technical note. J Neurosurg 1983;59:1100–1101.

686. Newman GC, et al. Dandy-Walker syndrome diagnosed in utero by ultrasonography. Neurology 1982;32:180–184.

687. Britton J, et al. MRI and hydrocephalus in childhood. Neuroradiology 1988;30:310–314.

688. Atlas SW, Mark AS, Fram EK. Aqueductal stenosis: evaluation with gradient-echo rapid MR imaging. Radiology 1988;169:449–453.

689. Barkovich AJ, Edwards MSB. Applications of neuroimaging in hydrocephalus. Pediatr Neurosurg 1992;18:65–83.

690. Nitz WR, et al. Flow dynamics of cerebrospinal fluid: assessment with phase-contrast velocity MR imaging performed with retrospective cardiac gating. Radiology 1992;183:395–405.

691. Ohara S, et al. MR imaging of CSF pulsatory flow and its relation to intracranial pressure. J Neurosurg 1988;69:675–682.

692. Schroth G, Klose U. Cerebrospinal fluid flow. III. Pathological cerebrospinal fluid pulsations. Neuroradiology 1992;35:16–24.

693. Quencer RM. Intracranial CSF flow in pediatric hydrocephalus: evaluation with cine-MR imaging. Am J Neuroradiol 1992;13:601–608.

694. Goumnerova LC, Frim DM. Treatment of hydrocephalus with third ventriculocisternostomy: outcome and CSF flow patterns. Pediatr Neurosurg 1997;27:149–152.

695. DiChiro G, Ashburn WL, Briner WH. Technetium Tc 99m serum albumin for cisternography. Arch Neurol 1968;19:218–227.

696. McCullough DC, et al. Prognostic criteria for cerebrospinal fluid shunting from isotope cisternography in communicating hydrocephalus. Neurology 1970;20:594–598.

697. McLone DG, Aronyk KE. An approach to the management of arrested and compensated hydrocephalus. Pedatr Neurosurg 1993;19:101–103.

698. Schain RJ. Carbonic anhydrase inhibitors in chronic infantile hydrocephalus. Am J Dis Child 1969;117:621–625.

699. Mealey J Jr, Barker DT. Failure of oral acetazolamide to advert hydrocephalus in infants with myelomeningocele. J Pediatr 1968;72:257–259.

700. Putnam TJ. Treatment of hydrocephalus by endoscopic coagulation of choroid plexuses: description of a new instrument and preliminary report of results. N Engl J Med 1934;210:1373–1376.

701. Cinalli G, et al. Failure of third ventriculostomy in the treatment of aqueductal stenosis in children. J Neurosurg 1999;90:448–454.

702. Matson DD. A new operation for the treatment of communicating hydrocephalus: report of a case secondary to generalized meningitis. J Neurosurg 1949;6:238–247.

703. Post EM. Shunt systems. In: Wilkins RH, Rengachary SS, eds. Neurosurgery, 2nd ed. New York: McGraw-Hill, 1996:3645–3653.

704. McLaurin RL. Ventricular shunts: complications and results. In: Section of Pediatric Neurosurgery, American Association of Neurological Surgeons, eds. Pediatric Neurosurgery. Surgery of the Developing Nervous System. 2nd ed. New York: Grune & Stratton, 1989:219–229.

705. Forslund M, Bjerre I, Jeppson JO. Cerebrospinal fluid protein in shunt-treated hydrocephalic children. Dev Med Child Neurol 1976;18:784–790.

706. Bayston R. Hydrocephalus shunt infections, London: Chapman and Hall, 1989.

707. Haines SJ, Walters BC. Antibiotic prophylaxis for cerebrospinal fluid shunts: a metanalysis. Neurosurgery 1994;34:87–92.

708. Meirovitch J, et al. Cerebrospinal fluid shunt infections in children. Pediatr Infect Dis J 1987;6:921–924.

709. Pople IK, Bayston R, Hayward RD. Infection of cerebrospinal fluid shunts in infants: a study of etiologic factors. J Neurosurg 1992;77:29–36.

710. Forward KR, Fewer HD, Stiver HG. Cerebrospinal fluid shunt infections: a review of 35 infections in 32 patients. J Neurosurg 1983;59:389–394.

711. Ronan A, Hogg GG, King GL. Cerebrospinal fluid shunt infections in children. Pediatr Infect Dis J 1995;14:782–786.

712. Vinchon M, et al. Cerebrospinal fluid eosinophilia in shunt infections. Neuropediatrics 1992;23:235–240.

713. Davidson RI. Peritoneal bypass in the treatment of hydrocephalus: historical review and abdominal complications. J Neurol Neurosurg Psychiatry 1976;39:640–646.

714. McComb JG. Comments. In: Abud-Dulu K, et al. Colonic complications of ventriculo-peritoneal shunts. Neurosurgery 1983;13:167–169.

715. Copeland GP, Foy PM, Shaw MD. The incidence of epilepsy after ventricular shunting operations. Surg Neurol 1982;17:279–281.

716. Laws ER, Niedermeyer E. EEG findings in hydrocephalic patients with shunt procedures. Electroenceph Clin Neurophysiol 1970;29:325.

716a. Baskin JJ, Manwaring KH. Rekate HL Ventricular shunt removal: the ultimate treatment of the slit ventricle syndrome *J Neurosurg* 1998;88:478–484.

717. Epstein FJ. Increased intracranial pressure in hydrocephalic children with functioning shunts: a complication of shunt dependency. *Concepts Pediatr Neurosurg* 1983;4:119–130.

718. Rekate HL. Classification of slit-ventricle syndromes using intracranial pressure monitoring. *Pediatr Neurosurg* 1993;19:15–20.

719. Saukkonen A, et al. Electroencephalographic findings and epilepsy in the slit ventricle syndrome of shunt treated hydrocephalic children. *Child's Nerv Syst* 1988;4:344–347.

720. Laurence KM, Coates S. Natural history of hydrocephalus: detailed analysis of 182 unoperated cases. *Arch Dis Child* 1962;37:345–362.

721. Laurence KM. Neurologic and intellectual sequelae of hydrocephalus. *Arch Neurol* 1969;20:73–81.

722. Riva D, et al. Intelligence outcome in children with shunted hydrocephalus. *Child's Nerv Syst* 1994;10: 70–73.

723. Hirsch JF. Consensus: long-term outcome in hydrocephalus. *Child's Nerv Syst* 1994;10:64–69.

724. Hemmer R, Böhm B. Once a shunt, always a shunt. *Dev Med Child Neurol* 1976;18[Suppl]:69–73.

725. Hayden PW, Shurtleff DB, Stuntz TJ. A longitudinal study of shunt function in 360 patients with hydrocephalus. *Dev Med Child Neurol* 1983;25:334–337.

726. Lorber J, Pucholt V. When is a shunt no longer necessary? An investigation of 300 patients with hydrocephalus and myelomeningocele: 11–22-year follow-up. *Z Kinderchir* 1981;34:327–329.

727. Lindenberg R, Swanson PD. "Infantile hydrancephaly." A report of five cases of infarction of both cerebral hemispheres in infancy. *Brain* 1967;90:839–850.

728. Fowler M, et al. Congenital hydrocephalus-hydrancephaly in five siblings with autopsy studies: a new disease. *Dev Med Child Neurol* 1972;14:173–188.

729. McElfresh AE, Arey JB. Generalized cytomegalic inclusion disease. *J Pediatr* 1957 51:146–156.

730. Myers RE. Brain pathology following fetal vascular occlusion: an experimental study. *Invest Ophthalmol* 1969;8:41–50.

731. Hockey A. Proliferative vasculopathy and an hydrancephalic-hydrocephalic syndrome: a neuropathological study of two siblings. *Dev Med Child Neurol* 1983; 25:232–239.

732. Lott IT, McPherson DL, Starr A. Cerebral cortical contributions to sensory evoked potentials: hydranencephaly. *Electroenceph Clin Neurophysiol* 1986;64: 218–223.

733. Hoffman J, Liss L. "Hydranencephaly." A case report with autopsy findings in a 7-year-old girl. *Acta Paediatr Scand* 1969;58:297–300.

734. Wang PJ, et al. Intracranial arachnoid cysts in children: related signs and associated anomalies. *Pediatr Neurol* 1998;19:100–104

735. Robertson SJ, Wolpert SM, Runge VM. MR imaging of middle cranial fossa arachnoid cysts: temporal lobe agenesis syndrome revisited. *Am J Neuroradiol* 1989;10:1007–1010.

736. Flodmark O. Neuroradiology of selected disorders of the meninges, calvarium and venous sinuses. *Am J Neuroradiol* 1992;13:483–491.

737. Aithala GJ, et al. Spinal arachnoid cyst with weakness in the limbs and abdominal pain. *Pediatr Neurol* 1999;20:155–156.

738. Rabb CH, et al. Spinal arachnoid cysts in the pediatric age group: an association with neural tube defects. *J Neurosurg* 1992;77:369–372,

739. Sato K, et al. Middle fossa arachnoid cyst: clinical, neuroradiological and surgical features. *Child's Brain* 1983;10:301–316.

740. Horton WA. Molecular genetic basis of the human chondrodysplasias. *Endocrin Metab Clin N Amer* 1996;25:683–697.

741. Shohat M, et al. Hearing loss and temporal bone structure in achondroplasia. *Am J Med Genet* 1993;45: 548–551.

742. Dandy WE. Hydrocephalus in chondrodystrophy. *Bull Johns Hopkins Hosp* 1921;32:5–10.

743. Reid CS, et al. Cervicomedullary compression in young patients with achondroplasia: value of comprehensive neurologic and respiratory evaluation. *J Pediatr* 1987;110:522–530.

744. Yamada Y, et al. Surgical management of cervicomedullary compression in achondroplasia. *Child's Nerv Syst* 1996;12:737–741.

745. Lundar T, Bakke SJ, Nornes H. Hydrocephalus in an achondroplastic child treated by venous decompression at the jugular foramen: case report. *J Neurosurg* 1990;73:138–140.

746. Ryken TC, Menezes AH. Cervicomedullary compression in achondroplasia. *J Neurosurg* 1994;81:43–48.

747. Nelson FW, et al. Neurological basis of respiratory complications in achondroplasia. *Ann Neurol* 1988;24:89–93.

748. Pauli RM, et al. Prospective assessment of risks for cervicomedullary-junction compression in infants with achondroplasia. *Am J Hum Genet* 1995;56:732–744.

749. Landau K, Gloor BP. Therapy-resistant papilledema in achondroplasia. *J Neuro Opthalmol* 1994;14:24–28.

750. Hahn YS, et al. Paraplegia resulting from thoracolumbar stenosis in a 7-month-old achondroplastic dwarf. *Pediatr Neurosci* 1989;15:39–43.

751. Rogers JG, Perry MA, Rosenberg LA. I.Q. measurements in children with skeletal dysplasia. *Pediatrics* 1979;63:894–897.

752. Rimoin DL. Cervicomedullary junction compression in infants with achondroplasia: when to perform neurosurgical decompression. *Am J Hum Genet* 1995;56: 824–827.

753. Pauli RM. Surgical intervention in achondroplasia. *Am J Hum Genet* 1995;56:1501–1502.

754. Elster AD, et al. Cranial imaging in autosomal recessive osteopetrosis. Part II. Skull base and brain. *Radiology* 1992;183:137–144.

755. Lehman RAW, et al. Neurological complications of infantile osteopetrosis. *Ann Neurol* 1977;2:378–384.

756. Patel PJ, et al. Osteopetrosis: brain ultrasound and computed tomography findings. *Eur J Pediatr* 1992;151:827–828.

757. Thompson DA, et al. Early VEP and ERG evidence of visual dysfunction in autosomal recessive osteopetrosis. *Neuropediatrics* 1998; 29: 137–144.

758. Ohlsson A, et al. Carbonic anhydrase II deficiency syndrome: recessive osteopetrosis with renal tubular acidosis and cerebral calcification. *Pediatrics* 1986;77: 371–381.

759. Al Rajeh S, et al. The syndromes of osteopetrosis, renal acidosis and cerebral calcification in two sisters. *Neuropediatrics* 1988;19:162–165.

760. Rees H, et al. Association of infantile neuroaxonal dystrophy and osteopetrosis: a rare autosomal recessive disorder. *Pediatr Neurosurg* 1995;22:321–327.

761. Harlan GC. Congenital paralysis of both abducens and both facial neres. *Trans Am Ophth Soc* 1880;3: 216–218.

762. Chisholm JJ. Congenital Paralysis of the sixth and seventh pairs of cranial nerves in an adult. *Arch Opthalmol* 1882;11:323–325.

763. Möbius PJ. Uber angeborene doppelseitige Abducens-Facialis-Lähmung. *München Med Wschr* 1888;35: 91,108.

764. Möbius PJ. Ueber infantilen Kernschwund. *München Med Wschr* 1892;39:17, 41, 55.

765. Thakkar N, et al. Möbius syndrome due to brain stem tegmental necrosis. *Arch Neurol* 1977;34:124–126.

766. Singh B, et al. Möbius syndrome with basal ganglia calcification. *Acta Neurol Scand* 1992;85:436–438.

767. O'Neill F, et al. Möbius syndrome: evidence for a vascular etiology. *J Child Neurol* 1993;8:260–265.

768. Sarnat HB. Ischemic brainstem syndromes of the fetus and neonate. *Eur J Paediatr Neurol* 1999 (*in press*).

769. Richter RB. Unilateral congenital hypoplasia of the facial nucleus. *J Neuropathol Exp Neurol* 1960;19: 33–41.

770. Pitner SE, Edwards JE, McCormick WF. Observations of pathology of Möbius syndrome. *J Neurol Neurosurg Psychiatry* 1965;28:362–374.

771. Henderson JL. The congenital facial diplegia syndrome: clinical features, pathology and etiology—a review. *Brain* 1939;62:381–403.

772. Meyerson MD, Foushee DR. Speech, language and hearing in Möbius syndrome. *Dev Med Child Neurol* 1978;20:357–365.

773. Sudarshan A, Goldie WD. The spectrum of congenital facial diplegia (Möbius syndrome). *Pediatr Neurol* 1985;1:180–185.

774. Konigsmark BW. Hereditary deafness in man. *N Engl J Med* 1969;281:713–720, 774–778, 827–832.

775. Steele MW. Genetics of congenital deafness. *Pediatr Clin North Am* 1981;28:973–980.

776. Das VK. Aetiology of bilateral sensorineural hearing impairment in children: a 10 year study. *Arch Dis Child* 1996;74:8–12.

777. Cohn ES, et al. Clinical studies of families with hearing loss attributable to mutations in the connexin 26gene (GJB2/DFNB1). *Pediatrics* 1999;103:546–550.

778. Waardenburg PJ. A new syndrome combining developmental anomalies of the eyelids, eyebrows and nose root with pigmentary defects of the iris and head hair and with congenital deafness. *Am J Hum Genet* 1951;3:195–253.

779. Baldwin CT, et al. An exonic mutation in the HuP2 paired domain gene causes Waardenburg's syndrome. *Nature* 1992;355:637–638.

780. DeStefano AL, et al. Correlation between Waardenburg syndrome phenotype and genotype in a population of individuals with identified PAX3 mutations. *Hum Genet* 1998;102:499–506.

781. Mills RP, Calver DM. Retinitis pigmentosa and deafness. *J Roy Soc Med* 1987;80:17–20.

782. Worster-Drought C. Suprabulbar paresis. *Dev Med Child Neurol* 1974[Suppl 30].

783. Kuzniecky R, Andermann F, Guerrini R. The epileptic spectrum in the congenital bilateral perisylvian syndrome. CBPS Multicenter Collaborative Study. *Neurology* 1994;44:379–385.

784. Fraser GR. The causes of profound deafness in childhood. In: Worstenholme GE, Knight J, eds. *Sensorineural hearing loss. A CIBA Foundation Symposium.* London: J. & A. Churchill, 1970:5–40.

785. Parker N. Congenital deafness due to a sex-linked recessive gene. *Ann Hum Genet* 1958;10:196–200.

786. Jervell A, Lange-Nielsen F. Congenital deaf-mutism, functional heart disease with prolongation of the -Q-T interval and sudden death. *Am Heart J* 1957; 54:59–68.

787. Wildervanck LS. Hereditary malformations of the ear in three generations. Marginal pits, preauricular appendages, malformations of the auricle and conductive deafness. *Acta Otolaryngol* 1962;54:553–560.

788. Falls HF, Kruse WT, Cotterman CW. Three cases of Marcus Gunn phenomenon in two generations. *Am J Ophthalmol* 1949;32(Part 2):53–59.

789. Duane A. Congenital deficiency of abduction, associated with impairment of abduction retraction movements, contractions of the palpebral fissure and oblique movements of the eye. *Arch Ophthalmol* 1905; 34:133–159.

790. Margalith D, et al. Clinical spectrum of congenital optic nerve hypoplasia: review of 51 patients. *Dev Med Child Neurol* 1984;26:311–322.

791. Skarf B, Hoyt CS. Optic nerve hypoplasia in children: association with anomalies of the endocrine and CNS. *Arch Ophthalmol* 1984;102:62–67.

792. Dickinson JT, Srisomboon P, Kamerer DB. Congenital anomaly of the facial nerve. *Arch Otolaryngol* 1968;88:357–359.

793. Nelson KB, Eng GD. Congenital hypoplasia of the depressor anguli oris muscle: differentiation from congenital facial palsy. *J Pediatr* 1972;81:16–20.

794. Pagon RA, et al. Coloboma, congenital heart disease, and choanal atresia with multiple anomalies: CHARGE association. *J Pediatr* 1981;99:223–227.

Chapter 5

Perinatal Asphyxia and Trauma

John H. Menkes and *Harvey B. Sarnat

*Departments of Neurology and Pediatrics, University of California, Los Angeles, UCLA School
of Medicine, and Department of Pediatric Neurology, Cedars-Sinai
Medical Center, Los Angeles, California 90048; and *Departments of Pediatric Neurology and
Neuropathology, University of Washington School of Medicine, and Children's Hospital and Regional
Medical Center, Seattle, Washington 98105*

"The name 'cerebral palsy' is thus nothing other than an invented word, the product of our nosographic classification, a label which we attach to a group of clinical cases: it should not be defined, rather it should be explained by reference to these clinical cases."

Sigmund Freud, *Infantile Cerebral Palsy*, Alfred Hoelder, Vienna 1897, p. 3.

Although more than 100 years have elapsed since the publication of Little's classic paper linking abnormal parturition, difficult labor, premature birth, and asphyxia neonatorum with a "spastic rigidity of the limbs" (1), the pathogenesis of cerebral birth injuries is far from completely understood. This is not because of lack of interest. The evolution and ultimate neurologic picture of cerebral palsy (i.e., the various syndromes of a persistent but not necessarily unchanging disorder of movement and posture resulting from a nonprogressive lesion of the brain acquired during development) have been recorded in innumerable papers. These include Little's 1843 paper on spastic diplegia and Cazauvielh's 1827 monograph on congenital hemiplegia (2), both also containing descriptions of childhood dyskinesia.

Investigations into the causes of cerebral palsy have taken various approaches. Prospective and retrospective studies have attempted to link the various neurologic abnor-malities to specific disorders of gestation or the perinatal period. Pathologic studies of the brain have produced careful descriptions of various cerebral abnormalities in patients with nonprogressive neurologic disorders and have led to attempts, often highly speculative, to formulate their causes. A third line of investigation has been to induce perinatal injuries in experimental animals and to correlate the subsequent pathologic and clinical pictures with those observed in children. These approaches have been supplemented by neuroimaging studies conducted during the perinatal period and in later life. Images have been correlated with neurologic or developmental outcome or with the pathologic examination of the brain.

The various investigations have demonstrated that a given clinical neurologic deficit can be caused by a cerebral malformation of gestational origin, by destructive processes of antenatal, perinatal, or early postnatal onset affecting a previously healthy brain, or by the various processes acting in concert. Developmental anomalies are discussed in Chapter 4 and intrauterine infections in Chapter 6. This chapter considers perinatal trauma, perinatal asphyxia, and the neurologic complications of prematurity.

The reader is referred to the excellent texts by Friede (3) on developmental neuropathology, by Rorke (4) on perinatal injuries, and by Volpe (5) on neonatal neurology. Additionally, the proceedings of a 1986 conference on perinatal events and brain damage are of considerable interest in that they provide the reader with a European point of view (6).

CRANIOCEREBRAL TRAUMA

Mechanical trauma to the central or peripheral nervous system is probably the insult that is understood best. Trauma to the fetal head can produce extracerebral lesions, notably molding of the head, caput succedaneum, subgaleal hemorrhage, and cephalhematoma.

The fetal head is often asymmetric owing to intrauterine or intravaginal pressure. The sutures override one another, the fontanelles are small or obliterated, and the tissues overlying the skull can be soft because of caput succedaneum. A caput usually appears at the vertex and is commonly accompanied by marked molding of the head. The hemorrhage and edema are situated between the skin and the aponeurosis. When the hemorrhage is beneath the aponeurosis, it is termed a *subgaleal hemorrhage*. As it does in a caput, blood crosses suture lines, but bleeding can continue after birth, and at times the blood loss is quite extensive.

Cephalhematoma and Subgaleal Hematoma

Cephalhematoma is a usually benign hemorrhage between the periosteum of the skull (pericranium) and the calvarium. It results from direct physical trauma or from the differential between intrauterine and extrauterine pressure. Vaginal delivery is not necessarily a prerequisite for its occurrence; it has been encountered in infants born by cesarean section. Neonatal cephalhematoma occurs in from 1.5% to 2.5% of deliveries. Approximately 15% occur bilaterally. A linear skull fracture is seen in 5% of unilateral and in 18% of bilateral cephalhematoma (7). A depressed skull fracture may underlie a minority of cephalhematomas and cannot be detected with certainty by palpation on physical examination, so that skull radiography may be indicated in infants with cephalhematoma and neurologic symptoms or signs. Routine ultrasound examination does not detect this lesion. Less commonly, a hematoma lies between the galea of the scalp and the periosteum. The subperiosteal hematoma is sharply delineated by the suture lines,

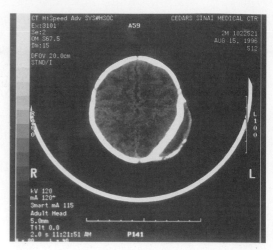

FIG. 5.1. Calcified cephalhematoma. (Courtesy of Dr. Franklin G. Moser, Division of Neuroradiology, Cedars-Sinai Medical Center, Los Angeles.)

whereas the subgaleal hematoma is not so limited and, therefore, is more diffuse. The hematoma is usually absorbed within 34 weeks, and aspiration, which can allow the introduction of infection, is contraindicated. On rare occasions, the scalp swelling is caused, not by a hematoma, but by cerebrospinal fluid (CSF) that leaked from the subarachnoid compartment via a dural tear and a skull fracture. Swelling from CSF does not usually disappear in 4 weeks, and diagnosis by aspiration becomes necessary, followed by operative repair, to avoid a *growing fracture*. Although occasionally a subperiosteal hematoma calcifies (Fig. 5.1), it should cause little concern, because calcium deposits are usually reabsorbed before the end of the first year, leaving no residual asymmetry.

Management of a cephalhematoma is fundamentally nonoperative. Underlying skull fractures do not create a management problem and need no specific therapy unless a significant depression of bone fragments occurs.

Large cephalhematomas can result in anemia or, more often, in hyperbilirubinemia owing to absorption of hemoglobin breakdown products (8). With the advent of the vacuum extractors, there has been an increased occurrence of subgaleal hematomas. In the experience of Chadwick and his group, 89% of neonates who had experienced a subgaleal hematoma had a vacuum extractor applied to their head at some time in the course of delivery (8a). Intracranial hemorrhage, skull fracture, and cerebral edema can complicate a subgaleal hematoma, as can hypovolemia, coagulopathy and jaundice, the latter consequences of extensive blood loss (9).

Skull Fractures

The skull of the newborn is poorly mineralized and extremely pliable. These factors permit considerable distortion of the head without injury to the skull itself. Nevertheless, a variety of skull fractures can be seen in the newborn. These can be incurred in utero, during labor, or secondary to the application of forceps.

The most common fracture is linear and is localized to the parietal or frontal regions. When no displacement is present, the fracture should heal spontaneously, and no treatment is indicated.

A depressed skull fracture can result from pressure of the head against the pelvis. Also, incorrect application of the obstetric forceps is often held responsible for the small, *ping-pong ball* depression.

Traumatic Intracranial Hemorrhage

Mechanical trauma to the infant's brain during delivery can induce lacerations in the tentorium or cerebral falx with subsequent subdural hemorrhage. With improved obstetric techniques, these injuries have become relatively uncommon, generally occurring only in large full-term infants delivered through an inadequate birth canal. In the series of Gröntoft published in 1953 (10), two-thirds of infants with tentorial lacerations weighed more than 4,500 g. Similar lesions can be seen in the premature infant (11).

Compression of the head along its occipitofrontal diameter, resulting in vertical molding, can occur with vertex presentations, whereas compression of the skull between the vault and the base, resulting in an anteroposterior elongation, is likely to be the outcome of face and brow presentations. Tears of the falx and tentorium can be caused by both forms of overstretch. In particular, the use of vacuum extraction can produce vertical stress on the cranium, with tentorial tears (12). Such hemorrhages are extremely common; in the series of Avrahami and colleagues pub-

lished in 1993, they could be demonstrated by computed tomography (CT) in everyone of ten infants delivered by vacuum extraction (13). Most of these are minor and inconsequential. In stretch injuries, damage usually occurs where the falx joins the anterior edge of the tentorium and the hemorrhage is usually infratentorial. Tears and thromboses of the dural sinuses and of the larger cerebral veins, including the vein of Galen, are accompanied commonly by subdural hemorrhages. These can be major and potentially fatal, or minor and clinically unrecognizable. The hemorrhages are mainly localized to the base of the brain; when the tears extend to involve the straight sinus and the vein of Galen, hemorrhages expand into the posterior fossa. The latter are poorly tolerated and can be rapidly fatal (14). Rarely, they can develop *in utero*, the consequence of motor vehicle accidents or other nonpenetrating trauma. *In utero* intracranial hemorrhage caused by unknown causes has been seen in infants born to Pacific Island mothers (15).

Overriding of the parietal bones occasionally produces a laceration of the superior sagittal sinus and a major fatal hemorrhage. Tearing of the superficial cerebral veins is probably relatively common. The subsequent hemorrhage results in a thin layer of blood over the cerebral convexity. Bleeding is often unilateral and usually is accompanied by a subarachnoid hemorrhage. This form of hemorrhage usually results in minimal or no clinical signs. Because the superficial cerebral veins of the premature infant are still underdeveloped, this hemorrhage is limited to full-term infants (16).

Subdural hemorrhage within the posterior fossa is being increasingly recognized by neuroimaging studies. The hemorrhage can be the result of a tentorial laceration or a traumatic separation of the cartilagenous joint between the squamous and lateral portions of the occiput in the course of delivery (11). Symptoms typically appear after a lag period of 12 hours to 4 days (17). They are relatively nonspecific and differ little from those seen with intracranial hemorrhage or hypoxic-ischemic encephalopathy (HIE). They include decreased responsiveness, apnea, bradycardia, opisthotonus, and seizures (18). As the subdural hematoma enlarges, the fourth ventricle is displaced forward and soon becomes obstructed, producing signs of increased intracranial pressure. Posterior fossa hemorrhage can be accompanied by intraventricular hemorrhage (IVH) or an intracerebellar hematoma (19). An intracerebral hemorrhage is a less common result of craniocerebral trauma. It is usually seen in conjunction with a major subdural or epidural hemorrhage (5).

Gross traumatic lesions to the brainstem are uncommon. Like spinal cord injuries, they are most likely to occur in the course of breech deliveries. Injury results from traction on the fetal neck during labor or delivery, with the force of excessive flexion, hyperextension, or torsion of the spine being transmitted upward. A compression injury can ensue, with the medulla being drawn into the foramen magnum. Other instances involve laceration of the cerebellar peduncles accompanied by local brainstem hemorrhage. Generally, death occurs during the course of labor or soon after birth as a consequence of damage to the vital medullary centers (20).

Spinal cord injuries are discussed in the section dealing with perinatal injuries to the spinal cord.

PERINATAL ASPHYXIA

Although in the past mechanical damage to the brain contributed significantly to mortality during the neonatal period and to subsequent persistent neurologic deficits, mortality and neurologic deficits are now more commonly the consequences of developmental anomalies and asphyxia, acting singly or in concert. Many definitions exist for the term *perinatal*. In the context of this chapter, we restrict it to the period extending from the onset of labor to the end of the first week of postnatal life.

No generally accepted definition exists for *asphyxia* (21). It can be inferred on the basis of indirect clinical markers: depressed Apgar scores, cord blood acidosis, or clinical signs in the neonate caused by HIE. From the physiologic viewpoint, asphyxia is a condition in which the brain is subjected not only to hypoxia, but also to ischemia and hypercarbia, which, in turn, can lead to cerebral edema and various circulatory disturbances (5). The incidence of postasphyxial encephalopathy in Leicester, England, from 1980 to 1984 was 6 in 1,000 full-term infants, with 1 in

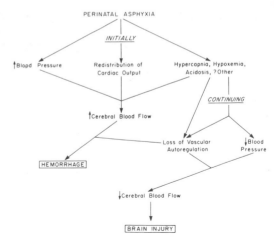

FIG. 5.2. Interrelationships between perinatal asphyxia, alterations in cerebral blood flow, and brain damage. In addition to the mechanisms depicted, acidosis can induce focal or generalized cerebral edema, which reduces cerebral blood flow. (From Volpe JJ. *Neurology of the newborn*, 3rd ed. Philadelphia: Saunders, 1995. With permission.)

1,000 infants dying or experiencing severe neurologic deficits as a consequence of the asphyxial insult (22,23). Asphyxia can occur at one or more times during intrauterine and extrauterine life. In the large series of asphyxiated infants studied by Brown and associates, the insult was believed to have occurred primarily antepartum in 51%, intrapartum in 40%, and postpartum in 9% (24). Low and coworkers who studied autopsies on perinatal deaths, found the insult to be antepartum in 10%, antepartum and intrapartum in 40%, intrapartum in 16%, and in the neonatal period in 34% (25). Comparable figures are presented by Volpe (5).

Pathogenesis

There are two facets to the pathogenesis of asphyxial brain damage: the pathophysiologic changes ensuing from asphyxia, and the mechanisms of hypoxic-ischemic cell damage and death within the central nervous system (CNS). The two aspects have been reviewed extensively (26–29).

Alterations in cerebral blood flow induced by asphyxia are of primary importance in understanding the genesis of birth injuries (Fig. 5.2). Following the onset of asphyxia, cardiac output is redistributed so that a large proportion enters the brain. This results in a 30% to 175% increase in cerebral blood flow. The increase in cerebral blood flow is induced locally by a reduction in cerebrovascular resistance, and systemically by hypertension. The severity and the speed of onset of the asphyxial insult determine the cerebrovascular response (30). When asphyxia is severe and develops rapidly, cerebral blood flow decreases rather than increases, probably due to by increased cerebrovascular resistance. When the hypoxic-ischemic insult is prolonged, these homeostatic mechanisms fail, cardiac output decreases, and systemic hypotension develops with reduced cerebral blood flow (31) (see Fig. 5.2).

Normal brain vasculature can compensate for the decreased cerebral perfusion by rapid dilation of the smaller vessels, so that cerebral blood flow is maintained relatively constant as long as blood pressure is kept within the normal range. The constancy of cerebral blood flow in the face of fluctuations in systemic blood pressure is termed *autoregulation*. The large cerebral blood vessels are believed to be more important for cerebral autoregulation in the neonate than the arterioles, with the response to changes in blood pressure being endothelium-dependent (32). A number of chemicals have been implicated in the control of cerebral arterial tone (33). Nitric oxide, by acting on the calcium-activated potassium channel of vascular endothelium, induces vascular dilatation. Endothelin-1 and prostanoids mediate vasoconstriction (32). Hypoxia, hypercarbia, and hypoglycemia all impair cerebral autoregulation. When autoregulation becomes defective as a result of hypoxia, cerebral arterioles fail to respond to changes in perfusion pressure and carbon dioxide concentrations, resulting in a pressure-passive cerebral blood flow. It is clear that in a clinical setting multiple factors can act in concert to cause cerebral vessels to become unresponsive to systemic blood pressure (34). Although in the preterm infant the lower limits of autoregulation are very close to the mean systemic arterial pressure, adequate cerebral perfusion can be maintained as long as the mean arterial blood pressure ranges between 24 and 39 mm Hg (35). When hypotension exceeds these lower limits, the preterm infant is unable to com-

pensate for the drop in blood pressure. With the arteriolar system unable to respond to decreased perfusion pressure by vasodilation, there is a striking reduction in cerebral blood flow (35).

Asphyxial brain injury is similar regardless whether the brain has incurred a global asphyxial insult as occurs in perinatal asphyxia, hypoperfusion as occurs after cardiac arrest (see Chapter 15), or focal ischemia as occurs after a vascular occlusion (see Chapter 12).

The mechanisms for brain damage in asphyxial brain injury are still not completely clear. Volpe, in reviewing the physiologic aspects of asphyxial injury, suggests that the loss of vascular autoregulation coupled with hypotension reduces cerebral blood flow to the point of producing tissue necrosis and subsequent cerebral edema (5). Combined clinical and imaging studies by Lupton and associates, in which intracranial pressure of asphyxiated term infants was correlated with their CT scan, corroborate Volpe's view that tissue necrosis precedes cerebral edema, rather than vice versa, with maximum abnormalities being seen between 36 and 72 hours after the insult (36). Nevertheless, it is still likely that tissue swelling can to some extent further restrict cerebral blood flow and cause secondary edema. The earliest phase of cerebral edema probably reflects a cytotoxic component, whereas a vasogenic component characterizes the edema that accompanies extensive tissue injury (37). In asphyxiated newborns, increased intracranial pressure after perinatal asphyxia is a relatively uncommon complication; in the series of Lupton and coworkers it was encountered in only 22% of asphyxiated infants (36).

Over the last few years increasing attention has been paid to the molecular and cellular aspects of cell death within the nervous system. Two distinct phases are recognized (38). The first phase occurs during the insult and the immediate period of reperfusion and reoxygenation. The second phase evolves after a period of some hours and extends for at least 72 hours. During the first phase, asphyxia rapidly results in the conversion of nicotinamide adenine dinucleotide (NAD) to reduced NADH. As the energy demands fail to be met, there is a shift from aerobic to anaerobic metabolism, causing acceleration of glycolysis and increased lactate production. In experimental animals, brain lactate increases within 3 minutes of induction of asphyxia (39). At the same time, the concentration of tricarboxylic acid cycle intermediates decreases, and the production of high-energy phosphates diminishes. These changes result in a rapid fall in phosphocreatine and a slower reduction in brain adenosine triphosphate concentrations. With reduction of adenosine triphosphate levels the various ion pumps, notably the Na^+-K^+ pump, the most important transporter for maintaining high intracellular concentrations of potassium and low intracellular concentrations of sodium, becomes inoperative. As ion pump function is lost, the neuronal membrane begins to change. Some neurons, such as the CA1 and the CA3 hippocampal neurons, hyperpolarize, whereas others, such as the dentate granule cells, depolarize. If anoxia persists, all cells undergo a rapid and marked depolarization with complete loss of membrane potential.

Decreases in intracellular and extracellular pH precede changes in membrane potential as hypoxia induces production of lactate and intracellular acidosis. The decrease in extracellular pH is believed to be the consequence of extrusion of intracellular hydrogen ions or intracellular lactate, or both. At the time when the neuronal membrane potential is abolished, there are a number of striking ionic changes. They include an influx into cells of sodium, chloride, and calcium and an efflux of potassium. Intracellular calcium rises, extracellular potassium increases markedly, and extracellular calcium, sodium, and chloride decrease. Notably, there is a massive increase in the extracellular concentration of glutamate a consequence of increased release of the neurotransmitter and impaired reuptake (40). The result is an excessive stimulation of the neuronal excitatory receptors. Several other mechanisms also have been implicated in the increase of excitatory amino acids. These have been reviewed by Martin and coworkers (41).

The aforementioned changes in lactate and high-energy phosphates can be documented in the asphyxiated infant by proton and ^{31}P magnetic resonance spectroscopy. These studies show an early increase in lactate (42). A decrease in phosphocreatine during the initial insult is reversed on resuscitation, but is followed by a slow secondary decline some 24 hours later. Intracellular pH and other indices of cellular energy status frequently remain normal for the first day of life (43,44).

Among the numerous factors responsible for asphyxial neuronal damage, excitotoxicity has received the most attention and is probably the most important. During hypoxia, the increase in extracellular glutamate results in overstimulation of glutamate receptors and cell death (45). How excitotoxins induce cell death is unclear. Rothman and Olney have proposed that prolonged neuronal depolarization induces both a rapid and a slowly evolving cell death (46,47). Rapid cell death is caused by an excessive influx of sodium through glutamate-gated ion channels. This leads to the entry of chloride into neurons. The increased intracellular chloride induces further cation influx to maintain electroneutrality, and the chloride and cation entry draws water into cells with ultimate osmotic lysis. Most important, calcium influx occurs. A sustained increase in intracellular calcium induces a "toxic cascade" whose end result is cell death by necrosis (28,48). The cascade includes the activation of a variety of catabolic enzymes, notably phospholipases, proteases, and endonucleases, with the consequent disruption of membrane phospholipids (48). Additionally, the activation of phospholipase A_2 and the release of polyunsaturated fatty acids, notably arachidonic acid, might stimulate tissue damage from the formation of free radicals (48). Calcium also activates nitric oxide synthase, and the increased formation of nitric oxide could contribute to cell death. A large number of strategies, aimed at blocking the postasphyxial events that lead to neuronal damage have been proposed, but at this point in time none have had any significant clinical application.

The second phase of asphyxial injury and cell death is marked by an inappropriate induction of apoptosis. Gluckman and coworkers believe that this stage can be recognized clinically by the appearance of postasphyxial seizures (38). The factors that promote postasphyxial apoptosis are under intense investigation. They are believed to include free radicals, increased expression and enhanced concentrations of inflammatory cytokines, and alterations in the concentrations or the response to endogenous growth factors (49). The observation that neurotropins, such as brain-derived neurotrophic factor, act as neuroprotectors after a hypoxic insult provides evidence for the importance of neurotropins in mediating postasphyxial brain injury (50). The activation of caspase, a key effector of apoptotic death, has been documented in animal models of perinatal asphyxia (51). Asphyxia also induces both rapid and delayed changes in the transcription of several genes, notably c-*fos*, c-*jun*, and some of the heat shock proteins (52–54). These substances are believed to have an important influence on the extent of apoptosis (53). Choi has proposed that a single insult might trigger both excitotoxic necrosis and apoptosis, with the severity and duration of the insult determining which death pathway predominates (48). The contributions of hypoglycemia, and intracellular acidosis, whether caused by accumulation of lactic acid or products of adenosine triphosphate (ATP) hydrolysis, to the extent and severity of asphyxial brain damage have still not been resolved (55).

With reoxygenation, cerebral perfusion rebounds. The role of postischemic impairment of microvascular perfusion (*no-reflow phenomenon*) and *luxury perfusion* in the genesis of tissue damage in the asphyxiated human neonate is still unclear (53).

A more extensive review of the role of excitotoxins in mediating hypoxic brain damage is beyond the scope of this text. The reader is referred to reviews by Monaghan and coworkers (56), Auer and Siesjö (57), and Choi and Rothman (58).

Pathology

Whatever the biochemical and physiologic mechanisms for brain damage, the relative resistance of the neonate's brain to hypoxia has been known for some time. Probably this phenomenon reflects a slower overall cerebral metabolism and smaller energy demands by the brain of the neonate compared with that of the adult. Total metabolism of the brain of a newborn mouse is approximately 10% that of the adult mouse's brain, and glycolysis also proceeds at a much slower rate (59). The cardiovascular system's relative resistance to hypoxic injury also can be operative.

The factors that determine the selective vulnerability of certain neuronal populations are still incompletely understood. In part, regional distribution of injury reflects the vascular supply to the brain, with the injury being maximal in the border zones between the major cerebral arteries. In addition, the topography of neuronal death is probably related to the density of excitatory receptors, with cells having a high density of glutamate receptors being the most vulnerable to asphyxia. Variations in the subunit composition of the receptor and changes in the expression of glutamate receptors with maturation may influence the sensitivity of neuronal to perinatal asphyxia. Thus, the increased expression of glutamate receptors in the globus pallidus during the perinatal period could be responsible for the susceptibility of this area to asphyxial damage (60). The striatal GABA-ergic medium-sized inhibitory neurons also are sensitive to asphyxia, whereas neurons containing the enzyme NAD diaphorase are resistant (61,62).

It is this combination of vascular and metabolic factors that results in the various distinct pathologic lesions that have been well described by classic pathologists over the course of the last century.

Multicystic Encephalomalacia

The neonatal brain responds to infarction differently than the mature brain. Rather than forming dense gliotic scars, pseudocysts are the usual long-term residual lesions. The reasons for the formation of cysts in the newborn brain are that areas of infarction tend to be relatively larger than in the adult because collateral circulation is less well developed and because the ability of neonatal brain to mobilize reactive gliosis is limited. The number of astrocytes per volume of neonatal brain is approximately one-sixth that of the adult brain in both gray and white matter, hence the response to injury is not nearly as effective, and the glial cells present are only able to form thin septa without neurons, compartmentalizing the empty space after macrophages have cleared away the necrotic tissue. These glial septa create the multiple pseudocysts of multicystic encephalomalacia. They are pseudocysts rather than true cysts because they are not lined by an epithelium, as are ependymal cysts. Multicystic encephalomalacia is therefore the end result of extensive cerebral infarcts.

When the primate fetus is subjected to acute total asphyxia, a reproducible pattern of brain disorders ensues (63,64). This pattern includes bilaterally symmetric lesions in the thalamus and in a number of brainstem nuclei, notably the nuclei of the inferior colliculi, superior olive, and lateral lemniscus. The neurons of the cerebral cortex, particularly the hippocampus, are especially vulnerable, as are the Purkinje cells of the cerebellum (4,65).

Soon after the initial insult, the first changes observed using electron microscopy are in the neuronal mitochondria, the internal structure of which becomes swollen and disrupted (66). Gradual widespread transneuronal degeneration follows. With progressively longer periods of total asphyxia, the destructive changes in the thalamus become more extensive, and damage begins to appear in the putamen and in the deeper layers of the cortex. In its extreme form, asphyxiated animals show an extensive cystic degeneration of both cortex and white matter. Connective tissue replaces the damaged areas in the forebrain, but a relative lack of cellular reaction occurs in the central nuclear areas (64).

This experimentally produced picture resembles cystic encephalomalacia (central porencephaly, cystic degeneration) of the human brain, a condition characterized by the formation of cystic cavities in white matter (Fig. 5.3). When small, the cysts are trabeculated and do not communicate with the ventricular system. In their most extensive form they can involve both hemispheres, leaving only small remnants of cortical tissue. The cavities are generally believed to be the products of insufficient glial reaction, perhaps the result of cerebral immaturity, or to reflect the sudden and massive tissue damage caused by the aforementioned circulatory or anoxic events. Lyen and associates have suggested that, in some instances, fetal viral encephalitis can induce a similar pathologic picture (67). The relationship of cystic degeneration to neonatal asphyxia was already established by Little (1), and infants surviving

this type of insult usually develop a severe form of spastic quadriparesis.

The pathologic differentiation between cystic degeneration and hydranencephaly is discussed in Chapter 4.

Periventricular Leukomalacia

The distribution of cerebral lesions induced by acute total asphyxia rarely reproduces the distribution of lesions found in infants who have survived partial but prolonged asphyxia. When prolonged partial asphyxia is induced experimentally, primates develop high carbon dioxide partial pressure (pCO_2) levels and mixed metabolic and respiratory acidosis (64,68). These are usually accompanied by marked brain swelling, which compresses the small blood vessels of the cerebral parenchyma. The resultant increase in vascular resistance superimposed on the systemic alterations leads to various focal cerebral circulatory lesions whose location is governed in part by vascular patterns and in part by the gestational age of the fetus at the time of the asphyxial insult (69,70).

One lesion that occurs with particular frequency in the premature infant is periventricular leukomalacia (PVL) (Figs. 5.4 and 5.5). First delineated by Banker and Larroche (71), this condition consists of a bilateral, fairly symmetric necrosis having a periventricular distribution. The two most common sites are at the level of the occipital radiation and in the white matter around the foramen of Monro (72,73). In addition, there can be diffuse cerebral white matter necrosis that usually spares the gyral cores (74). Preterm infants of 22 to 30 weeks' gestation tend to experience more widespread and confluent periventricular necrosis, whereas older premature infants exhibit more focal necrosis (75). Beta-amyloid precursor protein is deposited in axons around the zones of necrosis in PVL and in the neurons of the adjacent cerebral cortex (75).

The evolution of PVL has been studied by neuropathologic and neuroimaging methods. Within 6 to 12 hours of the suspected insult, coagulation necrosis occurs in the affected areas, accompanied by proliferation of astrocytes and microglia, loss of ependyma, and, in some cases,

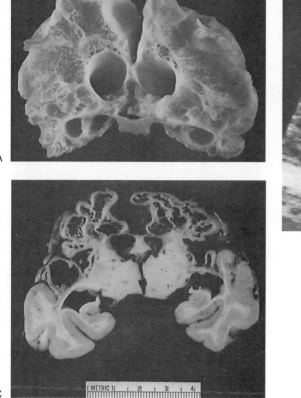

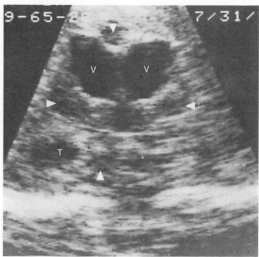

FIG. 5.3. Cystic encephalomalacia. **A:** Coronal section of the brain. The parenchyma of both hemispheres is replaced by a honeycomb of fine cavities. **B:** Coronal sonogram. Moderate ventriculomegaly and numerous poorly defined anechoic areas in periventricular parenchyma and in basal ganglia are visible (*arrowheads*). (V, lateral ventricles; T, temporal horn of lateral ventricle.) Ultrasonography was performed at 7 months of age, autopsy at 16 months. The infant had a history of seizures and profound developmental retardation. In this instance, the most likely cause for the condition appeared to have been a cytomegalovirus infection. **C:** Gross view of coronal section of the cerebral hemispheres in a case of extreme cystic encephalomalacia. The basal ganglia are mostly destroyed. The thalamus is pale and bilaterally sclerotic. The hippocampal formation, on the other hand, has a normal appearance, as does the adjacent temporal lobe cortex. This condition was the consequence of perinatal asphyxia. (**A** and **B**, from Stannard MW, Jimenez JF. Sonographic recognition of multiple cystic encephalomalacia. *AJNR Am J Neuroradiol* 1983;4:11. With permission. **C**, courtesy of Dr. Hideo H. Itabashi, Department of Pathology, Los Angeles County Harbor Medical

subcortical degeneration. Focal axonal disruption and death of oligodendroglia are some of the earliest signs of injury, with the developing oligodendroglia being especially vulnerable.

The pathogenesis of PVL remains uncertain and is most likely to be multifactorial. Four major factors are believed to be operative. The first is a failure in perfusion of the periventricular region. The distribution of PVL suggests inadequate circulatory perfusion and infarction of the vascular border zones "watershed areas" between the territories supplied by the ventriculopedal penetrating branches of the anterior, middle, and posterior cerebral arteries, and ventriculofugal arteries extending outward from striatal and choroidal branches (72,76). Nelson and colleagues, however, have questioned this widely accepted theory (77). They performed anatomic

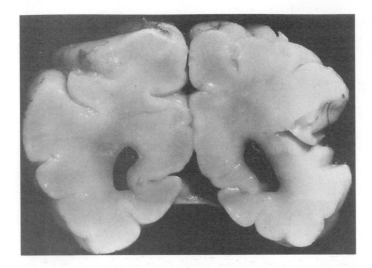

FIG. 5.4. Periventricular leukomalacia. Semicircular areas of malacia surround both lateral ventricles. (From Cooke RE. *The biologic basis of pediatric practice.* New York: McGraw-Hill, 1968. With permission.)

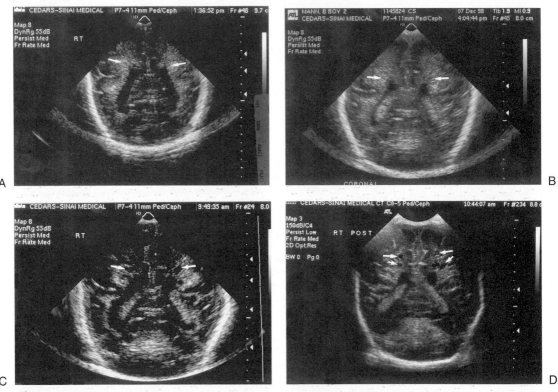

FIG. 5.5. Evolution of cystic periventricular encephalomalacia. Ultrasound, coronal views. **A:** At 4 days of age, there are focal echodense areas bilaterally in the periventricular white matter (*arrows*). **B:** At 9 days of age, the bilateral periventricular echogenicity is more clearly evident (*arrows*). **C:** At 23 days of age, early cystic changes are seen bilaterally in the periventricular region (*arrows*). These are more severe on the right. **D:** At 1 month of age, multiple periventricular cystic changes are seen (*arrows*). This boy was the 1,445-g product of a 30-week twin pregnancy. His neonatal course was complicated by recurrent apnea and bradycardia. A septic work-up was negative. Neurologic examination was unremarkable but for jerky movements of the extremities. At 5 months of age, this youngster has spastic diplegia most severe in the trunk and lower extremities. (Courtesy of Dr. Nancy Niparko, Cedars-Sinai Medical Center, Los Angeles.)

studies of the microvasculature of premature and term infants and were unable to find ventriculofugal arteries or the vascular border zone between ventriculofugal and ventriculopedal arteries previously described by de Reuck and colleagues (72) and Takashima and Tanaka (77).

A second factor in the pathogenesis of PVL is derived from the observation by Doppler ultrasound studies that cerebral vascular autoregulation is impaired in a substantial proportion of premature infants, with a propensity for pressure-passive circulation (78). Loss of autoregulation is particularly common in preterm infants who have experienced hypoxic ischemic events (78). Because even in healthy preterm infants white matter has an extremely low perfusion, the vulnerability of the periventricular watershed region to ischemia becomes readily explicable (34,79). Experimental work has demonstrated that hypotension induced by exsanguination or by administration of endotoxin results in reduced perfusion of periventricular white matter and occipital white matter. By contrast, these measures do not induce any significant reduction in blood flow to the cerebral cortex or to the deep gray matter nuclei (80). In substantiation of the clinical importance of impaired autoregulation in the induction of PVL, Volpe demonstrated that the subset of premature infants with pressure-passive cerebral circulation have an extremely high incidence of PVL (81).

A third factor in the pathogenesis of PVL pertains to the intrinsic vulnerability to excitatory neurotransmitters, such as glutamate, and to attack by free radicals of the early differentiating oligodendroglia (i.e., cells at a developmental stage before the acquisition of myelin) (82). This vulnerability may be the consequence of a lack of such antioxidant enzymes as catalase and glutathione peroxidase during a period when oligodendroglia undergo rapid iron acquisition (81,83).

Finally, an increasing amount of clinical and experimental evidence shows that cytokines play an important role in the induction of white matter damage. The administration of interferon-α2a to term infants as treatment for hemangiomas has resulted in spastic diplegia and delayed myelination. In some instances, diplegia did not resolve with discontinuation of cytokine therapy (84). Retrospective assays of neonatal blood have shown that pre-term and term children with spastic diplegia had higher blood levels of various cytokines, including interferon-α, interferon-γ, interleukin 6 (IL-6), IL-8, and tumor necrosis factor (TNF)–α, than did control children (85,86). In the study of Grether and colleagues, serum interferon levels were elevated in 78% of children with spastic diplegia, but only in 20% of children with hemiparesis, and in 42% of children who developed quadriparesis (86). It appears likely that cytokines such as interferon-α, interferon-γ, tumor necrosis factor-α, IL-6, or IL-8 might damage white matter by leading to hypotension, or by inducing ischemia through intravascular coagulation. Cytokines also could have a direct adverse effect on developing oligodendroglia or induce the product of other cytokines such as platelet-activating factor, which can further damage cells (87).

From a clinical point of view, spastic diplegia is the most common and most consistent sequel of PVL. It is nearly always bilateral although often asymmetric in severity. Because of the propensity of the periventricular necrotizing lesions to appear earliest and most prominently around the occipital horns of the lateral ventricles, optic radiation fibers may be involved and sometimes also result in cortical visual impairment.

A number of adverse perinatal events correlate with the development of PVL. Most important, PVL tends to occur in the larger premature infant, with the highest incidence by both neuropathologic and ultrasound criteria being between 27 and 30 weeks' gestational age (88,89) (Table 5.1). In the more recent French series of Baud and coworkers, published in 1999, the highest incidence (12.9%) was however seen in infants whose gestational age was 24 to 26 weeks (90). Other notable risk factors include prenatal factors such as premature, prolonged, or both premature and prolonged rupture of membranes, chorioamnionitis, and intrauterine infections (88,89,91). Several perinatal and postnatal factors also appear to be of importance. These include a low Apgar score, prolonged need for ventilatory assistance, hypercarbia, and recurrent episodes of apnea and bradycardia (92,93). In many instances, however, infants in whom PVL evolved have had a relatively benign postnatal course (89). Although systemic hypotension has been suggested as an important patho-

TABLE 5.1. *Incidence of periventricular leukomalacia according to gestational age*

Gestational age (weeks)	Ultrasound incidence of cystic periventricular leukomalacia (%)[a]
<27	7.2
27	12.93
28	15.7
29	10.5
30	12.4
31	6.5
32	4.3
Total	9.2

[a]The incidence of periventricular leukomalacia is calculated for infants surviving at least 7 days.

From Zupan V, et al. Periventricular leukomalacia: risk factors revisited. *Dev Med Child Neurol* 1996;38:1061. With permission.

genetic factor, several studies have failed to show an association between hypotension and PVL (94). In part, this lack of documentation reflects the lack of direct and continuous blood pressure recordings, or it might indicate that PVL results from a discrepancy between the metabolic requirements of periventricular white matter and its perfusion (95). We also should stress that in infants less than 31 weeks' gestation, relatively small reductions in systemic blood pressure (less than 30 mm Hg) for 1 hour or longer suffice to induce cerebral infarcts (96). This is particularly true in those whose autoregulation is defective or has been disrupted by asphyxia. As a rule, the less mature the periventricular vasculature, the less significant the clinical complications that accompany the evolution of PVL.

Several observational studies have reported that both maternal preeclampsia, and the prenatal administration of magnesium resulted in a lower incidence of spastic diplegia, and by inference of PVL in very-low-birth-weight infants (97–99). These observations could not be confirmed in a controlled, retrospective study (100), and randomized clinical trials will be necessary to determine the effectiveness of magnesium.

Newer imaging techniques such as ultrasonography and magnetic resonance imaging (MRI) permit the following of the evolution of PVL. In the series of infants autopsied by Iida and colleagues (74), the prenatal onset of PVL was observed in 20% of stillborn infants, and in 16.4% of infants who died by 3 days of age. These findings have

been confirmed by ultrasound studies showing the presence of cystic PVL as early as the third day of life (74,101). The evolution of PVL can be followed by ultrasonography. During the first week of life transient hyperechoic periventricular areas are frequent and probably represent a persistent germinal matrix (102). Persistent echogenic foci are pathologic, however. They too are seen during the first week of postnatal life. Within 1 to 3 weeks they are replaced with echolucent, cystic foci (cystic leukomalacia) (see Fig. 5.5C and D). As the intracystic fluid becomes resorbed, these cysts disappear and are replaced by gliosis (103). PVL can be accompanied by cystic lesions in the subcortical white matter and by delayed myelination (104). In some instances, gliosis becomes interspersed with areas of microcalcification (105). Calcification is more likely when lesions are not extensive. Periventricular echodensities can reflect several neuropathologic entities aside from PVL. They also are observed in hemorrhagic infarctions such as are seen in association with IVH and in ischemic edema (106).

PVL becomes hemorrhagic in up to 25% of infants (107), mostly a consequence of a hemorrhage into the ischemic area, the outcome of subsequent reperfusion (5).

Parasagittal Cerebral Injury

The most common site of brain damage in the term newborn is the cortex. Infarctions in this area are secondary to arterial or venous stasis and thromboses. One common pattern for the distribution of lesions, termed arterial "border zone" or "watershed lesions", usually results from a sudden decrease in systolic blood pressure and cerebral perfusion. Experimental studies have confirmed that the parasagittal cortex is the earliest and most severely damaged on prolonged asphyxia, with the amount of damage increasing geometrically with increasing duration of asphyxia (108). The lesions characteristically involve the territory supplied by the most peripheral branches of the three large cerebral arteries (Fig. 5.6) (109). Damage is maximal in the posterior parietal-occipital region, becoming less marked in the more anterior portions of the cortex. The lesions in the affected area can be located in the cortex or in the white matter. When gray matter is affected, damage usually

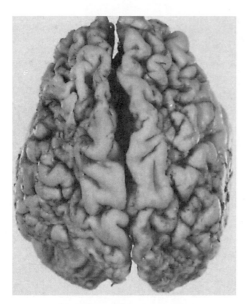

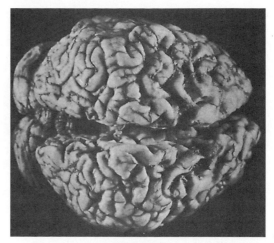

A

FIG. 5.6. Watershed pattern in a 10-year-old child with history of prolonged labor and spastic quadriparesis. Symmetric atrophy is seen in border zones of anterior, middle, and posterior cerebral arteries. (From Lindenberg R. Compression of brain arteries as pathogenetic factor for tissue necrosis and their areas of predilection. *J Neuropathol Exp Neurol* 1955;14:223. With permission.)

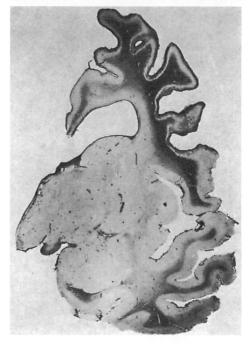

B

involves the portions around the depth of the sulci. In part, this distribution can reflect the effect of cerebral edema on the drainage of the cortical veins, and, in part, it can be the consequence of the impoverished vascular supply of this area in the healthy human newborn.

Ulegyria

Lesions involving damage to the deeper portions of gray matter have been termed *ulegyria* (mantle sclerosis, lobar sclerosis, nodular cortical sclerosis) (3). A common abnormality, ulegyria accounts for approximately one-third of clinical defects caused by circulatory disorders during the neonatal period (109). Its characteristic feature is the localized destruction of the lower parts of the wall of the convolution, with relative sparing of the crown. This produces a "mushroom" gyrus (Fig. 5.7). The margins of affected gray matter often contain abnormally dense aggregates of myelinated fibers, whereas adjacent white matter shows a considerable amount of myelin loss and

FIG. 5.7. A: Lobar sclerosis (ulegyria) in a 5-year-old child, mentally retarded and spastic since infancy. Sclerosis and distortion of the frontoparietal convolutions of the cerebrum are present. **B:** Coronal section of same brain showing shrunken and gliotic convolutions. The sulci are deepened and widened (Holzer's stain for myelin fibers). (From Towbin A. *The pathology of cerebral palsy.* Springfield, IL: Charles C Thomas, 1960. With permission.)

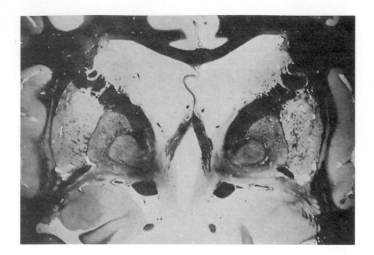

FIG. 5.8. Status marmoratus of basal ganglia. (From Merritt HH. *A textbook of neurology,* 6th ed. Philadelphia: Lea & Febiger, 1979. With permission.)

compensatory gliosis (110). Later on, coarse bundles of abnormally oriented, heavily myelinated fibers traverse the gliotic tissue, and the myelin sheaths enclose astrocytic processes as well as axons, similar to status marmoratus of the basal ganglia (111). Laminar necrosis of layer 3 often accompanies ulegyria.

Ulegyria can be extensive or so restricted that the gross appearance of the brain is normal. It most commonly occurs in major arterial watershed border zones, in a parasagittal distribution in the venous drainage territory of the superior sagittal sinus, or within the territory of a major cerebral artery with partial occlusion (112). The perisulcal topography of the necrosis is related to reduced perfusion as a consequence of impaired sulcal venous drainage, resulting from the compression of the stems of veins that ascend between gyri that have become edematous from previous hypoxic episodes (113). When ulegyria is widespread, an associated cystic defect in the subcortical white matter (porencephalic cyst) and dilatation of the lateral ventricles often occur. The meninges overlying the affected area are thickened and the small arteries occasionally can show calcifications in the elastica. Less often, ulegyria involves the cerebellum.

Abnormalities of Basal Ganglia

Abnormalities within the basal ganglia are seen in the majority of patients subjected to perinatal asphyxia (84% in the series of Christensen and Melchior) (114). One common lesion seen in this area has been termed *status marmoratus.* This picture was described first by Anton (115) in 1893, and later by the Vogts (116). Fundamentally, the pathologic picture is one of glial scarring corresponding to the areas of tissue destruction. It is characterized by a gross shrinkage of the striatum, particularly the globus pallidus, associated with defects in myelination. Although in some cases myelinated nerve fibers, probably of astrocytic origin (111), are found in coarse networks resembling the veining of marble (hence the name of the condition, status marmoratus) (Fig. 5.8), in other cases the principal pattern is one of a symmetric demyelination (status dysmyelinatus). Hypermyelination and demyelination probably represent different responses to the same insult. Hypermyelination probably results from oligodendrocytes becoming activated to produce excessive myelin and, lacking enough axons to ensheath, they envelop astrocytic processes. The number of nerve cells in the affected areas is usually conspicuously reduced, with the smaller neurons in the putamen and caudate nucleus appearing more vulnerable. Cystic changes within the basal ganglia were stressed by Denny-Brown but are rarely extensive (117). Although the abnormalities within the basal ganglia are often the most striking, a variety of associated cortical lesions can be detected in most instances.

It has been our experience, as well as that of others, that this condition is the result of an acute, severe hypoxic insult (118). As a rule, the asphyxia is not as prolonged as that which results in multicystic encephalomalacia, a condition in which there is also extensive damage to the cerebral cortex and white matter. The reason for the selective vulnerability of the basal ganglia to asphyxia is not fully understood. Given that these regions have a higher baseline oxygen consumption than other regions of the brain, as has been evidenced by positron emission tomography (PET) (119), other factors also must be operative to account for the particular vulnerability of the putamen and anterior thalamus (120). Experimental data have for a long time led one to suspect that the vulnerability of these regions is determined by the patterns of neurotransmitter receptors (60,121). In infants who suffer basal ganglia necrosis secondary to asphyxia, neuronal immunoreactivity to the various glutamate receptors was consistently decreased, with the areas of decreased immune reactivity corresponding to the damaged regions (122). These observations point to a primary role of glutamate excitotoxicity in basal ganglia neuronal damage, with the type of cell death induced by asphyxia (necrosis or apoptosis) being determined by the differential glutamate receptor phenotypes, neuronal maturity, and the severity and duration of asphyxia (123). Because astrocytes and oligodendroglia also express glutamate receptors, these cells may participate in basal ganglia injury (123). The importance of basal ganglia dopamine receptors in the expression and manifestations of asphyxial injury is still unclear (124).

The Myers model of "partial" versus "total" asphyxia, resulting in different sites of the principal lesions in neonatal monkeys, cannot be extrapolated to the human condition. This is because the monkey brain is more mature at birth, in terms not only of structure, synaptic organization, and myelination, but also in terms of better autoregulation of cerebral blood flow. In addition, the monkey brain is considerably smaller than the human brain, with a shorter distance for blood flow to reach terminal perfusion, and blood vessels are narrower than in the human neonate. Human cerebral arterioles do not acquire their muscular walls until near term, an anatomic prerequisite for autoregulatory function in cerebral blood flow, whereas the monkey already has mature cerebral vasculature for several weeks before birth.

Abnormalities of Cerebellum, Brainstem, and Pons

Occasionally, the major structural alterations resulting from perinatal injury are localized to the cerebellum. In the majority of instances, the involvement is diffuse, with widespread disappearance of the cellular elements of the cerebellar cortex, notably the Purkinje cells, and the dentate nucleus (3,125). As with the periventricular germinal matrix around the lateral ventricles, the external granular layer of the cerebellum is vulnerable to spontaneous hemorrhage, especially in preterm infants of young gestational age. However, in the vast majority of infants, selective cerebellar involvement is not the consequence of asphyxia (126).

In general, the human neonatal brainstem appears to be more resistant to ischemic and hypoxic insults than the cerebral cortex, but it is not invulnerable and sometimes lesions are more prominent in the brainstem than in supratentorial structures. The lesions are usually symmetric and involve both gray matter nuclei and adjacent white matter tracts, but the gray matter is more focally involved, perhaps because of its higher metabolic rate. Lesions may involve the inferior or superior colliculi almost selectively (3), or infarction may occur in the central core of the brainstem or selectively in the periaqueductal gray matter (3,112,127,128). Such multiple deep microinfarcts at times extend rostrally to involve deep supratentorial structures such as the thalamus and corpus striatum (129). Because of the microscopic size of many of the deep infarcts, particularly those of the brainstem, they are difficult to identify on neuroimaging.

Infarction in the nuclei of the brainstem and thalami, induced in experimental animals by total asphyxia of 10 to 25 minutes' duration, also can be seen in asphyxiated human infants with a history of acute profound asphyxial damage (130). Additionally, transient compression of the vertebral arteries in the course of rotation or hyperextension of the infant's head during delivery can be a cause for circulatory lesions of the brainstem (131,132).

One pattern of brainstem infarction is of particular importance because of its profound clinical implications. Bilateral symmetric or asymmetric infarcts of the pontine and medullary tegmentum may occur in midfetal to late fetal life and appear at birth as zones of necrosis surrounded by gliosis and calcification (133). This site is a watershed zone of the brainstem, between the territories of the segmental paramedian penetrating arteries and the long circumferential arteries. These vessels are branches of the basilar artery, hence vulnerable to even brief periods of systemic hypotension *in utero*. Should such lesions involve the abducens nucleus and the intramedullary loop of facial nerve around the abducens nucleus at the pontomedullary junction, an acquired form of Möbius syndrome may result. Tegmental infarcts often extend longitudinally in the pons and medulla to involve the tractus solitarius and nuclei solitarius and parasolitarius. The rostral fourth of these structures are gustatory in function, but the remainder is the neuroanatomic equivalent of the *pneumotaxic center* of neurophysiologists, and its involvement in ischemic lesions can result in loss of central respiratory drive, recurrent apnea, or neurogenic respiratory failure.

Pontosubicular Degeneration

Pontosubicular degeneration in isolation or accompanied by widespread cerebral damage has been described in premature and term infants (3,130,131). It is not a rare entity. It has been demonstrated in up to 59% of infants born before 38 weeks' gestation who died in the first month of postnatal life, suggesting it to be the most common cerebral lesion of preterm neonates, exceeding even germinal matrix hemorrhages (4,134–136).

The condition represents a unique topology of pathologic neuronal apoptosis in the fetal and neonatal brain, following hypoxia or ischemia. As its descriptive name implies, it selectively involves relay nuclei of the corticopontocerebel- lar pathway in the basis pontis and the subiculum, a transitional cortex between the three-layered hippocampus and the six-layered hippocampal gyrus. Although it may coexist with other hypoxic lesions in the cortex, thalamus, and cerebellum, these other regions are disproportionately less severely involved than the pontine nuclei and subiculum (112,134,137). Usually, there are no lesions in the tegmentum of the pons, although in rare instances symmetric microinfarcts have been described (133,138). Focal white matter infarcts also occur occasionally.

This distribution of infarcts is generally seen in infants older than 29 weeks' gestation, most commonly in infants of 32 to 36 weeks' gestation. The pattern can also occur in term infants and has occasionally been encountered in adult brains (139). The reason that pontosubicular degeneration is not better recognized by clinicians is that it is difficult to demonstrate during life and remains essentially a postmortem neuropathologic diagnosis.

The combination of infarcts in the basis pontis and the subiculum is difficult to explain, as these regions do not share common afferent or efferent fiber connections, use different neurotransmitters, have morphologically different types of neurons, arise from different embryologic primordia, and belong to different functional systems of the brain.

The pathogenesis of pontosubicular degeneration is poorly understood. Hyperoxemia in the presence of acidosis and hypoxia is described in some infants, suggesting that oxygen toxicity plays a role (135), but these cases represent only a small minority. Pontine neurons exhibiting karyorrhexis are immunoreactive to ferritin if accompanied by spongy changes and gliosis, suggesting that iron may be released to the damaged pontine neurons (140). *In situ* DNA fragmentation studies indicate apoptosis rather than frank necrosis as the mechanism of cellular death (141).

Pontosubicular degeneration has been described in stillborn fetuses, indicating that the lesions may result from intrauterine fetal distress and are not necessarily acquired intrapartum or postpartum (142,143). Sarnat has provided details of the histologic progression of changes in the degenerating neurons (112).

The spinal cord is also vulnerable to hypoxic-ischemic injuries, and damage to anterior horn cells results from hypoperfusion of the watershed area between the vascular distribution of the anterior spinal and the dorsal spinal arteries (144). The resultant hypotonia is generally attributed to cerebral injury, but electromyography (EMG) can demonstrate a lower motor neuron injury.

Infarcts

An infarct, the consequence of a focal or generalized disorder of cerebral circulation that occurs during the antenatal or early postnatal period and acts in isolation, is a relatively rare cause of brain damage. In the series of autopsies studied by Barmada and colleagues, arterial infarcts were seen in 5.4%, and infarcts of venous origin were found in 2.4% (145). Most commonly, the infarct is in the distribution of the middle cerebral artery. It is presumed to be the result of embolization arising from placental infarcts or of thrombosis caused by vascular maldevelopment, sepsis, or, as in the case of a twin to a macerated fetus, the exchange of thromboplastic material from the dead infant (3). In the series of Fujimoto and colleagues, 22% followed perinatal asphyxia; their onset was in the first 3 days of life (146). Infarcts can be asymptomatic, or present with convulsions. They are less common in the premature than the term infant, and compared with the term infant the premature infant has a better prognosis with regard to neurologic residua (147).

With increased use of neuroimaging studies, dural sinus thrombosis can be demonstrated as a consequence of severe perinatal asphyxia. The condition is also seen in a variety of other conditions which predispose the infant to a hypercoagulable state (147a,147b).

Porencephaly

A porencephalic cyst is a large intraparenchymal cyst that communicates with the ventricular system. Loculated cysts entirely within the subcortical white matter are not porencephalic and are pseudocysts rather than true cysts because they lack an epithelial lining. Porencephalic cysts are partly, though usually sparsely, covered by ependyma. Porencephaly results from infarction in the territory of a major artery, usually the middle cerebral artery, although at times it may be a sequel to a grade 4 IVH that extends the ventricle lumen into the empty parenchymal space left by the reabsorption of the hematoma. It is not a watershed infarct.

Porencephalic cysts often appear to communicate also with the overlying subarachnoid space, and such a communication may be reported by radiologists, but careful neuropathologic examination demonstrates that a thin pial membrane and sometimes arachnoidal tissue separate the porencephalic and subarachnoid compartments. The pia derives its vascular supply from meningeal rather than cerebral vessels. This membrane is too thin to resolve by CT or MRI, but is important during life in terms of fluid shifts and CSF flow.

The cerebral cortex immediately surrounding a porencephalic cyst often appears to be polymicrogyric. This is secondary to ischemia and atrophy of immature gyri and should not be misconstrued as a primary dysgenesis. These small gyri are gliotic and have extensive neuronal loss.

Porencephaly is usually limited to one hemisphere, and the clinical correlates are spastic hemiplegia, hemisensory deficits, and often hemianopia. Porencephalic cysts following grade 4 IVH are visualized in survivors 10 days to 8 weeks after the event (148). Although it is not a progressive lesion and does not obstruct the flow of CSF in the chronic phase, the porencephalic cyst occasionally enlarges and causes symptoms of intracranial hypertension. The reason for this phenomenon is the pulsation of the choroid plexus, which may induce a "waterhammer effect" because the force of the pulsations is transmitted to a larger surface area and the resistance to stretch is therefore less. The choroid plexus does not derive its blood supply from the middle cerebral artery, hence it usually survives the infarct. In some cases, a ventriculoperitoneal shunt may be required to prevent further enlargement of the porencephalic cyst, encroachment on functional brain, and midline shift.

TABLE 5.2. *Major types of neonatal intracranial hemorrhage and usual clinical setting*

Type of hemorrhage	Usual clinical setting
Subdural	Full-term > premature; trauma
Primary subarachnoid	Premature > full-term; trauma or "hypoxic" event(s)
Intracerebellar	Premature; "hypoxic" event(s); trauma (?)
Periventricular-intraventricular	Premature > full-term; "hypoxic" event(s)

From Volpe JJ. *Neurology of the newborn*, 3rd ed. Philadelphia: Saunders, 1995. With permission.

Intracranial Hemorrhage

Whereas mechanical trauma can be responsible for a subdural hemorrhage and, less commonly, a primary subarachnoid hemorrhage, it plays a relatively unimportant role in the evolution of periventricular (IVH), the most common form of neonatal intracranial hemorrhage (Table 5.2) (5,149,150). The various grades of hemorrhage are depicted in Figures 5.9, 5.10, and 5.11.

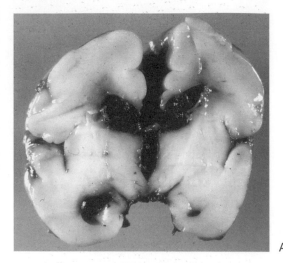

A

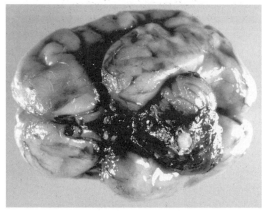

B

FIG. 5.10. A: Intraventricular hemorrhage, grade 3. More extensive intraventricular hemorrhage than in Figure 5.2, in a 28-week premature infant. Hemorrhage extends throughout the ventricular system and causes dilatation of the lateral ventricles bilaterally and the third ventricle; the original site of origin of the hemorrhage may be difficult to identify, but periventricular leukomalacia is seen around both frontal horns and the left side of the third ventricle. **B:** Blood from the lateral and third ventricles is seen in the subarachnoid space at the base of the brain, having exuded through the aqueduct and fourth ventricle and out the foramina of Luschka and Magendie during the course of cerebrospinal fluid flow.

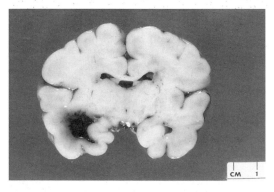

FIG. 5.9. Intraventricular hemorrhage, grade 2. Focal hemorrhage of the germinal matrix breaking through the ependyma and causing focal intraventricular hemorrhage that does not extend throughout or dilate the ventricular system. The coronal section of this brain of a 32-week premature infant shows hemorrhage into the left temporal horn and local dilatation of that horn, but blood does not extend into the frontal horn or across the midline, and the rest of the ventricular system is not dilated. In the dorsolateral periventricular region of the involved temporal horn, hemorrhage is seen in the parenchyma, but confined to that zone.

The site of the bleeding that results in an IVH is determined by the maturity of the infant. In the premature infant, bleeding originates in the capillaries of the subependymal germinal matrix, usually over the body of the caudate nucleus (150). With increasing maturation the germinal matrix involutes, so that in the term infant the choroid plexus becomes the principal site of the hemorrhage (93,150). Although Hayden and coworkers encountered IVH in 4.6% of term neonates (151), its incidence increases markedly with decreasing maturity, so that when ultrasonography is performed on infants with birth weights less than 1,500 g, a hemorrhage can be documented in as many as 50%. A high-grade hemorrhage is more common in this group than in infants with birth weights more than 1,500 g (152,153,154). At times, even premature infants of advanced gestational age may have extensive hemorrhages that can destroy the thalamus or basal ganglia (Fig. 5.11).

The pathogenesis of IVH is not completely understood. The predisposition of the premature infant to IVH in part is caused by the presence of a highly vascularized subependymal germinal matrix, to which a major portion of the blood supply of the immature cerebrum is directed. Furthermore, the capillaries of the premature infant have less basement membrane than those of the mature brain. Finally, abnormalities in the autoregulation of arterioles in premature and distressed term infants impair the infants' response to hypoxia and hypercarbia and thus permit transmission of arterial pressure fluctuations to the fragile periventricular capillary bed. Prenatal, as well as perinatal and postnatal, factors have been implicated in the evolution of IVH. As a rule, IVH that develops in the first 12 hours of life is associated with variables relating to labor and delivery, whereas IVH that starts later is associated with postpartum variables. Premature rupture of membranes and maternal chorioamnionitis increase the risk for the condition, suggesting that cytokines play a role in its evolution (154,155).

In most infants, acute fluctuations in cerebral blood flow and an impaired cerebral vascular autoregulation are more important than prenatal factors in the evolution of an IVH. Clinical studies have shown that infants with intact cerebrovascular autoregulation are at low risk for IVH. In contrast, a variety of adverse factors that disrupt autoregulation are associated with a high risk of IVH. These include low Apgar scores, respiratory distress, artificial ventilation, the presence of a patent ductus arteriosus, and

the various complications of perinatal and postnatal asphyxia (154–156). An elevation of venous pressure also has been implicated. Such an elevation can occur in the course of labor and delivery, or it can accompany positive-pressure ventilation, pneumothorax, hypoxic-ischemic myocardial failure, or hyperosmolality induced by administration of excess sodium bicarbonate (5). The importance of pneumothorax caused by positive-pressure ventilation in producing IVH was stressed by McCord and coworkers, who were able to reduce the incidence of respiratory distress syndrome by treatment with surfactant (157). This treatment was accompanied by a reduction of the incidence of IVH from 87% to 14%. Other surfactant trials have not been as convincing (156), and Leviton and colleagues conclude that the contribution of respiratory distress syndrome and pneumothorax to the evolution of IVH is relatively small (158). Other neonatal risk factors that predispose to the evolution of IVH include clotting disorders, and in the past, exposure to benzyl alcohol (159).

In the premature infant, the hemorrhage does not occur at the time of delivery, but tends to commence later, most commonly 24 to 48 hours after a major asphyxial insult, be it at the time of birth or subsequently (154,160). In the experience of Ment and associates, 74% of hemorrhages were detected by ultrasonography within 30 hours after birth (161) (Fig. 5.12). In the series of Trounce and colleagues, 15% of infants developed an IVH after 2 weeks of age (154). In some infants bleeding can be a slow process, rather than a sudden event (162). The extent of the hemorrhage can range from a slight oozing to a massive intraventricular bleed with an associated asymmetric periventricular hemorrhagic infarction and an extension of the blood into the subarachnoid space of the posterior fossa (see Figs. 5.9 and 5.10) (163).

Blood usually clears rapidly from the intraventricular and subarachnoid spaces. In fact, hemosiderin deposition, a reliable and permanent neuropathologic marker of old hemorrhage in the adult brain, is found rarely in children's brains after an IVH. Despite the resolution of the fresh blood, brain injury is a relatively common result of IVH. In part, injury can be the result of an antecedent asphyxial injury that pre-

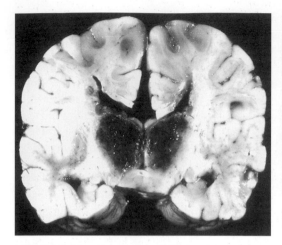

FIG. 5.11. Coronal section of brain of an infant of 36-weeks' gestation showing symmetric hemorrhagic infarction destroying the thalami. Periventricular focal hemorrhage is seen in the inferior walls of the frontal horns of the lateral ventricles, but the ventricular system is not dilated and contains no blood.

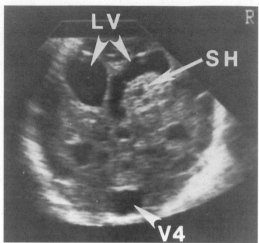

FIG. 5.12. Intraventricular hemorrhage in a 1,400-g infant of 30 weeks' gestation who suffered birth asphyxia. Coronal ultrasonographic scan reveals moderate hydrocephalus and a large subependymal hemorrhage (SH) in the wall of the right lateral ventricle. (LV, lateral ventricles; V4, fourth ventricle.) (From Babcock DS, Han BK. The accuracy of high-resolution, real-time ultrasonography of the head in infancy. *Radiology* 1981;139:665. With permission.)

disposed the infant to the bleeding. Other factors also are operative. As demonstrated by PET, cerebral blood flow becomes abolished in the area of an intraparenchymal hematoma and is reduced twofold to threefold over the entire affected hemisphere (164). How a hemorrhage induces such widespread vasospasm is unclear. Like the vasospasm encountered in older children and adults after a subarachnoid hemorrhage induced by the rupture of an aneurysm (see Chapter 12), the vasospasm could be related to the presence of high concentrations of blood in the CSF (165). Vasospasm may well have its major effect on the middle cerebral artery; as judged from the pulsatility index in the anterior cerebral artery, Perlman and Volpe have found no consistent effect of an IVH on flow in the anterior cerebral artery (166).

In addition to the vascular changes, metabolic alterations are responsible for subsequent neurologic abnormalities. Cerebral glucose metabolism is markedly reduced (167), and, as determined by MR spectroscopy, the brain phosphocreatine concentration is reduced for several weeks after the hemorrhage (168).

A fan-shaped hemorrhagic infarct, visualized by ultrasonography as an intracerebral periven-tricular, echodense lesion, is not unusual and can be demonstrated in approximately 15% of infants with IVH and in approximately one-third of those who harbor a severe hemorrhage (5,169) (Fig. 5.13). It is marked by a large region of hemorrhagic necrosis in the periventricular white matter at the point where the medullary veins become confluent and join the terminal vein in the subependymal region. The necrosis is usually markedly asymmetric; it is unilateral in the majority of instances (81). Approximately 80% of cases are accompanied by a large IVH, and in the past, the infarction was mistakenly described as a parenchymal extension of the IVH. Periventricular hemorrhagic infarction is believed to result from the IVH compressing and obstructing the terminal veins and interfering with their drainage (170). The periventricular hemorrhagic infarct produces tissue destruction and formation of cystic cavities and is associated with a poor functional outcome. Porencephalic cysts can develop in survivors and are visualized in 10 days to 8 weeks after the event (171).

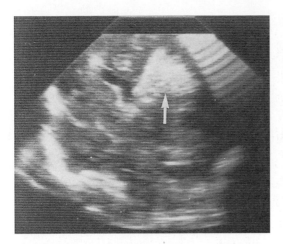

FIG. 5.13. Intracerebral hemorrhage in a neonate. Coronal ultrasonographic scan. The arrow indicates the presence of the hematoma. Displacement of the ventricular system occurred. (Courtesy of Dr. Eric E. Sauerbrei, Kingston General Hospital, Kingston, Ontario, Canada.)

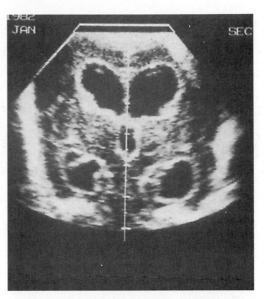

FIG. 5.14. Posthemorrhagic hydrocephalus in a 2-week-old premature infant. The lateral ventricles and the third ventricle are dilated; the fourth ventricle is not visualized. The increased echogenicity of the ventricular wall indicates posthemorrhagic hydrocephalus, as distinct from hydrocephalus resulting from a malformation, in which the hyperecho ring is absent. (Courtesy of Dr. W. Donald Shields, Division of Pediatric Neurology, University of California, Los Angeles.)

Progressive ventricular dilatation is a common sequel to IVH (Fig. 5.14). Evolving 1 to 3 weeks after the hemorrhage, it is caused by a fibrotic reaction that obliterates the subarachnoid spaces and induces ventricular dilatation with or without increased intracranial pressure (normal pressure hydrocephalus) (5). The factors responsible for normal pressure hydrocephalus in the neonate are poorly understood. Hill and Volpe attribute at least some of the brain damage in posthemorrhagic hydrocephalus to stretching or compression of the anterior cerebral artery, either by ventricular dilatation or by increased intracranial pressure with a consequent impairment of blood flow (172).

When an IVH occurs in term infants, it generally emanates from the choroid plexus, less frequently from the subependymal germinal matrix. The major causes are trauma and perinatal asphyxia (5). In the experience of Volpe, approximately one-half of term newborns with IVH have experienced difficult deliveries. The experience of Palmer and Donn is similar (173). In approximately 25%, the IVH is of unknown etiology. One cause that probably accounts for a large number of these cases is a cryptic hemangioma of the choroid plexus, well demonstrated at autopsy (174,175). The lesions range in size from thin-walled cavernous angiomas to fully formed arteriovenous malformations. They are sometimes difficult to show by imaging, in part because the hemorrhage may destroy the original vascular malformation or obscure its remains (175). Unruptured angiomas of the choroid villi are not uncommon as incidental findings at autopsy and must be distinguished from simple vascular congestion. One of us (H.S.) has found them to be more frequent in subjects with cerebral malformations or chromosomal abnormalities.

Term infants with IVH tend to become symptomatic at a later age, often not until the fourth week of life. Irritability, changes in alertness, and seizures are common presenting symptoms. In the series of Palmer and Donn, seizures were the first symptom in 69%; 23% of infants presented with apnea (173).

Extension of intracranial hemorrhage to the vertebral canal has received relatively little attention in the United States. Both epidural and sub-

TABLE 5.3. *Neuropathology in premature and full-term infants with cerebral palsy*

Birth weight (g)	Pathology	
	Birth injury (number of cases)	Central nervous system malformation (number of cases)
Less than 2,000	3	3
2,000–2,500	2	1
2,501–3,000	0	6
3,001–3,500	10	4
Greater than 3,500	7	7
Total known	22	21

From Malamud N, et al. An etiologic and diagnostic study of cerebral palsy. *J Pediatr* 1964;66:270. With permission.

dural bleeding have been encountered, the former being far more common. Epidural bleeding is associated not only with intracranial hemorrhage owing to asphyxia, but also with traumatic birth injuries (176,177). Although these hemorrhages either are asymptomatic or induce deficits that are obscured by the more obvious symptoms of an intracranial hemorrhage, diagnosis by MRI

of the spinal cord is now possible and was accomplished in one of our cases.

Primary and Secondary Malformations of the Central Nervous System

In addition to direct trauma, asphyxia, and circulatory disturbances, malformations of the CNS play an important part in the genesis of the lesions of perinatal asphyxia and trauma. Little doubt exists that in the premature infant, for instance, both faulty maturation of the nervous system and a greater vulnerability to perinatal trauma and asphyxia are responsible for the high incidence of neurologic deficits (Table 5.3) (178). The relative frequency of prenatal and perinatal brain lesions in moderately and severely retarded individuals can be determined from autopsy studies such as those by Freytag and Lindenberg (109) (Table 5.4).

Ischemic, hypoxic, and traumatic insults of the fetal brain in the second and third trimesters can induce malformations that are not primary defects of genetic programming. Because development is incomplete, lesions that interrupt or

TABLE 5.4. *Frequency of brain lesions*

Type of lesion	Number of patients with lesion[a]		Percentage of patients with demonstrable lesions	
Prenatal	150		50.5	
Malformations		93		31.3
Arnold-Chiari syndrome			23	
Microgyria, pachygyria, agyria			18	
Primary microcephaly			9	
Agenesis of corpus callosum			8	
Ectopic gray matter			6	
Abnormal convolutional pattern			6	
Other malformations			23	
Down syndrome		31		10.4
Hydrocephalus		23		7.7
Prenatal infections		2		0.7
Unclassified		1		0.3
Perinatal	47		15.8	
Circulatory lesions		42		14.1
Mechanical birth trauma		5		1.7
Postnatal [genetic disorders (e.g., leuko-dystrophies, lipidoses, tuberose sclerosis)]	27		9.1	
Postnatal owing to exogenous causes (meningitis, encephalitis)	44		14.8	
Unknown whether perinatal or prenatal	29		9.8	

[a]No morphologic lesions were detectable in another 62 autopsies.
Adapted from Freytag E, Lindenberg R. Neuropathological findings in patients of a hospital for the mentally deficient: a survey of 359 cases. *Johns Hopkins Med J* 1967;121:379. With permission.

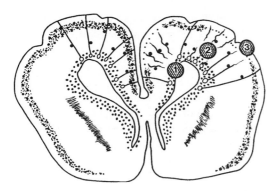

FIG. 5.15. Drawing of a coronal section of the cerebral hemisphere of a preterm infant to illustrate three possible sites where ischemic-hypoxic lesions might disrupt radial glial cells or their fibers to interfere with neuroblast and glioblast migration and thus cause secondary, acquired malformations as focal cortical dysplasias and subcortical heterotopia of incompletely migrated cells: (1) In the periventricular region, periventricular leukomalacia or grade 1 or 2 germinal matrix hemorrhage; (2) in the deep subcortical white matter, as either ischemic or hemorrhagic infarction; and (3) at the pial surface, where injury might cause retraction of radial glial end-feet. Examples of insults at the pial surface include contusions of the brain at delivery, subarachnoid hemorrhage, and neonatal meningitis. (From Sarnat HB. *Cerebral dysgenesis. Embryology and clinical expression.* New York: Oxford University Press, 1992. With permission.)

alter radial glial fibers, for example, can prevent further neuroblast and glioblast migration before the process is complete (Fig. 5.15) and may result in focal dysplasias of cortical lamination and in deep heterotopia of neurons arrested in migration. The abnormal synaptic relations that result from the abnormal anatomic positions of neurons may become a basis for later epilepsy.

Clinical Manifestations of Cerebral Perinatal Injuries

This section describes the clinical appearance of the neonate who has been subjected to perinatal asphyxia or trauma. It also traces the evolution of the spastic and extrapyramidal deficits and concludes with a discussion of the various syn-

TABLE 5.5. *Clinical features of hypoxic-ischemic encephalopathy*

Stage 1
Hyperalert
Normal muscle tone
Weak suck
Low threshold Moro
Mydriasis
No seizures
Stage 2
Lethargic or obtunded
Mild hypotonia
Weak or absent suck
Weak Moro
Miosis
Focal or multifocal seizures
Stage 3
Stuporous, responds to strong stimuli only
Flaccid
Intermittent decerebration
Absent suck
Absent Moro
Poor pupillary light response

Adapted from Sarnat HB, Sarnat MS. Neonatal encephalopathy following fetal distress. *Arch Neurol* 1976;33:696.

dromes of cerebral palsy, acknowledging that in many instances cerebral malformations play an etiologic role equaling or surpassing that of perinatal asphyxia and trauma.

The interested reader is referred to the pioneering studies by Paine on the evolution of tone and postural reflexes in neurologically damaged neonates (179,180).

Neonatal Period

The degree of a newborn's functional abnormality secondary to asphyxia incurred during labor and delivery depends on the severity, timing, and duration of the insult. (See the Introduction for a description of the essentials of a neurologic examination of the infant or small child.)

After birth, the infant subjected to perinatal asphyxia shows certain alterations in alertness, muscle tone, and respiration. These important clinical features of HIE were first graded by Sarnat and Sarnat (181) (Table 5.5). Several other grading schemes subsequently have been devised. In essence, they are similar to that of Sarnat and Sarnat; however, some schemes place infants with repetitive or prolonged seizures into grade 3, rather than grade 2 (21). The Sarnats specifically excluded seizures as a criterion for grading acute encephalopathy because of poor correlation with outcome in their experience and because some of the most severely involved infants in stage 3 do not have seizures because the cerebral cortex is so severely impaired that it can no longer generate epileptic activity. They did include electroencephalographic (EEG) criteria, however, as a measure of cerebral function rather than of paroxysmal activity. They also emphasized the importance of autonomic features, with sympathomimetic effects in stage 1 and strong parasympathetic (i.e., vagal) effects in stage 2.

In the experience of Levene and coworkers, 3.9 in 1,000 newborn term infants develop grade 1 HIE, 1.1 in 1,000 grade 2 HIE, and 1.0 in 1,000 develop grade 3 HIE (182).

Infants with grade 1 HIE are irritable with some degree of feeding difficulty, and are in a hyperalert state, in which their eyes are open with a "worried" facial appearance and a decreased frequency of blinking. They seem hungry and respond excessively to stimulation. Tremulousness, especially when provoked by abrupt changes of limb position or tactile stimulation, can resemble seizures. Mild degrees of hypotonia can be documented by a head lag and a lack of the normal biceps flexor tone in the traction response from the supine position. The Landau reflex is often abnormal, in that the infant's body tends to collapse into an inverted U shape.

A greater hypoxic insult results in the evolution of grade 2 HIE. Infants are lethargic or obtunded with delayed or incomplete responses to stimuli. Focal or multifocal seizures are common. Severely asphyxiated infants develop clinical signs of grade 3 HIE. The infant is markedly hypotonic. The sucking and swallowing reflexes are absent, producing difficulties in feeding. Palmar and plantar grasps are weak, the Moro reflex can be absent, and the placing and stepping reactions are impossible to elicit.

A variety of respiratory abnormalities can be encountered. These include a failure to initiate breathing after birth, which suggests a hypoxic depression of the respiratory reflex within the brainstem. Tachypnea or dyspnea in the absence of pulmonary or cardiac disease also suggests a neurologic abnormality. Periodic bouts of apnea are normal in the smaller premature infant. In larger infants, periodic apnea can result from a depression of the respiratory reflex or can indicate a seizure disorder (see Chapter 13).

The Apgar score has been used to measure the severity of the initial insult. Although a depressed score at 1 and 5 minutes implies the possibility of a hypoxic insult, the value of the score in terms of indicating asphyxia is limited. For instance, in the experience of Sykes and coworkers, only 20% of infants with a 5-minute Apgar score of less than 7 had an umbilical artery pH below 7.10 (183). However, virtually all of the infants of 35 to 36 weeks' gestation with a cord pH under 7.25 had a 5-minute Apgar score of 7 or more. In preterm infants the Apgar score is of even less value, and the more premature the infant, the more likely that the Apgar score will be low in the presence of a normal cord pH (184). The extended Apgar scores (Apgar scores taken at 10 and 20 minutes of life), however, are valuable in predicting neurologic outcome, in that the likelihood of ensuing cerebral palsy increases significantly once the Apgar score remains under 3 for 10 minutes or longer (185).

After 12 to 48 hours, the clinical picture of the previously hypotonic or flaccid infant (grade 3) can change to that of grade 2 or 1.5 (24). The infant becomes jittery, the cry is shrill and monotonous, the Moro reflex becomes exaggerated, and the infant has an increased startle response to sound. The deep tendon reflexes become hyperactive, and an increased extensor tone develops. Seizures can appear at this time. These signs of cerebral irritation also are noted in an infant who has experienced a major intracranial hemorrhage. In the series of Brown and associates (24), 24% of infants who were subjected to perinatal hypoxia demonstrated hypotonia progressing to extensor hypertonus. In the experience of DeSouza and Richards, this clinical course has an ominous prognosis, for none of the infants following it were ultimately free of neurologic deficits (186). In our experience, the greater the delay in emerging from grade 3 HIE, the worse the ultimate prognosis.

In other instances [24% in the series of Brown and associates (24)], an infant who has sustained perinatal asphyxia exhibits hypertonia and rigidity during the neonatal period. The clinical picture of spasticity in the neonate is modified by the immaturity of some of the higher centers. In the spastic infant, the deep tendon reflexes are not exaggerated, but can be depressed as a result of muscular rigidity. Hyperreflexia becomes evident only during the second half of the first year of life. A more reliable physical sign indicating spasticity is the presence of a sustained tonic neck response, which indicates a tonic neck pattern that can be imposed on the infant for an almost indefinite time and that the infant cannot break down. Such a response is never normal (see Fig. I.5). Spastic hemiparesis is manifest during the neonatal period in only 10% of infants (187), usually by a reduction of spontaneous movements or by excessive fisting in the upper extremity. Obvious paralyses during the neonatal period are rarely caused by cerebral damage; rather, they suggest a peripheral nerve or spinal cord lesion.

The evolution of IVH can go unrecognized clinically in more than 50% of infants (188,189). The remainder can have a sudden, sometimes catastrophic deterioration highlighted by alterations in consciousness, abnormalities of eye movements, and respiratory irregularities. Deterioration can continue over several hours, then stop, only to resume hours or days later (5). The presence of a full fontanel is noted in approximately one-third of asphyxiated infants (24). It can be the consequence of a massive intracranial hemorrhage, cerebral edema, or, less often, an acute subdural hemorrhage, the result of concomitant cerebral trauma.

Seizures secondary to perinatal asphyxia usually occur after 12 hours of age. However, when asphyxia is acute and profound, as can occur when a cord prolapse occurs, seizures can begin much earlier, and as a rule their onset cannot be used to time the asphyxial episode. The characterization and classification of seizures has been facilitated by the development of time-synchronized video and EEG/polygraphic monitoring. Generalized tonic-clonic convulsions are rare in the newborn. More often, one observes unifocal or multifocal clonic movements that tend to move from one part of the body to another. Generalized slow myoclonic jerks are another common neonatal seizure. EEG abnormalities do not accompany some behaviors previously considered to be neonatal seizures. These include a high percentage of tonic seizures, particularly those manifest by transient opisthotonos, and the various unusual forms of seizure activity ("subtle seizures"). Subtle seizures include paroxysmal blinking, changes in vasomotor tone, nystagmus, chewing, swallowing, or pedaling or swimming movements. These seizures probably represent primitive brainstem and spinal motor patterns, released from the normal tonic inhibition of forebrain structures (190). Apnea is not observed as the sole seizure manifestation. Seizures resulting from birth trauma or perinatal asphyxia often cease spontaneously within a few days or weeks, or they become relatively easy to control with adequate dosages of anticonvulsants. The topic of neonatal seizures is taken up in greater detail in Chapter 13.

Evolution of Motor Patterns

Infants who have suffered perinatal asphyxia experience various sequential changes of muscle tone and an abnormal evolution of postural reflexes.

Most often, there is a gradual change from the generalized hypotonia in the newborn period to spasticity in later life. In these subjects, the earliest sign of spasticity is the presence of increased resistance on passive supination of the forearm, or on flexion and extension of the ankle or knee. In spastic diplegia, this abnormal stretch reflex is first evident in the lower extremities and is often accompanied by the appearance of extension and scissoring in vertical suspension (see Fig. I.6), the late appearance or asymmetry of the placing response, a crossed adductor reflex that persists beyond 8 months of age, and the increased mobilization of extensor tone in the supporting reaction (180). In spastic hemiplegia, abnormalities first become apparent in the upper extremity. When five infants with unilateral hemispheric lesions detected by routine imaging studies during the first week of life were subjected to regular neurologic examinations, no abnormalities could be detected until 3 months of age, when one of the infants showed an asymmetric popliteal angle. Between 3 and 6 months of age the signs were subtle and usually consisted of asymmetric kicking in vertical suspension, which was seen in three infants by 6 months of age. Hand preference became apparent between 3 and 9 months of age (191). The more severe the hemiplegia, the earlier the abnormalities make their appearance. Other signs of hemiparesis include inequalities of muscle tone, asymmetry of fisting, and inequalities of the parachute reaction (see Fig. I.7). In many instances, parents also note poor feeding and frequent regurgitation.

Ingram has observed a remarkably constant sequence of neurologic manifestations in the progression from hypotonia to spasticity (192). The hypotonic stage lasts from 6 weeks to 17 months or longer. In general, the longer its duration, the more severely handicapped the child.

In a significant percentage of children, 1.3% in the series of Skatvedt (193), but 20% of the group with cerebral palsy at the Southbury Training School, Southbury, CT (194), the hypotonic state persists beyond the second or third year of life and, accordingly, the condition is designated as hypotonic (atonic) cerebral palsy, a term first proposed by Förster in 1910 (195). The differential diagnosis between hypotonic cerebral palsy and abnormalities in muscle function is discussed more fully in Chapter 14.

A stage of intermittent dystonia often becomes apparent when the infant is first able to hold up his or her head. At that time, abrupt changes in position, particularly extension of the head, elicit a response that is similar to extensor decerebrate rigidity. Probably, the frequency with which this intermediate dystonic stage is observed is a function of the care with which neurologic observations are performed. In the majority of children, dystonic episodes are present from 2 to 12 months of age. Ultimately, as rigidity appears, episodes become less frequent and more difficult to elicit. Transient dystonic posturing, notably torticollis or opisthotonos, has been associated with maternal use of cocaine (196).

TABLE 5.6. *Evolution of athetosis in infants with extrapyramidal cerebral palsy*

Age (months)	Cumulative percentage of patients showing athetosis in reaching for objects
6	0
9	12
12	36
15	56
18	64
21	64
24	72
27	76
30	84
33	88
36	92

From Paine RS, et al. Evolution of postural reflexes in normal infants and in the presence of chronic brain syndromes. *Neurology* 1964;14:1036. With permission.

In a smaller number of children with cerebral palsy, a transition occurs from the diffuse hypotonia seen in the neonatal period to an extrapyramidal form of cerebral palsy. Although a characteristic feature of the motor activity of the healthy premature and full-term infant is the presence of choreoathetoid movements of the hands and feet, the fully developed clinical picture of dyskinesia is not usually apparent until the second year of life (Table 5.6) (190). Until then, the neurologic picture is marked by persistent hypotonia accompanied by a retention of the immature postural reflexes. In particular, the tonic neck reflex, the righting response, and the Moro reflex are retained for longer periods in infants with extrapyramidal cerebral palsy than in those in whom a spastic picture predominates (180). In general, the earliest evidence of extrapyramidal disease is observed in the posturing of the fingers when the infant reaches for an object (Fig. 5.16). This can be noted as early as 9 months of age, and, as a rule, the early appearance of extrapyramidal movements indicates that the ultimate disability will be mild. In the child with dyskinesia, dystonic posturing can be elicited by sudden changes in the position of the trunk or limbs, particularly by extension of the head. Characteristically, when an infant with early extrapyramidal disease is placed with support in the sitting position, the

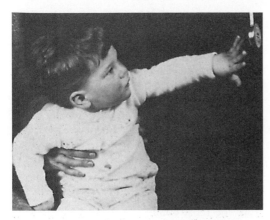

FIG. 5.16. Athetotic posture of the hand in an infant. The child is attempting to reach a proffered object. (From Cooke RE. *The biologic basis of pediatric practice.* New York: McGraw-Hill, 1968. With permission.)

TABLE 5.7. *Incidence of various forms of cerebral palsy*

Classification[a]	Crothers and Paine (161) (%)	Grether et al. (176) (%)
Spastic	64.6	82
Quadriplegia	19.0	22
Diplegia	2.8	41
Hemiplegia	40.5	19
Monoplegia	0.4	—
Triplegia	1.9	—
Extrapyramidal	22.0	5[b]
Mixed types	13.1	13

[a]Category of cerebral palsy as diagnosed by examining physician.
[b]Includes cases of ataxic cerebral palsy.

infant resists passive flexion of the neck and tends to retroflex the back and shoulders.

Every physician examining infants suspected of having sustained a cerebral birth injury has encountered a group of patients who appear to have clear-cut neurologic signs in early infancy but who, on subsequent examinations, have lost all of their motor dysfunction (197). Many of these have not escaped brain damage; follow-up studies show them to have delayed milestones, a high incidence of mental retardation (22%), abnormalities of extraocular movements (22%), and afebrile seizures (4.4%) (197). Still, approximately one-third appear normal, or, at worst, demonstrate mild perceptual handicaps or hyperkinetic behavior patterns (198).

Childhood

With the decline in neonatal mortality, the prevalence of cerebral palsy has risen significantly in most Western countries. In Northern California it was 1.23 in 1,000 3-year-old children born between 1983 and 1985 (199). In this group of children, 53% of children with cerebral palsy had birth weights of 2,500 g or less, and 28% had birth weights less than 1,500 g. In Sweden, 2.17 in 1,000 children born between 1979 and 1982 were diagnosed as suffering from cerebral palsy; 43% of these children were preterm (200). The increase in the incidence of cerebral palsy as a consequence of a decrease in neonatal mortality also has been reported from Australia, England, and Ireland (201).

In older children, the manifestations of cerebral birth injuries are so varied that it is difficult to devise an adequate scheme of classification. Yet the differences in cause, clinical picture, and prognosis require that cerebral palsy be subdivided into various entities based on the clinical picture. In this chapter, the following system is used:

Spastic cerebral palsy
  Spastic quadriparesis
  Spastic diplegia
  Spastic hemiparesis
Extrapyramidal cerebral palsy
Hypotonic cerebral palsy
Mixed and atypical forms

Table 5.7 shows the incidence of some of these forms of cerebral palsy. As many as one-seventh of children show a mixture of clear-cut pyramidal and extrapyramidal signs, and almost every child with spastic diplegia is found to have spastic quadriparesis on careful examination of the upper extremities. A number of authors have distinguished an ataxic form of cerebral palsy (192,193). In Skatvedt's series, published in 1958, this condition accounted for approximately 7% of children with cerebral palsy (193). Subsequent series do not distinguish this form of cerebral palsy. In most instances, neuropathologic studies on patients with cerebellar signs have revealed malformations of the cerebellum, often accompanied by even more conspicuous malformations of the cerebral hemispheres (125,126,131). Conversely, most patients with histologically verified lesions of the cerebellum attributable to perinatal trauma or asphyxia did not show cerebellar signs during their lifetime (111). Although Crothers and Paine (187) distinguished a condition termed *spastic monoplegia* (Table 5.7), this entity is probably rare. Most children fitting this designation have spastic hemiparesis revealed on subsequent examinations (187).

Spastic Quadriparesis

The heading Spastic Quadriparesis includes a group of children whose appearance corresponds to the description of spastic rigidity as given by Little (1) and contains some of the most severely damaged patients. In the Northern California series, spastic quadriparesis accounted for 22% of all children with cerebral palsy who were examined (202). This form of cerebral palsy was seen in 10% of Swedish children with cerebral palsy born at term, and 4% of children with cerebral palsy born preterm (200).

Although a mixed etiology exists for this form of cerebral palsy, abnormalities in delivery, particularly a prolonged second stage of labor, precipitate delivery, or fetal distress, are common causes. These abnormalities accounted for some 30% of cases in a 1989 Swedish series, whereas prenatal factors were thought to be responsible for some 55% (203). In the Australian series, intrapartum events were believed to be responsible in some 20% of children. It was higher in those children who had an associated athetosis (204).

In his classic pathologic studies, Benda noted the frequent occurrence of an extensive cystic degeneration of the brain (polycystic encephalomalacia, polyporencephaly) (see Fig. 5.3) (205). Other cerebral abnormalities included destructive cortical and subcortical lesions, PVL, and a variety of developmental malformations or residua of intrauterine infections.

Neuroimaging studies support the clinical and pathologic impressions of a multiplicity of

causes for this form of cerebral palsy. MRI studies on term infants with spastic quadriparesis demonstrate a mixture of polycystic encephalomalacia, parasagittal cortical lesions, and a variety of developmental abnormalities such as polymicrogyria and schizencephaly. It is of note that in a series of 26 term infants with spastic quadriparesis subjected to MRI, 12 (46%) demonstrated PVL (206). In term infants with spastic quadriparesis who suffered perinatal asphyxia, parasagittal cortical lesions, polycystic encephalomalacia, and basal ganglia lesions were the most common lesions (206). Several other studies, as well as our own clinical experience, corroborate these findings (207).

Patients with spastic quadriparesis demonstrate a generalized increase in muscle tone and rigidity of the limbs on both flexion and extension. In the experience of one of us (J.H.M.), the right side is more severely affected in the majority of children. In the most extreme form of spastic quadriparesis, the child is stiff and assumes a posture of decerebrate rigidity. Generally, impairment of motor function is more severe in the upper extremities. Few voluntary movements are present, and vasomotor changes in the extremities are common. Most children have pseudobulbar signs, with difficulties in swallowing and recurrent aspiration of food material. Optic atrophy and grand mal seizures are noted in approximately one-half of patients (192).

Intellectual impairment is severe in nearly all instances, and no child in Ingram's series was considered to be educable (192).

Spastic Diplegia

As defined by Freud, who coined the term *diplegia*, this condition is characterized by bilateral spasticity, with greater involvement of the legs than arms (208). Although the term *diplegia* inaccurately describes the clinical findings, we continue to use it for the sake of convenience. In the experience of Ford, spastic diplegia was the most common form of cerebral palsy encountered at Johns Hopkins Hospital (209). As is evident from Table 5.7, the incidence of spastic diplegia has increased in the decades between the 1950s and the 1990s. In Sweden, this form of cerebral palsy accounts for 18.7% of cerebral palsy in term infants and 71.3% of cases of cerebral palsy in preterm infants (210). The experience in Northern California is somewhat similar. Spastic diplegia is seen in 48% of those with birth weights less than 1,500 g, as contrasted with an incidence of 23% in children with cerebral palsy with birth weights of 1,500 to 2,499 g, and 28% of those with birth weights more than 2,500 g (202). In other studies, the frequency of prematurity is equally striking. In the classic series of Ingram, 44% of children with spastic diplegia had a birth weight of 2,500 g or less (192). Conversely, 81% of premature infants who develop the cerebral palsy syndrome have spastic diplegia (210).

Full-term and premature infants appear to differ with respect to the cause of this condition as determined by pathologic examination or neuroimaging studies. In premature infants, the most common finding is PVL (see Fig. 5.4). It was present in nearly all premature infants with spastic diplegia subjected to MRI (206,207,211). Most commonly, periventricular high-intensity areas are seen on T2-weighted images (Fig. 5.17). These are most marked in the white matter adjacent to the trigones and the bodies of the ventricles, and at times can be asymmetric. Additionally, a marked loss of periventricular white matter is seen, most striking in the trigonal region with compensatory ventricular dilatation (212). The distribution of the periventricular high-intensity areas corresponds to the anatomic distribution of PVL. The location of the white matter lesions produces an interruption of the downward course of the pyramidal fibers from the cortical leg area as they traverse the internal capsule, which explains the predominant involvement of the lower extremities. Lesions of the internal capsule and the thalamus also are noted on MRI. These usually are seen in the more severely affected children (213). Yokochi observed a paroxysmal downward deviation of the eyes in a large proportion of children with thalamic lesions (213).

In term infants with spastic diplegia PVL, as well as cortical abnormalities, porencephaly, and various congenital malformations of the gyri such as micropolygyria also have been seen

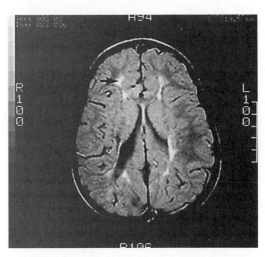

FIG. 5.17. Magnetic resonance imaging of spastic diplegia. Axial T2-weighted images show marked widening of occipital horns and markedly reduced occipitoparietal white matter, which is nearly absent on the right. Increased signal is seen in a periventricular distribution, particularly at the tips of the frontal horns (*arrow*), and in the occipital white matter. On sagittal views the corpus callosum was markedly thinned. This 7-year-old girl was the product of a 27-week twin pregnancy, with a birth weight of 1,022 g. Neonatal course was complicated by respiratory distress syndrome, which required ventilation for the first 2 months of life, and sepsis. The child now shows spastic quadriparesis that is more marked in the lower extremities, a seizure disorder, and severe mental retardation. The other twin died of sepsis during the first month of life.

(111) (see Chapter 4). A significant proportion of term infants with spastic diplegia has an apparently normal MRI result, suggesting that they might represent cases of familial spastic paraplegia with an early onset (see Chapter 2) (212).

The most striking physical finding in children with spastic diplegia is the increased muscle tone in the lower extremities. The severity of the spasticity varies from case to case. In the most involved patients, Ingram was able to distinguish a state in which rigidity predominates and the limbs tend to be maintained in extension (212). Thus, when a child is held vertically, the rigidity of the lower extremities becomes most evident, whereas the adductor spasm of the hips maintains the lower extremities in a scissored position (see Fig. I.6).

This stage is succeeded by the spastic phase, when flexion of the hips, knees, and, to a lesser extent, elbows becomes predominant. When the diplegia is less severe, patients show only impaired dorsiflexion of the feet, with increased tone at the ankles, which causes them to walk with the feet in the equinus position (toe walking). In such instances, the tone in the upper extremities is often normal to passive movement, but the child maintains the elbows flexed when walking (teddy-bear gait). In other instances, spasticity of the lower extremities is accompanied by impaired coordination of fine and rapid finger movements and by a slight weakness of the wrist extensors. Sensory impairment is rare. The deep tendon reflexes are hyperactive in all extremities, unless muscular rigidity makes them difficult to elicit. An ankle clonus and an extensor plantar response usually can be obtained. Dystonia, athetosis, and mixed types of involuntary movements occasionally are seen in more severe cases and can interfere considerably with muscular control.

After a variable period, usually more than 2 years, contractures appear. These tend to be more severe in the distal musculature, particularly at the ankles. As a consequence, feet tend to become fixed in plantar flexion, knees in flexion, and hips in flexion and adduction. Vasomotor changes and dwarfing of the pelvis and lower extremities are often striking and, in general, parallel the severity of the paresis. Optic atrophy, field defects, and involvement of the cranial nerves are relatively rare. A convergent strabismus is common, however, and was seen in 43% of Ingram's diplegic patients (192). Of the children in Ingram's series, 44% had a speech defect; most often, this was a matter of retarded speech development and an inability to pronounce consonants.

Seizures are a common accompaniment of spastic diplegia and were seen in 27% in Ingram's series (192) and in 16% of the patients reported by Veelken and colleagues (214). Most often these are grand mal seizures, and their incidence is unrelated to the severity of the motor handicap, although the presence of minor motor seizures is usually limited to patients with significant involvement of the upper extremities.

As a rule, the more severe the motor deficit, the more retarded the patient. Out of 29 children with little impairment of the upper extremities (spastic paraplegia), 6 had IQs above 100, but all of 27 children with major involvement of the upper extremities had an IQ below 100 (192). In the more recent series of Olsén and coworkers, preterm infants with MRI changes indicative of PVL tended to have visual motor and visuoperceptual deficits (215), although a significant proportion had grossly normal intelligence (206). The cognitive functions of premature infants are covered in Prematurity with Neurologic Complications, later in this chapter. When premature infants with minor neurodevelopmental deficits are subjected to MRI, a significant proportion exhibits PVL, which at times can be quite extensive. In the series of Olsén and colleagues 25% of infants with birth weights less than 1,750 g who had minor neurodevelopmental dysfunction at 8 years of age demonstrated PVL. Furthermore, 25% neurologically and developmentally normal ex-premature infants also demonstrated PVL that was generally considered mild (211).

Spastic Hemiparesis

Spastic hemiparesis is characterized by a unilateral paresis that nearly always affects the upper extremity to a greater extent than the lower and that ultimately is associated with some spasticity and flexion contractures of the affected limbs. It accounted for 19% of children with cerebral palsy in the series of Grether and coworkers (202). In the Swedish series of Hagberg and coworkers, spastic hemiparesis accounted for 56% of term infants with cerebral palsy, and 17% of preterm infants with cerebral palsy (200).

The correlation of congenital hemiparesis with cerebral abnormalities was established by Cazauvielh in 1827 (2); an antecedent history of abnormalities of labor and delivery was proposed by McNutt (216), Freud and Rie (217), and Ford (218). Since then it has become clear that the pathogenesis is multifactorial and that both morphogenetic and clastic lesions are

TABLE 5.8. *Incidence of abnormalities of pregnancy and delivery in patients with hemiparetic cerebral palsy*

Abnormality	Number of patients
Pregnancy	5
Delivery	20
Neither	27
Total	52

From Cohen ME, Duffner PK. Prognostic indicators in hemiparetic cerebral palsy. *Ann Neurol* 1981;9:353. With permission.

responsible, with the relatively low incidence of abnormalities of pregnancy and delivery in this form of cerebral palsy being quite striking (Table 5.8). In the majority of cases, the insult occurs during gestation (219,220). On the basis of fetal ultrasound studies coupled with pathologic examination of the brain, Larroche believes that intrauterine arterial ischemic lesions are frequent. These can be caused by maternal hemodynamic disturbances, emboli arising from the placenta, anomalies in the fetal circulation, or, in twin pregnancies, from the fetal transfusion syndrome (221). The role of these various intrauterine insults in the pathogenesis of hemiparetic cerebral palsy also is stressed by Nelson (222).

The pathologic picture in congenital hemiparesis is varied. Benda emphasized the frequency with which mantle sclerosis (ulegyria) can be found (205) (see Fig. 5.7), but a number of other abnormalities of the cerebral hemispheres also are encountered on MRI studies. In the series of Okomura and coworkers, bilateral lesions were seen in 35% of subjects with clinically evident hemiparesis (207). In term infants, these included cortical border zone infarcts, and basal ganglia lesions. PVL is a particularly important cause for hemiparesis in preterm infants. A variety of bilateral cortical malformations also have been recognized (223,224).

Of the various unilateral lesions seen in term infants with congenital hemiparesis, vascular infarcts are the most prominent. These are usually seen in the territory of the middle cerebral artery, with the left artery being more frequently affected than the right (225). As a rule, middle cerebral artery infarctions are more commonly

seen in infants older than 37 weeks' gestation (225,226). A variety of causes have been implicated in the focal infarction. These include perinatal asphyxia, thromboembolism, polycythemia, dehydration, cocaine abuse, extracorporeal membrane oxygenation, and a coagulopathy, notably a mutation in factor V Leiden (225,227). Other causes for hemiparesis include PVL, schizencephaly, pachygyria, unilateral hemimegalencephaly, and focal dysplasias of the cerebral cortex (228,229).

For unknown reasons, the hemiparesis is only rarely documented at birth, although some subsequently hemiparetic infants present with focal seizures during the first few days of life (230). As already stated in the section that deals with the evolution of motor patterns, even the most careful neurologic examination does not detect the hemiparesis for several months (191). The right side is more commonly affected. The incidence of right-sided involvement in three major series is 55% (231), 59% (192), and 66% (187).

The evolution of the hemiparesis from its appearance in the neonate to the spasticity seen in the older child has been traced by Byers (232). In older children, the extent of impaired voluntary function varies considerably from one patient to another. Generally, fine movements of the hand are the most affected, notably the pincer grasp of thumb and forefinger, extension of the wrist, and supination of the forearm. Proximal muscle power is well preserved, and function in the upper extremity relates to speed of movement and power in the distal musculature. In the lower extremity, dorsiflexion and eversion of the foot are impaired most frequently, with power in the proximal muscles being preserved. Increased flexor tone is invariable, leading to a hemiparetic posture, with flexion at the elbow, wrist, and knees, and an equinus position of the foot. Despite these abnormalities, most children with pure hemiparetic cerebral palsy walk by 20 months of age (233). Deep tendon reflexes are increased, and Babinski, and less often Hoffmann, reflexes can be elicited. In most children, the palmar grasp reflex persists for many years.

A large proportion of hemiparetic children has involuntary movements of the affected limbs. Goutieres and coworkers found dystonia in 12% and choreoathetosis in 9% of hemiparetic children (234). These disorders are seen most clearly in the hand, where the patient demonstrates an avoidance response and athetotic posturing of the hand, producing overextension of the fingers and occasionally of the wrist, as the child attempts to hold an object (235). This type of posture is similar to that of patients with parietal lobe lesions. Just as the grasp reflex in frontal lobe lesions reflects unopposed parietal lobe activity, this avoidance response reflects the unopposed frontal lobe activity (236). The affected side of the brain also participates in overflow movements, which are involuntary changes in position of the affected side associated with voluntary movements of the unaffected side. Before 10 years of age these movements are more evident in the unaffected hand; thereafter, they occur in both affected and unaffected hands (237). These changes are believed to reflect callosal inhibition of the uncrossed motor pathways and the organizational changes of the pyramidal motor system (238).

Sensory abnormalities of the affected limbs are common and were documented by Tizard and associates in 68% of patients with hemiparesis (239). Stereognosis is impaired most frequently; less often, two-point discrimination and position sense is defective. In addition to sensory impairment, frequently a neglect and unawareness of the affected side deficits aggravates considerably the handicap induced by the hemiparesis. In general, the severity of the sensory defect does not correlate with the severity of the hemiparesis.

Growth disturbances of the affected limbs are extremely common and, like the sensory defects, probably reflect damage to the parietal lobes. Failure of growth, most evident in the upper extremities and particularly in the terminal phalanges and in the size of the nail beds, is a result of underdevelopment of muscle and bone. Growth arrest is not always accompanied by sensory changes.

Between 17% and 27% of hemiparetic patients have homonymous hemianopia. When adequate testing of the visual fields is possible, sparing of the macula can often be demonstrated (187). Abnormalities in cranial nerve function

are frequent and usually the result of a supranuclear involvement of the muscles enervated by the lower cranial nerves. Facial weakness is probably the most common abnormality, being noted in approximately three-fourths of the patients (192,232). Deviation of the tongue and convergent strabismus are seen less often.

More than one-half of hemiparetic patients develop seizures, with the actual incidence probably being a function of the duration of follow-up (232,237,240). In 52%, seizures first appear before 18 months of age, and only 8% of hemiparetic children suffer their first attack after age 10 years. For those who had experienced seizures during the neonatal period, the likelihood of recurrence is high, being 100% in the series of Cohen and Duffner (237).

Seizures are usually in the form of major or focal motor attacks. A considerable proportion of children who, for months or even years, has only focal seizures can develop generalized convulsions (218). As a rule, anticonvulsant therapy is effective in reducing the frequency of attacks, but only a small proportion of children has remission of seizures for longer than 2 years. In these subjects, anticonvulsant withdrawal after 2 seizure-free years results in a high rate of relapse, 62% in the series of Delgado and coworkers (240). We, personally, would be most reluctant to ever discontinue anticonvulsant therapy in a seizure-free child with hemiparetic cerebral palsy. In a small group of seizure patients, attacks persist despite medication. These patients should be considered for surgical removal of the portion of the cerebral cortex from which the seizure originates, or for hemispherectomy, should there be more than one focus. The presurgical evaluation of such a patient is covered in Chapter 13.

The EEG and neuroimaging studies are of considerable prognostic value for a patient with hemiparetic cerebral palsy. A paroxysmal EEG almost invariably indicates the presence of a seizure disorder. Approximately one-half of hemiparetic children have average IQs, and 18% score above 100 (197). Nearly all of hemiparetic patients are educationally competitive and ultimately become at least partially independent economically (241). Neither the IQ nor the type of deficit, be it delayed language development or perceptual handicaps, depends on which hemisphere has sustained the major damage or the extent of structural damage, a reflection on hemispheric equipotentiality in the small infant. Neither is there a consistent relationship between the extent of the lesion, the severity of the hemiparesis, and the functional outcome (226). In our opinion, other developmental malformations of the brain undetectable by imaging studies probably determine the ultimate outcome.

Extrapyramidal Cerebral Palsies

Extrapyramidal cerebral palsies are characterized by the predominant presence of a variety of abnormal motor patterns and postures secondary to a defective regulation of muscle tone and coordination. Spasticity frequently accompanies the involuntary movements, and primitive reflex patterns can often be demonstrated.

This form of cerebral palsy is considered to be the result of damage to the extrapyramidal system. In contrast to spastic hemiparesis, whose cause is manifold, it appears to be caused by several fairly well-delineated insults acting singly, successively, or in concert. In the series reported from Hagberg's unit, 58% of children with extrapyramidal cerebral palsy had experienced perinatal asphyxia. A further 34% were of low-birth weight, and many of these were small for gestational age, with placental infarction and maternal toxemia being the most frequent prenatal risk factors (242). Kyllerman's group, studying a different Swedish population, came to similar conclusions (243,244). They distinguished two groups of extrapyramidal cerebral palsies: the hyperkinetic form characterized by choreiform and choreoathetoid movements, and the more severely involved dystonic form characterized by abnormal postures. The hyperkinetic group consisted of premature infants with asphyxia and hyperbilirubinemia; the dystonic group consisted of small-for-gestational-age infants who experienced asphyxia in the perinatal period or during the last trimester of their gestations. When extrapyramidal cerebral palsy affects term infants who are appropriate for gestational age, the characteristic antecedent event is a severe

but brief hypoxic stress late in labor, with a relatively mild degree of subsequent HIE (245).

An extrapyramidal syndrome caused exclusively by kernicterus is unusual nowadays and was not encountered in the large series of dyskinetic children reported in 1975 by Hagberg and colleagues (242). Kernicterus is discussed more fully in Chapter 9.

The clinical picture of extrapyramidal cerebral palsy evolves gradually from diffuse hypotonia with lively reflexes in infancy to choreoathetosis during childhood (246).

The onset of choreoathetosis usually occurs between the second and third years of life (see Table 5.6), with the most severely affected children continuing to manifest hypotonia for the longest time (180). Bobath has observed that hypotonic infants destined to develop extrapyramidal movements demonstrate a head lag when pulled into the sitting position. However, when pushed into the sitting position, their arms and shoulders press back. This resistance persists when the infant's body is pushed forward into flexion (247). One of us (J.H.M.) has termed this phenomenon the *Bobath response*. The onset of involuntary movements, almost invariably in the form of generalized or focal dystonia, can occur as late as the third decade of life (248). This delay in the clinical expression of a static cerebral lesion probably reflects changes with maturation in function and distribution of the various neurotransmitters.

A syndrome of transient dystonia characterized by hyperextension of the neck, hyperpronation of the forearm, and palmar transient flexion of the wrists has been reported (249). We have seen such children; as a rule, the dystonia subsides before the third year of life.

In the final stage of dyskinesia, a number of involuntary movements are recognized. Although collectively these have been termed *choreoathetosis*, the clinical picture is more complex. In most patients, a variety of involuntary movements, appearing discretely or in transitional forms, can be recognized. Their appearance and definition is discussed in the Introduction. These various dyskinesias combine with spasticity, which is seen in a large proportion of children, to interfere markedly with all types of voluntary movements.

TABLE 5.9. *Validity of early estimate of intelligence in two types of cerebral palsy*

Type of cerebral palsy	Original estimate		Estimate at follow-up		
	Range	Number of patients	Same	Higher	Lower
Hemiplegia	Superior	4	2	—	2
	Average	17	13	1	3
	Below average	19	11	1	7
	Inadequate or defective	27	25	2	—
Extrapyramidal	Superior	5	5	—	0
	Average	13	10	0	3
	Below average	6	6	0	0
	Inadequate or defective	27	16	11	—

From Crothers B, Paine RS. *The natural history of cerebral palsy.* Cambridge, MA: Harvard University Press, 1959. With permission.

Development of motor function is usually far more delayed than would be expected from the child's intelligence. Approximately one-half walk before the fourth year. In Ingram's series, the average age at which children walked unsupported was 2 years and 5 months (192). The delay in gait correlates well with delays in the other motor milestones. Crothers and Paine have shown that persistence of the obligatory tonic neck reflex (see Fig. I.5) suggests a bad prognosis in terms of the ability to walk without assistance and, to a lesser extent, the severity of athetosis (187). In their experience, walking is highly improbable as long as an obligatory tonic neck response can be elicited. Correlation of obligatory tonic neck response with intelligence was not uniform, and the persistence of the reflex does not necessarily indicate intellectual incompetence.

Skilled hand movements, such as those required for self-feeding, dressing, and writing, are equally impaired, and the disability in hand function can be severe enough to render a child virtually helpless. An occasional patient learns to perform these movements with the mouth or feet. Speech defects occur frequently in children with extrapyramidal cerebral palsy. In many, development of speech is retarded because of the uncoordinated movements of lips, tongue, palate, and respiratory muscles. In approximately two-thirds of children, incoordination of the muscles of respiration and speech is responsible for delayed speech (193); however, approximately one-half of patients begin to say intelligible words before 2 years of age (187), and almost all children who are not severely retarded are able to speak by 4 years of age.

A number of patients with moderately severe dyskinesia have impaired swallowing and control of saliva; drooling can persist for as long as 6 years of age. Cranial nerve involvement is less common than in the other forms of cerebral palsy. Strabismus is seen in approximately one-third of patients, however, and one-third have nystagmus (192). Seizures are encountered in approximately one-fourth of patients (198). Optic atrophy is rare. A sensorineural hearing loss can be documented in approximately one-half of children whose intelligence level permits adequate testing (243).

In a considerable proportion of children with extrapyramidal involvement, delayed language skills and gross motor handicaps can cause an erroneous underestimation of intelligence (Table 5.9) (187). In the experience of Crothers and Paine, 65% had IQs over 70, and 45% had IQs of 90 or better (187). The series of Kyllerman and associates, compiled in 1982, indicates that 78% of children with the choreoathetotic movement disorder demonstrate IQs of 90 or higher (243). Children with the dystonic form of cerebral palsy do not fare as well. A large proportion of children with normal or near normal intelligence, however, has an educational disability sufficiently severe to require their attendance at special schools.

On MRI, we have found a uniform picture of bilateral high intensity signals in the anterior lateral thalamus, posterior thalamus, and posterior

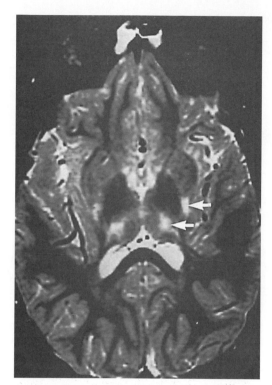

FIG. 5.18. Axial T2-weighted image (3,000/150/1) illustrating bilateral symmetric focal hyperintensities in the posterior putamen and the ventrolateral nucleus of the thalamus (*arrows*). The patient was a 6 ½-year-old boy who experienced severe shoulder dystocia. Birth weight was 4,230 g. Apgar scores were 1 and 0 at 1 and 5 minutes, respectively. Arterial pH was 6.84 at 4 hours and 20 minutes of age. The child demonstrated a mixed, but mainly extrapyramidal, form of cerebral palsy. He had low normal intelligence.

putamen in children with pure postasphyxial extrapyramidal cerebral palsy (120) (Fig. 5.18). The location of the changes corresponds with the location of glial scarring seen by Hayashi and colleagues in autopsied subjects who had experienced perinatal asphyxia (250). MRI abnormalities within the basal ganglia are seen in a variety of metabolic, genetic, and toxic disorders (251). These are summarized in Table 5.10.

Hypotonic (Atonic) Cerebral Palsy

Hypotonic (atonic) cerebral palsy, a relatively common condition, is characterized by general-ized muscular hypotonia that persists beyond 2 to 3 years of age and that does not result from a primary disorder of muscle or peripheral nerve. Characteristically, the deep tendon reflexes are normal or even hyperactive, and the electrical reactions of muscle and nerve are normal. Over the years, more than one-half of these children develop frank cerebellar deficits with incoordination, ataxia, and impaired rapid succession movements. Another one-third are profoundly retarded; the remainder develop minimal cerebral dysfunction syndrome (252). Hypotonic cerebral palsy also can be a forerunner to extrapyramidal cerebral palsy, but in the majority of children, the involuntary movements are apparent before 3 years of age (see Table 5.6).

The cause of hypotonia in this form of cerebral palsy is still a matter of considerable speculation. In many instances, muscle biopsy discloses a pattern termed *fiber type disproportion*, in which the type 1 muscle fibers are significantly smaller than type 2 fibers. Additionally, the number of type 1 fibers often is increased. This pathologic picture is nonspecific and is a manifestation of a delay in muscle maturation (253). In the fetus, type 1 fibers, which are rich in oxidative enzymes, form only a small proportion of total muscle fibers, whereas the type 2 fibers, which are rich in glycolytic enzymes, are predominant at 25 weeks' gestation, but not at term (253,254). Lesny suggested that the condition is a syndrome of extremely delayed brain development, with the generalized hypotonia representing the earliest sign of a cerebellar disorder (252). In the majority of his patients, prenatal factors, acting singly or in concert with other noxious influences, were presumably responsible. By contrast, perinatal asphyxia was believed responsible in less than 5% of children. Our own experiences are identical. We have found neuroimaging studies of little help in arriving at an anatomic diagnosis; some patients have a small cerebellum with a prominent fourth ventricle; a significant proportion of these children merely shows ventriculomegaly and gyral atrophy (126).

Cerebellar Cerebral Palsy

A small number of children experience a static neurologic disorder in which cerebellar signs

TABLE 5.10. *Basal ganglia abnormalities on magnetic resonance imaging in children with extrapyramidal movement disorders*

Condition	Caudate	Putamen	Globus pallidus	Thalamus
Perinatal asphyxia	+	+		+
Maple syrup disease	+	+		
Propionic acidemia	+	+		
Glutaric aciduria I	+	+		
Lesch-Nyhan disease	±			
Leigh syndrome	±	+	+	
Wilson disease	±	+		+
Methylmalonic acidemia		+	+	
Kernicterus			+	
Carbon monoxide			+	
3-Nitropropionic acid		+	+	

predominate. The majority of these has a developmental anomaly of the cerebellum. In others, generally children of normal intelligence, the symptoms appear to be the consequence of perinatal trauma or perinatal asphyxia.

Mixed Forms of Cerebral Palsy

In the experience of most physicians, a considerable proportion of children with cerebral palsy exhibits a mixture of spasticity and extrapyramidal movements (see Table 5.7). This combination can be manifested by minor amounts of athetotic posturing, as observed in a high percentage of children with spastic hemiparesis, or by the presence of extensor plantar responses in patients with predominantly extrapyramidal disease. When the mixed form is most obvious, the clinical picture is one of hyperreflexia, spasticity, and contractures in a child with frank dystonia or other extrapyramidal movements.

Diagnosis

The diagnosis of a neurologic disorder that has resulted from perinatal asphyxia incurred by a term infant is based on a history of intrauterine distress, a history of an abnormal neonatal course, and laboratory studies suggesting perinatal asphyxia.

Prenatal and Intrauterine Factors

Evidence of intrauterine distress includes an alteration of fetal heart rate pattern, the passage of meconium, and abnormalities in fetal acid–base status as determined by scalp or cord blood sampling. Although beat-to-beat variability and deceleration beginning after the start of a contraction and peaking well after the peak of the uterine contraction (late decelerations) are ominous in terms of fetal well-being, they do not seem to predict ultimate neurologic or intellectual deficits (255). In the experience of Valentin and coworkers, infants who demonstrated a pattern of reduced variability, reduced variability with late decelerations, or bradycardia with late decelerations had the most abnormal cord arterial pHs (256) and would therefore be at greatest risk for neurologic abnormalities. However, Nelson and coworkers in a retrospective study found that 37% of children with cerebral palsy showed none of the risk factors on prenatal fetal heart monitoring (257). Passage of large amounts of meconium after rupture of the fetal membranes also correlates with the subsequent presence of neurologic deficits (258). However, we should point out that infants with developmental abnormalities as well as those who have sustained neurologic injuries before the onset of labor are likely to demonstrate abnormal fetal heart rate patterns during labor (259). Mothers of infants whose neurologic handicaps were secondary to cerebral malformations have a statistically higher incidence of vaginal bleeding during pregnancy and a suggestively higher incidence of prenatal infections. Additionally, a breech presentation and the application of midforceps are significantly associated with both mechanical and asphyxial birth injury.

The relationship for arterial cord blood values and ultimate neurologic deficits has been the subject of several investigations. Infants with a complicated neonatal course tend to have a lower cord arterial pH and a significantly greater mean base deficit than those with an uncomplicated neonatal course (260,261). However, less than one-half of infants with an arterial cord pH of 7.00 or less have neonatal complications (262). Sehdev and coworkers found the additional presence of a high arterial base deficit and a low 5-minute Apgar score to be good predictors for neonatal morbidity (262). An arteriovenous pCO_2 difference of greater than 25 torr has been found to be a highly specific parameter for identifying asphyxiated infants who go on to develop HIE (263).

An infant small for gestational age (i.e., one whose birth weight is more than 2 standard deviations below the mean for any given week of gestation) is at a somewhat increased risk for developmental delay and possible neurologic deficits (264). Generally, the infant who is both underweight and short experienced an insult in early fetal life, whereas the infant who is underweight but of normal growth suffered an insult that was briefer and occurred later during gestation. Under both circumstances, brain growth, as inferred from head circumference, is less affected than body weight or length. Small-for-gestational-age infants are prone to perinatal asphyxia, the meconium aspiration syndrome, hypoglycemia, and the complications of polycythemia. In a survey of children with spastic cerebral palsy, 30.4% were below the tenth birth weight percentile, and 15.5% were below the third birth weight percentile. Small-for-gestational-age infants between 34 and 37 weeks' gestational age were at highest risk to develop spastic cerebral palsy (265). Amiel-Tison and Pettigrew suggest that intrauterine growth retardation is an adaptive response to placental insufficiency and that as judged from their physical examination and their brainstem-evoked responses, small-for-gestational-age infants are neurologically more mature than infants whose birth weights are appropriate for their gestational age (266). Whether small-for-gestational-age infants ultimately develop learning

disorders and minor cognitive and behavioral abnormalities beyond those caused by socioeconomic factors is a matter of dispute (267).

History of an Abnormal Neonatal Course

An abnormal neonatal course is the most important diagnostic feature of perinatal asphyxia that has been sufficiently severe to cause neurologic deficits. This includes delayed or impaired respiration requiring resuscitative measures such as endotracheal intubation and assisted ventilation. Additionally, depressed Apgar scores, particularly when the score is 3 or less for more than 10 minutes, correlate with subsequent development of neurologic complications, notably neonatal seizures, and the ultimate evolution of cerebral palsy (185,261). It must be remembered, however, that a low Apgar score does not by itself indicate perinatal asphyxia, because other causes, notably maternal drugs or anesthesia, can be responsible for the low score (268). Some of the other structural CNS lesions responsible for apnea at birth include a variety of CNS malformations and degenerative disorders (269). It therefore comes as no surprise that in the classic study of Sykes published in 1982, 73% of neonates with severe acidosis had a 1-minute Apgar score of 7 or higher, and only 21% of infants with a 1-minute Apgar score of less than 7 had severe acidosis (270). Other studies confirm this work. Thus, Socol and coworkers found that 60% of infants with a 5-minute Apgar score of 3 or less had an umbilical artery pH of greater than 7.0, and 54% had an arterial pH of greater than 7.10 (260). The results of Goldenberg and colleagues, are similar (184). Thus, neither scalp pH nor umbilical artery pH can provide more than inferential evidence for perinatal asphyxia and its severity.

Other abnormalities observed during the neonatal period include seizures, hypotonia, and a bulging fontanel; less obvious abnormalities are irritability, feeding difficulties, excessive jitters, or an abnormal cry. In addition, there may be clinical or laboratory evidence for asphyxial damage to organs other than the brain. In the experience of Perlman and colleagues, 67% of infants who had experienced asphyxial injury to the brain had evidence of injury to other organs (271). In 70% of children with brain and systemic injury, the injury was confined to one organ, most commonly the kidney.

The infant whose birth was complicated but whose neonatal period was uneventful (i.e., activity after the first day of life was normal, incubator care was not required beyond 3 days of age, and the infant did not have feeding problems, impaired sucking, respiratory difficulties, or neonatal seizures) is not at increased risk for neurologic damage (272,273).

Laboratory Studies Suggesting Perinatal Asphyxia

Examination of the CSF can provide some evidence for perinatal asphyxia in that the concentration of CSF protein can be elevated after perinatal asphyxia. In the term neonate, the mean protein concentration is 90 mg/dL; values more than 150 mg/dL are considered abnormal. In the premature neonate, the mean CSF protein is 115 mg/dL (274). The presence of blood from any source raises the total protein by 1.5 mg/dL of fluid for every 1,000 fresh red blood cells per μL (275). An elevation in the ratio of CSF lactate to pyruvate has been found to persist in asphyxiated infants for several hours after normal oxygenation has been reestablished (276), as does a striking elevation of blood creatine kinase-BB isoenzyme (277). A normal CSF does not exclude the possibility of perinatal asphyxia, however.

EEG is mainly of prognostic value. Several groups of French workers, however, have found the presence of positive rolandic sharp waves to be a specific and sensitive marker for PVL and white matter damage. In their experience EEG abnormalities can always be detected before the appearance of ultrasound abnormalities of cystic PVL (278,279).

Neuroimaging studies are invaluable in diagnosing the presence and the extent of tissue damage in the asphyxiated neonate and in determining the extent of an intracranial hemorrhage (280). The advantage of ultrasonographic scanning of the neonate is that examinations can be performed at the bedside and serially without harmful effects to the infant. In general, the brain is examined in two planes: coronal and sagittal. This technique provides excellent visualization of the ventricular system, basal ganglia, choroid plexus, and corpus callosum (163,281).

The location, extent, and course of an IVH can readily be followed by ultrasonography. IVHs produce strong echoes in the normally echo-free ventricles. Subependymal and intracerebral hemorrhages also are identified readily. Partridge and associates suggested that for their optimal detection, the scan be performed routinely at 4 to 7 days of age in all infants with birth weights less than 1,500 g (282). Follow-up scans for ventricular size should be done at 14 days of age and, in infants who demonstrate ventricular dilatation, at least weekly thereafter until ventricular size is stabilized, with a final examination being conducted at 3 months of age.

IVHs have been classified into three grades of severity: I, subependymal (germinal matrix) hemorrhage with minimal or no IVH; II, definite IVH but with neither lateral ventricle filled with blood; and III, IVH that completely fills and distends at least one lateral ventricle (283,284). As already mentioned in the section that deals with intracranial hemorrhage, parenchymal hemorrhagic necrotic lesions, the so-called grade IV hemorrhage seen in 15% of infants with IVH, probably result from a clot-induced impairment of venous flow and consequent venous infarction of brain tissue rather than representing an extension of an IVH (170).

Ultrasonography also has been used to demonstrate PVL, which initially presents as persistent periventricular echodense areas, and as echolucent cystic areas after the second week of life. These lesions are seen most commonly near the lateral ventricles, in front of the anterior horns, in the corona radiata, or posterior to the occipital horns (285,286).

Ultrasonography is of somewhat more limited value in the evaluation of the asphyxiated neonate. It is useful in the identification of asphyxial lesions in the basal ganglia and thalamus, and the detection of PVL (287). In the hands of Eken and coworkers, the use of a high-resolution transducer led to the detection of echogenicity in the cortex, which correlated well with the location of pathologic changes on autopsy (288). Although ultrasonography is inferior to CT scans in revealing details of brain anatomy, the procedure can be used to detect porencephalic cysts and other major structural lesions of the cerebrum.

The CT scan has wide diagnostic application to the newborn with neurologic disease. It is useful in diagnosing not only an intracranial hemorrhage, but also a variety of congenital malformations. For the first 48 to 72 hours after an asphyxial insult, the CT is more sensitive than MRI in demonstrating cortical changes because on MRI the edematous cortex is isodense with white matter. CT scans performed on asphyxiated infants 1 to 2 weeks after birth demonstrate local areas of hyperperfusion, with a dense network of proliferating capillaries that almost completely replaces the parenchyma. This alteration is most often observed in the basal ganglia, but it also can occur in the brainstem and cerebellum, the periventricular area, the depth of the cortical sulci, and the hippocampus. The *bright thalamus syndrome* probably represents an example of hyperperfusion as documented by cranial ultrasound (289). Shewmon and coworkers consider this hypervascularity a response to the antecedent hypoxia and reduced cerebral blood flow (290).

Whereas certain pathologic appearances (e.g., hemorrhage) are readily interpreted, difficulties are encountered in the CT analysis of parenchymal changes. These difficulties occur because of the frequent presence of alternating areas of high and low densities within the cerebral substance that lack adult equivalents. Both gray and white matter, however, have lower attenuation coefficients in neonates than in older children, and the difference in density between gray and white matter is greater than that in adults. Sulci and subarachnoid spaces are often prominent and should not be interpreted as cerebral atrophy (291,292).

In the preterm infant, interpretation of the CT scan is further complicated by the poor visualization of the ventricular system owing to its small volume in relation to brain parenchyma. Localized areas of low density in the periventricular region and hypodense parenchymal areas have little significance. In most instances, these changes are transient and can reflect a developmental stage (293).

Within 2 to 3 weeks following birth, MRI becomes the preferred neuroimaging study for delineating the extent and nature of asphyxial damage. Diffusion-weighted MRI in which the image contrast depends on differences in the molecular motion of water, allows detection of changes within minutes of the injury, and therefore much earlier than conventional MRI (294). MRI performed within the first 10 days of life on asphyxiated infants demonstrates four patterns of damage (295,296). In the largest group, abnormalities are confined to the thalamus and basal ganglia. In a second group, abnormalities are predominantly in the cerebral cortex and subcortical white matter. Periventricular white matter abnormalities are generally seen in preterm infants, or in infants believed to have sustained *in utero* asphyxial damage before 34 to 35 weeks' gestation (297). In some infants, imaging discloses a mixed pattern of abnormalities (295). Brainstem and cerebellar abnormalities are less common. Contrast enhancement of abnormalities in the thalamus and basal ganglia, in particular, correlates with tissue necrosis, and thus predicts a poor outcome (296,297). Focal parenchymal hemorrhages, mainly in a parietal or parieto-occipital distribution, were common in the series of Keeney and coworkers (298). These were unilateral or bilateral and generally resolved to be replaced by atrophy, thinning of myelin, or hemosiderin deposition. Basal ganglia hemorrhage occurred in 5% of asphyxiated infants; it was seen in 63% of term infants who had developed an IVH (299). On follow-up MRI studies, basal ganglia hemorrhage can resolve, or the hemorrhage is replaced by cysts or a calcification. For reasons as yet unknown, calcification can appear as early as 2 weeks after the asphyxial insult (300). MRI also assists in determining the extent and progress of myelination and can follow the loss of water from white matter with maturation (301). In the healthy newborn, white matter is lighter than gray matter when T2-weighted spin-echo pulse sequences are used (302,303). Areas of myelination are seen in the cerebellum and thalami, which, therefore, have a lower signal intensity. After perinatal asphyxia, there is a delay in myelination. This is best identified after 7 to 8 months of age. In the premature infant, PVL is accompanied by delayed myelination; IVH, as a rule, is not (304).

Measurements of cerebral blood flow and PET have been used experimentally for delineating regional cerebral blood flow and glucose metabolism during the acute stages of perinatal asphyxia. Discrepant results have been obtained. In the series of Lou and coworkers performed during the first few hours after birth, a low cerebral blood flow was associated with a poor outcome (305). Rosenbaum and coworkers, who performed the study during the first and second weeks of life, found that an abnormally high cerebral blood flow was followed by a poor outcome (306). The difference between the two studies probably reflects the timing when these were performed. A high cerebral blood flow after asphyxia is probably the result of impaired autoregulation. PET scanning performed shortly after birth can provide information as to the site of damage, by demonstrating areas of hypermetabolism (307). PET also has been used to study the functional anatomic correlations in children with long-standing cerebral palsy. In the latter group, abnormalities in glucose metabolism generally correspond to abnormalities of brain structure demonstrable by other neuroimaging studies, although metabolic impairment is usually more extensive than anatomic involvement (308).

Proton MR spectroscopy, which determines the relative amounts of various brain metabolites, is a noninvasive procedure that can provide information as to the severity of asphyxial brain damage, and by inference, its prognosis. The physical and chemical principles that form the basis of this technique are presented by Novotny and colleagues (309). When infants subjected to perinatal asphyxia are studied during the first 2 days of life, lactate is increased as is evidenced by the ratio of lactate to creatine and lactate to *N*-acetylaspartate (310). The magnitude of change appears to correlate with the severity of injury, and the neurodevelopmental outcome at 1 year of age (310). When MR spectroscopy is performed 1 to 2 weeks after birth, there usually is a reduced *N*-acetylaspartate to creatine ratio, and the lactate is generally normal. However, a persistently elevated basal ganglia lactate has been seen in some infants who have had a poor outcome from their asphyxial injuries

(311). In asphyxiated piglets the lactate increases sharply during the insult, then falls back to the baseline over the next few hours, only to experience a secondary increase by 24 to 48 hours after the insult. The secondary increase is unaccompanied by a decrease in intracellular pH. The reason for this increase as well as the reason for persistently elevated basal ganglia lactate in infants with asphyxial damage is unclear (311,312). On ^{31}P MR spectroscopy a reduction in the ratio of phosphocreatine MR signals to inorganic phosphate MR signals is considered an excellent indication of cerebral asphyxia, as is a decrease in brain intracellular pH (44,313). Techniques for spatial localization of these metabolic changes have been developed (314). These show that the metabolic derangement is most marked in the deeper layers of the cerebral cortex, an observation consistent with the known vulnerability of subcortical regions to hypoxic-ischemic injury (315).

Abnormalities in the brainstem auditory-evoked response and the visual-evoked response correlate well with the severity of the asphyxial insult. In infants who have experienced perinatal asphyxia, the brainstem auditory-evoked response can be completely abolished, or the interval between the auditory nerve action potential and the nerve action potential arising from the inferior colliculi can be prolonged (316). In the experience of Muttit and her group, a visual-evoked response that is absent or remains abnormal throughout the first week of life invariably predicts an abnormal neurologic outcome (317).

Cerebral Doppler studies have been used in some centers to evaluate infants with perinatal asphyxia and intracranial hemorrhage. Technical aspects, methodology, and clinical applications of this technique are reviewed by Raju (318).

In evaluating an older child with cerebral palsy, the best diagnostic tool is an MRI study, which can demonstrate abnormalities of myelination, areas of atrophy, cystic degeneration, and any anomalies in cortical architecture. Other diagnostic studies, notably CT, are of less help.

Treatment

The prevention of perinatal trauma and asphyxia is largely the task of the obstetrician and is, therefore, outside the scope of this text. Treatment of the asphyxiated neonate is also largely outside the domain of the neurologist. It is reviewed by Levene (182). Neither fluid restriction nor corticosteroids are effective in the management of postasphyxial cerebral edema. The value of hyperventilation or osmotic agents in improving the outcome of infants with cerebral edema is probably also minimal (182).

Experimental work suggests that there is a therapeutic window of 1 to 2 hours between the time the infant has been resuscitated successfully from perinatal asphyxia and the onset of the cascade of secondary changes that lead to necrotic and apoptotic neuronal death. Several pharmacologic agents are under current experimental investigations (319). N-methyl-D-aspartate (NMDA) antagonists, notably MK-801, have been found to protect the brain from experimentally induced asphyxial injuries, even when administered up to 1 hour after the insult. To date, none of them has been used in the human neonate. Calcium channel blockers, inhibitors of nitric oxide production, or oxygen-free radical inhibitors and scavengers such as allopurinol and indomethacin, also have been suggested, but have not received any clinical trials (319). Under experimental conditions, antisense oligodeoxynucleotides to one of the NMDA receptor channel complexes inhibit synthesis of the protein component of the channel and selectively reduce the expression of NMDA receptors, and the extent of focal ischemic infarctions. Although the use of antisense nucleotides represents a novel and exciting approach to the treatment of asphyxia, it has to date undergone no clinical trials (320).

Several regimens have been suggested to prevent IVH or to reduce its severity (321). The most extensively studied approach has been the prenatal administration of phenobarbital, which in combination with vitamin K does not appear to reduce the incidence of severe IVH (322,323). Treatment of the infant with phenobarbital appears to be ineffective in preventing IVH and could actually increase its incidence (5). Volpe has suggested that muscle paralysis with pancuronium can correct the fluctuating cerebral blood velocity and thus reduce the incidence of

large IVHs (5). Indomethacin (0.1 mg/kg) given at 6 to 12 hours and every 24 hours for two further doses lowered the incidence of the most extensive hemorrhages (324). Indomethacin reduces cerebral blood flow velocity and increases cerebral vascular resistance, and thus attenuates the adaptive vasodilatory response to asphyxia (325). It also reduces the formation of free radicals and accelerates maturation of the microvasculature in the germinal matrix (326). Ethamsylate administration also is associated with a lowered incidence of IVH, particularly the more extensive hemorrhages (327). The effectiveness of vitamin E in preventing the more extensive IVHs in the smaller preterm infants requires confirmation (5).

Our nurseries at Cedars-Sinai Medical Center use prenatal treatment of the fetus with corticosteroids to prevent respiratory distress syndrome, and thereby lessen the likelihood for IVH. Antenatal treatment with betamethasone is also associated with a decreased incidence of cystic PVL in very small premature infants (90). Infants with birth weights lower than 1,250 g are given prophylactic indomethacin. We believe that maintaining a good airway with a good cardiovascular support system and trying to prevent excessive swings in blood pressure and cardiac output reduce the likelihood of a large IVH. Additionally, allowing the pCO_2 to increase, but maintaining it below 55 mm Hg, appears to reduce the incidence of pneumothorax, which contributes to the evolution of IVH. Such factors as hypoxemia, acidemia, and rapid volume expansion all can lead to extension of the hemorrhage and should therefore be avoided.

In treating progressive ventricular enlargement, many centers suggest that lumbar punctures should be performed first, unless ultrasound or CT evidence exists of noncommunication between the ventricles and the spinal subarachnoid space. Acetazolamide or furosemide can be used as an adjunct to lumbar punctures. If these interventions fail to arrest the progressive ventricular enlargement, external ventricular drainage is indicated. A ventricular reservoir is inserted, and serial reservoir taps are performed until the ventricular fluid protein falls below 2,000 mg/dL, and there has been no resolution of the hydrocephalus, as indicated by serial ultrasounds. At that time, a ventriculo-peritoneal shunt replaces the reservoir. Serial monitoring with ultrasonography is recommended in all infants who have had an IVH, whatever treatment has been adopted.

Only a small proportion of patients undergoing a shunting procedure becomes neurologically and developmentally healthy adults. Several studies have demonstrated that in these subjects nonverbal skills are more impaired than verbal skills. The outlook for infants whose hydrocephalus responded to medical treatment with repeated lumbar punctures, osmotic diuretics, or acetazolamide is significantly better than it is for those who require a shunt (328). It is equally evident that the extent of parenchymal damage that attends IVH determines the ultimate prognosis (5,328).

The control of neonatal seizures is discussed in Chapter 13.

The treatment of children with cerebral palsy has been the subject of innumerable publications, most of them surprisingly uncritical and devoid of controls (329). At present, no evidence indicates that treatment programs that attempt to modify sensory input, to inhibit primitive reflexes, or to modify or inhibit abnormal movement patterns are ever successfully incorporated into the maturing nervous system with resulting improvement in motor function. Tizard proposes that before treatment is initiated, the following points should be considered (330): (a) Does the child need treatment? (b) What are the aims of treatment? (c) Do the family and child have the time required for treatment? (d) Will treatment disrupt family life?

Various means are available for the treatment of spasticity, which represents the most important disorder of motor control in children with cerebral palsy. Physiotherapy is the most traditional and principal nonsurgical form of treatment. Its aims are to prevent additional deformities and to promote functionally useful posture and movements. From the studies of Crothers and Paine (187) and Paine (331), it seems clear that to be most effective, the program must be determined by the nature of the handicap. Fixsen has divided orthopedic management into two aspects: the management of

the child who will ultimately become ambulatory, and the nonambulatory child (332).

Intensive physical therapy has been considered to be helpful for children with spastic hemiparesis and spastic diplegia. If possible, the effectiveness of the management should be monitored by gait analysis (332). Most children with these forms of cerebral palsy require regular physiotherapy as soon as they begin to walk, with special attention to the presence of contractures in the lower extremity. In evaluating the effectiveness of the physiotherapy for spastic children, Wright and Nicholson found no evidence that it improved the range of dorsiflexion of the ankle or abduction of the hip or that it affected the retention or loss of reflex automatisms (333). A controlled study of infants with spastic diplegia also found that the routine use of physical therapy offered no short-term advantages over an infant stimulation program (334). Bracing often is necessary. According to Tardieu and his group, bracing for 6 hours a day prevents contractures at the ankle (335). It is difficult to state categorically at what age treatment should be initiated. The controlled studies by Paine indicate that the eventual gait is better and contractures are fewer when physical therapy is begun before the age of 2 years (331).

Despite physical therapy, approximately one-half of the patients with spastic diplegia, spastic quadriparesis, or hemiparesis ultimately require some form of orthopedic procedure. Nonambulatory children, in particular, have a high incidence of spinal deformities, and more than 50% develop progressive displacement and dysplasia of the hips, and up to 20% ultimately develop frank dislocation (332). Park and Owen have divided surgical procedures into two categories: lengthening or release of muscles and tendons and procedures involving bones (336). The former procedures include tenotomy of the hip adductors, hamstring lengthening, lengthening of the heel cords, or the posterior tibial tendons. The majority of such operations is performed between 4 and 8 years of age. Surgery on bones is generally carried out in older individuals with the aim of correcting fixed deformities (337,338). The outcome of these procedures is not related to the age at surgery; rather the more severe the deficit, the greater the improvement. Long-term follow-ups, however, indicate that the greatest gains are seen 1 year after surgery; thereafter, function tended to return to preoperative levels (339). Much controversy surrounds the management of the hemiplegic hand. No differences in hand function, quality of upper extremity movement, or parents' perception of the child's hand function were noted when children received intensive neurodevelopmental therapy plus casting or regular occupational therapy. However, casting appears to be more effective in older children (340). Ultimate hand function is usually not improved by physical therapy or surgery, and when the hemiplegia is complicated by a hemisensory deficit, the affected hand will probably never do more than assist the good hand (341). Growth of the affected side is not improved by any mode of treatment. When the hemiplegia is mild, children achieve a good gait whether treated or not.

Few objective data indicate that either physiotherapy or orthopedic measures improve the disabilities of the child with a predominantly extrapyramidal disorder. In these subjects, hand function and the quality of the ultimate gait depend principally on the original severity of the disorder, and most children with extrapyramidal movements, particularly those with unimpaired intelligence, are able to teach themselves to assume certain positions and perform substitute movements by which involuntary movements are avoided. The substitute movements are often so complex that they could not possibly be invented by therapists. In all instances, coordination and function tend to improve with age. Various drugs have been tried for relief of the extrapyramidal movements. None of these has resulted in long-term benefit sufficient to outweigh the side effects (330).

Another type of surgical approach has been directed to correcting the pathophysiology underlying the spastic muscle. Normally, muscle tone results from a stream of impulses from the muscle spindles activating the motoneurons (the large motor neurons of the anterior horns). In spasticity, increased activity of the two types of small, γ-motoneurons results from an imbalance of two opposing influences, facilitation and inhibition. Facilitation is brought about by afferent fibers from the muscle spindles, and inhibition is mediated by the descending pyramidal tract fibers. When the descending pyramidal tract fibers have been damaged, inhibition is reduced. Stimulation of the cerebellum has been offered as a means of enhancing inhibition. However, neither chronic cerebellar stimulation nor the implantation of a subcutaneous dorsal column stimulator in the high cervical region of the spinal cord has been effective. Peacock and his group suggested a compensatory reduction of facilitation by selective sectioning of the posterior roots of the spinal cord (342). This procedure requires sectioning of those rootlets between the levels of L2 to S1 or S2 involved in spasticity-producing circuits, whose electrical stimulation induces either a tetanic muscle contraction or a diffusion of muscle contraction to muscle groups other than those being stimulated. This procedure is relatively free of complications, and any sensory loss induced by it appears to be minor and transient. Although the efficacy of the procedure and its neurophysiologic rationale have been questioned, several series have reported good results on patients who have severe spasticity in the lower extremities, but near normal intelligence, no major contractures, and no movement disorder. With good patient selection, significant improvement occurs in muscle tone, range of motion, and speed of walking, and the outcome is better than in children who are treated with intensive physiotherapy alone (343). In some instances upper limb function also improves (344). Rhizotomy should not be performed on patients whose spasticity enables them to maintain the erect position (345).

Various nonsurgical approaches have been tried for relief of spasticity. The most commonly used medications are baclofen, diazepam, and dantrolene. Doses are started at low levels and are increased until spasticity improves or side effects, notably drowsiness, occur. As a rule, these medications only have a small effect. The intrathecal administration of baclofen by continuous infusion is proving to be an effective means for treating spasticity in the lower extremities in a selected group of patients who have responded favorably to a trial dose of intrathecal baclofen (346). Complications of this procedure are relatively few, and in the experience of Armstrong and coworkers were limited to mechanical failures of the pump or the catheter (347). Side effects from the drug are usually temporary and can be managed by reducing the rate of infusion.

The injection of botulinum toxin A (Botox) into the gastrosoleus and hamstring group of muscles appears to improve gait for up to 6 months and may help to delay or obviate the need for serial casting or orthopedic surgery (348). The effect of the toxin becomes evident within 12 hours to 7 days, and the effect can last between 2 and 10 months (348,349). At this time no firm recommendations exist as to dosages and optimal sites for injection (349,350). Forssberg and Tedroff believe that treatment should be initiated at a time when children are still developing their motor control apparatus. This might prevent them from entering a vicious cycle in which CNS lesions affect the musculoskeletal system, thereby preventing the development of motor functions (351). In addition, experimental data on the formation of a cortical somatotopic map during early life indicate that the periphery plays an instructional role on the formation of central neuronal structures (352). The economics and effectiveness of this type of treatment also require further study.

Several authorities and parent groups have expressed their enthusiasm for infant stimulation programs. Even lacking objective evidence of their usefulness, they are apparently beneficial in controlling behavior and are here to stay (353,354).

A high incidence of ocular abnormalities is found in children with cerebral palsy. According to a survey taken in Scotland, some 60% show noteworthy defects (355). The most common abnormality encountered is strabismus, mainly caused by esotropia, which is found in approximately one-half of the patients with ocular problems (356). The condition is most common in children with spastic diplegia, and least common in those with extrapyramidal cerebral palsy. Strabismus that fluctuates from esotropia to exotropia, apparently unrelated to accommodative effort, is particularly common in children with extrapyramidal cerebral palsy and can be the first sign of this disorder (357). The cause for convergent strabismus is unknown, but because the alignment of the eye is often correctable under anesthesia, probably overactivity of the convergence center is at fault. Approximately one-third of patients have defects of horizontal conjugate gaze. Generally, surgical treatment of the eye muscles is deferred until the child has reached an age at which the degree of deviation is stable. Surgery is indicated when binocular vision is evident on sensory testing. If a surgical procedure is performed too early, the child, who has not yet achieved a fusion potential, does not maintain the correct alignment, and strabismus recurs. Only 10% to 15% of children with cerebral palsy ever achieve binocular vision. In the remainder, surgery serves only cosmetic purposes.

Asphyxiated infants can be cortically blind or can have delayed visual maturation. Delayed maturation can reflect delayed myelination and dendritic and synapse formation. The visual-evoked response in these children is usually abnormal, whereas the ERG is normal (358). Many of these cortically blind infants make a remarkable recovery, although often a residue of visual perceptual handicaps remains (358,359).

Impaired feeding and swallowing are relatively common. Symptoms result in part from an increased bite reflex and tongue thrust, and in part from incoordination of the swallowing mechanism (gastroesophageal reflux) (360). Dysfunctional problems can include drooling, coughing or aspiration, abnormal breathing patterns, uncoordinated swallowing, an absence of bilabial close on the spoon or cup, prolonged bottle feeding or impaired sucking, inadequate jaw or tongue movements, and rejection of textured foods. Additionally, dystonic hyperextension of the head allows liquids and foods to move into the trachea by gravity and causes aspiration and upper respiratory dysfunction.

Treatment for these problems is practical, but tedious. A major component in the treatment process is positioning (i.e., breaking up abnormal patterns such as hyperextension of the head by means of a hands-on technique in addition to the wheelchair headrest) (361).

The sequential steps for successful oral feeding intake are (a) tactile desensitization to allow oral intake of textured foods; (b) active feeding techniques to retrain lip and tongue movements, bilabial closure on the spoon and cup, and reduction of the tongue thrust; (c) active feeding techniques to encourage normal chewing skills; and (d) active feeding techniques to encourage automatic jaw closure, decrease drooling, and encourage normal breathing and swallowing patterns (362). Small amounts of benztropine (Cogentin) (0.5 to 6 mg per day) have been used successfully to reduce drooling (363). The neural control of swallowing has been reviewed by Miller (364).

Approximately one-third of children with cerebral palsy develop significant lower urinary tract symptoms, notably daytime urinary incontinence, urgency, and frequency. Videourodynamic studies disclose that the most common finding, seen in 74%, is hyperreflexia of the detrusor muscle of the bladder with reduced bladder capacity. Less often, 19% in the experience of Reid and Borzyskowski, detrusor sphincter dyssynergia occurs, which is a contraction of the detrusor concurrent with involuntary contraction of the external urethral sphincter. Treatment includes anticholinergic drugs, intermittent catheterization, antibiotic prophylaxis, and surgery. Reid and Borzyskowski review evaluation and management of these conditions (365).

In a large proportion of children with cerebral palsy, learning is impaired by defects in visual or auditory perception. The procedures by which these defects can be evaluated, and the educational aspects of visual and spatial and auditory and perceptual handicaps, are discussed in Chapter 16.

Because an effective treatment program requires considerable time and effort by the child's family and a large number of skilled personnel, deciding whether to advise treatment for the retarded child with cerebral palsy is difficult. Obviously, the goals for the cerebral palsy child and the time spent achieving them must be realistic. It is beyond the scope of this book to explore the emotional and social factors that need to be considered in the evaluation of each case.

From time to time a number of methods have been proposed for the treatment of cerebral palsy. Some of these are based on unproven or even false concepts of neuromuscular function, and claims for effectiveness are more a matter of bias than objective evaluation. Reviews by Dormans (366), Bleck (367), and Bobath and Bobath (368) can be consulted for further information on treatment programs, particularly with respect to orthopedic therapy, speech therapy, and handling of social and educational problems.

Prognosis

Perinatal Asphyxia

Underlying the prognosis of the asphyxiated infant is the unanswered question about whether asphyxia produces a continuum of brain damage (i.e., whether mild asphyxia causes a small amount of damage, and more severe asphyxia causes more severe damage), or whether a threshold exists beyond which the brain is damaged in an all or none manner. It is our opinion that there is a threshold of asphyxia beyond which there is a continuum of brain injury, and that below this threshold there is no damage.

It is clear that most infants who experience perinatal asphyxia do not exhibit abnormal neurologic signs or subsequent evidence of brain injury. It is also clear that unless clinical signs of neurologic abnormality are present during the neonatal period, the outcome of perinatal asphyxia is entirely favorable (272). In the experience of Dubowitz and Dubowitz all term infants who were healthy on neurologic examination were healthy at 1 year of age (369). Currently, the best predictor of outcome from a perinatal asphyxia is the clinical status of the infant during the neonatal period as assessed by the Sarnat scale (see Table 5.5). Numerous studies have confirmed the prognostic value of such an assessment (181,370). In terms of outcome, staging is best done according to the most severe signs, and according to the most severe stage of encephalopathy between 1 hour and 7 days of life (370). In the experience of Robertson and Finer, all infants with Stage 1 encephalopathy had a normal outcome, and their cognitive performance at 8 years of age did not differ from that of controls. The results of Handley-Derry and coworkers are similar (371). Infants with stage 3 encephalopathy fare poorly. Robertson and Finer found that 82% had died, and 18% were severely handicapped (370). The outcome of infants with stage 2 HIE is less certain. Robertson and Finer found that 80% were neurologically normal, 15% were neurologically disabled, and 5% died (370). Of the nondisabled survivors in this series as well as in several others a large proportion had significant cognitive dysfunction and poor school performance (370). In the study of Robertson and Finer, the presence of neonatal seizures did not appear to affect the prognosis. Temple and coworkers, however, found that infants who developed neonatal seizures after an asphyxial injury demonstrated significant cognitive deficits, even when the neurologic examination was normal (372). Renal injury, particularly prolonged oliguria when associated with asphyxia, also presages a poor neurologic outcome (373).

Other factors that influence the infant's response to an asphyxial insult, and thus its outcome include preexisting cerebral anomalies, fetal maturity, cerebral energy stores at the time of asphyxia, the adequacy of uteroplacental blood flow, and the fetal adaptive response to asphyxia. This adaptive response involves a redistribution of cardiac output so that blood flow to brain and heart is maintained at the expense of blood flow to kidney, the gastrointestinal tract, and the musculoskeletal system. Finally, experimental data indicate that not only can asphyxial injury cause neuronal loss, but it also can interfere with the normal subtractive processes including axon retraction and programmed cell death that may have been in progress at the time of injury (374).

In view of the interaction of these several factors, it should come as no surprise that many infants with severe and prolonged asphyxia recover without any neurodevelopmental deficits and an arterial cord pH as low as 6.60 is compatible with normal neurologic and cognitive examinations at a mean age of 47 months (260). Nevertheless, aggressive resuscitation of the newborn infant is not in order. Levene recommends that if an infant has no cardiac output after 10 minutes of effective resuscitation, treatment should be abandoned (182). The outcome of infants with good cardiac output who do not breathe spontaneously by 20 minutes is poor, and only 25% were left without significant neurologic deficits (375). These considerations are important in a time of medical cost control.

Several other methods have been used in an attempt to identify infants with a poor prognosis. The most traditional of these has been the Apgar score, even though it is now evident that a low Apgar score does not indicate the presence of asphyxia in either term or premature infants (184,185,270). Whereas the predictive value of the 1- and 5-minute Apgar scores in terms of subsequent neurologic deficits is limited, term infants with 5-minute Apgar scores of 6 or less are three times as likely to be neurologically abnormal at 1 year of age as those with scores of 6 to 10 (376). The likelihood of permanent brain damage increases even more significantly when depressed Apgar scores persist. Of infants with scores of 3 or less at 10 minutes of age, 68% die during the first year of life, and 12.5% of survivors are neurologically damaged. The prognosis is even worse when an Apgar score of 3 or less persists for 20 minutes. Of those infants, 87% die, and 36% of survivors have cerebral palsy (185). A poor outcome was seen in 30% of infants with a low Apgar score, but no significant acidosis (377).

Fetal blood sampling can provide somewhat better prognostic information, although there still are no absolute values of blood pO_2, pCO_2, or pH beyond which irreparable brain damage is certain to ensue. Studies designed to correlate the severity of acidosis in term infants at birth with outcome have failed to show any consistent relationship (378,379). When infants with umbilical cord pH of 7.0 or less are selected to be followed, the outcome is still unpredictable; however, when severe acidemia is associated with persistent bradycardia or seizures, the outcome is poor in 85% of cases (169). The predictive value of umbilical artery pH is somewhat better for preterm or for small-for-gestational-age infants (380). Because most of the asphyxial insults were believed to occur *in utero* during labor, electronic monitoring of the fetal heart rate was considered to be of prognostic value. Prospective studies have indicated otherwise.

Although one-fourth of high-risk infants whose fetal heart rate patterns showed severe variable decelerations or late decelerations were neurologically abnormal at 1 year of age, these abnormalities did not persist into later childhood (255,381). Erkert and coworkers have presented a model that can predict within 4 hours of birth a poor outcome from perinatal asphyxia (382). The three major adverse factors singled out by them were onset of spontaneous respirations after 10 minutes of life, administration of chest compression, and onset of seizures before 4 hours of age.

Because a significant proportion of infants with a neurologic examination consistent with Sarnat stage 2 fares well, prognosis in this group should be influenced by the results of neurodiagnostic tests (383).

The EEG is one of the commonly used means to evaluate the neonate with a history of perinatal asphyxia, and clinical evidence for moderate or severe HIE. Recovery is more likely to occur if the tracing is normal or if it demonstrates a single focus, rather than showing multifocal paroxysmal discharges or a burst-suppression pattern (384,385).

Ultrasonography can provide evidence for injury to the basal ganglia and for the presence of focal or multifocal ischemic parenchymal lesions, both predictors of ultimate major neurologic deficits. Consistent with the data obtained by CT scanning, small ventricles can be seen in a large proportion of control infants during the first week of life and do not predict neurologic damage (386).

CT scanning and MRI also can be used for prognostic purposes. The presence of areas of decreased density in brain parenchyma predicts a major neurologic handicap (387). This likelihood is particularly true when two or more focal areas of hypodensity exist, or when the density of the basal ganglia is reduced (388). Asphyxiated infants with normal CT rarely exhibit major neurologic residua. The presence of small ventricles does not correlate with ultimate outcome (389). Although the MRI provides more detail about the anatomic localization and severity of asphyxial injury, the practical problems associated with obtain-

ing such a study preclude it from being widely used in the early evaluation of asphyxiated infants (295,388,390). MR spectroscopy, although a potentially valuable prognostic tool, has a similar drawback (391).

Epidemiologically, severe mental retardation in the absence of other neurologic sequels is caused by asphyxia only rarely (185,392). In the experience of Hagberg, a perinatal cause could be assigned to only 18% of children with moderately severe mental retardation (IQ of 50 to 70) and to 15% of children with mild mental retardation. Perinatal asphyxia could not be implicated in any of the children with IQs between 70 and 75 (393). Nelson and Ellenberg have calculated that in the National Collaborative Perinatal Project, the proportion of cases of cerebral palsy owing to intrapartum asphyxia ranged between 3% and 13% and did not exceed 21% (394). In an Australian study, intrapartum asphyxia produced cerebral palsy in 4.9% to 8.2% in infants (395).

In this respect, it is important to note that Nelson and Ellenberg failed to find a statistically significant increase in mental retardation in children with low Apgar scores who did not also have cerebral palsy (185). They concluded that when mental retardation is a consequence of perinatal asphyxia, it is usually severe and accompanied by evidence of neurologic damage, notably spastic quadriparesis, athetosis, or both. The experience of Alberman and coworkers with low-birth-weight children developing severe educational subnormality is similar (396).

Prematurity with Neurologic Complications

Modern methods of perinatal care have brightened the outlook in terms of survival of even the smallest premature infant. However, concurrent with a decrease in neonatal mortality, there has been an increase in the incidence of neurologic handicaps in the smallest group of preterm infants (201). The incidence of neurologic disabilities in infants born from 1978 to 1979 as compared with infants born from 1988 to 1989 is depicted in Table 5.11 (397). The increased incidence of neurologic disability in the smallest preterm infants could result from

TABLE 5.11. *Survival and incidence of early*
childhood disability in infants
with birth weights of 500 to 1,250 g

	Birth year (%)			
	1978 to 1979		1988 to 1989	
One-year survival				
500–749 g	3		41	
750–999 g	21		64	
1,000–1,250 g	67		86	
Specific disabilities				
Cerebral palsy	17		10	
500–749 g		0		15
750–999 g		13		10
1,000–1,250 g		18		9
Mental retardation	11		7	
500–749 g		0		15
750–999 g		20		4
1,000–1,250 g		9		6

Adapted from Robertson CMT, et al. Population-based study of the incidence, complexity, and severity of neurologic disability among survivors weighing 500–1,250 grams at birth: a comparison of two birth cohorts. *Pediatrics* 1992;90:750.

postnatal damage owing to the complications of their extreme immaturity, and in part could reflect the fact that a significant proportion of premature infants are neurologically compromised prior to birth.

The neurodevelopmental outcome of prematurity is determined by three factors: the presence and severity of PVL, the presence and severity of periventricular and IVH, and the effects of premature delivery and neonatal complications on cerebral cortical organization.

The presence of PVL as detected on ultrasound or by neuroimaging studies, predicts the evolution of spastic diplegia over the ensuing months. In addition, children with PVL have a significantly curtailed intellect. In the study by Pharoah and colleagues, 68% of children with spastic diplegia had an IQ of 70 or higher, 15% had moderate mental retardation, and 17% had severe mental retardation (398). Visual perceptual deficits and other cognitive disorders are common in the group of children with PVL who appear to have grossly normal intelligence.

Several studies indicate that children who had sustained an uncomplicated IVH (grades I or II)

have subtle neurologic deficits. Most of these are not apparent during the first few years of life, but can be documented when follow-up examinations are performed between 5 and 7 years of age or later (399–401). The risk of developing neurologic deficits is significantly increased for infants who have sustained a major IVH. In the series of Fazzi and colleagues, only 20% of infants who sustained this lesion were considered to have developed normally at 2 years of age. By 5 to 7 years of age, this figure had declined to 8% (401). Other follow-up studies have yielded similar results (399,402).

The cause of the cognitive and attention deficits of premature infants who are grossly normal neurologically is not clear. Based on experimental work of Ghosh and Shatz (403), Volpe has postulated that neurons in the subependymal germinative zone, the subplate neurons, which are involved in cerebral cortical organization, are disrupted by the presence of even minor geminal matrix hemorrhages or PVL (404). Their injury could lead to the variety of cortical deficits that are so common in small premature infants.

Numerous follow-up studies have been done on small preterm infants. The earlier reports were relatively optimistic; more recent series published in the 1980s or 1990s have noted a significant incidence of cognitive and behavioral abnormalities that lead to learning disabilities. As a rule, these deficits are not apparent during the first 2 to 3 years of life. Hirata and colleagues found that in a group of infants with birth weights between 501 and 750 g, of the 40% who survived, 66% appeared normal, some 20% had borderline or low average IQs, and approximately 10% had significant neurologic sequelae (405). Kitchen and coworkers examined infants with birth weights between 500 and 999 g at 2 years of age. Their results were similar, with 68% of surviving infants born between 1985 and 1987 having no apparent functional handicap (406). The experience of Collin and coworkers who followed infants into their preschool years differs significantly. They observed a downward drift in performance between infancy and preschool, with only approximately one-third of infants who were deemed developmentally normal when seen between 12 and 25 months of age performing in the normal range when reassessed at approximately 4 years of age (407). Hack and coworkers believe that perinatal growth failure, as reflected in a subnormal head circumference at 8 months of age, predicts impaired cognitive function and academic achievement. Because most of these infants had a normal head circumference at birth, postnatal events are responsible for impairment in head growth, and, by inference, brain maturation (408). The studies more recently published continue to show similar results (409,410).

In most series, the risk of cerebral palsy appears to be greater in the small-for-date infant than in the preterm infant of comparable weight (411).

Child with Cerebral Palsy as an Adult

The ultimate social adjustment of the patient with cerebral palsy is determined primarily by the severity of the physical and mental handicap. Individuals who can be predicted to be unable to work are those with an IQ under 50, nonambulatory, and without communication skills, and who need assistance in using their hands. Those predicted for sheltered work are those with IQs between 50 and 79, who walk and have some communication skills (412). Generally, mental handicap is less of a barrier to useful employment than physical handicap. In the series of Sala and Grant, all children with spastic hemiparesis became ambulatory. Children with spastic diplegia became ambulatory in 86% to 91% of cases, with those who were able to sit independently by 2 years of age having the best prognosis for ambulation (413). Patients with hemiplegia are most often able to become competitive, approximately one-third of them being economically productive. One-fourth of patients with extrapyramidal disorders are ultimately able to work competitively (241). The outlook for patients with spastic quadriparesis is far worse. In the series of Crothers and Paine, published in 1959, none of the adult patients with spastic quadriparesis was gainfully employed (187). Also important in the ultimate prognosis is the presence or absence of

associated disabilities, including seizures, and impairment of vision or hearing. Adult subjects with cerebral palsy develop a variety of new functional disabilities. These include lower extremity contractures, scoliosis, cervical pain, and back pain (414). Finally, and most difficult to evaluate when first seeing a patient, is the attitude of the patient and his or her family to the disability, and the stability of the home in view of the severe and chronic emotional trauma caused by cerebral palsy (412).

Various estimates of life expectancy of children with cerebral palsy have been published. As a rule, life expectancy in the mildly to moderately disabled children is only slightly curtailed (415). Life expectancy for the profoundly handicapped and immobile child, however, is severely curtailed (416).

PERINATAL INJURY TO THE SPINAL CORD

Although spinal birth injuries were first described during the nineteenth century, much of the understanding of them can be attributed to the classic papers of Crothers (417), Ford (418), and Crothers and Putnam (419). Relatively common in the early 1900s, this type of birth injury has become less common with improved obstetric practice, and by 1959 it constituted only 0.6% of the series of children with cerebral palsy encountered by Crothers and Paine (187).

Pathogenesis and Pathology

Perinatal traumatic lesions of the spinal cord result more commonly from stretching of the cord than from compression or transection (420). Longitudinal or lateral traction to the infant's neck or excessive torsion, particularly in the course of a difficult breech delivery, stretches the cord, its covering meninges, the surface vessels, and the nerve roots. Lesions are most frequent in the lower cervical and upper thoracic regions (421). The most common gross pathologic findings are epidural hemorrhage, dural laceration with subdural hemorrhage, tears of the nerve roots, laceration and distortion of the cord, and focal hemorrhage and malacia within the cord (420). Ischemic lesions of the cord are less common. Gross or petechial hemorrhages also can be seen within the substance of the cord, and myelination of the tracts can be impaired above the transection (422).

Clinical Manifestations

Three-fourths of infants who suffer a spinal birth injury had a difficult breech delivery, with arrest of the aftercoming head. As a rule, children with cephalic presentation develop upper cervical lesions, whereas cervical cord damage resulting from breech delivery involves the lower cervical cord (423). When damage to the cord is severe, the neonate dies during labor or soon after. With a less extensive injury, infants show respiratory depression and generalized hypotonia, or flaccid paraplegia (424). Associated urinary retention and abdominal distention with paradoxic respirations occur (425). In addition to impaired motor function, sensation and perspiration are absent below the level of injury. The deep tendon reflexes usually cannot be elicited during the neonatal period, and mass reflex movements do not become apparent until later.

In approximately 20% of cases, damage to the brachial plexus also can be documented. In other cases, the lower brainstem is involved as well, with consequent bulbar signs.

The clinical picture after complete transection of the spinal cord is discussed in Chapter 8. A high percentage of survivors have normal intelligence.

Diagnosis

The presence of poor muscle tone and flaccid weakness involving all extremities or only the legs after a breech extraction should suggest a cord injury. Although not easy to demonstrate, loss of sensory function should always be sought.

Neuromuscular disorders, notably infantile spinal muscular atrophy (Werdnig-Hoffmann disease), are not associated with loss of sensory function or loss of sphincter control. Of the other neuromuscular disorders, congenital myasthenia gravis is diagnosed by reversibility of symptoms after injection of anticholinesterase drugs (see Chapter 14).

Occasionally, an infant with a congenital tumor of the cervical or lumbar cord presents a clinical picture akin to that of a spinal cord injury. Abnormalities of the skin along the posterior lumbosacral midline, including dimpling, hemangiomas, or tufts of hair, are commonly seen in congenital tumor of the lumbar cord (426). Neuroimaging studies are diagnostic.

Treatment and Prognosis

In most infants, fractures or fracture dislocations of the spine are absent, and the treatment is that outlined in Chapter 8 for spinal cord injuries of older children. Although the majority of clinically apparent spinal birth injuries are severe and irreversible, milder degrees of injury are potentially reversible.

PERINATAL INJURIES OF CRANIAL NERVES

Facial Nerve

The most common cranial nerve to be involved in birth trauma is the facial nerve. According to Hepner (427), some facial nerve injury is evident in 6% of neonates. The injury results from pressure of the sacral prominence of the maternal pelvis against the facial nerve distal to its emergence from the stylomastoid foramen (pes anserinus). Less often, compression results from forceps application. These insults are more likely to produce swelling of tissue around the nerve, than complete or partial anatomic interruption of the fibers.

The degree of facial paresis ranges from complete loss of function in all three main branches to weakness limited to a small group of muscles. One common picture is a mild paresis of the lower portion of the face, particularly the depressor muscle of the lower lip and the depressor muscle of the angle of the mouth, which is manifested most clearly when the infant cries by a failure in downward movement of the affected corner of the mouth. Because the mentalis muscle, innervated by the same nerve fibers as the depressor anguli oris, usually is unaffected, the condition probably reflects a maldevelopment rather than perinatal trauma (see Table 4.14) (428).

In most instances, the facial nerve palsy is mild, and some improvement becomes evident within a week. In the more severe cases, the start of recovery can be delayed for several months. Electrodiagnostic studies can be used to provide information on the extent and cause of nerve damage. The ability to produce contraction of the muscle by stimulating the nerve implies that the conductivity of the nerve is only partially interrupted and suggests a favorable prognosis. Good recovery is possible, however, even when electric reactions are completely absent (429). In traumatic facial nerve palsy, electrical studies performed within 48 hours of birth are normal and do not become abnormal until 72 or more hours. By contrast, the initial electrical study results are abnormal in congenital developmental weakness (430). Another less common traumatic cause for facial nerve palsy present at birth includes a basilar skull fracture. Möbius syndrome (see Chapter 4) generally involves a bilateral facial palsy, often accompanied by weakness of one or both abducens nerves or of other cranial nerves. Occasionally, Möbius syndrome is limited to one side of the face, or even one part of the face, and can be associated with the Poland syndrome (hypoplasia of the pectoralis major, and nipple and syndactyly of the hand). In Goldenhar syndrome hypoplasia of the facial musculature is associated with anomalies of the ear and vertebral anomalies.

Treatment of the facial nerve palsy is limited to protection of the eye by application of methylcellulose drops and by taping the paralytic lid. Electric stimulation of the nerve does not hasten recovery. Neurosurgical repair of the nerve should be considered only when evidence suggests that the nerve is severed.

Other Cranial Nerves

Conjunctival and retinal hemorrhages are common in the newborn infant, but birth injury involving the optic nerve exclusively is relatively rare. Unilateral and bilateral optic atrophy result from direct injury to the nerve through fracture of the orbit, or less often through the base of the skull (431,432).

A transient postnatal paralysis of the abducens and oculomotor nerves is occasionally encountered. Paralysis of the oculomotor nerve can take the form of a transient postnatal ptosis (433). Congenital suprabulbar paresis, as first delineated by Worster-Drought (434), is considered in Chapter 4. Symmetric tegmental infarcts of the brainstem sometimes extend as far caudally as the lower medulla and may involve the hypoglossal nuclei or the intramedullary course of their axons, causing atrophy and fasciculation of the tongue that may suggest spinal muscular atrophy (Werdnig-Hoffmann disease).

Hearing is impaired in approximately one-fourth of children with cerebral palsy. Perinatal asphyxia is accompanied by hemorrhages in the inner ear and damage to the auditory pathway within the brainstem (435). These injuries can be documented by the brainstem auditory-evoked potentials. An injury to the peripheral portion of the auditory pathway results in a heightened threshold and a prolonged latency of all responses, whereas an injury to the brainstem results in a prolonged latency of waves, which represents activity beyond the point of injury. Both types of abnormalities have been encountered in asphyxiated neonates (436,437). Hecox and Cone stress the prognostic value of a diminished amplitude of wave V, which reflects midbrain function relative to wave I, which reflects the activity of the VIII nerve. They have found that an abnormal amplitude ratio is an excellent predictor of a poor outcome of asphyxial injury to both premature and term infants (438).

PERINATAL INJURIES OF PERIPHERAL NERVES

Brachial Plexus

Although perinatal injuries of the peripheral nerves were first described by Smellie (439), the present-day understanding of the interrelationship between palsies of the upper extremity and injuries of the brachial plexus comes from a group of nineteenth century French neurologists. This includes Danyau (440) and Duchenne (441), who were the first to describe obstetric injuries to the fifth and sixth cervical roots (Erb-Duchenne palsy), and Klumpke (442), who described the lesion of the lower trunk of the cervical plexus that now bears her name.

Pathogenesis and Pathology

As a rule, brachial plexus injuries result from stretching of the plexus owing to turning the head away from the shoulder in a difficult cephalic presentation of a large infant. An injury also can be consequent to stretching of the brachial plexus owing to traction on the shoulder in the course of delivering the aftercoming head in a breech presentation (443,444). The condition has been reported in a few instances after delivery by cesarean section (445). However, to date whatever scant evidence exists for a classical brachial plexus injury resulting from intrauterine maladaptation is principally based on faulty interpretation of EMG (446,447). When intrauterine palsies do occur, they are characterized by limb atrophy and abnormal dermatoglyphics at birth (448).

In most instances, the brachial plexus is compressed by hemorrhage and edema within the nerve sheath. Less often, there is an actual tear of the nerves or avulsion of the roots from the spinal cord occurs, with segmental damage to the gray matter of the spinal cord (443). With traction, the fifth cervical root gives way first, then the sixth, and so on down the plexus. Thus, the mildest plexus injuries involve only C5 and C6, and the more severe involve the entire plexus (444).

Clinical Manifestations

The incidence of brachial plexus injury in 1994 as determined from the Swedish Medical Birth Registry was 2.2 per 1,000 births (449). This figure should be contrasted with an incidence of 1.3 per 1,000 births in 1980, a significant increase over the course of the past 15 years.

The incidence is 45 times greater in infants with birth weights more than 4,500 g, than at birth weights less than 3,500 g (449). In approximately 80% of infants, Erb-Duchenne paralysis is confined to the upper brachial plexus (450). Involvement was unilateral in approximately 95% of instances in the series of Eng and coworkers (448). One of us (J.H.M.) has seen an infant with what appeared to be bilateral brachial plexus injury who had agenesis of the biceps muscles. The right side is more frequently affected than the left, with the ratio in the series of Eng and coworkers being 51:45 (450). The weakness is recognized soon after delivery, with the involved arm assuming a characteristic posture. The shoulder is adducted and internally rotated, the elbow extended, the forearm pronated, and the wrist occasionally flexed. This position results from paralysis of the deltoid, the supraspinatus and infraspinatus, biceps, and brachioradialis muscles. The Moro reflex is absent or diminished on the affected side, but the grasp reflex remains intact. Unlike in the healthy neonate, the biceps reflex is abolished or is less active than the triceps reflex. In most infants, a sensory loss cannot be demonstrated, although occasionally cutaneous sensation is lost over the deltoid region and the adjacent radial surface of the upper arm.

Fractures of the clavicle or humerus, slippage of the capital head of the radius, and subluxation of the shoulder and the cervical spine often accompany a brachial plexus injury (444). When a significant degree of injury to the fourth cervical root is present, phrenic nerve paralysis can accompany injury to the upper brachial plexus (451). An affected infant can show signs of respiratory distress, including tachypnea, cyanosis, and decreased movement of the affected hemithorax. When the phrenic nerve palsy is unaccompanied by injury to the brachial plexus, as occurs occasionally, the condition can mimic congenital pulmonary or heart disease (452,453).

In the more severely involved infants, 12% in the series of Eng and colleagues (448), the entire brachial plexus is damaged, and the arm is completely paralyzed. The limb is flaccid, the Moro and grasp reflexes are unelicitable, deep tendon reflexes are absent, and sensory loss occurs over a portion of the extremity.

Isolated paralysis of the lower part of the brachial plexus (Klumpke paralysis) is relatively uncommon. It constituted only 2.5% of brachial plexus birth palsies in the experience of Ford (209), and a spinal cord lesion should be suspected whenever the paralysis involves the intrinsic muscles of the hand (448). The clinical picture of a lower plexus injury includes weakness of the flexors of the wrist and fingers, an absent grasp reflex, and a unilateral Horner syndrome caused by involvement of the cervical sympathetic nerves. Loss of sensation and sudomotor function over the hand can sometimes be demonstrated. Interference with the sympathetic innervation of the eye results in a delay or failure in pigmentation of the iris, and it is one of several causes for heterochromia iridis (454).

Diagnosis

The diagnosis of brachial plexus injury is usually readily apparent from the posture of the affected arm, and from the absence of voluntary and reflex movements. Radiographic examinations can detect associated fractures, usually of the clavicle, humerus, or both, whereas fluoroscopy can be used to ascertain any limitation of diaphragmatic movement. In severe injuries causing avulsion of the spinal roots and bleeding into the subarachnoid space, the CSF can be bloody. MRI can be used to visualize the brachial plexus and demonstrates root evulsions (455,456). EMG performed 2 to 3 weeks after the injury can confirm the extent of denervation. Because fibrillation potentials are seen in the proximal musculature of some healthy newborns during the first month of life and in the distal musculature during the first 3 months of life, an indication that the muscles are not completely innervated, both sides should always be studied (457). Repeated EMG examinations at 6-week intervals indicate the degree of recovery (448).

Congenital Horner syndrome can occur in the absence of trauma and can be associated with anomalies of the cervical vertebrae, enterogenous cysts, or congenital nerve deafness (458). The association of heterochromia iridis, congenital nerve deafness, white forelock, broad root of the nose, and lateral displacement of the medial canthi of the eyes and inferior lacrimal puncta is well recognized under the term *Waardenburg syndrome* (see Chapter 4) (458).

Treatment and Prognosis

Gentle passive exercises of the affected arm should be instituted at approximately 1 week after birth. The infant's sleeve should be pinned in a natural position, rather than in abduction and external rotation, as many texts suggest (209). Follow-up studies indicate that overimmobilization of the affected arm is conducive to contractures and deformities that can persist despite spontaneous recovery of nerve function (459).

Selection criteria for surgical intervention have not been established, and the good surgical results with early intervention should be tempered by reflecting on the high incidence of improvement with conservative management (460,461). In the series of Michelow and colleagues, 92% of infants recovered spontaneously (462). The presence of elbow flexion and elbow, wrist, and finger extension at 3 months of age was predictive of a good recovery. Eng and colleagues believe that if contraction occurs in the biceps and deltoid muscles by 2 months of age, shoulder function will recover almost completely. Mild sequelae, such as winging of the scapula, and limited shoulder flexion and abduction are common, however (448). If no improvement is noted in 3 to 6 months, surgical exploration of the brachial plexus should be considered, with repair of the damaged segment. In most instances in which poor recovery occurs, nerve damage is caused by avulsion of the spinal roots and surgical repair would, therefore, not be expected to result in any improvement.

In most cases, most of the recovery occurs between 2 and 14 months of age, with the condition becoming essentially stationary thereafter (449). Rossi and colleagues, however, believe that significant improvement is still possible up to the start of school (463).

As a rule, when the entire plexus is involved and an associated Horner syndrome exists, the outlook for full recovery is poor. Almost all children are left with hypoplasia of the limb and well-defined motor deficits, usually more marked in the proximal musculature. Contractures at the shoulder and elbow are common; approximately one-third have a clear-cut sensory deficit whose location is variable. Trophic changes involving the fingers are unusual (450,463). They were seen in 2% of children in the series of Eng and colleagues (448).

Some infants have an apparently good return of neuromuscular function and sensation, yet are unable to use the affected arm (450). Probably, transitory sensory motor deprivation in early life impairs the development of normal movement patterns and the organization of cortical body image. This would be in line with what has been observed with respect to the organization of the visual system after early deafferentation (464).

Other Peripheral Nerves

Birth injuries to the other peripheral nerves are relatively uncommon. Injury to the lumbosacral plexus can rarely occur after a frank breech delivery. Sciatic nerve palsy has been observed after injection of hypertonic glucose into the umbilical artery. It is caused by thrombosis of the inferior gluteal artery and is accompanied by circulatory changes in the buttock (465,466).

Palsies of the radial nerve (467) and obturator nerve (468) also have been recorded. The former is generally the consequence of intrauterine nerve compression.

Idiopathic Torticollis

Because idiopathic torticollis, a relatively common condition, is in some instances believed to be related to perinatal trauma, it is considered in this chapter.

Torticollis, meaning *twisted neck*, is a syndrome characterized by contracture of the sternocleidomastoid muscle accompanied by a tilt of the head to the affected side and a rotation of the neck so that the chin points to the opposite shoulder. Asymmetry of the skull and facial bones can be present.

The condition can be congenital, acquired, spasmodic, or intermittent.

Congenital muscular torticollis is encountered most frequently. It is characterized by the presence of a tumor in the affected sternocleidomastoid muscle. In the majority of cases, the tumor develops during the first few weeks of life, gradually disappearing by age 46 months. In the experience of Coventry and Harris (469), the tumor disappeared at a mean age of 14 weeks.

Considerable debate surrounds the cause of this condition. Although some instances are associated with congenital malformations of the cervical spine, abnormalities in the function of the extraocular muscles, and tumors of the brainstem or spinal cord, the majority of cases is truly idiopathic. The two most likely etiologic factors are restricted movement of the head owing to an unusual fetal posture or amniotic adhesions, and perinatal trauma to the sternocleidomastoid muscle (470). A relatively high incidence of breech deliveries (28% to 40%) is compatible with either cause.

Pathologic examination of the muscle usually reveals extensive fibrosis and nonspecific myopathic changes. When the condition is chronic, evidence exists for denervation and reinnervation, probably secondary to repeated episodes of minor trauma to the muscle, which results in an entrapment neuropathy of the accessory nerve. The innervation of the sternocleidomastoid is unique in the body because the accessory nerve to the clavicular head passes through the sternal head and may become entrapped or compressed by fibrosis, producing denervation of the clavicular head (470). Separate arterial supplies predispose to ischemia in the sternal head, resulting in focal myopathy with fibrosis (470). The sternocleidomastoid tumor is not a neoplasm, either benign or malignant; it is composed of actively proliferating fibroblastic tissue that surrounds fragments of atrophic or degenerating muscle fibers (471,472). The initial tumor is usually a hematoma.

Caputo and coworkers have noted that when torticollis is the consequence of disturbed function of the extraocular muscles it disappears when the infant is placed into the supine position, or when one eye is occluded (473).

Considerable debate surrounds the treatment of congenital torticollis. However, the majority of clinicians opts for early physical therapy measures such as stretching and massage, rather than surgical sectioning of the sternocleidomastoid muscle, removal of the tumor, or a combination of the two procedures (474). With physical therapy, the torticollis resolves in 70% of children by 12 months of age, regardless of its severity or the presence or absence of focal fibrosis (475).

Acquired torticollis most commonly is associated with an infratentorial tumor. It also can be seen with colloid cysts of the third ventricle, syringomyelia, and spinal cord tumors. On rare occasions, it develops in the course of a progressive muscular disease.

The association of torticollis with hiatus hernia and gastroesophageal reflux (Sandifer syndrome) was first reported by Kinsbourne (476). Torticollis can be present at birth; generally, no shortening of the sternocleidomastoid muscle occurs.

Spasmodic torticollis, occurring in isolation or progressing to a focal, segmental, or generalized dystonia, is rare during childhood. This condition is discussed to a greater extent in Chapter 2.

Paroxysmal torticollis is characterized by recurrent episodes of head tilting starting in infancy. These episodes are sometimes accompanied by vomiting and ataxia. Generally, symptoms subside within a few hours or days. Attacks occur at monthly intervals, and the condition remits spontaneously within a few years. The EEG and caloric tests during an attack are usually normal. A family history of similar attacks is not uncommon, and a number of children have ultimately developed migraine (477).

REFERENCES

1. Little WJ. Course of lectures on the deformities of human frame. *Lancet* 1843;1:318–322.
2. Cazauvielh JB. *Recherches sur l'agénése cérébrale et la paralysie congéniale*, Paris: Migneret, 1827.
3. Friede RL. *Developmental neuropathology*, 2nd ed. Berlin, New York: Springer-Verlag, 1989.
4. Rorke LB. *Pathology of perinatal brain injury*. New York: Raven Press, 1982.
5. Volpe JJ. *Neurology of the newborn*, 3rd ed. Philadelphia: WB Saunders, 1995.
6. Kubli F, et al., eds. *Perinatal events and brain damage in surviving children*. Berlin: Springer-Verlag, 1988.
7. Zelson C, Lee SJ, Pearl M. The incidence of skull fractures underlying cephalhematomas in newborn infants. *J Pediatr* 1974;85:371–373.
8. Kozinn PJ, et al. Massive hemorrhage–scalps of newborn infants. *Am J Dis Child* 1964;108:413–417.
9. Chadwick LM, Pemberton PJ, Kurinczuk JJ. Neonatal subgaleal haematoma: associated risk factors, complications and outcome. *J Paediatr Child Health* 1996;32:228–232.
10. Gröntoft O. Intracerebral and meningeal haemorrhages in perinatally deceased infants. II. Intracerebral haemorrhages: a pathologico-anatomical and obstetrical study. *Acta Obstet Gynecol Scand* 1953; 32:308–334.
11. Wigglesworth JS, Husemeyer RP. Intracranial birth trauma in vaginal breech delivery: the continued importance of injury to the occipital bone. *Br J Obstet Gynecol* 1977;84:684–691.
12. Hanigan WC, et al. Tentorial hemorrhage associated with vacuum extraction. *Pediatrics* 1990;85:534–539.
13. Avrahami E, Frishman E, Minz M. CT demonstration of intracranial haemorrhage in term newborn following vacuum extractor delivery. *Neuroradiology* 1993;35:107–108.
14. Menezes AH, Smith DE, Bell WE. Posterior fossa hemorrhage in the term neonate. *Neurosurgery* 1983;13:452–456.
15. Gunn TR, Mok PM, Becroft DMO. Subdural hemorrhage in utero. *Pediatrics* 1985;76:605–610.
16. Gröntoft O. Intracranial haemorrhage and blood-brain barrier problems in the newborn: pathologico-anatomical and experimental investigation. *Acta Pathol Microbiol Scand Suppl* 1954;100:1–109.
17. Blank NK, Strand R, Gilles FH. Posterior fossa subdural hematomas in neonates. *Arch Neurol* 1978;35:108–111.
18. Fishman MA, et al. Successful conservative management of cerebellar hematomas in term neonates. *J Pediatr* 1981;98:466–468.
19. Ravenel SD. Posterior fossa hemorrhage in the newborn. *Pediatrics* 1979;64:39–42.
20. Towbin A. Latent spinal cord and brain stem injury in newborn infants. *Dev Med Child Neurol* 1969;11:54–68.
21. Leviton A, Nelson KB. Problems with definitions and classifications of newborn encephalopathy. *Pediatr Neurol* 1992;8:85–90.
22. Levene MI, Kornberg J, Williams THC. The incidence and severity of post-asphyxial encephalopathy in full-term infants. *Early Hum Develop* 1985;11:21–26.
23. Levene MI, et al. Severe birth asphyxia and abnormal cerebral blood-flow velocity. *Dev Med Child Neurol* 1989;31:427–434.
24. Brown JK, et al. Neurological aspects of perinatal asphyxia. *Dev Med Child Neurol* 1974;16:567–580.
25. Low JA, Robertson DM, Simpson LL. Temporal relationships of neuropathologic conditions caused by perinatal asphyxia. *Am J Obstet Gynecol* 1989;160:608–614.
26. Volpe JJ. Hypoxic-ischemic encephalopathy: biochemical and physiologic aspects. In: Volpe JJ. *Neurology of the newborn*, 3rd ed. Philadelphia: WB Saunders, 1994:211–259.

27. Gluckman PD, Williams CE. When and why do brain cells die? *Dev Med Child Neurol* 1992;34: 1010–1021.

28. Dugan LL, Choi DW. Hypoxic-ischemic brain injury and oxidative stress. In: Siegel GJ, ed. *Basic neurochemistry: molecular, cellular and medical aspects.* 6th ed. Philadelphia: Lippincott–Raven Publishers 1999;711–729.

29. Hill A. Current concepts of hypoxic-ischemic cerebral injury in the term newborn. *Pediatr Neurol* 1991;7: 317–325.

30. Bennet L, et al. The cerebral hemodynamic response to asphyxia and hypoxia in the near-term fetal sheep as measured by near infrared spectroscopy. *Pediatr Res* 1998;44:951–957.

31. van Bel F, et al. Changes in cerebral hemodynamics and oxygenation in the first 24 hours after birth asphyxia. *Pediatrics* 1993;92:365–372.

32. Martínez-Orgado J, et al. Endothelial factors and autoregulation during pressure changes in isolated newborn piglet cerebral arteries. *Pediatr Res* 1998;44: 161–167.

33. Del Toro J, Louis PT, Goddard-Finegold J. Cerebrovascular regulation and neonatal brain injury. *Pediatr Neurol* 1991;7:3–12.

34. Pryds O. Control of cerebral circulation in the high-risk neonate. *Ann Neurol* 1991;30:321–329.

35. Tyszczuk L, et al. Cerebral blood flow is independent of mean arterial blood pressure in preterm infants undergoing intensive care. *Pediatrics* 1998;102: 337–341.

36. Lupton BA, et al. Brain swelling in the asphyxiated term newborn: pathogenesis and outcome. *Pediatrics* 1988;82:139–146.

37. Vannucci RC, Christensen MA, Yager JY. Nature, time-course, and extent of cerebral edema in perinatal hypoxic-ischemic brain damage. *Pediatr Neurol* 1993;9:29–34.

38. Gluckman PD, et al. Asphyxial brain injury—the role of the IGF system. *Mol Cell Endocrin* 1998;140: 95–99.

39. Vannucci RC, Duffy TE. Cerebral metabolism in newborn dogs during reversible asphyxia. *Ann Neurol* 1977;1:528–534.

40. Szatkowski M, Attwell D. Triggering and execution of neuronal death in brain ischemia: two phases of glutamate release by different mechanisms. *Trends Neurosci* 1994;17:359–365.

41. Martin RL, Lloyd HGE, Cowan AI. The early events of oxygen and glucose deprivation: setting the scene for neuronal death? *Trends Neurosci* 1994;17:251–257.

42. Hanrahan JD, et al. Cerebral metabolism within 18 hours of birth asphyxia: a proton magnetic resonance spectroscopy study. *Pediatr Res* 1996;39:584–590.

43. Hope PL, et al. Cerebral energy metabolism studied with phosphorus NMR spectroscopy in normal and birth-asphyxiated infants. *Lancet* 1984;2:366–370.

44. Azzopardi D, et al. Prognosis of newborn infants with hypoxic-ischemic brain injury assessed by phosphorus magnetic resonance spectroscopy. *Pediatr Res* 1989;25:441–451.

45. Delivoria-Papadopoulos M, Misbra OP. Mechanisms of cerebral injury in perinatal asphyxia and strategies for prevention. *J Pedatr* 1998;132:S30–S34.

46. Rothman SM, Olney JW. Glutamate and the pathophysiology of hypoxic-ischemic brain damage. *Ann Neurol* 1986;19:105–111.

47. Rothman SM, Olney JW. Excitotoxicity and the NMDA receptor: trends in neurosciences. 1987;10: 299–302.

48. Choi DW. Calcium still center-stage in hypoxic-ischemic neuronal death. *Trends Neurosci* 1995;18: 58–60.

49. Lindvall O, et al. Neurotrophins and brain insults. *Trends Neurosci* 1994;17:490–496.

50. Cheng Y, et al. Marked age-dependent neuroprotection by brain-derived neurotrophic factor against neonatal hypoxic-ischemic brain injury. *Ann Neurol* 1997;41: 521–529.

51. Cheng Y, et al. Caspase inhibitor affords neuroprotection with delayed administration in a rat model of neonatal hypoxic-ischemic brain injury. *J Clin Invest* 1998;101:1992–1999.

52. Blumenfeld KS, et al. Regional expression of cfos and heat shock protein-70 mRNA following hypoxia-ischemia in immature rat brain. *J Cereb Blood Flow Metab* 1992;12:987–995.

53. Fellman V, Raivio KO. Reperfusion injury as the mechanism of brain damage after perinatal asphyxia. *Pediatr Res* 1997;41:599–606.

54. Ringsted T, et al. Expression of c-*fos*, tyrosine hydroxylase, and neuropeptide mRNA in the rat brain around birth: effects of hypoxia and hypothermia. *Pediatr Res* 1994;37:15–20.

55. Vannucci RC, Yager JY. Glucose, lactic acid, and perinatal hypoxic-ischemic brain damage. *Pediatr Neurol* 1992;8:3–12.

56. Monaghan DT, Bridges RJ, Cotman CW. The excitatory amino acid receptors: their classes, pharmacology, and distinct properties in the function of the central nervous system. *Annu Rev Pharmacol Toxicol* 1989;29:365–402.

57. Auer RN, Siesjö BK. Biological differences between ischemia, hypoglycemia, and epilepsy. *Ann Neurol* 1988;24:699–707.

58. Choi DW, Rothman SM. The role of glutamate neurotoxicity in hypoxic-ischemic neuronal death. *Annu Rev Neurosci* 1990;13:171–182.

59. Thurston JH, McDougal DB. Effect of ischemia on metabolism of the brain of the newborn mouse. *Am J Physiol* 1969;216:348–352.

60. Greenamyre T, et al. Evidence for transient perinatal glutamatergic innervation of globus pallidus. *J Neurosc* 1987;7:1022–1030.

61. Ferriero DM, et al. Selective sparing of NADPH-diaphorase neurons in neonatal hypoxia-ischemia. *Ann Neurol* 1988;24:670–676.

62. Mallard EC, et al. Repeated asphyxia causes loss of striatal projection neurons in the fetal sheep brain. *Neuroscience* 1995;65:827–836.

63. Ranck JB, Windle WF. Brain damage in the monkey, macaca mulatta, by asphyxia neonatorum. *Exp Neurol* 1959;1:130–154.

64. Myers RE. Experimental models of perinatal brain damage: relevance to human pathology. In: Gluck L, ed. *Intrauterine asphyxia and developing fetal brain.* Chicago: Year Book Medical Publishers, 1977: 37–97.

65. Norman MG. Perinatal brain damage. *Perspect Pediatr Pathol* 1978;4:41–92.

66. Brown AW, Brierley JB. The earliest alterations in rat neurones and astrocytes after anoxia-ischaemia. *Acta Neuropathol* 1973;23:9–22.

67 Lyen KR, et al. Multicystic encephalomacia due to fetal viral encephalitis. *Eur J Pediatr* 1981;137: 11–16.

68. Brann AW, Myers RE. Central nervous system findings in the newborn monkey following severe in utero partial asphyxia. *Neurology* 1975;25:327–338.

69. Towbin A. Cerebral hypoxic damage in fetus and newborn: basic patterns and their clinical significance. *Arch Neurol* 1969;20:35–43.

70. Skov H, Lou H, Pederson H. Perinatal brain ischaemia: impact at four years of age. *Dev Med Child Neurol* 1984;26:353–357.

71. Banker BQ, Larroche J-C. Periventricular leukomacia of infancy. *Arch Neurol* 1962;7:386–410.

72. de Reuck J, Chatta AS, Richardson EP. Pathogenesis and evolution of periventricular leukomalacia in infancy. *Arch Neurol* 1972;27:229–236.

73. Shuman RM, Selednik LL. Periventricular leukomacia: a one-year autopsy study. *Arch Neurol* 1980;37: 231–235.

74. Iida K, et al. Neuropathologic study of newborns with prenatal-onset leukomalacia. *Pediatr Neurol* 1993;9:45–48.

75. Deguchi K, Oguchi K, Matsuura N, et al. Periventricular leukomalacia: relation to gestational age and axonal injury. *Pediatr Neurol* 1999;20:370–374.

76. Takashima S, Tanaka K. Development of cerebrovascular architecture and its relationship to periventricular leukomalacia. *Arch Neurol* 1978;35:11–16.

77. Nelson MD, Gonzalez-Gomez I, Gilles FH. Search for human telencephalic ventriculofugal arteries. *AJNR Am J Neuroradiol* 1991;12:215–222.

78. Blankenberg FG, et al. Impaired cerebrovascular autoregulation after hypoxic-ischemic injury in extremely low-birth-weight neonates: detection with power and pulsed wave Doppler US. *Radiology* 1997;205:563–568.

79. Börch K, Greisen G. Blood flow distribution in the normal human preterm brain. *Pediatr Res* 1998;43: 28–33.

80. Young RS, Hernandez MJ, Yagel SK. Selective reduction of blood flow to white matter during hypotension in newborn dogs: a possible mechanism of periventricular leukomalacia. *Ann Neurol* 1982; 12:445–448.

81. Volpe JJ. Neurologic outcome of prematurity. *Arch Neurol* 1998;55:297–300.

82. Yonezawa M, et al. Cystine deprivation induces oligodendroglial death: rescue by free radical scavengers and by a diffusible glial factor. *J Neurochem* 1996;67:566–573.

83. Kinney HC, Back SA. Human oligodendroglial development: relationship to periventricular leukomalacia. *Semin Pediatr Neurol* 1998;5:180–189.

84. Barlow CF, et al. Spastic diplegia as a complication of interferon Alfa-2a treatment of hemangiomas of infancy. *J Pediatr* 1998;132:527–530.

85. Nelson KB, et al. Neonatal cytokines and coagulation factors in children with cerebral palsy. *Ann Neurol* 1998;44:665–675.

86. Grether JK, et al. Interferons and cerebral palsy. *J Pediatr* 1999;134:324–332.

87. Damman O, Leviton A. Maternal intrauterine infection, cytokines, and brain damage in the preterm infant. *Pediatr Res* 1997;42:1–8.

88. Zupan V, et al. Periventricular leukomalacia: risk factors revisited. *Dev Med Child Neurol* 1996;38: 1061–1067.

89. Perlman JM, Risser R, Broyles RS. Bilateral cystic periventricular leukomalacia in the premature infant: associated risk factors. *Pediatrics* 1996;97:822–827.

90. Baud O, et al. Antenatal glucocorticoid treatment and cystic periventricular leukomalacia in very premature infants. *N Engl J Med* 1999;341:1190–1196.

91. Murphy DJ, et al. Case-control study of antenatal and intrapartum risk factors for cerebral palsy in very preterm singleton babies. *Lancet* 1995;346: 1449–1454.

92. Hesser U, et al. Diagnosis of intracranial lesions in very low-birth-weight infants by ultrasound: incidence and association with potential risk factors. *Acta Paediatr Suppl* 1997;419:16–26.

93. Trounce JQ, et al. Clinical risk factors and periventricular leucomalacia. *Arch Dis Child* 1988;63: 17–22.

94. Koppelman AE. Blood pressure and cerebral ischemia in very low-birth-weight infants. *J Pediatr* 1990;116:1000–1002.

95. Ment LR, et al. Beagle puppy model of perinatal infarction: acute changes in cerebral blood flow and metabolism during hemorrhagic hypotension. *J Neurosurg* 1985;63:441–447.

96. Miall-Allen VM, DeVries LS, Whitelaw AGL. Mean arterial blood pressure and neonatal cerebral lesions. *Arch Dis Child* 1987;62:1068–1069.

97. Gray PH, et al. Maternal hypertension and neurodevelopmental outcome in very preterm infants. *Arch Dis Child Fetal Neonatal Ed* 1998;79:F88–F93.

98. Sinillo A, et al. Preeclampsia, preterm delivery, and infant cerebral palsy. *Eur J Obstet Gynecol Reprod Biol* 1998;77:151–155.

99. Hirtz DG, Nelson K. Magnesium sulfate and cerebral palsy in premature infants. *Curr Opin Pediatr* 1998;10:131–137.

100. Wilson-Costello D, et al. Perinatal correlates of cerebral palsy and other neurologic impairment among very-low-birth-weight children. *Pediatrics* 1998;102:315–322.

101. Pidcock FS, et al. Neurosonographic features of periventricular echodensities associated with cerebral palsy in preterm infants. *J Pediatr* 1990;116: 417–422.

102. Van Wezel-Meijler G, et al. Magnetic resonance imaging of the brain in premature infants during the neonatal period: normal phenomena and reflection of mild ultrasound abnormalities. *Neuropediatrics* 1998;29:89–96.

103. Rodiguez J, et al. Periventricular leukomalacia: ultrasonic and neuropathological correlations. *Dev Med Child Neurol* 1990;32:347–355.

104. DeVries LS, et al. Neurological electrophysiological and MRI abnormalities in infants with extensive cystic leukomalacia. *Neuropediatrics* 1987;18:61–66.

105. Fawer CL, et al. Periventricular leukomalacia: a correlative study between real-time ultrasound and autopsy findings. *Neuroradiology* 1985;27:292–300.

106. Perlman JM, et al. Relationship between periventricular intraparenchymal echodensities and germinal matrix-intraventricular hemorrhage in the very-low-birth-weight neonate. *Pediatrics* 1993;91:474–480.

107. Armstrong D, Norman MG. Periventricular leucomalacia in neonates: complications and sequelae. *Arch Dis Child* 1974;49:367–375.

108. Williams CE, et al. Outcome after ischemia in the developing sheep brain: an electroencephalographic and histological study. *Ann Neurol* 1992;31:14–21.

109. Freytag E, Lindenberg R. Neuropathological findings in patients of a hospital for the mentally deficient: a survey of 359 cases. *Johns Hopkins Med J* 1967;121:379–392.

110. Norman RM, Urich H, McMenemey WH. Vascular mechanisms of birth injury. *Brain* 1957;80:49–58.

111. Borit A, Herndon RM. The fine structure of plaques fibromyeliniques in ulegyria and in status marmoratus. *Acta Neuropathol* 1970;14:304–311.

112. Sarnat HB. Perinatal hypoxic/ischemic encephalopathy: neuropathological features. In: García JH, ed. *Neuropathology: the diagnostic approach.* St. Louis: Mosby 1997:541–580.

113. Norman MG. On the morphogenesis of ulegyria. *Acta Neuropathol* 1981;53:331–332.

114. Christensen E, Melchior J. Cerebral palsy: a clinical and neuropathologic study. *Clin Dev Med* 1967;25.

115. Anton G. Ueber die Betheiligung der grossen basalen Gehirnganglien bei Bewegungsstörungen und insbesondere bei Chorea: Mit Demonstrationen von Gehirnschnitten. *Wien Klin Wchschr* 1893;6: 859–861.

116. Vogt C, Vogt O. Zur Lehre der Erkrankungen des striären Systems. *J Psychol Neuro* 1919–1920;25: 627–846.

117. Denny-Brown D. *The basal ganglia.* Oxford: Oxford University Press, 1962.

118. Paternak JF, Gorey MT. The syndrome of acute near-total intrauterine asphyxia in the term infant. *Pediatr Neurol* 1998;18:391–398.

119. Chugani HT, Phelps ME, Mazziotta JC. Positron emission tomography study of human brain functional development. *Ann Neurol* 1987;22:487–497.

120. Menkes JH, Curran J. Clinical and magnetic resonance imaging correlates in children with extrapyramidal cerebral palsy. *AJNR Am J Neuroradiol* 1994;15:451–457.

121. Silverstein FS, et al. Hypoxia-ischemia produces focal disruption of glutamate receptors in the developing brain. *Dev Brain Res* 1987;34:33–39.

122. Meng SZ, Ohyu J, Takashima S. Changes in AMPA glutamate and dopamine D_2 receptors in hypoxic-ischemic basal ganglia necrosis. *Pediatr Neurol* 1997;17:139–143.

123. Martin LJ, et al. Hypoxia-ischemia causes abnormalities in glutamate transporters and death of astroglia and neurons in newborn striatum. *Ann Neurol* 1997;42:335–348.

124. Chen Y, et al. Perinatal asphyxia induces long-term changes in dopamine D1, D2, and D3 receptor binding in the rat brain. *Exp Neurol* 1997;146:74–80.

125. Courville CB. Structural alterations in the cerebellum in cases of cerebral palsy: their relation to residual symptomatology in the ataxic-atonic group. *Bull Los Angeles Neurol Soc* 1959;24:148–165.

126. Sarnat HB, Alcala H. Human cerebellar hypoplasia: a syndrome of diverse causes. *Arch Neurol* 1980;37: 300–305.

127. Adams RD, Prodhom LS, Rabinowicz T. Intrauterine brain death: neuroaxial reticular core necrosis. *Acta Neuropathol* 1977;40:41–49.

128. Azarellli B, et al. Hypoxic-ischemic encephalopathy in areas of primary myelination: a neuroimaging and PET study. *Pediatr Neurol* 1996;14:108–116.

129. Natsume J, et al. Clinical, neurophysiologic, and neuropathological features of an infant with brain damage of total asphyxia type (Myers). *Pediatr Neurol* 1995;13:61–64.

130. Roland EH, et al. Selective brainstem injury in an asphyxiated newborn. *Ann Neurol* 1988;23:89–92.

131. Friede RL. Ponto-subicular lesions in perinatal anoxia. *Arch Pathol* 1972;94:343–354.

132. Yates PO. Birth trauma to vertebral arteries. *Arch Dis Child* 1959;34:436–441.

133. Leech RW, Alvord CE Jr. Anoxic-ischemic encephalopathy in the human neonatal period: the significance of brainstem involvement. *Arch Neurol* 1977; 34: 109–113.

134. Skullerud K, Westre B. Frequency and prognostic significance of germinal matrix hemorrhage, periventricular leukomalacia, and pontosubicular necrosis in preterm infants. *Acta Neuropathol* 1986; 70:257–261.

135. Ahdab-Barmada M, Moosey J, Painter M. Pontosubicular necrosis and hyperoxemia. *Pediatrics* 1989;66:840–847.

136. Paneth N, et al. *Brain damage in the preterm infant.* London: MacKeith Press and Cambridge University Press, 1994.

137. Skullerud K, Torvik A, Skaare-Botner L. Progressive degeneration of the cerebral cortex in infancy. *Acta Neuropathol* 1973;24:153–160.

138. Schneider H, et al. Anoxic encephalopathy with predominant involvement of basal ganglia, brainstem, and spinal cord in the perinatal period. *Acta Neuropathol* 1975;32:2878–2980.

139. Pullicino P, et al. Pontine ischemic rarefaction. *Ann Neurol* 1995;37:460–466.

140. Ozawa H, et al. Ferritin immunohistochemical study on pontine nuclei from infants with pontosubicular neuron necrosis. *Brain Dev* 1995;17:20–23.

141. Brück Y, et al. Evidence for neuronal apoptosis in pontosubicular neuronal necrosis. *Neuropathol Appl Neurobiol* 1996;22:23–29.

142. Skullerud K, Skjaeraasen J. Clinicopathological study of germinal matrix hemorrhage, pontosubicular necrosis, and periventricular leukomalacia in stillborn. *Child Nerv Syst* 1988;4:88–91.

143. Mito T, et al. Clinicopathological study of pontosubicular necrosis. *Neuropediatrics* 1993;24: 204–207.

144. Clancy RR, Sladky JT, Rorke LB. Hypoxic-ischemic spinal cord injury following perinatal asphyxia. *Ann Neurol* 1989;25:185–189.

145. Barmada MA, Moosey J, Shuman RM. Cerebral infarction with arterial occlusion in neonates. *Ann Neurol* 1979;6:495–502.

146. Fujimoto S, et al. Neonatal cerebral infarction: symptoms, CT findings, and prognosis. *Brain Dev* 1992;14:48–52.

147. DeVries LS, et al. Localized cerebral infarction in the premature infant: an ultrasound diagnosis correlated with computed tomography and magnetic resonance imaging. *Pediatrics* 1988;81:36–40.

147a. Shevell MI, et al. Neonatal dural sinus thrombosis. *Pediatr Neurol* 1989;5:161–165.

147b. Voorhies TM, et al. Occlusive vascular disease in asphyxiated newborn infants. *J Pediatr* 1984;105: 92–96.

148. Dykes FD, et al. Intraventricular hemorrhage: a prospective evaluation of etiopathogenesis. *Pediatrics* 1980;66:42–49.
149. Wigglesworth JS. Current problems in brain pathology in the perinatal period. In Pape KE, Wigglesworth JS. *Perinatal brain lesions*. Boston: Blackwell Scientific Publications, 1989:1–23.
150. Mitchell W, O'Tuama L. Cerebral intraventricular hemorrhages in infants: a widening age spectrum. *Pediatrics* 1980;65:35–39.
151. Hayden CK, et al. Subependymal germinal matrix hemorrhage in full-term neonates. *Pediatrics* 1985;75:714–718.
152. Bergman I, et al. Intracerebral hemorrhage in the full-term neonatal infant. *Pediatrics* 1985;75:488–496.
153. Trounce JQ, Rutter N, Levene MI. Periventricular leucomalacia and intraventricular haemorrhage in the preterm neonate. *Arch Dis Child* 1986;61:1196–1202.
154. Investigators DEN. The correlation between placental pathology and intraventricular hemorrhage in the preterm infant. *Pediatr Res* 1998;43:15–19.
155. Ment LR, et al. Risk factors for early intraventricular hemorrhage in low birth weight infants. *J Pediatr* 1992;121:776–783.
156. Perlman JM, et al. Reduction in intraventricular hemorrhage by elimination of fluctuating cerebral blood-flow velocity in preterm infants with respiratory distress syndrome. *N Engl J Med* 1985;312:1353–1357.
157. McCord FB, et al. Surfactant treatment and incidence of intraventricular haemorrhage in severe respiratory distress syndrome. *Arch Dis Child* 1988;63:10–16.
158. Leviton A, VanMarter L, Kuban KCK. Respiratory distress syndrome and intracranial hemorrhage: cause or association? Inferences from surfactant clinical trials. *Pediatrics* 1989;84:915–922.
159. Jardine DS, Rogers K. Relationship of benzyl alcohol to kernicterus, intraventricular hemorrhage, and mortality in preterm infants. *Pediatrics* 1989;83:153–160.
160. Tsiantos A, et al. Intracranial hemorrhage in the prematurely born infant: timing of clots and evaluation of clinical signs and symptoms. *J Pediatr* 1974;85:854–859.
161. Ment LR, et al. Intraventricular hemorrhage in preterm neonate: timing and cerebral blood flow changes. *J Pediatr* 1984;104:419–425.
162. Levene MI, de Vries LS. Extension of neonatal intraventricular haemorrhage. *Arch Dis Child* 1984;59:631–636.
163. Babcock DS, Han BK. The accuracy of high-resolution: real-time ultrasonography of the head in infancy. *Radiology* 1981;139:665–676.
164. Volpe JJ, et al. Positron emission tomography in the newborn: extensive impairment of regional cerebral blood flow with intraventricular hemorrhage and hemorrhagic intracerebral involvement. *Pediatrics* 1983;72:589–601.
165. Edvinsson L, Lou HC, Tvede K. On the pathogenesis of regional cerebral ischemia in intracranial hemorrhage: a causal influence of potassium? *Pediatr Res* 1986;20:478–480.
166. Perlman JM, Volpe JJ. Cerebral blood flow velocity in relation to intraventricular hemorrhage in the premature newborn infant. *J Pediatr* 1982;100:956–959.
167. Altman DI, Volpe JJ. Cerebral blood flow in the newborn infant: measurement and role in the patho-genesis of periventricular and intraventricular hemorrhage. *Adv Pediatr* 1987;34:111–138.
168. Younkin D. In vivo ^{31}P nuclear magnetic resonance measurement of chronic changes in cerebral metabolites following neonatal intraventricular hemorrhage. *Pediatrics* 1988;82:331–336.
169. Perlman JM, Risser R. Severe fetal acidemia: neonatal neurologic features and short-term outcome. *Pediatr Neurol* 1993;9:277–282.
170. Taylor GA. Effect of germinal matrix hemorrhage on terminal vein position and patency. *Pediatr Radiol* 1995;25:S37–S40.
171. Grant EG, et al. Evolution of porencephalic cysts from intraparenchymal hemorrhage in neonates: sonographic evidence. *Am J Roentgenol* 1982;138:467–470.
172. Hill A, Volpe JJ. Decrease in pulsatile flow in the anterior cerebral arteries in infantile hydrocephalus. *Pediatrics* 1982;69:47.
173. Palmer TW, Donn SM. Symptomatic subarachnoid hemorrhage in the term newborn. *J Perinatol* 1991;11:112–116.
174. Doe FD, Shuangshoti S, Netsky MG. Cryptic hemangioma of the choroid plexus. *Neurology* 1972;22:1233–1239.
175. Wakai S, Andoh Y, Nagai M, et al. Choroid plexus arteriovenous malformations in a full-term neonate. *J Neurosurg* 1990;72:127–129.
176. Volbert H, Schweitzer H. Ueber Häufigkeit, Lokalization und Aetiologie von Blutungen im Wirbelkanal bei unreifen Früchten und Frühgeburten. *Geburtsh Frauenh* 1954;11:1041–1048.
177. Coutelle C. Ueber epidurale Blutungen in den Wirbelkanal bei Neugeborenen und Säuglingen und ihre Beziehung zu anderen perinatalen Blutungen. *Z Geburtsh Gynakol* 1960;156:19–52.
178. Drillien CM. Aetiology and outcome in low-birth-weight infants. *Dev Med Child Neurol* 1972;14:563–574.
179. Paine RS, et al. Evolution of postural reflexes in normal infants and in the presence of chronic brain syndromes. *Neurology* 1964;14:1036–1048.
180. Paine RS. The evolution of infantile postural reflexes in the presence of chronic brain syndromes. *Dev Med Child Neurol* 1964;6:345–361.
181. Sarnat HB, Sarnat MS. Neonatal encephalopathy following fetal distress: a clinical and electroencephalographic study. *Arch Neurol* 1976;33:696–705.
182. Levene M. Management of the asphyxiated full-term infant. *Arch Dis Child* 1993;68:612–616.
183. Sykes GS, et al. Do Apgar scores indicate asphyxia? *Lancet* 1982;1:494–496.
184. Goldenberg RL, Huddleston JF, Nelson KG. Apgar scores and umbilical arterial pH in preterm newborn infants. *Am J Obstet Gynecol* 1984;149:651–654.
185. Nelson KB, Ellenberg J. Neonatal signs as predictors of cerebral palsy. *Pediatrics* 1979;64:225–232.
186. DeSouza SW, Richards B. Neurological sequelae in newborn babies after perinatal asphyxia. *Arch Dis Child* 1978;53:564–569.
187. Crothers B, Paine RS. *The natural history of cerebral palsy*, Cambridge: Harvard University Press, 1959.
188. Lazzara A, et al. Clinical predictability of intraventricular hemorrhage in preterm infants. *Pediatrics* 1980;65:30–34.

189. Dubowitz LMS, et al. Neurologic signs in neonatal intraventricular hemorrhage: a correlation with real-time ultrasound. *J Pediatr* 1981;99:127–133.
190. Mizrahi EM, Kellaway P. Characterization and classification of neonatal seizures. *Neurology* 1987;37:1837–1844.
191. Bouza H, et al. Evolution of early hemiplegic signs in full-term infants with unilateral brain lesions in the neonatal period: a prospective study. *Neuropediatrics* 1994;25:201–207.
192. Ingram TT. *Paediatric aspects of cerebral palsy,* Edinburgh: E & S Livingstone, 1964.
193. Skatvedt M. Cerebral palsy: a clinical study of 370 cases. *Acta Paediatr* Scand 1958;46[Suppl]:3.
194. Yannet H, Horton F. Hypotonic cerebral palsy in mental defectives. *Pediatrics* 1952;9:204–211.
195. Förster O. Der atonische-astatische Typus der infantilen Cerebrallähmung. *Dtsch Arch Klin Med* 1910;98:216–244.
196. Beltran RS, Coker SB. Transient dystonia of infancy: a result of intrauterine cocaine exposure? *Pediatr Neurol* 1995;12:354–356.
197. Nelson KB, Ellenberg JH. Children who "outgrew" cerebral palsy. *Pediatrics* 1982;69:529–536.
198. Taudorf K, et al. Spontaneous remission of cerebral palsy. *Neuropediatrics* 1986;17:19–22.
199. Cummins SK, et al. Cerebral palsy in four Northern California counties: births 1983 through 1985. *J Pediatr* 1993;123:230–237.
200. Hagberg B, et al. The changing panorama of cerebral palsy in Sweden. V. The birth year period 1979-82. *Acta Paediat Scand* 1989;78:283–290.
201. Stanley FJ. Survival and cerebral palsy in low-birth-weight infants: implications for perinatal care. *Paediatr Perinat Epidemiol* 1992;6:298–310.
202. Grether JK, Cummins SK, Nelson KB. The California cerebral palsy project. *Pediatr Perinat Epidemiol* 1992;6:339–351.
203. Edebol-Tysk K, Hagberg B, Hagberg G. Epidemiology of spastic tetraplegic cerebral palsy in Sweden. II. Prevalence, birth data and origin. *Neuropediatrics* 1989;20:46–52.
204. Stanley FJ, et al. Spastic quadriplegia in Western Australia: a genetic and epidemiological study. I: Case population and perinatal risk factors. *Dev Med Child Neurol* 1993;35:191–201.
205. Benda CE. *Developmental disorders of mentation and cerebral palsies,* New York: Grune & Stratton, 1952.
206. Krageloh-Mann I, et al. Bilateral spastic cerebral palsy—MRI pathology and origin analysis from a representative series of 56 cases. *Dev Med Child Neurol* 1995;37:379–397.
207. Okomura A, et al. MRI findings in patients with spastic cerebral palsy. II. Correlation with type of cerebral palsy. *Dev Med Child Neurol* 1997;39:369–372.
208. Freud S. Zur Kenntnis der cerebralen Diplegien des Kindesalters. Leipzig: Deuticke, 1893.
209. Ford FR. *Diseases of the nervous system in infancy, childhood and adolescence,* 5th ed. Springfield, IL: Charles C Thomas, 1966.
210. McDonald AD. Cerebral palsy in children of very low birth weight. *Arch Dis Child* 1963;38:579–588.
211. Olsén P, et al. Magnetic resonance imagine of periventricular leukomalacia and its clinical correlation in children. *Ann Neurol* 1997;41:754–761.
212. Yokochi K, et al. Magnetic resonance imaging in children with spastic diplegia: correlation with the severity of their motor and mental abnormality. *Dev Med Child Neurol* 1991;33:18–25.
213. Yokochi K. Thalamic lesions revealed by MR associated with periventricular leukomalacia and clinical profiles of subjects. *Acta Paediatr* 1997;86:493–496.
214. Veelken N, et al. Diplegic cerebral palsy in Swedish term and preterm children: differences in reduced optimality, relations to neurology and pathogenetic factors. *Neuropediatrics* 1983;14:20–28.
215. Olsén P, et al. Psychological findings in preterm children related to neurologic status and magnetic resonance imaging. *Pediatrics* 1998;102:329–336.
216. McNutt SJ. Apoplexia neonatorum. *Am J Obstet* 1885;18:73–81.
217. Freud S, Rie O. *Klinische Studie ueber die halbseitige Cerebrallähmung der Kinder,* Vienna: M. Perles, 1891.
218. Ford FR. Cerebral birth injuries and their results. *Medicine* 1926;5:121–194.
219. Michaelis R, Rooschuz B, Dopfer R. Prenatal origin of congenital spastic hemiparesis. *Early Hum Dev* 1980;4:243–255.
220. Molteni B, et al. Relationship between CT patterns, clinical findings and etiological factors in children born at term affected by congenital hemiparesis. *Neuropediatrics* 1987;18:75–80.
221. Larroche J-C. Fetal encephalopathies of circulatory origin. *Biol Neonate* 1986;50:61–74.
222. Nelson KB. Prenatal origin of hemiparetic cerebral palsy: how often and why? *Pediatrics* 1991;88:1058–1062.
223. Barkovich AJ. Subcortical heterotopia: a distinct clinicoradiologic entity. *AJNR Am J Neuroradiol* 1998;17:1315–1322.
224. Miller SP, et al. Congenital bilateral perisylvian polymicrogyria presenting as congenital hemiplegia. *Neurology* 1998;50:1866–1869.
225. De Vries LS, et al. Infarcts in the vascular distribution of the middle cerebral artery in preterm and full-term infants. *Neuopediatrics* 1997;28:88–96.
226. Bouza H, et al. Late magnetic resonance imaging and clinical findings in neonates with unilateral lesions on cranial ultrasound. *Dev Med Child Neurol* 1994;36:951–964.
227. Thorarenson O, et al. Factor V Leiden mutation: an unrecognized cause of hemiplegic cerebral palsy, neonatal stroke, and placental thrombosis. *Ann Neurol* 1997;42:372–375.
228. Wiklund LM, Uvebrant P, Flodmark O. Morphology of cerebral lesions in children with congenital hemiplegia. *Neuroradiology* 1990;32:179–186.
229. Barkovich AJ, Chuang SH. Unilateral megalencephaly: correlation of MR imaging and pathologic characteristics. *AJNR Am J Neuroradiol* 1990;11:523–531.
230. Lanska MJ, et al. Presentation, clinical course, and outcome of childhood stroke. *Pediatr Neurol* 1991;7:333–341.
231. Perlstein MA, Hood PN. Infantile spastic hemiplegia: incidence. *Pediatrics* 1954;14:436–441.
232. Byers RK. Evolution of hemiplegias in infancy. *Am J Dis Child* 1941;61:915–927.
233. Brown JK, et al. Neurophysiology of lower-limb function in hemiplegic children. *Dev Med Child Neurol* 1991;33:1037–1047.

234. Goutieres F, et al. Les hémiplégies congénitales: sémiologie, étiologie et prognostic. *Arch Franc Péd* 1972;29:839–851.

235. Twitchell TE. The grasping deficit in infantile hemiparesis. *Neurology* 1958;8:13–21.

236. Denny-Brown D, Chambers RA. The parietal lobe and behaviour. *Assoc Res Nerv Ment Dis Proc* 1958; 36:35–117.

237. Cohen ME, Duffner PK. Prognostic indicators in hemiparetic cerebral palsy. *Ann Neurol* 1981;9:353–357.

238. Nass R. Mirror movement asymmetries in congenital hemiparesis: the inhibition hypothesis revisited. *Neurology* 1985;35:1059–1062.

239. Tizard JP, Paine RS, Crothers B. Disturbances of sensation in children with hemiplegia. *JAMA* 1954;155: 628–632.

240. Delgado MR, et al. Discontinuation of antiepileptic drug treatment after two seizure-free years in children with cerebral palsy. *Pediatrics* 1996;97:192–197.

241. Cohen P, Kohn JG. Follow-up study of patients with cerebral palsy. *West J Med* 1979;130:6–11.

242. Hagberg B, Hagberg G, Olow I. The changing panorama of cerebral palsy in Sweden, 1954–1970. II. Analysis of the various syndromes. *Acta Paediatr Scand* 1975;64:187–200.

243. Kyllerman M, et al. Dyskinetic cerebral palsy. I. Clinical categories, associated neurologic abnormalities and incidences. *Acta Paediatr Scand* 1982;71: 543–550.

244. Kyllerman M, et al. Dyskinetic cerebral palsy. II. Pathogenetic risk factors and intrauterine growth. *Acta Paediatr Scand* 1982;71:551–558.

245. Rosenbloom L. Dyskinetic cerebral palsy and birth asphyxia. *Dev Med Child Neurol* 1994;36:285–289.

246. Polani PE. The clinical natural history of choreo athetoid cerebral palsy. *Guy Hosp Rep* 1959;108: 32–45.

247. Bobath KA Neurophysiological basis for the treatment of cerebral palsy. *Clinics Dev Med* 1991;75:73.

248. Saint Hilaire M-H, et al. Delayed-onset dystonia due to perinatal or early childhood asphyxia. *Neurology* 1991;41:216–222.

249. Deonna T-W, Ziegler A-L, Nielsen J. Transient idiopathic dystonia in infancy. *Neuropediatrics* 1991;22: 220–224.

250. Hayashi M, et al. Clinical and neuropathological findings in severe athetoid cerebral palsy: a comparative study of globo-luysian and thalamo-putaminal groups. *Brain Dev* 1991;13:47–51.

251. Malamud N, et al. An etiologic and diagnostic study of cerebral palsy. *J Pediatr* 1964;66:270–293.

252. Lesny IA. Follow-up study of hypotonic forms of cerebral palsy. *Brain Dev* 1979;1:87–90.

253. Fenichel GM. Cerebral influence on muscle fiber typing: the effect of fetal immobilization. *Arch Neurol* 1969;20:644–649.

254. Iannaccone ST, et al. Type 1 fiber size disproportion: morphometric data from 37 children with myopathic, neuropathic, or idiopathic hypotonia. *Pediatr Pathol* 1987;7:395–419.

255. Painter MJ, et al. Fetal heart rate patterns during labor: neurologic and cognitive development at six to nine years of age. *Am J Obstet Gynecol* 1988;159: 854–858.

256. Valentin L, et al. Clinical evaluation of the fetus and neonate: relation between intra-partum cardiotocography, Apgar score, cord blood acid-base status and neonatal morbidity. *Arch Gynecol Obstet* 1993;253: 103–115.

257. Nelson KB, et al. Uncertain value of electronic fetal monitoring in predicting cerebral palsy. *N Engl J Med* 1996;334:613–618.

258. Meis PJ, et al. Meconium passage: a new classification for risk assessment during labor. *Am J Obstet Gynecol* 1978;131:509–513.

259. Painter MJ. Fetal heart rate patterns, perinatal asphyxia, and brain injury. *Pediatr Neurol* 1989;5: 137–144.

260. Socol ML, Garcia PM, Riter S. Depressed Apgar scores, acid-base status, and neurologic outcome. *Am J Obstet Gynecol* 1994;170:991–998.

261. Perlman JM, Risser R. Can asphyxiated infants at risk for neonatal seizures be rapidly identified by current high-risk markers? *Pediatrics* 1996;97: 456–462.

262. Sehdev HM, et al. Predictive factors for neonatal morbidity in neonates with an umbilical arterial cord pH less than 7.00. *Am J Obstet Gynecol* 1997;177: 1030–1034.

263. Belai Y, et al. Umbilical arteriovenous pO_2 and pCO_2 differences and neonatal morbidity in term infants with severe acidosis. *Am J Obstet Gynecol* 1998;178:13–19.

264. Markestad T, et al. Small-for-gestational-age (SGA) infants born at term: growth and development during the first year of life. *Acta Obstet Gynecol Scand* 1997;[Suppl]165:93–101.

265. Blair E, Stanley F. Intrauterine growth and spastic cerebral palsy. I. Association with birth weight for gestational age. *Am J Obstet Gynecol* 1990;162:229–237.

266. Amiel-Tison C, Pettigrew AG. Adaptive changes in the developing brain during intrauterine stress. *Brain Devel* 1991;13:67–76.

267. Allen MC. Developmental outcome and follow-up of the small for gestational age infant. *Semin Perinatol* 1984;8:123–156.

268. Committee on Fetus and Newborn, American Academy of Pediatrics. Use and abuse of the Apgar score. *Pediatrics* 1996;98:141–142.

269. Brazy JE, Kinney HC, Oakes WJ. Central nervous system structural lesions causing apnea at birth. *J Pediatr* 1987;111:163–175.

270. Sykes GS, et al. Do Apgar scores indicate asphyxia? *Lancet* 1982;1:494–496.

271. Perlman JM, et al. Acute systemic organ injury in term infants after asphyxia. *Am J Dis Child* 1989;143:617–620.

272. Nelson KB, Ellenberg JH. The asymptomatic newborn and risk of cerebral palsy. *Am J Dis Child* 1987;141:1333–1335.

273. Freeman JM, Nelson KB. Intrapartum asphyxia and cerebral palsy. *Pediatrics* 1988;82:240–249.

274. Volpe JJ. Neonatal intracranial hemorrhage. *Clin Perinatol* 1977;4:77–102.

275. Tourtellotte WW, et al. A study on traumatic lumbar punctures. *Neurology* 1958;8:159–160.

276. Svenningsen NW, Siesjö BK. Cerebrospinal fluid lactate/pyruvate ratio in normal and asphyxiated neonates. *Acta Paediatr Scand* 1972;61:117–124.

277. Walsh P, et al. Assessment of neurologic outcome in asphyxiated term infants by use of serial CK-BB isoenzyme measurement. *J Pediatr* 1982;101: 988–992.

278. Baud O, et al. The early diagnosis of periventricular leukomalacia in premature infants with positive rolandic sharp waves on serial electroencephalography. *J Pediatr* 1998;132:813–817.

279. Marret S, et al. Prognostic value of neonatal electroencephalography in premature newborns less than 33 weeks of gestational age. *Electroencephalogr Clin Neurophysiol* 1997;102:178–185.

280. Blickman JG, Jaramillo D, Cleveland RH. Neonatal cranial ultrasonography. *Curr Probl Diagn Radiol* 1991;20:91–119.

281. Levene MI, Williams JL, Fawer C-L. *Ultrasound of the infant brain. Clin Dev Med* 92, Oxford: Blackwell Scientific Publications (Spastics International Medical Publications), Oxford, 1985.

282. Partridge JC, et al. Optimal timing for diagnostic cranial ultrasound in low-birth-weight infants: detection of intracranial hemorrhage and ventricular dilation. *J Pediatr* 1983;102:281–287.

283. Papile LA, et al. Incidence and evolution of subependymal and intraventricular hemorrhage: a study of infants with birth weights less than 1,500 g. *J Pediatr* 1978;92:529–543.

284. Guzzetta F, et al. Periventricular intraparenchymal echo-densities in the premature newborn: critical determinant of neurologic outcome. *Pediatrics* 1986;78:995–1006.

285. Graham M, et al. Prediction of cerebral palsy in very low-birth-weight infants: prospective ultrasound study. *Lancet* 1987;2:593–596.

286. Fawer C-L, Deibold P, Calame A. Periventricular leucomalacia and neurodevelopmental outcome in preterm infants. *Arch Dis Child* 1987;62:30–36.

287. Seigal MJ, et al. Hypoxic-ischaemic encephalopathy in term infants: diagnosis and prognosis evaluated by ultrasound. *Radiology* 1984;152:395–399.

288. Eken P, et al. Intracranial lesions in the full-term infant with hypoxic ischaemic encephalopathy: ultrasound and autopsy correlation. *Neuropediatrics* 1994;25:301–307.

289. Shen EY, et al. Sonographic finding of the bright thalamus. *Arch Dis Child* 1986;61:1096–1099.

290. Shewmon DA, et al. Postischemic hypervascularity of infancy: a stage in the evolution of ischemic brain damage with characteristic CT scan. *Ann Neurol* 1981;9:358–365.

291. Hope PL, et al. Precision of ultrasound diagnosis of pathologically verified lesions in the brains of very preterm infants. *Dev Med Child Neurol* 1988;30:457–471.

292. Fitzhardinge PM, et al. The prognostic value of computed tomography of the brain in asphyxiated premature infants. *J Pediatr* 1982;100:476–481.

293. Picard L, et al. Cerebral computed tomography in premature infants with an attempt at staging developmental features. *J Comput Assist Tomogr* 1980;4:435–444.

294. Cowan FM, et al. Early detection of cerebral infarction and hypoxic ischemic encephalopathy in neonates using diffusion-weighted magnetic resonance imaging. *Neuropediatrics* 1994;25:172–175.

295. Barkovich AJ. Perinatal asphyxia: MR findings in the first 10 days. *AJNR Am J Neuroradiol* 1995;16:427–438.

296. Westmark KD, et al. Patterns and implications of MR contrast enhancement in perinatal asphyxia: a preliminary report. *AJNR Am J Neuroradiol* 1995;16: 685–692.

297. Barkovich AJ, Truwit CL. Brain damage from perinatal asphyxia: correlation of MR findings with gestational age. *AJNR Am J Neuroradiol* 1990;11:1087–1096.

298. Keeney SE, et al. Prospective observations of 100 high-risk neonates by high field (1.5 Tesla) magnetic resonance imaging of the central nervous system. II. Lesions associated with hypoxic-ischemic encephalopathy. *Pediatrics* 1991;87:431–438.

299. Roland EH, Flodmark O, Hill A. Thalamic hemorrhage with intraventricular hemorrhage in the full-term newborn. *Pediatrics* 1990;85:737–742.

300. Michoni G, Willinsky R. Rapid postanoxic calcification of the basal ganglia. *Neurology* 1992;42: 2144–2146.

301. Byrne P, et al. Serial magnetic resonance imaging in neonatal hypoxic-ischemic encephalopathy. *J Pediatr* 1990;117:694–700.

302. Holland BA, et al. MRI of normal brain maturation. *AJNR Am J Neuroradiol* 1986;7:201–208.

303. Johnson MA, et al. Serial imaging in neonatal cerebral injury. *AJNR Am J Neuroradiol* 1987;8:83–92.

304. van de Bor M, et al. Early detection of delayed myelination in preterm infants. *Pediatrics* 1989;84: 407–411.

305. Lou HC, Skov H, Henricksen L. Intellectual impairment with regional cerebral dysfunction after low neonatal cerebral blood flow. *Acta Paediatr Scand* 1989;[Suppl]36:72–82.

306. Rosenbaum JL, et al. Higher neonatal cerebral blood flow correlates with worse childhood neurologic outcome. *Neurology* 1997;49:1035–1041.

307. Blennow M, et al. Early [^{18}F] FDG positron emission tomography in infants with hypoxic-ischemic encephalopathy shows hypermetabolism during the postasphyctic period. *Acta Paediatr* 1995;84: 1289–1295.

308. Kerrigan JF, Chugani HT, Phelps ME. Regional cerebral glucose metabolism in clinical subtypes of cerebral palsy. *Pediatr Neurol* 1991;7:415–425.

309. Novotny E, Ashwal S, Shevell M. Proton magnetic resonance spectroscopy: an emerging technology in pediatric neurology research. *Pediatr Res* 1998;44:1–10.

310. Hanrahan JD, et al. Relation between proton magnetic resonance spectroscopy within 18 hours of birth asphyxia and neurodevelopment at 1 year of age. *Dev Med Child Neurol* 1999;41:76–82.

311. Hanrahan JD, et al. Persistent increases in cerebral lactate concentration after birth asphyxia. *Pediatr Res* 1998;44:304–311.

312. Penrice J, et al. Proton magnetic resonance spectroscopy of the brain in normal preterm and term infants, and early changes after perinatal hypoxia-ischemia. *Pediatr Res* 1996;40:6–14.

313. Hamilton PA, et al. Impaired energy metabolism in brains of newborn infants with increased cerebral echo-densities. *Lancet* 1986;1:1242–1246.

314. Gadian DG, et al. NMR spectroscopy: current status and future possibilities. *Acta Neurochir* 1993; 57[Suppl]:18.

315. Moorcraft J, et al. Spatially localized magnetic resonance spectroscopy of the brains of normal and asphyxiated newborns. *Pediatrics* 1991;87:273–282.

316. Despland PA, Galambos R. The auditory brain stem response (ABR) is a useful diagnostic tool in the intensive care nursery. *Pediatr Res* 1980;14:154–158.

317. Muttit SC, et al. Serial visual evoked potentials and outcome in term birth asphyxia. *Pediatr Neurol* 1991;7:86–90.

318. Raju TNK. Cerebral Doppler studies in the fetus and newborn infant. *J Pediatr* 1991;119:165–174.

319. Vanucci RC, Perlman JM. Interventions for perinatal hypoxic-ischemic encephalopathy. *Pediatrics* 1997; 100:1004–1014.

320. Wahlestedt C, et al. Antisense oligodeoxynucleotides to NMDA-R1 receptor channel protect cortical neurons from excitotoxicity and reduce focal ischaemic infarctions. *Nature* 1993;363:260–263.

321. Kuban KCK. Intracranial hemorrhage. In: Cloherty JP, Stark AR. *Manual of neonatal care*. Philadelphia: Lippincott-Raven Publishers, 1998:505–515.

322. Thorp JA, et al. Combined antenatal vitamin K and phenobarbital therapy for preventing intracranial hemorrhage in newborns less than 34 weeks gestation. *Obstet Gynecol* 1995;86:1–8.

323. Shankaran S, et al. The effects of antenatal phenobarbital therapy on neonatal intracranial hemorrhage in preterm infants. *N Engl J Med* 1997;337: 466–471.

324. Ment LR, et al. Low-dose indomethacin and prevention of intraventricular hemorrhage: a multicenter randomized trial. *Pediatrics* 1994;93:543–550.

325. Yanowitz TD, et al. Effects of prophylactic low-dose indomethacin on hemodynamics in very low-birth-weight infants. *J Pediatr* 1998;132:28–34.

326. Volpe J. Brain injury caused by intraventricular hemorrhage: is indomethacin the silver bullet for prevention? *Pediatrics* 1994;93:673–677.

327. Benson JWT, et al. Multicentre trial of ethamsylate for prevention of periventricular hemorrhage in very low-birth-weight infants. *Lancet* 1986;2:1297–1300.

328. Fletcher JM, et al. Effects of intraventricular hemorrhage and hydrocephalus on the long-term neurobehavioral development of preterm very-low-birth-weight infants. *Dev Med Child Neurol* 1997;39:596–606.

329. Sutherland DH. Research objectives. *Dev Med Child Neurol* 1984;26:567–568.

330. Tizard JPM. Cerebral palsies: treatment and prevention. The Croonian lecture 1978. *J Roy Coll Physicians Lond* 1980;14:72–77.

331. Paine RS. On the treatment of cerebral palsy: the outcome of 177 patients, 74 totally untreated. *Pediatrics* 1962;29:605–616.

332. Fixsen JA. Orthopedic management of cerebral palsy. *Arch Dis Child* 1994;71:396–397.

333. Wright T, Nicholson J. Physiotherapy for the spastic child: an evaluation. *Dev Med Child Neurol* 1973; 15:146–163.

334. Palmer FB, et al. The effects of physical therapy on cerebral palsy: a controlled trial in infants with spastic diplegia. *N Engl J Med* 1988;318:803–808.

335. Tardieu C, et al. For how long must the soleus muscle be stretched each day to prevent contracture? *Dev Med Child Neurol* 1988;30:3–10.

336. Park TS, Owen JH. Surgical management of spastic diplegia in cerebral palsy. *N Engl J Med* 1992; 326:745–749.

337. Banks HH. The foot and ankle in cerebral palsy. In: Samilson RL, ed. *Orthopaedic Aspects of Cerebral Palsy. Clin Dev Med, Vol. 52-53*. Philadelphia: JB Lippincott Co, 1975.

338. Ruda R, Frost HM. Cerebral palsy: spastic varus and forefoot adductus treated by intramuscular posterior tibial tendon lengthening. *Clin Orthop* 1971; 79:61–70.

339. Damron T, Breen AL, Roecker E. Hamstring tenotomies in cerebral palsy: long-term analysis. *J Pediatr Orthoped* 1991;514–519.

340. Law M, et al. A comparison of intensive neurodevelopmental therapy plus casting and a regular occupational therapy program for children with cerebral palsy. *Dev Med Child Neurol* 1997;39:664–670.

341. Goldner JL. The upper extremity in cerebral palsy. In: Samilson RL, ed. *Orthopaedic Aspects of Cerebral Palsy. Clin Dev Med Vol. 52-53*. Philadelphia: JB Lippincott Co, 1975.

342. Peacock WJ, Arens LJ, Berman B. Cerebral palsy spasticity: selective posterior rhizotomy. *Pediatr Neurosci* 1987;13:61–66.

343. Steinbok P, et al. A randomized clinical trial to compare selective posterior rhizotomy plus physiotherapy with physiotherapy alone in children with spastic diplegic cerebral palsy. *Dev Med Child Neurol* 1997;39:178–184.

344. Peacock WJ, Staudt LA. Spasticity in cerebral palsy and the selective posterior rhizotomy procedure. *J Child Neurol* 1990;5:179–185.

345. Bleck EE. Posterior rootlet rhizotomy in cerebral palsy. *Arch Dis Child* 1993;68:717–719.

346. Gersztein PC, Albright AL, Johnstone GF. Intrathecal baclofen infusion and subsequent orthopedic surgery in patients with spastic cerebral palsy. *J Neurosurg* 1998;88:1099–1013.

347. Armstrong RW, et al. Intrathecally administered baclofen for treatment of children with spasticity of cerebral origin. *J Neurosurg* 1997;87:409–414.

348. Cosgrove AP, Corry IS, Graham HK. Botulinum toxin in the management of the lower limb cerebral palsy. *Dev Med Child Neurol* 1994;36:386–396.

349. Wong V. Use of botulinum toxin injection in 17 children with spastic cerebral palsy. *Pediatr Neurol* 1998;18:124–131.

350. Corry IS, et al. Botulinum toxin compared with stretching casts in the treatment of spastic equinus: a randomized prospective trial. *J Pediatr Orthop* 1998; 18:304–311.

351. Forssberg H, Tedroff KB. Botulinum toxin treatment in cerebral palsy: intervention with poor evaluation. *Dev Med Child Neurol* 1997;39:635–640.

352. Killackey HP, Rhades RW, Bennett-Clarke CA. The formation of a cortical somatotopic map. *Trends Neurosci* 1995;18:402–407.

353. Ferry PC. Infant stimulation programs: a neurologic shell game? *Arch Neurol* 1986;43:281–282.

354. Russman BS. Are infant stimulation programs useful? *Arch Neurol* 1986;43:282–283.

355. Douglas AA. Ophthalmological aspects of cerebral palsy. *Spastics' Quart* 1962;11:37–47.

356. Black P. Visual disorders associated with cerebral palsy. *Br J Opthalmol* 1982;66:46–52.

357. Buckley E, Seaber JH. Dyskinetic strabismus as: a sign of cerebral palsy. *Am J Ophthalmol* 1981;91:652–657.

358. Fielder AR, et al. Delayed visual maturation. *Trans Ophthalmol Soc U K* 1985;104:653–661.

359. Foley J, Gordon N. Recovery from cortical blindness. *Dev Med Child Neurol* 1985;27:383–387.

360. Menkes JH, Ament ME. Neurologic disorders of gastroesophageal function. *Adv Neurol* 1988;49: 409–416.

361. Reilly S, Skuse D. Characteristics and management of feeding problems of young children with cerebral palsy. *Dev Med Child Neurol* 1992;34:379–388.

362. Yossen F. Personal communication, 1989.

363. Camp-Bruno JA, et al. Efficacy of benztropine therapy for drooling. *Dev Med Child Neurol* 1989;31:309–319.

364. Miller AJ. Deglutition. *Physiol Rev* 1982;62: 129–184.

365. Reid CJD, Borzyskowski M. Lower urinary tract dysfunction in cerebral palsy. *Arch Dis Child* 1993;68:739–742.

366. Dormans JP. Orthopedic management of children with cerebral palsy. *Pediatr Clin North Am* 1993;40: 645–657.

367. Bleck EE. *Orthopaedic Management of Cerebral Palsy. Orthopaedic Aspects of Cerebral Palsy Clin Dev Med*, 99/100, Philadelphia: JB Lippincott Co, 1987.

368. Bobath B, Bobath K. *Motor development in the different types of cerebral palsy*, London: Heineman, 1975.

369. Dubowitz L, Dubowitz V. The neurological assessment of the preterm and full-term newborn infant. *Clinics in Devel Med* 1981;79.

370. Robertson CMT, Finer NN. Long-term follow-up of term neonates with perinatal asphyxia. *Clin Perinatol* 1993;20:483–500.

371. Handley-Derry M, et al. Intrapartum fetal asphyxia and the occurrence of minor deficits in 4- to 8-year-old children. *Dev Med Child Neurol* 1997;39:508–514.

372. Temple CM, et al. Neonatal seizures: long-term outcome and cognitive development among "normal" survivors. *Dev Med Child Neurol* 1995;37:109–118.

373. Perlman JM, Tack ED. Renal injury in the asphyxiated newborn: relationship to neurologic outcome. *J Pediatr* 1988;113:875–879.

374. Janowsky JS, Finlay BL. The outcome of perinatal brain damage: the role of normal neuron loss and axon retraction. *Dev Med Child Neurol* 1986;28:375–389.

375. Ergander U, Eriksson M, Zetterstrom R. Severe neonatal asphyxia: incidence and prediction of outcome in the Stockholm area. *Acta Paediatr Scand* 1983;72:321–325.

376. Drage JS, et al. The Apgar score as an index of infant morbidity: a report from the collaborative study of cerebral palsy. *Dev Med Child Neurol* 1966;8:141–148.

377. Dennis J, et al. Acid-base status at birth and neurodevelopmental outcome at four-and-one-half years. *Am J Obstet Gynecol* 1989;161:213–220.

378. Dijxhoorn MJ, et al. Apgar score, meconium, and acidaemia at birth in relation to neonatal neurological morbidity in term infants. *Brit J Obstet Gynaecol* 1986;93:217–222.

379. Fee SC, et al. Severe acidosis and subsequent neurologic status. *Am J Obstet Gynecol* 1990;162:802–806.

380. Huisjes HJ, et al. Obstetrical-neonatal neurologic relationships: a replication study. *Eur J Obstet Gynaecol Reprod Biol* 1980;10:247–256.

381. Painter MJ, Depp R, O'Donoghue MN. Fetal heart rate patterns and development in the first year of life. *Am J Obstet Gynecol* 1978;132:271–277.

382. Ekert P, et al. Predicting the outcome of postasphyxial hypoxic-ischemic encephalopathy within 4 hours of birth. *J Pediatr* 1997;131:613–617.

383. Majnemer A, Mazer B. Neurologic evaluation of the newborn infant: definition and psychometric properties. *Develop Med Child Neurol* 1998;40:708–715.

384. Rose AL, Lombroso CT. A study of clinical, pathological, and electroencephalographic features in 137 full-term babies with a long follow-up. *Pediatrics* 1970;45:404–425.

385. Holmes G, et al. Prognostic value of the electroencephalogram in neonatal asphyxia. *Electroencephalogr Clin Neurophysiol* 1982;53:60–72.

386. Siegel MJ, et al. Hypoxic-ischemic encephalopathy in term infants: diagnosis and prognosis evaluated by ultrasound. *Radiology* 1984;152:395–399.

387. Lipp-Zwalen AE, et al. Prognostic value of neonatal CT scans in asphyxiated term babies: low-density score compared with neonatal neurological signs. *Neuropediatrics* 1985;16:209–217.

388. Roland EH, et al. Perinatal hypoxic-ischemic thalamic injury: clinical features and neuroimaging. *Ann Neurol* 1998;44:161–166.

389. Adsett DB, Fitz CR, Hill A. Hypoxic-ischaemic cerebral injury in the term newborn: correlation of CT findings with neurologic outcome. *Dev Med Child Neurol* 1985;27:155–160.

390. Rutherford MA, et al. Abnormal magnetic resonance signal in the internal capsule predicts poor neurodevelopmental outcome in infants with hypoxic-ischemic encephalopathy. *Pediatrics* 1998;102:323–328.

391. Martin E, et al. Diagnostic and prognostic value of cerebral 31P magnetic resonance spectroscopy in neonates with perinatal asphyxia. *Pediatr Res* 1996;40:749–758.

392. Paneth N, Stark RI. Cerebral palsy and mental retardation in relation to indicators of perinatal asphyxia: an epidemiologic overview. *Am J Obstet Gynecol* 1983;147:960–966.

393. Hagberg B, et al. Mild mental retardation in Swedish school children. II. Etiologic and pathogenetic aspects. *Acta Paediatr Scand* 1981;70:445–452.

394. Nelson KB, Ellenberg JH. Antecedents of cerebral palsy: multivariate analysis of risk. *N Engl J Med* 1986;315:81–86.

395. Blair E, Stanley FJ. Intrapartum asphyxia: a rare cause of cerebral palsy. *J Pediatr* 1988;112:515–519.

396. Alberman E, Benson J, McDonald A. Cerebral palsy and severe educational subnormality in low-birth-weight children: a comparison of birth in 1951–53 and 1970–73. *Lancet* 1982;1:606–608.

397. Robertson CMT, et al. Population-based study of the incidence, complexity, and severity of neurologic disability among survivors weighing 500–1,250 grams at birth: a comparison of two birth cohorts. *Pediatrics* 1992;90:750–755.

398. Pharoah PO, et al. Effects of birth weight, gestational age, and maternal obstetrical history on birth prevalence of cerebral palsy. *Arch Dis Child* 1987;62:1035–1040.

399. Lowe J, Papile LA. Neurodevelopmental performance of very-low-birth-weight infants with mild periventricular, intraventricular hemorrhage: outcome at 5–6 years of age. *Am J Dis Child* 1990; 144:1242–1245.

400. van de Bor M, et al. Outcome of periventricular-intraventricular haemorrhage at 5 years of age. *Dev Med Child Neurol* 1993;35:33–41.

401. Fazzi E, et al. Neurodevelopmental outcome in very low-birth-weight infants at 24 months and 5 to 7 years of age: changing diagnosis. *Pediatr Neurol* 1997;17:240–248.

402. Jongmans M, et al. Duration of periventricular densities in preterm infants and neurological outcome at 6 years of age. *Arch Dis Child* 1993;69[Spec No. 1]:9–13.

403. Ghosh A, Shatz CJ. A role for subplate neurons in the patterning of connections from thalamus to neocortex. *Development* 1993;117:1031–1047.

404. Volpe JJ. Subplate neurons—missing link in brain injury of the premature infant? *Pediatrics* 1996;97:112–113.

405. Hirata T, et al. Survival and outcome of infants 501 to 750 gm: a six-year experience. *J Pediatr* 1983;102:741–748.

406. Kitchen WH, et al. Changing two-year outcome in infants weighing 500–999 grams at birth: a hospital study. *J Pediatr* 1991;118:938–943.

407. Collin MF, Halsey CL, Anderson CL. Emerging developmental sequelae in the "normal" extremely low-birth-weight infant. *Pediatrics* 1991;88:115–120.

408. Hack M, et al. Effect of very low-birth-weight and subnormal head size on cognitive abilities at school age. *N Engl J Med* 1991;325:231–237.

409. Piecuch RE, et al. Outcome of extremely low-birth-weight infants (500 to 999 grams) over a 12-year period. *Pediatrics* 1997;100:633–639.

410. Hack M, et al. School-age outcomes in children with birth weights under 750 g. *N Engl J Med* 1994;331:753–759.

411. Sabel KG, Olegard R, Victorin L. Remaining sequelae with modern perinatal care. *Pediatrics* 1976;57:652–658.

412. O'Grady RS, Crain LS, Kohn J. The prediction on long-term functional outcomes of children with cerebral palsy. *Dev Med Child Neurol* 1995;37:997–1005.

413. Sala DA, Grant AD. Prognosis for ambulation in cerebral palsy. *Dev Med Child Neurol* 1995;37:1020–1026.

414. Murphy KP, Molnar GE, Lankasky K. Medical and functional status of adults with cerebral palsy. *Dev Med Child Neurol* 1995;37:1075–1084.

415. Hutton JL, et al. Life expectancy in children with cerebral palsy. *Brit Med J* 1994;309:431–435.

416. Crichton JU, Mackinnon M, White CP. The life expectancy of persons with cerebral palsy. *Dev Med Child Neurol* 1995;37:567–576.

417. Crothers B. Injuries of the spinal cord in breech extractions as an important cause of fetal death and paraplegia in childhood. *Am J Med Sci* 1923;165:94–110.

418. Ford FR. Breech delivery in its possible relations to injury of the spinal cord with special reference to infantile paraplegia. *Arch Neurol & Psychiat* 1925;14:742–750.

419. Crothers B, Putnam MC. Obstetrical injuries of spinal cord. *Medicine* 1927;6:4–126.

420. Towbin A. Latent spinal cord and brain stem injury in newborn infants. *Dev Med Child Neurol* 1969;11:54–68.

421. Byers RK. Spinal cord injuries during birth. *Dev Med Child Neurol* 1975;17:103–110.

422. Hedley-Whyte ET, Gilles FH. Observations on myelination of human spinal cord and some effects of parturitional transection. *J Neuropathol Exp Neurol* 1974;33:436–445.

423. Rossitch E, Oakes WJ. Perinatal spinal cord injury: clinical, radiographic, and pathologic features. *Pediatr Neurosurg* 1992;18:149–152.

424. Bucher HU, et al. Birth injury to the spinal cord. *Helv Paediatr Acta* 1979;34:517–527.

425. Melchior JC, Tygstrup I. Development of paraplegia after breech presentation. *Acta Paediatr Scand* 1963;52:171–176.

426. Schwartz HG. Congenital tumors of spinal cord in infants. *Ann Surg* 1952;136:183–192.

427. Hepner WR Jr. Some observations on facial paresis in the newborn infant: etiology and incidence. *Pediatrics* 1951;8:494–497.

428. Nelson KB, Eng GD. Congenital hypoplasia of the depressor anguli oris muscle: differentiation from congenital facial palsy. *J Pediatr* 1972;81:16–20.

429. Douglas DB, Kessler RE. Significance of electrical reactions in facial palsy of newborn: a case report. *Behav Neuropsychiatry* 1971;2:67.

430. Shapiro NL, et al. Congenital unilateral facial paralysis. *Pediatrics* 1996;97:261–265.

431. Vannas M. Zur Sehnervenatrophie nach Geburtsverletzung. *Acta Ophthalmol* 1933;11:514–525.

432. Gifford H. Congenital defects of abduction and other ocular movements and their relation to birth injuries. *Am J Ophthalmol* 1926;9:3–22.

433. Cogan DG. *Neurology of the ocular muscles*, 2nd ed. Springfield: Charles C Thomas, 1975.

434. Worster-Drought C. Suprabulbar paresis. *Dev Med Child Neurol* 1974;[Suppl]:30.

435. Spector GJ, et al. Fetal respiratory distress causing CNS and inner ear hemorrhage. *Laryngoscope* 1978;88:764–784.

436. Galambos R, Despland PA. The auditory brain stem response (ABR) evaluates risk factors for hearing loss in the newborn. *Pediatr Res* 1980; 14:159–163.

437. Henderson-Smart DJ, Pettigrew AG, Campbell DJ. Clinical apnea and brain-stem neural function in preterm infants. *N Engl J Med* 1983;308:353–357.

438. Hecox KE, Cone B. Prognostic importance of brainstem auditory evoked responses after asphyxia. *Neurology* 1981;31:1429–1434.

439. Smellie WA. *Treatise on the theory and practice of midwifery: a collection of preternatural cases and observations in midwifery*, 3rd ed. Vol 3. London: D. Wilson & T. Durham, 1766.

440. Danyau N. Un cas de paralysie du bras, chez un enfant nouveau né. *Bull Soc Chir Paris* 1851;2:148–151.

441. Duchenne GB. *De l'Electrisation Localisée*, Paris: Bailliere et fils, 1872.

442. Klumpke A. Contribution a l'étude des paralysies radiculaires du plexus brachial; paralysies radiculaires totales; paralysies radiculaires inférieres; de la participation des filets sympathiques oculopupillaries dans ces paralysies. *Rev Méd Paris* 1885; 5:591–596.

443. Shoemaker J. Ueber die Aetiologie der Entbindungslähmungen, speziell der Oberarmparalysen. *Z Geburtsh Gynaek* 1899;41:33–53.

444. Clark LP, Taylor AS, Prout FP. A study on brachial birth palsy. *Am J Med Sci* 1905;130:670–707.

445. McFarland LV, et al. Erb/Duchenne palsy: a consequence of fetal macrosomia and method of delivery. *Obstet Gynecol* 1986;68:784–788.

446. Jennet RJ, Tarby TJ, Kreinick CJ. Brachial plexus palsy: an old problem revisited. *Am J Obstet Gynecol* 1992;166:1673–1677.

447. Dunn DW, Engle WA. Brachial plexus palsy: intrauterine onset. *Pediatr Neurol* 1985;1:367–369.

448. Eng GD, et al. Obstetrical brachial plexus palsy (OBPP) outcome with conservative management. *Muscle Nerve* 1996;19:884–891.

449. Bager B. Perinatally acquired brachial plexus palsy—a persisting challenge. *Acta Paediatr* 1997; 86:1214–1219.

450. Eng GD. Brachial plexus palsy in newborn infants. *Pediatrics* 1971;48:18–28.

451. Schifrin N. Unilateral paralysis of the diaphragm in the newborn infant due to phrenic nerve injury: with and without associated brachial palsy. *Pediatrics* 1952;9:69–121.

452. Adams FH, Gyepes MT. Diaphragmatic paralysis in the newborn infant simulating cyanotic heart disease. *J Pediatr* 1971;78:119–121.

453. Smith BT. Isolated phrenic nerve palsy in the newborn. *Pediatrics* 1972;49:449–451.

454. Robinson GC, Dikranian DA, Roseborough GF. Congenital Horner's syndrome and heterochromia iridium: their association with congenital foregut and vertebral anomalies. *Pediatrics* 1965;35:103–107.

455. Urabe F, et al. MR imaging of birth brachial palsy in a two-month-old infant. *Brain Dev* 1991;13: 130–131.

456. Posniak HV, et al. MR imaging of the brachial plexus. *Am J Roentgenol* 1993;161:373–379.

457. Eng GD. Spontaneous potentials in premature and full-term infants. *Arch Phys Med Rehabil* 1976;57: 120–121.

458. DiGeorge AM, Olmsted RW, Harley RD. Waardenburg's syndrome: syndrome of heterochromia of irides, lateral displacement of medial canthi and lacrimal puncta, congenital deafness and other characteristic associated defects. *Trans Amer Acad Opthal Otolaryng* 64:816–839.

459. Adler JB, Patterson RL. Erb's palsy: long-term results of treatment in eighty-eight cases. *J Bone Joint Surg* 1967;49A:1052–1064.

460. Laurent JP, et al. Neurosurgical correction of upper brachial plexus birth injuries. *J Neurosurg* 1993;79: 197–203.

461. Greenwald AG, Shute P, Shively J. Brachial plexus birth palsy: a 10-year report on the incidence and prognosis. *J Pediatr Orthoped* 1984;4:689–692.

462. Michelow BJ, et al. The natural history of obstetrical brachial plexus palsy. *Plast Reconstruct Surg* 1994;93:675–680.

463. Rossi LN, Vassella F, Mumenthaler M. Obstetrical lesions of the brachial plexus: natural history in 34 personal cases. *Eur Neurol* 1982;21:1–7.

464. Schlaggar BL, Fox K, O'Leary DDM. Postsynaptic control of plasticity in developing somatosensory cortex. *Nature* 1993;364:623–626.

465. Penn A, Ross WT. Sciatic nerve palsy in newborn infants: report of case. *S Afr Med J* 1955;29:553–554.

466. San Agustin M, Nitowsky HM, Borden JN. Neonatal sciatic palsy after umbilical vessel injection. *J Pediatr* 1962;60:408–413.

467. Escolar DM, Jones HR. Pediatric radial mononeuropathies: a clinical and electromyographic study of sixteen children with review of the literature. *Muscle Nerve* 1996;19:878–883.

468. Craig WS, Clark JMP. Obturator palsy in the newly born. *Arch Dis Child* 1962;37:661–662.

469. Coventry MB, Harris LE. Congenital muscular torticollis in infancy: some observations regarding treatment. *J Bone Joint Surg (Amer)* 1959;41:815–817.

470. Sarnat HB, Morrissy RT. Idiopathic torticollis: sternocleidomastoid myopathy and accessory neuropathy. *Muscle Nerve* 1981;4:374–380.

471. Sanerkin NG, Edwards P. Birth injury to the sternomastoid muscle. *J Bone Joint Surg (Brit)* 1966;48:441–447.

472. Lidge RT, Bechtol RC, Lambert CN. Congenital muscular torticollis: etiology and pathology. *J Bone Joint Surg (Am)* 1957;39:1165–1182.

473. Caputo AR, et al. The sit-up test: an alternative clinical test for evaluating pediatric torticollis. *Pediatrics* 1990;90:612–615.

474. Morrison DL, MacEwen GD. Congenital muscular torticollis: observations regarding clinical findings, associated conditions and results of treatment. *J Pediatr Orthop* 1982;2:500–505.

475. Binder H, et al. Congenital muscular torticollis: results of conservative management with long-term follow-up in 85 cases. *Arch Phys Med Rehabil* 1987;68:222–225.

476. Kinsbourne M. Hiatus hernia with contortions of the neck. *Lancet* 1964;1:1058–1061.

477. Deonna T, Martin D. Benign paroxysmal torticollis in infancy. *Arch Dis Child* 1981;56:956–959.

Chapter 6

Infections of the Nervous System

*Marvin Lee Weil, †Elaine Tuomanen, ‡Victor Israele,
§Robert Rust, and ‖John H. Menkes

Departments of Pediatrics and Neurology, University of California, Los Angeles, UCLA School of Medicine, Los Angeles, California 90048, and Department of Biochemistry, University of Oxford, Oxford, England OX1 1SU; †Department of Pediatrics, University of Tennessee, Memphis, College of Medicine, and Department of Infectious Diseases, St. Jude Children's Research Hospital, Memphis, Tennessee 38105; ‡Department of Pediatrics, Fundación Centro de Estudios Infectiológicos (FUNCEI), Buenos Aires, Argentina 1425; §Department of Neurology, University of Virginia School of Medicine, Charlottesville, Virginia 22908; and ‖Departments of Neurology and Pediatrics, University of California, Los Angeles, UCLA School of Medicine, and Department of Pediatric Neurology, Cedars-Sinai Medical Center, Los Angeles, California 90048

The central nervous system (CNS) responds to injury in a limited number of ways. Regardless of the nature of the invading organism, infectious diseases share many clinical and pathologic features, with unique symptom complexes being caused by tropism or virulence of the particular invading organism and variable expression of host defense mechanisms. Whereas, on clinical grounds bacterial CNS infections generally can be distinguished from viral infections, it is difficult to distinguish between bacterial and fungal infections, and between chronic granulomatous diseases and viral, spirochetal, and protozoan infections solely from the physical examination of the patient. Diagnosis requires laboratory studies, including isolation and propagation of the suspected organism or identification of distinctive cellular, serologic, or molecular indicators.

MENINGITIS

By common usage, the various types of meningeal inflammation are classified into two syndromes: septic or purulent meningitis and aseptic meningitis. Septic meningitis is caused by bacterial or fungal organisms. The aseptic meningitis syndrome refers to meningitis or meningeal irritation caused by viral, spirochetal, protozoal, metazoal, neoplastic, or other nonseptic causes.

Acute Purulent Meningitis

In the United States, approximately 25,000 cases of meningitis are seen each year. Most cases are caused by one of three organisms: *Streptococcus pneumoniae*, *Neisseria meningitidis*, and *Haemophilus influenzae*.

Pathology and Pathophysiology

Anatomic Considerations

Bacterial organisms reach the meningeal region by one of four routes: direct hematogenous spread, passage through the choroid plexus, rupture of superficial cortical abscesses, or contiguous spread of an adjacent infection.

Direct hematogenous spread can occur by passive transfer as organisms are carried by diapedetic leukocytes. Organisms also can spread from damaged or malformed blood vessels or as a consequence of neurosurgical procedures. Additionally, meningitis can result from open (compound) fractures of the skull and can complicate congenital defects of the coverings of the brain or cord, such as myelomeningocele or dermal sinus. Infection of the leptomeninges from foci in the underlying cerebral or choroid parenchyma has been postulated in tuberculosis of the nervous system (1). Other sites where contiguous infection is prone to spread directly to the meninges include the skull and the spine. Such a spread can occur in the course of an abscess, osteomyelitis, or thrombophlebitis of the bridging and penetrating vessels. Spread by thrombophlebitis is particularly common in otitis media and sinusitis with resultant epidural or subdural empyema as well as meningitis (2).

In healthy animals, the subarachnoid space resists infection. Seeding of the meninges by induced bacteremia is difficult to produce in laboratory animals; it occurs more readily if the cerebrospinal fluid (CSF) pressure is altered during bacteremia (3).

Meningitis also can develop after bacterial attachment and invasion of the nasopharyngeal mucosa (4). The incidence of meningeal infection correlates with the magnitude and duration of the bacteremia, which in turn is directly related to the amount of the intranasal inoculum. *S. pneumoniae*, *H. influenzae*, and *N. meningitidis* secrete IgA proteases that neutralize IgA. These organisms also impair the mucosal ciliary defense mechanisms. In the case of *N. meningitidis* and *S. pneumoniae*, invasion across the nasopharyngeal mucosal epithelium can occur by endocytosis with transport across the cell in membrane-bound vacuoles. In the case of *H. influenzae* infections, invasion follows the separation of tight junctions between columnar epithelial cells (4). Once in the bloodstream, organisms have various methods for avoiding lysis by circulating complement (5). It is unclear how most organisms breach the blood–brain barrier (6). This barrier, which is composed of the arachnoid membrane, the choroid plexus epithelium, and the endothelial cells of the cerebral microvasculature, separates the intravascular compartment from the brain and CSF. Pneumococci have been shown to use a surface protein to bind to the receptor for platelet activating factor on cytokine-activated cerebral endothelial cells. By corrupting this host chemokine receptor pathway bacteria enter the cell, and the receptor is recycled for subsequent reuse (7). In meningitis, the blood–brain barrier is injured perhaps as a consequence of the separation of intercellular tight junctions, primarily in the endothelial cells of the cerebral microvasculature, and, to a lesser degree, in the endothelium of the choroid plexus (5,6,8). Matrix metalloproteinases (MMP) contribute to this disruption as does nitric oxide, reactive oxygen species, and metabolites of the arachidonic pathway (9). Gelatinase B (MMP-9) is upregulated in the cerebrospinal fluid of patients acutely ill with bacterial and viral meningitis. In experimental inflammation induced by injection of heat-killed meningococcus into the cisterna magna of rats, some MMPs are upregulated (collagenase-3 and stromelysin-1), whereas others are not (stromelysin-2 and -3, gelatinase A, matrilysin) (9a). Having entered the CSF, organisms meet little humoral defense because antibody, complement, and opsonic activity is minimal in that compartment.

Bacterial infection of the meninges also can result from various developmental anomalies (10), or from penetrating injuries of the skull. Both establish continuity between the external environment and the CNS. Nosocomial bacterial meningitis after general or neurosurgical procedures has been reported.

Microbiological and Immunologic Aspects: Invasion of Micro-Organisms and the Inflammatory Response

Almost any of the bacteria can induce meningitis. Unique antigens, often capsular polysaccharides, are associated with the more pathogenic strains in some species of bacteria (5,11). Table 6.1 presents the frequency of the most common forms (12). The clinical and pathologic aspects of meningitis were summarized by Adams and coworkers (13), and current understanding of its pathogenesis by Saez-Llorens and coworkers (14), Smith (15), and Tunkel and Scheld (16,17).

The fundamental process in bacterial meningitis is an inflammation of the leptomeninges, the first stage being hyperemia of the meningeal vessels, and the next, migration of neutrophils into the subarachnoid space (Fig. 6.1). The subarachnoid exudate rapidly increases over hours and extends into the sheaths of blood vessels and

TABLE 6.1. *Frequency of the common forms of acute meningitis in infancy and childhood[a]*

	<1 Month	1–23 Months	2–18 Years	19–59 Years	>60 Years
Haemophilus influenzae[b]	—	5	10	15	5
Streptococcus pneumoniae	10	45	30	60	60
Neisseria meningitidis	—	30	60	20	5
β-Hemolytic *Streptococcus*	70	20	5	5	5
Listeria monocytogenes	20	—	—	10	15

[a]Figures are percentage of total cases within a given age group.

[b]Immunization against *Haemophilus influenzae* has significantly reduced the proportion of this type of meningitis in selected regions of the world.

Modified from Schuchat A, et al., for the Active Surveillance Team. Bacterial meningitis in the United States in 1995. *N Engl J Med* 1997;337:970.

along cranial and spinal nerves. Initially, polymorphonuclear leukocytes that often contain phagocytized bacteria predominate. The number of lymphocytes and histiocytes increases over the subsequent days if the patient survives. Neutrophilic leukocytes begin to degenerate and are removed by macrophages derived from meningeal histiocytes or monocytes. During this time, fibrinogen and other blood proteins are exuded and more plasma cells appear. By this time, the exudate beneath the arachnoid consists of an outer layer of neutrophils and fibrin, and an inner layer next to the pia composed largely of lymphocytes, macrophages, and plasma cells. Fibroblasts, which appear early, are not conspicuous until later when they participate in the organization of exudate, fibrosis of the arachnoid, and walling off of pockets of exudate.

Once established, the meningeal infection spreads for a short distance along the leptomeningeal investments of penetrating cortical vessels in the Virchow-Robin spaces. The adventitia of these vessels is formed by an investment of the arachnoid membrane and is invariably involved in even the initial stages of meningitis. The subarachnoid arteries also are affected. Endothelial cells swell, proliferate, and crowd into the vessel lumen in 48 to 72 hours. The adventitial connective tissue becomes infiltrated by neutrophils, and a layer of inflammatory cells also appears beneath the arterial intima. Foci of necrosis of the arterial walls can develop and occasionally induce arterial thrombosis with infarction. Such vascular changes can be demonstrated by neuroimaging studies in children with meningitis (18).

A similar process occurs in the veins (19). Focal necrosis and mural thrombi develop that partially or totally occlude the lumen. In bacterial meningitis, venous thrombosis is much more frequent than arterial thrombosis (Fig. 6.2). Venous thrombosis is particularly common in subdural empyema, where the thrombus forms on the outer side of the vein next to the subdural infection.

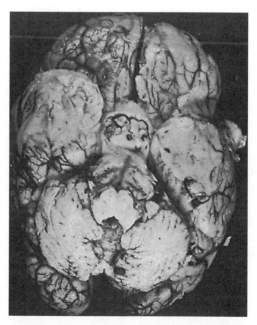

FIG. 6.1. *Haemophilus influenzae* meningitis. The brain is swollen with flattening of the gyri. The meninges are thickened, and purulent material lies along the bases and over the temporal and frontal poles. (Courtesy of Dr. P. Cancella, Department of Pathology, University of California, Los Angeles.)

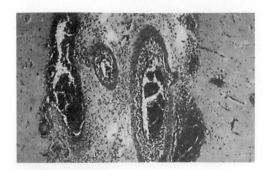

FIG. 6.2. *Haemophilus influenzae* meningitis. A purulent exudate is seen in the subarachnoid space surrounding the venules, which are partially or completely thrombosed (hematoxylin and eosin stain, ×25). (Courtesy of Dr. P. Cancella, Department of Pathology, University of California, Los Angeles.)

Direct damage to either the meningeal and dural bridging veins or the arachnoid itself can result in preferential transudation of low-molecular-weight protein into the subarachnoid and subdural spaces.

The perineural sheaths and blood vessels along the spinal and cranial nerves become infiltrated by inflammatory cells only after several days, although they are surrounded by purulent exudate from the beginning of the infection. The endoneurium occasionally is infiltrated, and degenerating myelinated fibers become evident with fat-laden macrophages and proliferating Schwann cells and fibroblasts.

With resolution of meningitis, cells disappear in the order in which they appeared. The number of neutrophils diminishes after a few weeks, whereas lymphocytes, plasma cells, and macrophages can persist for months. The completeness of resolution depends on the stage at which infection is arrested. If infection is controlled early, residua can be minimal, but an infection lasting several weeks produces permanent fibrous overgrowth of the meninges, which results in a cloudy arachnoid membrane and, sometimes, in adhesions between the arachnoid and dura.

The inflammatory response elicited by bacteria and by bacterial cell wall fragments is responsible for much of the tissue injury that results from infection of the nervous system (20,21). Indeed, initial therapy with bactericidal drugs can result in transient exacerbation of inflammation owing to fragmentation of bacteria. Low doses of bacterial lipopolysaccharide, which produce a brisk inflammatory response in the choroid plexus and ventricles, produce little response in brain parenchyma. Higher doses elicit a monocytic response in the parenchyma after a 48-hour delay, whereas even higher doses result in a full-blown inflammatory response with a delay in mononuclear response of up to 1 week (22). Treatment at the initiation of antibiotic therapy with steroidal or nonsteroidal anti-inflammatory agents can minimize the inflammatory response (23), as can therapeutic methods that involve nonlytic antibiotics, capture of cell wall pieces, blockade of leukocyte adhesion to the vessel endothelium, and inhibition of host mediators of inflammation (24).

More than 40 chemokines, chemotactic cytokines that mediate inflammation and are important in the pathogenesis of the disease process, have been identified (25). Cytokines are soluble proteins that are released by host cells in response to bacterial products such as endotoxin, cell walls, and toxins. They both amplify and inhibit meningeal inflammation. In excess amounts they contribute to parenchymal injury (26,27). Cytokines can directly affect the function of endothelial cells so as to increase blood–brain barrier permeability, decrease autoregulation of cerebral blood flow, and induce cytotoxic edema (28). Most important, however, they induce recruitment of leukocytes into the infected compartment. Proinflammatory cytokines include tumor necrosis factor-alpha (TNF-α), interleukin-1β (IL-1β), interleukin-6 (IL-6), and IL-8. IL-10 and transforming growth factor β (TGF-β) are examples of anti-inflammatory cytokines (29). TNF-α, also known as cachectin, is a low-molecular-weight protein secreted by activated macrophages, leukocytes, endothelial cells, microglia (23), and astrocytes (24). Although less potent than IL-1, TNF-α increases the permeability of the blood–brain barrier (30–32), induces cell lysis (33), and mediates myelin and oligodendrocyte damage (34). Levels of TNF-α are transiently elevated to more than 200 pg/mL in CSF in the majority of patients in the first 24 to 48 hours of purulent meningitis (35). CSF concentrations of TNF-α usually remain normal in patients with viral meningitis (36,36a).

TABLE 6.2. *Cytokines that increase in response to meningitis*

Cytokine	Serum	Cerebrospinal fluid		References
		Viral	Bacterial	
IL-1	+	+	++	Lopez-Cortes et al. (35), Ramilo et al. (42), Mustafa et al. (28)
IL-6	++	++	++	Rusconi et al. (48), Kanoh et al. (45a), Hashim et al. (144)
IL-8		+	++	Lopez-Cortes et al. (35)
IL-9	−	+		Gallo et al. (51)
Tumor necrosis factor	+	+	+	Arditi et al. (45b), Glimaker et al. (45c), Moller et al. (46a)
Tumor growth factor-β			+	Ossege et al. (47a)
Platelet-activating factor	−	−	+	Arditi et al. (45b)
C-reactive protein	+	+	++	Kanoh et al. (45a)
α_2-Microglobulin		−	+	Kanoh et al. (45a)

IL, interleukin.

IL-1β is a highly potent inducer of neutrophil accumulation and is a procoagulant promoting vessel thrombosis (32). It also stimulates the release of other cytokines such as TNF and IL-6 and of hypothalamic corticotrophin-releasing factor, which, in turn, causes increased levels of adrenocorticotrophic hormone (ACTH) (37). ACTH can increase blood–brain barrier permeability for albumin with augmentation of edema (38). Peak concentrations of CSF IL-1β more than 100 pg/100 mL correlate significantly with poor outcome for neonatal gram-negative meningitis and childhood pyogenic meningitis (35); no correlation exists between outcome and CSF concentrations of TNF-α (39). IL-1β and TNF-α secretion by astrocytes is temperature dependent; pyrexia reduces production (40). This effect is augmented by dexamethasone. Thus, fever may serve a beneficial role in bacterial meningitis. Intracisternal injection of IL-1β induces neutrophil emigration into CSF and increases blood–brain barrier permeability (32,41,42). This is inhibited by antibody or induction of neutropenia (43,44). Intracisternal injection of TNF-α results in less dramatic changes in CSF inflammatory parameters, but does produce a monophasic febrile response (41). IL-1 and TNF-α act synergistically to produce both inflammation and disruption of the blood–brain barrier (41). Additionally, they stimulate human vascular endothelial cells to promote transendothelial passage of neutrophils (41,45).

IL-1 is one of at least 18 interleukins produced by leukocytes, endothelial cells, fibroblasts, and glia (Table 6.2). Another interleukin, IL-2, in conjunction with interferon-γ, a glycosylated protein produced principally by T cells, can induce the generation of cytotoxic T cells that exhibit specificity for virus-infected cell targets (46). IL-6 plays a role in the induction and propagation of inflammatory responses; it also is a pyrogen. Increased levels of IL-6 are detected in CSF of patients with bacterial meningitis, and IL-6 is exceptional in that serum concentrations also are elevated in contrast to the compartmentalization of the responses of other cytokines in meningitis (36a,47,48). IL-8, a leukocyte chemotactic agent that promotes leukocyte adherence (49), is increased in CSF of patients with meningococcal meningitis but not aseptic meningitis (50). IL-10 is not present in serum but is elevated in CSF in the first 48 to 72 hours of viral meningitis. It is believed to downregulate inflammation and may contribute to chronicity of disease (51). Systemic administration of IL-10 attenuates the development of an inflammatory response in experimental meningitis (52).

Cytokines released from damaged cells serve to initiate leukocyte chemotaxis from blood into CSF, a response that is more pronounced in the

TABLE 6.3. *Therapeutic interventions against the inflammatory response*

Intervention	Action
Anti-CD-18 monoclonal antibodies to adhesion glycoproteins	Inhibit cytokine-induced leukocytosis and brain edema (26)
Pentoxifylline	Inhibits release from microglia of tumor necrosis factor, interleukin-1 (26a)
Transforming growth factor-β	Inhibits cytokine production, adhesion of granulocytes to endothelium (26b)
Dexamethasone	Inhibits cytokine-induced exudation of neutrophils in CSF (26)
	Inhibits secretion of interleukin-1β (40)
	Inhibits secretion of tumor necrosis factor-α (40)
	Inhibits phospholipase A_2, decreases release of free arachidonic acid, decreases production of prostanoids, leukotrienes (14)
Dexamethasone and nifedipine	Inhibit production of nitric oxide synthetase (26c)
Anticytokine antibody, interleukin-1, receptor antagonist soluble tumor necrosis factor receptor	Block cytokine action (44)
Nonsteroidal anti-inflammatory drug	Inhibits production of variety of cytokines (29)
Thalidomide	Inhibits tumor necrosis factor production (29a)
Interleukin-10	Downregulation of macrophage activation (52)
Fucoidin	Competitive inhibition of selectin, mediated leukocyte adhesion (52a)

juvenile than in the adult brain (53). Chemokines include diverse agents such as platelet-activating factor, IL-β, families of cysteine-containing chemokines, and the macrophage inhibitory proteins (MIP). Ectopic expression of chemokines in the CNS leads to dramatic accumulation of circulating leukocytes in brain parenchyma and CSF with accompanying pathology (54). Conversely, inhibition of leukocyte trafficking to the brain attenuates inflammation and tissue damage indicating that leukocytes are an important mediator of neuronal injury (43). This inhibition can occur at the level of the leukocyte integrins that serve as adhesion molecules or at the level of the endothelial adhesion receptors, such as selectins and intercellular adhesion molecules (55).

Reactive oxygen and nitrogen species are potent antimicrobial agents that also can damage host cells. Research has demonstrated that microglia, when activated with interferon-β and bacterial lipopolysaccharide, cause neuronal cell injury by a nitric oxide mechanism (56,57). Nitric oxide, a gas with a half-life of seconds, is responsible for regulation of vascular tone and perfusion pressure. In excess amounts, as generated in the CSF during infec-

tion, nitric oxide induces blood–brain barrier permeability and leukocytosis (58). Administration of inhibitors of inducible nitric oxide synthase decreases the bystander damage to host cells during meningitis. It is of note that the mean concentration of nitric oxide is significantly elevated in CSF taken in early stages of septic but not aseptic meningitis (59). In addition, nitric oxide is inhibitory to the replication of several pox viruses and herpes simplex, but has no effect against tick-borne encephalitis virus (60).

A number of therapeutic interventions have been introduced to prevent the injury induced by the various cytokines. These are summarized in Table 6.3.

Unique to established bacterial meningitis is the presence of elevated concentrations of complement C3 and factor β in the CSF. This elevation, which does not occur in aseptic meningitis of viral origin, can be of diagnostic value (59).

In addition to these inflammatory responses, the meninges also can manifest delayed hypersensitivity in the form of an acute exudative reaction, as occurs in the severe exudative meningitis produced by tuberculoprotein in animals, and by visceral tuberculosis in humans (61).

Because the arachnoid membrane is an effective barrier to the spread of infection, massive subdural empyema is infrequent in meningitis. Generally, only small amounts of fibrinous exudate are found in microscopic sections of the spinal or cranial dura. When fibrinopurulent exudate accumulates in large quantities around the spinal cord, the spinal subarachnoid space becomes obstructed. In the later stages of meningitis, noncommunicating hydrocephalus can be produced by exudate in the foramina of Luschka and Magendie or in the aqueduct of Sylvius. Communicating hydrocephalus results from inflammation or exudate in the subarachnoid space around the midbrain and pons or over the cerebral convexity. This exudate interferes with the flow of CSF from the cisterna magna and lateral recesses to the basal cisterns, or with the subsequent resorption of CSF by arachnoid granules (Fig. 6.3). An infrequent late sequela of bacterial meningitis is chronic adhesive arachnoiditis.

A mild inflammatory reaction in the vicinity of the perivascular spaces is soon followed by edema of the superficial cortex, which can become extensive.

Changes in cerebral function can occur because of occlusion of meningeal and cerebral vessels, direct interference with cerebral metabolism by invading organisms and their products, cellular damage owing to lymphokine production within the nervous system, inhibition of essential enzyme reactions, or cerebral edema.

Perfusion of blood can be impeded by acute increases in intracranial pressure (62,63), changes in the vascular bed, or acute hydrocephalic dilatation of the ventricles. Brain metabolism changes to glycolysis with increased glucose oxidation and lactate production and the depletion of high-energy compounds, such as phosphocreatine and adenosine triphosphate (ATP).

Brain edema in meningitis can be vasogenic, the result of increased permeability of the blood–brain barrier, or cytotoxic. Both vasogenic and cytotoxic edema can be caused by constituents of the neutrophil membrane (64). Cytotoxic brain edema is marked by increased brain water, cellular swelling, increased intracellular sodium, and loss of intracellular potassium (64). This edema can lead to depolarization of neuronal membranes and predispose to seizure activity. These changes are mediated in part by polyunsaturated fatty acids, released from leukocytes and possibly brain cell membranes (65). Vasogenic edema is caused by the opening of tight junctions between cerebral capillary endothelial cells, and increased micropinocytosis across endothelial cells. It can result from the presence of bacteria as well as inflammation (16). Additionally, there are concomitant increases in superoxide and lipid peroxidation, believed to result from inhibition of superoxide dismutase activity (66). Arachidonic acid, formed in part by cleavage of phospholipids by phospholipase A2, not only accumulates in meningitis, but also in other pathologic insults such as ischemia, hypoxia, and trauma. Dexamethasone, which inhibits phospholipase A2 and is said to be a membrane stabilizer, is effective in reducing arachidonic acid–induced brain edema *in vivo* but not *in vitro* (see Table 6.3) (65). Bacterial cells or cell fragments also induce cerebral arteriolar vasodilatation by formation of oxygen free radicals. Pretreatment with superoxide dismutase prevents the vasodilatation and edema (67).

If the inflammatory process continues unchecked for several days, glial proliferation occurs. The changes in the nerve cells can be slight or there can be widespread destruction of both cortical cells and myelinated fibers. Cortical and subcortical abscesses are rare. The breakdown of the nervous tissue can, by itself, induce a cellular response, which augments that caused by the infectious agent.

Fibrous encapsulation of a cerebral infection is limited because the only available supply of fibroblasts arises from blood vessel walls and from dural mesodermal elements. Thrombophlebitis of the cerebral veins can produce ischemic necrosis of the cortex, although extensive cortical necrosis can be observed without any demonstrable venous thrombosis. Focal areas of wedge-shaped cortical infarction or widespread areas of infarction have been demonstrated by neuroimaging in one-third of children with meningitis complicated by seizures, hemiparesis, or coma. This necrosis,

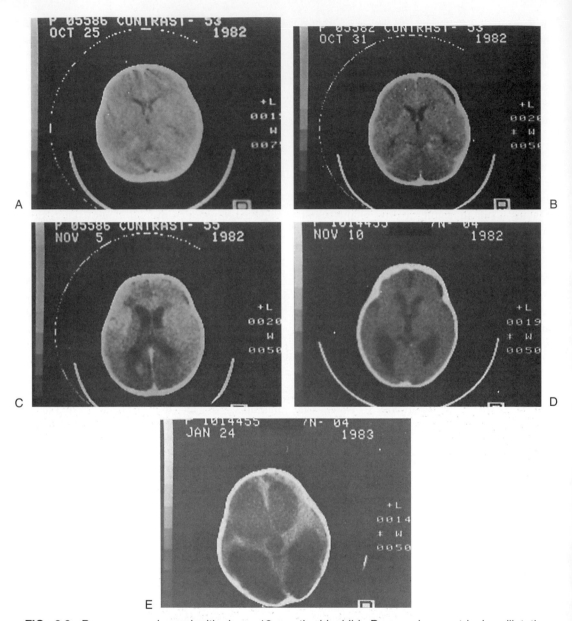

FIG. 6.3. Pneumococcal meningitis in a 12-month-old child. Progressive ventricular dilatation resulted from atrophy and subsequent hydrocephalus. **A:** Treatment day 1. Computed tomographic (CT) scan with contrast. Ventricles are small. The child is having seizures during syndrome of inappropriate secretion of antidiuretic hormone. **B:** Treatment day 6. CT scan with contrast. An infarct is seen in the territory of the left middle cerebral artery and a right subdural effusion. Additionally, early ventricular dilatation is seen. **C:** Treatment day 11. CT scan with contrast. Contrast enhancement is in the region of the infarct. The ventricular dilation has increased, even though intracranial pressure is 6–8 mm Hg, a normal value. **D:** Treatment day 16. CT scan without contrast. There has been progressive hydrocephalus with enlargement of the cranium. Atrophy of brain substance is greatest in the region of the left middle cerebral artery infarct. **E:** Three months after onset of meningitis. Ventricular enlargement is now massive with little cortical mantle. A subsequent ventriculoperitoneal shunt arrested head enlargement, but failed to reconstitute the cortical mantle. (Photography by Mr. Edgar Davis.)

which is best visualized by contrast-enhanced CT scans or MRI, can occur as early as the second day of illness (see Fig. 6.3) (68).

In one-third of the patients, meningitis is associated with ventriculitis, and involvement of the ependyma, choroid plexus, and subependymal tissues can result. Ependyma and subependymal tissues change little early in meningitis, but cellular infiltration of the subependymal perivascular spaces and glial proliferation can occur in severe or prolonged meningitis and result in overgrowth of the ependymal lining and obliteration of the aqueduct of Sylvius.

Gram-negative endotoxin within the ventricular system can induce systemic alterations with resultant respiratory and circulatory failure (69,70). Symptoms include pulmonary edema, which develops from an intense systemic vasoconstriction; subendocardial hemorrhages; myocardial necrosis; hemorrhagic lesions in the adrenal corticomedullary junction; and ulcerations of the intestinal mucosa. McCracken found that the endotoxin concentrations in CSF correlate with clinical severity and neurologic outcome of *H. influenzae* type B meningitis (71).

Obstructive hydrocephalus can result from ependymal or glial proliferation with aqueductal obstruction. A block of the fourth ventricular foramina can result from creamy or gelatinous pus at the base of the brain (see Fig. 6.1). Communicating hydrocephalus can result from involvement of the basilar meninges, the absorptive surfaces, the arachnoid villi, or the dural sinuses.

Vascular Consequences of Meningitis

In early meningitis, regional cerebral blood flow is increased; however, in severe meningitis cerebral blood flow is reduced (72,73). Doppler blood flow studies document that an increase in intracranial pressure decreases cerebral blood flow by lowering end-diastolic blood flow velocity, with little change in peak systolic blood flow velocity. Survivors of bacterial meningitis have a significant increase in end-diastolic cerebral blood flow velocity relative to the initial value in comparison with nonsurvivors, and there is a reduction in the use of available oxygen (73). In

the study of Paulson and associates, cerebral blood flow was reduced to 72% of normal, and the cerebral arteriovenous oxygen difference to 63% of normal, with a consequent decrease in oxygen consumption to 42% of normal. Additionally, the physiologic independence of cerebral arterial blood flow from the systemic circulation was lost in two-thirds of subjects (74). This loss of cerebrovascular autoregulation, which in some cases was restored by hypocapnia, is believed to be caused by tissue acidosis (74) or by increased intracranial pressure (75). Although autoregulation is lost in experimental meningitis, its importance in the evolution of meningitic symptoms is not clear. In the study of Ashwal and associates, autoregulation of cerebral blood flow was preserved in all children with bacterial meningitis (76). Cerebral blood flow can be substantially decreased globally, with considerable regional variability. Ashwal and coworkers found that the response of cerebral blood flow to changes in carbon dioxide partial pressure (pCO_2) varied between patients and between different regions of the brain, and that hyperventilation could reduce cerebral blood flow below ischemic thresholds (76). For this reason they advised caution in the routine use of hyperventilation to reduce intracranial pressure in meningitis. Mortality in infections of the nervous system correlates with decreased cerebral perfusion pressure, increasing to 100% if the cerebral perfusion pressure cannot be maintained above 30 mm Hg (77).

Regional alterations in cerebral blood flow also can be induced by local vasospasm. Neuropeptide Y is a neuromodulator in sympathetic nerves where it acts in cooperation with norepinephrine for regulation of vascular tone (78). It is abundant in the brain and the peripheral nervous system. It is increased threefold in the medulla, and an increase in neuropeptide Y immunoreactive fibers surrounding small vessels occurs after 48 hours of infection in experimental pneumococcal meningitis (79).

Disorder of cortical neurons with a change in mental state or seizures occurs in some patients as much as several days before microscopic alterations are demonstrable. This disorder is not the result of bacteria within the substance of the brain, but represents a metabolic or toxic encephalopathy (64). Excitatory amino acids such as glutamate, which is increased in the CSF of patients with bacterial meningitis but not viral meningitis, may contribute to neuronal death. The concentration of glutamate and the duration of its elevation in the CSF of patients with meningitis correlate with the severity of the disease as measured by the Glasgow Coma Score and with a poor neurologic outcome (80).

The leptomeningeal inflammation increases vascular permeability for fluid and at the same time reduces bulk absorption. The result is an increase in intracranial pressure, which progressively impedes cerebral perfusion and produces further tissue hypoxia. The pathophysiology of pulmonary edema associated with increased intracranial pressure in some cases of meningitis is not completely understood, but it not only is associated with vasoconstriction, but also with an increase in pulmonary artery pressure, increased lung vascular permeability, and, occasionally, elevation in left atrial pressure (81).

Clinical Manifestations

Occult bacteremia often precedes bacterial meningitis. In a review of literature by Baraff and associates, the mean probability of subsequent meningitis for children who had fever caused by occult bacteremia and who did not receive antibiotics was 9.8%, for those who received oral antibiotic it was 8.2%, and for those who received parenteral antibiotic it was only 0.3% (82).

Signs and symptoms associated with the fully developed picture of acute purulent meningitis include fever, headache, nausea and vomiting, nuchal and spinal rigidity, alterations of sensorium, convulsions, cranial nerve palsies, disturbances in vision, and occasionally papilledema (83–85).

Headache results from inflammation of the meningeal vessels and from increased intracranial pressure. It is often accompanied by photophobia and hyperesthesia. Head retraction, neck stiffness, and spinal rigidity are caused by irritation of the meninges and spinal roots, which elicits protective reflexes intended to shorten the spinal axis and immobilize the irritated tissue (86). With lengthening of the spine, nerve roots are stretched, and the resulting pain and reflex spasm is the basis of Kernig sign, as well as of the neck and leg Brudzinski signs. Spinal rigidity is a more sensitive sign of meningeal irritation than nuchal rigidity, especially in young children. Nuchal stiffness is most readily demonstrated with the child in the sitting position with the legs extended (87).

Alterations in sensorium are related to a toxic and metabolic encephalopathy or can be postictal.

Seizures can be both generalized and focal. In the series of Dodge and Swartz seizures occurred in 44% of patients with *H. influenzae* meningitis, 25% of *S. pneumoniae* infections, 10% of meningococcal infections, and 78% of patients with streptococcal meningitis (85). Focal seizures can be the result of localized involvement of the cerebral hemispheres. In a study by Samson and associates (88), 18% of patients had their first febrile convulsion in the course of meningitis. Significantly, 40% of these patients, all younger than 16 months of age, had no clinical evidence of meningitis. A lumbar puncture, therefore, is advised at the time of the first febrile convulsion and might be advisable in subsequent febrile convulsions in children younger than 18 months, even in the absence of nuchal rigidity, as long as meningitis is strongly suspected (89) or the seizure has atypical features (90).

Cranial nerve involvement is caused by local inflammation of the perineurium, as well as by impaired vascular supply to the nerves. Cranial nerves VI, III, and IV are most commonly affected. Transient opsoclonus can occur (91). Cochlear and vestibular deficits occur owing to septic involvement of the endolymphatic and perilymphatic systems of the scala tympani (92) or are caused by cytolytic toxins elaborated by bacteria (93). Conductive hearing loss that results from middle ear dysfunction following meningitis should not be confused with sensorineural deafness (94). Fortnum and Davis found no difference in the incidence of hearing loss depending on the infecting pathogen. However, they found a significantly increased risk for children aged younger than 1 month or more than 5 years of age, children with hydrocephalus, those in hospital longer than 16 days, and those with a decreased CSF glucose (95). Jiang and coworkers suggest that a slightly depressed amplitude of the brainstem auditory potential wave V is the most sensitive indicator of brainstem dysfunction in children recovered from meningitis (96). Otoacoustic emissions are another effective way to detect hearing loss due to meningitis (96a).

Focal lesions of the brainstem can occur. These include discrete bilateral lesions in the region of the mesencephalic-diencephalic junction, with resultant selective downward gaze paralysis (97). In a few rare instances, acute cerebellar ataxia can be the presenting symptom in *H. influenzae* or *Neisseria meningitidis* (98,99). Cortical blindness also has been encountered (100).

Sustained increased intracranial pressure only rarely results in papilledema, unless the acute meningitis is associated with mass lesions such as abscesses or subdural collections. Widened sutures can occur within 2 days after onset of meningitis in young children (101); however, progressive ventricular enlargement can develop without excessive head growth during or after a bout of meningitis (102). This enlargement results from cerebral destruction or from the effects of increased intraventricular pressure on already compromised brain parenchyma. In young infants, the low water content of brain parenchyma, lack of myelin, and relatively large subarachnoid space also permit ventricular enlargement without increasing the head circumference.

Focal cerebral signs are usually secondary to cortical necrosis or occlusive vasculitis, most commonly thrombosis of the cortical veins. Focal signs also may occur with cerebral vasculitis, cerebritis, or abscess formation. Hemiparesis or seizures that appear after the tenth day of the infection can signify delayed vascular thrombosis.

Cranial bruits over the anterior fontanel and the posterior temporal areas are more common in children with purulent meningitis than in both febrile and afebrile controls (103). Tache cérébrale is a common, but not pathognomonic, finding in meningitis (104).

Complications

Complications of bacterial meningitis include ventriculitis, subdural effusion, electrolyte disturbances, and recurrent bacterial meningitis.

Ventriculitis

Infections of the ventricular system can be primary or can develop secondary to the spread of organisms from the subarachnoid space caused by the ebb and flow of CSF or by the migration of motile bacteria. This complication is particularly common in neonates and has been reported in 92% of neonates with fatal meningitis (105). When ventriculitis is accompanied by an obstruction of the aqueduct of Sylvius, the infection becomes localized and can behave as an abscess. Rapid increase in intraventricular pressure can induce brainstem herniation and impair perfusion of the periventricular structures. Additionally, intraventricular toxins can produce remote effects. Ventriculitis is treated with massive parenteral antibiotics, but in addition, it can require periodic irrigation and drainage (106).

Subdural Effusion and Subdural Empyema

Although these complications were noted in cases occurring in the last century, they are now more easily diagnosed as the result of the availability of neuroimaging studies. Most subdural effusions occur over the frontoparietal region, although localized collections can develop over the occipital region. Subdural effusion is caused by the increased efflux of intravascular fluids as a consequence of thrombophlebitis of the veins bridging the subdural space, abnormal vascular permeability at the arachnoid–dura interface, or spread of the infection from an arachnoiditis. The effusion is usually bilateral. Its incidence has varied considerably from one series to another and is probably proportional to the

TABLE 6.4. *Indications for suspecting a sub-dural effusion in infants with purulent meningitis*

1. Failure of temperature curve to show progressive decline after 72 hours of adequate antibiotic and supportive treatment
2. Persistent positive spinal culture results after 72 hours of appropriate antibiotic therapy
3. Occurrence of focal or persistent convulsions
4. Persistence or recurrence of vomiting
5. Development of focal neurologic signs
6. An unsatisfactory clinical course, particularly evidence of increased intracranial pressure after 72 hours of antibiotic therapy

From Matson DD. *Neurosurgery of infancy and childhood*, 2nd ed. Springfield, IL: Charles C Thomas, 1969. With permission.

vigor with which this complication is sought. The condition is more likely to develop in younger infants, and most cases are seen in children younger than 2 years of age. Other factors that favor the evolution of a subdural effusion include a rapid onset of illness, low peripheral white blood count, and high levels of CSF protein and bacterial antigen. Although patients with effusion are more likely to have neurologic abnormalities at the time of admission and at completion of therapy and are more likely to have seizures during the course of treatment, no greater incidence of seizures, hearing loss, neurologic deficits, or developmental delay is seen on long-term follow-up (107).

Subdural empyema represents an infectious process in the subdural space. The term *subdural abscess* has been applied to the condition when the infection is localized to the subdural space. By contrast to subdural effusion, subdural empyema is a rare complication of bacterial meningitis (108). Subdural effusions are seen in bacterial meningitis caused by a variety of organisms. They are most common when meningitis results from *H. influenzae* (45% of all effusions). Less often, pneumococcus (30% of all effusions) and meningococcus (9% of all effusions) are the responsible bacteria.

Indications for suspecting a subdural effusion or subdural empyema in the presence of meningitis are presented in Table 6.4 (109). The criteria set forth by Matson more than 30 years ago are still applicable; in particular, the presence of fever that lasts more than 3 to 5 days

after the start of antibiotic therapy should prompt initiation of diagnostic studies for these complications. Clinically, the differentiation between a subdural effusion and subdural empyema is difficult. The conditions can best be diagnosed by neuroimaging studies, with either ultrasound or gadolinium-enhanced MRI assisting in the distinction between subdural effusions and subdural empyema (110). Although the electroencephalogram (EEG) can reveal focal slowing or voltage depression, the result is too often normal to be a reliable diagnostic tool.

In a subdural effusion the fluid is xanthochromic or blood tinged initially and can become less yellow with repeated taps. The protein content ranges between 50 and 1,000 mg/dL and is always higher than the CSF protein obtained simultaneously. Compared with serum, subdural fluid has a disproportionately high albumin to globulin ratio. MRI generally shows the fluid to be isointense relative to CSF on both T1- and T2-weighted images (110). In subdural empyema the fluid shows a markedly elevated white count and protein concentration, with the glucose concentration being generally less than in CSF (110). On MRI the subdural empyema is hyperintense relative to CSF on proton density-weighted and T2-weighted images (110).

Currently, most centers recommend a conservative treatment of subdural effusions, and multiple subdural aspirations or surgical intervention are no longer recommended, because most collections resorb spontaneously (107). Snedeker and colleagues recommend a noninvasive approach to subdural effusion if the patient is improving, even though fever persists, and recommend that subdural taps be reserved for patients suspected of subdural empyema (107). Surgical intervention also is indicated if the effusion becomes hemorrhagic, or if it is large enough to result in a significant ventricular shift. The technique for a subdural tap is described by Matson (109). Should the decision be to remove the subdural fluid, the effusions are treated with repeated taps, removing no more than 30 mL of fluid on each occasion to relieve increased intracranial pressure. When the fluid condition fails to respond to a 2-week trial of repeated aspiration, a limited trial of closed extradural drainage of the subdural space can reduce the subdural fluid protein content to tolerable levels for a subdural-peritoneal shunt. This procedure is recommended when there is considerable loss of brain parenchyma and it is desired to convert a loculated subdural accumulation of fluid into a subarachnoid space occupied by CSF. Stripping of the subdural membrane is of doubtful efficacy and is no longer practiced. The persistence of subdural effusions reflects underlying cortical damage, for a normal cerebrum would sooner or later obliterate the subdural space (111).

Fluid and Electrolyte Disturbances

Compromise of intracranial intravascular volume in association with impaired cerebrovascular autoregulation and the presence of inflammation results in lower mean arterial blood pressure, lowered cerebral blood flow, and higher CSF lactate in human and experimental meningitis (112). Children with meningitis have an initial increase in total body water, almost all of which is in the extracellular compartment. The excess correlates with the severity of the illness and reverts to normal with recovery (112a).

Disturbance in sodium metabolism, usually with hyponatremia, is seen in approximately 20% of patients with meningitis (113). Hyponatremia can be the result of an intracellular shift of sodium with an extracellular shift of potassium as a consequence of the inflammation, syndrome of inappropriately high secretion of antidiuretic hormone (SIADH), or increased release of atrial natriuretic peptide (114). Inappropriate ADH release, which can occur with or without clinical hyponatremia (115), occurs in almost every case of bacterial meningitis, and in approximately 60% of cases of viral meningitis (116). It leads to hypervolemia, oliguria, and increased urinary osmolality, despite low serum osmolality. The symptoms are those of water intoxication and include restlessness, irritability, and convulsions, all of which can be ascribed to meningitis. The diagnosis can be made by repeated measurements of body weight, serum electrolytes, and serum osmolality, and by determinations of urinary volume, specific gravity, and urinary osmolality. The condition is treated by restricting

water intake, administering diuretics such as furosemide, and in severe cases, administering small amounts of additional sodium (117). In some of the chronic meningitides, inappropriate ADH secretion can induce a secondary diminution in aldosterone or increase in third factor effect with increased urinary sodium loss.

Children with tuberculous meningitis and laboratory evidence of inappropriate ADH secretion have significantly higher intracranial pressure than children without laboratory evidence of SIADH. In these children, the plasma level of arginine vasopressin (AVP) correlates with mean arterial pressure, but no correlation exists between plasma or CSF levels of AVP and increased intracranial pressure (118). Serum vasopressin levels can become elevated because of hypovolemia secondary to fluid restriction in patients with meningitis, and levels can normalize after treatment with maintenance plus replacement fluid therapy. We agree with Powell and associates that patients with meningitis can be given maintenance plus replacement fluid therapy, but should be monitored for the development of SIADH (119).

Recurrent Meningitides

Recurrent bacterial meningitis can be caused by acquired or congenital gross anatomic defects, foci of infection, or disorders in immune mechanism.

Gross anatomic defects that allow continuity between the nervous system and the exterior can allow frank leakage of CSF; other defects are minute and difficult to find. Skull fractures, especially those affecting the base of the brain and extending to the sinuses and petrous pyramids, are the most common cause of recurrent meningitis. They are discussed in Chapter 8. Congenital defects include myelomeningoceles, neurenteric cysts, midline or spinal dermal sinuses, and anomalies of the labyrinthine capsule and stapes foot plate. These conditions are covered in Chapter 4. Neuroschisis also can occur in the anterior portion of the pharynx as an anterior encephalocele or in the cribriform or orbital plate as a fine defect. Meningitis caused by these defects can first occur late in childhood (120).

Recurrent meningeal infections secondary to defects in the immune response can occur after

TABLE 6.5. *Major complications seen in 71 children after recovery from meningitis*

Complication	Number of cases
Mental retardation	3
Seizures	3
Hemiparesis or quadriparesis	1
Bilateral deafness	4
Vestibular disturbance	1
Hydrocephalus	1
Total	13 (18%)

Modified from Dodge PR, Swartz MN. Bacterial meningitis: a review of selected aspects. II. Special neurologic problems, postmeningitic complications and clinicopathological correlations. *N Engl J Med* 1965;272:954.

splenectomy or in the various immunopathies, including infection with the human immunodeficiency virus (HIV) and disorders of immunoglobulin production. Children with leukemia and lymphoma have a particularly high incidence of recurrent purulent and fungal meningitis (see Chapter 15). Recurrence caused by the same organism can be seen if therapy was inadequate or the organism is relatively resistant to treatment (121).

The incidence of chronic complications of meningitis is listed in Table 6.5 (85).

Diagnosis

The diagnosis of meningitis requires prompt examination and culture of the CSF (122,123). The technique of lumbar puncture and the interpretation of CSF findings are discussed in the Introduction chapter of this book. Like Archer, we do not believe that CT of the brain is indicated before performing a lumbar puncture in acute meningitis unless the patient shows atypical features such as an atypical history or findings on physical examination, particularly focal neurologic findings or coma (124). Inability to visualize the optic disc on funduscopic examination is not an indication for CT. For patients with papilledema, the risks associated with lumbar puncture are 10 to 20 times lower than the risks associated with bacterial meningitis alone (124). When a CT is indicated, blood culture and empiric therapy should be instituted before performing the imaging study. A 2-hour delay between antibiotic therapy and lumbar puncture does not interfere with isolation and culture of the causative organism if CSF culture is done along with blood cultures and tests for bacterial antigens in the CSF (125).

Characteristically, the fluid is under increased pressure and is cloudy. During the acute stage, the cells are predominantly polymorphonuclear, whereas a mononuclear response appears in the later stages. The cell counts generally range between 1,000 and 10,000 per μL, but in approximately 6% of cases they are normal during the earliest stage of the infection (126). Much higher counts suggest meningitis secondary to rupture of a brain abscess. Organisms can be seen intracellularly and extracellularly in smears, and occasionally they can be visualized or cultured in the absence of pleocytosis (127).

Eosinophilic granulocytes can be seen in the CSF of patients with parasitic infestations of the CNS, including cysticercosis, trichinosis, toxocariasis, toxoplasmosis, ascariasis, angiostrongyliasis, echinococcosis, and gnathostomiasis. Eosinophilic meningitis also can occur with coccidiomycosis (128).

Characteristic for bacterial and tuberculous meningitis is a decrease in the CSF glucose content. First observed by Lichtheim (129), the decrease was initially attributed to consumption of glucose by bacteria growing in the CSF. This explanation, along with many subsequent ones, has been abandoned in view of conflicting experimental evidence, and the mechanism of the low CSF sugar remains uncertain. Leukocyte fragments have been shown to have a direct effect on brain metabolism (64); however, hypoglycorrhachia and elevated lactate levels occur in CSF of leukopenic rabbits with experimental pneumococcal meningitis (16). Prockop and Fishman found that the facilitated diffusion of glucose from blood to CSF and from CSF to blood is impaired in bacterial meningitis, although the increase in nonspecific bulk transport of glucose more than makes up for the deficit (130). Some evidence also points to a significant decrease in cerebral glucose oxidation and an increase in glycolysis, so that a combination of these metabolic alterations can be responsible (131). Low CSF sugars also are seen in sarcoidosis, mumps leptomeningitis, herpes zoster meningitis, CNS leukemia, and meningeal carcinomatosis (132). In bacterial meningitis, the CSF to blood glucose ratio is usually below 0.40 (133).

CSF protein is elevated in 80% to 92% of patients (83), and there is a significant direct correlation between mortality and increased CSF protein (134). Blood–brain barrier permeability is increased in meningitis but not in aseptic meningitis. The serum to CSF ratio of albumin is approximately 100:1 in healthy children and those with aseptic meningitis, whereas it is approximately 15 to 50:1 in bacterial meningitis. Normal permeability is reestablished approximately 3 weeks after therapy is initiated (135). CSF lactate is significantly increased in bacterial meningitis, although brain tissue lactate can remain normal (136). An elevation of CSF lactate has been considered to be useful in the diagnosis of bacterial meningitis by some (137), but not all, authorities. CSF lactate is normal in aseptic meningitis unless cerebral hypoxia or edema has activated the glycolytic pathways (138,139). The slow decrease of CSF lactate to normal with a 3-day course of antibiotic therapy can be useful in the diagnosis of partially treated bacterial meningitis (140) and cerebral abscesses (138) and can aid in differentiating bacterial meningitis from aseptic meningitis (141). The decrease in CSF pH, which also occurs in bacterial meningitis, is more transient than the elevation of CSF lactate, and therefore, is less reliable for diagnostic purposes (140). The concentration of free amino acids and the activities of a variety of CSF enzymes, notably L-lactic dehydrogenase (142) and glutamic-oxaloacetic transaminase (143), are increased in bacterial meningitis, but their measurement is of little diagnostic value. The chloride level, once thought to differentiate between bacterial and tuberculous meningitis, also is of little value, because the low CSF chloride levels, common in chronic meningitis, reflect low systemic chloride levels.

Many of the cytokines, including TNF, IL-1β, IL-6, IL-8, and IL-10, have been investigated in the search for a practical marker to distinguish bacterial from viral infection. Thus far, no single measure has achieved sufficient sensitivity and specificity. IL-6 and C-reactive protein appear to be the most promising, with IL-6 levels having up to 86% specificity for bacterial infection (144). Serum C-reactive protein is elevated after 12 hours in bacterial, but not often in viral infections of the nervous system (145). It is more useful for the diagnosis of bacterial meningitis than determination of CSF TNF-α, or IL-1β when there is a low CSF leukocyte count (146). Determination of CSF ferritin levels appears promising as a marker for the diagnosis of partially treated bacterial meningitis. In the study by Katnik, CSF ferritin levels were elevated in 98% of cases with bacterial meningitis and ventriculitis, and in 20% of cases with nonhemorrhagic aseptic meningitis. Among 441 control patients, elevation of ferritin (more than 18 ng/mL) occurred in two cases of leukemia in relapse and 12 with sepsis (147).

Counterimmunoelectrophoresis, useful in demonstrating bacterial antigens in the CSF, has largely been replaced by latex agglutination for the diagnosis of *H. influenzae* (148), *Escherichia coli* (149), and other types of bacterial meningitis.

The polymerase chain reaction (PCR) has been used for the diagnosis of meningitis and recognition of the causative agent by identification in the CSF of DNA fragments from *N. meningitidis* (150), *H. influenzae*, and *Mycobacterium tuberculosis* (151). It also has been useful in the diagnosis of meningitis caused by *Mycoplasma* (152,153), spirochetes (154), and a large variety of viral organisms (155–157). This highly sensitive technique, however, can give false-positive results unless proper laboratory controls are employed (158). Because antigen concentration is closely related to bacterial count, a positive correlation exists between the concentration of bacterial antigen in the CSF and the presence of neurologic sequelae (159). Persistence of antigen for longer than 48 hours after the start of therapy is ominous and can indicate the need for a change of antibiotic therapy (160).

Partial treatment of bacterial meningitis or prior administration of intravenous antibiotics reduces the incidence of positive bacteriologic identification by culture or smear from 97% to 73% (161), but does not otherwise alter the diagnostic validity of the changes seen on examination of CSF (162).

Leptomeningeal carcinomatosis can be difficult to recognize because symptoms and CSF findings can simulate granulomatous meningitis. Levels of carcinoembryonic antigen are frequently elevated in leptomeningeal carcinomatosis and occasionally may be increased with epidural or parenchymal metastases. α-Glucuronidase levels can be elevated in lymphomatous and leukemic meningitis, but occasional mild elevations have been reported in acute and chronic or infectious or inflammatory meningitis (163).

On rare occasions, bacterial meningitis can be complicated by a simultaneous viral infection of the CNS (164).

The role of neuroimaging studies in the diagnosis of meningitis is relatively limited. However, they are of considerable assistance in the diagnosis of the various complications of bacterial meningitis.

During the course of therapy, indications for neuroimaging studies include prolonged, depressed level of consciousness, prolonged, partial or late seizures, focal neurologic abnormalities, enlarging head circumference, evidence of continuing infection, progressive neurologic signs, or recurrence of disease (122–124,165).

In the series of Rennick and colleagues, cerebral herniation occurred in 4.3% of children with meningitis (166). When ventricular dilatation is significant, it is sometimes prudent to reduce the intracranial pressure before lumbar puncture to diminish the risk of herniation (167). This is particularly true if the child has a Glasgow Coma Score of 7 or less (168). Severe cerebral edema complicating neonatal meningitis has been associated with uncal herniation (169,170).

Treatment

Treatment of purulent meningitis falls into two categories: antibacterial chemotherapy and specific measures designed to prevent or reverse systemic and neurologic complications (171). The management of the pediatric patient with meningitis is reviewed by Quagliarello and Scheld (125) and Feigin and colleagues (123), with an update by Wubbel and McCracken (172).

The following fundamental principles apply to the management of meningitis without regard for cause.

1. Antibiotic therapy should be prompt and appropriate.
2. Cerebral metabolism should be protected.
3. Increased intracranial pressure should be monitored by clinical signs, intracranial sensors, or by serial measurements of head circumference.
4. Seizures should be prevented or controlled.
5. Fluid management should strive for normovolemia, avoiding the hypervolemia of SIADH and the hypovolemia of dehydration.
6. Hyperpyrexia, which increases cerebral metabolic demand, should be controlled.

The principal aim of antibiotic therapy is to use the proper antibiotic in a dosage high enough to maintain effective CSF concentrations. The choice of the antibiotic depends on the causative organism (Table 6.6). Details of currently recommended schedules for antibiotics in the treatment of the more common forms of bacterial meningitis are presented in the 1997 Report of the Committee on Infectious Diseases, American Academy of Pediatrics (172).

Antibiotics vary in their ability to cross the noninflamed meninges depending on lipid solubility, protein binding, and degree of ionization. Antibiotics are metabolized or removed by bulk or facilitated transport (173). The ratio of brain level to blood level corrected for serum contamination was found to be 9:1 for chloramphenicol, 1:7 for cephalothin, 1:20 for cephaloridine, 1:23 for penicillin, and 1:56 for ampicillin (174). This ratio is altered by inflammation, which disrupts the blood–brain barrier of the meninges, and by the protein-binding property of each antibiotic.

Cefotaxime (175) or ceftriaxone (176) is effective in childhood bacterial meningitis caused by *H. influenzae*, meningococcus, or pneumococcus and has been recommended for empiric therapy of meningitis for children out of the neonatal

TABLE 6.6. *General recommendations regarding treatment of meningitis*

Known organisms	Primary treatment for susceptible organisms	Alternative treatment
Streptococcus pneumoniae	Third-generation cephalosporin	Vancomycin
Neisseria meningitidis	Penicillin	Cefotaxime
Haemophilus influenzae	Ceftriaxone	Cefotaxime
Staphylococci	Nafcillin, oxacillin	Vancomycin (if methicillin resistance is suspected)
Listeria monocytogenes	Ampicillin and aminoglycoside	Trimethoprim-sulfa
Usual gram-negative rods	Cefotaxime, ceftizoxime, ceftriaxone	Ampicillin and aminoglycoside
Resistant gram-negative rods (especially *Pseudomonas*)	Ceftazidime and aminoglycoside (intravenous, intrathecal)	Ticarcillin, mezlocillin, and aminoglycoside
Anaerobes (including *Bacteroides fragilis*)	Penicillin and metronidazole	Chloramphenicol
Unknown pyogenic organism in neonates (younger than 2 months of age)	Ampicillin and aminoglycoside	Ampicillin and third-generation cephalosporin (e.g., cefotraxime)
Unknown pyogenic organism in children	Ampicillin and chloromycetin	Third-generation cephalosporin and penicillin

Adapted from Wubbel L, McCrackcn GH Jr. Management of bacterial meningitis. *Pediatr Rev* 1998;19:78; and Kennedy SS, Zacharski LR, Beck JR. Thrombotic thrombocytopenic purpura: analysis of 48 unselected cases. *Semin Thromb Hemost* 1980;6:341.

age range. Ceftriaxone offers an advantage because it can be administered as a single daily dose. With rare exception (1 in 81) both produce negative CSF cultures within 24 hours of the beginning of therapy (177). The antibiotics should be supplemented with ampicillin in infants younger than 3 months of age (125).

Although there is no generally accepted standard exists for duration of treatment (178), current recommendations of the American Academy of Pediatrics are 7 to 10 days for *H. influenzae*, 10 to 14 days for pneumococcus, and 5 to 7 days for meningococcus. We suggest that patients with bacterial meningitis should have parenteral therapy for at least 5 days after the fever has subsided. We also recommend an intravenous route of administration, with the infusion extended over several hours to achieve the high blood and CSF levels of antibiotics needed to overcome reconstitution of the blood–brain barrier as healing progresses (179,180). The oral route creates considerable uncertainty with respect to blood levels, and the subcutaneous and intramuscular routes can incite severe local reaction. The oral use of chloramphenicol, a route that gives more effective levels than the parenteral route, is allowable during the latter part of therapy.

We recommend that treatment be continued for at least 5 days after CSF cultures have become sterile. Other authors do not consider that a repeat lumbar puncture to verify a sterile CSF is required for older infants and children who have responded promptly to antibiotic therapy. Although experimental data suggest that certain combinations of antibiotics are antagonistic, clinical evidence does not offer support. Increasing the number of antibiotics, however, increases the incidence of toxic reaction.

The use of steroids in the management of the child with meningitis has received considerable attention. Clinical trials with dexamethasone, in addition to antibiotics, for the treatment of meningitis demonstrate a significantly lower incidence of profound hearing loss in the dexamethasone-treated group (181). The clinical experience in several studies of cephalosporins in combination with dexamethasone for the treatment of meningitis caused by *H. influenzae*, *N. meningitidis*, and *S. pneumoniae*, demonstrated a similar beneficial effect of combined antibiotic and corticosteroid therapy (182–185). A modification of the steroid regimen to shorten it to 2 days beginning with the first dose of antibiotics is currently recommended by the American Academy of Pediatrics. This recommendation is based on the work of Syro-giannopoulous (186). One important caveat arises when considering these results. Most of the cases of meningitis were caused by *H. influenzae*, in contrast to the predominance of *S. pneumoniae* in the current postvaccine era (187,188). The strength of the recommendation to use steroids broadly in the adjunctive therapy of meningitis hinges on the extensive experimental animal data that indicate that various anti-inflammatory agents generally improve outcome (189).

The action of corticosteroids on the various cytokines is outlined in Table 6.3.

Indications for repeat lumbar punctures depend on the clinical course of the patient. A patient with uncomplicated purulent meningitis who responds well to treatment might not need a second lumbar puncture before termination of therapy because the wide range of glucose and protein values and cell counts encountered in the CSF precludes interpretation (190). Persistence of a positive CSF culture result 24 hours after initiation of therapy is considered a poor prognostic sign (191).

The increase in intracranial pressure, noted early in meningitis, can cause significant alterations in consciousness. Reduction in intracranial pressure can be accomplished by slow repeated removal of CSF, by the use of hyperosmolar agents such as mannitol or furosemide, or by diuretics. These agents can result in prompt improvement in the sensorium. Mannitol can be of short-term use to reduce intracranial pressure. Mannitol is effective for the cytotoxic edema, but not for the vasogenic edema of meningitis. Loculation of infection within the ventricles can require ventricular taps (106). This procedure, however, can promote brain abscess by intracerebral seeding of bacteria, a complication preventable by antibiotic therapy. In such situations, repeated taps can be avoided by the use of a reservoir.

Intracranial pressure exceeding 20 mm Hg is abnormal. Intracranial pressure can be reduced by elevating the head of the patient's bed by 30 degrees. Hyperflexion, hyperextension, or turning the neck, which can elevate intracranial pressure, as can inordinately tight tracheostomy ties, should be avoided. Increase in intracranial pressure with suctioning can be minimized with intravenous lidocaine. The use of hyperventilation to reduce intracranial pressure by reduction of pCO_2 is controversial and may be detrimental in some cases (76), because it can cause augmentation of increased intracranial pressure or cerebral anoxia.

When seizures complicate meningitis, their prompt treatment is imperative. Lorazepam or diazepam is effective for emergency use. Phenytoin, which does not have the depressant effects of barbiturates, should be considered for the acute treatment period.

In general, fluid deficit should be replaced. Thereafter, the amount of intravenous fluid administered to a patient with meningitis should be on the low side of the daily maintenance and replacement requirements (1,200 to 1,400 mL/m^2 per day) to avoid the complications of hypervolemia and hyponatremia induced by an inappropriate ADH output (113). Careful monitoring of cardiovascular status is important because overzealous restriction of fluid can result in hypovolemia with hypotension and tachycardia, and a resultant hypoperfusion of the inflamed brain.

A secondary increase in temperature after 4 days of antibiotic therapy can be caused by phlebitis at the site of intravenous therapy, or it can indicate drug fever (192). Prolonged fever can be the result of persistence of the organism, an inappropriate antibiotic, subdural effusions or empyema, brain abscess, purulent arthritis, pneumonia, pericarditis, otitis media, mastoiditis, or ophthalmitis (193). A second infection, such as pulmonary tuberculosis or tuberculous meningitis, also can be encountered.

Recurrent infections with the same organism can be seen after inadequate therapy or when relative resistance to antibiotics permits the organism to remain dormant in a cryptic focus. Complement deficiency or other immunodeficiency also can result in recurrence of infection, as can any congenital or acquired communication between the CSF spaces and the exterior.

The management of bacterial meningitis complicating skull fractures is considered in

Chapter 8. The management of shunt infections is considered in Chapter 4.

Prognosis

The following four factors influence the outcome of meningitis:

1. The nature of the infectious agent and the severity of the initial process.
2. The age of the patient. As a rule, the younger the child, the poorer the prognosis.
3. The duration of symptoms before diagnosis and institution of intensive antibiotic therapy. In some studies (194) but not in others (125,195), the incidence of residua is higher in children whose diagnosis and treatment are delayed. Thus, Kresky and colleagues observed residua in 12% of children whose treatment was started less than 24 hours after the onset of symptoms, in contrast to 59% in those treated after 3 or more days of symptoms (196). However, in the experience of Kilpi and collaborators, an acute onset of symptoms was associated with a higher mortality than an insidious onset, which can delay diagnosis and treatment for more than 2 days (197).
4. The type and amount of antibiotic used. Bactericidal drugs are more effective than bacteriostatic ones. Patients with pneumococcal or gram-negative bacillary meningitis have poorer outcomes when treated with bacteriostatic drugs. The bactericidal activity of antibiotics in CSF depends on the ability of the antibiotic to penetrate into the fluid, its CSF concentration, and its intrinsic activity (125). Bactericidal drugs act somewhat more rapidly than bacteriostatic ones, but are associated with the release of bacterial cell constituents, which can cause a brief exacerbation of inflammation.

In the study by Chang and coworkers, the causes of early death from meningitis are hemodynamic in approximately two-thirds of patients and neurologic in one-third. Clinical parameters present on hospital admission that associate significantly with risk of death within the next 3 days are tachycardia, tachypnea, hypothermia, poor skin perfusion, metabolic acidosis, leukopenia, thrombocytopenia, and low cerebrospinal leukocyte count (198).

In the study by Grimwood and colleagues, published in 1995, one in four school-aged meningitis survivors had serious and disabling sequelae, a functionally important behavior disorder, or neuropsychological or auditory dysfunction that adversely affected academic performance (199). Children who survive meningitis contracted before 12 months of age are at greatest risk for sequelae (200).

In the experience of Thomas, published in 1992, residual deficits included a sensorineural hearing loss (8.5%), which was bilateral and severe in 5.6%, learning difficulties (12%), motor problems (7%), speech delay (7%), hyperactivity (4.2%), blindness (2.8%), obstructive hydrocephalus (2.8%), and recurrent seizures (2.8%) (201). Baraff and coworkers, in a meta-analysis of reports on meningitis in children 2 months to 19 years of age and published between 1955 and 1993, found that not surprisingly children from developed countries had a lower mortality (4.8% versus 8.1%) and lower likelihood of sequelae (17.5% versus 26.1%) than those from underdeveloped countries (202). Mortality was highest for meningitis caused by *S. pneumoniae* (15.3%) and less for *N. meningitis* (7.5%) and *H. influenzae* (3.8%) (202).

After bacterial meningitis, the 20-year risk for subsequent unprovoked seizures is 13% for those patients with early seizures, and 2.4% for those without early seizures. These figures contrast with the incidence of seizures after viral encephalitis. In the series of Annegers and colleagues, published in 1988, the 20-year risk for seizures was 22% for patients with early seizures, and 10% for those without early seizures. The 20-year risk for seizures was not increased after aseptic meningitis. When seizures did develop, their incidence was highest during the first 5 years after infection, but remained elevated over the next 15 years (203). Patients who develop intractable seizures after meningitis or encephalitis incurred before 4 years of age have a high incidence of neocortical seizure foci or mesial temporal sclerosis. The latter group of patients can respond to surgical intervention should seizures not respond to anticonvulsants (204).

The incidence of minimal residua after meningitis depends in part on the care with which reevaluation of survivors is performed. In long-term follow-up studies on survivors of *H. influenzae* meningitis, published in 1983, 29% were found to have significant handicaps, and only 48% were apparently free of sequels on neurologic examination. Children in the latter group, however, functioned at a significantly lower level than their peers (205). The incidence of sequelae does not depend on whether children were treated with antibiotics for 7 days or for 10 to 14 days (206). In the study by Moura-Ribeiro, published in 1992, the EEG was normal 2 to 6 months after meningitis in 17% of children, whereas 34% of EEGs were normal 2 years later (207). In the prospective study by Pike and colleagues, focal or generalized suppression on the EEG was associated with poor outcome. Cerebral infarction and edema demonstrated by CT were also predictive of a poor outcome; enlarged ventricles, enlarged subarachnoid spaces, and subdural effusions were not (208).

As documented by the various follow-up studies, a significant proportion of children, particularly those whose meningitis is caused by pneumococci, have bilateral conductive or sensorineural hearing loss (209). In the experience of MacDonald and Feinstein, hearing loss developed during the first 48 hours of the illness (210). Hearing loss is the consequence of labyrinthitis with involvement of the cochlea and, on occasion, the semicircular canals. Less often, deafness is caused by an arachnoiditis of the eighth nerve or damage to the auditory projection areas. If recovery occurs, it usually does so during the first 2 weeks, but improvement can continue for as long as 6 months (191). These results, obtained by brainstem auditory-evoked responses, underline the value of this procedure (211). We recommend such an examination in any child who has recovered from meningitis (209,212). In addition, audiometric examinations are indicated for older children who have recovered from septic meningitis.

The outcome of pediatric bacterial meningitis between 1979 and 1989 was reviewed by Thomas (201). The neurologic sequelae of meningitis have been reviewed by Smith (213).

Common Forms of Meningitis

With the introduction of immunization against *H. influenzae* and prophylaxis of group B streptococcal infections, the incidence of bacterial meningitis in children in the United States has undergone a significant change (see Table 6.1) (214).

Several forms of purulent meningitis present sufficiently distinctive clinical pictures to warrant separate discussions.

Meningococcal Meningitis and Other Neisserial Meningitides

Infections with *N. meningitidis* can assume three distinct clinical courses: meningitis; septicemia, which can precede invasion of the nervous system or can appear in an isolated, but fulminant form accompanied by a variety of skin lesions (Waterhouse-Friderichsen syndrome); and chronic meningococcemia, in which an equilibrium between bacteria and host appears to have become established (215). Susceptibility to meningococcal disease has a hereditary component. Families with low TNF production have a 10-fold increased risk for fatal outcome, whereas high IL-10 production increases the risk 20-fold. IL-10 is a potent inhibitor of TNF (216).

The epidemiology of meningococci has changed. Until 1962, sulfonamide-sensitive group A organisms were predominant. Since then, the overwhelming majority of both endemic and epidemic meningitis has been caused by group B organisms, and since 1985 groups Y and W135, and especially group C organisms have become more common. None of these groups responds to sulfonamide therapy. Although clinical and laboratory findings are similar for meningitis caused by groups A and C organisms, patients with group C infection carry a greater risk for arthritis, cutaneous vasculitis, septicemic manifestations, and death than do infections with organisms from other serogroups (217,218). Children with meningitis caused by nongroupable meningococci and

Neisseria-related bacteria should be studied for complement deficiency (219).

The meningococcus produces distinctive skin lesions in approximately 75% of patients. The rash can be petechial, maculopapular, or morbilliform. Petechiae also are occasionally seen in patients with *H. influenzae*, pneumococcal, or streptococcal meningitis. Septicemia can result in local tissue sensitization leading to purpura fulminans as a consequence of intravascular coagulation. Purpura fulminans also has been seen in septicemia and meningitis caused by other Neisseria, including *N. catarrhalis* (220), *N. subflava* (221), and *N. gonorrhoeae* (222).

Meningococcal septicemia can cause a rapidly evolving fulminant illness with high rates of morbidity and mortality. Two pathogenic mechanisms have been distinguished: bacterial embolization and the effects of gram-negative endotoxin and gram-negative endotoxin-induced shock (223,224). Bacterial embolization and shock result in widespread pulmonary microvascular thromboses. These thrombi, composed largely of platelets and leukocytes, can cause severe cor pulmonale. Meningococcal endotoxin activates the cascades of procoagulation, anticoagulation, and fibrinolysis, as well as the cytokine network and the complement system (224). Meningococcal endotoxin also produces disseminated intravascular coagulation, a response similar to the Schwartzman phenomenon, in which there is rapid consumption of fibrinogen and formation of fibrin thrombi in adrenal glands and renal glomeruli (225). The fibrin thrombi cause hemorrhagic infarction of the adrenal glands and renal cortical necrosis (226). Bilateral adrenal hemorrhages are seen in two-thirds of fatal cases.

Gram-negative endotoxic shock (septic shock) in meningococcemia is similar to that caused by other gram-negative organisms (227). Septic shock has been extensively reviewed by Astiz and Rackow (228) and by Parrillo (229), who point out the harmful role of cardiovascular dysfunction with myocardial depression and dilatation, vasodilatation and subsequent vasoconstriction, leukocyte aggregation, endothelial cell dysfunction, and multiorgan failure. Septic shock takes place in two phases. Vasodilation occurs first (hyperdynamic phase), with high cardiac output and low peripheral resistance. Later, hypovolemia results from extensive capillary leakage. The initial manifestations of inflammation are followed by a period of immune depression (228). Corticosteroid therapy is of no benefit when treatment is started after the onset of endotoxemia (229,230). Mortality correlates with the serum level of TNF (231) and with reduction in serum protein-C levels (232). The incidence of fatalities from meningococcemia gram-negative endotoxic shock and bacteremia can be reduced with a combination of protein-C concentrate, heparin, and hemodia filtration (224). Other modes of therapy that appear to be beneficial include infusion of recombinant amino-terminal fragment of bactericidal and permeability-increasing protein (233), and treatment with recombinant tissue plasminogen activator (234). Extracorporeal membrane oxygenation in support of intractable cardiorespiratory failure for patients unresponsive to conventional therapy in meningococcemia has been of benefit in the experience of Goldman and coworkers (235). Treatment of gram-negative endotoxemia with human antiserum to the lipopolysaccharide endotoxin core (236) or by the use of monoclonal IgM antibody against endotoxin (237) has been ineffective in human trials. The use of early hemodiafiltration therapy for meningococcemia remains controversial (238).

Chronic meningococcemia is associated with intermittent and relatively mild episodes of chills, fleeting rashes, joint pain or swelling, or joint effusions. Symptoms can regress without specific therapy or can recur over several days or weeks. They can be in the form of petechiae, erythema nodosum, papulonecrotic tuberculids, macules, or maculopapules. The severity of the accompanying fever varies. Recurrent neisserial infections of the nervous system are rare, but they occur with increased frequency in patients with deficiencies of IgG subclass (239) or complement (240).

Complications of meningococcal bacteremia can be seen with or without meningitis. Pericarditis has been reported in up to 1.6% of cases, arthritis in 2.7% to 5.8% of cases, and eye involvement in 0.4% to 3.1% of cases (241). Eye lesions include hypopyon and panophthalmitis. Autopsy of 200 fatal cases of meningococcal infection revealed acute interstitial myocarditis with focal necrosis and hemorrhage in 78% (242). Deafness after meningococcal meningitis is more frequent with infections by the uncommon serogroups (W135, X, Y, 29E) than with meningitis caused by serogroup B (243).

Specific therapy for meningococcal meningitis is outlined in the Report of the Committee on Infectious Diseases of the American Academy of Pediatrics (244). Supportive therapy is of prime importance in meningococcemia. It includes the use of colloids, α-adrenergic blocking agents (phenoxybenzamine) or β-adrenergic drugs (isoproterenol), and hypothermia. The hemorrhagic adrenal glands found in many of the fatal cases of meningococcemia suggest adrenal insufficiency, and studies by Migeon and associates have demonstrated a diminished adrenal stress response in severe meningococcal meningitis (245). Adrenal insufficiency might only contribute to the circulatory collapse, however. Even so, pharmacologic doses of cortisol in combination with administration of plasma reduce mortality in experimental endotoxic shock. Although heparin can attenuate intravascular coagulation, it did not affect the pulmonary microthrombi or the mortality and survival time in experimental models (246).

Chemoprophylaxis of extended family and other intimate contacts is recommended (244,247). Meningococcus group A capsular polysaccharide vaccine is effective in preventing meningitis when given to children aged 3 months to 5 years (248,249). However, antibody titers decrease with or without a 2-year booster to prevaccination levels after 5 years (250). Group B outer membrane vaccine is effective for children aged 4 years or older; group C vaccine is effective for children aged 2 years or older (251).

Several scoring systems have been developed to predict the outcome of meningococcal infections. These rely on the presence or absence of shock, altered mental status, rapid onset of symptoms, peripheral and CSF leukocyte count, erythrocyte sedimentation rate, and the presence of signs of meningeal irritation (252,253). A close correlation exists between the prognosis of meningococcal infections and the presence of a consumption coagulopathy. Unfavorable prognostic features include presence of petechiae for more than 12 hours before admission to a hospital, presence of shock, absence of meningitis, a normal or low blood leukocyte count, and a normal or low erythrocyte sedimentation rate. In the experience of Kornelisse and coworkers, a low CRP level, a low platelet count, a high serum potassium, and a high serum base deficit were associated with a high mortality (253a).

Haemophilus *Meningitis*

Before the availability of *H. influenzae* vaccine, *H. influenzae* was the leading cause of meningitis in the United States, resulting in 8,000 to 11,000 cases annually. Between the years 1985 and 1991, after the widespread introduction of the vaccine, the incidence of *H. influenzae* meningitis in the United States decreased by 82% (254,255) (see Table 6.1). *H. influenzae* vaccines consist of Hib capsular polysaccharide covalently linked to a carrier protein. They are not effective against virulent nonencapsulated organisms that are capable of CNS disease (256). *H. influenzae* meningitis almost always occurs in children, most commonly it is caused by *H. influenzae* type B, and occurs in 56% of cases of invasive *H. influenzae* infection (257). Less often, *Haemophilus* meningitis is caused by types A through F or nontypable organisms, *H. parainfluenzae* or *H. aphrophilus* (257,258).

Meningitis caused by *H. influenzae* occurs almost exclusively in children younger than 6 years of age (83). After the age of 6 years, the incidence is so low that when it occurs one should suspect defects in resistance or parameningeal infection. Cases have been described in apparently healthy adults, however (259).

Symptoms of influenzal meningitis in the older child are those associated with any acute meningitis infection. Most fatal cases are characterized by a fulminating meningitis, marked by neurologic deterioration within 24 hours of onset of symptoms. These symptoms include increased intracranial pressure, seizures, coma, and respiratory arrest. Ischemic cerebrovascular lesions develop in 90% of children in the course of the acute illness (260). Carotid artery occlusion (261), pericarditis, myocarditis, atrioventricular block (262), epiglottitis, cellulitis, and septic arthritis can accompany influenzal meningitis (263).

The most commonly recommended antibiotic treatment of *H. influenzae* meningitis is intravenous ceftriaxone (100 mg/kg per 24 hours) (182). Intravenous cefotaxime (200 mg/kg per 24 hours) is an acceptable alternative. These third-generation cephalosporins have blood–brain barrier penetration that is superior to their first- or second-generation predecessors (264). Pretreatment with corticosteroids such as dexamethasone is recommended to avoid sudden worsening of inflammatory manifestations caused by the transient increase in release of bacterial constituents. The risk for gastrointestinal bleeding as a consequence of corticosteroid use in infants with bacterial meningitis appears to be less than 1% (265). Ceftriaxone can cause reversible biliary pseudolithiasis and either drug may significantly alter the gastrointestinal flora, promoting overgrowth of such potentially pathogenic organisms as *Clostridium difficile*.

The combination of intravenous ampicillin (300 mg/kg per 24 hours; maximum, 10 g/day) and chloramphenicol (100 mg/kg per 24 hours), formerly the preferred form of therapy, has proven less reliable because 12% to 40% of *H. influenzae* isolates are resistant to these drugs. Chloramphenicol rarely causes the shocklike "gray baby syndrome". In addition, bone marrow suppression makes this drug less attractive as primary therapy.

Selection of the most effective antibiotic is based on bacterial sensitivity. Sensitivity of organisms in the CSF may not coincide with that in the blood, hence bacterial isolation from the CSF is preferable.

The mortality did not change much during the 1980s and 1990s, ranging from 2.8% to 3.8% (266). Approximately 15% of survivors have significant neurologic defects (267). Hearing loss is the most common neurologic sequela and is more common in children who have not been treated earlier than 24 hours after the onset of illness (268). This study is at variance with that of MacDonald and Feinstein who found that hearing loss developed during the first 48 hours of *H. influenzae* meningitis (210). Deficits ranging from moderate hearing loss to total deafness are found in approximately 11% of cases. In approximately one-half of the instances the hearing loss is bilateral.

Taylor and coworkers studied a group of children with a mean age of 17 months who contracted *H. influenzae* meningitis between 1972 and 1984 (269). Persistent neurologic sequelae occurred in 14%, with sensorineural hearing loss in 11% (unilateral in approximately one-half), seizure disorder in 2%, and hemiplegia with mental retardation in 1%. Children with acute neurologic complications (42%) scored slightly below their siblings in reading ability and IQ; no difference was found for children without acute neurologic complications. In the study by Taylor, sequelae were associated with lower socioeconomic status and with a lower CSF to blood glucose ratio (269). Other residua include visual and speech deficits, awkwardness, incoordination, transient cortical blindness (270), and facial paresis. Craniocervical myelopathy with permanent brainstem dysfunction can occur (271). Postmeningitic sequelae can result in selective cognitive dysfunction with lowered performance IQ but preservation of verbal IQ (269,272). Delay in motor maturation can be directly related to vestibular or cerebellar dysfunction. Residual EEG abnormalities can be present in as many as one-fourth of patients who recover, and psychological interviews and testing can disclose residual anxiety related specifically to the hospital experience in as many as 50% of older children (205,269).

Factors associated with poor prognosis include young age (younger than 1 year of age), illness duration of more than 3 days before therapy, more than 10 organisms per milliliter of CSF, a finding that correlates with high antigen concentrations, a severe inappropriate ADH level, focal neurologic findings unrelated to postictal state, and onset or persistence of seizures after 3 days of treatment (268).

Risk of disease in household contacts is increased 600-fold during the month after exposure to the index case. Of these cases, 50% occur within 3 days of onset of meningitis in the index case, and 75% occur within 7 days. Attack rates decrease with increasing age: rates are 3.8%

among children younger than 2 years of age, 1.5% among children 2 to 3 years of age, and 0.1% in children 4 to 5 years of age. Clusters of cases have been encountered in day care centers.

Rifampin prophylaxis (20 mg/kg per day in one dose for 4 days to a maximum of 600 mg per day) of *H. influenzae* type B disease has been recommended for index cases during their hospitalization, usually just before discharge, and for adult and pediatric household contacts when an unvaccinated child younger than 4 years of age lives in the household (273). It should be given as soon as possible, because 54% of secondary cases occur in the first week after hospitalization of the index case (274).

Pneumococcal Meningitis

The most common cause of meningitis for all age groups is *S. pneumoniae*. Predisposing factors for pneumococcal meningitis in the pediatric age group include an upper respiratory infection, acute or chronic otitis media, purulent conjunctivitis, and CSF rhinorrhea secondary to developmental abnormalities or trauma (83).

The pathogenesis of pneumococcal meningitis differs from that of meningitis caused by other organisms because a gram-positive pathogen does not harbor endotoxin. Pneumococci adhere specifically to cerebral capillaries using a surface protein, CbpA, which recognizes carbohydrates (7). The absence of CbpA completely eliminates invasion of human cells. Once attached, the invasive step involves bacterial recognition of the receptor for the chemokine, platelet-activating factor (PAF) (274). Both PAF and the pneumococcus contain choline, allowing the bacteria to subvert the endocytosis/recycling pathway of the PAF receptor for cellular transmigration. Once in the CSF, a variety of pneumococcal components, including the cell wall, lipoteichoic acid, and several cytotoxins, incite the inflammatory response (275). Interestingly, the potent cytotoxin, pneumolysin, contributes to loss of cochlear cells in meningitic hearing loss, but does not contribute to cell damage or inflammation in the brain itself (276,277). Cytochemical and pathophysiologic differences occur in experimental meningitis

caused by different strains of *S. pneumoniae* depending on their ability to release various surface components.

Diseases that alter splenic function (e.g., sickle cell disease) and splenectomy considerably increase the risk for pneumococcal or *H. influenzae* meningitis (278). Conversely, the immune reaction of the host may actually play an important role in enhancing bacterial virulence. Thus, the host's complement activation may worsen injury to the nervous system, as has been suggested by careful studies of meningococcal disease (279). It is even less well understood how invasive strains of blood-borne bacteria succeed in passing through the blood–brain barrier (6).

Pneumococcal meningitis is seen more often in children with sickle cell disease, particularly those younger than 5 years of age than in control populations (280). This difference results from the decrease in heat-labile opsonins (281), and the functional asplenia of children with sickle cell disease (282).

The general clinical signs and symptoms of pneumococcal meningitis are similar to those of the other bacterial meningitides. Cranial nerve palsies, as in tuberculous meningitis, may be a significant feature of basilar exudate (283). Mortality, greatest in children younger than age 1 year, is higher in patients with fulminating disease than in those whose infection develops more slowly (284,285). In the experience of Kornelisse and coworkers, approximately one-third of children who survive pneumococcal meningitis have sequelae; 19% had hearing loss and 25% neurologic sequelae; mortality was 17%. Presence on admission of coma, respiratory distress, shock, a CSF protein level of 250 mg/dL or greater, a peripheral white count of less than 5,000 per μL, and a serum sodium of less than 135 mEq/L were associated with mortality. Sequelae were associated with the presence of coma and a CSF glucose level of less than 11 mg/100 mL (286). The experiences of Arditi and coworkers are similar. Of the surviving children in his series, 25% had significant neurologic sequelae, and 32% were left with unilateral or bilateral hearing loss. It is of note that in this group of children the incidence of hearing loss was significantly higher in those who had received dexamethasone than in those who did not (286a).

The diagnosis of *S. pneumoniae* is best made by Gram's stain of the CSF. The success of this technique is volume-dependent, with 0.5 mL or more of CSF being optimal. In our experience, turnaround time for CSF Gram's stain result is approximately 1 hour. When antibiotics have been given before obtaining a CSF specimen, the organisms can appear bizarre or may not be present at all. The diagnosis also can be made by culturing the organism from the CSF or the blood. Blood culture results are positive in 50% of patients, whereas nasopharyngeal and ear culture results are positive in only 24% and, therefore, are less reliable for diagnosis (83). Otitis media is seen in 22% of children with pneumococcal meningitis, but the organisms isolated from the middle ear do not always coincide with those isolated from the CSF (285). When pneumococcal meningitis is accompanied by pneumococcal pneumonia, the prognosis is poorer.

Penicillin given by constant intravenous infusion is the preferred treatment because it produces sustained CSF concentrations between 4 and 6 hours after the start of the infusion. By contrast, single intravenous injections produce CSF levels that are high, but much less sustained. Therapy with penicillin is more effective early in the infection. *In vitro* and *in vivo* experiments have demonstrated rapid killing of bacteria when penicillin is added 4 hours after the beginning of an experimental infection, but little effect is seen when treatment is withheld for 12 hours. The prevalence of strains with decreased susceptibility to penicillin has increased dramatically, approaching 50% in some areas of the United States (287). Since the clinical presentation of children infected with penicillin-sensitive and penicillin-resistant organisms is similar, it is widely recommended that initial antibiotic therapy for childhood meningitis include vancomycin plus a third-generation cephalosporin (286,286a,288). Moxifloxacin, or some of the other quinolones that have good CSF penetrance, appears to be of promise in the treatment of penicillin-resistant pneumococci (289).

Organisms that are resistant to third-generation cephalosporin have been reported (290).

The pneumococcal polysaccharide vaccine can play a role in preventing infections caused by such bacteria (291), but the vaccine currently available commercially is poorly immunogenic in children younger than 24 months of age.

Staphylococcal Meningitis

Staphylococcus aureus is the cause of 0.8% to 8.8% of meningitis in several series encompassing patients of all ages. Approximately 20% of cases occurred in neonates, 10% in children, and 70% in adults (292). As many as 90% of cases occur in association with predisposing abnormalities of the CNS; in particular they can be a sequela to recent neurosurgery and head trauma. *S. aureus* is second only to *S. epidermidis* as a cause of CSF shunt-related infections, accounting for between 12% and 36% of such cases. Meningitis may develop from staphylococcal abscesses within the brain parenchyma or from spinal epidural abscesses. More remote staphylococcal infection, such as oral or abdominal abscesses, sinusitis, osteomyelitis, pneumonia, cellulitis, infected shunts or intravascular grafts, decubitus ulcers, and even abdominal abscesses, also have been implicated in the etiology of *S. aureus* meningitis, sometimes through the intermediate stage of brain or paraspinal abscesses. *S. aureus* is the organism most likely to cause meningitis in the setting of infective endocarditis. Meningitis caused by this organism may occasionally complicate cavernous sinus thrombosis. Other predisposing factors include various forms of immunocompromise, diabetes mellitus, renal failure, or malignancy (293,294). *S. aureus* meningitis related to surgery or shunts has a better prognosis than *S. aureus* that develops as a consequence of hematogenous seeding of the meninges. Thus, the overall mortality for children may be closer to 25% as compared with a 50% mortality for adults. Mortality for meningitis related to infective endocarditis, however, can be more than 80%. Other unfavorable prognostic factors include the development of shock, infection with type 95, and greater age (295).

Coagulase-negative staphylococcus infections, especially those with slime-producing variants (296), have been responsible for an indolent meningitic complication of ventriculoatrial and ventriculoperitoneal shunts (297, 298). In ventriculoatrial shunts, the location of the distal end of the shunt is an important factor in the frequency of shunt infections and meningitis. Location below T7 often results in bacteremia, whereas location at a level of T4 or higher is less likely to be associated with an infection (299). In some cases, more than one staphylococcal subgroup can colonize the shunt, each having a different antibiotic spectrum. This multiplicity is important in selecting an antibiotic because single-colony antibiotic sensitivities might not be sufficient (see Chapter 4 for a discussion of shunt-related infections).

Acute Purulent Meningitis in the Neonate

Neonatal meningitis has an incidence of 0.2 to 0.32 cases per 1,000 live births (300). It differs from meningitis in older infants and children in its clinical manifestations, the high incidence of gram-negative organisms, and the generally poor prognosis.

Meningitis occurs more often in male infants (68% to 76%) (301), except for group B streptococcus meningitis, which has a female preponderance (55% to 88%) (302). In the series of Bates and coworkers, reported in 1965, 38% of infections were caused by *E. coli*, 31% by group B β-hemolytic streptococci, 5% by *Listeria monocytogenes*, and 25% by one or more of 16 different pathogens (303). The latter include rare organisms, such as *Pasteurella multocida* (303), *Flavobacterium*, and *Pseudomonas cepacia* (304). Organisms uncommon in the newborn, such as *Salmonella* (305) and *N. meningitidis* (306), also can be encountered.

In a review published in 1993 by Unhanand and coworkers of children younger than age 2 years with gram-negative enteric bacillary meningitis, the median age for the onset of meningitis was 10 days (307). Predisposing factors were present in 26%, the most common being neural tube defects and urinary anomalies. The principal causative agents in their series were *E. coli* (53%), *Klebsiella-Enterobacter* species (16%), *Citrobacter diversus* (9%), and *Salmonella* species (9%).

Proteus species account for a large proportion of brain abscesses found in neonates (308).

In part, this spectrum of invaders results from virulence factors of the organism or from alterations in the immune state during the neonatal period. The various immune deficiencies of the normal newborn have been reviewed by Cole (309).

Additionally, the character of the invader can determine the evolution of the infection and its severity. S-fimbriated *E. coli* bind to human brain endothelial cells threefold greater than nonfimbriated organisms (310). *E. coli* K1 capsular antigen has been found in 84% of the *E. coli* colonies isolated from neonates with meningitis, which suggests that the presence of this antigen is associated with the organism's virulence (311). K1 strains account for approximately 40% of all *E. coli* meningitis in children younger than 2 years of age (312). Both mortality and morbidity in *E. coli* meningitis are greater when it is caused by K1 strains as compared with non-K1 strains.

Complications during pregnancy, labor, and delivery, especially if associated with fetal distress, are associated with an increased incidence of neonatal meningitis. Maternal infections, particularly of the genitourinary tract, also predispose to infection. The same agent can be isolated from the site of infection in the mother and from the CSF of her infant. Premature rupture of the membranes, when associated with peripartum infection and chorioamnionitis, can contribute to the susceptibility to meningitis (313,314).

In addition, infections of the fetus, particularly those of the respiratory tract and skin, predispose to meningitis. Bacterial meningitis complicates 20% to 30% of neonatal septicemia (300). Negative blood culture in early onset neonatal meningitis are seen in up to one-third of cases (300,315).

The paucity of clinical signs in neonatal meningitis makes the diagnosis extremely difficult. The major signs and symptoms are presented in Table 6.7. Classic signs of meningitis are rare; a bulging fontanel was observed in only 30% of patients, and nuchal rigidity in only 18%. Rather, the most common abnormalities are fever, poor activity and poor feeding, a gray

TABLE 6.7. *Signs and symptoms in 39 infants with neonatal meningitis*

	Premature infants		Full-term infants	
	Initial	Overall	Initial	Overall
Anorexia or vomiting	4	10	4	15
Lethargy	3	12	1	13
Irritability	0	0	4	15
Jaundice	3	10	2	3
Respiratory distress	5	11	1	5
Diarrhea	1	3	1	4
Bulging fontanelle	0	0	0	13
Convulsions	0	2	1	9
Nuchal rigidity	0	1	0	6
Fever	0	2	8	19
Pyoderma	0	0	1	6
Total	16		23	

From Groover RV, Sutherland JM, Landing BH. Purulent meningitis of newborn infants: eleven year experience in the antibiotic era. *N Engl J Med* 1961;264:1115. With permission.

appearance, and seizures (316). In preterm infants with respiratory distress but no other signs, bacterial culture of the CSF diagnoses meningitis in 0.3% (317). CSF findings can be confusing in neonatal meningitis. White blood counts of less than 32 per μL occur in 29% of group B streptococcal and 4% of gram-negative neonatal meningitis; protein concentrations of less than 170 mg/dL occur in 47% and 23%; and CSF to blood glucose ratios of more than 0.44 occur in 45% and 15%, respectively (318). CSF values for healthy term and preterm infants are presented in the Introduction.

In the 1980s and 1990s, group B streptococcal meningitis has assumed increasing importance (319). Two clinically and epidemiologically distinct forms of illness have been recognized. In one, symptoms begin within 10 days of birth. The incidence of obstetric complications is high (92%), infants are seriously ill at the time of diagnosis, and the mortality is high (58%). In this form of infection, the organisms are isolated from both CSF and other tissue fluids.

In the second form of group B streptococcal meningitis, the illness begins later than 10 days of age. The incidence of maternal complications is low (19%), infants are less severely ill, and

mortality and permanent neurologic sequelae are uncommon (19%). Organisms are usually isolated from only CSF and blood (320). Infants acquiring this form of meningitis are born to mothers with low levels of anticapsular polysaccharide antibody. In contrast to adults, these infants fail to produce polysaccharide antibodies on convalescence from the infection (321).

The diagnosis of neonatal meningitis can be made only by lumbar puncture. Specific CSF culture of organisms is the most reliable test. Primary cultures onto agar plates have a sensitivity of 81%. Broth enrichment cultures do not improve the sensitivity and frequently give false-positive results (322). Even in the CSF, the response to infection can be atypical, with only a minimal pleocytosis. Blood cultures are positive in 50% to 90% of infants with early onset meningitis, and usually yield the same organism as the CSF (323). Culture of the nasopharynx yields the same organism as the CSF in 40% of cases. The presence of bacterial antigens demonstrated by counterimmunoelectrophoresis in the CSF or by limulus lysate test also confirms neonatal meningitis. Demonstration of specific bacterial antigens in the serum or urine suggests meningitis.

The prognosis is poor. In the series of Hristeva and coworkers, published in 1993, the mortality was 26% with significant neurologic sequelae in 27% of survivors (323a). Not surprisingly, the degree of EEG abnormality correlates with outcome. Infants with normal or mildly abnormal background activity have favorable outcomes, whereas those with markedly abnormal patterns either die or have severe neurologic sequelae (324). In infants, mortality owing to CNS infections also correlates closely with the degree of decrease of cerebral perfusion pressure (77,325).

Therapy should be specific for the invading organism and instituted as early as possible. Choice of antibiotic is similar to that for older children (see Table 6.6). For group B streptococci, a combination of ampicillin and gentamicin is recommended (172,326). Therapy for gram-positive bacteria should last approximately 14 to 21 days (326). In infections caused by gram-negative pathogens, therapy should be continued for 2 weeks after sterilization of the

CSF or for a minimum of 3 weeks total. A combination of ampicillin (150 mg/kg per day in three divided doses for infants younger than 7 days of age; 200 mg/kg per day in four divided doses for infants 1 to 4 weeks old) and gentamicin (5 mg/kg per day in two divided doses for infants younger than 1 week old; 7.5 mg/kg per day in three divided doses for infants 1 to 4 weeks old) is rational therapy for most gram-negative rod infections (327). Kanamycin or netilmicin can be substituted for gentamicin (300). Third-generation cephalosporins, particularly cefotaxime, have been advocated for the therapy of gram-negative meningitis caused by ampicillin-resistant organisms, in view of the poor CSF penetration of aminoglycosides.

Although the use of intrathecal (328) or intraventricular gentamicin (329) has not resulted in any significant improvement in mortality, morbidity, or duration of positive CSF culture results, some authorities advocate these means of drug delivery in gram-negative neonatal meningitis.

Ventriculitis in association with meningitis is common in the neonate. Access of organisms to the ventricles is by direct retrograde movement, hematogenous spread through the choroid plexus, or direct passage from the leptomeninges via the transverse or choroidal fissure. Demonstration of ventriculomegaly, intraventricular echogenic material, echogenic ependymal regions, and ventricular strands and membranes by real-time ultrasound examination can assist in the diagnosis of ventriculitis. The presence of cells or products of inflammation renders the ventricular CSF echogenic so that a to-and-fro flow in the aqueduct of Sylvius can be visualized by Doppler flow imaging (330). Periventricular edema associated with ventriculitis can be demonstrated by neuroimaging studies. Culture results of ventricular fluid can remain positive after CSF culture results from the lumbar theca become negative (331).

In neonatal meningitis, unlike in meningitis developing in older children, lumbar puncture should be repeated after 48 hours of therapy, and regularly thereafter until the CSF becomes sterile, to monitor the response to therapy (332).

Candida species meningitis can be present without neurologic impairment in infants with systemic *Candida* involvement. In such cases a routine diagnostic lumbar puncture is recommended (333). It also can be a complication of indwelling peripheral venous catheters.

Chronic and Granulomatous Bacterial Meningitis

Tuberculous Meningitis

Despite advances in chemotherapy, meningitis caused by *Mycobacterium tuberculosis* remains a serious worldwide pediatric problem, and even in the United States, tuberculous meningitis causes more deaths than any other form of tuberculosis. In England and Wales, tuberculous meningitis occurred in 4.4% of children reported during 1983 to have tuberculosis (334).

Pathology and Pathophysiology. In children, tuberculous meningitis almost always accompanies generalized miliary tuberculosis. In some of the older clinical series published in 1997 (335), 68% of children with meningitis had miliary tuberculosis, and conversely, 81% of children with miliary disease developed tuberculous meningitis. In a Turkish series published in 1998, miliary tuberculosis was seen by chest radiography in 20% (335a).

In the majority of cases in the United States, infection is caused by the human type of mycobacteria. Bovine tuberculosis has become uncommon because of the widespread pasteurization of milk. The human form also is more common in tropical countries because of the relative inaccessibility of non-human milk and milk products.

Involvement of the meninges is probably secondary to a small tuberculoma in the cortex or the leptomeninges (1), and the brains of most patients who die of tuberculous meningitis demonstrate older superficial foci. Tuberculomas of the choroid plexus are a less common site for the infection.

At autopsy, the meninges look gray and opaque, and a gelatinous exudate fills the basal cisterns, particularly the anterior portion of the pons. Small tubercles can appear over the convexity of the brain or the periventricular area. The basal ganglia and thalamus in the region of the lenticulostriate and thalamo-perforating arteries are involved in 46% of cases (336).

Microscopic examination shows the exudate to consist of lymphocytes, plasma cells, and large histiocytes with typical caseation. Langhans giant cells are rare. The meningeal arteries are inflamed and thrombosed, and secondary infarctions of the superficial cortex are common. Tuberculomas are now relatively rare in Western countries, but were at one time one of the most common causes for a posterior fossa mass in children (337). They occur most commonly in the cerebellum, and less often within the brainstem.

Clinical Manifestations. The most common form of tuberculous meningitis, constituting approximately 70% of all cases, is a caseous meningitis that results from direct invasion of the meninges. In approximately 75% of children, this invasion occurs while the primary focus is fresh (i.e., less than 6 months old). The illness is often precipitated by an acute infectious disease, commonly measles. Before 1955, its incidence in the United States was highest in the spring. When tuberculous meningitis is part of the initial attack, its incidence is highest among children between the ages of 1 and 2 years. When it is a complication of systemic tuberculosis, it is more likely to affect older children.

Untreated, tuberculous meningitis rapidly progresses to death, with an average duration of only 3 weeks. Lincoln distinguished three stages of the illness, each lasting approximately a week (338).

In the initial stage (stage I), gastrointestinal symptoms predominate, and no definite neurologic manifestations are seen. The child can be apathetic or irritable with intermittent headache, but the results of the neurologic examination are negative. In approximately 10% of patients, commonly in infants, a febrile convulsion is the most significant symptom of this stage.

During stage II, the child develops drowsiness and disorientation, with signs of meningeal irritation. The deep tendon reflexes are hyperactive, abdominal reflexes disappear, and ankle and patellar clonus can be present. Cranial nerve signs are evident, with involvement of cranial nerves VII, VI, and III, in that order of frequency (335a). Choroid tubercles are present in 10% of patients.

During stage III, the patient is comatose, although periods of intermittent wakefulness can occur. The pupils are fixed, and recurrent clonic spasm of the extremities, irregular respiration, and a rising fever are present. Hydrocephalus develops in approximately two-thirds of patients whose illness lasts longer than 3 weeks. It was present at presentation in 80% of patients in the Turkish series of Yaramis and coworkers (335a). It is particularly common when treatment is delayed or inadequate.

A serous form of tuberculous meningitis is encountered less commonly. In children known to have active primary tuberculosis, the presenting symptom is meningeal irritation. Unlike in tuberculous meningitis, the CSF is normal.

A third form of tuberculous meningitis, seen in 17% of instances, consists of cases with primary spinal cord infection. These children can have major problems with blockage of the spinal canal that can be associated with Pott disease. Spinal tuberculosis can be differentiated from the other types by its history and laboratory findings. The symptoms usually last longer, often existing for 6 months before meningitis is considered. A fall often produces back pain and staggering or clumsy gait. Abdominal pain, presumably of root origin, is common. Nuchal or spinal rigidity can develop while the sensorium remains clear. CSF can be scant and show marked elevation in protein.

Recognition of tuberculous meningitis can be difficult because the characteristic signs and symptoms of meningitis can be absent during the early stages of the illness. In the series of Idriss and coauthors, nuchal rigidity occurred in 77%, apathy in 72%, fever in 47%, vomiting in 30%, drowsiness in 23%, headache in 21%, coma in 14%, convulsions, sweating, facial palsy, optic atrophy, and abducens and oculomotor palsies each in 9%, hemiparesis in 5%, and eighth nerve palsy and diabetes insipidus each in 2% (339).

Metabolic disturbances during tuberculous meningitis include metabolic alkalosis, hyponatremia, hypochloremia, and hypotonic expansion of extracellular fluid. Intracellular potassium concentration is normal or decreased, whereas sodium concentration within red cells and skeletal muscle generally increases. No evidence exists for a salt-losing renal lesion in tuberculous meningitis, although hypervolemia can result in secondary hypoaldosteronism and increased secretion of atrial natriuretic peptide factor (340). The hyponatremic syndrome in tuberculous meningitis is associated with elevations in atrial naturietic peptide more often (65%) than elevation of vasopressin (3%) (340). Vomiting often tends to aggravate electrolyte disturbances.

The presence of focal neurologic signs in a patient with tuberculous meningitis and with hypoglycorrhachia persisting beyond 12 weeks should suggest a tuberculous brain abscess or tuberculoma (341,342). Tuberculomas or vascular occlusions can develop weeks or months after active therapy is instituted (343). However, they were seen in only 2% of patients in the series of Yaramis and colleagues (335a). The presence of these complications indicates the need for revision of chemotherapy. Paradoxic expansion of intracranial tuberculomas can occur during therapy (344).

Tuberculous spinal arachnoiditis, which occurs in 7% to 42% of cases, can cause paraplegia or quadriplegia (345). Sensory loss can occur with a sensory level, root distribution pattern, bladder or bowel involvement, or root pain (346).

Diagnosis. The diagnosis of tuberculous meningitis depends on the clinical picture of a subacute meningitis, a history of exposure to the disease, often from an otherwise asymptomatic older relative, a positive skin test result, and the CSF changes.

Anergy to tuberculosis can occur in up to 36% of patients (346). In the experience at Bellevue Hospital, New York City, 85% of patients had positive reactions. Another 10% were inadequately tested or died before tuberculin tests could be completed (338,347). In the Turkish series, only 30% had a positive skin test result (335a). In the series of Kent and coworkers, which comprised both children and adults, 75% of patients reacted positively to 100 U or less of purified protein derivative (346a). A decreased humoral immune response can occur in the presence of intact cell-mediated immunity (348). The

chest radiograph is not always reliable; in the series of Zarabi and colleagues children with tuberculous meningitis had normal chest radiograph results in 43% of cases, signs of disseminated miliary tuberculosis in 23%, and calcifying primary intrathoracic tuberculosis in 10% (349). In the more recent series of Yaramis and colleagues, the chest radiograph result was abnormal in 87%; a hilar adenopathy was the most common abnormality, being present in 34% (335a).

The CSF findings are characteristic. The fluid has a ground glass appearance and when spun down forms a pellicle in which the organisms can occasionally be visualized. In 85% of cases the total CSF cell counts was less than 500 cells per μL (335a). The cells are composed of reactive mononuclear and ependymal cells with few polymorphonuclear cells. CSF protein is invariably increased (335a,346a). Of tuberculous meningitis patients reported from Turkey, 83% showed a sugar of 40 mg/dL or less (335a). In the Australian series of Kent and colleagues, the initial CSF glucose was normal in 60%, but in the majority of patients (74%) who initially had a normal CSF glucose level, subsequent values fell below normal (346a). Tuberculous meningitis can be diagnosed rapidly by means of the polymerase chain reaction (PCR), enzyme-linked immunosorbent assay (ELISA), and latex particle agglutination detection of mycobacterial antigen (152,350,351). ELISA detection of IgG and IgM antibodies and identification of tuberculostearic acid in CSF with gas chromatography and mass spectrometry also can assist in arriving at a diagnosis of tuberculous meningitis (352). CSF culture results for mycobacteria are positive in less than one-half of instances (335a). Repeated lumbar punctures, and obtaining large volumes of CSF, markedly enhance the likelihood of obtaining a positive culture result (352a). The PCR for early detection of *Mycobacterium tuberculosis* in CSF has a sensitivity of only 48%; microscopy has a sensitivity of 9% (152). Fatal *Mycobacterium avium* meningitis has been confused with meningitis caused by *Mycobacterium tuberculosis* in immunocompetent children (353).

Diffuse or focal EEG abnormalities occur in approximately 80% of cases (354). Neuroimaging is of relatively little assistance in the diagnosis of tuberculous meningitis. Cranial CT within 1 week of initial symptoms can reveal basilar enhancement, ventricular dilatation, or infarction (335a,355). MRI with gadolinium enhancement also can demonstrate meningeal inflammation. Mild to marked third ventricular enlargement is extremely common and was invariably present in one study (356). Severe hydrocephalus was demonstrable by CT scans in 87% of children with tuberculous meningitis, but in only 12% of adults. Visible infarcts are present in 28% to 40% of cases, usually involving the territory of the middle cerebral artery. Patients with nonenhancing lesions have a good prognosis, whereas those with enhancing lesions are likely to die or have irreversible sequelae despite medical therapy or shunting (334,356).

The appearance of tuberculomas revealed by neuroimaging studies differs from that of abscesses, metastases, and gliomas. MRI of tuberculomas show large, ring-enhancing lesions with low intensity on T2-weighted images and intermediate intensity on T1-weighted images. Small lesions with ring enhancement on CT scan show a central bright signal on T2-weighted images with a peripheral low-intensity rim, surrounded by high-intensity edema (357).

Treatment. Therapy for tuberculous meningitis must be prompt and adequate (358). It includes appropriate chemotherapy, correction of fluid and electrolyte disturbances, and relief of increased intracranial pressure.

Treatment of tuberculous meningitis, as recommended by the Committee on Infectious Diseases of the American Academy of Pediatrics (359), should include daily doses of four drugs for 2 months: isoniazid (INH), rifampin, pyrazinamide, and streptomycin. This is followed by INH and rifampin administered daily or twice weekly under direct observation for 10 months. For patients who may have acquired tuberculosis in geographic locales where resistance to streptomycin is common, capreomycin (15 to 30 mg/kg per day) or kanamycin (15 to 30 mg/kg per day) may be used instead of streptomycin. Treatment of tuberculomas should be similar to that for tuberculous meningitis. CSF penetration of INH (89%) and pyrazinamide (91%) changes little during the course of therapy for tuberculous meningitis; penetration of rifampin (5%)

and streptomycin (20%) can decline to result in subtherapeutic levels. Corticosteroids have little effect on the penetration of these drugs (360).

INH (10 to 15 mg/kg per day up to a maximum dosage of 300 mg/day, 20 to 40 mg/kg per dose twice weekly up to a maximum of 900 mg per dose) is a bactericidal and bacteriostatic drug that interacts with nucleic acid synthesis and inhibits production of cell wall mycolic acid (361). Peak serum concentrations usually range from 6 to 20 µg/mL. The optimal duration of treatment with INH is not known, but therapy should be continued for at least 1 year. Peripheral neuritis can complicate the use of INH in some patients. This complication can be prevented or relieved by pyridoxine (25 to 50 mg/day). Adding pyridoxine is probably not necessary for infants or children unless they are malnourished, but it is recommended for adolescents (358). Other adverse reactions can include gastrointestinal and hematologic hypersensitivity and lupus-like reactions. Hepatitis is rare in children younger than 11 years of age. When INH is used together with rifampin, the incidence of hepatotoxicity increases if the INH dose exceeds 10 mg/kg per day.

Rifampin (10 to 20 mg/kg up to 600 mg daily or twice weekly) is a bactericidal drug that inhibits RNA synthesis by binding to bacterial DNA-dependent RNA polymerase. Rifampin is recommended for children with resistant organisms. Adverse reactions include gastrointestinal and hematologic hypersensitivity, most often thrombocytopenia, flu-like symptoms, and hepatitis. Birth control pills may be rendered ineffective.

Pyrazinamide (20 to 40 mg/kg per day or 50 to 70 mg/kg twice weekly up to 2,000 mg/day) is a bacteriostatic drug used for drug-resistant organisms. It can cause hepatotoxicity, hyperuricemia, arthritis, skin rash, or gastrointestinal upset.

Streptomycin (20 mg/kg intramuscularly daily or twice weekly up to 1,000 mg/day) is a bactericidal drug that blocks protein synthesis. Adverse reactions include ototoxicity with greater incidence of vestibular than auditory involvement, hypersensitivity, and rarely, nephrotoxicity. Streptomycin toxicity usually develops after 12 weeks of therapy.

Ethambutol (15 to 25 mg/kg per day or 50 mg/kg per dose twice weekly up to 2,500 mg per day) is a bacteriostatic drug that has replaced para-aminosalicylic acid in older individuals. It is usually reserved for children older than 5 years of age because of the risk of optic neuritis or optic atrophy in younger children. These complications are rare if the recommended dose is not exceeded. Impairment of visual acuity or color vision may occur, as well as rashes, gastrointestinal symptoms, and fever.

Para-aminosalicylic acid (200 mg/kg per day in three divided doses up to 12 g per day) reduces the emergence of drug-resistant strains. Gastrointestinal side effects can be intolerable.

In the United States, the incidence of drug-resistant strains has been low, but is becoming an increasing problem, and in some regions of the world resistance to INH can be as high as 30%. This percentage makes a laboratory evaluation of drug susceptibility imperative. Ethionamide, cycloserine, kanamycin, amikacin, ofloxacin, ciprofloxacin, and capreomycin should be considered in multidrug-resistant tuberculosis (362).

Spinal arachnoiditis is a common complication of tuberculous meningitis. Intrathecal hyaluronidase has been reported in a nonrandomized trial to reduce the mortality and disability of patients with tuberculous meningitis when compared with a control group (345).

Adjuvant treatment with corticosteroids such as prednisone remains controversial. In the study of Schoeman and coworkers, prednisone improved the survival rate and intellectual outcome of patients with tuberculous meningitis (359,363); it did not affect the incidence of motor deficits, blindness, deafness, increased intracranial pressure, or basal ganglia infarction (363). Its use has been recommended for seriously ill patients (359,364). In other studies, corticosteroids reduced intracranial pressure, basal exudate, and cerebral edema without altering morbidity or mortality (360,365), and relieved pulmonary symptoms in miliary tuberculosis (358). The neurologic state of patients sometimes deteriorates shortly after the initiation of therapy. Corticosteroid treatment can benefit this condition and can favorably influence mortality, if started before the onset of

coma (364,366). Most experts consider 1 to 2 mg/kg per day of prednisone or its equivalent given for 6 to 8 weeks to be appropriate (359).

Intracranial pressure above 400 mm of CSF significantly impairs perfusion of cerebral tissue, and patients who have consistent severe elevations of intracranial pressure require short courses of dexamethasone (6 mg/m^2 every 4 to 6 hours) to reduce edema, or neurosurgical intervention with ventriculo-external or ventriculoperitoneal shunts to relieve acute hydrocephalus (367,368). Hydrocephalus becomes more marked at pressures up to 600 mm CSF, by which point hemoperfusion has fallen to approximately 40% of normal. Peacock and Deenny observed that ventriculoperitoneal shunting of patients with tuberculous meningitis resulted in a better outcome than was seen in matched nonshunted children (369).

The treatment of tuberculoma has been considered by Bhagwati and Parulekar. In their experience some 60% of the patients responded to drugs alone, and 23% required surgical intervention for failure to respond or mass effect (370). Infratentorial tuberculomas associated with hydrocephalus should receive ventriculoperitoneal shunts.

Prognosis. Untreated tuberculous meningitis was invariably fatal. With the newer treatment regimens, fewer survivors have major sequelae than were observed several decades ago (371). Even so, in the experience of Deeny and coworkers, reported in 1985, only 18% of survivors were neurologically and intellectually normal (372). As a rule, the prognosis is good for patients presenting with stage 1 disease, and generally poor for those presenting with stage 3 disease. In the series of Kent and colleagues 25% of patients presenting with stage 2 disease died or were left with sequelae (346a). With treatment, CSF glucose returns to normal within 1 to 2 months, and CSF protein becomes normal within 4 to 26 months (346a).

Major neurologic sequelae include hydrocephalus, spastic pareses, seizures, paraplegia, and sensory disturbances of the extremities. Late ophthalmologic complications include optic atrophy and blindness. Hearing and vestibular residua can occur both as a conse-

TABLE 6.8. *Some rarer organisms responsible for meningitis*

Organism (references)	Clinical features	Treatment of choice
Listeria monocytogenes (377–379)	Primary meningitis in newborn infants, or later in first month of life, rhombencephalitis	Ampicillin (150–250 mg/kg/day) IV, alone or in combination with trimethoprim-sulfamethoxazole or aminoglycosides
Proteus spp. (380)	Neonatal meningitis or secondary to otitis media, genitourinary tract infection; hydrocephalus, hemorrhagic necrosis of brain are common complications; CSF culture results may be negative with ventricular culture results positive	Variable sensitivities: usually penicillin, kanamycin, ampicillin, chloramphenicol
Mima polymorpha (381)	Neonatal meningitis	Variable: sensitivities necessary (usually sensitive to ampicillin or gentamicin)
Salmonella	Neonatal meningitis	Third-generation cephalosporins, chloramphenicol
Klebsiella pneumoniae	Secondary to middle ear or respiratory tract, wound infections; usually younger than age 1, high mortality	Variable: sensitivities necessary
Bacillus anthracis (382)	Secondary to septicemia from primary cutaneous or visceral lesion; fulminant course, trismus common; meningitis often hemorrhagic	Penicillin, corticosteroids
Yersinia pestis (304)	Regional adenopathy, meningitis; may have primary cutaneous lesion	Chloramphenicol, gentamicin IV and IT, streptomycin, tetracycline
Pasteurella ureae (383)	Basal skull fracture with otorrhea	Ampicillin
Pasteurella pneumotropica	Seizures, contact with animals	Sensitivities necessary
Citrobacter (384)	Meningitis in newborn infant; abscesses form in most patients	Sensitivities necessary
Brucella spp. (385–389)	Chronic meningitis with increased intracranial pressure, prolonged indolent course; encephalitis, meningoencephalitis; parenchymatous dysfunction without direct evidence of infection (e.g., cerebellum)	Tetracyclines, sulfonamides, (trimethoprimsulfamethoxazole), streptomycin, rifampin in some combination
Yersinia enterocolitica (388)	Enterocolitis, meningitis	Trimethoprim-sulfamethoxazole, cefotaximes, aminoglycoside, doxicillin (in children older than 9 years of age)

quence of streptomycin therapy and the disease process itself. Minor neurologic sequelae include cranial nerve palsies, nystagmus, ataxia, mild disturbances of coordination, and spasticity.

Intellectual defects occur in approximately two-thirds of survivors (372). These patients have a high incidence of encephalographic abnormalities, which correlate with the persistence of sequelae such as convulsions and mental subnormality. Intracranial calcifications develop in approximately one-third of children who recover from tuberculous meningitis (373). Panhypopituitarism has been reported after cured tuberculous meningitis (374). One-fifth of survivors have such selective pituitary hypothalamic disturbances as sexual precocity, hyperprolactemia, and deficiencies in ADH, growth hormone, corticotropin, and gonadotropin (375).

Children younger than 3 years of age have a poorer prognosis for survival than do older children, a fact that might relate to the easier recognition of the disorder in older children (372,376).

Meningitis Caused by Unusual Organisms

Table 6.8 summarizes the essential clinical features of the various meningeal infections produced by some of the less common organisms and indicates the currently recommended forms of treatment (304,377–388).

BRAIN ABSCESSES

A brain abscess consists of localized free or encapsulated pus within the brain substance. Although the condition has been known for more than 200 years, and its association with cyanotic congenital heart disease was described more than 100 years ago, the absence of classic signs and symptoms hinders its early clinical diagnosis and treatment.

Etiology and Pathogenesis

Predisposing conditions are always present. In the experience of Ersahin and coworkers, reported in 1994, the cause of the abscess was meningitis in 36% of cases, otitis in 27%, head injury in 16%, and congenital heart disease in 9%. Multiple abscesses occurred in 29% of the children (389). Pyogenic organisms gain access to the brain substance by one of three routes. The first is through the bloodstream either from a remote infection, as a consequence of sepsis, or in association with a cardiopulmonary malfunction, most commonly, cyanotic congenital heart disease with a right-to-left shunt. The second is by extension of contiguous infections such as leptomeningitis, infections of the middle ear, or infections of the paranasal sinuses either directly or as a result of septic thrombophlebitis of bridging veins. The third is as a complication of a penetrating wound. Children with chronic bacterial infection are more prone to this complication, in that they can develop an infected infarct (390).

The most common causative organisms in order of frequency are anaerobic and microaerophilic streptococci, *Fusobacterium* species, β-hemolytic streptococci, *S. aureus*, and pneumococci. *Actinomyces* (gram positive), as well as *Bacteroides* and other gram-negative rods, particularly *Haemophilus* species, are seen less often (391,392). Abscesses caused by *Aspergillus* and *Nocardia* (393) or protozoa such as *Toxoplasma* (394), are even rarer in the nonimmunocompromised host. Anaerobic organisms alone cause approximately 56% of brain abscesses, aerobic bacteria alone cause approximately 18%, and mixed aerobic and anaerobic bacteria cause approximately 26% (395). Frequently, the organism cannot be identified, often owing to failure to perform the appropriate cultures or the use of antibiotics before securing cultures.

Pathology

The earliest stage of an abscess is cerebritis (septic encephalitis). This is usually localized in the white matter even when infection has to pass through the cortex. It is an edematous area with softening and congestion of brain tissue, often with numerous petechial hemorrhages. The center becomes liquefied, thus forming the abscess cavity (Fig. 6.4). Initially, its wall is poorly defined and irregular. Gradually, a firmer, thicker wall develops, which ultimately can become a thick, firm, concentric capsule of fibrous tissue. The adjacent brain tissue is infiltrated with polymorphonuclear leukocytes and plasma cells near the abscess, with lymphocytes in the more peripheral zones, and heavy lymphocytic cuffing of vessels in the area. In more chronic abscesses, a border of granulation tissue merges gradually into a collagenous capsule. Abscesses enlarge within the softer and less vascular white matter, and extend toward the ventricles, rupturing into this space rather than into the subarachnoid fluid. Seeding of the leptomeninges and subsequent meningitis results from local thrombophlebitis more often than from actual rupture.

Abscesses resulting from hematogenous spread can be localized within any part of the brain, but most commonly in the distribution of the middle cerebral artery at the junction of gray and white matter of the cerebral hemispheres. By contrast, abscesses derived from contiguous sources tend to be superficial and close to the infected bone or dura. Multiple abscesses occur in 6% of patients, usually when sepsis or congenital heart disease is the predisposing cause.

Clinical Manifestations

During initial stages of the brain abscess, the clinical picture can be nonspecific. The patient,

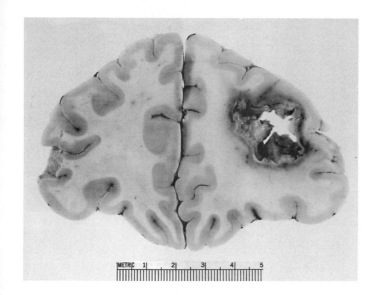

FIG. 6.4. Anterior frontal lobe abscess in a child with cyanotic congenital heart disease. The brain is edematous and flattening of the gyri is seen. Gross representation of coronal section. (Courtesy of Dr. Hideo H. Itabashi, Department of Pathology, Los Angeles County Harbor Medical Center.)

who can have cyanotic congenital heart disease or a primary infection, develops the complex of headache, vomiting, and convulsions, either partially or in its entirety. As the abscess progresses, the neurologic signs, which initially were minimal or completely absent, become readily apparent. As indicated in Table 6.9 (396), they include papilledema, lateralizing signs, notably hemiparesis or homonymous hemianopia, and more obvious indications of increased intracranial pressure. Focal percussion tenderness often aids in the localization of the lesion. Untreated, the condition is usually fatal, either as a consequence of decompensated increased intracranial pressure or from sudden rupture of the abscess into the ventricular system. Sudden rupture is marked by a sudden high fever, meningeal signs, and deterioration of consciousness (397).

Cerebellar abscesses are most commonly seen in association with mastoid infections and occur most frequently during the second and third decades of life. Symptoms and neurologic signs are those associated with any posterior fossa mass lesion. Mastoid infections also give rise to abscesses of the temporal lobe. Abscesses of the pituitary fossa can have a prolonged course that simulates a slow-growing tumor (398).

Intramedullary abscesses of the spinal cord have been observed in infants as young as 8 days of age. In a review of 73 cases, 17% occurred before the age of 5 years (399).

TABLE 6.9. *Incidence of symptoms and neurologic findings in 19 cases of brain abscess with congenital heart disease*

Symptoms	Number of patients
Headache, vomiting, or both	15
Seizures	7
Fever (101° F or more)	6
Listlessness	4
Disorientation	4
Neck pain	4
Neurologic sign	
Lateralizing signs	15
Papilledema	13
Hemiparesis	12
Increased deep tendon reflexes	12
Extensor plantar responses	9
Pupillary changes	7
Stupor	6
Neck stiffness	5
Aphasia	5
Homonymous hemianopia	4
Localized percussion tenderness of skull	a

[a]Although not cited, this is a common neurologic sign and is valuable in localizing the abscess.

Adapted from Raimondi AJ, Matsumoto S, Miller RA. Brain abscess in children with congenital heart disease. I. *J Neurosurg* 1965;23:588.

Diagnosis

Peripheral blood counts are usually of little value in establishing the diagnosis of brain abscess. Peripheral white blood cell counts of greater than 11,000 per µL occur in only one-third of patients (400). The erythrocyte sedimentation rate is normal in 11% of patients. The CSF leukocyte count in patients without congenital heart disease is greater than 5 per µL in 80% of cases. In patients with congenital heart disease, the CSF cell count is normal in 47% and the CSF protein is normal in 67% (400). Generally, the more striking the CSF pleocytosis, the closer the abscess is to the ventricular lining. Hypoglycorrhachia of less than 45 mg/dL occurs in approx-

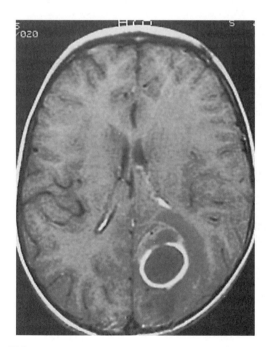

FIG. 6.5. Brain abscess. Magnetic resonance imaging study after gadolinium contrast. The axial T1-weighted image demonstrates an abscess in the occipital region. The rim of the abscess enhances, and some surrounding edema has caused a slight midline shift. A small daughter abscess is also noted. A second occipital lobe abscess is not visualized in this cut. This was a 5-year-old boy with pulmonary atresia and hypoplastic right ventricle, who presented with a seizure. He was afebrile, and neurologic examination was unremarkable, although visual fields could not be performed.

imately 30% of cases. Bacterial culture results of CSF are usually negative unless the abscess is leaking into the ventricular system (400). As a rule, a lumbar puncture should be avoided in children with brain abscess because the procedure results in neurologic deterioration in 15% to 33% of cases and the information is of little use in management (400).

The EEG almost always shows a focal slowing, which corresponds closely to the location of the abscess. Neuroimaging studies are the preferred diagnostic methods (401) (Fig. 6.5). These reveal a focal process that rapidly assumes the character of a mass lesion with a contrast-enhanceable margin (401). If MRI is not available, CT or cerebral arteriography is the preferred procedure when the abscess requires further delineation (402). Focal arterial displacement and the presence of the ripple sign, a concentric, curvilinear displacement of opacified sulci in the late arterial phase caused by perifocal edema, are helpful arteriographic findings (403).

In patients with cyanotic congenital heart disease, a brain abscess must be differentiated from intracranial vascular accidents and hypoxic attacks. Thromboses of arteries, veins, and dural sinuses are particularly common in severely cyanotic infants. Although dehydration and stasis play a minor role in the evolution of cerebral vascular thromboses, in the series of Tyler and Clark virtually every infant who experienced a thrombosis had an arterial oxygen saturation of 10 volumes percent or less (404). Except for a more abrupt onset of symptoms, the clinical picture can mimic that of an abscess; however, the patient's age is of considerable importance in the differential diagnosis. Brain abscesses are rare before 2 years of age, whereas vascular thromboses are rare in patients older than 2 years (404). Emboli in patients with congenital heart disease are highly unusual, and when present they are precipitated by cardiac or other surgery. The differential diagnosis of these two entities, and their distinction from hypoxic attacks, which are often accompanied by headaches, is further covered in the section on Neurologic Complications of Cardiac Disease in Chapter 15.

A partially treated meningitis also should be considered in the differential diagnosis of a brain abscess. It lacks the neurologic and EEG evidence of focal central involvement, and, of course, neuroimaging studies are diagnostic.

Clark has pointed out that old focal neurologic signs, which are often present in the patient with cyanotic congenital heart disease, are aggravated by stress, including a recent infection (405). The ensuing picture simulates a progressive lesion.

Treatment

Treatment of any brain abscess should include a diligent search for the source of infection (406,407). In a child without congenital heart disease, the presence of multiple brain abscesses should raise the question of immunodeficiency. Once the diagnosis has been made, a massive antibiotic regimen is instituted. Initial therapy should include coverage for anaerobic as well as aerobic organisms. The antibiotics of choice are generally intravenous penicillin G, chloramphenicol, or metronidazole. Oxacillin or methicillin also should be started until it is established that a β-lactamase–producing organism is not involved. Ampicillin can be used, but is not as effective as penicillin against anaerobic organisms. If surgical intervention is indicated and can be performed without delay, antibiotic therapy should be withheld until immediately after cultures have been obtained (400). Subsequent therapy is guided by laboratory determination of antibiotic sensitivity and by neuroimaging studies. It is continued for a minimum of 3 weeks and often for 4 to 6 weeks. Intravenous fluid is usually limited to 1,500 mL/m^2 to minimize cerebral edema.

Controversy still surrounds the indications for surgical therapy and the various surgical methods. These methods include tapping of the abscess, with or without excision of the shrunken abscess capsule, and operative removal of the acute abscess (408). Generally, surgical therapy is indicated when the patient does not improve after 24 hours of antibiotic therapy, when clinical status deteriorates, or when there is life-threatening displacement of cerebral structures. Sinusitis or mastoiditis contiguous to a brain abscess should be treated vigorously, usually with prompt surgery. A short

course of corticosteroids to reduce life-threatening edema can be used safely.

When an abscess is fully established, surgical treatment is usually necessary. Mampalam and Rosenblum compared treatment by surgical excision with treatment by aspiration (400). Excision resulted in a shorter course of antibiotic therapy, but there was no difference in morbidity or mortality. Wright and Ballantine recommend total excision of brain abscesses, having had no deaths with this approach (409), whereas significant mortality was associated with drainage or medical treatment alone. Berlit and coworkers recommend burr hole aspiration plus antibiotic treatment of brain abscesses. In their study, mortality for this group was 9%, as opposed to 62% for the subgroup treated with antibiotics alone (410). The affected region is aspirated and the aspirate examined for aerobic and anaerobic bacteria, mycobacteria, fungi, and parasites, notably *Toxoplasma*. Patients with increased intracranial pressure should not receive halothane, trichloroethylene, or methoxyflurane, as these agents can cause considerable increase in intracranial pressure (411). Because seizures can occur owing to the cortical injury produced by the brain abscess or its surgical therapy, anticonvulsant medication should be used during the acute phase.

Brain abscess in the early phase of cerebritis may respond to antimicrobial therapy without surgical drainage (412,413).

Complications

Residual defects include seizure activity, localized neurologic abnormalities, mental retardation, and hydrocephalus. Seizures can appear at any time between 1 month and 15 years after a supratentorial abscess, with the latent period being somewhat shorter when the abscess occurs in the temporal lobe. In 40% of patients, seizures develop within 1 year, and the mean time of onset is 3.3 years. No relationship exists between the development of seizures and the age of the patient or the mode of surgical therapy (414).

The overall mortality has declined from 30% in the pre-CT era to almost none in the past few years. The prognosis remains poor in infants with brain abscesses, with mortality approaching 50% (415).

Subdural Abscesses

Subdural abscesses or subdural empyema result from sepsis, from a direct extension of an infection such as an osteomyelitis, or from bacterial contamination of a subdural effusion in meningitis or a post-traumatic subdural hematoma. Presently, approximately two-thirds occur subsequent to a prior craniotomy. Otitis media and pneumococcal meningitis are other sources of organisms for subdural abscesses in children, whereas sinusitis is a more common antecedent in adults. Approximately 9% of children with brain abscesses develop subdural empyemas. These lesions generally occur over the convexity of the brain, but 12% are found interhemispherically.

Signs and symptoms are those of a space-occupying lesion in association with evidence of infection. Increased intracranial pressure and focal neurologic findings, notably focal seizures, are common (416,417).

The presence of subdural abscesses is demonstrated by neuroimaging (18). Sinusitis-induced subdural empyemas may not become apparent on CT scan until 1 or 2 weeks after symptoms develop, hence they may be missed on initial CT scans (418). Enhancement of membranes with gadolinium on MRI can occur when no enhancement is seen on CT (419). Early diagnosis and prompt chemotherapy and surgical drainage are imperative (392). Subdural infections are caused by the same spectrum and distribution of bacteria as those causing brain abscesses (392).

Epidural Abscesses

Epidural abscesses can develop from contiguous infection of structures that surround the brain and spinal cord. They can arise from local infection or can be secondary to congenital anomalies such as dermal sinuses (420,421). Bacteremia and trauma also have been implicated. Approximately one-third of cases involve staphylococcal organisms (422).

Infection of the spinal epidural space, though extremely rare in childhood, produces a devastating neurologic picture. The infection is limited to the dorsal surface of the cord except in the cord's lower sacral portion, where the abscess completely surrounds the cord. The anatomy of the epidural space limits extension to vertical spread and produces extradural compression. Epidural infections can result from the use of epidural catheters for prolonged postoperative analgesia in children (422a).

The clinical course can be acute and rapidly progressive or chronic. The acute form, more common in children, is usually the result of a metastatic infection, whereas chronic lesions are commonly caused by a direct extension of a spinal osteomyelitis. The classic case of spinal epidural abscess follows a fairly typical pattern of development. Within 1 to 2 weeks of an infection, backache develops; this backache is enhanced by jarring or straining and is accompanied by local spinal tenderness. Within a few days, tenderness progresses to radicular pain followed by symptoms of cord involvement, including weakness of voluntary movements and impaired sphincter control. Paraplegia can be complete within a few hours or days.

In many patients, the history and neurologic signs are impossible to differentiate from those of acute transverse myelitis. Intradural extramedullary tumors can produce a similar clinical picture.

A history compatible with infection, in association with focal pain in the region of the spine, especially when accompanied by neurologic symptoms of spinal cord or root involvement, should suggest the diagnosis, which can be confirmed by neuroimaging studies (18). Prompt blood cultures can reveal the causative organism. Lumbar puncture should not be performed because of the risk of spreading the infection to the subdural or subarachnoid space. Aspiration can be performed with a large-gauge needle, but only under radiographic guidance. If the CSF is examined, it shows pleocytosis and an elevated protein level.

An epidural abscess that has produced neurologic deficit is treated by laminectomy with decompression and drainage. In view of the rapid progression of potentially irreversible symptoms, this condition is a surgical emergency. Antibiotic therapy is secondary. If tuber-

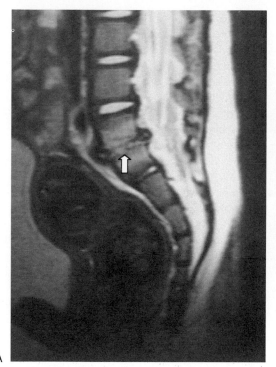

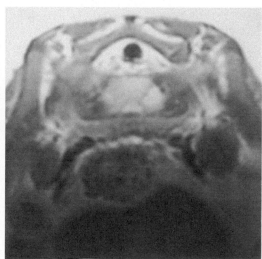

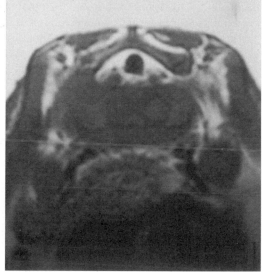

FIG. 6.6. Septic discitis. Magnetic resonance imaging scan of the lumbar spine of a 14-month-old child who stopped cruising. **A:** Sagittal T2-weighted scan showing reduced signal in the L5/S1 intervertebral disc (*arrow*), and high signal in the end plate and adjacent medullary bone. **B:** Axial T1-weighted scan after contrast demonstrated intense contrast enhancement of the disc. **C:** Axial T1-weighted scan showing nerve roots surrounded by fat. (Courtesy of Dr. Philip Anslow, Department of Radiology, Radcliffe Infirmary, Oxford, England.)

culosis of the spine is suspected, antituberculous therapy should be instituted pending identification of the causative organisms.

Intramedullary Abscesses

Approximately 27% of intramedullary abscesses occur before age 10 years, and 40% occur during the first two decades of life (423). The abscess develops by spread from infected contiguous dermal sinuses or, less often, from suppurative foci at other sites. In some instances, particularly since the advent of antibiotics, the disease can be insidious, and in approximately one-fourth of cases, the infection has been present for at least 4 months before diagnosis. The thoracic cord is involved in most instances. Symptoms generally simulate an intramedullary tumor.

Infections of Intervertebral Disc Space

Self-limited intervertebral disc space infections can occur in children. These infections can be caused by *S. aureus* or diphtheroids, but often no organism can be isolated. Infections of the disc space are characterized by back pain with or without fever, a variable incidence of hip pain or abdominal pain, radiographic evidence of narrowing of the intervertebral space, enhanced radionuclide uptake, and an elevated sedimentation rate (424). Cross-sectional MRI is probably the most useful diagnostic procedure (425) (Fig. 6.6). Treatment by immobilization relieves pain. Antibiotics have been used, but are not always needed. Scoliosis and complete interbody ankylosis can occur (426,427). In a follow-up of 35 children on average 17 years after discitis, flexion of the low back was normal in 90% but extension was markedly restricted in 86%, 80% had narrowing of the vertebral canal, 74% had a block vertebrae, and 43% still complained of backache (428). Nonspecific discitis without bacterial cause can occur in young children. It is characterized by restriction of spinal mobility and an elevated sedimentation rate. Biopsy usually reveals chronic or subacute inflammation although approximately one-third of the biopsies yield normal tissue. The disease is usually self-limiting in most cases with only minor residual radiographic changes (428a).

Intraventricular Shunt Infections

The management of infected cerebrospinal shunts is covered in Chapter 4.

CONGENITAL INFECTIONS OF THE NERVOUS SYSTEM

Infections of the fetal nervous system differ from those of older children and adults in that, by causing significant damage to development and to the elaboration of neural relationships, they produce multiple defects. The induction of congenital anomalies in the infected developing embryo depends on when the teratogen acts (429). Before entering the blastula stage, the embryo is resistant to the action of teratogens, and damage results either in death or in recovery without malfunction. When the primary germ layers have become established, and during organogenesis, the embryo becomes vulnerable to infectious agents. Congenital malformations occasionally have resulted from infections

incurred during the second trimester (430). After the second trimester, congenital malformations become increasingly uncommon. For these reasons, the fetal brain is highly susceptible to some infectious agents that are of little consequence to older children.

Another feature of prenatal infections is the altered biological response to injury. The immature fetal brain is unable to repair damage, remove abnormal cells, and compensate for missing tissue. The inflammatory response, which often contributes to the damage produced by viruses at a later age, is absent or less marked in the fetus (431).

The two main pathways for transmission of infection to the fetus are the ascending cervical amniotic route and the transplacental route. Bacteria invade usually by the ascending route, whereas toxoplasmosis, syphilis, rubella, cytomegalovirus (CMV), and other viruses generally assume the transplacental route (432). Placental changes have been demonstrated in most of these conditions (433). The pathogenesis of prenatal viral infections has been reviewed by Volpe (434).

During the first 3 weeks of gestation, virus spreads through the human embryo by cell contiguity because no circulation is established. In the older fetus, virus spreads similarly to that seen in adults.

The invading virus can kill fetal cells or stop cell growth and division. Thus, a fetus infected with rubella and CMV has a subnormal number of cells but a normal cytoplasmic mass. Certain viruses, notably rubella, produce lesions in the endothelium of chorionic and fetal blood vessels. These lesions, by themselves, can result in maldevelopment secondary to ischemia and faulty tissue proliferation. Subependymal germinolysis, forming the subependymal cysts seen in the region of the striatothalamic junction, is probably caused by viral destruction of the telencephalic subependymal germinal matrix. This destruction occurs in the same regions as hypoxic hemorrhage in premature infants, and it also can disrupt subsequent cytoarchitectural development. During the neonatal period, visualization by sonography of the lenticulostriate arteries as echogenic stripes in the basal ganglia is highly suggestive of cerebral infection. This finding can be seen in viral infections, bacterial meningitis, or syphilis (435), but is not encountered normally, and only rarely in babies with noninfectious intracranial disorders (436).

The course of fetal infection can be influenced by the specific immune response. IgG antibodies, mainly of maternal origin, have been demonstrated in the blood of 3- to 4-month-old fetuses. Specific fetal IgM and IgG antibodies can be produced from the twentieth week on, so that inordinately high IgM levels at birth are often indicative of a prenatal infection. Some 34% of newborns with IgM levels above 19.5 mg/dL can be shown to have infections, as compared with only 0.8% of infants with IgM values below this level (437,438).

In some instances, congenital malformations result from unrecognized viral infection. This topic is covered more extensively in Chapter 4. Experimental evidence in animals shows that a variety of viruses can induce cerebral malformations, including neural tube defects, encephalocele, cerebellar hypoplasia, hypomyelination, hydranencephaly, porencephaly, and hydrocephalus. More applicable to humans is the demonstration that involvement of the ependyma by mumps, influenza, and parainfluenza 2 virus results in aqueductal stenosis, obstruction of the foramina of Monro, and hydrocephalus (439,440).

Five organisms that affect the fetal brain are discussed more extensively. They are rubella, CMV, varicella, toxoplasma, and herpes simplex.

Rubella

Rubella was first noted to produce congenital malformations by Gregg in 1941 (441). Severe CNS involvement can accompany congenital rubella, the incidence and severity of the malformations depending on the time of maternal infection. Congenital rubella, occurring after maternal infection with rash, is present in more than 80% of infants during the first 12 weeks of pregnancy, in 54% at 13 to 14 weeks, and in 25% at the end of the second trimester. The infection rate increases again during the last month. Rubella-induced defects, principally congenital heart disease and deafness, occur in almost all infants infected before the eleventh week; deafness alone occurs in 35% of those infected at 13 to 16 weeks (442). Congenital rubella after maternal disease during the second

trimester results in more subtle abnormalities, notably disorders in communication and delayed mental development in some two-thirds of infants (429,443). Intrauterine growth retardation occurs in the fetus who contracts rubella during gestation. Growth retardation persists for at least 2 years when rubella is contracted in early gestation, but not when it is contracted in late gestation (442).

Pathology

The histopathologic abnormalities of rubella infection of the nervous system are of two types: those resulting from retardation or inhibition of cell growth, observed in 6% of cases studied by autopsy, and those resulting from cellular necrosis caused by a variety of vascular lesions (444). These vascular lesions include focal destruction of vessel walls, focal defects of internal elastic lamina with adjacent proliferation of subintimal fibrous tissue, pericapillary granular deposits, and endothelial proliferation. As a consequence of these lesions, the parenchyma of the brain demonstrates multiple small areas of liquefactive necrosis and gliosis with vasculitis and perivascular calcification. The lesions can be in the periventricular white matter, basal ganglia, or, less frequently, midbrain, pons, or spinal cord (445). Additionally, usually a chronic leptomeningitis occurs with round cell infiltration. Impairment of cellular immunity also has been reported (446). The virus can be isolated from affected tissues (447).

Clinical Manifestations

The clinical picture of the congenital rubella syndrome is summarized in Table 6.10. Cataracts, glaucoma, and cardiac malfunctions occur when the infant is infected during the first 2 months of gestation; hearing loss and psychomotor retardation can result from infection any time in the first trimester and, rarely, as late as 16 weeks' gestation (448,449). In approximately 80% of rubella-infected infants, symptoms referable to the nervous system can be observed during the first year of life (448–450).

In 72% of the cases, the clinical picture at birth is marked by lethargy, hypotonia, and a large, full, or bulging fontanel. Later, between

TABLE 6.10. *Clinical manifestations of congenital rubella infections*

Findings	Percentage of patients
Deafness	67.0
Heart disease	48.5
Bilateral cataracts	15.4
Unilateral cataract	13.4
Glaucoma	3.2
Chorioretinitis	39.1
Psychomotor retardation	45.2
Mild	22.4
Moderate	10.6
Severe	12.2
Thrombocytopenia	22.5
Spasticity	12.2

From Cooper LZ, et al. Rubella: clinical manifestations and management. *Am J Dis Child* 1969;118:1829. With permission.

ages 1 and 4 months, irritability, restlessness, constant movements, vasomotor instability, and photophobia become the most prominent clinical features. Opisthotonic posturing and a marked developmental delay are common. Approximately one-half of congenitally infected infants improve between ages 6 and 12 months and begin to develop (448–450).

Of affected infants, 16% are small, hypotonic, and nonreactive, with little evidence of irritability. In 11%, convulsions start shortly after birth or symptoms of meningitis are present. Seizures occur in 25% of affected children. Lennox-Gastaut syndrome or abrupt vasomotor changes are the most common forms of seizures (448).

When the CNS is involved during prenatal life, congenital malformations including microcephaly, hydrocephalus, and spina bifida can develop (451), but they might not be recognized until developmental or speech retardation becomes obvious. Retarded language development can be caused by a peripheral hearing loss (44%), central auditory imperception (42%), or mental retardation (452).

The most common ocular abnormality in congenital rubella is chorioretinitis. It is characterized by areas of discrete, patchy, black pigmentation interspersed with similar patchy depigmentation, the so-called salt and pepper appearance. No evidence exists that this defect of retinal pigmentation interferes with vision. Microphthalmia, nuclear cataracts, glaucoma, and severe myopia also are common.

In approximately one-third of affected children, a variety of abnormal EEG tracings, including hypsarrhythmia, can be obtained.

In most patients, the CSF protein content is abnormally high at birth, diminishing to normal levels by age 3 months.

Diagnosis

Congenital rubella can be diagnosed by an elevated IgM level at birth identified as specific rubella antibody. The virus can be isolated from nasopharynx, urine or stool. It also can be isolated from CSF for as long as 18 months after birth (449). In older children, the diagnosis of congenital rubella is difficult. Viral isolation is rarely successful, serology is frequently not diagnostic, and by age 5, hemagglutination-inhibition antibody is seronegative in 18.5% of patients. Administration of rubella vaccine can be of diagnostic assistance. In seronegative children with congenital rubella, only 10% respond with an increase in the titer of hemagglutination-inhibition antibodies, in contrast to 98% of nonimmune healthy children (453).

Treatment

No specific treatment for rubella exists. The control of congenital rubella infections rests on the prevention of maternal viremia by vaccination with attenuated viral strains. Rubella vaccine given to a pregnant woman has resulted in intrauterine infection by the vaccine virus (454). Infants with congenital rubella are a potential source of viral infection for nursing personnel.

Prognosis

Nearly all long-term survivors of congenital rubella are deaf (451). Cataracts and chorioretinopathy are common (455). Severe mental retardation (24%) and spasticity (20%) occur, but most patients who have sustained severe neurologic damage die during the early years of life (449,455).

Cytomegalovirus

CMV is ubiquitous and can be isolated from the urine of approximately 11.4% of asymptomatic newborn infants (456,457). Prenatal (congenital) infections are characterized by the presence of virus in the tissue and urine of the infant at birth. Only 19% of these infants are symptomatic at birth (458,459). The factors responsible for a clinically apparent infection are unclear, but Hanshaw and coworkers have pointed out that in symptomatic patients the infection occurs during the second or third trimester of pregnancy, in contrast to rubella infections, which tend to occur during the first trimester (456,458,459). The risk of congenital infection is greatest when the mother has a primary infection (460). Congenitally acquired infections have been observed, however, in consecutive pregnancies (461). Reactivation of a latent infection without involvement of the fetus occurs in 0.7 to 2.9% of pregnancies.

CMV has an affinity for the rapidly growing subependymal cells lining the cerebral ventricles. Multiplication of the virus and subsequent deposition of calcium in this area result in periventricular or diffuse calcifications and subsequent failure of brain growth. Microgyria, commonly found with congenital infections caused by CMV, can result from vascular changes as well as disturbances in neurogenesis (462). Intranuclear inclusion bodies appear within endothelial cells, neurons, and cells surrounding the cerebral vasculature. CMV infections of the inner ear involve the organ of Corti and spiral ganglion, the striae vascularis, and Reissner membrane (463). Generally, the longer the intrauterine infection lasts, the more severe the fetal involvement (464).

Clinical Manifestations

Clinical manifestations of congenital CMV are usually seen during the early neonatal period in infants who are premature or small for gestational age (Table 6.11) (465).

The classic picture of congenital CMV infection is low birth weight, persistent jaundice, hepatosplenomegaly, thrombocytopenia, and severe anemia. Neurologic abnormalities include microcephaly and, on rare occasions, hydrocephalus. Microgyria and other cortical malformations, cerebellar aplasia, subdural effusions, polycystic encephalomalacia, porencephaly, and

TABLE 6.11. *Clinical and laboratory manifestations in 19 children with congenital cytomegalovirus infections*

Finding	Number of patients
Hepatomegaly	17
Splenomegaly	16
Jaundice	13
Low birth weight (less than 2,500 g)	12
Thrombocytopenia	11
Petechiae	10
Cerebral calcifications	5
Microcephaly	5
Hemolytic anemia	4
Chorioretinitis	2
Hydrocephalus	1

From Shinefield HR. Prenatal and perinatal infections. In: Eichenwald HF, ed. *Prevention of mental retardation through control of infectious diseases.* Publ. no. 1692. Washington, DC: US Government Printing Office, 1968:65.

calcifications of the cerebral arteries also can be encountered (see Figs. 5.3A, B, and C and Fig. 6.7). Progressive hydrocephalus also can be seen (466). Of symptomatically infected neonates, 50% are microcephalic and 12% to 30% have chorioretinitis by 4 years of age (463). Approximately 10% to 35% of children with congenital microcephaly have CMV infections, contrasted with a 4% to 7% incidence in controls (456).

Some evidence also indicates that congenital CMV infections can produce milder neurologic manifestations, including mental retardation (467). On long-term follow-up evaluations only 59% of newborn infants with neuroradiographic abnormalities caused by CMV have an IQ of greater than 70. Almost one-half have an IQ less than 50. Ninety percent of children with abnormal CT scans in the newborn period develop at least one neurologic sequelae compared with 29% of children with normal scans (468). Residual ocular abnormalities include chorioretinitis, anomalies of the optic disc, microphthalmia, cataracts, optic atrophy, retinal calcifications, and other malformations (459).

Inapparent congenital infections have been found in 7% to 14% of neonates with cord IgM antibody levels over 19 mg/dL (469,470). In this group of children, 17% had increased CSF leukocyte or protein levels and 6% had an elevation of both. Subsequent hearing assessment

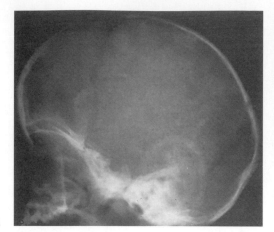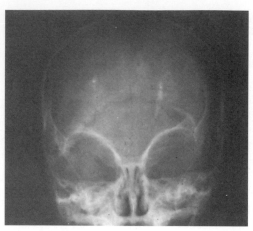

A   B

FIG. 6.7. Cytomegalic inclusion disease. Extensive periventricular calcifications are present. **A:** Lateral view of the skull. **B:** Anteroposterior view of the skull. (Courtesy of Dr. G. Wilson, Department of Radiology, University of California, Los Angeles.)

demonstrated hearing loss in 56% of infected subjects, in contrast to 17% of the control population. In some instances, the hearing deficit became more severe with time (471). In the study by Fowler and coworkers, 7% of children born with asymptomatic CMV infection have sensorineural hearing loss, whereas hearing loss of delayed onset occurred in 18% (472).

In 16% of cases, an infection that was clinically inapparent during the newborn period progressed as the children grew older, producing microcephaly, mental retardation, hypotonia, and profound deafness (473,474). Specific language disorders also can occur (475).

Whether congenital or acquired, the CMV infection can persist for months despite high antibody levels, and the presence of maternal antibodies does not protect the fetus against congenital infections (476). Viruria can still be demonstrated after 2 years of age (477). The virus also can be found in saliva and leukocytes up to 4 years after congenital infection (471). Infant-to-infant transmission resulting in inapparent infections can occur in nurseries (478).

The diagnosis of CMV infection rests on the demonstration of inclusion bodies in cells from the urinary sediment, or on the isolation of the virus from the infant at birth. The presence of viruria in an infant is not necessarily diagnostic of congenital CMV infection because CMV can

be acquired in the perinatal period. Isolation of the virus from the CSF, urine, or blood or demonstration of IgM antibodies to CMV at birth confirms a congenital infection (479). IgM antibody can develop as the result of infection acquired at the time of birth and can be present in the first week of life. The acquired IgM antibody can persist for 11 months (480).

The paraventricular calcifications seen in approximately one-third of subjects with cytomegalic inclusion disease (see Fig. 6.7) are not specific for this condition, and a similar radiologic appearance has been reported in toxoplasmosis (481).

At present, no proven effective therapy is available for human infections, although ganciclovir or phosphonoformate has been used in the CMV-infected immunocompromised host (482). The ability of ganciclovir to limit the effects of CMV on congenitally infected infants is under investigation.

Varicella

Multiple neurologic defects, including mental retardation, microcephaly, abnormalities of the ocular fundus, seizures, and dilated ventricles, vocal cord paresis, porencephaly, and cerebral calcifications are associated with congenital varicella (483–486). The patient also can have hypotonia, areflexia, muscle wasting, sphincter disturbances, limb contractures, and an electromyogram showing widespread denervation (484,487). The risk of embryopathy is approximately 2% after maternal varicella infection during the first 20 weeks of gestation (484).

Toxoplasma

The protozoan *Toxoplasma gondii*, a parasite first found in the gondii, a North African rodent, causes toxoplasmosis. It infects a wide range of birds and mammals and is an obligatory intracellular parasite, lacking host and tissue specificity (488). Humans usually acquire the infection by ingesting oocysts in uncooked meat or from cat feces (489).

Toxoplasma infection in the human infant was first described by Wolf and associates in 1939 (490). In the human, congenital infections have been estimated to occur in 1 in 1,000 to 10,000 live births. If stillbirths are included, it occurs in approximately 1% of all pregnancies (488,491).

The intrauterine infection results from fetal transmission of an infection incurred during the last 7 months of pregnancy. Infection of the placenta occurs before fetal infestation (488). If maternal antibodies develop, they modify the course of the fetal infection. Of mothers who give birth to children with toxoplasmosis, 15% have a history of respiratory illness. Only an infection newly acquired by the mother during her pregnancy seems to endanger the fetus; chronic infection does not produce fetal toxoplasmosis. The most dangerous period is from the second to sixth month of pregnancy (492). In mothers who seroconvert before 13 weeks of gestation, risk of fetal transmission is low, but becomes high should mothers develop an infection (492a). Maternal infections before the second month are more severe than those that occur later and generally result in fetal death. Infections incurred during the third trimester are more common and usually result in subclinical disease. Initially, these are relatively benign, with the infection being latent for at least the first few years of life (492,493). In mothers who seroconvert at 36 weeks' gestation or later, risk of transmission of infection is high, but infants are unlikely to have clinical features of the disease (492a).

Pathology

Cerebral lesions are of three types: large granulomatous areas with a necrotic center, diffuse inflammation, and small miliary granulomas. Miliary granulomas, most common in the cerebral cortex, consist of large epithelioid and round cells. Adherent overlying meninges are congested and densely infiltrated. Organisms can be found free in the most recent lesions and in the subarachnoid space. Although they are mainly extracellular, they also can exist within large epithelioid cells. As the infection progresses, areas of necrosis develop, and calcium salts become deposited in amorphous masses with predilection for the ventricular walls.

Hydrocephalus is frequent, most often caused by ependymitis or by abscesses occluding the aqueduct (494). Cerebral atrophy or hydranencephaly also can occur (488).

Clinical Manifestations

The most severe forms of congenital toxoplasmosis are the most familiar, but cases with few symptoms are common (491,495). The severe form can be apparent at birth or can remain asymptomatic for a few days or weeks. Chorioretinitis complicating congenital toxoplasmosis may not appear for several years. It ultimately develops in the majority of subjects, hence periodic ophthalmologic examinations are mandatory for all cases of congenital toxoplasmosis (491). Clinical manifestations are summarized in Table 6.12. Symptoms can be generalized or concentrated in the nervous system. In both severe and mild types, the principal findings are a chorioretinitis (Fig. 6.8), which in 85% of patients is bilateral (496), an abnormal CSF, anemia, and seizures. When the nervous system bears the major impact of toxoplasmosis, the incidence of cerebral calcifications and hydrocephalus also is higher (see Table 6.12). Serial examinations of infants detected by neonatal serologic screening programs indicate that 60% of neonates have a normal initial clinical examination (491).

TABLE 6.12. *Clinical and laboratory manifestations in infants with congenital toxoplasmosis*

	Generalized form	Neurologic form
Chorioretinitis	66	94
CSF pleocytosis, elevated protein	84	55
Anemia	77	51
Convulsions	—	50
Intracranial calcifications	—	50
Jaundice	79	29
Hydrocephalus	—	28
Fever	77	25
Splenomegaly	90	21
Lymphadenopathy	68	17
Hepatomegaly	77	17
Vomiting	48	17
Microcephaly	—	13
Cataracts	—	4.6
Optic atrophy	—	1.9
Pneumonitis	41	—

Adapted from Eichenwald HF. *Human toxoplasmosis: proceedings of the conference on clinical aspects and diagnostic problems of toxoplasmosis in pediatrics.* Baltimore: Williams & Wilkins, 1956.

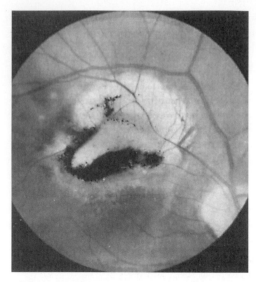

FIG. 6.8. Chorioretinitis in toxoplasmosis. (Courtesy of Dr. John Chang, Department of Ophthalmology, University of California, Los Angeles.)

Postnatally acquired toxoplasmosis is a common, generally inapparent infection. Infection of the choroid plexus, especially in the immunosuppressed patient, precedes CSF and cerebral dissemination (497). Clinical manifestations include hepatomegaly, lymphadenopathy, pneumonia, and, occasionally, a mild encephalitis (498). Less often a patient develops an isolated facial palsy (499), generalized seizures (500), or a condition that mimics a space-occupying lesion (501). The CSF in acquired toxoplasmosis usually shows an elevated protein and a variable degree of mononuclear pleocytosis. Cerebral abscesses caused by *Toxoplasma gondii* have been encountered in immunocompromised hosts.

The widespread use of serologic tests for toxoplasmosis has revealed incomplete forms of the disease. Positive serologic reactions are more frequent in patients with isolated chorioretinitis than in controls (493), and toxoplasmosis is a leading cause of chorioretinitis. Toxoplasmosis also is responsible for isolated cerebral calcifications in approximately 50% of patients (496). Rarely, toxoplasmosis causes seizures or psychomotor retardation in otherwise unaffected children (502).

Diagnosis

Because the clinical picture of congenital toxoplasmosis can be identical to that seen in CMV infection, syphilis, prenatal sepsis, and hemolytic disease of the newborn, serologic tests become the primary means of diagnosis (503).

The presence of IgG-specific antibodies is measured by the indirect immunofluorescence test or by enzyme immunoassay. The highly sensitive double-sandwich IgM ELISA, which detects antibody in 75% of babies with congenital toxoplasmosis, or the detection of antitoxoplasmic IgA antibody are more specific indicators of a recently acquired infection (504). The isolation of the parasite by inoculation of mice can be extremely difficult, as well as hazardous to laboratory workers. However, identification of *Toxoplasma gondii* in lymph nodes by immunofluorescence has been successful.

CSF in patients with toxoplasmosis can contain 500 to 1,000 mg/dL protein. Pleocytosis is often in the range of 30 to 60 white blood cells per µL. Rarely, congenital toxoplasmosis also can present with eosinophilic meningitis (505). Cerebral calcifications, although suggestive of toxoplasmosis, are not pathognomonic. The radiologic features of the intracranial calcifications have been reviewed by Mussbichler (506). The deposits are scattered irregularly throughout the brain and tend to cluster in the caudate nucleus, meninges, choroid plexus, and subependymal region. None is found in the subtentorial region or spinal cord, although toxoplasmosis can rarely affect the spinal cord predominantly (507). It is of note that the presence of intracerebral calcifications is not predictive of outcome in infants treated with pyrimethamine and sulfadiazine (508).

Treatment

The combination of pyrimethamine with triple sulfa or sulfadiazine has been reported to be beneficial in the acute illness (488). This treatment eliminates trophozoites, but not encysted forms. A regimen with oral clindamycin and pyrimethamine has proven effective for *Toxoplasma* encephalitis (509). The progressive nature of congenital *Toxoplasma* infections dictates that the patient begin treatment as early as possible (510).

Therapy of infants with congenital infection consists of sulfadiazine (100 mg/kg per day) and pyrimethamine (1 mg/kg) given twice a week. Folinic acid (5 mg) also is given twice weekly. In some centers, this regimen is alternated with spiramycin (100 mg/kg per day) given in 6-week cycles. Therapy for small children consists of sulfadiazine or trisulfapyrimidine (100 to 150 mg/kg per day in divided doses), and pyrimethamine (1 mg/kg per day in divided doses; a double dose is used for the first 3 days). Older children and adults receive the usual dosage of sulfadiazine up to a maximum of 8 g per day, together with 25 mg of pyrimethamine. Because sulfadiazine is no longer marketed in the United States, the drug has to be obtained from the Centers for Disease Control and Prevention in Atlanta (511). Folinic acid (but not folic acid) also is given (5 to 10 mg/day) to avoid hematologic toxicity. Treatment should be continued for 1 to 6 months for both congenital and acquired toxoplasmosis (489,511). Because of the risk of treatment failure, some experts recommend that treatment be continued for 1 year. Because pyrimethamine is a folic acid antagonist, platelet and leukocyte counts are done twice weekly during therapy, and the drug is discontinued if one or both are significantly reduced. Clindamycin can be used together with pyrimethamine in patients who do not tolerate sulfanamides. Atovaquone has been advocated for patients intolerant to standard therapies (512).

Prognosis

The prognosis for infants with generalized congenital toxoplasmosis, or toxoplasmosis affecting the nervous system primarily, is poor. In one study, overall mortality for patients with apparent early neurologic disease was 11.1%, whereas mortality for the group with generalized disease was 13.6%. Major sequelae were found in a large majority of survivors (495). A 4-year follow-up of the group with apparent neurologic disease in infancy disclosed mental retardation (89%), convulsions (83%), spasticity (69%), severely impaired vision (42%), hydrocephalus and microcephaly (44%), and deafness (17%); only 9% were healthy. The group with generalized involvement had only a slightly better long-term picture, with mental retardation (81%), convulsions (77%), spasticity (58%), and hydrocephalus and microcephaly (10%); 16.1% were healthy. In the experience of Roizin and colleagues, the outcome was poor when the neonatal period was marked by apnea and bradycardia, hypoglycemia, and hydrocephalus with a CSF protein greater than 1 g/dL (513). As is the case for some of the other congenital infections, chorioretinitis and neurologic symptoms might not be present at birth but can appear later in infancy or childhood. In such instances, neurologic involvement is less severe and resolves with therapy. The outcome for these children is quite good, and in the series of Roizin and colleagues 67% had an IQ in the average range (513).

Herpes Simplex

Infection of the fetus with herpes simplex virus can result in a fatal generalized disease. In most instances of congenital herpes, the infection is recognized between ages 1 and 3 weeks and is usually caused by type 2 strains. Transplacental infection has been demonstrated only when the mother has acquired a primary herpetic infection while pregnant (514).

Congenital infection of the fetus with herpes simplex type 2 virus can result in microcephaly, intracranial calcifications, microphthalmia, and retinal dysplasia. Cutaneous lesions with vesicles can be present (515).

Most cases of herpes infection develop in the neonatal period. They are considered in another section of this chapter (see Human Herpesvirus Types 6 and 7, later in this chapter).

Although a number of chemotherapeutic agents, including vidarabine and acyclovir, have been used with some benefit in the treatment of herpes encephalitis in neonates and older children, their effect in congenital infections is doubtful.

Postinfectious and Postvaccinal Encephalomyelitis

The neurologic complications encountered in the course of the various exanthems, notably measles, chickenpox, and rubella, and mumps, are considered in Chapter 7. The complications of prophylactic immunization, particularly those associated with pertussis vaccination and rabies prophylaxis, also are discussed in Chapter 7.

VIRAL INFECTIONS

Viral infections of the CNS are usually benign and self-limited with a good clinical outcome. A subset of viruses, however, can result in a severe clinical course with a high morbidity and mortality. Acute encephalitis is more common in children (more than 16 cases per 100,000 patient-years) than in adults (between 3.5 and 7.4 cases per 100,000 patient-years) (516). The number of annual cases of primary and postinfectious encephalitis reported to the Centers for Disease Control and Prevention from 1989 to 1994 has ranged from 717 to 1,341 and from 82 to 170, respectively. Since 1995, these clinical entities are no longer nationally notifiable.

Pathogenesis

Viruses can cause CNS damage through direct invasion of central nervous tissues (primary or infectious encephalitis) or through the generation of an immune response to a systemic viral infection (postinfectious encephalomyelitis) (517).

In a naturally acquired infection, virus spreads to the CNS through two main mechanisms: hematogeneous and neuronal. These two mechanisms are not mutually exclusive and can occur concurrently to spread a virus.

Hematogenous Spread

The most common pathway for spread of virus to the CNS is by way of the bloodstream. Viral growth generally begins in extraneural tissue: poliomyelitis in the gut or regional lymphatics; herpes simplex in the respiratory tract or gastrointestinal mucosa; arbovirus in the vascular epithelium; and coxsackievirus, reovirus, rabies, and variola in brown fat. The viremia is maintained by shedding of the virus, absorption into red blood cells, or growth within leukocytes. Virus in blood can enter the CSF by either passing through or growing through the choroid plexus. Growth of virus in the choroid plexus might explain the ease with which echovirus and coxsackievirus can be isolated from the CSF. Migration of infected phagocytes through cerebral vessels and replication of virus in the endothelial cells with growth or passive transfer through the blood–brain barrier also can occur.

Once within the nervous system, the virus can spread by direct contiguity or through the limited extracellular space. Neurovirulent viruses that lack the neuroinvasive ability to cross the blood–brain barrier are able to produce infection once the barrier is breached by bacterial lipopolysaccharide (517).

Neuronal Spread

Less commonly, neuronal spread occurs from peripheral and cranial nerves. Viruses can enter the nervous system tissue by centripetal spread along the endoneurium, perineural Schwann cells, and fibrocytes of peripheral nerves. Once the virus has gained access to the spinal cord by this route, it can spread randomly along the endoneurium or the interstitial space within the nerve. Spread within the nerve is significant for rabies and for some herpes simplex infections. Penetration at sensory or motor nerve endings with transport to specific sensory ganglion cells or motor neurons by retrograde axoplasmic flow has been demonstrated for herpes simplex, polio viruses, and rabies virus.

Spread by way of the olfactory system has been demonstrated in herpes simplex, poliomyelitis, and arbovirus infections. These viruses spread along olfactory rods and nerve fibers to the mitral cell neurons of the olfactory bulb, or along the interstitial spaces, endoneurium, and perineurium of the olfactory nerves to the parenchymal cells of the olfactory bulb, and from there along the subarachnoid cuffs to the meninges (518).

Pathology

Cells of the CNS vary in their susceptibility to viral infection. Thus, herpes simplex seems to infect all cell types, whereas poliomyelitis has a predilection for the larger motor cells, Purkinje cells, and cells of the reticular formation. Susceptibility is determined by cell receptor sites and by the route of entry.

The reactions of brain tissue to viral invasion are similar in all forms of encephalitis. The most obvious histologic lesion is a cellular infiltration. Initially, this consists largely of polymorphoneutrophils; later, round cells predominate. Proliferation of microglial cells can be diffuse or focal. With diffuse proliferation, the cells accumulate around degenerated or dying nerve cells, a phenomenon associated with neuronophagia. Most commonly, alterations within nerve cells consist of a loss of Nissl granules and eosinophilia of the cytoplasm. Inclusion bodies within neurons and glial cells, such as the Negri bodies seen in rabies, can be typical of the disease or can represent nonspecific degeneration products.

Arteritis and other alterations of the vessel walls are observed in a number of conditions, notably in the equine encephalitides. Demyelination can result from the loss of cortical nerve cells or can occur independently, as in subacute sclerosing panencephalitis (SSPE) or other slow virus infections.

Viral infections are characterized by intrathecal production of oligoclonal immunoglobulin within the CNS. Viral-specific IgM is produced during the early stage of infection, with specific IgG and IgA produced slightly later.

The patient's humoral and cellular immune response to infection can contribute to the disease picture. For instance, in experimental lymphocytic choriomeningitis, the virus causes severe meningeal infiltrates only in immunologically mature and competent animals. TNF, the cytokine associated with inflammation in bacterial infections, is not demonstrable in many viral infections of the nervous system (519,520). Leukotriene B4, a potent chemotactic factor for leukocytes, and leukotriene C4, which increases vascular permeability and causes smooth muscle contraction, are increased in the CSF of children with aseptic meningitis and encephalitis (521). Suppression of the immune response with dexamethasone may have no benefit or can even be deleterious (522). For a review of T-cell activation, critical to activation of the immune response to viruses, see the publication by Reiser and Stadecker (523).

Apoptosis is a common pathway to virus-induced cell death. It can result from viral infection of cells or from the action of leukocytes and their products. This subject has been extensively reviewed by Razvi and Welsh (524).

Clinical Manifestations

Viruses can cause encephalitis (inflammation of the brain) and meningitis (inflammation of the meninges). These processes can be seen independently as well as concurrently.

Acute Encephalitis

The initial clinical picture can be protean, manifesting as a systemic infection without neurologic symptoms or findings. Fever, irritability, headaches, nausea, vomiting, poor appetite, and restlessness precede neurologic symptoms. In Finnish studies, the most characteristic neurologic symptoms of viral encephalitis during the acute phase were lowered consciousness manifested by disorientation, confusion, somnolence, or coma. These symptoms were recorded in 58% of patients. Ataxia was seen in 58%; an altered mental status, notable aggressiveness, and apathy were seen in 40%. Seizures, either generalized (32%), focal (5%), or both, were encountered less commonly. Neurologic findings were generally nonspecific, and meningeal symptoms and signs were not always present (525,526). The CSF examination was often frequently normal early in the disease (527). As a general rule, the initial CSF pleocytosis is characterized by a rapidly decreasing proportion of granulocytes. The transient elevation in CSF granulocyte colony-stimulating factor observed during the initial stages of aseptic meningitis is associated with this change (528). Young age, disorientation, or loss of consciousness are serious prognostic signs in encephalitis, especially if the encephalitis is caused by herpes simplex. In the study by Klein and coworkers, focal signs on neurologic examination and abnormal neuroimaging studies were the only two factors present at admission that predicted a poor short-term outcome (529). Unilateral hyperperfusion demonstrated by single photon emission CT (SPECT) also is associated with a poor prognosis in encephalitis (530).

Viral Meningitis (Aseptic Meningitis)

This is a clinical syndrome characterized in children by fever, abrupt onset of headaches, vomiting, irritability, and physical findings of meningeal irritation such as Kernig and Brudzinski signs. Infants present with a mild syndrome without the physical findings found in older children. The spinal fluid reveals less than 1,000 white blood cells with a mononuclear predominance, although early in the course of the illness, a polymorphonuclear predominance may be observed. CSF glucose is normal or slightly decreased, and CSF protein is slightly elevated. The Gram's stain is universally negative as are bacterial, mycobacterial, and fungal cultures.

Diagnosis

The diagnosis of a presumptive CNS viral infection starts with a thorough and meticulous history looking for significant exposures within the previous 2 to 3 weeks. The exposure of the patient to sick humans or animals (especially horses), travel history and exposure to mosquitoes, rodents, and ticks helps to ascertain potential etiologies. The physical examination provides useful information about the extent of the disease and guides the choice of diagnostic studies required.

The analysis of the CSF is crucial in the search of the etiologic diagnosis. The cytochemical analysis combined with specific virologic (PCR and cultures) and serologic tests (specific IgM, IgG, or both) can assist in confirming the etiology. CSF also helps to rule out other treatable infectious or noninfectious causes, which could mimic a viral process. Thus, it is important in a child with a clinical picture of aseptic meningoencephalitis to rule out fungal, mycobacterial, and parasitic infections by performing appropriate stains and cultures. Bacterial infections of the CNS need to be ruled out by Gram's stains, rapid antigen tests, and cultures. Viral cultures of blood, stool, and throat serve as a useful diagnostic tool. Blood obtained in the beginning of the clinical course as well as 2 to 3 weeks later can be used for the serologic confirmation of diseases through the observation of a fourfold increase in the specific antibody titer.

The value of neuroimaging studies lies not in determining the etiology of the viral encephalitis or meningitis, but in assessing the degree of CNS damage. For this purpose, MRI has been found to be more helpful than CT (531).

By the combined use of the various diagnostic studies, the etiology of viral meningitis or encephalitis can be determined in approximately 60% of patients (526).

This section considers the various types of viral infections according to etiology. A survey of their relative frequencies, as derived from data of Koskiniemi and Vaheri, is presented in Table 6.13 (532). Table 6.14 compiles the etiologic agents, type of disease, mechanism of acquisition, frequency, fatality rates, and laboratory confirmation, as derived from data from Cassady and Whitley (533) and Johnson (534). Table 6.15 lists some of the more uncommon viral pathogens that have been associated with CNS disease.

Enterovirus Infections

Enterovirus infections, a group of RNA viruses, include poliomyelitis (three types), coxsackie groups A (22 serotypes) and B (six serotypes), and the echovirus group (31 serotypes). Viruses isolated after the original classification are sim-

TABLE 6.13. *Known reported causes of encephalitis in 412 children 16 years or younger (1968 through 1987)*

Pathogen	Percent of known agents
Measles, mumps, rubella group[a]	30.4
Measles	12.8
Mumps	16.0
Rubella	1.6
Herpes group	24.1
Varicella	15.4
Herpes simplex virus	6.4
Cytomegalovirus	1.3
Epstein-Barr virus	1.0
Respiratory group	18.3
Adenovirus	8.7
Parainfluenza virus and respiratory syncytial virus	4.2
Influenza A and B viruses	5.4
Enterovirus group	9.7
Enteroviruses	7.7
Rotavirus	1.0
Reovirus	1.0
Mycoplasmal pneumonia	13.1
More than one virus	2.9
Postvaccination encephalitis (measles-mumps-rubella, polio)	1.0
Agent unknown	32.0

[a]No case of mumps, measles, or rubella encephalitis was encountered after 1982.

Adapted from Koskiniemi M, Vaheri A. Effect of measles, mumps, rubella vaccination on pattern of encephalitis in children. *Lancet* 1989;1:31.

ply assigned an enterovirus number (serotypes 68 to 72) (535).

Organisms enter the body through the oral or respiratory tracts, replicate and extend to the regional lymphoid tissue, induce a minor viremia, and subsequently can invade multiple sites, including the nervous system. The clinical picture produced by these agents depends on factors such as type and virulence of the virus, the site of CNS invasion, and, as is the case for poliomyelitis, host factors such as degree of susceptibility and recent inoculations or trauma (536).

Enterovirus infection is transmitted principally by direct or indirect contamination through infected fecal material. Organisms can be isolated from the oropharynx, stool, blood, or CSF. Isolation of virus from CSF confirms the cause of a specific episode (536). Diagnosis by isolation of an enterovirus from stool can be misleading because virus can be excreted for 12 to 17 weeks after infection. In such a situation, only a definite increase in the titer of antibodies to the isolated agent can confirm a recent significant infection.

The clinical manifestations of an enterovirus infection of the nervous system can take several forms.

In aseptic meningitis, children usually have an infection associated with epidemic disease caused by coxsackievirus A9 and B2, 4, and 5 or echoviruses 4, 6, 9, 11, 16, 30, and 33; other types are less common. Febrile infants infected with coxsackievirus group B, and echovirus 11 and 30 were more likely to have aseptic meningitis than those infected with other serotypes (537). Berlin and coworkers were able to identify the viral pathogen in 62% of children younger than 2 years of age with aseptic meningitis; group B coxsackievirus or echoviruses were implicated in 92% of the laboratory-diagnosed cases (538). In 63.5% of cases, the infection developed at 8 weeks of age or earlier (539). Fever, pharyngitis, or other respiratory symptoms are common. Abdominal pain can occur. Rash is common but its incidence depends on the specific viral agent; one-third to one-half of patients with echovirus 9 meningitis have exanthem. This rash is variable in appearance, but can be petechial and simulate the rash of meningococcemia. Herpangina, pleurodynia, or myocarditis are associated findings that suggest enterovirus infection (539a). SIADH occurs in approximately 9% of children with enteroviral meningitis. It usually lasts less than 2 days (536,538). Multiple attacks of enteroviral aseptic meningitis occasionally have occurred in the same individual.

Enterovirus encephalitis is most commonly caused by echovirus type 9, less commonly by echoviruses 4, 6, 11, and 30, and coxsackievirus B5. Outbreaks of encephalitis have been associated with enterovirus 71 (539a). Three neurologic syndromes have been observed. Most commonly, there is a rhombencephalitis marked by myoclonic jerks, ataxia, and various brainstem signs; less often there is an aseptic meningitis, or an acute flaccid paralysis (539b). Enteroviruses account for approximately 10% to 20% of the cases of encephalitis of proven viral

TABLE 6.14. *Common viral infections of the central nervous system*

Viral agent	Disease	Transmission	Incidence	Fatality rate	Laboratory confirmation
Herpesvirus					
Herpes simplex	Encephalitis Meningoencephalitis Aseptic meningitis	Human	Common	>70% if untreated	PCR has become method of choice
Varicella zoster	Cerebellitis	Human	Rare Uncommon	<1% None	Culture of CSF, brain biopsy Clinical picture, culture of skin lesions, DFA of skin or brain tissue, serology
	Encephalitis Aseptic meningtitis Transverse myelitis Reye syndrome		Rare Rare Very rare Very rare	>40%	
Cytomegalovirus	Encephalitis	Human	Uncommon	Rare	Culture of CSF, brain, PCR becoming gold standard, serology
Epstein-Barr Virus	Meningitis Encephalitis	Human Rare	Rare Uncommon	Rare	Serology is most useful, PCR of CSF
	Meningitis Transverse myelitis Guillain-Barré syndrome				
Human herpesvirus type 6	Encephalitis	Human	Uncommon	No	Culture PBMC, saliva, PCR on CSF, serology
	Meningitis Encephalomyelitis				
Human herpesvirus type 7	Acute hemiplegia	Human	?	?	Culture PBMC, saliva, PCR on CSF, serology
	Seizures				
Enteroviruses					
Polio virus	Meningitis	Human	None in United States, clinical disease in developing countries	5% to 50%	Culture, PCR
	Paralytic polio		Very common	None	Culture of stool, CSF, PCR of CSF very useful, serology
Coxsackievirus (C) and echovirus (E)	Meningitis Encephalitis Paralytic disease Guillain-Barré syndrome Transverse myelitis Cerebellitis Peripheral neuritis	Human	Rare (C), uncommon (E) Common (C), rare (E)[a] Uncommon (C), rare (E) Rare Rare Rare		

	Clinical manifestations	Reservoir/vector	Frequency	Mortality	Diagnosis
Newer enteroviruses	Meningitis Encephalitis Paralytic disease Encephalomyelitis	Human	Uncommon	Rarely fatal	Viral culture, serology not useful
Arboviruses[b]					
Western equine encephalitis virus[c]	Meningitis Encephalitis	Mosquitoes/birds	Common	10% in infants	Serology, antigen detection in brain
Eastern equine encephalitis virus[d]	Meningitis	Mosquitoes/birds	Uncommon	50% in all ages	Serology, IgM, ELISA, culture and antigen in brain
Venezuelan equine encephalitis virus[e]	Encephalitis Meningitis Encephalitis	Mosquitoes/horses	Uncommon	<1%	Serology, IgM, ELISA
Japanese encephalitis virus[f]	Meningitis Encephalitis	Mosquitoes/swine/birds	Very common	25%	ELISA, serology, CSF antigen
St. Louis encephalitis virus[g]	Meningitis Encephalitis Febrile headache	Mosquitoes/birds	Common	7–20%	Serology, CSF IgM, ELISA
West Nile fever virus[h]	Meningitis Encephalitis Myelitis	Mosquitoes/birds	Common	10%	Serology, CSF IgM, ELISA
Murray Valley virus[i]	Encephalitis	Mosquitoes/birds	Uncommon	20%	Serology
Tick-borne encephalitis virus[j]	Meningitis Encephalitis Myelitis Radiculoneuritis	Tick/rodents	Uncommon	1%	Serology, CSF IgM, ELISA
California (La Crosse) encephalitis virus[k]	Meningitis Encephalitis	Mosquitoes/chipmunks Squirrels	Common	<1%	Serology, culture, CSF IgM, ELISA
Paramyxoviruses					
Measles virus	Encephalitis Subacute sclerosing panencephalitis	Human	Uncommon Rare	<5% 100% fatal	Serology Elevated CSF globulin
Mumps virus	Meningitis Encephalitis	Human	Common in unvaccinated	<1%	Serology, culture of CSF
Togaviruses					
Rubella virus	Encephalitis Guillain-Barré Optic neuritis Myelitis Progressive panencephalitis	Human	Rare	<1%	Serology

Continued

519

TABLE 6.14. *Continued.*

Viral agent	Disease	Transmission	Incidence	Fatality rate	Laboratory confirmation
Orthomyxoviruses					
Influenza virus	Encephalitis	Human	Uncommon	<1%	Culture of respiratory secretions, serology
	Transverse myelitis			<1%	
	Reye syndrome			>40%	
Rabdoviruses					
Rabies virus	Encephalitis	Bats, raccoons, skunks, dogs, squirrels, cats	Common	>99%	Antigen detection in brain, culture, serology
	Encephalomyelitis				
Adenoviruses					
Adenovirus	Meningitis	Human	Rare	<1%	Culture of CSF, brain
	Encephalitis				
Retroviruses					
Human immuno-deficiency virus	Encephalitis	Human	Uncommon	100% fatal	Serology, culture of CSF, PCR of CSF
	Transverse myelitis				
	Leukoencephalopathy				
Arenaviruses					
Lymphocytic choriomeningitis virus	Meningitis	Mice/hamsters	Rare	<2%	CSF, blood, urine cultures, serology
	Encephalitis				

DFA, direct fluorescent antibody; ELISA, enzyme-linked immunosorbent assay; PBMC, peripheral blood mononuclear cells; PCR, polymerase chain reaction.

[a] Incidence varies according to serotypes.
[b] Incidence depends on geographic region.
[c] Seen in United States west of Mississippi River.
[d] Seen in United States Atlantic and Gulf Coast states.
[e] Seen in southwestern United States, Florida, and Central and South America
[f] Seen in Southeast Asia, India, and Nepal.
[g] Seen in all of United States.
[h] Seen in Africa, Middle East, Southeast Asia, India, Australia, areas of Europe, and the northeastern United States.
[i] Seen in Australia.
[j] Seen in Central Europe and Russia.
[k] More than 90% of cases seen in Midwest of United States.

TABLE 6.15. *Viruses that have been rarely associated with central nervous system disease*

Virus	Disease
Parainfluenza	Aseptic meningitis
	Guillain-Barré syndrome
	Demyelinating disease
	Encephalomyocarditis
	Aseptic meningitis
Rotavirus	Aseptic meningitis
	Encephalitis
Coronavirus	Aseptic meningitis
	Polyradiculitis
	Multiple sclerosis?
Parvovirus B19	Aseptic meningitis
	Encephalitis
Rhinoviruses	Aseptic meningitis

etiology. Neurologic symptoms can be diffuse or focal (540). Clinical manifestations of the diffuse form of encephalitis range from mild changes of mental status to coma, whereas focal neurologic symptoms include focal seizures, hemichorea, or ataxia. Although the general prognosis is favorable, fatal cases of enterovirus encephalitis involving coxsackievirus B3 and B6, echoviruses 2, 9, 17, and 25, and enterovirus 70 have been reported (536,538).

Coxsackievirus and echoviruses can on rare occasions cause paralytic syndromes that are clinically indistinguishable from paralytic poliomyelitis. The course is less severe, however, and of shorter duration. Acute paralytic syndromes also can occur after acute epidemic conjunctivitis caused by enterovirus type 70 (541). The three patterns most commonly seen are limb involvement only (43%), involvement of nerves and limbs (33%), and involvement of one or more cranial nerves only (24%). Severe, diffuse pain that does not conform to root or nerve distribution and that is sometimes associated with muscle tenderness usually precedes the onset of paralysis (542). Approximately one-half of patients have fasciculations during the acute paralytic stage. In some instances, radiculitis, myelitis, or radiculomyelitis can occur (543).

Coxsackieviruses and echoviruses have been associated with a variety of other neurologic conditions, notably Guillain-Barré syndrome, transverse myelitis, dermatomyositis, polymyositis,

cerebellar ataxia, and the syndrome of opsoclonus-myoclonus (538,544,545). Pulmonary edema, thought to be neurogenic in origin, has been associated with enterovirus 71 (546). Cardiopulmonary failure occurs in the absence of severe neurologic signs but is accompanied by severe, widespread inflammation of the brainstem and spinal cord (547).

Enterovirus infections of neonates are a serious and potentially fatal condition. Vertical transmission of enteroviruses can occur transplacentally, during delivery, and during the postpartum period. Whereas the presence of a primary maternal infection during late pregnancy can lead to stillbirth and severe neonatal disease manifested within the first 2 days of life, this is not a common occurrence. The majority of children manifest symptoms between the third and tenth day of life. This reflects the transmission of the virus by genital, respiratory, and gastrointestinal secretions during the immediate perinatal period. Enteroviruses reported to cause neonatal disease include coxsackieviruses B1 through 5, and echoviruses 5, 7, 9, 11, 17, 19, and 22 (548).

Signs and symptoms suggestive of severe CNS involvement include extreme lethargy, flaccid paralysis, and coma. These symptoms usually are associated with a multisystem organ involvement that includes liver, heart, and lungs with hypocoagulability and bleeding, a picture suggestive of neonatal sepsis (549). In the experience of Rorabaugh and associates, only 8.7% of infants younger than 16 weeks of age show meningeal irritation when first examined (539). A more benign picture of isolated aseptic meningitis also has been seen. Because of the decline in neonatal bacterial meningitis, enteroviruses have become the most common cause of meningitis in neonates older than 7 days and are currently responsible for one-third of all cases of neonatal meningitis (550). Repeat episodes of meningitis caused by different strains of enterovirus can occur within 1 month of each other (551).

A long-term follow-up study suggests that approximately 10% to 15% of infants who recover from enterovirus infections incurred during the first year of life have motor deficits or subnormal intelligence (552–554). Enterovirus infections in infants younger than 3 months of age can cause subtle deficits in language skills, particularly in receptive language. These children, therefore, should be monitored carefully for language development (555). When infection is incurred after the first year of life, no residua are usually demonstrable.

Persistent and fatal enteroviral CNS infections can occur in patients with agammaglobulinemia (540,556).

The diagnosis of enteroviral infections is based in the recovery of the virus in feces, urine, blood, CSF, or from cultures obtained on biopsy specimen during the acute episode of the disease. The PCR technique is highly sensitive and specific for the detection of virus-specific DNA. Its speed, accuracy, and 100% sensitivity make it particularly useful in CNS infections (557).

Poliomyelitis

Although poliomyelitis caused by wild virus has been eradicated from the Western hemisphere since 1994, it remains a problem in developing countries. An extensive discussion is warranted because it serves as a prototype for viral infections of the nervous system.

Poliomyelitis is an acute infectious disease first described by Heine in 1840 (558). It affects the motor neurons of the spinal cord and brain and results in an asymmetric flaccid paralysis of the voluntary muscles. The severity of the illness varies; asymptomatic or mild cases are approximately 100 times more common than the classic paralytic disease. Poliomyelitis can occur throughout the world. It is contracted earlier in life and is less likely to be symptomatic in areas with inadequate sanitation, because poor sanitation is conducive to exposure at an age when lingering transferred maternal immunity can attenuate the clinical picture.

With widespread immunization, poliomyelitis has become preventable, and the recurrent major epidemics are no longer encountered. Approximately 8 to 10 cases per year have been reported in the United States. All of these have been associated with the use of the oral polio vaccine (OPV). These cases are more commonly associated with the administration of the first dose of vaccine (1 per 720,000 recipients of OPV). Based on the lack of wild cases and the occurrence of vaccine-associated paralytic polio (VAPP), the Advisory Committee on Immunization Practices voted to recommend a sequential schedule of inactivated polio vaccine (IPV) and OPV for polio immunization, with either all OPV or all IPV as acceptable alternatives (559).

Pathology

Alterations within the CNS depend on the stage of the disease at the time of death. In the early days of the illness, neurons undergo a variety of nonspecific microscopic changes that vary in severity and result directly from viral invasion. These changes are accompanied by an initial polymorphonuclear reaction, which later becomes mononuclear. As the illness progresses, motor neurons degenerate, become surrounded by inflammatory cells, and undergo neuronophagia. The distribution of lesions is characteristic of poliomyelitis. Lesions are usually mild and restricted to layers 3 and 5 in the precentral gyrus and adjacent cortex, thalamus, and globus pallidus (560). Neuronal necrosis can be caused by toxic levels of neurotransmitters such as quinolinic acid that occur in areas of the brain affected by the virus, as well as from direct viral damage to neurons (561).

Cerebellar vermis and deep cerebellar nuclei are often severely involved, whereas the cerebellar hemispheres are usually free of lesions (562). Also, marked involvement of motor and sensory cranial nuclei of the medulla occurs, especially the vestibular and ambiguous nuclei and throughout the reticular formation. The basis pontis and inferior olivary nuclei are usually spared.

In the spinal cord, lesions usually are restricted to the anterior horn cells, although some cases also show spotty involvement of the neurons in the intermediate, intermediolateral, and posterior gray columns. Extension of lesions to the sensory spinal ganglia is the rule in more extensive cord involvement. The cervical and lumbar cord tend to be more affected than the thoracic region.

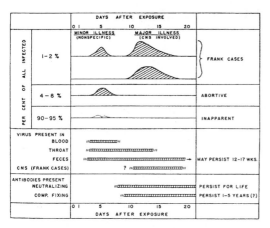

FIG. 6.9. Schematic diagram of the clinical and subclinical forms of poliomyelitis, showing presence of virus and antibodies in relation to development and subsidence of infection. (From Horsfall FL, Tamm I. *Viral and rickettsial infections of man.* 4th ed. Philadelphia: Lippincott, 1965. With permission.)

TABLE 6.16. *Distribution of paralysis in 5,784 cases of acute anterior poliomyelitis*

Location	Percentage of cases
Leg	78.6
Arm	41.4
Trunk	27.8
Throat and neck	5.8
Cranial nerves	13.8
Facial muscles	40.9
Pharyngeal	31.9
Ocular	30.1
Palatal	15.8
Glossal	5.6
Masticatory	2.9

Modified from Wernstedt W. Epidemiologische Studien Über die zweite grosse Poliomyelitisepidemie in Schweden 1911–1913. *Ergebn Inn Med Kinderheilk* 1924;26:248.

Clinical Manifestations

The clinical picture of poliomyelitis ranges from a nonspecific mild febrile illness to a severe and potentially fatal paralytic disease. An inapparent infection is estimated to occur in 90% to 95% of infected individuals, a minor nonparalytic illness in 4% to 8%, and paralytic poliomyelitis in 1% to 2% (Fig. 6.9). The incubation period ranges between 3 and 35 days, with an average of 17 days (563).

The minor illness coincides with the period of viremia and the appearance of virus in the stool. It lasts 24 to 48 hours and is manifested by nonspecific symptoms of headache, vomiting, sore throat, and gastrointestinal disturbances.

The major illness can follow in 2 to 5 days of recovery from the minor illness. When mild, it produces aseptic meningitis with fever, headache, vomiting, and meningeal irritation. The disease might not advance any further, or it might progress to the paralytic stage.

The clinical course and picture of paralytic poliomyelitis varies with the age of the patient and the site of maximal involvement. The classic diphasic course is more common in children than in adults. It was noted in 37% of children aged 2

to 9 years, but only in 11% of adolescents 15 years or older (564). In the remaining cases, the preparalytic stage is mild or inapparent. Infants show relatively little fever and lack meningeal signs despite extensive and often symmetric paralysis. Paralysis occurs in 90% of infants younger than 1 year of age who develop symptomatic infections with poliomyelitis virus (565).

The presenting symptom of paralytic poliomyelitis is pain, often severe and localized to the lower back. It usually is accompanied by hyperesthesia, drowsiness, or irritability. The initial indications of paralysis are localized muscular pain, fasciculation, twitching, and diminution or loss of the deep tendon reflexes. The paralysis appears during the first or second day of the major illness. Often it reaches its maximum within a few hours, and, less commonly, it can advance for 4 to 5 days. The fever that generally accompanies the paralysis falls by lysis.

Table 6.16 shows the distribution of paralysis, as encountered in an early epidemic (566). Curiously, when an infected child had received an injection before the onset of symptoms, the illness more likely involves the injected limb. A similar problem has been encountered when intramuscular injections are given within 30 days of immunization with oral poliovirus vaccine (566a). These observations can be explained by the upregulation of the poliovirus receptor consequent to trauma. The poliovirus receptor is an integral membrane protein with structural characteristics of the immunoglobulin superfamily of proteins (567,567a).

Spinal, bulbar, and encephalitic forms of poliomyelitis have been recognized. Spinal paralytic poliomyelitis is characterized by an asymmetric, scattered, flaccid paralysis that more frequently involves the lower extremities. On examination, the weakness is accompanied by muscle tenderness and spasm. Deep tendon reflexes in the affected area are usually absent. Autonomic involvement can be manifested by excessive sweating and vasomotor disturbances. Some 10% to 20% of patients have bladder involvement, notably sphincter spasm and overflow incontinence (568). Pyramidal tract and segmental sensory involvement are extremely rare.

The bulbar form of poliomyelitis generally evolves with explosive rapidity. Other areas of the neuraxis, most often the cervical cord, also are affected in 90% of cases.

The clinical picture of bulbar poliomyelitis reflects the site of involvement. Most commonly, the paralysis affects the facial, pharyngeal, and ocular muscles (see Table 6.16) (566,569). Involvement of the reticular formation can lead to respiratory and cardiovascular irregularities (570). Pulmonary edema is regarded as a manifestation of extensive damage to both the dorsal nuclei of the vagus and the medial reticular (vasomotor) nuclei of the medulla (571). When the tenth cranial nerve is involved, there is impairment of swallowing and faulty innervation of the larynx. This presents a serious threat to life by obstruction of the airway and is an indication for early elective tracheotomy. Fatal involvement of the respiratory center or the circulatory center may occur. Hypertension can develop secondary to medullary involvement or hypocapnia. Hypothalamic dysfunction is manifested by impaired temperature regulation and hypertension (572). Papilledema results from carbon dioxide retention caused by inadequate pulmonary ventilation. It also is associated with a high CSF protein, which interferes with normal CSF absorption.

In as many as one-third of cases, poliomyelitis is accompanied by symptoms and signs of encephalitis, including changes in consciousness, anxiety, irrationality, and restlessness or hyperac-tivity, muscular tremors, and twitching. These signs should first be considered as caused by hypoxia even in the absence of cyanosis. Only when these symptoms persist after adequate oxygenation can they be attributed to viral involvement of the cortex. Other complications of the acute stage of poliomyelitis include infections of the respiratory tract and atelectasis.

Paralytic ileus with gastric atony can result from viral damage to the vegetative centers or altered serum potassium concentrations.

Diagnosis

The blood is usually normal, although leukopenia can be found in the early stages of the illness. The CSF is almost always abnormal. CSF pressure is normal but can become elevated with carbon dioxide retention. The cell count is highest in the preparalytic stage, when polymorphonuclear cells predominate. The average count of 185 cells per μL decreases to 50 cells per μL 1 week after the onset of paralysis. By then there is a predominantly monocytic response. The protein content is normal in the early stages of the illness. In the experience of Merritt and Fremont-Smith, it reached a maximum 25 days after the onset of paralysis (573). Thereafter, the protein content decreased gradually, remaining elevated long after the pleocytosis had disappeared. The sugar content is normal.

The virus is best isolated from the stool and oropharynx. Poliovirus has been isolated from the stool as early as 19 days before onset of illness and as late as 3 months after onset. The mean duration of virus excretion is approximately 5 weeks after onset of clinical illness. Poliovirus is rarely isolated from the CSF. The PCR technique performed on CSF (574), stool, blood, and throat specimens (575) is a sensitive, specific, and rapid technique for the diagnosis of enteroviral infections. It also has been used to differentiate wild poliovirus infections from vaccine strains and from other enteroviral infections (576). Serologic diagnosis is impractical but can be made by demonstrating an elevation in the specific complement fixation or neutralizing antibody titers. The etiologic diagnosis of inapparent, abortive, or nonparalytic poliomyelitis can be made only by laboratory studies.

Currently, poliomyelitis occurs rarely, and no confirmed case of wild-type polio virus infection has been reported in this country since 1991 (577). Since then, all cases encountered in the United States have been associated with vaccination (578,579). All patients who develop poliomyelitis soon after oral vaccine administration should be evaluated for humoral and cellular immunosuppression (580). In the survey of Nkowane and coworkers, 33% of cases of poliomyelitis encountered between 1973 and 1984 were seen in recipients of OPV, 48% in contacts of such recipients, and 13% in immunodeficient subjects (578). Virus reversion to the neurovirulent form involves point mutations at a single or several nucleotide positions (581).

On rare occasions, children who have been previously vaccinated with OPV present with an ascending paralysis simulating Guillain-Barré syndrome in association with a subsequent poliomyelitis type 1 infection (582,583).

Differential Diagnosis

In patients who are not immunodeficient and who have not been exposed to the vaccine, the diagnosis of poliomyelitis has become difficult. A number of other enteroviruses, notably coxsackieviruses and echoviruses, can produce a flaccid paralysis. When these conditions are unassociated with an exanthem, their diagnosis rests on PCR, viral isolation, or serologic confirmation. An illness resembling acute poliomyelitis also has been observed after infection with Epstein-Barr virus (583a), as well as with an agent of the Russian spring-summer louping ill group of viruses (584).

Poliomyelitis must be differentiated from infectious polyneuritis, whose presenting symptom is symmetric paralysis, usually progresses for more than 3 days, and is unaccompanied by fever. When sensory deficits can be documented, they confirm the diagnosis of polyneuritis. The absence of pleocytosis in the presence of a progressive paralysis also argues for polyneuritis.

A poliomyelitis-like paralysis (Hopkins syndrome) can occur during recovery from an asthma-like respiratory tract disease (585). In some instances this syndrome can result from

enterovirus or herpesvirus type I infections (586). Other conditions that mimic poliomyelitis include epidemic motor polyradiculoneuritis, insect and snake bites, schistosomiasis of the spinal cord, ingestion of chemicals such as arsenic and organic phosphates, trichinosis, and tetanus (587–589).

Prognosis

Recovery from nonparalytic forms of poliomyelitis is complete. The degree of disability that results from paralytic poliomyelitis depends on the extent of involvement. Function generally improves as pain and spasm recede after the acute phase. Overall mortality for the paralytic disease is approximately 4%. Spontaneous recovery of muscle function begins within a few weeks. Some involved neurons recover, but muscles totally paralyzed 1 month after the onset of the illness become completely normal only 1.4% of the time (590). Muscles severely paralyzed at the end of the acute period regain functional strength in 50% of cases and become normal in 20%. Moderately paralyzed muscles recover in 90% of cases. One-half the affected muscles continue to improve after 1 year. Three-fourths of functional recoveries occur in the first year, slightly less than one-fourth during the second year, and 5% during the third year. In general, prognosis is best for the proximal muscles in the lower extremities; it is poorest for the opponens pollicis and abdominal muscles (591).

Children with severe paralytic disease have developed a progressive neurologic disorder marked by increased weakness, fatigualility, and pain some 30 to 40 years after the initial infection. Several explanations for this postpolio syndrome have been proposed. Sharief and colleagues suggest that it results from a chronic progression of the infection because there is intrathecal production of detectable IgM oligoclonal bands specific for poliovirus in the CSF and elevated CSF levels of IL-2 (592). Mononuclear perivascular cuffs occur in postpolio patients dying as long as 38 years after poliomyelitis (593). Late decompensation also could result from the combination of an abnormal enlargement of the motor units, resulting from the loss of the anterior horn cells, and the increased end-plate complexity seen with aging (593,594). Another factor that could cause post-polio syndrome is chronic muscle overuse, because 40% of children with severe residual paralytic disease have elevated creatine kinase levels (594). Patients with residual leg weakness are twice as likely to report symptoms in those limbs as those with residual arm weakness (595). Sleep apnea can be a late complication of the postpolio syndrome (596). Relapses and second attacks of poliomyelitis are extremely rare. Other than a continued exercise program there is no effective treatment for this condition (596a).

Treatment

Control of poliomyelitis has been achieved by the use of orally administered live attenuated virus vaccine. Because of the vaccine-associated paralytic polio, changes in the poliovirus vaccine schedule occurred in 1997. Details of the currently advised vaccination schedules are presented in the 1997 Report of the Committee on Infectious Diseases, American Academy of Pediatrics (597).

Oral attenuated poliomyelitis vaccine should not be given to individuals with altered immunocompetence. Inactivated poliomyelitis vaccine is recommended for adults 18 years or older because of the increased risk of vaccine paralysis in that age group (578,579), and for immunization of HIV-positive children (597). For a detailed discussion of the response to vaccination, the characteristics of immunity, and the complications of vaccination, the reader is referred to Salk and Salk (598).

During the acute phase of the illness, treatment is solely symptomatic.

Coxsackievirus

An increasing number of coxsackievirus strains have been reported as causing infections of the human nervous system. The clinical pictures produced by the various strains of coxsackievirus are indistinguishable. Neurologic manifestations include aseptic meningitis, encephalitis, acute flaccid paralysis, Guillain-Barré syndrome, transverse myelitis, cerebellar ataxia, opsoclonus-myoclonus, and epidemic pleurodynia (599). These occur with both group A and B infections.

The clinical picture of aseptic meningitis caused by infection with coxsackievirus is nonspecific. The illness is preceded by a prodromal phase manifested by malaise and gastrointestinal disturbances, during which time viremia can be demonstrated. Neurologic symptoms can develop in association with pleurodynia, particularly in older children infected with B1 and B3 viruses. Exanthems are rare.

Coxsackieviruses B5, 1, 2, and 4, and A9 have been associated with the development of a clinical picture of encephalitis. The outcome is usually favorable. Serotypes A5, A9, and B2 have been associated with focal encephalitis (600).

Group A viruses also can cause acute lymphonodular pharyngitis, acute parotitis, hand-foot-and-mouth disease, polymyositis, chronic myopathies, and respiratory infections. Group B viruses have been associated with pleurodynia (Bornholm disease or epidemic pleurodynia) and diarrhea. Both types have been associated with pericarditis and myocarditis.

Anatomic alterations within the CNS are slight and nonspecific. They include meningeal inflammation and focal glial infiltration of gray and white matter of cerebrum, brainstem, and cerebellum (601).

A mild paralytic disease has been reported (602,603), as well as acute cerebellar ataxia, unilateral paralysis of the oculomotor nerve, palatal paralysis, and a postencephalitic parkinsonian picture (603,604). Focal necrotizing encephaloclastic lesions with subsequent porencephalic cyst formation also can occur.

Coxsackievirus infection is diagnosed by recovering the virus from blood or CSF, feces, and oropharyngeal swabbings, by detection of viral DNA by PCR in CSF or in brain biopsies, and by demonstrating an at least fourfold increase in neutralizing antibodies against the isolated virus.

The prognosis for recovery is usually excellent, and treatment is purely symptomatic.

Echovirus

Echoviruses are the most frequent cause of enterovirus infection of the nervous system. Sporadic infections have been described for 25 members of the group, whereas outbreaks usually occur with types 4, 6, 9, 11, 16, 18, and 30.

The clinical manifestations vary. Most common is an aseptic meningitis. All echovirus serotypes except 24, 26, 29, and 32 are associated with this entity (605). The illness is biphasic and generally self-limited. It presents a nonspecific picture of fever, headache, signs of meningeal irritation, sore throat, neck and back pain, and, occasionally, myalgia. In some cases, symptoms simulate basilar migraine (606). The illness usually resolves in 7 to 10 days. Certain viral strains can produce an illness associated with exanthematous or petechial rashes that can antecede or be associated with the period of central nervous involvement.

Although most patients have no paralytic residua, a few patients have been left with impaired strength in the anterior neck muscles. Rarely, a paralytic disease indistinguishable from poliomyelitis can occur with echovirus infections. Paralysis can be mild and transient or so severe as to be permanent or fatal. In the latter case, the virus has been isolated from CNS tissue.

Encephalitis manifested by focal or generalized seizures, disorders of sensorium, tremor, cranial nerve deficits, disorders of ocular movement, choreiform movements, paresthesias, and other signs of cerebral dysfunction have been associated with echovirus infections (607). Cerebellar ataxia of short duration (608) and acute ascending polyradiculomyelitis also have been described (609), as has muscular hypotonia in association with bilateral edema of the basal ganglia (610). Encephalitis with white matter necrosis can occur in the neonatal period (611). Persistent and fatal CNS infections with echoviruses can occur in patients with agammaglobulinemia (612). The course of these infections can be ameliorated by repeated administration of intravenous infusions of gamma-globulin, and intrathecal administration of gamma-globulin prepared for intravenous use (612,613).

The diagnosis of echovirus infection usually rests on laboratory tests. IgG echovirus antibody elevation has been demonstrated in CSF of individuals with and without meningeal involvement. Because antibody titers to other viruses also are elevated, IgG echovirus antibody elevation reflects a nonspecific transport of IgG-associated viral antibodies from the serum to the CSF, or reflects endogenous production of multiple antibodies within the CNS (614). PCR of CSF and a four-fold rise of specific antibodies confirm the etiologic agent.

Newer Enteroviruses

Four new enteroviruses (serotypes 68 through 71) have been recognized. These viruses can cause sporadic or epidemic infections of hand-foot-and-mouth disease, and they have been recognized throughout the world. Serotypes 70 and 71 have been associated with CNS infections such as aseptic meningitis, encephalitis, and encephalomyelitis. Serotype 71 is responsible for more serious CNS disease, leading to acute paralytic manifestations indistinguishable from poliomyelitis and fatal encephalomyelitis (539a,539b,615).

The diagnosis is based on the virus isolation from skin vesicles, CSF, and brain tissue, using a monoclonal fluorescent antibody technique. At present no specific serologic diagnosis exists. Treatment of these infections is supportive.

Reovirus

Reovirus type 1 can cause meningitis in young infants (616).

Adenoviruses

Adenovirus infections usually cause an acute respiratory disease associated with conjunctivitis or keratoconjunctivitis. In a small percentage of cases, these symptoms are associated with involvement of the nervous system, notably a severe encephalitis or meningoencephalitis (617,618). Neonatal infections usually are generalized. In fatal cases with neonatal encephalitis the CSF has been reported to be normal (619).

The diagnosis of these infections can be made through the isolation of the virus from the CSF or brain. A four-fold rise in adenoviral antibodies can provide a retrospective diagnosis. The prognosis of the CNS manifestations of adenoviruses is difficult to ascertain, because of the few reported cases. No specific treatment for these infections is available.

Human Herpesvirus Types 6 and 7

Exanthem Subitum (Roseola Infantum)

Roseola, the most common exanthem of infancy, is characterized by the relative absence of prodromal symptoms, a rapid increase in body temperature, and conspicuously little listlessness or irritability. The temperature remains elevated for 3 to 5 days and subsides with the appearance of maculopapular rash. A bulging fontanel, the result of increased intracranial pressure, occurs during the second to fifth day of fever in about one-third of children (620). The condition occurs at a median age of 9 months when caused by human herpesvirus-6 (HHV-6), and at a median age of 26 months when caused by human herpesvirus-7 (HHV-7) (621). Other viral agents also are believed to be responsible for this condition (622).

CNS involvement can occur from 1 day before the onset of fever to day 2 of the illness (620). Neurologic complications include aseptic meningitis, acute disseminated encephalomyelitis (623,624), and acute encephalitis (625).

The incidence of seizures varies considerably from one series of cases to the next (626). In the prospective study of Hall and coworkers, HHV-6 infection accounted for one-third of all febrile seizures under the age of two years (626a). Persistent neurologic complications and death have been reported. The former include hemiparesis, recurrent seizures, and mental retardation. The cause of the residual encephalopathy is unknown (623).

HHV-6 DNA has been detected in the CSF of children who had three or more febrile seizures. This observation suggests that in some instances recurrence of febrile convulsions is associated with reactivation of the virus (626a,627).

Approximately one-fifth of children have CSF with either a pleocytosis of more than 5 white blood cells per μL or a protein more than 45 mg/dL; CSF glucose is normal. Approximately one-fourth of children have encephalopathy or encephalitis; all of these have an abnormal EEG. Transient periodic complexes can occur over the temporal lobes similar to those described for herpes simplex virus encephalitis (623). Unilateral or bilateral CT changes usually begin as hypodense areas that can progress to irregular cerebral atrophy or become hemorrhagic (623).

The association of HHV-6 with the neurologic complications is suggested by the concomitant isolation of virus, the identification of DNA by PCR in the CSF (628), and by the fourfold increase in specific neutralizing antibodies.

HHV-7 has been associated with febrile seizures, a severe encephalopathy, and in two instances with acute hemiplegia by the isolation of HHV-7 through viral culture and PCR (628a,629). The diagnosis of HHV-7 is based on the methods described for HHV-6.

Many strains of HHV-6 are sensitive *in vitro* to ganciclovir and foscarnet (630). Doses of 10 mg/kg per day in two divided doses of ganciclovir, or 180 mg/kg per day in three divided doses of foscarnet can be given in cases of serious CNS infections caused by HHV-6.

Arboviruses

Arthropod-borne (arbo) viruses are RNA viral agents transmitted between susceptible vertebrate hosts by means of blood-sucking arthropods (631). Approximately 200 viruses have been tentatively classified into this group, and approximately 150 of these have been assigned to 21 groups that share common antigens. At least 51 have been associated with human disease. The epidemiology of these infections is largely determined by the nature and lifestyle of the vector. Most of the infections are sustained in sylvan hosts, with transmission through humans and domestic animals being usually incidental and insignificant in the natural history of the virus. Of greatest significance in the United States are the La Crosse (LAC) strain of the California encephalitis group, St. Louis encephalitis (SLE), western equine encephalitis (WEE), eastern equine encephalitis (EEE), Venezuelan equine encephalitis (VEE), Colorado tick fever, and Powassan encephalitis. In this section we also include Dengue virus and Japanese encephalitis virus.

In humans, these viruses can be asymptomatic or can produce a mild generalized illness. The full-blown diseases, which are discussed in this section, are the least common manifestations of infection.

The nonspecificity of symptoms necessitates diagnosis by means of laboratory studies. Viral-specific IgM antibodies appear in serum in the first week of illness, and serologic tests on paired samples, taken several weeks apart, can suggest a recent infection (632). The detection of virus-specific IgM in the CSF is diagnostic. Virus can be isolated from blood or from nervous tissue by means of biopsies or autopsies.

La Crosse Encephalitis

LAC, a member of the California serogroup of Bunyavirus, is the most commonly reported cause of mosquito-borne disease in the United States (633). This disease, originally encountered most frequently in midwestern states, also has become endemic in the mid-Atlantic region. *Aedes triseriatus*, the principal mosquito vector, transmits the virus during the summer and early fall. Tree holes that contain water as well as discarded automobile tires that hold rainwater serve as the breeding habitat for the mosquito.

In 99% of instances LAC virus infection is asymptomatic. The symptomatic disease can be mild or severe (634).

Pathology

The alterations within the brain are largely microscopic. They are those of an acute encephalitis without distinctive findings (634).

Clinical Manifestations

The peak incidence of LAC is between July and October. There is a strong association between rural outdoor exposure and the presence of antibodies and clinical illness; the incidence of antibodies is 26.8% in rural populations and 15.3% in urban areas. Significant increases in antibody titer occur between ages 5 and 9 years among rural populations and between ages 10 and 19 years among urban populations living in endemic areas (635). Male subjects are affected three times as often as female subjects.

The clinical picture is that of a meningoencephalitis with fever, changes in consciousness, headache, and meningeal irritation (634,636,637). Balfour and associates define two clinical patterns (638). A mild form begins with a 2- to 3-day prodromal stage characterized by fever, headache, malaise, and gastrointestinal symptoms. An increase in temperature on approximately the third day is associated with lethargy and evidence of meningeal irritation. Symptoms abate over 7 or 8 days without overt neurologic residua.

The severe form begins abruptly with fever and headache, followed in 12 to 24 hours by sudden onset of focal or generalized seizures. These have been reported in 40% to 50% of patients with neurologic symptoms (638).

The CSF shows pleocytosis, which in 85% of cases is mainly mononuclear. The protein content is mildly elevated in 20% of the patients and the glucose content is normal. Presence of the SIADH is common. The EEG is always abnormal, with abnormalities persisting for months or years in 55% of cases (639).

Diagnosis

In contrast to infections caused by enteroviruses, LAC is not biphasic and is not obviously associated with upper respiratory signs or symptoms. Familial outbreaks are extremely rare. EEG and neuroimaging demonstrate a focal process in 15% to 40% of subjects (638). Such focal involvement also is observed in herpes simplex encephalitis; in both conditions, the CSF can be hemorrhagic. Specific IgM and IgG serologies in CSF and serum confirm the viral etiology. A fourfold increase in these antibodies provides a retrospective diagnosis. If a brain biopsy is performed, infected brain cells can be detected by a monoclonal antibody technique (640).

Prognosis

LAC is a relatively mild illness with a case fatality rate in symptomatic cases of less than 1% (633). Permanent neurologic residua are uncommon, but patients can have a variety of neurologic and behavioral residua (637,641). Older children and adolescents tend to show emotional lability, difficulty in learning, and personality problems. Later, difficulties in processing visual and auditory information become apparent, and some children develop behavior that resembles the organic hyperkinetic syndrome (642). However, a controlled assessment of 29 children who recovered from encephalitis failed to demonstrate significant personality changes when compared with the premorbid state (642).

Treatment

The treatment of neurologic manifestations of LAC has changed over the past few years. Ribavirin, which is active *in vitro* against LAC (643,644), was given for 10 days to a child for a severe, biopsy-proven case of LAC encephalitis, with a good outcome (643). Future studies will determine the need for its routine use.

St. Louis Encephalitis

SLE was first recognized in St. Louis in the summer of 1932 during an epidemic of encephalitis that originated in Paris, Illinois. Since then, sporadic outbreaks have occurred in the St. Louis area, California, the Rio Grande valley, Florida, and the central river valleys and western coastal regions of the United States. The vector for this virus is the *Culex* mosquito, and the virus has been isolated from overwintering mosquitoes (645,646).

Pathology

Diffuse vascular congestion and edema occur with meningeal and perivascular infiltration, petechiae, and glial nodules. Lesions predominate in the thalamus and substantia nigra. The cortex, anterior horns of the spinal cord, molecular and Purkinje cell layers, and dentate nucleus of the cerebellum also are involved (647).

Clinical Manifestations

Most commonly, this virus produces a clinically inapparent infection, and the ratio of asymptomatic to symptomatic cases has ranged from 19:1 to 427:1 in various outbreaks (648). Most cases occur in late summer and early fall; boys are affected three times more often than girls in some epidemics. Generally, the severity of the encephalitis and the extent of residua are greater in the higher age groups (649).

The clinical manifestations of SLE range from a nonspecific flulike illness to fatal cases of encephalitis. In the 1964 Houston epidemic, most children had fever, headache, and meningeal irritation. Ataxia was noted in 27%, and fine tremors of the upper extremity in 19%. Cranial nerve palsies were encountered in 12% (648). Occasionally, the virus is responsible for transient parkinsonism (649a), the syndrome of opsoclonus and myoclonus (650), and for acute cerebellar ataxia (651). The latter two conditions are covered in Chapter 7.

Abnormalities in the CSF are those expected for a viral encephalitis, namely pleocytosis, which initially is predominantly polymorphonuclear, but later becomes mononuclear, a mild elevation of protein levels, and a normal sugar content (652). The EEG is often abnormal. Electromyographic studies have shown fasciculations in 59% of cases, fibrillations in 8%, and excessive insertional potentials in 54%. In some cases, these abnormalities have persisted for more than 1 month (648). The diagnosis is confirmed by specific IgM serology in the CSF or blood. When obtained within 4 days of the clinical onset of the disease, the serology has been positive in 75% of cases. Fourfold increases in specific IgG antibodies in blood can provide a retrospective diagnosis. Viral isolation should be pursued when a brain biopsy or autopsy is obtained.

Prognosis

SLE is intermediate in severity between California encephalitis and the equine encephalitides. The mortality in the 1964 St. Louis epidemic was 8% in children younger than 10 years of age. In more recent epidemics, it has ranged from 0% to 22%. Major sequelae occur less frequently than after EEE or WEE, but have been observed in 7.7% to 10.0% of survivors. Most commonly, they involve disturbances of gait and equilibrium, difficulties in speech and vision, and changes in personality

(652,653). Children and young adults are much less prone to long-term motor disability than older adults (652).

Treatment

Treatment is symptomatic and supportive. No specific antiviral therapy or vaccines are available.

Western Equine Encephalitis

WEE is caused by a group A arbovirus from the family Togaviridae. It occurs in the western United States and in the central states west of the Mississippi Valley. The virus was first isolated in 1930 in California from horses with encephalitis. The chief vectors are several *culex* mosquitoes, notably *Culex tarsalis* in the United States. The enzoonotic cycle is kept between mosquitoes, birds, and other vertebrate hosts. Horses and humans become dead-end hosts.

Pathology

The alterations within the nervous system in WEE are similar to those seen in the other encephalitides caused by arboviruses. The greatest damage is usually in the basal ganglia and cerebral white matter, with foci of demyelination and necrosis. The subcortical white matter is more extensively damaged than the cortex in the majority of fatal cases (654). White matter subjacent to cortex is more involved than deeper white matter in some children. Striking involvement of the substantia nigra might explain the relatively frequent appearance of parkinsonism as a late sequel of WEE (655,656). Extensive cystic degeneration of white matter can occur in infants.

A striking finding, noted as late as 5 years after onset of the acute illness, is the presence of both chronic inactive areas of destruction and active foci of glial proliferation and perivascular cuffing. This finding suggests that a slow progressive form of the disease can continue for years (657).

Chronic cases can have a significant endothelial proliferation with a vasculitis producing almost complete occlusion of small vessels. Scattered areas of focal necrosis often contain phagocytic elements. In some cases, extensive cavities replace brain tissue (653,658).

Clinical Manifestations

Clinically inapparent infections far outnumber overt infections, although infants younger than 1 year of age have an equal incidence of apparent and inapparent infections (659).

In infants younger than 1 year of age, one common clinical picture is that of a sudden onset of high fever, seen in 92% of patients, accompanied by focal or generalized seizures, seen in 77% of patients (660). Older children have a severe encephalitis with fever, headache, vomiting, changes in consciousness, and meningeal signs. Convulsions develop in approximately 50% of children aged 1 to 4 years, and in 9% of children aged 5 to 14 years.

Symptoms usually persist for approximately 10 days, then gradually subside. In fatal cases, the course is rapidly progressive. The CSF findings resemble those encountered in the other arbovirus infections (660).

The mortality in different epidemics has ranged from 9% to 23%. Sequelae are frequent and are most severe in very young infants; 56% of infants who contracted the illness when they were younger than 1 month of age had major sequelae (653). These include microcephaly, pyramidal or extrapyramidal motor impairment, seizures, and developmental retardation (657). Follow-up studies conducted on survivors reveal that the younger the patient is at the time of illness, the greater are the incidence and severity of sequelae (657,658). In older infants and in children, the sequelae are less severe. In Finley's series, no patient contracting the illness between ages 1 and 2 years developed motor or behavior problems; 25%, however, developed seizures (657). Such seizures represent persistence of convulsions that first appeared during the acute illness.

The diagnosis is based on the detection of specific IgM and IgG in CSF and blood. The virus can be isolated rarely from blood or CSF. When brain tissue is obtained, the virus can be easily cultured.

No vaccine or specific treatment is available.

Eastern Equine Encephalitis

EEE is a group A arbovirus from the family Togaviridae first isolated in 1933 from brain tissue of infected horses. It is distributed along the Atlantic coast from the northeastern United States to Argentina. Small epidemics have been encountered in Massachusetts, New Jersey, Florida, Texas, and, more recently, Jamaica. The virus is transmitted by a variety of mosquitoes, *Culiseta melanura* being the most common in the United States. Birds are the amplifying host and horses and humans dead-end hosts (632).

Pathology

The outstanding feature of EEE is the predominance of neutrophilic leukocytes in the infiltrates, which undoubtedly reflects the rapid demise of most fatally infected patients. Focal or diffuse accumulations of neutrophils and histiocytes are prominent in the leptomeninges and in the cerebral cortex, particularly the occipital and frontal lobes and hippocampus (661).

Foci of tissue damage with rarefaction necrosis permeated by neutrophilic leukocytes and pleomorphic ameboid cells are often found. Neuronolysis, often with adjacent neutrophilic leukocytes and microglial cells, is common in fulminant cases. Large perivascular collections of neutrophils, histiocytes, and other ameboid cells are detected in the white matter in regions of cortical involvement. Other sites of predilection are the basal ganglia and brainstem. Edema and congestion are prevalent early. Vascular lesions characterized by numerous small thrombi in arterioles and venules can occur. Many vessels show complete involvement of their walls with neutrophilic infiltration and fibrin deposition. As the disease progresses, the dominant cell type changes to mononuclear lymphocytes and macrophages (653,661).

Clinical Manifestations

Infected children have a subclinical to clinical ratio of 2:1 to 8:1; adults have a ratio of 4:1 to 50:1 (662). For this reason, EEE is particularly common in infants, with two-thirds of the clinical cases being younger than 2 years old. It is usually fulminant with an abrupt onset, high fever, stupor or coma, convulsions, and signs of meningeal irritation. Patients can die within 48 hours of their initial symptoms or can survive for a few days, dying from damage of the vital medullary centers, dural sinus thrombosis, or subarachnoid hemorrhage. Survivors can remain comatose for several days or weeks before becoming responsive.

Laboratory studies are not diagnostic. The peripheral blood can show a prominent leukocytosis. The increase in CSF pressure can be striking. Initial CSF cell counts range between 250 and 2,000 white blood cells per µL, often containing almost 100% polymorphonuclear cells. The pleocytosis diminishes rapidly, and mononuclear cells predominate after 3 days in surviving patients (661). The EEG almost invariably shows generalized slowing and disorganization of the background activities, with the occasional patient demonstrating epileptiform discharges. The confirmation of the diagnosis is obtained through specific serology in CSF (IgM), a fourfold increase in the titer of serum antibodies, and/or the isolation of EEE virus from CSF or brain tissue (663).

Neuroimaging study results can be normal, show diffuse edema, or a variety of focal lesions. In the review by Deresiewicz and coworkers, abnormal findings include focal lesions in the basal ganglia, thalami, and brainstem. Cortical lesions, meningeal enhancement, and periventricular white matter changes were less common. The presence of large radiographic lesions did not predict a poor outcome (663).

Prognosis

Infection with the virus of EEE has the most serious prognosis of all virus infections prevalent in the United States. The mortality in EEE in patients younger than 10 years is approximately 60% (662). The case fatality rate for all patients reported to the Centers for Disease Control and

Prevention between 1988 and 1994 was 36%, with 35% of surviving patients showing moderate to severe sequelae. These include mental retardation, motor dysfunction, deafness, and seizures. Complete neurologic recovery is seen in only a small proportion of survivors. A high CSF white count, or severe hyponatremia were predictive of a poor outcome (663).

Venezuelan Equine Encephalomyelitis

Although VEE, a group A arbovirus, is indigenous to Colombia, Venezuela, and Panama, it was responsible for the 1971 Texas encephalitis epidemic. The organism was also responsible for an outbreak of encephalitis in 1995 in Colombia and Venezuela that involved 75,000 to 100,000 cases (664). The organism has been isolated from many wild rodents, as well as from *Aedes* and *Culex* mosquitoes (665).

VEE is much more benign than California (La Crosse) encephalitis, SLE, EEE, and WEE. It is marked by sudden onset of malaise, chills and fever, nausea and vomiting, headache, myalgia, and bone pain. The fever lasts from 24 to 96 hours, then abruptly drops. A period of 2 to 3 weeks of marked asthenia can follow. In contrast to other arboviruses, whose ratios of inapparent to apparent infections range from 23:1 to 500:1, in VEE a ratio of 11:1 has been reported.

The CSF findings are as in the other arbovirus infections. Virus can be isolated from serum during the first 3 days of the illness in 75% of confirmed cases (665).

PCR provides a fast, sensitive, and specific method for the detection of viral DNA in infected blood. The detection of specific IgM in CSF and serum, and the observation of a fourfold increase in specific IgG in serum provide serologic confirmation of the disease.

Prognosis is good and, with good care, fatalities are rare.

Japanese Encephalitis

Japanese encephalitis virus is transmitted by culicine mosquitoes between birds and humans.

Histologic changes are most marked in the thalamus and brainstem. Patients who die rapidly can have no histologic signs of inflammation, yet have immunohistochemical evidence of viral antigen in morphologically normal neurons. Clinical features of this condition are much like those of the other encephalitides (666,667). Fever, headache, and vomiting are followed by meningism and coma. Convulsions have been reported in 85% of children. A characteristic masklike facies with a vacant stare, or grimacing or lip-smacking can occur, as can a paralytic disease that mimics acute poliomyelitis. Pyramidal tract signs, a rare complication in poliomyelitis, should suggest the diagnosis of Japanese encephalitis in endemic areas (668,669). In the 1986 Nepal epidemic, children accounted for the majority of all hospitalized cases. The fatality rate in children was markedly less than that in adults (670). In the Indian epidemic studied by Kumar and colleagues, of children with proven Japanese encephalitis, the case fatality rate was 32%; major sequelae occurred in 45%; only 29% were healthy on follow-up (671). Sequelae of the disease were more severe when the initial illness was prolonged or was associated with focal neurologic deficits. A tumor necrosis factor (TNF) concentration over 50 pg/mL in serum correlated significantly with a fatal outcome, whereas high levels of Japanese encephalitis virus–IgM antibodies (more than 500 units) in the CSF were associated with a nonfatal outcome (671a).

The MRI in Japanese encephalitis patients shows lesions in the thalamus, cortex, midbrain, cerebellum, and spinal cord. Classically, the lesions are hyperintense in T2-weighted images and hypodense in T1-weighted images (671b). In some 70% of cases these are hemorrhagic. According to Kumar and coworkers bilateral thalamic involvement, especially hemorrhagic, can be considered to be characteristic of Japanese encephalitis in endemic areas (671c).

A specific diagnosis can be made by detecting a fourfold increase in specific IgG antibodies in acute and convalescent sera, and by measuring Japanese encephalitis virus IgM in serum and CSF by ELISA. IgM can be

TABLE 6.17. *Distribution of neurotropic arboviruses*

Name	Distribution	Vector	Reference
Japanese	Eastern Siberia, China, Korea, Taiwan	Mosquito	653,1365,1366
Toscana virus	Tuscany, Italy	Sandfly	1363
Murray Valley encephalitis	Eastern Australia, Northern Territory, New Guinea	Mosquito	1364,1367,1368
Tick-borne encephalitides			
European	Europe	Tick *(Ixodes ricinus)*	653,1369
Far Eastern (Russian spring-summer encephalitis)	Siberia, Far East	Tick *(Ixodes persulcatus)*	1370
Kyasanur Forest disease	India	Tick	1371
Powassan virus	Ontario, Canada	Tick	1372
Colorado tick fever	Western United States	Wood tick	653,1373,1374
Kumlinge disease		Tick	1375
Louping III	Scotland	Tick *(Ixodes ricinus)*	1369,1376,1377

detected 1 week after the onset of clinical symptoms. Virus isolation can be performed but needs to be done during the first 7 days of the disease prior to the mounting of an immune response.

No effective treatment exists, and high-dose dexamethasone treatment has been of no benefit. Interferon-α has been used in a small number of patients and bigger trials are being awaited to assess its efficacy. A Japanese encephalitis vaccine is now available in the United States (632).

Powassan Encephalitis

Powassan encephalitis is a virus within the tick-borne flaviviruses. In North America it is transmitted by ticks to small mammals. Human infections are related to outdoor activities and tick bites. Canada and the northeastern, north central, and western United States are the geographic areas of distribution of this disease.

The incubation period ranges from 4 to 21 days, after which, fevers, headache, lethargy, vomiting, and photophobia appear as early signs, followed by an increase in the intracranial pressure reflected by alterations of the consciousness, seizures, and motor impairment. The disease tends to be similar to the CNS disease caused by the mosquito-borne viral meningoencephalitis. Mortality approximates 1%, and sequelae such as

hemiplegia, quadriplegia, aphasia, and chronic convulsive disorders have been reported.

The diagnosis is based on the detection of specific IgM antibodies in serum, CSF, or both. Powassan encephalitis can be isolated from brain tissue in biopsies and autopsies. No specific therapy for Powassan encephalitis is available.

Dengue Fever

Dengue is unique among flaviviruses in that humans are the most important natural host, and infections are frequently symptomatic. *Aedes aegypti* mosquitoes are the most common vectors. Neurologic complications referred to as dengue encephalopathy can occur secondary to the two forms of the disease, dengue hemorrhagic fever or an acute febrile illness with facial flushing, headache, arthralgia, myalgia, retro-orbital pain, petechiae, and a fine maculopapular rash. Dengue fever is caused by four distinct viral species. Immunity to a heterologous dengue serotype predisposes to Dengue hemorrhagic fever (672). In most cases neurologic manifestations are thought to be manifestations secondary to severe disease. Intracranial hemorrhages and cerebral edema can occur. A Reye-like metabolic encephalopathy secondary to hepatic failure can occur. Occasionally there can be, direct invasion of the CNS. Lethargy, confusion, convulsions, and coma are the most common clinical features, but meningism, paresis, and cranial nerve palsies can occur (672a). CSF can be normal or show mild pleocytosis (672a).

Other Arboviruses

The distribution of encephalitides caused by other arboviruses is summarized in Table 6.17.

Rift Valley Fever

Rift Valley fever is caused by a virus of the phlebotomus fever serogroup. It has an ever widening distribution in Africa and is capable of widespread epizootics and epidemics such as the Egyptian outbreak of 1977, which had an estimated morbidity of 200,000 and a mortality of 600. The disease is characterized by sudden onset of fever, occasionally with one early recurrence (saddleback fever), severe myalgia, especially in the lower back, headache, retro-orbital pain, conjunctival suffusion, vomiting, and anorexia. The disease usually lasts 4 to 7 days.

Three forms of complications occur. Retinal complications can develop 7 to 20 days after the onset of other symptoms, with decrease in visual acuity that can result in permanent loss of central vision in the more severe cases owing to edema, exudates, hemorrhage, and vasculitis. Meningoencephalitis can occur during convalescence from a febrile illness lasting 5 to 10 days, often beginning with hallucinations, disorientation, and vertigo. Residual neurologic deficits can occur, but fatalities are infrequent. Hemorrhagic Rift Valley fever with jaundice and hemorrhagic phenomena can develop in 2 to 4 days. This is the chief cause of mortality; in 3 to 6 days, the patient either dies or begins a slow convalescence (673).

Mumps

Mumps virus was the most common cause of CNS involvement by any of the contagious diseases of childhood before the widespread use of mumps immunization. It is now much less common in countries with effective vaccination programs. It remains a frequent complication in nonimmunized populations and vaccine failures can occur. The most common complication of mumps is an aseptic meningitis syndrome; meningoencephalitis is a much rarer manifestation. Mumps virus involvement of the nervous system can occur with or without signs of clinical parotitis. The incidence of neurologic involvement is difficult to estimate, but CFS pleocytosis has been demonstrated in 56% of patients with parotitis. Meningoencephalitis is far less common, developing in 0.2% of cases (674). In approximately one-third of children, CNS symptoms occur in the absence of clinical parotitis, although subclinical parotitis usually can be documented by elevations in serum amylase. More commonly CNS symptoms accompany the swelling or develop from 8 days before to 20 days after the appearance of clinical parotitis (675). Male subjects are three or four times more likely to have neurologic symptoms than female subjects. Signs of meningeal irritation may or may not be present; headache, nausea, and vomiting are associated with the benign leptomeningeal form of the disease. In this entity recovery is complete.

Mumps meningoencephalitis is a far more serious condition. Signs and symptoms in order of observed frequency include fever, vomiting, nuchal rigidity, lethargy, headache, convulsions, and delirium. Vertigo, ataxia, facial nerve palsy, and optic atrophy also have been reported (676,677). Sequelae are relatively common. They were seen in 25% of survivors in the Finnish series of Koskiniemi and coworkers (678) and were most common when children presented with seizures or altered consciousness. Interestingly, the prognosis was worse in those patients without salivary gland swelling. Behavioral disturbances and persistent headache are the most common sequelae. Other residua include ataxia, extrapyramidal disorders, optic neuritis and atrophy, facial palsy, impairment of extraocular muscles, neurogenic deafness, and a seizure disorder (679,680). Hydrocephalus related to ependymal changes in the aqueduct of Sylvius is a rare sequela (680).

Facial nerve paralysis can be caused by swollen parotid gland compression of the nerve or by cranial neuritis. Labyrinthine and vestibular nerve involvement can result in neurogenic vertigo. Transverse myelitis can occur. In rare instances, there is chronic progressive encephalitis (681).

Mumps infection also can result in muscle weakness, which is most marked in the neck flexors and becomes evident at the end of the acute phase. Muscle weakness can persist for as long as 5 months.

The CSF usually shows an early granulocytic pleocytosis that soon has a lymphocytic predominance and an elevated protein count. Hypoglycorrhachia is present in approximately 10% of cases (677,678,682). Serum amylase is elevated in patients with clinical as well as many with subclinical parotitis. After mumps meningitis, CSF pleocytosis may persist for months, and mumps virus-specific oligoclonal IgG can persist for more than a year (683). Rapid direct diagnosis of mumps meningitis is possible by demonstration of mumps virus antigen in CSF (684).

MRI is more reliable than CT in confirming involvement of the brain parenchyma in mumps encephalitis (685). The reactions to measles, mumps, and rubella immunization are described in Chapter 7.

Herpes Simplex

Herpes simplex viruses are widespread organisms that commonly infect humans. They produce a protean picture that only rarely results in neurologic manifestations. Prenatal herpes infection is referred to in the section on Congenital Infections of the Nervous System in this chapter.

Etiology

Herpes simplex viruses are a member of the herpesvirus family, whose genomes consist of a single double-stranded DNA molecule. They occur in two distinct serotypes that are distinguishable by serologic and cultural means (686,687). Individual strains can be characterized by restrictive endonucleases so that epidemiologic studies can identify sources of contact. Type 1 virus, generally associated with orofacial herpes infections, is identified in most cases of herpes simplex encephalitis in patients 6 months of age or older. Type 2 virus is identified in genital herpes and causes most of the congenital or perinatally acquired infections (688).

Pathology

Experimental virus invasion of the nervous system has been demonstrated after intranasal inocu-

lation. The virus spreads by infection of mucosal and submucosal cells, ultimately crossing the cribriform plate, or by infection of endoneural and perineural cells of the olfactory fibers to involve the parenchymal cells of the olfactory bulb (689). The first neurons to be infected are usually constituents of the peripheral nervous system. Viral infection then spreads by continuity to other neurons through synaptic contact. For an extensive review of the biology of the herpes viruses in infections of the nervous system, see the review by Enquist and co-authors (689a).

CNS infection by herpes simplex virus shows the usual microscopic picture of viral encephalitis: lymphocytic infiltration of the meninges, perivascular aggregates of lymphocytes and histiocytes in the cortex and subjacent white matter, and proliferation of microglia with formation of glial nodules.

Several pathologic features are distinctive, however. One feature is the severity of the process. Necrosis is unusually severe in the areas of greatest involvement, with gross softening, destruction of architecture, hemorrhage, and in severe cases, loss of all nervous and glial elements. Another feature is the topography of lesions. Lesions are generally widespread with many foci of hemorrhage and necrosis, but the mediotemporal and orbital regions are the most severely damaged. A final feature is inclusion bodies. Intranuclear Cowdry type A inclusion bodies are recognized in neurons, oligodendroglia, and astrocytes (690).

Persistence of herpesvirus type 1 in trigeminal ganglia (691) and type 2 in sacral ganglia (692) leads to recurrent cutaneous or mucosal infections by means of axonal spread. Latent herpes virus type 1 infection of the trigeminal ganglia occurs in 18% of individuals newborn to 20 years of age (693).

Clinical Manifestations

Encephalitis can occur as part of a systemic herpes infection or as an isolated phenomenon. It can develop from a primary infection or from reactivation of a preexisting infection (694). Encephalitis also has developed after long-term corticosteroid therapy, and experimentally after injection of adrenaline or induction of anaphylactic shock (695).

Cases of neonatal herpes meningoencephalitis caused by type 2 generally are associated with disseminated herpes infection. When the infection is contracted during the perinatal period, an event usually associated with primary infection of the mother, symptoms can begin as early as the first few days of life (696).

In another group of type 2 infections, infants become symptomatic at 4 months of age or later in association with serologic evidence of probable reinfection or reactivation. When first seen, these infants' IgG antibody to herpes simplex virus is already elevated, suggesting maternal transfer of considerable antibody or a prior infection.

Specific IgM and IgG responses occur in serum and CSF during the acute disease. Localization of the type 2 infection tends to be frontoparietal rather than temporal, as occurs in type 1 infection. The association of type 2 virus with diffuse meningoencephalitis rather than with a hemorrhagic or necrotizing focal disease can reflect in part its greater incidence in young infants (697).

The incidence of CNS involvement in herpes simplex infections is uncertain, but the virus probably accounts for approximately 10% of all viral infections of the CNS and herpes simplex virus is the most common cause of sporadic, fatal meningoencephalitis in the United States. Of all herpes cases, 31% occur in patients younger than 20 years of age, and 12% occur in patients between 6 months and 10 years of age (698). In general, the incidence of herpes is lowest between the ages of 5 and 15 years (699). Herpes encephalitis has no clear seasonal incidence (698).

Prodromal symptoms unrelated to CNS disease occur in approximately 60% of patients. Fever and malaise are most common; symptoms of respiratory infection are present in one-third of patients. This prodromal period usually lasts 1 to 7 days.

Neurologic involvement includes aseptic meningitis and a diffuse or focal encephalitis (699). Aseptic meningitis is relatively benign and is encountered in approximately 20% of cases. Patients experience an acute febrile illness with headache and stiff neck, occasionally with orchitis or pneumonitis, and recover uneventfully in 4 to 7 days. CSF pleocytosis is common, ranging from 300 to 1,000 cells with a protein concentration from 50 to approximately 200 mg/dL. In

12% of cases, the initial CSF examination is normal (700). Though the condition is asymptomatic, CSF changes can persist for months.

More often, herpes is associated with encephalitis. The clinical findings are of two kinds: nonspecific changes of encephalitis, including fever, papilledema, meningeal irritation, and global confusion; and changes referable to focal necrosis, usually of the orbital or temporal regions of the brain, including anosmia, memory loss, disordered behavior, and olfactory or gustatory hallucinations (690). Only 22% of patients have a history of recurrent herpes simplex lesions (698).

Focal symptoms and neurologic findings are not unusual. They include focal seizures, seen in 28% of patients, and hemiparesis, seen in 33%. In the series of Whitley and associates, ataxia was seen in 40% of patients, cranial nerve deficits in 32%, papilledema in 14%, and visual field loss in 14% (698).

Initial signs of herpes encephalitis are frequently referable to the CNS. The most common early symptoms are alterations in consciousness (97%), fever (90%), headache (81%), personality change (71%), generalized, but often partial, motor seizures (67%), vomiting (46%), and hemiparesis (33%). The most common neurologic findings include changes in personality (85%), dysphasia (76%), autonomic dysfunction (60%), ataxia (40%), hemiparesis (38%), seizures (38%, of which 74% were focal, 26% generalized, and 13% mixed), cranial nerve defects (32%), papilledema (14%), and visual field loss (14%). Essentially, similar histories and neurologic findings were obtained from a group of patients who did not have biopsy evidence of herpes simplex encephalitis and no signs are pathognomonic for herpes simplex encephalitis (698).

Herpes simplex encephalitis can occasionally present as apyrexial, with focal seizures and normal neuroimaging studies. Less commonly, it can present as an opercular syndrome with anarthria and impairment of mastication and swallowing. This is caused by focal, bilateral cortical involvement of the anterior opercular regions (701). In other cases, expressive aphasia or paresthesias precede the more severe CNS signs.

The mortality from herpes simplex encephalitis is still considerable, and approximately one-half of the survivors aged 5 to 11 have major residual deficits (694). These include severe disturbances in mental function, either diffuse cerebral damage or isolated damage to memory or speech areas. Selective cognitive deficits, mental retardation, personality changes, incoordination, hyperkinetic movement disorders, seizures, or hemiparesis also can persist (702).

Diagnosis

The clinical picture of herpes encephalitis or herpes aseptic meningitis can be indistinguishable from that produced by other viral organisms. However, localizing signs, mostly focal seizures and paralyses, are found in approximately three-fourths of patients. When present, focal temporal lobe or limbic symptoms suggest the diagnosis, as can the presence of a bloody or xanthochromic CSF. A history of preceding herpetic infection or the presence of mucocutaneous herpes is present in fewer than 50% of patients. In neonates, the differential diagnosis is principally between group B streptococcal meningitis and enteroviral meningoencephalitis.

The CSF can be normal in the first hours of encephalitis, but virtually all patients develop CSF abnormalities. The CSF is under increased pressure and shows pleocytosis. In 92% of cases, the cell count is less than 500 cells per μL, in 22% of cases there are less than 50 cells per μL. The CSF protein elevation can persist for months. In other cases, a hemorrhagic encephalitis produces a xanthochromic or bloody CSF, usually with less than 500 red cells per μL. Infants younger than 1 month of age tend to have a mild hypoglycorrhachia (703).

The EEG is of considerable diagnostic aid. The result is usually diffusely abnormal, although in some patients it demonstrates a focal temporal or frontal lesion, or focal centrotemporal spike complexes, recurring every 1 to 2 seconds against a slow-wave background (704,705). A burst-suppression pattern is considered to be characteristic for this condition. Neuroimaging studies also are of considerable diagnostic assistance. The MRI can demonstrate unilateral or bilateral inflammation of the temporal lobe on T2-weighted images (Fig. 6.10).

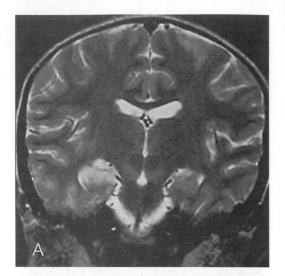

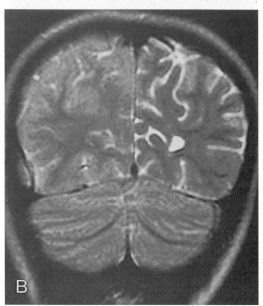

FIG. 6.10. Herpes simplex encephalitis in an 8-year-old child. Coronal T2-weighted magnetic resonance images. **A:** Focal involvement of right hippocampus and inferior temporal region. **B:** Focal involvement of right parieto-occipital region. (Courtesy of Dr. Philip Anslow, Department of Radiology, Radcliffe Infirmary, Oxford, United Kingdom.)

These abnormalities can be seen in the presence of a normal CSF (706,707). They also are noted before any detectable abnormality on CT scan, which does not become evident until the third to the eleventh day of illness (707).

Rapid diagnosis of herpesvirus encephalitis can best be achieved by demonstration of viral DNA in the CSF by PCR (708). This test has largely replaced brain biopsy as the major diagnostic procedure. When DNA primers with sequences common to herpes simplex viruses 1 and 2 have been used, a sensitivity greater than 95% and specificity of 100% has been reported in patients with brain biopsy proven herpes simplex encephalitis (708a). Viral culture of CSF has a relatively high yield in neonates (30% to 50%); in older children the viral culture is positive in only 1% of the cases. No clear correlation exists between the viral load as measured from the number of infected cells in the CSF and the patient's morbidity (709). Viral DNA also can be detected in the serum in neonatal infections, but not in the serum of older children (710). Serum serologic diagnosis has not been satisfactory for herpes encephalitis. Fourfold increases in titer can occur from herpes infection at other sites. A prior herpesvirus infection can cause elevations in titer that do not change significantly during neurologic involvement. However, a simultaneous serum-CSF herpes antibody titer ratio of 20 or less is diagnostic of herpes encephalitis (711). This change is usually found after the second week of illness (712). A rise in CSF or serum IgM herpes antibody correlates best with an active herpetic process (713). Some acute cases of herpes encephalitis can represent reactivation of latent infection or reinfection, rather than new infection.

If the clinical picture and neurodiagnostic procedures are at all suggestive of herpes simplex encephalitis, treatment with acyclovir, as discussed later, should be instituted immediately. If the clinical picture and the neuroimaging studies are not diagnostic, or if progress during treatment with acyclovir is unsatisfactory, a brain biopsy is recommended (714,715). For histologic confirmation or virus isolation, the biopsy should be obtained early in the course of the illness and must be taken from the involved area either by needle aspiration or direct surgical approach. Histopathologic changes can be missed if the biopsy is taken from the wrong site, or it can be misinterpreted because Cowdry type A inclusion bodies can be absent or can occur in other diseases such as subacute sclerosing panencephalitis. Even in proven cases, attempts at viral isolation from brain tissue can be unsuccessful. In their series published in 1982, Nahmias and coworkers correlated the histologic, serologic, and clinical findings on patients undergoing brain biopsy for suspected herpes encephalitis (716).

Of patients in their series with negative brain biopsy findings, 23% had diseases requiring other forms of therapy. Conditions that mimic focal encephalitis caused by herpes simplex include other forms of encephalitis, bacterial abscess, and tuberculosis (717). Mesenrhomboencephalitis, which can be established as caused by herpes simplex virus in approximately 30% of cases, also can be caused by agents such as *Listeria monocytogenes* (718). Focal EEG and CT findings during an acute episode of encephalomyelopathy caused by mitochondrial encephalopathy lactic acidosis stroke (MELAS) syndrome can lead to the erroneous presumptive diagnosis of herpes encephalitis (719).

Treatment

Untreated, the disease pursues an unremitting downhill course. Currently accepted treatment for herpes encephalitis involves acyclovir (714). Treatment should start as soon as possible after the onset of infection if permanent brain damage is to be minimized, although early therapy is not the only determinant of a satisfactory outcome. The quantity of virus produced, as well as the extent and site of brain involvement, also influences the outcome (717).

Acyclovir is given in a dose of 10 mg/kg (500 mg/m^2 of body surface area for children younger than 12 years of age) every 8 hours, in the form of a 20 mg/mL solution, administered over 1 hour for a 14- to 21-day course (720). Caution should be exercised because extravasation of the drug may cause a marked local bullous inflammatory reaction. Toxic side effects of acyclovir include renal tubular crystalluria with elevation of serum creatinine or, less commonly, an encephalopathy (721).

Strains of herpes simplex types 1 and 2 resistant to acyclovir have been isolated from patients treated with several courses of the drug (722). These resistant strains have evolved after 7 days of acyclovir therapy, and most have been isolated from immunocompromised individuals (723,724). Should acyclovir therapy fail to arrest the disease, a trial of intravenous foscarnet is recommended (724). The drug is given at a dosage of 60 mg/kg every 8 hours intravenously for 14 days.

Generally, mortality and morbidity are less in younger patients, especially when treatment is initiated early in the course of the disease and before consciousness deteriorates. Approximately one-half of patients recover completely. Such recovery occurs more often when therapy is instituted before the onset of stupor. When encephalitis is accompanied by seizures and coma, the outcome is generally poor. Only 10% of patients in whom therapy is delayed to that stage recover (725). These results stress the need for early therapy whenever herpes simplex encephalitis is suspected. Surviving patients usually improve in 10 to 25 days. They do not experience persistent chronic encephalitis.

Some 7% of patients have relapses after a dramatic initial response to therapy, usually 1 to 3 months after treatment (717,726). Involuntary movement disorders such as choreoathetosis or chorea can occur 1 to 18 days after relapse (727). They are much more often associated with relapse than with the primary illness. In some instances of relapses, viral DNA can be demonstrated in CSF (728), although brain biopsy does not reveal any evidence of recrudescent infection or demyelination (717).

In neonatal herpes simplex encephalitis, the outcome generally depends on the type of virus responsible. Neonates have a low risk of herpes simplex virus infection if virus exposure occurs at the time of delivery to mothers with recurrent genital herpes simplex virus infection. This is because of placental transfer of maternal specific neutralizing antibody. The risk is much greater if the mother has acute genital herpes and lacks neutralizing antibody at the time of delivery (728). In the experience of Corey and coworkers, all infants with type 1 virus had normal results on follow-up during the second year of life, compared with 28% of infants surviving type 2 herpesvirus infection (729). Even infants treated promptly for type 2 herpes have a poor outcome. In the various reported series the overall mortality for neonatal herpesvirus infection of the CNS ranges between 15% and 27% (730,731). Malm and associates found that, of the survivors, 48% were healthy whereas 39% had severe disabilities such as severe mental retardation and quadriparesis (731). Of children surviving with severe or mild neurologic impairment, 94% had ophthalmologic abnormalities (731).

Influenza Virus

Influenza viruses are classified as orthomyxoviruses. They are RNA viruses of three major antigenic types: A, B, and C. Influenza viruses are responsible for an acute respiratory infection of worldwide distribution, but can attack any portion of the neuromuscular system.

Encephalomyelitis can be attended by changes in consciousness, opisthotonos, ataxia, or a transverse myelopathy. Seizures are not infrequent, although in some cases they represent activation of a preexisting epileptic focus. Although neurovirulent influenza A virus demonstrates a predilection for the substantia nigra in experimental animals, no clear association with postencephalitic parkinsonism has been demonstrated (734). Two forms of influenza virus–induced acute infectious polyneuritis have been recognized. In the first, seen only in children, the course is mild and lasts 2 to 10 days. Weakness usually is limited to the lower extremities. The second form resembles classic Guillain-Barré syndrome (see Chapter 7).

Myositis caused by one of several strains of influenza viruses and involving primarily the gastrocnemius and soleus muscles also has been encountered. Symptoms appear as the respiratory phase of the illness wanes. They include muscle pain and tenderness that is exaggerated by bedrest. Symptoms last from a few days to several weeks. An elevation of serum creatine phosphokinase levels is often noted (735,736).

The CSF in influenza meningoencephalitis can be normal or can reveal a mild pleocytosis. Mild pleocytosis has been noted also in patients with the respiratory form of influenza who lack overt CNS symptoms. Virus isolation has been successful only rarely (737).

MRI during acute influenza A encephalitis reveals multifocal areas of involvement in the cortex and subcortical white matter that can persist for long periods (736). Pontine lesions also may occur (737). The involved areas have decreased blood flow by single photon emission CT (SPECT). This is in distinction from the increased blood flow usually noted in the focal lesions of acute herpes simplex encephalitis (736). Symmetric hypodense lesions within the thalami and pons can be the major findings on CT (737).

Parainfluenza virus type 3 can cause encephalitis with periodic breathing, opsoclonus-myoclonus, or a clinical picture resembling herpes simplex encephalitis. These patients have recovered without neurologic residuc (738,739). Parainfluenza virus type 4 can cause aseptic meningitis in children (740).

Varicella Zoster Virus

Varicella zoster virus (VZV) reaches the CNS through the bloodstream or by direct spread from sensory ganglia where they are harbored latently.

The virus causes two diseases: varicella (chickenpox) and herpes zoster (shingles). Varicella is the manifestation of the primary VZV infection, whereas herpes zoster, more commonly seen in adults, is the result of the reactivation of a VZV infection. Both may lead to neurologic infection and disease. VZV can lead to neurologic disease through direct viral invasion (infectious) or by the development of a specific immune response (postinfectious). The occurrence of neurologic symptoms in some chickenpox-infected children before the onset of the rash points to the former type of disease mechanism (741). In addition, some of the symptoms are the result of a vasculopathy that involves large and small cerebral vessels (742–747). Despite their multifactorial etiologies, the various neurologic complications of varicella are considered in Chapter 7.

Herpes Zoster

Clinical, epidemiologic, and virologic evidence has established that herpes zoster results from varicella virus that is localized to cranial sensory and dorsal root ganglia and their connections, and to the skin area corresponding to the distribution of the involved sensory nerves (745). It is believed that the initial varicella exposure results in viral invasion of neuronal and glial tissue, and any subsequent reversion to generalized infection is suppressed by persistent immunity. During latency, the viral genomes are found in nonneuronal cells, only spreading to neuronal cells on reactivation of the virus (746). Gradual attenuation of the resistance, or immune suppression as a consequence of intrinsic or extrinsic factors, can lower cellular immunity to a level that permits the virus to activate. The observation that immune individuals show immunologic evidence of reinfection with VZV indicates that herpes zoster also can become symptomatic through reacquisition of virus (747). Serologic and viral studies do not distinguish between varicella virus and herpes zoster, although zoster patients carry a higher immune titer for varicella. Zoster vesicle fluid can produce typical varicella lesions in susceptible children, and in children with leukemia, live attenuated varicella vaccine can cause herpes zoster in immunized children (748).

Pathology

Pathologic changes in herpes zoster are usually limited to one dorsal root or sensory ganglion, and the corresponding nerve (749). Infiltration with lymphocytes, plasma cells, and polymorphonuclear cells occurs around a central area of congestion and hemorrhage caused by intense inflammation and hemorrhagic necrosis. Nerve cells in the area demonstrate degeneration and neuronophagia. Involvement often extends to the spinal cord where microglial cells abound in the dorsal horns, in Clarke's column, as well as in the lateral and ventral horns. Anterior horn cells can show chromatolysis and neuronophagy. Similar involvement in the brainstem accompanies infection of the trigeminal or glossopharyngeal nerves.

Pathologic lesions in varicella zoster encephalomyelitis include focal areas of necrosis and perivascular demyelination. These are mainly seen in cortex and peripheral white matter. Gliosis and astrocytic proliferation also are present. Cowdry's type A inclusion bodies with VZV particles are most abundant in oligodendroglia near the focus of necrosis, but can be found in ganglial cells, damaged nerve roots, vasa nervorum, peripheral nerve endo, perineurium, epineurium, and in Schwann cells of peripheral nerves (750). In trigeminal herpes zoster, tissue damage in the brainstem can extend to the spinal and principal nucleus of the trigeminal nerve and mildly disseminate to the bulbo-ponto-mesencephalic region. The mesencephalic trigeminal nucleus is spared. Myositis with demonstrable VZV in the masseter muscle can complicate trigeminal herpes zoster (751).

Clinical Manifestations

The incidence of herpes zoster increases steadily with increasing age. The condition occurs in approximately 0.74 in 1,000 children up to 9 years of age, in 1.38 in 1,000 children 10 to 19 years of age, and approximately 2.5 in 1,000 individuals through age 49 (752). Neonatal cases have been described. Generally, children older than age 2 years who develop herpes zoster have had a previous attack of varicella; those younger than 2 years of age might have been exposed during gestation or infancy without clinical disease. Incidence of second attacks is 3 to 5 per 1,000 (752). Rarely, children develop segmental symptoms of herpes zoster during an attack of varicella.

Essential to the diagnosis of herpes zoster are grouped vesicular lesions distributed over one or more dermatomes. Systemic reactions, usually fever, nuchal rigidity, headache, and enlargement of the regional lymph nodes, are common in children. In 89% of patients younger than age 12 years, the lesion is localized to the thoracolumbar area (Fig. 6.11). Cervical herpes is seen in 8% and maxillary lesions in 3% of children. Ophthalmic herpes and geniculate herpes are extremely rare.

The skin lesions first appear as erythematous papules that progress to vesicles in 12 to 24 hours and to pustules in 72 hours. Lesions often appear in the proximal area of the dermatome and spread peripherally. When pustulation

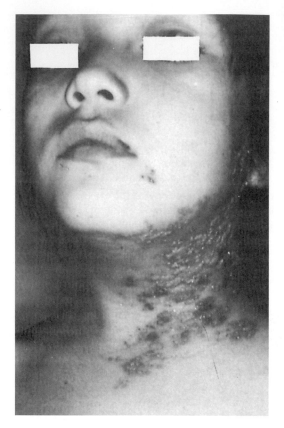

FIG. 6.11. Herpes zoster showing the skin eruption over the third and fourth cervical dermatome.

appears, the surrounding erythema begins to subside, and in 7 to 8 days pustules begin to dry up. Crusts form in 10 to 12 days and fall off in 2 or 3 weeks. Unilateral involvement is the rule, with bilateral involvement occurring in only 0.5% of cases.

Pain, noted by approximately two-thirds of children, can be a prodrome, can occur during the acute infection, or can develop after the skin inflammation has subsided. The pain is evanescent in some and persistent in others; it bears no relationship to the severity of cutaneous lesions. Patients describe it as pruritic, aching, stabbing, or burning.

The most common adult complication of herpes zoster, postherpetic neuralgia, is unusual in children (753). Although in the series of Kost and Straus, 18% of patients younger than 19 years of age developed postherpetic neuralgia, the pain lasted less than 1 month in almost all of them, and lasted longer than 1 year in only 4% (754). Sensory deficits and tactile allodynia coexist in the involved dermatomes.

There has been considerable interest in the cause of the persistent pain. The observation that the number of nerve endings in unilateral postherpetic neuralgia is reduced in both the ipsi- and contralateral dermatomes suggests a central process (755). Kost and Straus have postulated that after their injury peripheral nerves discharge spontaneously and have lower activation thresholds and an exaggerated response to stimuli (754). In addition, axonal regrowth after injury produces nerve sprouts that are prone to unprovoked discharges. The increased peripheral activity leads to hyperexcitability of the dorsal horns and an exaggerated central response to all input (756).

Localized paralysis and atrophy of muscles after an attack of herpes zoster are not unusual, and in some instances are permanent. Ascending myelitis and diffuse encephalomyelitis have been reported also (757).

Hemiparesis, ipsilateral to ophthalmic herpes zoster, can occur after a delay of several weeks to 6 months. It usually involves a territory of the middle cerebral artery. VZV antigen has been demonstrated in the media of the middle cerebral artery ipsilateral to the site of the infection and contralateral to the hemiparesis (758,759). Hemiparesis also can develop some 3 weeks to 2 months after primary chickenpox. The vascular lesions are usually in the basal ganglia, internal capsule, or both, with occasional involvement of the cortex. Children usually recover without recurrences (760,761).

Disseminated herpes zoster occurs in 2% to 5% of cases. Widespread lesions involving the skin, mucous membranes, and lungs, and a clinical syndrome with many characteristics of varicella, can develop in 2 to 12 days, usually by 6 days after the onset of herpes zoster (762). Viremia has been documented just before dissemination of dermal lesions. The more severe cases of disseminated herpes zoster correlate positively with prolonged viremia (763).

Neurologic complications of herpes zoster can occur when the rash is present or months thereafter and are more common in immunocompro-

mised hosts. They include encephalitis, leukoencephalitis, herpes zoster ophthalmicus with delayed contralateral hemiparesis, myelitis, and cranial and peripheral nerve palsies (636). The most common neurologic complication is postherpetic neuralgia, which fortunately is rare in children.

Herpes zoster encephalitis is diffuse and can occur from the start of the appearance of the rash to up to 1 year later. It is seen more frequently in immunocompromised hosts. The clinical symptoms are acute or subacute delirium with few or no focal findings. The presence of viral particles as well as the rapid clinical improvement when acyclovir is administered, speaks of the likely infectious pathogenesis.

Patients with acquired immunodeficiency syndrome (AIDS) and with other immunodeficiencies have been found to develop other VZV-induced neurologic disorders such as multifocal leukoencephalitis, ventriculitis, myelitis, and focal brainstem lesions (764,764a). Because the patients with AIDS have to be severely immunosuppressed to develop these entities, they have been reported mainly in adult subjects. With the development of effective therapies and prolongation of life for pediatric HIV infections, these entities will probably begin to surface in the pediatric population.

An acute aseptic meningitis syndrome (765), acute polyneuritis, myelitis, and encephalitis (766) also have been described in serologically proven varicella zoster infection, in some instances without demonstrable skin lesions (767,768).

The appearance of herpes zoster lesions in preadolescent children can be the first manifestation of HIV infection acquired in the neonatal period (769). Once established, this exacerbation of infection elicits an anamnestic immune response too late to abort the process (753).

The association of herpes zoster with leukemia and Hodgkin disease has been well documented. Treatment of the underlying malignancy with corticosteroids, antimetabolites, and alkylating agents does not appear to have an adverse effect on the course of herpes (770).

Herpes zoster of the geniculate ganglion is a rare cause of facial nerve palsy in the pediatric population. In some instances, herpetic lesions are seen on the tympanic membrane and in the auricular sensory distribution of the facial nerve (771). VZV DNA can be demonstrated by PCR in the auricular lesions (772). The diagnosis can best be made by gadolinium-enhanced MRI of the facial nerve. This demonstrates discrete or, in the more severe cases, diffuse enhancement of the facial and vestibulocochlear nerves in the internal auditory canal and labyrinth (773). Early treatment with acyclovir and prednisone has been recommended (774).

Diagnosis

VZV infections can cause CNS disease with or without the presence of characteristic skin eruptions. When present, the clinical characteristics of the skin rash in children with chickenpox and herpes zoster are cardinal in the diagnosis of these clinical entities (see Fig. 6.10). In the differential diagnosis of facial palsy, herpetic lesions of the tympanic membrane and external auditory canal should be sought for. The isolation of VZV from skin lesions as well as the detection of specific antigens within epithelial cells by the use of fluorescent monoclonal antibodies by direct fluorescent antibody provide confirmation of the etiologic diagnosis. The direct fluorescent antibody monoclonal test is much more sensitive than Tzank smear in the diagnosis of VZV infections.

In the CSF a mild pleocytosis occurs with mononuclear predominance and a protein elevation; hypoglycorrhachia can occur (132). IgG and IgA varicella zoster antibodies are found in CSF when neurologic complications are present (765,775). Early diagnosis can be established by the detection of virus-specific DNA sequences in the CSF (775a,775b). Viral isolation in cell culture is considered the gold standard, but is difficult to perform and usually too slow to prove of diagnostic assistance.

Treatment

As a rule, antiviral treatment of children with uncomplicated chickenpox or shingles and normal immune status is not warranted. However,

secondary skin lesions should be prevented. Oral acyclovir for 7 days reduces the duration of the acute phase of herpes zoster; a further 14 days of therapy is of only slight additional benefit (776). Maximum benefit is obtained when acyclovir is started within the first 24 hours of the disease, and treatment is ineffective if delayed beyond 72 hours after the onset of the illness (777). Acyclovir-resistant zoster myelitis has responded to famciclovir (778). The concurrent use of a short course of prednisolone can accelerate healing and reduce the severity of pain in herpes zoster during the first 2 weeks of therapy, but is associated with an increased incidence of adverse reactions. Neither drug seems to influence the incidence or severity of postherpetic neuralgia (776,777).

Treatment with intravenous acyclovir (500 mg/m^2 every 8 hours for a minimum of 7 days) is reserved for children with a normal immune status who develop CNS manifestations of varicella before the appearance of the rash or who develop severe encephalitis within the first week of the rash. Treatment also is indicated for children who develop shingles with neurologic or ophthalmologic complications and for immunocompromised children who develop either chickenpox or herpes zoster. Controlled studies have shown that intravenous acyclovir reduces the risk for cutaneous and visceral dissemination of VZV in immunocompromised hosts (777a), and that it improves the clinical outcome of neurologic complications (777b).

Little experience has accrued in the management of prolonged herpetic pain in the pediatric population. In adults, persistent pain has been treated with topical lidocaine preparations. Amitriptyline or desipramine give moderate to complete relief in approximately one-half of the patients. Carbamazepine and gabapentin also have been recommended (755,779), as well as ketamine, and a variety of antiviral agents, including acyclovir, famciclovir, and valacyclovir (755).

Rabies

Rabies is an acute infection of the nervous system caused by an RNA virus with a predilection for exocrine glands, kidneys, and the nervous system. The virus is present in the saliva of infected mammals and is transmitted by bite. The disease was well described by Greek and Roman clinicians. Pasteur's study of the disease led to his 1885 development of a modified virus vaccine, which is still the basis for immunization (780).

Etiology and Pathology

At least six antigenically distinct strains of rabies virus affect animals in the United States (781). Of these, four affect humans (782). Worldwide, the dog is the principal vector of human infection. The virus carried in saliva is transmitted when the dog bites or causes a skin abrasion. Of the 18 cases of rabies reported in the United States between 1980 and 1993, only eight were acquired in the United States. Virus isolates suggest that six of these were acquired from the reservoir in bats, one from the reservoir in dogs, and one from the reservoir in skunks (781). A number of other mammals have been found to be responsible for human infections (781,783). The disease also has been contracted by indirect exposure, probably by inhalation of virus particles in a bat-infested cave, or after corneal transplants. In one series, no history of animal bite was obtained in 39% of cases (784). A heavy inoculum accompanying considerable tissue damage, such as occurs with a wolf bite, is much more likely to cause fatality than a lesser bite. Bites around the face and neck are the most dangerous; a fatal clinical illness is 10 times more likely after a face bite than a bite on the upper extremity, and 28 times more likely after a face bite than a bite on a lower extremity (785).

The virus enters the nervous system through the nicotinic acetylcholine receptor of the neuromuscular junction (781,786) and reaches the CNS along peripheral nerves (787). The essential pathology of rabies is that of a generalized encephalomyelitis. When the bite occurs on the extremities, the corresponding posterior horn of the spinal cord shows hyperemia, neuronophagia, and cellular infiltrations. Intracytoplasmic eosinophilic inclusions (Negri bodies) (Fig. 6.12), demonstrated in the neurons in most cases, consist of many aggregated viral particles and are pathognomonic for the disease (788). Negri bodies are most numerous in the forebrain. Usually, they abound in the pyramidal layer of the hippocampus, but they are common also in the cerebral cortex and the cerebellar Purkinje cells. These inclusions are seen after infection only with street or "wild" virus, not with fixed or adapted virus. Another eosinophilic cytoplasmic body, the lyssa body, is seen not only in rabies, but also in a variety of other degenerative conditions not related to virus infection. Van Gehuchten and Nelis lesions, in which ganglion cells are pushed further and further apart because of dense proliferation of capsular cells, occur in the cranial nerve and spinal ganglia.

Centrifugal spread of the virus from the CNS occurs and results in infection of acinar cells in the salivary and submaxillary glands with secretion of virus in the saliva. Spread of virus to muscles of the head and neck and to the cornea make these sites useful for diagnosis by biopsy of the nape of the neck or by corneal smear.

Microscopic lesions are distributed differently in the two clinical types of disease. In the classic form after a dog bite and characterized clinically by restlessness and dysphagia, the chief lesions are in the brainstem, notably in the jugular, gasserian, and dorsal root ganglia, and in the lower two-thirds of the medulla. Infiltrations can be seen also in the substantia nigra, hypothalamic nuclei, peripheral nerves, spinal cord, and cerebral and cerebellar hemispheres.

The paralytic form after bat bites results in congestion of the cord and a striking softening of the lower cord. Neuronal degeneration is marked in both anterior and posterior horns and extends up into the medulla. Microglial infiltration is marked, but Negri bodies are often sparse or absent. Paralytic rabies appears to correlate with absence of significant immune response to the infection (789).

Clinical Manifestations

The highest incidence of rabies in humans occurs in children younger than age 15 years. The incubation period usually ranges from 1 to 3 months, but it can be as short as 4 days (783), or as long as 4 years (790).

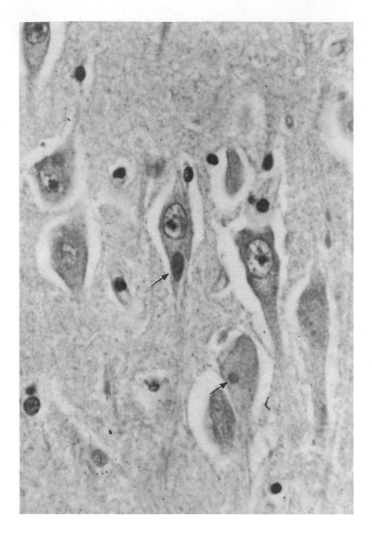

FIG. 6.12. Rabies. Photomicrograph shows Negri bodies (*arrows*) in neuronal cytoplasm of the dorsal cell band of the hippocampus (original magnification ×160). (Courtesy of Dr. Hideo H. Itabashi, Department of Pathology, Los Angeles County Harbor Medical Center.)

Rabies infection has three phases: the initial phase, excitement phase, and paralytic phase. Once symptoms develop, progression to death is usually relentless over the course of 7 to 14 days (781). The initial or premonitory phase, lasting 2 to 4 days, is characterized by fever, headache, anorexia, malaise, and sore throat. Gastrointestinal and upper respiratory symptoms, and subtle changes in mental status, can occur (791). The body temperature can be mildly elevated, but it is seldom higher than 102° F. The most striking symptom during this period is numbness or paresthesia in the region of the bite. Numbness occurs in approximately 80% of cases and has been ascribed to the direct action of the virus on sensory neurons. Decreased sensitivity to local pain can be demonstrated, yet, paradoxically,

patients complain of drafts and bedclothes that cause general stimulation of the skin.

Symptoms of the second or excitement phase usually have a gradual onset. Hyperacusis and photophobia can occur. Signs include hyperactive deep tendon reflexes, increased muscle tone, and tics. Facial expression becomes overactive. Signs referable to the autonomic system can be prominent; they include pupillary dilatation, lacrimation, excessive salivation, priapism, and increased perspiration. SIADH and diabetes insipidus have been reported, but the secretion of anterior pituitary hormones does not seem to be affected (792). A combination of hypoxia, hypocapnia, and respiratory alkalosis early in the disease gradually changes to hypoventilation and increasing periods of respiratory arrest (792).

As the excitement phase progresses, the patient becomes increasingly nervous, sleepless, anxious, and apprehensive. The outstanding clinical sign of rabies is related to the act of swallowing. When fluid comes in contact with the fauces, it is expelled with considerable violence. The patient experiences painful spasmodic contractions of the muscles of deglutition and of the accessory muscles of respiration. Subsequently, the sight, smell, or sound of liquids can precipitate spasm. Drooling of bloody saliva can be prominent at this time (793). Choking from attempts at swallowing can result in such severe spasm of the respiratory muscles that prolonged apnea develops with cyanosis and anoxia. The term *hydrophobia* was derived from this phenomenon.

Convulsions are common, as is maniacal behavior, such as tearing of clothes and bedding. Periods of intense excitement are interspersed with relative quiet, during which the patient is oriented and responds intelligently.

Patients can die in the acute excitement stage in the course of a convulsion, often before the paralytic phase becomes evident. Depressive or paralytic symptoms can dominate the disease picture from its onset or can supervene at any time. Weakness of muscle groups in the vicinity of the bite can become apparent early in the disease. If the patient survives the acute excitement stage, muscle spasms often cease within 1 to 3 days and the patient becomes quiet. The patient might be able to swallow with difficulty. The face becomes expressionless; anxiety and excitement are replaced by apathy, stupor, and coma. Bowel and bladder control can be lost. For a few hours the patient can seem to improve, but this apparent remission is rapidly followed by progressive paralysis.

In rare instances, ascending paralysis begins in the muscles of the legs and progresses without relationship to the original site of infection. Rabies in humans caused by the bite of the vampire bat, as described in Trinidad, is uniformly of the paralytic type (794).

Death can result from heart failure as well as hypoxia. Myocarditis has been reported (795). The disease has been uniformly fatal, but several survivors have been reported after prolonged intensive care unit support.

The white blood count is increased and can range from 20,000 to 30,000 white blood cells per µL with a polymorphonuclear preponderance. Proteinuria, glycosuria, and acetonuria are frequently minimal. CSF cell count usually is within normal limits, but mononuclear pleocytosis of more than 100 cells has been encountered (784,796).

Diagnosis

The diagnosis of rabies in humans is based on the history, clinical features, and laboratory tests. The long incubation periods often make the history of a bite unreliable, and laboratory test results, including serum antibodies, can be negative for long periods of time. Fluorescent antibody tests on saliva can be equally disappointing (797). The diagnosis is confirmed by fluorescence microscopy or virus isolation using corneal smears, or skin or muscle biopsies from the nape of the neck, or by examination of saliva or CSF. Serologic diagnosis of rabies is possible by serum-virus neutralization tests, indirect fluorescent antibody titration, or the complement fixation test (798). Presence of rabies antibodies in the CSF, serum, or both is indicative of rabies. Examination of the brain of the animal involved also can be helpful.

Prevention and Treatment

Once symptoms are present, rabies progresses inexorably and is generally fatal. Only three symptomatic persons have been known to survive; all received some form of rabies vaccine (799,800). The recommended procedure for preventing the disease in the exposed child has been summarized (781,783). Immediate and thorough washing with soap and water of all bite wounds and scratches markedly reduces the likelihood of rabies (781). Among infectious diseases, rabies is unique in that the long incubation period allows the induction of active, as well as passive, immunity before the onset of illness. Active immunity is achieved by use of one of several types of rabies vaccines. In the United States the most widely used of these is the human diploid cell culture vaccine. This provides better protection than other types of killed virus vaccines and causes fewer adverse reactions (801). Deltoid injection is recommended because it produces a better immune response and fewer vaccine failures than gluteal injection (802). A combination of rabies immune serum (40 IU/kg body weight for equine antirabies serum, or 20 IU/kg body weight for human rabies immune globulin) and human diploid cell vaccine has proved extremely effective in preventing the disease (801). Details of the immunization regimen are given in the *Red Book* of the American Academy of Pediatrics (783).

Passive immunization by means of hyperimmune antirabies serum should be administered concurrently with the first dose of rabies vaccine, except if the child has been previously vaccinated against rabies. The recommended dose is 20 IU/kg of body weight. Approximately one-half of the dose is used to infiltrate the wound; the remainder is given intramuscularly. Human rabies immune globulin should be used whenever possible, and if not available, purified equine globulin at a dose of 40 IU/ kg is the recommended choice. Passive antibody can inhibit the response to vaccine; therefore, the recommended dose should not be exceeded. One case of complex partial seizures immediately after treatment with human diploid cell rabies vaccine and human rabies immune globulin has been reported (803). Prophylactic immunization with human diploid cell vaccine or rhesus rabies vaccine (absorbed) should be considered for persons in high-risk groups, such as veterinarians, animal handlers, certain laboratory workers, children living in areas where rabies is a constant threat, and persons traveling to areas where rabies is common (781,783).

The complications of rabies vaccination are discussed in Chapter 7.

Lymphocytic Choriomeningitis Virus

Lymphocytic choriomeningitis virus (LCMV) is an arenavirus that causes human disease ranging from a mild flulike illness to meningitis. It also is associated with a congenital viral infection. LCMV is a chronic infection of mice and hamsters. Humans become infected through the inhalation or ingestion of dust or food contaminated by the virus in urine, feces, blood, or secre-

tions of infected animals. No human-to-human transmission has been reported.

Etiology and Pathology

LCMV is a relatively common infection, with a frequency comparable with that of mumps. The overall prevalence in North America ranges from 3.5% (804) to 4.0% (804a). The prevalence of antibody in persons younger than 30 years of age was 0.3%, whereas in those older than 30 years it was 5.4% (804). Female subjects were found to be more likely to be seropositive (804a). In the United States, hamsters have been described as vectors in several reports, including outbreaks in families.

Although transmission has been postulated to occur through inhalation or ingestion of dried mouse urine or feces, the high prevalence of the disease suggests the existence of other infectious routes. The benign nature of the illness has precluded extensive pathologic studies. Meningeal reactions can be present, but the most constant lesion is a perivascular accumulation of glial cells, lymphocytes, and fat granules (805,806).

Clinical Manifestations

Infections by the LCMV virus can result in a number of clinical forms. The disease is often inapparent. In other cases, a flulike picture develops after an incubation period of 1 to 3 weeks. The course can be biphasic, or symptoms of meningitis or meningoencephalomyelitis can begin abruptly without antecedent prodrome.

When evident, the initial phase can be influenza-like, with retro-orbital headache, photophobia, severe myalgia, malaise, chills, anorexia, and aching nonpleuritic chest pains. Fever ranges from 100° to 104° F. This period lasts from 5 days to 3 weeks (807). In one reported case, parotitis with isolation of virus antedated the onset of symptoms of meningitis by 9 days (808). The initial phase can pass without signs of meningeal involvement.

Of cases with definite signs of meningeal involvement, 50% have a prodromal period as described previously. The remainder has an abrupt onset of meningeal signs similar to those seen in acute purulent meningitis (809). Moderately severe nuchal rigidity can be noted with presence of Kernig and Brudzinski signs in approximately 75% of patients. Consciousness is impaired in approximately two-thirds of cases, and patients occasionally complain of syncope, vertigo, abdominal pain, tremor, or insomnia (809). Recovery from the meningitic form of LCMV can be prompt or can take several weeks or as long as 4 months.

In a few children, encephalitic symptoms predominate. These include alterations of sensorium, seizures, hemiplegia, extrapyramidal signs, cranial nerve palsies, and cerebellar dysfunction (805). Cases simulating bulbar poliomyelitis or infectious polyneuritis also have been reported (810).

The CSF findings in LCMV are characteristic of the disease. The cell count is almost always elevated and can be as high as 6,000 cells per μL. Except for the first few days of the illness, the response is predominantly mononuclear. Cell counts and CSF protein tend to remain elevated for several weeks to months. The concentration of CSF glucose remains normal (810).

During the convalescent period, arthralgia of the hands and shoulders is common. In rare instances, arthralgia is associated with nonmigratory pain and swelling of the small joints of the fingers. Mild generalized alopecia 2 to 3 weeks after the onset of the illness and a delayed orchitis also have been described (807). Hydrocephalus caused by posterior fossa arachnoiditis, which produces headache and prolonged increased intracranial pressure, represents a more serious delayed complication of LCMV (809).

A congenital LCMV syndrome, which resembles congenital toxoplasmosis, has been reported. It is manifested by chorioretinitis, which was present in 88% of infants in the series of Wright and colleagues, macrocephaly, microcephaly, and intracranial calcifications, the last observed in 19% of infants (811). The disease had a 35% mortality and 63% of survivors had severe neurologic residua. Approximately one-half of mothers experienced an illness compatible with LCMV during pregnancy.

Diagnosis

Although the clinical picture of LCMV is not characteristic, the diagnosis can be suspected from a history of exposure to rodents and the CSF findings, particularly from the persistent and marked monocytic pleocytosis. LCMV can be confirmed by virus isolation. Viremia can persist until approximately the fifteenth day of the disease. Virus titers in CSF are lower and are present for a shorter period despite the prolonged abnormalities in cell and protein content. Pharyngeal secretions and urine also can yield the virus. Indirect fluorescent or complement fixation antibodies appear 2 to 3 weeks after the onset of the illness, reach their maximum titers 5 to 6 weeks after the onset of the illness, and decrease to low or undetectable levels in several months. Neutralizing antibodies appear later, 2 to 6 weeks after the onset of symptoms, but persist for 6 months to 5 years (804). Acute and convalescent sera can be tested for increases in antibody titers. An increase in the specific IgM in blood and CSF is diagnostic. A nested reverse transcription–PCR assay has been developed for the detection of LCMV RNA in CSF (811a).

LCMV can be distinguished from bacterial infections, particularly from tuberculous meningitis, in that in the latter the CSF sugar is almost invariably depressed. Mycotic and spirochetal infections, when associated with normal CSF sugar, can be excluded by isolating the infecting organisms. In meningeal carcinomatosis, the CSF sugar is usually normal. Differential diagnosis rests on the microscopic examination of a cell block prepared from the centrifuged CSF.

Treatment

No specific treatment or vaccine is available.

Epstein-Barr Virus (Infectious Mononucleosis)

Epstein-Barr virus (EBV) is a herpesvirus responsible for infectious mononucleosis. In the United States infectious mononucleosis is seen mainly in adolescents and young adults, whereas in developing countries the primary infection with EBV occurs in the first 2 years of life. The younger the child, the more likely the infection will be asymptomatic. The most common clinical findings include fevers, lymphadenopathy, pharyngitis, splenomegaly, and hepatomegaly. The laboratory hallmarks are a lymphocytosis with more than 10% of atypical lymphocytes, transaminitis, and neutropenia. Specific serologic diagnosis is easily made from serum.

Minor neurologic disturbances, such as headache and nuchal rigidity, are common in infectious mononucleosis, but serious neurologic complications occur in only 1% to 7% of cases (812,813). These include, in order of frequency, an aseptic, lymphocytic meningitis, polyneuritis, encephalomyelitis, and mononeuritis. Seizures, subtle corticospinal tract signs, vertical nystagmus, confusion, disorientation, or coma can occur (813). A poliomyelitis-like syndrome also has been reported (813a). In some cases, neurologic symptoms are the first or the only clinical manifestations of the disease (813).

The pathogenesis of EBV-associated neurologic disease can be immune mediated, infectious, or both. Whereas some studies have found no traces of EBV in CSF or brain tissue (814), others have recovered EBV from the CSF (815).

Neurologic symptoms can occur as early as a week before the onset of systemic manifestations, or they can be delayed until several weeks after recovery from systemic manifestations (696,816).

The presenting symptoms of lymphocytic meningitis and other aseptic meningitides are usually headache, malaise, and nuchal rigidity. Peripheral neuritis can be mild or severe. Motor and sensory functions are usually impaired, and CSF changes similar to those in acute infectious polyneuritis (Guillain-Barré syndrome) have been reported (583,817).

Presenting symptoms of encephalomyelitis involve the cerebrum, cerebellum, brainstem, or spinal cord, singly or in combination (816,818,819). Menigoencephalitis with a lymphoma-like response can occur in immunocompetent individuals (819a). Generalized or myoclonic seizures or metamorphopsia "Alice in Wonderland syndrome" can be evident (819b). Localized brainstem encephalitis and mononeuritis of a variety of nerves also have been reported (819). These mononeuritides include an olfactory and an optic neuritis, the latter with papillitis (820). Palsies of one or more cranial nerves have been encountered

(821,822), as well as that of the nerve to the serratus anterior muscle (823). An undulating course with exacerbations and remissions of encephalitic signs has been described (824). Because the manifestations of EBV infection of the nervous system can be protean, all acute neurologic diseases of undetermined origin should be screened for EBV (817).

Approximately 30% of patients with infectious mononucleosis have 5 or more cells per µL in the CSF (825). These alterations can persist for months, often after complete clinical recovery. EEG abnormalities have been noted in a large proportion of children (816,825).

The diagnosis of EBV encephalitis can be made by detecting the viral genome in CSF through PCR (826). EBV serology can be determined by virus-specific immunofluorescence or by a variety of spot tests (827). Patients usually recover from the neurologic sequelae within a few days to several months. In some cases, a poor correlation exists between the severity of the neurologic disorder and the clinical course, prognosis, and laboratory findings.

The role played by EBV in the development of nasopharyngeal carcinoma, Hodgkin disease, systemic lupus, and lymphoma in immunosuppressed patients is outside the scope of this text.

Treatment

No specific therapy or vaccine is available.

Rotavirus Encephalitis

Afebrile benign convulsions can occur during the course of rotavirus gastroenteritis. CSF increases in leukocytes have been minimal (15 white blood cells per µL); protein and sugar are unchanged. Rotavirus genome and antivirus IgG in the CSF and changes in CT have been demonstrated. No sequelae have been reported (828).

Cytomegalovirus

CMV involvement of the nervous system most often is a complication of the immunocompromised host, but it can also occur in immunocompetent young children and adolescents.

CMV infections are common among young children. If the child is an immunocompetent host, CMV causes in the great majority of cases an asymptomatic infection and in a small minority a clinical picture that resembles infectious mononucleosis (828a).

Neurologic complications are seen in 5% of normal hosts during CMV mononucleosis. They include encephalitis (828b), acute idiopathic polyneuritis (828c), Guillain-Barré syndrome (732,828d), and a potential association with Rasmussen syndrome (828e). Immunocompromised hosts, such as patients with AIDS and children who are receiving immunosuppressant drugs, have a much higher likelihood of developing disseminated CMV infections with neurologic compromise than immunocompetent subjects. In some instances activation of a latent infection may be caused by enterovirus infection (583,733).

The diagnosis of CMV CNS infections is best made by PCR of CSF (828f), or, if available, by tissue obtained at brain biopsy. The CSF reveals pleocytosis with high protein content and hypoglycorrhachia. Serologic studies have little diagnostic value in these patients.

Whereas the treatment of CMV chorioretinitis has been extensively studied and found to be efficacious, no double-blinded, placebo-controlled studies of anti-CMV therapy in patients with neurologic compromise have been reported. Treatment of adult patients with CMV neurologic disease with ganciclovir has given mixed results, ranging from lack of clinical response to clinical improvement.

Cat-Scratch Disease

Cat-scratch disease is an infectious illness, first described by Debré in 1950 (829), and contracted by a scratch from a cat. It is characterized by fever, a primary cutaneous lesion with regional lymphadenitis, and occasional neurologic complications.

Etiology

Cat-scratch disease is a syndrome caused by members of the alpha-proteobacteria, most commonly, *Bartonella henselae*. Less commonly,

Afipia felis and *Bartonella quintana* have been implicated (830,831,832). These agents are small gram-negative rods that can be visualized only with difficulty in lymph node sections (833). They have been successfully cultivated (834). *B. henselae*, although serologically cross-reactive with *A. felis*, differs from it in its genetic structure. It is responsible for the majority of cases seen in the United States (831).

Clinical Manifestations

Neurologic manifestations are encountered in approximately one-third of cases of cat-scratch fever. They follow the initial symptoms of the illness, usually by 1 to 5 weeks (830,835). In the series of Carithers and Margileth, encephalitis accounted for 80% of neurologic complications, whereas seizures were present in 46%, and combative behavior in 40% of children. Twenty percent had cranial nerve palsies or peripheral nerve involvement. Optic neuritis was seen in 13% (836). Cerebral arteritis and a transverse myelitis also have been reported (835,837,838).

The onset of the encephalitic phase is usually precipitous, with convulsions, confusion, lethargy, stupor, and coma. Status epilepticus lasting up to several hours can occur (839). Despite the apparent severity of the picture, the patient improves rapidly and generally returns to consciousness in 2 to 10 days. Varieties of transient neurologic sequelae have been encountered, and an occasional patient has died from the encephalitis.

The CSF is usually normal. Rarely, a mild to moderate mononuclear pleocytosis occurs. The EEG is almost uniformly abnormal during the acute phase of the illness. Focal or generalized abnormalities can persist for several years, even after an apparently complete clinical recovery.

Diagnosis

A history of contact with cats, a cat scratch, or a primary dermal lesion is obtainable in 90% of cases (835). The diagnosis is suggested by positive serology against *B. henselae* or *B. quintana*, or by lymph node biopsy with demonstration of necrotizing granulomatous lymphadenitis and visualization of *B. henselae* organisms. False-negative serologic diagnosis may occur because antigenic variability results in distinct serogroups that do not cross-react (840). The organism can be cultivated with difficulty. Eighty-eight percent of patients with suspected cat-scratch disease have serum antibodies that react with *B. henselae* antigen. This assay also can be useful for diagnosis of cat-scratch disease in the immunocompromised host (841,842). The most sensitive test available to detect the presence of *B. henselae* DNA sequences is the PCR. This test can be performed on sterile fluids and from tissues obtained at biopsy.

Treatment

No immunization is available. A variety of antibiotics, notably aprofloxacin and azithromycin, have been suggested but no controlled trials have been described (836).

SLOW VIRUS INFECTIONS AND RELATED DISORDERS

Although scrapie, a chronic spongiform encephalopathy of sheep, was first described by Sigurdsson in 1954 (843), the concept that an infectious transmissible agent can modify normal gene products and continue to propagate within the host for several months to years, and ultimately produce a progressive debilitative disease of the nervous system, is relatively new (844). These agents, called *prions*, have been implicated in animal and human disease. Although they differ from all other conventional infectious agents they are included in this section (845).

In humans, three forms of prion disease are manifest as transmissible, sporadic, and inherited disorders (844). Transmissible forms require B lymphocytes to become neuroinvasive (846). These include Creutzfeldt-Jakob disease (CJD), bovine spongiform encephalopathy, Gerstman-Strõussler-Scheinker syndrome, fatal familial insomnia, kuru, and iatrogenic CJD (844,847,848). New variant CJD (nvCJD), described in Europe, is caused by the same prion strain as bovine spongiform encephalopathy (849). All entities involve the aberrant metabolism and resulting accumulation of the prion protein. The conversion of the normal cellular protein (PrP^c) to the abnormal disease-causing isoform (PrP^{Sc}) involves a conformational change in the protein. PrP^C and PrP^{Se} are membrane-bound phosphatidylinositol sialoglycoproteins (849a). The conformational change renders the protein more resistant to protease digestion and nondenaturing detergents. The mechanism whereby transmission of abnormal prion protein induces changes in normal prion protein of susceptible hosts is unknown (850). PrP^{Sc} is the source of plaques and amyloid found in the transmissible spongiform encephalopathies (846). Inherited prion diseases in humans are associated with at least 20 different mutations of the *PrP* gene. These different mutations account for the conformational changes that confer diversity to prion diseases (848). However, a few sporadic cases of CJD, and possibly a few cases of sporadic Gerstman-Strõussler-Scheinker syndrome, have no demonstrable mutation of the *PrP* gene. In scrapie, these glycosylated, phosphatidylinositol glycosylated prion proteins result in the production of protease-resistant filaments that differ from normal, protease-susceptible neurofilaments. In scrapie, PrP^{Sc} reaches concentrations 20 times that of PrP^c which remains unchanged during scrapie. In normal animals PrP^{Sc} is distributed in the cell bodies and proximal dendrites of many neurons with much less in the neuropil. In experimental scrapie, PrP is lost from most cell bodies, but high concentrations of PrP are found in the neuropil (851). The gene that encodes the precursor of an amyloid protein (PrP) involved in the pathogenesis of spongiform encephalopathies is located on the short arm of human chromosome 20. A different gene appears to control the incubation time for scrapie. The molecular basis of neurologic dysfunction is unknown, although cellular receptor-mediated responses are altered (852,853). For a more complete discussion of this rapidly evolving field, the reader is referred to reviews by Prusiner (844,845), Prusiner and DeArmont (847), and Pablos-Mindez and colleagues (854).

Slowly progressive infections can also be caused by lentiviruses (e.g., AIDS, HIV), or by conventional agents. Examples of conventional agents include SSPE caused by measles virus, progressive rubella panencephalitis, progressive multifocal leukoencephalopathy (papovavirus), subacute encephalitis (herpes simplex), chronic mumps encephalitis (855), progressive bulbar palsy with epilepsy (Russian spring-summer encephalitis) (856), recurrent Japanese encephalitis virus (857), and CMV brain infection. Only slow infections that become clinically symptomatic during childhood are discussed here.

Human Immunodeficiency Virus/Acquired Immunodeficiency Syndrome

The AIDS virus (also called HIV) has an affinity for the CD4 receptor, a membrane protein of T4 lymphocytes (858,859). When complexed with antibody the virus binds to Fc receptors. It also binds to galactosylceramide on brain and bowel cells, and the chemokine receptors CXCR4 and CCR5 (860). Several mechanisms have been proposed to account for the effects of the virus on the CNS. These include a direct effect of the virus, the effects of viral products on neurons and other cells of the nervous system (861), macrophage expression of cytokines (859,862), and upregulation of unique monocyte subsets to induce neuronal apoptosis (863). In addition, neurologic symptoms can arise as a result of complications of an immunodeficient state, or through a combination of these factors (861,864–866). Brain involvement can occur soon after infection because infected microglia have been identified in brain parenchyma as early as 7 days after transfusion with infected blood (867).

Neurologic disorders that result from primary infections of the nervous system include congenital or neonatal infections that can produce early signs of mental retardation and developmental delay (868) or produce mental deterioration of delayed onset (869,870). Metabolic changes demonstrable by MR spectroscopy can occur in newborn children of HIV-seropositive mothers (865). Postnatal infections in children or young adults result from parenteral injection of blood products or from sexual transmission or intravenous drug use.

Productive HIV-1 infection of the CNS is probably limited to macrophages, microglia, and astrocytes. High levels of plasma virus and low CD4 counts relatively early in HIV infection are associated with increased risk of neurologic disease (870a). Most studies fail to localize HIV antigen to nerve cells (871,872). The HIV viral load of the nervous system is low in presymptomatic AIDS. With the onset of symptomatic HIV infection of the nervous system, the brain and spinal cord have high viral loads, which correlates with the presence of giant cell encephalitis or myelitis (872).

Inflammatory cell infiltrates, multinucleated cells, microglial nodules, white matter pallor, and calcification mainly in the vessels of the basal ganglia and deep cerebral white matter characterize the autopsy findings (871,873). Encephalitic changes are focally distributed in the brain where in severe cases they are associated with multinucleated cell encephalitis. There is preferential involvement of the diencephalic structures, particularly the globus pallidus, but also the substantia nigra, deeper white matter, with less frequent infection of the cerebral cortex. Patients with only mild AIDS dementia have pathologic findings usually restricted to central gliosis and white matter pallor with limited inflammatory response (874,875). Brains from children have fewer HIV-1 infected macrophages, multinucleated giant cells, and microglia than brains from adults (876). Cellular changes are numerous in the globus pallidus, and less so in the corpus striatum and thalamus. Infratentorial involvement is most prevalent in the ventral midbrain, especially the substantia nigra and the dentate nucleus. Lower levels of infection, often patchy, occur in the cerebral and cerebellar white matter and the pontine base. HIV-1 positive cells are usually less numerous in the cerebral cortex, medulla, and spinal cord (872,876). Although the cerebral cortex is relatively preserved in most cases, massive and diffuse destruction of the cerebral cortex with severe neuronal loss caused by HIV has been reported (877).

With primary brain involvement, oligoclonal antibody to HIV is synthesized within the blood–brain barrier. Viral particles, viral DNA, RNA, and other viral antigens can be demonstrated in CNS tissue or CSF. However, lack of correlation between the amount of viral antigen present and the extent of the lesion suggests that one or more additional factors such as cytokines or cytokine activation of nitric oxide, blood–brain barrier dysfunction, blockage of neurotrophic factors, disturbance of ion channels by viral proteins, or direct damage to neurons and glial cells play a role in the disease (878–880).

Clinical Manifestations

Maternal-to-infant transmission of HIV-1 occurs in 13% to 40% of pregnancies (881). Mothers who transmit infection to their offspring have higher mean concentrations of IgG_1 antibodies to a portion of the viral envelope (gp160) than nontransmitters (881). Infants born to mothers with more advanced disease before delivery have a greater risk of serious manifestations of disease or early death than those whose mothers have less advanced disease (882). In the experience of Sperling and coworkers, infants born to untreated mothers with HIV-1 infections have a 22% chance of acquiring HIV-1, whereas the risk was 7.6% for zidovudine-treated mothers (883). The rate of HIV transmission by untreated mothers to newborn infants is 25% when membranes are ruptured more than 4 hours before delivery, and 14% when membranes are ruptured for less than 4 hours (884). Among infants with maternally transmitted HIV infection, approximately one-fifth have rapid progression to profound immunodeficiency, whereas the remainder have much slower progression (882). On rare occasions postnatal infection appears to have been acquired by way of breast milk (885). The incubation period is generally shorter in congenital infections than in acquired ones.

During the clinically latent period, DNA provirus is active and progressive in lymphoid tissue (886,887). After an intrauterine HIV-1 infection, neurologic signs can appear as early as 3 weeks of age. After a perinatal infection, approximately 50% of patients develop signs or symptoms by 12 months of age, 78% by 2 years

of age, and 82% by 3 years of age (888). Belman and coworkers found neurologic problems in 90% of prenatally and perinatally infected infants followed for an average of 18 months (889). In a subsequent study, the same workers found that uninfected children with antibody passively transferred from infected mothers did not differ from controls in neurologic status or growth (889a). Infected children who remain free from AIDS-defining illnesses for the first 2 years of life have only a slightly increased frequency of neurologic abnormalities, which, when these do develop, are often transient or mild. In the original study by Roy and coworkers, 71% of the affected children presented with progressive encephalopathy characterized by developmental delay with loss of acquisitions and cognitive decline, impaired growth, microcephaly, and corticospinal dysfunction (890). Cerebral atrophy was present in all cases, and basal ganglia calcification could be demonstrated in 29%. Cooper and coworkers (890a) reported that encephalopathy represented the first AIDS-defining condition in 67% of HIV-infected children and was diagnosed in 21% of HIV-infected children by age 2 years. Encephalopathy was correlated with a high viral load in infancy and with a median survival of 14 months after the diagnosis was made.

An acute meningoencephalitis syndrome can present during acute HIV-1 infection. This syndrome must be considered in the differential diagnosis of aseptic meningitis (891). Childhood infection also can result in acute or subacute dementia, chronic aseptic meningitis, acute encephalopathy, or granulomatous angiitis involving the CNS. Pediatric HIV-1 infection frequently involves the corticospinal tract with involvement of myelin alone, or both myelin and axons (888). Spinal cord involvement has been associated with vacuolar myelopathy in adults, but this is rare in children (888). Peripheral nerve involvement has been associated with distal symmetric sensorimotor neuropathy, mononeuritis multiplex, chronic inflammatory demyelinating polyradiculoneuropathy, and a polyneuritis simulating the Guillain-Barré syndrome (583). Progressive multifocal leukoencephalopathy has been reported in HIV-infected children (891a). Clinical deterioration can be acute, chronic, or characterized by intermittent decline. Intellectual deterioration is often accompanied by progressive corticospinal or corticobulbar signs, ataxia, or disturbance of tone. Microcephaly can result from involvement of the developing brain (873). Seizures or myoclonus are an uncommon occurrence (888).

Bale and coworkers found that on admission to a longitudinal study of HIV-positive hemophiliacs, 11% had cranial nerve dysfunction, 17% had abnormal deep tendon reflexes, 23% had abnormal strength, 25% had abnormal coordination, and 31% had abnormal tone bulk or range of motion. Less than 2% demonstrated abnormal movements, or had abnormalities of sensation or mental status (892). A subsequent follow-up of this group showed that there was a progressive increase in the incidence of behavior change, gait disturbance, and muscle atrophy (893).

The EEG shows diffuse background slowing. CSF can be normal or have mild pleocytosis or an elevation in protein (873). Neuroimaging studies are relatively insensitive to the primary changes of HIV encephalitis during the early stages of the disease. In the series of DeCarli and associates, who studied, by CT, children with symptomatic, but untreated AIDS who did not have cerebral complications from other causes, ventricular enlargement was seen in 78%, cortical atrophy in 69%, white matter attenuation in 26%, and cerebral calcification in 19% (893a). All children with intracerebral calcifications were encephalopathic. CT abnormalities were present in some children during the presymptomatic stage before onset of encephalopathy. MRI demonstrates focal or multifocal areas of demyelination that appear as progressive, high-intensity T2-weighted images, usually in the periventricular white matter and centrum semiovale (894). Central atrophy, primarily affecting the subcortical white matter or the basal ganglia regions in MRI of children can be suggestive of AIDS encephalopathy (895).

Other neuroimaging findings include cerebrovascular complications such as arterial ectasia and arterial fibrosing sclerosis (896). MR spectroscopy of the basal ganglia has been used before and after antiretroviral therapy to show a normalization of the *N*-acetylaspartate/creatinine and lactate levels, an indication of decreased inflammation (897). Salvan and coworkers (898) used *in vivo* proton MR spectroscopy to study the cerebral metabolism of HIV-infected children with and without encephalopathy. Children with progressive encephalopathy had an abnormal profile consisting of an increased proportion of lipid signals, decreased proportion of *N*-acetylaspartate, and increased proportion of the *myo*-inositol signal. None of the children without encephalopathy had these changes.

Secondary opportunistic infections of the brain accompanying HIV infection include CMV encephalitis, toxoplasmosis, CMV viral lymphoma, progressive multifocal leukoencephalopathy, and, less commonly, viral encephalitis owing to VZV or herpes simplex virus. Myelitis has resulted from VZV, herpes simplex, and CMV. Meningitis can result from typical and atypical mycobacteria, especially *Mycobacterium avium intracellulare*, cryptococcal, and other fungal meningitides. Cerebral infection with *Bartonella henselae*, the agent implicated in cat-scratch disease, has been associated with AIDS encephalopathy (841,899). Radiculitis has been caused by varicella zoster, or by CMV.

Diagnosis

Diagnosis of HIV infection in an infant relies on the performance of virologic assays. The HIV DNA PCR is the method of choice for the diagnosis of HIV infection during the first 6 months of life. This test result is positive in 38% of prenatally HIV-infected children within the first 48 hours of life (899a). After 2 weeks of age, 93% of the HIV-infected neonates had a positive PCR assay result. The majority of HIV-infected infants has a positive DNA PCR by 1 month of age, and all infants are positive by 6 months of age. Whereas the HIV-1 culture is as sensitive as the HIV DNA PCR (899b), it is more cumbersome to perform and more expensive. The initial testing ideally should be performed within the first 48 hours of life. A positive test result indicates an intrauterine acquisition of HIV and predicts rapid progression of the infection (899c). Passively acquired maternal IgG antibody to HIV detectable by ELISA or Western blot declines slowly: 60% of uninfected children have negative test results at 12 months of age, 80% at 15 months, and 100% by 18 months. Indications of neonatal infection include prolonged persistence of IgG antibody or a fourfold increase in titer, the presence of IgG subclasses that differ from that of the mother, appearance of new bands on Western blot, or specific anti-HIV IgM or IgA antibody (899,899d). The serologic diagnosis of HIV infection by ELISA and Western blot analysis is reliable in infants 18 months and older. In neonates serologic detection of HIV infection is complicated by the presence of HIV antigens complexed to passively transferred maternal antibody. Early detection of HIV infection in neonates can be achieved by serologic testing with immune-complex–dissociated HIV p24 antigen (899). Detection of p24 antigen in the neonate predicts the development of early and severe HIV-related disease (899d). Viral culture at birth can identify only approximately one-half of HIV-infected newborns, probably because infections acquired late in pregnancy or during delivery may be missed (899d).

HIV DNA, HIV RNA, and HIV-1 culture have been performed on CSF and brain tissues from children with HIV infection and encephalopathy. Sei and coworkers (899e) have evaluated the levels of HIV RNA in CSF in children with HIV encephalopathy. They found that the levels were highest in children with severe encephalopathy, intermediate when the encephalopathy was moderate, and the lowest in nonencephalopathic children. These findings speak about the potential role of increased viral replication within the CNS in the progression of HIV encephalopathy.

The diagnosis of an acute postnatally acquired HIV-1 infection cannot be made with standard serologic tests. Serologic tests first become positive 22 to 27 days after infection. Earlier diagnosis must rely on detection of p24 antigen in serum or plasma (891).

Treatment

Every HIV-infected infant younger than 12 months of age, independent of clinical, immunologic, and virologic status should receive combination antiretroviral therapy. The majority of the experts agrees that the same criteria apply to children older than 1 year (894b). Aggressive antiretroviral therapy using three drugs is preferred. The combination of two nucleoside reverse transcriptase inhibitors and a protease inhibitor is the combination of choice. This combination of drugs has led to a significant decrease in the mortality of patients with HIV infection and an accompanying significant improvement in the quality of life.

Antiretroviral therapy improves and even reverses the course of the HIV encephalopathy in children. For CNS disease, zidovudine, stavudine, and lamivudine are preferred over didanosine, because of their better CNS penetration. The protease inhibitors are highly bound to serum proteins with low penetration in the CNS. Ongoing trials will determine which is the best combination of drugs to fight HIV within the CNS.

A more extensive discussion of treatment, complications of treatment, and control measures for AIDS is beyond the scope of this text.

HUMAN T-LYMPHOTROPIC VIRUS MYELONEUROPATHIES

Four different neurologic diseases are related to infection with human T-lymphotropic virus types I and II (HTLV-I and HTLV-II): tropical spastic paraparesis/HTLV-I associated myelopathy (TSP/HAM), polymyositis, progressive neurologic abnormalities without immune reactivity against the virus, and tropical ataxic neuropathy (900–903).

TSP/HAM usually occurs in high HTLV-I endemic areas such as southern Japan, equatorial Africa, and the Seychelles, as well as in high endemic foci in Central and South America, Melanesia, and South Africa. Sporadic cases have been described in the United States and Europe.

Neuropathologic changes in TSP/HAM consist most notably of chronic inflammatory changes in the spinal cord that are prominent as a meningomyelitis of the lower thoracic region. Radiculitis, leptomeningitis, and pial thickening can occur. With time the inflammatory changes predominate in the perivascular region and are accompanied by hyalinosis of blood vessels, meningeal fibrosis, glial scars, and progressive atrophy of the spinal cord. Early lesions usually demonstrate destruction of myelin; later, both myelin and axons are destroyed (901). Both immunologic response and viral load play a role in the development of symptoms. Symptomatic patients have an activated immune response and as much as 50 times more HTLV-I proviral DNA in peripheral blood lymphocytes than do seropositive asymptomatic persons. HTLV-I RNA is present in CD4$^+$ lymphocytes and astrocytes (904). These lymphocytes are thought to enter the nervous system where they evoke local expansion of virus-specific CD8$^+$ cytotoxic T lymphocytes, which together with cytokines cause the pathologic lesions (905).

Symptoms may appear as early as 6 years of age, although onset before the age of 20 years is uncommon (901). The onset is insidious without prodromata or provocation. Symptoms include stiffness or weakness in one or both legs, often associated with lumbar pain, and various sensory symptoms in the legs including numbness, burning, and "pins and needles." Urinary frequency and urgency are common. The disease progresses at a variable rate, but usually reaches a plateau. After 10 years, 30% of patients are bedridden and 45% cannot walk unaided. Complete paralysis can occur within 2 years (901). Early onset has been associated with more rapid progression.

The clinical presentation is one of spastic paraparesis or paraplegia. Minor sensory involvement of the posterior columns and spinothalamic tract are found in the lower extremities. Cerebellar signs limited to intention tremor have been reported in 20% of patients. Cranial nerves are usually spared, but optic neuropathy can develop occasionally. Cognitive functions remain normal (901).

MRI of the spinal cord can be normal or show atrophy of the thoracic spinal cord with a diffuse high signal on T2-weighted images. Approximately one-half of patients have non-specific lesions of the brain, which consist of increased signal on T2-weighted images and decreased signal on T1-weighted images, either contiguous with the ventricles or scattered throughout deep cerebral white matter (901). EEGs are abnormal in up to 64% of patients, and visual-evoked responses are abnormal in approximately 30% of cases (901). Somatosensory-evoked potentials are abnormal in the legs in two-thirds of patients and in the arms in one-third of patients (901). Conduction velocities can be reduced in the spinothalamic tracts and posterior columns without clinical impairment of sensation (903).

The CSF usually demonstrates a mild pleocytosis, elevated IgG, and intrathecal production of oligoclonal antibodies against HTLV-I (901). Rarely, TSP/HAM coexists with adult T-cell leukemia.

The pathologic features of polymyositis associated with HTLV-I are indistinguishable from polymyositis in noninfected individuals. Specific diagnosis is made by demonstration of virus in inflammatory lymphocytes or HTLV-I–positive endomysial macrophages of the involved tissue by PCR (900). HTLV-I and HTLV-I–positive lymphocytes do not infect muscle. Virus, which persists in tissues other than muscle, triggers T-cell–mediated and major histocompatibility complex I–restricted cytotoxicity (906)

Chronic progressive myelopathy without detectable HTLV-I antibodies is observed most frequently in HTLV-I endemic areas. HTLV-I related DNA sequences have been demonstrated in peripheral blood mononuclear cells of these patients by PCR. Patients have a clinical disease similar to TSP/HAM, except that the onset of disease is at a younger age and little or no sphincteric or sensory disturbance occurs (901).

Interferon-α is of benefit in HTLV-I–associated myelopathy, although the therapy has a considerable incidence of side effects (907).

HTLV-II causes a myelopathy similar to HTLV-I except that it is associated with more prominent ataxia and mental changes (tropical ataxic neuropathy) (902,903).

Creutzfeldt-Jakob Disease

Transmitted CJD has occurred in young adults 10 to 17 years after inoculation of prion protein by injection of human growth hormone (908–910). The disease also develops in older patients after corneal transplantation and after implantation of cerebral electrodes. Spontaneous CJD can develop in adolescence as early as 16 years of age with dementia progressing to severe disability within 12 months, and death within 28 months (911). Some 5% to 10% of spongiform encephalopathies are familial (912).

PrPCJD, an abnormal isoform of prion protein that accumulates in the brain in parallel with development of the disease, differs in location in iatrogenic and in spontaneous CJD. PrPCJD is found in high concentrations in the cerebellum of iatrogenic CJD cases in comparison with sporadic cases; conversely PrPCJD amounts are greater in the forebrain of sporadic CJD than of iatrogenic cases (913).

The condition is marked by dementia, accompanied by pyramidal tract disease, extrapyramidal signs, and myoclonus, which is often stimulus sensitive. Initial symptoms also can be highlighted by cerebellar signs, which are followed by mental deterioration and myoclonus, with death ensuing within a few months (911). The EEG is characteristic: it demonstrates periodic complexes of spike or slow wave activity at intervals of 0.5 to 2.0 seconds (914).

Conventional laboratory studies of CSF are usually unremarkable. Elevations in neuron-specific enolase and demonstration of 14-3-3 brain protein in CSF have been associated with early diagnosis of CJD (915,916). CSF 14-3-3 protein also is elevated in herpes simplex encephalitis and stroke, but rarely in other neurologic conditions.

Kuru

Kuru, first described by Berndt in 1954 (917), is a progressive degenerative disease of the CNS with predominantly cerebellar features. The disease is limited to the Fore tribe of the eastern highlands of central New Guinea, in a population that until recently practiced cannibalism (918).

Pathologic changes are seen only on microscopy (919). They include widespread neuronal degeneration that is most marked within the cerebellum, proliferation of astroglia and microglia, and minimal demyelination. The disease has been transmitted experimentally to the chimpanzee, in which it develops after incubation periods ranging from 18 to 30 months (920). It is now believed to have passed from human to human by cutaneous inoculation during the cannibalistic ingestion of infected human brain, although one well-documented case was seen in a visitor to the endemic area (921).

The clinical course is remarkably uniform. In boys, the mean age of onset is approximately 14 years of age. In female subjects, the age of onset has a bimodal distribution, with one mode occur-

ring at approximately 8 years of age and the other at 33 years of age. The earliest case of kuru occurred in a child 5 years of age. The initial symptom is ataxia, which is progressive and accompanied by a fine tremor of the trunk, extremities, and head. During the second to third month of illness, the tremor becomes more coarse and severe, and choreiform movements can appear. Intelligence is preserved, although alterations in mood are common. In most children, the disease is fatal within 6 to 9 months of onset (922).

Laboratory studies have been unremarkable and in particular have shown no abnormalities of the CSF (910).

Although no therapy has been effective once symptoms have become apparent, abolition of cannibalism among the Fore tribe has led to disappearance of the illness.

New-Variant Creutzfeldt-Jakob Disease

nvCJD or bovine spongiform encephalopathy has occurred in adolescents as young as 14 years of age. Involvement of lymphoid tissue as early as 8 months before the onset of symptoms (923), as well as early involvement of nervous tissue, has been demonstrated (924). This variant has clinical features that help distinguish it from other phenotypes. Psychiatric symptoms, most often depression, are common. Ataxia and involuntary movements occur in all cases, and akinetic mutism is often a late occurrence. One-third of patients develop persistent and often painful sensory symptoms (925,926). These symptoms, except for their early age of onset, may overlap with atypical cases of sporadic CJD. For epidemiologic aspects of this disorder, see the review by Collee and Bradley (927).

Fatal familial insomnia, a rare prion disease usually seen only in adults, has caused death in a 13-year-old child (928).

Subacute Sclerosing Panencephalitis

SSPE is a slow virus infection, first encountered in Tennessee children by Dawson in 1933 (929), and caused by measles virus, which presents a clinical picture of CNS degeneration characterized by myoclonic seizures, involuntary movements, and mental deterioration. Although

SSPE was once a relatively common condition, its frequency has been decreased significantly by the widespread use of measles immunization. This topic is reviewed in a book by Bergamini and coworkers (930).

Etiology and Pathology

The alterations within the brain are usually evident on both gross and microscopic examination. They consist of a subacute encephalitis that is accompanied by demyelination.

Lesions generally involve the cerebral cortex, hippocampus, thalamus, brainstem, and cerebellar cortex. In the cerebral cortex, the histologic picture is a nonspecific one of subacute encephalitis with cell loss that is sometimes accompanied by neuronophagia and meningeal and perivascular infiltration. Perivascular cells are predominantly CD4$^+$ T cells, whereas the parenchymal inflammatory infiltrate are B cells (931). Inclusions are seen within both the nucleus and the cytoplasm of neurons and glial cells. Characteristically, they consist of homogeneous eosinophilic material (Cowdry type A); less often, the inclusions are small and multiple (Cowdry type B). They are almost always found in the brainstem (932). Older aged patients often show neurofibrillary tangles in neurons and fibrillary tangles in oligodendroglia (931).

The demyelination is particularly evident in the more chronic cases. It is sudanophilic with astrocytic and fibrillary gliosis and is independent of the loss of cortical neurons. In its early stages, SSPE affects the occipital areas primarily; subsequently, it spreads to the anterior portions of the cerebral hemispheres, subcortical structures, brainstem, and spinal cord (933). The presence of measles virus antigen has been convincingly demonstrated by several methods, including *in situ* hybridization to nucleic acid sequences from the measles virus matrix (M) protein (934).

The interplay between viral mutation and abnormal host response to the virus that results in SSPE is not clear. At one time it was thought that the pathogenesis of SSPE involved an abnormality in the host synthesis in brain of the M protein, one of the nonglycosylated polypeptides of the measles virus involved in the assembly of viral nucleocapsid with the viral glycoproteins in the cell membrane. It is now clear that multiple viral mutations, rather than host factors, cause defective measles virus gene expression in SSPE (935,936). Although strains of SSPE measles virus can code for matrix (M) protein, the conformation of the protein is defective and it is unable to bind to nucleocapsids (937).

Host factors are probably also important. Patients with SSPE have low titers of antibody to the M protein, even though they have high titers of antibody to the other measles virus polypeptides (935). Oligoclonal IgG in the sera of patients with SSPE is only partially specific for measles antigens (938).

SSPE patients have an increased CSF to serum ratio of β_2-microglobulin, and higher than normal levels of serum soluble IL-2 receptor, and CSF-soluble CD8. During clinical worsening of the disease, the level of CSF-soluble CD8 increases, whereas the level of serum β_2-microglobulin decreases (939).

Clinical Manifestations

SSPE is more common in rural than in urban populations. The age of onset ranges from 5 to 15 years, and boys are more frequently affected than girls by a factor of 3 to 5. Occasional cases begin in adult life. Children with SSPE are more likely to have been infected with natural measles than with a live vaccine strain. The risk of SSPE after measles is 4.0 in 100,000 cases compared with a risk after measles vaccine of 0.14 in 100,000 doses. Children with early measles infection are more prone to the disease. When measles is contracted in children younger than 1 year of age, the risk for SSPE is 16 times greater than when measles is contracted in children older than 5 years of age. Receipt of measles vaccine subsequent to natural measles does not increase the incidence of SSPE. During the period 1980 through 1986, 36.6% of SSPE was vaccine associated, with SSPE developing after a latency of 7.7 years. The median interval between natural measles and the onset of SSPE is 8 years (940).

Initially, personality changes and an insidious deterioration of intellect occur. Seizures, usually appearing within 2 months, characteristically are myoclonic jerks, initially of the head and subsequently of the trunk and limbs. Muscular contraction is followed by 1 to 2 seconds of relaxation associated with a decrease in muscle action potentials or complete electric silence. The myoclonic jerks do not interfere with consciousness but may be a troublesome cause of falling episodes. They are exaggerated by excitement and disappear during sleep. Although initially they are infrequent and might be regarded as stumbling, clumsiness, or possibly ataxia, later in the course of the illness they occur every 5 to 15 seconds. Patients can present with intractable simple partial seizures (941).

Spontaneous speech and movements decrease, although comprehension seems relatively well preserved.

With further progression of the illness, extrapyramidal dyskinesia and spasticity become more prominent. The former includes athetosis, chorea, ballismus, and dystonic movements with transient periods of opisthotonus. Swallowing difficulties can develop at this stage. Progressive vision loss associated with focal chorioretinitis, cortical blindness, and, occasionally, optic atrophy also has been noted (942,943).

In the terminal stages of the disease, a progressive unresponsiveness is associated with increasing extensor hypertonus and decerebrate rigidity. Respirations become irregular and stertorous, and the patient has a variety of signs of hypothalamic dysfunction. These include vasomotor instability, hyperthermia, profuse sweating, and disturbances of pulse and blood pressure.

Ocular involvement is present in 56% of patients with SSPE. When present, it is bilateral in approximately 80% of patients. Optic neuritis occurs in 72% of involved eyes, retinitis in 35%, and macular pigment disturbances in 9%. Visual agnosia can occur but is rare. Ophthalmologic involvement precedes the neurologic signs in approximately 10% of patients (944).

The clinical course is characterized by slowly progressive deterioration or variable periods of remission, with the mean duration of the disease being approximately 12 months (945). Patients have lived for as short as 6 weeks after the onset of symptoms, or as long as 20 years. Patients with remissions that last up to 25 years have been encountered (946).

A fulminant disease that can be as brief as 1 month, has been described after acquired measles (947). It is probably related to measles inclusion body encephalitis, which is encountered in immunocompromised children.

Cerebral metabolism during SSPE has been studied by positron emission tomography. During the initial active period of disease progression, inflammation in the basal ganglia appears to lead to neuronal excitation accompanied by hypermetabolism. This is followed by widespread functional inhibition of cortical metabolism. Striatal inflammation ends with necrosis and hypometabolism. Later, deep midbrain and brainstem structures become hypermetabolic. No such changes are found during clinical remission (948). CT scans obtained during the early stages of SSPE show small ventricles and obliteration of hemispheric sulci and interhemispheric fissures. Atrophy of white and gray matter can be seen after a prolonged course, but tomograms are normal, sometimes for as long as 5 years after onset of the disease (949).

MRI shows abnormal signal in gray and white matter, which reflects the inflammatory process, and occasionally mimics a neoplasm. These abnormalities can resolve during progression of the disease (950). Two types of MRI abnormalities are observed: focal areas of increased signal intensity on T2-weighted images (hypointense or isointense on T1-weighted images) and atrophy (951). Although the cortical and subcortical lesions seen on MRI have some correlation with clinical findings, the extent of the periventricular white matter lesions and cortical atrophy generally do not correlate with the neurologic status (952). Typically, the CSF contains a normal or slightly elevated protein concentration, but the concentration of gamma globulin, predominantly oligoclonal IgG, is always increased to amounts that can vary from slightly above normal to 60% of the total protein concentration. Antibodies against measles virus can be demonstrated in both serum and CSF by a variety of techniques. Almost invariably, the ratio of the IgG and IgA antibody content in the CSF compared with that in serum is disproportionately high because of

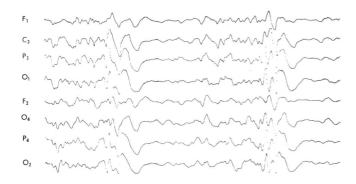

FIG. 6.13. Subacute sclerosing panencephalitis. Electroencephalogram in a 5-year-old boy, showing characteristic suppression bursts. Unipolar leads, F1, C3, P3, O1, left frontal, central, parietal, and occipital leads; F2, C4, P4, O2, right frontal, central, parietal, and occipital leads.

intrathecal production of antibody. CSF pleocytosis can be absent or minimal, with a variable proportion of mononuclear cells.

The EEG is characteristic. Paroxysmal bursts of high-voltage diphasic activity 2- to 3-seconds duration occur synchronously throughout the tracing and are often associated with spike discharges. They are followed by a short period of flattened activity. The entire pattern, termed a *suppression burst* (Fig. 6.13), occurs in approximately 80% of patients (953). These discharges are believed to arise from the mesencephalic activating system or the subcortical area adjacent to the thalamus (954). The background activity can be normal initially; later, it becomes disorganized. These EEG abnormalities can be seen as early as 4 years before the clinical appearance of myoclonus (955). Terminally, paroxysmal activity can decrease, or it can disappear completely with periods of hyperpyrexia. The myoclonic contractions can coincide with the paroxysmal bursts observed by EEG, or they can be disassociated from them. During sleep, the myoclonic discharges disappear, but the paroxysmal EEG bursts continue.

Diagnosis

The clinical picture of intellectual deterioration associated with myoclonic seizures and the presence of suppression bursts suggests SSPE. The diagnosis is confirmed by the strikingly elevated levels of measles antibodies in the serum and CSF.

SSPE should be distinguished from subacute measles encephalitis with immunosuppression

measles inclusion body encephalitis (MIBE), which occurs in children with immunocompromised cellular immunity. One to 6 months after exposure to measles virus, a neurologic disorder can develop with seizures, neurologic deficits, stupor, coma, and death over a period of a few days to a few weeks. Seizures, often severe, may take the form of epilepsia partialis continua. The CSF can have no abnormalities and no elevation in measles antibody titers, although measles virus can be demonstrated in the brain. Eosinophilic inclusions occur in the neurons and glia. Variable degrees of necrosis and a paucity of inflammation are found in the brain (956,957). Quantitative differences occur in the pattern of measles mRNA expression in brain tissue with restricted expression of envelope proteins (M, F, and H) (958).

SSPE also should be differentiated from the group of late infantile or juvenile lipidoses (see Chapter 1), progressive rubella panencephalitis, and the various degenerations of white matter. Affected children frequently have a history of recent falls, which suggests cerebral trauma or akinetic seizures. Occasionally, patients can demonstrate lateralizing neurologic signs, or less commonly, papilledema, findings that can lead to an erroneous diagnosis of an intracranial space-occupying lesion.

Treatment

No adequate therapy is currently available. Non-randomized studies suggest, but by no means confirm, that isoprinosine can prolong life in patients with SSPE (959). Anlar and coworkers recommend intraventricular interferon and oral isoprinosine, especially for those with slowly progressive disease (960). Administration of human interferon alone to patients with SSPE has been of uncertain benefit in cases of mild progression and did not alter the course of patients with rapid deterioration (961). Carbamazepine is of some benefit for myoclonus-induced falling episodes (962).

Progressive Rubella Panencephalitis

A chronically progressive panencephalitis, appearing after congenital or acquired rubella, has been described in some 12 children and young adults, all male (963,964). The brain shows diffuse destruction of white matter with perivascular mononuclear and plasma cells and with fibrillary astrocytosis. Moderate neuronal loss occurs, and microglial nodules are present. Inclusion bodies have not been found. Cerebellar involvement is prominent (965).

Symptoms appear 4 to 14 years after the rubella infection. Initially, an insidiously progressive dementia occurs, followed by progressive pyramidal and extrapyramidal deficits. Truncal ataxia and myoclonic seizures are often prominent. The condition progresses over several years and is ultimately fatal.

The EEG demonstrates high-voltage slow-wave activity without the periodicity characteristic of SSPE (963). Examination of the CSF reveals mononuclear pleocytosis and an elevation of protein. Oligoclonal IgG constitutes 30% to 52% of the total CSF protein, indicating considerable antibody production within the brain (863). Oligoclonal IgG antibodies to rubella virus also are present in serum (966).

Rubella virus has been isolated from brain and peripheral leukocytes (967). The persistence of circulating interferon and IgM antibody to rubella, the presence of circulating immune complexes in serum, and the presence in serum of a possible blocking factor of lymphocyte cytotoxicity for rubella-infected target cells imply that unusual immune responses play a role in this disorder (968). A serum inhibitor of interferon production by normal donor lymphocytes is present on stimulation with rubella antigen (969).

Diagnosis is suggested by the presence of high rubella antibody titers in serum and CSF, and a reduced serum to CSF antibody ratio when compared with other viral agents. Management is symptomatic.

LEPROSY

More than 5.5 million patients suffer from leprosy worldwide, with an incidence of approximately 1 million new patients per year (970). A majority of affected patients live in underdeveloped countries, but increasing numbers of affected patients live in North America and Europe, largely because of increasing immigration and travel. Although drug treatment is now effective in achieving microbiological cure and reducing transmission, approximately 25% of survivors are left with chronic disability (971).

Infection with *Mycobacterium leprae* is probably only acquired from contact with infected individuals discharging viable organisms. Infection rates are highest in children living in close proximity to patients with lepromatous leprosy who excrete large numbers of bacilli. A naturally occurring leprosy-like disease among wild armadillos and the detection of living *M. leprae* in mosquitoes suggest that non-human reservoirs of leprosy may exist, and that in some instances an intermediate host is involved (972).

The spectrum of clinical disease is broad and depends on the individual's immune response to the bacillus. The disease can be classified clinically and histologically into five stages: full lepromatous, borderline lepromatous, borderline, borderline tuberculoid, and full tuberculoid (973). Patients with lepromatous leprosy have extensive disease that is often bilateral, with large numbers of bacilli present in the lesions and nasal secretions and associated with multiple erythematous macules, papules, or nodules. Nerve involvement in lepromatous disease is diffuse but less severe than in tuberculoid cases. Palpable nerve thickening is uncommon and sensory loss is patchy, typically a mononeuritis multiplex (974). In these lesions messenger RNAs coding for IL-4, IL-5, and IL-10 predominate (975).

Tuberculoid leprosy is characterized by isolated disease, with large erythematous plaques that have sharply demarcated outer edges. The center of the plaques is flattened and the area is anesthetic. Hypopigmented macules can be present. Peripheral nerves can be visibly swollen. In tuberculoid leprosy, bacilli are seldom seen within the lesions and are not present in the nasal secretions. In these lesions, messenger RNAs for IL-2 and interferon-γ are most evident (975). Patients with borderline lepromatous and borderline tuberculoid disease have features between those of lepromatous and tuberculous forms. In all forms of the disease, T cells are Ia-positive, which is evidence for an activated state (976,977).

The histologic features of lepromatous and borderline lepromatous leprosy are poorly formed granulomata that are largely comprised of foamy macrophages (978). Epithelioid cell formation is poorly developed, only scanty lymphocytes are seen, and Langerhans-type giant cells are absent. Large numbers of mycobacteria are visible within the granuloma. Bacilli can be seen extensively proliferating within Schwann cells and perineural cells of nerve bundles, but structural preservation of axons is better than in tuberculoid disease (979). In tuberculoid leprosy, a well-developed granulomatous process has histologic features similar to the lesions of sarcoidosis. Epithelioid cells are prominent, as are Langerhans giant cells. Extensive lymphocyte infiltrates are seen, but bacilli are infrequently seen. Nerve bundles are grossly swollen and infiltrated with mononuclear inflammatory cells. In late cases, there is extensive fibrous replacement of the most distal segments of peripheral nerves, and fibrous plaques can prevent regenerating axons from reaching cutaneous nerves (979).

Immunologic mechanisms underlie the different clinical manifestations of the disease. Patients with lepromatous leprosy are anergic to *M. leprae* and have a generalized impairment of delayed T-cell hypersensitivity responses (980). Immunoglobulin levels are markedly increased, indicating a polyclonal proliferative response, and a variety of autoimmune phenomenon may be present including a false-positive VDRL test, autoantibodies to testicular germinal cells and thyroglobulin, and positive antinuclear factor or rheumatoid factor (980,981). Patients with tuberculoid leprosy have positive lepromin reactions and exhibit normal delayed T-cell hypersensitivity tests to other antigens (982).

Reversal reactions are seen when patients with borderline leprosy are treated and probably present an increasing inflammatory response caused by the acquisition of T-cell immunity to the mycobacteria (983). Lepromatous skin lesions may rapidly develop brawny, raised induration, and in some cases ulceration. There is worsening of the neuritis, with swelling of the nerve and loss of motor function. Reversal reactions entail a reduction in the number of bacilli, extensive edema formation, and an increase in the number of lymphocytes in the inflammatory infiltrate.

The neurologic consequences of leprosy range from isolated anesthetic areas caused by denervation, to severe peripheral neuropathy with loss of both sensory and motor functions (984). The neurologic lesions of leprosy are of three types (985,986). Purely sensory polyneuritis results in loss of light touch, light pain, and temperature sense in a glove-and-stocking distribution, whereas deep pressure and deep pain, vibration, and joint sense are preserved. Sensory polyneuritis can occur without characteristic skin lesions. A less common lesion is a mixed sensory polyneuritis and mononeuritis with paralysis in a peripheral nerve distribution and sensory loss more widely distributed than in sensory polyneuritis (987). Rarely, a myositis occurs, or a pure mononeuritis, which results in a motor deficit with a peripheral nerve distribution (988,989).

Symptoms can begin abruptly or develop insidiously. Peripheral nerve trunks can become enlarged, hard, and tender. The most commonly involved nerves include the ulnar nerve just above the elbow, the lateral popliteal nerve at the neck of the fibula, the posterior tibial nerve behind the internal malleolus, and the great auricular nerve. Intense neuralgia or shooting pains can precede impairment of sensation (987). In addition to the sensory loss, sudomotor dysfunction with anhidrosis is commonly seen in the absence of evidence of vasomotor abnormality. Ocular complications are extremely common and approximately 2% of infected patients are blind (990). Reversal reactions occurring in borderline leprosy, often during the initial months of treatment, may result in damage to trigeminal and facial nerves. Facial nerve dysfunction causes inability to close the eyes fully. This causes exposure keratitis and progressive scarring over the lower half of the cornea, which may ultimately result in blindness. Involvement of the trigeminal nerve also may cause hypoanesthesia, and traumatic damage to the cornea may result. The eye may be directly involved by acute uveitis and episcleritis as a component of erythema nodosum leprosum, or by the presence of ocular lepromas. Dysfunctional and anesthetic limbs are extremely susceptible to damage, and serious deformities with destruction to limbs and digits are often the result.

The diagnosis of leprosy should be considered in patients presenting with dermatologic, neurologic, or multisystem complaints, who have come from parts of the world where the disease is endemic. Hypoesthesic or anesthetic skin lesions, with or without associated nerve thickenings, are important diagnostic clues. The diagnosis can be confirmed by skin biopsy, which should include both a central and peripheral area of the lesion, and which should be examined histologically, including with mycobacterial stains.

The management of leprosy remains difficult. The treatment regimen and the adverse reactions to treatment are beyond the scope of this text. The interested reader is referred to reviews by Jacobson and Krahenbuhl (973), Nations and colleagues (991), and Willcox (992).

Damage to nerves frequently progresses or worsens after the initiation of treatment, particularly in patients with lepromatous or borderline lepromatous disease. Patients undergoing reversal reactions are treated with corticosteroids to reduce the inflammatory response.

SPIROCHETAL INFECTIONS

Leptospirosis

Leptospirosis, caused by *Leptospira icterohaemorrhagiae*, *L. canicola*, *L. pomona*, or *L. grippotyphosa*, is an uncommon cause of meningitis. It is characterized by sudden onset of fever, muscle

pain, articular symptoms, epigastric pain, and headache. Hemorrhagic symptoms can occur. Jaundice, hepatosplenomegaly, and renal damage are common. Single or multiple relapses occur, but almost all patients recover.

Signs of meningeal irritation occur in approximately 10% of patients (993,994). These commence between the fifth and fourteenth days of the illness, most often by the end of the first week. Symptoms are of variable severity and do not correlate with the severity of other manifestations of the infection. Symptoms subside in 1 to 14 days.

CSF pleocytosis is usually below 500 white blood cells per L, with a progressive increase in the proportion of mononuclear cells. It can persist for several weeks. Protein can range from normal to 140 mg/dL. Leptospiral meningitis is regarded as an antigen-antibody reaction; this explains the absence of early CSF pleocytosis, the abrupt onset of meningeal symptoms toward the end of the first week of illness, the rapid disappearance of leptospires after the onset of meningitis, and the uniformly good prognosis (995). A severe form of encephalitis, myelitis, and peripheral neuritis caused by leptospirosis, has been seen on rare occasions (996). CNS involvement can occur without evidence of renal dysfunction or jaundice (996).

Leptospirosis is diagnosed by isolation of the organism or by antibody studies. Penicillin is the drug of choice. It is given for 7 days and appears to be effective, even when started late in the course of the illness (997).

Syphilis

The resurgence of syphilis throughout the world gives added importance to congenital and acquired cases of neurosyphilis seen in infancy or childhood.

Pathology and Pathogenesis

The pathology of congenital neurosyphilis resembles that of the acquired forms (998). Syphilitic infection can be transmitted to the fetus any time during gestation, but it usually is transmitted during the fourth through seventh months. Of the children of untreated syphilitic mothers, 25% to 80% develop syphilis; clinical signs of congenital neurosyphilis occur in 2% to 16% of these.

Neurosyphilis takes either the meningovascular or the parenchymatous form. In both forms, the infectious process begins in the meninges as a widespread diffuse arachnoiditis with inflammation concentrated around the meningeal vessels and the branches that penetrate into the cortex. Small meningeal vessels can show thickening and infiltration of the adventitia, as well as intimal proliferation; syphilitic phlebitis is less common, although both can result in infarction with localized lesions of the brain or spinal cord.

Obstructive or communicating hydrocephalus can result from meningeal fibrosis and obliteration of the subarachnoid spaces.

Diffuse meningeal inflammation of the secondary stage can be carried over into the tertiary stage with increased fibrosis of the meninges and the formation of small, often miliary gummas.

In parenchymatous congenital syphilis, as in juvenile paresis, diffuse degeneration occurs with cerebral and cerebellar atrophy. Microscopic changes include round cell meningeal and perivascular infiltration, loss and degenerative changes in the nerve cells with an increase in microglia and astroglia, a disturbance of normal cytoarchitecture, deposition of iron pigment, and presence of spirochetes.

Clinical Manifestations

The CNS becomes involved during the first few months or years of life. In 50% to 80% of cases of congenital neurosyphilis, one or more of the stigmata of congenital syphilis are present. These include interstitial keratitis, chorioretinitis, defective teeth, malformed or "saddle" nose, frontal bossing of the skull, saber shins, Clutton joints, and rhagades, either singly or in combination. Nerve deafness, which when seen with dental deformities and interstitial keratitis forms the classic Hutchinson triad, is infrequent. Painful bone involvement can cause pseudoparalysis. Syphilitic meningitis is more common during the first few months of postnatal life,

whereas vascular syndromes are prevalent during the first 2 years of life.

Syphilitic meningitis usually appears between ages 3 and 12 months with a sudden onset of convulsions, listlessness, apathy, vomiting, feeding difficulties, or progressive enlargement of the head. Nuchal rigidity, a full fontanel, head retraction, various cranial nerve palsies with optic atrophy, or strabismus can develop in the course of the illness.

Chronic syphilitic meningitis can give rise to hydrocephalus. Rarely present at birth, hydrocephalus usually develops progressively at 9 to 12 months, sometimes accompanied by cranial nerve deficits. Congenital cerebrovascular syphilis can result in diverse vascular syndromes because of arteritis and thrombosis of cerebral vessels (998,999).

Mental deficiency, mental subnormality, and behavior disorders are more common in subjects with congenital syphilis than in the general population, not because of the infection itself, but because of other hereditary and environmental factors (1000).

Tertiary congenital syphilis begins after some 5 to 25 years of infection, the same interval as for acquired syphilis. Juvenile paresis is the most common form of congenital tertiary neurosyphilis. It usually begins between ages 6 and 21 years, the average age of occurrence being 13 years. Male and female subjects are affected equally often. The onset of juvenile paresis in children with marked mental retardation is vague and impossible to date. When the children are moderately retarded or of normal intelligence, onset of juvenile paresis is marked by loss of previous accomplishments.

Patients with juvenile paresis most commonly have simple mental deterioration characterized by regression, confusion, flattened affect, and restless, purposive behavior. The neurologic syndromes of juvenile paresis are more diverse and advanced than those of acquired paresis, and in 25% of cases, cerebellar deficits are conspicuous. In 50% of children, one or more limbs are spastic. Seizures occur in 30% to 40%. Spinal cord involvement indicating taboparesis is present in 10% to 15% of cases. Optic atrophy with or without chorioretinitis is present in 12% to 18%, compared with an incidence of 5% in the acquired form of disease. The facial nerve is involved in 10% of cases, the auditory nerve in 2%, and the hypoglossal nerve in approximately 10% to 15%. Other deficits and multiple cranial nerve deficits can occur also. Untreated, the disease steadily progresses to death in 2 to 5 years.

Tabes dorsalis is rare in congenital syphilis and eventually develops in only 1.5% to 9.0% of those afflicted. Its age of onset corresponds to that of congenital paretic neurosyphilis. Often the first symptom is failing vision or urinary incontinence, which is often nocturnal. Approximately one-half of the cases have cranial nerve palsies; strabismus is common. Pupillary abnormalities are almost always present; the pupils are usually dilated and fixed, although Argyll Robertson pupils can occur. Lightning pains and gastric crises are relatively uncommon, and ataxia and arthropathies are rare.

The clinical course of tabes dorsalis is mild, and many of the cases are discovered during routine examination of syphilitic children.

Diagnosis

The diagnosis of active neurosyphilis is based on serologic evidence of treponemal infection, demonstration of *Treponema pallidum* DNA by PCR or by rabbit infectivity testing (1001). Serum and CSF treponema antibody tests provide evidence of past infection, but give no information about CNS activity (1002). The CSF in paretic neurosyphilis shows a mononuclear pleocytosis ranging from 10 to 100 cells per μL, with the degree of pleocytosis being an indicator of disease activity. In 80% of cases, the protein content is elevated, with a disproportionate rise in γ-globulin and the presence of oligoclonal banding (1002). Contamination of CSF with as little as 0.008 μL/mL of fluorescent treponemal antibody absorption test (FTA-ABS)–reactive blood (equivalent to adding 43 red blood cells to 1 mL of CSF) can result in a false-positive FTA reaction (1003). The specificity of the CSF VDRL in diagnosing probably active neurosyphilis is 100%, but its sensitivity is only 27%. The insensitivity of the CSF VDRL limits its usefulness as a screening test for neurosyphilis. The CSF FTA-ABS is more sensitive for screening, but its lack of specificity in distinguishing active neurosyphilis from past syphitic infections necessitates the use of clinical judgment based on clinical history, clinical findings, and CSF evaluation (1004). The presence of maternal reagin or immunoglobulins passively transferred to the newborn renders early diagnosis of congenital syphilis more difficult. The presence of elevated IgM levels in the newborn is indirect evidence of prenatal infection. Assay for both specific neonatal IgM antibody and *T. pallidum* DNA in the serum and CSF is recommended for the diagnosis of asymptomatic infected neonates (1005). Demonstration of IgM FTA reactivity is specific for fetal infection (1006), but is positive in only approximately 40% of asymptomatic infected neonates (1001).

Inadvertent partial therapy can render the VDRL test result negative, whereas the serum FTA or treponema pallidum immobilization (TPI) test result remains positive.

The differential diagnosis of juvenile paresis is that of any progressive degenerative disease of the nervous system with onset in childhood (see Chapter 1). Thus, leukodystrophies and the various lipid storage disorders should be among possible conditions to be considered.

Treatment

Penicillin G is the drug of choice for treatment of all stages of neurosyphilis (1002). Details of treatment are beyond the scope of this text. The reader is referred to the *Red Book* of the American Academy of Pediatrics (1007).

Recommended follow-up for children younger than age 2 years is clinical examination and quantitative VDRL titer at 2, 4, 6, 12, and 24 months. Quantitative VDRL titers should be followed until they become nonreactive. CSF should be rechecked 1 year after completion of treatment.

If CSF serologies are nonreactive in children with congenital syphilis older than 2 years, qualitative serologic tests for syphilis should be done at 6-month intervals for 2 years. If CSF serology is reactive, quantitative serologic tests for syphilis and CSF examinations should be done quarterly for 1 year, then semiannually for two additional years. The disease is regarded as inactive in the nervous system when the cell count and protein level have returned to normal. Serofast cases should be observed carefully. Persistence of serologic titer does not necessarily mean that previous therapy was inadequate or that additional treatment is indicated.

Lyme Disease

Lyme disease is caused by a spirochete, *Borrelia burgdorferi*. At least four genospecies are recognized throughout the world, each with its own degree of virulence (1008). The organism can be isolated from blood, skin lesions, brain, or CSF of infected patients. It also has been isolated from the nymphal and adult forms of its vectors, *Ixodes scapularis* and *I. pacificus* (1008–1010). In Europe, another common vector is *I. ricinus* (1011). A bimodal age of distribution of Lyme disease occurs in the United States, with the highest incidence rates in children aged 5 to 9 years and in adults older than 30 (1008). Lyme neuroborreliosis occurs once in every 620 infected children (1012).

The pathology of neuroborreliosis is highlighted by an inflammatory thrombotic vasculopathy that can cause axonal degeneration of the peripheral nerves through involvement of vasa nervorum and causes ischemic lesions of the CNS (1012). Large areas of demyelination in periventricular white matter as well as lymphocytic vasculitis has been found in fatal cases (1013). Cellular and humoral autoimmune mechanisms also are important, and the serum of infected patients contains IgM antibodies that cross-react with an axonal component (1014).

Three stages of Lyme disease have been distinguished. The first stage is highlighted by the presence of a unique skin lesion, erythema chronicum migrans, which can be accompanied by fatigue (54%), myalgia (44%), arthralgia (44%), fever, chills, or both (39%), arthralgias, malaise, fatigue, myalgia, lymphadenopathy, and symptoms that suggest meningeal irritation: headache (42%) and neck stiffness (35%). The rash may not occur in some 10% to 20% of patients (1008,1010,1011,1015). The second

stage features systemic involvement. A variety of neurologic complications develop during this stage in some 15% to 20% of patients. The third stage is seen in untreated patients 1 to 3 years after the initial infection. It is marked by chronic arthritis, but a variety of neurologic complications also can be encountered.

The neurologic symptoms and signs of neuroborreliosis are protean and can involve any portion of the neuraxis. In Europe, more than 80% of childhood neuroborreliosis manifests as facial palsy or an aseptic meningitis (154,1012). A predominantly mononuclear CSF pleocytosis occurs in 95% of children with neuroborreliosis (1012). Oligoclonal IgG antibodies are found in the CSF in only one-third of children (1012). Facial palsy usually occurs ipsilateral to a tick bite on the head or neck, but it can be bilateral (1016). It may develop during the first week of treatment, but this does not constitute treatment failure (1008). Additionally, one encounters a variety of cranial neuropathies other than that of the facial nerve (1012,1017,1018), a spastic or flaccid paralysis, chorea, cerebellar dysfunction, seizures, and a radiculoneuritis (1019,1020). A predominantly mononuclear CSF pleocytosis occurs in 95% of children with neuroborreliosis (1012). A chronic lymphocytic meningitis has been seen in approximately 6% of children. It can last up to 6 years. Meningeal signs are rare despite significant CSF changes (1021). A clinical picture similar to Guillain-Barré clinical picture occurs in 1.8% of children (1006,1010). It is atypical in that it can have CSF pleocytosis in the range of 35 to 120 cells per μL, with 60% to 100% mononuclear cells (1022). Rarely, cases present with pseudotumor cerebri (1023). Painful lymphocytic meningoradiculoneuritis (Bannwarth syndrome) has been associated serologically with Lyme disease (1024). This expression of the disease is much more common in Europe than in the United States where headache and stiff neck and subtle encephalitic signs with less radiculopathy are more likely (1011). On rare occasions, an acute focal meningoencephalitis (1025) or an acute psychosis (1026) can be the first signs of the disease. Lyme neuroborreliosis can be difficult to distinguish from viral meningitis. The presence of cranial neuropathies, papilledema, or erythema migrans are characteristics that should suggest Lyme disease (1026a).

A chronic course occurs in 6% of children. A wide spectrum of abnormalities also are seen during this, the third stage of Lyme disease. A subacute encephalopathy is the most common neurologic complication. It is characterized by cognitive deficits and disturbances of mood and sleep (1010,1027). A destructive chronic meningoencephalitis can progress over many years in untreated individuals (1028). A chronic lymphocytic meningitis or a subacute encephalitis also can accompany this stage of the disease (1026,1027). Chronic meningoradiculomyelitis has been associated with persistent intrathecal secretion of oligoclonal *Borrelia burgdorferi*-specific IgG (1029,1030). However, radiculitis with pathologic changes of peripheral neuropathy can occur without intrathecal synthesis of specific antibody (1031). In addition to arthritis, an occasional case can present as Shulman syndrome (eosinophilic fasciitis) (1032).

In comparison with adults, children with neuroborreliosis have less common and milder radicular pain, less facial diplegia, but more often have headache, clinical signs of meningitis, and fever. Monosymptomatic paresis, usually facial paresis, without concomitant pain, fever, or neck stiffness occurs almost exclusively in children (1033).

EEG changes, usually in the form of moderate generalized slowing, occur in approximately one-third of children with Lyme neuroborreliosis. Children with facial palsy caused by Lyme disease have abnormal EEGs more often than those with idiopathic facial palsy, or facial palsy caused by other causes. It also is of diagnostic significance that nearly all children with facial palsy caused by Lyme disease have CSF pleocytosis, or intrathecal production of antibodies to *B. burgdorferi* (whereas only 11.7% of children with facial palsy caused by unknown causes have CSF pleocytosis) (1034).

MRI scans can show punctate areas of increased signal in white matter of the cerebral hemispheres on both T1- and T2-weighted images (1020,1029,1035).

The diagnosis of acute childhood Lyme neuroborreliosis is most reliably made by demonstrating the presence of IgM antibodies to *B. burgdorferi* (1012), or by PCR, a more sensitive method. Tests on CSF may give false-negative results because of strain variation or false-positive results in the absence of active infection (154). In some cases the comparison of antibody content for equal amounts of serum and CSF IgG confirms intrathecal *Borrelia* antibody production (1021). Oligoclonal IgG antibodies are found in the CSF in only one-third of children (1012). Serologic diagnosis is not always reliable because seronegative Lyme disease can occur in patients with vigorous T-cell proliferative responses to whole *B. burgdorferi* organisms (1029,1036). After effective therapy the presence of specific activated IgM class B cells, an indication of acute disease, is the earliest marker to disappear (1037). Although in some cases Western blot and ELISA may be discordant, positive results from both tests strongly support the diagnosis of Lyme disease (1038).

The paradox of the difficulty in demonstrating the causative agent within the neuraxis in the face of significant neurologic dysfunction can perhaps be explained by the presence of neuroactive kyurenines elicited by immune stimulation. Levels of quinolinic acid, an excitotoxin and an N-methyl-D-aspartate agonist, are substantially elevated in CSF of patients with CNS Lyme disease and correlate with CSF leukocytosis (1039). Direct invasion of the CNS has been confirmed by demonstration of *B. burgdorferi* DNA in areas with inflammatory changes (1013).

For early disease, doxycycline (100 mg twice daily) is the preferred drug for children 8 years of age or older; for younger children, penicillin V or amoxicillin (25 mg to 50 mg/kg per day in three divided doses, maximum 1 g to 2 g per day) is recommended (1040). Treatment is recommended for 14 to 21 days (1040). Treatment for 21 to 28 days is recommended for isolated facial palsy (1040). In the later stages of the disease, high-dose intravenous penicillin is used. Ceftriaxone (75 mg to 100 mg/kg, intravenously or intramuscularly once daily, maximum 2 g per day), cefotaxime, or intravenous penicillin G (300,000 U/kg per day given in divided doses every 4 hours for 14 to 21 days, maximum 20 million U/d) are recommended for the treatment of meningitis or encephalitis (1041,1042). Treatment within the first year of infection results in a more favorable clinical response than later therapy, and probably reduces the incidence of neurologic complications attributable to the disease (1012,1043). Lyme radiculoneuritis has responded to intravenous gamma globulin (1044).

Lyme borreliosis can cause long-term residual cognitive deficits in verbal memory, mental flexibility, verbal associative functions, and articulation (1045).

Tick-Borne Relapsing Fever

Tick-borne relapsing fever is caused by spirochetes of the genus *Borrelia* that can vary their surface antigens extensively. Neurologic involvement occurs in 5% to 10% of patients (1046).

Mycoplasma Infections

Although *Mycoplasma* species, usually *M. pneumoniae*, are generally implicated in pneumonia and other respiratory tract infections, the organisms also produce neurologic disease in up to 0.1% of infections and in 7% of *Mycoplasma*-infected subjects treated in hospitals (1047). CNS disease can be caused by direct CNS invasion, microthromboembolism, or an immune-mediated disseminated encephalomyelitis (583,1048).

Male subjects are more commonly affected by a factor of 4 (1049). Neurologic complications of *M. pneumoniae* infections can be divided into seven categories: encephalitis, myelitis, meningitis or meningoencephalitis, encephalomyelitis, cranial neuritis or radiculitis, Guillain-Barré syndrome, and vascular problems. Meningeal, cerebral, brainstem, spinal cord, and nerve root involvement can occur singly or in combination (1050).

Cerebral involvement with an altered mental state and a nonfocal or focal encephalitis is the most common neurologic manifestation of a *Mycoplasma* infection. Symptoms include seizures, somnolence, or changes in consciousness. Encephalitis can be focal and involve principally the putamen and head of the caudate nucleus

with symptoms of drowsiness, seizures, bradykinesia, dysarthria, ocular movement disorders, and dysphagia. Convulsions occur in 51% of children. Status epilepticus can develop with tonic-clonic seizures that often last for hours, sometimes for days. Ataxia was noted in 19% of children in a Finnish series (1047). An encephalitis lethargica-like illness also has been seen (1051). Other, less common manifestations of CNS involvement with *Mycoplasma* include cranial nerve dysfunction (1052), an ascending paralysis (Guillain-Barré syndrome) (583), and stroke resulting from occlusion of the internal carotid artery (1052). Myalgias and arthralgias are encountered in 15% to 45% of cases. Neonatal infections of the CNS can occur (1053,1054) and can complicate a severe intraventricular hemorrhage (1055).

An EEG obtained in the first week after onset of illness shows severe generalized disturbance in 58% of children. During the second to fourth week after onset, the EEG abnormality becomes worse in 25% of patients (1047). Serial EEGs initially may show bilateral periodic lateralized epileptiform discharges that subsequently are replaced by other abnormalities (1056).

Myelitis can be symptomatic (1057) or can be associated with clinically silent lesions demonstrable by MRI (1058).

In the meningitis-meningoencephalitis group the CSF can be normal or show a marked pleocytosis of up to 4,000 white blood cells per μL. In the Finnish series of pediatric patients with *Mycoplasma* encephalitis, the CSF was normal during the first week of illness in 70% of patients. CSF protein ranged from normal to 164 mg/dL (1047). The cranial neuritis-radiculitis group is characterized by a more modest CSF pleocytosis that decreases more slowly. Although symptoms usually remit in 4 to 10 weeks, pleocytosis of up to 60 white blood cells per μL can persist for 6 to 24 weeks, but rarely longer. CSF IgM elevation occurs in all patients except those with Guillain-Barré syndrome. Blood–brain barrier disruption, which is demonstrated by elevation in lipoprotein, albumin, or α_2-microglobulin, occurs in most cases (1059).

The diagnosis of a *Mycoplasma* infection rests on elevation of the *M. pneumoniae* complement fixation (1060) or specific IgG or IgM antibody titers (1061). The increase in titer commences 7 to 9 days after the onset of symptoms and peaks at 3 to 4 weeks. IgM antibody persists for approximately 15 months, whereas CF and IgG antibodies persist for approximately 3 years (1060,1061). A fourfold rise in titer is necessary for diagnosis. An increase in cold agglutinin titers is less reliable. CNS infection can be confirmed by demonstration of *Mycoplasma pneumoniae* DNA in CSF using the method of nested PCR (1062). Isolation of organisms from CSF is rarely successful.

Antimicrobial therapy has been ineffective in modifying the course of neurologic complications (1060).

Recovery is often slow and can require many months of hospitalization. Patients having focal encephalitis or nerve root involvement run the greatest risk for residua. In the Finnish series, the mortality was 10%. Severe neurologic damage such as psychomotor retardation, movement disorders, choreoathetosis, or recurrent convulsions occurred in 24% of patients. Only 52% of patients had recovered completely by 2 to 26 weeks after discharge (1047). One-third of patients who recover have permanent or persistent defects.

MYCOTIC INFECTIONS OF THE NERVOUS SYSTEM

Mycotic infections of the nervous system lead to a chronic granulomatous meningitis or abscesses. The infection can be primary, or more commonly, secondary to diabetes or other chronic illnesses, immune deficiency, debilitation, or an infection elsewhere in the body that requires antibiotic therapy (1063).

Candidiasis

Candida albicans can produce candidemia and subsequent meningitis in infants born with major congenital anomalies such as intestinal malrotation and meconium ileus, or it can complicate ventriculoatrial shunt created for hydrocephalus (1064). *Candida* meningitis also is an uncommon complication of prolonged antibiotic or corticosteroid therapy, irradiation,

immune suppression, total parenteral alimentation, surgery, or extensive burns (1065,1066). When *Candida* is the primary invader of the nervous system, it usually progresses to gross abscess formation; patients in whom it is a secondary invader complicating antibiotic therapy can develop diffuse cerebritis with widespread microabscesses (1067). These microabscesses are found throughout the brain in association with other granulomalike lesions containing epithelioid and giant cells. Meningeal inflammation also can occur. *Candida* can invade the walls of blood vessels, with granulomatous vasculitis and resulting thrombi formation producing necrosis and hemorrhages (1067). Because candidal infection cannot be reliably diagnosed from CSF changes, culture of the organism from the CSF or from biopsies is needed for diagnosis. The subacute course, lack of a characteristic clinical picture, variable CSF findings, difficulty in recovering the organism from the CNS and its slow *in vitro* growth, and misinterpretation of positive cultures as representing contaminants all contribute to a delay in diagnosis (1066).

The combination of amphotericin B and 5-flucytosine is the treatment of choice (1068). This combination takes advantage of a synergistic effect and permits lower and less toxic doses of amphotericin (1065,1068). Fluconazole, an oral antifungal drug, is better tolerated than 5-fluorocytosine and has been advocated as an alternative for amphotericin B in immunocompetent patients with candidemia (1069).

Coccidioidomycosis

Coccidioides immitis can produce a chronic meningitis, usually by inhalation of the spore form. The disease is endemic to the southwestern United States. The infection rate is particularly high in California's southern San Joaquin Valley, southern Nevada, central and southern Arizona, southern New Mexico, and throughout western Texas along the Mexican border. Outside of the United States, a high infection rate also exists in the northern states of Mexico, Honduras, Venezuela, and the Chaco region of Bolivia, Paraguay, and Argentina (1070).

Symptoms are mainly headache, low-grade fever, weight loss, progressive obtundation, and minimal meningeal signs (1071). Multiple sites of obstruction can develop, particularly at the outlets of the fourth ventricle and the upper parts of the spinal cord, leading to hydrocephalus and isolation of these regions from therapy (1072). Patients with active or untreated disease usually have hydrocephalus and intense enhancement of the cervical subarachnoid space, basilar, sylvian, and interhemispheric cisterns on postcontrast MRI scans. Focal areas of ischemia or infarction are common (1073).

The CSF is almost always abnormal. Mononuclear pleocytosis ranges up to more than 1,000 cells per μL. The protein is usually elevated, whereas the glucose concentration is reduced in approximately 75% of cases (1070). *Coccidioides* spherules can be recognized in the CSF by direct examination using lactophenol cotton blue or India ink preparations, or after culture.

The diagnosis of coccidioidomycosis is suggested by the presence of pulmonary lesions. A skin test result is usually positive, but can be misleading because some disseminated cases are nonreactive. The complement fixation and precipitin tests assist in the diagnosis. The precipitin test result becomes negative after approximately 3 to 4 months, however, regardless of the progression of the disease (1074).

Amphotericin B has traditionally been the recommended antibiotic for the treatment of coccidioidal meningitis. Details of treatment are given in the *Red Book* of the American Academy of Pediatrics (1075). Fluconazole, one of a series of antifungal azoles, is an effective and well-tolerated drug, which is successful in arresting the progress of the disease (1069,1076). According to Kauffman, it has replaced amphotericin as the drug of choice (1077). In addition, several lipid formulations of amphotericin that are less nephrotoxic came on the market in the late 1990s (1078). Most improvement occurs within 4 to 8 months after the start of therapy. Relapses can occur after discontinuation of prolonged therapy (1069,1079).

Coccidioidomycosis meningitis is rarely completely eradicated. Intensive follow-up is necessary, and repeated courses of antifungal therapy are required to suppress the infection.

Histoplasmosis

Histoplasmosis, caused by *Histoplasma capsulatum*, is endemic to the northeastern, central, and south-central United States (1070). CNS involvement is seen only after disseminated involvement, although clinical signs of dissemination may be lacking. It occurs in approximately one-fourth of cases with signs of clinical dissemination, and in 7.6% of all *Histoplasma* infections (1080).

Infants and children younger than age 3 years can have systemic signs, including fever, anemia, or hepatosplenomegaly, and, less often, weight loss, adenopathy, or cough. Neurologic symptoms are usually absent. Older children can have tetany or pyramidal tract signs (1080). The CSF is abnormal in all age groups. Hyperactive T-suppressor cells in CSF can suppress proliferative responses to *Histoplasma* antigen, whereas T cells from blood do not. This difference can result in a selective lack of cellular and humoral response in some patients (1081).

Brain changes include the formation of granulomas within the parenchyma or in the perivenous regions, a meningitis that most often involves the basilar regions, and the formation of isolated abscesses. Cerebral or spinal mass lesions may resemble neoplasms (1082).

Skin tests or complement fixation tests are generally used for the diagnosis of *Histoplasma* infections. The results are often negative in patients with CNS disease, however, and a bone marrow biopsy is probably the best diagnostic procedure currently available (1080).

Treatment with amphotericin B is similar to the treatment for coccidioidomycosis. Fluconazole, itraconazole, and to a lesser extent, other azoles, have proven effective alternatives to amphotericin B for *Histoplasma* meningitis (1069,1077,1083).

Cryptococcosis

Cryptococcosis is one of the most common fungal infections of the nervous system. It is caused by *Cryptococcus neoformans*, an organism that is

TABLE 6.18. *Characteristics of rarer fungal infections of the nervous system*

Organism (disease)	Major central nervous system symptoms	Therapy	Reference
Actinomyces bovis (actinomycosis)	Chronic low-grade meningitis, abscesses	Penicillin, tetracycline, surgical drainage	1095
Aspergillus niger (aspergillosis)	Multiple brain abscesses, vascular thromboses	Amphotericin B	1063,1096
Aspergillus fumigatus	Meningoencephalitis, single or multiple brain abscesses, granulomas, myelopathy	Amphotericin B	1097,1098
Blastomyces dermatitidis (blastomycosis)	Meningitis	Amphotericin B, ketoconazole	1099
Cephalosporium granulomatis	Meningitis	Amphotericin B	1100
Phycomycetes rhizopus (mucormycosis)	Thromboses of cerebral and meningeal arteries	Amphotericin B	1101,1102
Nocardia asteroides (nocardiosis)	Meningitis, multiple focal abscesses	Sulfadiazine or trimethoprim-sulfamethoxazole	1103–1105

widely distributed and is often isolated from soil, particularly in the vicinity of pigeon nests (1063).

The pathologic changes in the brain vary. Some areas have only minimal inflammation, whereas others have pseudotubercles composed of giant cells, epithelioid cells, and lymphocytes. Patients with cryptococcal meningitis have significantly lower natural killer cytotoxic activity of their peripheral blood mononuclear leukocytes. This can be fully reconstituted *in vitro* with IL-2, but not with interferon-γ (1084).

The infection is rare in children. Adults are more commonly involved because of greater exposure, and because of the predilection of cryptococcal infection for debilitated or immunocompromised individuals.

Symptoms usually reflect meningeal involvement, although, occasionally, neurologic signs or alterations in mental status predominate. Spinal arachnoiditis can occur without meningitis (1085).

The diagnosis is difficult. Approximately one-half of patients with active cryptococcal disease have a negative cryptococcal antigen skin test result. Complement fixation tests, latex agglutination, fluorescent antibody, and hemagglutination tests also have been employed (1086).

The CSF in patients with cryptococcal meningitis resembles the CSF of tuberculous meningitis, with a moderate lymphocytic pleocytosis, increased protein content, and decreased sugar content. The diagnosis depends on culture of organisms from the fluid, or demonstration in CSF of the cryptococcal polysaccharide by latex agglutination tests. Culture-negative meningitis occurs frequently, even in experienced laboratories, although the chance of obtaining a positive culture result is higher if the CSF is dripped directly into the culture medium (1087). India ink preparations are positive in 71% of cases (1088). A latex agglutination test result can be positive, even when organisms cannot be demonstrated by other methods (1089).

Untreated cryptococcal meningitis is fatal within a few months. In immunocompetent patients, combined therapy with amphotericin B and flucytosine is the treatment of choice (1090,1091). Amphotericin B nephrotoxicity can be minimized by use of amphotericin B lipid emulsion, although anaphylaxis has been reported (1092,1093). Plasma levels of flucytosine should be monitored because of the potential for bone marrow suppression (1069). Fluconazole is as effective as amphotericin B for treatment of cryptococcal meningitis in the immunocompromised host (1069,1077,1091,1094).

Some of the rarer fungal infections of the nervous system are summarized in Table 6.18 (995–1105).

RICKETTSIAL INFECTIONS

A number of rickettsial organisms invade the nervous system and produce neurologic symptoms. Based on serologic and clinical characteristics, six major rickettsial entities have been recognized.

The epidemic louse-borne form of typhus fever is caused by *Rickettsia prowazekii*; the endemic murine type is caused by *R. typhi*. Rocky Mountain spotted fever is caused by *R. rickettsii* in the western hemisphere. Scrub typhus is caused by *R. tsutsugamushi* and found in Australasia (Japan, India, and Australia). Q fever is caused by *Coxiella burnetii*. Rickettsialpox is caused by *R. akari*, with the agent being transmitted to humans by the mouse mite. Finally, trench fever is transmitted to humans by the louse and is caused by *R. quintana*.

Rocky Mountain Spotted Fever

In the United States, the most common rickettsial disease is Rocky Mountain spotted fever. This condition has been reported from almost all parts of the United States, notably the Appalachian and the western Rocky Mountain areas. The main vectors for humans are the Rocky Mountain wood tick (*Dermacentor andersoni*); the dog tick (*Dermacentor variabilis*), which is more prevalent in the eastern United States; and the Lone Star tick (*Amblyomma americanum*), which is prevalent in the Gulf states (1106).

The rickettsial organisms invade the human by way of a tick bite followed by contamination by tick feces. Thus, early removal of the tick can prevent the disease. One can best remove a tick by grasping its body with a pair of tweezers and applying gentle traction until it releases its hold in 30 to 60 seconds. This method also reduces the chance of leaving behind the head with biting mouth.

Rickettsia first enter the nuclei of the capillary endothelial cells, where they multiply and destroy the cells. The lesions extend along the blood vessels to the arterioles, where smooth muscle cells of the media are invaded and destroyed. Vascular lesions result in scattered thrombosis and extravasation of blood, producing microinfarcts. Alterations within the nervous system are more striking in Rocky Mountain spotted fever than in any of the other rickettsial diseases. The patient has areas of petechial hemorrhages, perivascular infiltration, glial nodules, and minute sites of focal necrosis. Patches of demyelination are seen throughout the brain (1107).

Clinical Manifestations

Neurologic symptoms are prominent in Rocky Mountain spotted fever. Meningoencephalitis, a major manifestation of the disease, evolves after an incubation period of 4 to 8 days (1108). The acute phase begins with headache, myalgia, fever, and shaking chills. Meningeal signs can be prominent (1109). Mental confusion, hallucination, or delirium can appear and progress to coma. Muscular twitchings, fibrillary tremors, fasciculations, and convulsions are common. Focal motor seizures can occur. A variety of neurologic signs, including diffuse hyperreflexia, choreoathetosis, sixth nerve palsies, alteration in pupillary size and reflexes, cerebellar signs, and neurogenic bladder can develop (1110). Deafness often develops during the acute illness (1111). A variety of ophthalmologic signs have been noted, including retinal edema, papilledema, and choroiditis. Choked discs can be observed in the presence of normal intracranial pressure as a consequence of vasculitis (1112). Intracranial hemorrhage can result from thrombocytopenia and hypofibrinogenemia secondary to intravascular coagulation (1113).

After several days of fever, the rash usually begins over the extremities. It spreads centripetally and in 2 to 3 days changes from a macular to a maculopapular petechial eruption. Hemorrhagic areas can coalesce to form ecchymotic lesions. At this point, myocardial involvement can lead to cardiac failure with hypotension, tachycardia, and shock. Renal and hepatic involvements result in oliguria and hypoproteinemia with generalized edema.

Residual neurologic deficits might not be immediately apparent. At reevaluation after 1 to 8 years, 16% of survivors showed definite neurologic abnormalities, although one-half of this group had no objective changes during the acute phase of the illness. A variety of neurologic residua were observed, including mental retardation, behavioral disturbances, impairment of coordination, and hypotonia. In one-third of subjects, the EEG was persistently abnormal (1113). Perceptuomotor deficits also have been observed as a late sequela (1114).

Diagnosis

The diagnosis of Rocky Mountain spotted fever rests in part on a history of exposure and the development of the characteristic rash. The CSF is normal in 56% of cases. In the remainder, white blood cells can range from 11 to 300 per μL; only one-fourth of these have more than 50% polymorphonuclear cells. Modest elevations in protein content occur in approximately 33% of cases; the sugar content remains normal. Laboratory diagnosis can be made by complement fixation, rickettsial agglutination, Felix-Weil reaction, or by indirect fluorescent antibody studies (1115).

Treatment

Chloramphenicol or a tetracycline is the preferred antibiotic. They are continued until at least 1 week after the patient has become afebrile. Intravenous tetracycline should be avoided because it can cause hepatic necrosis (1116).

For a discussion of the neurologic complications of typhus and the other rickettsial infections, the reader is referred to the classic papers by Noad and Haymaker on the complications of scrub typhus (tsutsugamushi fever) (1117) and by Herman on typhus fever (1118). Chloramphenicol-resistant and doxycycline-resistant strains of scrub typhus have been reported (1119).

Q Fever

Although Q fever usually presents as a febrile illness with mild to moderate pneumonia, headache is the most common neurologic manifestation of *Coxiella burnetii* infection. Lymphocytic

meningitis and encephalitis can occur with minimal changes in the CSF (1120).

PROTOZOAL AND PARASITIC INFECTIONS OF THE NERVOUS SYSTEM

Aside from toxoplasmosis and cysticercosis, no protozoal and parasitic organisms commonly invade the nervous system of children in the United States and Western Europe (1121).

Generally, parasitic infestations of the CNS can produce diffuse symptoms of meningoencephalitis, a space-occupying lesion, or lesions caused by the migration of larvae through brain substance.

Cysticercosis

Cysticercosis of the CNS has become a relatively common entity in those areas of the United States settled by immigrants from various Latin American countries. The condition is not unusual in Chile, Mexico, Peru, India, and the Middle East. In Mexico, for instance, cysticercosis accounts for approximately 25% of intracranial tumors. The infection is almost always caused by the encysted form of *Taenia solium*. In the parenchymatous form of cysticercosis, the organisms encyst within the parenchyma of the brain. They also can seed into the ventricles or cisterns, thus producing chronic inflammation of the leptomeninges and ependyma. The inflammation becomes much worse after the death of the organisms (1122). Serial CT scans demonstrate that cysts can disappear in a few months or can progress to residual calcified lesions (1123).

The most common symptoms are focal or generalized seizures, found as the presenting feature in up to 90% of subjects (1124,1125), increased intracranial pressure, found in 44% to 75% of cases (1124–1126), and cranial nerve palsies. Tumor and encephalitic and basilar meningitic forms of infestation also have been described (1122,1127).

Cysts, sometimes free floating, can occur in the CSF. These can cause acute neurologic symptoms by obstructing the aqueduct if they are in the third ventricle. Cysts can cause spinal cord compression if they are in the spinal canal. CT visualization may require CSF contrast media.

The racemose form of cyst can invade the ventricular or subarachnoid spaces and persist there for many years. Intermittent rupture of cysts contiguous to CSF can cause a marked inflammatory response with transient high fevers. In approximately one-third to two-thirds of cases, CSF eosinophilia is present. Approximately one-half of patients show intracranial calcification by CT scan (1126). Kramer and associates documented the natural history of cerebral cysticercosis with serial CT scans. In the early acute stage, they found focal nonenhancing areas of edema that progress to homogeneously enhancing lesions. In the chronic phase, beginning a few months after infestation, nonenhancing cysts occur that later demonstrate ring enhancement. Lesions can completely resolve then, or they can resolve totally or partially before developing punctate calcifications (1123). Positive CSF serology results are diagnostic. For a detailed review of the neurologic aspects of cysticercosis, see the publication by Garg (1128).

Praziquantel is effective against the parenchymatous form of the disease, but has limited usefulness against the racemose form. The treatment of cysticercosis with praziquantel and albendazole is reviewed by Liu and coworkers (1129). When cysts produce CSF obstruction, they must be removed surgically (1122).

In the United States, parenchymatous cerebral cysticercosis has a good prognosis. Seizures are usually easily controlled and the disease is self-limited and does not require therapy (1130). Albendazole is recommended for the treatment of persistent, solitary cysticercosis granulomas in patients with seizures (1131).

Trichinosis

Trichinosis is caused by a nematode, *Trichinella spiralis*, that most often infests live pigs and is ingested when pork is raw or poorly cooked. The encysted larvae escape to all parts of the body by the bloodstream, but survive and grow only in skeletal muscle.

Microscopy reveals parasites within the muscle fibers, where they set up a focal inflammation and ultimately become calcified. Within the CNS, filiform larvae are found in the capillaries and in parenchyma, where they cause a focal inflammatory response (1132).

The clinical picture is highlighted by fever, myalgia, and abdominal pain. Muscles innervated by the cranial nerves, including the extraocular and masticatory muscles, can be involved. In 10% to 20% of infestations, the nervous system also is invaded within the first weeks of the onset of infection. CNS damage can be caused by larval migration, vascular obstruction, toxic parasite antigens, as well as inflammatory and eosinophile infiltration (1133). Encephalitis or meningeal signs can be present along with papilledema and focal neurologic abnormalities including bilateral facial palsies (1134,1135). Sagittal sinus thrombosis can occur (1136), and the disease can be fatal (1137).

The most striking laboratory findings include eosinophilia and occasional electrocardiographic abnormalities compatible with a myocarditis. The diagnosis rests on a history of potential exposure, persistent eosinophilia, increasing serum antibody titer, and positive muscle biopsy result. In approximately one-fourth of patients, larvae are seen in the CSF (1134).

Mebendazole is the recommended treatment (1138). Thiabendazole (25 mg/kg twice a day for 5 to 7 days) kills adult worms in the intestine, but seems ineffective against encysted larvae. Corticosteroids are recommended for severe symptoms to reduce inflammation and edema, but improvement is generally not dramatic.

When the infection has not been extensive, the prognosis for survival is good, but weakness and electrocardiographic abnormalities can persist for long periods after apparent clinical recovery. In chronic infections, radiography of the muscles, particularly those of the gastrocnemius, reveal the calcified filarial cysts.

Cerebral Malaria

Malaria remains one of the most important causes of childhood mortality and morbidity worldwide. The World Health Organization has estimated that at least 1 million children die of malaria annually in Africa alone (1139). The vast majority of deaths from malaria is caused by cerebral malaria, which is the most common, severe, and potentially fatal complication of *Plasmodium falciparum* infection.

In malarial endemic countries, cerebral malaria most commonly affects young children. However, in nonendemic areas and in nonimmune travelers who acquire malaria, cerebral malaria can occur at any age (1140,1141). In the past, it was assumed that most patients who recover from acute cerebral malaria have no sequelae of the illness. However, increasingly it is recognized that a significant proportion of survivors are left with long-term neurologic sequelae (1142,1143). Cerebral malaria is, therefore, an important cause of long-term childhood neurologic disability in many countries.

Pathophysiology

A major impediment to improving the prognosis of cerebral malaria is the inadequate understanding of the pathophysiology of the disorder. Early neuropathologic studies indicated that cerebral malaria was associated with preferential sequestration of parasitized erythrocytes within the cerebral microvasculature (1144). These observations led to the hypothesis that sequestration of parasitized cells in the cerebral capillary bed is a key initial step in the pathogenesis of cerebral malaria (1145,1146). Although more recent studies in fatal cases have confirmed that there are indeed large numbers of parasitized red blood cells within capillaries, a number of features argue against simple mechanical occlusion of the vasculature by parasitized erythrocytes as the prime cause of the disorder (1140,1146). Diffuse encephalopathy, rather than focal neurologic abnormalities, is the usual manifestation of cerebral malaria. Furthermore, complete recovery of neurologic function occurs in a majority of patients, including those who have been in deep coma. Such a course would be unlikely if thrombotic occlusion of the vasculature had occurred.

Adherence of parasitized red cells to the endothelium occurs through a specific, receptor-mediated interaction. Many different endothelial receptors for infected red cells have been identified (1147). Some, notably CD 36 and thrombospondin, are used by all strains of malaria parasites, others, such as intercellular adhesion molecule-1 (ICAM-1), are specific for certain parasite strains (1148). Binding to ICAM-1 is highest in patients with cerebral malaria, with the degree of binding correlating with the severity of the illness (1148). Genetic factors also appear to play a role in the degree of binding of parasitized red cells in cerebral vascular endothelium. Individuals homozygous for certain mutations in the gene coding for ICAM-1 have an increased susceptibility to develop severe cerebral malaria (1149).

Intact parasitized red cells can modulate the immune system by adherence to dendritic cells, thereby inhibiting their maturation and their capacity to stimulate T cells (1149a). Cytokines such as TNF, released during malaria infection, may increase expression of ICAM-1 and facilitate increased adherence of parasitized cells within the cerebral circulation (1150,1151). The mechanisms by which parasitized red cells within the cerebral circulation alter brain function remain unclear. Candidate toxic mediators include malaria-derived cytokines such as TNF, and nitric oxide (1144,1151,1152). TNF levels are increased in children with severe malaria and are higher in those who die in comparison with survivors (1153). Increased IL-1 levels also correlate positively with outcome (1153–1155). It is unclear, however, whether TNF is a specific mediator of the inflammatory process in cerebral malaria or simply a marker of the severity of that process. Anti-TNF therapy, however, inhibits fever in cerebral malaria (1156).

Metabolic factors also have been implicated in the pathophysiology of cerebral malaria. Hypoglycemia is found in almost one-third of children with cerebral malaria, and children who are hypoglycemic on admission are at significantly greater risk of death from the development of neurologic sequelae (1157,1158). Hypoglycemia is accompanied by elevated plasma lactate levels, with acidosis and lactate concentrations in plasma and CSF being significantly higher in patients with a poor outcome than in those who make a full recovery (1157). Plasma insulin concentrations are appropriately low, suggesting that inhibition of gluconeogenesis is the most likely mechanism responsible for hypoglycemia (1157,1159). Competition between parasites and host cells for essential nutrients may contribute to the metabolic derangement. Release of toxic metabolites that impair brain cell metabolism also may occur (1140). An association between some cases of fatal cerebral malaria and inducible nitric oxide synthase polymorphism (NOS2 locus) has been reported (1160).

Little evidence exists to suggest cerebral edema plays a significant role in the pathophysiology of cerebral malaria, even though MRI shows brain volume to be increased during the acute phase of cerebral malaria. Rather, this results from an increase in the volume of intracerebral blood, probably the consequence of the sequestration of parasitized erythrocytes (1161). Turner and Miller and coworkers have reviewed the pathophysiology of cerebral malaria (1144,1162).

Clinical Manifestations

The clinical features of cerebral malaria are those of an acute encephalopathic illness, and overlap other infective and metabolic causes of childhood encephalopathy (1163,1164). In the series of Newton and Warrell, 82% of children with cerebral malaria developed seizures before hospitalization (1165). Another 15% were deeply unconscious with a Glasgow Coma Score of less than 6. Hypoglycemia was seen in 23% and metabolic acidosis in 42%. Retinal hemorrhage was noted in 6% (1165). In children younger than 5 years of age, the disease typically presents with fever, headache, malaise, anorexia, and vomiting. Neurologic signs are those of a diffuse encephalopathy with symmetric upper motor neuron signs and brainstem disturbances, including dysconjugate gaze, palsies, hypotonicity or hypertonicity, extensor plantar responses, absent abdominal reflexes, and stertorous breathing. Retinal hemorrhages can be present, and decorticate and decerebrate posturing are seen in severe cases (1157,1166).

Diagnosis

In malaria endemic areas, two difficulties exist in the diagnosis of cerebral malaria. First, malaria parasitemia in a child with neurologic abnormalities does not exclude the possibility of other diagnoses such as bacterial meningitis. Second is the converse: Occasionally, patients with cerebral malaria may not have detectable *P. falciparum* in the peripheral blood, either caused by sequestration of the parasitized cells within the vasculature or due to previous antimalarial treatment. In such cases, treatment for cerebral malaria must always be commenced without awaiting definite confirmation of the diagnosis (1163,1164). In children with malaria who have experienced febrile convulsions, the possibility of cerebral malaria must always be considered if neurologic abnormality persists or progresses 30 minutes after convulsions have stopped. Lumbar puncture is generally required to exclude the possibility of bacterial meningitis. The CSF in cerebral malaria contains normal numbers of white blood cells, and normal or minimally elevated concentrations of protein. CSF glucose may be depressed and CSF lactate increased (1157,1167). All of the clinical features of cerebral malaria can be seen in other bacterial and viral infections of the CNS or in a variety of metabolic disorders (1163,1164,1167).

Treatment

In childhood malaria, death can occur within hours of the onset of illness. Antimalarial drugs are the only specific therapy known to arrest the infection, and children suspected of having cerebral malaria must receive the best available antimalarials by the parenteral route as quickly as possible. Specific therapy should not be delayed if cerebral malaria is suspected but cannot be ruled out by appropriate investigations. Parenteral quinine is recommended in most countries for patients with cerebral malaria because of the worldwide spread of chloroquine-resistant *P. falciparum*. In countries with low levels of chloroquine resistance, chloroquine is often given to patients with uncomplicated malaria, with quinine being reserved for those with severe malaria. Even with parenteral administration, quinine may take up to 48 hours to achieve desirable plasma concentrations and a loading dose is frequently recommended (1168). Quinine dihydrochloride is given in a dose of 20 mg salt (16.7 mg base) per kg body weight by intravenous infusion over 4 hours as a loading dose, followed by 10 mg of salt (8.3 mg base) per kg infused over 4 hours, every 12 hours until the patient has regained consciousness. Quinidine gluconate is used as an alternative to quinine in some countries (1169). Quinine may be given by intramuscular route if intravenous access is difficult. Careful monitoring of blood glucose is required, although hyperinsulinemia has rarely been documented during treatment of children with cerebral malaria. Quinine does not result in rapid parasite clearance, and many regimes use additional antimalarial agents such as pyrimethamine sulfadoxine or mefloquine to ensure parasite killing once consciousness has been regained.

A number of new antimalarial agents have been evaluated for use in cerebral malaria, particularly in regions where multidrug resistant parasites are increasingly found. The artemethrin derivative artemetha, developed in China from the traditional remedy Qinghausu, is among the most promising antimalarial drugs (1170). In studies in Malawi, artemetha was found to clear parasitemia more rapidly than quinine and was associated with more rapid recovery from coma (1171). Mortality for children treated with artemether (20.5%) is similar to that for children treated with quinine (21.5%) (1172). Further trials are required to establish whether this agent is associated with improved mortality. In areas of the world such as the Thai–Burmese border, where an increasing resistance of organisms to quinine has occurred, combination regimes of quinine with tetracycline cotrimoxazole or Artemisinin or its derivatives may be required. In some areas of Africa combined therapy of Artemisinin or its derivatives and pyrimethamine-sulphadoxine has been recommended (1172a). Some of the less prevalent antiparasitic drugs (1173) are available from the Parasitic Disease Drug Service of the Centers for Disease Control and Prevention in Atlanta.

As in any comatose patients, successful outcome of patients with cerebral malaria also depends on control of convulsions, with particular attention to fluid and electrolyte balance, maintenance of the airway, and good nursing care. The vast majority of patients with cerebral malaria is treated in hospitals with minimal facilities for intensive medical support. Patients with cerebral malaria in more developed countries are treated with full intensive care support, including elective ventilation to optimize cerebral perfusion. A wide number of adjunctive agents have been suggested as being beneficial in the treatment of cerebral malaria. These include corticosteroids, heparin, mannitol, low-molecular-weight dextran, prostacyclin, TNF antibodies, and desferrioxamine. Most of these agents have not been subjected to controlled clinical trials or clinical trials have shown no benefit. However, a randomized double-blind placebo-controlled trial of iron chelation therapy with desferrioxamine documented more rapid resolution of coma and increased parasite clearance in patients receiving desferrioxamine (1174). Further trials of this and other experimental agents such as anti-TNF antibodies are required before any specific recommendations can be made. Parecetamol significantly delays the clearance time of Plasmodium falciparum in children; its role in the treatment of malaria is uncertain (1174a).

Prognosis

The mortality for patients admitted with cerebral malaria ranges from 6% to 30% in different series. Some of the variation in mortality is explained by differences in the criteria for diagnosis (1157). A number of clinical and laboratory features that are present on admission of children with cerebral malaria are predictive of severe disease and a poor outcome. These include profound coma, signs of decerebration, absence of corneal reflex, and convulsions at the time of admission. Laboratory findings predictive of a poor outcome are hypoglycemia, leukocytosis, hyperparasitemia, elevated concentrations of alanine and 5-nucleotidase, and elevated plasma or CSF lactate (1157).

Although in the past survivors of cerebral malaria were thought to have an excellent prognosis for full neurologic recovery, more recent studies from several countries have documented a significant rate of long-term neurologic sequelae (1142,1157). Approximately 10% to 30% of survivors experience neurologic deficits including hemiplegia, ataxia, generalized motor deficits, with spasticity or hypotonia (1165). No detailed studies are available of long-term effects on intellect or later development. It is likely that an even greater proportion of survivors have experienced subtle long-term residua (1143). Persistence of neurologic abnormalities is associated with the same poor prognostic features that are predictive of increased mortality.

A postmalaria neurologic syndrome occurs rarely in patients who have recovered from *P. falciparum* malaria. It occurs more often after treatment with mefloquine, but also occurs in patients who have not received this drug. This syndrome usually occurs within 2 months after recovery from malaria and usually lasts 1 to 10 days. It is characterized by one or more of the following: psychosis or acute confusional episodes, generalized convulsions, tremors, or fever. At the time of this complication, blood smear results for malaria parasites are negative. CSF can show a mild pleocytosis (8 to 80 white blood cells) with lymphocyte predominance and a mild elevation in protein (1175).

Prophylaxis

Chloroquine can no longer be recommended for prophylaxis because of widespread resistance to the drug, especially in Africa. Resistance to sulfadoxine/pyrimethamine also has been reported in Africa. A combination of atovaquone plus proguanil prophylaxis has been recommended in children (1176).

Trypanosomiasis

The CNS can be involved in both African and American trypanosomiasis. African trypanosomiasis is caused by *Trypanosoma brucei* of which there are two subspecies, *gambiense* and *rhodesiense*. CNS involvement is the major clinical complication of African trypanosomiasis and is fatal if untreated.

Pathogenesis and Pathology

African trypanosomiasis is transmitted to humans by the bite of blood-sucking flies of the genus *Glossina* (Tsetse fly). Gambiense occurs in West and central sub-Sahara Africa, and *T. rhodesiense* occurs in east and south East Africa. Although 25 to 50 million people live in areas of Africa where the disease is endemic, the disease is distributed in patches in approximately 200 known hyperendemic foci. The official incidence figures of 20,000 to 25,000 cases annually are probably a substantial underestimate, considering that over 7,000 cases were diagnosed in 1987 alone in an epidemic in Uganda (1177,1178).

The pathogenesis of trypanosomiasis is not completely understood. Parasites enter the body after the bite of the infected fly. Active parasite replication and invasion of local tissues occurs, leading to an inflammatory nodule at the site of the bite. The trypanosomes enter the lymphatics causing lymphadenopathy and the bloodstream causing parasitemia. During the hemolymphatic stage of the illness, recurrent episodes of fever and constitutional symptoms occur, which remit spontaneously and are followed by intervening periods of well-being (1179). The trypanosomes are coated with a glycoprotein called the variant surface glycoprotein, which shields underlying structures from host antibodies. Each parasite has more than 1,000 different genes for this protein, only one form of which is expressed on the surface of the parasite at a particular point in time (1179,1180). The production of host antibodies to this antigenic surface results in clearance of the parasite from the blood and cessation of symptoms. However, a new wave of parasitemia follows, resulting from the growth of a population of parasites with a new antigenically distinct surface glycoprotein. This cycle of parasite proliferation and humeral immune response may be repeated for months or years and is associated with a marked elevation in immunoglobulins. Eventually, the parasite invades the brain, probably via the choroid plexus and induces a lymphocytic/plasmacytic meningoencephalitis. An interaction of the parasite with the cytokine network of the host is believed to play a role in the proliferation of the parasite and in evoking the inflammation (1180,1180a). Inflammatory lesions occur predominantly in a perivascular distribution with sparing of neuronal elements. In some fatal cases, demyelination and choroid plexus involvement occur. An acute hemorrhagic encephalopathy with discrete and confluent hemorrhages also can occur (1181,1182). The mechanisms by which trypanosomes damage the brain are unclear. It has been suggested that toxins produced by the trypanosomes induce vascular injury or induce a CNS metabolic derangement (1180,1180a). Alternatively, brain injury may be caused by the host inflammatory response, and evidence of autoantibodies directed against brain myelin proteins can be detected in a high proportion of cases (1183). Immunofluorescent studies have shown deposition of complement and immunoglobulins in brain tissue suggesting immune complex deposition as a mechanism of vascular injury (1184).

Clinical Manifestations

Clinical features of the East African and West African forms of trypanosomiasis differ, with *T. rhodesiense* causing a much more acute and fulminant disease. In *T. rhodesiense* infection, the CNS involvement occurs early, with death occurring within weeks to months in untreated cases. The Gambian disease is indolent and is characterized by prominent lymphadenopathy, a gradual onset, and late CNS involvement. The illness may last months to years. The hemolymphatic stage of both diseases is associated with constitutional symptoms, such as weakness, joint pains, weight loss, and headache (1185). Major CNS symptoms include headache, alterations in mentation and behavior, abnormal sleep patterns, and progressive deterioration of consciousness. Psychological and behavioral changes, including personality disorder, psychosis, and major affective disorders, are common (1186). Excessive sleeping increases as the disease progresses. Extrapyramidal symptoms and signs, with cerebellar ataxia, parkinsonian rigidity, and convulsions appear as the disease progresses, as does papilledema. Stupor and coma ultimately develop and the mortality in untreated cases approaches 100% (1187).

Diagnosis

Diagnosis depends on the demonstration of parasites in fluid aspirates from chancre or lymph nodes, or in blood, bone marrow, or CSF. Repeated examinations may be necessary because of the cyclic nature of parasitemia (1188). CSF abnormality is always present in severe disease, with pleocytosis and elevated protein. Microscopically visible trypanosomes are found in less than 20% of cases. CSF immunoglobulin, particularly IgM, is increased markedly. Serologic methods are now available to detect antibodies against the parasite in both the blood and CSF (1188).

Treatment

Treatment of cerebral trypanosomiasis is difficult. Intravenous suramin is effective in the lymphatic stage of the disease, but is ineffective once CNS invasion occurs (1179,1189). Pentamidine can be used in early cases of *T. gambiense* infection, but is ineffective against *T. rhodesiense* disease. The only agent that can penetrate the CNS and is effective in CNS disease is melarsoprol, which is given as a single daily intravenous injection of 3.6 mg/kg for 3 days and is repeated three times with a rest period of 7 days between courses (1189,1190). Patients with severe disease also should receive a short course of suramin before receiving melarsoprol. Of treated patients 10% to 18% experience severe complications of treatment with symptoms of arsenical encephalopathy, which may be fatal (1189). A number of other agents are under investigation that may prove to be less toxic, including difluoromethyl ornithine (DFMO) (1191).

American Trypanosomiasis

CNS disease is extremely rare in adult Chagas disease, but is seen as a complication of congenital infection with *Trypanosoma cruzi* (1192). Transmission to the fetus occurs in 2% of pregnancies if the mother is seropositive. The majority of cases of Chagas disease with CNS involvement are in children younger than 1 year of age. Parasites can be found in the CSF after acute infection at any age, but clinical or pathologic meningoencephalitis is rare. It is usually fatal when it does occur. Histologic findings are those of scattered granulomas in which amastigote forms of the parasite can be found (1193).

Acute chagasic encephalitis manifests with a range of signs from tremor to spasticity, coma, and convulsions (1194). Infants with congenital infection show delayed development or regression. Diagnosis can be established by finding parasites in the blood, tissues, or CSF. Serologic testing can be helpful. Treatment is with the trypanocides, nifurtimox and benznidazole.

CESTODE INFECTIONS

Echinococcosis (Hydatid Disease)

Hydatid cysts in the CNS produce symptoms of space-occupying lesions. In children, they are found in the brain (77%), spine (18%), and skull (8%) (1195,1196). The preferred management is surgical extirpation (1195,1197). Prolonged courses of mebendazole or albendazole have been used in inoperable cases (1197).

Amoebic Infections of the Central Nervous System

Amoebic infections of the CNS caused by both pathogenic and free living amoebae occur infrequently. Cerebral amoebiasis occurs when *Entamoeba histolytica* spreads from its normal site of infection in the bowel to cause amoebic abscesses within the CNS (1198). Considering that in any year more than 400 million people are infected with *E. histolytica*, CNS infection is remarkably rare. Most patients with amoebic brain abscesses are young adults, and the disease affects male subjects much more than female subjects. The majority of reported patients has died, possibly because the diagnosis is seldom made during life (1199). At necropsy, the brain is swollen with areas of focal meningitis. Multiple focal, hemorrhagic necrotic lesions are usually found, the walls of which are infiltrated by mononuclear cells. Amoebae may be identified within these necrotic lesions. The presenting features are indistinguishable from those of brain abscesses or tumors. CSF may be normal or show nonspecific changes, and biopsy of the lesions may be required to establish the diagnosis. It is likely that prompt treatment with metronidazole coupled with surgical aspiration or exci-

sion of accessible lesions may improve the prognosis of what has been up to now a largely fatal illness (1200).

Primary amoebic meningoencephalitis is caused by free-living amoebae belonging to two genera, *Naegleria* and *Acanthamoeba*. The organisms flourish in warm moist conditions, and infection in children is usually acquired while swimming in unchlorinated freshwater sources (1201). *N. fowleri* is the most common species associated with acute primary amoebic meningoencephalitis, whereas *Acanthamoeba* may cause a more chronic granulomatous amoebic encephalitis. The amoebae enter the nasal cavity during swimming or diving and, in some patients, invade the roof of the nasal cavity, crossing the olfactory epithelium and ascending into the anterior cranial fossa through the cribriform plate. The amoebae reach the meninges surrounding the frontal lobes where they multiply, spread, and destroy the brain substance (1202). Less commonly, bloodstream invasion can occur. *Acanthamoeba* species also can invade the CNS from a primary corneal infection of the eye (1202).

The histologic findings are severe meningoencephalitis and necrosis (1203). An intense polymorphonuclear infiltrate occurs, with areas of hemorrhage and necrosis. In cases of *Acanthamoeba* infection, single or multiple brain abscesses can be found and histologic findings of a granulomatous meningitis can be present.

The acute form of primary amoebic meningoencephalitis presents with sudden onset of high fever, photophobia, headache, and progression to coma (1204). The initial features are indistinguishable from those of acute bacterial meningitis. Subacute or chronic meningoencephalitis can present more insidiously with symptoms suggesting a brain tumor or abscess. Most cases are diagnosed initially as having bacterial meningitis. The CSF is consistent with findings of bacterial meningitis with pleocytosis, hypoglycorrhachia, and elevated protein concentration. The diagnosis can be made before death by examination of fresh, warm specimens of CSF to detect amoeboid movements of the motile trophozoites. Identification of organisms by PCR is under investigation (1205). After death, the parasite can be visualized with light or electron microscopy within the brain. In the chronic form of the disorder, no trophozoites are found in the CSF and the diagnosis can only be made by biopsy of a necrotic lesion detected by neuroimaging.

The free-living amoebae are sensitive to a variety of antimicrobial agents, including amphotericin B, pentamidine, tetracycline, and rifampicin. Most of the reported cases have been fatal, but treatment with intravenous pentamidine or with amphotericin and rifampicin may reduce the mortality if diagnosis is made early (1206,1207).

NEMATODE INFECTIONS

Angiostrongyliasis

The nematode *Angiostrongylus cantonensis* is a common cause of eosinophilic meningitis in many countries, including Thailand, Malaysia, Vietnam, and the Pacific Islands. Additional cases have been reported from the Middle East and Africa (1208). Rats are the definitive host of the parasite, and human infection follows ingestion of the larvae present in contaminated foods such as mollusks. The larvae migrate to the CNS where they die and initiate an intense inflammatory process. Symptoms begin 6 to 30 days after ingesting raw mollusks and include headache, stiff neck, paresthesias, and vomiting. The CSF characteristically shows leukocytosis with a high proportion of eosinophils, and elevated protein concentration.

The prognosis is generally good. Most patients recover within 1 or 2 weeks, but full resolution of symptoms may take considerably longer (1209). The treatment is symptomatic, although thiabendazole may hasten clearance of the parasite. The neurologic complications of strongyloidiasis have been reviewed by Lowichik and Ruff (1210).

Gnathostomiasis

Gnathostoma spinigerum may cause a serious CNS infection acquired by ingestion of raw or partially cooked animal flesh. The parasite is widely distributed in the Far East, and although most cases have been reported from Thailand and Japan, the disease has now been recognized in various parts of Mexico (1211). The parasite causes a variety of neurologic syndromes including radiculomyelitis, encephalitis, and subarachnoid or intracerebral hemorrhage (1212). Highly motile larvae or worms invade nerve roots and migrate to the spinal canal or the spinal cord itself from which they migrate to the brain. This explains the diverse clinical findings of radicular pain, radicular myelitis, eosinophilic meningitis, or encephalitis. In endemic areas, painless migratory subcutaneous edema is highly suggestive of the subcutaneous form of the disease. CNS involvement is suggested by sudden onset of severe radicular pain followed by CNS signs (1213). Typical CSF findings are a moderate leukocytosis with a high percentage of eosinophils, elevated protein, and elevated blood cells.

No specific drug treatment has been shown to be of benefit, and patients have to be treated symptomatically. Corticosteroids may be used to reduce inflammation and edema.

Toxocariasis

Nematodes of the genus *Toxocara* are common parasites of dogs and cats, and humans become infected through ingestion of soil containing ova, which hatch in the small intestine to produce larvae that pass through the intestinal wall and migrate into the tissues. Visceral larvae migrans refers to the disorder produced during migration of the larvae through the organs. The larvae elicit granulomatous inflammation associated with eosinophilia. When the larvae come to rest in the tissues, necrosis develops in the surrounding area with infiltration of polymorphonuclear cells, eosinophils, and histiocytes. Focal granuloma with multinucleated giant cells may develop. Because toxocariasis is rarely fatal, only a few descriptions of CNS pathology in this disorder are found (1214).

Seroprevalence studies indicate that *Toxocara* infection is common in young children, with a majority of the infections being asymptomatic. The usual manifestations of visceral larvae migrans are of abdominal pain, anorexia, nausea, vomiting, behavior disturbance, cough, wheeze, and fever. Striking eosinophilia is usually present and should suggest the diagnosis. The most common CNS symptom is headache, which is present in a high proportion of cases, but may be unrelated to direct CNS invasion. Encephalopathy with seizures can occur (1215). Children with idiopathic epilepsy have antitoxocaral antibodies more often than controls. This association has led to the suggestion that in some instances toxocariasis can be a precipitant of epilepsy (1216).

CENTRAL NERVOUS SYSTEM DISEASE CAUSED BY TREMATODES

Schistosomiasis

Schistosomiasis is one of the most important parasitic diseases, occurring in more than 200 million people worldwide. Of the various schistosomal species, *S. mansoni*, *S. haematobium*, and *S. japonicum* are the most common disease-causing organisms (1217). CNS schistosomiasis usually follows migration of adult worms to the CNS with eggs being laid in the spinal cord or brain vasculature. In other cases, eggs are embolized from the portal mesenteric system to the brain and spinal cord (1217). The size of the eggs produced by the different species determines the site of CNS involvement (1218). *S. japonicum* eggs are more likely to reach the brain, whereas the larger eggs of *S. mansoni* cause mostly spinal lesions. *S. haematobium* also causes mainly spinal cord disease. The presence of eggs within the CNS can elicit an inflammatory reaction characterized by infiltration of lymphocytes, eosinophils, and macrophages and lead to a florid granulomatous reaction (1217).

Acute schistosomiasis occurs predominantly in children, adolescents, and young adults. Neurologic syndromes can occur in nonimmune individuals with Katayama fever, which probably results from an immunologic reaction to cercaria, schistosomula, and eggs (1218). Mental confusion, seizures, coma, visual defects, and signs of increased intracranial pressure can occur. Occasionally, hemiplegia or other focal neurologic signs can occur. Schistosomal myelopathy is more commonly symptomatic than cerebral schistosomiasis (1219,1220). Symptoms, which depend on the site of involvement, include paraplegia, sphincter dysfunction, areflexia, radiculopathy, and a rapidly progressive transverse myelitis usually affecting the lumbosacral segments of the spinal cord. These reflect the presence of single or multiple granulomata in the spinal cord with cord compression and necrosis (1217). Examination of the CSF in acute schistosomiasis can show an increase in protein concentration and lymphocytosis with eosinophilia (1221).

Neurologic symptoms occurring in chronic schistosomiasis include headache, confusion, seizures, and incoordination.

The diagnosis of schistosomiasis depends on a history of potential exposure and a high index of suspicion. In some cases, blood and CSF eosinophilia are seen. *Schistosoma* eggs can be detected in feces, urine, or by rectal snips, and serologic tests can indicate previous exposure. Intracerebral and spinal cord lesions can be demonstrated by neuroimaging studies (1222). The presence in CSF of an immunoglobulin G specific for schistosome-soluble egg antigen is highly specific but not very sensitive for the diagnosis (1223).

Treatment of schistosomiasis depends on a combination of drug therapy with praziquantel to eradicate the infection and measures to reduce inflammation (1224). Neurologic disease during Katayama fever responds to corticosteroids. Surgical decompression may be required for lesions that compress the spinal cord. The effectiveness of a vaccine is under investigation (1225).

Paragonimiasis

Infestation with paragonimiasis, a common condition in Southeast Asia and in certain parts of Africa and South America, generally causes pulmonary symptoms. Occasionally, the organism can cause serious neurologic disease. *Paragonimus westermani*, the oriental lung fluke, is the most common etiologic agent, although other species also can cause CNS infection. Infection is acquired through ingestion of seafood or contaminated water. The metacercaria excyst in the small intestine, penetrate the bowel wall, and migrate into the tissues. Larval flukes migrate to the lung and, occasionally, elsewhere in the body. Flukes can migrate from the lung through the jugular and carotid foramina at the base of the skull to reach the temporal and occipital lobes of the brain, where they cause necrosis and an eosinophilic, granulomatous reaction. The spinal cord can be invaded through the intervertebral disc. Adult flukes can invade muscle, usually the psoas.

Common symptoms include headache, nausea and vomiting, seizures, visual disturbance, focal motor defects, and other neurologic signs. These symptoms can have features suggestive of meningitis, meningoencephalitis, encephalopathy, brain tumor, or brain abscess (1226–1228). Diagnosis of cerebral paragonimiasis is based on an epidemiologic history of exposure. Eosinophilia may be present, but all other features overlap with those of other CNS disorders, including tuberculosis. CT scanning may show calcification and ventricular dilatation. Contrast-enhanced MRI can be used to assess the extent of the inflammatory activity (1229). Biopsy of a CNS lesion may be required to confirm the diagnosis. The disease is treated by praziquantel or bithionol to eradicate the parasite. Convulsion and coma can occur as complications of treatment for cerebral paragonimiasis. The dosage may require adjustment, and corticosteroids should be given as in cysticercosis. Surgery may be required for focal lesions.

OTHER NEUROLOGIC DISORDERS OF PRESUMED INFECTIOUS ETIOLOGY

Sarcoidosis

Nervous system sarcoidosis is unusual in children. The cause of the disease is still problematic, but for convenience it is classified with infectious diseases. Although sarcoidosis occurs throughout the world, it is particularly common in the southeastern portions of the United States, where it predominates among blacks. Genetic factors have been implicated (1230). Most affected children are between 9 and 15 years old.

Pathologically, the disease is characterized by widely disseminated epithelioid cells, tubercles with little or no necrosis, and giant cells. The predominant lymphocyte at the site of disease is the T4-helper/inducer cell. Locally, the T4 to T8 ratio is increased, whereas it is reduced in the peripheral circulation (1231). Tissues most frequently involved are the lymph nodes, lungs, skin, eyes, and bones. In adults, any part of the nervous system can be affected, in particular the cranial nerves, meninges, and musculature (1232,1233). In children, neurologic symptoms are most commonly associated with uveoparotid fever. This syndrome, first described by Heerfordt (1234), is characterized by ocular disturbances, most commonly uveitis and less commonly optic neuritis, swelling of the parotid gland, and facial nerve palsy. Facial nerve palsy usually follows a subacute course; it appears after the parotid swelling and subsides with it. It occurs in 4% of children with sarcoidosis (1235). Meningeal signs, peripheral neuritis, papilledema, and diabetes insipidus are other rare findings associated with childhood CNS sarcoidosis (1235). Intramedullary spinal cord involvement can occur (1236). The CSF protein content can show an elevation with evidence of intrathecal production of oligoclonal IgM and IgG (1237). Other cases demonstrate intrathecal production of polyclonal IgG. However, only 24% of cases have either an elevated IgG index or an increased synthesis rate (1238). Cranial MRI evaluation should be done on all children with systemic sarcoidosis since clinically inapparent neurosarcoidosis can occur (1238a).

Sarcoidosis has a slowly progressive course, with a tendency to undergo partial or complete spontaneous remissions.

The diagnosis of sarcoidosis depends on the clinical and radiologic features along with histologic evidence of epithelioid cell granulomas on biopsy of the lung or other tissue. Because facial weakness is rare in mumps, the association of parotid swelling and facial palsy should suggest sarcoidosis. In the rare condition, termed *Melkersson syndrome*, recurrent facial nerve palsy is accompanied by edema of the face or lips. This condition is covered in Chapter 7. The MRI is not characteristic in CNS sarcoidosis. It can resemble multiple sclerosis with periventricular and multifocal lesions in the white matter (1239). A fuller discussion of the diagnostic problems is beyond the scope of this text; the reader is referred to reviews by Scott (1240) and Newman and colleagues (1230).

Treatment with corticosteroids tends to improve cerebral, ocular, and facial nerve involvement. Other immunosuppressive drugs can be of benefit should corticosteroid therapy fail. Surgical intervention may be required for hydrocephalus or expanding mass lesions (1230).

Encephalopathy and Fatty Degeneration of the Viscera (Reye Syndrome)

Reye syndrome, which was first described by Reye and coworkers in 1963 (1241), is an acute illness after a viral infection, characterized by a progressive encephalopathy, hypoglycemia, and disordered hepatic function (1242). The disease, once relatively common, has almost completely disappeared, so most currently encountered cases are atypical (1243).

Etiology and Pathology

The cause of Reye syndrome is unknown; the essential pathophysiology consists of a generalized impairment of mitochondrial function (1244). Reye syndrome has accompanied a large number of viral illnesses, notably varicella, influenza, and parainfluenza (1241,1244,1245). In northern Thailand, a condition resembling Reye syndrome has been associated with a toxin from *Aspergillus flavus* (1246). Most importantly, the association between the disease and administration of salicylates used to treat the fever accompanying the antecedent illnesses has been established by epidemiologic studies (1247). The incidence of Reye syndrome has decreased dramatically with the decreased use of salicylates as an antipyretic in childhood infections. At present, a significant proportion of cases are caused by a variety of inborn errors of metabolism.

The serum from patients with Reye syndrome contains an inhibitor of mitochondrial function capable of inducing in normal mitochondria morphologic changes similar to those seen in patients with Reye syndrome. The

inhibitor's properties resemble those of a dicarboxylic acid, and analysis of serum from patients with Reye syndrome demonstrates a marked increase in both medium- and long-chain dicarboxylic acids. The clinical similarity of Reye syndrome to Jamaican vomiting sickness and the various inborn errors of fatty acid metabolism, in which dicarboxylic acids accumulate, suggests that dicarboxylic acids indeed play a crucial role in the disease. These conditions are more fully discussed in the section on organic acidurias in chapter 1.

In fatal cases, the brain shows severe edema and brainstem herniation. The histopathologic changes are nonspecific. The cortical neurons are either swollen or shrunken and deeply staining. Astrocytes and oligodendroglia are swollen without microglial proliferation. Some cells are laden with sudanophilic granules. Brain mitochondria are usually grossly deformed and swollen. Their matrix is rarefied, and its materials are coarsely granular. Cristae are fragmentary, widely spaced, and few in number.

The liver is enlarged and yellow with fatty infiltration observed in every cell. This extensive fatty change is unassociated with necrosis. Electron microscopy reveals the most striking abnormalities to be in mitochondria, which are swollen and pleomorphic (1248). Similar changes are seen in the kidney, occasionally in the myocardium, and in pancreatic acinar cells.

Clinical Manifestations

Reye syndrome is primarily a disease of childhood and more than 90% of reported cases have been in persons younger than 15 years of age.

A variety of antecedent illnesses are associated with Reye syndrome. In order of their frequency, these are respiratory, varicella, and gastrointestinal illnesses, the last with diarrhea as the main symptom. Prodromal symptoms of Reye syndrome can be mild or can consist of nonspecific complaints such as malaise, cough, rhinorrhea, or sore throat. The child rapidly deteriorates, usually after 1 to 3 days, but sometimes as late as 2 to 3 weeks, with vomiting and the onset of stupor or coma, which is sometimes followed by convulsions. Wild delirium and unusual restlessness have been noted in approximately one-half of patients as the level of consciousness declines. Various types of seizures occur in approximately 85% of cases (1249).

With coma, the child develops changes in muscle tone, decorticate and decerebrate status, or opisthotonus. The pupils become dilated, unresponsive to light, or unequal. Central neurogenic hyperventilation or shallow breathing can occur. Symptoms often correlate with metabolic disturbances or brainstem herniation. The liver is frequently enlarged.

The clinical course of Reye syndrome is rapid, and in one series, 61% of deaths occurred within 24 hours of the onset of CNS manifestations. The cause of death in most cases is encephalopathy with cerebral edema leading to increased intracranial pressure and brainstem compression. Reye syndrome can stop progressing at any stage, with complete recovery in 5 to 10 days.

EEG changes correlate with the severity of Reye syndrome and with prognosis. Aoki and Lombroso have characterized the EEG changes (1250).

Diagnosis

A bout of vomiting followed by the sudden onset of a profound disturbance of consciousness associated with hepatic dysfunction and hypoglycemia should suggest the diagnosis of Reye syndrome. This is supported by abnormal liver function test results, such as elevated serum transaminases, prolonged prothrombin times, and high arterial blood ammonia with or without hypoglycemia. Hypoglycemia and impaired gluconeogenesis are not the only signs of disturbed glucose metabolism; blood lactate, pyruvate, acetoacetate, glycerol, glucose, glucagon, insulin, and growth hormone can be elevated. The CSF is normal. Biopsy of the liver confirms the diagnosis (1251). A variety of toxic substances, notably ethanol, and salicylates can produce a similar picture.

Treatment

Reye syndrome can be a mild, self-limited disease, or a rapidly progressive, relentless, fatal illness (1248). Control of intracranial hypertension is one of the most critical issues in the care

of patients with Reye syndrome (1252). An important adjunct to therapy is the monitoring of intracranial pressure. If possible, all patients with Reye syndrome should receive care in a setting where intracranial pressure can be monitored if coma evolves. Careful attention to metabolic and physiologic disturbances can be life saving in severe cases.

Generally, the residual neurologic deficit is proportional to the severity of the disease (1253,1254). Among survivors of Reye syndrome, 30% of those developing decerebrate posturing or seizures during hospitalization had serious neurologic sequelae when discharged. Evidence of increased intracranial pressure and a blood ammonia level greater than 300 g/dL was associated with a significantly greater mortality, as was hyperkalemia, hyperpnea, and hematemesis (1244). Disorders of voice and speech can be the major disabling handicaps in survivors of Reye syndrome (1255).

Hemorrhagic Shock and Encephalopathy Syndrome

This syndrome, first described by Levin and coworkers in 1983 (1256), affects previously healthy infants and young children. It manifests with a sudden onset of fever, watery diarrhea, shock, disseminated intravascular coagulation, and renal and hepatic dysfunction (1256,1257). The encephalopathy is characterized by seizures and coma. Neuroimaging studies demonstrate cerebral edema with relative sparing of cerebellum and basal ganglia (1258). The majority of survivors has significant neurologic deficits. Bacterial culture results have been uniformly negative, and the etiology of hemorrhagic shock and encephalopathy syndrome remains unknown. Sofer and coworkers suggest that the condition is the result of hyperpyrexia in genetically susceptible infants (1259).

Behçet Disease

Behçet disease is a chronic and relapsing condition characterized by keratitis, uveitis, recurrent ulcerations of the mouth and genitalia, and a variety of skin lesions (1260,1261). Although the disease largely affects adults, it may occur in children as young as 2 years of age, and transient ulcerative manifestations have been observed in newborns of mothers with Behçet disease (1262). The nervous system is involved in approximately one-fifth of patients (1263a).

Although reports of viral isolation from affected subjects have prompted classification of this disease with infectious illnesses, as yet no convincing evidence exists for such an etiology, and bacterial, autoimmune, and environmental factors also have been suggested (1264). Allen has proposed that an underlying genetic predisposition coupled with a triggering event leads to alterations in immune function and response (1265). Brain pathology is not specific. Multiple foci of necrotizing lymphocytic perivenular and pericapillary inflammatory cuffing are found in gray and white matter, and thrombosis of small vessels or of the large veins and dural sinuses occurs (1266).

In most patients, neurologic manifestations of Behçet disease include aseptic meningitis, or a recurrent meningoencephalitis (1267). Less often an episodic progressive brainstem syndrome occurs (1267,1268). Dural sinus thrombosis or pseudotumor cerebri also can develop with subsequent increase in intracranial pressure (1269). A mild CSF pleocytosis is common, with most patients having fewer than 60 white blood cells per μL. The MRI shows scattered areas of high signal intensity on T2-weighted images, with a predilection for central structures of the cerebrum, cerebral peduncles, and basis pontis during the acute illness. This evolves to atrophy of posterior fossa structures with signal attenuation suggestive of hemosiderin deposits (1270). The condition is rare in the United States, but appears to be relatively common in Turkey and Japan (1271). Patients with an Asian heritage have been associated with HLA-B5 haplotype (1263). As with most inflammatory diseases that involve the CNS, the neurologic manifestations are not specific, and the diagnosis rests on the presence of systemic manifestations. These include a marked cutaneous sensitivity to trauma, recurrent aphthous stomatitis, recurrent genital aphthous ulcers, and ocular manifestations, notably anterior

uveitis. Devlin and coworkers recommend performing contrast-enhanced MRI and CSF analysis in any patient who fulfills the criteria for systemic Behçet disease and who has a history of altered mental status, recurrent headache, or altered neurologic examination (1261).

The neurologic complications are generally treated with corticosteroids, although immunomodulators or chlorambucil also have been used (1263,1272). Interferon-α2b can benefit refractory ocular disease (1273). Colchicine is said to prevent relapses (1263).

Uveomeningoencephalitic Syndrome (Vogt-Koyanagi-Harada Syndrome)

Another cause for uveomeningitic disease in the pediatric population is Vogt-Koyanagi-Harada syndrome. This is an uncommon condition characterized by the association of uveitis, a meningoencephalitis of variable severity, occasional loss of skin and hair pigmentation, and auditory disturbances (1274).

The condition is presumed to be a class II major histocompatibility complex autoimmune inflammatory disease primarily directed at the antigens of melanocytes with particular injury to pigmented structures of the eye (1275,1276). The condition is more frequently encountered in the Japanese population in whom a strong association exists with HLA-DR4 (1275). A secondary association to HLA-DR1 also exists, involving a sequence that is linked with susceptibility to rheumatoid arthritis (1275). An inflammatory process similar to that found in the ocular choroid but directed at melanocytes of the inner ear may account for the frequent finding of auditory disturbance in Vogt-Koyanagi-Harada syndrome (1277). Melanin-laden macrophages may constitute a significant portion of the pleocytic cells found in CSF of patients with Vogt-Koyanagi-Harada syndrome (1278). It is unclear what provokes the autoimmune response in Vogt-Koyanagi-Harada syndrome.

The onset of Vogt-Koyanagi-Harada syndrome is typically one of a subacute onset of bilateral anterior, posterior, or both, uveitis associated with ocular pain. This may be followed by abrupt onset of aseptic meningitis or meningoencephalitis. Meningeal signs may be the first sign of disease and are found at some stage in approximately 60% of cases of Vogt-Koyanagi-Harada syndrome (1279). In the series of Beniz and coworkers, symptoms included meningismus, predominantly headache (67%), tinnitus (17%), dysacusis (13%), alopecia (13%), vitiligo (10%), and poliosis (6%) (1280). Ocular findings included iridocyclitis, vitreitis, diffuse swelling of the choroid, serous retinal detachment, or optic disc hyperemia (1280). Most cases occur during adult life, and in the series of Belfort and coworkers only 12% were younger than age 20 years (1281), the youngest being 4 years of age (1282). Waxing and waning abnormalities of cranial nerve function may be noted, especially of the third, seventh, and eighth cranial nerves. Tonic pupils, dysfunction of ocular accommodation, and corneal anesthesia are additional possible features (1283). The development of areas of depigmentation (poliosis) involving eyebrows and eyelashes, alopecia, and of dermal vitiligo are other common late manifestations.

A lymphocytic CSF pleocytosis is typical. MRI studies can show multiple focal lesions or increased T2 signal in the periventricular area (1284,1285).

Treatment with high doses of corticosteroids has been advocated. In patients whose neurologic symptoms do not respond, intravenous immune globulin can be of benefit (1285). Recovery takes place gradually over several months but is usually incomplete, with both visual and auditory system sequelae (1274). In children, the outcome for visual acuity is poor, and in the series of Tabbara and colleagues, 61% of children required cataract surgery, and 61% had a final visual acuity of 20/200 or worse (1286).

Mollaret Meningitis

A recurrent, benign, lymphocytic meningitis, probably of diverse causes (1287,1288), but presumed to be infectious, was first described by Mollaret (1289). Mollaret meningitis's association with herpes simplex types 1 and 2 has been suggested by the demonstration of viral DNA in the CSF (1287,1290). Symptoms recur at intervals of weeks or months over the course of several years,

and as many as five or more attacks can occur (1291). Seizures or coma have been reported, but focal neurologic signs are uncommon. Episodes are often associated with fever. Large mononuclear cells can be found in the CSF early in the course of an exacerbation (1292), but a CSF protein elevation is not invariable. The EEG can be normal or can demonstrate focal accentuations without spikes (1293). The long-term prognosis is good with spontaneous recovery and no residua.

Mollaret meningitis should be distinguished from chronic granulomatous infections of the nervous system, from an aseptic meningitis syndrome induced by trimethoprim therapy (1294), and from an intracranial epidermoid cyst (1288). Yamamoto and colleagues recommend acyclovir prophylaxis for those patients with detectable herpes simplex virus DNA in the CSF (1295).

Benign Paroxysmal Vertigo

Benign paroxysmal vertigo is characterized by recurrent attacks of vertigo associated with vomiting, pallor, nystagmus, and profuse sweating. Although benign paroxysmal vertigo is unaccompanied by loss of consciousness, children are known to fall during an attack. Episodes can last a few minutes to several hours or can recur for many weeks or even months, gradually decreasing in severity. A similar condition, epidemic vertigo, has occurred in epidemics, with more than one case appearing in the same family (1296). The preservation of consciousness during an attack and abnormalities in labyrinthine function distinguish benign paroxysmal vertigo from complex partial seizures with a vertiginous component and from vestibulogenic epilepsy, in which an attack is triggered by labyrinthine stimulation (1297–1299). In some children, recurrent attacks of vertigo are ultimately replaced by typical migraine (see Chapter 13). Benign paroxysmal vertigo also should not be confused with vestibular neuronitis or Ménière vertigo, a condition that is almost exclusively limited to the adult years (1300).

Epidemic Encephalitis

Epidemic encephalitis, first described by von Economo in 1917, attained epidemic proportions throughout Europe and the United States over the subsequent few years (1301). Since then, it has become progressively less common, although sporadic cases still occur (1302). Al-Mateen and coworkers encountered one such case, confirmed by the presence of increased signal intensity on MRI from the basal ganglia and substantia nigra and associated with *Mycoplasma* encephalitis (1051).

Epidemic encephalitis presented as an acute encephalitis that was often marked by somnolence and oculomotor palsies. The encephalitis cleared completely or left a variety of residua, including mental disturbances and disorders of eye movements. After a quiescent interval of months or years, many of the survivors developed a chronic progressive extrapyramidal disorder marked by parkinsonism, oculogyric crises, tremors, and dystonia (1303).

A common residual finding in children was a postencephalitic behavior syndrome marked by hyperkinesia, shortened attention span, and impaired fine motor function (1304). This picture resembled attention deficit hyperactivity disorder (ADHD). As a consequence, many children with this condition used to be regarded as postencephalitic without having any history of encephalitis (see Chapter 16).

Kawasaki Disease (Mucocutaneous Lymph Node Syndrome)

Kawasaki disease is a triphasic illness, possibly related to superantigen expansion and activation of T cells (1305) by bacterial (1306) or viral infection (1307,1308). T-cell autoreactivity for antibodies to antigenic determinants of human heat shock protein that develop during the course of the disease has been related to susceptibility to this condition (1309).

Kawasaki disease has an acute phase lasting approximately 2 weeks. In typical cases, this phase is marked by a febrile period of more than 5 days, an erythematous rash, conjunctival injection, erythema and crusting of lips and mouth, a strawberry tongue, swelling of hands and feet, and lymph node enlargement. After approximately 10 days, the fever subsides and the subacute phase begins. Arthritic manifestations, cardiac disease with coronary obstruction

or aneurysms, and thrombocytosis can occur during this period, as well as desquamation of the fingers and toes. Sterile pyuria or proteinuria, diarrhea, abdominal distress, hepatitis, or hydrops of the gallbladder also is encountered. The convalescent phase can last for several months. If death occurs, it is usually caused by cardiac complications.

Nearly all patients with Kawasaki disease demonstrate some degree of CNS involvement. Irritability, mood lability, and sleep disturbances are common. Semicoma or coma can occur for several days. Approximately one-fourth of children have an aseptic meningitis with severe lethargy and nuchal rigidity. Severe myositis can occur (1310). Facial palsy is a rare complication (1311). In up to 40% of patients the CSF shows a mononuclear pleocytosis of up to 320 cells. Protein and glucose are usually normal (1312,1313).

Treatment with intravenous gamma globulin (2 g/kg as a single dose given over 10 to 12 hours; a second infusion may be needed of 400 mg/kg per day for 4 days) and aspirin decreases the cardiac sequelae and leads to rapid resolution of sequelae (1314–1316). Plasma exchange also can be of benefit (1317).

Chronic Focal Encephalitis (Rasmussen Encephalitis)

Chronic focal encephalitis (Rasmussen syndrome), first described in 1958, is characterized by uncontrollable focal seizures associated with focal inflammation in cerebral tissue (1318). The current concept is that the condition represents a syndrome with a heterogeneous etiology (1319). Evidence exists for a viral etiology in that in some cases CMV and herpes simplex virus genomes can be demonstrated in brain tissue (1320–1322). In other instances, serum autoantibodies to glutamate receptor GluR3 are seen (1323). Elevated serum antinuclear antibody titers, CSF evidence of endogenous production of IgG, and immunofluorescent staining of brain tissue for IgG, IgM, IgA, C3, and C1q also have been described (1321a).

On pathologic examination of brain, the cortex of the affected side is thinned and scarred. Microscopically, perivascular lymphocytic infiltrates are seen with vascular injury and astrogliosis. Microglial nodules can occur; leptomeningeal infiltration is rare. Neuronal loss and cortical atrophy can be marked (1324). The contralateral side is generally normal.

Typically, patients develop simple partial seizures before age 10 years. An antecedent febrile illness is usually absent. In more than one-half of children, these seizures progress to epilepsia partialis continua. Complex partial seizures or secondary generalized seizures also can occur. As a result of the disease process, most patients experience a developmental arrest or regression. Neuropsychological deficits or behavioral disturbances can result, in part from the persistent seizure activity or from large doses of anticonvulsants (1325).

Hart and coworkers have described a form of chronic encephalitis with onset of seizures in adolescence without apparent cause and pathologic features of chronic encephalitis. These cases differ from classical Rasmussen encephalitis in that the course is more benign, an increased incidence of occipital involvement occurs, and the response to surgery is variable (1326).

EEG in Rasmussen encephalitis demonstrates broadly distributed but lateralized spike foci with underlying slow-wave disturbances, usually in the centrotemporal region (1325). CSF changes can include a mild pleocytosis or elevation of protein.

Neuroimaging studies generally show the progressive evolution of focal or hemispheric atrophy (1327). Regional hypoperfusion and interictal hypometabolism can be demonstrated by PET scanning. Proton MR spectroscopy is more sensitive than MRI in that it provides evidence for progressive neuronal damage at a stage when the MRI shows normal results. Even this sensitive study fails to show any abnormalities on the contralateral side (1328).

The sudden onset in a previously healthy youngster of an intractable unilateral seizure disorder, particularly one that manifests with epilepsia partialis continua, points to the diagnosis. The progressive nature of the condition, and the progressive changes on neuroimaging confirm the diagnosis.

Therapy with anticonvulsant drugs is usually unsuccessful, but hemispherectomy has proved beneficial in the majority of patients (1329, 1330). Selected cases have responded to chronic corticosteroid therapy (1331), intravenous gamma globulin (1332), or plasmapheresis (1333). Ganciclovir therapy also has been reported to be of benefit (1334). In the majority of children hemispherectomy is required. The response to the procedure is generally satisfactory. The use of hemispherectomy in the treatment of intractable focal seizures is covered more extensively in Chapter 13.

Thrombotic Thrombocytopenic Purpura and Hemolytic-Uremic Syndrome

Thrombotic thrombocytopenic purpura (TTP) and hemolytic-uremic syndrome (HUS) are two closely related conditions that may in fact represent differing clusters of manifestations of a single disease process. TTP is marked by the combination of fever, hemolytic anemia, renal failure, and neurologic dysfunction in association with widespread hyaline thrombosis of small blood vessels. HUS may have any or all of these same findings. In fact, no objective criteria except age distinguish these two illnesses. When the patient is younger (e.g., younger than 5 years of age) and renal abnormalities are predominant, HUS is usually diagnosed. When the patient is older and neurologic findings are predominant, TTP is usually diagnosed.

TTP and HUS appear to have common mechanisms, and it is not known why there is age-related variation in organ involvement. Patients with recurrent illness may have manifestations suggesting HUS on one exacerbation and TTP on another (1335).

Both illnesses appear to be mediated by inflammatory or toxic vascular endothelial injury. Antiendothelial antibodies may play a role in TTP (1336), whereas circulating bacterial toxins may mediate injury in HUS (1137,1338). The epidemic form of HUS has been associated with a verocytotoxin-producing *E. coli*, notably *E. coli* O157:H7, or *Shigella dysenteriae* type 1 infection (1339). This toxin kills mammalian cells by inhibiting protein synthesis and is thought to initiate HUS by damaging vascular endothelial cells (1340). Verocytotoxin is composed of five B subunits and one A subunit. The B subunits bind to Gb_3 ganglioside in the cell membrane. After endocytosis the A unit enzymatically inactivates the 60S ribosomal subunit, thus blocking protein synthesis (1340). The mechanism by which vero-cytotoxins produce disease are not fully understood (1339). An overwhelming amount of unusually large multimeric forms of von Willebrand factor is produced (1341). TNF and IL-1 induce expression of the verocytotoxin receptor globotriaosylceramide in human endothelial cells (1342). Shiga lipopolysaccharide (endotoxin) and TNF, but not IL-1, augment the cytotoxicity of Shiga toxin (1343). Other factors also may be involved because female gender, use of antimotility drugs, and increased hemoglobin level are associated with an increased risk for developing a neurologic manifestation, whereas prior administration of a blood product is associated with a decreased risk (1344). In addition, it is possible that patients are rendered more vulnerable to either HUS or TTP because they are deficient in a plasma factor that regulates endothelial prostacyclin synthctase. Circulating factors related to platelet adhesion that also may be of importance include a calcium-activated cysteine protease, or unusually large von Willebrand factor multimers. The von Willebrand multimers, produced by megakaryocytes or endothelial cells, may react with circulating adenosine diphosphate, calcium, or abnormalities of fluid shear forces and result in platelet aggregation. Some patients may lack a component of plasma that is involved in the reduction of large circulating multimers of von Willebrand factor. Persistence of these multimers in circulation may be of particular importance in recurrence of TTP or HUS (1345,1346).

Although TTP is often idiopathic, it can develop in association with a variety of inflammatory diseases (e.g., rheumatoid arthritis, polyarteritis nodosa, systemic lupus erythematosus, Sjögren syndrome), lymphoma, endocarditis, puerperium, and drugs and poisons (i.e., sulfa, cyclosporine A, iodine, birth control pills) (1347,1348). TTP is slightly more common in girls than in boys (ratio 3:2).

HUS develops in approximately 1% of patients treated with cyclosporine. On rare occasions the condition is associated with *Salmo-*

nella typhi infection, pneumococcal sepsis caused by neuraminidase-producing organisms, and *Campylobacter* enteritis (1349). It also is seen as a complication of pneumococcal meningitis or pneumococcal pneumonia (1350).

Although the peak incidence of TTP is in the third decade, it can occur in neonates and young children (1351). The illness may be monophasic or may recur. The tendency to recur is not predictable on either a clinical or laboratory basis. Some studies have suggested an autosomal recessive trait that predisposes patients to TTP, conceivably genetic deficiency of one of the factors noted previously, such as prostacyclin synthetase (1352).

By contrast, HUS develops in infants and young children. It is manifested by a prodromal period of vomiting, bloody diarrhea, and abdominal pain lasting an average of 1 week. Occasionally, an antecedent urinary tract infection occurs (1353). Then, after a silent period of several days, children have acute renal insufficiency, hemolytic anemia, and thrombocytopenia.

Neurologic symptoms, which can be the presenting feature, appear during the third phase in as many as 20% to 50% of patients (1341,1354,1355). They are believed in part to be caused by azotemia, hyponatremia, and hypocalcemia. In addition, a thrombotic microangiopathy occurs, with areas of reduced cerebral perfusion seen on single photon emission CT (1356). Some 3% to 5% of subjects develop focal areas of infarction surrounded by edema and necrosis. Thrombi are usually located in arterioles and capillary-postcapillary venular complexes. Two patterns can be distinguished. One is a loose fibrin meshwork with entrapped leukocytes and erythrocytes, and the other is a course granular aggregation of eosinophilic material that is often acellular (1357). Large thrombotic strokes also have been reported (1358).

Neurologic manifestations include changes in consciousness and generalized or partial seizures (1349,1355,1356). Seizures can occur in the absence of uremia or hypertension (1357). Less common are transient or permanent hemipareses, decerebrate or dystonic posturing, cortical blindness, or transient hallucinations (1356,1359). CNS symptoms can be aggravated by complica-

tions of systemic involvement such as hyponatremia, uremia, or severe hypertension (1360).

The EEG can show a unique pattern with
epochs of diffuse slowing alternating with epochs
of classic burst suppression. Infusion of fresh
frozen plasma improves this tracing before any
clinical improvement (1361). Neuroimaging studies disclose large vessel infarctions or multiple
small infarcts, often in conjunction with diffuse
cerebral edema or multiple hemorrhages (1355).

Treatment of the neurologic symptoms
requires correction of any electrolyte imbalance
and cerebral edema and control of seizures.
Hemolysis can cause significant anemia and
hyperkalemia. Seizures, which may be caused
by cerebral structural damage, electrolyte
imbalance, hypertension, or severe azotemia,
require specific therapy but generally respond to
diazepam and phenytoin (1349).

In the majority of children, neurologic symptoms recede, and the prognosis is that of renal
insufficiency, which is usually self-limiting.
Factors associated with a poor prognosis are elevated polymorphonuclear leukocyte count, short
duration of prodrome, bloody diarrhea, hypocalcemia, and oliguria detected within 48 hours of
hospital admission (1341). Children with neurologic involvement are more likely to develop
residual hypertension or chronic renal failure, or
to die, suggesting that neurologic involvement is
associated with increased severity of the syndrome (1362). Coma and increased CSF protein
are more common in patients with a poor outcome (1354). However, even prolonged coma
can be compatible with good outcome (1363).

REFERENCES

1. Rich AR, McCordock HA. The pathogenesis of tuber-culous meningitis. *Bull Johns Hopkins Hosp* 1933;52:5–37.
2. Rosenfeld EA, Rowley AH. Infectious intracranial complications of sinusitis, other than meningitis in children: 12-year review. *Clin Infect Dis* 1994;18:750–754.
3. Harter DH, Petersdorf RG. A consideration of the pathogenesis of bacterial meningitis. Review of experimental and clinical studies. *Yale J Biol Med* 1960;32:280–309.
4. Stephens DS, Farley MM. Pathogenic events during infection of the human nasopharynx with *Neisseria meningitidis* and *Haemophilus influenzae*. *Rev Infec Dis* 1991;13:22–33.
5. Quagliarello V, Scheld WM. Bacterial meningitis: pathogenesis, pathophysiology, and progress. *N Engl J Med* 1992;327:864–872.
6. Tunkel AR, Scheld WM. Alterations in the blood-brain barrier in bacterial meningitis: in vivo and in vitro models. *Pediatr Infect Dis J* 1989;8:911–912.
7. Ring A, Weiser JN, Tuomanen EI. Pneumococcal trafficking across the blood-brain barrier: molecular analysis of a novel bi-directional pathway. *J Clin Invest* 1998;102:347–360.
8. Wispelwey B, Hansen EJ, Scheld WM. *Haemophilus influenzae* outer membrane vesicle-induced blood-brain barrier permeability during experimental meningitis. *Infect Immun* 1989;57:2559–2562.
9. Paul R, et al. Matrix metalloproteinases contribute to the blood-brain barrier disruption during bacterial meningitis. *Ann Neurol* 1998;44:592–600.
9a. Kieseier BC, et al. Differential expression of matrix metalloproteinases in bacterial meningitis. *Brain* 1999;122: 1579–1587.
10. Hemphill M, et al. A new, treatable source of recurrent meningitis: basioccipital meningocele. *Pediatrics* 1982;70:941–943.
11. Schiffer MS, et al. A review: relation between invasiveness and the K-1 capsular polysaccharide of *Escherichia coli*. *Pediatr Res* 1976;10:82–87.
12. Schuchat A, et al., for the Active Surveillance Team. Bacterial meningitis in the United States in 1995. *N Engl J Med* 1997;337:970–976.
13. Adams RD, Kubik CS, Bonner FJ. The clinical and pathological aspects of influenzal meningitis. *Arch Ped* 1948;65:354–376, 408–441.
14. Saez-Llorens X, et al. Molecular pathophysiology of bacterial meningitis: current concepts and therapeutic implications. *J Pediatr* 1990;116:671–684.
15. Smith AL. Bacterial meningitis. *Pediatr Rev* 1993;14: 11–18.
16. Tunkel AR, Scheld WM. Pathogenesis and pathophysiology of bacterial meningitis. *Ann Rev Med* 1993;44:103–120.
17. Tunkel AR, Scheld WM. Acute bacterial meningitis. *Lancet* 1995;346:1675–1680.
18. Sze G, Zimmerman RD. The magnetic resonance imaging of infections and inflammatory diseases. *Radiol Clin North Am* 1988;26:839–859.
19. Smith JF, Landing BH. Mechanism of brain damage in *Haemophilus influenzae* meningitis. *J Neuropathol Exp Neurol* 1960;19:248–265.
20. Gallin GI, Goldstein IM, Snyderman R. *Inflammation. Basic principles and clinical correlates*, 2nd ed. New York: Raven Press, 1992.
21. Syrogiannopoulos GA, Hansen EJ, Erwin AL. *Haemophilus influenzae* type B lipooligosaccharide induces meningeal inflammation. *J Infect Dis* 1988;157:237–244.
22. Perry VH, Gordon S. Microglia and macrophages. In: Keane RW, Hickey WF (eds) *Immunology of the nervous system*. Oxford: Oxford University Press, 1997: 155–172.
23. Mustafa MM, et al. Prostaglandins E2 and I2, interleukin 1-β and tumor necrosis factor in cerebrospinal fluid in infants and children with bacterial meningitis. *Pediatr Infect Dis J* 1989;8:921–922.
24. Tuomanen E. Partner drugs: a new outlook for bacterial meningitis. *Ann Intern Med* 1988;109:690–692.

25. Liles WC, Van Voorhis WC. Review: nomenclature and biologic significance of cytokines involved in inflammation and the host immune response. *J Infect Dis* 1995;172:1573–1580.

26. Saukkonen K, et al. The role of cytokines in the generation of inflammation and tissue damage in experimental gram-positive meningitis. *J Exp Med* 1990; 171:439–448.

26a. Chao CC, et al. Cytokine release from microglia: differential inhibition by pentoxifylline and dexamethasone. *J Infect Dis* 1992;166:847–853.

26b. Pfister HW, et al. Transforming growth factor-β-2 inhibits cerebrovascular changes and brain edema formation in the tumor necrosis factor-α-independent early phase of experimental pneumococcal meningitis. *J Exp Med* 1992;176:265–268.

26c. Szabó, C, et al. Nifedipine inhibits the induction of nitric oxide synthase by bacterial lipopolysaccharide. *J Pharmacol Exp Ther* 1993;265:674–680.

27. Ramilo, O. et al. Tumor necrosis factor-α, cachectin, and interleukin 1-β initiate meningeal inflammation. *J Exper Med* 1990;172:497–507.

28. Mustafa MM, et al. Cerebrospinal fluid prostaglandins, interleukin 1 beta, and tumor necrosis factor in bacterial meningitis. Clinical and laboratory correlations in placebo-treated and dexamethasone-treated patients. *Am J Dis Child* 1990;144:883–887.

29. Van Furth AM, Roord JJ, van Furth R. Roles of proinflammatory and anti-inflammatory cytokines in pathophysiology of bacterial meningitis and effect of adjunctive therapy. *Infect Immun* 1996;64:4883–4890.

29a. Burroughs M, et al. Effect of thalidomide on the inflammatory response in cerebrospinal fluid in experimental meningitis. *Microb Pathog* 1995;19:245–255.

30. Sawada M, et al. Production of tumor necrosis factor-α by microglia and astrocytes in culture. *Brain Res* 1989;491:394–397.

31. Chung IY, Benveniste EN. Tumor necrosis factor-α production by astrocytes. Induction by lipopolysaccharide, IFN-gamma, and IL-1-β. *J Immunol* 1990;144: 2999–3007.

32. Quagliarello VJ, et al. Recombinant human interleukin-1 induces meningitis and blood-brain barrier injury in the rat. Characterization and comparison with tumor necrosis factor. *J Clin Invest* 1991;87: 1360–1366.

33. Laster SM, Wood JS, Gooding LR. Tumor necrosis factor can induce both apoptic and necrotic forms of cell lysis. *J Immunol* 1988;141:2629–2634.

34. Selmaj KW, Raine CS. Tumor necrosis factor mediates myelin and oligodendrocyte damage in vitro. *Ann Neurol* 1988;23:339–346.

35. Lopez-Cortes LF, et al. Measurement of levels of tumor necrosis factor-alpha and interleukin-1 beta in the CSF of patients with meningitis of different etiologies: utility in the differential diagnosis. *Clin Infect Dis* 1993;16:534–539.

36. Glimaker M, et al. Tumor necrosis factor (TNF)-α in cerebrospinal fluid from patients with meningitis of different etiologies. High levels of TNF-α indicate bacterial meningitis. *J Infect Dis* 1993;167:882–889.

36a. Dulkerian S, et al. Cytokine elevations in infants with bacterial and aseptic meningitis. *J Pediatr* 1995;126: 872–876.

37. Sapolsky R, et al. Interleukin-1 stimulates the secretion of hypothalamic corticotropin-releasing factor. *Science* 1987;238:522–524.

38. Long JB, Holaday JW. Blood-brain barrier: endogenous modulation by adreno-cortical function. *Science* 1985;227:1580–1583.

39. McCracken GH, et al. Cerebrospinal fluid interleukin 1-β and tumor necrosis factor concentrations and outcome from neonatal gram-negative enteric bacillary meningitis. *Pediatr Infect Dis J* 1989;8:155–159.

40. Velasco S, et al. Temperature-dependent modulation of lipopolysaccharide-induced interleukin-1-β and tumor necrosis factor-α in cultured human astroglial cells by dexamethasone and indomethacin. *J Clin Invest* 1991;87:1674–1680.

41. Scheld WM, Quagliarello VJ, Wispelwey B. Potential role of host cytokines in *Haemophilus influenzae* lipopolysaccharide-induced blood-brain barrier permeability. *Pediatr Infect Dis J* 1989;8:910–911.

42. Ramilo O, et al. Tumor necrosis factor alpha/cachectin and interleukin 1 beta initiate meningeal inflammation. *J Exp Med* 1990;172:497–507.

43. Saukkonen K, et al. The role of cytokines in the generation of inflammation and tissue damage in experimental gram-positive meningitis. *J Exp Med* 1990; 171:439–448.

44. Paris MM, et al. Effect of interleukin-1 receptor antagonist and soluble tumor necrosis factor receptor in animal models of infection. *J Infect Dis* 1995;171:161–169.

45. Moser R, et al. Interleukin-1 and tumor necrosis factor stimulate human vascular endothelial cells to promote transendothelial neutrophil passage. *J Clin Invest* 1989;83:444–455.

45a. Kanoh Y, Ohtani H. Levels of interleukin-6, CRP, and alpha 2 macroglobulin in cerebrospinal fluid (CSF) and serum as indicator of blood-CSF barrier damage. *Biochem Mol Biol Int* 1997;43:269–278.

45b. Arditi M, et al. Cerebrospinal fluid cachectin/tumor necrosis factor-alpha and platelet-activating factor concentrations and severity of bacterial meningitis. *Microb Pathog* 1995;19:245–255.

45c. Glimaker M, et al. Tumor necrosis factor-alpha (TNF alpha) in cerebrospinal fluid from patients with meningitis of different etiologies: high levels of TNF alpha indicate bacterial meningitis. *J Infect Dis* 1993;167: 882–889.

46. Mizel SB. The interleukins. *FASEB J* 1989;3: 2379–2388.

46a. Moller B, et al. Bioactive and inactive forms of tumor necrosis factor-alpha in spinal fluid from patients with meningitis. *J Infect Dis* 1991;163:886–889.

47. Torre D, et al. Cerebrospinal fluid levels of IL-6 in patients with acute infections of the central nervous system. *Scand J Infec Dis* 1992;24:787–791.

47a. Ossege LM, et al. Detection of transforming growth factor beta 1 mRNA in cerebrospinal fluid cells of patients with meningitis by non-radioactive in situ hybridization. *J Neurol* 1994;242:14–19.

48. Rusconi F, et al. Interleukin 6 activity in infants and children with bacterial meningitis. The collaborative study on meningitis. *Ped Infect Dis* 1991;10:117–121.

49. St. Georgiev V, Albright JF. Cytokines and their role as growth factors and in regulation of immune responses. In: St. Georgiev V, Yamaguchi H, eds. Immunomodulating drugs. *Ann NY Acad Sci* 1993;685:586–602.

50. Ostergaatrd C, et al. Interleukin-8 in cerebrospinal fluid from patients with septic and aseptic meningitis. *Eur J Clin Microbiol Infect Dis* 1996;15:166–169.

51. Gallo P, et al. Intrathecal synthesis of interleukin-10 (IL-10) in viral and inflammatory diseases of the central nervous system. *J Neurol Sci* 1994;126:48–53.

52. Koedel U, et al. Systemically (but not intrathecally) administered IL-10 attenuates pathophysiologic alterations in experimental pneumococcal meningitis. *J Immunol* 1996;157:5158–5191.

52a. Granert C, et al. Inhibition of leukocyte rolling with polysaccharide fucoidin prevents pleocytosis in experimental meningitis in the rabbit. *J Clin Invest* 1994;93:929–936.

53. Anthony D, et al. CXC chemokines generate age-related increases in neutrophil-mediated brain inflammation and blood-brain barrier breakdown. *Curr Biol* 1998;923–926.

54. Tani M, et al. Neutrophil infiltration, glial reaction, and neurological disease in transgenic mice expressing the chemokine N51/KC in oligodendrocytes. *J Clin Invest* 1996;98:529–539.

55. Tang T, et al. Cytokine-induced meningitis is dramatically attenuated in mice deficient in endothelial selectins. *J Clin Invest* 1996;97:2485–2490.

56. Lipton SA, et al. A redox based mechanism for the neuroprotective and neurodestructive effects of nitric oxide and related nitroso-compounds. *Nature* 1993;364:626–632.

57. Moncada S, Higgs A. The L-arginine-nitric oxide pathway. *N Engl J Med* 1993;329:2002–2012.

58. Buster BL, et al. Potential role of nitric oxide in the pathophysiology of experimental bacterial meningitis in rats. *Infect Immun* 1995;63:3835–3839.

59. Stahel PF, et al. Complement C3 and factor B cerebrospinal fluid concentrations in bacterial and aseptic meningitis. *Lancet* 1997;349:1886–1887.

60. Kreil TR, Eibi MM. Nitric oxide and viral infection: NO antiviral activity against a flavivirus in vitro, and evidence for contribution to the pathogenesis in experimental infection *in vivo*. *Virology* 1996;219: 304–306.

61. Burn CG, Finley KH. The role of hypersensitivity in the production of experimental meningitis. *J Exp Med* 1932;56:203–221.

62. Goitein KJ, Tamir I. Cerebral perfusion pressure in central nervous system infections of infancy and childhood. *J Pediatr* 1983;103:40–43.

63. Tureen JH, et al. Loss of cerebrovascular autoregulation in experimental meningitis in rabbits. *J Clin Invest* 1990;85:577–581.

64. Fishman RA, Sligar K, Hake RB. Effects of leukocytes on brain metabolism in granulocytic brain edema. *Ann Neurol* 1977;2:89–94.

65. Chan PH, et al. Induction of brain edema following intracerebral injection of arachidonic acid. *Ann Neurol* 1983;13:625–632.

66. Chan PH, Fishman RA. Transient formation of superoxide radicals in polyunsaturated fatty acid-induced brain swelling. *J Neurochem* 1980;35:1004–1007.

67. McNight AA, et al. Oxygen-free radicals and the cerebral arteriolar response to Group B streptococci. *Pediatr Res* 1992;31:640–644.

68. Snyder RD, et al. Cerebral infarction in childhood bacterial meningitis. *J Neurol Neurosurg Psychiatry* 1981;44:581–585.

69. Raetz CR, et al. Gram-negative endotoxin: an extraordinary lipid with profound effects on eukaryocytic signal transduction. *FASEB J* 1991;5:2652–2660.

70. Ducker TB, Simmons RL. The pathogenesis of meningitis: systemic effects of meningococcal endotoxin within the cerebrospinal fluid. *Arch Neurol* 1968;18: 123–128.

71. McCracken GH Jr. Endotoxin concentrations in cerebrospinal fluid correlate with clinical severity and neurologic outcome of *Haemophilus influenzae* type B meningitis. *Am J Dis Child* 1991;145: 1099–1103.

72. Pfister HW, et al. Microvascular changes during the early phase of experimental bacterial meningitis. *J Cereb Blood Flow Metab* 1990;10:914–922.

73. Goh D, Minns RA. Cerebral blood flow velocity monitoring in pyogenic meningitis. *Arch Dis Child* 1993;68:111–119.

74. Paulson OB, et al. Cerebral blood flow, cerebral metabolic rate of oxygen and CSF acid-base parameters in patients with acute pyogenic meningitis and with acute encephalitis. *Acta Neurol Scand Suppl* 1972;51: 407–408.

75. Guerra Romero L, Tureen JH, Tauber MG. Pathogenesis of central nervous system injury in bacterial meningitis. *Antibiot Chemother* 1992;45:18–29.

76. Ashwal S, et al. Cerebral blood flow and carbon dioxide reactivity in children with bacterial meningitis. *J Pediatr* 1990;117:523–530.

77. Goitein KJ, Amit Y, Mussaffi H. Intracranial pressure in central nervous system infections and cerebral ischaemia of infancy. *Arch Dis Child* 1983;58: 184–186.

78. Shigeri Y, Mihara S-I, Fujimoto M. Neuropeptide Y receptor in vascular smooth muscle. *J Neurochem* 1991;56:852–859.

79. Tauber MG, et al. Brain levels of neuropeptide Y in experimental pneumococcal meningitis. *Mol Chem Neuropathol* 1993;18:15–26.

80. Spranger M, et al. Excess glutamate levels in the cerebrospinal fluid predict clinical outcome in bacterial meningitis. *Arch Neurol* 1996;53:992–996.

81. Colice GL, et al. Neurogenic pulmonary edema. *Am Rev Respir Dis* 1984;130:941–948.

82. Baraff LJ, Oslund S, Prather M. Effect of antibiotic therapy and etiologic microorganism on the risk of bacterial meningitis in children with occult bacteremia. *Pediatrics* 1993;92:140–143.

83. Swartz MH, Dodge PR. Bacterial meningitis: a review of selected aspects. I. General clinical features, special problems and unusual meningeal reactions mimicking bacterial meningitis. *N Engl J Med* 1965;272: 725–731, 779–787, 842–848, 898–902.

84. Durand ML, Calderwood SB, Webber DJ, et al. Acute bacterial meningitis in adults. A review of 493 episodes. *N Engl J Med* 1993;328:21–28.

85. Dodge PR, Swartz MN. Bacterial meningitis: a review of selected aspects. II. Special neurologic problems, post-meningitic complications and clinicopathological correlations. *N Engl J Med* 1965;272:954–960, 1003–1010.

86. O'Connell JE. The clinical signs of meningeal irritation. *Brain* 1946;69:9–21.

87. Vincent J, Thomas K, Mathew O. An improved clinical method for detecting meningeal irritation. *Arch Dis Child* 1993;68:215–218.

88. Samson JH, Apthorp J, Finley A. Febrile seizures and purulent meningitis. *JAMA* 1969;10:1918–1919.
89. Rutter N, Smales OR. Lumbar puncture in children with convulsions. *Lancet* 1977;2:190–191.
90. Green SM, et al. Can seizures be the sole manifestation of meningitis in febrile children? *Pediatrics* 1993;92:527–534.
91. Rivner MH, et al. Opsoclonus in *Haemophilus influenzae* meningitis. *Neurology* 1982;32:661–663.
92. Eavey RD, et al. Otologic features of bacterial meningitis of childhood. *J Pediatr* 1985;106:402–407.
93. Comis SD, et al. Cytotoxic effects on hair cells of guinea pig cochlea produced by pneumolysin, the thiolactivated toxin of *Streptococcus pneumoniae*. *Acta Otolaryngol Stockh* 1993;113:152–159.
94. Jeffery H, et al. Deafness after bacterial meningitis. *Arch Dis Child* 1977;52:555–559.
95. Fortnum H, Davis A. Hearing impairment in children after bacterial meningitis: incidence and resource implications. *Br J Audiol* 1993;27:43–52.
96. Jiang ZD, et al. Long-term impairments of brain and auditory functions of children recovered from purulent meningitis. *Dev Med Child Neurol* 1990;32:473–480.
96a. Richard MP, et al. Otoacoustic emissions as a screening test for hearing impairment in children recovering from acute bacterial meningitis. *Pediatrics* 1998;102:1364–1368.
97. Green JP, Newman NJ, Winterkorn JS. Paralysis of downward gaze in two patients with clinical-radiologic correlation. *Arch Ophthalmol* 1993;111:219–222.
98. Schwartz JF. Ataxia in bacterial meningitis. *Neurology* 1972;22:1071–1074.
99. Yabek SM. Meningococcal meningitis presenting as acute cerebellar ataxia. *Pediatrics* 1973;52:718–720.
100. Thun-Hohenstein L, et al. Cortical visual impairment following bacterial meningitis: magnetic resonance imaging and visual evoked potentials findings in two cases. *Eur J Pediatr* 1992;15:779–782.
101. Holmes RD, Kuhns LR, Oliver WJ. Widened sutures in childhood meningitis, unrecognized sign of an acute illness. *Am J Roentgenol* 1977;128:977–979.
102. Snyder RD. Ventriculomegaly in childhood bacterial meningitis. *Neuropediatrics* 1984;15:136–138.
103. Mace JW, Peters ER, Mathies AW Jr. Cranial bruits in purulent meningitis in childhood. *N Engl J Med* 1968;278:1420–1422.
104. Gellis S, Feingold M, Steinhoff MC. Picture of the month. Tache cerebrale. *Am J Dis Child* 1977;131:709–710.
105. Berman PH, Banker BQ. Neonatal meningitis: a clinical and pathological study of 29 cases. *Pediatrics* 1966;38:6–24.
106. Salmon JH. Ventriculitis complicating meningitis. *Am J Dis Child* 1972;124:35–40.
107. Snedeker JD, et al. Subdural effusion and its relationship with neurologic sequelae of bacterial meningitis in infancy: a prospective study. *Pediatrics* 1990;86:163–170.
108. Bok AP, Peter JC. Subdural empyema: burr hole or craniotomy?—a retrospective computerized tomography-era analysis of treatment in 90 cases. *J Neurosurg* 1993;78:574–578.
109. Matson DD. *Neurosurgery of infancy and childhood*, 2nd ed. Springfield, IL: Charles C Thomas, 1969.
110. Chen CY, et al. Subdural empyema in 10 infants: US characteristics and clinical correlates. *Radiology* 1998;207:609–617.
111. Rabe EF, Flynn RE, Dodge PR. Subdural collections of fluids in infants and children: a study of 62 patients with special reference to factors influencing prognosis and efficacy of various forms of therapy. *Neurology* 1968;18:559–570.
112. Tureen JH, Täuber MG, Sande MA. Effect of hydration status on cerebral blood flow and cerebrospinal fluid lactic acidosis in rabbits with experimental meningitis. *J Clin Invest* 1992;89:947–953.
112a. Kumar V, Singhi P, Singhi S. Changes in body water compartments in children with acute meningitis. *Pediatr Infect Dis J* 1994;13:299–303.
113. Kaplan SL, Feigin RD. The syndrome of inappropriate secretion of antidiuretic hormone in children with bacterial meningitis. *J Pediatr* 1978;92:758–761.
114. Fuyong J, et al. Concentrations of atrial naturietic peptide of plasma and CSF neurologic diseases [Abstract]. *Pediatr Neurol* 1992;8:3–46.
115. Padilla G, et al. Vasopressin levels in pediatric head trauma. *Pediatrics* 1989;83:700–705.
116. Fajardo JE, et al. Inappropriate antidiuretic hormone in children with viral meningitis. *Pediatr Neurol* 1989;5:37–40.
117. Decaux G, et al. Treatment of the syndrome of inappropriate secretion of antidiuretic hormone with furosemide. *N Engl J Med* 1981;304:329–330.
118. Cotton MF, et al. Raised intracranial pressure, the syndrome of inappropriate antidiuretic hormone secretion, and arginine vasopressin in tuberculous meningitis. *Childs Nerv Syst* 1993;9:10–15.
119. Powell KR, et al. Normalization of plasma arginine vasopressin concentrations when children with meningitis are given maintenance plus replacement fluid therapy. *J Pediatr* 1990;117:515–522.
120. Lieb G, et al. Recurrent bacterial meningitis. *Eur J Pediatr* 1996;155:26–30.
121. Cherry JD, Sheenan CP. Bacteriologic relapse in *Haemophilus influenzae* meningitis: inadequate ampicillin therapy. *N Engl J Med* 1968;278:1001–1003.
122. Klein JO, Feigin RD, McCracken GH Jr. Report of the task force on diagnosis and management of meningitis. *Pediatrics* 1986;78:959–982.
123. Feigin RD, McCracken GH Jr, Klein JO. Diagnosis and management of meningitis. *Pediatr Infect Dis J* 1992;11:785–814.
124. Archer BD. Computed tomography before lumbar puncture in acute meningitis: a review of the risks and benefits. *Can Med Assoc J* 1993;148:961–965.
125. Quagliarello VJ, Scheld WM. Treatment of bacterial meningitis. *N Engl J Med* 1997;336:708–716.
126. Rosenthal J, Golan A, Dagan R. Bacterial meningitis with initial normal cerebrospinal fluid findings. *Isr J Med Sci* 1989;25:186–188.
127. Milne A, Hamilton W. Developing or normocellular meningitis. *NZ Med J* 1976;84:6–8.
128. Ismail Y, Arsura EL. Eosinophilic meningitis associated with coccidioidomycosis. *West J Med* 1993;158:300–301.
129. Lichtheim L. Bei Gehirnkrankheiten durch die Punction der Subarachnoidalräume auf der Höhe des dritten Lendenwirbels und Entziehung von Liquor cerebrospinalis therapeutish enizugreifen [Abstract]. *Dtsch Med Wochenschr* 1893;19:12–34.

130. Prockop LD, Fishman RA. Experimental pneumococcal meningitis. Permeability changes influencing the concentration of sugars and macromolecules in the cerebrospinal fluid. *Arch Neurol* 1968;19: 449–463.

131. Menkes JH. The causes for low spinal fluid sugar in bacterial meningitis—another look. *Pediatrics* 1969; 44:1–3.

132. Wolf SM. Decreased cerebrospinal fluid glucose level in herpes zoster meningitis. Report of a case. *Arch Neurol* 1974;30:109.

133. Donald PR, Malan C, van der Walt A. Simultaneous determination of cerebrospinal fluid glucose and blood glucose concentrations in the diagnosis of bacterial meningitis. *J Pediatr* 1983;103:413–415.

134. Shaaban SY, et al. Prognostic value of cerebrospinal fluid protein content and leukocyte count in infants and childhood bacterial meningitis. *J Egypt Public Health Assoc* 1991;66:345–355.

135. Anagnostakis D, et al. Blood-brain barrier permeability in "healthy" infected and stressed neonates. *J Pediatr* 1992;121:291–294.

136. Lindquist R, et al. Experimental meningitis in the rabbit. II. Cerebral energy metabolism in relation to increased cerebrospinal fluid concentrations of lactate. *Acta Neurol Scand* 1987;75:405–409.

137. Lindquist L, et al. Value of cerebrospinal fluid analysis in the differential diagnosis of meningitis—a study of 710 patients with suspected central nervous system infection. *Eur J Clin Microbiol Infect Dis* 1988;7:374–380.

138. Controni G, et al. Cerebrospinal fluid lactic acid levels in meningitis. *J Pediatr* 1977;91:379–384.

139. Gould IM, Irwin WJ, Wadhwani RR. The use of cerebrospinal fluid lactate determination in the diagnosis of meningitis. *Scand J Infect Dis* 1980;12:185–188.

140. Bland RD, Lister RC, Ries JP. Cerebrospinal fluid lactic acid levels and pH in meningitis. AIDS in differential diagnosis. *Am J Dis Child* 1974;128: 151–156.

141. Converse GM, et al. Alteration of cerebrospinal fluid findings by partial treatment of bacterial meningitis. *J Pediatr* 1973;83:220–225.

142. Feldman WE. Cerebrospinal fluid lactic acid dehydrogenase activity. Levels in untreated and partially antibiotic-treated meningitis. *Am J Dis Child* 1975; 127:77–80.

143. Belsy MA. CSF glutamic oxaloacetic transaminase in acute bacterial meningitis. *Am J Dis Child* 1969;117: 288–293.

144. Hashim IA, et al. Cerebrospinal fluid interleukin-6 and its diagnostic value in the investigation of meningitis. *Ann Clin Biochem* 1995;32:289–296.

145. Hansson LO, et al. Serum C-reactive protein in the differential diagnosis of acute meningitis. *Scand J Infect Dis* 1993;25:625–630.

146. Roine I, et al. Serum C-reactive protein vs. tumor necrosis factor α and interleukin-1-β of the cerebrospinal fluid in diagnosis of bacterial meningitis with low cerebrospinal fluid cell count. *Pediatr Infect Dis J* 1992;11:1057–1058.

147. Katnik RA. A persistent biochemical marker for partially treated meningitis/ventriculitis. *J Child Neuro* 1995;10:93–99.

148. O'Reilly RJ, et al. Circulating polyribophosphate in *Haemophilus influenzae*, type B meningitis. Correlation with clinical course and antibody response. *J Clin Invest* 1975;56:1012–1022.

149. McCracken GH Jr, et al. Relation between *Escherichia coli* K-1 capsular polysaccharide antigen and clinical outcome in neonatal meningitis. *Lancet* 1974; 2:246–250.

150. Ni H, et al. Polymerase chain reaction for diagnosis of meningococcal meningitis. *Lancet* 1992;340: 1432–1434.

151. Narita M, et al. Nested amplification protocol for the detection of *Mycobacterium tuberculosis*. *Acta Paediatr* 1992;81:997–1001.

152. Kox LFF, Ing SK, Kolk AHJ. Early diagnosis of tuberculous meningitis by polycerase chain reaction. *Neurology* 1995;45:2228–2232.

153. Seth P, et al. Evaluation of polymerase chain reaction for rapid diagnosis of clinically suspected tuberculous meningitis. *Tuber Lung Dis* 1996;77: 353–357.

154. Hansen K. Lyme neuroborreliosis. Improvements of the laboratory diagnosis and a survey of epidemiological and clinical features in Denmark 1985–1990. *Acta Neurol Scand* 1994;89[Suppl 151]:6–44.

155. Casas I, et al. Two different PCR assays to detect enteroviral RNA in CSF from patients with acute aseptic meningitis. *J Med Virol* 1995;47:378–85.

156. Troendle-Atkins J, Demmler GJ, Buffone GJ. Rapid diagnosis of herpes simplex virus encephalitis by using the polymerase chain reaction. *J Pediatr* 1993;123: 376–380.

157. Jeffery KJM, et al. Diagnosis of viral infections of the central nervous system: clinical interpretation of PCR results. *Lancet* 1997;349:313–317.

158. Noordhoek GT, van Embden JDA, Kolk AHJ. Questionable reliability of the polymerase chain reaction in the detection of *Mycobacterium tuberculosis* [Letter]. *N Engl J Med* 1993;329:20–36.

159. Mertsola J, et al. Endotoxin concentrations in cerebrospinal fluid correlate with clinical severity and neurologic outcome of *Haemophilus influenzae* type B meningitis. *Am J Dis Child* 1991;145: 1099–1103.

160. Denis F, et al. Bacterial antigen concentrations in cerebrospinal fluid and prognosis of purulent meningitis [Letter]. *Lancet* 1981;1:1361.

161. Mandal BK. The dilemma of partially treated bacterial meningitis. *Scand J Infect Dis* 1976;8:185–188.

162. Talan DA, et al. Role of empiric parenteral antibiotics prior to lumbar puncture in suspected bacterial meningitis: state of the art. *Rev Infect Dis* 1988;10: 365–376.

163. Balm M, Hammack J. Leptomeningeal carcinomatosis. *Arch Neurol* 1996;53:626–632.

164. Squadrini F, et al. Simultaneous bacterial and viral meningitis [Letter]. *Lancet* 1977;1:1371.

165. Riordan FAI, et al. Does computed tomography have a role in the evaluation of complicated acute bacterial meningitis in childhood? *Dev Med Child Neurol* 1993;35;275–276.

166. Rennick G, Shann F, de Campo J. Cerebral herniation during bacterial meningitis in children. *BMJ* 1993; 306:953–955.

167. Brown K, Steer C. Strategies in the management of children with acute encephalopathies. In: Gordon N, McKinlay I, eds. *Children with neurological diseases*. Book 2. Boston: Blackwell, 1986:219–293.

168. Benjamin CM, Newton RW, Clark MA. Risk factors for death from meningitis. *BMJ* (Clin Res Ed) 1988; 296:20.
169. Feske SK, et al. Uncal herniation secondary to bacterial meningitis in a newborn. *Pediatr Neurol* 1992;8: 142–144.
170. Lambert HP. Meningitis. *J Neurol Neurosurg Psychiatry* 1994;57:405–415.
171. Kaplan SL, Fishman MA. Supportive therapy for bacterial meningitis. *Pediatr Infec Dis J* 1987;6:670–677.
172. Wubbel L, McCracken GH Jr. Management of bacterial meningitis. *Pediatr Rev* 1998;19:78–84.
173. Roos KL, Tunkel AR, Scheld WM. Acute bacterial meningitis in children and adults. In: Scheld WM, Whitley RJ, Durack DT, eds. *Infections of the central nervous system.* New York: Raven Press, 1991: 335–409.
174. Kramer PW, Griffith RS, Campbell RL. Antibiotic penetration of the brain—a comparative study. *J Neurosurg* 1969;31:295–302.
175. Peltola H, Anttila M, Renkonen OV. Randomized comparison of chloramphenicol, ampicillin, cefotaxime, and ceftriaxone for childhood bacterial meningitis. *Lancet* 1989;1:1281–1287.
176. Craig JC, Abbott GD, Mogridge NB. Ceftriaxone for paediatric bacterial meningitis. *NZ Med J* 1992;105: 441–444.
177. Scholz H, et al. Prospective comparison of ceftriaxone and cefotaxime for the short-term treatment of bacterial meningitis in children. *Chemotherapy* 1998;44: 142–147.
178. Radetsky M. Duration of treatment in bacterial meningitis: a historical inquiry. *Pediatr Infect Dis J* 1990; 9:2–9.
179. Plorde JJ, Garcia M, Petersdorf RG. Studies on the pathogenesis of meningitis. IV. Penicillin levels in the cerebrospinal fluid in experimental meningitis. *J Lab Clin Med* 1964;64:960–969.
180. Hieber JP, Nelson JD. A pharmacologic evaluation of penicillin in children with purulent meningitis. *N Engl J Med* 1977;297:410–413.
181. Lebel MH, et al. Dexamethasone therapy for bacterial meningitis. Result of two double-blind, placebo-controlled trials. *N Engl J Med* 1988;319: 964–971.
182. Schaad UB, et al. Dexamethasone therapy for bacterial meningitis in children. Swiss meningitis study group. *Lancet* 1993;342:457–461.
183. Jafari HS, McCracken GH Jr. Update on steroids for bacterial meningitis. *Rep Pediatr Infect Dis* 1993;3:5–6.
184. Kanra GY, et al. Beneficial effects of dexamethasone in children with pneumococcal meningitis. *Pediatr Infect Dis J* 1995;14:490–494.
185. Kaplan S. Pneumococcal meningitis: an evolving approach to management. *Rep Pediatr Infect Dis* 1995;5:13–14.
186. Syrogiannopoulos GA, et al. Dexamethasone therapy for bacterial meningitis in children: 2- versus 4-day regimen. *J Infect Dis* 1994;169:8553–8858.
187. Schaad UB, Kaplan SL, McKracken GH Jr. Steroid therapy for bacterial meningitis. *Clin Infect Dis* 1995;20:685–690.
188. Spellerberg B, Tuomanen EI. The pathophysiology of pneumococcal meningitis. *Ann Med* 1994;26: 411–418.
189. Bhatt SM, Cabellos C, Nadol JB Jr. The impact of dexamethasone on hearing loss in experimental pneumococcal meningitis. *Pediatr Inf Dis J* 1995;14:93–96.
190. Durack DT, Spanos A. End-of-treatment spinal tap in meningitis. *JAMA* 1982;248:75–78.
191. Feigin RD, Pearlman E. Bacterial meningitis beyond the neonatal period. In: Feigin RD, Cherry JD, eds. *Textbook of pediatric infectious diseases,* 4th ed. Philadelphia: WB Saunders Co, 1998:400–429.
192. Balagtas RC, et al. Secondary and prolonged fevers in bacterial meningitis. *J Pediatr* 1970;77:957–964.
193. Lin TY, Nelson JD, McCracken GH Jr. Fever during treatment for bacterial meningitis. *Pediatr Infect Dis* 1984;3:319–322.
194. Dodge PR. Sequelae of bacterial meningitis. *Pediatr Infect Dis J* 1986;5:618–620.
195. Radetsky M. Duration of symptoms and outcome in bacterial meningitis: an analysis of causation and the implications of a delay in diagnosis. *Pediatr Infect Dis J* 1992;11:694–698.
196. Kresky B, Buchbinder S, Greenberg IM. The incidence of neurologic residua in children after recovery from bacterial meningitis. *Arch Pediatr* 1962;79: 63–71.
197. Kilpi T, et al. Length of prediagnostic history related to the course and sequelae of childhood bacterial meningitis. *Pediatr Infect Dis J* 1993;12:184–188.
198. Chang YC, et al. Risk factors for early fatality in children with acute bacterial meningitis. *Pediatr Neurol* 1998;18:213–217.
199. Grimwood K, et al. Adverse outcomes of bacterial meningitis in school-age survivors. *Pediatrics* 1995; 95:646–656.
200. Anderson V, et al. Childhood bacterial meningitis: impact of age at illness and acute medical complications on long term outcome. *J Int Neuropsychol Soc* 1997;3:147–158.
201. Thomas DG. Outcome of paediatric bacterial meningitis 1979–1989. *Med J Aust* 1992;157:519–520.
202. Baraff LJ, Lee SI, Schriger DL. Outcomes of bacterial meningitis in children: a meta-analysis. *Pediatr Infect Dis J* 1993;12:389–394.
203. Annegers JF, et al. The risk of unprovoked seizures after encephalitis and meningitis. *Neurology* 1988; 38:1407–1410.
204. Marks DA, et al. Characteristics of intractable seizures following meningitis and encephalitis. *Neurology* 1992;42:1513–1518.
205. Sell SH. Long-term sequelae of bacterial meningitis in children. *Pediatr Infect Dis* 1983;2:90–93.
206. Jadavji T, et al. Sequelae of acute bacterial meningitis in children treated for seven days. *Pediatrics* 1986;78: 21–25.
207. Moura-Ribeiro MVL. Serial EEG studies in bacterial meningitis in children [Abstract]. *Pediatr Neurol* 1992;8:402.
208. Pike MG, et al. Electrophysiologic studies, computed tomography, and neurologic outcome in acute bacterial meningitis. *J Pediatr* 1990;116:702–706.
209. Bhatt SM, et al. Progression of hearing loss in experimental pneumococcal meningitis: correlation with cerebrospinal fluid cytochemistry. *J Infect Dis* 1993; 167:675–683.
210. MacDonald JT, Feinstein S. Hearing loss following *Haemophilus influenzae* meningitis in infancy. Diag-

nosis by evoked response audiometry. *Arch Neurol* 1984;41:1058–1059.

211. Bao X, Wong V. Brainstem auditory-evoked potential evaluation in children with meningitis. *Pediatr Neurol* 1998;19:109–112.

212. Dodge PR, et al. Prospective evaluation of hearing impairment as a sequela of acute bacterial meningitis. *N Engl J Med* 1984;311:869–874.

213. Smith AL. Neurologic sequelae of meningitis. *N Engl J Med* 1988;319:1012–1014.

214. Schuchat A, et al. Bacterial meningitis in the United States in 1995. *N Engl J Med* 1997;337:970–976.

215. Wehrle PF, Leedom JM, Mathies AW. Treatment of meningococcal meningitis. *Mod Treatment* 1967;4:929–938.

216. Westendorp RGJ, et al. Genetic influences on cytokine production and fatal meningococcal disease. *Lancet* 1997;349:170–173.

217. Erickson L, De Wals P. Complications and sequelae of meningococcal disease in Quebec, Canada, 1990–1994. *Clin Infect Dis* 1998;26:1159–1164.

218. Whalen CM, et al. The changing epidemiology of invasive meningoccal disease in Canada, 1985–1992. Emergence of a virulent clone of *Neisseria meningitidis*. *J Am Med Assoc* 1995;273:390–394.

219. Fijen CA, et al. Complement deficiency predisposes to meningitis due to nongroupable meningococci and *Neisseria*-related organisms. *Clin Infect Dis* 1994;18:780–784.

220. Feigin RD, San Joaquin VS, Middlekamp JN. *Purpura fulminans* associated with *Neisseria catarrhalis* septicemia and meningitis. *Pediatrics* 1969;44:120–123.

221. Demmler GJ, Couch RS, Taber LH. *Neisseria subflava* bacteremia and meningitis in a child: report of a case and review of the literature. *Pediatr Infect Dis* 1985;4:286–288.

222. Swierczewski JA, et al. Fulminating meningitis with Waterhouse-Friderichsen syndrome due to *Neisseria gonorrhoeae*. *Am J Clin Pathol* 1970;54:202–203.

223. Dalldorf FG, Jennette JC. Fatal meningococcal septicemia. *Arch Pathol Lab Med* 1977;101:6–9.

224. Smith OP, et al. Use of protein-C concentrate, heparin, and haemodiafiltration in meningococcus-induced purpura fulminans. *Lancet* 1997;350:1590–1593; and comments, Protein-C concentrate for meningococcal purpura fulminans. *Lancet* 1997;351:986–989.

225. Margaretten W, McAdams AJ. An appraisal of fulminant meningococcemia with reference to the Shwartzman phenomenon. *Am J Med* 1958;25:868–876.

226. Evans RW, et al. Fatal intravascular consumption coagulopathy in meningococcal sepsis. *Am J Med* 1969;46:910–918.

227. Glauser MP, et al. Septic shock: pathogenesis. *Lancet* 1991;338:732–736.

228. Astiz ME, Rackow EC. Septic shock. *Lancet* 1998;351:1501–1505.

229. Parrillo JE. Pathogenetic mechanisms of septic shock. *N Engl J Med* 1993;328:1471–1477.

230. Cohen J, Glauser MP. Septic shock: treatment. *Lancet* 1991;338:736–739.

231. Waage A, Halstensen A, Espevik T. Association between tumor necrosis factor in serum and fatal outcome in patients with meningococcal disease. *Lancet* 1987;1:355–357.

232. Fijnvandraat K, et al. Coagulation activation and tissue necrosis in meningococcal septic shock: severely reduced protein C levels predict a high mortality. *Thromb Haemost* 1995;73:15–20.

233. Giror BP, et al. Preliminary evaluation of recombinant amino-terminal fragment of human bacteriocidal/permeability-increasing protein in children with severe meningococcal sepsis. *Lancet* 1997;350:1439–1443.

234. Zenz W, et al. Recombinant tissue plasminogen activator treatment in two infants with fulminant meningococcemia. *Pediatrics* 1995;96:144–148.

235. Goldman AP, et al. Extracorporeal support for intractable cardiorespiratory failure due to meningococcal disease. *Lancet* 1997;349:466–469.

236. Ziegler EJ, et al. Treatment of gram-negative bacteremia and shock with human antiserum to a mutant *Escherichia coli*. *N Engl J Med* 1982;307:1225–1230.

237. Ziegler EJ, et al. Treatment of gram-negative bacteremia and septic shock with HA-1A human monoclonal antibody against endotoxin. A randomized, double-blind, placebo-controlled trial. *N Engl J Med* 1991;324: 429–436.

238. Best C, et al. Early haemo-diafiltration in meningococcal septicemia. *Lancet* 1995;347:202; and comments, Veno-venous haemodiafiltration in meningococcal septicaemia. *Lancet* 1996 611–615.

239. Bass JL, et al. Recurrent meningococcemia associated with IgG2-subclass deficiency [Letter]. *N Engl J Med* 1983;309:430.

240. Davis CA, et al. Neutrophil function in a patient with meningococcal meningitis and C7 deficiency. *Am J Dis Child* 1983;137:404–406.

241. Williams DN, Geddes AM. Meningococcal meningitis complicated by pericarditis, panophthalmitis, and arthritis. *Brit Med J* 1970;2:93.

242. Hardman JM, Earle KM. Myocarditis in 200 fatal meningococcal infections. *Arch Pathol* 1969;87:318–325.

243. Mayatepek E, Grauer M, Sonntag HG. Deafness after meningococcal meningitis. *Lancet* 1991;338:13–31.

244. American Academy of Pediatrics. Meningococcal infections. In: Peter G, ed. *1997 Red Book: Report of the Committee on Infectious Diseases*, 24th ed. Elk Grove Village, IL: American Academy of Pediatrics, 1997:357–362.

245. Migeon CJ, et al. Study of adrenal function in children with meningitis. *Pediatrics* 1967;40:163–183.

246. Gaskins RA Jr, Dalldorf FG. Experimental meningococcal septicemia. Effect of heparin therapy. *Arch Pathol Lab Med* 1976;100:318–324.

247. Cuevas L, Hart CA. Chemoprophylaxis of bacterial meningitis. *J Antimicrob Chemother* 1993;31[Suppl B]:79–91.

248. Lepow MI, Gold R. Meningococcal A and other polysaccharide vaccines. A five-year progress report. *N Engl J Med* 1983;308:1158–1160.

249. Frasch CE. Vaccines for prevention of meningococcal disease. *Clin Microbiol Rev* 1989;2[Suppl1]:S134–S138.

250. Ceesay SJ, et al. Decline in meningococcal antibody levels in African children 5 years after vaccination and the lack of effect of a booster immunization. *J Infect Dis* 1993;167:1212–1216.

251. de Moraes JC, et al. Protective efficacy of serogroup B meningococcal vaccine in Sao Paulo, Brazil. *Lancet* 1992;340:1074–1078.

252. Sinclair JF, Skeoch CH, Hallworth D. Prognosis of meningococcal septicemia. *Lancet* 1987;ii:38.

253. Tesoro LJ, Selbst SM. Factors affecting outcome in meningococcal infections. *Am J Dis Child* 1991;145:218–220.

253a. Kornelisse, RF, et al. Meningococcal septic shock in children: clinical and laboratory features, outcome, and the development of a prognostic score. *Clin Infect Dis* 1997;25:640–646.

254. Adams WG, et al. Decline of childhood *Haemophilus influenzae* type B (Hib) disease in the Hib vaccine era. *JAMA* 1993;269:221–226.

255. Schoendorf KC, et al. National trends in *Haemophilus influenzae* meningitis mortality and hospitalization among children 1980 through 1991. *Pediatrics* 1994;93:663–668.

256. Nizet V, et al. A virulent nonencapsulated *Haemophilus influenzae*. *J Infect Dis* 1996;173:180–186.

257. A survey of invasive *Haemophilus influenzae* infections—England and Wales. *Can Comm Dis Rep* 1992;18:42–47.

258. Falla TJ, et al. Population-based study of non-typable *Haemophilus influenzae* invasive disease in children and neonates. *Lancet* 1993;341:851–854.

259. Smith ER. An adult with *Haemophilus meningitis*: case report. *NZ Med J* 1976;83:367–368.

260. Dunn DW, et al. Ischemic cerebrovascular complications of *Haemophilus influenzae* meningitis. The value of computed tomography. *Arch Neurol* 1982;39:650–652.

261. Headings DL, Glasgow LA. Occlusion of the internal carotid artery complicating *Haemophilus influenzae* meningitis. *Am J Dis Child* 1977;131:854–856.

262. Morriss JH, Gillette PC, Barrett FF. Atrioventricular block complicating meningitis: treatment with emergency cardiac pacing. *Pediatrics* 1976;58:866–868.

263. Granoff DM, Nankervis GA. Cellulitis due to *Haemophilus influenzae* type B. Antigenemia and antibody responses. *Am J Dis Child* 1976;130:1211–1214.

264. Steele RW, Bradsher RW. Comparison of ceftriaxone with standard therapy for bacterial meningitis. *J Pediatr* 1983;103:138–141.

265. Ioannidis JPA, et al. Risk of gastrointestinal bleeding from dexamethasone in children with bacterial meningitis. *N Engl J Med* 1994;343:792.

266. Koskiniemi M, et al. *Haemophilus influenzae* meningitis. A comparison between chloramphenicol and ampicillin therapy with special reference to impaired hearing. *Acta Paediatr Scand* 1978;67:17–24.

267. Coggins A, Shepherd CW, Cockburn F. Epidemiology of *Haemophilus* type B invasive disease in children in Glasgow. *Scott Med J* 1993;38:1820.

268. Granoff DM, Squires JE. *Haemophilus meningitis*: new developments in epidemiology, treatment and prophylaxis. *Semin Neurol* 1982;2:151–165.

269. Taylor HG, et al. Intellectual, neuropsychological, and achievement outcomes in children six to eight years after recovery from *Haemophilus influenzae* meningitis. *Pediatrics* 1984;74:198–205.

270. Tepperberg J, Nussbaum E, Feldman F. Cortical blindness following meningitis due to *Haemophilus influenzae* type B. *J Pediatr* 1977;91:434–435.

271. Miller V. Craniocervical myelopathy associated with *Haemophilus influenzae* meningitis: MRI findings. *Neurology* 1992;42:1121–1122.

272. Taylor HG, Schatschneider C. Academic achievement following childhood brain disease: implications for the concept of learning disabilities. *J Learn Disabil* 1992;25:630–638.

273. American Academy of Pediatrics. *Haemophilus influenzae* infections. In: Peter G, ed. *1997 Red Book: Report of the Committee on Infectious Diseases*, 24th ed. Elk Grove Village, IL: American Academy of Pediatrics, 1997:220–231.

274. Tuomanen E, Masure R. The molecular and cell biology of pneumococcal infection. *Microb Drug Resist* 1997;3:297–308.

275. Tuomanen E, et al. The induction of meningeal inflammation by components of the pneumococcal cell wall. *J Infect Dis* 1985;151:859–868.

276. Friedland I, et al. Limited role of pneumolysin in the pathogenesis of pneumococcal meningitis. *J Infect Dis* 1995;172:805–809.

277. Winter A, et al. A role for pneumolysin but not neuraminidase in the hearing loss and cochlear damage induced by experimental pneumococcal meningitis in guinea pigs. *Infect Immun* 1997;65:4411–4418.

278. Scheld WM. Bacterial meningitis in the patient at risk: intrinsic risk factors and host defense mechanisms. *Am J Med* 1984;76:193–207.

279. Brandtzaeg P, Mollnes TE, Kierulf P. Complement activation and endotoxin levels in systemic meningococcal disease. *J Infect Dis* 1989;160:58–65.

280. Griesemer DA, Winkelstein JA, Luddy R. Pneumococcal meningitis in patients with a major sickle hemoglobinopathy. *J Pediatr* 1978;92:82–84.

281. Winkelstein JA, Drachman RH. Deficiency of pneumococcal serum opsonizing activity in sickle-cell disease. *N Engl J Med* 1968;279:459–466.

282. Pearson HA, Spencer RP, Cornelius EA. Functional asplenia in sickle cell anemia. *N Engl J Med* 1969;281:923–926.

283. Chu MLY, et al. Cranial nerve palsies in *Streptococcus pneumoniae* meningitis. *Pediatr Neurol* 1990;6:209–210.

284. Baird DR, Whittle HC, Greenwood BM. Mortality from pneumococcal meningitis. *Lancet* 1976;2:1344–1346.

285. Laxer RM, Marks MI. Pneumococcal meningitis in children. *Am J Dis Child* 1977;131:850–853.

286. Kornelisse RF, et al. Pneumococcal meningitis in children: prognostic indicators and outcome. *Clin Infect Dis* 1995;21:1390–1397.

286a. Arditi M. et al. Three-year multicenter surveillance of pneumococcal meningitis in children: clinical characteristics, and outcome related to penicilline susceptibility and dexamethasone use. *Pediatrics* 1998;102: 1087–1097.

287. Friedland IR, McCracken GH Jr. Management of infections caused by antibiotic-resistant *Streptococcus pneumoniae*. *N Engl J Med* 1994;331:377–382.

288. American Academy of Pediatrics Committee on Infectious Diseases. Therapy for children with inva-

sive pneumococcal infections. *Pediatrics* 1997;99: 289–299.

289. Ostergaard C, et al. Evaluation of moxifloxacin, a new 8-methoxyquinolone, for treatment of meningitis caused by a pencillin-resistant pneumococcus in rabbits. *Antimicrob Agents Chemother* 1998;42: 1706–1712.

290. Klugman KP, Saunders J. Pneumococci resistant to extended-spectrum cephalosporins in South Africa [Letter]. *Lancet* 1993;341:1164.

291. Anonymous. Pneumococcal polysaccharide vaccine. *MMWR* 1978;27:25.

292. Kim JH, et al. *Staphylococcus aureus* meningitis: review of 28 cases. *Rev Infect Dis* 1989;11:698–706.

293. Givner LB, Kaplan SL. Meningitis due to *Staphylococcus aureus* in children. *Clin Infect Dis* 1993;16: 766–771.

294. Ziment I. Nervous system complications in bacterial endocarditis. *Am J Med* 1969;47:593–607.

295. Jensen AG, et al. *Staphylococcus aureus* meningitis. A review of 104 nation-wide, consecutive cases. *Arch Int Med* 1993;153:1902–1908.

296. Diaz-Mitoma F, et al. Clinical significance of a test for slime production in ventriculoperitoneal shunt infections caused by coagulase-negative staphylococci. *J Infect Dis* 1987;156:555–560.

297. Holt R. The classification of staphylococci from colonized ventriculo-atrial shunts. *J Clin Pathol* 1969;22: 475–482.

298. Shurtleff DB, Christie D, Faltz EL. Ventriculoauriculostomy-associated infection. A 12-year study. *J Neurosurg* 1971;35:686–694.

299. Becker DP, Nulsen FE. Control of hydrocephalus by valve-regulated venous shunt: avoidance of complications in prolonged shunt maintenance. *J Neurosurg* 1968;28:215–226.

300. deLouvois J. Acute bacterial meningitis in the newborn. *J Antimicrob Chemother* 1994;34[Suppl A]:61–73.

301. Dyggve H. Prognosis in meningitis neonatorum. *Acta Pediatr Scand* 1962;51:303–312.

302. McCrory JH, et al. Recurrent group B streptococcal infection in an infant: ventriculitis complicating type Ib meningitis. *J Pediatr* 1978;92:231–238.

303. Bates HA, et al. Septicemia and meningitis in a newborn due to *Pasteurella multocida*. *Clin Pediatr* 1965;4:668–670.

304. Mann JM, Shandler L, Cushing AH. Pediatric plague. *Pediatrics* 1982;69:762–767.

305. Kostiala AA, Westerstrahle M, Muttilainen M. Neonatal salmonella Panama infection with meningitis. *Acta Paediatr* 1992;81:856–858.

306. Jones RN, Slepack J, Eades A. Fatal neonatal meningococcal meningitis. Association with maternal cervical-vaginal colonization. *JAMA* 1976;236:2852–2853.

307. Unhanand M, et al. Gram-negative enteric bacillary meningitis: a twenty-one-year experience. *J Pediatr* 1993;122:15–21.

308. Renier D, et al. Brain abscesses in neonates. A study of 30 cases. *J Neurosurg* 1988;69:877–882.

309. Cole FS. Immunology. In: Taeusch HW, Ballard RA, Avery ME, eds: *Diseases of the newborn*. Philadelphia: WB Saunders, 1991:305–320.

310. Stins MF, et al. Binding characteristics of S fibriated *Escherichia coli* to isolated microvascular endothelial cells. *Am J Pathol* 1994;145:1228–1236.

311. Glode MP, et al. Neonatal meningitis due to *Escherichia coli* K-1. *J Infect Dis* 1977;136[Suppl]: S93–S97.

312. Siitonen A, et al. Invasive *Escherichia coli* infections in children: bacterial characteristics in different age groups and clinical entities. *Pediatr Inf Dis J* 1993;12:606–612.

313. Overall JC Jr. Neonatal bacterial meningitis. Analysis of predisposing factors and outcome compared with matched control subjects. *J Pediatr* 1970;76: 499–511.

314. St. Geme JW Jr, et al. Perinatal bacterial infection after prolonged rupture of membranes. Analysis of risk and management. *J Pediatr* 1984;104:608–613.

315. Visser VE, Hall RT. Lumbar puncture in the evaluation of neonatal sepsis. *J Pediatr* 1980;96:1063–1067.

316. Groover RV, Sutherland JM, Landing BH. Purulent meningitis of newborn infants: eleven year experience in the antibiotic era. *N Engl J Med* 1961;264: 1115–1121.

317. Weiss MG, Ionides SP, Anderson CL. Meningitis in premature infants with respiratory distress: role of admission lumbar puncture. *J Pediatr* 1991;119: 973–975.

318. Sarff LD, Platt LH, McCracken GH Jr. Cerebrospinal fluid evaluation in neonates: Comparison of high-risk infants with and without meningitis. *J Pediatr* 1976;88:473–477.

319. Baker CJ, et al. Suppurative meningitis due to streptococci of Lancefield group B. A study of 33 infants. *J Pediatr* 1973;82:724–729.

320. Haslam RH, et al. The sequelae of group B β hemolytic meningitis in early infancy. *Am J Dis Child* 1977;131: 845–849.

321. Baker CJ, Kasper DL. Immunological investigation of infants with septicemia or meningitis due to group B streptococcus. *J Infect Dis* 1977;136:[Suppl]: S98–S104.

322. Hristeva L, et al. Value of cerebrospinal fluid examination in the diagnosis of meningitis in the newborn. *Arch Dis Child* 1993;69:514–517.

323. Booy R, Kroll S. Bacterial meningitis in children. *Curr Opin Pediatr* 1994;6:29–35.

323a. Hristeva L, et al. Prospective surveillance of neonatal meningitis. *Arch Dis Child* 1993;69[1 Spec No]:14–18.

324. Chequer RS, et al. Prognostic value of EEG in neonatal meningitis: retrospective study of 29 infants. *Pediatr Neurol* 1992;8:417–422.

325. Goitein KJ, Tamir I. Cerebral perfusion pressure in central nervous system infections of infancy and childhood. *J Pediatr* 1983;103:40–43.

326. American Academy of Pediatrics. Group B Streptococcal infections. In: Peter G, ed. *1997 Red Book: Report of the Committee on Infectious Diseases*, 24th ed. Elk Grove Village, IL: American Academy of Pediatrics, 1997:494–501.

327. American Academy of Pediatrics. Antibacterial drugs for newborn infants. In: Peter G, ed. *1997 Red Book: Report of the Committee on Infectious Diseases*, 24th ed. Elk Grove Village, IL: American Academy of Pediatrics, 1997:607–608.

328. McCracken GH Jr, Mize SG. A controlled study of intrathecal antibiotic therapy in gram-negative enteric meningitis of infancy. Report of the neonatal

meningitis cooperative study group. *J Pediatr* 1976; 89:66–72.

329. McCracken GH Jr, Mize SG, Threlkeld N. Intraventricular gentamycin therapy in gram-negative bacillary meningitis of infancy. Report of the Second Neonatal Meningitis Cooperative Study Group. *Lancet* 1980;1:787–791.

330. Tatsuno M, Motohiro H. Okuyama K. Ventriculitis in infants: diagnosis by color Doppler flow imaging. *Pediatr Neurol* 1993;9:127–130.

331. Gilles FH, Jammes JL, Berenberg W. Neonatal meningitis—The ventricle as a bacterial reservoir. *Arch Neurol* 1977;34:560–562.

332. Isaacs D, Moxon ER. *Neonatal infections.* Oxford: Butterworth–Heinemann 1991:67.

333. Isaacs D, Moxon ER. *Neonatal infections.* Oxford: Butterworth–Heinemann 1991:143.

334. Medical Research Council Tuberculosis and Chest Diseases Unit. Tuberculosis in children: a national survey of notifications in England and Wales in 1983. *Arch Dis Child* 1988;63:266–276.

335. Kopanoff DE. A continuing survey of tuberculosis primary drug resistance in the United States: March 1975 to November 1977. A United States Public Health Service cooperative study. *Am Rev Respir Dis* 1978;118:835–842.

335a. Yaramis A, et al. Central nervous system tuberculosis in children: a review of 214 cases. *Pediatrics* 1998; 102:E49.

336. Dastur DK, et al. The brain and meninges in tuberculous meningitis: gross pathology in 100 cases and pathogenesis. *Neurology* (India) 1970;18:86–100.

337. Critchley M. Brain tumors in children: their general symptomatology. *Br J Child Dis* 1925;22:251–264.

338. Lincoln EM. Tuberculous meningitis in children. I. Tuberculous meningitis. *Am Rev Tuberc Pulm Dis* 1946:56:75–94.

339. Idriss ZH, Sinno AA, Kronfol NM. Tuberculous meningitis in childhood. Forty-three cases. *Am J Dis Child* 1976;130:364–367.

340. Narotam PK, et al. Hyponatremic natriuretic syndrome in tuberculous meningitis: the probable role of atrial natriuretic peptide. *Neurosurgery* 1994;34: 982–98(discussion 988).

341. Whitener DR. Tuberculous brain abscess. Report of case and review of the literature. *Arch Neurol* 1978;35:148–155.

342. Lees AJ, McLeod AF, Marshall J. Cerebral tuberculomas developing during treatment of tuberculous meningitis. *Lancet* 1980;1:1208–1211.

343. Teoh R, Humphries MJ, O'Mahoney G. Symptomatic intracranial tuberculoma developing during treatment of tuberculosis: a report of 10 patients and a review of the literature. *QJM* 1987;63:449–460.

344. Chambers ST, et al. Paradoxical expansion of intracranial tuberculomas during chemotherapy. *Lancet* 1984;2:181–184.

345. Gourie-Devi M, Satishchandra P. Hyaluronidase as an adjuvant in the management of tuberculous spinal arachnoiditis. *J Neurol Sci* 1991;102:105–111.

346. Davis LE, et al. Tuberculous meningitis in the southwest United States: a community-based study. *Neurology* 1993;43:1775–1778.

346a. Kent SJ, et al. Tuberculous meningitis: a 30-year review. *Clin Infect Dis* 1993;17:987–994.

347. Lincoln EH, Sewell EM. *Tuberculosis in children.* New York: McGraw-Hill, 1963.

348. Seth V, et al. Tuberculous meningitis in children: manifestation of an immune compromised state. *Indian Pediatr* 1993;30:1181–1186.

349. Zarabi M, Sane S, Girdany BR. The chest roentgenogram in the early diagnosis of tuberculous meningitis in children. *Am J Dis Child* 1971;121: 389–392.

350. Narita M, et al. Nested amplification protocol for the detection of *Mycobacterium* tuberculosis. *Acta Paediatr* 1992;81:997–1001.

351. Hernandez R, Muñoz O, Guiscafre H. Sensitive enzyme immunoassay for early diagnosis of tuberculous meningitis. *J Clin Microbiol* 1984;20:533–535.

352. Larsson L, et al. Use of selected ion monitoring for detection of tuberculostearic and C32 mycocerosic acid in mycobacteria and in five-day-old cultures of sputum specimens from patients with pulmonary tuberculosis. *Acta Pathol Microbiol Scand [B]* 1981; 89:245–251.

352a. Hinman AR. Tuberculous meningitis at Cleveland Metropolitan General Hospital 1959–1963. *Am Rev Respir Dis* 1975;670–673.

353. Weiss IK, et al. Fatal *Mycobacterium avium* meningitis after mis-identification of *M. tuberculosis.* Lancet 1995; 305:991–992.

354. Chandra B. Some aspects of tuberculous meningitis in Surabaya. *Proc Aust Assoc Neurol* 1976;13:73–81.

355. Shanley DJ. Computed tomography and magnetic resonance imaging of tuberculous meningitis. *J Am Osteopathic Assoc* 1993;93:497–501.

356. Bhargava S, Gupta AK, Tandon PN. Tuberculous meningitis—a CT study. *Br J Radiol* 1982;55: 189–196.

357. Gupta RK, et al. Intracranial tuberculomas: MRI signal intensity correlation with histopathology and localised proton spectroscopy. *Magn Reson Imaging* 1993;11: 443–449.

358. Durfee NL, et al. The treatment of tuberculosis in children. *Am Rev Resp Dis* 1969;99:304–307.

359. American Academy of Pediatrics. Tuberculosis. In: Peter G, ed. *1994 Red Book: report of the committee on infectious diseases*, 24th ed. Elk Grove Village, IL: American Academy of Pediatrics, 1997:541–562.

360. Kaojarern S, et al. Effect of steroids on cerebrospinal fluid of antituberculous drugs in tuberculous meningitis. *Clin Pharmacol Ther* 1991;49:6–12.

361. Rozwarski DA, et al. Modification of the NADH of the isoniazid target (InhA) from *Mycobacterium tuberculosis. Science* 1998;279:99–102.

362. Iseman MD. Treatment of multidrug-resistant tuberculosis. *N Engl J Med* 1993;329:784–791.

363. Schoeman JF, et al. Effect of corticosteroids on intracranial pressure, computed tomographic findings, and clinical outcome in young children with tuberculous meningitis. *Pediatrics* 1997;99: 226–231.

364. Alzeer AH, Fitzgerald JM. Corticosteroids and tuberculosis: risks and use as adjunct therapy. *Tuber Lung Dis* 1993;74:6–11.

365. O'Toole RD, et al. Dexamethasone in tuberculous meningitis. Relationship of cerebrospinal fluid effects to therapeutic efficacy. *Ann Intern Med* 1969;70: 39–48.

366. Watson JD, Schnier RC, Seale JP. Central nervous system tuberculosis in Australia: a report of 22 cases. *Med J Aust* 1993;158:408–413.
367. Damany BJ. Surgery in tuberculous meningitis. *Prog Pediatr Surg* 1982;15:181–185.
368. Bullock MR, Van Dellen JR. The role of cerebrospinal fluid shunting in tuberculous meningitis. *Surg Neurol* 1982;18:274–277.
369. Peacock WJ, Deenny JE. Improving the outcome of tuberculous meningitis in childhood. *S Afr Med J* 1984;66:597–598.
370. Bhagwati SN, Parulekar GD. Management of intracranial tuberculomas in children. *Childs Nerv Syst* 1986;2:232–234.
371. Todd RM, Neville JG. Sequelae of tuberculous meningitis. *Arch Dis Child* 1964;39:213–225.
372. Deeny JE, et al. Tuberculous meningitis in children in the Western Cape. Epidemiology and outcome. *S Afr Med J* 1985;68:75–78.
373. Lorber J. Long-term follow up of 100 children who recovered from tuberculous meningitis. *Pediatrics* 1961;28:778–791.
374. Drury MI, O'Lochlainn S, Sweeney E. Complications of tuberculous meningitis. *BMJ* 1968;1:842.
375. Lam KS, et al. Hypopituitarism after tuberculosis in childhood. *Ann Intern Med* 1993;118:701–706.
376. Lorber J. The results of treatment of 549 cases of tuberculous meningitis. *Am Rev Tuberc Pul Dis* 1954;69:13–25.
377. Lavetter A, et al. Meningitis due to *Listeria monocytogenes*. A review of 25 cases. *N Engl J Med* 1971;285:598–603.
378. Brook I. *Listeria monocytogenes* meningitis. *NY State J Med* 1980;80:1845–1846.
379. Armstrong RW, Fung PC. Brainstem encephalitis (rhombencephalitis) due to *Listeria monocytogenes*: case report and review. *Clin Infect Dis* 1993;16:689–702.
380. Levey HL, Ingall D. Meningitis in neonates due to *Proteus mirabilis*. *Am J Dis Child* 1967;14:320–324.
381. Graber CD, Higgins LS, Davis JS. Seldom-encountered agents of bacterial meningitis. *JAMA* 1965;192:956–960.
382. Tahernia AC, Hashemi G. Survival in anthrax meningitis. *Pediatrics* 1972;50:329–333.
383. Kolyvas E, et al. *Pasteurella ureae* meningoencephalitis. *J Pediatr* 1978;92:81–82.
384. Foreman SD, et al. Neonatal *Citrobacter* meningitis: pathogenesis of cerebral abscess formation. *Ann Neurol* 1984;16:655–659.
385. Omar FZ, Zuberi S, Minns RA. Neurobrucellosis in childhood: six new cases and a review of the literature. *Dev Med Child Neurol* 1997;39:762–765.
386. Lubani MM, et al. Neurobrucellosis in children. *Pediatr Infect Dis* 1989;8:79–82.
387. McLean DR, Russel N, Khan MY. Neurobrucellosis: clinical and therapeutic features. *Clin Infect Dis* 1992;15:582–590.
388. Cover TL, Aber RC. *Yersinia enterocolitica*. *N Engl J Med* 1989;321:16–24.
389. Ersahin Y, Mutluer S, Guzelbag E. Brain abscess in infants and children. *Childs Nerv Syst* 1994;10:185–189.
390. Fischer EG, Schwachman H, Wepsic JG. Brain abscess and cystic fibrosis. *J Pediatr* 1979;95:385–388.
391. Jadavji T, Humphreys RB, Prober CG. Brain abscesses in infants and children. *Pediatr Infect Dis* 1985;4:394–398.
392. Tekkok IH, Erbengi A. Management of brain abscess in children: review of 130 cases over a period of 21 years. *Childs Nerv Syst* 1992;8:411–416.
393. Byrne E, Brophy BP, Perrett LV. Nocardial cerebral abscess: new concepts in diagnosis, management, and prognosis. *J Neurol Neurosurg Psychiatry* 1979;11:1038–1045.
394. McLeod R, et al. Toxoplasmosis presenting as brain abscesses. Diagnosis by computerized tomography and cytology of aspirated purulent material. *Am J Med* 1979;67:711–714.
395. Brook I. Aerobic and anaerobic bacteriology of intracranial abscesses. *Pediatr Neurol* 1992;8:210–214.
396. Raimondi AJ, Matsumoto S, Miller RA. Brain abscess in children with congenital heart disease. I. *J Neurosurg* 1965;23:588–595.
397. Fischer EG, McLennan JE, Suzuki Y. Cerebral abscess in children. *Am J Dis Child* 1981;135:746–749.
398. Domingue JN, Wilson CB. Pituitary abscesses. Report of seven cases and review of literature. *J Neurosurg* 1977;46:601–608.
399. Candon E, Frerebeau P. Abcès bactériens de la moelle épinière. Revue de la littérature (73 cas). *Rev Neurol (Paris)* 1994;150:370–376.
400. Mampalam TJ, Rosenblum ML. Trends in the management of bacterial brain abscess: a review of 102 cases over 17 years. *Neurosurgery* 1988;23:451–458.
401. Smith RR. Neuroradiology of intracranial infection. *Pediatr Neurosurg* 1992;18:92–104.
402. Segall HD, et al. Neuroradiology in infections of the brain and meninges. *Surg Neurol* 1973;1:178–186.
403. Heinz ER, Cooper RD. Several early angiographic findings in brain abscess including the "ripple sign." *Radiology* 1968;90:735–739.
404. Tyler HR, Clark DB. Cerebrovascular accidents in patients with congenital heart disease. *Arch Neurol Psychiatr* 1957;77:483–489.
405. Clark DB. Brain abscess and congenital heart disease. *Clin Neurosurg* 1966;14:274–287.
406. Rosenblum ML, et al. Nonoperative treatment of brain abscesses in selected high-risk patients. *J Neurosurg* 1980;52:217–225.
407. Hirsch JF, et al. Brain abscess in childhood. A study of 34 cases treated by puncture and antibiotics. *Childs Brain* 1983;10:251–265.
408. Editorial. Treatment of brain abscess. *Lancet* 1988;1:219–220.
409. Wright RL, Ballantine HT Jr. Management of brain abscesses in children and adolescents. *Am J Dis Child* 1967;114:113–122.
410. Berlit P, et al. Bacterial brain abscess: a review of 67 patients in Germany. *Forschritte der Neurologie Psychiatrie* 1996;64:297–306.
411. Jennett WB, et al. Effect of anaesthesia on intracranial pressure in patients with space-occupying lesions. *Lancet* 1969;1:61–64.
412. Berg B, et al. Non-surgical cure of brain abscess. Early diagnosis and follow-up with computerized tomography. *Ann Neurol* 1978;3:474–478.
413. Boom WH, Tauazon CU. Successful treatment of multiple brain abscess with antibiotic alone. *Rev Infect Dis* 1985;7:189–199.

414. Legg NJ, Gupta PC, Scott DF. Epilepsy following cerebral abscess. *Brain* 1973;96:259–268.
415. Tekkok IH, Erbengi A. Management of brain abscess in children: review of 130 cases over a period of 21 years. *Childs Nerv Syst* 1992;8:411–416.
416. Galbraith JG, Barr VW. Epidural abscess and subdural empyema. *Adv Neurol* 1974;6:257–267.
417. Farmer TW, Wise GR. Subdural empyema in infants, children and adults. *Neurology* 1973;23:254–261.
418. Skelton R, Maixner W, Isaacs D. Sinusitis induced subdural hematoma. *Arch Dis Child* 1992;67:1478–1480.
419. Ogilvy CS, Chapman PH, McGrail K. Subdural empyema complicating bacterial meningitis in a child: enhancement of membranes with gadolinium on magnetic resonance imaging in a patient without enhancement on computed tomography. *Surg Neurol* 1992;37:138–141.
420. Nielsen H, Gyldensted C, Harmsen A. Cerebral abscess. Aetiology and pathogenesis, symptoms, diagnosis and treatment. A review of 200 cases from 1935–1976. *Acta Neurol Scand* 1982;65:609–622.
421. Smith HP, Hendrick EB. Subdural empyema and epidural abscess in children. *J Neurosurg* 1983;58:392–397.
422. Baker AS, et al. Spinal epidural abscess. *N Engl J Med* 1975;293:463–468.
422a. Kost-Byerly S, et al. Bacterial colonization and infection rate of continuous epidural catheters in children. *Anesth Analg* 1998;86:712–716.
423. DiTullio MV Jr. Intramedullary spinal abscess: a case report with a review of 53 previously described cases. *Surg Neurol* 1977;7:351–354.
424. Leahy AL, et al. Discitis as a cause of abdominal pain in children. *Surgery* 1984;95:412–414.
425. Garcia FF, et al. Diagnostic imaging of childhood spinal infection. *Orthop Rev* 1993;22:321–327.
426. Boston HC Jr, Bianco AJ Jr, Rhodes KH. Disc space infections in children. *Orthop Clin North Am* 1975;6:953–964.
427. Spiegel PG, et al. Intervertebral disc-space inflammation in children. *J Bone Joint Surg* 1972;54A:284–296.
428. Jansen BR, Hart W, Schreuder O. Discitis in childhood. 12–35-year follow-up of 35 patients. *Acta Orthop Scand* 1993;64:33–36.
428a. Ryoppy S, et al. Nonspecific diskitis in children, a nonmicrobial disease? *Clin Orthop* 1993;297:95–99.
429. Reynolds DW, Stagno S, Alford CA. Chronic congenital and perinatal infections. In: Avery GB, ed. *Neonatology: pathophysiology and management of the newborn*, 3rd ed. Philadelphia: JB Lippincott, 1987:874–916.
430. Hardy JB, et al. Adverse fetal outcome following maternal rubella after the first trimester of pregnancy. *JAMA* 1969;207:2414–2420.
431. Töndury G, Smith DW. Fetal rubella pathology. *J Pediatr* 1966;68:867–879.
432. Dudgeon JA. Fetal infections. *J Obstet Gynaec Br Comm* 1968;75:1229–1233.
433. Overall JC Jr, Glasgow LA. Virus infections of the fetus and newborn infant. *J Pediatr* 1977;7:315–333.
434. Volpe JJ. Viral, protozoan, and related intracranial infections. In: Volpe JJ. *Neurology of the newborn*, 3rd ed. Philadelphia: WB Saunders, 1995:675–729.
435. Ben Ami T, et al. Lenticulostriate vasculopathy in infants with infections of the central nervous system sonographic and Doppler findings. *Pediatr Radiol* 1990;20:575–579.
436. Hughes P, Weinberger E, Shaw DW. Linear areas of echogenicity in the thalami and basal ganglia of neonates: an expanded association. *Radiology* 1991;179:103–105.
437. Alford CA Jr, et al. Subclinical central nervous system disease of neonates: a prospective study of infants born with increased levels of IgM. *J Pediatr* 1969;75:1167–1178.
438. Dudgeon JA, Marshall WC, Soothill JF. Immunological responses to early and later intrauterine virus infections. *J Pediatr* 1969;75:1149–1166.
439. Sarnat HB. Ependymal reactions in injury. A review. *J Neuropath Exp Neurol* 1995;54:1–15.
440. Lahat E, et al. Hydrocephalus due to bilateral obstruction of the foramen of Monro: a "possible" late complication of mumps encephalitis. *Clin Neurol Neurosurg* 1993;95:151–154.
441. Gregg N. Congenital cataract following German measles in the mother. *Trans Ophthalmol Soc Aust* 1941;3:35–46.
442. Miller E, Craddock-Watson JE, Pollock TM. Consequences of confirmed maternal rubella at successive stages of pregnancy. *Lancet* 1982;2:781–784.
443. Hardy JB. Clinical and developmental aspects of congenital rubella. *Arch Otolaryngol* 1973;98:230–236.
444. Rorke LB. Nervous system lesions in the congenital rubella syndrome. *Arch Otolaryngol* 1973;249–251.
445. Plotkin SA, et al. Some recently recognized manifestations of the rubella syndrome. *J Pediatr* 1965;67:182–191.
446. Fuccillo DA, et al. Impaired cellular immunity to rubella virus in congenital rubella. *Infect Immun* 1974;9:81–84.
447. Alford CA, Neva FA, Weller TH. Virologic and serologic studies on human products of conception after maternal rubella. *N Engl J Med* 1964;271:1275–1281.
448. Cooper LZ, et al. Rubella: clinical manifestations and management. *Am J Dis Child* 1969;118:18–29.
449. Desmond MM, et al. Congenital rubella encephalitis. Course and early sequelae. *J Pediatr* 1967;71:311–331.
450. Desmond MM, et al. Congenital rubella encephalitis: effects on growth and early development. *Am J Dis Child* 1969;118:30–31.
451. Tartakow IJ. The teratogenicity of maternal rubella. *J Pediatr* 1965;66:380–391.
452. Ames MD, et al. Central auditory imperception—a significant factor in congenital rubella deafness. *JAMA* 1970;213:419–421.
453. Cooper LZ, et al. Loss of rubella hemagglutination antibody in congenital rubella. Failure of seronegative children to respond to HPV-77 rubella vaccine. *Am J Dis Child* 1971;122:397–403.
454. Phillips CA, et al. Intrauterine rubella infection following immunization with rubella vaccine. *JAMA* 1970; 213:624–625.
455. Forrest JM, Menser MA. Congenital rubella in school children and adolescents. *Arch Dis Child* 1970;45:63–69.

456. Hanshaw JB. Congenital cytomegalovirus infection: a fifteen year perspective. *J Infect Dis* 1971;123:555–561.
457. Melish ME, Hanshaw JB. Congenital cytomegalovirus infection. Developmental progress of patients by routine screening. *Am J Dis Child* 1973;126:190–194.
458. Ho M. Cytomegalovirus. *Biology and infection*, 2nd ed. New York: Plenum Medical Book Co, 1991:205–227.
459. Stagno S. Cytomegalovirus. In: Remington JS, Klein JO, eds. *Infectious disease of the fetus and newborn infant*, 4th ed. Philadelphia: WB Saunders Co, 1995:312–354.
460. Fowler KB, et al. The outcome of congenital cytomegalovirus infection in relation to maternal antibody status. *N Engl J Med* 1992;326:663–667.
461. Editorial. Congenital cytomegalovirus infection—more problems. *Lancet* 1974;1:845–846.
462. Marques-Dias MJ, et al. Prenatal cytomegalovirus disease and cerebral microgyria: Evidence for perfusion failure, not disturbance of histogenesis, as the major cause of cytomegalovirus encephalopathy. *Neuropediatrics* 1984;15:18–24.
463. Pass RF, et al. Outcome of symptomatic congenital cytomegalovirus infection: Results of long-term longitudinal follow-up. *Pediatrics* 1980;66:758–762.
464. Monif GR, et al. The correlation of maternal cytomegalovirus infection during varying stages in gestation with neonatal involvement. *J Pediatr* 1972;80:17–20.
465. Shinefield HR. Prenatal and perinatal infections. In: Eichenwald HF, ed. *Prevention of mental retardation through control of infectious diseases*. Pub. #1692. Washington, DC: U.S. Government Printing Office, 1968:65.
466. Bale JF Jr, Bray P, Bell WE. Neuroradiographic abnormalities in congenital cytomegalovirus infection. *Pediatr Neurol* 1985;1:42–47.
467. Stern H, et al. Microbial causes of mental retardation. The role of prenatal infections with cytomegalovirus, rubella virus, and toxoplasma. *Lancet* 1969;2:443–448.
468. Boppana SB, et al. Neuroradiographic findings in the newborn period and long-term outcome in children with symptomatic cytomegalovirus infection. *Pediatrics* 1997;99:409–414.
469. Stagno S, et al. Auditory and visual defects resulting from symptomatic and subclinical congenital cytomegaloviral and toxoplasma infections. *Pediatrics* 1977;59:669–678.
470. Reynolds DW, et al. Inapparent congenital cytomegalovirus infection with elevated cord IgM levels. Causal relation with auditory and mental deficiency. *N Engl J Med* 1974;290:291–296.
471. Brookhouser PE, Bordley JE. Congenital rubella deafness. Pathology and pathogenesis. *Arch Otolaryngol* 1973;98:252–257.
472. Fowler KB, et al. Progressive and fluctuating sensorineural hearing loss in children with asymptomatic congenital cytomegalovirus infection. *J Pediatr* 1997;130:624–630.
473. Hanshaw JB, et al. School failure and deafness after "silent" congenital cytomegalovirus infection. *N Engl J Med* 1976;295:468–470.
474. Williamson WD, et al. Progressive hearing loss in infants with asymptomatic congenital cytomegalovirus infection. *Pediatrics* 1992;90:862–866.
475. Williamson WD, et al. Symptomatic congenital cytomegalovirus. Disorders of language, learning, and hearing. *Am J Dis Child* 1982;136:902–905.
476. Stagno S, et al. Congenital cytomegalovirus infection. *N Engl J Med* 1977;296:1254–1258.
477. McCracken GH Jr, et al. Congenital cytomegalic inclusion disease. A longitudinal study of 20 patients. *Am J Dis Child* 1969;117:522–539.
478. Medearis DN Jr. Observations concerning human cytomegalovirus infection and disease. *Bull Johns Hopkins Hosp*;1964;114:181–211.
479. Jamison RM, Hathorn AW Jr. Isolation of cytomegalovirus from cerebrospinal fluid of a congenitally infected infant. *Am J Dis Child* 1978;132:63–64.
480. The TH, Langenhuysen MM. Antibodies against membrane antigens of cytomegalovirus infected cells in sera of patients with a cytomegalovirus infection. *Clin Exp Immunol* 1972;11:475–482.
481. Molloy PM, Loriwman RM. The lack of specificity of the neonatal intracranial paraventricular calcifications. *Radiology* 1963;80:98–102.
482. Crumpacker CS. Ganciclovir. *N Engl J Med* 1996;335:721–729.
483. Paryani SG, Arvin AM. Intrauterine infection with varicella-zoster virus after maternal varicella. *N Engl J Med* 1986;314:1542–1546.
484. Pastusxak AL, et al. Outcome after maternal varicella infection in the first 20 weeks of pregnancy. *N Engl J Med* 1994;330:901–905.
485. Wheatley R, Morton RE, Nicholson J. Chickenpox in mid-trimester pregnancy: always innocent? *Dev Med Child Neurol* 1996;38:455–466.
486. Randel RC, et al. Vocal cord paralysis as a presentation of intrauterine infection with varicella-zoster virus. *Pediatrics* 1996;97:127–128.
487. Harding B, Baumer JA. Congenital varicella-zoster. A serologically proven case with necrotizing encephalitis and malformation. *Acta Neuropathol* 1988;76:311–315.
488. Wong S-W, Remington JS. Biology of *Toxoplasma gondii*. *AIDS* 1993;7:299–316.
489. Krick JA, Remington JS. Current concepts in parasitology. Toxoplasmosis in the adult—an overview. *N Engl J Med* 1978;298:550–553.
490. Wolf A, Cowen D, Paige B. Human toxoplasmosis: occurrence in infants as an encephalomyelitis—verification by transmission to animals. *Science* 1939;89:226–227.
491. Guerina NG, Hsu H-W, Meissner HC. Neonatal serologic screening and early treatment for congenital *Toxoplasma gondii* infection. *N Engl J Med* 1994;330:858–863.
492. Desmonts G, Couvreur J. Congenital toxoplasmosis. *N Engl J Med* 1974;290:1110–1116.
492a. Dunn D, et al. Mother-to-child transmission of toxoplasmosis; risk estimates for clinical counselling. *Lancet* 1999;353:1829–1833.
493. Couvreur J, Desmonts G. Congenital and maternal toxoplasmosis. A review of 300 congenital cases. *Dev Med Child Neurol* 1962;4:519–530.
494. Hall EG, et al. Congenital toxoplasmosis in the newborn. *Arch Dis Child* 1953;28:117–124.

495. Eichenwald HF. *Human toxoplasmosis: proceedings of the Conference on Clinical Aspects and Diagnostic Problems of Toxoplasmosis in Pediatrics.* Baltimore: Williams & Wilkins, 1956.

496. Feldman HA. Congenital toxoplasmosis. Study of one hundred three cases. *Am J Dis Child* 1953;86: 487–489.

497. Falangola MF, Petito CK. Choroid plexus infection in cerebral toxoplasmosis in AIDS patients. *Neurology* 1993;43:2035–2040.

498. Hafström T. Toxoplasmic encephalopathy: a form of meningo-encephalomyelitis in adult toxoplasmosis. *Acta Psychiatr Neurol Scand* 1959;34:311–321.

499. Fondu P, DeMeuter F. Facial palsy, a manifestation of acquired toxoplasmosis. *Helv Paediatr Acta* 1969;24: 208–211.

500. Khanna KK, et al. Acute acquired toxoplasmosis encephalitis in an infant. *Can Med Assoc J* 1969;100: 343–345.

501. Koeze TH, Klingon GH. Acquired toxoplasmosis: case with focal neurologic manifestations. *Arch Neurol* 1964;11:191–197.

502. von Thalhammer O. Oligosymptomatische toxoplamose. *Helv Paediatr Acta* 1954;9:50–58.

503. Baine AD, et al. Congenital toxoplasmosis simulating haemolytic disease of the newborn. *J Obstet Brit Empire* 1956;63:826–832.

504. Brooks RG, McCabe RE, Remington JS. Role of serology in the diagnosis of toxoplasmic lymphadenopathy. *Rev Infect Dis* 1987;9:775–782.

505. Woods CR, Englund J. Congenital toxoplasmosis presenting with eosinophilic meningitis. *Pediatr Infect Dis J* 1993;12:347–348.

506. Mussbichler H. Radiologic study of intracranial calcifications in congenital toxoplasmosis. *Acta Radiol [Diagn]* 1968;7:369–379.

507. Vasquez A, Gonzalez V, Augilar J. P. Acute toxoplasmic myelitis in the newborns. *Bol Med Hosp Infant Mex* 1979;36:885–892.

508. McAuley J, Boyer KM, Patel D. Early and longitudinal evaluations of treated infants and children and untreated historical patients with congenital toxoplasmosis: the Chicago collaborative treatment trial. *Clin Infect Dis* 1994;18:38–72.

509. Luft BJ, et al. Toxoplasmic encephalitis in patients with the acquired immunodeficiency syndrome. *N Engl J Med* 1993;329:995–1000.

510. Saxon SA, et al. Intellectual deficits in children born with subclinical congenital toxoplasmosis: a preliminary report. *J Pediatr* 1973;82:792–797.

511. American Academy of Pediatrics. *Toxoplasma gondii* infections (Toxoplasmosis). In: Peter G, ed. *1997 Red Book: report of the Committee on Infectious Diseases*, 24th ed. Elk Grove Village, IL: American Academy of Pediatrics, 1997:531–535.

512. Kovacs JA, NIAID-Clinical Center Intramural AIDS Program. Efficacy of atovaquone in treatment of toxoplasmis in patients with AIDS. *Lancet* 1992;340: 637–638.

513. Roizin N, et al. Neurologic and developmental outcome in treated congenital toxoplasmosis. *Pediatrics* 1995;95:11–20.

514. Brown ZA, et al. Effects on infants of a first episode of genital herpes during pregnancy. *N Engl J Med* 1987;317:1246–1251.

515. South MA, et al. Congenital malformation of the central nervous system associated with genital type (type 2) herpesvirus. *J Pediatr* 1969;75:13–18.

516. Koskiniemi M, et al. Epidemiology of encephalitis in children: a 20-year survey. *Ann Neurol* 1991;29: 492–497.

517. Johnson RT. The pathogenesis of acute viral encephalitis and postinfectious encephalomyelitis. *J Infect Dis* 1987;155:359–364.

518. Gonzalez-Scarano F, Tyler KL. Molecular pathogenesis of neurotropic viral infections. *Ann Neurol* 1987;22:565–574.

519. Leist TP, et al. Tumor necrosis factor in the cerebrospinal fluid during bacterial, but not viral meningitis. Evaluation in murine model infections and in patients. *J Exp Med* 1988;167:1743–1748.

520. Ramilo O, et al. Detection of interleukin-1-β but not tumor necrosis factor-α in the cerebrospinal fluid of children with aseptic meningitis. *Am J Dis Child* 1990;144:349–352.

521. Matsuao M, et al. Leukotriene B4 and C4 in cerebrospinal fluid from children with meningitis and febrile seizures. *Pediatr Neurol* 1996;14:121–124.

522. Hoke CH Jr, et al. Effect of high-dose dexamethasone on the outcome of acute encephalitis due to Japanese encephalitis virus. *J Infect Dis* 1992;165:631–637.

523. Reiser H, Stadecker MJ. Costimulatory B7 molecules in the pathogenesis of infectious and autoimmune diseases. *N Engl J Med* 1996;335:1369–1377.

524. Razvi ES, Welsh RM. Apoptosis in viral infections. *Adv Virus Res* 1995;45:1–60.

525. Rantala H, et al. Outcome after childhood encephalitis. *Dev Med Child Neurol* 1991;33:858–867.

526. Rotenone J, Koskiniemi M, Vaheri A. Prognostic factors in childhood acute encephalitis. *Pediatr Infect Dis J* 1991;10:461–466.

527. Berlin LE, et al. Aseptic meningitis in infants <2 years of age: diagnosis and etiology. *J Infect Dis* 1993;169: 888–892.

528. Fukushima K, Ishiguro A, Shimbo T. Transient elevation of granulocyte-stimulating factor levels in cerebrospinal fluid at the initial stage of aseptic meningitis in children. *Pediatr Res* 1995;37:160–164.

529. Klein SK, et al. Predictive factors of short-term neurologic outcome in children with encephalitis. *Pediatr Neurol* 1994;11:308–312.

530. Launes J, et al. Unilateral hyperperfusion in brain-perfusion SPECT predicts poor prognosis in acute encephalitis. *Neurology* 1997;48:1347–1351.

531. Koelfen W, et al. MRI of encephalitis in children: comparison of CT and MRI in the acute stage with long-term follow-up. *Neuroradiology* 1996;38: 73–79.

532. Koskiniemi M, Vaheri A. Effect of measles, mumps, rubella vaccination on pattern of encephalitis in children. *Lancet* 1989;1:31–34.

533. Cassady KA, Whitley RJ. Pathogenesis and pathophysiology of viral infections of the central nervous system. In: Scheld WM, Whitley RJ, Durack DT, eds. *Infections of the central nervous system*. Philadelphia: Lippincott–Raven Publishers, 1997:7–22.

534. Johnson RT. Acute encephalitis. *Clin Infect Dis* 1996;23:219–226.

535. Modlin JF. Update on enterovirus infections in infants and children. In: Aronoff SC, Hughes WT, Kohl S,

Wald ER, eds. *Advances in pediatric infectious diseases*. St Louis: Mosby, 1996;12:155–180.

536. Cherry JD. Enteroviruses: coxackieviruses, echoviruses, and polioviruses. In: Feigin RD, Cherry JD, eds. *Textbook of pediatric infectious diseases*, 4th ed. Philadelphia:WB Saunders, 1998:1787–1839.

537. Dagan R, et al. Association of clinical presentation, laboratory findings, and virus serotypes with the presence of meningitis in hospitalized infants with enterovirus infections. *J Pediatr* 1988;113:975–978.

538. Berlin LE, et al. Aseptic meningitis in infants <2 years of age: diagnosis and etiology. *J Infect Dis* 1993;169:888–892.

539. Rorabaugh ML, et al. Aseptic meningitis in infants younger than 2 years of age: acute illness and neurologic complications. *Pediatrics* 1993;92:206–211.

539a. Komatsu I, et al. Outbreak of severe neurologic involvement associated with enterovirus 71 infection. *Pediatr Neurol* 1999;20:17–23.

539b. Huang CC, et al. Neurological complications in children with enterovirus 71 infection. *N Engl J Med* 1999;341:936–942.

540. Modlin JD, et al. Focal encephalitis with enterovirus infections. *Pediatrics* 1991;88:841–845.

541. Wadia NH, et al. A study of the neurological disorder associated with acute hemorrhagic conjunctivitis due to enterovirus 70. *J Neurol Neurosurg Psychiatry* 1983;46:599–610.

542. Katiyar BC, et al. Neurological syndromes after acute epidemic conjunctivitis. *Lancet* 1981;2:866–867.

543. Wadia NH, Irani PF, Katrak SM. Lumbosacral radiculomyelitis associated with pandemic acute hemorrhagic conjunctivitis. *Lancet* 1973;1:350–352.

544. Bowles NE, et al. Dermatomyositis, polymyositis, and Coxsackie-B-virus infection. *Lancet* 1987;1:1004–1007.

545. Jadoul C, Van Goethem J, Martin JJ. Myelitis due to Coxsackie-virus B infection. *Neurology* 1995;45:1626–1627.

546. Chang L-Y, Huang Y-C, Lin T-Y. Fulminant neurogenic pulmonary oedema with hand, foot, and mouth disease. *Lancet* 1998;352:367–368.

547. Lum LCS, et al. Neurogenic pulmonary oedema and enterovirus 71 encephalomyelitis [Letter]. *Lancet* 1998;352:13–91.

548. Modlin JD. Neonatal enterovirus infections. In: Feigin RD, ed. *Seminars in pediatric infectious diseases*, Vol. 5., no. 1. Philadelphia: WB Saunders, 1994:70–77.

549. Lake AM, et al. Enterovirus infections in neonates. *J Pediatr* 1976;89:787–791.

550. Shattuck KE, Chonmaitree T. The changing spectrum of neonatal meningitis over a fifteen-year period. *Clin Pediatr Phila* 1992;31:130–136.

551. Aintablian N, Pratt RD, Sawyer MH. Rapidly recurrent enteroviral meningitis in non-immunocompromised infants caused by different viral strains. *J Med Virol* 1995;47:126–129.

552. Sells CJ, Carpenter RL, Ray CG. Sequelae of central-nervous-system enterovirus infections. *N Engl J Med* 1975;293:1–4.

553. Wilfert CM, et al. Longitudinal assessment of children with enteroviral meningitis during the first three months of life. *Pediatrics* 1981;67:811–815.

554. Bergman I, et al. Outcome in children with enteroviral meningitis during the first year of life. *J Pediatr* 1987;110:705–709.

555. Baker RC, et al. Neurodevelopmental development of infants with viral meningitis in the first three months of life. *Clin Pediatr Phila* 1996;35:295–301.

556. Wilfert CM, et al. Persistent and fatal central-nervous-system echovirus infections in patents with agammaglobulinemia. *N Engl J Med* 1977;296:1485–1489.

557. Rotbart HA, et al. Diagnosis of enterovirus infection by polymerase chain reaction of multiple specimen samples. *Pediatr Infect Dis J* 1997;16:409–411.

558. Heine J. Beobachtungen über Lähmungszustände der unteren Extremitäten und deren Behandlung. Stuttgart: Kohler, 1840.

559. Center for Disease Control. MMWR Poliomyelitis prevention in the United States: introduction of a sequential vaccination schedule of inactivated poliovirus vaccine followed by oral polio vaccine. Recommendations of the Advisory Committee on Immunization Practices (ACIP) 1997;46[Suppl RR-3]:1–25.

560. Baker AB, Cornwell S, Tichy F. Poliomyelitis IX. The cerebral hemispheres. *Arch Neurol Psychiatr* 1954;71:435–454.

561. Heyes MP, et al. A mechanism of quinolinic acid formation by brain in inflammatory neurological disease. Attenuation of synthesis from l-tryptophan by 6-chlorotryptophan and 4-chloro-3 hydroxyanthranilate. *Brain* 1993;116:1425–1450.

562. Baker AB, Cornwell S, Tichy F. Poliomyelitis X. The cerebellum. *Arch Neurol Psychiatr* 1954;71:455–465.

563. Horstmann DM, Paul JR. The incubation period in human poliomyelitis and its implications. *JAMA* 1947;135:11–14.

564. Horstmann DM. Poliomyelitis: severity and type of disease in different age groups. *Ann NY Acad Sci* 1955;61:956–967.

565. Abramson H, Greenberg M. Acute poliomyelitis in infants under one year of age: epidemiological and clinical features. *Pediatrics* 1955;16:478–487.

566. Wernstedt W. Epidemiologische Studien über die zweite grosse Poliomyelitisepidemie in Schweden 1911–1913. *Ergebn Inn Med Kinderheilk* 1924;26:248–350.

566a. Strebel PM, et al. Intramuscular injections within 30 days of immunization with oral poliovirus vaccine— risk factor for vaccine-associated paralytic poliomyelitis. *N Engl J Med* 1995;332:500–506.

567. Hill AB, Knowelden J. Inoculation and poliomyelitis: statistical investigation in England and Wales in 1946. *BMJ* 1950;2:16.

567a. Leon-Monzon ME, Illa I, Dulakas MC. Expression of poliovirus receptor in human spinal cord and muscle. *Ann NY Acad Sci* 1995;753:48–57.

568. Lawson RB, Garvey FK. Paralysis of the bladder in poliomyelitis. *JAMA* 1947;135:93–94.

569. Minnesota Poliomyelitis Research Commission. The bulbar form of poliomyelitis. Diagnosis and the correlation with physiologic and pathologic manifestations. *JAMA* 1947;134:757–762.

570. Baker AB, Matzke HA, Brown JR. Poliomyelitis III. Bulbar poliomyelitis: a study of medullary function. *Arch Neurol Psychiatr* 1950;63:257–281.

571. Baker AB. Poliomyelitis: a study of pulmonary edema. *Neurology* 1957;7:743–751.

572. Baker AB, Cornwell S, Brown IA. Poliomyelitis VI. The hypothalamus. *Arch Neurol Psychiatr* 1952;68:16–36.

573. Merritt HH, Fremont-Smith F. *The cerebrospinal fluid*. Philadelphia: WB Saunders, 1937.

574. Rotbart HA. Enteroviral infections of the central nervous system. *Clin Infect Dis* 1995;20:971–981.

575. Sharland M, et al. Enteroviral pharyngitis diagnosed by reverse transcriptase-polymerase chain reaction. *Arch Dis Child* 1996;74:462–463.

576. Chezzi C. Rapid diagnosis of poliovirus infection by PCR amplification. *J Clin Microbiol* 1996;34: 1722–1725.

577. Centers for Disease Control and Prevention. Recommendation of the international task force for disease eradication. *MMWR* 1993;42:10.

578. Nkowane RM, et al. Vaccine-associated paralytic poliomyelitis. United States: 1973–1984. *JAMA* 1987; 257:1335–1340.

579. Gaebler JW, et al. Neurologic complications in oral polio vaccine recipients. *J Pediatr* 1986;108:878–881.

580. Groom SN, et al. Vaccine-associated poliomyelitis. *Lancet* 1994;343:609–610.

581. Otelea D, et al. Genomic modifications in naturally occurring neurovirulent revertants of Sabin 1 polioviruses. *Dev Biol Stand* 1993;78:33–38.

582. Yohannan MD, Ramia S, al-Frayh AR. Acute paralytic poliomyelitis presenting as Guillain-Barré syndrome. *J Infect* 1991;22:129–133.

583. Halm AF. Guillain-Barré Syndrome. *Lancet* 1998;352: 635–641.

583a. Wong M, Connolly AM, Noetzel MJ. Poliomyelitis-like syndrome associated with Epstein-Barr infection. *Pediatr Neurol* 1999;20:235–237.

584. Likar M, Dane DS. An illness resembling acute poliomyelitis caused by a virus of the Russian spring-summer encephalitis louping ill group in Northern Ireland. *Lancet* 1958;1:456–458.

585. Hopkins IJ. A new syndrome: poliomyelitis-like illness associated with acute asthma in childhood. *Aust Paedatr* 1974;10:273–276.

586. Kyllerman MG, et al. PCR diagnosis of primary herpesvirus type I in poliomyelitis-like paralysis and respiratory tract disease. *Pediatr Neurol* 1993;9:227–229.

587. Sabin AB. My last will and testament on rapid elimination and ultimate eradication of poliomyelitis and measles. *Pediatrics* 1992;90[Suppl]:162–169.

588. McKhann GM, et al. Clinical and electrophysiological aspects of acute paralytic disease of children and young adults in northern China. *Lancet* 1991;338: 593–597.

589. Gear JH. Nonpolio causes of polio-like paralytic syndromes. *Rev Infect Dis* 1984;6[Suppl 2]:S379–S384.

590. Bodian D, Howe HA. Experimental non-paralytic poliomyelitis. Frequency and range of pathological involvement. *Bull Johns Hopkins Hosp* 1945;76:1–17.

591. Bukh N. Muscle recovery of poliomyelitis. *Acta Orthop Scand* 1968;39:579–592.

592. Sharief MK, Hentges R, Ciardi M. Intrathecal immune response in patients with the post-polio syndrome. *N Engl J Med* 1991;325:749–755.

593. Dalakas MC, Bartfeld H, Kurland LT, eds. *The post-polio syndrome. Advances in the pathogenesis and treatment. Annals of the New York Academy of Sciences*. Vol. 753. New York: The New York Academy of Sciences, 1995.

594. Waring WP, Davidoff G, Werner R. Serum creatine kinase in the post-polio population. *Am J Phys Med Rehabil* 1989;68:86–90.

595. Windebank AJ, et al. Late effects of paralytic poliomyelitis in Olmsted County, Minnesota. *Neurology* 1991;41:501–507.

596. Dean AC, et al. Sleep apnea in patients with postpolio syndrome. *Ann Neurol* 1998;43:661–664.

596a. Dalakas MC. Why drugs fail in postpolio syndrome. Lessons from another clinical trial. *Neurology* 1999; 53:1166–1167.

597. American Academy of Pediatrics. Poliovirus infections. In: Peter G, ed. *1997 Red Book: report of the Committee on Infectious Diseases*, 24th ed. Elk Grove Village, IL: American Academy of Pediatrics, 1997:424–433.

598. Salk J, Salk D. Control of influenza and poliomyelitis with killed virus vaccines. *Science* 1977;195:834–847.

599. Kuban KC, et al. Syndrome of opsoclonus-myoclonus caused by Coxsackie B3 infection. *Ann Neurol* 1983; 13:69–71.

600. Chalhub EG, et al. Coxsackie A9 focal encephalitis associated with acute infantile hemiplegia and porencephaly. *Neurology* 1977;27:574–579.

601. Moossy J, Geer JC. Encephalomyelitis, myocarditis and adrenal cortical necrosis in Coxsackie B3 virus infection. Distribution of the central nervous system lesions. *Arch Pathol* 1960;70:614–622.

602. Walker SH, Togo Y. Encephalitis due to group B, type 5 coxsackievirus. *Am J Dis Child* 1963;105.209–212.

603. Walters JH. Post-encephalitic Parkinson syndrome after meningoencephalitis due to coxsackievirus Group B, Type 2. *N Engl J Med* 1960;263:744–747.

604. Casals J, Clarke DH. Arboviruses: group A. In: Horsfall FL, Tamm I, eds. *Viral and rickettsial infections of man*, 4th ed. Philadelphia: JB Lippincott, 1965: 583–605.

605. Modlin JF. Coxsackieviruses, echoviruses, and newer enteroviruses. In: Mandell G, Bennett J, Dolin R, eds. *Principles and practice of infectious diseases*, 4th ed. New York: Churchill Livingstone, 1995:1620–1636.

606. Casteels-van Daele M,et al. Basilar migraine and viral meningitis [Letter]. *Lancet* 1981;1:13–66.

607. Karzon DT, et al. An epidemic of aseptic meningitis syndrome due to ECHO virus type 6. II. A clinical study of ECHO 6 infection. *Pediatrics* 1962;29: 418–431.

608. Marzetti G, Midulla M. Acute cerebellar ataxia associated with Echo 6 infection in two children. *Acta Paediatr Scand* 1967;56:547–551.

609. Forbes SJ, Brumlik J, Harding HB. Acute ascending polyradiculomyelitis associated with ECHO 9 virus. *Dis Nerv Syst* 1967;28:537–540.

610. Freund A, et al. Bilateral oedema of the basal ganglia in echovirus type 21 infection: complete clinical and radiological normalization. *Dev Med Child Neurol* 1998;40:421–423.

611. Haddad J, et al. Neonatal echovirus encephalitis with white matter necrosis. *Neuropediatrics* 1990;21: 215–217.

612. Roberton DM, et al. Failure of intraventricular gamma-globulin and α-interferon for persistent

encephalitis in congenital hypogammaglobulineamia. *Arch Dis Child* 1988;63:948–952.

613. Kondoh H, et al. Successful treatment of echovirus meningoencephalitis in sex-linked agammaglobulinaemia by intrathecal and intravenous injection of high titer gamma-globulin. *Eur J Pediatr* 1987;146: 610–612.

614. Ogra PL. Distribution of echovirus antibody in serum, nasopharynx, rectum, and spinal fluid after natural infection with echovirus type 6. *Infect Immun* 1970;2: 150–155.

615. Lum LCS, et al. Fatal enterovirus 71 encephalomyelitis. *J Pediatr* 1998;133:795–798.

616. Johansson PJ, et al. Reovirus type 1 associated with meningitis. *Scand J Infect Dis* 1996;28:117–120.

617. Davis D, Henslee PJ, Markesbery WR. Fatal adenovirus meningoencephalitis in a bone marrow transplant patient. *Ann Neurol* 1988;23:385–389.

618. Kim KS, Gohd RS. Acute encephalopathy in twins due to adenovirus type 7 infection. *Arch Neurol* 1983;40: 58–59.

619. Osamura T, et al. Isolation of adenovirus type 11 from the brain of a neonate with pneumonia and encephalitis. *Eur J Pediatr* 1993;152:496–499.

620. Suga S, et al. Clinical and virological analyses of 21 infants with exanthem subitum (roseola infantum) and central nervous system complications. *Ann Neurol* 1993;33:597–603.

621. Caserta MT, et al. Primary human herpesvirus 7 infection: a comparison of human herpesvirus 7 and human herpesvirus 6 infections in children. *J Pediatr* 1998; 133:386–389.

622. Cherry JD. Contemporary infectious exanthems. *Clin Infect Dis* 1993;16:199–207.

623. Huang LM, et al. Meningitis caused by human herpesvirus-6. *Arch Dis Child* 1991;66:1443–1444.

624. Kamei A, et al. Acute disseminated demyelination due to primary herpesvirus-6 infection. *Eur J Pediatr* 1997;156:709–712.

625. Huang LM, et al. Meningitis caused by human herpesvirus-6. *Arch Dis Child* 1991;66:1443–1444.

626. Asano Y, et al. Clinical features of infants with primary human herpesvirus 6 infection (Exanthum subitum, Roseola infantum). *Pediatrics* 1994;93:104–108.

626a. Hall CB, et al. Human Herpesvirus-6 infection in children —a prospective study of complications and reactivation. *N Engl J Med* 1994;331:432–438.

627. Kondo K, et al. Association of human herpesvirus 6 infection of the central nervous system with recurrence of febrile convulsions. *J Infect Dis* 1993;167: 1197–1200.

628. Yoshikawa T, et al. Human herpesvirus-6 DNA in cerebrospinal fluid of a child with exanthem subitum and meningoencephalitis. *Pediatrics* 1992;89: 888–890.

628a. van den Berg JSP, et al. Neuroinvasion by human herpesvirus type 7 in a case of exanthem subitum with severe neurologic manifestations. *Neurology* 1999;52: 1077–1079.

629. Torigoe S, et al. Human herpesvirus 7 infection associated with central nervous system manifestations. *J Pediatr* 1996;129:301–305.

630. Agut H, et al. In vitro sensitivity of human herpesvirus-6 to antiviral drugs. *Res Virol* 1989,140:219–228.

631. Rehle TM. Classification, distribution, and importance of arboviruses. *Trop Med Parisitol* 1989;40:391–395.

632. American Academy of Pediatrics. Arboviruses. In: Peter G, ed. *1997 Red Book: report of the Committee on Infectious Diseases*, 24th ed. Elk Grove Village, IL: American Academy of Pediatrics, 1997;137–141.

633. *MMWR Morb Mortal Wkly Rep* 1999;47:1119.

634. Chun RW, et al. California arbovirus encephalitis in children. *Neurology* 1968;18:369–375.

635. Monath TP, et al. Studies on California encephalitis in Minnesota. *Am J Epidemiol* 1970;92:40–50.

636. Johnson KP, Lepow ML, Johnson RT. California encephalitis. I. Clinical and epidemiological studies. *Neurology* 1968;18:250–254.

637. Tsai TF. Arboviral infections in the United States. *Infect Dis Clin North Am* 1991;5:73–102.

638. Balfour HH Jr, et al. California arbovirus (La Crosse) infections. I. Clinical and laboratory findings in 66 children with meningoencephalitis. *Pediatrics* 1973;52:680–691.

639. Grabow JD, et al. The electroencephalogram and clinical sequelae of California arbovirus encephalitis. *Neurology* 1969;19:394–404.

640. Chun RW. Clinical aspects of La Crosse encephalitis: neurological and psychological sequelae. *Prog Clin Biol Res* 1983;123:193–200.

641. Matthews CG, et al. Psychological sequelae in children with California arbovirus encephalitis. *Neurology* 1968;18:1023–1030.

642. Rie HE, Hilty MD, Cramblett HG. Intelligence and coordination following California encephalitis. *Am J Dis Child* 1973;125:824–827.

643. McJunkin JE, et al. Treatment of severe La Crosse encephalitis with intravenous Ribavirin following diagnosis by brain biopsy. *Pediatrics* 1997;99:261–267.

644. Cassidy LF, et al. Mechanism of La Crosse virus inhibition by ribavirin. *Antimicrob Agents Chemother* 1989;33:2009–2011.

645. Bailey CL, et al. Isolation of St. Louis encephalitis virus from overwintering culex pipiens mosquitoes. *Science* 1978;199:1346–1349.

646. McCordock HA, Collier W, Gray SH. The pathologic changes of the St. Louis type of acute encephalitis. *JAMA* 1934;103:822–825.

647. Barrett FF, Yow MD, Phillips CA. St. Louis encephalitis in children during the 1964 epidemic. *JAMA* 1965;193:381–385.

648. Powell KE, Blakey DL. St. Louis encephalitis. The 1975 epidemic in Mississippi. *JAMA* 1977;237: 2294–2298.

649. Estrin WJ. The serologic diagnosis of St. Louis encephalitis in a patient with the syndrome of opsoclonia, body tremulousness, and benign encephalitis. *Ann Neurol* 1977;1:596–598.

649a. Pranzatelli MR, et al. Clinical spectrum of secondary parkinsonism in childhood: a reversible disorder. *Pediatr Neurol* 1994;10:131–140.

650. Kaplan AM, Koveleski JT. St. Louis encephalitis with particular involvement of the brain stem. *Arch Neurol* 1978;35:45–46.

651. Zentay PJ, Basman J. Epidemic encephalitis type B in children. *J Pediatr* 1939;14:323–332.

652. Azar GJ, et al. Follow-up studies of St. Louis encephalitis in Florida. Sensorimotor findings. *Am J Public Health* 1966;56:1074–1081.

653. Smadel JE, Bailey P, Baker AB. Sequelae of the arthropod-borne encephalitides. *Neurology* 1958;8: 873–896.

654. Rozdilsky B, Robertson HE, Chorney J. Western encephalitis: a report of eight fatal cases. *Can Med Assoc J* 1965;98:79–86.
655. Herzon H, Shelton JT, Bruyn HG. Sequelae of western equine and other arthropod-borne encephalitides. *Neurology* 1957;7:535–548.
656. Schultz DR, Barthal JS, Garrett C. Western equine encephalitis with rapid onset of Parkinsonism. *Neurology* 1977;27:1095–1096.
657. Finley KH, et al. Western encephalitis and cerebral ontogenesis. *Arch Neurol* 1967;16:140–164.
658. Noran HH, Baker AB. Western equine encephalitis: the pathogenesis of the pathological lesions. *J Neuropathol Exp Neurol* 1945;4:269–276.
659. Reeves WC, Hammon WM. Epidemiology of the arthropod-borne viral encephalitides in Kern County, California 1943–1952. Berkeley, CA: University of California Press, 1962. *Univ Calif Publ Public Health* 1962;4:1257.
660. Kokernot RH, Shinefield HR, Longshore WA Jr. The 1952 outbreak of encephalitis in California: differential diagnosis. *Calif Med* 1953;79:73–77.
661. Feemster RF. Equine encephalitis in Massachusetts. *N Engl J Med* 1957;257:701–704.
662. Johnson RT. Eastern encephalitis virus. In: Johnson RT, ed. *Viral infections of the nervous system*. New York: Raven Press, 1982:109.
663. Deresiewicz RL, et al. Clinical and neuroradiographic manifestations of eastern equine encephalitis. *N Engl J Med* 1997;336:1867–1874.
664. Weaver SC et al. Re-emergence of epidemic Venezuelan equine encephalomyelitis in South America. *Lancet* 1996;348:436–440.
665. Bowen GS, Calisher CH. Virological and serological studies of Venezuelan equine encephalomyelitis in humans. *J Clin Microbiol* 1976;4:22–27.
666. Chaudhuri N, et al. Epidemiology of Japanese encephalitis. *Indian Pediatr* 1992;29:861–865.
667. Poneprasert B. Japanese encephalitis in children in northern Thailand. *Southeast Asian J Trop Med Public Health* 1989;20:599–603.
669. Arya SC. Japanese encephalitis virus and poliomyelitis-like illness. *Lancet* 1998;351:1964.
670. McCallum JD. Japanese encephalitis in southeastern Nepal: clinical aspects in the 1986 epidemic. *J R Army Med Corps* 1991;137:8–13.
671. Kumar R, et al. Clinical sequelae of Japanese encephalitis in children. *Indian J Med Res* 1993; 97: 9–13.
671a. Ravi V, et al. Correlation of tumor necrosis factor levels in the serum and cerebrospinal fluid with clinical outcome in Japanese encephalitis patients. *J Med Virol* 1997;51:132–136.
671b. Abe T, et al. Japanese encephalitis. *J Magn Reson Imagining* 1998;8:755–761.
671c. Kumar S, et al. MRI in Japanese encephalitis. *Neuroradiology* 1997;39:180–184.
672. White, NJ. Variation in virulence of dengue virus. *Lancet* 1999;354:1401–1402.
672a. Monath TP. Early indicators in acute dengue infection. *Lancet* 1997;350:1719–1720.
673. Meegan JM, Shope RE. Emerging concepts on Rift Valley fever. In: *Perspectives in neurology*. Vol. II. New York: Alan R. Liss, 1981:267.
674. Russell RR, Donald JC. The neurological complications of mumps. *BMJ* 1958;2:27–30.
675. Levitt LP, et al. Central nervous system mumps. A review of 64 cases. *Neurology* 1970;20:829–834.
676. Azimi PH, Cramblett HG, Haynes RE. Mumps meningoencephalitis in children. *JAMA* 1969;207:509–512.
677. Wilfert CM. Mumps meningoencephalitis with low cerebrospinal fluid glucose, prolonged pleocytosis and elevation of protein. *N Engl J Med* 1969;280:855–859.
678. Koskiniemi M, Donner M, Pettay O. Clinical appearance and outcome in mumps encephalitis in children. *Acta Paediatr Scand* 1983;72:603–609.
679. Oldfelt V. Sequelae of mumps meningoencephalitis. *Acta Med Scand* 1949;134:405–415.
680. Leheup BP, et al. Lésions des noyeaux gris centraux au cours des oreillons. Evolution clinique et neuroradiologique d'un cas. *Rev Neurol* 1987;143:301–303.
681. Haginoya K, et al. Chronic progressive mumps virus encephalitis in a child. *Lancet* 1995;346:50.
682. Murray H, Fuld CM, McLeod W. Mumps meningoencephalitis. *BMJ* 1960;1:1850–1853.
683. Vandvik B, et al. Mumps meningitis: prolonged pleocytosis and occurrence of mumps virus-specific oligoclonal IgG in the cerebrospinal fluid. *Eur Neurol* 1978;17:13–22.
684. Chomel JJ, et al. Rapid direct diagnosis of mumps meningitis by ELISA capture technique. *J Virol Methods* 1997;68:97–104.
685. Tarr RW, et al. MRI of mumps encephalitis: comparison with CT evaluation. *Pediatr Radiol* 1987;17:59–62.
686. Nahmias AJ, Roizman B. Infections with herpes simplex viruses 1 and 2. *N Engl J Med* 1973;289:667–674, 719–725, 781–789.
687. Plummer G, et al. Type 1 and type 2 herpes simplex viruses: serological and biological differences. *J Virol* 1970;5:51–59.
688. Dowdle WR, et al. Association of antigenic type of herpes-virus hominis with site of viral recovery. *J Immunol* 1967;99:974–980.
689. Johnson RT, Mims CA. Pathogenesis of viral infections of the nervous system. *N Engl J Med* 1968;278: 23–30, 84–92.
689a. Enquist LW, et al. Infection and spread of alpha-herpesviruses in the nervous system. *Advances in Virus Research* 1999;51:237–347.
690. Drachman DA, Adams RD. Herpes-simplex and acute inclusion-body encephalitis. *Arch Neurol* 1962;7: 45–63.
691. Baringer JR, Swoveland P. Recovery of herpes-simplex virus from human trigeminal ganglions. *N Engl J Med* 1973;228:648–650.
692. Baringer JR. Recovery of herpes-simplex virus from sacral ganglions. *N Engl J Med* 1974;291:828–830.
693. Liedtke W, et al. Age distribution of latent herpes simplex virus 1 and varicella-zoster virus genome in human nervous tissue. *J Neurol Sci* 1993;116:6–11.
694. Leider W, et al. Herpes-simplex-virus encephalitis: its possible association with reactivated latent infection. *N Engl J Med* 1965;273:341–347.
695. Crompton MR, Teare RD. Encephalitis after reduction of steroid maintenance therapy. *Lancet* 1965;2: 1318–1320.
696. Prober CG, et al. Use of routine viral cultures at delivery to identify neonates exposed to herpes simplex virus. *N Engl J Med* 1988;318:887–891.
697. Craig CP, Nahmias AJ. Different patterns of neurologic involvement with herpes simplex virus types 1 and 2: isolation of herpes simplex virus 2 from the

buffy coat of two adults with meningitis. *J Infect Dis* 1973;127:365–372.

698. Whitley RJ, et al. Herpes simplex encephalitis. Clinical assessment. *JAMA* 1982;247:317–320.

699. Olson LC, et al. Herpesvirus infections of the human central nervous system. *N Engl J Med* 1967;277: 1271–1277.

700. Illis LS, Gostling JV. *Herpes simplex encephalitis.* Bristol, PA: Scientechnica, 1972.

701. van der Poel JC, Haenggeli CA, Overweg-Plandsoen WCB. Operculum syndrome: unusual feature of herpes simplex encephalitis. *Pediatr Neurol* 1995;12: 246–249.

702. Shanks DE, Blasco PA, Chason DP. Movement disorder following herpes simplex encephalitis. *Dev Med Child Neurol* 1991;33:348–352.

703. Mikati M, Krishnamoorthy KS. Hypoglycorrhachia in neonatal herpes simplex meningoencephalitis. *J Pediatr* 1985;107:746–748.

704. Upton A, Gumpert J. Electroencephalography in diagnosis of herpes-simplex encephalitis. *Lancet* 1970;1: 650–652.

705. Smith JB, et al. A distinctive clinical EEG profile in herpes simplex encephalitis. *Mayo Clin Proc* 1975;50: 469–474.

706. Kowal-Vern A, et al. Magnetic resonance imaging in an unusual presentation of herpes encephalitis. *Neuropediatrics* 1988;19:49–51.

707. Schroth G, et al. Early diagnosis of herpes simplex encephalitis by MRI. *Neurology* 1987;37:179–183.

708. Troendle-Atkins J, Demmler GJ, Buffone GJ. Rapid diagnosis of herpes simplex virus encephalitis by using the polymerase chain reaction. *J Pediatr* 1993;123: 376–380.

708a. Lakeman FD, Whitley RJ. The National Institute of Allergy and Infectious Diseases Collaborative Antiviral Study Group. Diagnosis of herpes simplex encephalitis: application of polymerase chain reaction to cerebrospinal fluid from brain-biopsied patients and correlation with disease. *J Infect Dis* 1995;171: 857–863.

709. Wildemann B, et al. Quantitation of herpes simplex virus type 1 DNA in cells of cerebrospinal fluid of patients with herpes simplex virus encephalitis. *Neurology* 1997;48:1341–1346.

710. Kimura H, et al. Detection of viral DNA in neonatal herpes simplex virus infections: frequent and prolonged presence in serum and cerebrospinal fluid. *J Infect Dis* 1991;164:289–293.

711. Levine DP, Lauter CB, Lerner AM. Simultaneous serum and cerebrospinal fluid antibodies in herpes simplex virus encephalitis. *JAMA* 1978;240: 356–360.

712. Koskiniemi M, Vaheri A, Taskinen E. Cerebrospinal fluid alterations in herpes simplex virus encephalitis. *Rev Infect Dis* 1984;6:608–618.

713. Hanada N, et al. Non-invasive method for early diagnosis of herpes simplex encephalitis. *Arch Dis Child* 1988;63:1470–1473.

714. Arvin AM, et al. Consensus: management of the patient with herpes simplex encephalitis. *Pediatr Infect Dis* 1987;6:2–5.

715. Anderson NE, et al. Brain biopsy in the management of focal encephalitis. *J Neurol Neurosurg Psych* 1991;54: 1001–1003.

716. Nahmias AJ, et al. Herpes simplex virus encephalitis: laboratory evaluations and their diagnostic significance. *J Infect Dis* 1982;145:829–836.

717. Whitley RJ, et al. Herpes virus encephalitis. Vidarabine therapy and diagnostic problems. *N Engl J Med* 1981;304:313–318.

718. Soo MS, et al. Mesenrhomboencephalitis: MR findings in nine patients. *Am J Roentgenol* 1993;160: 1089–1093.

719. Johns DR, Stein AG, Wityk R. MELAS syndrome masquerading as herpes simplex encephalitis. *Neurology* 1993;43:2471–2473.

720. Whitley RJ, Gnann JW Jr. Acyclovir: a decade later. *N Engl J Med* 1992;327:782–789.

721. Wade JC, Meyers JD. Neurologic symptoms associated with parenteral acyclovir treatment after marrow transplantation. *Ann Int Med* 1983;98:921–925.

722. Erlich KS, et al. Acyclovir-resistant herpes simplex infections in patients with the acquired immunodeficiency syndrome. *N Engl J Med* 1989;320: 293–296.

723. Burns WH, et al. Isolation and characterisation of resistant herpes simplex virus after acyclovir therapy. *Lancet* 1982;1:421–423.

724. Wutzler P. Antiviral therapy of herpes simplex and varicella-zoster virus infections. *Intervirology* 1997;40:343–356.

725. Kohl S. Effectiveness of adenine arabinoside therapy for herpes simplex infections. *J Infect Dis* 1984;150: 777–778.

726. Pike MG, et al. Herpes simplex encephalitis with relapse. *Arch Dis Child* 1991;66:1242–1244.

727. Hargrave DR, Webb DW. Movement disorders in association with herpes simplex virus encephalitis in children: a review. *Dev Med Child Neurol* 1998;40: 640–642.

728. Prober CG, et al. Low risk of herpes simplex virus infections in neonates exposed to the virus at the time of vaginal delivery to mothers with recurrent genital herpes simplex virus infections. *N Engl J Med* 1987;316:240–244.

729. Corey L, et al. Difference between herpes simplex virus type 1 and type 2 neonatal encephalitis in neurologic outcome. *Lancet* 1988;1:1–4.

730. Whitley RJ. Neonatal herpes simplex virus infections: pathogenesis and therapy. *Pathol Biol Paris* 1992; 40:729–734.

731. Malm G, et al. A follow-up study of children with neonatal herpes simplex virus infections with particular regard to late nervous disturbances. *Acta Paediatri Scand* 1991;80:226–234.

732. Takahashi, M, et al. The substantia nigra is a major target for neurovirulent influenza A virus. *J Exp Med* 1995;181:2161–2169.

733. Middleton PJ, Alexander RM, Szymanski MT. Severe myositis during recovery from influenza. *Lancet* 1970;2:533–535.

734. Stevens D, et al. Temporary paralysis in childhood after influenza B. *Lancet* 1974;2:1354–1355.

735. Paisley JW, et al. Type A2 influenza viral infections in children. *Am J Dis Child* 1978;132:34–36.

736. Fujii Y, et al. MRI and SPECT in influenzal encephalitis. *Pediatr Neurol* 1992;8:133–136.

737. Protheroe SM, Mellor DH. Imaging of influenza A encephalitis. *Arch Dis Child* 1991;66:702–705.

738. McCarthy VP, Zimmerman AW, Miller CA. Central nervous system manifestations of parainfluenza virus type 3 infections in childhood. *Pediatr Neurol* 1990; 6:197–201.

739. Craver RD, et al. Isolation of parainfluenza virus type 3 from cerebrospinal fluid associated with aseptic meningitis. *Am J Clin Pathol* 1993;99:705–707.

740. Lindquist SW, et al. Parainfluenza virus type-4 infections in pediatric patients. *Pediatr Infect Dis J* 1997;16: 34–38.

741. Tsolia M, et al. Pre-eruptive neurologic manifestations associated with multiple cerebral infarcts in varicella. *Pediatr Neurol* 1995;12:165–168.

742. Yilmaz, K, et al. Acute childhood hemiplegia associated with chickenpox. *Pediatr Neurol* 1998; 18:256–261.

743. Tsolia, M, et al. Pre-eruptive neurologic manifestations associated with multiple cerebral infarcts in varicella. *Pediatr Neurol* 1995;12:165–168.

744. Amlie-Lefond, C, et al. The vasculopathy of varicella-zoster virus encephalitis. *Ann Neurol* 1995;37: 784–790.

745. Downie AW. Chickenpox and zoster. *Br Med Bull* 1959;15:197–200.

746. Croen KD, Straus SE. Varicella-zoster virus latency. *Ann Rev Microbiol* 1991;45:265–282.

747. Arvin AM, Koropchak CM, Wittek AE. Immunologic evidence of reinfection with varicella-zoster virus. *J Infect Dis* 1983;148:200–205.

748. Hardy I, et al. Varicella Vaccine Collaborative Study Group. The incidence of zoster after immunization with live attenuated varicella vaccine. A study of children with leukemia. *N Engl J Med* 1991;325: 1545–1550.

749. Denny-Brown D, Adams RD, Fitzgerald PJ. Pathologic features of herpes zoster. A note on "geniculate herpes." *Arch Neurol Psychiatry* 1944;51:216–231.

750. McCormick WF, et al. Varicella zoster encephalomyelitis—a morphologic and virologic study. *Arch Neurol* 1969;21:559–570.

751. Schmidbauer M, et al. Presence, distribution and spread of productive varicella zoster virus infection in nervous tissues. *Brain* 1992;115:383–398.

752. Hope-Simpson RE. The nature of herpes zoster. A long-term study and a new hypothesis. *Proc R Soc Med* 1965;58:9–20.

753. DeMorgas JM, Kierland RR. The outcome of patients with herpes zoster. *Arch Dermatol* 1957;75: 193–196.

754. Kost RG, Straus SE. Drug therapy: postherpetic neuralgia—pathogenesis, treatment, and prevention. *N Engl J Med* 1996;335:32–42.

755. Oaklander AL, et al. Unilateral postherpetic neuralgia is associated with bilateral sensory neural damage. *Ann Neurol* 1998;44:789–795.

756. Baron R, Saguer M. Postherpetic neuralgia. *Brain* 1993;116:1477–1496.

757. Rose FC, Brett EM, Burston J. Zoster encephalomyelitis. *Arch Neurol* 1964;11:155–172.

758. Rosenfeld J, Taylor CL, Atlas SW. Myelitis following chickenpox: a case report. *Neurology* 1993;43: 1834–1836.

759. Eidelberg D, et al. Thrombotic cerebral vasculopathy associated with herpes zoster. *Ann Neurol* 1986;19: 7–14.

760. Reshef E, Greenberg SB, Jankovic J. Herpes Zoster ophthalmicus followed by contralateral hemiparesis: report of two cases and review of the literature. *J Neurol Neurosurg Psychiatry* 1985;48:122–127.

761. Bodensteiner JB, Hille MR, Riggs JE. Clinical features of vascular thrombosis following varicella. *Am J Dis Child* 1992;146:100–102.

762. Merselis JG Jr, Kaye D, Hooke EW. Disseminated herpes zoster: a report of 17 cases. *Arch Intern Med* 1964;113:679–686.

763. Feldman S, et al. A viremic phase for herpes zoster in children with cancer. *J Pediatr* 1977;91:557–560.

764. Horten B, Price RW, Jiminez D. Multifocal varicella-zoster virus leukoencephalitis temporally remote from herpes zoster. *Ann Neurol* 1981;9: 251–266.

764a. Gnann JW, Whitley RJ. Neurologic manifestations of varicella and herpes zoster. In: Scheld WM, Whitley RJ, Durack DT, eds. Infections of the Central Nervous System, 2nd ed. Philadelphia: Lippincott–Raven Publishers, 1997:91–105.

765. Echevarria JM, et al. Aseptic meningitis due to varicella-zoster virus: serum antibody levels and local synthesis of specific IgG, IgM, and IgA. *J Infect Dis* 1987;155:959–967.

766. Peterslund NA. Herpes zoster associated encephalitis: clinical findings and acyclovir treatment. *Scand J Infect Dis* 1988;20:583–592.

767. Mayo DR, Booss J. Varicella zoster-associated neurologic disease without skin lesions. *Arch Neurol* 1989;46:313–315.

768. Silliman CC, et al. Unsuspected varicella-zoster virus encephalitis in a child with acquired immunodeficiency syndrome. *J Pediatr* 1993;123:418–422.

769. Persaud D, et al. Delayed recognition of human immunodeficiency virus infection in preadolescent children. *Pediatrics* 1992;90:688–691.

770. Keidan SE, Mainwaring D. Association of herpes zoster with leukemia and lymphoma in children. *Clin Pediatr* 1965;4:13–17.

771. Hunt JR. On herpetic inflammations of the geniculate ganglion: a new syndrome and its complications. *J Nerv Ment Dis* 1907;34:73–96.

772. Terada K, et al. Detection of varicella-zoster virus DNA in peripheral mononuclear cells from patients with Ramsay Hunt syndrome or zoster sine herpete. *J Med Virol* 1998;56:359–363.

773. Berrettini S, et al. Herpes zoster oticus: correlations between clinical and MRI findings. *Eur Neurol* 1998;39:26–31.

774. Murakami S, et al, Treatment of Ramsay Hunt syndrome with acyclovir-prednisone: significance of early diagnosis and treatment. *Ann Neurol* 1997;41: 353–357.

775. Gershon A, et al. Varicella-zoster-associated encephalitis: detection of specific antibody in cerebrospinal fluid. *J Clin Microbiol* 1980;12:764–769.

775a. Casas I, et al. Viral diagnosis of neurological infection by RT multiplex PCR: a search for entero- and herpesviruses in a prospective study. *J Med Virol* 1999; 57:145-51.

775b. Echevarria JM, et al. Infections of the nervous system caused by varicella-zoster virus: a review. *Intervirology* 1997;40:72–84.

776. Wood MJ, et al. A randomized trial of acyclovir for 7 or 21 days with and without prednisolone for treat-

ment of acute herpes zoster. *N Engl J Med* 1994; 330:896–900.

777. Hay J, Arvin AM. Varicella-zoster virus infection: new insights into pathogenesis and post-herpetic neuralgia. *Ann Neurol* 1994;35[Suppl]:S1–S72.

777a. Whitley RJ, et al. Disseminated herpes zoster in the immunocompromised host: a comparative trial of acyclovir and vidarabine. *J Infect Dis* 1992;165: 450–455.

777b. Otero J, et al. Response to acyclovir in two cases of herpes zoster leukoencephalitis and review of the literature. *Eur J Clin Microbiol Infect Dis* 1998;17: 286–289.

778. de Silva SM, et al. Zoster myelitis: improvement with antiviral therapy in two cases. *Neurology* 1996;47: 929–931.

779. Segal AZ, Rordorf G. Gabapentin as a novel treatment for post herpetic neuralgia. *Neurology* 1996;46: 1175–1176.

780. Pasteur L. Méthode pour prevenir la rage après morsure. *CR Acad Sci (Paris)* 1885;101:765–774.

781. Fishbein DB, Robinson LE. Rabies. *N Engl J Med* 1993;329:1632–1638.

782. Plotkin SA, Clark HF. Rabies. In: Feigin RD, Cherry JD, eds. *Textbook of pediatric infectious diseases*, 4th ed. Philadelphia: WB Saunders, 1998:2111–2125.

783. American Academy of Pediatrics. Rabies. In: Peter G, ed. *1997 Red Book: report of the Committee on Infectious Diseases*, 24th ed. Elk Grove Village, IL: American Academy of Pediatrics, 1997:435–442.

784. Dupont JR, Earle K. Human rabies encephalitis. A study of forty-nine fatal cases and a review of the literature. *Neurology* 1965;15:1023–1034.

785. McKendrick AG. A ninth analytical review of reports from Pasteur Institutes on the results of anti-rabies treatment. *Bull Health Organ League of Nations* 1940;9:31–78.

786. Lentz TL, et al. The acetylcholine receptor as a cellular receptor for rabies virus. *Yale J Biol Med* 1983;56: 315–322.

787. Schindler R. Studies on the pathogenesis of rabies. *Bull WHO* 1961;25:119–126.

788. Gonzalez-Angulo A, et al. The ultrastructure of Negri-bodies in Purkinje neurons in human rabies. *Neurology* 1970;20:323–328.

789. Mrak RE, Young L. Rabies encephalitis in humans: pathology, pathogenesis and pathophysiology. *J Neuropathol Exp Neurol* 1994;53:1–10.

790. Anonymous. Human rabies: strain identification reveals lengthy incubation period [Editorial]. *Lancet* 1991;337: 822–823.

791. Anderson LJ, et al. Human rabies in the United States, 1960–1979: epidemiology, diagnosis and prevention. *Ann Int Med* 1984;100:728–735.

792. Bhatt DR, et al. Human rabies. *Am J Dis Child* 1974;127:862–869.

793. Blatt ML, Hoffman SJ, Schneider M. Rabies: report of twelve cases, with a discussion of prophylaxis. *JAMA* 1938;111:688–691.

794. Blattner RJ. Bats and rabies. *J Pediatr* 1955;46: 612–614.

795. Cheetham HD, et al. Rabies with myocarditis. Two cases in England. *Lancet* 1970;1:921–922.

796. Perl DP, Good PF. The pathology of rabies in the central nervous system. In: Baer GM, ed. *The natural his-*

tory of rabies*, 2nd ed. Boca Raton: CRC Press, 1991:164–190.

797. Cereghino JJ, et al. Rabies: a rare disease but a serious pediatric problem. *Pediatrics* 1970;45:839–844.

798. Johnson HN. Rabies virus. In: Lennette EH, Schmidt NJ, eds. *Diagnostic procedures for viral, rickettsial and chlamydial infections*, 5th ed. Washington, DC: American Public Health Association 1979:843–877.

799. Whitley RJ. Rabies. In: Scheld WM, Whitley RJ, Durack DT, eds. *Infections of the central nervous system*. New York: Lippincott–Raven Press, 1997: 181–198.

800. Hattwick MA, et al. Recovery from rabies. A case report. *Ann Intern Med* 1972;76:931–942.

801. Vodopija I, Soreau P, Smerdel S. Current issues in human rabies immunization. *Rev Infect Dis* 1988;10[Suppl 4]:S758–S763.

802. Fishbein DB, et al. Administration of human diploid-cell rabies vaccine in the gluteal area [Letter]. *N Engl J Med* 1988;318:124–125.

803. Mortiere MD, Falcone AL. An acute neurological syndrome temporally associated with postexposure treatment of rabies. *Pediatrics* 1997;100:720–721.

804. Park JY, Saron MF. Age distribution of lymphocytic choriomeningitis virus serum antibody in Birmingham, Alabama: evidence of a decreased risk of infection. *Am J Trop Hyg* 1997;57:37–41.

804a. Marrie TJ, Saron MF. Seroprevalence of lymphocytic choriomeningitis virus in Nova Scotia. *Am J Trop Hyg* 1998;58:47–49.

805. Howard ME. Infection with the virus of choriomeningitis in man. *Yale J Biol Med* 1940;13:161–180.

806. Baker AB. Chronic lymphocytic choriomeningitis. *J Neuropathol Exp Neurol* 1947;6:253–264.

807. Baum SG, et al. Epidemic non-meningitic lymphocytic-choriomeningitis-virus infection. An outbreak in a population of laboratory personnel. *N Engl J Med* 1966;274:934–936.

808. Lewis JM, Utz JP. Orchitis, parotitis and meningoencephalitis due to lymphocytic-choriomeningitis virus. *N Engl J Med* 1961;265:776–780.

809. Green WR, Sweet LK, Prichard RW. Acute lymphocytic choriomeningitis: a study of 21 cases. *J Pediatr* 1949;35:688–701.

810. Adair CV, Gauld RL, Smadel JE. Aseptic meningitis, a disease of diverse etiology: clinical and etiologic studies on 854 cases. *Ann Intern Med* 1953;39: 675–704.

811. Wright R, et al. Congenital lymphocytic meningitis virus syndrome: a disease that mimics congenital toxoplasmosis or cytomegalovirus infection. *Pediatrics* 1997;100:E9 (on line).

811a. Park JY, et al. Development of a reverse transcription-polymerase chain reaction assay for the diagnosis of lymphocytic choriomeningitis virus infection and its use in a prospective surveillance study. *J Med Virol* 1997;51:107–114.

812. Gautier-Smith PC. Neurological complications of glandular fever (infectious mononucleosis). *Brain* 1965;88:323–334.

813. Silverstein A, Steinberg G, Nathanson M. Nervous system involvement in infectious mononucleosis. The heralding and/or major manifestation. *Arch Neurol* 1972;26:353–358.

813a. Wong M, Connolly AM, Noetzel MJ. Poliomyelitis-like syndrome associated with Epstein-Barr virus infection. *Pediatr Neurol* 1999;20:235–237.

814. Pedneault L, et al. Detection of Epstein-Barr virus in the brain by polymerase chain reaction. *Ann Neurol* 1992;32:184–192.

815. Halsted CC, et al. Infectious mononucleosis and encephalitis: recovery of EB virus from spinal fluid. *Pediatrics* 1979;64:257–258.

816. Domachowske JB, et al. Acute manifestations and neurologic sequelae of Epstein-Barr virus encephalitis in children. *Pediatr Infect Dis J* 1996;15: 871–875.

817. Grose C, et al. Primary Epstein-Barr infections in acute neurologic diseases. *N Engl J Med* 1975;292: 392–395.

818. Erzurum S, Kalavsky SM, Watanakunakorn C. Acute cerebellar ataxia and hearing loss as initial symptoms of infectious mononucleosis. *Arch Neurol* 1983;40: 760–762.

819. North K, de Silva L, Procopis P. Brain-stem encephalitis caused by Epstein-Barr virus. *J Child Neurol* 1993;8:40–42.

819a. Connelly PD, DeWitt LD. Neurologic complications of infectious mononucleosis. *Pediatr Neurol* 1994;10: 181–184.

819b. Schellinger PD, et al. Epstein-Barr virus meningoencephalitis with a lymphoma-like response in an immunocompetent host. *Ann Neurol* 1999;45: 659–662.

820. Shechter FR, Lipsius EI, Rasansky HN. Retrobulbar neuritis. A complication of infectious mononucleosis. *Am J Dis Child* 1955;89:58–61.

821. Gross C, et al. Bell's palsy and infectious mononucleosis. *Lancet* 1973;2:231–232.

822. Parano E, et al. Reversible palsy of the hypoglossal nerve complicating infectious mononucleosis in a young child. *Neuropediatrics* 1998;29:46–47.

823. Erwin W, Weber RW, Manning RT. Complications of infectious mononucleosis. *Am J Med Sci* 1959;238: 699–712.

824. Walsh FC, Poser CM, Carter S. Infectious mononucleosis encephalitis. *Pediatrics* 1954;13:536–543.

825. Pejme J. Infectious mononucleosis. A clinical and hematological study of patients and contacts, and a comparison with healthy subjects. *Acta Med Scand* 1964;413[Suppl]:183.

826. Tselis A, et al. Epstein-Barr virus encephalomyelitis diagnosed by polymerase chain reaction: detection of the genome in the CSF. *Neurology* 1997;48: 1351–1355.

827. Gerber MA, et al. Evaluations of enzyme-linked immunosorbent assay procedure for determining specific Epstein-Barr virus serology and of rapid test kits for diagnosis for infectious mononucleosis. *J Clin Microbiol* 1996;34:3240–3241.

828. Hongou K, et al. Rotavirus encephalitis mimicking afebrile benign convulsions in infants. *Pediatr Neurol* 1998;18:354–357.

828a. Lajo A, et al. Mononucleosis caused by Epstein-Barr virus and cytomegalovirus in children: a comparative study of 124 cases. *Pediatr Infect Dis J* 1994;13:56–60.

828b. Studahl M, et al. Cytomegalovirus encephalitis in four immunocompetent patients. *Lancet* 1992;340: 1045–1046.

828c. Kabins S, et al. Acute idiopathic polyneuritis caused by cytomegalovirus. *Arch Intern Med* 1976;136:100–101.

828d. Schmitz H, et al. Cytomegalovirus as a frequent cause of Guillain-Barré syndrome. *J Med Virol* 1977;1: 21–27.

828e. Power C, et al. Cytomegalovirus and Rasmussen's encephalitis. *Lancet* 1990;336:1282–1284.

828f. Cinque P, et al. Cytomegalovirus infection of the central nervous system in patients with AIDS: diagnosis by PCR amplification from cerebrospinal fluid. *J Infect Dis* 1992;166:1408–1411.

829. Debré R, et al. La maladie des griffes de chat. *Sem Hop Paris* 1950;26:1895–1904.

830. Parrot JH, Dure L, Sullender W. Central nervous system infection with *Bartonella quintana*: a report of two cases. 1997;100:403–408.

831. Zangwill KM, et al. Cat scratch disease in Connecticut. Epidemiology, risk factors and evaluation of a new diagnostic test. *N Engl J Med* 1993;329:8–13.

832. Adal KA, Cockerell CJ, Petri WA Jr. Cat scratch disease, bacillary angiomatosis, and other infections due to rochalimaea. *N Engl J Med* 1994;330: 1509–1515.

833. Wear DJ, et al. Cat scratch disease: a bacterial infection. *Science* 1983;221:1403–1405.

834. Regnery RI, Andersen BE, Clarridge JE III. Characterization of a novel *Rochalimaea* species, *R. Henselae* sp. nov., isolated from blood of a febrile, human immunodeficiency virus-positive patient. *J Clin Microbiol* 1992;30:265–274.

835. Carithers HA, Margileth AM. Cat-scratch disease: acute encephalopathy and other neurologic manifestations. *Am J Dis Child* 1991,145:98–101.

836. Margileth AM. Cat scratch disease. *Adv Pediatr Infect Dis* 1993;8:1–21.

837. Lewis DW, Tucker SH. Central nervous system involvement in cat scratch disease. *Pediatrics* 1986;77: 714–721.

838. Carithers H.A. Cat-scratch disease: an overview based on a study of 1,200 patients. *Am J Dis Child* 1985;139:1124–1133.

839. Tsao CY. Generalized tonic-clonic status epilepticus in a child with cat-scratch disease and encephalopathy. *Clin Electroencephalogr* 1992;23:65–67.

840. Drancour M, et al. New serotype of *Bartonella henselae* in endocarditis and cat-scratch disease. *Lancet* 1996;347:441–443.

841. Patnaik M, et al. Possible role of *Rochalimaea henselae* in pathogenesis of AIDS encephalopathy. *Lancet* 1992;340:971.

842. Regnery RL, et al. Serological response to "*Rochalimaea henselae*" antigen in suspected cat-scratch disease. *Lancet* 1992;339:1443–1445.

843. Sigurdsson B. Rida, a chronic encephalitis of sheep. With general remarks on infections which develop slowly and some of their special characteristics. *Br Vet J* 1954;110:341–358.

844. Prusiner SB. Prions. *Proc Nat Acad Sci USA*. 1998;95:13363–13383.

845. Prusiner SB. The prion diseases. *Brain Pathol* 1998;8:499–513.

846. Klein MA, et al. A role for B cells in neuroinvasive scrapie. *Nature* 1997;390:687–690.

847. Prusiner SB, DeArmond SJ. Prion diseases and neurodegeneration. *Annu Rev Neurosci* 1994;17:311–339.

848. Prusiner SB. Prion diseases and the BSE crisis. *Science* 1997;278:245–251.

849. Hill AF, et al. The same prion strain causes vCJD and BSE. *Nature* 1997;389:448–450.

849a. Haywood AM. Transmissible spongiform encephalopathies. *N Engl J Med* 1997;337:1821–1828.

850. Mestel R. Putting prions to the test. *Science* 1996;273:184–189.

851. DeArmond SJ, et al. Changes in the localization of brain prion proteins during scrapie infection. *Neurology* 1987;37:1271–1280.

852. Kristensson K, et al. Scrapie prions alter receptor-mediated calcium responses in cultured cells. *Neurology* 1993;43:2335–2341.

853. Collinge J, et al. Prion protein is necessary for synaptic function. *Nature* 1994;370:295–297.

854. Pablos-Mindez A, Netto EM, Defendini R. Infectious prions or cytotoxic metabolites? *Lancet* 1993;341:159–161.

855. Ito M, et al. Chronic mumps virus encephalitis. *Pediatr Neurol* 1991;7:467–470.

856. Ogawa M, et al. Chronic progressive encephalitis occurring 13 years after Russian spring-summer encephalitis. *J Neurol Sci* 1973;19:363–373.

857. Sharma S, et al. Japanese encephalitis virus latency in peripheral blood lymphocytes and recurrence of infection in children. *Clin Exp Immunol* 1991;85:85–89.

858. Pantaleo G, Graziosi C, Fauci AS. The immunopathogenesis of human immunodeficiency virus infection. *N Engl J Med* 1993;328:327–335.

859. Greene WC. The molecular biology of human immunodeficiency virus type 1 infection. *N Engl J Med* 1991; 324:308–317.

860. Levy JA. Infection by human immunodeficiency virus—CD4 is not enough. *N Engl J Med* 1996;335:1528–1530.

861. Human immunodeficiency virus. In: Johnson RT. *Viral infections of the nervous system*, 2nd ed. Philadelphia: Lippincott–Raven, 1998:287–313.

862. Merril JE, Jonakait M. Interactions of the nervous and immune systems in development, normal brain homeostasis, and disease. *FASEB* J 1995;9:611–618.

863. Pulliam L, et al. Unique monocyte subset in patients with AIDS dementia. *Lancet* 1997;349:692–695.

864. Tyor WR, et al. Cytokine expression of macrophages in HIV-1-associated vacuolar myelopathy. *Neurology* 1993;43:1002–1009.

865. Kolson DL, Lavi E, González-Scarano F. The effects of human immunodeficiency virus in the central nervous system. *Adv Virus Res* 1998;50:1–47.

866. Lipton SA, Gendelman HE. Dementia associated with the acquired imunodeficiency syndrome. *N Engl J Med* 1995;332:934–944.

867. Davis LE, et al. Early viral brain invasion in iatrogenic human immunodeficiency virus infection. *Neurology* 1992;42:1736–1739.

868. Chamberlain MC, Nichols SL, Chase CH. Pediatric AIDS: comparative cranial MRI and CT scans. *Pediatr Neurol* 1991;7:357–362.

869. Epstein LG, et al. Neurologic manifestations of human immunodeficiency virus infection in children. *Pediatrics* 1986;78:678–687.

870. Brown MM. Retroviruses and diseases of the nervous system. *J R Soc Med* 1989;82:306–309.

870a. Childs EA, et al. Plasma viral load and CD4 lymphocytes predict HIV-associated dementia and sensory neuropathy. *Neurology* 1999;52:607–613.

871. Dickson DW, et al. Central nervous system pathology in pediatric AIDS: an autopsy study. *APMIS* 1989; 8[Suppl]:40–57.

872. Donaldson YK, Bell JE, Ironside JW. Redistribution of HIV outside the lymphoid system with onset of AIDS. *Lancet* 1994;343:382–385.

873. Falloon J, et al. Human immunodeficiency virus infection in children. *J Pediatr* 1989;114:1–30.

874. Spencer DC, Price RW. Human immunodeficiency virus and the central nervous system. *Annu Rev Microbiol* 1992;46:655–693.

875. Petito CK. What causes brain atrophy in human immunodeficiency virus infection? *Ann Neurol* 1993; 34:128–129.

876. Kure K, et al. Morphology and distribution of HIV-1 gp41-positive microglia in subacute AIDS encephalitis. Pattern of involvement resembling a multisystem degeneration. *Acta Neuropathol* 1990;80:393–400.

877. Giangaspero F, et al. Massive neuronal destruction in human immunodeficiency virus (HIV) encephalitis. A clinico-pathological study of a pediatric case. *Acta Neuropathol* 1989;78:662–665.

878. Evans BK, Donley DK, Whitaker JN. Neurological manifestations of infection with the human immunodeficiency viruses. In: Scheld WM, Whitley RJ, Durack DT, eds. *Infections of the central nervous system*. New York: Raven Press, 1991:201–232.

879. Gray F, et al. Neuropathology of early HIV-1 infection. *Brain Pathology* 1996;6:1–15.

880. Adamson DC, et al. Immunologic NO synthase: elevation in severe AIDS dementia and induction by HIV-1 gp41. *Science* 1996;274:1917–1921.

881. Markham RB, et al. Maternal IgG1 and IgA antibody to the V3 loop consensus sequence and maternal-infant HIV-1 transmission. *Lancet* 1994;343:390–391.

882. Blanche S, et al. Relation of the course of HIV infection in children to the severity of the disease in their mothers at delivery. *N Engl J Med* 1994;330:308–312.

883. Sperling RS, et al. Maternal viral load, zidovudine treatment, and the risk of transmission of human immunodeficiency virus type 1 from mother to infant. *N Engl J Med* 1996;335:1621–1629.

884. Landesman SH, et al. Obstetrical factors and the transmission of human immunodeficiency virus type 1 from mother to child. *N Engl J Med* 1996;334:1617–1623.

885. Newell M-L. Mechanisms and timing of mother-to-child transmission of HIV-1. *AIDS* 1998;12:831–837.

886. Pantaleo G, Graziosi C, Demarest JF. HIV infection is active and progressive in lymphoid tissue during the clinically latent stage of disease. *Nature* 1993;362:355–358.

887. Fauci AS. Multifactorial nature of human immunodeficiency virus disease: implications for therapy. *Science* 1993;262:1011–1018.

888. Civitello LA. Neurologic complications of HIV infection of children. *Pediatr Neurosurg* 1991;17:104–112.

889. Belman AL, et al. Pediatric acquired immunodeficiency syndrome: neurologic syndromes. *Am J Dis Child* 1988;142:29–35.

890. Roy S, et al. Neurological findings in HIV-infected children: a review of 49 cases. *Can J Neurol Sci* 1992;19:453–457.

890a. Cooper ER, et al. Encephalopathy and progression of human immunodeficiency virus disease in a cohort of children with perinatally acquired human immunodeficiency virus infection. Women and Infants transmission study group. *J Pediatr* 1998;132:808–812.

891. Kahn JO, Walker BD. Acute human immunodeficiency virus type 1 infection. *N Engl J Med* 1998;339:33–39.

891a. Morriss MC, et al. Progressive multifocal leukoencephalopathy in an HIV-infected child. *Neuroradiology* 1997;39:142–144.

892. Bale JF Jr, et al. Neurologic history and examination results and their relationship to human immunodeficiency virus type 1 serostatus in hemophilia subjects: results from the hemophilia growth and development study. *Pediatrics* 1993;91:736–741.

893. Mitchell WG, et al. Longitudinal follow-up of a group of HIV-seropositive and HIV-seronegative hemophiliacs: results from the hemophilia growth and development study. *Pediatrics* 1997;100:817–824.

893a. DeCarli C, et al. The prevalence of computerized tomographic abnormalities of the cerebrum in 100 consecutive children symptomatic with the human immunodeficiency virus. *Ann Neurol* 1993;34: 198–205.

894. Post MJ, et al. CT, MR, and pathology in HIV encephalitis and meningitis. *Am J Roentgenol* 1988; 151:373–380.

895. Scarmato V, et al. Central brain atrophy in childhood AIDS encephalopathy. *AIDS* 1996;10:1227–1231.

896. States LJ, Zimmerman RA, Rutstein RM. Imaging of pediatric central nervous system HIV infection. *Neuroimaging Clin N Am* 1997;7:321–339.

897. Pavlakis SG, et al. Brain lactate and N-acetylaspartate in pediatric AIDS encephalopathy. *Am J Neuroradiol* 1998;19:383–385.

898. Salvan AM, et al. Localized proton magnetic resonance spectroscopy of the brain in children infected with human immunodeficiency virus with and without encephalopathy. *Pediatr Res* 1998;44:755–762.

899. Miles SA, et al. Rapid serologic testing with immune-complex-dissociated HIV p24 antigen for early detection of HIV infection in neonates. *N Engl J Med* 1993;328:297–302.

899a. Dunn DT, et al. The sensitivity of HIV-1 DNA polymerase chain reaction in the neonatal period and the relative contributions of intra-uterine and intra-partum transmission. *AIDS* 1995;9:7–11.

899b. McIntosh K, et al. Blood culture in the first 6 months of life for diagnosis of vertically transmitted human immunodeficiency virus infection. The woman and infant study group. *J Infect Dis* 1994; 170:996–1000.

899c. Public Health Service Task Recommendations. Guidelines for the use of antiretroviral agents in pediatric HIV infection. *MMWR Morb Mortal Wkly Rep* 1998;47(RR-4):1–34.

899d. Burgard M, et al. The use of viral culture and p24 antigen testing to diagnose human immunodeficiency virus infection in neonates. *N Engl J Med* 1992;327: 1192–1197.

899e. Sei S, et al. Evaluation of human immunodeficiency virus (HIV) type 1 RNA levels in cerebrospinal fluid and viral resistance to zidovudine in children with HIV encephalopathy. *J Infect Dis* 1996;174: 1200–1206.

900. McFarlin DE. Neurological disorders related to HTLV-I and HTLV-II. *J Acquir Immune Defic Syndr* 1993;6: 640–644.

901. Gessain A, Gout O. Chronic myelopathy associated with human T-lymphotropic virus type I (HTLV-I). *Ann Intern Med* 1992;117:933–946.

902. Harrington WJ Jr, et al. Spastic ataxia associated with human T-cell lymphotropic virus type II infection. *Ann Neurol* 1993;33:411414.

903. Sheremata, WA, et al. Association of '(tropical) ataxic neuropathy' with HTLV-II. *Virus Res* 1993;29:71–77.

904. Levin MC, et al. Immunologic analysis of a spinal cord biopsy specimen from a patient with human T-cell lymphotropic virus type I-associated neurologic disease. *N Engl J Med* 1997;336:839–845.

905. Moritoyo T, et al. Human T-lymphotrophic virus type I myelopathy and tax gene expression in CD4+ T lymphocytes. *Ann Neurol* 1996;40:84–86.

906. Leon-Monzon M, Illa I, Dalakas MC. Polymyositis in patients infected with human T-cell leukemia virus type I: the role of virus in the cause of the disease. *Ann Neurol* 1994:36;643–649.

907. Izumo S, et al. Interferon-alpha is effective in HTLV-I-associated myelopathy: a multicenter, randomized, double-blind, controlled trial. *Neurology* 1996;46: 1016–1021.

908. Gibbs CJ Jr, et al. Clinical and pathological features and laboratory confirmation of a Creutzfeldt-Jakob disease in a recipient of pituitary-derived human growth hormone. *N Engl J Med* 1985;313:734–738.

909. Rappaport EB, Graham DJ. Pituitary growth hormone from human cadavers: neurologic disease in ten recipients. *Neurology* 1987;37:1211–1213.

910. Brown P, et al. Human spongiform encephalopathy: the National Institutes of Health series of 300 cases of experimentally transmitted disease. *Ann Neurol* 1994;35:513–529.

911. Monreal J, et al. Creutzfeldt-Jakob disease in an adolescent. *J Neurol Sci* 1981;52:341–350.

912. Brown P, et al. Iatrogenic Creutzfeldt-Jakob disease: an example of the interplay between ancient genes and modern medicine. *Neurology* 1994;44:291–293.

913. Deslys J-P, Lasmizas C, Dormont D. Selection of specific strains in iatrogenic Creutzfeldt-Jakob disease. *Lancet* 1994;343:848–849.

914. Hayashi R, et al. Serial computed tomographic and electroencephalographic studies in Creutzfeldt-Jakob disease. *Acta Neurol Scand* 1992;85:161–165.

915. Zerr I, et al. Diagnosis of Creutzfeldt-Jakob disease by two-dimensional gel electrophoresis of cerebrospinal fluid. *Lancet* 1996;348:846–849.

916. Hsich G, et al. The 14-3-3 Protein in cerebrospinal fluid as a marker for transmissible spongiform encephalopathies. *N Engl J Med* 1996;335:924–930.

917. Berndt RM. Reaction to contact in the eastern highlands of New Guinea. *Oceania* 1954;24:206.

918. Gajdusek DC. Unconventional viruses and the origin and disappearance of Kuru. *Science* 1977;197: 943–960.

919. Gajdusek DC, Zigas V. Kuru. *Am J Med* 1959;26: 442–469.
920. Gajdusek DC, Gibbs CJ Jr. Transmission of Kuru from man to Rhesus monkey *(Macaca mulatta)* eight and one-half years after inoculation. *Nature* 1972; 240:351.
921. Grabow JD, et al. A transmissible subacute spongiform encephalopathy in a visitor to the eastern highlands of New Guinea. *Brain* 1976;99:637–658.
922. Gajdusek DC, Zigas V. Degenerative disease of the central nervous system in New Guinea: the endemic occurrence of "Kuru" in the native population. *N Engl J Med* 1957;257:974–978.
923. Hilton DA, et al. Prion immunoreactivity in appendix before clinical onset of variant Creutzfeldt-Jakob disease. *Lancet* 1998;352:703–704.
924. Aguzzi A. Neuro-immune connection in spread of prions in the body? *Lancet* 1997;349:742–743.
925. Zeidler M, et al. New variant Creutzfeldt-Jakob disease: neurological features and diagnostic tests. *Lancet* 1997;350:903–907.
926. Zeidler M, et al. New variant Creutzfeldt-Jakob disease: psychiatric features. *Lancet* 1997;350:908–910.
927. Collee JG, Bradley R. BSE: a decade on—part 1 and 2. *Lancet* 1997;349:636–641, 715–721.
928. Medori R, et al. Fatal familial insomnia, a prion disease with a mutation at codon 178 of the prion protein gene. *N Engl J Med* 1992;326:444–449.
929. Dawson JR Jr. Cellular inclusions in cerebral lesions of epidemic encephalitis. *Arch Neurol Psychiatr* 1934;31: 685–700.
930. Bergamini F, Defanti CA, Ferrante P. *Subacute sclerosing panencephalitis: a reappraisal.* New York: Elsevier Science Publishers, 1986:440.
931. Case 15-1998 Case records of the Massachusetts General Hospital. *N Engl J Med* 1998;338:1448–1456.
932. Herndon RM, Rubinstein LJ. Light and electron microscopy observation on the development of viral particles in the inclusions of Dawson's encephalitis (subacute sclerosing panencephalitis). *Neurology* 1968;18:8–20.
933. Ohya T, et al. Subacute sclerosing panencephalitis: correlation of clinical, neurophysiologic and neuropathologic findings. *Neurology* 1974;24:211–218.
934. Shapshak P, et al. Subacute sclerosing panencephalitis: measles virus matrix protein nucleic acid sequences detected by in situ hybridization. *Neurology* 1985;35: 1605–1609.
935. Hirano A, et al. The matrix proteins of neurovirulent subacute sclerosing panencephalitis virus and its acute measles progenitor are functionally different. *Proc Natl Acad Sci U S A* 1992;89:8745–8749.
936. Schmid A, et al. Subacute sclerosing panencephalitis is typically characterized by alterations in the fusion protein cytoplasmic domain of the persisting measles virus. *Virology* 1992;188:910–915.
937. Hirano A, et al. Functional analysis of matrix proteins expressed from cloned genes of measles virus variants that cause subacute sclerosing panencephalitis reveals a common defect in nucleocapside binding. *J Virol* 1993;67:1848–1853.
938. Mehta PD, Thormar H, Wisniewski HM. Oligoclonal IgG bands with and without measles antibody activity in sera of patients with subacute sclerosing panencephalitis (SSPE). *J Immunol* 1982;129: 1983–1985.
939. Mehta PD, et al. Increased levels of β_2-microglobulin, soluble interleukin-2 receptor, and soluble CD8 in patients with subacute sclerosing panencephalitis. *Clin Immunol Immunopathol* 1992;65: 53–59.
940. Miller C, Farrington CP, Harbert K. The epidemiology of subacute sclerosing panencephalitis in England and Wales 1970–1989. *Int J Epidemiol* 1992;21: 998–1006.
941. Kornberg AJ, Harvey AS, Shield LK. Subacute sclerosing panencephalitis presenting as simple partial seizures. *J Child Neurol* 1991;6:146–149.
942. Robb RM, Watters GV. Ophthalmic manifestations of sub-acute sclerosing panencephalitis. *Arch Ophthalmol* 1970;83:426–435.
943. Jabbour JT, et al. Subacute sclerosing panencephalitis: a multidisciplinary study of eight cases. *JAMA* 1969;207:2248–2254.
944. Cochereau-Massin I, et al. Changes in the fundus in subacute sclerosing panencephalitis. Apropos of 23 cases. *J Fr Ophthalmol* 1992;15:255–261.
945. Freeman JM. The clinical spectrum and early diagnosis of Dawson's encephalitis. *J Pediatr* 1969;75: 590–603.
946. Grünewald T, et al. A 35-year-old bricklayer with myoclonic jerks. *Lancet* 1998;351:1926.
947. PeBenito R, et al. Fulminating subacute sclerosing panencephalitis: case report and literature review. *Clin Pediatr* 1997;36:149–154.
948. Huber M, et al. Changing patterns of glucose metabolism during the course of subacute sclerosing panencephalitis as measured with ^{18}FDG-positron-emission tomography. *J Neurol* 1992;293: 157–161.
949. Pedersen H, Wulff CH. Computed tomographic findings in early subacute sclerosing panencephalitis. *Neuroradiology* 1982;23:31–32.
950. Winer JB, et al. Resolving MRI abnormalities with progression of subacute sclerosing panencephalitis. *Neuroradiology* 1991;33:178–180.
951. Anlar B, et al. MRI findings in subacute sclerosing panencephalitis. *Neurology* 1996;47:1278–1283.
952. Brismar J, et al. Subacute sclerosing panencephalitis: evaluation with CT and MR. *AJNR Am J Neuroradiol* 1996;17:761–772.
953. Wulff CH. Subacute sclerosing panencephalitis: serial electroencephalographic studies. *J Neurol Neurosurg Psychiatry* 1982;45:418–421.
954. Yagi S, et al. The origin of myoclonus and periodic synchronous discharges in subacute sclerosing panencephalitis. *Acta Paediatr Jpn* 1992;34:310–315.
955. Giminez-Roldan S, et al. Preclinical EEG abnormalities in subacute sclerosing panencephalitis. *Neurology* 1981;31:763–767.
956. Johnson RT. Subacute measles encephalitis with immunosuppression. In: Johnson RT, ed. *Viral infections of the nervous system.* New York: Raven Press, 1982:247.
957. Kim TM, et al. Delayed acute measles body encephalitis in a 9-year-old girl: ultrastructural, immunohistochemical, and in situ hybridization studies. *Mod Pathol* 1992;5:348–352.

958. Baczko K, et al. Restriction of measles virus gene expression in measles inclusion body encephalitis. *J Infect Dis* 1988;158:144–150.

959. DuRant RH, Dyken PR. The effect of inosiplex on the survival of subacute sclerosing panencephalitis. *Neurology* 1983;33:1053–1055.

960. Anlar B, et al. Long-term follow-up of patients with subacute sclerosing panencephalitis treated with intraventricular gamma-interferon. *Neurology* 1997; 48:526–528.

961. Yoshioka H, et al. Administration of human leukocyte interferon to patients with subacute sclerosing panencephalitis. *Brain Dev* 1989;11:302–307.

962. Hayashi T, et al. Carbamazepine and myoclonus in SSPE subacute sclerosing panencephalitis. *Pediatr Neurol* 1996;346:346.

963. Weil ML, et al. Chronic progressive panencephalitis due to rubella virus simulating subacute sclerosing panencephalitis. *N Engl J Med* 1975;292:994–998.

964. Wolinsky J. Subacute sclerosing panencephalitis, progressive rubella panencephalitis, and multifocal leukoencephalopathy. *Res Publ Assoc Res Nerv Ment Dis* 1990;68:259–268.

965. Townsend JJ, et al. Neuropathology of progressive rubella panencephalitis after childhood rubella. *Neurology* 1982;32:185–190.

966. Vandvik B, et al. Progressive rubella panencephalitis: synthesis of oligoclonal virus-specific antibodies and free light chains in the central nervous system. *Acta Neurol Scand* 1978;57:53–64.

967. Wolinsky JS, Berg BO, Maitland CJ. Progressive rubella panencephalitis. *Arch Neurol* 1976;33:722–723.

968. Weil ML, et al. Chronic progressive panencephalitis due to rubella virus. *Arch Neurol* 1975;32:501.

969. Wolinsky JS, et al. Progressive rubella panencephalitis: immunovirological studies and results of isoprinosine therapy. *Clin Exp Immunol* 1979;35: 397–404.

970. Noorden SK, Lopez-Bravo L, Sundaresan TK. Estimated number of leprosy cases in the world. *Bull World Health Organ* 1992;70:7–10.

971. Smith WCS. The epidemiology of disability in leprosy including risk factors. *Lep Rev* 1992;63[Suppl]:23–30.

972. Centers for Disease Control. Public health service. Veterinary public health notes. Mosquitoes carry Hansen's disease. US Dept HEW 1975;90:183.

973. Jacobson RR, Krahenbuhl JL. Leprosy. *Lancet* 1969; 353:655–660.

974. Pfaltzgraff RE, Bryceson A. Clinical leprosy. In: Hastings RC, ed. *Leprosy*. Edinburgh: Churchill Livingstone, 1985:134–176.

975. Yamamura M, Uyemura K, Deans RJ. Defining protective responses to pathogens: cytokine profiles in leprosy lesions. *Science* 1991;254:277–279.

976. van Voorhis WC, et al. The cutaneous infiltrates of leprosy. Cellular characteristics and the predominant T-cell phenotypes. *N Engl J Med* 1982;307: 1593–1597.

977. Wallach D, Cottenot F, Bach M. Imbalance in T cell subpopulations in lepromatous leprosy. *Int J Lepr* 1982;50:282–290.

978. Job CK, Desikan KV. Pathological changes and their distribution in peripheral nerves in lepromatous leprosy. *Int J Lepr* 1968;36:257–270.

979. Miko TL, Maitre CL, Kinfu Y. Damages and regeneration of peripheral nerves in advanced treated leprosy. *Lancet* 1993;3442:521–525.

980. Bullock WE. *Mycobacterium leprae*. In: Mandel CL, Douglas RG, Bennett JE, eds. *Principles and practice of infectious diseases*, 3rd ed. New York: Churchill Livingstone, 1990:1906–1914.

981. Wall JR, Wright DM. Antibodies against testicular germinal cells in lepromatous leprosy. *Clin Exp Immunol* 1974;17:51–54.

982. Bullock WE. Studies of immune mechanisms in leprosy. Depression of delayed allergic responses to skin test antigens. *N Engl J Med* 1968;278:298–301.

983. Flaguel B, Wallach D, Vignon-Pennamer M. Late onset reversal reaction in borderline leprosy. *J Am Acad Dermatol* 1989;20:857–860.

984. Pearson JMH, Ross WX. Nerve involvement in leprosy: pathology, differential diagnosis and principles of management. *Lepr Rev* 1975;46:199–207.

985. Crawford CL. Neurological lesions in leprosy. *Lepr Rev* 1968;39:9–13.

986. Monrad-Krohn GH. *The neurological aspect of leprosy*. Chicago: Chicago Medical Book Co, 1923.

987. Browne SG. Some less common neurological findings in leprosy. *J Neurol Sci* 1965;2:253–261.

988. Dash MS. A study of the mechanisms of cutaneous sensory loss in leprosy. *Brain* 1968;91:379–392.

989. Job CK, et al. Leprous myositis—a histopathological and electron microscopic study. *Lepr Rev* 1969; 40:9–16.

990. Editorial. Ocular complications of leprosy. *Lancet* 1992;340:642–643.

991. Nations SP, et al. Leprous neuropathy: an American perspective. *Semin Neurol* 1998;18:113–124.

992. Willcox ML. The impact of multiple drug therapy on leprosy disabilities. *Lepr Rev* 1997;68:350–366.

993. Hubbert WT, Humphrey GL. Epidemiology of leptospirosis in California: a cause of aseptic meningitis. *Calif Med* 1968;108:113–117.

994. Lecour H, et al. Human leptospirosis: a review of 50 cases. *Infection* 1989;17:10–14.

995. Edwards GA, Domm BM. Human leptospirosis. *Medicine* 1960;39:117–156.

996. Watt G, Manaloto C, Hayes CG. Central nervous system leptospirosis in the Philippines. *Southeast Asian J Trop Med Public Health* 1989;20:265–269.

997. American Academy of Pediatrics. Leptospirosis. In: Peter G, ed. *1997 Red Book: report of the Committee on Infectious Diseases*, 24th ed. Elk Grove Village, IL: American Academy of Pediatrics, 1997:326–327.

998. Merritt HH, Adams RD, Solomon HC. *Neurosyphilis*. New York: Oxford University Press, 1946.

999. Marcus JC. Congenital neurosyphilis: a re-appraisal. *Neuropediatrics* 1982;13:195–199.

1000. Hallgren B, Hollström E. Congenital syphilis: a follow-up study with reference to mental abnormalities. *Acta Psychiatr Neurol Scand* 1954;93[Suppl]:1–81.

1001. Sanchez PJ, et al. Evaluation of molecular methodologies and rabbit infectivity testing for the diagnosis of congenital syphilis and neonatal central nervous system invasion by *Treponema pallidum*. *J Infect Dis* 1993;167:148–157.

1002. Jordan KG. Modern neurosyphilis—a critical analysis. *West J Med* 1988;149:47–157.

1003. Davis LE, Sperry S. The CSF-FTA test and the significance of blood contamination. *Ann Neurol* 1979;6: 68–69.

1004. Davis LE, Schmitt JW. Clinical significance of cerebrospinal fluid tests for neurosyphilis. *Ann Neurol* 1989;25:50–55.

1005. Burstain JM, et al. Sensitive detection of *Treponema pallidum* by using the polymerase chain reaction. *J Clin Microbiol* 1991;29:62–69.

1006. Rosen EU, Richardson NJ. A reappraisal of the value of the IgM fluorescent treponemal antibody absorption test in the diagnosis of congenital syphilis. *J Pediatr* 1975;87:38–42.

1007. American Academy of Pediatrics. Syphilis. In: Peter G, ed. *1997 Red Book: report of the Committee on Infectious Diseases*, 24th ed. Elk Grove Village, IL: American Academy of Pediatrics, 1997:504–514.

1008. Pfister H-W, Wilske B, Weber K. Lyme borreliosis: basic science and clinical aspects. *Lancet* 1994;343: 1013–1016.

1009. Steere AC, et al. The spirochetal etiology of Lyme disease. *N Engl J Med* 1983;308:733–740.

1010. Spach DH, et al. Tick-borne diseases in the United States. *N Engl J Med* 1993;329: 936–947.

1011. Reik L, Burgdorfer W, Donaldson JO. Neurological abnormalities in Lyme disease without erythema chronicum migrans. *Am J Med* 1986;81:73–78.

1012. Christen H-J, et al. Epidemiology and clinical manifestations of Lyme borreliosis in childhood. A prospective multicentre study with special regard to Neuroborreliosis. *Acta Paediatr* 1993;386[Suppl]: 176.

1013. Oksi J, et al. Inflammatory brain changes in Lyme borreliosis: a report of three patients and review of literature. *Brain* 1996;119:2143–2154.

1014. Sigal LH, Tatum AH. Lyme disease patients' serum contains IgM antibodies to *Borrelia burgdorferi* that cross-react with neuronal antigens. *Neurology* 1988;38:1439–1442.

1015. Szer IS, Taylor E, Steere AC. The long-term course of Lyme arthritis in children. *N Engl J Med* 1991; 325:159–163.

1016. Glasscock ME III, et al. Lyme disease. A cause of bilateral facial paralysis. *Arch Otolaryngol* 1985; 111:47–49.

1017. Darras BT, Annunziato D, Leggiadro RJ. Lyme disease with neurologic abnormalities. *Ped Infect Dis* 1983;2:47–49.

1018. Krejcova H, et al. Otoneurological symptomatology in Lyme disease. *Adv Otorhinolaryngol* 1988;42: 210–212.

1019. Belman AL, et al. Neurologic manifestations in children with North American Lyme disease. *Neurology* 1993;43:2609–2614.

1020. Jörbeck HJ, et al. Tick-borne *Borrelia*-meningitis in children. An outbreak in the Kolmar area during the summer of 1984. *Acta Paediatr Scand* 1987;76: 228–233.

1021. Hansen K, Lebech AM. The clinical and epidemiological profile of Lyme neuroborreliosis in Denmark 1985–90. A prospective study of 187 patients with *Borrelia burgdorferi* specific intrathecal antibody production. *Brain* 1992;115:399–423.

1022. Sterman AB, Nelson S, Barclay P. Demyelinating neuropathy accompanying Lyme disease. *Neurology* 1982;32:1302–1305.

1023. Kan L, Sood SK, Maytal J. Pseudotumor cerebri in Lyme disease: a case report and review of the literature. *Pediatr Neurol* 1998;18:439–441.

1024. Ryberg B, et al. Antibodies to Lyme-disease spirochaete in European lymphocytic meningoencephalitis (Bannwarth's syndrome) [Letter]. *Lancet* 1983;2:519.

1025. Feder HM, Zalneraitis EL, Reik L Jr. Lyme disease: acute focal meningoencephalitis in a child. *Pediatrics* 1988;82:931–934.

1026. Pfister H-W, et al. Catatonic syndrome in acute severe encephalitis due to *Borrelia burgdorferi* infection. *Neurology* 1993;43:433–435.

1026a. Eppes SC, et al. Characterization of Lyme meningitis and comparison with viral meningitis in children. *Pediatrics* 1999;103:957–960.

1027. Ackermann R, et al. Chronic neurologic manifestations of erythema migrans borreliosis. *Ann NY Acad Sci* 1988;539:16–23.

1028. Bensch J, Olcen P, Hagberg L. Destructive chronic *Borrelia* meningoencephalitis in a child untreated for 15 years. *Scand J Infect Dis* 1987;19:697–700.

1029. Halperin JJ, Volkman DJ, Wu P. Central nervous system abnormalities in Lyme neuroborreliosis. *Neurology* 1991;41:1571–1582.

1030. Martin R, et al. Persistent intrathecal secretion of oligoclonal, *Borrelia burgdorferi*-specific IgG in chronic meningoradiculomyelitis. *J Neurol* 1988; 235:229–233.

1031. Halperin JJ, et al. Lyme neuroborreliosis: central nervous system manifestations. *Neurology* 1989;39: 753–759.

1032. Hirai K, et al. *Borrelia burgdorferi* and Shulman syndrome [Letter]. *Lancet* 1992;340:1472.

1033. Hansen K, Lebech A-M. The clinical and epidemiological profile of Lyme neuroborreliosis in Denmark 1985–1990. A prospective study of 187 patients with *Borrelia burgdorferi* specific intrathecal antibody. *Brain* 1992;115:399–423.

1034. Albisetti M, et al. Diagnostic value of cerebrospinal fluid examination in children with peripheral facial palsy and suspected Lyme borreliosis. *Neurology* 1997;49:817–824.

1035. Belman AL, et al. MRI findings in children infected by *Borrelia burgdorferi*. *Pediatr Neurol* 1992;8:428–431.

1036. Dattwyler RJ, et al. Seronegative Lyme disease. Dissociation of specific T- and B-lymphocyte responses to *Borrelia burgdorferi*. *N Engl J Med* 1988;319: 1441–1446.

1037. Tumani H, Nölker G, Reiber H. Relevance of cerebrospinal fluid variables for early diagnosis of neuroborreliosis. *Neurology* 1995;45:1663–1670.

1038. Rose CD, et al. Use of Western blot and enzyme-linked immunosorbent assay in the diagnosis of Lyme disease. *Pediatrics* 1991;88:465–470.

1039. Halperin JJ, Heyes MP. Neuroactive kynurenines in Lyme borreliosis. *Neurology* 1992;42:43–45.

1040. Karlssen M, et al. Comparison of intravenous penicillin G and oral doxycycline for treatment of Lyme neuroborreliosis. *Neurology* 1994;44:1203–1207.

1041. American Academy of Pediatrics. Lyme disease. In: Peter G, ed. *1997 Red Book: report of the Committee on Infectious Diseases*, 24th ed. Elk Grove Village, IL: American Academy of Pediatrics, 1997:329–333.

1042. Weber K, Pfister H-W. Clinical management of Lyme borreliosis. *Lancet* 1994;343:1016–1017.

1043. Salazar JC, Gerber MA, Goff CW. Long-term outcome of Lyme disease in children given early treatment. *J Pediatr* 1993;122:591–593.

1044. Crisp D, Ashby P. Lyme radiculoneuritis treated with intravenous immunoglobulin. *Neurology* 1996;46:1174–1175.

1045. Benke T, et al. Lyme encephalopathy: long-term neuropsychological deficits years after neuroborreliosis. *Acta Neurol Scand* 1995;91:353–357.

1046. Southern PM Jr, Sanford JP. Relapsing fever: a clinical and microbiological review. *Medicine* 1969;48:129–149.

1047. Lehtokoski-Lehtiniemi E, Koskiniemi ML. *Mycoplasma pneumoniae* encephalitis: a severe entity in children. *Pediatr Inf Dis J* 1989;8:651–653.

1048. Pellegrini M, et al. *Mycoplasma pneumoniae* infection associated with an acute brainstem syndrome. *Acta Neurol Scand* 1996;93:203–206.

1049. Cherry JD, Hurwitz ES, Welliver RC. *Mycoplasma pneumoniae* infections and exanthems. *J Pediatr* 1975;87:369–373.

1050. Lerer RJ, Kalavsky SM. Central nervous system disease associated with *Mycoplasma pneumoniae* infection: report of five cases and review of literature. *Pediatrics* 1973;52:658–668.

1051. Al-Mateen M, et al. Encephalitis lethargica-like illness in a girl with mycoplasma infection. *Neurology* 1988;38:1155–1158.

1052. Pongsakdi V, Chiemchanya S, Sirinavin S. Internal carotid artery occlusion associated with *Mycoplasma pneumoniae* infection. *Pediat Neurol* 1992;8:237–239.

1053. Siber GR, et al. Neonatal central nervous system infection due to *Mycoplasma hominis*. *J Pediatr* 1977;90:625–627.

1054. McDonald JC, Moore DL. *Mycoplasma hominis* meningitis in a premature infant. *Pediatr Infect Dis J* 1988;7:795–798.

1055. Gilbert GL, et al. Chronic *Mycoplasma hominis* infection complicating severe intraventricular hemorrhage, in a premature neonate. *Pediatr Infect Dis J* 1988;7:817–818.

1056. Hulihan JF, Bebin EM, Westmoreland BF. Bilateral periodic lateralized epileptiform discharges in *Mycoplasma* encephalitis. *Pediatr Neurol* 1992;8:292–294.

1057. MacFarlane PI, Miller V. Transverse myelitis associated with *Mycoplasma pneumoniae*. *Arch Dis Child* 1984;59:80–82.

1058. Francis DA, et al. MRI appearances of the CNS manifestations of *Mycoplasma pneumoniae*: a report of two cases. *J Neurol* 1988;235:441–443.

1059. Maida E, Kristoferitsch W. Cerebrospinal fluid findings in *Mycoplasma pneumoniae* infections with neurological complications. *Acta Neurol Scand* 1982;65:524–538.

1060. Murray HW, et al. The protean manifestations of *Mycoplasma pneumoniae* infection in adults. *Am J Med* 1975;58:229–242.

1061. Vikerfors T, et al. Detection of specific IgM antibodies for the diagnosis of *Mycoplasma pneumoniae* infections: a clinical evaluation. *Scand J Infec Dis* 1988;20:601–610.

1062. Narita M, et al. DNA diagnosis of central nervous system infection by *Mycoplasma pneumoniae*. *Pediatrics* 1992;90:250–253.

1063. Fetter BF, Klintworth GK, Hendry WS. *Mycoses of the central nervous system*. Baltimore: Williams & Wilkins, 1967.

1064. Kozinn PJ, et al. *Candida* meningitis successfully treated with amphotericin B. *N Engl J Med* 1963;268:881–884.

1065. Chesney PJ, et al. Successful treatment of *Candida* meningitis with amphotericin B and 5-fluorocytosine in combination. *J Pediatr* 1976;89:1017–1019.

1066. Kourtopoulos H, Holm SE. Treatment of *Candida* ventriculitis and septicemia with 5-fluoro-cytosine. Combined peroral and intraventricular administration. *Neuropaediatrie* 1976;7:356–361.

1067. Roessmann U, Friede RL. Candidal infection of the brain. *Arch Pathol* 1967;84:495–498.

1068. Chesney PJ, Justman RA, Bogdanowicz WM. *Candida* meningitis in newborn infants: a review and report of combined amphotericin B-flucytosine therapy. *Johns Hopkins Med J* 1978;142:155–160.

1069. Como JA, Dismukes WE. Oral azole drugs as systemic antifungal therapy. *N Engl J Med* 1993;330:263 272.

1070. Conant NF. Medical mycology. In: Dubos RJ, Hirsch JG, eds. *Bacterial and mycotic infections of man*. Philadelphia: JB Lippincott, 1965:825–885.

1071. Caudill RG, Smith CE, Reinarz JA. Coccidioidal meningitis. A diagnostic challenge. *Am J Med* 1970;49:360–365.

1072. McCullough DC, Harbert JC. Isotope demonstration of CSF pathways. Guide to antifungal therapy in coccidioidal meningitis. *JAMA* 1969;209:558–560.

1073. Wrobel CJ, et al. MR findings in acute and chronic coccidioidomycosis meningitis. *Am J Neuroradiol* 1992; 13:1241–1245.

1074. Reeves DL. Chronic coccidioidal meningitis. Report of two cases. *J Neurosurg* 1968;28:383–386.

1075. American 63 of Pediatrics. Systemic treatment with amphotericin B. In: Peter G, ed. *1997 Red Book: report of the Committee on Infectious Diseases*, 24th ed. Elk Grove Village, IL: American Academy of Pediatrics, 1997:630–631.

1076. Galgiani JN, et al. Fluconazole therapy for coccidioidal meningitis. The NIAID-mycosis study group. *Ann Int Med* 1993;119:28–35.

1077. Kauffman CA. Role of azoles in antifungal therapy. *Clin Infect Dis* 1996;22[Suppl 2]:S148–S153.

1078. Patel R. Antifungal agents. Part I. Amphotericin B preparations and flucytosine. *Mayo Clin Proc* 1998;73:1205–1225.

1079. Tucker RM, et al. Itraconazole therapy for chronic coccidiodal meningitis. *Ann Intern Med* 1990;112:108–112.

1080. Cooper RA Jr, Goldstein E. Histoplasmosis of the central nervous system. Report of two cases and review of the literature. *Am J Med* 1963;35:45–57.

1081. Couch JR, Abdou NI, Sagawa A. Histoplasma meningitis with hyperactive suppressor T cells in cerebrospinal fluid. *Neurology* 1978;28:119–123.

1082. Wheat LJ, Batteiger BE, Sathapatayavongs B. Histoplasma capsulatum infections of the central nervous system. A clinical review. *Medicine* 1990;69:244–260.

1083. Rivera IV, et al. Chronic progressive CNS histoplasmosis presenting in childhood: response to fluconazole therapy. *Pediatr Neurol* 1992;8:151–153.

1084. Gonzalez-Amaro R, et al. Natural killer cell-mediated cytotoxicity in cryptococcal meningitis. *Rev Invest Clin* 1991;43:133–138.

1085. Woodall WC III, et al. Spinal arachnoiditis with *Cryptococcus neoformans* in a nonimmunocompromised child. *Pediatr Neurol* 1990;6:206–208.

1086. Gordon MA, Vedder DK. Serologic tests in diagnosis and prognosis of cryptococcosis. *JAMA* 1966;197:961–967.

1087. McIntyre HB. Cryptococcal meningitis. A case successfully treated by cisternal administration of amphotericin B with a review of the recent literature. *Bull Los Angeles Neurol Soc* 1967;32:213–219.

1088. Sarosi GA, Parker JD, Doto IL. Amphotericin B in cryptococcal meningitis: long-term results of treatment. *Ann Intern Med* 1969;71:1079–1087.

1089. Goodman JS, Kaufman L, Koenig MG. Diagnosis of cryptococcal meningitis. Value of immunologic detection of cryptococcal antigen. *N Engl J Med* 1971;285:434–436.

1090. Dismukes WE, et al. Treatment of cryptococcal meningitis with combination amphotericin B and flucytosine for four as compared with six weeks. *N Engl J Med* 1987;317:334–341.

1091. American Academy of Pediatrics. *1997 Red Book: report of the Committee on Infectious Diseases*, 24th ed. Elk Grove Village, IL: American Academy of Pediatrics, 1997:184–185.

1092. Leake HA, Appleyard MN, Hartley JP. Successful treatment of resistant cryptococcal meningitis with amphotericin B lipid emulsion after neurotoxicity with conventional intravenous amphotericin B. *J Infect* 1994;28:319–322.

1093. Laing RB, et al. Anaphylactic reactions to liposomal amphotericin [Letter]. *Lancet* 1994;344:682.

1094. Saag MS, et al. Comparison of amphotericin B with fluconazole in the treatment of acute AIDS-associated cryptococcal meningitis. *N Engl J Med* 1992;326:83–89.

1095. Barter AP, Falconer MA. Actinomycosis of the brain. *Guy Hosp Rep* 1955;104:135–145.

1096. Iyer S, Dodge PR, Adams RD. Two cases of *Aspergillus* infection of the central nervous system. *J Neurol Neurosurg Psychiatry* 1952;15:152–163.

1097. Mukoyama M, Gimple AB, Poser CM. Aspergillosis of the central nervous system. Report of a brain abscess due to A. *fumigatus* and a review of the literature. *Neurology* 1969;19:967–974.

1098. Koh S, et al. Myelopathy resulting from invasive Aspergillosis. *Pediatr Neurol* 1998;19:135–138.

1099. Gonyea EF. The spectrum of primary blastomycotic meningitis: a review of central nervous system blastomycosis. *Ann Neurol* 1978;3:26–39.

1100. Papadatos C, Pavlatou M, Alexiou D. Cephalosporium meningitis. *Pediatrics* 1969;44:749–751.

1101. Landau JW, Newcomer VD. Acute cerebral phycomycosis (mucormycosis). Report of a pediatric patient successfully treated with amphotericin B and cycloheximide and review of the pertinent literature. *J Pediatr* 1962;61:363–385.

1102. Blodi FC, Hannah FT, Wadsworth JA. Lethal orbitocerebral phycomycosis in otherwise healthy children. *Am J Ophthalmol* 1969;67:698–705.

1103. Smego RA Jr, Moeller MB, Gallis HA. Trimethoprim-sulfamethoxazole therapy for *Nocardia* infections. *Arch Intern Med* 1983;143:711–718.

1104. Ballenger CN Jr, Goldring D. Nocardiosis in childhood. *J Pediatr* 1957;50:145–169.

1105. Lope ES, Gutierrez DC. *Nocardia asteroides* primary cerebral abscess and secondary meningitis. *Acta Neurochir* 1977;37:139–145.

1106. Spach DH, et al. Tick-borne diseases in the United States. *N Engl J Med* 1993;329:936–947.

1107. Miller JQ, Price TR. The nervous system in Rocky Mountain fever. *Neurology* 1972;22:561–566.

1108. Horney LF, Walker DH. Meningoencephalitis as a major manifestation of Rocky Mountain spotted fever. *South Med J* 1988;81:915–918.

1109. Bell WE, Lascari AD. Rocky Mountain spotted fever. Neurological symptoms in the acute phase. *Neurology* 1970;20:841–847.

1110. Hornaday CA, Kernodle DS, Curry WA. Neurogenic bladder in Rocky Mountain spotted fever. *Arch Intern Med* 1983;143:365.

1111. Miller JQ, Price TR. Involvement of the brain in Rocky Mountain spotted fever. *South Med J* 1972;65:437–439.

1112. Raab EL, Leopold IH, Hodes HL. Retinopathy in Rocky Mountain spotted fever. *Am J Ophthalmol* 1969;68:42–46.

1113. Rosenblum MJ, Masland RL, Harrell GT. Residual effects of rickettsial disease on the central nervous system. Results of neurologic examinations and electroencephalograms following Rocky Mountain spotted fever. *Arch Intern Med* 1952;90:444–455.

1114. Wright L. Intellectual sequelae of Rocky Mountain spotted fever. *J Abnormal Psychol* 1972;80:315–316.

1115. Haynes RE, Sanders DY, Cramblett HG. Rocky Mountain spotted fever in children. *J Pediatr* 1970;76:685–693.

1116. American Academy of Pediatrics. Rocky mountain spotted fever. In: *1997 Red Book: report of the Committee on Infectious Diseases*, 24th ed. Elk Grove Village, IL: American Academy of Pediatrics. 1997:452–454.

1117. Noad KB, Haymaker W. Neurological features of tsutsugamushi fever with special reference to deafness. *Brain* 1953;76:113–131.

1118. Herman E. Neurological syndromes in typhus fever. *J Nerv Ment Dis* 1949;109:25–36.

1119. Watt G, et al. Scrub typhus infections poorly responsive to antibiotics in northern Thailand. *Lancet* 1996;348:86–89.

1120. Case records of the Massachusetts General Hospital. Case 38-1996. *N Engl J Med* 1996;335:1829–1834.

1121. Most H. Treatment of common parasitic infections of man encountered in the United States. *N Engl J Med* 1972;287:495–498, 698–702.

1122. Brown WJ. Cysticercosis. In: Brown WJ, Voge M, eds. *Neuropathology of parasitic infections*. New York: Oxford University Press, 1982:108.

1123. Kramer LD, et al. Cerebral cysticercosis: documentation of natural history with CT. *Radiology* 1989;171:459–462.

1124. Virmani V, Roy S, Kamala G. Periodic lateralised epileptiform discharges in a case of diffuse cerebral cysticercosis. *Neuropädiatrie* 1977;8:196–203.

1125. Kalra V, Sethi A. Childhood neurocysticercosis—epidemiology, diagnosis and course. *Acta Paediatr Jpn* 1992;34:365–370.
1126. Lopez-Hernandez A, Garaizar C. Childhood cerebral cysticercosis: clinical features and computed tomographic findings in 89 Mexican children. *Can J Neurol Sci* 1982;9:401–407.
1127. Thompson AJG. Neurocysticercosis: experience at the teaching hospitals of the University of Cape Town. *S Afr Med J* 1993;83:332–334.
1128. Garg RS. Neurocysticercosis. *Postgrad Med J* 1998;74:321–326.
1129. Liu LX, Weller PF. Antiparasitic drugs. *N Engl J Med* 1996;334:1178–1184.
1130. Mitchell WG, Crawford TO. Intraparenchymal cerebral cysticercosis in children: diagnosis and treatment. *Pediatrics* 1988;82:76–82.
1131. Rajshekhar V. Albendazole therapy for persistent, solitary cysticercosis granulomas in patients with seizures. *Neurology* 1993;43:1238–1240.
1132. Dalessio DJ, Wolff HG. *Trichinella spiralis* infection of the central nervous system. Report of a case and review of the literature. *Arch Neurol* 1961;4:407–417.
1133. Tatatuto AL, Venturiello SM. Trichinosis. *Brain Pathology* 1997;7:663–672.
1134. Kramer MD, Aita JF. Trichinosis with central nervous system involvement. A case report and review of the literature. *Neurology* 1972;22:485–491.
1135. Lopez-Lozano JJ, Garcia-Merino JA, Liano H. Bilateral facial paralysis secondary to trichinosis. *Acta Neurol Scand* 1988;78:194–197.
1136. Evans RW, Pattern BM. Trichinosis associated with superior sagittal sinus thrombosis. *Ann Neurol* 1982;11:216–217.
1137. Gay T, et al. Fatal CNS trichinosis. *JAMA* 1982;127:1024–1025.
1138. American Academy of Pediatrics. Trichinosis (Trichinella spiralis). In: Peter G, ed. *1997 Red Book: report of the Committee on Infectious Diseases*, 24th ed. Elk Grove Village, IL: American Academy of Pediatrics, 1997:535–536.
1139. Zucker JR, Campbell CC. Malaria: principles of prevention and treatment. *Infect Dis Clin North Am* 1993;7:547–567.
1140. Phillips RE, Solomon T. Cerebral malaria in children. *Lancet* 1990;336:1355–1360.
1141. Warrell DA. Cerebral malaria. *QJM* 1989;71:369–371.
1142. Brewster DR, Kwiatkowski D, White NJ. Neurological sequelae of cerebral malaria in children. *Lancet* 1990;336:1039–1043.
1143. van Hensbroek MB, et al. Residual neurologic sequelae after childhood cerebral malaria. *J Pediatr* 1997;131:125–129.
1144. Turner G. Cerebral malaria. *Brain Pathol* 1997;7:569–582.
1145. MacPherson GG, et al. Human cerebral malaria. A quantitative ultrastructural analysis of parasitized erythrocyte sequestration. *Am J Pathol* 1985;119:385–401.
1146. Aikawa M, et al. The pathology of human malaria. *Am J Trop Hyg* 1990;43:30–37.
1147. Nakamura K, et al. Plasmodium falciparum-infected erythrocyte receptor(s) for CD36 and thrombospondin are restricted to knobs on the erythrocyte surface. *J Histochem Cytochem* 1992;40:1419–1422.
1148. Newbold C, et al. Receptor-specific adhesion and clinical disease in Plasmodium falciparum. *Am J Trop Med Hyg* 1997;57:389–398.
1149. Fernandez-Reyes D, et al. A high frequency African coding polymorphism, in the N-terminal domain of ICAM-1 predisposing to cerebral malaria in Kenya. *Hum Mol Genet* 1997;6:1357–1360.
1149a. Urban BC, et al. *Plasmodium falciparum*—Infected erythrocytes modulate the maturation of dendritic cells. *Nature* 1999;400:73–77.
1150. Johnson JK, et al. Cytoadherence of *Plasmodium falciparum*-infected erythrocytes to microvascular endothelium is regulatable by cytokines and phorbol ester. *J Infect Dis* 1993;167:698–703.
1151. Clark IA, Chaudhri G, Cowden WB. Roles of tumor necrosis factor in the illness and pathology of malaria. *Trans R Soc Trop Med Hyg* 1989;83:436–440.
1152. Clark IA, Rockett KA, Cowden WB. Possible central role of nitric oxide in conditions clinically similar to cerebral malaria. *Lancet* 1992;340:894–896.
1153. Kwiatkowski D, et al. TNF concentration in fatal malaria, non-fatal cerebral, and uncomplicated *Plasmodium falciparum* malaria. *Lancet* 1990;336:1201–1204.
1154. Grau GE, et al. Tumor necrosis factor and disease severity in children with falciparum malaria. *N Engl J Med* 1989;320:1586–1591.
1155. Grau GE, et al. Tumor necrosis factor and other cytokines in cerebral malaria. Experimental and clinical data. *Immunol Rev* 1989;112:49–70.
1156. Kwiatkowski D, et al. Anti-TNF therapy inhibits fever in cerebral malaria. *QJM* 1993;86:91–98.
1157. Molyneux ME, et al. Clinical features and prognostic indicators in paediatric cerebral malaria: a study of 131 comatose Malawian children. *QJM* 1989: 71:441–459.
1158. Jaffar S, et al. Predictors of a fatal outcome following childhood cerebral malaria. *Am J Trop Med Hyg* 1997;57:20–24.
1159. Taylor TE, Borgstein A, Molyneux ME. Acid-base status in paediatric *Plasmodium falciparum* malaria. *QJM* 1993;86:99–109.
1160. Burgner D, et al. Inducible nitric oxide synthase polymorphism and fatal cerebral malaria. *Lancet* 1998;232:1193–1194.
1161. Looareesuwan S, et al. Magnetic resonance imaging of the brain in patients with cerebral malaria. *Clin Infect Dis* 1995;21:300–309.
1162. Miller LH, Good MF, Milon G. Malaria pathogenesis. *Science* 1994;264:1878–1883.
1163. Wright PW, et al. Initial clinical assessment of the comatose patient: cerebral malaria vs. meningitis. *Pediatr Infect Dis J* 1993;12:37–41.
1164. White NJ, Krishna S, Looareesuwan S. Encephalitis, not cerebral malaria, is likely cause of coma with negative blood smears. *J Infect Dis* 1992;166:1195–1196.
1165. Newton CRJC, Warrell DA. Neurological manifestations of falciparum malaria. *Ann Neurol* 1998;43:695–702.
1166. Lewallen S, et al. Ocular fundus findings in Malawian children with cerebral malaria. *Ophthalmology* 1993;100:857–861.

1167. White NJ, et al. Severe hypoglycemia and hyperinsulinemia in falciparum malaria. *N Engl J Med* 1983; 309: 61–66.

1168. White NJ, et al. Quinine loading dose in cerebral malaria. *Am J Trop Med Hyg* 1983;332:1–5.

1169. Phillips RE, et al. Intravenous quinidine for the treatment of severe falciparum malaria. Clinical and pharmacokinetic studies. *N Engl J Med* 1985;312: 1273–1278.

1170. Shwe T, et al. Clinical studies on treatment of cerebral malaria with artemether and mefloquine. *Trans R Soc Trop Med Hyg* 1989;83:489.

1171. Taylor TE, et al. Rapid coma resolution with artemether in Malawian children with cerebral malaria. *Lancet* 1993;341:661–662.

1172. Van Hensbroek MB, Onyiorah E, Jaffar S. A trial of artemether or quinine in children with cerebral malaria. *N Engl J Med* 1996;335:69–75.

1172a. White NJ, et al. Averting a malaria disaster. *Lancet* 1999;353:1965–1967.

1173. White NJ. The treatment of malaria. *N Engl J Med* 1996;335:800–806.

1174. Gordeuk V, et al. Effect of iron chelation therapy on recovery from deep coma in children with cerebral malaria. *N Engl J Med* 1992;327:1473–1477.

1174a. Brandts CH, et al. Effect of paracetamol on parasite clearance time in *Plasmodium Falciparum* malaria. *Lancet* 1997;350:704–709.

1175. Mai NTH, et al. Post-malaria neurological syndrome. *Lancet* 1996;348:917–921.

1176. Lell B, et al. Randomised placebo-controlled study of atovaquone plus proguanil for malaria in children. *Lancet* 1998;351:709–713.

1177. Power J. Sleeping sickness research and control. *TDR News* 1989:28:3.

1178. Kuzoe FA. Current knowledge on epidemiology and control of sleeping sickness. *Ann Soc Belg Med Trop* 1989;69:217–220.

1179. Hajduk SL, Englund PT, Smith DH. African trypanosomiasis. In: Warren KS, Mahmoud AAF, eds. *African trypanosomiasis*. New York: McGraw-Hill, 1990: 268–281.

1180. Mhlanga JD, Bentivoglio M, Kristensson K. Neurobiology of cerebral malaria and African sleeping sickness. *Brain Res Bull* 1997;44: 579–589.

1180a. Bentivoglio M, et al. *Trypanosoma brucei* and the nervous system. *Trends Neurosci* 1994;17: 325–329.

1181. Poltera AA, Owor R, Cox JN. Pathological aspects of human African trypanosomiasis in Uganda. A postmortem survey of 14 cases. *Virchows Arch* 1976;373: 249–265.

1182. Adams JH, Hallen L, Boa FY. African trypanosomiasis: a study of 16 fatal cases with some observations on acute reactive arsenical encephalopathy. *Neuropathol Appl Neurobiol* 1986;12:81–94.

1183. Asongonyi T, Lando G, Ngu JL. Serum antibodies against human brain myelin proteins in Gambian trypanosomiasis. *Ann Soc Beg Med Trop* 1989;69: 213–221.

1184. Poltera AA. Immunopathological and chemotherapeutic studies in experimental trypanosomiasis with special reference to the heart and brain. *Trans R Trop Med Hyg* 1980;74:706–715.

1185. Wellde BT, Chumo DA, Hockmeyer WT. Sleeping sickness in the Lambwe Valley in 1978. *Ann Trop Med Parasitol* 1989;83:21–27.

1186. Lambo TA. Neuropsychiatric syndromes associated with human trypanosomiasis in tropical Africa. *Acta Psychiatrica Scand* 1966;42:474–484.

1187. Calwell HG. The pathology of the brain in Rhodesian trypanosomiasis. *Trans R Soc Trop Med Hyg* 1937; 30:611–624.

1188. Van Meirvenne N, Le Ray D. Diagnosis of African and American trypanosomiasis. *Br Med Bull* 1985;41: 156–161.

1189. Gutteridge WE. Trypanosomiasis: existing chemotherapy and limitations. *Br Med Bull* 1985;41: 162–168.

1190. Arroz JO. Melarsoprol and reactive encephalopathy in *Trypanosoma brucei* rhodesiense infection. *Trans R Soc Trop Med Hyg* 1987;81:192.

1191. McCann PP, Bitoniti AJ, Bacchi CJ. Use of difluoromethylornithine (DFMO, eflornithine) for late stage trypanosomiasis. *Trans R Soc Trop Med Hyg* 1987; 81:701–702.

1192. Pitella JEH. Brain involvement in the chronic cardiac form of Chagas disease. *J Trop Med Hygiene* 1985; 88:313–317.

1193. Cegielski JP, Durack DT. Protozoal infections of the central nervous system. In: Scheld WM, Whitley RJ, Durack DT, eds. *Infections of the central nervous system*. New York: Raven Press, 1991: 767–800.

1194. Leiguarda R, Roncoroni A, Taratuto AI. Acute CNS infection by *trypanosoma cruzi* in immunosuppressed patients. *Neurology* 1990;40:850–851.

1195. Carrea R, Dowling E Jr, Guevara JA. Surgical treatment of hydatid cysts of the central nervous system in the pediatric age (Dowling's technique). *Child's Brain* 1975;1:4–21.

1196. Boles DM. Cerebral echinococciasis. *Surg Neurol* 1981;16:280–282.

1197. Radford AJ. Hydatid disease. In: Weatherall DJ, Ledingham JGG, Warrell DA, eds. *Oxford textbook of medicine*, 2nd ed. Oxford: Oxford University Press, 1988:561–565.

1198. Banerjee AK, Bhatnagar RK, Bhusnurmath SR. Secondary cerebral amoebiasis. *Trop Geogr Med* 1993; 35:333–336.

1199. Cegielski JP, Durack DT. Protozoal infections of the central nervous system. In: Scheld WM, Whitley RJ, Durack DT, eds. *Infections of the central nervous system*. New York: Raven Press, 1991:767–800.

1200. Becker GL, Knep S, Lance KP. Amoebic abscess of the brain. *Neurosurgery* 1980;6:192–194.

1201. Barnett ND, et al. Primary amoebic meningoencephalitis with *Naegleria fowleri*: clinical review. *Pediatr Neurol* 1996;15:230–234.

1202. Visuesuara GS, Callaway CS. Light and electron microscopic observation on the pathogenesis of *Naeglaria fowleri* in mouse brain and tissue culture. *J Protozool* 1990;21:239–250.

1203. Thong YH, Ferrante A. Migration patterns of pathogenic and non-pathogenic *Naegleria* spp. *Infect Immun* 1986;51:177–180.

1204. Rutherford GS. Amoebic meningo-encephalitis due to free living amoeba. *S Afr Med J* 1986;69: 52–55.

1205. Kilvington S, Beeching J. Identification and epidemiological typing of *Naegleria fowleri* with DNA probes. *Appl Environ Microbiol* 1995;61: 2071–2078.

1206. Brown RL. Successful treatment of primary amoebic meningo-encephalitis. *Arch Intern Med* 1991;151: 1201–1202.

1207. Slater CA, et al. Brief report: successful treatment of disseminated acanthamoeba infection in an immunocompromised patient. *N Engl J Med* 1994; 331:85–87.

1208. Koo J, Dien F, Kliks MM. Angiostrongylus eosinophilic meningitis. *Rev Infect Dis* 1988;10:1155–1162.

1209. Kliks MM, Kroenke K, Handman JM. Eosinophilic radiculomyelo-encephalitis. *J Trop Med Hyg* 1982; 31:1114–1122.

1210. Lowichik A, Ruff AJ. Parasitic infections of the central nervous system in children. Part II: disseminated infections. *J Child Neurol* 1995;10:77–87.

1211. Diaz Camacho SP, et al. Clinical manifestations and immunodiagnosis of gnathostomiasis in Culiacan, Mexico. *Am J Trop Med Hyg* 1998;59:908–915.

1212. Chitanondh H, Rosen L. Fatal eosinophilic encephalomyelitis caused by the nematode *Gnathostoma spinigerum*. *Am J Trop Med Hyg* 1967;16: 638–645.

1213. Schmutzhand E, Boorgind P, Veijjava A. Eosinophilic meningitis in Thailand caused by CNS invasion of *Gnathostoma spinigerum* and *Angiostrongylus cantonensis*. *J Neurol Neurosurg Psych* 1988;51:80–87.

1214. Hill IR, Denham DA, Scholtz CL. *Toxocara canis* larvae in the brain of a British child. *Trans R Soc Trop Med Hyg* 1985;79:351–354.

1215. Mikhael NZ, Montpetit UJA, Orizaga M. *Toxocara canis* infestation with encephalitis. *Can J Neurol Sci* 1974;1:114–120.

1216. Glickman L, et al. *Toxocara* infection and epilepsy in children. *J Pediatr* 1979;94:75–78.

1217. Pitella JE. Neuroschistosomiasis. *Brain Pathol* 1997;7:649–662.

1218. Scrimgeour EM, Gajdusek DC. Involvement of the central nervous system in *Schistosoma mansoni* and *S. haematobium* infection. *Brain* 1985;108:1023–1038.

1219. Anonymous. Acute schistosomiasis with transverse myelitis in American students returning from Kenya. *MMWR* 1984;33:445–447.

1220. Boyce TG. Acute transverse myelitis in a 6-year-old girl with schistosomiasis. *Pediatr Infect Dis J* 1990;9: 279–284.

1221. Pitella JE, Lana-Peixoto MA. Brain involvement in hepatosplenic *Schistosomiasis mansoni*. *Brain* 1981; 104:621–632.

1222. Bennett G, Provenzale JM. Schistosomal myelitis: finding at MR imaging. *Eur J Radiol* 1998;27: 268–270.

1223. Ferrari TC, et al. The value of an enzyme-linked immunosorbent assay for the diagnosis of *schistosomiasis mansoni* myeloradiculopathy. *Trans R Soc Trop Med Hyg* 1995;89:496–500.

1224. Watt E, et al. Praziquantel in the treatment of cerebral schistosomiasis. *Lancet* 1986;2:529–532.

1225. Jankovic D, et al. Optimal vaccination against *Schistosoma mansoni* requires the induction of both B cell- and IFN-gamma-dependent effector mechanisms. *J Immunol* 1999;162:345–351.

1226. Higashi K, et al. Cerebral paragonimiasis. *J Neurosurg* 1971;34:515–527.

1227. Oh SJ. Spinal paragonimiasis. *J Neurol Sci* 1968; 6:125–140.

1228. Oh SJ. Ophthalmological signs in cerebral paragonimiasis. *Trop Geogr Med* 1968;20:13–20.

1229. Chang KH, Han MH. MRI of CNS parasitic diseases. *J Magn Reson Imaging* 1998;8:297–307.

1230. Newman LS, Rose CS, Maier LA. Sarcoidosis N. *Engl J Med* 1997;336:1224–1234.

1231. Johns CJ, Scott PP, Schonfeld SA. Sarcoidosis. *Annu Rev Med* 1989;40:353–371.

1232. Jefferson M. Sarcoidosis of the nervous system. *Brain* 1957;80:540–556.

1233. Symonds C. Recurrent multiple cranial nerve palsies. *J Neurol Neurosurg Psychiatry* 1958;21:95–100.

1234. Heerfordt CF. Über eine, "Febris uveoparotidea sub chronica" an der Glandula parotis und der Uvea des Auges lokalisiert und häufig mit Paresen cerebrospinaler Nerven kompliziert. *Arch Ophthalmol (Leipz)* 1889;70:254–273.

1235. McGovern JP, Merritt DH. Sarcoidosis in childhood. *Adv Pediatr* 1956;8:97–135.

1236. Rubinstein I, Hiss J, Baum GL. Intramedullary spinal cord sarcoidosis. *Surg Neurol* 1984;21: 272–274.

1237. Kinnman J, Link H. Intrathecal production of oligoclonal IgM and IgG in CNS sarcoidosis. *Acta Neurol Scand* 1984;69:97–106.

1238. Borucki SJ, et al. Cerebrospinal fluid immunoglobulin abnormalities in neurosarcoidosis. *Arch Neurol* 1989;46:270–273.

1238a. Koné-Paut I, et al. The pitfall of silent neurosarcoidosis. *Pediatr Neurol* 1999;20:215–218.

1239. Miller DH, et al. Magnetic resonance imaging in central nervous system sarcoidosis. *Neurology* 1988;38: 378–383.

1240. Scott TF. Neurosarcoidosis: progress and clinical aspects. *Neurology* 1993;43:8–12.

1241. Reye RD, Morgan G, Baral J. Encephalopathy and fatty degeneration of the viscera. A disease entity in childhood. *Lancet* 1963;2:749–752.

1242. Pollack JD, ed. *Reye's syndrome*. New York: Grune & Stratton, 1975.

1243. Hardie RM, et al. The changing clinical pattern of Reye's syndrome 1982–1990. *Arch Dis Child* 1996;74: 400–405.

1244. Jenkins R, Dvorak A, Patrick J. Encephalopathy and fatty degeneration of the viscera associated with chickenpox. *Pediatrics* 1967;39:769–771.

1245. Powell HC, Rosenberg RN, McKellar B. Reye's syndrome: isolation of parainfluenza virus. Report of three cases. *Arch Neurol* 1973;29:135–139.

1246. Olson LC, et al. Encephalopathy and fatty degeneration of the viscera in northeastern Thailand. Clinical syndrome and epidemiology. *Pediatrics* 1971;47: 707–716.

1247. Editorial. Reye's syndrome and aspirin. Epidemiological associations and inborn errors of metabolism. *Lancet* 1987;2:429–431.

1248. Partin JC, Schubert WK, Partin JS. Mitochondrial ultrastructure in Reye's syndrome. *N Engl J Med* 1971;285:1339–1343.

1249. Lovejoy FH Jr, et al. Clinical staging in Reye's syndrome. *Am J Dis Child* 1974;128:36–41.

1250. Aoki Y, Lombroso CT. Prognostic value of electroencephalography in Reye's syndrome. *Neurology* 1973;23:333–343.

1251. Ey JL, Smith SM, Fulginiti VA. Varicella hepatitis without neurologic symptoms or findings. *Pediatrics* 1981;67:285–287.

1252. Venes JL, Shaywitz BA, Spencer DD. Management of severe cerebral edema in the metabolic encephalopathy of Reye-Johnson syndrome. *J Neurosurg* 1978;48:903–915.

1253. Brunner RL, et al. Neuropsychologic consequences of Reye's syndrome. *J Pediatr* 1979;95:706–711.

1254. Benjamin PY, et al. Intellectual and emotional sequelae of Reye's syndrome. *Crit Care Med* 1982;10:583–587.

1255. Reitman MA, et al. Motor disorders of voice and speech in Reye's syndrome survivors. *Am J Dis Child* 1984;138:1129–1131.

1256. Levin M, et al. Haemorrhagic shock and encephalopathy: a new syndrome with a high mortality in young children. *Lancet* 1983;2:64–67.

1257. Whittington LK, Roscelli JD, Parry WH. Hemorrhagic shock and encephalopathy: further description of a new syndrome. *J Pediatr* 1985;106:599–602.

1258. Jardine DS, Winters WD, Shaw DW. CT scan abnormalities in a series of patients with hemorrhagic shock and encephalopathy syndrome. *Pediatr Radiol* 1997;27:540–544.

1259. Sofer S, et al. Possible aetiology of haemorrhagic shock and encephalopathy syndrome in the Negev area of Israel. *Arch Dis Child* 1996;75:332–334.

1260. Behçet H. Über rezidivierende Aphthöse durch ein Virus verursachte Geschwüre am Mund, am Auge, und an den Genitalien. *Dermatol Monatsschr* 1937;105:1152–1157.

1261. Devlin T, et al. Neuro-Behçet's disease: factors hampering proper diagnosis. *Neurology* 1995;45:1754–1757.

1262. Lewis MA, Priestley BL. Transient neonatal Behcet's-disease. *Arch Dis Child* 1986;61:805–806.

1263. Rakover Y, et al. Behçet disease: long-term follow-up of three children and review of the literature. *Pediatrics* 1989;83:986–992.

1263a. Sakane T, et al. Behçet's disease. *N Engl J Med* 1999;341:1284–1291.

1264. Arbesfeld SJ, Kurban AK. Behçet's disease. New perspectives on an enigmatic syndrome. *J Am Acad Dermatol* 1988;19:767–779.

1265. Allen NB. Miscellaneous vasculitic syndromes including Behcet's disease and central nervous system vasculitis. *Curr Opin Rheumatol* 1993;5:51–56.

1266. Martinez JM, et al. Anatomo-clinical study of Behçet's syndrome with involvement of the central nervous system. *Rev Neurol (Paris)* 1988;144:130–135.

1267. Wolf SM, Schotland DL, Phillips LL. Involvement of nervous system in Behçet syndrome. *Arch Neurol* 1965;12:315–325.

1268. Iseki E, et al. Two necropsy cases of chronic encephalomyelitis: variants of neuro-Behcet's syndrome? *J Neurol Neurosurg Psychiatry* 1988;51:1084–1087.

1269. Wechsler B, et al. Cerebral venous thrombosis in Behçet's syndrome. A clinical study and long term follow-up of 25 cases. *Neurology* 1992;42:614–618.

1270. Al-Kawi MZ, Bohlega S, Banna M. MRI findings in neuro-Behçet's disease. *Neurology* 1991;41:405–408.

1271. Yurdakul S, et al. The prevalence of Behçet's syndrome in a rural area in northern Turkey. *J Rheumatol* 1988;15:820–822.

1272. Hatzinikolaou P, et al. Adamantiadis–Behçet's syndrome: central nervous system involvement. *Acta Neurol Scand* 1993;87:290–293.

1273. Feron EJ, et al. Interferon-α-2b for refractory ocular Behçet's disease [Letter]. *Lancet* 1994;343:14–28.

1274. Riehl JL, Andrews JM. The uveomeningoencephalitic syndrome. *Neurology* 1966;16:603–609.

1275. Goldberg AC, et al. HLA-DRB1*0405 is the predominant allele in Brazilian patients with Vogt-Koyanagi-Harada disease. *Hum Immunol* 1998;59:183–188.

1276. Moorthy RS, Inomata H, Rao NA. Vogt-Koyanagi-Harada syndrome. *Surv Ophthalmol* 1995;39:265–292.

1277. Kimura R, et al. Swollen ciliary processes as an initial symptom in Vogt-Koyanagi-Harada disease. *Am J Ophthalmol* 1983;95:402–403.

1278. Takeshita T, et al. A patient with long standing melanin laden macrophages in cerebrospinal fluid in Vogt-Koyanagi-Harada syndrome. *Br J Ophthalmol* 1997;81:11–14.

1279. Ohno C, et al. Vogt-Koyanagi-Harada syndrome. *Am J Ophthalmol* 1977;83:735–740.

1280. Beniz J, Forster DJ, Lean JS, Smith RE, Rao NA. Variations in clinical features of the Vogt-Koyanagi-Harada syndrome. *Retina* 1991;11:275–280.

1281. Belfort R Jr, et al. Vogt-Koyanagi-Harada's disease in Brazil. *Jpn J Ophthalmol* 1988;32:344–347.

1282. Gruich MJ, et al. Vogt-Koyanagi-Harada syndrome in a 4-year-old child. *Pediatr Neurol* 1995;13:50–51.

1283. Brouzas D, et al. Corneal anesthesia in a case with Vogt-Koyanagi-Harada syndrome. *Acta Ophthalmol Scand* 1997;75:464–465.

1284. Ikeda M, Tsukagoshi H. Vogt-Koyanagi-Harada disease presenting meningoencephalitis. Report of a case with magnetic resonance imaging. *Eur Neurol* 1992;32:83–85.

1285. Helveston WR, Gilmore R. Treatment of Vogt-Koyanagi-Harada syndrome with intravenous immunoglobulin. *Neurology* 1996;46:584–585.

1286. Tabbara KF, Chavis PS, Freeman WR. Vogt-Koyanagi-Harada syndrome in children compared to adults. *Acta Ophthalmol Scan* 1998;76:723–726.

1287. Picard FJ, et al. Mollaret's meningitis associated with herpes simplex type 2 infection. *Neurology* 1993;43:1722–1727.

1288. Achard J-M, Lallement P-Y, Veyssier P. Recurrent aseptic meningitis secondary to intracranial epidermoid cyst and Mollaret's meningitis: two distinct entities or a single disease? A case report and a nosologic discussion. *Am J Med* 1990;89:807–810.

1289. Mollaret P. La meningite endothelioleucocytaire multiricurrente binigne. Syndrome nouveau ou maladie nouvelle? Documents humoraux et microbiologiques. *Ann Inst Pasteur (Paris)* 1945;71:1–17.

1290. Cohen BA, Rowley AH, Long CM. Herpes simplex type 2 in a patient with Mollaret's meningitis: demonstration by polymerase chain reaction. *Ann Neurol* 1994;35:112–116.

1291. Hermans PE, Goldstein NP, Wellman WE. Mollaret's meningitis and differential diagnosis of recurrent meningitis. Report of case, with review of literature. *Am J Med* 1972;52:128–150.

1292. Haynes BF, Wright R, McCracken JP. Mollaret meningitis—a report of three cases. *JAMA* 1976;236: 1967–1969.
1293. Iivanainen M. Benign recurrent aseptic meningitis of unknown aetiology (Mollaret's meningitis). *Acta Neurol Scand* 1973;49:133–138.
1294. Blumenfeld H, Cha J-H, Cudkowicz ME. Trimethoprim and sulfonamide-associated meningoencephalitis with MRI correlates. *Neurology* 1996;46: 556–558.
1295. Yamamoto LJ, et al. Herpes simplex virus type 1 DNA in the cerebrospinal fluid of a patient with Mollaret's meningitis. *N Engl J Med* 1991;325:1082–1085.
1296. Pederson E. Epidemic vertigo. Clinical picture, epidemiology and relation to encephalitis. *Brain* 1959;82:566–580.
1297. Basser LS. Benign paroxysmal vertigo of childhood. (A variety of vestibular neuronitis.) *Brain* 1964;87: 141–152.
1298. Koenigsberger MR, et al. Benign paroxysmal vertigo of childhood. *Neurology* 1968;18:301–302.
1299. Eviatar L, Eviatar A. Vertigo in children: differential diagnosis and treatment. *Pediatrics* 1977;59:833–838.
1300. Morgon A. Vertigo in children. *Ann Pediatr (Paris)* 1992;39:519–522.
1301. von Economo C. *Encephalitis lethargica: its sequelae and treatment.* London: Oxford University Press, 1931.
1302. Rail D, Scholtz C, Swash M. Post-encephalitic parkinsonism: current experience. *J Neurol Neurosurg Psychiatry* 1981;44:670–676.
1303. Association for Research in Nervous and Mental Disease. *Acute epidemic encephalitis.* New York: Paul B. Hoeber, 1921.
1304. Hohman LB. Post-encephalitic behavior disorders in children. *Bull Johns Hopkins Hosp* 1922;33:372–375.
1305. Sissons JGP. Superantigens and infectious disease. *Lancet* 1993;341:1627–1629.
1306. Leung DYM, et al. Toxic shock syndrome toxin-secreting *Staphylococcus aureus* in Kawasaki disease. *Lancet* 1993;342:1385–1388.
1307. Nigro G, Zerbini M, Krzysztofiak A. Active or recent parvovirus B19 infection in children with Kawasaki disease. *Lancet* 1994;343:1260–1261.
1308. Kuijpers TW, et al. A boy with chickenpox whose fingers peeled. *Lancet* 1998;351:1782.
1309. Yokota S, et al. Presence in Kawasaki disease of antibodies to mycobacterial heat-shock protein HSP65 and autoantibodies to epitopes of human HSP65 cognate antigen. *Clin Immunol Immunopathol* 1993;67: 163–170.
1310. Gama C, Breeden K, Miller R. Myositis in Kawasaki disease. *Pediatr Neurol* 1990;6:135–136.
1311. Bushara K, Wilson A, Rust RS. Facial palsy in Kawasaki syndrome. *Pediatr Neurol* 1997;17: 362–364.
1312. Melish ME. Kawasaki syndrome (the mucocutaneous lymph node syndrome). *Annu Rev Med* 1982;33: 569–585.
1313. Dengler LD, et al. Cerebrospinal fluid profile in patients with acute Kawasaki disease. *Pediatr Infect Dis J* 1998;17:478–481.
1314. American Academy of Pediatrics. Kawasaki disease. In: Peter G, ed. *1997 Red Book: report of the Committee on Infectious Diseases*, 24th ed. Elk Grove Village, IL: American Academy of Pediatrics, 1997: 316–319.
1315. Takei S, Arora YK, Walker SM. Intravenous immunoglobulin contains specific antibodies inhibitory to activation of T cells by staphylococcal toxin superantigens. *J Clin Invest* 1993;91: 603–607.
1316. Newburger JW. Treatment of Kawasaki disease. *Lancet* 1996;347:11–28.
1317. Takagi, N, et al. Plasma exchange in Kawasaki disease. *Lancet* 1995;346:1307.
1318. Rasmussen T, Olszewski J, Lloyd-Smith D. Focal seizures due to chronic localized encephalitis. *Neurology* 1958;8:435–445.
1319. Antel JP, Rasmussen T. Rasmussen's encephalitis and the new hat. *Neurology* 1996;46:9–11.
1320. Power C, et al. Cytomegalovirus and Rasmussen's encephalitis. *Lancet* 1990;336:1282–1284.
1321. Andrews JM, et al. Chronic encephalitis, epilepsy and cerebrovascular immune complex deposits. *Ann Neurol* 1990;28:88–90.
1321a. Whitney KD, Andrews PL, McNamara JO. Immunoglobulin G and complement immunoreactivity in the cerebral cortex of patients with Rasmussen's encephalitis *Neurology* 1999;53:699–708.
1322. Jay V, et al. Chronic encephalitis and epilepsy (Rasmussen's encephalitis): Detection of cytomegalovirus and herpes simplex virus 1 by the polymerase chain reaction and in situ hybridization. *Neurology* 1995; 45:108–117.
1323. Rogers SW, et al. Autoantibodies to glutamate receptor GluR3 in Rasmussen's encephalitis. *Science* 1994;265:648–651.
1324. Aguilar MJ, Rasmussen T. Role of encephalitis in pathogenesis of epilepsy. *Arch Neurol* 1960;2: 663–676.
1325. Piatt JH Jr, et al. Chronic focal encephalitis (Rasmussen's syndrome): six cases. *Epilepsia* 1988;29: 268–279.
1326. Hart YM, et al. Chronic encephalitis and epilepsy in adults and adolescents: a variant of Rasmussen's syndrome? *Neurology* 1997;48:418–424.
1327. Tien RD, et al. Rasmussen's encephalitis: neuroimaging findings in four patients. *Am J Roentgenol* 1992;158:1329–1332.
1328. Cendes F, et al. Imaging of axonal damage in vivo in Rasmussen's syndrome. *Brain* 1995;118:753–758.
1329. Vining EP, et al. Why would you remove half a brain? The outcome of 58 children after hemispherectomy—the Johns Hopkins experience. *Pediatrics* 1997;100: 163–171.
1330. Vining EP, et al. Progressive unilateral encephalopathy of childhood (Rasmussen's syndrome): a reappraisal. *Epilepsia* 1993;34:639–650.
1331. Krauss GL, et al. Chronic steroid-responsive encephalitis without antibodies to glutamate receptor GluR3. *Neurology* 1996;46:247–249.
1332. Wise MS, Rutledge SL, Kuzniecky RI. Rasmussen syndrome and long-term response to gamma globulin. *Pediatr Neurol* 1996;14:149–152.
1333. Andrews PI, et al. Plasmapheresis in Rasmussen's encephalitis. *Neurology* 1996;46:242–246.
1334. McLachlan RS, Levin S, Blume WT. Treatment of Rasmussen's syndrome with ganciclovir. *Neurology* 1996;47:925–928.

1335. Ruggenenti P, Remuzzi G. Thrombotic microangiopathies. *Crit Rev Oncol Hematol* 1991;11:243–265.
1336. Wall RT, Harker LA. The endothelium and thrombosis. *Annu Rev Med* 1980;31:361–371.
1337. Karmali MA, et al. Sporadic cases of haemolyticuraemic syndrome associated with faecal cytotoxin and cytotoxin-producing *Escherichia coli* in stools. *Lancet* 1983;1:619–620.
1338. Akashi, S, et al. A severe outbreak of haemorrhagic colitis and haemolytic uraemic syndrome associated with *Escherichia coli* O157:H7 in Japan. *Eur J Pediatr* 1994;153:650–655.
1339. Rondeau E, Peraldi M-N. *Escherichia coli* and the hemolytic-uremic syndrome. *N Engl J Med* 1996;335:660–662.
1340. Mead PS, Griffin PM. *Escherichia coli* O157:H7. *Lancet* 1998;352:1207–1212.
1341. Moake JL. Haemolytic-uremic syndrome: basic science. *Lancet* 1994;343:393–397.
1342. van de Kar NC, et al. Tumor necrosis factor and interleukin-1 induce expression of the verocytotoxin receptor globotriaosylceramide on human endothelial cells: implications for the pathogenesis of the hemolytic uremic syndrome. *Blood* 1992;80:2755–2764.
1343. Louise CB, Obrig TG. Shiga toxin-associated hemolytic uremic syndrome: combined cytotoxic effects of shiga toxin and lipopolysaccharide (endotoxin) on human vascular endothelial cells in vitro. *Infect Immun* 1992;60:1536–1543.
1344. Cimolai N, Morrison BJ, Carter JE. Risk factors for the central nervous system manifestations of gastroenteritis-associated hemolytic-uremic syndrome. *Pediatrics* 1992;90:616–621.
1345. Moake JL. The role of von Willebrand factor (vWF) in thrombotic thrombocytopenic purpura (TTP) and the hemolytic-uremic syndrome (HUS). *Prog Clin Biol Res* 1990;337:135–140.
1346. Moake JL. Recent observations on the pathophysiology of thrombotic thrombocytopenic purpura and the hemolytic-uremic syndrome. *Hematol Pathol* 1990;4:197–201.
1347. Remuzzi G. HUS and TTP; variable expression of a single entity. *Kidney Int* 1987;32:292–308.
1348. Teshima T, Miyoshi T, Ono M. Cyclosporine-related encephalopathy following allogeneic bone marrow transplantation. *Int J Hematol* 1996;63:161–164.
1349. Siegler RL. Management of hemolytic-uremic syndrome. *J Pediatr* 1988;112:1014–1020.
1350. Cabrera GR, et al. Hemolytic uremic syndrome associated with invasive *Streptococcus pneumoniae* infection. *Pediatrics* 1998;101:699–703.
1351. Kennedy SS, Zacharski LR, Beck JR. Thrombotic thrombocytopenic purpura: analysis of 48 unselected cases. *Semin Thromb Hemost* 1980;6:341–349.
1352. Fuchs WE, et al. Thrombotic thrombocytopenic purpura. Occurrence two years apart during late pregnancy in two sisters. *J Am Med Assoc* 1976;235:2126–2127.
1353. Tarr PI, et al. Hemolytic-uremic syndrome in a six-year old girl after a urinary tract infection with shigatoxin-producing *Escherichia coli* 0103:H2. *N Engl J Med* 1996;335:635–638.
1354. Bale JF Jr, Brasher C, Siegler RL. CNS manifestations of the hemolytic-uremic syndrome: relationship to metabolic alterations and prognosis. *Am J Dis Child* 1980;134:869–872.
1355. Hahn JS, et al. Neurological complications of hemolytic-uremic syndrome. *J Child Neurol* 1989;4:108–113.
1356. Siegler RL. Spectrum of extrarenal involvement in postdiarrheal hemolytic-uremic syndrome. *J Pediatr* 1994;125:511–518.
1357. Upadhyaya K, et al. The importance of nonrenal involvement in the hemolytic-uremic syndrome. *Pediatrics* 1980;65:115–120.
1358. Travathan E, Dooling EC. Large thrombotic strokes in hemolytic-uremic syndrome. *J Pediatr* 1987;111:863–866.
1359. Gianantonio C, et al. The hemolytic-uremic syndrome. *J Pediatr* 1964;64:478–491.
1360. Neild GH. Haemolytic-uraemic syndrome in practice. *Lancet* 1994;343:398–401.
1361. Pascual-Leone A, et al. EEG correlation of improvement in hemolytic-uremic syndrome after plasma infusion. *Pediatr Neurol* 1990;6:269–271.
1362. Martin DL, et al. The epidemiology and clinical aspects of the hemolytic-uremic syndrome in Minnesota. *N Engl J Med* 1990;323:1161–1167.
1363. Steele BT, et al. Recovery from prolonged coma in hemolytic-uremic syndrome. *J Pediatr* 1983;102:402–404.
1364. Mackenzie JS, et al. Australian encephalitis in Western Australia. *Med J Aust* 1993;158:591–595.
1365. Richter RW, Shimojyo S. Neurologic sequelae of Japanese B encephalitis. *Neurology* 1961;11:553–559.
1366. Ishii T, Matsushita M, Hamada S. Characteristic residual neuropathological features of Japanese B encephalitis. *Acta Neuropathol (Berl)* 1977;38:181–186.
1367. Burrow JN, et al. Australian encephalitis in the Northern Territory: clinical and epidemiological features, 1987–1996. *Aust N Z J Med* 1998;28:590–596.
1368. Robertson EG. Murray Valley encephalitis: pathological aspects. *M J Australia* 1952;1:107–110.
1369. Hloucal L. Tick-borne encephalitis as observed in Czechoslovakia. *J Trop Med Hyg* 1960;63:293–296.
1370. Gesikova M, Kaluzova M. Biology of tick-borne encephalitis virus. *Acta Virol* 1997;41:115–124.
1371. Pavri K. Clinical, clinicopathologic, and hematologic features of Kyasanur Forest disease. *Rev Infect Dis* 1989;11[Suppl 4]:S854–S859.
1372. Kolski H, et al. Etiology of acute childhood encephalitis at The Hospital for Sick Children, Toronto, 1994–1995. *Clin Infect Dis* 1998;26:398–409.
1373. Silver HK, Meiklejohn G, Kempe CH. Colorado tick fever. *Am J Dis Child* 1961;101:30–36.
1374. Johnson AJ, Karabatsos N, Lanciotti RS. Detection of Colorado tick fever virus by using reverse transcriptase PCR and application of the technique in laboratory diagnosis. *J Clin Microbiol* 1997;35:1203–1208.
1375. Wahlberg P, Saikku P, Brummer-Korvenkontio M. Tick-borne viral encephalitis in Finland. The clinical features of Kumlinge disease during 1959–1987. *J Intern Med* 1989;225:173–177.
1376. Braito A, et al. *Toscana* virus infections of the central nervous system in children: a report of 14 cases. *J Pediatr* 1998;132:144–148.
1377. Davidson MM, Williams H, Macleod JA. Louping ill in man: a forgotten disease. *J Infect* 1991;23:241–242.

Chapter 7

Autoimmune and Postinfectious Diseases

Robert Rust and *John H. Menkes

*Department of Neurology, University of Virginia School of Medicine, Charlottesville,
Virginia 22908; and *Departments of Neurology and Pediatrics, University of California,
Los Angeles, UCLA School of Medicine, and Department of Pediatric Neurology,
Cedars-Sinai Medical Center, Los Angeles, California 90048*

This chapter considers several groups of neurologic diseases believed to result from a failure of the normal mechanisms of self-tolerance. One group consists of the primary demyelinating illnesses of the central nervous system (CNS), the second the immunologically mediated diseases affecting CNS gray matter, the third the immunologically mediated demyelinating diseases of the peripheral nervous system, and the last group includes the primary and secondary systemic vasculitides with nervous system manifestations. Myasthenia gravis, another autoimmune condition, is discussed in Chapter 14. The paraneoplastic processes are so uncommon in the pediatric age group that they do not warrant discussion here.

EXPERIMENTAL ALLERGIC ENCEPHALOMYELITIS

Experimental allergic encephalomyelitis (EAE) has served for many years as a useful animal model in the study of the evolution of autoimmune diseases that affect the nervous system. Departing from the postulate that the neuroparalytic accidents observed after the use of a rabies vaccine prepared from neural tissue were allergies, Rivers and Schwentker observed that the repeated injection of cerebral tissue into monkeys produced an inflammatory demyelinating encephalomyelitis (1).

Similar lesions have been produced consistently in other mammalian species; their appearance is enhanced by the addition of Freund's adjuvant, a commonly used emulsion of water, oil, and killed acid-fast organisms added to the antigenic material. Its mode of action is unknown, but is believed to be a slow release of antigen and the induction of an inflammatory reaction that attracts mononuclear cells. In the original studies of Wolf and associates (2), 90% of monkeys developed EAE in 2 to 8 weeks after the first of an average of three weekly subcutaneous inoculations. The characteristic clinical features of this monophasic disease included paresis of the extremities, ataxia, nystagmus, and blindness. The disease was usually fatal, but some animals had mild symptoms that often subsided. A chronic disease and a relapsing disease marked by exacerbations and remissions reminiscent of the clinical picture of multiple sclerosis (MS) were produced subsequently in several animal species, including non-human primates (3,4).

Pathologic examination of animals dying from EAE shows multiple focal perivascular areas of demyelination throughout the neuraxis. Microscopically, these lesions show an extensive infiltration by round cells, mainly lymphocytes and microglial cells, small perivascular hemorrhages, and myelin degeneration with preservation of the axon cylinders.

The first pathologic alteration observed in experimental lesions is the perivenous appearance of hematogenous cells. These are initially seen in areas where the blood–brain barrier has been damaged or where lack of a barrier allows serum proteins to enter the nervous tissue (5). At the same time, primary and secondary (wallerian) demyelination can occur. Electron microscopic examination reveals a focal disruption of the myelin lamellae, and processes of the invading cells extend between the lamellae. Additionally, vesiculation of myelin occurs.

In older lesions, the patches of demyelination are well defined and marked by varying degrees of gliosis. It is still unclear how perivascular demyelination develops in EAE.

Myelin basic protein (MBP) is the substance in the injected cerebral tissue that initiates the evolution of the demyelinating process (6). This encephalitogenic protein has been isolated in relatively pure condition from the brain of a number of species. A component of normal myelin sheath, it contributes approximately 40% of total myelin proteins of adult white matter. *In vivo*, it is bound to acidic lipids or proteins. The gene coding for it is located on chromosome 18. The complete amino acid sequence has been determined, and the encephalitogenic activity resides in several peptides.

As a consequence of the injection of MBP, T cells carrying gene-specified MBP receptors on their surface lose their immunologic tolerance to neural antigens by an unknown mechanism and escape from the host immunoregulatory restraints to develop into clones of cytotoxic cells. These bind to native MBP within the brain of the host, resulting in the deposition of an immune complex. The mechanism by which activated T cells enter the CNS is as yet unknown. Both encephalitogenic and nonencephalitogenic cells are able to enter the CNS, but only the encephalitogenic cells remain; nonencephalitogenic cells are cleared within a few days (7). It is believed that in the course of a systemic immune response, antigen-specific T cells adhere to the brain endothelial cells. Research indicates that EAE is almost exclusively mediated by Th1 cells, which produce interleukin-2 (IL-2) and interferon-γ. Multiple other cytokines produced by astrocytes and microglial cells also play major roles in inflammation and tissue destruction. T-cell adherence to endothelial cells is further enhanced by the class II major histocompatibility complex antigens, molecules induced by interferon-γ. Other factors, notably endoglycosidases, guide the T cells through the blood–brain barrier. Once within the CNS, these immune complexes can attract hematogenous mononuclear cells and induce the release of chemotactic factors to initiate the ensuing inflammation. Macrophages are believed to play an important role in myelin destruction by their release of myelinolytic proteases (8).

The passive transfer of EAE can be accomplished by CD4$^+$ T lymphocytes, but not by serum. Other characteristics of EAE are that the disease can be blocked by antibodies against CD4$^+$ T cells, by treatment of susceptible animals with a synthetic peptide, structurally related to the encephalitogenic portion of the MBP, or by irradiation (9,10). The development of EAE also can be suppressed by the administration of corticosteroids, nitrogen mustard, or 6-mercaptopurine.

Susceptibility to the induction of the condition depends on a number of host factors. Immature animals are relatively more resistant to EAE than adult animals; diets inadequate in vitamin B_{12}, biotin, or folic acid decrease susceptibility. Most important, both highly susceptible and highly resistant genetic lines have been segregated in a number of mammalian species.

MBP also is the encephalitogen responsible for the encephalomyelitis after rabies immunization. Antibodies to MBP can be demonstrated in serum and in the cerebrospinal fluid (CSF) at the onset of symptoms, and a T-cell response to CNS myelin can be demonstrated in vaccinated subjects who develop encephalitis (11). A T-cell response and circulating antibodies to MBP also have been found in postmeasles encephalitis.

The role, if any, of MBP in the other autoimmune disorders is not as clear. Whether the antigen responsible for MS is similar to the MBP that induces EAE, or whether the antigen is derived from a virus or viruses remains to be answered. In any case, the sequence of events leading to demyelination in MS appears to be morphologically similar to that observed in EAE (12), and, for the time being, this condition still serves as the best available laboratory model for the pathogenesis of some of the autoimmune and postinfectious disorders.

Much work has concentrated on the effects of soluble factors (cytokines) on activated T cells. IL-2 is thought to play a particularly important role in the propagation of the activated T cells that may mediate EAE (12a). Human interferon-γ and tumor necrosis factor (TNF) can induce the plasminogen activator of lymphocytes from patients with acute disseminated encephalomyelitis (ADEM) and MS, but not from control subjects, possibly indicating a role for these cytokines in the mediation of demyelination (12b).

PRIMARY DEMYELINATING DISEASES OF THE CENTRAL NERVOUS SYSTEM

In the northern hemisphere, ADEM, MS, and optic neuritis are the three most frequently encountered primary demyelinating illnesses of the CNS. The first is more common in children younger than age 12 years; the second is more common in adolescents and adults. Difficulty in distinguishing ADEM from the first bout of MS is among the most important reasons for the requirement of a second distinct episode occurring at least 1 month after the first for diagnosis of MS. It remains controversial as to whether "recurrent ADEM" should be distinguished from MS, but it appears likely that this distinction is valuable in prepubertal children. Optic neuritis and the combination of optic neuritis and transverse myelitis (Devic disease) usually occur as manifestations of ADEM or MS, but may result from other types of illness.

An area of semiologic overlap exists between ADEM and Gullain-Barré syndrome (GBS). This area of overlap includes some or possibly all patients who manifest the clinical findings of Miller-Fisher syndrome. It also includes the minority of ADEM cases that manifest diminished or absent muscle stretch reflexes in combination with weakness and sensory changes referable to peripheral nerve dysfunction. The designation encephalomyeloradiculoneuropathy (EMRN) may be applied to cases exhibiting this overlap of central and peripheral demyelinative

manifestations. Other much rarer primary demyelinative conditions that may occur in children and are difficult to accurately classify are acute (Marburg type) MS, Schilder disease, and Balo disease (concentric sclerosis). Infants younger than 2 years of age may experience a single bout of severe demyelination with edema that could be termed acute MS or, perhaps more appropriately, severe ADEM.

The etiology and pathogenesis of these various primary demyelinating illnesses are as yet incompletely understood and it is not known whether MS, ADEM, and such related illnesses as optic neuritis, transverse myelitis, and others share exactly the same mechanism. Both MS and ADEM involve autoimmune responses that are directed, at least in part, against myelin antigens, but it is as yet unknown whether this represents a primary or secondary aspect of the inflammatory process of either illness. The onset of MS does not have a clear etiologic relationship to preceding infection and bouts are typically associated with detectable and abnormal production of immunoglobulin within the CNS. ADEM appears in many cases to be provoked by an immediately preceding infectious illness and only a minority of cases exhibit elevated CSF concentrations of immunoglobulin or immunoglobulin oligoclonality. Normal CSF immunoglobulin studies are characteristic of recurrences of ADEM, as compared with a greater than 94% likelihood of abnormality in association with an MS recurrence.

A small minority of individuals who have experienced typical cases of ADEM in early childhood ultimately satisfies the clinical criteria for diagnosis of MS during adolescence. It is not known why some individuals experience one or more bouts of postinfectious demyelination but achieve stable remission (ADEM or recurrent ADEM) before adolescence, whereas others satisfy criteria for the diagnosis of MS with either relapsing-remitting or steadily progressive manifestations of primary central demyelination. No completely reliable diagnostic test exists for either illness, and in every case a number of other illnesses must be excluded before assigning either of these labels. It may be particularly difficult to distinguish ADEM and related forms of inflammation from encephalitis. Indeed, some forms of encephalitis (such as those caused by herpes or measles viruses) may manifest pathologic abnormalities of ADEM in combination with those of encephalitis.

Multiple Sclerosis

Historical Aspects

MS is the principal immune-mediated demyelinating illness of humans (13). The pathologic lesions of MS were described by Cruveilhier and Carswell early in the nineteenth century. Frerichs was the first to make a clinical diagnosis of MS in 1849. Charcot's extensive studies of the clinical manifestations and natural history of MS resulted in diagnostic criteria for a coherent clinical entity designated disseminated sclerosis or *sclerose en plaques* that also is and quite justifiably termed *Charcot disease* (14). Although the particular prevalence of this illness among young adults was recognized at the outset, subsequent clinical experience and confirmatory pathologic studies have demonstrated that MS may occur in infants and children (15,16).

Pathogenesis

MS occurs more frequently in certain parts of the world, and in regions of greater endemicity, certain subpopulations are at greater risk. Thus, in both Europe and North America, the risk is roughly proportional to the distance from the equator of the latitude in which a given individual has spent the first few decades of life. A particularly significant increase in prevalence exists in North America above the 38th parallel, whereas in Europe this increase occurs above the 46th parallel. Not all populations in these regions of high prevalence (30 to 100 cases per 100,000) partake of this enhanced risk, however. Thus, for example, the risk for Hungarian gypsies is 15- to 25-fold lower than that for the predominantly Magyr population of that country. However, the clear demonstration of regionally determined risk has been one of several lines of evidence advanced in support of the widely held

concept that MS is initially provoked by an infectious agent. This line of reasoning has been supported by the development of MS epidemics in certain sheltered populations suddenly exposed to an influx of people from areas of relatively high endemic risk for MS. The appearance of MS on the Faroe Islands when British troops were stationed there during World War II is an important example of this phenomenon. Genetic susceptibility also may have played a role in this epidemic (17).

Among the most important data supporting a direct etiologic role of infection or some other childhood experience are those obtained in studies of families migrating either from temperate or subarctic regions of the northern hemisphere to Israel or from Israel to these northerly latitudes. These studies demonstrate that the risk for MS is strongly influenced by the latitude, or perhaps even more specifically by the climate in which individuals live during the first two decades of life. This suggests the possibility that MS is caused by infection, incurred early in life, with an agent that is more prevalent in more northern latitudes. It is not known whether any possible directly infectious neurologic dysfunction might chiefly affect oligodendrocytes or myelin. Despite considerable effort and the identification of candidate viruses that are capable of provoking CNS demyelination (visna, JHM virus—a corona virus,—canine distemper, Theiler murine encephalomyelitis virus, measles, herpes simplex virus), a direct etiologic role for viruses or other infectious agents remains unproven (18). It remains possible that an intermittently activated *MS virus* resides undetected in oligodendrocytes.

A second hypothesis suggests that infection with a virus or other agent serves indirectly to provoke MS because of the induction of immunodysregulation and autoimmunity. This hypothesis suggests that any of a number of viral or bacterial organisms possess the capacity to produce this unfavorable host response in susceptible individuals. By extension, the increased risk for MS in northern latitudes would be explained by greater prevalence of candidate micro-organisms within the temperate and subarctic ecological niche. The disturbance in immunoregulation might result from (a) abrogation of blood–brain barrier caused by inflammatory injury to blood vessels with secondary exposure of *privileged* antigens, (b) disturbance of self-tolerance caused by infectious alteration in host antigens, or (c) sensitization to autoantigens because antigens of invading organism happen to closely resemble them. The existence of a limited degree of normal immunosurveillance of the CNS by lymphocytes capable of passing through the intact blood–brain barrier may be permissive of the second and third mechanisms.

The third mechanism is termed *molecular mimicry*. This hypothesis further suggests that the mediation of host autosensitization involves the activity of a trimolecular complex consisting of a cell-surface antigen of an invading organism, phagocytic antigen-presenting cells (macrophages or possibly microglial cells), and T-helper cells. As the result of the interaction between the foreign antigens and these cells, insufficiently specific clonal stimulation of cytotoxic T cells occurs, and inflammatory consequences are experienced by host tissues with similar antigenic determinants. It also is possible that the nonspecific clonal stimulation simply increases the number of activated cells in circulation and that these activated cells incite a poorly regulated inflammatory response directed at epitopes expressed on the surface of endothelial tissues or privileged nervous system tissues that are not similar to those of the foreign organism. The vascular, humoral, and cellular aspects of autoimmunity are discussed in further detail in the following section on ADEM.

Support for the notion that MS is provoked indirectly by infection is provided by the characteristic occurrence of pathologically and clinically similar ADEM in the wake of one of a wide variety of febrile infectious illnesses. A novel, and as yet unsubstantiated, third hypothesis suggests attempts to explain the enhancement of MS risk in proportion to distance of early life residence from the equator on the basis of limited cumulative childhood sun exposure and the associated effects on vitamin D metabolism. More than one of these mechanisms or indeed others may contribute to MS or by extension ADEM pathogenesis. It is probable that if any of these mechanisms contribute to MS

pathogenesis, the likelihood that such indirect effects will occur is genetically regulated.

It is clear that the risk for MS is influenced by the immunologic constitution of the individual, represented in part by the human leukocyte antigen (HLA) genes that control the immune system. Although the HLA genes may play only a minor role in MS pathogenesis (19), the expression of certain HLA haplotypes appears to increase the risk for MS by 10- to 20-fold or more within certain populations. Among these *permissive* haplotypes are DRw15, DRw2 or DQw6 (North American and northern European whites), DR4 (Italians and Arabs), DR6 (Japanese and Mexicans), and A3, B7, or DR. Diminished rates of expression of the HLA haplotypes A2, B12, and DR7 are found in northern hemisphere whites with MS (20–22).

The genetic aspect of MS risk also is demonstrated by the disparity observed among genetically distinct populations living within the same latitude. Genetic influence on susceptibility for MS is strongly supported by studies of families of patients with MS. Prevalence rates for MS among first-degree relatives of individuals with MS are approximately 20-fold greater than those of other individuals from the same region. Approximately 10% to 15% of patients with MS report another blood relative with this disease. Identical twins have a 25% to 35% concordance rate for MS, as compared with 0.5% for offspring (possibly much higher for daughters of mothers with MS), 0.6% for parents, 1.2% for siblings, and 2% to 4% for dizygotic twins (23–25). Genetic studies have further suggested that T-cell receptor germline polymorphisms may participate in the determination of risk for MS, but these data remain inconclusive (26–28). The lack of 100% concordance for identical twins makes it clear that MS is not caused solely by a single gene defect. It has been estimated that as many as 10 to 15 interacting genes may be involved, in addition to environmental factors (29).

Pathology

The pathognomonic lesion of MS is the plaque. Histopathologically, the typical acute plaques are areas of venulocentric demyelination with relative

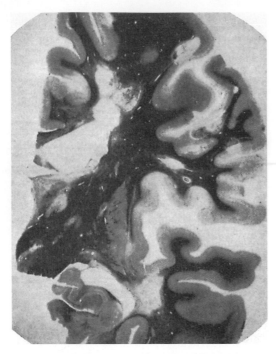

FIG. 7.1. Multiple sclerosis. Disseminated area of demyelination in white and gray matter of cerebral hemispheres. Myelin stain. (From Merritt HH. *Textbook of neurology*, 5th ed. Philadelphia: Lea & Febiger, 1973. With permission.)

preservation of axis cylinders. Recent plaques and the margins of "active" plaques contain a mixture of inflammatory cells, primarily lymphocytes, microglia, and macrophages. Older plaques become gliotic and contain astrocytes. Plaques may be found anywhere in brain or spinal cord. They are largely, but not entirely, confined to white matter, with particular abundance in the periventricular zones (30) (Fig. 7.1). The histopathology closely resembles that of ADEM and of the experimental system that has been developed as a model for both MS and ADEM, EAE. On the other hand, MS plaques tend to have more discrete margins than those of ADEM.

Because plaques may be located in almost any portion of the CNS, the clinical manifestations of MS are remarkably diverse. Larger plaques are clearly visible with appropriate brain imaging and may in some instances occupy locations that explain signs or symptoms of disease. However, often no clear clinico-anatomic associ-ation exists for any individual plaque. Moreover, clinical improvement may occur before observable resolution of plaques, suggesting that the nervous system dysfunction of MS is caused by more than just demyelination.

Immunology

An enormous amount of information has accumulated concerning immune system abnormalities found in patients with MS. Much of this information falls beyond the scope of this text. Information particularly relevant to MS is considered in this section, whereas information particularly relevant to the other autoimmune conditions is reviewed in other sections of this chapter. It is clear that patients with MS as a class do not have immune dysfunction such as might result in systemic immunodeficiency or autoimmunity, vasculitis, or susceptibility to malignancy (31,32). Systemic antibody responses and delayed-type hypersensitivity are normal. The primary disease is restricted to the CNS, within which no increase in susceptibility to unusual infections or any evidence for vasculitis occurs. Within the CNS and particularly within the demyelinating plaque, there is clear evidence for disturbances of both humoral and cellular immunity (26,33).

Abnormal modulation of the humoral immune system is a consistent finding in patients with MS. It is represented by the almost universal presence in CSF of (a) electrophoretically detectable oligoclonal immunoglobulin, (b) elevated rates of synthesis and concentration in CSF of intrathecally generated immunoglobulin G (IgG) and IgM with varied or unknown epitopic specificity, and (c) increased levels of immunoglobulin components such as kappa chains (26,34–36). Although IgG_1 subclass elevation is the most common, other classes and subclasses of immunoglobulin also are elevated. As noted, the antigenic specificity of these immunoglobulins is various, including reactivity to a wide variety of viruses or other microbes, but in most cases the specificity is unknown.

Abnormalities of cellular immunity include loss of T-suppressor/cytotoxic cells with resulting increases in the circulating CD4$^+$ T-helper/inducer to CD8$^+$ T-suppressor/cytotoxic cell ratio during MS relapses in children and adults (31,37–39a). The prominence of lymphocytic infiltration within an active MS plaque suggests the importance of these cells to MS pathogenesis. CD4$^+$ T cells are predominant at the leading edges of active demyelinating lesions, whereas CD8$^+$ T cells are more frequently encountered in less active plaque regions. Most of the T cells found within MS plaques bear the TCR (T-cell receptor) $\alpha\beta$ chains, although within chronic lesions a number of T cells bear TCR$\gamma\delta$ chains. It has been speculated that TCR$\alpha\beta$ T cells initiate inflammation, whereas TCR$\gamma\delta$ T cells downregulate the initial response but perpetuate the inflammatory activity of chronic active lesions (33).

The considerably diminished cadre of oligodendroglial cells found within chronic active plaques express a particular 65-kD heat shock protein (hsp 65), which is a known stimulus for TCR$\gamma\delta$ T-cell clones. This suggests some relationship of this protein either to the elimination (40) or less likely to the preservation of these oligodendroglia. Enhanced expression of the major histocompatibility antigens also is found within active MS plaques. This expression is found on the surfaces of microglial cells and macrophages and especially involves the class II major histocompatibility complex antigens with which CD4$^+$ T cells characteristically interact (33,41). Astrocytes within plaques are involved to a lesser extent in the expression of major histocompatibility complex antigens, but oligodendroglial cells are not.

Data obtained in the EAE experimental model suggest that activated lymphocytes mediate demyelination, because both the monophasic and chronic relapsing forms of EAE can be transferred passively by lymphocytes but not by serum. Moreover, demyelination in the coronavirus–induced experimental demyelination model requires the presence of splenic Thy1+ cells (42). In EAE, myelin antigens such as MBP are of considerable importance in cell-mediated demyelination. The particular target antigens of MS are unknown but may include myelin epitopes, viruses, and heat-shock proteins (43). Cellular immunity to myelin in MS has not been conclusively proven (33). It is possible that the importance of the MBP sensitization is of greater importance in ADEM than MS. The roles of T-cell activation and T-cell receptor specificity in MS are the subjects of several detailed reviews (26,27,33,39a,43,44).

Enhanced expression of adhesion molecules and cytokines also is found within MS plaques (26,33,43). Among the adhesion molecules of greatest importance are intercellular adhesion molecule-1 (ICAM-1) found on endothelial membranes and leukocyte function-associated antigen-1 (LFA-1) found on lymphocytes. Both appear to facilitate the trafficking of inflammatory cells into MS plaques. Among the proinflammatory cytokines found within MS lesions are IL-2, tumor necrosis factor-α (TNF-α), and interferon-γ (IFN-γ). Circulating systemic lymphocytes from patients with MS show increased production of these proinflammatory cytokines and subnormal production of such anti-inflammatory cytokines as transforming growth factor-β (TGF-β) (45,46).

Clinical Manifestations of Multiple Sclerosis in Children and Adolescents

MS is primarily a disease of young adults (47). The peak age of onset is 25 to 30 years, and onset before puberty is uncommon. In a series of some 5,000 cases of MS, less than 0.2% presented before 11 years of age. In the same series, only 2.5% of cases presented between 11 and 16 years of age (48). In our experience, most adolescent cases present at or after 13 years of age. Thereafter, the prevalence increases with each additional year of age. In the pediatric population, girls are affected 2.2 times as frequently as boys, and whites are at greater risk than blacks (48a). The symptoms of the initial attack of MS in childhood are listed in Table 7.1 (48b–48d).

For reasons as yet unknown, childhood MS is more common in China than in the West. In a series compiled in 1982, 3.5% of Chinese MS patients experienced the onset of their illnesses before age 10 years, and 22% developed it before age 20 years (49). This age distribution contrasts with 1.5% and 2.7%, with onset before

TABLE 7.1. *Symptoms during the initial episode of multiple sclerosis in 56 children*

Symptoms	Number of patients
Ataxia or muscle weakness	31
Disturbance of vision (blurring, diplopia, blindness)	19
Numbness or paresthesia	13
Dizziness, headache, vomiting	10
Vertigo	6
Urinary incontinence	2
Facial weakness	1
Hearing loss	1
Focal jacksonian seizures	1

Compiled from Low and Carter (48b), Isler (48c), and Gall et al. (48d).

10 and 16 years, respectively, for a series compiled in Canada (50). In China, MS is characterized by a rapidly progressive course, with lesions most frequently localized to the optic nerve and spinal cord. A similar distribution of lesions, corresponding to what has been designated as neuromyelitis optica (Devic disease), has been observed in Japan (51).

Among the most common initial manifestations of MS in adolescents and young adults are such monosymptomatic deficits as pure sensory disturbances, optic neuritis, diplopia, or pure motor paresis. In the series of Duquette and colleagues these symptoms accounted, respectively, for 26%, 14%, 11%, and 11% of initial manifestations (48). In the same series, ataxia, gait abnormalities, visual blurring, and combinations of sensorimotor and visual difficulties accounted for an additional 27% of presentations. Myelitis, sphincter disturbances, vestibular problems, and other manifestations accounted for only 12%. Ataxia and vestibular abnormalities are rather more commonly documented in adult MS than childhood-onset MS (52).

Many of the initial manifestations of MS are subtle and transient. They are often unreported or ascribed to some other cause, and their true significance is ascertained only retrospectively. The common paraparetic presentation of young adult MS usually is associated with abnormalities of posterior column sensory dysfunction, which in our experience is often overlooked in adolescent cases because of an inadequate exam-ination. This posterior column dysfunction may be more common in early MS than in ADEM.

Prepubertal children may be more likely to manifest unusual clinical features during their first or even during subsequent bouts of MS. Acute encephalopathy, seizures, and prominent pyramidal tract abnormalities are among these unusual presentations. Some young children develop acute MS with rapid and profound psychomotor deterioration (53,54). The clinical signs and symptoms of MS typically progress over hours to days, although some patients have gradual worsening for as long as several months. Transient paroxysmal signs and symptoms may occur in MS, lasting variably from seconds to minutes. These include Lhermitte's and Uhthoff's signs, constricting truncal band sensations, and momentary exacerbation of weakness or sensory disturbance. Lhermitte's sign consists of a sudden, electriclike sensation spreading down the body and into the limbs on sudden flexion of the neck. Uhthoff sign consists of the transient appearance of signs or worsening of existing signs in association with exercise or when exposed to hot ambient temperatures (atmospheric or during bathing). It is thought to be the result of heat-induced impairment of conduction through already demyelinated axons. These various paroxysmal phenomena may occur as patients are improving or between bouts of MS and are not regarded either as evidence for recurrence or progression of illness or as separate bouts.

In the experience of Cole and Stuart, only 14% of patients whose symptoms appeared before 16 years of age developed primary progressive MS, whereas the majority of children developed the relapsing-remitting form of MS, with 71% of this group being entirely well between relapses (55,56).

Diagnosis

MS is primarily a clinical diagnosis and one of exclusion. Remission, exacerbation, and CNS multifocality were recognized as key diagnostic features in Charcot's original description. Thus, the criteria for what is usually termed *clinically definite MS* require evidence for appropriate deficits "separated in both space and time." It is

TABLE 7.2. *Rose research criteria for the clinical diagnosis of multiple sclerosis*

Clinically definite	Consistent course
	Relapsing-remitting: two bouts separated by at least 1 month
	Slow or stepwise progression for at least 6 months
	Documented neurologic signs of lesions ascribable to more than one site in white matter of brain or spinal cord
	Onset of symptoms between 10 and 50 years of age
	No better etiologic explanations
Clinically probable	History of relapsing-remitting symptoms but signs not documented and only one current sign commonly associated with multiple sclerosis
	Documented single bout of symptoms with signs of more than one white matter lesion; good recovery, then variable signs or symptoms
	No better etiologic explanation
Clinically possible	History of relapsing-remitting symptoms without documented signs
	Objective signs insufficient to establish presence of lesions at more than one site in central nervous system white matter
	No better etiologic explanation

From Rose AS, et al. Criteria for the clinical diagnosis of multiple sclerosis. *Neurology* 1976;26(6 PT 2):20–22. With permission.

essential that at least two bouts whose signs persist for more than 24 hours occur with an intervening period of at least 30 days, and that a recurrence manifests at least one novel clinical or paraclinical lesion as compared with the initial bout. The interval between first and second bouts may be longer than 10 years in some children. Relapses occurring during the taper of corticosteroid therapy must be distinguished from true MS relapses. The diagnostic criteria for MS are summarized in Table 7.2.

The demonstration of multifocality of lesions can in part be satisfied by paraclinical evidence such as neurophysiologic tests and CSF and brain imaging studies. Such studies can prove informative in the common childhood monosymptomatic presentations of MS, including optic neuritis, or purely sensory, spinal, or hemiplegic illnesses. The CSF is abnormal at some time in more than two-thirds of patients. In Freedman and Merritt's study, which included patients of all ages, mild pleocytosis (6–40 cells/mm^3) was seen in 28% of patients and the total protein content was elevated in 24% (57). In the series of Sindern and colleagues, the mean CSF cell count obtained some 6 years after the onset of the disease was 10.5 ± 9.2 (58). CSF glucose and protein abnormalities are uncommon in childhood MS; they are more common in ADEM.

More specific CSF examinations include tests that reflect endogenous CNS production of immunoglobulin. Some of these tests are quantitative, such as the CSF/serum IgG index, the IgG synthetic rate, and free kappa or lambda light chains. Others are qualitative, such as detection of oligoclonal bands. In our experience, the CSF IgG ratio, CSF/serum IgG index, and oligoclonal band determinations are abnormal in 82% of children with MS (50). With MS recurrences this number increases to greater than 90%. This compares with abnormalities in approximately 20% of children and adolescents experiencing ADEM. An increased synthesis of IgG within the CNS is seen in 85% to 95% of patients (59). MBP can be demonstrated in CSF by radioimmunoassays in 70% to 93% of patients during an acute exacerbation of the illness, and its level correlates with the severity of the demyelinating process with the highest elevations observed in ADEM cases (60).

None of these tests is totally specific for MS. Oligoclonal IgG can be seen in some patients with infectious polyneuropathy, herpes encephalitis, and subacute sclerosing panencephalitis (SSPE) (61). Similarly, MBP in CSF indicates merely demyelination. Accordingly, it is found in a variety of leukodystrophies and after vascular accidents.

Abnormalities of visual-, auditory-, and somatosensory-evoked potentials provide information about the multiplicity of demyelinating lesions within the CNS, and, by inference, may help confirm the diagnosis. Among the available tests, the latency of the P100 potential of the visual-evoked response, the I–III or III–IV inter-

TABLE 7.3. *Rate of positivity for paraclinical tests in patients with clinically definite multiple sclerosis*

	Clinically definite multiple sclerosis
Cerebrospinal fluid IgG index	
Cerebrospinal fluid IgG synthetic rate	84–92%
Light chains	
Oligoclonal bands	91–95%
Myelin basic protein	
Visual-evoked potentials	81%
Somatosensory-evoked potentials	70%
Brainstem auditory-evoked response	57%
Magnetic resonance imaging	93%

IgG, immunoglobulin G.
From Paty DW, et al. MRI in the diagnosis of MS: a prospective study with comparison of clinical evaluation, evoked potentials, oligoclonal banding, and CT. *Neurology* 1988;38:180. With permission.

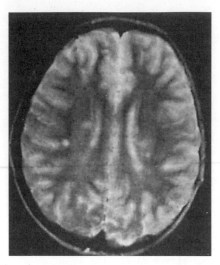

FIG. 7.2. Childhood multiple sclerosis. T2-weighted magnetic resonance imaging study showing multiple, discrete areas of increased signal intensity in white matter, particularly in the periventricular region. The patient, a 9-year-old boy, presented with intranuclear ophthalmoplegia, followed by an attack of left hemiparesis. Visual-evoked responses and somatosensory-evoked responses were abnormal. There were oligoclonal bands in the cerebrospinal fluid. The computed tomographic scan was normal. The youngster is currently asymptomatic. (Courtesy of Dr. Laura Flores de Sarnat, Instituto National de Pediatria, Mexico City.)

wave latency of the brainstem auditory-evoked response, or the central component latencies of somatosensory-evoked potentials are particularly likely to be abnormal in patients with MS (62). Sensitivity of the various tests for the diagnosis of MS is shown in Table 7.3.

Magnetic resonance imaging (MRI) is a sensitive and important diagnostic tool for demonstrating dissemination in space in children as well as in adults (63). Lesions are seen as round or elongated areas of increased signal with sharp margins in the periventricular white matter, less commonly in the brainstem on both proton-density and T2-weighted images. These lesions correspond to plaques, and it is believed that during the acute phase edema is responsible for the increased signal, whereas gliosis causes the abnormal signal during the chronic phase. Demyelinating lesions as small as 3 to 4 mm can be identified by MRI; most are asymptomatic (Fig. 7.2). The presence of gadolinium enhancement indicates that the lesion is acute and suggests an impairment of the blood–brain barrier, a consistent finding in new lesions. In the majority of instances, gadolinium enhancement does not persist beyond 3 to 5 weeks (64). MRI abnormalities are noted in 70% to 92% of patients with possible, probable, or definite MS. The criteria as established by Paty for the MRI-based diagnosis of MS of four or more lesions, are probably too stringent for the pediatric age group, since the specificity of the MRI findings declines with increasing age (65,65a).

These MRI characteristics of MS plaques tend to distinguish them from the T2-bright lesions of ADEM. The latter are typically more amorphous, less sharply defined, more likely to be centered on the inner margin of the cerebral cortical ribbon involving both white and gray matter, and less likely to show contrast enhancement. Symmetric and fairly extensive bilateral areas of abnormality involving gray or white matter may be found in some ADEM cases (66). On the other hand, lesions that closely resemble MS plaques may be produced by human T-cell lymphotropic virus (HTLV-1) infection (67), cerebral vasculitis (68), or certain neoplastic lesions. Parasitic lesions, brain abscesses, and metastatic lesions occasion-

TABLE 7.4. *Differential diagnosis for multiple sclerosis*

	Symptoms and signs	
	Recurrent unifocal	Multifocal
Acute disseminated encephalomyelitis	X	X
Angiomata	X	
Arachnopathy	X	X
Brain abscess/abscesses	X	X
Embolic disease	X	X
Granulomatous disease	X	X
Malignancy	X	X
Meningitis/meningo-encephalitis	X	X
Metabolic diseases	X	X
Migraine	X	
Mollaret encephalitis	X	
Orthopedic abnormalities	X	
Parasitic disease	X	X
Slow viral diseases	X	X
Syringomyelia/syringobulbia	X	
Vasculitides/vasculopathies	X	X

ally resemble MS plaques, but are less likely to be confused if edematous.

MRI of optic nerves and spinal cord with T2 weighting can disclose abnormalities in patients with MS-related manifestations suggesting disease in those locations (69,70). Proton MR spectroscopy has been performed in children with MS and could become an important means to follow the activity and progression of the disease (71).

Other causes of recurrent neurologic manifestations are summarized in Table 7.4. Differentiation of MS from ADEM can be difficult during the initial bout of demyelinating illness in prepubertal children. MS is more likely when there are recurrences, or when the initial bout or recurrence occurs after 12 years of age. The diagnosis of ADEM is much more likely in prepubertal patients in general, and the likelihood of ADEM becomes near certain if multifocal central neurologic dysfunction follows a clearly defined infectious prodrome or is accompanied by fever, constitutional symptoms, lethargy, disturbances of consciousness, seizures, or a movement disorder. The MS risk for patients with any of these manifestations is less than 10%.

Infectious, parainfectious or postinfectious, vasculitic, and granulomatous inflammatory

conditions are other conditions to be considered in the differential diagnosis of MS. Syphilis, Lyme encephalomyelitis/neuroborreliosis, cysticercosis, echinococcosis, toxoplasmosis, tropical spastic paraparesis (HTLV-1–associated myelopathy), SSPE, and progressive multifocal leukoencephalopathy also can show clinical fluctuation and tend to improve with immunosuppressive therapy. Almost all of the vasculitides also must be considered. The recurrent hemiplegic manifestations of moyamoya disease or mitochondrial disorders also can suggest MS. Certain chronic intoxications may resemble MS. These include toluene sniffing, subacute myeloopticoneuropathy, and chronic excessive use of barbiturates, diphenylhydantoin, or bromium.

Important factors in assigning diagnosis or estimating risk for ultimate diagnosis of MS are the child's age, clinical findings, distribution of changes on MRI scan, and the CSF immune profile. Based on our experience, the risk for MS for children younger than 12 years of age who have had a single bout of acute idiopathic demyelinating illness is less than 6%. The MS risk for children who have had one to three relapses of otherwise unexplained inflammatory demyelination before 12 years of age increases to 15% to 33%, with the remainder probably having a recurrent form of ADEM. Children with more than three recurrences before 12 years of age are more likely to have vasculitic or other inflammatory illnesses. A single bout of otherwise unexplained demyelinating illness in an individual older than 11.9 years of age implies at least a 50% risk for the diagnosis of MS within 9 years, whereas additional recurrences increase that risk to the range of 80% to 100%.

Failure to achieve clinical remission, especially in young patients, weighs against the diagnosis of MS. This last qualification includes patients who improve on corticosteroid therapy but cannot be weaned from that form of treatment without relapse. In such instances a vasculitic illness must be considered.

Treatment

Because MS is so variable in its manifestations and so unpredictable in its course, it is extremely difficult to evaluate the efficacy of the various proposed forms of therapy, and many patients show some clinical improvement after the introduction of a new agent, whatever its nature. It is clear that there is value in limiting or eliminating exacerbating circumstances such as heat or fatigue, improving nutrition and hydration, and preventing or promptly treating complications such as urinary tract infections. Appropriate forms of supportive treatment, including physical, occupational, and speech therapy, should be started.

Currently, initial bouts of MS and most relapses are generally treated with high doses of intravenous corticosteroids that should probably be followed by slowly tapering doses of oral corticosteroids (72). Although corticosteroids appear to shorten the latency to onset of improvement in individual bouts and may shorten the interval to full remission, it is less clear that they improve the degree of recovery and they do not significantly influence the long-term course of the disease (73).

If corticosteroid therapy is elected, it is our practice to administer intravenous corticosteroids, 10 to 20 mg/kg (maximum 1 g) as a single early morning dose for 3 to 5 days, followed by an oral taper (initially at 2 mg/kg per day, maximum 80 mg of prednisone or methylprednisolone) over the ensuing 3 weeks. In our experience, this form of management results in an onset of improvement within three days and sometimes within a few hours. We do not know whether intravenous administration of immunoglobulin (IVIG) confers any advantage. Side effects, notably meningismus or vomiting, are more common with immunoglobulin, and treatment is much more expensive. The effectiveness of plasmapheresis in childhood MS is still unproven (73a).

With more frequent or severe relapses, continuous immunomodulatory treatment is currently favored in the hope that one of these agents might modify the natural course of MS by minimizing ongoing disease activity, including subclinical disease progression, and preventing recurrences or the accumulation of deficits. Three choices are currently available: interferon-β (Betaseron), glycosylated interferon-β (Avonex), and a random polymerized mixture of myelin-related amino acids (glatirameracetate) (Copaxone). Limited data suggest that each may be beneficial, although as yet no rational guidelines exist for their use.

At present, many clinicians favor interferon-β for severe MS with frequent exacerbations and rapidly progressive disability (73b). It is administered on alternate days and relatively often gives rise to skin lesions at injection sites and provokes antibodies that can reduce efficacy. Glycosylated interferon-β may be preferable in children and adolescents because it is administered weekly and is less likely to generate the skin reactions. Alternatively, it is argued that copaxone may be the best drug for young patients with MS because it has few side effects and is well tolerated. However, daily subcutaneous injections are necessary.

When patients are intolerant of interferon-β, continuous treatment with azathioprine or cyclophosphamide may be considered. Cyclophosphamide should be reserved for those children or adolescents who exhibit severe, frequently relapsing MS with progressive disability, or who manifest a secondary chronic progressive demyelination. Continuous monthly bolus therapy, with or without induction, may be beneficial to some of the younger patients (74).

Other forms of therapy for severe MS include methotrexate, mitoxantrone, and 2-chlorodeoxyadenosine. Cyclosporin A provides no advantage over interferon-β, azathioprine, or cyclophosphamide and has little if any role in the treatment of the mild relapsing and remitting MS to which children and adolescents are subject.

Prognosis

The majority of children develops the relapsing-remitting form of MS, with most patients in this group being entirely well between relapses (55). Most authors consider childhood-onset MS to be less aggressive than its adult counterpart and adolescents who develop MS generally have a more favorable prognosis than individuals who develop MS at later ages (55,56).

Initial bouts of demyelination in children who are subsequently proven to have MS tend to last

6 to 10 weeks. This includes days to weeks of maximal affliction, which is shorter for patients with vague sensory and mild motor complaints than those with hemiparesis. It is longest for subjects with significant spinal cord syndrome, such as transverse myelitis, in whom improvement may require months to years. The manifestations most likely to remit completely include sensory changes, optic neuritis, and other abnormalities of cranial nerve function, whereas weakness and abnormalities of the cerebellar, dentatorubral, or autonomic systems are less likely to recover completely. It is possible that patients who would otherwise have recovered from their bout of spinal cord disease do not do so because swelling during the acute phase of illness has compromised regional circulation and therefore cord necrosis has occurred. As in adult patients, the recurrences of adolescents tend to be clinically similar to previous occurrences and patients with fixed deficits usually demonstrate worsening of those deficits with ensuing bouts, followed by recovery either to the preexisting level of deficit or to a somewhat lesser functional state. Perhaps one-fifth of recurrences manifests new signs or symptoms.

Some adolescent patients appear to have a form of MS that recurs for a number of bouts, followed by a prolonged period of quiescence during which the illness appears to partially or entirely burn out. Unusual courses include fulminant cases of acute MS that may cause death within weeks, to clinically silent MS discovered only at autopsy (75).

Less often childhood MS follows a chronic progressive pattern. The progressive form may present primarily, or more commonly secondarily, after several years of relapsing-remitting illness (76). Most progressive cases have myelopathic initial presentations with little recovery and slow rates of deterioration thereafter. Curiously, some children manifest an initial bout suggesting the diagnosis of MS but do not experience their second bout until 10 years or more have elapsed. The overall prognosis is not necessarily worse for individuals whose second bout occurs within a few weeks of the first.

Relapses may be provoked by acute febrile viral illnesses. Bacterial infections, typically involving the urinary tract of girls or women with MS, may provoke a relapse, but it is more likely that they worsen the degree of already existing disease activity. Although concerns have been expressed about the possibility that attenuated or live virus vaccines (hepatitis B, polio virus, and others) may initiate MS or provoke relapses, as yet no proof exists. Influenza vaccine does not appear to pose any risk.

Other factors that may be associated with a relapse include stress, physical trauma, and surgery. Spinal anesthesia can provoke relapse of MS, whereas epidural or inhalation anesthetics do not. As greater numbers of relapses occur, patients tend to recover less completely and deficits may become cumulative. As a rule, the longer a given bout lasts, the more likely that recovery will be incomplete.

Not all patients become significantly handicapped. Slightly more than one-third do not develop permanent disability of a degree sufficient to significantly impair personal or professional function. Perhaps 25% of adolescent-onset cases with a severe course develop significant permanent disability and a small fraction of these have a rapidly malignant course of deterioration culminating in early death. The remainder, perhaps 40% of cases, develop moderate permanently handicapping deficits. It is not clear what life-span can be expected of individuals who develop MS in childhood or adolescence.

Variants of Multiple Sclerosis

Three variants of MS that attracted considerable attention among neurologists of past generations are Schilder disease (myelinoclastic diffuse cerebral sclerosis), Balo disease (encephalitis periaxialis concentrica), and Devic disease (neuromyelitis optica).

Schilder Disease (Myelinoclastic Diffuse Cerebral Sclerosis, Encephalitis Periaxialis Diffusa)

Diffuse cerebral sclerosis was first described in 1912 by Schilder (77), who termed it *diffuse periaxial encephalitis*. In the intervening years, the term *Schilder disease* has become consider-

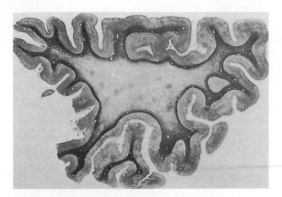

FIG. 7.3. Diffuse cerebral sclerosis. Myelin preparation of frontal lobe demonstrating demyelination. The arcuate fibers are characteristically spared. (Courtesy of the late Dr. D. B. Clark, University of Kentucky, Lexington.)

ably confused, in that two of Schilder's three original cases represented an adrenoleukodystrophy and SSPE. Also, Poser and van Bogaert (78), in analyzing the cases compiled by Bouman in his extensive monograph on the disease (79), found that more than one-half were leukodystrophies, perinatal encephalopathies, or subacute sclerosing encephalopathy. Schilder disease is now considered to be an inflammatory demyelinating disease of cerebral white matter of unknown etiology, possibly a variant of MS (80,81). The condition is distinguished by two features. First, a peculiar tendency exists to produce one or several often fairly symmetric large plaques of demyelination in the deep frontal central cerebral hemispheric white matter with sparing of the subcortical U-fibers and relative sparing of axis cylinders (81a). Second, there is an exquisite sensitivity to treatment with corticosteroids (81b).

In the sectioned brain, the most striking alteration is the gross demyelination of the central white matter. The plaques are fewer and larger than in MS, and their deep location with sparing of the gray–white junction distinguishes them from ADEM. The lesions are most common in the occipital lobe, but can involve any part of the cerebral hemispheres, brainstem, and cerebellum. Even in the most severely affected brain, a small band of subcortical white matter is usually spared (Fig. 7.3). The histopathology is indistin-

guishable from MS (81c) or ADEM, except a tendency to central necrosis and cavitation within large plaques exists.

The illness tends to present in children between the ages of 4 and 13 years. Onset is often subacute, with some combination of headache, lethargy, behavioral and intellectual disturbances, changes in personality, progressive clumsiness, or ataxia. Most cases exhibit hemiparesis or asymmetric double hemiparesis, variously combined with aphasia, visual disturbances, dysarthria, oropharyngeal dysfunction, bilateral pyramidal signs, ataxia, or pseudobulbar manifestations (81a,81d,81e). Increased intracranial pressure with papilledema is occasionally encountered. Unlike ADEM, there is usually no clear history of prodromal illness or fever.

The CSF protein is generally normal, as is the ratio of T-helper to T-suppressor cells. Oligoclonal bands are found in some samples (81c). The CT scan demonstrates extensive hypodense areas. The MRI shows massive single or multiple areas of demyelination in the subcortical white matter of the cerebral hemispheres. The typical large plaques are usually clearly visible as areas of intense bright signal on T2-weighted MRI. There is no special predilection for the periventricular area or the brainstem. Some lesions have a cystic appearance, with the edges enhancing with gadolinium (81a,81f).

Diagnosis

The subacute onset of focal neurologic signs and increased intracranial pressure initially suggests a space-occupying lesion. Neuroimaging studies exclude this diagnosis, however, and point to a demyelinating process. The diagnosis of diffuse cerebral sclerosis can be made with considerable certainty because no other demyelinating condition progresses with sufficient rapidity to produce massive cerebral edema. Adrenoleukodystrophy, which occasionally can progress relatively rapidly, can be distinguished by the presence of very-long-chain fatty acids in serum. In addition, ring enhancement on contrast administration distinguishes Schilder lesions from the demyelination observed in adrenoleukodystrophy, which is usually found in parieto-occipital white matter (81g). Occasionally, the diagnosis requires aspiration or stereotactic biopsy of a lesion to exclude abscess and tumor.

Treatment

Immunosuppression with corticosteroids or with a combination of cyclophosphamide and adrenocorticotropic hormone (ACTH) has been reported to induce rapid and unequivocal improvement in the majority of cases, with complete or nearly complete resolution of the MRI lesions (81d). In the series of Barth and coworkers, all five pediatric patients did well after corticosteroid therapy (81e).

The rapid early improvement of clinical manifestations and radiographic changes with the administration of corticosteroids is a characteristic feature of Schilder disease. Maximal recovery, however, may require weeks or months and can be incomplete. It is unclear whether corticosteroids merely promote earlier onset of recovery, exert some influence on duration and extent of maximal recovery, or prevent progression to MS. Although some uncertainty exists about dosage, it is likely true that high doses should be administered intravenously for 3 to 5 days followed by an oral taper. The MRI appearance usually improves, but abnormalities may persist for years, especially if there is necrosis and cavitation of a large lesion.

The majority of patients appears to experience prolonged remission after treatment. Occasionally, there are recurrences (81d). It is important to distinguish exacerbation caused by corticosteroid taper from true recurrences.

Encephalitis Periaxialis Concentrica (Balo Disease)

Encephalitis periaxialis concentrica (Balo disease) is now considered to be a variant of MS, the only distinguishing feature being the bizarre concentric zones of demyelination in central white matter (82). In the few reported cases, the clinical picture has been indistinguishable from that of ADEM. The diagnosis can be made by the characteristic findings on MRI (83).

Neuromyelitis Optica (Devic Disease)

Neuromyelitis optica is relatively rare in the western world but not uncommon in Asia (84). It is characterized clinically by optic neuritis and acute transverse myelitis (ATM) appearing simultaneously or within several weeks or months, with no neuroimaging evidence of white matter lesions in the brain, brainstem, or cerebellum. Pathologically, the process is particularly marked in white matter of the spinal cord and the optic nerves (85). MRI studies have confirmed the distribution of the lesions in brain and spinal cord (86,87). Probably neuromyelitis optica is a form of MS, modified by histocompatibility antigens or by one or more external factors. Long-term treatment with prednisone and azathioprine has been suggested (88).

ACUTE DISSEMINATED ENCEPHALOMYELITIS

ADEM is an immunologically mediated, acute inflammatory demyelinating disease marked by the onset of neurologic symptoms in close temporal relationship to a viral disease or immunization. As a rule, the condition occurs just once, or at the most, up to three times with its highest prevalence in prepubertal children. Only in a minority of these children does the disease either evolve into MS or prepubertal MS that closely resembles ADEM.

Historical Aspects

Illnesses recognizable as ADEM were first described in the late nineteenth century by Osler and others, who were particularly struck by the occasional child who showed remarkable recovery from severe, acute, multifocal encephalitic illnesses. Many cases occurred in association with epidemics of viral illnesses that spread through Europe in the wake of the First World War. The characteristic pathology was described almost simultaneously in the late 1920s and early 1930s in children who had died from

ADEM after measles, chickenpox, influenza, smallpox, and vaccinations (89).

Pathology

The cardinal pathologic features of ADEM are a relatively symmetric perivenular inflammatory infiltration and periaxial demyelination (i.e., destruction of myelin with relative preservation of nerve fiber axons) (90). These pathologic changes occur in a particular sequence. These stages are (a) venular hyperemia; (b) perivascular/subendothelial inflammatory cell infiltration and edema; (c) vascular necrosis; (d) demyelination with or without hemorrhage; and (e) astrocytic response with remyelination and gliosis.

The early inflammatory infiltrate is made up of polymorphonuclear leukocytes, but over time lymphocytes become predominant. As demyelinative changes occur, microglial cells become admixed with lymphocytes, as do phagocytes containing the lipid by-products of myelin degradation. Although microscopic changes resemble those of MS, as well as those of SSPE, the plaquelike areas of ADEM-related demyelination are macroscopically unlike those of MS. Meningeal inflammation also may be found. Severe cases may show disseminated hemorrhages, a syndrome that has been designated acute hemorrhagic encephalopathy (91–93).

Pathogenesis

A number of theories have been proposed to explain the mechanism and the target of the process that leads to demyelination in ADEM. These include (a) direct or indirect effects of virus within the nervous system; (b) nonspecific effects of vascular inflammation; (c) humoral (immune complex) mediation; and (d) cell-mediated immune mediation. The possible targets for injury include vascular endothelium, myelin, microglia, or oligodendrocytes. The last two are the least likely targets.

The notion that a viral infection of the nervous system induces ADEM is suggested by three lines of evidence: (a) occurrence of most cases in the setting of recent viral infection; (b) clinical and pathologic resemblance to the changes that occur in viral encephalitis; and (c) experimental induction of encephalomyelitis with viruses. Before widespread immunization, measles was the most common prodromal illness, with ADEM developing in 1 of 1,000 cases (94). ADEM arises as a complication of various other exanthematous diseases, notably rubella (95) and varicella. In approximately 10% of patients it is a manifestation of herpes simplex virus encephalitis (96). Infections with herpesvirus-6 infection, Epstein-Barr, and a variety of other viruses (97) can precede ADEM. In other instances, ADEM occurs in the wake of respiratory or gastrointestinal illnesses that are presumed to be viral; in these a specific viral agent is rarely identified.

ADEM can develop after vaccination with a wide variety of killed or attenuated organisms. These include rabies vaccines grown in brain or spinal cord (98), Japanese encephalitis (99), and influenza vaccines. Leptospiral, mycoplasmal, *Campylobacter*, and streptococcal infections also have been associated with ADEM (100–102).

Direct effects of virus within the nervous system could include viral killing of endothelial cells, resulting in an impairment of the blood–brain barrier, or injury to myelin or myelin-producing oligodendrocytes or other glial cells. These forms of injury also could be produced as "bystander effects" caused by immune responses directed at the virus within the nervous system (103,104). Thus, viruses might expose or alter CNS antigens to which an immune response would be directed.

The notion that vascular events are important in ADEM is based on the pathologic observation that subtle vascular changes precede the accumulation of an inflammatory perivenular exudate or demyelination. These changes are similar to those observed in serum sickness and immune-complex disease. In immune-complex disease insufficient antibody production and sustained antigen excess produce circulating immune complexes that become lodged in the vascular endothelium. This stimulates complement activation and release of vasoactive substances. Injury to vascular endothelial cells, particularly at the capillary level, may then result in blood–brain barrier impairment and result in extravasation of protein and fluids into the tissues. Blood–brain barrier changes also may expose antigens, permitting inflammatory response to be directed against otherwise immunologically privileged tissues. Early impairment of blood–brain barrier function has been demonstrated in EAE, as discussed previously. The blood–brain barrier changes are associated with reduced numbers of mitochondria and increased numbers of transcytotic vesicles within the capillary endothelium. These effects could be blocked, in some cases, by the administration of prazosin, an α_1-adrenoreceptor antagonist, possibly acting at the level of the capillary pericytes (105). The transcytotic vesicles are thought to be associated with the development of inflammatory edema.

Research has focused on the possible role of adhesion molecules, expressed on the surface of CNS capillaries, in mediation of the proposed vascular phase of immune dysregulation. Adhesion molecules may be capable of selectively recruiting inflammatory cells on the basis of sialyl moieties on the surface of the circulating cells. Such an interaction might have either positive or negative consequences depending on whether it results in clearance of regional infection or impaired blood–brain barrier function with inflammatory demyelination (106). Evidence has been advanced for the upregulated expression of adhesion molecules during experimental relapsing autoimmune dysregulation (107). This vascular concept has been advanced as a unifying concept (vasculinomyelopathies) for postinfectious neurologic illnesses of both the peripheral nervous system and CNS (108).

The possibility that ADEM is mediated by humoral immunity is supported by the fact that the illness is monophasic, multifocal, and may be provoked by a wide variety of antigenic precipitants (109). It is further supported by evidence for circulating immune complexes in at least some children with ADEM and by pathologic resemblance to immune-complex injury in other organ systems (110). Moreover, signs and symptoms suggesting immune-complex–mediated processes in other organ systems, such as myalgia, arthral-

gia, rash, proteinuria, and glomerulonephropathy, are found in many patients.

The role of cellular immunology in the pathogenesis of ADEM is supported by the similarity of the pathologic changes to EAE, which is believed to be a T-cell–mediated condition. The frequency of T-cell lines reacting to MBP is 10-fold higher in patients with ADEM as compared with healthy subjects or patients with viral encephalitis, with the IL-4 being the predominant cytokine secreted by these cell lines (110a).

One unifying hypothesis for the pathogenesis of ADEM suggests that viral antigens form a complex with phagocytic cells (macrophages or microglial cells) and T-helper cells (111). This so-called trimolecular complex then results in nonspecific T-cell activation, including clonal stimulation of cytotoxic T cells. These activated cells then enter the CNS either because of the vascular changes induced by the interaction of T cells with microvascular adhesion molecules, because the increased numbers of circulating autoreactive T cells overwhelm some threshold that normally contains the activity of cellular-mediated immunity, or because T cells engage in regular traffic into the nervous system as part of host immune surveillance. These clones of stimulated cells attack one of the targets noted previously (i.e., an exposed antigen, myelin, or a particular CNS cellular population). The myelin injury thus produced may be nonspecific ("bystander effect") (112). Thus, the occurrence of ADEM appears to require the conjunction of genetically determined susceptibility (cellular immune locus) with sufficient antigenic stimulus and other poorly understood conditions.

Clinical Manifestations

Typical cases of ADEM arise 2 to 20 days after a febrile childhood illness, although some 15% to 20% of cases have no clearly defined prodrome (113–115a). ADEM is more common in winter months, a period during which childhood respiratory and gastrointestinal viral illnesses tend to be particularly prevalent. The mean age at presentation is 7.4 years. The male to female ratio is approximately 1.3:1 and the white to black ratio may be as high as 6:1.

Typically, children recovering from the viral prodrome abruptly develop irritability and lethargy. In the Turkish series of Apak and coworkers, ataxia was the most common presenting complaint, followed by optic neuritis, cranial nerve palsies, and seizures (115a). Most children are febrile during prodrome; fever at onset of ADEM is variable. Occasionally, ADEM may occur after a prolonged fever of unknown origin. Over the course of minutes to days, diffuse neurologic signs develop. Changes in mental status and long tract signs are commonly observed in ADEM.

Diagnosis

Evaluation of children with ADEM is aimed primarily at excluding other causes of diffuse CNS dysfunction, particularly intoxications, infections, and such vasculitic conditions as systemic lupus erythematosus (SLE). MRI is the diagnostic test of choice, demonstrating discrete areas of increased signal on T2 weighting, particularly at the gray-white junction (66,116). ADEM most commonly shows plaquelike lesions throughout the neuraxis; unlike MS plaques, the margins are often indistinct and they tend to be found at the gray-white junction more commonly than in periventricular white matter. Lesions in brainstem and cerebellum are not uncommon, and many of the lesions have no clear clinical concomitant. Rarely, symmetric, linear, posteriorly emphasized white matter changes on T2 weighting suggestive of leukodystrophy are found in ADEM. The clinical course usually distinguishes ADEM from tumor or leukodystrophy, but not necessarily from SLE. ADEM rarely affects the hearing or causes pseudobulbar changes; where these are found, leukodystrophy is more likely.

ADEM may be either associated with or in some cases confused with Lyme disease, acquired immunodeficiency syndrome, and tropical spastic paraparesis (see Chapter 6). Where appropriate, specific serologic studies should be undertaken. A few cases have been mistaken for diffuse metazoa or parasitic diseases, such as cysticercosis. The absence of any considerable degree of edema usually distinguishes ADEM from tumor or parasitic disease.

When spinal manifestations predominate, MRI of spine with T2 weighting often distinguishes the acute presentation of an extramedullary tumor, stroke, or hemorrhage. Some cases of ADEM with prominent myelitis have peripheral nerve signs, representing clinical overlap with GBS. This overlap is particularly prominent in patients with acquired immunodeficiency syndrome. Tumors with involvement of the cauda equina or nerve roots also must be considered.

The electroencephalography (EEG) results can be normal and can exhibit disturbances of normal sleep rhythms and slowing during the waking state in patients with the early stages of ADEM, a finding that helps to distinguish ADEM from MS (115a). In the experience of one of us (R.S.R.), the absence of such EEG abnormalities during the first bout of acute disseminated demyelinating illness in a child significantly increases the risk for the ultimate diagnosis of MS. CSF immune studies are positive in a minority of cases of ADEM; MBP is more frequently elevated. Moderate elevations of these studies occur in some children with monosymptomatic ADEM (117); strongly positive results are seen in SSPE, neurosyphilis, neuroborreliosis, and in some cases of heritable leukodystrophy.

Treatment

Given abundant evidence for immune-mediation of ADEM, it is quite logical to consider anti-inflammatory therapy. Many agents have been used, including corticosteroids, ACTH, IVIG, and cyclosporine. Corticosteroid treatment is the most common therapy, and most patients appear to be responsive (115a,118). Often clinical response is observable within hours of initiation of intravenous corticosteroids, particularly after high intravenous doses (15 to 20 mg/kg of methylprednisolone). Unfortunately, no systematic data exist regarding appropriate dosage or length of therapy. Corticosteroid dependency, similar to that observed in some patients with GBS, may occur during the taper of corticosteroids. These children usually respond well to a slower taper, but a few chronic relapsing cases, resembling MS, are seen in young children who may require corticosteroid therapy for many months or years.

In cases resistant to high doses of corticosteroids, IVIG or cyclosporine may be tried. Patients in coma from ADEM have been successfully treated with plasma exchange or plasmapheresis (119).

Prognosis

The outlook for recovery is generally excellent. Although some older series suggest up to 10% mortality, in the experience of one of us (R.S.R.) only 1.5% of our 60 cases died of ADEM-related complications. Recovery is unrelated to severity of illness, and complete recovery may be observed even in children who become blind, comatose, and quadriparetic. Recovery is poorest in children younger than age 2 years, a population in whom long-term motor and intellectual deficits are fairly common.

OPTIC NEURITIS

The term *optic neuritis* refers to a variety of lesions of one or both optic nerves, be they inflammatory, toxic, or demyelinating, that share a clinical picture of diminution of visual acuity. When optic neuritis develops during childhood it is more likely to be bilateral. In part, this tendency might reflect the ability of small children to ignore unilateral vision loss, even though it has developed abruptly.

Clinical Manifestations

In most children symptoms appear suddenly, and in approximately 70% they follow an acute infectious illness, notably exanthematous diseases such as measles, mumps, and varicella (120–123). Vision loss can occur over a few hours or days and can progress to complete blindness in days. In some instances, one eye becomes affected a few days or weeks after the other. In a minority, vision loss develops over weeks to months. The patient can experience headache or pain when moving the eyes, but clear-cut neurologic deficits are rare, although some patients can have transient extensor plan-

tar responses. Involvement is bilateral in approximately 60% of children (124,125). In the vast majority of children, more than 90% in the series of Meadows (126) and 76% in the Finnish series of Riikonen and colleagues (125), the appearance of the disc is abnormal, with swelling and hemorrhages, a picture that at times is indistinguishable from that seen in papilledema. In papilledema, the visual field defect is minimal, however, usually an enlargement of the blind spot, whereas in optic neuritis the field defect is extensive, usually a central scotoma. When the optic nerve is involved proximal to the optic disc, the fundus appears normal (retrobulbar neuritis). Striking abnormalities, including fiber layer hemorrhages at the optic nerve margin, vascular tortuosity, or sheathing of veins are readily observable on funduscopy in many cases (125). vision loss may be preceded by headache (frontal or ocular), scintillating scotomata, or by painful eye movements.

The frequency with which optic neuritis in the pediatric age group is an antecedent to MS varies widely from one series to the other. In the Mayo Clinic series of Lucchinetti and colleagues, 26% of subjects who had experienced optic neuritis before 16 years of age developed MS by age 40 (127). Approximately one-half of the children developed frank MS within 1 year of their optic neuritis (127). The risk for MS with unilateral optic neuritis was less than for simultaneous bilateral optic neuritis, and only 5% of children with unilateral optic neuritis went on to develop MS (127). This is in contrast to data on adult patients, in whom unilateral optic neuritis is followed by MS in up to 87% (124–126). When bilateral optic neuritis is sequential, that is if the second eye is involved more than 2 weeks after the first eye, the likelihood for MS is approximately 50%. The presence of abnormal MRI results and oligoclonal bands in the CSF is particularly ominous in that more than 80% of patients demonstrating the oligoclonal bands go on to develop full-blown MS (128,129). The complaint of transient blurring of vision with exertion (Uhthoff symptom) also correlates with early development of MS (130). In unilateral optic neuritis, visual-evoked potentials and, to a lesser extent, MRI can demonstrate abnormalities in the apparently unaffected optic nerve (131).

Diagnosis

The diagnosis of optic neuritis is made on the basis of a combination of clinical and laboratory findings. In subtle cases, diagnosis can be clinically supported by loss of red-vision (*red desaturation*), or by loss of duration or variety of the *flight of colors* that occurs when the eye is closed after a period of bright illumination of the retina. When greater visual impairment occurs, loss of the reflexive constriction of the contralateral pupil occurs when the retina of the affected eye is illuminated. Visual-evoked responses (VERs) are particularly useful where the diagnosis is uncertain; optic neuritis results in increased latency of the positive component of this cortical response (132). This delay in VER may persist for several years in patients who have shown excellent clinical recovery. MRI demonstrates swelling of the optic nerve in most cases; the extent of optic nerve enlargement may be alarming in some children who experience good recovery (133). Imaging also excludes lesions that compress the optic nerve and result in vision loss. Disseminated bright lesions on T2-weighted images may be found by MRI elsewhere in brain in as many as 70% of patients (125). In children these lesions do not necessarily indicate MS, and their interpretation is difficult. Where such abnormalities are at the gray-white junction and the patients are younger, they suggest ADEM; periventricular plaques in adolescents are more indicative of MS. SSPE, intoxications (e.g., methanol), leukodystrophies, and stroke must occasionally be considered. Malingering may be excluded on the basis of inconsistencies on clinical examination or by VER testing.

Treatment and Prognosis

No clear-cut evidence indicates that oral or intravenous corticosteroid therapy is of any benefit. Intravenous methylprednisolone has been recommended for patients whose visual acuity is worse than 20/40 (134). These recommendations, based on experience with adult patients with mainly uniocular disease, may not be applicable to children who have generally bilateral disease, and it is not known whether corticosteroids affect the natural history of the disease in the pediatric population (135). In adult populations, treatment with intravenous methylprednisolone does not affect visual outcome although it appears to speed recovery from acute exacerbations (136).

Although recovery may be slow (137), the prognosis of childhood optic neuritis, particularly when it is bilateral, is excellent, and the overwhelming majority of children recover vision completely within weeks or months. The most common residua include optic nerve atrophy and impairments of color and stereoscopic vision (138). Permanent severe vision loss is quite exceptional.

ACUTE TRANSVERSE MYELITIS

ATM is characterized by the sudden onset of rapidly progressive weakness of the lower extremities, accompanied by loss of sensation and sphincter control, and often preceded by a respiratory infection. The condition has been recognized for more than 100 years; an excellent description of the clinical picture is that of Gowers in 1886 (139). Before then, many diseases of the spinal cord were termed *myelitis*; only subsequent to the description of MS by Cruveilhier, tabes by Duchenne, Todd, and Romberg, and syringomyelia by Gull and Hallopeau, did this entity gain recognition. Its first description in this century is that by Foix and Alajouanine (140).

Pathology and Pathogenesis

ATM is an acute disorder that presents with CNS dysfunction referable to a discrete portion of the rostrocaudal extent of the spinal cord and involving tracts on both sides of the cord.

The condition occurs in association with a number of factors. These include such autoimmune diseases as GBS, ADEM, or MS, bacterial, viral, or spirochetal infections, notably Lyme disease, and vascular malformations.

On pathologic examination, the spinal cord is generally softened, with the most striking changes occurring in the thoracolumbar region. The lesion can be focally transverse or can extend over several cord segments. In the affected area, the spinal cord is often completely necrotic; all nervous elements are lost, replaced by a cellular infiltrate or by cavitation. Microscopic examination shows perivenular inflammatory changes with demyelination, closely resembling those of ADEM; in severe cases myeloclasia with cavitation is seen.

Although the exact pathogenesis is unknown, in most cases a cell-mediated autoimmune response is believed responsible. This concept is supported by the observation that lymphocytes from 70% of transverse myelitis patients responded to bovine MBP and to human peripheral nerve myelin P2 protein (141). In some instances, the acute onset of symptoms and the distribution of the clinical and pathologic deficits suggest that the vascular supply to the spinal cord has been compromised, possibly as a result of an occlusion of the anterior spinal artery caused by an autoimmune or postinfectious vasculitis (142,143).

Clinical Manifestations

Transverse myelitis can occur in isolation or in association with or as a sequel to a multiplicity of conditions. These include herpes simplex and herpes zoster, Epstein-Barr virus, the echoviruses, hepatitis B virus, influenza, Lyme disease, *Mycoplasma pneumoniae*, and the various exanthematous diseases, notably measles, mumps, and varicella (144–146). It also can be seen after rabies or tetanus toxoid immunization, in conjunction with SLE, and with the antiphospholipid syndrome, and after *Mycoplasma pneumoniae* infections (147,148). Approximately two-thirds of affected children have a history of a recent or a concurrent acute infection, and the condition has been noted to cluster around the summer months (142,149). The presence or absence of an infection does not alter the clinical course of the disease. Occasionally, cases are preceded by relatively trivial blunt trauma to the spine.

Most cases occur in children older than 5 years of age (150). The earliest symptom is sensory loss or pain in the back, extremities, or abdomen (151). This symptom is followed by a rapidly progressive paraparesis, which usually involves the legs, but occasionally can ascend to affect legs and arms sequentially. Fever is present in approximately one-half of the children, and neck stiffness in approximately one-third. At first, the weakness is flaccid, but gradually evidence of pyramidal tract involvement can be elicited with spasticity, increased deep tendon reflexes, ankle clonus, and extensor plantar responses that usually become obvious by the end of the second week of illness (142). Sphincter tone was lost in 86% of cases in the Australian series of Dunne and coworkers (149); sensory impairment, usually with a well-defined level, can be documented in most instances (in 80% of cases in the series of Paine and Byers) (142).

The onset of paraplegia, sensory loss, and sphincter dysfunction may develop over days to weeks or have a paroxysmal onset over hours. In more than one-half of patients, the maximum deficit occurs within 3 days of the onset of symptoms (149). As a rule, the rate of onset is often proportional to the intensity of the initial discomfort. Intense pain may foreshadow hyperacute presentation with abrupt and severe onset of myelitis. Cervical ATM can compromise breathing and may occasionally present in cardiopulmonary arrest. Rarely, ATM presents with the isolated complaint of urinary retention (152).

In all cases the neurologic examination should be directed at detecting bilateral weakness and a sensory level. The weakness is initially flaccid and the involved extremities may be areflexic. Pyramidal tract signs such as increased tendon reflexes and extensor plantar reflexes develop after a number of days. Superficial reflexes (abdominal, cremasteric, bulbocavernosis) are usually absent. In most children who can be examined adequately, pain and temperature sensations are affected primarily, whereas posterior column function (vibration and proprioception) is generally spared. A sensory level is present in almost all cases and is best determined in children by examining cold sensation. The sensory level is located between T5 and T10. In approximately 20% of patients it is located in the cervical region, and in 5% to 10% in the lumbar region (149,151). Maximal deficits occur in hours to days in hyperacute and acute cases, and days to weeks in subacute cases.

Approximately one-half of affected children have pleocytosis and an elevated protein content in the CSF. CSF MBP is elevated in postinfectious cases (142,151,153). Although many times neuroimaging is normal, MRI demonstrates enlargement of the cord in approximately one-half of the cases (146), and increased signal on T2-weighted MRI with gadolinium enhancement has been noted in a few cases (154). MRI scanning of the head may disclose clinically silent T2 bright lesions (155); the significance of such findings in children is uncertain and, as in optic neuritis, should not necessarily indicate a diagnosis of MS.

Diagnosis

ATM should be distinguished from acute infectious polyneuritis and from spinal cord symptoms caused by a space-occupying lesion. The diagnosis of acute polyneuritis is not easy, particularly in the small child, whose sensory examination is not reliable. In acute polyneuritis, loss of pain sensation is generally not as complete as it is in transverse myelitis, and proprioception is the sensory modality most involved. Loss of sphincter function and the appearance of clear-cut pyramidal tract signs argue strongly for ATM. Neither electric studies nor examination of the CSF are of much assistance in the differential diagnosis, although abnormal visual-evoked responses suggest the diagnosis of MS (149). Linssen and colleagues believe that an elevation of CSF MBP argues for the diagnosis of ATM (153). If the posterior columns are interrupted, somatosensory-evoked potentials with lower limb stimulation are abolished. In the experience of Wilmshurst and colleagues, electrophysiologic evidence for anterior horn cell involvement is associated with poor recovery (156). ATM also should be differentiated from compressive injuries, arteri-

ovenous malformations, hemorrhage, stroke, and radiation injury. Tropical spastic paraparesis, a progressive myelopathy caused by HTLV-1 infection, does occur in children, and may produce MRI changes indistinguishable from ATM, although the changes may be disseminated throughout the cord (see Chapter 6). The progression of neurologic symptoms in HTLV-1 is generally much slower than that of ATM.

Treatment and Prognosis

Treatment with high-dose (1 g/1.73 m^2) intravenous methylprednisolone may be effective in children with ATM (157). In the experience of Lahat and colleagues, published in 1998, all of 10 children treated in this manner within 5 to 16 days of the onset of symptoms had a good outcome or were normal (158). Other studies, however, have not found any significant effect on the outcome of the illness (149).

The prognosis of ATM in children is usually good. Approximately 60% of patients have good return of function, and only 15% fail to show any significant improvement. Return of function usually starts within 1 month; in the series of Dunne and colleagues (149), it began between 2 and 17 days after the onset of symptoms and was essentially complete by 6 months. Dunne and coworkers and Wilmshurst and colleagues found that the more acute the onset of the myelitis, the worse the outcome (149,156). Whereas some 20% of adult patients with transverse myelitis ultimately develop MS, children do not. In a retrospective Canadian study, only 3% of MS patients whose symptoms became apparent before 16 years of age had presented with transverse myelitis (50). Normal cranial MRI and normal visual-evoked potentials tend to exclude the diagnosis of MS. These study results are positive in almost all patients who go on to develop MS after an attack of transverse myelitis.

ACUTE CEREBELLAR ATAXIA

Acute cerebellar ataxia is a relatively common condition that was first described by Batten in 1907 (159). It is characterized by the sudden onset of ataxia, often after a nonspecific infectious illness.

Pathology and Etiology

Because acute cerebellar ataxia is not a fatal condition, its pathology is unknown. The cause of the condition is probably heterogeneous, with a number of infectious agents being directly or indirectly responsible. Cases after infection with polio virus type 1, influenza A, and influenza B have been reported. In other patients, echovirus type 9 (160) and coxsackievirus type B have been isolated from CSF. Ataxia with an acute onset and an identical clinical picture also is seen after a variety of exanthematous diseases, most commonly varicella, less often rubella (161,162). Acute and transient cerebellar ataxia can be the presenting symptom of childhood MS also (see Table 7.1).

The association of acute cerebellar ataxia with occult neuroblastoma has been observed on numerous occasions (163,164). One can, therefore, conclude that in some instances acute cerebellar ataxia is caused by direct viral invasion of the cerebellum, whereas in others it is the result of an autoimmune response to a variety of agents. It also is uncertain whether the site of injury within the nervous system is neuronal or whether fiber tracts are affected.

Clinical Manifestations

Acute cerebellar ataxia is seen in children of all ages, although in the experience of Weiss and Carter (165), it occurred most commonly between 1 and 2 years of age. By definition, the onset of ataxia is always acute, although approximately one-half of the children experience a nonspecific infectious illness within 3 weeks before the onset of neurologic symptoms (165). In the largest reported series, acute cerebellar ataxia was preceded by varicella in 26%. Epstein-Barr virus infections were seen in 2.6% (166). In 49% other presumed viral illnesses occurred, with respiratory illnesses more common than gastrointestinal. There was no prodrome in 19.2%, and 2.6% developed acute cerebellar ataxia after immunization.

The clinical picture is marked by severe truncal ataxia resulting in rapid deterioration of gait. Hypotonia and tremor of the extremities, head, and trunk are seen less often. Nystagmus is encountered in 45% of patients, whereas a number of other children have sudden random motions of the eyes during voluntary movements. Speech is often affected. Other neurologic signs are usually absent, although headache, dizziness, photophobia, and myoclonic movements of the head and arms have been reported occasionally. Brainstem signs are present occasionally. Constitutional symptoms, including fever, are absent, and nuchal rigidity is rare.

The CSF is usually normal, although a mild pleocytosis is found in 25% of cases (165,167). The CSF protein content can be normal on initial taps but may become elevated late in the course of the illness (165). Neuroimaging studies have shown swelling of the cerebellum, and a transiently increased signal in the cerebellar cortex or the brainstem (168,169,170). When MRI abnormalities are confined to the brainstem, the condition resembles brainstem encephalitis, except that in the latter disease cerebellar symptoms are accompanied by clinical evidence of widespread CNS involvement. The SPECT scan has shown decreased blood flow to the cerebellum (171).

In the majority of cases, the disease is self-limiting. In approximately two-thirds of children, the ataxia clears completely, with an average duration of cerebellar signs of approximately 2 months. Some mildly affected children recover completely within 1 week. Nearly 90% of children recover completely over weeks to months. More than 2 months are required for recovery of 18% to 33% of children with viral prodromata, and 50% of those without prodromata. Persistence of major neurologic deficits is noted in approximately one-third of children. These deficits include ataxia of trunk and extremities, speech impairment, mental retardation, and behavioral abnormalities.

One of us (J.H.M.) has encountered at least two children whose cerebellar ataxia recurred over several years, with exacerbations often preceded by a mild respiratory illness. These bouts could be distinguished from the aggravation of ataxia expected in any uncoordinated patient experiencing an acute febrile episode. Both patients were left with mental retardation.

Diagnosis

Acute cerebellar ataxia is diagnosed by excluding other conditions that produce sudden onset of ataxia. The most important of these are the posterior fossa tumors, occult neuroblastoma, acute labyrinthitis, and drug intoxications. Although the onset of ataxia in a posterior fossa tumor is rarely sudden, imaging studies to exclude a mass lesion are indicated. The presence of papilledema and a history of headache or vomiting point to a posterior fossa tumor.

Catecholamine metabolites, notably homovanillic acid and vanillylmandelic acid, are excreted in amounts higher than normal by patients harboring a neuroblastoma. Analysis of urinary homovanillic acid and vanillylmandelic acid can be done on random and 24-hour urine collections. Tuchman and coworkers analyzed random urine specimens in a large series of patients, with no false-positive and some 7% false-negative results (172).

In a significant percentage of children who develop MS, ataxia is the first sign of the disease. Diagnostic studies to exclude this entity are therefore indicated.

Ataxia can develop in the course of acute viral diseases of the CSF, notably varicella, mumps, and poliomyelitis. The distinction between these cases and the usual cases of acute cerebellar ataxia is difficult and might well be semantic (i.e., if a causative agent can be proven, the condition is termed *cerebellar encephalitis*, but otherwise it is termed *acute cerebellar ataxia of unknown cause*).

Acute labyrinthitis (vestibular neuronitis or epidemic vertigo) is not easily distinguished from ataxia, particularly in an uncooperative youngster. It is usually associated with nausea, intense vertigo, and abnormal tests of labyrinthine function (173), particularly an absence of caloric responses (174,175).

Acute cerebellar ataxia also can be seen after the ingestion of a variety of toxins, particularly alcohol, thallium, and organic mercurials (see Chapter 9).

Acute cerebellar ataxia, often precipitated by a respiratory infection, accompanies a number of metabolic disorders, including various mitochondrial disorders, Hartnup disease, and the intermittent forms of maple syrup urine disease (see Chapter 1). Recurrent attacks of ataxia can be transmitted as a dominant trait. Two forms of this condition have been delineated, with defects in the voltage-gated potassium channel gene, and one of the calcium channel genes, respectively. These entities have been reviewed by Baloh and colleagues (176) and are covered more extensively in Chapter 2.

Ataxia also can develop as a consequence of heatstroke, a result of hyperthermia-induced cerebellar degeneration (177).

Some children with minor motor seizures suddenly develop ataxia that probably results from frequent transitory impairment of consciousness. EEG signs of a seizure disorder should readily distinguish this entity.

Ataxia associated with the various cerebellar degenerations develops gradually and should cause little diagnostic confusion. Apparent ataxia can be the consequence of generalized weakness (e.g., in acute infectious polyneuritis). In acute cerebellar ataxia, hypotonia is associated with normal or increased deep tendon reflexes, whereas in polyneuritis, the reflexes are reduced or absent.

Treatment

Acute cerebellar ataxia is a self-limiting disease, and no specific treatment, including adrenocortical corticosteroids, has been found convincingly effective.

OPSOCLONUS-MYOCLONUS SYNDROME (MYOCLONIC ENCEPHALOPATHY)

A syndrome of myoclonic encephalopathy has been noted in infants and young children (178) (Kinsbourne syndrome). It is characterized by acute or subacute onset of polymyoclonus, often after a respiratory infection, cerebellar ataxia, and a chaotic irregularity of eye movements in which the globes are in a state of constant agitation with rapid and unequal movements that usually take place in the horizontal plane (opsoclonus). The abnormal eye movements are most prominent at the onset of each attempt to alter the position of the eyes. In addition to opsoclonus, shock-like myoclonic contractions persist when the affected part is at rest and produce total disorganization of willed movements. In approximately one-half of patients this entity represents a post-infectious process, and thus is related to acute cerebellar ataxia. In the remainder it is a neuroimmunologic complication of neural crest tumors, most commonly, neuroblastoma (179).

IgM and IgG autoantibodies from sera derived from patients with myoclonic encephalopathy, regardless of its cause, bind to cerebellar Purkinje cells' cytoplasm and axons. A high-molecular-weight subunit of neurofilaments appears to be one of the major targets (179).

The condition is self-limiting, and in a substantial proportion of children, corticosteroids induce a dramatic improvement (164). Nevertheless, the long-term outcome is not totally favorable, and more than one-half of the children are left with intellectual deficits and abnormalities in motor performance, speech, and behavior (164,180).

In some 50% of patients with myoclonic encephalopathy, a malignant tumor can be demonstrated, most commonly a neuroblastoma. The tumor is often inapparent at the onset of the illness and is uncovered only after persistent diagnostic studies (181). Palpation of the abdomen, rectal examination, and tomography or ultrasonography of the chest and abdomen are the most useful procedures. In the experience of Boltshauser and coworkers, bone marrow examinations, skeletal surveys, and urinary vanillylmandelic acid (VMA) assays were rarely helpful (164).

The clinical course, response to corticosteroid therapy, and long-term prognosis of myoclonic encephalopathy associated with neuroblastoma are the same as in children with myoclonic encephalopathy who do not harbor a tumor. For reasons as yet unknown, the survival rate of children with myoclonic encephalopathy and neuroblastoma is far better than that of the general population of children with neuroblas-

toma (180,182). Aside from neuroblastoma, myoclonic encephalopathy has many other causes. In the majority of cases, the syndrome is caused by a viral infection, notably polio virus, coxsackievirus B3, and St. Louis encephalitis virus (183) (see Chapter 6). Intracranial tumors, various intoxications, and hydrocephalus are other, considerably rarer, causes.

SPASMUS NUTANS

Spasmus nutans is an unusual, but generally benign, condition described in 1897 by Raudnitz (184). It commences in late infancy (aged 1 to 15 months), often in late winter or early spring, and is marked by anomalous head positions, head nodding, and small-amplitude, rapid nystagmus, which can be conjugate, dysconjugate, or uniocular (185). When visual targets such as a picture book are presented, children start to nod or the amplitude of the nystagmus becomes larger. Straightening the tilted head or fixing the head also increases the amplitude of the nystagmus. For these reasons, Gottlob and colleagues believe that head nodding is compensatory to the nystagmus (186). Neuroimaging studies are invariably normal. The condition is self-limiting, clearing after a period of 4 months to several years and is unassociated with any visual deficits. In most children a subclinical nystagmus persists for many years (187). In the majority of instances the cause remains unknown; it might be the sequel to a viral illness (188,189). For unknown reasons, the condition appears to be far more common in the eastern United States than in the southwest of the country.

Spasmus nutans should be differentiated from congenital nystagmus, in that the latter usually starts before 6 months of age, and that visual acuity is abnormal in approximately 90% of children with congenital nystagmus.

An increasing number of reports have linked spasmus nutans to gliomas of the optic nerve and chiasm (190). In other cases, the condition has been associated with arachnoid or porencephalic cysts (191). MRI studies of the optic nerves and of the CNS, therefore, are indicated.

IMMUNOLOGICALLY MEDIATED DISEASES AFFECTING CENTRAL NERVOUS SYSTEM GRAY MATTER

Rheumatic Fever (Sydenham Chorea)

The principal neurologic manifestation of rheumatic fever is Sydenham chorea (chorea minor; for many years the term *chorea magna* was used to designate chorea of hysterical nature). This condition was first defined by Sydenham in 1684 (192).

> Chorea Sancti Viti is a sort of Convulsion, which chiefly invades Boys and Girls, from ten Years of Age to Puberty: First it shews its self by a certain Lameness, or rather Instability of one of the Legs, which the Patient drags after him like a Fool; afterward it appears in the hand of the same side; which he that is affected with this Disease, can by no means keep in the same Posture for one moment, if it be brought to the Breast, or any other Part, but it will be distorted to another Position or Place by a certain Convulsion, let the Patient do what he can. If a Cup of Drink be put into his Hand he represents a thousand Gestures, like Juglers, before he brings it to his Mouth in a right line, his Hand being drawn hither and thither by the Convulsion, he turns it often about for some time, till at length happily raching his Lips, he flings it suddenly into his Mouth, and drinks it greedily, as if the poor Wretch designed only to make sport. For as much as this Disease seems to me to proceed from some Humour rushing in upon the Nerves, which provoke such Preternatural Motions, I think the curative Indications are first to be directed to the lessening of those Humours by bleeding and purging, and then to the strengthening the Genus Nervosum, in order to which I use this method: I take seven Ounces of Blood from the Arm, more or less, according the Age of the Patient; the next Day I prescribe half, or somewhat more, (according to the Age, or the more or less disposition of the Body to bear purging) of the common purging Potion above-described, of Tamarinds, Sena etc. In the Evening I give the following Draught:
>
> Take of Black-cherry-water one Ounce, of Langius's Epileptick-water three Drachms, of old Venice-Treacle one Scruple, of Liquid Laudanum eight Drops; make a Draught.

Etiology and Pathology

The relationship of Sydenham chorea to rheumatic fever was first suggested by Stoll in 1780 (193) and gained general acceptance by the medical profession in the nineteenth century. Most cases of chorea are preceded by a streptococcal infection or rheumatic fever; however, the interval between the bacterial infection and the onset of neurologic symptoms is between 2 and 7 months, so that in one study, serologic evidence of the streptococcal infection was no longer demonstrable in 27% of the children who had chorea as the only clinical manifestation of rheumatic disease (194). In approximately one-third of choreic patients, rheumatic heart disease or other major manifestations of rheumatic fever develop after the onset of chorea (195). Conversely, Sydenham chorea has been seen in approximately one-third of rheumatic fever cases (196). In a series of patients from Brazil, reported in 1997, chorea was seen in 26% (197).

Using immunofluorescent staining techniques, Husby and coworkers demonstrated that sera from 46% of children with Sydenham chorea contain IgG antibodies that react with neuronal cytoplasmic antigens located preferentially in the region of the caudate and subthalamic nuclei. Staining of neurons probably represents a cross-reaction between neuronal cytoplasm and antigens present in the membrane of group A streptococci. These antibodies are less prevalent and are of lower titer in children with active rheumatic fever without chorea and in control subjects (198). Antiphospholipid antibodies are found in some 80% of patients with Sydenham chorea. It is not known whether these antibodies contribute to the pathogenesis of the condition or whether they merely reflect stimulation by the streptococcal M protein of T-cells directed against self-antigens (199).

Genetic factors also operate in inducing rheumatic fever. A family history of rheumatic fever can be elicited in 26% of choreic patients, and Sydenham chorea is found in 3.5% of parents and in 2.1% of siblings of choreic patients

(195). Emotional trauma also can be important in the development of chorea, for the onset of neurologic symptoms is sometimes closely correlated with experiences that cause obvious psychic trauma (200,201).

Neuropathologic studies have been singularly uninformative. The few persons who have died during the illness, often because of other rheumatic manifestations, have shown an arteritis with a mild perivascular cellular infiltration and a diffuse loss of nerve cells not only from the basal ganglia, but also from the cortex and cerebellum. No typical Aschoff bodies have been found in the brain (202).

These findings do not explain the pathophysiology of chorea, and it has been postulated that immunoglobulin or complement deposition on cells within the basal ganglia alters the metabolism of various neurotransmitters.

Clinical Manifestations

Up to the last 10 to 20 years, Sydenham chorea had become a rare condition in the western world (203); in the 1980s and 1990s the number of cases of acute rheumatic fever increased greatly. This increase has occurred against a backdrop of no particular increase in the rate of group A streptococcal pharyngitis. The microbiological and host reasons for this resurgence are not completely understood; they are reviewed by Kaplan (204). In part, the resurgence is believed to result from the appearance of certain serologic types of group A streptococci that produce pyrogenic exotoxin, particularly toxin A, which had been uncommon for many years. In a 1987 report from Ohio, some 17% of children with acute rheumatic fever presented with choreic manifestations. Many of these patients came from middle- or upper-middle-class homes, making invalid the previously noted predisposition for occurrence in low-income groups and crowded housing (205).

The condition begins between ages 3 and 13 and is somewhat more common in girls. In the Brazilian series the mean age of onset was 9.2 years, and the female to male ratio was 1.16:1 (197). An adage, cited by Wilson (206), is that the child with Sydenham chorea is punished

three times before the diagnosis is made: once for general fidgetiness, once for breaking crockery, and once for making faces at his grandmother. In part, this adage illustrates the three major clinical features of Sydenham chorea: spontaneous movements, incoordination of voluntary movements, and muscular weakness.

The involuntary movements affect mainly the face, hands, and arms. At first inconspicuous and usually best observed when the patient is under stress, they are abrupt and short, but gradually they become more frequent and extensive, ultimately being almost continuous, disappearing only during sleep and sedation. Chorea interrupts the voluntary movements and is particularly prominent during skilled motor acts and speech. Muscular weakness can be profound and is sometimes the most prominent aspect of the disorder.

The child with pronounced Sydenham chorea is not difficult to recognize. The child is restless and emotional. Involuntary movements are continuous, quick, and random. They involve mainly the face and the distal portion of the extremities. Speech is jerky, indistinct, and at times completely absent. Willed acts also are performed abruptly; as quickly as the tongue is protruded, it returns into the mouth ("chameleon tongue"). Muscular hypotonia and weakness result in the characteristic pronator sign: When the patient holds the arms above the head, the palms turn outward. Hypotonia also can be demonstrated when the arms are extended in front of the body. The wrist is flexed, and the metacarpophalangeal joints are overextended ("choreic hand") (Fig. 7.4). The child is unable to maintain muscular contraction, and the grip waxes and wanes abruptly ("milkmaid's grip"). The deep tendon reflexes are usually normal, but the patellar reflex is often "hung up." With the legs hanging down, the contraction of the quadriceps elicited by the tap is maintained, causing the leg to be briefly held outstretched before it falls back down.

Occasional variants of chorea provide a diagnostic problem. The most common is hemichorea, in which the movements are confined to or are more marked on one side of the body. Hemichorea was seen in 18% of choreic patients reviewed by Aron and associates (195). In paralytic chorea, the hypotonia and muscular

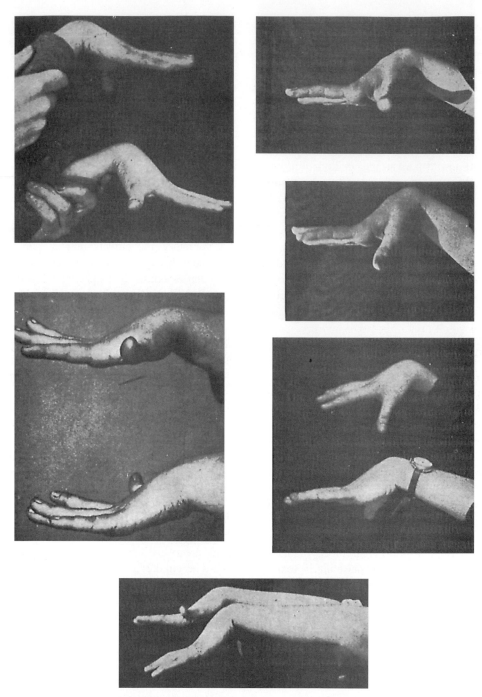

FIG. 7.4. Sydenham chorea. Hand in various characteristic choreiform positions. (From Wilson SAK, Bruce AN. *Neurology,* 2nd ed. London: Butterworth, 1969. With permission.)

weakness are sufficiently pronounced to obscure the presence of choreiform movements.

MRI studies often show increased signal on T2-weighted images in the head of the caudate, and in other portions of the basal ganglia, notably the putamen (207). Quantitative MRI demonstrates an increase in the size of the caudate, putamen, and globus pallidus, consistent with the presence of an antibody-mediated inflammation of this region (208). These abnormalities resolve with clinical improvement. SPECT has shown a marked increase in perfusion of the thalamus and striatum during the stage of active chorea. This abnormality resolves as the movements subside (209).

Chorea lasts from 1 month to 2 years. Approximately one-third of patients have a single attack; the remainder have up to five or even more recurrences, despite adequate penicillin prophylaxis. It is not clear whether these recurrences represent exacerbations of chronic low-grade choreiform activity, the response to transient, mild streptococcal infections, or the response to other nonstreptococcal stimuli (210). If the patient has been free of symptoms for 1 to 2 years, there is little likelihood of relapse.

Complications of Sydenham chorea are rare. Occlusion of the central retinal artery and pseudotumor cerebri are unusual associated conditions (211). Although complete recovery without gross neurologic residua is the rule in Sydenham chorea, minor neurologic signs, notably tics or other adventitious movements, tremor, and impaired coordination, can persist (200). Some of the signs, such as an unusual abruptness of voluntary movements, can be apparent long after the chorea has disappeared. Furthermore, convalescents can develop choreic reactions to a variety of drugs, notably methylphenidate, phenylethylamines, and dextroamphetamine (212). Behavioral disturbances, notably obsessive-compulsive disorder (OCD), are common; in many instances, these had been noted before the onset of chorea.

Diagnosis

The major causes for chorea are presented in Table 7.5. Chorea must be differentiated from tics and from a variety of other movement disorders (see Introduction). Additionally, Sydenham chorea should be distinguished from chorea that results from a variety of other causes, notably perinatal asphyxia, Huntington disease, SLE, and chorea which is an expression of the motor

TABLE 7.5. *Major causes of chorea*

	Reference
Onset before 3 years of age	
Physiologic chorea of infancy	Freud (432)
Perinatal asphyxia	Chapter 5
Kernicterus	Chapter 9
Postcardiopulmonary bypass	Chapter 15
Onset in childhood	
"Minimal brain dysfunction"	Prechtl (433)
Genetic	
Disorders of intermediary metabolism	
Glutaric acidemia type I	Chapter 1
δ-Glyceric acidemia	
Sulfite oxidase deficiency	
GM_1 gangliosidosis	
GM_2 gangliosidosis	
Lesch-Nyhan syndrome	
Leigh syndrome	
Heredodegenerative disorders	
Ataxia-telangiectasia	Chapter 11
Familial nonprogressive choreoathetosis	Chapter 2
Paroxysmal dyskinesia	Chapter 2
Toxic	
Neuroleptics (tardive dyskinesia)	Chapter 2
Anticonvulsants (phenytoin, carbamazepine)	Chapter 13
Metals (thallium, manganese)	Chapter 9
Isoniazid, reserpine	
Metabolic	
Hepatic encephalopathy	Chapter 15
Renal encephalopathy	Chapter 15
Hypoparathyroidism	Chapter 15
Pseudohypoparathyroidism	Chapter 15
Hyponatremia and hypernatremia	Chapter 15
Post protein-calorie malnutrition	Chapter 9
Infectious	
Viral encephalitis	Chapter 6
Behçet disease	
Immunologic	
Systemic lupus erythematosus	Chapter 7
Sydenham chorea	
Trauma	Chapter 8
Onset in adolescence	
Heredodegenerative diseases	
Wilson disease	Chapter 1
Huntington disease	Chapter 2
Hallervorden-Spatz disease	Chapter 2
Pelizaeus-Merzbacher disease	Chapter 2
Toxic	
Metabolic	
Infectious	
Immunologic	
Trauma	

impersistence of sensorimotor and cognitive immaturity (minimal brain dysfunction).

Tics, unlike true chorea, are abrupt, repetitive, and patterned, involving the same muscle groups repeatedly. They do not interfere with coordination and are not associated with muscular hypotonia. To complicate the differentiation between chorea and tics, preexisting motor tics can merge into Sydenham chorea after a streptococcal infection (213). Sydenham chorea also should be distinguished from the various pediatric autoimmune neuropsychiatric diseases associated with streptococcal infection (PANDAS) (see Pediatric Autoimmune Neuropsychiatric Diseases Associated with Streptococcal Infection, later in this chapter). The differentiation of chorea that develops as a symptom of SLE and Sydenham chorea rests on the presence of antinuclear and anti-DNA antibodies in the former entity. Antibodies against streptococcal DNAase are particularly useful for the diagnosis of Sydenham chorea because they tend to remain elevated for some 6 months after a streptococcal infection. Additionally, increased expression of the D8/17 B-cell alloantigen is seen in patients with Sydenham chorea, rheumatic fever, but not in SLE (214).

Choreic movements resulting from perinatal asphyxia generally become apparent between the first and the third years of life (see Chapter 5), an earlier age than in Sydenham chorea. The movements are usually slower and tend to be more evident in the larger proximal musculature. Like the involuntary movements of Sydenham chorea, they are exaggerated by fatigue and emotion. In most cases, choreiform movements are accompanied by other involuntary movements, principally athetosis.

The differential diagnosis between children with mild choreiform movements owing to Sydenham chorea and those whose choreiform movements are based on minimal brain dysfunction (see Chapter 16) is difficult, because children with Sydenham chorea also have a high incidence of preexisting learning and personality problems. Resolution of the chorea in a matter of months suggests Sydenham chorea, as does the absence of clear-cut cognitive immaturities.

Huntington disease is rarely seen in children (see Chapter 2). The involuntary movements predominantly involve the proximal musculature, and, although abrupt, they are more extensive than those of Sydenham chorea. In particular, twisting movements of the shoulders and trunk are characteristic of Huntington disease. Mental deterioration or seizures, commonly found in Huntington disease and not observed in Sydenham chorea, and a history of autosomal dominant transmission are further clinical diagnostic aids.

Numerous drugs, notably haloperidol, isoniazid, reserpine, phenytoin, or phenothiazines such as prochlorperazine also can induce choreiform movements. The various forms of paroxysmal choreoathetosis, a subgroup of the paroxysmal dyskinesias, can be distinguished by the sudden onset of choreiform movements in a child who has few, if any, involuntary movements between attacks (see Chapter 2). Familial benign choreoathetosis is a rare condition that begins in the first two decades of life. It is characterized by choreiform movements of the hands, shoulders, arms, and legs, and by a combined resting and intention tremor (see Chapter 2). The disorder is transmitted in an autosomal dominant manner.

Treatment

Since Sydenham in 1684 recommended bleeding, purges, and Laudanum (alcoholic tincture of opium) for the treatment of chorea, a large number of therapeutic regimens have been suggested. The variability in the duration of untreated chorea makes evaluation difficult, and the effectiveness of salicylates, cortisone, or ACTH in shortening the length of the illness has not been proved.

Currently, the optimal form of treatment is bedrest in a darkened, quiet room. For children whose movements are severe, drug therapy is necessary. In the past, phenobarbital, chlorpromazine, or haloperidol has been used. Sodium valproate (15 to 25 mg/kg per day) appears to be equally efficacious and controls the involuntary movements in 5 to 10 days (215). The mechanism by which it works remains a matter of speculation. The drug is gradually withdrawn after 2 to 6 months. Should symptoms recur, it is restarted.

Even when streptococci cannot be isolated from throat cultures, a course of penicillin is indicated as soon as the diagnosis of Sydenham chorea is made. The patient is given a single intramuscular dose of 1.2 million U of benzathine penicillin, or an oral penicillin dose of 200 to 250 mg given four times daily for 10 days.

The subsequent occurrence of rheumatic complications in many patients with Sydenham chorea dictates the prophylactic use of antimicrobial agents: the oral administration of penicillin (200,000 U two or three times daily) or clindamycin (75 mg two or three times daily) (216). The antibiotic is given for several years, or at least until the patient has completed high school.

Pediatric Autoimmune Neuropsychiatric Diseases Associated with Streptococcal Infection

The term *PANDAS* has been used to designate a group of neuropsychiatric disorders, notably tic disorders, Tourette syndrome, and OCD, which are believed to be related to an antecedent streptococcal infection, and for which an autoimmune pathogenesis has been postulated.

The condition began to be recognized in the early 1990s. Whether it had been present before then and not recognized, or whether it is of new onset, is unknown. Serum antineuronal antibodies that cross-react with caudate nucleus and other brain tissue have been found in Tourette syndrome and OCD (217). In the study by Kiessling and colleagues, a strong positive response to antibody was found in 53% of children with choreiform movements, 43% of children with tic disorders, but only in 21% of children without a movement disorder (217). Patients with OCD or Tourette syndrome are frequently positive for B-lymphocytes that express an epitope reactive with a D8/17 monoclonal antibody, the same antibody whose expression is increased in rheumatic fever and Sydenham chorea (218).

The clinical characteristics for the diagnosis of PANDAS have been listed by Swedo and colleagues (219). They are (a) presence of OCD, a tic disorder, or both; (b) onset between 3 years of age and puberty; (c) episodic course with abrupt onset, or dramatic exacerbation of symptoms;

(d) symptom exacerbations temporally related to group A beta hemolytic streptococcal infections, as demonstrated by a positive throat culture result, elevated antistreptococcal antibody titers, or both; and (e) association with neurologic abnormalities, notably choreiform movements.

PANDAS is not a rare disorder, and the characteristic patient demonstrates a combination of choreiform movements and a tic disorder, which has had an abrupt onset, or a marked worsening in the wake of a streptococcal infection. The diagnosis is suggested by a positive throat culture result or by positive antistreptococcal antibodies. Many questions about this disorder remain, notably how to treat it, and most important, well-controlled studies are required to verify the relationship between streptococcal infection and the movement disorder (220,221).

Various treatments have been proposed. These include antibiotics directed against the putative inciting streptococcal organisms, serotonin reuptake blockers, intravenous immunoglobins (IVIG) (1 gm/kg for two consecutive days), and plasmapheresis (5 to 6 procedures performed on alternate days). When children are given IVIG, improvement is seen 3 weeks after treatment or even later, and persists for 1 or more years (221a). With plasma exchange, symptom improvement is noted toward the end of the first week of treatment, and persists for 1 year or longer (221a). In the experience of Perlmutter and colleagues, tic symptoms are more effectively treated with plasma exchange, whereas IVIG and plasma exchange appear almost equally effective for symptoms of OCD (221a).

Rasmussen Syndrome

Rasmussen syndrome is a rare, progressive, gray matter disease of children. It is marked by an onset in the first decade of life with intractable focal epilepsy, progressive hemiparesis, atrophy of the contralateral cerebral hemisphere, and dementia. The presence of serum GluR3 antibodies in some patients with Rasmussen syndrome but not in a control group suggests that this condition represents an immune-mediated disease. Rasmussen syndrome is more fully described in Chapter 6.

IMMUNOLOGICALLY MEDIATED DEMYELINATING DISEASES OF THE PERIPHERAL NERVOUS SYSTEM

Guillain-Barré Syndrome

In the past, GBS was considered as a single pathologic and clinical entity. The condition can be subdivided into several diverse disorders. These are classified as follows: (a) sporadic GBS, which is most common, accounting for some 85% to 90% of cases has been termed acute inflammatory demyelinating polyneuropathy (AIDP); (b) acute motor-sensory axonal neuropathy (AMSAN); (c) acute motor-axonal neuropathy (AMAN); (d) Miller Fisher syndrome; and (e) chronic inflammatory demyelinative polyneuropathy (CIDP). AIDP or GBS (the terms are still used interchangeably) is by far the most common cause of immune-mediated peripheral nerve disease in children, and with the near disappearance of poliomyelitis, is responsible for the great majority of cases of acute flaccid, areflexic paralysis. The condition is characterized by progressive weakness, which usually appears a few days to weeks after a nonspecific infection and is accompanied by mild sensory disturbances and an albuminocytologic dissociation (high protein but normal cell count) in the CSF.

The first cases were recorded in 1859 by Landry (222), who noted that the disorder can produce both motor and sensory symptoms (especially motor), that it involves the distal parts of the limbs, and that in some instances it can become generalized by a sequential ascent of the neuraxis. Guillain, Barré, and Strohl stressed the presence of albuminocytologic dissociation (223).

Pathology

The pathologic findings are characterized by a marked segmental demyelination. In the majority of cases, GBS is marked by a mononuclear, predominantly T-lymphocytic and macrocytic inflammatory infiltration of all levels of the peripheral nervous system, from the anterior and posterior roots to the terminal twigs (224,225) and involving at times also the sympathetic chain and ganglia and the cranial nerves. Cells are usually clustered around the endoneurial and epineurial vessels, particularly the small veins. T-lymphocyte infiltration appears to be preceded by a complement-mediated Schwann cell damage and vesicular demyelination (226). Segmental demyelination occurs in the areas infiltrated by inflammatory cells, whereas interruption of the axonal cylinders with subsequent wallerian degeneration is less extensive, usually occurring only where an intense inflammation occurs. The number of Schwann cell nuclei is increased, possibly representing a reparative response. Ultrastructural studies reveal that macrophages are the major effectors of demyelination, and that neither Schwann cells nor myelin sheaths show any damage, except where they are in contact with macrophages (227). In a minority of cases, macrophage-associated demyelination occurs despite a paucity of lymphocytes (228).

In the CNS, the alterations are secondary to secondary axonal degeneration. Most common is chromatolysis involving the anterior horn cells and the cells in the motor nuclei of the cranial nerves. Long-standing cases show some degeneration of the posterior columns (225).

Pathogenesis

The morphologic alterations in GBS resemble those induced in experimental animals by immunization with peripheral nerve homogenates (229), or more specifically, by a peptide (P2) derived from the basic protein of peripheral nerves (230). As is the case for GBS, the earliest event in the induction of experimental allergic neuritis is the presentation of antigen to "naive" T cells resulting in their activation. The activated T cells circulate in the blood and attach to the venular endothelium of peripheral nerves. T cells then migrate through the endothelial lining to a perivascular location. There they enlarge, their ribosomes increase in number, and RNA production accelerates. The now sensitized lymphocytes contact myelin, and after a lag of at least several hours, they produce segmental demyelination (231,232). Cytokines, released by inflammatory cells and by Schwann cells contribute to demyelination, and to changes in Schwann cells that have deleterious effects on myelin and axons (233). Tumor necrosis factor-α and IL-1β, medi-

TABLE 7.6. *Infectious organisms associated with Gullain-Barré syndrome or acute disseminated encephalomyelitis*

	Envelope	Gullain-Barré syndrome	Acute disseminated encephalomyelitis	Encephalitis
DNA viruses				
Adenoviridae				
Adenovirus		X	X	X
Herpesviridae				
Cytomegalovirus	X	X	X	X
Epstein-Barr virus	X	X	X	X
Herpes simplex I, II	X	X	X	X
Human herpesvirus 6	X	X	?	X
Varicella zoster	X	X	X	
Poxviridae				
Vaccinia	X	X		
Variola	X	X		
RNA viruses				
Flaviviridae				
Japanese encephalitis virus		X		X
Orthomyoxoviridae				
Influenza viruses A and B	X	X		X
Paramyxoviridae				
Measles virus		X	X	X
Mumps virus		X	X	X
Picornaviridae (enteroviruses)				
Coxsackievirus		X		X
Echovirus		X		X
Retroviridae				
Human immunodeficiency viruses	X	X		X
Coronavirus				
Hepatitis viruses A, B, C				
Parainfluenza viruses I, II, III			X	
Parvovirus B19			X	
Respiratory syncytial virus				

ators of inflammation, are secreted by activated macrophages and by antigen-activated T-lymphocytes. Their serum levels correlate with neurophysiologic evidence of demyelination (234). The role of integrins, a family of cell adhesion molecules, in the development of inflammation in experimental allergic neuritis and GBS, and subsequent remyelination is reviewed by Archelos and colleagues (235).

The consensus of evidence indicates that the GBS represents an interaction between an infectious agent and a cell-mediated immune response directed against the myelin-producing Schwann cells, the peripheral myelin, or one of the components of myelin (232). The antigen on the Schwann cell membrane that is involved in GBS is believed to be a glycoconjugate, which is carried on the bacterial or viral organism that is responsible for the antecedent infection, and which generates an immune response. Antibodies directed against the foreign glycoconjugate target similar epitopes on nerve fibers. This process has been termed *molecular mimicry*.

An antecedent acute infectious illness has been documented in approximately two-thirds of children who develop GBS. Most commonly, it is a respiratory tract infection or a gastroenteritis. Several agents have been implicated in these infections (236–238). Of these, *Campylobacter jejuni* infection has become recognized as the most common bacterial antecedent of GBS. In various series it accounted 26% to 41% of sporadic cases (239,240). Other responsible agents include cytomegalovirus, which has been implicated in 10% to 22% of GBS cases (240), and the Epstein-Barr virus, which is responsible for some 10% of cases. Primary infection with herpes zoster has been noted in nearly 5% of childhood cases of GBS in some series (237). Other viruses implicated in the evolution of GBS are listed in Table 7.6. The chief feature shared by most of these is that they have a viral envelope.

Several vaccines have been implicated in the evolution of GBS. Of these the best substantiated is the rabies vaccine as prepared from brain tissue and probably contaminated with myelin antigens (240a). The swine-flu influenza vaccine, as administered in 1976 and 1977, also was responsible for numerous cases of GBS (240b). The association of GBS with other immunizations, notably tetanus, oral polio vaccine, other influenza vaccines, and measles vaccine has been more difficult to establish. The best that can be said at this time is that such an association cannot be excluded (240,240c). The association of GBS with trauma or surgical procedures is probably anecdotal.

Considerable work has been directed at establishing the connection between an antecedent *C. jejuni* infection and GBS. The lipopolysaccharide of *C. jejuni* contains a GM_1 epitope, which induces a high production of IgG anti-GM_1 antibodies that are believed to react with epitopes located mainly on axons, but also, to a lesser degree on myelin. Patients whose sera have anti-GM_1 antibodies tend to develop the acute motor axonal neuropathy form of GBS (241,242). *C. jejuni* also has been implicated in the demyelinating form of GBS (242a). It has now become apparent that the antigenic structure of the antecedent infectious agent determines the clinical manifestations of GBS. Thus, patients with the Miller-Fisher syndrome are likely to have serum antibodies against the ganglioside GQ_{1b} (243), whereas antibodies directed against GalNAc-GD_{1a} gangliosides carried on *C. jejuni* tend to induce a clinical picture marked by distal weakness, no sensory loss, and a normal cranial nerve examination (244).

Unlike MS, genetic factors appear to play little or no role in the evolution of GBS, and the appearance of the disease is not influenced by genes associated with the HLA-A or HLA-B locus (245). Furthermore, no abnormalities exist in the subsets of the T-cell population. The pathogenesis of GBS is reviewed in greater detail by Ho and colleagues (232).

Clinical Manifestations

Acute Inflammatory Demyelinating Polyneuropathy

Clinical symptoms result from disturbed saltatory conduction through myelinated axons (con-

TABLE 7.7. *Clinical characteristics of 56 children with acute infectious polyneuritis*

Characteristic	Percent
Antecedent infection	70
Distal weakness predominantly	44
Proximal weakness predominantly	14
Cranial nerve weakness	43
Facial nerve	32
Spinal accessory nerve	21
Papilledema	5
Paresthesia and pain	43
Loss of vibratory or position sense or both	34
Meningeal irritation	17
Cerebrospinal fluid protein more than 45 mg/dL	88
Mortality	4
Full recovery or mild impairment	77
Relapses	7
Asymmetry of involvement	9

Data from Low NL, Schneider J, Carter S. Polyneuritis in children. *Pediatrics* 1958;22:972; and Peterman AF, et al. Infectious neuronitis (Guillain-Barré syndrome) in children. *Neurology* 1959;9:533.

duction block). GBS can occur at any time during childhood, but is most frequent between ages 4 and 9 years (246). A prodromal respiratory illness or gastroenteritis occurs in approximately two-thirds of the patients, usually within 2 weeks before the onset of weakness (Table 7.7) (246,247).

Neurologic symptoms usually appear fairly suddenly. In a large proportion of cases, 89% of adult patients in the series of Moulin and colleagues (248), paralysis was accompanied by pain or paresthesia. In 47%, pain was severe and was described as a deep aching pain in back and legs. Visceral pain was noted in 20%.

The paralysis usually begins in the lower extremities, then ascends. Characteristically, it is symmetric, although minor differences between the sides are not rare. In approximately 50% of patients, the weakness is mostly distal, whereas in approximately 15%, the proximal musculature is more extensively involved (see Table 7.7). Cranial nerve palsies can appear at any time during the illness. The facial nerve is involved most commonly; it was involved in more than one-half of patients in the series of Winer and colleagues (249). Papilledema is relatively rare. Although its appearance correlates well with increased intracranial pressure (250), papilledema is not invariably accompanied by elevation in CSF protein, and its pathogenesis remains unexplained (251).

Paralysis of the respiratory muscles is a common complication in severely involved patients, but even in the absence of respiratory symptoms, vital capacity can be impaired with consequent carbon dioxide retention. Involvement of the sympathetic nervous system can produce a variety of circulatory abnormalities, including profuse sweating, hypertension, or postural hypotension, which often are predictors of a fatal cardiac arrhythmia (252). Sphincter disturbances are noted in up to one-third of patients (249).

Position sense is the sensory function most frequently impaired, followed by vibration, pain, and touch, in descending order of frequency. The deep tendon reflexes are generally absent, although increased reflexes and extensor plantar responses are occasionally recorded during the initial days of the illness.

An elevation in the CSF protein content is characteristic. This exceeds 45 mg/dL in 88% of affected children (see Table 7.7) and increases to its maximum by 4 to 5 weeks, thereafter gradually returning to normal (Fig. 7.5). The CSF cell count is usually normal, although significant pleocytosis (100+ cells/mL) occurs in approximately 5% of patients.

Electromyography (EMG) reveals a picture compatible with involvement of the lower motor neurons or peripheral nerves. Abnormalities in nerve conduction are the most specific electrophysiologic findings. The most characteristic is the presence of conduction block. This is a reduction in amplitude of the muscle action potential after stimulation of the distal, as compared with the proximal, portion of the nerve. Approximately 80% of patients have nerve conduction block or slowing at some time during the illness. The conduction velocity often does not become abnormal until several weeks into the illness (253,254).

This neurologic picture evolves rapidly, and paralysis can be maximal within a few hours of the initial symptoms. More commonly, however, the paralysis becomes more extensive over 1 to 2 weeks, often, as in the classic Landry type of paralysis, progressively affecting the trunk,

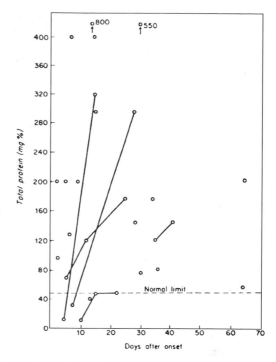

FIG. 7.5. Acute infectious polyneuritis. Protein content of the cerebrospinal fluid at various intervals after onset of symptoms. Determinations performed on the same patient are connected by a line. [From Peterman AF, Daly DD, Dion FR, et al. Infectious neuronitis (Guillain-Barré syndrome) in children. *Neurology* 1959;9:533. With permission.]

upper extremities, and cranial nerves. After the paralysis reaches a plateau, clinical improvement is usually first noted by the second to fourth week of the illness, and the majority of children experience complete recovery. Recovery usually is achieved within 2 months, although it can take as long as 18 months.

Some children, approximately 10% of the Dublin series of Briscoe and coworkers (255), experience one or more relapses over the subsequent 2 months to several years. Such patients are considered to have CIDP. This condition is covered in a subsequent section.

Acute Motor-Sensory Axonal Neuropathy

Feasby and others first described a subgroup of patients who developed a fulminant, extensive, and severe weakness with delayed and incomplete recovery. Electrophysiologic studies in these patients suggested a primary axonal degeneration, which was confirmed by nerve biopsy performed on patients who died shortly after the onset of their illness (256,257). This demonstrated severe axonal degeneration with little demyelination, and scanty lymphocytic infiltration, an indication that in this condition the primary insult is to motor and sensory nerve axons (258). In these patients the earliest identifiable changes are in the nodes of Ranvier of motor fibers (259). Patients with this form of neuropathy are much more likely to have experienced an antecedent *C. jejuni* infection than control populations and are more likely to have high titers of serum anti-GD_{1a} antibodies (242,260).

Acute Motor-Axonal Neuropathy

A pure motor axonal neuropathy has been reported from China and India. In the Chinese cases, the disease appeared in annual summer epidemics and manifested as a severe motor neuropathy, with involvement of the proximal portion of the motor neurons or cell bodies and good recovery. Electrophysiologic studies indicate that the motor fibers are lost selectively, and that neither involvement of the sensory fibers nor demyelination occur (232). In the Indian paralytic disease, fever and a hemorrhagic conjunctivitis occur at the onset of the illness, the weakness is asymmetric, and the CSF demonstrates a pleocytosis. This form of neuropathy also is closely associated with a *C. jejuni* infection (261).

Miller Fisher Syndrome

Another variant of GBS was first described by Fisher in 1956 (262). It is characterized by the evolution, within approximately a week, of external ophthalmoplegia, ataxia, and areflexia. The first symptom is usually diplopia, with bilateral facial paresis being present in approximately one-half of the affected children (263). Internal ophthalmoplegia is present in approximately two-thirds. The CSF shows a mild protein content elevation and, occasionally, pleocytosis. Peripheral motor and sensory conduction times and the EMG are generally normal. The EEG can show excessive slow-wave

activity or can be normal (264). Neuroimaging studies exclude a mass lesion (265,266).

Symptoms remain severe for 1 to 2 weeks before recovery commences. Recovery proceeds at a variable rate, but generally is complete.

The Miller Fisher syndrome is associated with strains of *C. jejuni* that have the ability to induce antibodies against ganglioside GQ_{1b} (243,267). Such antibodies can be demonstrated in 96% of patients with Miller Fisher syndrome, and their titers parallel the course of the disease. These antibodies have the ability to block the release of acetylcholine from motor nerve terminals, with oculomotor fibers having the highest concentration of GQ_{1b}-reactive antigens (232,268). The effect resembles that induced by α-latrotoxin (268a) (see Table 9.6).

At present, it is still a matter of dispute whether Miller Fisher syndrome should be distinguished from brainstem encephalitis, as delineated by Bickerstaff and others (see Chapter 10) (269). According to some, ataxia in Miller Fisher syndrome is caused entirely by peripheral nerve involvement, and pathologic changes are restricted to the peripheral nervous system (270). Others believe that the CNS also is involved and that in some cases a combined central and peripheral demyelination exists. MRI studies do not appear to help in the differential diagnosis. Whereas the MRI is normal in some cases of Miller Fisher syndrome, in others T2-weighted images demonstrate areas of increased signal in the brainstem. Conversely, there are several instances of clinically diagnosed brainstem encephalitis in whom electrophysiologic evidence exists for involvement of the peripheral nerves (271). Miller Fisher syndrome also must be distinguished from posterior fossa tumors. Before neuroimaging studies this differentiation was difficult. However, the constellation of a severe and sometimes complete external ophthalmoplegia, ataxia, and loss of deep tendon reflexes in a fairly alert child is unique.

Chronic Inflammatory Demyelinating Polyradiculoneuropathy

CIDP has some of the clinical features of GBS, but the evolution of the neurologic symptoms is slower, being a matter of weeks or months,

TABLE 7.8. *Differential diagnosis of chronic polyneuritis of childhood*

Condition	Diagnostic features
Lead poisoning	Blood lead levels; basophilic stippling of erythrocytes
Arsenic poisoning	Elevated arsenic in hair, nails
Thiamine deficiency	Transketolase deficiency
Polyarteritis nodosa	Muscle biopsy
Systemic lupus erythematosus	Antinuclear antibodies
	Antiphospholipid antibodies
	Familial history
Hereditary motor and sensory neuropathies	Sural nerve biopsy; motor and sensory conduction times on patient and on parents
Refsum disease (ataxia polyneuritiformis)	Elevated blood phytanic acid
Metachromatic leukodystrophy	Intellectual deterioration; absent urinary and tissue arylsulfatase
Globoid cell leukodystrophy (Krabbe)	Early onset, intellect deteriorates, nerve biopsy, galactocerebroside galactosidase assays in serum
Chronic polyneuritis of unknown cause	Exclusion of above

Modified from Byers RK, Taft LT. Chronic multiple neuropathy in childhood. *Pediatrics* 1957;20:517.

rather than days. Some patients have a chronic fluctuating course without complete recovery between exacerbations (272,273). In the few children thus affected, the motor component of the picture is usually predominant (274), and weakness is greatest in the distal muscles. On biopsy the peripheral nerves show a segmental demyelination and increased numbers of Schwann cells. Their processes are arranged in whorls around the demyelinated axons. Termed *onion bulbs*, they are characteristic of not only the hereditary peripheral neuropathies, but also of most chronic recurrent neuropathies, and their presence correlates with the duration of symptoms (275). Table 7.8 shows the differential diagnosis of CIDP of childhood, together with some salient diagnostic features of each of the major entities. The initiating factor responsible for CIDP remains unknown in most children. Unlike GBS, in which no association with histocompatibility antigens has been established, CIDP has been shown to be associated with haplotypes B8, DR3, and Dw3 (276). Antibodies directed at GM_1, GD_{1b}, and asialo-GM_1 glycolipids have been identified in some cases, suggesting that the galactosyl (beta 1 → 3) N-acetogalactosaminyl moiety of myelin may be an important target antigen in some cases (277).

Diagnosis

The criteria for the clinical diagnosis of classical GBS were established in 1978 by the National Institute of Neurologic and Communicative Disorders and Stroke (278) and were updated in 1990 by Asbury and Cornblath (279). They are presented in Table 7.9. In essence they rest on the gradual development of symmetric muscular weakness, which is often worse over the distal portion of the lower extremities, the presence of areflexia, and the aforementioned CSF and electrodiagnostic abnormalities. In the presence of sensory changes, usually little doubt exists about the diagnosis. When sensory changes are absent, however, a number of other entities must be con-

TABLE 7.9. *Guillain-Barré syndrome study group diagnostic criteria*

Required for diagnosis
    Progressive motor weakness involving more than one extremity
    Areflexia or marked hyporeflexia
    No more than 50 monocytes or two granulocytes per µL cerebrospinal fluid
Strongly supportive of diagnosis
    Initial absence of fever
    Progression over days to a few weeks
    Onset of recovery 2 to 4 weeks after cessation of progression
    Relatively symmetric weakness
    Mild sensory signs and symptoms
    Cranial nerve signs
    Elevation of cerebrospinal fluid protein after 1 week of symptoms
    Slowed nerve conduction velocity or prolonged f-waves
    Autonomic dysfunction

From National Institute of Neurologic and Communicative Disorders and Stroke. Ad hoc Committee. Criteria for diagnosis of Guillain-Barré syndrome. *Ann Neurol* 1978;3:565. With permission.

sidered. In poliomyelitis, the onset of paralysis is accompanied by fever and evidence of a systemic illness. The paralysis is rarely symmetric, and CSF pleocytosis is common during the initial stages of the illness (see Chapter 6).

Polymyositis can be confused with GBS. The distribution of muscular weakness in polymyositis tends to be proximal, and the CSF protein content remains normal. The presence of hypokalemia in the occasional patient with GBS requires the differential diagnosis of hypokalemic paralysis. This condition usually carries a family history, and the ECG is abnormal during a paralytic attack (280). The differential diagnosis of ATM and GBS has been noted already. Other less common conditions that induce progressive muscular weakness of rapid onset are described in Chapter 14.

Treatment

Treatment of GBS should be proactive. The neuropathy can progress rapidly, so that the potential for paralysis of the respiratory muscles should be considered in each patient, and facilities for tracheostomy and mechanical ventilation should be readily available. Generally, these measures should be instituted when impaired vital capacity first becomes apparent, rather than after embarrassment of respiration is obvious and the patient has difficulty breathing. A reduction of vital capacity to approximately one-half the norm for the age calls for immediate consideration of tracheostomy. Fluctuations in blood pressure, hemodynamic instability, autonomic dysfunction, and oropharyngeal weakness are common.

Several large controlled trials have shown that neither oral nor intravenous corticosteroids are beneficial for the various forms of GBS and possibly are contraindicated (281). However, many patients who experience CIDP show a clear-cut response to corticosteroids (282).

Plasmapheresis and IVIG have been used extensively. Controlled studies have confirmed that in pediatric patients plasmapheresis shortens the interval to independent ambulation (283) and the duration of mechanical ventilation (284). One study, involving patients older than 16 years, indicated that for mild cases of GBS two exchanges are better than none. For moderate or severe cases, four exchanges, conducted in the course of 1 week, are better than two. More than four exchanges do not confer additional benefits (285).

High-dose IVIG is another effective means of treating GBS. In a double-blind study a clear difference existed in favor of IVIG over plasmapheresis in adult and pediatric patients. More patients improved with IVIG, median time to improvement was shorter, there were fewer complications, and less need for ventilation (286). Furthermore, IVIG treatment is safer and less traumatic to children, and is, therefore, in our opinion, the preferred form of intervention for the child who has a major deficit during the first week of the disease. High-dose IVIG also has been effective in the treatment of CIDP (287). Although there are few adverse reactions to IVIG, several groups have reported significant relapses in GBS patients treated in this fashion (288). Other adverse reactions include an allergic response to γ-globulin and a chemical meningitis. The mechanism of action of IVIG is poorly understood. The most likely is that it modulates the immune response in GBS by selective suppression of the proinflammatory cytokines (289).

Because with good supportive care the long-term outcome for even those children who require ventilation is excellent, supportive treatment still finds its adherents for all but the most severely affected.

An important part of the general support of the child with GBS is the use of physiotherapy. This should be instituted during convalescence, and both active and passive exercises should be graduated as recovery progresses.

Prognosis

In general, the outlook for life and recovery is better in children than in adults. The greatest danger during the acute phase of GBS is respiratory paralysis and cardiac arrhythmias. Cardiac arrhythmias can be brought on by manipulation of the patient, such as from changing a tracheotomy tube (290). Early tracheostomy and the availability of mechanical ventilation should eliminate a considerable proportion of fatalities. In the pediatric age group, there is generally no correlation between the severity of the illness and the long-term outcome (290). Several studies suggest that evidence for an antecedent *C. jejuni* infection correlates with a disease in which there is axonal degeneration and a poor outcome (291).

BELL'S PALSY

An acute paralysis of the face, often after a mild infection, was first described by Bell in 1829 (292).

> Cases of this partial paralysis must be familiar to every medical observer. It is very frequent for young people to have what is vulgarly called a blight, by which is meant a slight palsy of the muscles on one side of the face, and which the physician knows is not formidable. Inflammations of glands seated behind the angle of the jaw will sometimes produce this. . . . The patient has a command over the muscles of the face; he can close the lips, and the features are duly balanced; but the slightest smile is immediately attended with distortion, and in laughing and crying the paralysis becomes quite distinct.

Pathology and Pathogenesis

Because the process is often partly or wholly reversible, little is known about the acute pathology or pathophysiology, which is assumed to be inflammatory. The essential anatomic changes of the seventh nerve in Bell's palsy are still under considerable dispute. Most authors agree that during the acute phase of the illness, patients have considerable edema of the nerve and venous congestion in the facial canal. A few microscopic hemorrhages occur, but little inflammatory reaction.

In 73% of patients, there is an antecedent upper respiratory infection or exposure to cold drafts; these causes were the most frequently implicated during the nineteenth century (293). Currently, a variety of infectious agents have been suggested. On the basis of antibody levels,

the list includes Epstein-Barr virus (in some 20% of patients) (294), mumps, and possibly herpes simplex and herpes zoster. Facial palsy caused by Lyme disease is particularly frequent in Scandinavia and other endemic areas. In one series, 60% of children with Bell's palsy had specific IgM antibodies for the spirochete in CSF (295). Lymphocytes from subjects with Bell's palsy have been found to respond specifically to a basic protein (P1) isolated from human peripheral myelin. No response could be elicited to the P2 protein implicated in GBS (296). Additionally, T-lymphocytes, mainly T-helper cells, are depressed during the first 2 weeks of the disease (297). A genetic predisposition also appears to be important (298).

Clinical Manifestations

Any aspects of facial nerve function may be involved. This includes the facial motor movement, notably facial expression and lid closure; the tensor tympani resulting in impaired dampening of eardrum reaction to loud noises; taste sensation of the anterior two-thirds of the tongue; and autonomic regulation of lachrymal and salivary glands. The site of dysfunction determines which modalities are involved. Although potential sites include any point from the pontine nucleus to distal portions of nerve within canaliculi of the skull, the most common site is within the facial canal of the temporal bone.

Bell's palsy occurs in 2.7 in 100,000 children younger than 10, and 10.1 in 100,000 children older than 10 years of age. As is the case for GBS and ADEM, Bell's palsy commonly follows an upper respiratory illness. Whereas most childhood cases are unilateral, asymmetric bilateral Bell's palsy occasionally is encountered; usually this is a manifestation of GBS.

In many cases, pain localized in the ear or surrounding area is the initial symptom. This is followed by a rapid evolution of the paralysis, which reaches its full extent in a few hours. Characteristically, paralysis involves the musculature of the forehead, cheek, and perioral region. Approximately one-half of patients lose taste sensation. Lacrimation is retained in the great majority of children (299). Auditory-evoked potentials and trigeminal nerve-evoked potentials indicate that in a considerable proportion of subjects, Bell's palsy is not a mononeuropathy, but is accompanied by subclinical involvement of the trigeminal and auditory pathways (300). The pain, which can reflect trigeminal nerve involvement, usually disappears quickly. In most children, recovery begins within a few weeks and reaches its maximum in 1 to 9 weeks (299). The CSF is usually normal or shows a slight pleocytosis. In cases that evolve as a complication of Lyme disease, pleocytosis is often striking (295,301). MRI demonstrates enhancement of the intra-meatal segment of the facial nerve on T1-weighted images. On T2-weighted images enlargement of the intra-meatal segment can be seen with three-dimensional imaging (302).

The patient can be expected to recover completely when the palsy is partial, as is the case in 80% of children (303), or when evoked EMG shows an incomplete denervation of the facial nerve. When denervation is complete, the onset of recovery is delayed for approximately 6 weeks, and its maximal extent is not achieved until 6 months (304). In such instances, return of muscle function is usually incomplete. In 7% of children facial paralysis recurs (305). In some, it is part of Melkersson syndrome. This condition is characterized by recurrent facial palsy that is often associated with swelling of the lips, tongue, cheeks, or eyelids, and, less commonly, with furrowing of the tongue (306). With each attack of Melkersson syndrome, facial nerve function becomes progressively more impaired, and paralysis ultimately can be nearly complete (307). Treatment with methylprednisolone has been suggested (308).

Rarely, there is a familial predisposition to facial nerve palsy; in these cases, facial nerve weakness can be accompanied by oculomotor paralyses (309).

Diagnosis

The diagnosis of Bell's palsy rests on the exclusion of other causes of isolated facial paralysis (Table 7.10).

TABLE 7.10. *Causes of isolated facial paralysis, 1957 through 1972*

Cause	Paine (299)	Manning and Adour (304)
Congenital		
Congenital anomaly	15	2
Birth trauma	18	5
Postnatal		
Idiopathic (Bell's)	19	37
With upper respiratory infection	9	
Without upper respiratory infection	10	
Otitis media	16	6
Surgical trauma	2	
Other trauma	3	2
Intracranial tumor	2	
Extracranial tumor	1	
Hypertension	2	
Polymyelitis	2	
Histiocytosis X		2
Varicella		1
Herpes zoster (Ramsay Hunt)		1
Mumps		1
Postimmunization (diphtheria-pertussis-tetanus and polio)		1

Facial nerve palsy caused by otitis media, with or without mastoiditis, is still relatively common (304). A number of intracranial neoplasms, particularly those involving the brainstem, can result in the sudden onset of facial weakness (see Chapter 10). In some instances, transient improvement can be observed before other neurologic signs appear. Isolated facial nerve palsy can be seen with a variety of viral encephalitides, notably mumps, varicella, and the enteroviruses (see Chapter 6). It also is a concomitant to osteomyelitis of the skull, pseudotumor cerebri, and systemic hypertension (310,311). The cause of the facial palsy in systemic hypertension is not clear, but is believed to be induced by hemorrhages within the facial canal. The facial palsy can be the presenting feature of hypertension, and it is often intermittent and unrelated to the level of hypertension. In children, facial palsy is rarely caused by herpes zoster of the geniculate ganglion (Ramsay Hunt syndrome) (304). Another unusual cause for facial nerve palsy is the presence of an intra-aural tick. The salivary gland of the tick secretes a toxin that interferes with the synthesis or liberation of acetylcholine at the motor end-plates of facial muscle fibers (311a).

Treatment and Prognosis

A number of therapeutic approaches have been suggested. Administration of corticosteroids to reduce the edema within the facial canal has been used for several years. In view of the high recovery rate of untreated children, its evaluation is difficult. An analysis of all available studies led Huizing and coworkers to conclude that therapy was ineffective (312). In many instances, however, one has the clinical impression that treatment with corticosteroids within several days of the onset of symptoms is beneficial. Late treatment is certainly of no value.

Decompression of the facial nerve from the stylomastoid foramen through its pyramidal portion has been advised for patients who show complete denervation on evoked EMG, although no evidence indicates this procedure to be effective in either children or adults (313).

In children whose facial function recovers only partially, contractures can be expected. Misdirection of growth results in facial mass action in which attempted activity of one muscle group produces movements in several different muscle groups (synkinesis). Misdirection of growth also can result in tics or in the syndrome of crocodile tears. In this syndrome, food in the mouth or the smell of food is followed by lacrimation rather than salivation (314).

Varieties of cosmetic surgical procedures have been described, but these should be deferred until facial growth is complete. Artificial tears and eye patches should be supplied to all children whose Bell's palsy results in incomplete eye closure, particularly during sleep.

Generally, the younger the patient, the more likely there will be a good recovery. Other favorable factors include the absence of hyperacusis, and relatively normal minimal excitability values for the affected facial nerve. These values are obtained by electrical stimulation of the branches of the nerve just anterior to the ear and measurement of the minimal current required to effect a visible contraction of the muscle. The excitability study must be done within the first few days of the onset of paralysis; if corticosteroid therapy has been chosen, the dosage of corticosteroids can be modified according to the values obtained (315).

POSTINFECTIOUS ABDUCENS PALSY

A painless palsy of the abducens nerve that clears without residua can develop in children of any age, 7 to 21 days after a nonspecific febrile illness or upper respiratory infection. The paralysis is often complete but unassociated with any other cranial nerve palsy or neurologic signs. Improvement becomes evident in 3 to 6 weeks, and the palsy clears completely in 2 to 3 months. Except for the CSF, which can occasionally show a mild lymphocytosis, all laboratory and radiologic study results are normal (316).

Postinfectious abducens palsy is diagnosed by exclusion of abducens palsy secondary to increased intracranial pressure, tumors of the brainstem, brainstem encephalitis, and Gradenigo syndrome (317). The last, caused by an osteomyelitis of the apex of the petrous bone, is characterized by an abducens palsy after otitis media; it is accompanied by pain in the distribution of the homolateral trigeminal nerve.

Rarely, abducens palsy may recur, with the episodes occurring on the same side. A variety of events can precede the palsy. These include a febrile illness, trauma, and diphtheria-pertussis-tetanus (DPT) immunization (318).

OTHER POSTINFECTIOUS CRANIAL NEUROPATHIES

An isolated temporary paralysis of the glossopharyngeal nerve has been reported. The presenting symptoms in children were dysphagia and nasal speech. CSF examination was normal, and the condition cleared completely within 1 to 2 months (319).

Other postinfectious cranial neuropathies include an isolated hypoglossal nerve palsy, asymmetric palatal paresis, and involvement of the trigeminal sensory nerve (320–323).

SYSTEMIC VASCULITIDES WITH NERVOUS SYSTEM MANIFESTATIONS

Primary Systemic Vasculitides (Collagen Vascular Diseases, Rheumatic Diseases)

Vasculitic conditions are those diseases in which histologically evident injury to the endothelium of blood vessels contained within nervous tissues constitutes the primary process that leads to injury to surrounding nervous tissues. They are variously labeled as vasculitic, collagen-vascular, and rheumatic diseases. There are two important pathologic hallmarks of vasculitis. The first is the presence of inflammatory cells or the deposition of such humoral immune system elements as immunoglobulin and complement components within vascular endothelium or other layers of the vascular wall. The second is the development of necrotic changes of the vascular wall with associated luminal compromise and secondary downstream ischemia of tissues subserved by the involved vessel (324,325). Vasculitides are primary (i.e., without identifiable etiology or pathogenesis) or secondary, arising on the basis of some known toxic, infectious, neoplastic, or other etiology.

A great deal remains to be learned about the mechanisms of these diseases. This includes factors that determine susceptibility, the nature of the vascular process and of any associated inflammatory reaction that imperils nervous tissues, and the triggers of the immunologic and inflammatory response that becomes deleterious to the host.

Considerable pathophysiologic overlap exists between the vasculitic conditions that arise primarily in the nervous system. Thus, when neurologic abnormalities of a systemic vasculitic condition become evident before abnormalities of other systems, laboratory tests and subsequent clinical developments must often be relied on to distinguish systemic from such primarily neurologic inflammatory illnesses.

Because vasculitic and nonangiitic vasculopathic conditions have clinical and radiographic similarities that may cause diagnostic difficulties, the diagnosis of vasculitis usually rests on the pathologic examination of biopsy specimens obtained from skin, muscle, or kidney. In some cases, biopsy of other organs, including brain or meninges, are required to establish the diagnosis. In some instances even the biopsy of tissues may not distinguish the various illnesses, because the pathologic changes are often quite nonspecific. A general classification of vasculitides and other vasculopathic conditions is shown in Table 7.11.

General Pathogenetic Mechanisms of Vasculitic Diseases

The general categories of inflammatory vasculitis include those that are antibody mediated, immune-complex–mediated, and cell mediated. An increasingly complex array of soluble factors, such as cytokines, and cellular elements, such as adhesion molecules, have been shown to be of importance in mediating vasculitic conditions. Although one of these several mechanisms may predominate, there are many instances in which the other elements become secondarily involved in injury either to the vascular endothelium or to those secondarily involved tissues that are exposed to the immune response as the result of endothelial injury. Antiendothelial antibodies produced either because of exposure of antigens or molecular mimicry appear in many instances to invoke a cellular destructive response that involves tumor necrosis factor, interferon-γ, IL-1, and possibly other substances. The complex vascular response to injury may subsequently involve vasospasm, localized vascular contraction, luminal obliteration, and events that are mediated by calcium, prostaglandins, or inhibition of release of endothelium-derived relaxing factor (326–28).

The critical unifying feature is that the normally well-controlled and regulated immune response somehow goes out of control. The reason for this exuberant loss of control is unknown, but it may involve the type or persistence of a particular antigenic stimulus or some hidden flaw in the regulatory apparatus that is either inherited or acquired.

In many instances clear evidence exists that circulating immune complexes attach to the vascular endothelium, leading to complement activation, polymorphonuclear chemotaxis, and

TABLE 7.11. *Systemic vasculopathic conditions associated with neurologic disease*

Primary vasculitides
  Behçet disease
  Churg-Strauss angiitis
  Cogan syndrome
  Eales disease
  Giant cell arteritis
    Takayasu arteritis (Pulseless disease)
    Temporal arteritis (Horton disease)
  Hypersensitivity vasculitides
    Cryoglobulinemia
    Cutaneous vasculitis
    Henoch-Schönlein purpura
    Hypersensitivity angiitis of Zeek
    Hypocomplementemic vasculitis
    Hypersensitivity vasculitides caused by infection, malignancy, or connective tissue diseases
      Allergic granulomatous angiitis
      Granulomatous angiitis
    Serum sickness
  Kawasaki disease/infantile polyarteritis nodosa
  Peripheral nervous system vasculitis
  Polyarteritis nodosa
  Primary angiitis of the central nervous system
  Vogt-Koyanagi-Harada syndrome
  Wegener's granulomatosis
Secondary vasculitides
  Collagen vascular diseases
    Acute rheumatic fever
    Juvenile rheumatoid arthritis
    Mixed connective tissue disease
    Sjögren syndrome
    Systemic lupus erythematosus
    Systemic sclerosis (scleroderma)
  Autoimmune endocrinopathies
  Infectious vasculitis
  Neoplastic vasculitis
  Toxic vasculitis
    Immunosuppressive drugs
Other vasculopathic conditions
  Acute hypertension
  Amphetamine vasculopathy
  Amyloid angiopathy
  Fibromuscular dysplasia
  Köhlmeier-Degos disease
  Lymphomatoid granulomatosis
  Microangiopathy of the brain, ear, and retina
  Moyamoya disease
  Necrotizing sarcoid granulomatosis
  Sarcoidosis
  Sneddon syndrome

phagocytosis of immune complexes with release of chemicals harmful to vessel wall constituents. The type of blood vessel and organ system that contains that vessel, and the degree immune dysregulation dictate the type and severity of disease.

Few examples of vasculitic conditions are primarily antibody mediated. Kawasaki disease and infantile periarteritis nodosa, which probably are the same disease, and Wegener's granulomatosis are representative examples. In Kawasaki disease, circulating cytokines such as IL-1 and tumor necrosis factor either alter existing endothelial antigens or induce the formation of new antigenic epitopes, to which antiendothelial antibodies then respond with ensuing endothelial lysis associated with induction of thrombosis. Other forms of vasculitic inflammation may then be provoked. Wegener's granulomatosis is mediated by antineutrophilic and monocytic cytoplasmic component antibodies. These antibodies may directly injure vascular endothelium, possibly because of molecular mimicry. Alternatively, they may in their interaction with the target inflammatory cells provoke degranulation and release of lysosomal enzymes, oxidants, cytokines, or other substances that can alter endothelial antigens, directly injure the endothelium, or incite further inflammatory responses that injure the vascular endothelium.

Immune complex–mediated vasculitis is best exemplified by systemic (serum sickness) or focal (Arthus reaction) formation and circulation of antigen-antibody complexes that occur in the context of antigen excess. The complexes become deposited on vascular endothelium, where complement activation and recruitment of granulocytes and macrophages then occur. Inflammatory injury to the endothelium develops, followed by necrosis. In many cases this is associated with thrombosis, luminal occlusion, and hemorrhage within the vascular wall. These mechanisms appear to be the cause of hypersensitivity vasculitis and polyarteritis nodosa (PAN), conditions in which circulating immune complexes have been detected.

Various populations of activated T cells may be involved in cell-mediated vasculitis. These cells have in some fashion become sensitized to tissue specific antigens expressed in target cells or tissues such as myelin. Examples may include primary angiitis of the CNS, or vasculitis of peripheral nerves. Sensitization of the T cells is likely to require the formation of a tri-

TABLE 7.12. *Vasculitides affecting the nervous system*

Disease	Systemic manifestations	Characteristic laboratory features	Neurologic symptoms
Churg-Strauss syndrome	Lungs primarily	Peripheral hypereosinophilia	Peripheral neuropathy
Cogan syndrome	Interstitial keratitis, aortic valvulitis	Cerebrospinal fluid pleocytosis	Progressive deafness, vestibular abnormalities, encephalopathy
Takayasu disease	Aortic arch affected predominantly, female subjects affected mainly	Elevated erythrocyte sedimentation rate	Vascular accidents, vision loss
Temporal arteritis	In pediatric population affects temporal arteries and external carotids	Elevated serum levels of elastin peptide	Headaches, painful nodule of superficial temporal artery, vision loss
Wegener's granulomatosis	Small vessels of respiratory tract and kidneys	Elevated erythrocyte sedimentation rate, thrombocytosis	Peripheral neuropathy
Mixed connective tissue disease	Skin lesions of dermatomyositis, scleroderma	Antibodies directed at the ribonucleases-sensitive component of extractable nuclear antigen	Headache, seizures, aseptic meningitis

molecular complex with antigen and antigen-presenting cell, as is discussed for GBS and ADEM. Promotion of the inflammatory process involves the release of various cytokines from T cells, endothelial cells, macrophages, or other cells. T-cell release of interferon-γ prompts the formation of adhesion molecules on the endothelial surface, molecules that recruit or retain additional T cells that are not specific for the initiating antigen.

CNS vasculitis tends to present with one or more of the following: encephalopathy, stroke, or seizure. The primary mechanism for neurologic dysfunction in patients with vasculitis is presumed to be ischemia caused by angiitic luminal compromise (324,325,329). In some cases vasospasm, embolization from necrotic areas of vascular endothelial compromise, secondary propagation of the inflammatory response within nervous tissues, or other mechanisms contribute to neurologic dysfunction. Moreover, patients with systemic vasculitides may experience neurologic dysfunction as the secondary result of the impaired function of other organs, such as heart, lung, liver, or kidney. Vasculitides that affect the peripheral nervous system may produce mononeuropathy multiplex, radiculopathy, plexopathy, or polyneuropathy. Nerves of various size and function may be involved, resulting variously in neuropathies that

are primarily motor, primarily sensory, autonomic, or a mixture of these elements.

Primary Systemic Vasculitides

Of the various primary systemic vasculitides, Behçet disease, Kawasaki disease, and Vogt-Koyanagi-Harada syndrome are covered in Chapter 6. Giant cell arteritis, Churg-Strauss vasculitis, Takayasu disease, and Cogan syndrome are rarely seen in the pediatric population. These conditions are summarized in Table 7.12.

Primary Angiitis of the Central Nervous System

Primary angiitis of the CNS (PACNS) is a rare entity whose manifestations are confined to the CNS. The disorder is mainly seen in adults and presents with a wide spectrum of severity. Although PACNS is diagnosed most frequently in middle age, reports have included patients with ages ranging from 3 to 78 years. Slightly more than two-thirds of cases have occurred in male subjects. There is no clear regional or racial predilection. The pathologic manifestations consist of a prominent vasculitic mononuclear cell infiltrate that almost invariably affects small vessels; medium-sized vessels are involved in approximately three-fourths of cases. Multinucleated giant cells are commonly seen; for this reason the condition also has been termed *granulomatous angiitis* (329a). No vascular deposition of immunoglobulin can be found, supporting the view that PACNS is a cell-mediated vasculitis (329,330).

The most common clinical presentation is that of encephalopathy with headache. Mental status may range from normal with irritability to various degrees of confusion and obtundation. Almost any focal manifestation of dysfunction of the encephalon may be found in association. In some cases strokes, single or multiple cranial neuropathies, or spinal cord syndromes are the predominant or sole manifestations of PACNS (331). CSF pleocytosis or mild elevation of CSF protein is found in approximately one-half the cases of PACNS (330,332,333).

PACNS is a diagnosis of exclusion. In almost all instances cerebral angiography is abnormal and shows vascular irregularities and luminal narrowing in multiple vessels producing a beaded appearance (332). MRI changes include widespread, small, and irregular tufts of T2 bright signal that suggest a vasculitis rather than ADEM; the plaquelike lesions at the gray-white junction that are so characteristic of ADEM are usually not present. The sedimentation rate is almost invariably normal, whereas various autoantibodies are absent. These findings, which are suggestive of the diagnosis, can only be confirmed by brain biopsy.

Untreated, PACNS can be fatal. However, remission or even cure may be attained in patients who are treated with the combination of oral prednisone and cyclophosphamide, as outlined by Woolfenden and colleagues (332). The combination therapy should be continued for at least 1 year. Thereupon, if angiographic evaluation of patients who formerly displayed angiographic abnormalities shows resolution, cyclophosphamide can be discontinued and the prednisone tapered over 3 to 6 months. PACNS should be suspected in children who are thought to have corticosteroid-responsive forms of ADEM that relapse as long-term corticosteroid monotherapy is weaned to low dosages. The usual threshold for relapse is at prednisone equivalents of approximately 12 to 16 mg administered every other day (333).

Polyarteritis Nodosa

PAN accounts for approximately 15% of all cases of systemic vasculitis (334). The incidence is approximately 0.7 to 1.8 in 100,000 per year, prevalence is approximately 5 in 100,000, and boys are approximately 2.5 times as likely to have PAN. Most cases occur in adults and most childhood cases occur in older children and adolescents. However, the disease has been described in children as young as 6 years of age.

The pathologic changes of PAN are necrotizing arteriopathic vasculitis. The inflammatory angiocentric exudate is predominantly granulocytic, tending to involve small and medium-sized muscular arteries and occasional arterioles. Obliterative and necrotizing endarteritis may develop and microaneurysm formation and rupture may complicate the disease (335).

PAN is caused by a multiplicity of causes. At least one-half of the cases of PAN appear to be an immune complex–mediated vasculitic condition with detectable circulating immune complexes. Up to 40% of adults with PAN are chronic carriers of hepatitis B antigen, and circulating immune complexes involving the hepatitis B antigen could be involved in the pathogenesis of this disease in some patients (336). Familial Mediterranean fever, an autosomal-recessive illness characterized by recurrent but self-limited fever and polyserositis, is another disease that has been associated with the development of PAN. In such cases the Mediterranean fever tends to manifest before 12 years of age and PAN shortly thereafter (337,338).

Clinical Manifestations

PAN is uncommon in the pediatric population, though two distinct syndromes have been recognized. An infantile form has a predilection for the coronary arteries and is probably the same as Kawasaki disease. This variant can be associated with seizures and aseptic meningitis (339). Kawasaki disease is more fully considered in Chapter 6.

In older children, PAN resembles the clinical picture seen in adults. In the Turkish series of Ozen and coworkers, severe myalgia unresponsive to analgesics was seen as the presenting complaint in 77% of children (340). Peripheral nerve involvement marked by numbness and paresthesias was seen in 13%. Encephalitic symptoms including seizures, cranial nerve palsies, and hemiplegia also were encountered (341). Multiple mononeuropathies (mononeuritis multiplex) are said to be characteristic of the condition. Mononeuritis multiplex refers to involvement of several or many individual nerves simultaneously or at different times in the course of the disease (342). The peripheral nerves most frequently affected are the branches of the lateral popliteal nerve (343). Remissions and relapses of neuropathy are common. Coalescence of the multiple nerve lesions, usually seen at a late stage of the illness, results in a symmetric polyneuritis. Practically every cranial nerve has been reported involved.

Asymmetric shrinkage of visual fields, scotomata, and loss of acuity may occur as consequences of proliferative retinitis and retinal hemorrhage. Appropriate funduscopic changes should be evident. Papilledema may develop in patients with intracranial hypertension; these patients and those with significant systemic hypertension are at greater risk for retinal hemorrhage (344).

Diagnosis

The diagnosis of PAN should be considered in patients whose obscure febrile illness is linked with disease of the CNS or peripheral nervous system and in whom antinuclear and anti-DNA antibodies are negative. In the series of Ozen and colleagues, hepatitis B antigen was only present in 10% (340). Neuroimaging studies of brain may be normal, but can demonstrate bland or hemorrhagic infarction, focal or generalized encephalomalacia, or intraparenchymal or subarachnoid blood. Cerebral angiography may be normal early in the course of illness, but segmental narrowing of small and medium-sized vessels is often found after weeks or months of illness. Areas of microaneurysmal dilatation involving superficial or deep small or medium-sized arteries are less commonly seen (340).

Diagnosis usually requires angiography of liver, kidney, and gut in combination with biopsy of symptomatic organs, especially kidney, as well as skin or muscle and its supplying nerve. The pathognomonic findings on renal angiography are segmental vasculitis of medium-sized renal arteries with microaneurysmal dilatation and focal hypoperfusion. Kidney biopsy demonstrates necrotizing arteritis or diffuse glomerulonephritis. Because the distribution of the characteristic necrotizing arteritis is irregular, a negative biopsy result by no means excludes the diagnosis.

Several other vasculitic syndromes can affect the CNS. Most of these are uncommon in childhood. They are summarized in Table 7.12. Those most likely to be encountered in children include Takayasu's arteritis, granulomatous angiitis of the nervous system, Cogan syndrome, and Wegener's granulomatosis. Takayasu's arteritis tends to affect the aortic arch and its major branches, but reduced cerebral blood flow can result in neurologic symptoms, notably transient loss of vision, vertigo, syncope, and cerebral infarction (345). Primary angiitis of the nervous system tends to present with a global dysfunction of the nervous system, marked headache, weakness, and confusion. Cogan syndrome, which can be seen in adolescence, presents with episodes of acute interstitial keratitis occasionally accompanied by a meningoencephalitis or a cranial neuropathy (345). In Wegener's granulomatosis, granulomatous lesions of the upper respiratory tract and lungs are accompanied by an inflammatory process of the small and medium-sized arteries and veins. Neurologic symptoms were seen in 17% of children in the series of Rottem and colleagues. The symptoms included a peripheral neuropathy, multiple cranial nerve palsies, and seizures (346). The presence of antineutrophil cytoplasmic antibodies indicates the diagnosis. Mixed connective tissue disease combines the features of progressive systemic sclerosis with those of polymyositis and SLE. It is usually not seen in children. The most common significant neurologic complication of this condition is myositis. Other neurologic complications of childhood mixed connective tissue disease include headache, seizures, elevation of CSF protein, and aseptic meningitis (347).

Treatment

Evaluation of therapy is complicated by the natural fluctuations of the disease. Corticosteroid therapy combined with immunosuppressant drugs is the preferred treatment (336). Adult PAN patients have been treated successfully with the combination of corticosteroids and plasmapheresis, but no information exists concerning the efficacy of this combination in children with PAN. The prognosis of childhood cases is poor, and the disease tends to assume a steady, downhill course (339). In the series of Ozen and coworkers, complete remission was achieved in only 13% of children (340).

SECONDARY SYSTEMIC VASCULITIDES

Collagen Vascular Diseases

Acute Rheumatic Fever

The characteristic pathologic lesion of acute rheumatic fever is a rheumatic proliferative endarteritis. Neuropathologic descriptions of patients with acute rheumatic fever are not abundant. Proliferative endarteritis of smaller cerebral cortical and meningeal blood vessels has been described. Patches of cortical encephaloclasia also have been noted, presumably caused by obliterative endarteritis (348).

Infantile Multisystem Inflammatory Disease

A multisystem inflammatory syndrome has been described during the first year of life. It is marked by the onset of arthritis and intermittent fever and is associated with adenopathy, an evanescent maculopapular rash, CSF pleocytosis, a persistently open fontanelle, papilledema, and seizures. Development may slow, and cerebral atrophy may be apparent on brain imaging. A relationship to juvenile rheumatoid arthritis (JRA) has been suggested but remains unproven. The condition must be differentiated from early onset JRA and from Behçet syndrome (349).

Juvenile Rheumatoid Arthritis

Except for fatigue, irritability, myalgia, or disuse amyotrophy, neurologic dysfunction is uncommon in JRA. Focal neurologic disturbances that do occur are produced most commonly as the secondary consequence either of inflammatory processes that involve soft tissues or bone, or of the treatments for JRA (350). Some 6% of patients with JRA develop encephalopathy (351). This can take the form of meningismus and seizures. In a milder form, it is marked by irritability, drowsiness, and a diffusely abnormal electroencephalographic result. Progression to decorticate posturing and coma also has been noted.

A symmetric, ascending, sensorimotor polyneuropathy has been seen in some children with rheumatoid arthritis or scleroderma (352). This polyneuropathy is probably caused by an arteritis of the vasa nervorum and generally carries a poor prognosis. The CSF can show increased protein content and, less commonly, mild pleocytosis.

Rarely, patients with JRA develop other immune-mediated diseases that involve the neuromuscular system, notably myositis, myasthenia gravis, or inflammatory neuropathy (353).

Most neurologic complications of JRA improve once the underlying systemic JRA is brought under control. Many cases respond to aspirin or nonsteroidal antiinflammatory agents. In other instances corticosteroids, IVIG, parenteral gold salts, penicillamine, or immunosuppressive agents are required (354). Appropriate physical and occupational therapy can alleviate pain and assist in the management of spinal and muscular dysfunction or peripheral nerve entrapment (355).

Scleroderma

Two forms of scleroderma occur in childhood: focal scleroderma and childhood progressive systemic sclerosis. Both are chronic systemic diseases that involve integument and connective tissues as well as joints and visceral organs. Typical dermal histologic features include increased thickness and density of subepidermal collagen associated with scattered foci of perivascular mononuclear infiltrate.

The chief manifestations of focal scleroderma, peculiarly a disease of childhood and adolescence, are morphea and linear scleroderma. Both of these lesions initially present with edema and induration with subsequent sclerotic atrophy and the development of associated hyperpigmentation. Focal scleroderma is associated with abnormalities of esophageal peristalsis, chronic recurrent sinusitis, and hemiatrophy. Renal and cardiac abnormalities often remain subclinical. Neurologic complications include headache, seizures, and a variety of ophthalmologic disturbances that range from diplopia to indistinct or diminished vision. Some of these cases have developed vasculitic changes in the small or medium-sized cerebral or meningeal vessels underlying linear scleroderma or morphea of the face or scalp. Contralateral hemiatrophy, hemiparesis, and focal seizures may develop in such cases (356). Peripheral neuropathy, possibly the result of involvement of endoneurial blood vessels, and inflammatory myopathy resembling polymyositis also may develop (357).

Sjögren Syndrome

Sjögren syndrome, characterized by xerostomia, recurrent lymphocytic inflammation of the salivary glands, and keratoconjunctivitis sicca rarely afflicts children (358). No neurologic complications have been noted in the few childhood cases that have occurred primarily in adolescent girls.

Systemic Lupus Erythematosus

SLE is an inflammatory disease affecting blood vessels and connective and other bodily tissues. The annual incidence in North America is approximately 5 in 100,000; the prevalence is approximately 45 to 50 in 100,000 (359). Neurologic complications, occurring either as presenting symptoms or sometime in the course of the illness, occur in 10% to 45% of children affected by SLE (360,361).

Pathology and Pathogenesis

Genetic and hormonal factors may render certain individuals more vulnerable to a poorly regulated immune response to infection or other environmental factors that develops into a self-sustaining autoimmune disease. At least five genes have been implicated in determining genetic predisposition. Individuals who develop the disease can make pathogenic subsets of autoantibodies and immune complexes and cannot regulate their production or clearance.

Within the CNS, lesions of SLE are focal, diffuse, or both and are produced by several mechanisms (362).

A true vasculitis is relatively rare; it is seen in only 8% to 16% of patients with CNS manifestations (363). More characteristic is a noninflammatory vasculopathy that induces intimal proliferation of the small cerebral and meningeal arteries and induces multiple ischemic lesions (364,365). Embolic brain infarcts, generally arising from the heart, were encountered in 20% of the autopsy series of Devinsky and coworkers (366). Additionally, thrombotic thrombocytopenic purpura and a variety of bacterial or mycotic infections also can produce abnormalities in SLE. Gross hemorrhages are seen in some 10% of reported cases with CNS lupus. They are believed to arise from aneurysmal dilatations of the arteries induced by lupus angiitis.

In many instances, the extent of the microvascular lesions and the severity of the clinical picture correlate poorly. For this reason, brain-reactive antibodies–antineuronal antibodies, antiglial antibodies, anti-GM_1 ganglioside, and antiribosomal P protein have been implicated in the pathogenesis of the neurologic symptoms, with the antibodies being able to enter the CNS as a consequence of a disruption in the normal blood–brain barrier (367–369). Supporting this suggestion are the observations that immunoglobulins adhere to neurons in postmortem material, and that the concentration of antineuronal antibodies is elevated in the CSF of patients with CNS lupus, but not in those who have SLE without neurologic complications. Antiribosomal P antibodies are more likely to be elevated in pediatric SLE patients with psychosis, than in those SLE patients without psychosis (370). Furthermore, the presence of circulating antiphospholipid antibodies is associated with cerebral arterial and venous thromboses, producing transient ischemic attacks or vascular accidents (371). Antiphospholipid antibodies interfere with the protein C pathway, resulting in prolonged activation of the coagulation system after small vessel damage and thrombosis. Additionally, antiphospholipid antibodies can cause endocardial and cardiac valvular disease and thrombocytopenia (372). Mackworth-Young has reviewed the multiple effects of the antiphospholipid antibodies (373).

Despite the multiplicity of abnormal serologic reactions against many different tissue components, especially nuclear proteins, the pathogenesis of SLE remains uncertain, as does the manner in which autoantibodies produce tissue damage. The disease is currently believed to result from multiple events that begin as interactions between susceptibility genes and environmental stimuli to create an abnormal CD4+ T-cell driving force, which results in the production of autoantibodies and immune complexes that cause tissue damage. Hahn provides a more extensive discussion of the pathogenesis of the disease (374).

Clinical Manifestations

Female subjects are susceptible to SLE more than male subjects by a ratio as high as 9:1, with onset in the second decade of life. CNS manifestations can occur at any time in the course of the illness. Neuropsychiatric complications develop in more than one-half and other neurologic complications in 20% to 45% of patients with SLE and are the first manifestations of SLE in approximately 5% of cases (360,361).

Two neurologic syndromes can be distinguished as based on information derived from serologic data and neuroimaging (375). The first, and more common, entity is a diffuse, toxic encephalopathy that results in an organic psychosis, behavioral disorders, generalized seizures, or migrainelike headaches. Virtually every form of psychiatric disturbance has been described, ranging from disorders of mood or personality to psychosis. Anxiety or depression may be acute or intermittent and is a common early complaint in SLE, as are irritability and episodes of unusual elation. Episodic or progressive confusion, memory disturbance, and other forms of cognitive disability can occur and in some cases progressive dementia ensues. These symptoms can be caused by cerebral lesions (vascular or immunologic), and in as many as 80% of cases they are accompanied by

high titers of antineuronal antibodies, antineurofilament antibodies, antiribosomal P, or other autoantibodies. The role, if any, of these autoantibodies in the evolution of CNS symptoms is still uncertain (376). Patients who develop neurologic complications usually do so within the first year of illness. The prevalence of neurologic complications such as neuropsychiatric, cerebrovascular, peripheral neuromuscular, nonspecific encephalopathy, and seizures increases with increasing chronicity of SLE. MRI often demonstrates increased signal on T2-weighted images in the occipital lobes and in subcortical white matter that does not correspond to any vascular distribution (377). Increased signal on T2-weighted images also can be seen in the periventricular region. In the series of Stimmler and coworkers, the latter type of abnormality was associated frequently with lupus nephritis and hypertension (378).

A diffuse encephalopathy also can be induced by electrolyte disturbances, the result of impaired renal tubular function, or, rarely, by corticosteroid therapy. Much more commonly, a psychotic reaction is seen during acute exacerbations of the disease, and symptoms improve as systemic manifestations of SLE are corrected with corticosteroid therapy (363,379).

The second syndrome involves focal neurologic symptoms, which can take the form of focal seizures, cranial nerve palsies, and cerebral infarctions. Less commonly, a myelopathy, polyneuritis, and movement disorders, notably chorea, can develop (380). This syndrome is the result of thrombotic or embolic CNS disease and is associated with a high incidence of antiphospholipid antibodies (381). Several antiphospholipid antibodies have been described. These include anticardiolipin antibodies and the lupus anticoagulant. Antiphospholipid antibodies are strongly associated with cerebrovascular disease, not only in the framework of CNS lupus, but also in young individuals who lack clinical or serologic evidence for lupus (see Chapter 12). Antiphospholipid antibodies also are present in chorea, not only when chorea develops as part of the clinical picture of SLE, but also in choreic patients with the primary antiphospholipid antibody syndrome. The clinical appearance of these

TABLE 7.13. *Neurologic symptoms and signs in 16 children with systemic lupus erythematosus*

Symptom or sign[a]	Number of patients
Headache	7
Lethargy	7
Acute organic brain syndrome	6
Seizures	5
Cranial nerve palsies	3
Ataxia	3
Papilledema	2
Basal ganglia involvement	2

[a]No cases of chorea were encountered in this particular series.

From Yancey CL, Doughty RA, Athreya BH. Central nervous system involvement in childhood systemic lupus erythematosus. Reprinted from *Arthritis and Rheum* 1981;24:1389. With permission of the American College of Rheumatology.

TABLE 7.14. *Neuropsychiatric symptoms encountered in systemic lupus erythematosus*

Central nervous system
  Aseptic meningitis
  Cerebrovascular disease
  Demyelinating syndrome
  Headache (including migraine and benign intracranial hypertension)
  Movement disorder (chorea)
  Myelopathy
  Seizure disorders
  Acute confusional state
  Anxiety attacks
  Cognitive dysfunction
  Mood disorder
  Psychosis
Peripheral nervous system
  Guillain-Barré syndrome (acute inflammatory demyelinating polyneuropathy)
  Autonomic disorder
  Motor neuropathy, single/multiplex
  Myasthenia gravis
  Neuropathy, cranial
  Plexopathy
  Polyneuropathy

From The American College of Rheumatology. Nomenclature and case definitions for neuropsychiatric lupus syndromes. *Arthritis Rheum* 1999;42:599. With permission.

forms of chorea is indistinguishable from that of Sydenham chorea (382). The MRI features in patients with SLE and focal neurologic signs resemble those of cerebral infarctions (377). MRI changes consistent with major arterial territory infarction in patients with lupus have been associated with elevated cardiolipin and lupus anticoagulant titers rather than the various other brain tissue-specific antibodies that may develop in patients with lupus (383).

The most common neurologic symptoms and signs of childhood SLE are listed in Table 7.13 (361). In 35% of patients, neurologic involvement, most commonly headache, lethargy, an organic brain syndrome, and seizures, was the presenting manifestation. Seizures are usually self-limited. When antiepileptic drugs are administered, early discontinuation should be considered, especially in cases in which primary disease activity or a specific complication has been effectively ameliorated. Of those 35% who had CNS lupus, 81% presented with evidence for SLE. Although chorea was not encountered in this particular series, it occurs in up to 4% of childhood SLE and occasionally precedes the development of other clinical manifestations of SLE by months or, rarely, years (384,385). Transient visual abnormalities are experienced by at least 5% of children with systemic SLE. These include sudden or gradual vision loss, optic neuritis, or pseudotumor cerebri. Funduscopy may disclose papilledema, more likely caused by pseudotumor cerebri than caused by increased intracranial pressure, although cerebral vein thrombosis, related to the presence of antiphospholipid antibodies has been reported (386,387). Patients also may develop diplopia, ophthalmoplegia, or ptosis, along with such other brainstem or cerebellar manifestations as facial sensory or motor dysfunction, acute hearing loss, vertigo, vocal cord paralysis, or ataxia (380,388). Transverse myelopathy, the consequence in at least some cases of ischemic spinal cord infarction, has been encountered (389). Peripheral neuropathy and myositis also have been described (388). A standardized nomenclature for the neuropsychiatric syndromes has been developed (390) and is presented in Table 7.14.

The progression of childhood SLE varies. Spontaneous exacerbations and remissions are common; the ultimate prognosis, although still not good, has improved considerably since the 1970s (361,379). In the experience of Yancey and associates, reported in 1981, 12% of children died in the course of a 5-year follow-up; the majority of survivors was able to return to school (361). Although pre-illness IQs were generally unavailable, many children appeared to experience a decline in intelligence during the course of their disease.

Diagnosis

The diagnosis of SLE in the presence of exclusively neurologic symptoms is difficult and rests on either the intermittency of symptoms or evidence of systemic involvement including renal abnormalities, notably hematuria and albuminuria. No single laboratory tool can make a definite diagnosis of CNS lupus. Tests that confirm the diagnosis include the immunofluorescent antinuclear antibody test, which has a positive result in almost every patient with presenting neurologic symptoms owing to SLE [97% in the series of Yancey and coworkers (361)]. This test result also is positive, however, in rheumatoid arthritis, in a small percentage of patients with dermatomyositis, and in chronic active hepatitis. It quickly becomes negative with corticosteroid therapy.

The presence of antibodies against DNA is the most specific laboratory test. The test result was positive in 86% of patients in the series of Yancey and colleagues (361), and it also provides information about the activity of the disease. Measurements of antibodies against ribonucleoprotein and Sm antigen, a soluble nucleoprotein antigen, also are being used clinically.

Lupus erythematosus (LE) cells are detectable in the bone marrow or in the buffy coat of peripheral blood at some time during the course of the disease. They occasionally can be seen in the CSF. The LE cells are formed when IgG antideoxyribonucleoprotein antibodies react with cell nuclei to form altered nuclear material that is taken up by phagocytes. The LE cell test is, therefore, a method of detecting IgG antinuclear antibodies to deoxyribonucleoproteins. It is rarely positive in the absence of a positive antinuclear antibody test result, but it frequently becomes negative when the patient enters a clinical remission.

CSF pleocytosis has been documented in 10% to 30% of patients with CNS lupus. CSF protein is elevated in 50%, and occasionally low CSF glucose occurs.

MRI and CT scans are generally abnormal in subjects with focal neurologic signs or seizures. The abnormalities in subjects with diffuse CNS involvement are often transient and may resolve spontaneously or with corticosteroid therapy. Cerebral atrophy can correlate with corticosteroid therapy, as this finding has been encountered in patients receiving systemic corticosteroid therapy but lacking CNS involvement (391,392). PET scans can show areas of focal hypometabolism even when the MRI is normal. This is particularly true for patients in whom seizures are a manifestation of CNS lupus (393).

SLE also can be induced by a variety of drugs. The most important group, from the viewpoint of the pediatric neurologist, is the anticonvulsants, particularly hydantoins, trimethadione, ethosuximide, and possibly carbamazepine (394). Symptoms include fever, migratory polyarthritis, a malar rash, and widespread lymphadenopathy (395,396). These symptoms usually subside when the offending medication is discontinued, but continued exposure to the drug once symptoms have developed can induce irreversible SLE. It is not clear whether these isolated cases represent instances of idiopathic systemic lupus that were unmasked by the anticonvulsant. Approximately 20% of children attending a seizure clinic were found to have antinuclear antibodies. Because none of these children developed symptoms of SLE after a prolonged follow-up, the presence of these antibodies need not prompt the physician to discontinue anticonvulsant medication (396).

Treatment

A full discussion of the management of SLE is beyond the scope of this text, because it is rather more of an art than a science (397). As with systemic manifestations, oral corticosteroids, high-dose intravenous corticosteroids, immunosuppressants, and, in some instances, plasmapheresis can control neurologic symptoms without curing the disease (398,399). In particular, the combination of intravenous methylprednisolone and cyclophosphamide appears to be of considerable benefit for children with severe neuropsychiatric symptoms (400). Seizures and an organic mental syndrome can be induced by hormone therapy, but more commonly are part of the disease process itself, and their appearance should not be an indication to discontinue therapy; rather, they should suggest increases in corticosteroid dosage. Thromboembolization in the presence of elevated antiphospholipid antibodies can be treated with antiplatelet drugs or anticoagulation. Intravenous gammaglobulin also has been suggested (363). Increases in serum complement levels or reversion of a positive DNA antibody test result correlate well with changes in the activity of the disease (401).

NEUROLOGIC COMPLICATIONS OF IMMUNIZATIONS

Postvaccinal Encephalomyelitis

Although no longer encountered, the neurologic complications after smallpox vaccination can be considered as a prototype for complications encountered after various other immunizations in which a live organism is introduced into the human host. Neurologic complications were seen after either primary or repeat vaccination. Their average incidence was 2.9 in 1,000,000 vaccinations, with the highest frequency in the younger vaccinated subjects.

Two clinical pictures were observed. Postvaccinal encephalomyelitis was an acute illness that began during the second week after the successful vaccination of a nonimmune subject (402,403). Its pathologic picture was highlighted by perivascular demyelination and is identical to the postexanthematous encephalitides.

The other postvaccinal complication was termed *postvaccinal encephalopathy*. It commonly affected infants younger than 2 years old and followed a variable incubation period of 1 to 24 days. The condition was heralded by a prolonged generalized convulsion. The CSF was normal, and aside from cerebral edema, no striking pathologic alterations were encountered.

Postrabies Vaccination Encephalopathy

Because rabies immunization by the use of either a duck embryo vaccine or vaccines grown in human diploid cell culture (preparations with a low content of nervous tissue antigen) has become common practice in western countries, the incidence of postvaccinal complications has fallen markedly. The current estimated rate is less than 1 in 100,000 individuals, contrasted with 1 in 300 to 1 in 7,000 at a time when the neural vaccines were being used (404). In third-world countries, vaccines grown in brain or spinal cord are still in vogue, and the most recently reported incidence of encephalomyelitis was 1 in 220, with a 17% mortality (405).

Neurologic symptoms appear 8 to 21 days after the first injection of the vaccine. Their onset is marked by chills, fever, headache, myalgia, vomiting, and changes in mental status. The most common neurologic complications are encephalitis and meningitis. Each of these was encountered in one-third of subjects in a series from Thailand (98). Less frequently, patients develop transverse myelitis, usually involving the thoracic or lumbar segments of the spinal cord, or neuritis of the peripheral, and less often of the cranial nerves (98,405). A postvaccination GBS also has been encountered (240a). High titers of IgG and IgM antibodies to GM_1 and GD_{1a} ganglioside have been detected in patients with neuroparalytic complications, suggesting that these antibodies play a pathogenetic role in postvaccine demyelination (405a). Genetic susceptibility also may play a role in the pathogenesis of the encephalopathy (405b).

The CSF usually shows lymphocytic pleocytosis and increased protein content. CSF MBP is elevated within 1 day after the onset of the neurologic symptoms, and lymphocytes demonstrate a positive response to purified myelin in approximately one-half of the patients (98). The MRI demonstrates multiple white matter lesions in the cerebrum, cerebellar peduncles, and brainstem, which resolve in parallel with clinical improvement (405c). Although relapses occur occasionally, the disease is usually monophasic. Treatment with dexamethasone has been recommended. Patients usually recover in 1 to 2 weeks. In the Thailand series, recovery was complete in 83% of patients.

Postinfluenza Vaccination

Before 1976, when a federal program of immunization against swine flu was initiated, complications of influenza immunization were rare. The incidence of postinfluenza vaccination encephalitis is uncertain. In the cases reported to the surveillance group, almost all patients developed systemic and neurologic symptoms in 5 hours to 4 days after the immunization. The neurologic picture was characterized by a change in consciousness and occasionally by brainstem dysfunction. The CSF showed significant pleocytosis in approximately one-half the instances. In the majority of cases, recovery was reported to be complete.

A GBS-like polyneuropathy was observed more often, occurring in 1 in 100,000 immunizations. It began between 5 and 10 weeks after the immunization (406). The clinical course of this complication was similar to that seen after viral infections.

Other reported complications included brachial plexus neuropathy, transverse myelitis, optic neuritis, and other cranial neuropathies (406).

Encephalopathy after Pertussis Vaccination

Hardly any other subject in pediatric neurology has evoked more controversy in both professional and lay groups than the neurologic complications after immunization with the whole-cell vaccine.

Although the earliest reports date back to 1933, Byers and Moll were the first to document a severe encephalopathy after prophylactic pertussis vaccination in infants (407). Between that time and up to the introduction of acellular vaccine numerous reports were made of children who experienced seizures and encephalopathy soon after their pertussis immunization. A variety of neurologic complications have been recorded.

Febrile seizures and a hypotonic hyporesponsive state are temporary neurologic complications. In the prospective study of Cody and coworkers, both were encountered with a frequency of 1 in 1,750 immunizations, or approximately in 1 in 650 infants immunized (408). Although some of the infants who experienced a febrile seizure within 48 hours of their vaccination were younger than 5 to 6 months of age, and below the age range during which simple febrile seizures are generally encountered (see Chapter 13), the failure to document seizure recurrence or any permanent adverse effects in the majority of these infants suggests that a pyrogen in the whole-cell vaccine preparation evoked the seizure response. Approximately 10% of children who experience seizures within 48 hours of diptheria, pertussis, and tetanus (DPT) vaccination have afebrile convulsions (409).

Hypotonic hyporesponsive episodes occur within 24 hours, with a mean interval of 12 hours from immunization. Approximately one-half of infants are febrile, and the episode subsides in minutes to at most 4 hours, leaving no apparent residua (409). Additionally, persistent or high-pitched crying was seen in 3.2% of DPT-immunized infants, and drowsiness was seen in approximately 32%. These complications were far less common following the use of a diptheria tetanus (DT) vaccine (403). A smaller study, conducted in the United Kingdom using aluminum hydroxide-adsorbed DPT, failed to demonstrate any difference between DPT and DT vaccines with respect to the incidence of convulsions and other neurologic complications (410). Follow-up studies on the infants initially reported by Cody and associates did not uncover any apparent evidence of major neurologic damage (411). A transient increase in intracranial pressure, manifested by a bulging fontanelle, has been encountered after both whole-cell DPT and DT immunizations. Its mechanism is unknown (412). No long-term follow-up studies of infants with "minor" neurologic complications after whole-cell DPT administration have been carried out, but they would be important to determine whether such complications are precursors to hyperactivity, learning disorders, or perceptual handicaps.

Several seemingly permanent neurologic syndromes develop soon after whole-cell pertussis immunization. An encephalopathy characterized by generalized febrile or nonfebrile convulsions, altered consciousness, and serious neurologic or neuropsychological residua can occur within 72 hours of immunization. The encephalopathy's incidence has been estimated at 1 in 165,000 immunizations (413). The prognosis for survival is good, but most children, 77% in the series of Miller and colleagues, are left with major neurologic residua, retardation, or recurrent seizures (414,415). A similar high incidence of these complications was found in the older series of Byers and Moll (407) and Kulenkampff and coworkers (416). More commonly, the first seizure, febrile or afebrile, occurs within 24 hours of immunization, and the infants, usually without fully recovering to their preimmunization levels of functioning, develop a chronic mixed major and minor motor seizure disorder clinically related to Brett's epileptogenic encephalopathy, severe myoclonic epilepsy, or the Lennox-Gastaut syndrome (see Chapter 13). In the experience of Miller and associates 85% of children who developed afebrile seizures and 44% of children who developed prolonged febrile convulsions within 7 days of their vaccination died or were left with neurologic dysfunction. A serious seizure disorder commencing within 24 hours of immunization was recorded in 1 in 106,000 patients in a retrospective study conducted by Walker and coworkers (417).

Pathologic examination of the brain in infants who have died shortly after their pertussis immunization has not been helpful. Some have a diffuse neuronal destruction with gliosis; in others, the changes were minimal beyond cerebral edema. An acute encephalitis, perivascular infiltration, and demyelination were not seen (418). The picture thus differs from that seen in the encephalopathy that followed smallpox vaccination.

Experimental data indicate that pertussis toxin can attach itself to neuronal membrane receptors and, by ADP-ribosylation, modify the adenylate cyclase system so that the action of inhibitory neurotransmitters is impaired, and the action of excitatory neurotransmitters is enhanced (419,420). Whereas in the vast majority of cases the blood–brain barrier prevents entry of the toxin into the brain, its temporary disruption with a concurrent viral disease or fever or as a response to the endotoxin present in the vaccine, could well facilitate access of pertussis toxin to the nerve cells. Such a disruption has been seen in pertussis encephalopathy, in which high CSF antibody titers to pertussis toxin have been demonstrated (421).

None of the numerous epidemiologic studies has exonerated or implicated pertussis vaccine in these more serious adverse responses (422).

All are confounded by the relatively low incidence of these complications and by the differences in whole-cell pertussis vaccines as used at different times and in different countries. Whole-cell vaccines were not only not standardized between manufacturers, but also, one suspects, varied with the same manufacturer from one lot to the next. This is reflected in the marked differences in antibody response to pertussis vaccination (423).

From the wealth of case reports and studies attempting to understand the relationship, if any, between whole-cell pertussis immunization and permanent brain damage, the Institute of Medicine has offered three conclusions: (a) DPT administration causes a serious acute neurologic illness, and subsequent permanent neurologic dysfunction in children who otherwise would not have experienced either acute or chronic neurologic illness; (b) DPT vaccination triggers an acute and subsequently a chronic neurologic illness in children with an underlying brain abnormality; and (c) DPT vaccination causes an acute neurologic illness in children with underlying brain abnormalities, which would eventually have led to chronic neurologic disease even in the absence of the acute, DPT-initiated neurologic illness.

Choosing between these three alternatives depends a great deal on whether one sets out from the proposition that whole-cell pertussis vaccine can or cannot cause permanent neurologic damage in previously healthy children. There is of course no reason why the same alternative should be operative for all children with suspected vaccine reactions.

No major neurologic reactions to acellular pertussis vaccine have been reported to date.

Other Immunizations

Neurologic adverse reactions to the other immunizations are less controversial. The most common reaction to measles, mumps, and rubella immunization is mumps meningoencephalitis. Depending on the strain of vaccine used, its incidence ranges from 1 in 11,000 to 1 in 100,000 doses, with symptoms beginning between 15 and 35 days after immunization (424). Like meningitis induced by the wild mumps virus, the outcome is generally excellent (425).

Acute encephalopathy can follow immunization with live attenuated monovalent measles vaccine, or measles vaccine in combination with mumps vaccine, rubella vaccines, or both (426). The condition develops between 2 and 15 days after immunization, with the peak onset of encephalopathy on days 8 and 9. It is marked by seizures, altered behavior or consciousness, and ataxia. Death or mental regression is common. No cases of encephalopathy have been identified after administration of monovalent mumps or rubella vaccines (426). The association of measles, mumps, and rubella vaccination and autism or pervasive developmental disorders and Crohn disease (427) has not been confirmed; in fact, there was no sudden increase of autism in the United Kingdom after the introduction of measles, mumps, and rubella vaccine (427a). The administration of tetanus toxoid has been reported to be followed by some 10 to 14 days by polyneuritis, transverse myelitis, optic neuritis, or an encephalopathy (406,428).

The anterior horn disease that follows immunization with attenuated oral polio virus is covered in Chapter 6. In some children recovering from an acute episode of asthma, a flaccid paralysis resembling poliomyelitis has been encountered. This condition, first reported from Australia in 1974 (429), has been termed *Hopkins syndrome*. No consistent virus has been cultured from such patients, who generally have been successfully vaccinated against poliomyelitis. The disorder primarily involves the anterior horn cells. A rapid progression of paralysis usually affects one limb, leaving the child with a severe and permanent weakness. No sensory involvement occurs. The CSF usually shows moderate mononuclear pleocytosis, and the protein content can be slightly elevated (430). Some of the children have evidence for an underlying immune deficiency (431).

REFERENCES

1. Rivers TM, Schwentker FF. Encephalomyelitis accompanied by myelin destruction experimentally produced in monkeys. *J Exp Med* 1935;61:689–702.
2. Wolf A, Kabat EA, Bezer AE. The pathology of acute disseminated encephalomyelitis produced experimentally in the Rhesus monkey and its resemblance to human demyelinating disease. *J Neuropathol Exp Neurol* 1947;6:333–359.
3. Ferraro A, Cazullo CL. Chronic experimental allergic encephalomyelitis in monkeys. *J Neuropathol Exp Neurol* 1948;7:235–260.
4. Shaw C-M, Alvord EC, Hruby S. Chronic remitting relapsing experimental allergic encephalomyelitis induced in monkeys with homologous myelin basic protein. *Ann Neurol* 1988;24:738–748.
5. Wisniewski HW. Immunopathology of demyelination in autoimmune diseases and virus infections. *Br Med Bull* 1977;33:54–59.
6. Paterson PY. Molecular and cellular determinants of neuroimmunologic inflammatory disease. *Fed Proc* 1982;41:2569–2576.
7. Barbarese E, et al. Comparison of CNS homing pattern among murine TH cell lines responsive to myelin basic protein. *J Neuroimmunol* 1992;39:151–162.
8. Cammer W, et al. Degradation of basic protein in myelin by neutral proteases secreted by stimulated macrophages: a possible mechanism of inflammatory demyelination. *Proc Natl Acad Sci U S A* 1978; 75:1554–1558.
9. Ben Nun A, Wekerle H, Cohen IR. Vaccination against autoimmune encephalomyelitis with T-lymphocyte line cells reactive against myelin basic protein. *Nature* 1981;292:60–61.
10. Shaw MK, et al. A combination of adoptive transfer and antigenic challenge induces consistent murine experimental autoimmune encephalomyelitis in C57BL/6 mice and other reputed resistant strains. *J Neuroimmunol* 1992;39:139–149.
11. Hemachudha T, et al. Myelin basic protein as an encephalitogen in encephalitis and polyneuritis following rabies vaccination. *N Engl J Med* 1987;316:369–374.
12. Adams CW. The onset and progression of the lesion in multiple sclerosis. *J Neurol Sci* 1975;25:165–182.
12a. Matsumoto Y, et al. In situ inactivation of infiltrating T cells in the central nervous system with autoimmune encephalomyelitis: the role of astrocytes. *Immunology* 1993;79:381–390.
12b. Sugita K, et al. Involvement of cytokines in *N*-methyl-*N*-nitro-*N*-nitrosoguanidine-induced plasminogen activator activity in acute disseminated encephalomyelitis and multiple sclerosis lymphocytes. *Eur Neurol* 1993;33:358–362.
13. Matthews WB. *McAlpine's multiple sclerosis*, Edinburgh: Churchill Livingstone, 1991.
14. De Jong RN. Multiple sclerosis: history, definition and general considerations. In: Vinken PJ, Bruyn GW, eds. *Handbook of clinical neurology*. Amsterdam: North Holland Publishing Co., 1970:45–62.
15. Shaw CM, Alvord EC, Jr. Multiple sclerosis beginning in infancy. *J Child Neurol* 1987;2:252–256.
16. Hanefeld FA, et al. Childhood and juvenile multiple sclerosis. In: Bauer HJ, Hanefeld FA, eds. *Multiple sclerosis: its impact from childhood to old age*. Philadelphia: WB Saunders, 1993:14–52.
17. Sadovnick AD, Baird PA, Ward RH. Multiple sclerosis: updated risks for relatives. *Am J Med Genet* 1988;29:533–541.

18. Dal Canto MC, Rabinowitz SG. Experimental models of virus-induced demyelination of the central nervous system. *Ann Neurol* 1982;11:109–127.
19. Hillert J. Human leukocyte antigen studies in multiple sclerosis. *Ann Neurol* 1994;36:S15–S17.
20. Visscher BR, et al. HLA types and immunity in multiple sclerosis. *Neurology* 1979;29:1561–1565.
21. Oger JF, Arnason BGW. Immunogenetics of multiple sclerosis. In: Panayi GS, David CS, eds. *Immunogenetics*. London: Butterworth, 1984:177–206.
22. Tiwari JL, Terasaki PI. *HLA and disease associations*, New York: Springer-Verlag, 1985.
23. Mumford CJ, et al. The British Isles survey of multiple sclerosis in twins. *Neurology* 1994;44:11–15.
24. Ebers GC. Genetics and multiple sclerosis: an overview. *Ann Neurol* 1994;36:S12–S14.
25. Compston DAS. Genetic susceptibility to multiple sclerosis. In: Matthews WB, ed. *McAlpine's multiple sclerosis*. Edinburgh: Churchill Livingstone, 1991: 301–319.
26. Olsson T. Immunology of multiple sclerosis. *Curr Opin Neurol Neurosurg* 1992;5:195–202.
27. Utz U, McFarland HF. The role of T cells in multiple sclerosis: implications for therapies targeting the T cell receptor. *J Neuropathol Exp Neurol* 1994;53: 351–358.
28. Vandevyver C, et al. HLA and T-cell receptor polymorphisms in Belgian multiple sclerosis patients: no evidence for disease association with the T-cell receptor. *J Neuroimmunol* 1994;52:25–32.
29. Phillips JT. Genetic susceptibility models in multiple sclerosis. In: Rosenberg RN, ed. *The molecular and genetic basis of neurological disease* 2. Boston: Butterworth–Heinemann, 1993:41–46.
30. Prineas JW. Pathology of multiple sclerosis. In: Cook SD, ed. *Handbook of multiple sclerosis*. New York: Marcel Dekker, 1990:187–218.
31. Reder AT, Arnason BGW. Immunology of multiple sclerosis. In: Koetsier JC, ed. *Handbook of clinical neurology*. Amsterdam: Elsevier Science, 1985: 337–395.
32. Allen IV. Pathology of multiple sclerosis. In: Matthews WB, ed. *McAlpine's multiple sclerosis*. Oxford: Churchill Livingstone, 1991:341–378.
33. Raine CS. The Dale E. McFarlin Memorial Lecture: the immunology of the multiple sclerosis lesion. *Ann Neurol* 1994;36:S61–72.
34. Miller JR, Burke AM, Bever CT. Occurrence of oligoclonal bands in multiple sclerosis and other CNS diseases. *Ann Neurol* 1983;13:53–58.
35. Mehta PD. Diagnostic usefulness of cerebrospinal fluid in multiple sclerosis. *Crit Rev Clin Lab Sci* 1991;28:233–251.
36. Rudick RA, et al. Relative diagnostic value of cerebrospinal fluid kappa chains in multiple sclerosis: comparison with other immunoglobulin tests. *Neurology* 1989;39:964–968.
37. Hauser SL, et al. Childhood multiple sclerosis: clinical features and demonstration of changes in T cell subsets with disease activity. *Ann Neurol* 1982;11: 463–468.
38. Hauser SL, et al. Immunoregulatory T-cells and lymphocytotoxic antibodies in active multiple sclerosis: weekly analysis over a six-month period. *Ann Neurol* 1983;13:418–425.
39. Allen IV. Aetiological hypotheses for multiple sclerosis: evidence from human and experimental diseases. In: Matthews WB, ed. *McAlpine's multiple sclerosis*. Oxford: Churchill Livingstone, 1991: 379–390.
39a. Gran B, et al. Molecular mimicry and multiple sclerosis: degenerate T-cell recognition and the induction of autoimmunity. *Ann Neurol* 1999;45:559–567.
40. Selmaj K, Brosnan CF, Raine CS. Colocalization of lymphocytes bearing gamma delta T-cell receptor and heat shock protein hsp65+ oligodendrocytes in multiple sclerosis. *Proc Natl Acad Sci USA* 1991;88: 6452–6456.
41. Ransohoff RM, Estes ML. Astrocyte expression of major histocompatibility complex gene products in multiple sclerosis brain tissue obtained by stereotactic biopsy. *Arch Neurol* 1991;48:1244–1246.
42. Fleming JO, et al. Interaction of immune and central nervous systems: contribution of anti- viral Thy-1+ cells to demyelination induced by coronavirus JHM. *Reg Immunol* 1993;5:37–43.
43. Ffrench-Constant C. Pathogenesis of multiple sclerosis. *Lancet* 1994;343:271–275.
44. Luccchinetti CF, Rodriguez M. The controversy surrounding the pathogenesis of the multiple sclerosis lesion. *Mayo Clin Proc* 1997;72:665–678.
45. Mokhtarian F, et al. Defective production of anti-inflammatory cytokine TGF-beta by T cell lines of patients with active multiple sclerosis. *J Immunol* 1994;152:600–6010.
46. Link J, et al. Increased transforming growth factor-beta, interleukin-4, and interferon-gamma in multiple sclerosis. *Ann Neurol* 1994;36:379–386.
47. McFarlin DE, McFarland HF. Multiple sclerosis (second of two parts). *N Engl J Med* 1982;307: 1246–1251.
48. Duquette P, et al. Multiple sclerosis in childhood: clinical profile in 125 patients. *J Pediatr* 1987;111: 359–363.
48a. Ghezzi A, et al. Multiple sclerosis in childhood: clinical features of 149 cases. *Mult Scler* 1997;3:43-46.
48b. Low NL, Carter S. Multiple sclerosis in children. *Pediatrics* 1956;18:24–30.
48c. Isler W. Multiple Sklerose im Kindesalter. *Helv Paediatr Acta* 1961;16:412–431.
48d. Gall JC, et al. Multiple sclerosis in children: a clinical study of 40 cases with onset in childhood. *Pediatrics* 1958;21:703–709.
49. Baoxun Z, et al. Multiple sclerosis in China: a clinical study of 256 cases. In: Kuroiwa Y, Kurland LT, eds. *Multiple sclerosis East and West*. Fukuoka: Kyushu Univ Press, 1982:71–81.
50. Duquette P, et al. Multiple sclerosis in childhood: clinical profile in 125 patients. *J Pediatr* 1987:111: 359–363.
51. Kuroiwa Y, et al. Nationwide survey of multiple sclerosis in Japan. *Neurology* 1975;25:845–851.
52. Haslam RHA. Multiple sclerosis: experience at the hospital for sick children. *Int Pediatr* 1987;2: 163–167.
53. Bye AME, Kendall B, Wilson J. Multiple sclerosis in childhood: a new look. *Dev Med Child Neurol* 1985; 27:215–222.
54. Shaw CM, Alvord EC, Jr. Multiple sclerosis beginning in infancy. *J Child Neurol* 1987;2:252–256.

55. Cole GF, Stuart CA. A long perspective on childhood multiple sclerosis. *Dev Med Child Neurol* 1995;37: 661–666.
56. Pinhas-Hamiel O, et al. Juvenile multiple sclerosis: clinical features and prognostic characteristics. *J Pediatr* 1998;132:735–737.
57. Freedman DA, Merritt HH. The cerebrospinal fluid in multiple sclerosis. *Ass Res Nerv Ment Dis Proc* 1950;28:428–439.
58. Sindern E, et al. Early onset MS under the age of 16: clinical and paraclinical features. *Acta Neurol Scand* 1992;86:280–284.
59. Hart RG, Sherman DG. The diagnosis of multiple sclerosis. *JAMA* 1982;247:498–503.
60. Kohlschutter A. Myelin basic protein in cerebrospinal fluid from children. *Eur J Pediatr* 1978;127:155–161.
61. Johnson KP, Nelson BJ. Multiple sclerosis: diagnostic usefulness of cerebrospinal fluid. *Ann Neurol* 1977;2:425–431.
62. Evoked potentials in multiple sclerosis. [Editorial.] *Lancet* 1982;1:1445–1446.
63. Golden GS, Woody RC. The role of nuclear magnetic resonance imaging in the diagnosis of MS in childhood. *Neurology* 1987;37:689–693.
64. Miller DH, et al. Serial gadolinium enhanced magnetic resonance imaging in multiple sclerosis. *Brain* 1988;111:927–939.
65. Offenbacher H, et al. Assessment of MRI criteria for a diagnosis of MS. *Neurology* 1993;43:905–909.
65a. Paty DW, et al. MRI in the diagnosis of MS: a prospective study with comparison of clinical evaluation, evoked potentials, oligoclonal banding, and CT. *Neurology* 1988;38:180–185.
66. Kesselring J, et al. Acute disseminated encephalomyelitis: MRI findings and the distinction from multiple sclerosis. *Brain* 1990;113:291–302.
67. Jacobson S, et al. Immunological studies in tropical spastic paraparesis. *Ann Neurol* 1990;27:149–156.
68. Ormerod IE, et al. NMR in multiple sclerosis and cerebral vascular disease [letter]. *Lancet* 1984;2:1334–1335.
69. Millner MM, et al. Multiple sclerosis in childhood: contribution of serial MRI to earlier diagnosis. *Dev Med Child Neurol* 1990;32:769–777.
70. Koopmans RA, et al. The lesion of multiple sclerosis: imaging of acute and chronic stages. *Neurology* 1989; 39:959–963.
71. Bruhn H, et al. Multiple sclerosis in children: cerebral metabolic alterations monitored by localized proton magnetic resonance spectroscopy in vivo. *Ann Neurol* 1992;32:140–150.
72. Troiano R, Cook SD, Dowling PC. Steroid therapy in multiple sclerosis: point of view. *Arch Neurol* 1987;44:803–807.
73. Milligan NM, Newcombe R, Compston DA. A double-blind controlled trial of high-dose methylprednisolone in patients with multiple sclerosis: clinical effects. *J Neurol Neurosurg Psychiatry* 1987;50: 511–516.
73a. Takahashi I, et al. Childhood multiple sclerosis treated with plasmapheresis. *Pediatr Neurol* 1997;17: 83–87.
73b. Adams AB, Tyor WR, Holden KR. Interferon beta-1b and childhood multiple sclerosis. *Pediatr Neurol* 1999;21:481–483
74. Weiner HL, et al. Intermittent cyclophosphamide pulse therapy in progressive multiple sclerosis: final report of the Northeast Cooperative Multiple Sclerosis Treatment Group. *Neurology* 1993;43:910–918.
75. Aicardi J. *Diseases of the nervous system in childhood*, London: MacKeith Press, 1992:705.
76. Koopmans RA, et al. Chronic progressive multiple sclerosis: serial magnetic resonance brain imaging over six months. *Ann Neurol* 1989;26:248–256.
77. Schilder P. Zur Kenntniss der sogenannten diffusen Sklerose. *Z Ges Neurol Psychiat* 1912;10:1–60.
78. Poser CM, van Bogaert L. Natural history and evolution of the concept of Schilder's diffuse sclerosis. *Acta Psychiatr Neurol Scand* 1956;31:285–331.
79. Bouman L. *Diffuse sclerosis*, Bristol: John Wright and Co, 1934.
80. Leuzzi V, et al. Childhood demyelinating diseases with a prolonged remitting course and their relation to Schilder's disease: report of two cases. *J Neurol Neurosurg Psychiatr* 1999;63:407–408.
81. Poser CM, et al. Schilder's myelinoclastic diffuse sclerosis. *Pediatrics* 1986;77:107–112.
81a. Mehler MF, Rabinowitz L. Inflammatory myelinoclastic diffuse sclerosis. *Ann Neurol* 1988;23:413–415.
81b. Pretorius ML, et al. Demyelinating disease of Schilder type in three young South African children: dramatic response to corticosteroids. *J Child Neurol* 1998;13:197–201.
81c. Poser CM, et al. Schilder's myelinoclastic diffuse sclerosis. *Pediatrics* 1986;77:107–112.
81d. Konkol RJ, Bousonis F, Kuban KC. Schilder's disease: additional aspects and a therapeutic option. *Neuropediatrics* 1987;18:149–152.
81e. Barth PG, et al. Schilder's diffuse sclerosis: case study with three years' follow-up and neuro-imaging. *Neuropediatrics* 1989;20:230–233.
81f. Kepes JJ. Large focal tumor-like demyelinating lesions of the brain: intermediate entity between multiple sclerosis and acute disseminated encephalomyelitis? A study of 31 patients. *Ann Neurol* 1993;33:18–27.
81g. Aicardi J. *Diseases of the nervous system in childhood*, London: MacKeith Press, 1992:709.
82. Balo J. Encephalitis periaxialis concentrica. *Arch Neurol Psychiatr* 1928;19:242–264.
83. Murakami Y, et al. Balo's concentric sclerosis in a 4-year-old Japanese infant. *Brain Dev* 1998;20:250–252.
84. Kuroiwa Y, et al. Multiple sclerosis in Asia. *Neurology* 1977;27:188–192.
85. Walsh FB. Neuromyelitis optica: an anatomical-pathological study of one case; clinical studies of three additional cases. *Bull Johns Hopkins Hosp* 1935;5 6:183–210.
86. Leys D, et al. Neuromyélite optique de Devic. Quatre cas. *Rev Neurol* 1987;143:722–728.
87. O'Riordan JI, et al. Clinical, CSF, and MRI findings in Devic's neuromyelitis optica. *J Neurol Neurosurg Psychiatry* 1996;60:382–387.
88. Mandler RN, Ahmed W, Dencoff JE. Devic's neuromyelitis optica: a prospective study of seven patients treated with prednisone and azathioprine. *Neurology* 1998;51:1219–1220.
89. Greenfield JG. Acute disseminated encephalomyelitis and sequel to influenza. *J Pathol Bacteriol* 1930;33:453–462.
90. Adams RD, Kubik CS. The morbid anatomy of the demyelinative diseases. *Am J Med* 1952;12:510–546.

91. Hurst EW. Acute hemorrhagic leukoencephalitis: a previously undefined entity. *Med J Austral* 1947;2:1–6.
92. Byers RK. Acute hemorrhagic leukoencephalitis: report of three cases and review of the literature. *Pediatrics* 1975;56:727–735.
93. Seitelberger F, Sluga E. Acute hemorrhagic leukoencephalitis of herpes simplex-virus type: histological and electronmicroscopical findings. *J Neuropathol Exp Neurol* 1967;26:124–125.
94. Johnson RT. *Viral infections of the nervous system*, New York: Raven Press, 1982.
95. Bitzan M. Rubella myelitis and encephalitis in childhood: a report of two cases with magnetic resonance imaging. *Neuropediatrics* 1987;18:84–87.
96. Kaji M, et al. Survey of herpes simplex virus infections of the central nervous system, including acute disseminated encephalomyelitis, in the Kyushu and Okinawa regions of Japan. *Mult Scler* 1996;2:83–87.
97. Kamei A, et al. Acute disseminated demyelination due to primary human herpesvirus-6 infection. *Eur J Pediatr* 1997;156:709–712.
98. Hemachudha T, et al. Neurologic complications of Semple-type rabies vaccine: clinical and immunologic studies. *Neurology* 1987;37:550–556.
99. Ohtaki E, et al. Acute disseminated encephalomyelitis after treatment with Japanese B encephalitis vaccine (Nakayama-Yoken and Beijing strains). *J Neurol Neurosurg Psychiatry* 1995;59:316–317.
100. Munn R, Farrell K, Cimolai N. Acute encephalomyelitis: extending the neurological manifestations of acute rheumatic fever? *Neuropediatrics* 1992;23:196–198.
101. Kornips HM, Verhagen WI, Prick MJ. Acute disseminated encephalomyelitis probably related to a *Mycoplasma pneumoniae* infection. *Clin Neurol Neurosurg* 1993;95:59–63.
102. Nasralla CA, et al. Postinfectious encephalopathy in a child following *ampylobacter jejuni* enteritis. *AJNR Am J Neuroradiol* 1993;14:444–448.
103. Kennedy CR, Webster AD. Measles encephalitis [letter]. *N Engl J Med* 1984;311:330–331.
104. Johnson RT, et al. Measles encephalomyelitis—clinical and immunologic studies. *N Engl J Med* 1984;310:137–141.
105. Claudio L, Brosnan CF. Effects of prazosin on the blood-brain barrier during experimental autoimmune encephalomyelitis. *Brain Res* 1992;594:233–243.
106. Simmons RD, Cattle BA. Sialyl ligands facilitate lymphocyte accumulation during inflammation of the central nervous system. *J Neuroimmunol* 1992;41:123–130.
107. Cannella B, Cross AH, Raine CS. Upregulation and coexpression of adhesion molecules correlate with relapsing autoimmune demyelination in the central nervous system. *J Exp Med* 1990;172:1521–1524.
108. Reik L, Jr. Disseminated vasculomyelinopathy: an immune complex disease. *Ann Neurol* 1980:7:291–296.
109. Johnson AB, Bornstein MB. Myelin-binding antibodies in vitro: immunoperoxidase studies with experimental allergic encephalomyelitis, anti-galactocerebroside and multiple sclerosis sera. *Brain Res* 1978;159:173–182.
110. Stricker RB, Miller RG, Kiprov DD. Role of plasmapheresis in acute disseminated (postinfectious) encephalomyelitis. *J Clin Apheresis* 1992;7:173–179.
110a. Pohl-Koppe A, et al. Myelin basic protein reactive Th2 T cells are found in acute disseminated encephalomyelitis. *J Neuroimmunol* 1998;91:19–27.
111. Sedgwick JD, et al. Central nervous system microglial cell activation and proliferation follows direct interaction with tissue-infiltrating T cell blasts. *J Immunol* 1998;160:5320–5330.
112. Wisniewski HW. Immunopathology of demyelination in autoimmune diseases and virus infections. *Br Med Bull* 1977;33:54–59.
113. Miller HG, Stanton JB, Gibbons JL. Acute disseminated encephalomyelitis and related syndromes. *Br Med J* 1957;1:668–671.
114. de Vries E. *Postvaccinial perivenous encephalitis*, Amsterdam: Elsevier Science, 1960.
115. Scott TF. Postinfectious and vaccinal encephalitis. *Med Clin North Am* 1967;51:701–717.
115a. Apak RA, et al. Acute disseminated encephalomyelitis in childhood: report of 10 cases. *J Child Neurol* 1999;14:198–201.
116. Epperson LW, Whitaker JN, Kapila A. Cranial MRI in acute disseminated encephalomyelitis. *Neurology* 1988;38:332–333.
117. Rust RS Jr, Dodson WE, Trotter JL. Cerebrospinal fluid IgG in childhood: the establishment of reference values. *Ann Neurol* 1988;23:406–410.
118. Straub J, Chofflon M, Delavelle J. Early high-dose intravenous methylprednisolone in acute disseminated encephalomyelitis: a successful recovery. *Neurology* 1997;49:1145–1147.
119. Kanter DS, et al. Plasmapheresis in fulminant acute disseminated encephalomyelitis. *Neurology* 1995;45: 824–827.
120. Kazarian EL, Gager WE. Optic neuritis complicating measles, mumps, and rubella vaccination. *Am J Opthalmol* 1978;86:544–547.
121. Kline LB, Margulies SL, Oh SJ. Optic neuritis and myelitis following rubella vaccination. *Arch Neurol* 1982;39:443–444.
122. Purvin V, Hrisomalos N, Dunn D. Varicella optic neuritis: neurology 1988;38:501–503.
123. Riikonen R. The role of infection and vaccination in the genesis of optic neuritis and multiple sclerosis in children. *Acta Neurol Scand* 1989;80:425–431.
124. Kennedy C, Carroll FD. Optic neuritis in children. *Arch Ophthalmol* 1960;63:747–755.
125. Riikonen R, Donner M, Erkkila H. Optic neuritis in children and its relationship to multiple sclerosis: a clinical study of 21 children. *Dev Med Child Neurol* 1988;30:349–359.
126. Meadows SP. Retrobulbar and optic neuritis in childhood and adolescence. *Trans Ophthalmol Soc UK* 1969;89:603–638.
127. Lucchinetti CF, et al. Risk factors for developing multiple sclerosis after childhood optic neuritis. *Neurology* 1997;49:1413–1418.
128. Link H, Stendahl-Brodin L. Optic neuritis and multiple sclerosis. *N Engl J Med* 1983;308:1294–1295.
129. Tumani H, et al. Acute optic neuritis: combined immunological markers and magnetic resonance imaging predict subsequent development of multiple sclerosis: The Optic Neuritis Study Group. *J Neurol Sci* 1998;155:44–49.
130. Scholl GB, Song H-S, Wray SH. Uhthoff's symptom in optic neuritis: relationship to magnetic resonance imaging and development of multiple sclerosis. *Ann Neurol* 1991;30:180–184.
131. Miller DH, et al. Magnetic resonance imaging of the optic nerve in optic neuritis. *Neurology* 1988;38: 175–179.

132. Hely MA, et al. Visual evoked responses and ophthalmological examination in optic neuritis: a follow-up study. *J Neurol Sci* 1986;75:275–283.

133. Cornblath WT, Quint DJ. MRI of optic nerve enlargement in optic neuritis. *Neurology* 1997;48:821–825.

134. Beck RW, et al. Corticosteroid treatment of optic neuritis: a need to change the treatment practices. *Neurology* 1992;42:1133–1135.

135. Shetty T. Corticosteroids and optic neuritis [Letter]. *Neurology* 1993;43:632.

136. Kapoor R, et al. Effects of intravenous methylprednisolone on outcome in MRI-based prognostic subgroups in acute optic neuritis. *Neurology* 1998;50: 230–237.

137. Good WV, et al. Optic neuritis in children with poor recovery of vision. *Aust N Z J Ophthalmol* 1992;20:319–323.

138. Parkin PJ, Hierons R, McDonald WI. Bilateral optic neuritis: a long-term follow-up. *Brain* 1984;107:951–964.

139. Gowers WR. *A manual of disease of the nervous system*, London: J.A. Churchill, 1886:213–232.

140. Foix C, Alajouanine T. La myelite necrotique subaguë. *Rev Neurol* 1926;33:1–42.

141. Abramsky O, Teitelbaum D. The autoimmune features of acute transverse myelopathy. *Ann Neurol* 1977;2:36–40.

142. Paine RS, Byers RK. Transverse myelopathy in childhood. *Am J Dis Child* 1953;85:151–163.

143. Hoffman HL. Acute necrotic myelopathy. *Brain* 1955;78:377–393.

144. Tyler KL, Gross RA, Cascino GD. Unusual viral causes of transverse myelitis. Hepatitis: a virus and cytomegalovirus. *Neurology* 1986;36:855–858.

145. Huisman TA, et al. Unusual presentations of neuroborreliosis (Lyme disease) in childhood. *J Comput Assist Tomogr* 1999;23:39–42.

146. Knebusch M, Strassburg HM, Reiners K. Acute transverse myelitis in childhood: nine cases and review of the literature. *Dev Med Child Neurol* 1998;40: 631–639.

147. Mills RW, Schoolfield L. Acute transverse myelitis associated with *Mycoplasma pneumoniae* infection: a case report and review of the literature. *Pediatr Infect Dis J* 1992;11:228–231.

148. Penn AS, Rowan AJ. Myelopathy in systemic lupus erythematosus. *Arch Neurol* 1968;18:337–349.

149. Dunne K, et al. Acute transverse myelopathy in childhood. *Dev Med Child Neurol* 1986;28:198–204.

150. Berman M, et al. Acute transverse myelitis: incidence and etiologic considerations. *Neurology* 1981;31: 966–971.

151. Altrocchi PH. Acute transverse myelopathy. *Arch Neurol* 1963;9:111–119.

152. Ropper AH, Poskanzer DC. The prognosis of acute and subacute transverse myelopathy based on early signs and symptoms. *Ann Neurol* 1978;4:51–59.

153. Linssen WHJP, Gabreëls FJM, Wevers RA. Infective acute transverse myelopathy: report of two cases. *Neuropediatrics* 1991;22;107–109.

154. Sanders KA, Khandji AG, Mohr JP. Gadolinium MRI in acute transverse myelopathy. *Neurology* 1990;40: 1614–1616.

155. Miller DH, et al. Magnetic resonance imaging in isolated noncompressive spinal cord syndromes. *Ann Neurol* 1987;22:714–723.

156. Wilmshurst JM, Walker MC, Pohl KR. Rapid onset transverse myelitis in adolescent: implications for pathogenesis and prognosis. *Arch Dis Child* 1999;80:137–142.

157. Sebire G, et al. High-dose methylprednisolone in severe acute transverse myelopathy. *Arch Dis Child* 1997;76:167–168.

158. Lahat E, et al. Rapid recovery from transverse myelopathy in children treated with methylprednisolone. *Pediatr Neurol* 1998;19:279–282.

159. Batten FE. Case of acute ataxia. *Trans Clin Soc London* 1907;40:276–277.

160. McAllister RM, Hummeler K, Correll LL. Acute cerebellar ataxia: report of case with isolation of type 9 ECHO virus from cerebrospinal fluid. *N Engl J Med* 1959;261:1159–1162.

161. Boughton CR. Varicella-zoster in Sydney. II. Neurological complications of varicella. *Med J Aust* 1966;2:444–447.

162. Margolis FJ, Wilson JL, Top FH. Post-rubella encephalomyelitis. *J Pediatr* 1943;23:158–165.

163. Bray PF, et al. Coincidence of neuroblastoma and acute cerebellar encephalopathy. *J Pediatr* 1969;75:983–990.

164. Boltshauser E, Deonna T, Hirt HR. Myoclonic encephalopathy of infants or "dancing eyes syndrome." *Helv Paediatr Acta* 1979;34:119–133.

165. Weiss S, Carter S. Course and prognosis of acute cerebellar ataxia in children. *Neurology* 1959;9:711–721.

166. Connolly AM, et al. Course and outcome of acute cerebellar ataxia. *Ann Neurol* 1994;35:673–679.

167. Cotton DG. Acute cerebellar ataxia. *Arch Dis Child* 1957;32:181–188.

168. Maggi G, Varone A, Aliberti F. Acute cerebellar ataxia in children. *Childs Nerv Syst* 1997;13:542–545.

169. Groen RJM, et al. Acute cerebellar ataxia in a child with transient pontine lesions demonstrated by MRI. *Neuropediatrics* 1991;22:225–227.

170. Bakshi R, et al. Magnetic resonance imaging findings in acute cerebellitis. *Clin Imaging* 1998;22:79–85.

171. Nagamitsu S, et al. Decreased cerebellar blood flow in postinfectious acute cerebellar ataxia. *J Neurol Neurosurg Psychiatry* 1999;67:109–112.

172. Tuchman M, et al. Three years of experience with random urinary homovanillic and vanillylmandelic acid levels in the diagnosis of neuroblastoma. *Pediatrics* 1987;79:203–205.

173. Basser LS. Benign paroxysmal vertigo of childhood. *Brain* 1964;87:141–152.

174. Pedersen E. Epidemic vertigo: clinical picture, epidemiology and relation to encephalitis. *Brain* 1959; 82:566–580.

175. Eviatar L, Eviatar A. Vertigo in children: differential diagnosis and treatment. *Pediatrics* 1977;59:833–838.

176. Baloh RW, et al. Familial episodic ataxia: clinical heterogeneity in four families linked to chromosome 19p. *Ann Neurol* 1997;41:8–16.

177. Freedman D, Schenthal J. A parenchymatous cerebellar syndrome following protracted high body temperature. *Neurology* 1953;3:513–516.

178. Kinsbourne M. Myoclonic encephalopathy of infants. *J Neurol Neurosurg Psychiatr* 1962;25:271–276.

179. Connolly AM, et al. Serum autoantibodies in childhood opsoclonus-myoclonus syndrome: an analysis of antigenic targets in neural tissues. *J Pediatr* 1997;130:878–884.

180. Koh PS, et al. Long-term outcome in children with opsoclonus-myoclonus and ataxia and coincident neuroblastoma. *J Pediatr* 1994;125:712–716.
181. Bellur SN. Opsoclonus: its clinical value. *Neurology* 1975;25:502–507.
182. Altman AJ, Bachner RL. Favorable prognosis for survival in children with coincident opsomyoclonus and neuroblastoma. *Cancer* 1976;37:846–852.
183. Kuban KC, et al. Syndrome of opsoclonus-myoclonus caused by Coxsackie B3 infection. *Ann Neurol* 1983;13:69–71.
184. Raudnitz RW. Zur Lehre vom Spasmus nutans. *Jahrb Kinderh* 1897;45:145–176.
185. Weissman BM, et al. Spasmus nutans: a quantitative prospective study. *Arch Ophthalmol* 1987;105:525–528.
186. Gottlob I, et al. Head nodding is compensatory in spasmus nutans. *Ophthalmology* 1992;99:1024–1031.
187. Gottlob I, Wizov SS, Reinecke RD. Spasmus nutans: a long-term follow-up. *Invest Ophthalmol Vis Sci* 1995;36:2768–2771.
188. Norton WD, Cogan DG. Spasmus nutans: clinical study of 20 cases followed two years or more since onset. *AMA Arch Ophthalmol* 1954;52:442–446.
189. Hoefnagel D, Biery B. Spasmus nutans. *Dev Med Child Neurol* 1968;10:32–35.
190. Farmer J, Hoyt CS. Monocular nystagmus in infancy and early childhood. *Am J Ophthalmol* 1984;98:504–509.
191. King RA, Nelson LB, Wagner RS. Spasmus nutans: a benign clinical entity? *Arch Ophthalmol* 1986;104:1501–1504.
192. Sydenham T. *The whole works of that excellent practical physician Dr. Thomas Sydenham*. The fourth edition corrected from the original Latin by John Pechey, M.D. London: printed for R. Wellington, 1705:422–423.
193. Stoll M. *Rationis medendi, in Nosocomio practico Vindobonensis, pars tertia*, Vol. 7:6. Viennae: sumptibus A. Bernardi, 1780.
194. Taranta A, Stollerman GH. Relationship of Sydenham's chorea to infection with group A streptococci. *Am J Med* 1956;20:170–175.
195. Aron AM, Freeman JM, Carter S. The natural history of Sydenham's chorea. *Am J Med* 1965;38:83–95.
196. Westlake RM, Graham TP, Edwards KM. An outbreak of acute rheumatic fever in Tennessee. *Pediatr Infect Dis J* 1990;9:97–100.
197. Cardoso F, et al. Chorea in fifty consecutive patients with rheumatic fever. *Mov Disord* 1997;12:701–703.
198. Husby G, et al. Antibodies reacting with cytoplasm of subthalamic and caudate neurons in chorea and acute rheumatic fever. *J Exp Med* 1976;144:1094–1110.
199. Figueroa F, et al. Anticardiolipin antibodies in acute rheumatic fever. *J Rheumatol* 1992;19:1175–1180.
200. Freeman JM, et al. The emotional correlates of Sydenham's chorea. *Pediatrics* 1965;35:42–49.
201. Bird MT, Palkes H, Prensky AL. A follow-up study of Sydenham's chorea. *Neurology* 1976;26:601–606.
202. Buchanan DN. Pathologic changes in chorea. *Am J Dis Child* 1941;62:443–445.
203. Nausieda PA, et al. Sydenham's chorea: an update. *Neurology* 1980;30:331–334.
204. Kaplan EL. Recent epidemiology of Group A streptococcal infections in North America and abroad: an overview. *Pediatrics* 1996;97:945–948.
205. Hosier DM, et al. Resurgence of acute rheumatic fever. *Am J Dis Child* 1987;141:730–733.
206. Wilson SK, ed. *Neurology*, 2nd ed. New York: Hafner Press, 1969.
207. Heye N, et al. Sydenham chorea: clinical, EEG, MRI and SPECT findings in the early stage of the disease. *J Neurol* 1993;240:121–123.
208. Giedd JN, et al. Sydenham's chorea: magnetic resonance imaging of the basal ganglia. *Neurology* 1995;45:2199–2202.
209. Lee PH, et al. Serial brain SPECT images in a case of Sydenham chorea. *Arch Neurol* 1999;56:237–240.
210. Berrios X, et al. Are all recurrences of "pure" Sydenham's chorea true recurrences of acute rheumatic fever? *J Pediatr* 1985;107:867–872.
211. Chun RW, Smith NJ, Forster FM. Papilledema in Sydenham's chorea. *Am J Dis Child* 1961;101:641–644.
212. Nausieda PA, et al. Chronic dopaminergic sensitivity after Sydenham's chorea. *Neurology* 1983;33:750–754.
213. Kerbeshian J, Burd L, Pettit R. A possible post-streptococcal movement disorder with chorea and tics. *Develop Med Child Neurol* 1990;32:642–644.
214. Feldman BM, et al. Diagnostic use of B-cell alloantigen D8/17 in rheumatic chorea. *J Pediatr* 1993;123: 84–86.
215. Dhanaraj M, et al. Sodium valproate in Sydenham's chorea. *Neurology* 1985;35:114–115.
216. Massell BF. Prophylaxis of streptococcal infections and rheumatic fever: a comparison of orally administered clindomycin and penicillin. *JAMA* 1979;241:1589–1594.
217. Kiessling LS, Marcotte AC, Culpepper L. Antineuronal antibodies in movement disorders. *Pediatrics* 1993;92:39–43.
218. Swedo SE, et al. Identification of children with pediatric autoimmune neuropsychiatric disorders associated with streptococcal infections by a marker associated with rheumatic fever. *Am J Psychiatry* 1997;154:110–112.
219. Swedo SE, et al. Pediatric autoimmune neuropsychiatric disorders associated with streptococcal infections: clinical description of the first 50 cases. *Am J Psychiatry* 1998;155:264–271.
220. Kurlan R. Tourette's syndrome and 'PANDAS': will the relation bear out? Pediatric autoimmune neuropsychiatric disorders associated with streptococcal infection. *Neurology* 1998;50:1530–1534.
221. Shulman ST. Pediatric autoimmune neuropsychiatric disorders associated with streptococci (PANDAS). *Pediatr Infect Dis J* 1999;18:281–282.
221a. Perlmutter SJ, et al. Therapeutic plasma exchange and intravenous immunoglobin for obsessive-compulsive disorder and tic disorders in childhood. *Lancet* 1999;354:1153–1158.
222. Landry O. Note sur la paralysie ascendante aiguë. *Gaz Hebd Med Chir* 1859;6:472–474.
223. Guillain G, Barré JA, Strohl A. Sur un syndrome de radiculo-névrite avec hyperalbuminose du liquide céphalorachidien sans réaction cellulaire: remarques sur les caractères cliniques et graphiques des réflexes tendineux. *Bull Soc Med Hop Paris* 1916;40:1462–1470.
224. Haymaker W, Kernohan JW. The Landry-Guillain-Barré syndrome: a clinical pathologic report of 50 fatal cases and a review of the literature. *Medicine* 1949;28:59–141.

225. Asbury AK, Arnason BG, Adams RD. The inflammatory lesion in idiopathic polyneuritis: its role in pathogenesis. *Medicine* 1969;48:173–215.

226. Hafer-Macko CE, et al. Immune attack on the Schwann cell surface in acute inflammatory demyelinating polyneuropathy. *Ann Neurol* 1996;39:625–635.

227. Prineas JW. Pathology of the Guillain-Barré syndrome. *Ann Neurol* 1981;9 [Suppl]:S6–S19.

228. Honavar M, et al. A clinicopathological study of the Guillain-Barré syndrome. *Brain* 1991;114:1245–1269.

229. Waksman BH, Adams RD. Allergic neuritis: an experimental disease of rabbits induced by the injection of peripheral nervous tissue and adjuvants. *J Exp Med* 1955;102:213–236.

230. Rostami A, et al. The role of myelin P_2 protein in the production of experimental allergic neuritis. *Ann Neurol* 1984;16:680–685.

231. Astrom KE, Webster H de F, Arnason BG. The initial lesion in experimental allergic neuritis: a phase and electron microscopic study. *J Exp Med* 1968;128:469–495.

232. Ho TW, McKhann GM, Griffin JW. Human autoimmune neuropathies. *Ann Rev Neurosci* 1998;21: 187–226.

233. Lisak RP, et al. The role of cytokines in Schwann cell damage, protection, and repair. *J Infect Dis* 1997;176:[Suppl 2]S173–S179.

234. Sharief MK, et al. Circulating tumor necrosis factor-α correlated with electrodiagnostic abnormalities in Guillain-Barré syndrome. *Ann Neurol* 1997;42:68–73.

235. Archelos JJ, Previtali SC, Hartung H-P. The role of integrins in immune-mediated diseases of the nervous system. *Trends Neurosci* 1999;22:30–38.

236. Beghi E, Kurland LT, Mulder DW, Wiederholt WC. Guillain-Barré syndrome: clinico-epidemiologic features and effect of influenza vaccine. *Arch Neurol* 1985;42:1053–1057.

237. Rantala H, Uhari M, Niemela M. Occurrence, clinical manifestations, and prognosis of Guillain-Barré syndrome. *Arch Dis Child* 1991;66:706–708.

238. Hart DE, et al. Childhood Guillain-Barré syndrome in Paraguay: 1990 to 1991. *Ann Neurol* 1994;36:859–863.

239. Rees JH, et al. *Campylobacter jejuni* infections and Guillain-Barré syndrome. *N Engl J Med* 1995;333: 1374–1379.

240. Hahn AF. Guillain-Barré syndrome. *Lancet* 1998; 352:635–641.

240a Hemachudha T, et al. Immunologic studies of rabies vaccination-induced Guillain-Barré syndrome. *Neurology* 1988;38:375–378.

240b. Safranek TJ, et al. Reassessment of the association between Guillain-Barré syndrome and receipt of swine influenza vaccine in 1976–1977: results of a two-state study. *Am J Epidemiol* 1991;133:940–951.

240c. Hughes R, et al. Vaccines and Guillain-Barré syndrome. *BMJ* 1996;312:1475–1476.

241. Yuki N. Molecular mimicry between gangliosides and lipopolysaccharides of *Campylobacter jejuni* isolated from patients with Guillain-Barré syndrome and Miller Fisher syndrome. *J Infect Dis* 1997;176[Suppl 2]:S150–S151.

242. Ho TW, et al. Anti-GD1a antibody is associated with axonal but not demyelinating forms of Guillain-Barré syndrome. *Ann Neurol* 1999;45:168–173.

242a. Vriesendorp FJ, et al. Serum antibodies to GM_1 GD_{1b}, peripheral nerve myelin, and *Campylodacter jejuni* in patients with Guillain-Barré syndrome and controls: correlation and prognosis. *Ann Neurol* 1993;34:1301–135.

243. Willison HJ, et al. Miller-Fisher syndrome is associated with serum antibodies to GN1b ganglioside. *J Neurol Neurosurg Psychiatry* 1993;56:204–206.

244. Hao Q, et al. Anti-GalNAc-GD1a antibody-associated Guillain-Barré syndrome with a predominantly distal weakness without cranial nerve impairment and sensory disturbance. *Ann Neurol* 1999;45:758–768.

245. Adams D, et al. HLA antigens in Guillain-Barré syndrome. *Lancet* 1977;2:504–505.

246. Low NL, Schneider J, Carter S. Polyneuritis in children. *Pediatrics* 1958;22:972–990.

247. Peterman AF, et al. Infectious neuronitis (Guillain-Barré syndrome) in children. *Neurology* 1959;9:533–539.

248. Moulin DE, et al. Pain in Guillain-Barré syndrome. *Neurology* 1997;48:328–331.

249. Winer JB, Hughes RAC, Osmond C. A prospective study of acute idiopathic neuropathy. I. Clinical features and their prognostic value. *J Neurol Neurosurg Psychiatr* 1988;51:605–612.

250. Morley JB, Reynolds EH. Papilledema and Landry-Guillain-Barré syndrome: case reports and review. *Brain* 1966;89:205–222.

251. Sullivan RL, Reeves AG. Normal cerebrospinal fluid protein, increased intracranial pressure and the Guillain-Barré syndrome. *Ann Neurol* 1977;1:180–184.

252. Winer JB, Hughes RAC. Identification of patients at risk for arrhythmia in the Guillain-Barré syndrome. *QJM* 1988;68:735–739.

253. Asbury AK, Cornblath DR. Assessment of current diagnostic criteria for Guillain-Barré syndrome. *Ann Neurol* 1990;27[Suppl]:S21–S24.

254. Ropper AH. Current concepts: the Guillain-Barré syndrome. *N Engl J Med* 1992;326:1130–1136.

255. Briscoe DM, McMenamin JB, O'Donohoe NV. Prognosis in Guillain-Barré syndrome. *Arch Dis Child* 1987;62:733–735.

256. Feasby TE, et al. An acute axonal form of Guillain-Barré polyneuropathy. *Brain* 1986;109:1115–1126.

257. Feasby TE, et al. Severe axonal degeneration in acute Guillain-Barré syndrome: evidence of two different mechanisms? *J Neurol Sci* 1993;116:185–192.

258. Griffin JW, et al. Pathology of the motor-sensory axonal Guillain-Barré syndrome. *Ann Neurol* 1996;39:17–28.

259. Griffin JW, et al. Early nodal changes in the acute motor axonal neuropathy pattern of the Guillain-Barré syndrome. *J Neurocytol* 1996;25:33–51.

260. Hughes RAC, Rees JH. Clinical and epidemiologic features of Guillain-Barré syndrome. *J Infect Dis* 1997;176[Suppl 2]S92–S98.

261. Rees JH, et al. A prospective case control study to investigate the relationship between *Campylobacter jejuni* infection and Guillain-Barré syndrome. *N Engl J Med* 1995;333:1374–1379.

262. Fisher M. An unusual variant of acute idiopathic polyneuritis (syndrome of ophthalmoplegia, ataxia and areflexia). *N Engl J Med* 1956;255:57–65.

263. Becker WJ, Watters GB, Humphreys P. Fisher's syndrome in childhood. *Neurology* 1981;31:555–560.

264. Bell W, Van Allen M, Blackman J. Fisher's syndrome in childhood. *Dev Med Child Neurol* 1970;12:758–766.

265. Shuaib A, Becker WJ. Variants of Guillain-Barré syndrome: facial diplegia and multiple cranial nerve palsies. *Can J Neurol Sci* 1987;14:611–616.

266. Landau WM, Glenn C, Dust G. MRI in Miller Fisher variant of Guillain-Barré syndrome. *Neurology* 1987;37:14–31.

267. Jacobs BC, et al. Serum anti-GQ1b antibodies recognize surface epitopes on *Campylobacter jejuni* from patients with Miller Fisher syndrome. *Ann Neurol* 1995;37:260–264.

268. Roberts M, et al. Serum factor in Miller Fisher variant of Guillain-Barré syndrome and neurotransmitter release. *Lancet* 1994;343:454–455.

268a. Plomp JJ, et al. Miller Fisher antiGQ1b antibodies: α-Latrotroxin-like effect on motor endplate. *Ann Neurol* 1999;45:189–199.

269. Bickerstaff ER. Brain stem encephalitis: further observations on a grave syndrome with a benign prognosis. *BMJ* 1957;1:1384–1387.

270. Jamal GA, Ballantyne JP. The localization of the lesion in patients with acute ophthalmoplegia, ataxia and areflexia (Miller Fisher syndrome). *Brain* 1988; 111:95–114.

271. Petty RK, et al. Brain stem encephalitis and the Miller Fisher syndrome. *J Neurol Neurosurg Psychiatry* 1993;56:201–203.

272. Tasker W, Chutorian AM. Chronic polyneuritis of childhood. *J Pediatr* 1969;74:699–708.

273. McCombe PA, Pollard JD, McLeod JG. Chronic inflammatory demyelinating polyradiculoneuropathy: a clinical and electrophysiological study of 92 cases. *Brain* 1987;110:1617–1630.

274. Byers RK, Taft LT. Chronic multiple neuropathy in childhood. *Pediatrics* 1957;20:517–537.

275. Pleasure DE, Towfighi J. Onion bulb neuropathies. *Arch Neurol* 1972;26:289–301.

276. Tiwari JL, Terasaki PI. *HLA and disease associations*, New York: Springer-Verlag, 1985.

277. Yoshino H, Inuzuka T, Miyatake T. IgG antibody against GM1, GD1b and asialo-GM1 in chronic polyneuropathy following *Mycoplasma pneumoniae* infection. *Eur Neurol* 1992;32:28–31.

278. National Institute of Neurological and Communicative Disorders and Stroke. Ad Hoc Committee. Criteria for diagnosis of Guillain-Barré syndrome. *Ann Neurol* 1978;3:565–566.

279. Asbury AK, Cornblath DR. Assessment of current diagnostic criteria for Guillain-Barré syndrome. *Ann Neurol* 1990;27[Suppl]:S21–S24.

280. Livingstone IR, Cumming WJK. Hyperkalemic paralysis resembling Guillain-Barré syndrome. *Lancet* 1979;963–964.

281. Guillain-Barré Syndrome Steroid Trial Group. Double-blind trial of intravenous methylprednisolone in Guillain-Barré syndrome. *Lancet* 1993;341:586–590.

282. Austin JH. Recurrent polyneuropathies and their corticosteroid treatment with 5-year observations of a placebo-controlled case treated with corticotrophin, cortisone, and prednisone. *Brain* 1958;81:157–192.

283. Epstein MA, Sladky JT. The role of plasmapheresis in childhood Guillain-Barré syndrome. *Ann Neurol* 1990;28:65–69.

284. Jansen PW, Perkin RM, Ashwal S. Guillain-Barré syndrome in childhood: natural course and efficacy of plasmapheresis. *Pediatr Neurol* 1993;9:16–20.

285. The French Cooperative Group on Plasma Exchange in Guillain-Barré syndrome. Appropriate number of plasma exchanges in Guillain-Barré syndrome. *Ann Neurol* 1997;41:298–306.

286. van der Meché FGA, et al. A randomized trial comparing intravenous immune globulin and plasma exchange in Guillain-Barré syndrome. *N Engl J Med* 1992;326:1123–1129.

287. van Doorn PA, et al. High-dose intravenous immunoglobulin treatment in chronic inflammatory demyelinating polyneuropathy: a double-blind, placebo-controlled, crossover study. *Neurology* 1990;40: 209–212.

288. Bleck TP. IVIg for GBS: potential problems in the alphabet soup. *Neurology* 1993;43:857–858.

289. Sharief MK, et al. IV immunoglobulin reduces circulating proinflammatory cytokines in Guillain-Barré syndrome. *Neurology* 1999;52:1833–1838.

290. Cole GF, Matthew DJ. Prognosis in severe Guillain-Barré syndrome. *Arch Dis Child* 1987;62:288–291.

291. Rees JH, Hughes RAC. *Campylobacter jejuni* and Guillain-Barré syndrome. *Ann Neurol* 1994;35:248–249.

292. Bell C. On the nerves of the face, being a second paper on that subject. *Phil Trans* 1829;111:317–339.

293. Zülch KJ. Idiopathic facial paresis. In: Vinken PJ, Bruyn GW, eds. *Handbook of clinical neurology*. Vol. 8. *Diseases of nerves*, Pt. 2. Amsterdam: Elsevier Science, 1968:241–302.

294. Grose C, et al. Primary Epstein-Barr virus infections in acute neurologic diseases. *N Engl J Med* 1975;292:392–395.

295. Christen H-J, et al. Peripheral facial palsy in childhood-Lyme borreliosis to be suspected unless proven otherwise. *Acta Paediatr Scand* 1990;79:1219–1224.

296. Abramsky O, et al. Cellular immune response to peripheral nerve basic protein in idiopathic facial paralysis (Bell's palsy). *J Neurol Sci* 1975;26:13–20.

297. Jonsson L, Sjöberg O, Thomander L. Activated T cells and Leu-7+ cells in Bell's palsy. *Acta Otolaryngol* 1988;105:108–113.

298. Alter M. Familial aggregation of Bell's palsy. *Arch Neurol* 1963;8:557–564.

299. Paine RS. Facial paralysis in children: review of the differential diagnosis and report of ten cases treated with cortisone. *Pediatrics* 1957;19:303–316.

300. Hanner P, et al. Trigeminal dysfunction in patients with Bell's palsy. *Acta Otolaryngol* 1986;101:224–230.

301. Roberg M, et al. Acute peripheral facial palsy: CSF findings and etiology. *Acta Neurol Scand* 1991;83: 55–60.

302. Sartoretti-Schefer S, et al. T2-weighted three-dimensional fast spin-echo MR in inflammatory peripheral facial nerve palsy. *Am J Neuroradiol* 1998;19: 491–495.

303. Salam EA, Ekyahky WS. Evaluation of prognosis and treatment of Bell's palsy in children. *Acta Paediat Scand* 1968;57:468–472.

304. Manning JJ, Adour KK. Facial paralysis in children. *Pediatrics* 1972;49:102–109.

305. Park HW, Watkins AL. Facial paralysis: analysis of 500 cases. *Arch Phys Med* 1949;30:749–762.

306. Wadlington WB, Riley HD, Lowbeer L. The Melkersson-Rosenthal syndrome. *Pediatrics* 1984;73:502–506.

307. Stevens H. Melkersson's syndrome. *Neurology* 1965;15:263–266.

308. Kesler A, Vainstein G, Gadoth N. Melkersson-Rosenthal syndrome treated by methylprednisolone. *Neurology* 1998;51:1440–1441.

309. Rousseau JJ, Godfoi ME, Husquinet H. Paralysie faciale idiopathique familiale recurrente. *Acta Neurol Belg* 1983;83:23–28.

310. Chutorian AM, Gold AP, Brown CW. Benign intracranial hypertension and Bell's palsy. *N Engl J Med* 1977;296:1214–1215.

311. Sigler RL, et al. Hypertension first seen as facial paralysis: case reports and review of the literature. *Pediatrics* 1991;87:387–389.

311a. Indudharan R, Dharap AS, Ho TM. Intra-aural tick causing facial palsy. *Lancet* 1996;348:6–13.

312. Huizing EH, Michelse K, Staal A. Treatment of Bell's palsy: analysis of the available studies. *Acta Otolaryngol* 1981;92:115–121.

313. May M, Klein SR, Taylor FH. Idiopathic (Bell's) facial palsy: Natural history defies steroid or surgical treatment. *Laryngoscope* 1985;95:406409.

314. Ford FR. Paroxysmal lacrimation during eating as a sequel of facial palsy (syndrome of crocodile tears): report of 4 cases with possible interpretation and comparison with auriculotemporal syndrome. *Arch Neurol Psychiatr* 1933;29:1279–1288.

315. Devi S, et al. Prognostic value of minimal excitability of facial nerve in Bell's Palsy. *J Neurol Neurosurg Psychiatr* 1978;41:649–652.

316. Knox DL, Clark DB, Schuster FF. Benign VI nerve palsies in children. *Pediatrics* 1967;40:560–564.

317. Gradenigo G. Über circumscripte Leptomeningitis mit spinalen Symptomen und über Paralyse des N. abducens ototischen Ursprungs. *Arch f Ohrenh* 1904;51:255–270.

318. Afifi AK, et al. Recurrent lateral rectus palsy in childhood. *Pediatr Neurol* 1990;6:315–318.

319. Edin M, et al. Isolated temporary pharyngeal paralysis in childhood. *Lancet* 1976;1:1047–1049.

320. Wright GDS, Lee KD. An isolated right hypoglossal nerve palsy in association with infectious mononucleosis. *Postgrad Med J* 1980;56:185–186.

321. Robertson DM, Mellor DH. Asymmetrical palatal paresis in childhood: a transient cranial mononeuropathy. *Dev Med Child Neurol* 1982;24:842–846.

322. Auberge C, et al. Les hemiparalysies velopalatines isolées et acquises chez l'enfant. *Arch Franc Pediatr* 1979;36:283–286.

323. Blau JN, Harris M, Kennett S. Trigeminal sensory neuropathy. *N Engl J Med* 1969;281:873–876.

324. Kissel JT. Neurologic manifestations of vasculitis. *Neurol Clin* 1989;7:655–673.

325. Lie JT. Diagnostic histopathology of major systemic and pulmonary vasculitic syndromes. *Rheum Dis Clin North Am* 1990;16:269–292.

326. Miller WL, Burnett JC Jr. Blood vessel physiology and pathophysiology. *Rheum Dis Clin North Am* 1990;16:251–260.

327. Cines DB. Disorders associated with antibodies to endothelial cells. *Rev Infect Dis* 1989;11[Suppl 4]:S705–711.

328. Conn DL. Polyarteritis. *Rheum Dis Clin North Am* 1990;16:341–362.

329. Fieschi C, et al. Central nervous system vasculitis. *J Neurol Sci* 1998;153:159–171.

329a. Younger DS, et al. Granulomatous angiitis of the brain: an inflammatory reaction of diverse etiology. *Arch Neurol* 1988;45:514–518.

330. Moore PM. Diagnosis and management of isolated angiitis of the central nervous system. *Neurology* 1989;39:167–173.

331. Caccamo DV, Garcia JH, Ho KL. Isolated granulomatous angiitis of the spinal cord. *Ann Neurol* 1992;32:580–582.

332. Woolfenden AR, et al. Angiographically defined primary angiitis of the CNS: is it really benign? *Neurology* 1998;51:183–188.

333. Vollmer TL, et al. Idiopathic granulomatous angiitis of the central nervous system: diagnostic challenges. *Arch Neurol* 1993;50:925–930.

334. Hunder GG, et al. The American College of Rheumatology 1990 criteria for the classification of vasculitis. introduction. *Arthritis Rheum* 1990;33:1065–1067.

335. Malamud N. A case of periarteritis nodosa with decerebrate rigidity and extensive encephalomalacia in a five-year-old child. *J Neuropathol Exp Neurol* 1945;4:88–92.

336. Ronco P, et al. Immunopathological studies of polyarteritis nodosa and Wegener's granulomatosis: a report of 43 patients with 51 renal biopsies. *QJM* 1983;52:212–223.

337. Ozdogan H, et al. Vasculitis in familial Mediterranean fever. *J Rheumatol* 1997;241;323–327.

338. Said R, et al. Spectrum of renal involvement in familial Mediterranean fever. *Kidney Int* 1992;41:414–419.

339. Ettlinger RE, et al. Polyarteritis nodosa in childhood: a clinical pathological study. *Arthritis Rheum* 1979;22:820–825.

340. Ozen S, et al. Diagnostic criteria for polyarteritis nodosa in childhood. *J Pediatr* 1992;120:206–209.

341. Engel DG, et al. Fatal infantile periarteritis nodosa with predominant central nervous system involvement. *Stroke* 1995;26:699–701.

342. Ford RG, Siekert RG. Central nervous system manifestations of periarteritis nodosa. *Neurology* 1965;15:114–122.

343. Bleehen SS, Lovelace RE, Cotton RE. Mononeuritis multiplex in polyarteritis nodosa. *QJM* 1963;32:193–209.

344. Magilavy DB, Petty RE, Cassidy JT, Sullivan DB. A syndrome of childhood polyarteritis. *J Pediatr* 1977;91:25–30.

345. Sigal LH. The neurologic presentation of vasculitic and rheumatologic syndromes. *Medicine (Baltimore)* 1987;66:157–180.

346. Rottem M, et al. Wegener granulomatosis in children and adolescents: clinical presentation and outcome. *J Pediatr* 1993;122:26–31.

347. Oetgen WJ, Boice JA, Lawless OJ. Mixed connective tissue disease in children and adolescents. *Pediatrics* 1981;67:333–337.

348. Halbreich U, et al. Rheumatic brain disease: a disease in its own right. *J Nerv Ment Dis* 1976;163:24–28.

349. Yarom A, Rennebohm RM, Levinson JE. Infantile multisystem inflammatory disease: a specific syndrome? *J Pediatr* 1985;106:390–396.

350. Yamashita Y, et al. Atlantoaxial subluxation: radiography and magnetic resonance imaging correlated to myelopathy. *Acta Radiol* 1989;30:135–140.

351. Jan JE, Hill RH, Low MD. Cerebral complications in juvenile rheumatoid arthritis. *Can Med Assoc J* 1972;107:623–625.

352. Sundelin F. Investigations of the cerebrospinal fluid in cases of rheumatoid arthritis. *Am J Med* 1947;2:579–587.

353. Carbajal-Rodriguez L, et al. Neurologic involvement in juvenile rheumatoid arthritis. *Bol Med Hosp Infant Mex* 1991;48:502–508.

354. Fink CW. Medical treatment of juvenile arthritis. *Clin Orthop* 1990:60–69.

355. Rhodes, VJ. Physical therapy management of patients with juvenile rheumatoid arthritis. *Phys Ther* 1991;71:910–919.
356. Kornreich HK, et al. Scleroderma in childhood. *Arthritis Rheum* 1977;20:343–350.
357. Clements PJ, et al. Muscle disease in progressive systemic sclerosis: diagnostic and therapeutic considerations. *Arthritis Rheum* 1978;21:62–71.
358. Deprettere AJ, et al. Diagnosis of Sjögren's syndrome in children. *Am J Dis Child* 1988;142:1185–1187.
359. Brown MM, Swash M. Polyarteritis nodosa and other systemic vasculitides. In: Toole JF, ed. *Handbook of clinical neurology*. Amsterdam: Elsevier Science, 1989:353–368.
360. King KK, et al. Clinical spectrum of systemic lupus erythematosus in childhood. *Arthritis Rheum* 1977;20:287–294.
361. Yancey CL, Doughty RA, Athreya BH. Central nervous system involvement in childhood systemic lupus erythematosus. *Arthritis Rheum* 1981;24:1389–1395.
362. Moore PM, Lisak RP. Systemic lupus erythematosus: immunopathogenesis of neurologic dysfunction. *Springer Semin Immunopathol* 1995;17:43–60.
363. Wallace DJ, Metzger AL. Systemic lupus erythematosus and the nervous system. In: Wallace DJ, Hahn BH, eds. Dubois' lupus erythematosus. Philadelphia: Lea & Febiger, 1993:370–385.
364. Malamud N, Saver G. Neuropathologic findings in disseminated lupus erythematosus. *Arch Neurol Psychiatr* 1954;71:723–731.
365. Ellis SG, Verity MA. Central nervous system involvement in systemic lupus erythematosus: a review of neuropathologic findings in 57 cases, 1955–1977. *Semin Arthritis Rheum* 1979;8:212–221.
366. Devinsky O, Petito CK, Alonso DR. Clinical and neuropathologic findings in systemic lupus erythematosus: the role of vasculitis, heart emboli, and thrombotic thrombocytopenic purpura. *Ann Neurol* 1988;23:380–384.
367. Kelly MC, Denburg JA. Cerebrospinal fluid immunoglobulins and neuronal antibodies in neuropsychiatric systemic lupus erythematosus and related conditions. *J Rheumatol* 1987;14:740–744.
368. Zvaifler NJ, Bluestein HG. The pathogenesis of central nervous system manifestations of systemic lupus erythematosus. *Arthritis Rheum* 1982;25:862–866.
369. Bonfa E, et al. Association between lupus psychosis and anti-ribosomal P protein antibodies. *N Engl J Med* 1987;317:265–271.
370. Press J, et al. Antiribosomal P antibodies in pediatric patients with systemic lupus erythematosus and psychosis. *Arthritis Rheum* 1996;39:671–676.
371. Levine SR, et al. Cerebral venous thrombosis with lupus anticoagulants: report of two cases. *Stroke* 1987;18:801–804.
372. van Dam AP. Diagnosis and pathogenesis of CNS lupus. *Rheumatol Int* 1991;11:1–11.
373. Mackworth-Young C. Antiphospholipid antibodies: more than just a disease marker. *Immunol Today* 1990;11:60–64.
374. Hahn BH. An overview of the pathogenesis of systemic lupus erythematosus. In: Wallace DJ, Hahn BH, eds. *Dubois' lupus erythematosus*. Philadelphia: Lippincott, Williams & Wilkins, 5th ed. 1997:69–76.
375. Sewell KL, et al. Magnetic resonance imaging vs. computed tomographic scanning in neuropsychiatric systemic lupus erythematosus. *Am J Med* 1989;86: 625–626.
376. Schneebaum AB, et al. Association of psychiatric manifestations with antibodies to ribosomal P proteins in systemic lupus erythematosus. *Am J Med* 1991;90:54–62.
377. Bell CL, et al. Magnetic resonance imaging of central nervous system lesions in patients with lupus erythematosus. *Arthritis Rheumat* 1991;34:432–441.
378. Stimmler MM, Coletti PM, Quismorio FP. Magnetic resonance imaging of the brain in neuropsychiatric systemic lupus erythematosus. *Semin Arthritis Rheum* 1993;22:335–349.
379. O'Connor JF, Musher DM. Central nervous system involvement in systemic lupus erythematosus. *Arch Neurol* 1966;14:157–164.
380. Gold AP, Yahr MD. Childhood lupus erythematosus. *Trans Am Neurol Assoc* 1960;85:96–102.
381. Asherson RA, et al. Cerebrovascular disease and antiphospholipid antibodies in systemic lupus erythematosus; lupus-like disease, and the primary antiphospholipid syndrome. *Am J Med* 1989;86:391–399.
382. Asherson RA, et al. The primary antiphospholipid syndrome: major clinical and serologic features. *Medicine* 1989;68:366–374.
383. Bell CL, et al. Magnetic resonance imaging of central nervous system lesions in patients with lupus erythematosus: correlation with clinical remission and antineurofilament and anticardiolipin antibody titers. *Arthritis Rheum* 1991;34:432–441.
384. Bruyn GW, Padberg G. Chorea and systemic lupus erythematosus: a critical review. *Eur Neurol* 1984;23: 278–290.
385. Groothuis JR, et al. Lupus-associated chorea in childhood. *Am J Dis Child* 1977;131:1131–1134.
386. Cassidy JT, et al. Lupus nephritis and encephalopathy: prognosis in 58 children. *Arthritis Rheum* 1977;20:315–322.
387. Uziel Y, et al. Cerebral vein thrombosis in childhood systemic lupus erythematosus. *J Pediatr* 1995;126: 722–727.
388. McAbee GN, Barasch ES. Resolving MRI lesions in lupus erythematosus selectively involving the brainstem. *Pediatr Neurol* 1990;6:186–189.
389. Waga S, et al. Myelopathy, ascites and pleural effusion in systemic lupus erythematosus. *Acta Paediatr Jpn* 1989;31:78–84.
390. The American College of Rheumatology nomenclature and case definitions for neuropsychiatric lupus syndromes. *Arthritis Rheum* 1999;42:599–608.
391. Carette S, et al. Cranial computerized tomography in systemic lupus erythematosus. *J Rheumatol* 1982;9:855–859.
392. McCune WJ, et al. Identification of brain lesions in neuropsychiatric systemic lupus erythematosus by magnetic resonance scanning. *Arthritis Rheum* 1988; 31:159–166.
393. Stoppe G, et al. Positron emission tomography in neuropsychiatric lupus erythematosus. *Neurology* 1990;40:304–308.
394. Rubin RL. Drug-induced lupus. In: Wallace DJ, Hahn BH, eds. *Dubois' lupus erythematosus*. Philadelphia: Lippincott, Williams & Wilkins, 5th ed. 1997: 871–901.
395. Jacobs JC. Systemic lupus erythematosus in childhood. *Pediatrics* 1963;32:257–264.

396. Singsen BH, Fishman L, Hanson V. Antinuclear antibodies and lupus-like syndromes in children receiving anticonvulsants. *Pediatrics* 1976;57:529–534.

397. Decker JL. The management of systemic lupus erythematosus. *Arthritis Rheum* 1982;25:891–894.

398. Pisetsky DS. Systemic lupus erythematosus. *Med Clin North Am* 1986;70:337–353.

399. Manolios N, Schrieber L. Current concepts in the etiopathogenesis and treatment of systemic lupus erythematosus (SLE). *Aust NZ J Med* 1986;16:729–743.

400. Baca V, et al. Favorable response to intravenous methylprednisolone and cyclophosphamide in children with severe neuropsychiatric lupus. *J Rheumatol* 1999;26:432–439.

401. Singsen BS, Bernstein BH, Koster King K. Systemic lupus erythematosus in childhood: correlations between changes in disease activity and serum complement levels. *J Pediatr* 1976;89:358–369.

402. Adams RD, Kubik CS. The morbid anatomy of the demyelinative diseases. *Am J Med* 1952;12:510–546.

403. Spillane JD, Wells CE. The neurology of Jennerian vaccination. *Brain* 1964;87:1–44.

404. Cereghino JJ, et al. Rabies: rare disease but serious pediatric problem. *Pediatrics* 1970;45:839–844.

405. Mozar HN, et al. Myelopathy after duck embryo rabies vaccine. *JAMA* 1973;224:1605–1607.

405a. Laouini D, et al. Antibodies to human myelin proteins and gangliosides in patients with acute neuroparalytic accidents induced by brain-derived rabies vaccine. *J Neuroimmunol* 1998;91:63–72.

405b. Piyasirisilp S, et al. Association of HLA and T-cell receptor gene polymorphisms with Semple rabies vaccine–induced autoimmune encephalomyelitis. *Ann Neurol* 1999;45:595–600.

405c. Murthy JM. MRI in acute disseminated encephalomyelitis following Semple antirabies vaccine. *Neuroradiology* 1998;40:420–423.

406. Fenichel GM. Neurological complications of immunization. *Ann Neurol* 1982;12:119–128.

407. Byers RK, Moll FC. Encephalopathies following prophylactic pertussis vaccine. *Pediatrics* 1948;1:437–457.

408. Cody CL, et al. Nature and rates of adverse reactions associated with DPT and DT immunizations in infants and children. *Pediatrics* 1981;68:650–660.

409. Blumberg DA, et al. Severe reactions associated with diphtheria-tetanus-pertussis vaccine: detailed study of children with seizures, hypotonic-hyporesponsive episodes, high fevers, and persistent crying. *Pediatrics* 1993;91:1158–1165.

410. Pollock TM, et al. Symptoms after primary immunisation with DTP and with DT vaccine. *Lancet* 1984;2:146–149.

411. Baraff LJ, et al. Infants and children with convulsions and hypotonic-hyporesponsive episodes following diphtheria-tetanus-pertussis immunization: follow-up evaluation. *Pediatrics* 1988;81:789–794.

412. Gross TP, Milstien JB, Kuritsky JN. Bulging fontanelle after immunization with diphtheria-tetanus-pertussis vaccine and diphtheria-tetanus vaccine. *J Pediatr* 1989;114:423–425.

413. Stewart GT. Vaccination against whooping-cough: efficacy versus risks. *Lancet* 1977;1:234–237.

414. Murphy JV, Sarff LD, Marquardt KM. Recurrent seizures after diphtheria, tetanus, and pertussis vaccine immunization: onset less than 24 hours after vaccination. *Am J Dis Child* 1984;138:908–911.

415. Miller D, et al. Pertussis immunization and serious acute neurological illnesses in children. *BMJ* 1993; 307:1171–1176.

416. Kulenkampff M, et al. Neurological complications of pertussis inoculation. *Arch Dis Child* 1974;49:46–49.

417. Walker AM, et al. Neurologic events following diphtheria-tetanus-pertussis immunization. *Pediatrics* 1988;81:345–349.

418. Corsellis JAN, Janota I, Marshall AK. Immunization against whooping cough: a neuropathological review. *Neuropathol Appl Neurobiol* 1983;9:261–270.

419. Dolphin AC. Nucleotide binding proteins in signal transduction and disease. *Trends Neurosci* 1987;10: 53–57.

420. Black WJ, et al. ADP-ribosyltransferase activity of pertussis toxin and immunomodulation by *Bordatella pertussis*. *Science* 1988;240:656–659.

421. Grant CC, et al. Pertussis encephalopathy with high cerebrospinal fluid antibody titers to pertussis toxin and filamentous hemagglutinin. *Pediatrics* 1998;102: 986–990.

422. Howson CP, Howe CJ, Fineberg HV. *Adverse effects of pertussis and rubella vaccines*, Washington, DC: National Academy Press, 1991.

423. Edwards KM, Decker MD, Halsey NA, et al. Differences in antibody response to whole-cell pertussis vaccines. *Pediatrics* 1991;88:1019–1023.

424. Miller E, et al. Risk of aseptic meningitis after measles, mumps and rubella vaccine in UK children. *Lancet* 1993;341:979–982.

425. Gray JA, Burns SM. Mumps meningitis following measles, mumps and rubella immunization. *Lancet* 1989;2:98.

426. Weibel RE, et al. Acute encephalopathy followed by permanent brain injury or death associated with further attenuated measles vaccines: a review of claims submitted to the National Vaccine Injury Compensation Program. *Pediatrics* 1991;101:383–387.

427. Wakefield AJ, et al. Ileal-lymphoid-nodular hyperplasia, non-specific colitis, and pervasive developmental disorder in children. *Lancet* 1998;351:637–641.

427a. Taylor B, et al. Autism and measles, mumps, and rubella vaccine: no epidemiological evidence for a causal association. *Lancet* 1999;353:2026–2029.

428. Read SJ, Schapel GJ, Pender MP. Acute transverse myelitis after tetanus toxoid vaccination. *Lancet* 1992;339:1111–1112.

429. Hopkins IJ. A new syndrome: Poliomyelitis-like illness associated with acute asthma in childhood. *Austral Paediatr J* 1974;10:273–276.

430. Beede HE, Newcomb RW. Lower motor neuron paralysis in association with asthma. *Johns Hopkins Med J* 1980;147:186–187.

431. Manson JI, Thong YH. Immunological abnormalities in the syndrome of poliomyelitis-like illness associated with acute bronchial asthma (Hopkin's syndrome). *Arch Dis Child* 1980;55:26–32.

432. Freud S. Die infantile Cerebrallähmung. In: Nothnagel H, ed. Spezielle Pathologie und Therapie. Vol 9, part 3. Wien: Alfred Holder, 1897:253–254.

433. Prechtl HFR, Stemmer CJ. The choreiform syndrome in children. *Dev Med Child Neurol* 1962;4:119–127.

Chapter 8

Postnatal Trauma and Injuries by Physical Agents

John H. Menkes and *Richard G. Ellenbogen

*Departments of Neurology and Pediatrics, University of California, Los Angeles, UCLA School of Medicine, and Department of Pediatric Neurology, Cedars-Sinai Medical Center, Los Angeles, California 90048; and *Department of Neurological Surgery, University of Washington School of Medicine, Children's Hospital and Regional Medical Center, Seattle, Washington 98105*

CRANIOCEREBRAL TRAUMA

In the western world, accidents constitute the major cause of death of children between the ages of 5 and 19 years (Table 8.1) (1). From 1951 to 1971, the number of children with head injuries admitted to hospitals in Newcastle-upon-Tyne, United Kingdom, increased sixfold, until it reached 13.9% of all admissions to pediatric wards (2). This increase probably is partially caused by a change in policy, such that more apparently minor injuries are admitted for observation. In the United States, the situation is similar; cranial and major facial injuries are responsible for 3.6% of hospital admissions and 3.3% of days spent in the hospital, and they are the most common neurologic conditions requiring hospital admission for patients younger than 19 years of age (3). Head injury is now the most common cause of death and disability of children in the United States, causing death in approximately 7,000 children each year (3a). It is also the cause of significant cognitive and motor-sensory dysfunction in the pediatric population, with an estimated economic burden approximating $10 billion a year in the United States alone (3b).

A high proportion of head injuries cause death at the site of the accident or on the way to the hospital, so admission figures reflect only part of the incidence. In the San Diego Prospective Survey, as many as 85% of fatalities occurred at these times (4). Since the 1980s, child abuse has been recognized increasingly. The incidence of reported cases has risen from 10.1 in 1,000 children in 1976 compared with 39 in 1,000 children in 1990 (5), with one of the more recent estimates of the incidence of fatal abuse in children younger than 4 years of age being at least 10 in 100,000 (6). As the reported frequency of maltreatment has risen, it has become an important cause of head injury. In infants younger than age 1 year, 36% of all head injuries and 95% of injuries resulting in intracranial hemorrhage or other major cerebral complications were, in one series, caused by child abuse (7). In older children, the proportion of injury from abuse is lower, but still significant.

Although no accurate data exist, cranial trauma commonly occurs in childhood sports. Brain concussion occurs in an estimated 19 in 100 American football players per year. Bicycling is probably the second most common sport leading to head injury. In an Australian series, bicycling was responsible for more than 20% of all head injuries in children (8).

TABLE 8.1. *Causes of death in children in 1986*

Cause of Death	Age			
	Less than 5 years	5–9 years	10–14 years	15–19 years
All causes	46,371	4,082	4,706	16,224
Accidents	5.5%	20.6%	18.3%	10.8%
Motor vehicle accidents	2.6%	26.2%	27.2%	43.1%
Influenza and pneumonia	0.9%	1.2%	0.9%	0.5%
Congenital anomalies	19.7%	6.3%	0.1%	1.6%
Malignant neoplasms	2.3%	21.3%	15.8%	7.1%

From Vital Statistics of the United States. U.S. Department of Health, Education and Welfare, Public Health Service, Washington, DC, 1986.

This chapter presents only postnatal injuries; perinatal injuries are described in Chapter 5. This chapter discusses the diagnosis and nonsurgical management of head injuries and considers their pathophysiology and pathology based on the severity of the craniocerebral trauma, and the complications and sequelae of head injuries.

Dynamics and Pathophysiology

Physical forces, mainly acceleration and deceleration, act on the brain through shear-strain deformation, which is a change in shape without a change in volume, and through compression-rarefaction strain, which consists of a change in volume without a change in shape. The brain is injured through these two mechanisms acting alone, in combination, or in succession (9–11).

Shear-Strain Deformation

The injury from shearing or tearing is responsible for most lesions (12), especially in an infant or young child, whose skull is more easily deformed than an adult's. Deformation absorbs much of the energy of impact, reducing the ill effects of acceleration and deceleration, but adding to the risk of tearing of blood vessels. Because of its elasticity and ability to undergo a greater degree of deformation, the skull of an infant absorbs the energy of the physical impact and protects the brain better than the skull of an older person.

The relationship between stress waves and deformity depends mainly on the momentum of the head and of the object at the instant of impact. In a child with intact reflexes, a free fall probably causes more injury to the brain than an aimed object striking the head with even greater speed. Approximately 70% of shear-strain deformation skull fractures are linear and single; the rest are depressed fractures. The faster the blow, the more likely that a depressed fracture will result; a lower velocity impact with the same momentum tends to produce deformity and linear fracture, sometimes distant from the point of impact, but at a weak part of the cranial vault where distortion can occur. A linear fracture is usually not important in management of the child, because outcome of the injury and its complications are determined by damage to the intracranial contents at the moment of impact; an injury can be fatal in the absence of a fracture.

Compression-Rarefaction Strains

In an acceleration injury, in which the momentary compression is greatest, the effects of compression-rarefaction strains are usually maximal at the point of impact; at the same time, an area of low pressure or rarefaction occurs contralaterally (13,14), the site of the familiar contrecoup injury. Thus, a blow to the occiput can result in the major damage occurring in the frontal and temporal regions. Contrecoup injuries are relatively rare in infants and young children, presumably because skull distortion rather than pressure waves dominates (15). Contrecoup injuries are most likely to occur when the impact is to the side of the head (16). Distortion of the brainstem is particularly likely in deceleration injuries such as those that occur in falls;

TABLE 8.2. *Classification of traumatic intracranial lesions*

Primary lesions
  Intraaxial
    Diffuse axonal injury
    Cortical contusion
    Subcortical matter injury
    Primary brainstem injury
  Extraaxial hematomas
    Extradural
    Subdural
  Diffuse hemorrhage
    Subarachnoid
    Intraventricular
  Primary vascular injuries
Secondary lesions
  Pressure necrosis (secondary to brain displacement and herniations)
  Tentorial arterial infraction
  Diffuse hypoxic injury
  Diffuse brain swelling
  Boundary and terminal zone infarction
  Others
    Fatty embolism
    Secondary hemorrhage
    Infection

From Gentry LR, Godersky JC, Thompson B. MR imaging of head trauma: review of the distribution and radiopathologic features of traumatic lesions. *AJR Am J Roentgenol* 1988;15:663. With permission.

TABLE 8.3. *Expected injury types associated with accidental mechanisms in young children*

Mechanism	Injury types
Fall <4 ft	Concussion/soft tissue injury
	Linear fracture
	Epidural hematoma
	Ping-pong fracture
	? Depressed fracture[a]
Fall >4 ft	Injuries listed for fall <4 ft plus the following:
	Depressed fracture
	Basilar fracture
	Multiple fractures
	Subarachnoid hemorrhage
	Contusion
	? Subdural hematoma[a]
	? Stellate fracture[a]
Motor vehicle accident	Injuries listed for fall < and >4 ft plus the following:
	Subdural hematoma
	Diffuse axonal injury

[a]Injury types are uncommonly associated with the given mechanism.
From Dumaine AC. Head injury in very young children. *Pediatrics* 1992;90:184. With permission.

any resulting loss of function in this area is liable to have serious consequences.

Magnetic resonance imaging (MRI) has allowed a better understanding of the lesions that can result from head injury. These have been grouped into primary and secondary lesions by Gentry and coworkers (17) (Table 8.2). The injuries expected from various accidental mechanisms are depicted in Table 8.3.

Axonal Injury

The term *axonal injury* refers to a clinical-radiologic entity whose pathologic correlates match well with the MRI findings. As viewed on MRI, the most common primary lesion is diffuse axonal injury. Diffuse axonal injury generally is not caused by a fall, except a fall from a considerable height. Rather, it results from severe angular acceleration-deceleration forces (18) and can induce coma through disconnection of the cortex from the lower centers. It is responsi-

ble for severe, irreversible, and potentially fatal brain damage occurring at the moment of injury. Diffuse axonal lesions are frequently unaccompanied by skull fracture, increased intracranial pressure, or cerebral contusion (18). The most characteristic sign for diffuse axonal injury is loss of consciousness.

Postmortem examinations have demonstrated axonal lesions in the inferior portion of the corpus callosum, and the dorsolateral quadrant of the rostral brainstem, notably in the region of the superior cerebellar peduncles, and throughout the cerebral hemisphere and cerebellum (19–21). Damage to the superior cerebellar peduncles, which are particularly vulnerable to rotational injuries, is responsible for the ataxia commonly observed after major head injuries (22). The microscopic picture of axonal lesions was first described by Strich (23), who proposed that the shearing forces sustained during injury cause stretching of axons, which might be sufficient to prevent them from functioning. The more subtle changes that precede this final state have been studied in animals by electron microscopy and through the use of immunocytochemical labeling techniques. Although the exact time course for humans has not been determined, in animals an alteration in the structure of the nodes of Ranvier occurs within 15 minutes of the injury (24). This is followed, some 12 to 24 hours later, by an interruption of antegrade and retrograde axonal transport, the loss of microtubules, and the gradual development of axonal swelling. When axonal swelling exceeds a certain critical level, effective transection of the axon occurs, although without evident tearing or damage to adjacent blood vessels. It is unclear how mechanical forces induce the instantaneous perturbation of the cell membrane that in turn initiates these axonal changes. The most likely explanation is that membrane channels are opened at the moment of injury, with an influx of calcium, activation of calmodulin, and an increase of extracellular potassium at the damaged node (25). Intracellular calcium, in turn, increases the activity of proteolytic enzymes that disrupt axonal cytoarchitecture. Over time, the swollen axons either degenerate or undergo regenerative changes, as shown by sprouting and growth cones (26).

The neuropathologic picture correlates well with the appearance on MRI. By this technique diffuse axonal injury appears as small, oval, focal abnormalities in white matter tracts, usually adjacent to cortical gray matter, but sometimes in the splenium of the corpus callosum (17). Proton magnetic resonance spectroscopy can provide further information on the extent of axonal injury. A lowered N-acetylaspartate (NAA) to creatine ratio is believed to be indicative of axonal injury, but there does not appear to be any elevation of tissue lactate (27).

Cortical Contusion

The second most common type of brain injury visualized by MRI of patients with severe head trauma is cortical contusion, which tends to be multiple. As verified by both imaging and pathologic studies, points of predilection for contusions are the crests of gyri on the orbital surfaces of the frontal lobes and the inferolateral aspect of the temporal lobes (10,17). Contusions consist mainly of petechial hemorrhages in the superfi-

cial cortical layers, occurring at the site of impact (coup injuries) or at contrecoup areas (Fig. 8.1). Impact on the forehead or vertex can send the initial pressure wave caudally, leading to downward displacement of the brain toward and into the tentorial opening. This displacement can result in contusions of the hippocampal gyrus, particularly the uncus, the basal ganglia, and the upper part of the brainstem (28). The severity of brain damage caused by contusion depends on the extent of vascular injury. Damage tends to be less common and less severe in infants and small children than in older children or adults subjected to comparable trauma (16). One of the major clinical issues in the management of contusions is the tendency for them to increase in size, coalesce, or cause a mass effect, especially after the first day following injury. Therefore, a follow-up imaging study is often useful.

Cerebral Laceration

Cerebral lacerations are usually the result of damage from penetrating wounds or depressed skull fractures, but they can occur without fracture in small children, whose skulls tend to become more grossly distorted at the moment of injury. Lacerations frequently involve the frontal and temporal poles and are associated primarily with tears of the dura and tears or other injuries of the major vessels, and secondarily with thromboses, hemorrhages, or focal cerebral ischemia. Tears in the white matter are seen commonly in infants after blunt trauma even without fracture (29) (Fig. 8.2). They result from the soft consistency of the poorly myelinated cerebrum and from the pliancy of the immature skull.

MRI has demonstrated that macroscopic traumatic injuries to subcortical structures such as the thalamus and to the brainstem are rare. Rather, the pathologic change that results in the clinical picture generally attributed to primary brainstem damage is diffuse axonal injury.

Concussion

The physical processes within the skull caused by trauma induce numerous changes within the

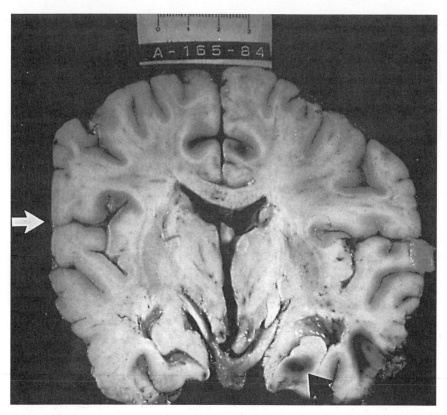

FIG. 8.1. Contrecoup injury. A left-sided epidural hematoma not seen in the picture caused severe compression of the left cerebral hemisphere (*white arrow*). Hemorrhage in the right inferior temporal lobe (*black arrow*) probably represents a contrecoup injury. (Courtesy of Dr. Harry V. Vinters, Division of Neuropathology, UCLA Center for the Health Sciences, Los Angeles.)

brain. The most common is concussion. According to one widely accepted definition, concussion is a transient but instant widespread loss of neural function. It is usually followed by permanent amnesia for the moment of injury and for a variable period before it (retrograde amnesia). The pathogenesis of concussion is still under debate. From a structural viewpoint, concussion is believed to result from minor degrees of diffuse axonal injury. In addition, there appears to be a loss of cerebral autoregulation in a significant proportion of patients with minor head injuries (30). With more severe concussive injuries, a massive release of excitatory neurotransmitters occurs, notably glutamate. As a result, neuronal membranes depolarize with subsequent increase of extracellular potassium (31). This is accompanied by the entry of calcium into nerve terminals

and is followed by further glutamate release and potassium flux. At the same time, arachidonic acid is released, which in turn induces a cascade of reactions with the ultimate formation of free radicals (32). These changes are accompanied by increased energy demands, as brain cells attempt to reinstate normal ionic membrane balance (33). With an increase in energy consumption there is a rapid decrease in adenosine triphosphate (ATP) and an increase in lactic acid (34). These biochemical alterations, which suggest impaired mitochondrial function, are confirmed by the electron microscopic observations of swollen neuronal mitochondria and an increased permeability of the organelles' outer membranes (35). Compounding the imbalance between energy demands and supply is the loss of autoregulation, the presence of vasospasm, and a global increase

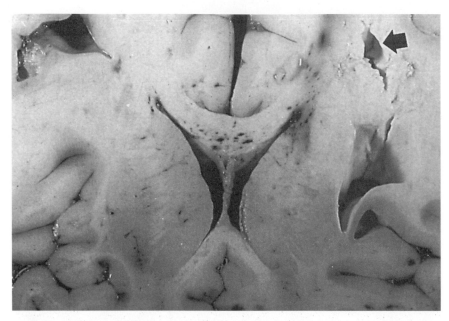

FIG. 8.2. Closed head injury. Note the petechial hemorrhages in the corpus callosum and a tear in the white matter of the right centrum semiovale (*arrow*). (Courtesy of Dr. Harry V. Vinters, Division of Neuropathology, UCLA Center for the Health Sciences, Los Angeles.)

in intracranial pressure, which reduce the supply of substrates to the tissue.

Secondary Effects of Brain Trauma

Secondary effects of trauma develop as a consequence of circulatory disorders and shifts of water and ions in and out of neurons, glia, and intercellular space. Of primary importance is the evolution of cerebral swelling (brain edema). This condition has been defined as an increase in volume caused by an increase in brain water and sodium content (36). Fishman distinguishes three major categories of brain edema: vasogenic edema, cytotoxic or cellular edema, and interstitial edema (36). Vasogenic edema is characterized by increased permeability of brain capillary endothelial cells. This results from defects in the tight endothelial cell junctions, and an increased number of pinocytic vesicles, which are responsible from the transport of macromolecules across the blood–brain barrier. Vasogenic edema occurs around brain tumors, after cerebral infarction, and in lead encephalopathy. Cytotoxic edema is marked by swelling of all cellular elements of the brain with reduction in the vol-

ume of extracellular fluid. This form of edema is characteristic of energy depletion such as occurs during the initial stages of cerebral hypoxia. Fishman postulates a third form of brain edema in which there is an increase in water and sodium content of periventricular white matter (36). This condition is seen in obstructive hydrocephalus.

In brain trauma the prominence of astrocytic swelling, the integrity of the interepithelial tight junctions, and the relative paucity of protein-rich fluid suggest that edema is mainly cytotoxic (37). This is confirmed by diffusion-weighted MRI performed on experimental animals. These studies demonstrate that immediately after injury, there is predominantly vasogenic edema that, over the next few hours to days, becomes superseded and overshadowed by cytotoxic edema (38). Additionally, massive swelling of perivascular astrocytic foot processes can compress the microvasculature and reduce tissue perfusion, inducing secondary vasogenic edema. The molecular mechanisms that induce astrocytic swelling are believed to be those responsible for the alterations in neuronal function associated with concussion (39).

The pathophysiologic mechanisms after head trauma are depicted in Figure 8.3.

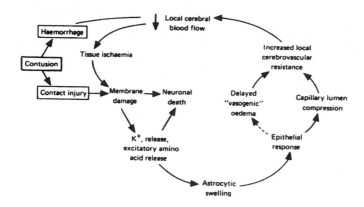

FIG. 8.3. Possible pathophysio-logic mechanisms after cere-bral contusions. (From Bullock R, et al. Glial swelling following human cerebral contusion: an ultrastructural study. *J Neurol Neurosurg Psychiatry* 1991;54: 427. With permission.)

A number of biochemical changes follow severe traumatic head injury. In both clinical and experimental settings, good correlation exists between the severity of traumatic brain injury and the amount of neuroexcitatory amino acids, such as glutamate and aspartate that are released (40). In addition, there is a local inflammatory response with complement and microglial activation and an increased release into cerebrospinal fluid (CSF) of a variety of cytokines (interleukin-1, interleukin-6, and interleukin-10) (41). These substances contribute to the evolution of diffuse cerebral edema.

The effects of traumatic brain injury on cerebral blood flow are critical to the development of cerebral edema. Early after severe traumatic brain injury, marked hypoperfusion develops with reduction in oxygen delivery and cerebral ischemia (42). Some 24 hours later cerebral blood flow increases, and there is uncoupling of cerebral blood flow and oxidative cerebral metabolism (1). Post-traumatic hyperemia is more common in infants and children than in adults and is probably the consequence of a loss of cerebral autoregulation. Hyperemia in turn contributes to the massive brain swelling, which is not uncommon in infants and young children, and has been termed *malignant brain edema* (43).

Anatomically, cerebral edema involves principally the subcortical white matter and the centrum semiovale. Less often, cerebral edema surrounds an area of contusion or an intracerebral hematoma. Brain swelling also can occur in response to the evacuation of a large extracerebral clot or after other major intracranial surgery (44).

When the additive effects of injury and brain swelling are severe, a self-perpetuating sequence develops, which can lead to further increases of intracranial pressure, with collapse of cerebral venules. This collapse in turn reduces cerebral perfusion and causes tissue hypoxia. This leads to further cerebral edema (45). A loss of selective permeability of cell membranes results, with increased loss of fluid from the vascular compartment into the parenchyma, thereby increasing cerebral swelling. Recovery has not been seen when intracranial pressure equals or exceeds mean systemic arterial pressure, at which point cerebral perfusion ceases.

Numerous changes occur secondary to cerebral edema. Herniation of the uncus over the tentorial edge compresses the midbrain and often occludes the posterior cerebral arteries. Edema and infarction of the occipital poles can occur, contributing further to supratentorial pressure and thus to herniation. Petechial hemorrhages develop in the midbrain and pons, with infarctions in the areas of the basal ganglia supplied by the anterior choroidal artery. A decrease in blood pressure, commonly seen with a severe injury, potentiates the vicious circle.

Clinical Conditions

Closed Head Injury

More than 90% of major pediatric head injuries are nonpenetrating and closed (i.e., no scalp wound exists). The clinical picture is highlighted by alterations in consciousness (9). As is the case for head injuries at all ages, boys are involved three times more often than girls.

Clinical Manifestations

When the injury is mild, initial unconsciousness is brief and is followed by confusion, somnolence, and listlessness. Vomiting, pallor, and irritability are common, and particularly in infants can occur in the apparent absence of an initial loss of consciousness. By definition, except for transient nystagmus or extensor plantar responses, neurologic signs are not observed in concussion. As a rule, a computed tomography (CT) scan clarifies the differential diagnosis of contusion, cerebral laceration, or other complications of closed head injury, and a lumbar puncture is not warranted without specific indications.

From 7% to 40% of children with mild head injuries have associated linear fractures of the skull (46). These fractures are most common in the parietal region. According to most authorities, such fractures do not, by themselves, affect the clinical course or prolong the period of morbidity; children with and without simple fractures have the same incidence of serious sequelae (9,46,47).

Electroencephalography (EEG), when performed soon after injury, can reveal striking abnormalities, such as generalized and focal slowing, prolonged reaction to hyperventilation, and even hypsarrhythmia. In milder head injuries, these changes tend to be transient. Taking into account the time elapsed between injury and recording, Mizrahi and Kellaway found that the degree of EEG abnormality correlated with the severity of the injury (48). Nevertheless, the EEG does not predict the development of post-traumatic epilepsy, and there is no correlation between the appearance of the EEG immediately after the head injury and development of early post-traumatic epilepsy (49,50).

In major closed head injuries, consciousness is interrupted more profoundly and for longer periods than in minor head injuries, and focal neurologic signs point to localized brain contusion. The clinical picture in such cases is outlined in Table 8.4 (51). Generally, the greatest neurologic deficit is found at the time of injury. New neurologic signs appearing subsequently indicate progressive brain swelling, or, if localized, indicate secondary intracranial hemorrhage, vasospasm, or thrombosis. The duration of coma depends on the site and severity of injury.

TABLE 8.4. *Clinical findings in 4,465 children with major closed head injuries*[a]

Finding	Percent
Initial level of consciousness	
Normal	56.0
Drowsy, confused	30.2
Major impairment	13.8
Vomiting	30.3
Skull fractures	26.6
Linear	72.8
Depressed	27.2
Compound	19.7
Seizures	7.4
Paralyses	3.8
Retinal hemorrhages	2.3
Pupillary abnormalities	3.6
Papilledema	1.5
Extradural hematoma	0.9
Subdural hematoma	5.2
Mortality	5.4
Major neurologic residua	5.9

[a]This series includes 243 infants with major birth injuries. This group had 50% mortality and a higher incidence of paralyses, retinal hemorrhages, and major residua.
From Hendrick EB, Harwood-Nash DC, Hudson AR. Head injuries in children: a survey of 4465 consecutive cases at the Hospital for Sick Children, Toronto, Canada. *Clin Neurosurg* 1963;11:46. With permission.

The clinical picture can follow one of several courses (52). Many children die without recovering consciousness. In a smaller group of patients, coma can persist. Prognosis for survival is relatively good in children alive 48 hours after injury. In one-half of the surviving children, consciousness is regained in less than 24 hours. Recovery is often complete or nearly complete, although transient sequelae are not unusual. These include CSF leakage often complicated by secondary meningitis, post-traumatic epilepsy, and the development of a carotid artery–cavernous sinus fistula. Communicating hydrocephalus resulting from subarachnoid bleeding more commonly follows perinatal trauma and is discussed in Chapters 4 and 5.

Nonsurgical Treatment

Major Head Injury

A recommended sequence consists of the following four steps: a rapid initial evaluation,

TABLE 8.5. *Pediatric coma scale*

Eyes open	
Spontaneously	4
To speech	3
To pain	2
Not at all	1
Best verbal response	
Oriented	5
Words	4
Vocal sounds	3
Cries	2
None	1
Best motor response	
Obeys commands	5
Localizes pain	4
Flexion to pain	3
Extension to pain	2
None	1
Normal aggregate score	
Birth to 6 months	9
6–12 months	11
1–2 years	12
2–5 years	13
Older than 5 years	14

Modified from Simpson D, Reilly P. Pediatric coma scale. *Lancet* 1982;2:450.

resuscitation, a more extensive secondary evaluation, including radiologic assessment, and definitive treatment (1,53). In many instances of major closed head injury, diagnosis of the injury is performed in parallel with emergency treatment.

Because in children the clinical condition can change rapidly and frequently, a high degree of alertness and preparedness is required by both medical and nursing attendants.

Neurologic Examination

Careful, but not elaborate, neurologic examination must be made and recorded, with particular emphasis on the state of consciousness; pupillary size, equality, and response to light; the extent and symmetry of spontaneous movements; and the reflex responses. Recording of blood pressure, pulse, and respiration is likewise essential. Caloric and optokinetic responses are useful for evaluating brainstem function. Some or all of these observations, especially the level of consciousness and motor activity, are principally of value when made serially at intervals that can be as often as every 5 minutes. Such examinations allow trends away from or toward normal func-

tioning to be detected, thus providing warning of any need to intervene surgically.

Several pediatric modifications of the Glasgow Coma Scale (54), which is widely used for the assessment of head-injured adults, have been proposed. One example is presented in Table 8.5 (55).

The Glasgow Coma Scale measures three neurologic responses: eye opening, verbal response, and limb movement. Each response is given a score; the higher the score, the better the condition of the patient.

Additionally, the extent of retrograde and post-traumatic amnesia should be recorded when possible. Spontaneous or provoked episodes of decerebrate activity or hypotonia are associated with a poor outcome (56); the length of pre- and post-traumatic amnesia is a useful indicator of the severity of the head injury (57).

Maintenance of Airway and Circulation

After the immediate evaluation of the child's general condition, an adequate airway should be established and maintained. Airway obstruction is the most frequent cause of respiratory failure. Maintenance of patency requires suction of mouth or pharyngeal contents, or endotracheal intubation followed, when necessary, by artificial respiration. Tracheostomy may be indicated to bypass mechanical obstruction of the airway caused by facial or mandibular injuries. Because an injury to the cervical spine must be presumed until proven absent, the neck must be stabilized while an airway is established. Arterial pressure is monitored by cannulation of a peripheral artery and maintained by administration of crystalloid, colloid, or blood products (58). Gas exchange also must be monitored.

Shock in closed head injuries is usually caused by blood loss elsewhere in the body. Rarely, it indicates damage to the medullary cardiovascular centers. Infants and young children have a higher incidence of shock than older age groups (1). In infants, in particular, subgaleal, subperiosteal, subdural, or extradural, hemorrhages can be sufficiently extensive to induce shock. The injured brain is highly susceptible to episodes of systemic hypotension, in part because cerebral edema in conjunction with sys-

TABLE 8.6. *Management strategy for radiographic imaging in pediatric patients with head trauma*

Low-risk group	Moderate-risk group	High-risk group
Possible findings	Possible findings	Possible findings
Asymptomatic	Change of consciousness at time of injury or subsequently	Depressed or decreasing level of consciousness
Headache	Unreliable history	Focal neurologic signs
Dizziness	Younger than 2 years of age	Penetrating skull injury
Scalp laceration	Post-traumatic seizure	Depressed fracture
Scalp hematoma	Vomiting	
	Signs of basilar skull fracture	
	Fracture into an air sinus	
	Possible depressed fracture	
	Suspected child abuse	
Recommendations	Recommendations	Recommendations
Observation	Hospitalization	Emergency CT scan
Discharge with head injury information sheet, and have family observe child	Close observation	Neurosurgical consultation
	CT scan and neurosurgical consultation	

CT, computed tomography.
Adapted from Masters SJ, et al. Skull x-ray examinations after head trauma. Recommendations by a multidisciplinary panel and validation study. *N Engl J Med* 1987;316:84.

temic hypotension lowers cerebral blood flow, and perhaps because an impairment of autoregulation of cerebral blood flow also occurs. Whatever the physiologic mechanism, when head injury is accompanied by systemic hypotension, the outcome is significantly worse (59).

After the initial emergency measures have been completed, the child's neurologic status should be reevaluated. The importance of repeated observations of vital signs and neurologic status cannot be overemphasized. Slowing of the pulse rate and widening of pulse pressure often accompany an increase of intracranial pressure (Cushing effect) (see Chapter 10). An irregular respiratory pattern is also common after severe head injuries (60).

Neuroimaging Studies

CT of the head has revolutionized the clinical assessment of head injuries, and it is the most appropriate study for the assessment of intracranial complications, taking precedence over skull radiography and MRI (61). The need for and timing of such imaging studies depends mainly on the clinical findings. A suggested strategy is outlined in Table 8.6 (62). Some centers suggest that in children who show signs of brainstem compression and a Glasgow coma score of 3,

precious time can be saved by foregoing CT and proceeding directly with exploratory surgery to remove a hematoma. Although emergency trephination may benefit the occasional patient, scanning is still the most important diagnostic study for the majority of children (63).

CT can delineate the presence and the extent of fractures and can demonstrate the presence of diffuse cerebral swelling and hyperemia of the brain (64), hemorrhages in the epidural and subdural space, and intracerebral hemorrhages (Fig. 8.4) (65). Hobbs found that some features of skull fracture point to the presence of child abuse. In his experience with children younger than 2 years old, he found that abused children were more likely to have multiple or complex fractures; depressed, wide, and growing fractures; involvement of more than a single cranial bone; and a nonparietal fracture (66).

In some injuries, the condition of the sinuses should be noted for evidence of a fracture, which makes the injury compound, or the presence of blood. Ethmoid and maxillary sinuses are pneumatized at birth, the sphenoid sinuses become pneumatized at approximately 5 years of age, and the frontal sinuses, the last to develop, are not visualized until 4 to 6 years of age (67).

MRI usually contributes little to the initial management of major closed head injury. It is,

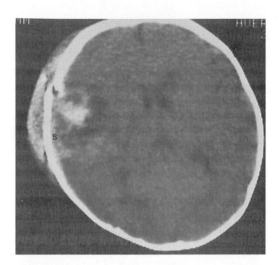

FIG. 8.4. Computed tomographic scan after head trauma. Head injury shown by computed tomographic scan without contrast. The soft tissue swelling and the left parietal skull fracture are readily evident. An intracerebral hematoma is seen with surrounding cerebral edema resulting in ventricular compression and shift. A small subdural hematoma (s) is also evident.

however, more sensitive than CT in detecting an extra-axial hematoma and thin collections of fluid (68). Additionally, MRI provides better visualization of subacute and chronic contusions and of shearing lesions of the white matter such as result from child abuse (69). MR angiography (MRA), performed at a subsequent time, can be of use in delineating such vascular abnormalities as arteriovenous fistulae, venous sinus occlusion, and arterial occlusions (58).

One must guard against excessive complacency on the basis of a single normal CT obtained in the early hours after an injury, because hemorrhagic complications can evolve subacutely after an interval of several hours or days. A repeat CT is indicated under the following circumstances: (a) when doubt exists about the presence of a mass lesion, (b) when intracranial pressure monitoring demonstrates an increase in pressure, (c) when a patient is unconscious despite an initial benign appearing CT, and (d) when a contusion is accompanied by a neurologic deficit. A normal CT result also does not exclude the presence of cerebral edema. In the series of O'Sullivan and cowork-

ers, 88% of head-injured patients with a Glasgow Coma Scale of 8 or less and no evidence of cerebral edema by CT had increased intracranial pressure when recorded directly (70).

Fluid and Electrolytes

The appropriate fluid management of the hypovolemic head-injured patient is still controversial, although both clinical and experimental studies indicate that the most important goals are to correct any hypovolemia and prevent reduction of osmolality. A period of hyponatremia with natriuresis is a common response to brain injury (71). Hyponatremia can result from either a cerebral salt-wasting syndrome characterized by hypovolemia, or from an inappropriate excess of antidiuretic hormone that causes water retention. Whereas the cerebral salt-wasting syndrome is treated by fluid and salt supplementation, the syndrome of inappropriate output of antidiuretic hormone requires fluid restriction. In the majority of patients, hyponatremia during the first week after a head injury is caused by excessive antidiuretic hormone, whereas hyponatremia that develops later probably results from chronic salt-wasting (72). There are no simple means to distinguish between the two syndromes, although Sivakumar and colleagues advocate the measurement of central venous pressure to determine whether a given patient is hypovolemic or hypervolemic (71).

The relationship between fluid load, sodium balance, and intracranial pressure is still unclear. The traditional view is that during the early posttraumatic period, there is danger of overloading the patient with fluids, which can increase intracranial pressure and thus diminish the level of consciousness. Therefore, fluid intake for the first 2 to 4 days should be between 35% and 50% of the average normal daily fluid requirements, as long as urine volume remains adequate (73). This view has been challenged, and more recent work indicates that rapid infusion of hypertonic saline or lactated Ringer solution have no effect on cerebral edema or neurologic outcome in experimental animals (73a). Even though fluid restriction increases the likelihood of cerebral infarction, Schmoker and coworkers found that in adult patients with severe head injury, there was no significant correlation between fluid balance, total sodium intake, and either intracranial pressure or outcome (74). However, to avoid cerebral ischemia most neurosurgeons currently recommend that hypertonic crystalloid solutions be given intravenously to maintain a normal intravascular volume and adequate cerebral perfusion pressure (74a). Both clinical and experimental studies suggest that glucose-containing solutions should be avoided because these tend to increase cerebral lactic acidosis (73a).

Despite the evidence of sodium retention in the early post-traumatic period, salt should be administered to avoid hypotonicity of extracellular fluids. A total of 30 mEq of sodium chloride per liter of calculated fluid requirements meets the usual electrolyte requirements. As a result of a catecholamine-induced intracellular potassium shift, hypokalemia can accompany severe head injuries (75). Although hypokalemia also is seen in less severe head injuries, extra potassium generally is not required (76).

Less commonly, hypernatremia and dehydration follow closed head injury. These are occasionally seen in a subfrontal injury that has caused hypothalamic damage and diabetes insipidus, or they are the result of a failure in the thirst response or inadequate hydration of an unconscious patient.

Coagulation Defects

A significant proportion of patients with head injuries severe enough to result in destruction of brain tissue shows clinical and laboratory evidence of impaired coagulation. These patients have low fibrinogen levels, diminished amounts of factors V and VIII, and thrombocytopenia. Treatment can require emergency replacement of hemostatic factors (77). Disseminated intravascular coagulation was seen in approximately one-third of children evaluated within 2 hours of major head injury (78).

Seizures

Seizures can occur shortly after the injury or can appear after an interval of days to years.

Seizures appearing during the acute stage can increase intracranial pressure by Valsalva effects, increasing cerebral blood flow, the release of neuroexcitatory transmitters, and aggravating any preexisting hypoxia. They generally are managed with intravenous phenytoin (5 mg/kg loading dose). Intramuscular phenytoin, which can crystallize within muscles, is unreliable. Diazepam (0.1 to 0.3 mg/kg) or lorazepam (0.05 to 0.25 mg/kg) are suitable alternatives. Some authorities are loath to administer phenytoin to infants and toddlers, preferring carbamazepine. EEG monitoring is desirable to detect electrical seizures even when paralysis of the patient prevents overt seizures. The role of anticonvulsants in the treatment of post-traumatic seizures is discussed in Chapter 13. In view of the relative rarity of post-traumatic seizures, we do not advocate preventive anticonvulsant therapy, except in the presence of a major brain laceration. For this purpose, phenytoin, the traditional drug, appears to be inferior to carbamazepine, probably because therapeutic blood levels of phenytoin are difficult to achieve and maintain (79,80).

Increased Intracranial Pressure

Children tend to have a lower incidence of surgically treatable mass lesions than adults (less than 10% in a CT-verified series), but a higher incidence of increased intracranial pressure (81). Therefore, in the infant or child who has sustained a severe head injury, control of increased intracranial pressure becomes the most important problem of medical management. For this purpose, continuous pressure monitoring is necessary for the more seriously injured patients and for infants who are more likely to experience increased intracranial pressure (1,73,82). A variety of monitoring techniques are currently in use, each with its advantages and disadvantages. These include an indwelling ventriculostomy with direct monitoring from the ventricular system; monitoring from the subarachnoid, subdural, and epidural spaces (82,83); and fiber-optic monitoring by placement of a device into the frontal parenchyma (84). Of these methods, subdural monitoring using the Camino or Codman fiberoptic pressure transducer is currently preferred at the University of California, Los Angeles, and the University of Washington. This allows an indirect, continuous measurement of intracranial pressure, which, when combined with the value of mean arterial blood pressure, permits calculation of cerebral perfusion pressure (cerebral perfusion pressure = mean systemic arterial blood pressure – intracranial pressure). When possible, estimation or measurement of cerebral blood flow allows detection of global cerebral ischemia, which generally worsens the clinical course and outcome (85). Focal cerebral ischemia is more difficult to assess. After major head injuries, some regions of the brain may require higher levels of cerebral perfusion pressure to maintain adequate cerebral blood flow.

In some head-injured children CSF drainage via a ventriculostomy is a useful adjunct for controlling elevated intracranial pressure in those subjects whose ventricles can safely be cannulated. Ventriculostomy remains the most effective way to monitor intracranial pressure and treat elevated pressure via continuous or intermittent CSF drainage. In selected patients who do not have mass lesions, but with elevated intracranial pressures that are refractory to all other therapies, treatment with controlled lumbar CSF drainage has been encouraging (85a).

Continuous monitoring of jugular venous oxygen saturation using an indwelling fiberoptic catheter also has been suggested but the usefulness of this technique in the pediatric population has yet to be assessed (1). Venous oxygen saturation in the adult should lie between 55% and 85% and values below 45% indicate global cerebral ischemia (86).

Intracranial pressure is usually maintained below 15 mm Hg, although temporary increases to 20 mm Hg are often unavoidable and can occur in the course of nursing procedures. The initial step in lowering intracranial pressure is to induce hypocarbia by hyperventilation and reduce the carbon dioxide partial pressure (pCO_2) to between 25 and 30 mm Hg. With profound hyperventilation and pCO_2 values below 25 mm Hg, cerebral ischemia can develop (87).

Should hyperventilation be ineffective in reducing increased intracranial pressure, other measures must be undertaken.

Historically, the use of hyperventilation has been part of the treatment algorithm for trauma patients with elevated intracranial pressures. This maneuver causes cerebral vasoconstriction, thereby decreasing cerebral blood flow and volume. The response to hyperventilation is rapid but short-lived, and hyperventilation must be continued or increased to remain effective. Studies show that the prolonged and routine use of hyperventilation may be deleterious in some patients by exacerbating ischemic brain injuries. Therefore, in the absence of elevated intracranial pressure, we no longer recommend the routine use of hyperventilation. Substantial beneficial effects can be realized when refractory elevated intracranial pressure is treated by moderate hyperventilation, accomplished by maintaining the arterial carbon dioxide pressure between 28 and 35 mm Hg. This therapy can be administered safely, with careful monitoring to avoid the complications associated with prolonged, profound hyperventilation, notably cerebral ischemia (87a,87b).

Raising the head between 0 and 30 degrees in the neutral, midline position is commonly performed after severe head injury. This maneuver facilitates cerebral venous drainage and thus theoretically decreased intracranial pressure. Feldman and coworkers showed in their randomized study of head position of the trauma patient that by elevating the head from 0 to 30 degrees, the intracranial pressure decreased without a decrease in cerebral perfusion pressure of cerebral blood flow (87c). When the head is raised approximately 60 degrees there appears to be a deleterious effect on cerebral blood flow. However, these studies have not been confirmed for children. Thus, the most advantageous head position in a child with an intracranial pressure monitor (i.e., the best way to maximize cerebral perfusion pressure) can be determined by raising the head and observing the concomitant change in intracranial pressure and cerebral perfusion pressure.

Diuretics have been used in a number of centers. Mannitol and urea are the most commonly used osmotic diuretics. Mannitol, given in amounts of 1.5 to 2.0 g/kg body weight in the form of a 20% solution, has a slower effect than urea, but maintains the lowered intracranial pressure at its minimum level for 2 to 4 hours. It has the disadvantage of leaking into the brain through areas where injury has damaged the blood–brain barrier and thus inducing local edema. Also, by slowly diffusing into the intercellular space, mannitol carries water with it, thereby inducing a rebound effect. For these reasons diuretics are used mainly as a temporary measure to gain time while the patient and operating room are readied for surgery, while diagnostic studies are performed, or for acute control of elevated intracranial pressure. Mannitol, furosemide, or both are currently favored in most institutions. One appropriate dosage for furosemide is 0.5 to 1.0 mg/kg, administered every 4 to 6 hours.

Numerous well-controlled clinical studies have failed to demonstrate any significant effectiveness of corticosteroids in counteracting brain swelling in head-injured children, although methylprednisolone might have a neuroprotective effect when given within 6 hours of severe injury, and in extremely high dosages (30 mg/kg) (88). In summary, the effectiveness of corticosteroids has been extensively investigated in head-injured adults. The agents did not improve outcome or lower intracranial pressure and may, in some cases, have been deleterious. For these reasons corticosteroids are not routinely employed in the treatment of pediatric head injuries (88a).

The clinical effectiveness of various oxygen-derived free radical scavengers, when given to patients with severe head injuries within 8 to 12 hours of the injury, has not been established in terms of improving neurologic outcome (89).

High doses of barbiturates, generally pentobarbital, have been advocated whenever intracranial pressure does not respond to other forms of therapy. However, there is no convincing evidence that barbiturate coma improves outcome, and the initial enthusiasm for this form of treatment has waned because barbiturates can cause myocardial depression (1,90). For this reason barbiturates require cau-

tious use in children, especially those with hemodynamic instability. Currently, barbiturates are used as a last resort to help control intractable elevations of intracranial pressure and to help place patients who are in status epilepticus into EEG burst suppression. Under these circumstances, bedside EEG monitoring is mandatory.

Sedation with pharmacologically induced paralysis is often used in the treatment of the severely head-injured child. This reduces the increase in intracranial pressure associated with agitation, suctioning, and ventilation. In our institutions, sedation and paralysis is titrated with intracranial pressure. Intravenous narcotics in small doses by continuous or bolus infusion, short-acting benzodiazepines, and nondepolarizing muscle relaxants are used effectively for this purpose. Titration of short-acting drugs permits intermittent examinations, and rapid reversal, when necessary. In nonventilated, awake, but intermittently confused patients, medication is used sparingly, because the neurologic examination is the most important parameter for the management of the head-injured patient. Small boluses of narcotics and short-acting benzodiazepines are used in some institutions to sedate the agitated pediatric patient without a mass lesion, but this issue remains controversial among neurosurgeons and critical care physicians.

Induced mild hypothermia (cooling to 32° to 33° C) in conjunction with hyperventilation (pCO_2 between 25 and 30 mm Hg) and barbiturates (4 to 6 mg/kg intravenous thiopental, followed by 6 to 8 mg/kg per hour of continuous thiopental) has reemerged as another measure to lower increased intracranial pressure and increase cerebral perfusion by lowering metabolic demands (91). Preliminary results suggest that this method can improve neurologic outcome (91,92).

Neurogenic pulmonary edema is a rare and potentially fatal complication of head injury. Its pathogenesis is unknown, but focal brainstem lesions, particularly in the region of the nucleus solitarius, can increase pulmonary arterial pressure and capillary permeability. Symptoms appear within the first day after injury and are managed with diuretics and positive end-expiratory pressure (93).

More detailed treatment schedules for the child with a major closed head injury are given by Jennett and Teasdale (94), and by Pascucci (94a). All infants with head injuries and all older children with severe head injuries, as defined by a Glasgow coma score of 8 or less, or who have sustained a major skull fracture should be seen by a neurosurgeon.

Minor Head Injury

No consensus exists with respect to the diagnostic workup or the management of the child with a minor head injury. Considerable judgment is required to avoid unnecessary hospitalization and expensive diagnostic studies, at the same time keeping in mind the possibility of post-traumatic complications that require emergency surgery. In general, children who have experienced only a momentary loss of consciousness are better managed at home. Parents are instructed to note at regular intervals the child's state of alertness and ability to move his or her extremities. The parents should be told to contact the physician if diminished consciousness or limb weakness occurs.

The role of routine CT in the management of the child with minor head injuries continues to be controversial. As indicated in Table 8.6, the infant younger than 2 years of age, or the child who sustains loss of consciousness, should undergo CT. The cost effectiveness of CT as a screening for safe discharge as compared with hospitalization for observation has been affirmed in a number of centers both in the United States and Europe (95–97). The use of skull radiography as a screening device for children with minor head injuries has serious limitations and should no longer be used inasmuch as a CT with bone windows to show the presence of fractures is superior diagnostically (95). According to some authorities, the presence of a linear skull fracture should not influence the decision about whether to send the child home; others suggest that a child found to have a skull fracture is at increased risk for an extradural hematoma and, therefore, should be observed in

the hospital (98). We believe that whenever the fracture line crosses the groove of the middle meningeal artery or crosses the path of the sagittal or other major venous sinus, the possibility of an extradural hemorrhage is increased, so that the child should be hospitalized for the initial 24 hours. If the fracture involves an air sinus, checking for the next 10 days for signs of intracranial infection is recommended even if the child is not hospitalized.

The rehabilitation of a child with a major head injury is summarized in Table 8.7. A more detailed discussion is presented in a book edited by Ylvisaker (99).

Prognosis

There has been continuing improvement in terms of mortality and ultimate neurologic status in the outcome of severely brain-injured infants and children as defined by a postresuscitation Glasgow coma score of 8 or less (100). The outlook for full intellectual function in children experiencing minor head injuries (i.e., head injuries without associated neurologic manifestations) is generally excellent (101). The prognosis for major head injuries, although less certain, is far better in children than in infants or adults. As a rule, prediction of outcome with respect to the severity of ultimate disability is accurate in only 70% by the end of the first week after the injury (102). In the experience of the Traumatic Coma Data Bank, children younger than age 4 years, who have sustained a severe head injury have a cumulative mortality of 62% during the first year after their injury. This compares with a mortality during the same period of 22% in children aged 5 to 10, and 48% in adults (103). In this series, only one in five infants had a favorable outcome. These figures, published in 1992, should be contrasted with a mortality of 10% in a cohort gathered in the years 1994 to 1996 (100). A low postresuscitation Glasgow coma score and the presence of cerebral swelling, particularly when it is accompanied by a shift of midline structures, are indices for a poor outcome. These indices have not changed in the last few decades. The poor outcome in infants in all series probably reflects

TABLE 8.7. *Rehabilitation of head injuries at each level of consciousness*

Level[a]	Neurologic characteristic	Therapeutic intervention
V	No response to stimuli Glasgow coma score = 3	Keep patient in intensive care unit
IV	Responds to pain by flexor withdrawal or increased extensor tone. No visual response to light or threat. Glasgow coma score = 4–6	Maintain clear airway and prevent pulmonary complications Control hypertension and tachycardia Institute seizure prophylaxis Institute nasogastric tube feeding Prevent contractures (range of motion, casting, splinting, medication to reduce spasticity) Get child out of bed; provide sensory stimulation Continue crisis intervention counseling with family
III	Responds to visual stimuli by blinking to light or threat or tracking Shows nonpurposeful movements of extremities Glasgow coma score = 8–10	Decrease agitation (do not use drugs) Stimulate visual and auditory responses Facilitate purposeful movements Improve head and trunk control Begin feeding program (delay gastronomy, try nasogastric tube feeding) Continue family support
II	Coma ends Demonstrates purposeful movements Follows commands, imitates gestures, responds verbally Glasgow coma score = 12–14	Reinforce appropriate behavior and decrease agitation Improve gross and fine motor skills Begin transfers and ambulation training Start self-care and self-feeding program Evaluate for developmental and perceptual deficits Improve child's speech, language, and cognitive performance: auditory processing, orientation, attention span Continue family support Plan discharge
I	Is oriented to person, time, and place; may still have cognitive and perceptual deficits Glasgow coma score = 15	Refine motor skills, community ambulation Increase independence in self-care and community living skills Improve orientation, verbal expression, and cognitive and perceptual skills Assess vision and hearing Perform neuropsychological assessment Complete discharge planning Continue family preparation and training, adaptive equipment, outpatient medical and therapy follow-up, school placement, involvement with community agencies

[a]Depending on the severity of the injury, progress can stop at any of these levels.
Adapted from Brink J. *Case management of head injuries.* With permission of the author.

the higher incidence of child abuse and multiple injuries during the first year of life. Hobbs found that 95% of fatal head injuries incurred by infants younger than 2 years of age were caused by child abuse (66).

In a series of children treated for major head injuries at the Johns Hopkins Hospital and reported in 1983, 29% were normal on follow-up, and 53% had returned to school with mild behavioral or cognitive problems. In the latter group, however, 61% had shown evidence of significant language delay, minimal cerebral dysfunction, and learning problems before the accident (104). The outcome tended to be worse in children who sustained prolonged coma. When outcome is stratified according to age, all studies show that morbidity as well as mortality is greater when the injury is experienced in infancy or in early childhood.

Generally, children with only behavioral abnormalities during the early post-traumatic period later achieve normal functioning. No significant improvement in cognitive function can be expected after the first 6 to 12 months after injury. Improvement in speech and motor function, however, can continue for several years (105,106). Decerebrate rigidity during the early postinjury phase, although associated with an early mortality in 25% to 50% of patients, by itself does not preclude functional survival; approximately one-half of survivors have a fairly good quality of life (106). Excessive daytime sleepiness is fairly common after head trauma, especially in adolescents. In some of these, notably when there has been an associated whiplash injury, sleep apnea is responsible; in others, the condition resembles narcolepsy (see Chapter 13) (107). In the experience of Guilleminault and coworkers, daytime sleepiness can persist for months to years, and its duration correlates with the severity of the initial head trauma (107). Methylphenidate and amphetamine appear to be the most effective medications. A significant postural and intention tremor affecting primarily the upper extremities has been observed in a substantial number of children recovering from a serious head injury. In the series of Johnson and Hall, the tremor appeared within 2 months of the injury in 49% of their patients, and between 2 and 12 months of the injury in 40%. It subsided spontaneously in 54%. The cause of this complication is unknown, but probably reflects an injury to the midbrain (108).

A substantial proportion of survivors from major head injuries experience subsequent emotional and psychiatric disorders. These are covered in another section of this chapter.

Skull Fractures

Linear Fractures

The immature and more flexible skull of the child can sustain a greater degree of deformation than that of an adult. Most skull fractures are linear and asymptomatic and, in the older child, are readily diagnosed by CT using bone windows. In infants, fractures tend to be irregular, so that on plain skull films they are sometimes confused with a suture or wormian bone

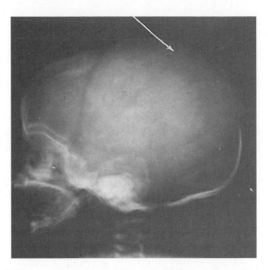

FIG. 8.5. Depressed frontal fracture and linear parietal fracture (*arrow*) on plain skull films of a newborn infant who had undergone a difficult forceps delivery. Associated left-sided epidural hematoma was demonstrated at angiography.

(Fig. 8.5). In early childhood the fracture can be diastatic and usually involves the lambdoid suture. The separation of the bones indicates that the intracranial pressure increased at the moment of impact.

Often a subperiosteal or subgaleal hematoma, termed *cephalhematoma* in the newborn infant, accompanies a linear skull fracture. Palpation of the hematoma may falsely lead the examiner to think a depressed skull fracture exists. Imaging studies disclose the underlying linear fracture. A small number of these hematomas calcify (see Fig. 5.1). There rarely is an indication for aspiration of a traumatic hematoma, and insertion of a needle or drain only increases the risk of introducing an infection into the hematoma cavity. (See Chapter 5 for further discussion of this complication.)

Closed linear fractures generally heal in 3 to 4 months and, except for breaks crossing the path of major vessels or entering the paranasal sinuses, do not require special therapy or observations.

An infrequent complication of a closed head injury with a linear fracture in an infant is the diastatic or *growing* fracture (109). It occurs in less than 1% of all fractures and usually represents a complication of a serious head injury (109a). Rare after age 3 years, it is thought to be more common in victims of child abuse, but its appearance is not confined to victims of nonaccidental trauma (66,109a). Dural tears responsible for a growing fracture occur mostly in the parietal area; their presence, unrecognized because the scalp is intact, leads to the development of a CSF-filled cyst between the cortex and the overlying bone. At the same time, the bone edges along the fracture do not unite, apparently prevented by their direct contact with fluid. The bone is resorbed, so that plain skull radiography or CT scans taken after an interval of several months show an irregular bone defect with scalloped edges that is an elliptical erosive cranial defect (109).

In many instances an associated cortical injury occurs and beneath the area of the cyst there is usually a porencephalic diverticulum of the lateral ventricle, producing a palpable and sometimes visible bone defect, and, occasionally, leading to seizures and progressive hemiparesis. Leptomeningeal cysts should be differentiated from an encephalocele, which is congenital, usually located in the occipital midline, and associated with a regular bone defect. A growing fracture does not resolve spontaneously and must be treated surgically. Treatment, which should be begun as early as possible, involves the surgical separation of the bone from underlying arachnoid, dural repair or replacement, and closure of the bone defect with autologous bone, bone source, or cranioplasty. In rare cases, normal pressure hydrocephalus develops, which requires a ventriculoperitoneal shunt.

Basal Skull Fractures

Basal skull fractures are uncommon in children. Their presence can be suspected when the child has signs of bleeding from the nasopharynx or the middle ear, or if the child has postauricular ecchymoses (Battle's sign) (110). Epistaxis is frequent in childhood head injury, however, because of the high incidence of nasal fractures.

Fractures of the base of the anterior fossa can lead to hemorrhage into the orbit. Under these circumstances a subconjunctival hemorrhage represents a forward extension of blood behind the optic globe, in contrast to an anterior hemorrhage, which arises from a direct blow to the eye. Exophthalmos and subconjunctival hemorrhage occur in conjunction with "raccoon eyes." Fractures of the mastoid portion of the temporal bone result in postauricular ecchymoses.

Distinctive unilateral fresh purpuric hemorrhages in the antitragus, triangular fossa, and helix of the ear have been termed the "tin ear syndrome." The condition can be associated with retinal hemorrhages and an ipsilateral subdural hematoma, a syndrome considered to be pathognomonic of child abuse. Rotational acceleration of the head produced by blunt trauma to the ear is believed to produce this syndrome (111).

CSF rhinorrhea can accompany a fracture of the floor of the anterior fossa that has involved the cribriform plate. It represents a rare complication of head trauma in children, but the high risk of intracranial infections (20% to 37% as reported by Wilson and coworkers) makes its recognition imperative (112).

CSF rhinorrhea usually appears within the first 2 days after the injury, but it may not become apparent for up to several years. In 70% of cases, it ceases within 1 week, and in a large proportion of the remainder, it ends within 6 months. It is accompanied by anosmia in approximately 75% of cases (113). Because the glucose content of nasal discharge (40 mg/dL) differs little from that of CSF, glucose determinations are of no value in distinguishing CSF rhinorrhea from ordinary nasal discharge (114).

Several imaging modalities have been evaluated for their ability to pinpoint the site of CSF leakage. High-resolution CT and MR cisternography, using a water-soluble nonionic contrast medium, appear to be equally accurate in localizing the site and the extent of the CSF fistula (115,116) and are superior to CT cisternography (117). In our institutions, high-resolution CT or CT cisternography have proven adequate for pinpointing the site of CSF leakage.

When rhinorrhea has not ceased within a week to 10 days, surgical repair of the dural and bony defect is usually indicated, inasmuch as any CSF leak, particularly one that results in

CSF rhinorrhea, predisposes to meningitis (112). The infecting agents are a variety of gram-positive cocci and gram-negative bacilli (118). Conservative management of CSF fistulas is successful in most instances. Bedrest with the head of the bed elevated is usually sufficient. Continuous lumbar or ventricular drainage often works in persistent CSF fistulas. If conservative treatment fails, surgical repair (intradural, extradural, or both) is required.

Whether chemoprophylaxis should be used on all patients with basal skull fractures has been the subject of considerable debate. Prospective studies have shown that prophylactic ampicillin does not reduce the risk of meningitis, but can change the flora so that gram-negative organisms become the infecting agents (119). We, therefore, prefer to withhold antibiotics until careful observation has revealed evidence of infection. Lumbar puncture to obtain CSF and ascertain the presence of an infection is unwise because it can facilitate the entry of organisms into the anterior fossa by lowering intracranial pressure. The patient should be observed carefully, with therapy undertaken only when indicated by symptoms and subsequently by the CSF examination.

Injury to the cranial nerves, particularly the olfactory, facial, and acoustic nerves, can accompany basal fractures. Complete loss of the sense of smell is usually permanent; 90% of facial nerve injuries recover spontaneously (120). Deafness can be a temporary or permanent sequela to temporal bone fractures.

Labyrinthine disorders, notably vertigo and spontaneous or positional nystagmus, are common. In the experience of Eviatar and coworkers, more than 50% of children who had experienced a head injury complained of dizziness, headache, or both (121). The condition is usually transient. In approximately one-half of the cases, electronystagmography provides objective evidence of the presence of an injury to the labyrinth (121). Less commonly, one may encounter episodic vertigo that resembles Ménierè disease. It can result either from fistulization of the bony labyrinth with disturbed perilymph-endolymph pressure

relationship, or from direct injury to the membranous labyrinth or to the endolymphatic draining system (122).

CSF otorrhea is seen in approximately 0.5% of childhood head injuries, but in approximately 95% of cases it stops spontaneously within 7 to 10 days. Unlike CSF rhinorrhea, recurrence of leakage is rare (120). Rarely, transient total blindness can follow an apparently mild blunt head injury. The child may not complain of vision loss, but can appear restless and disoriented and have an unsteady gait. The cause for blindness is uncertain, but the intact pupillary light reflexes suggest it to be cortical. In some children the event may recur (123,124).

The diagnosis of basal fractures often depends on the clinical findings, because in many instances, the fracture is not readily demonstrated by imaging studies. As a rule, the child with a basal fracture associated with hematotympanum or Battle's sign is hospitalized and observed. However, when the neurologic examination is normal and imaging studies do not show an intracranial injury, hospitalization might not be required (125). Because the incidence of meningitis in children with basilar skull fractures is only 1%, antibiotics should be withheld.

When meningitis is associated with a CSF leak, antibiotic treatment should be continued well after the leak stops.

Air within the cranial cavity (pneumocele) or air within the brain (pneumocephalus) rarely complicates head injury (126). When it does occur, it most commonly follows a fracture into the frontal sinuses and is usually an incidental finding on radiography. Pneumocephalus can denote either extradural or intradural air. Intradural air is of concern because it signifies a dural tear that can require surgical repair. Extradural air often denotes an air sinus disruption that may well resolve spontaneously. However, follow-up imaging is essential in all cases of pneumocephalus. Because meningitis develops occasionally, some centers suggest prophylactic antibiotic therapy until the air has resolved. Tension pneumocephalus is even more rare; it presents a neurosurgical emergency because of the rapid increase in intracranial pressure (127).

Depressed Fractures

Depressed fracture is a common consequence of perinatal injury, often the result of a difficult forceps delivery (ping-pong fracture; see Chapter 5). It also can occur with any localized skull trauma in later childhood and is often associated with a break in the skin (compound fracture) and localized cerebral injury. The extent of the bony injury is best diagnosed by CT. In the past, elevation and examination of the underlying dura was recommended if the depression was greater than approximately 3 mm and the fracture did not reduce spontaneously. Steinbok and coworkers adopt a more conservative approach, reserving surgery for infants with compound depressed fractures or those with focal neurologic signs. The outcome appears to be the same with or without surgery (128). We believe that a case can be made for elevating on cosmetic grounds a deep or unsightly depression, particularly when it is located in the frontal region.

Compound Fractures

Compound fractures of the skull are seen in approximately 20% of children with major head trauma (51). In this kind of injury, medical treatment is limited to an initial cleansing of the scalp, institution of antibiotics, and tetanus prophylaxis. Anticonvulsant therapy is used routinely when the bony fragments have penetrated beyond the dura. Traditionally, phenytoin has been the preferred drug. Its use requires an intravenous loading dose of 10 mg/kg and subsequent oral doses to maintain a blood level between 12 and 20 µg/mL. In children, maintaining this level is usually difficult and requires careful, repeated determinations of blood levels and adjustments of dosage (129). Because of the unreliability of phenytoin in infants and small children and its relatively high incidence of side reactions, we

prefer to use carbamazepine as a maintenance anticonvulsant.

Scalp Lacerations

Scalp lacerations can cause considerable blood loss. If any doubt exists about the presence of a scalp injury, the child's hair should be clipped, and the area around the wound widely shaved. If examination and radiography do not show an underlying fracture, the wound should be closed in anatomic layers after careful débridement with strict adherence to aseptic techniques. Closure of the galeal layer to stem hemorrhage and protect from infection is optimal. Tetanus immunization should be administered.

Complications

Extradural Hematoma

An extradural or epidural hematoma is a localized accumulation of blood between the skull and the dura. It occurs in approximately 1.0% to 3.4% of children hospitalized for head trauma (51,130). According to Matson, nearly one-half of childhood cases occur during the first 2 years of life (131). In this age group, the injury is usually the result of a fall less than 4 to 5 feet, and no other significant injuries are seen (132,133). In the experience of Shugerman and coworkers, 47% of children who developed an epidural hematoma had falls of 6 feet or less and skull fractures were seen in only 18%. Abuse was diagnosed in only 6% (133).

Pathogenesis

An extradural hematoma develops at or near the point of traumatic impact, usually in the temporoparietal region, less commonly in the frontal region. It is nearly always unilateral. In adults, the hematoma is almost invariably caused by a laceration of the middle meningeal artery or one of its branches. In children, extradural bleeding can be the consequence of even mild injury that has produced a tear in the dural veins [15% of patients in Matson's series (131)], in the meningeal artery or its branches, in the accom-

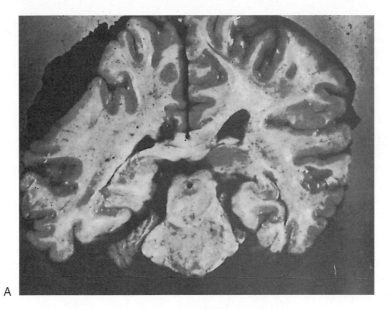

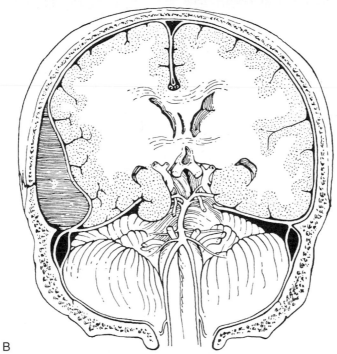

FIG. 8.6. Cerebral compression and tentorial pressure cone owing to extradural hematoma. **A:** Coronal section of brain. **B:** Diagram illustrating the swelling and displacement of the involved cerebral hemisphere with distortion of brainstem structures. (From Mealey J. *Pediatric head injuries.* Springfield, IL: Charles C Thomas, 1968. With permission.)

panying middle meningeal veins (60% of cases), or in the smaller emissary veins of the dural sinuses (15%). The stripping of the dura from the skull successively tears more vessels, contributing to the enlargement of the hematoma. This successive tearing of dural vessels is probably why Mazza and coworkers were unable to identify a source in some 20% of their cases (134). Arterial bleeding results in a rapidly evolving deterioration of the clinical condition as the hematoma enlarges and produces acute cerebral compression (Fig. 8.6A and B). The severity of symptoms depends on the size of the hematoma, the speed of its evolution, and the development of transtentorial herniation. Transtentorial herniation is more likely when cerebral edema accompanies the hematoma. When bleeding arises from veins, neurologic symptoms progress gradually, a feature more common to the extradural hematomas of childhood than to those of adult life (135). Rarely, the hematoma can stop growing; it can then resolve or ultimately calcify.

The effects of transtentorial herniation accompanying an epidural hematoma are similar to those seen with other space-occupying lesions and are considered in Chapter 10.

Clinical Manifestations

In adults, an extradural hematoma characteristically is preceded by a temporary loss of consciousness, followed by partial or full recovery, with subsequent deterioration of sensorium and appearance of focal neurologic signs. This sequence is rare in children; it did not appear in any of Mealey's 20 children with extradural hematoma (9), and it appeared in only one-third of 125 cases reported by McKissock and colleagues (135), and in 40% of Mazza's 62 cases (134). More commonly, the child appears little affected by the initial injury, or, at worst, has a brief period of unconsciousness. After an interval of minutes to several days, a progressive impairment of consciousness develops, and neurologic signs appear. Of the children reported by McKissock and colleagues, 67% took this course (135). In general, the younger the child, the longer the latency. In Mealey's series, 50% of children younger than 6 years remained asymptomatic for

TABLE 8.8. *Common clinical features of extradural hematoma*

Symptom[a]	Percent of patients
Vomiting	62.5
Unequal pupils	55.0
Delayed loss of consciousness	48.7
Skull fracture, all types	40.0
Hemiparesis	25.0
Papilledema	22.5
Depressed skull fracture	20.0
Third nerve paresis, other than pupillary dilation	17.5
Retinal hemorrhages	12.5

[a]Symptoms listed occur with a significantly greater frequency in children with extradural hematomas than in the general head trauma series.

Modified from Hendrick EB, Harwood-Nash DC, Hudson AR. Head injuries in children: a survey of 4465 consecutive cases at the Hospital for Sick Children, Toronto, Canada. *Clin Neurosurg* 1963;11:46.

12 hours or longer (9). The clinical picture of extradural hematoma is summarized in Table 8.8.

Aside from the delayed progressive impairment of consciousness, the most significant neurologic signs are pupillary inequality, hemiparesis, papilledema, and changes in vital signs. As the hematoma enlarges, signs of transtentorial herniation appear. The earliest of these signs is a dilated pupil, which soon becomes unreactive to light and, in approximately 90% of instances, is on the side of the lesion (135). This dilation is followed by hemiparesis, usually contralateral to the hematoma, and finally by decerebrate rigidity and cardiovascular signs of decompensated increased intracranial pressure. Ipsilateral hemiparesis can develop caused by compression of the cerebral peduncle against the tentorial edge by a contralateral mass, and in the days before neuroimaging, resulted in a false localizing sign (Kernohan sign) (136). Blood loss in infants can be sufficient to produce shock. When the latency period in infants is as long as days or weeks, progressive anemia can provide a clue to the diagnosis. Seizures resulting from an epidural hematoma are rare and were present in only 7.5% of children seen by Hendrick and colleagues (51).

Occasionally, an extradural hematoma develops in the posterior fossa (137,138). Bleeding usually arises from the lateral dural sinuses, and fracture lines crossing the lateral sinus are seen nearly always. The history includes a severe fall on the occiput, followed by persistent impairment of consciousness, headache, vomiting, and neck stiffness. Only approximately one-half of the children have such posterior fossa signs as nystagmus, cerebellar ataxia, and cranial nerve palsies. Evacuation of a posterior fossa hematoma generally constitutes an emergency procedure.

Diagnosis

The diagnosis of an extradural hematoma rests principally on the clinical picture, and in some cases surgical treatment is so urgent that there is no time for imaging studies (63). Extradural hematoma must be differentiated from an acute subdural hematoma, an intracerebral hematoma, and severe brain swelling with or without contusion. Because both an acute extradural hematoma and an acute subdural hematoma require immediate surgical evacuation, the distinction between these two entities is academic. CT almost always detects the hematoma, except when the collection of blood is very thin (Fig. 8.7). MRI is equal or superior to CT, but is rarely indicated because of the time constraints associated with treating an acute injury. In 20% to 40% of children with extradural hematoma, a skull fracture is not detectable by radiographic examination or even at operation (9), so that time should not be spent on searching for the fracture. EEG and MRI, which are also time-consuming procedures, should not be used to further delineate the hematoma.

Posterior fossa extradural hematomas are more difficult to recognize. The biconvex and more focal configuration of the extradural hematoma frequently permits the CT to distinguish between extradural and subdural accumulations (see Fig. 8.7). Repeat CTs also are useful in assessing a patient after surgical evacuation of a hematoma.

Treatment

Operative removal of the clot can be performed occasionally through burr holes, but usually requires a craniotomy for complete removal and arrest of the bleeding. If the child's condition does not allow time for imaging studies, a low tempo-

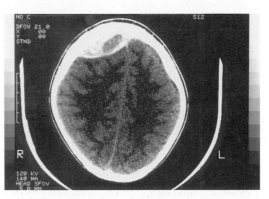

FIG. 8.7. Extradural hematoma in a victim of child abuse. The lentiform shape of the hematoma and the fact that the collection of blood crosses to the opposite side are consistent with the presence of an extradural hematoma. Bone films (not shown) disclosed an underlying skull fracture. (Courtesy of Dr. Franklin G. Moser, Division of Neuroradiology, Cedars-Sinai Medical Center, Los Angeles.)

ral burr hole is made for confirmation of the diagnosis and rapid removal of the clot. Further burr holes or craniectomy might then be needed. For details of the neurosurgical procedure, see Marshall (139) or Jennett and Teasdale (94).

Prognosis

Although the majority of patients shows dramatic improvement, the general prognosis of extradural hematoma remains grave, if the condition is not treated in a timely fashion. Surgery for a large acute extradural hematoma is a life-saving procedure when performed within the first few hours of injury. In Matson's series, published in 1969, the mortality was nearly 10%, with another 20% of patients being left with major neurologic residua (131). Generally, infants fare worse than older children. In a 1986 series of children younger than 2 years reported by Choux and coworkers, 68% were left without apparent sequelae, some 10% died, and 12% had major residua (140). As a rule, the likelihood for sequelae increases if the child deteriorates acutely, or had a depressed level of consciousness or neurologic abnormalities by the time of surgery. Posterior fossa extradural hematomas also have a grave prognosis, partly because they tend to progress rapidly (141). Despite the ready availability of imaging, the mortality in one series was 35%, and 20% of patients were left with a moderate disability (138). Both the prognosis for survival and the extent of the neurologic deficit are related to the early diagnosis of this complication and the presence of associated brain damage.

Subdural Hematoma

A subdural hematoma is a collection of bloody fluid between the dura and the arachnoid over the cerebral mantle. It is a relatively common complication of recognized and unrecognized head trauma of childhood and represents one of the two major neurosurgical problems of infancy. In the series of Choux and coworkers, this complication was seen in 4.3% of children with head trauma; 73% of cases occurred in children younger than 2 years of age (140). A subdural hematoma should be distinguished from a postmeningitic subdural effusion containing clear or xanthochromic fluid with a high protein concentration. The etiology and the course of treatment of a postmeningitic subdural effusion differ from that of a subdural hematoma and are discussed in Chapter 6.

Pathogenesis

Subdural bleeding usually arises from veins that pass from the cerebral cortex to the dural sinuses, bridging the potential subdural space. Skull distortion at the moment of injury, particularly in infants, and possibly the relative movement of the brain within the skull, can so stretch these veins that they rupture and bleed beneath the dura, separating the dura from the underlying arachnoid membrane. It is also likely that a tear of the arachnoid allows CSF to leak into the subdural space. Venous bleeding also can arise from a laceration of the dura, or from a direct injury to a dural sinus, as can happen with depressed fractures. Less often, the bleeding originates from cortical arteries and is associated with cerebral contusion. In 80% to 85% of infants, the hematoma is bilateral and located in the frontoparietal region. In a large percentage of infants whose hematomas result from postnatal trauma, parental abuse can be suspected from evidence of soft tissue bruising and radiographic evidence of multiple episodes of skeletal trauma (134,142–144).

The appearance of the hematoma varies with the age of the lesion (Fig. 8.8). In the acute stage, the fluid can be dark red or can even consist of clotted blood. Subsequently, the formed elements break down, producing a fluid that changes in color from chocolate to straw. It contains few red cells, but large amounts of methemoglobin and bilirubin. The former can be detected by MRI, the latter spectrophotometrically. Within approximately 1 week, a membrane forms from the inner surface of the dura and ultimately envelops the clot or fluid collection. Eventually, the lesion can enlarge, probably from the leakage of albumin from the thin-walled and abnormally permeable vessels of the outer subdural membrane (145). The accumulation of albumin in the subdural pocket increases the osmotic pressure and causes an influx of water. Although the enlarging subdural hematoma can produce symptoms of increased intracranial pressure, no evidence exists that the presence of either a hematoma or the membranes interfere with brain development. Rather, any permanent neurologic deficit results from the original trauma that caused the hematoma. Additionally, often a diffuse damage occurs secondary to increased intracranial pressure and diminished cerebral perfusion. Single photon emission CT (SPECT) scanning has been of assistance in demonstrating both regional and diffuse abnormalities in cerebral perfusion (146). Focal ischemic damage in the hemisphere underlying the subdural hematoma is believed to result from the release of vasogenic substances from the hematoma that enhance vasoconstriction and attenuate vasodilatation (147). The focal ischemia, in turn, induces localized cytotoxic edema and the release of free radicals (148). The biochemical changes of the underlying parietal white matter show an accumulation of lactate and a loss of *N*-acetylaspartate. The severity of these alterations is believed to be prognostic of the outcome (149).

Unlike subdural hematomas in older children and in adults, the post-traumatic subdural

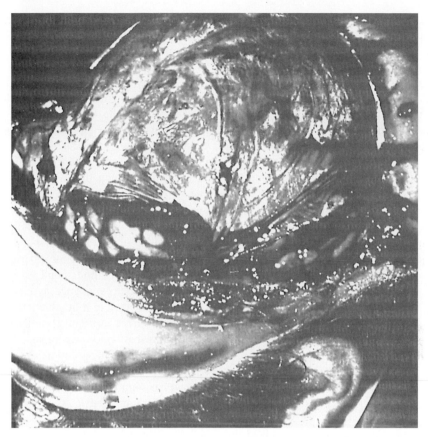

FIG. 8.8. Subacute subdural hematoma. Gross appearance of brain. Note blood oozing from the subdural compartment. (Courtesy of Dr. Harry V. Vinters, Division of Neuropathology, UCLA Center for the Health Sciences, Los Angeles.)

hematoma of infants tends to recollect repeatedly, even after total evacuation. Mealey attributes the reaccumulation of fluid to the disproportion between the enlarged skull and the previously compressed brain (9). Although it is unlikely that a subdural hematoma inhibits brain growth, it produces an enlargement of the skull and creates a pocket that tends to refill with blood. A similar disproportion between the volume of the brain and the skull increases the incidence of subdural hematomas in infants with congenital or acquired cerebral atrophy (9).

Clinical Manifestations

To a great extent, clinical manifestations depend on the patient's age. In older children, as in adults, the disorder can be acute or chronic. In both groups, symptoms of increased intracranial pressure predominate.

When a subdural hematoma after a serious head injury takes an acute course, symptoms develop within the first day or two. Venous bleeding usually does not produce symptoms unless it is accompanied by a major cerebral contusion or laceration. In these conditions, the hematoma is only one of several components of the injury, and its evacuation is not usually followed by rapid recovery (150). In part, the poor outlook reflects the aforementioned reduction of cerebral blood flow and metabolic rate throughout the hemisphere underlying the hematoma. Brain injury, usually in the form of an acute subdural hematoma, is seen in a significant proportion of battered babies, and an acute subdural hematoma is the most common cause of death or physical disability in infants; it must, therefore, be sought in all victims of child abuse.

Chronic subdural hematomas are rare in children older than age 2 years; they are more frequent during adolescence (151). In this age group, the clinical picture is one of a gradual change in personality and alertness, headaches, and, ultimately, seizures or rapid deterioration of consciousness. Often, there is no history of antecedent head trauma. The hematoma is unilateral in 80% of instances, and its differentiation from a tumor of the cerebral hemispheres is difficult clinically. The diagnosis is usually made by imaging studies. MRI permits better delineation of small subdural hematomas, hematomas that are adjacent to the falx or the tentorium, and isodense accumulations. MRI also delineates any associated cerebral injuries and assists in timing the lesion (69). On CT, the subdural hematoma can appear hyperdense, isodense, or hypodense, depending on the age of the lesion. Acute lesions tend to be hyperdense, and lesions that have produced symptoms for more than 3 weeks are usually hypodense; when symptoms have been present for 1 to 3 weeks, the fluid collection tends to be isodense. Under these circumstances the hematoma is recognized by ventricular compression and distortion (152).

Far more common is the chronic subdural hematoma of infancy, usually encountered between ages 2 and 6 months, the average age at admission being 4 months. In this age group, the lesions are bilateral in approximately 80% of cases. In some 60% of infants, the environmental history or other evidence of recent unreported physical trauma suggests child abuse (132,152). The more serious the head injury, the greater the likelihood of abuse. Of 45 infants younger than 1 year of age who sustained a skull fracture, only 11% were victims of child abuse, whereas of 19 infants who had a subdural hematoma or other forms of serious intracranial injury, 95% were abused (7). In the experience of Bruce and Zimmerman, 80% of traumatic deaths occurring in children younger than 2 years of age were nonaccidental; in fact, infants rarely sustain an accidental injury that is sufficiently severe to render them unconscious (153). Harcourt and Hopkins observed that intraocular hemorrhages in the absence of subdural effusions and external evidence of ocular trauma are commonly encountered in battered children. They postulate that these hemorrhages result from the gravitational effects of swinging the infant around by its feet (154). Additionally, compression of the thorax inducing an abrupt increase in intracranial pressure can play a role. Whether the abused infant is injured by these means or by violent to and fro shaking has since been disputed: Much greater gravitational forces can be generated by striking the infant's head against a mattress (153).

CT and MRI can be of considerable assistance in confirming that a child has been battered (65,155,156). An interhemispheric subdural hematoma in the sub-temporal or the parieto-occipital region accompanied by a skull fracture can be documented in more than 50% of abused children, whereas in trauma unrelated to abuse, bleeding in this region accompanied by a skull fracture is seen in only 13% (155,157). Additionally, the presence of both acute and chronic hematomas supports the diagnosis of child abuse.

An interhemispheric subdural hematoma should be distinguished from an interhemispheric subarachnoid hemorrhage (falx sign), which can be seen after perinatal trauma. In interhemispheric subarachnoid hemorrhage, the hemorrhage tends to extend along the entire interhemispheric fissure (158).

Although in infancy a chronic subdural hematoma lacks a characteristic clinical picture, certain features should suggest the condition. Lethargy and seizures are the most common presenting features. Seizures occur in approximately one-half of the patients; they are focal or, more commonly, generalized. Vomiting, fever, and hyperirritability or lethargy are other common clinical features (Table 8.9) (159,160). Most often, the infant's history includes failure to gain weight; refusal of feedings, followed by frequent episodes of vomiting, some of which might be projectile; irritability; progressive enlargement of the head; and, ultimately, a seizure. Often, symptoms are present for several months before a diagnosis is made.

On examination, the infant can be febrile as a result of dehydration or blood within the cranial

TABLE 8.9. *Clinical features of 116 cases of infantile subdural hematoma*

Symptom of finding	Percentage of infants
Tense anterior fontanelle	73
Vomiting	70
Seizures	60
Retinal or subhyaloid hemorrhages	54
Abnormal skull circumference	40
Impaired consciousness	22
Papilledema	12
Skull fracture	13
Other fractures	17

Modified from Till K. Subdural haematoma and effusion in infancy. *BMJ* 1968;2:400.

cavity. The head is enlarged, with a prominent parietal or biparietal bulge. The fontanelle is full, and a setting sun sign of the eyes might be noted. Funduscopy can reveal retinal hemorrhages, subhyaloid hemorrhages, or less commonly, papilledema (161,162). Retinal hemorrhages have been found in more than 50% of infants with a subdural hematoma, and almost invariably indicate a nonaccidental injury (131,143). Focal neurologic signs, including hemiparesis or facial palsy, are present in 15% to 25% of patients.

Laboratory studies are usually of little help in establishing the diagnosis, although approximately 50% of the infants are anemic. It is important to exclude a bleeding disorder, and various inborn errors of metabolism, notably kinky hair disease (Menkes disease), a sex-linked disorder of copper transport, and glutaric aciduria type I, which can present with a subdural hematoma and subperiosteal bleeding (see Chapter 1 and Fig. 1.11) (163). Lumbar puncture can reveal grossly bloody or xanthochromic fluid, evidence of an associated cerebral injury. The protein level can be elevated, and a pleocytosis can be present if the hematoma has been long-standing. The EEG is of little assistance in either the diagnosis or localization of a subdural hematoma and frequently fails to show any focal abnormality.

Diagnosis

A chronic subdural hematoma should be suspected in an irritable infant who has failed to gain weight and has developed an enlarged head and a tense fontanelle. Characteristically, the head assumes a biparietal bulge that differs from the frontal bulge of early hydrocephalus. Confirmation of the diagnosis and determination of the size of the hematoma and of any associated brain damage rest on CT and, if necessary, MRI.

Treatment

Several regimens have been proposed for the treatment of post-traumatic infantile subdural hematoma. Based on the classic work of Sherwood (164) and Ingraham and Heyl (165), Litovsky and coworkers have outlined a course of therapy (152). Initially, the subdural fluid is removed at regular intervals by subdural tapping. If the subdural hematoma does not dry up, the taps are performed daily on alternate sides for approximately 2 to 3 weeks. This waiting period allows the general condition of the infant to become stabilized. Because of the anemia and the recurrent loss of high-protein fluid, transfusions or other supportive therapy may be required.

We have found that with serial subdural taps the collection of fluid dries up completely in selected patients, thus eliminating the need for a surgical procedure. When fluid reforms between tapping, or when imaging studies reveal the presence of a subdural clot, surgical intervention must be considered. This occurs in approximately 50% of cases. In the remainder of instances, fluid formation gradually decreases and the membranes disappear. However, this does not happen when the brain and skull are disproportionate, as is the case in cerebral atrophy. The operative removal of subdural membranes can never be complete. It is no longer practiced except when craniotomy is being performed for the removal of a large blood clot, which seldom is present in the chronic stage of infantile subdural hematoma. Instead, a subdural-peritoneal shunt (94) using simple tubes without valves, allows the drainage of fluid and reduces the volume of dead space, allowing it to be obliterated by the growing brain. A unilateral shunt is sufficient in many cases (160). Subdural membranes completely disappear and the vascularity becomes reduced with time, as long as the subdural space is adequately drained. Improvement can be confirmed by repeated imaging studies (166). Continuous external subdural drainage is also useful in selected patients before subdural-peritoneal shunting because in approximately one-half of the children the procedure makes it possible to avoid shunt placement (167).

Chronic subdural hematomas occurring in older children and adolescents are drained through burr holes (168). At this age, too, the fluid collection is frequently bilateral.

Prognosis

The prognosis for an infant with a subdural hematoma correlates with the extent of damage sustained by the brain, rather than with the volume of subdural fluid itself. If brain injury has been extensive, the brain does not expand, and the hematoma can calcify or ossify. Removal of a calcified subdural hematoma is of no advantage (169).

The prognosis for children whose subdural hematoma resulted from nonaccidental trauma has been shown to be relatively poor (170,171). Even when no gross neurologic deficits are present, abused children have a higher incidence of neurologic residua, significantly lower IQ scores, growth failure, and a significantly higher incidence of emotional handicaps than children with accidental subdural hematoma (172,173). In part, these differences may result from the repetitive rotational forces experienced by the brain during shaking, and in part from the socioeconomic environment of children who have experienced abuse (170,172).

Post-Traumatic Epilepsy

Seizures associated with trauma have been classified according to their time of onset into immediate, early, and late types (49,173). A few patients experience seizures in 1 or 2 seconds after their head trauma. Such immediate seizures are most probably the result of direct mechanical stimulation of cerebral tissue having a low seizure threshold.

Seizures can appear during the first week after major cerebral trauma (early post-traumatic seizures). These arise from cerebral edema or from intracranial hemorrhage, contusion, laceration, or necrosis. The convulsions are usually generalized, but unilateral seizures and focal twitching (epilepsia partialis continua) can be seen. Generally, early post-traumatic epilepsy is more common in children than in adults, and in the experience of Jennett it was encountered in approximately 10% of head-injured children, aged 5 years or younger (173). A history of prior seizures or developmental abnormalities is seen in approximately one-half (174). Status epilepticus occurs in approximately one-fifth of children and is most likely to occur during the first hour after trauma (49). In the experience of Hendrick and his group, 7.4% of children with head trauma requiring hospitalization had seizures during the early post-traumatic period (51). The incidence was highest in infants younger than 1 year of age; those subjected to perinatal injury were particularly susceptible (see Chapter 5).

In the experience of Hendrick and colleagues, 24% of patients with early post-traumatic seizures had an associated skull fracture (51). Closed and compound depressed fractures are particularly common, together accounting for approximately one-half the fractures seen in patients with early post-traumatic epilepsy. Seizures, and even status epilepticus, are far more likely to occur in children who have sustained relatively minor head trauma than in adults with similar trauma.

Late post-traumatic seizures tend to develop within the first 2 years after the injury. Approximately 75% of children with late post-traumatic seizures had no significant deficits at the time of the injury (175). In approximately 50% of cases, seizures appear during the first 12 months after trauma (49). Anatomic and EEG studies indicate that the seizures originate from a cerebromeningeal scar, with the epileptic focus localized to grossly normal tissue (176). The overall incidence of late post-traumatic epilepsy is difficult to estimate, as the figure is lowered by the inclusion of mild head injuries in any prospective series. In the series of Annegers and colleagues, which included both children and adults, the 5-year and 30-year cumulative incidence after severe head injury was 10% and 16.7%, respectively. It is of note that after severe injury the incidence of new-onset seizures remained elevated throughout the follow-up period, an indication that the interval between serious head injury and the onset of post-traumatic seizures can be many years (177).

According to Jennett, the likelihood of late post-traumatic epilepsy is increased by the presence of any of three factors: an acute hematoma, a depressed skull fracture, or early epilepsy (49). This conclusion, derived from his experience with a mixed adult and pediatric population, needs some amplification. Annegers and colleagues found that in children the presence of early post-traumatic epilepsy did not predict late post-traumatic epilepsy (174), and Jennett noted that when early focal seizures occur in children, the incidence of late post-traumatic seizures did not increase significantly (49). It is not clear whether the location of brain injury, as judged from the fracture site, affects the likelihood of late epilepsy. Most authorities agree, however, that injuries to the parietal lobe and to the anterior and medial parts of the temporal lobe are most likely to be followed by late post-traumatic epilepsy.

In Jennett's data, only 2% of children who did not lose consciousness after head trauma developed post-traumatic epilepsy (49). The percentage rose to 5% to 10% when consciousness was lost for 1 hour or longer. By comparison, children who sustained brain laceration had a 30% incidence of post-traumatic epilepsy. In general, if the dura is penetrated, the incidence of post-traumatic epilepsy increases at least twofold. Another factor that influences the incidence of late epilepsy is the duration of post-traumatic amnesia; late epilepsy is twice as common in children with more than 24 hours of post-traumatic amnesia.

Seizures can take several clinical forms. They can be generalized or focal with secondary generalization. Focal seizures can be preceded by an aura consisting of motor phenomena such as clonic movements of an extremity or by somatosensory phenomena. The seizures also

can be focal without secondary generalization, but petit mal (absence) attacks do not occur as a result of trauma (49,178). The EEG has proved to be uniformly unsuccessful in predicting post-traumatic epilepsy in children (49,179).

The diagnosis of post-traumatic epilepsy depends on the antecedent history of head trauma and the absence of any pretraumatic seizure history. The possibility of an intracranial hematoma should always be excluded using imaging studies.

Treatment of post-traumatic epilepsy is similar to that used for focal or generalized seizures of unknown cause (see Chapter 13). No evidence exists that prophylactic phenytoin or other anticonvulsants help prevent either early or late post-traumatic seizures inasmuch as these studies are confounded by poor compliance.

Generally, the prognosis of post-traumatic seizures is good. The clinical impression that seizures that begin within 2 years of trauma have a better likelihood of subsiding than those with a later onset has not been proven by more recent studies. Jennett and Teasdale concluded that once a patient has developed late post-traumatic epilepsy, the patient will always remain prone to a seizure disorder, even though the patient can experience remissions of 2 years or longer (94). In approximately 20% to 50% of all patients, seizures gradually become less frequent after the third year and finally cease completely (49,180). In all instances, medical therapy should be used first, but surgery for excision of the meningocerebral scar and any underlying cysts or gliosis should be considered in patients whose seizures persist for 2 or more years despite adequate anticonvulsant therapy (181).

Some children are subject to profound but temporary alterations of consciousness after relatively mild head trauma. The attacks, similar to complicated migraine, are marked by a scotoma or other visual symptoms, including cortical blindness, hemianopsia, brainstem signs, confusion or depression of consciousness, headache, nausea, and vomiting (182). Convulsions can develop after the onset of the migraine-like symptoms, as can a hemiparesis. Attacks do not develop immediately after head trauma, but rather after a symptom-free interval of several minutes to an hour. The great majority of attacks resolves completely within 24 hours. During an attack, EEG tracings show symmetric or asymmetric slowing, whereas cerebral angiography and neuroimaging are generally normal. The mechanism for the attacks is still unknown (183).

Major Vascular Injuries

Blunt or penetrating injuries to the major vessels of the head or neck are relatively uncommon in children who have experienced trauma to that area. Blunt carotid injuries can result in a contusion or tear of the wall of the internal carotid artery, with a subsequent dissecting aneurysm, or in a carotid-cavernous fistula (184). Traumatic thrombosis of the internal carotid artery has been reported in children as a result of relatively minor injuries to the head or neck, or after puncture of the soft palate by a lollipop stick (185) (see Fig. 12.3). Symptoms of an internal carotid artery dissection can appear immediately after the accident. More commonly, they develop a few hours, days, or even years later (186). Symptoms include focal ischemia or a headache accompanied by an objective and subjective bruit and by Horner syndrome. Internal carotid artery dissection is treated by anticoagulation and early thrombectomy if the site of obstruction is accessible (187). A traumatic carotid-cavernous fistula is usually the result of a sphenoid bone fracture, which lacerates the internal carotid artery as it passes through the cavernous sinus. Symptoms include unilateral pulsating exophthalmos, an intracranial bruit, and paralysis of the cranial nerves, most commonly the sixth (188).

Trauma to the cervical spine can produce stretching of the vertebral arteries, with disruption of the endothelium and subsequent arterial dissection. Symptoms of intermittent brainstem and cerebellar dysfunction can develop and last for months or years. When, as often occurs, the patient has no history of antecedent trauma, cervical spinal trauma is difficult to differentiate from complicated migraine (189,190). MRI of the upper cervical spine and foramen magnum region and MR angiography can assist in the diagnosis (190a). Basilar artery migraine is covered in Chapter 13.

Delayed Deterioration after Mild Head Injury

A relatively common, potentially fatal complication of head injury in the pediatric age group is one of rapid secondary deterioration occurring within minutes or hours after relatively minor trauma, and after a lucid interval or a period of improved consciousness (191). A significant proportion of children with this symptom complex has early post-traumatic seizures, sometimes with focal or generalized status epilepticus. The syndrome also has been encountered in youngsters who have experienced repeated concussive injuries in sports ("second impact syndrome") (192).

The mechanism underlying this phenomenon is not fully understood, but is probably secondary to brain swelling that can occur after a relatively minor head injury. In the series of Bruce and colleagues, it was encountered in 15% of children and adolescents whose Glasgow coma scores on admission were 8 or better (193). Most likely, the swelling results from vasodilation and hyperemia, which is probably the consequence of a loss of cerebral vascular autoregulation, with a subsequent increase in brain bulk. Treatment, directed at constricting brain vascular volume, is accomplished by prolonged (24 to 48 hours) hyperventilation of the intubated youngster, coupled with the treatment scheme for cerebral edema described elsewhere in this chapter.

Post-Traumatic Mental Disturbances

During recovery from a major head injury, almost every child shows some abnormality of behavior or intellect that often is more disturbing to the child and family than any physical handicap (194–196). Although it is said that because of its greater plasticity the child's brain recovers more fully after injury than the adult's brain, this is true only in terms of gross neurologic function. When higher cognitive skills are examined, the converse appears to be the case, and a variety of significant deficits are uncovered that affect the way the child functions in society. In the experience of Koskiniemi and colleagues, who studied the long-term outcome of severe head injury incurred by preschool children, 30% had a below normal IQ when tested in adulthood (197). Only 21% of those with normal IQ were able to work full time outside the home. None of the children who experienced the head injury before 4 years of age was able to work independently.

As a rule, the capacity for new learning is more affected than retention of previously learned information. Even an apparently normal neuropsychological profile does not preclude permanent changes in behavior and personality (198). One must conclude that a child is better able to compensate for focal brain injury than an adult, but tolerates diffuse injury less well. This difference results in subtle long-term learning difficulties that often are not apparent to family, teacher, or physician, but are detected by a neuropsychological evaluation (195). Neuroimaging studies, notably positron emission tomography and single photon emission CT scans, can corroborate the neurocognitive deficiencies by showing areas of hypoperfusion, but these tests do not assist in prognosis (199).

One of the most obvious cognitive deficits is post-traumatic amnesia, an inability to recall events as a result of injury. In most cases, the length of post-traumatic amnesia is proportional to the severity of brain damage (57,200). One of the common features of concussion injuries is a failure to recall events that occurred just before the injury (retrograde amnesia). Here, too, a relationship exists between the length of time before the accident for which memory is impaired and the severity of the brain injury. Post-traumatic amnesia is usually more extensive than retrograde amnesia. When a patient has unusually extensive retrograde amnesia, trauma to the limbic system, particularly the hippocampal formation and the mamillary bodies, should be suspected. Generally, the rate of recovery is faster in children than in adults; however, in the experience of Harris, major post-traumatic psychological difficulties persisted in one-half of the 13% of children who manifested prolonged retrograde amnesia (201).

Deficits in verbal and visual recognition memory are particularly evident in younger children and are proportional to the duration of impaired consciousness (202). These tests are relatively easy to administer in an office setting and are described by Hannay and coworkers (203).

These observations point to the relatively low threshold for neuropsychological dysfunction in younger children. In many instances, however, the appearance of major psychiatric disorders after head injury, including lability of mood, outbursts of anger, increased aggressiveness, sleep disturbances, nightmares, and enuresis, is unrelated to the injury itself, but reflects the child's family and social environment. In this respect, it is undoubtedly significant that a large proportion of children showing these post-traumatic behavior disturbances had a history of previous accidents requiring medical treatment, and that approximately 25% were either mentally retarded or had required psychiatric therapy before their head injury. Shaffer and associates believe that several factors are responsible for these observations (194). In their experience, a high percentage (40%) of children with head trauma came from broken homes, and an equally high percentage had emotionally disturbed mothers. Also, it appears that head injury increases a child's vulnerability to subsequent environmental stresses (204). It is also significant that when head injuries are incurred during sports, the clinical picture of the postconcussion syndrome, although similar to that seen after potentially litigious injuries, is strikingly brief (205). This observation lends support to the view that the postconcussion syndrome results from environmental, psychological, and physiologic factors. These are reviewed by McClelland and colleagues (206). In the experience of Mahoney and colleagues (104), Shaffer and colleagues (194), and Hjern and Nylander (207), the overwhelming majority of children with persistent psychiatric symptoms had similar problems before their accident, which only served to aggravate symptoms. A more recent series confirms these observations, with a prior history of emotional cognitive disturbances in 45% of children who experienced severe head injuries (106). Conversely, none of the children who had been free of psychiatric symptoms before their accident displayed permanent post-traumatic mental disturbances.

Psychiatric symptoms of head injury can frequently be avoided by giving parents, particularly mothers, reassurance or extensive supportive therapy at an early stage, preferably as soon as the child is admitted to the hospital (207). We have most of our patients return to school as soon as feasible, but recommend limiting academic demands, increasing them gradually as warranted by the child's adjustment and school performance. Based on the considerable evidence that the effects of repeated concussion are additive, children who have had two or more episodes of head injury associated with loss of consciousness or amnesia should not be allowed to participate in contact sports (192).

In summary, the long-term outcome of severe head injuries is poor when incurred in infancy or during the preschool years in terms of both gross neurologic deficits and developmental delays. In infants, the results of the ocular examination, part of the pediatric Glasgow coma score assessed on admission, appear to be most predictive of the outcome. Additionally, when an initial CT scan demonstrates cerebral swelling and a midline shift, a poor outcome can be expected. The outcome for older children is better; it is a function of the condition of the child on admission to the hospital, the severity of increased intracranial pressure, and the duration of coma. Even prolonged coma is consistent with recovery without major neurologic deficits. For instance, in one study, 26% of children who were in coma longer than 24 hours died and 61% had a good outcome from a gross neurologic standpoint (104).

PERSISTENT VEGETATIVE STATE

Persistent vegetative state (PVS) is a relatively rare sequela to major head trauma in the pediatric population. As defined by Jennett and Plum (208), in this state the patient exhibits periods of apparent wakefulness during which the eyes open and move, and responsiveness is limited to primitive postural and reflex movements of the limbs.

In the majority of instances, patients blink in response to painful stimuli, exhibit spontaneous eye movements, and show a sleep-wake periodicity. Less often, yawning, chewing, and eye-

following movements occur. Meaningless laughter or weeping are not unusual. Decerebrate rigidity is seen in approximately one-half of cases and reflects damage to the midbrain and pons. This is confirmed by MRI studies that show diffuse axonal injury localized in the majority of instances to the corpus callosum and the dorsolateral aspect of the rostral brainstem (209).

Higashi and coworkers have proposed three levels of PVS (210). Level I is marked by the presence of a sleep-wake cycle and emotional expression, level II is marked by a sleep-wake cycle without emotional expression, and level III is marked by the absence of the sleep-wake cycle. The EEG does not correspond to the severity of damage, or to changes in the clinical status; in fact, 25% of patients demonstrate a significant amount of activity.

The prognosis of PVS in the pediatric patient when it follows head trauma is significantly better than when it follows hypoxic brain injury (211). In the experience of Heindl and Laub, 84% of children who had been in post-traumatic PVS for at least 30 days had left PVS 19 months after the injury. Of all children in post-traumatic PVS, 16% were able to become independent. However, after 9 months in PVS less than 5% were able to leave this state (211). Survival in PVS is conditional on the age of the youngster, with infants younger than 1 year of age having a mean survival of 2.6 years, as contrasted with 5.2 years in children aged 2 to 6 years and 7.0 years in children aged 7 to 18 years (212). The same group found that life expectancy doubled between the 1980s and 1993 to 1996, so that in 1993 life expectancy for a 15-year-old in PVS was 10.5 to 12.2 years. For a 1-year-old it was 7.2 years (212a). See Chapter 15 for a discussion of the diagnosis of brain death in infants and children.

SPINAL CORD INJURIES

Because of the spinal cord's protected location, a considerable amount of direct trauma is required to injure it. In children, therefore, injuries to the spinal cord are relatively uncommon. Most frequently, they are the result of indirect trauma. This is seen in accidents marked by sudden hyperflexion or hyperextension of the neck, or by vertical compression of the spine resulting from falls on the head or buttocks, as can occur from surfing, diving into shallow water, falling from a horse, or various other athletic accidents (213). In physically abused infants, spinal cord injuries can be induced by violent shaking of the head. Obstetric spinal cord injuries are covered in Chapter 5.

Common sites for childhood spinal cord injuries are the second cervical vertebra (27%), followed by the tenth thoracic vertebra (13%), seventh thoracic vertebra (6%), and first lumbar segment (6%) (214). Fractures of the twelfth thoracic and first lumbar vertebrae are relatively common and can produce a conus medullaris and cauda equina syndrome.

In the experience of Hamilton and Myles, fracture of the vertebral body or posterior elements without subluxation was the most common pediatric spinal injury. It was seen in 56% of patients (213). Fracture with subluxation was seen in 29%, and subluxation without fracture in only 2%. Major spinal cord injury without any radiologic abnormalities was seen in 13% of children. It was the most common form of spinal injury in children younger than 9 years of age, being encountered in 42% of spinal cord injuries.

With the increased use of lap belts in cars, children can incur a horizontal splitting of the spine, also known as a Chance fracture in the course of a motor vehicle accident. The typical fracture involves L1 with a transverse fracture through the vertebra, with compression of the anterior portion of the body, and vertical distraction posteriorly. Intra-abdominal injuries are common, but the spinal canal can be compromised with resultant spinal cord injury and paraplegia (214a). The radiographic findings are often subtle and are best visualized on lateral lumbar spine views (214b).

Because of the mobility of the neck, the lower cervical region is particularly prone to fracture and dislocation injuries. Direct violence along the axis of the vertebral column can produce fractures of the vertebral bodies, and the spinal cord can be injured by fragments of bone that enter the vertebral canal.

Pathology and Pathophysiology

Discussion of the acute and chronic pathophysiologic responses of the spinal cord to injury, in particular, the contributions of oxygen radical formation and lipid peroxidation to cell damage and death, are beyond the scope of this text. This topic is reviewed by Hall and Braughler (215) and Banik and colleagues (216).

In many patients in whom an accident produced early paraplegia, the spinal cord does not show any gross pathologic abnormality. Termed *spinal concussion*, this condition is characterized by transient loss of spinal cord function (217). The mechanism inducing spinal concussion is not clear, but is believed to involve changes in the microvasculature and in neurotransmitters.

In other instances, the spinal cord, when examined shortly after the injury, is swollen over several segments, and microscopic examination shows numerous punctate hemorrhages. More extensive confluent hemorrhage is common, particularly after injuries to the lower cervical region. The major hemorrhages are generally central and extend in the form of a column cephalad and caudad from the site of injury. Extensive damage to the cord can be caused by direct compression from without by bone and intervertebral disc or from within by hematoma, or it can be caused by interference with the cord's vascular supply. The importance of vascular changes in the induction of spinal cord injury has only recently become evident. In particular, post-traumatic ischemia is of major importance in the evolution of spinal cord lesions (218). The anterior spinal artery and its sulcal branches seem particularly vulnerable; the vascular shed in the upper thoracic cord and the ventral radicular artery (artery of Adamkiewicz), which usually feeds the cord at approximately the tenth thoracic vertebra, are other favorite sites for interruption of the blood supply (219). Relatively minor trauma to this area or to the cervical spine can, on occasion, result in an infarction of the spinal cord, with ensuing paraparesis or quadriparesis, respectively (220). Such injuries constituted 8% of spinal cord injuries at the Toronto Hospital for Sick Children (221). Symptoms do not appear immediately, but after a latent period of some 2 hours to 4 days. Paraplegia or tetraplegia is usually profound and recovery is unlikely. Imaging study results are generally normal, although spinal angiography occasionally visualizes an occlusion of the anterior spinal artery (221).

When the patient survives major spinal cord injury for a long time, the damaged area is found to be softened, gray and white matter are poorly delineated, the myelin sheaths are destroyed, and all cellular elements are lost extensively. Replacement by cavities or fibrous gliosis occurs ultimately. In less than 5% of paraplegics, this leads to post-traumatic syringomyelia with worsening of symptoms starting one to several years after the initial injury. There is dispute as to the mechanism of the syringomyelic cavity (222). It can arise from a hematoma at the site of the original injury, or from softening of the cord and liquefaction, or it may result from the cord being pulled open by meningeal fibrosis or arachnoiditis. If symptomatic and of significant diameter, most authorities advise syringo-subarachnoid or syringo-pleural drainage, although others prefer a wide opening of the subarachnoid spaces to allow free CSF movement past the area of cord damage (223).

Clinical Manifestations

The clinical picture depends on the severity of the injury and its location. Concussion can result from apparently minor falls on the back and is characterized by a temporary and completely reversible loss of function below the injured segment. With more extensive injuries, recovery is only partial and permanent residua can be expected.

Evaluation of the patient who has sustained injury to the spinal cord has been facilitated by a grading system devised by Frankel and coworkers (224). This scheme describes four levels: (a) no sensory or motor function; (b) incomplete sensory function, no motor function; (c) incomplete sensory function, no useful motor function; and (d) normal function with some spasticity.

When the cord is seriously compromised, the clinical picture is highlighted by spinal shock. Spinal shock is described in the classic experimental studies of Sherrington (225) and their clinical application by Riddock (226). The condition is marked by the loss of all reflex function distal to the injury, with the segments closest to the injury being the most severely affected.

Spinal shock represents a transient decrease of synaptic excitability of neurons distal to the injury. It is caused by loss of supraspinal impulses, which normally produce a background of partial depolarization of the spinal neurons. Clinically, spinal shock can persist for days or weeks and can be prolonged by sepsis, particularly urinary tract infection. The ultimate return of reflexes, and progression to spasticity probably reflects a reorganization of receptors (226a).

Immediately after the injury, the patient experiences complete loss of motor and sensory function in the segments caudal to the injury (227). The patient has complete areflexia of variable duration, usually for at least 2 to 6 weeks. Should reflex activity not return, probably the distal spinal cord has been destroyed as the result of vascular insufficiency.

During the first stage of spinal shock, the stage of flaccidity, complete bladder paralysis and urinary retention occur (226,227). Gradually, a muscular response of the lower extremities can be elicited in response to stimulation of the skin or the deeper structures. The earliest movements occur in the legs and are flexor. The deep tendon reflexes reappear and soon become hyperactive. Abdominal reflexes also can return. A typical extensor plantar response can be induced and is often accompanied by flexor withdrawal movements of the foot, ankle, and, subsequently, the knee, and hips. Contraction of the extensor muscles of the crossed limb frequently accompanies the mass flexion reflex (226,228). During this stage, the bladder empties automatically, although never completely.

In the majority of patients, extensor reflexes involving the quadriceps and other extensor muscles ultimately appear, becoming the dominant reflex activity. Stimuli eliciting the extensor reflex are more complicated than those inducing the flexion response. They include extension of the thigh, as is seen when the patient shifts from a sitting to a supine position, and squeezing of the thigh.

Depending on the severity of the spinal cord injury, the ultimate result can be purely reflex activity of the isolated cord. With less extensive injuries, muscular function or subjective sensation can return over the course of the next few months up to 1 year.

The neurologic picture of the most common spinal cord injuries is summarized in Table 8.10.

An unusual clinical picture, which occurs exclusively in children, is a transient apparent subluxation of the atlantoaxial joint, which often follows an upper respiratory infection or trauma, especially sports-related trauma (229,229a). It is called *rotary atlantoaxial luxation*. Children present with a head tilt to the affected side, the "cock robin sign", after its similarity to the appearance of the bird. The neck is tender laterally and posteriorly over C1 and C2. The bulge of the anterior dislocation can be felt by the examiner through the posterior pharyngeal wall, but is best diagnosed by cine CT scan. This study demonstrates that the subluxed axis and atlas move as a unit during neck rotation (229a). The condition is associated only rarely with root or cord signs and usually resolves with traction and immobilization. When the subluxation is persistent or recurrent, as happens in the occasional patient, surgical immobilization is required.

Dislocation of the atlantoaxial joint and an increased atlantoaxial interval are seen with particular frequency in Down syndrome (see Chapter 3).

Diagnosis

The history of trauma is usually readily elicitable, and the most common diagnostic problem is to establish the site and extent of the injury. In small children, the physician can best perform a sensory examination by demonstrating impairment of autonomic response. Shortly after the injury, the dermatomes below the lesion are dry and often have a defective vasomotor response. Evaluation of reflexes and motor function should not be particularly difficult because reflex withdrawal is not seen during the acute phase of spinal shock.

The patient with a suspected cervical spinal cord injury must be moved to the radiography unit with utmost care. After plain films of the spine, including lateral films of the cervical spine, are evaluated, it is usually necessary to establish the presence or absence of a subarachnoid block, which can be caused by bone fragments, disc material, hematoma, or swelling of neural tissues

TABLE 8.10. *Clinical features of spinal cord injuries*

Injury	Neurologic features
Transverse injuries	
T12–1.1	Flaccid paralysis of lower extremities
	Loss of sphincter control
	Loss of sensation below inguinal ligament
C5–6	Flaccid quadriparesis
	Sparing of diaphragmatic movements
	Sensory level at second rib, with preservation of sensation over upper lateral aspect of arm
	Bilateral Horner syndrome
	Loss of sphincter control
C1–4	Respiratory paralysis, complete quadriplegia
	Rapid death
Conus medullaris	
Cauda equina syndrome	Urinary retention
	Disturbance of renal sphincter
	Loss of sensation over lumbosacral dermatomes
	Flaccid paralysis of lower extremities
Brown-Séquard syndrome	Unilateral muscular paresis
	Contralateral disturbances of superficial sensitivity, especially pain and temperature
	Incomplete forms far more common than classic syndrome
Central cord lesion	Disproportionately more motor impairment of upper extremities (caused by involvement of the more medial segments of the lateral corticospinal tracts)
	Lower motor neuron lesion of upper extremities: upper motor neuron lesion of lower extremities: upper motor neuron lesion of lower extremities
	Bladder dysfunction (usually urinary retention)
	Varying degrees of sensory loss, usually pain and temperature below level of lesion
	Relatively good prognosis
	Motor power returns first to lower extremities

(Fig. 8.9). CT or MRI of the involved and adjacent spinal levels provides the most complete information on the status of the spinal column, and on the extent to which the spinal cord and canal have been compromised by the injury (230).

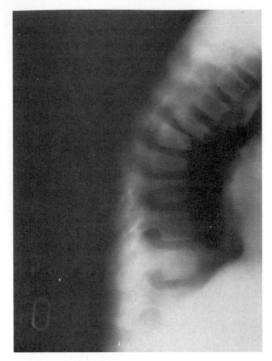

FIG. 8.9. Compression fracture of thoracic spine (T6, T7, and T8) with anterior displacement of T6 on T7. This patient was a 9-year-old girl who fell from a tree and had an immediate total motor and sensory paralysis below the level of the injury.

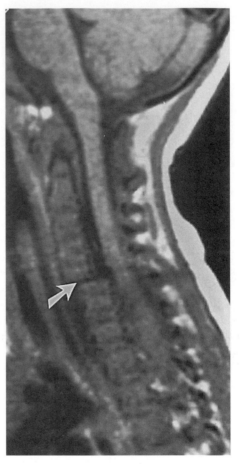

FIG. 8.10. Spinal cord trauma. A sagittal T1-weighted magnetic resonance image (600/15/2) demonstrates vertebral subluxation at the C4–5 level (*arrow*). The cord at and below the bony injury is expanded and hypointense. This 2-year-old boy was wrenched from his mother's lap and thrown around the vehicle in a motor vehicle accident. He was rendered quadriparetic. (Courtesy of Dr. John Curran, Department of Radiology, UCLA Center for the Health Sciences, Los Angeles.)

Generally, MRI centers are not equipped to image patients with multisystem injuries and needing complex life support systems, so that this procedure is usually deferred until the patient is stabilized. Each imaging study has its advantages. CT provides a better picture of fractures and of trauma to the osseous elements, whereas MRI is better suited to view disc protrusions and the spinal cord itself, and any associated bleeding or edema (Fig. 8.10). MRA can be used to screen the status of the vasculature, in particular, the vertebral arteries, although angiography remains the definitive diagnostic procedure.

Analogous to the changes seen in craniocerebral trauma, three types of abnormalities of the cord can be distinguished. The most common is hyperintensity on T2-weighted images, represented by edema of the cord. Less often, one sees a central hypointensity on T1-weighted images, which evolves to a hypointensity on T2-weighted images surrounded by a ring of hyperintensity. This finding is consistent with an intramedullary hemorrhage and is a poor prognostic sign. In some 16% to 21% of children, all imaging study results are completely normal (213,214,231).

The radiologic diagnosis of a dislocated cervical spine has many pitfalls (232). A marked anterior displacement of C2 on C3 can be seen in 20% of all children younger than 7 years of age. This variant is particularly common during the first 3 years of life. Displacement of C3 on C4 is also common, as is an apparent hypermobility of the atlas on the axis.

The severity of the injury often cannot be determined immediately. An early return of reflex activity, particularly of extensor movements, is encouraging. In general, sensory changes give a clearer indication of the level of the lesions than do motor changes. In cervical cord injuries, bilateral meiosis is a bad prognostic sign because it indicates extensive cord damage (233). Prognosis is better when the cord lesion is incomplete. For instance, in the experience of Hamilton and Myles, 74% of children with a physiologically incomplete spinal cord deficit improved by one or two Frankel levels, with 59% experiencing complete recovery (213). When the spinal cord injury was physiologically complete, only 10% improved by one or two Frankel levels. In this study, the absence of radiologic abnormalities did not influence the outcome.

Treatment

Treatment of the child with a spinal cord injury is essentially surgical, but not always operative, and involves a multidisciplinary approach. Intravenous fluids, colloids, and vasopressors are administered to maintain arterial blood pressure. The late Sir Ludwig Guttman advanced the conservative, postural treatment of the patient with spinal cord injury and believed that operative procedures for decompression and stabilization should be used only in selected cases (234). Because excessive movement is likely to aggravate spinal cord injury, special care is required in the handling of the patient, and only the absolutely essential diagnostic studies should be done. In injuries of the cervical spine, the head should be maintained in neutral position (235,236). Skeletal traction, usually by means of tongs inserted into the skull, is required for hyperflexion injuries of the cervical spine, whereas mild traction using a canvas sling is used in hyperextension injuries. The management of cervical spine injuries is reviewed by Sypert (237). Injuries of the lumbar spine and thoracolumbar junction are best stabilized in slight hyperextension.

A number of treatments have been proposed to reverse secondary pathophysiologic processes such as ischemia, excitotoxicity, and lipid peroxidation. High doses of methylprednisolone, a synthetic glucocorticoid drug, given within 8 hours of the injury as a 30 mg/kg bolus, followed by 5.4 mg/kg per hour for 23 hours, induce greater improvement in motor and sensory functions than does placebo in patients with complete and incomplete spinal cord deficits (238). At these doses, methylprednisolone may act as an antioxidant or as a free radical scavenger. The monosialoganglioside GM_1, which experimentally has been observed to increase neurite outgrowth and to prevent cell death by inhibiting glutamate-induced neuronal excitotoxicity, has been found to improve lower limb function after spinal cord injury. The drug is started within 19 to 72 hours after the injury, and administered at 100 mg/day for 18 to 32 days (239). Optimal dosages of these drugs, their optimal initiation time, and duration of therapy are still not known. Many other drugs, notably calpain, other free radical inhibitors, and tirilazad mesylate, a 21-amino corticosteroid that acts as a potent antioxidant with no glucocorticoid receptor activity, await preclinical and clinical investigations (216,240).

There has been considerable interest in the prospects of functional spinal cord regeneration. Although axons of injured spinal neurons cannot regrow within the spinal cord, they can grow long distances in peripheral nerves outside the cord. The reason for this discrepancy is the presence within spinal cord of myelin-associated neurite growth inhibitors (241). The various interventional strategies and the problems that prevent their current clinical applications have been reviewed (242).

All patients with open wounds of the spine, with injuries in which imaging studies reveal bony fragments within the spinal canal, and with an apparent total block in the presence of an incomplete transection of the cord should undergo surgery, including débridement, removal of bone fragments, laminectomy, and dural repair, if necessary. Any patient whose neurologic deficit increases after initial assessment, either by extending cephalad or by becoming more complete, also should have the benefit of an exploratory laminectomy. Surgical intervention is needed for dislocations of the spine that cannot be reduced adequately by traction and immobilization, and for injuries of the spine, known by past experience to be unstable; the surgical intervention often need not be immediate. Reduction of dislocations and internal stabilization are then carried out as indicated.

The long-term care of the paraplegic child is beyond the scope of this book. It is reviewed by Guttman (234), Short and colleagues (243), and Piepmeier (244). The management of the quadriplegic patient has been considered by Whiteneck (245). Generally, the patient requires care of the skin overlying the paralyzed part and prevention of decubitus lesions. Also needed is care of the urinary system (246). During the acute phase, urinary retention is treated by intermittent catheterization or insertion of an indwelling catheter, preferably one with a separate irrigating arm (three-way Foley). Additionally, the child needs regular enemas to treat fecal retention; automatic sphincter function can develop. Ileus, when present, can be relieved with neostigmine or with an indwelling rectal tube.

The ultimate outlook for spinal cord function after injury depends on the extent of the injury. The immediate loss of function is caused by both anatomic alteration and impaired physiologic function of the cord. In general, much of the improvement occurs during the first 6 months after the injury, and at a much slower pace from 6 months to 2 years after the injury. As a rule, muscles with no initial motor power have a longer period of recovery than those in which there was some initial motor power. The mechanisms underlying the improvement are not clear; certainly, resolution of edema cannot account for the slow recovery. In rare instances, a progressive myelopathy can be caused by a nonunited or malunited dens fracture (247).

Herniated Intervertebral Disc

Although common in the adult, this entity is rare in children, with most cases occurring during adolescence, usually after trauma.

Injuries at L4–5 and L5–S1 occur with approximately equal frequency. Many affected children have an underlying malformation of the vertebral column, most often spondylolisthesis or spina bifida. Herniation of intervertebral discs also has been noted in achondroplasia (248). Because the presenting symptoms of extradural neoplasms can be similar, MRI is indicated for all suspected disc lesions.

INJURIES TO THE CRANIAL NERVES

Injury to the cranial nerves is a relatively common complication of head injuries. The mechanisms of cranial nerve paralysis are multiple. As listed by Friedman and Merritt (249), they include injury to the nerve by bony fragments, laceration of the nerve when a fracture involves the canal by which the cranial nerve leaves the cranial cavity, tears or stretching, compression by hemorrhage, edema or arachnoiditis, contusion, and injury to the motor cells in the brainstem. Injuries to the olfactory nerves are the most common and are generally bilateral. They are believed to be caused by trauma to the frontal poles or by tearing of the olfactory filaments. Facial and abducens nerve injuries are also encountered, as are palsies of the trochlear nerve. They are generally accompanied by evidence of fracture of middle fossa. Seventh and eighth nerve palsies result from a fracture of the petrous ridge. In children, trauma is the most common cause of isolated, acquired, unilateral, or bilateral trochlear nerve palsy (250). In the experience of Friedman and Merritt, the onset of cranial nerve palsy was immediate in 68%, and delayed for several days in the remainder (249). In the majority of instances, dysfunction is permanent when the palsy is immediate. The likelihood for recovery is significantly greater when the palsy is delayed (250a).

INJURIES TO THE PERIPHERAL NERVES

Peripheral nerve injuries are relatively uncommon in childhood. The most common postnatal injuries are of the brachial plexus and are caused by severe trauma to the shoulder or sudden traction to the arm. Other injuries include division of the ulnar and median nerves at the wrist, the result of pushing the hand through a pane of glass; division of the radial nerve in the upper arm, associated with fracture of the humerus; division of the ulnar nerve with fracture or dislocation of the medial epicondyle; injury of one or both branches of the sciatic nerve as a consequence of injections into the buttocks; and division of the common peroneal nerve in fractures at the neck of the fibula. Peripheral neuropathies are relatively common in Ehlers-Danlos syndrome, with both brachial plexus palsy and lumbosacral plexus palsies developing because of increased ligament laxity (251).

Pathology

The pathologic changes in an injured peripheral nerve depend on whether the axon remains intact. When the axon is destroyed at the site of injury, wallerian degeneration is induced in the peripheral segment of the nerve. The pathologic, neurophysiologic, and biochemical alterations accompanying wallerian degeneration are beyond the scope of this book.

Stretch injuries of the peripheral nerves result from damage to the perineurium and the blood vessels (vasa nervorum). Ischemic peripheral nerve injuries also are produced by impairment of the blood supply to the nerves via these vessels. Regeneration of the injured nerve starts from the proximal end of the axon and begins shortly after injury, proceeding in children at approximately 2.5 to 3.0 mm/day. The speed and extent of recovery depend on whether the sheaths of the nerve remain intact; these provide a continuous channel for the young neurites sprouting from the proximal axonal end. When the gap between nerve ends is wide, and particularly when the ends are separated by fibrous tissue, a neuroma can form proximally, and spontaneous anastomosis can be delayed or prevented.

Clinical Manifestations

The salient clinical features of the most frequent peripheral nerve lesions of childhood are presented in Table 8.11. In general, symptoms consist of weakness and sensory disturbances in the area supplied by the individual nerve. Muscular weakness and wasting are characteristic for peripheral nerve injuries. Contractures develop through overaction of unopposed muscle groups.

When a nerve regenerates, manual pressure on the nerve at the level to which axons have regrown can induce a tingling pain referred distally to an area that is still anesthetic (Tinel's sign). Pain and paresthesia can be generalized or can be referred to one site along the course of the nerve. These symptoms are aggravated by touch or muscular contractions.

Deep tendon reflexes are diminished or abolished in the affected area. A number of vasomotor symptoms, including mottling and thinning of the skin, edema, cyanosis, and impaired sweating, also are observed.

Diagnosis

Examination of the child with a peripheral nerve injury is directed toward determining the cause and the anatomic site of the injury. Several manuals detail the neurologic examination of such a patient (252). Generally, evaluation of motor function and sensory deficits is more important in the diagnosis of peripheral nerve injuries than is the status of reflexes, because the presence or absence of reflexes does not depend on the integrity of a single nerve.

Tinel's sign, which originally was believed to be evidence of regeneration, does not have much prognostic significance during the first month of injury, unless the most distal point at which it can be elicited moves further down the nerve trunk on progressive examinations.

Electric studies can delineate the extent of the nerve injury. Somatosensory-evoked potentials can delineate the extent of the injury and distinguish between peripheral nerve and spinal cord injuries (253). Electromyography indicates fibrillation potentials of denervated muscles. Nerve conduction times are either impossible to elicit or reduced. The ability of the nerve below the lesion to respond to direct electric stimulation despite motor paralysis indicates absence of wallerian degeneration and is a favorable prognostic sign. In the course of regeneration, the conduction times, which initially are impossible to determine, are slow at first, and subsequently

TABLE 8.11. *Clinical features of common peripheral nerve injuries*

Nerve injury	Predisposing factors	Clinical features
Brachial plexus upper root (Erb-Duchenne)	Sudden traction to arm	Arm internally rotated at shoulder, pronated at forearm Paralysis of spinati, deltoid, biceps, brachialis, brachioradialis, extensor carpi radialis Sensory disturbance minimal or absent Biceps and supinator jerks lost, triceps preserved
Lower root (Klumpke paralysis)	Violent upward pull of shoulder	Arm flexed at elbow, forearm supinated, fingers extended, edema and cyanosis of hand Paralysis of small muscles of hand, finger flexors Sensory loss of ulnar aspects of fingers, hand, and forearm Horner syndrome if root avulsed
Long thoracic nerve	Carrying heavy weights on shoulder Postimmunization	Paralysis of serratus magnus with or without trapezius No sensory symptoms
Circumflex nerve	Fracture of humerus (crutch palsy)	Paralysis of deltoid Sensory loss of upper and outer part of arm
Radial nerve	Fracture of humerus (Saturday night palsy)	Paralysis of triceps uncommon, only if nerve damaged in axilla Paralysis of brachioradialis, extensors of wrist and fingers Sensory loss inconstant
Median nerve (276)	Cuts at wrist, mucolipidosis III	Atrophy of thenar eminence Paralysis of pronation beyond midposition Paralysis of flexor of index finger, impaired flexion, and opposition of thumb Sensory loss of radial aspect of palm
Ulnar nerve	Fractures at lower end of humerus Pressure palsy at elbow	Flattened hypothenar eminence, claw hand Paralysis of ulnar flexors at wrist and fingers, interossei, adductor of thumb Sensory loss of ulnar side of arm, hand
Sciatic nerve [common peroneal and posterior tibial nerve (277)]	Intramuscular injuries (common peroneal component injured more frequently)	Foot drop, paralysis of peronei, anterior tibialis, extensors of toe Sensory loss of anterior aspect of lower leg and foot Absent ankle jerk
Femoral nerve (278)	Hemorrhagic disease (hemophilia)	Paralysis and atrophy of quadriceps Defective sensation, anterior and anterior medial aspect of thigh
Common peroneal nerve	Fracture at neck of fibula	Stepping gait Loss of dorsiflexion (anterior tibialis) eversion at ankle (peronei), extensors of toe
	Incorrectly fitted leg cast	Sensory deficit, dorsum of foot and outer side of leg Achilles tendon reflex lost or reduced

regain as much as 60% of the original velocity (254). CT myelography and MRI have been used for the diagnosis of cervical root evulsion in brachial plexus injury (255). MR neurography has shown great promise in the diagnosis and management of patients with peripheral nerve pathology (255a).

Treatment

Surgical treatment may not be required during the early phase of peripheral nerve injuries.

Clean lacerations of a nerve are suitable for early repair. In other types of nerve injury, nothing is gained by immediate exploration of the site. If the nerve presents readily in the wound, a single stainless-steel marking suture can facilitate subsequent repair. Secondary disability, such as contractures or injury of the paralyzed muscles by excess stretching, should be prevented by splinting the affected limb. Electrostimulation of the paralyzed muscles is of no advantage. A severed nerve should be explored and reapproximated 3 weeks after injury, provided the wound is healed. At this time, the extent of nerve injury can be defined more clearly, and suturing is technically more satisfactory. A nerve that is known to have been traumatized but not severed, should be explored if recovery of motor and sensory functions does not take place or is less complete than anticipated. External and internal neurolysis of such a nerve trunk can allow further recovery of function. A neuroma in continuity can require resection and reanastomosis if nerve function is absent or poor.

Prognosis

The prognosis depends on the extent and nature of the nerve injury. Pressure palsies almost invariably recover. If electric studies indicate wallerian degeneration of the distal segment, recovery is delayed until the regenerating fibers reach the muscles they innervate. If no recovery can be documented after 3 months by either clinical or electric examinations, the ultimate prognosis is poor, and few patients benefit from surgical exploration. Different nerves have different capacities for regeneration. Generally, radial nerve injuries fare best, and sciatic, worst. Spontaneous recovery from sciatic nerve injuries can be extremely slow, but can continue for 1 to 2 years.

REFLEX SYMPATHETIC DYSTROPHY

Reflex sympathetic dystrophy (causalgia; complex regional pain syndrome), which is an occasional sequela to nerve injury and which was first defined in adults by Mitchell (256), also has been encountered in children, predominantly in girls (257,258). The condition is characterized by constant burning pain and hyperesthesia in an extremity. Most often, the lower extremities, notably the ankle and foot, are affected. Pain is accompanied by swelling, sweating, vasomotor instability, and sometimes trophic changes. There may not be a history of antecedent trauma or the injury may have been considered minor. Psychological disturbances are common and can become the most important part of the clinical picture. An important early sign of reflex sympathetic dystrophy is piloerection over the

hairy aspect of the affected limb (259). Often associated muscle spasms, myoclonus, or focal dystonia occur (260). When dystonia is part of the condition, it can appear at the same time as the causalgia, or up to many months later. Many theories exist as to etiology, none of them has been well supported by clinical evidence. A disorder of the sympathetic system, release of a pain substance, or supersensitivity to neurotransmitters are the most likely (258). Pathologic examination of nerve and muscle taken from the affected limb suggest a microangiopathy (260a). Symptoms of causalgia can last a few days to as long as a year. A number of therapies have been suggested; none is infallible. The response to intensive physical therapy is often excellent in children (259). Analgesics, nonsteroidal inflammatory drugs, antidepressants, narcotics, and corticosteroids all have their advocates. Blockage of the sympathetic chain with paravertebral or epidural anesthetics has been tried, as has surgical sympathectomy (261). No treatment for the movement disorder has been effective; an occasional patient recovers spontaneously after a few years (260).

INJURIES BY PHYSICAL AGENTS

Injuries of the Nervous System by X-Ray Irradiation

Radiation damage to the central nervous system can occur before birth and can result in a variety of gross and microscopic malformations of the brain. These are discussed in Chapter 4.

The neurologic complications of therapeutic irradiation for intracranial tumors are discussed in Chapter 10.

Heatstroke (Sunstroke)

Heatstroke results from prolonged exposure to direct sunlight and heat, with subsequent failure of the body's heat-regulating mechanism. Presence of hyperpyrexia distinguishes it from symptoms resulting from sodium loss caused by excessive sweating.

The clinical and pathologic picture of heatstroke results from a combination of hyperpyrexia and shock. Sunlight contributes to the heat load, but probably does not affect the brain directly. In fatal cases, examination of the brain reveals generalized edema and degeneration of cerebellar neurons, particularly the Purkinje cells and the cells of the dentate nucleus, with lesser degrees of neuronal loss in other areas of the neuraxis (262,263).

Clinically, the patient has sudden onset of coma, cyanosis, impaired sweating, generalized or focal seizures, and hyperpyrexia (264). Rhabdomyolysis, hyperkalemia, and metabolic acidosis can complicate the picture. Clinical heatstroke can be associated with an underlying abnormality of skeletal muscle similar to that of malignant hyperthermia (265). Cerebellar symptoms can be evident with recovery. They usually improve considerably in time.

Treatment of the acute condition involves removing the child from the sun, reducing body temperature, and providing intravenous fluids.

Electric Injuries of the Nervous System

Electric injuries to children can be caused by household current or lightning. Lightning is responsible for approximately one-fourth of all fatal electric accidents. Generally, the patient either dies at once as a result of cardiac arrest or recovers without neurologic sequelae (266). A few patients develop a variety of delayed or progressive neurologic signs, including hemiparesis, cerebellar deficits, paraplegia, cranial nerve palsies, and other focal neurologic signs. Increased intracranial pressure also has been observed (267,268). Long-term behavioral changes, including disturbances in affect, memory, and mood, are not unusual and can last for months, out of proportion to the duration of any cardiorespiratory arrest (266). Kotagal and colleagues suggest they are the consequence of a direct injury to the limbic system (269).

Neurologic Complications of Burns

Currently, approximately 5% of children develop encephalitic symptoms within the first few weeks after they sustain severe burns. As a rule, these represent complications of a compli-

cation from the burn. These symptoms include changes in level of consciousness, seizures, aphasia, extrapyramidal disorders, and impaired intellectual function, which result from infections, metabolic encephalopathies, and cerebrovascular accidents. Neurologic symptoms during the first 3 days after the burn are generally caused by shock and derangements of electrolytes. Infections are responsible for neurologic symptoms after the first week after the burn in what is essentially an immunocompromised host. They are most common during the second to third week after the injury. Three organisms are usually responsible: *Candida*, *Pseudomonas aeruginosa*, and *Staphylococcus aureus*. Almost invariably they enter the nervous system from a systemic source. Microabscesses of the brain are most likely to be caused by candidiasis, with *Staphylococcus aureus* a less common culprit. Meningitis or septic infarcts are caused by *P. aeruginosa*. Intracranial hemorrhages are less common than infarcts and generally result from disseminated intravascular coagulation or serum hyperosmolarity. Central pontine myelinolysis and cerebral edema also can develop, the latter generally caused by anoxia (270,271).

Despite the number of potentially irreversible neurologic complications, the majority of children experiences full neurologic recovery (272).

Neurologic Injury from Undersea Diving

Underwater diving places the teenager or young adult at risk for two major types of neurologic injuries.

The most common is decompression sickness that results from a too rapid decompression on ascent. It mainly affects the spinal cord and results in a unique multilevel spinal cord disease, with deficits consisting of pain, sensory loss, and motor weakness (273). The condition usually resolves with administration of oxygen and recompression, although there may be a residual patchy sensory loss. Arterial gas embolism, a much rarer condition, is the most serious complication of self-contained underwater breathing apparatus (scuba) diving. It results from pulmonary overpressure on ascent with extravasation of air into the arterial system and occlusion of a major cerebral artery. The first sign of the condition is usually a seizure. This can be quickly followed by an acute, strokelike picture marked by hemiparesis, aphasia, and cortical blindness. It is the major cause of death in diving accidents. MRI studies of the head show ischemic changes in a vascular distribution (274). By contrast, imaging study of brain and spinal cord are usually normal in decompression sickness, although on rare occasion studies demonstrate a swollen spinal cord with increased signal posteriorly on T2-weighted images (275).

REFERENCES

1. Adelson PD, Kochanek PM. Head injuries in children. *J Child Neurol* 1998;13:2–15.
2. Craft AW, Shaw DA, Cartlidge NE. Head injuries in children. *BMJ* 1972;4:200–203.
3. North AF. When should a child be in the hospital? *Pediatrics* 1976;57:540–543.
3a. Kraus JF, Rock A, Hemyari P. Brain injuries among infants, children, adolescents and young adults. *Am J Dis Child* 1990;144:684–691.
3b. Frankowski RF, Annegers JF, Whitman S. Epidemiological and descriptive studies. Part 1. The descriptive epidemiology of head trauma in the U.S. In: Becker DP, Povlishok JT, eds. *Central nervous system trauma, status report 1985*. Bethesda, MD: N.I.H., N.I.N.C.D.S., 1985:33–43.
4. Klauber MR, et al. The epidemiology of head injury: a prospective study of an entire community—San Diego County, CA, 1978. *Am J Epidemiol* 1981;113:500–509.
5. Leventhal JM, et al. Maltreatment of children born to teenage mothers: a comparison between the 1960s and 1980s. *J Pediatr* 1993;122:314–319.
6. McClain PW, et al. Estimates of fatal child abuse and neglect, United States, 1979 through 1988. *Pediatrics* 1993;91:338–343.
7. Billmire ME, Myers PA. Serious head injury in infants: accident or abuse. *Pediatrics* 1985;75:340–342.
8. O'Rourke NA, et al. Head injuries to children riding on bicycles. *Med J Aust* 1987;146:619–621.
9. Mealey J. *Pediatric head injuries*. Springfield, IL: Charles C Thomas, 1968.
10. Courville CB. *Forensic neuropathology*. Mundelein, IL: Callaghan and Co, 1964.
11. Gurdjian ES, et al. Mechanism of head injury. *Clin Neurosurg* 1964;12:112–128.
12. Holbourn AHS. The mechanics of brain injuries. *Br Med Bull* 1945;3:147–149.
13. Stålhammar D. Experimental models of head injury. *Acta Neurochirurg* 1986;36[Suppl]:33–46.
14. Gross AG. A new theory on the dynamics of brain concussion and brain injury. *J Neurosurg* 1958;15:548–561.
15. Berney J, Froidevaux AC, Favier J. Paediatric head trauma: influence of age and sex. II. Biomechanical

and anatomo-clinical correlations. *Childs Nerv Syst* 1994;10:517–523.
16. Courville CB. Contrecoup injuries of the brain in infancy. *Arch Surg* 1965;90:157–165.
17. Gentry LR, Godersky JC, Thompson B. MR imaging of head trauma: review of the distribution and radiopathologic features of traumatic lesions. *Am J Roentgenol* 1988;15:663–672.
18. Adams JH, et al. Diffuse axonal injury in nonmissile head injuries. *J Neurol Neurosurg Psychiatr* 1991;54:481–483.
19. Adams JH, et al. Diffuse brain damage of immediate impact. *Brain* 1977;100:489–502.
20. Adams JH, et al. Diffuse axonal injury due to non-missile head injury in humans. An analysis of 45 cases. *Ann Neurol* 1982;12:557–563.
21. Yamaki T, et al. Pathological study of diffuse axonal injury patients who died shortly after impact. *Acta Neurochir* 1992;119:153–158.
22. Chester CS, Reznick BR. Ataxia after severe head injury: the pathological substrate. *Ann Neurol* 1987;22.77–79.
23. Strich SJ. Diffuse degeneration of the cerebral white matter in severe dementia following head injury. *J Neurol Neurosurg Psychiat* 1956;19:163–174.
24. Maxwell WL, et al. Focal axonal injury: the early axonal response to stretch. *J Neurocytol* 1991;20:157–164.
25. Maxwell WL, Povlishock JT, Graham DL. A mechanistic analysis of nondisruptive axonal injury: a review. *J Neurotrauma* 1997;14: 419–440.
26. Povlishock JT, Becker DP. Fate of reactive axonal swellings induced by head injury. *Lab Invest* 1985;52: 540–552.
27. Cecil KM, et al. Proton magnetic resonance spectroscopy for detection of axonal injury in the splenium of the corpus callosum of brain-injured patients. *J Neurosurg* 1998;88:795–801.
28. Lindenberg R. Significance of the tentorium in head injuries from blunt forces. *Clin Neurosurg* 1964;12: 129–142.
29. Calder IM, Hill I, Scholtz CL. Primary brain trauma in nonaccidental injury. *J Clin Pathol* 1984;37: 1095–1100.
30. Junger EC, et al. Cerebral autoregulation following minor head injury. *J Neurosurg* 1997;86:425–432.
31. Katayama Y, et al. Massive increases in extracellular potassium and the indiscriminate release of glutamate following concussive brain injury. *J Neurosurg* 1990;73:889–900.
32. Becker DP, et al. Brain cellular injury and recovery—horizons for improving medical therapies in stroke and trauma. *West J Med* 1988;148:670–684.
33. Kawamata T, et al. Administration of excitatory aminoacid antagonists via microdialysis attenuates the increase in glucose utilization seen following concussive brain injury. *J Cereb Blood Flow Metab* 1992;12:12–24.
34. Hovda DA, Becker DP, Katayama Y. Secondary injury and acidosis. *J Neurotrauma* 1992;9[Suppl 1]:S47–S60.
35. Bakay L, et al. Experimental cerebral concussion. Part I: An electron microscopic study. *J Neurosurg* 1977;47:525–531.
36. Fishman RA. *Cerebrospinal fluid in diseases of the nervous system*, 2nd ed. Philadelphia: WB Saunders, 1992:116–138.

37. Bullock R, et al. Glial swelling following human cerebral contusion: an ultrastructural study. *J Neurol Neurosurg Psychiatry* 1991;54:427–434.

38. Barzo P, et al. Contribution of vasogenic and cellular edema to traumatic brain swelling measured by diffusion-weighted imaging. *J Neurosurg* 1997;87:900–907.

39. Kimelberg HK. Astrocytic edema in CNS trauma. *J Neurotrauma* 1992;9[Suppl 1]:S71–S81.

40. Baker AJ, et al. Excitatory amino acids in cerebrospinal fluid following traumatic brain injury in humans. *J Neurosurg* 1993;79:369–372.

41. Bell MJ, et al. Comparison of the interleukin-6 and interleukin-10 response in children after severe traumatic brain injury or septic shock. *Acta Neurochir Suppl (Wien)* 1997;70:96–97.

42. Adelson PD, et al. Cerebrovascular response in infants and young children following severe traumatic brain injury: a preliminary report. *Pediatr Neurosurg* 1997;26:200–207.

43. Bruce DA, et al. Diffuse cerebral swelling following head injuries in children. The syndrome of "malignant brain edema." *J Neurosurg* 1981;54:170–178.

44. Langfitt TW, et al. Prospects for the future in the diagnosis and management of head injury: pathophysiology, brain imaging, and population based studies. *Clin Neurosurg* 1982;29:353–376.

45. Cruz J, et al. Continuous monitoring of cerebral hemodynamic reserve in acute brain injury: relationship to changes in brain swelling. *J Trauma* 1992;32:629–635.

46. Choux M. Incidence, diagnosis and management of skull fractures. In: Raimondi AS, Choux M, DiRocco C, eds. *Head injuries in the newborn and infant*. New York: Springer Verlag, 1986:163–182.

47. Lloyd DA, et al. Predictive value of skull radiography for intracranial injury in children with blunt head injury. *Lancet* 1997;349:821–824.

48. Mizrahi EM, Kellaway P. Cerebral concussion in children: assessment of injury by electroencephalography. *Pediatrics* 1984;73:419–425.

49. Jennett B. *Epilepsy after nonmissile head injuries*, 2nd ed. Chicago: Year Book Medical Publishing, 1975.

50. Chiafalo N, Madsen J, Basauri L. Perinatal and posttraumatic seizures. In: Raimondi AJ, Choux M, DiRocco C, eds. *Head injuries in the newborn and infant*. New York: Springer-Verlag, 1986:217–232.

51. Hendrick EB, Harwood-Nash DC, Hudson AR. Head injuries in children: a survey of 4465 consecutive cases at the Hospital for Sick Children, Toronto, Canada. *Clin Neurosurg* 1963;11:46–65.

52. Raimondi AJ, Hirschauer J. Head injury in the infant and toddler—coma scoring and outcome scale. *Childs Brain* 1984;11:12–35.

53. Jaffe D, Wesson D. Current concepts: emergency management of blunt trauma in children. *N Engl J Med* 1991;324:1477–1482.

54. Teasdale G, Jennett B. Assessment of coma and impaired consciousness. A practical scale. *Lancet* 1974;2:81–84.

55. Simpson D, Reilly P. Pediatric coma scale. *Lancet* 1982;2:450.

56. Overgaard J, et al. Prognosis after head injury based on early clinical examination. *Lancet* 1973;2:631–635.

57. Russell WR. *The traumatic amnesias*. London: Oxford University Press, 1971.

58. Pfenninger, J, et al. Treatment and outcome of the severely head injured child. *Intensive Care Med* 1983;9:13–16.

59. Chesnut RM, et al. The role of secondary brain injury in determining outcome from severe head injury. *J Trauma* 1993;34:216–222.

60. Plum FB, Posner JB. *Diagnosis of stupor and coma*, 3rd ed. Philadelphia: FA Davis Co, 1980.

61. White RJ, Likavec MJ. The diagnosis and initial management of head injury. *N Engl J Med* 1992;327:1507–1511.

62. Masters SJ, et al. Skull x-ray examinations after head trauma. Recommendations by a multidisciplinary panel and validation study. *N Engl J Med* 1987;316:84–91.

63. Johnson DL, Duma C, Sivit C. The role of immediate operative intervention in severely head-injured children with a Glasgow Coma Scale score of 3. *Neurosurgery* 1992;30:320–324.

64. Zimmerman RA, et al. Computed tomography of pediatric head trauma: acute general cerebral swelling. *Radiology* 1978;126:403–408.

65. Johnson MH, Lee SH. Computed tomography of acute cerebral trauma. *Radiol Clin North Am* 1992;30:325–352.

66. Hobbs CJ. Skull fractures and the diagnosis of abuse. *Arch Dis Child* 1984;59:246–252.

67. Ginsburg CM. Frontal sinus fractures. *Pediatr Rev* 1997;18:120–121.

68. Sklar EML, et al. Magnetic resonance applications in cerebral injury. *Radiol Clin North Am* 1992;30:353–356.

69. Kelly AB, et al. Head trauma: comparison of MR and CT-experience in 100 patients. *Am J Neuroradiol* 1988;9:699–708.

70. O'Sullivan MG, et al. Role of intracranial pressure monitoring in severely head-injured patients without signs of intracranial hypertension on initial computerized tomography. *J Neurosurg* 1994;80:46–50.

71. Sivakumar V, Rajshekhar V, Chandy MJ. Management of neurosurgical patients with hyponatremia and natriuresis. *Neurosurgery* 1994;34:269–274.

72. Vingerhoets F, de Tribolet N. Hyponatremia hypoosmolarity in neurosurgical patients. "Appropriate secretion of ADH" and "cerebral salt-wasting syndrome." *Acta Neurochir* 1988;91:50–54.

73. Pascucci RC. Head trauma in the child. *Intensive Care Med* 1988;14:185–195.

73a. Feldman Z, et al. Brain edema and neurological status with rapid infusion of lactated Ringer's or 5% dextrose solution following head trauma. *J Neurosurg* 1995;83:1060–1066.

74. Schmoker JD, Zhuang J, Shackford SR. Hypertonic fluid resuscitation improves cerebral oxygen delivery and reduces intracranial pressure after hemorrhagic shock. *J Trauma* 1991;31:1607–1613.

74a. Zornow MH, Prough DS. Fluid management in patients with traumatic brain injury. *New Horizons* 1995;3:488–498.

75. Schaefer M, et al. Excessive hypokalemia and hyperkalemia following head injury. *Intensive Care Med* 1995;21:235–237.

76. Lazar L, et al. Brain concussion produces transient hypokalemia in children. *J Pediatr Surg* 1997;32:88–90.

77. Goodnight SH, et al. Defibrination after brain-tissue destruction. *N Engl J Med* 1974;290:1043–1047.
78. Miner ME, et al. Disseminated intravascular coagulation fibrinolytic syndrome following head injury in children: frequency and prognostic implications. *J Pediatr* 1982;100:687–691.
79. Young B, et al. Failure of prophylactically administered phenytoin to prevent early posttraumatic seizures. *J Neurosurg* 1983;58:231–235.
80. Young B, et al. Failure of prophylactically administered phenytoin to prevent late posttraumatic seizures. *J Neurosurg* 1983;58:236–241.
81. Zimmerman RA, Bilaniuk LT. Computed tomography in pediatric head trauma. *J Neuroradiol* 1981;8:257–271.
82. Saul TG. ICP monitoring worthwhile? *Clin Neurosurg* 1988;34:560–571.
83. Kanter MJ, Narayan RK. Intracranial pressure monitoring. *Neurosurg Clin North Am* 1991;2:257–265.
84. Jensen RL, Hahn YS, Ciro E. Risk factors of intracranial pressure monitoring in children with fiberoptic devices: a critical review. *Surg Neurol* 1997;47:16–22.
85. Bouma GJ, et al. Cerebral circulation and metabolism after severe traumatic brain injury: the elusive role of ischemia. *J Neurosurg* 1991;75:685–693.
85a. Levy DI, et al. Controlled lumbar drainage in pediatric head injury. *J Neurosurg* 1995;83:453–460.
86. Miller JD. Head injury. *J Neurol Neurosurg Psychiatr* 1993;56:440–447.
87. Muizelaar JP, et al. Adverse effects of prolonged hyperventilation in patients with severe head injury: a randomized clinical trial. *J Neurosurg* 1991;75:731–739.
87a. Marion DW, Firlik A, McLaughlin MR. Hyperventilation therapy for severe traumatic brain injury. *New Horizons* 1995;3:439–447.
87b. Cruz J, et al. Cerebral oxygen monitoring. *Crit Care Med* 1993;21:1242–1246.
87c. Feldman Z, et al. Effect of head elevation on intracrnial pressure, cerebral perfusion pressure, and cerebral blood flow in head-injured patients. *J Neurosurg* 1992;76:207–211.
88. Hall ED. The neuroprotective pharmacology of methylprednisolone. *J Neurosurg* 1992;76:13–22.
88a. Saul TG, et al. Steroids in severe head injury. A prospective, randomized clinical trial. *J Neurosurg* 1981;54:596–600.
89. Young B, et al. Effects of pegorgotein on neurologic outcome of patients with severe head injury. A multicenter, randomized controlled trial. *J Am Med Assoc* 1996;276:538–543.
90. Ward JD, et al. Failure of prophylactic barbiturate coma in the treatment of severe head injury. *J Neurosurg* 1985;62:383–388.
91. Shiozaki T, et al. Effect of mild hypothermia on uncontrollable intracranial hypertension after severe injury. *J Neurosurg* 1993;79:363–368.
92. Marion DW, et al. Treatment of traumatic brain injury with moderate hypothermia. *N Engl J Med* 1997;336:540–546.
93. Milley JR, Nugent SK, Rogers MC. Neurogenic pulmonary edema in childhood. *J Pediatr* 1979;94:706–709.
94. Jennett B, Teasdale G. *Management of head injuries*. Philadelphia: FA Davis, 1981.
94a. Pascucci RC. Head trauma in the child. *Intensive Care Med* 1988;14:185–195.
95. Stein SC, O'Malley KF, Ross SE. Is routine computed tomography scanning too expensive for mild head injury? *Ann Emerg Med* 1991;20:1286–1289.
96. Davis RL, et al. The use of cranial CT scans in the triage of pediatric patients with mild head injury. *Pediatrics* 1995;95:345–349.
97. Ingebrigtsen T, Romner B. Routine early CT-scan is cost saving after minor head injury. *Acta Neurol Scand* 1996;93:207–210.
98. Rosenthal BW, Bergman I. Intracranial injury after moderate head trauma in children. *J Pediatr* 1989;115:346–350.
99. Ylvisaker M, ed. *Traumatic brain injury rehabilitation: children and adolescents*, 2nd ed. Boston: Butterworth–Heinemann, 1997.
100. Levi L, et al. Severe head injury in children—analyzing the better outcome over a decade and the role of major improvements in intensive care. *Childs Nerv Syst* 1998;14:195–202.
101. Bijur PE, Haslum M, Golding J. Cognitive and behavioral sequelae of mild head injury in children. *Pediatrics* 1990;86:337–344.
102. Hall DMB, Johnson SL, Middleton J. Rehabilitation of head injured children. *Arch Dis Child* 1990;65:553–556.
103. Levin HS, et al. Severe head injury in children: experience of the Traumatic Coma Data Bank. *Neurosurgery* 1992;31:435–443.
104. Mahoney WJ, et al. Long-term outcome of children with severe head trauma and prolonged coma. *Pediatrics* 1983;71:756–762.
105. Hjern B, Nylander I. Late prognosis of severe head injuries in childhood. *Arch Dis Child* 1962;37:113–116.
106. Costeff H, Groswasser Z, Goldstein R. Long-term follow up review of 31 children with severe closed head trauma. *J Neurosurg* 1990;73:684–687.
107. Guilleminault C, et al. Posttraumatic excessive daytime sleepiness: a review of 20 patients. *Neurology* 1983;33:1584–1589.
108. Johnson SL, Hall DM. Posttraumatic tremor in head injured children. *Arch Dis Child* 1992;67:227–228.
109. Kingsley D, Till K, Hoare RD. Growing fractures of the skull. *J Neurol Neurosurg Psychiatr* 1978;41:312–318.
109a. Muhonen MG, Piper JG, Menezes AH. Pathogenesis and treatment of growing skull fractures. *Surg Neurol* 1995;43:367–373.
110. Battle WH. *Hunterian lectures*. London: Royal College of Surgeons of England, 1890.
111. Hanigan WC, Peerson RA, Njus G. Tin ear syndrome: rotational acceleration in pediatric head injuries. *Pediatrics* 1987;80:618–622.
112. Wilson NW, Copeland B, Bastian JF. Posttraumatic meningitis in adolescents and children. *Pediatr Neurosurg* 1990–1991;16:17–20.
113. Ommaya AK. Spinal fluid fistulae. *Clin Neurosurg* 1976;23:363–392.
114. Hull HF, Morrow G. Glucorrhea revisited: prolonged promulgation of another plastic pearl. *JAMA* 1975;234:1052–1053.
115. El Gammal T, et al. Cerebrospinal fluid fistula: detection with MR cisternography. *Am J Neuroradiol* 1998;19:627–631.
116. Shetty PG, et al. Evaluation of high-resolution CT and MR cisternography in the diagnosis of cere-

brospinal fluid fistula. *Am J Neuroradiol* 1998;19: 633–639.

117. Eberhardt KE, et al. MR cisternography: a new method for the diagnosis of CSF fistulae. *Eur Radiol* 1997;7:1485–1491.

118. Baltas I, et al. Posttraumatic meningitis: bacteriology, hydrocephalus, and outcome. *Neurosurgery* 1994;35: 422–426.

119. Rathore MH. Do prophylactic antibiotics prevent meningitis after basilar skull fracture? *Pediatr Infect Dis J* 1991;10:87–88.

120. Hughes BJ. The results of injury to special parts of the brain and skull. In: Rowbotham GF, ed. *Acute injuries of the head: their diagnosis, treatment, complications and sequels.* Baltimore: Williams & Wilkins, 1964:406.

121. Eviatar L, Bergtraum M, Randel RM. Posttraumatic vertigo in children: a diagnostic approach. *Pediatr Neurol* 1986;2:61–66.

122. Shea JJ, Ge X, Orchik DJ. Traumatic endolympathic hydrops. *Am J Otol* 1995;16:235–240.

123. Griffith JF, Dodge PR. Transient blindness following head injury in children. *N Engl J Med* 1968;278: 648–651.

124. Eldridge PR, Punt JAG. Transient traumatic cortical blindness in children. *Lancet* 1988;1:815–816.

125. Kadish HA, Schunk JE. Pediatric basilar skull fracture: do children with normal neurologic findings and no intracranial injury require hospitalization? *Ann Emerg Med* 1995;26:37–41.

126. Dandy WE. Pneumocephalus (intracranial pneumatocele or aerocele). *Arch Surg* 1926;12:949–982.

127. Keskil S, et al. Clinical significance of acute traumatic intracranial pneumocephalus. *Neurosurg Rev* 1998;21:10–13.

128. Steinbok P, et al. Management of simple depressed skull fractures in children. *J Neurosurg* 1987;66: 506–510.

129. Foy PM, et al. Do prophylactic anticonvulsants alter the pattern of seizures after craniotomy? *J Neurol Neurosurg Psychiatry* 1992;55:753–757.

130. Dhellemmes P, et al. Traumatic extradural hematoma in infancy and childhood. *J Neurosurg* 1985;62: 861–864.

131. Matson DD. Extradural hematoma. In: Matson DD. *Neurosurgery of infancy and childhood,* 2nd ed. Springfield, IL: Charles C Thomas, 1969:316.

132. Duhaime AC, et al. Head injury in very young children: mechanisms, injury types, and ophthalmologic findings in 100 hospitalized patients younger than 2 years of age. *Pediatrics* 1992;90:179–185.

133. Shugerman RP, et al, Epidural hemorrhage: is it abuse? *Pediatrics* 1996;97:664–668.

134. Mazza, C, et al. Traumatic extradural haematoma in children: experience with 62 cases. *Acta Neurochir* 1982;65:67–80.

135. McKissock W, et al. Extradural haematoma: observations on 125 cases. *Lancet* 1960;2:167–172.

136. Kernohan JW, Woltman HW. Incisura of the crus due to contralateral brain tumor. *Arch Neurol Psychiatr* 1929;21:274–278.

137. Lemmen LJ, Schneider RC. Extradural hematomas of the posterior fossa. *J Neurosurg* 1952;9:245–253.

138. Holtzschuh M, Schuknecht B. Traumatic epidural haematomas of the posterior fossa: 20 new cases and

a review of the literature since 1961. *Br J Neurosurg* 1989;3:171–180.

139. Marshall LF. Surgical treatment of extracerebral lesions in head injury. In: Pitts LH, Wagner FC, eds. *Craniospinal trauma.* New York: Thieme Medical Publishers, 1990:37–48.

140. Choux M, Lena G, Genitori L. Intracranial hematomas. In: Raimondi AJ, Choux M, DiRocco C, eds. *Head injuries in the newborn and infant.* New York: Springer-Verlag, 1986:203–216.

141. Neubauer UJ. Extradural hematoma of the posterior fossa. Twelve years experience with CT-scan. *Acta Neurochir* 1987;87:105–111.

142. Helfer BE, Kempe RS. *The battered child,* 4th ed. Chicago: University of Chicago Press, 1987.

143. Duhaime AC, et al. The shaken baby syndrome. A clinical, pathological, and biomechanical study. *J Neurosurg* 1987;66:409–415.

144. Wilkins B. Head injury—abuse or accident? *Arch Dis Child* 1997;76:393–396.

145. Rabe EF, Flynn RC, Dodge PR. A study of subdural effusions in an infant with particular reference to the mechanisms of their persistence. *Neurology* 1962;12: 79–92.

146. Provencale J. The current role of SPECT in imaging subdural hematoma. *J Nucl Med* 1992;33:248–250.

147. Yakubu MA, Leffler CW. 5-Hydroxytryptamine-induced vasoconstriction after cerebral hematoma in piglets. *Pediatr Res* 1997;41:317–320.

148. Miller JD, et al. Ischemic brain damage in a model of acute subdural hematoma. *Neurosurgery* 1990;27: 433–439.

149. Haseler LJ, et al. Evidence from proton magnetic resonance spectroscopy for a metabolic cascade of neuronal damage in shaken baby syndrome. *Pediatrics* 1997;99:4–14.

150. McLaurin RL, Tutor FT. Acute subdural hematoma: review of ninety cases. *J Neurosurg* 1961;18:61–67.

151. Rahme ES, Green D. Chronic subdural hematoma in adolescence and early adulthood. *JAMA* 1961;176: 424–426.

152. Litovsky NS, Raffel C, McComb JG. Management of symptomatic chronic extra-axial fluid collections in pediatric patients. *Neurosurgery* 1992;31:445–450.

153. Bruce DA, Zimmerman RA. Shaken impact syndrome. *Pediatr Ann* 1989;18:482–494.

154. Harcourt B, Hopkins D. Ophthalmic manifestations of the battered-baby syndrome. *BMJ* 1971;3:398–401.

155. Barlow KM, et al. Magnetic resonance imaging in acute non-accidental head injury. *Acta Paediatr* 1999;88:734–740.

156. Harwood-Nash DC. Abuse to the pediatric central nervous system. *Am J Neuroradiol* 1992;13:569–575.

157. Zimmerman RA, et al. Computed tomography of craniocerebral injury in the abused child. *Radiology* 1979;130:687–690.

158. Dolinskas CA, Zimmerman RA, Bilaniuk LT. A sign of subarachnoid bleeding on computed tomograms of pediatric head trauma patients. *Radiology* 1978;126: 409–411.

159. Parent AD. Pediatric chronic subdural hematoma: a retrospective comparative analysis. *Pediatr Neurosurg* 1992;18:266–271.

160. Till K. Subdural haematoma and effusion in infancy. *BMJ* 1968;2:400–402.

161. Hollenhorst RW, et al. Subdural hematoma, subdural hygroma and subarachnoid hemorrhage among infants and children. *Neurology* 1957;7:813–819.
162. Wilkinson WS, et al. Retinal hemorrhage predicts neurologic injury in the shaken baby syndrome. *Arch Ophthalmol* 1989;104:1509–1512.
163. Hoffmann GF, Naughten ER. Abuse or metabolic disorder? *Arch Dis Child* 1998;78:199.
164. Sherwood D. Chronic subdural hematoma in infants. *Am J Dis Child* 1930;39:980–1021.
165. Ingraham FD, Heyl HL. Subdural hematoma in infancy and childhood. *JAMA* 1939;112:198–204.
166. Aoki N. Chronic subdural hematoma in infancy: clinical analysis of 30 cases in the CT era. *J Neurosurg* 1990;73:201–205.
167. Ersahin Y, Mutluer S, Koraman S. Continuous external subdural drainage in the management of infantile subdural collections: a prospective study. *Childs Nerv Syst* 1997;13:526–529.
168. Tabaddor K, Shulman K. Definitive treatment of chronic subdural hematoma by twist-drill craniostomy and closed-system drainage. *J Neurosurg* 1977;46:220–226.
169. McLaurin RL, McLaurin KS. Calcified subdural hematomas in childhood. *J Neurosurg* 1966;24:648–655.
170. Haviland J, Russell RI. Outcome after severe non-accidental head injury. *Arch Dis Child* 1997;77:504–507.
171. Martin HP, et al. The development of abused children. *Adv Pediatr* 1974;21:25–73.
172. Elmer E. A follow-up study of traumatized children. *Pediatrics* 1977;59:273–279.
173. Jennett WB. Trauma as a cause of epilepsy in childhood. *Dev Med Child Neurol* 1973;15:56–62.
174. Annegers JF, et al. Seizures after head trauma: a population study. *Neurology* 1980;30:683–689.
175. Hendrick E, Harris L. Posttraumatic epilepsy in children. *J Trauma* 1968;8:547–556.
176. Grand W. The significance of posttraumatic status epilepticus in childhood. *J Neurol Neurosurg Psychiatry* 1974;37:178–180.
177. Annegers J, et al. A population-based study of seizures after traumatic brain injuries. *N Engl J Med* 1998;338:20–24.
178. Caveness WF, et al. The nature of posttraumatic epilepsy. *J Neurosurg* 1979;50:545–553.
179. Walton JW, Barwick DD, Longley BP. The electroencephalogram in brain injury. In: Rowbotham GF, ed. *Acute injuries of the head: their diagnosis, treatment, complications and sequels.* Baltimore: Williams & Wilkins, 1964.
180. Walker AE. Posttraumatic epilepsy: an inquiry into the evolution and dissolution of convulsions following head injury. *Clin Neurosurg* 1958;6:69–103.
181. Babb TL, Pretorius JK. Pathological substrates of epilepsy. In: Wyllie E, ed. *The treatment of epilepsy: principles and practice,* 2nd ed. Baltimore: Williams & Wilkins, 1997:106–121.
182. Jan MS, et al. Vomiting after mild head injury is related to migraine. *J Pediatr* 1997;130:134–137.
183. Haas DC, Lourie H. Trauma-triggered migraine: an explanation for common neurological attacks after mild head injury. *J Neurosurg* 1988;68:181–188.
184. Dandy WE, Follis RH Jr. On the pathology of carotid-cavernous aneurysms (pulsating exophthalmos). *Am J Ophthalmol* 1941;24:365–385.
185. Pitner SE. Carotid thrombosis due to intraoral trauma: an unusual complication of a common childhood accident. *N Engl J Med* 1966;274:764–767.
186. Mokri B, Piepgras DG, Houser OW. Traumatic dissections of the extracranial internal carotid artery. *J Neurosurg* 1988;68:189–197.
187. Bruetman ME, et al. Cerebral hemorrhage in carotid artery surgery. *Arch Neurol* 1963;9:458–467.
188. Desal H, et al. Fistule carotido-caverneuse directe, études clinique, radiologique et thérapeutique. Á propos de 49 cas. *J Neuroradiol* 1997;24:141–154.
189. Lewis DW, Berman PH. Vertebral artery dissection and alternating hemiparesis in an adolescent. *Pediatrics* 1986;78:610–613.
190. Khurana DS, et al. Vertebral artery dissection: issues in diagnosis and management. *Pediatr Neurol* 1996;14:255–258.
190a. Auer A, et al. Magnetic resonance angiographic and clinical features of extracranial vertebral artery dissection. *J Neurol Neurosurg Psychiatry* 1998;64:474–481.
191. Snoek JW, Minderhoud JM, Wilmink JT. Delayed deterioration following mild head injury in children. *Brain* 1984;107:15–36.
192. McCrory PR, Berkovic SF. Second impact syndrome. *Neurology* 1998;50:677–683.
193. Bruce DA, et al. Diffuse cerebral swelling following head injuries in children: the syndrome of malignant brain edema. *J Neurosurg* 1981;54:170–178.
194. Shaffer D, Chadwick O, Rutter M. Psychiatric outcome of localized head injury in children. In: *Outcome of severe damage to the nervous system.* Ciba Foundation Symposium 34. Amsterdam: Elsevier–North Holland Publishing Co, 1975:191–213.
195. Fuld PA, Fisher P. Recovery of intellectual ability after closed head injury. *Dev Med Child Neurol* 1977;19:495–502.
196. Black P, et al. The posttraumatic syndrome in children. In: Walker AE, Caveness WF, Critchley M, eds. *The late effect of head injury.* Springfield, IL: Charles C Thomas, 1969:142.
197. Koskiniemi M, et al. Long-term outcome after severe head injury in preschoolers is worse than expected. *Arch Pediatr Adolesc Med* 1995;149:249–254.
198. Miner ME, Fletcher JM, Ewing-Cobbs L. Recovery versus outcome after head injury in children. In: Miner ME, Wagner KA, eds. *Neurotrauma: treatment, rehabilitation and related issues.* Boston: Butterworths, 1986:233–240.
199. Mitchener A, et al. SPECT, CT, and MRI in head injury: acute abnormalities followed up at six months. *J Neurol Neurosurg Psychiatry* 1997;62:633–636.
200. Symonds C. Disorders of memory. *Brain* 1966;89:625–644.
201. Harris P. Head injuries in childhood. *Arch Dis Child* 1957;32:488–491.
202. Levin HS, et al. Memory and intellectual ability after head injury in children and adolescents. *Neurosurgery* 1982;11:668–673.
203. Hannay HJ, Levin HS, Grossman PG. Impaired recognition memory after head injury. *Cortex* 1979;15:269–283.
204. Chadwick O. Psychological sequelae of head injury in children. *Dev Med Child Neurol* 1985;27:72–75.
205. Cook JB. The effects of minor head injuries sustained in sport and the postconcussion syndrome. In: Walker

AE, Caveness WF, Critchley M, eds. *The late effects of head injury*. Springfield, IL: Charles C Thomas, 1969.

206. McClelland RJ, Fenton GW, Rutherford W. The post-concussional syndrome revisited. *J Roy Soc Med* 1994;87:508–510.

207. Hjern B, Nylander I. Acute head injuries in children: traumatology, therapy and prognosis. *Acta Paediatr* 1964;[Suppl]:152.

208. Jennett B, Plum F. Persistent vegetative state after brain damage. A syndrome in search of a name. *Lancet* 1972;1:734–737.

209. Kampfl A, et al. The persistent vegetative state after closed head injury: clinical and magnetic resonance imaging findings in 42 patients. *J Neurosurg* 1998;88:809–816.

210. Higashi K, et al. Epidemiological studies on patients with a persistent vegetative state. *J Neurol Neurosurg Psychiatry* 1977;40:876–885.

211. Heindl UT, Laub MC. Outcome of persistent vegetative state following hypoxic or traumatic brain injury in children and adolescents. *Neuropediatrics* 1996;27:94–100.

212. Ashwal S, Eyman RK, Call TL. Life expectancy in a persistent vegetative state. *Pediatr Neurol* 1994;10: 27–33.

212a. Strauss DJ, Shavelle RM, Ashwal S. Life expectancy and median survival time in the permanent vegetative state. *Pediatr Neurol* 1999;21:626–631.

213. Hamilton MG, Myles ST. Pediatric spinal injury: review of 174 hospital admissions. *J Neurosurg* 1992;77:700–704.

214. Ruge JR, et al. Pediatric spinal injury: the very young. *J Neurosurg* 1988;68:25–30.

214a. Greenwald TA, Mann DC. Pediatric seatbelt injuries: diagnosis and treatment of lumbar flexion-distraction injuries. *Paraplegia* 1994;32:743–751.

214b. Taylor GA, Eggli KD. Lap-belt injuries of the lumbar spine in children: a pitfall in CT diagnosis. *Am J Roentgenol* 1988;150:1355–1358.

215. Hall ED, Braughler JM. Free radicals in CNS injury. *Res Publ Assoc Res Nerv Ment Dis* 1993;71:81–105.

216. Banik NL, et al. Role of calpain in spinal cord injury: effects of calpain and free radical inhibitors. *Ann NY Acad Sci* 1998;844:131–137.

217. Zwimpfer TJ, Bernstein M. Spinal cord concussion. *J Neurosurg* 1990;72:894–900.

218. Tator CH, Fehlings MG. Review of the secondary injury theory of acute spinal cord trauma with emphasis on vascular mechanisms. *J Neurosurg* 1991;75: 15–26.

219. Bischof W, Nittner K. Zur Klinik und Pathogenese der vaskular bedingten Myelomalazien. *Neurochirurgie* 1965;8:215–231.

220. Ahmann PA, et al. Spinal cord infarction due to minor trauma in children. *Neurology* 1975;25:301–307.

221. Choi JU, et al. Traumatic infarction of the spinal cord in children. *J Neurosurg* 1986;65:608–610.

222. Williams B. Pathogenesis of posttraumatic syringomyelia. *Br J Neurosurg* 1992;6:517–520.

223. La Haye PA, Batzdorf U. Posttraumatic syringomyelia. *West J Med* 1988;148:657–663.

224. Frankel HL, et al. The value of postural reduction in the initial management of closed injuries of the spine with paraplegia and tetraplegia. *Paraplegia* 1969;7:179–192.

225. Sherrington CS. *The integrative action of the nervous system*. New York: Charles Scribner Sons, 1906.

226. Riddock G. The reflex functions of the completely divided spinal cord in man, compared with those associated with less severe lesions. *Brain* 1917;40: 264–402.

226a. Atkinson PP, Atkinson JLD. Spinal shock. *Mayo Clin Proc* 1996;71:384–389.

227. Chiles BW, Cooper PR, Acute spinal injury. *N Engl J Med* 1996;514–520.

228. Kuhn RA. Functional capacity of the isolated human spinal cord. *Brain* 1950;73:1–51.

229. Sullivan AW. Subluxation of atlanto-axial joint. *J Pediatr* 1949;35:451–464.

229a. Menezes AH, Mohonen M. Management of occipito-cervical instability. In: Cooper PR, ed. *Neurosurgical topics*, Vol. 1. Baltimore: Williams & Wilkins, 1990:65–76.

230. Controversies in imaging acute cervical spine trauma. *Am J Neuroradiol* 1997;18:1866–1868.

231. Hadley MN, et al. Pediatric spinal trauma. Review of 122 cases of spinal cord and vertebral column injuries. *J Neurosurg* 1988;68:18–24.

232. Cattell HS, Filtzer DL. Pseudosubluxation and other normal variations in the cervical spine in children. *J Bone Joint Surg* 1965;47A:1295–1309.

233. Jefferson G. Concerning injuries of the spinal cord. *BMJ* 1936;2:1125–1130.

234. Guttman L. *Spinal cord injuries*, 2nd ed. Oxford: Blackwell Scientific Publications, 1976.

235. Sonntag VKH, Hadley MN. Nonoperative management of cervical spine injuries. *Clin Neurosurg* 1988;34:630–649.

236. Vale FL, et al. Combined medical and surgical treatment after acute spinal cord injury: results of a prospective pilot study to assess the merits of aggressive medical resuscitation and blood pressure management. *J Neurosurg* 1997;87:239–246.

237. Sypert GW. Stabilization and management of cervical injuries. In: Pitts LH, Wagner FC, eds. *Craniospinal trauma*. New York: Thieme Medical Publishers, 1990:171–185.

238. Bracken MB, et al. Methylprednisolone or naloxone treatment after acute spinal cord injury: 1-year follow-up data. Results of the Second National Acute Spinal Cord Injury Study. *J Neurosurg* 1992;76:23–31.

239. Geisler FH, Dorsey FC, Coleman WP. Recovery of motor function after spinal cord injury—a randomized, placebo-controlled trial with GM_1 ganglioside. *N Engl J Med* 1991;324:1829–1838.

240. Geisler FH. Clinical trials of pharmacotherapy for spinal cord injury. *Ann N Y Acad Sci* 1998;845: 374–381.

241. Kapfhammer JP. Axon sprouting in the spinal cord: growth promoting and growth inhibitory mechanisms. *Anat Embryol* 1997;196:417–426.

242. Bregman BS, et al. Intervention strategies to enhance anatomical plasticity and recovery of function after spinal cord injury. *Adv Neurol* 1997;72:257–275.

243. Short DJ, Frankel HL, Bergström EMK. Injuries of the spinal cord in children. In: Vinken GW, Bruyn GW, Klawans HL, Frankel HL, eds. *Spinal Cord trauma, handbook of clinical neurology*. Rev Ser, 17, Vol. 61. Amsterdam: Elsevier Science Publishers, 1992:233–252.

244. Piepmeier JM. Late sequelae of spinal cord injury. In: Narayan RK, Wilberger JE Jr, Povlikshock JT, eds. *Neurotrauma.* New York: McGraw-Hill, 1996:1237–1244.

245. Whiteneck G, et al., eds. *The management of high quadriplegia.* New York: Demos Medical Publishing, 1989.

246. Lightner DJ. Contemporary urologic management of patients with spinal cord injury. *Mayo Clin Proc* 1998;73:434–438.

247. Crockard HA, Heilman AE, Stevens JM. Progressive myelopathy secondary to odontoid fractures: clinical, radiological and surgical features. *J Neurosurg* 1993;78:579–586.

248. Epstein JA, Lavine LS. Herniated lumbar intervertebral disks in teenage children. *J Neurosurg* 1964;21: 1070–1075.

249. Friedman AP, Merritt HH. Damage to cranial nerves resulting from head injury. *Bull Los Angeles Neurol Soc* 1944;9:135–139.

250. Brazis PW. Palsies of the trochlear nerve: diagnosis and localization—recent concepts. *Mayo Clin Proc* 1993;68:501–509.

250a. McKennan KX, Chole RA. Facial paralysis in temporal bone trauma. *Am J Otol* 1992;13:167–172.

251. Galan E, Kousseff BG. Peripheral neuropathy in Ehlers-Danlos syndrome. *Pediatr Neurol* 1995;12:242–245.

252. Medical Research Council. *Aids to the examination of peripheral nerve injuries.* London: Balliere Tindall, 1986.

253. Fagan ER, Taylor MJ, Logan WJ. Somatosensory evoked potentials. Part II. A review of the clinical applications in pediatric neurology. *Pediatr Neurol* 1987;3:189–196.

254. Hodes R, Larrabee MG, German W. The human electromyogram in response to nerve stimulation and the conduction velocity of motor axons: studies on normal and on injured peripheral nerves. *Arch Neurol Psychiatry* 1948;60:340–365.

255. Carvalho GA, et al. Diagnosis of root avulsions in traumatic brachial plexus injuries: value of computerized tomography myelography and magnetic resonance imaging. *J Neurosurg* 1997;86:69–76.

255a. Filler AG, et al. Application of magnetic resonance neurography in the evaluation of patients with peripheral nerve pathology. *J Neurosurg* 1996;85:299–309.

256. Mitchell SW. *Injuries of nerves and their consequences.* Philadelphia: JB Lippincott Co, 1872.

257. Bernstein BH, et al. Reflex neurovascular dystrophy in childhood. *J Pediatr* 1978;93:211–215.

258. Gordon N. Reflex sympathetic dystrophy. *Brain Dev* 1996;18:257–262.

259. Hannington-Kiff JG. Reflex sympathetic dystrophy. *J R Soc Med* 1987;80:605.

260. Bhatia KP, Bhatt MH, Marsden CD. The causalgia-dystonia syndrome. *Brain* 1993;116:843–851.

260a. van der Laan L, et al. Complex regional pain syndrome type I (RSD). Pathology of skeletal muscle and peripheral nerve. *Neurology* 1998;51:20–25.

261. Honjyo K, et al. An 11-year-old girl with reflex sympathetic dystrophy successfully treated by thoracoscopic sympathectomy. *Acta Paediatr* 1997;86: 903–905.

262. Malamud N, Haymaker W, Custer RP. Heat stroke: a clinicopathologic study of 125 fatal cases. *Milit Surg* 1946;99:397–449.

263. Freedman D, Schenthal J. A parenchymatous cerebellar syndrome following protracted high body temperature. *Neurology* 1953;3:513–516.

264. Chavez-Carballo E, Bouchama A. Fever, heatstroke, and hemorrhage shock and encephalopathy. *J Child Neurol* 1998;13:286–287.

265. Hopkins PM, Ellis FR, Halsall PJ. Evidence for related myopathies in exertional heat stroke and malignant hyperthermia. *Lancet* 1991;338:1491–1492.

266. Cherington M. Central nervous system complications of lightning and electrical injuries. *Semin Neurol* 1995;15:233–240.

267. Critchley M. Neurologic effects of lightning and electricity. *Lancet* 1934;1:68–72.

268. Silversides J. The neurological sequelae of electrical injury. *Can Med Assoc J* 1964;91:195–204.

269. Kotagal S, et al. Neurologic, psychiatric and cardiovascular complications in children struck by lightning. *Pediatrics* 1982;70:190–192.

270. Winkelman MD, Galloway PG. Central nervous system complications of thermal burns. A postmortem study of 139 patients. *Medicine* 1992;71: 271–283.

271. Mohnot D, Snead OC, Benton JW. Burn encephalopathy in children. *Ann Neurol* 1982;12:42–47.

272. Antoon AY, Volpe JJ, Crawford JD. Burn encephalopathy in children. *Pediatrics* 1972;50:609–616.

273. Greer HD. Neurologic consequences. In: Bove AA, ed. *Diving medicine*, 3rd ed. Philadephia: WB Saunders Co, 1997:258–269.

274. Reuter M, et al. MR imaging of the central nervous system in diving-related decompression illness. *Acta Radiol* 1997;38:940–944.

275. Manabe Y, et al. Presumed venous infarction in spinal decompression sickenss. *Am J Neuroradiol* 1998;19: 1578–1580.

276. Deymeer F, Jones HR. Pediatric median mononeuropathies: a clinical and electromyelographic study. *Muscle Nerve* 1994;17:755–762.

277. Gilles FH, French J. Postinjection sciatic nerve palsies in infants and children. *J Pediatr* 1961;58: 195–204.

278. DeBolt WL, Jordan JC. Femoral neuropathy from heparin hematoma: report of two cases. *Bull Los Angeles Neurol Soc* 1966;31:45–50.

Chapter 9

Toxic and Nutritional Disorders

John H. Menkes

Departments of Neurology and Pediatrics, University of California, Los Angeles,
UCLA School of Medicine, and Department of Pediatric Neurology, Cedars-Sinai
Medical Center, Los Angeles, California 90048

TOXIC DISORDERS

Neurotoxins are endogenous or environmental. Various sections of this text consider the endogenous neurotoxins, notably the excitatory neurotransmitters. These substances are implicated in cell death from asphyxia and hypoglycemia, after uncontrolled seizures, and possibly in some of the heredodegenerative disorders. This chapter discusses environmental toxins. Almost all environmental toxins induce neurologic symptoms if ingested in sufficient quantity. This chapter considers only those that are encountered in clinical practice commonly and for which the nervous system is a primary site of action. They are discussed in ascending order of their chemical complexity.

Drug intoxications that are encountered less commonly by the practitioner are not considered in detail. The reader is referred to Table 9.1 for a summary of their neurologic complications and treatment.

In addition, the reader is directed to the comprehensive text on medical toxicology edited by Ellenhorn and colleagues (23), a book on neurotoxicology edited by Spencer and Schaumburg (24), and a series of capsule presentations of the most common intoxications in a pediatric practice written by Mack and published in the *North Carolina Journal of Medicine* (25).

The incidence of the various drug intoxications in an Australian pediatric population during the years 1977 through 1981 is depicted in Table 9.2 (26). A series compiled from the Children's Hospital of the University of Antwerp for the years 1980 through 1988 shows a similar distribution (27).

Metallic Toxins

Lead

Although some of the toxic actions of lead have been known since antiquity, the understanding of the clinical picture of lead poisoning is based on the classic studies of Tanquerel des Planches (28), Blackfan (29), and Holt (30). As a result of the considerable advances in the prevention of lead exposure, cases of acute lead encephalopathy have all but disappeared from the United States. Nevertheless, children with increased blood lead levels are still being encountered with considerable frequency.

Pharmacology

One of the major sources of lead continues to be exterior and, to a lesser extent, interior lead-based paint, which remains as an environmental hazard in some 3.8 million homes in the United States housing children 7 years of age or younger (31). Lead can be absorbed by water with a low mineral content as it passes through lead pipes or lead-soldered copper pipes. It also

TABLE 9.1. Neurotoxic complications of some drugs

Drug	Neurologic symptoms	Reference
Antihistamine	Tonic-clonic seizures	Hestand and Tesky (1), Goetz, et al. (1a)
Atropine (jimson weed, thornapple, deadly nightshade)	Dilated pupils, slurred speech, ataxia, seizures	Priest (Down syndrome) (2), Amitai et al. (3)
Boric acid	Seizures	Valdez-Dapena and Arey (4), Cheng (5)
Codeine	Respiratory depression	von Muhlendahl et al. (6)
Dextromethorphan	Dystonia	Warden et al. (7)
Diphenoxylate (Lomotil)	Excitement, hypotonia, rigidity, cortical blindness, cerebral edema	McCarron et al. (8)
Ferrous sulfate	Vomiting, diarrhea, seizures, lethargy	Robotham and Leitman (9), Mann et al. (10)
Hexachlorophene	Seizures, blindness, spastic paraparesis	Martinez et al. (11), Martin-Bouyer et al. (12)
Hydroxyquinolines (clioquinol)	Optic neuritis, myelitis, peripheral neuropathy	Oakley (13), Selby (14), Shigematsu and Yanagawa (15)
Imipramine and other tricyclic antidepressants	Clonic movements, seizures, coma	Saraf et al. (16), Greene and Cromie (17)
Phenylpropanolamine	Cerebral vasculitis, intracranial hemorrhage	Foreman et al. (18)
Piperazine	Impaired coordination, chorea, encephalopathy	Parsons (19)
Propoxyphene (Darvon)	Lethargy, seizures	Lovejoy et al. (20)
Sympathomimetics (dextroamphetamine)	Agitation, seizures	Espelin and Done (21), Alldredge et al. (22)

can be ingested when water is boiled in soldered electric kettles. Until recently, organic lead also was ingested from roadside dust contaminated with automobile emissions, or by habitual sniffing of leaded gasoline. Less common sources of lead include lead arsenate insecticides, lead solder, which in the United States has been virtually eliminated from the seams of food and beverage cans, ancient pewter, imperfectly glazed ceramics, painted jewelry, and eye shadow, which in some developing countries is applied to infant boys and girls. One form of lead poisoning, once relatively common in nursing infants, was caused by prolonged use of lead nipple shields.

The gastrointestinal tract of infants and children absorbs approximately 40% of ingested lead, with the remainder being excreted. Approximately 90% of inhaled lead is absorbed. Iron deficiency and constipation encourage absorption; diarrhea has the reverse effect. Lead and calcium compete for a common transport mechanism; reduced calcium intake and low serum levels of 25-hydroxy vitamin D_1 increase lead absorption. After absorption, lead is distributed into three compartments: Some enters a rapidly exchangeable pool in the liver and kidney, and from there binds to a low-molecular-

TABLE 9.2. Agents accidentally ingested by children (0 through 12 years) resulting in hospital admission

Agent	Number of patients	Percent of accidental ingestions
Petroleum distillates	255	13
Antihistaminics	186	9
Benzodiazepines	182	9
Bleach, detergents	142	7
Aspirin, acetaminophen	117	6
Camphor, mothballs	117	6
Barbiturates	97	5
Caustic soda	69	3
Painting chemicals	61	3
Noxious plants	49	2
Tricyclics	45	2
Phenytoin	40	2
Iron tablets	36	2
Sympathomimetics	36	2

Data from Brisbane, Australia, 1977–1981. From Pearn J, et al. Accidental poisoning in childhood. Five year urban population study with 15 year analysis of fatality. *BMJ* 1984;288:45. With permission.

weight protein of erythrocytes (32); some enters a rapidly exchangeable pool in soft tissue and is loosely bound to bone; and the major portion (60% to 90%) is tightly bound as the insoluble and nontoxic lead triphosphate in the skeleton, notably in the epiphyseal portion of growing bone. Lead also is deposited in hair and nails and crosses the placenta. Only a small amount of lead enters the brain; the major portion is found in gray matter and the basal ganglia (33,34). High phosphate and high vitamin D intakes favor skeletal storage of lead, whereas parathormone, low phosphate intake, and acidosis promote its release into the bloodstream. Almost all the absorbed lead is excreted in urine; fecal lead represents the unabsorbed fraction. The half-life of lead in blood is 1 to 2 months; it is 20 to 30 years in bone. Excretion is so slow that even a slight increase in the average daily intake above 0.3 mg/day, the maximum permissible level for adults, can ultimately induce poisoning.

The levels of lead in blood and urine are an index of the degree of exposure to the toxin. The concentration of blood lead tends to peak approximately 2 years of age. Although blood lead levels below 30 µg/dL were once considered acceptable, δ-aminolevulinic acid dehydratase (ALAD) activity is significantly inhibited at blood lead levels of 5 to 10 µg/dL (35), and ferrochelatase, the enzyme that inserts iron into hemoglobin, is inhibited in a dose-related fashion at levels between 15 and 18 µg/dL (36). Measurement of hair lead is an unreliable indicator of the severity of lead exposure, whereas the reliability of tooth lead content is still under debate (37). As yet, the threshold level for neurotoxicity is unknown. The American Academy of Pediatrics has stated that concentrations of 25 µg/dL or higher are certain to be toxic, and the average blood lead level in American children is 2.6 µg/dL (38).

Pathology

Almost all organs are affected by lead poisoning, with damage caused by heavy metal inhibition of numerous sulfhydryl enzymes. One of the earliest manifestations of lead intoxication is anemia, induced by a disturbance in heme synthesis and by shortening of red cell life span. Lead impairs heme synthesis at several points, with globin synthesis also being disrupted at higher lead levels (39,40).

Within the central nervous system (CNS), lead acts primarily on capillary endothelium. It causes extravasation of plasma, followed by endothelial, microglial, and astrocytic proliferation and widespread interstitial edema (41). Widespread neuronal degeneration occurs, with the neocortex and cerebellum being affected most prominently; neocortical degeneration also can reflect agonal anoxia, rather than a direct effect of lead. Experimental work suggests that the immature cerebral vasculature is particularly sensitive to lead, and that neurotoxicity is the result of multifactorial events. Lead interrupts the cellular calcium pump in mitochondria with a resultant calcium-mediated cell death in the cerebrovascular endothelium (42). Chronic exposure to lead interferes with calmodulin-dependent processes resulting in abnormal post-translational modifications of cytoskeletal proteins. In addition, lead inhibits acetylcholine release and enhances the release of dopamine and norepinephrine (43).

In peripheral nerves, axonal degeneration occurs with loss of large myelinated fibers, but with no demyelination (44). Occasionally, the anterior horn cells also are degenerated. Chronic, low-level exposure, as is seen in industrial workers, can produce paranodal demyelination and internodal remyelination (45). No explanation exists for the preferential involvement of nerves in the upper extremity.

Pathologic changes within other organs, notably the liver and kidney, have been described in a classic publication by Blackman (46).

Clinical Manifestations

Neurologic symptoms of lead poisoning form a continuum from the most minor to the most severe (47). In the classic form of severe lead encephalopathy, symptoms progress insidiously, first becoming apparent in late summer in some 80% of cases. Before then, there is usually a prodromal period of several weeks or months during

TABLE 9.3. *Signs and symptoms of overt lead poisoning in children (Chicago, 1955–1957)*

Prodromal symptoms	Number of cases	Overt symptom	Number of cases
Irritability	20	Convulsions	11
Pallor	16	Lethargy	7
Vomiting	16	Sixth nerve palsy	7
Constipation	11	Ataxia	2
Weight loss	7		
	2-Year follow-up of 14 patients		
	13/46	Fatal	
	3/14	Retarded motor development	
	7/14	Retarded language development	

Adapted from Mellins RB, Jenkins CD. Epidemiologic and psychological study of lead poisoning in children. *JAMA* 1955;158:15; and Jenkins CD, Mellins RB. Lead poisoning in children. *Arch Neurol Psychiatry* 1957;77:70.

which the child is pale, irritable, listless, and without appetite. Epigastric pain, vomiting, and constipation are common. These nonspecific symptoms are often interrupted by the sudden onset of a series of generalized convulsions or by depression of consciousness (Table 9.3) (48,49).

Seizures are common and resist anticonvulsant therapy. They can be followed by hemiplegia or other neurologic sequelae.

The child with lead encephalopathy demonstrates increased intracranial pressure. Less frequent is cerebellar ataxia and palsies of the sixth and seventh cranial nerves. Nuchal rigidity is fairly common and can be related to tonsillar herniation. Patients in some parts of the world have a high incidence of optic neuritis with profound vision loss, acute communicating hydrocephalus, and tremors (50).

In children, peripheral neuritis caused by lead poisoning is rare. When seen, it almost invariably occurs in subjects with sickle cell anemia (51).

Anemia and deranged renal tubular function usually accompany the neurologic symptoms. Red cells in peripheral blood and bone marrow can show basophilic stippling, and the presence of a large number of such cells is almost invariable in chronic poisoning caused by inorganic lead, although not in poisoning with organic (tetraethyl) lead. Basophilic stippling, however, is not specific for lead intoxication.

Radiologic findings in acute lead encephalopathy are characteristic (52). Most prominent is the presence of a dense, radiopaque band at the metaphyses of numerous long bones. Less commonly,

radiopaque particles are found within the gastrointestinal tract as evidence of recent plaster ingestion.

Although lead encephalopathy and peripheral neuritis represent the classic forms of lead intoxication, neurobehavioral symptoms are now far more common, and have, in the last few years, become a contentious issue for health care workers.

A large number of epidemiologic studies designed to examine the effects of low-level lead exposure on the nervous system differ with respect to the measures selected to reflect the amount of lead to which the developing brain has been exposed. They also differ in the areas of cognitive and neurologic performance chosen to measure the effects of lead intoxication. In almost every study, the results have been confounded by the association between increased lead intake and disadvantaged family and home environment. Smith (53) and Pocock and colleagues (37) have extensively and dispassionately reviewed these issues.

I concur with their conclusions that from the current state of knowledge one is unable to say whether low-level lead exposure affects performance or behavior of children, or whether a reverse causality exists (i.e., children with lower IQs or aberrant behavior patterns have increased lead uptake). In either case, in cases in which effects of environmental lead are found, they are likely to be small and overshadowed by the effects that result from the child's socioeconomic status, quality of home environment, and parental intelligence (37,53,54). Additionally, there is no evidence as yet for a threshold blood lead level above which there is a clear effect on IQ (53). We also do not know what role, if any, intrauterine exposure to lead plays in cognitive deficits (37,54). Thus, in the Australian study of Baghurst and coworkers, no significant relation existed between IQ at 57 months of age and antenatal or perinatal blood lead concentrations (54).

A further discussion on the interrelation between lead exposure and cognitive function can be found in Chapter 16.

Diagnosis

Seizures and increased intracranial pressure should always suggest the diagnosis of lead encephalopathy. Posterior fossa tumors rarely produce seizures, and tumors of the cerebral hemispheres are rare in toddlers. Lead lines on radiographic examination and basophilic stippling in a blood smear offer a presumptive diagnosis even in the absence of a history of pica.

The differential diagnosis between a sickle cell crisis that produces neurologic symptoms and lead poisoning can be difficult because both can produce cramping abdominal pains and seizures. Generally, neurologic signs in sickle cell crisis are caused by cerebrovascular occlusion and thus result in lateralizing findings, which are generally absent in lead encephalopathy.

Several tests are available to detect chronic but low-grade exposure to lead:

- *Blood lead levels*: A capillary blood test is obtained for screening purposes. A finger stick value of 15 µg/dL or higher should be confirmed by a venous sample.
- *Elevation of free erythrocyte protoporphyrins*: The elevation of free erythrocyte protoporphyrins persists long after cessation of lead exposure. A level of higher than 25 µg/dL indicates excess lead exposure (55). Because of the poor sensitivity of this test at lower blood lead concentrations, this test has largely been abandoned for screening purposes.
- *Inhibition of δ-aminolevulinic acid dehydratase activity*: This is probably the most sensitive indicator of lead exposure (56).
- *An elevation of hair lead level*: This has been proposed as an indicator for the timing of increased exposure to lead. This measure-

ment, however, is unreliable in that hair lead concentrations can vary in different hairs from the same individual. It also is difficult to remove surface contaminants without removing lead from within the hair.

- *Increased lead content of deciduous teeth* (57): Lead is unevenly distributed within a tooth, and there also are significant differences in lead content between incisors and canines and teeth removed from the maxilla and the mandible (53).
- *Estimation of urinary coproporphyrins* (58): A striking increase in coproporphyrin excretion also is seen in hepatocellular injury, inborn errors of porphyrin metabolism, bulbar poliomyelitis, rheumatic fever, and various febrile illnesses.
- *Zinc protoporphyrin levels*: Assays for zinc protoporphyrin have been recommended as a means to screen large populations for lead toxicity (38). However, in the presence of an acute and massive lead load, there frequently is no increase in zinc protoporphyrin levels (59).

Because peripheral nerve conduction times are slowed in many youngsters with even inapparent neuropathy, peripheral nerve conduction studies can provide an ancillary indication of subclinical lead intoxication (51).

Treatment and Prognosis

Because recurrent exposure is common, and because neurologic damage caused by lead poisoning is probably progressive rather than all or none, the source of the ingested lead must be ascertained and eliminated before the child returns home from the hospital. The recommended practice is to forego treatment for children whose blood lead level is less than 25 µg/dL. Children with blood lead levels between 25 and 45 µg/dL require their immediate removal from lead exposure. Chelation therapy is indicated for patients with blood lead levels over 45 µg/dL. Two parenteral and two oral chelation agents are currently available. The former are dimercaprol and calcium disodium ethylenediaminetetraacetic acid (EDTA). Oral chelation agents are succimer, a water-soluble analogue of dimercaprol, and D-penicillamine.

A full discussion of dosages, duration of therapy, and adverse reactions is beyond the scope of this text. They are detailed in the treatment guidelines prepared by the American Academy of Pediatrics, Committee on Drugs (60) and in a publication by Piomelli and colleagues (61). Case management and pitfalls in the treatment of children with severe lead poisoning are discussed by Friedman and Weinberger (62).

Even with the best therapy, the prognosis for complete recovery in children with lead encephalopathy is not good, and by the time symptoms become overt, lasting CNS damage has already been incurred. The mortality from lead encephalopathy varies from 5% to 50% depending on the severity of the cases in the various series. Recurrent convulsions are seen in 40% of children recovering from encephalopathy, and another 20% have other permanent neurologic damage, such as hemiplegia, blindness, and bilateral spasticity.

Thallium

Children can accidentally ingest thallium-containing pesticides. How the metal damages the nervous system is still unknown. In fatal cases, one sees white matter edema and degenerative changes in the nerve cells of cerebral and cerebellar cortex, hypothalamus, olivary nuclei, and corpus striatum. In peripheral nerves, there is a loss of myelinated fibers and degeneration of the central axons of sensory ganglion cells (63).

Depending on the dose ingested, intoxication can be fatal during the acute phase by causing renal and cardiac failure. In less severe intoxications, neurologic symptoms appear 2 to 6 days after ingestion, including a motor neuropathy that principally affects the lower extremities. Hair fibers in the growing stage, which constitute between 80% and 90% of scalp hair, and large diameter fibers are most vulnerable to thallium intoxication (64). Subsequently, cerebellar ataxia can develop, accompanied by somnolence or seizures. A characteristic depilation resembling that seen after vincristine therapy, begins within 2 weeks. Less commonly, there is retrobulbar neuritis and cranial nerve palsies (65,66).

Approximately one-half of the survivors have persistent neurologic deficits, most commonly mental retardation and ataxia. The diagnosis suggested by neurologic symptoms in the presence of depilation can be confirmed by the detection of thallium in urine using atomic absorption spectroscopy and emission spectrography (67).

Chelating agents such as diethyl dithiocarbamate are ineffective in the treatment of thallium poisoning. Although they increase thallium excretion, the chelate formed is lipophilic and crosses the blood–brain barrier. As a consequence, neurologic symptoms worsen (68). Prussian blue, however, does have some value, having induced clinical improvement in a number of patients.

Arsenic

At present, arsenic poisoning in the pediatric population most commonly results from the accidental ingestion of pesticides, notably ant poison (69). The pathologic changes in the brain have been reviewed in a classic paper by Russell (70). They include generalized edema and pericapillary hemorrhages within white matter, with foci of demyelination. Nerve biopsies show axonal degeneration (71). The toxicity of arsenic probably lies in the ability of the trivalent form to inactivate a number of sulfhydryl enzymes, notably the pyruvate dehydrogenase complex. Additionally, the pentavalent form of arsenic uncouples mitochondrial oxidative phosphorylation (72).

Symptoms of arsenic poisoning in the pediatric population are more likely to be gastrointestinal than neurologic (73). After acute arsenic ingestion, they can take the form of a violent attack of vomiting and bloody diarrhea. Chronic arsenic intake induces intermittent gastrointestinal upsets. In children, anemia is not unusual. Neurologic symptoms are mainly those of a peripheral sensory neuritis; numbness and severe paresthesias of the distal portion of the extremities predominate. Distal weakness of the lower extremities follows and can extend to involve the upper extremities.

The neurologic complications of the therapeutic use of organic arsenicals (Jarisch-Herxheimer reactions) are too rare nowadays to warrant discussion (74).

Drugs of choice in the treatment of arsenic poisoning are dimercaprol and D-penicillamine. Their mode of administration to children is described by Cullen and colleagues (73) and Peterson and Rumack (75).

Mercury

Mercury poisoning can result from exposure to elemental mercury in the form of its vapor, inorganic mercury salts, and organic mercury, most commonly as methylmercury. All forms of intoxication are unusual in children.

Mercury vapor poisoning has been reported to induce seizures. Pink disease (acrodynia), once relatively common owing to ingestion of calomel (mercuric chloride) teething powders (76), is now much rarer, but has been observed after exposure to latex paint, which up to 1990 contained phenylmercuric acetate. Mercury is released from surfaces coated with this paint, after it has dried (77). Only a small proportion of exposed infants and young children become symptomatic. Clinical manifestations are marked by erythema, most intense over the fingertips and toes, profound weakness of all extremities, hyperesthesia, extreme irritability, and changes in consciousness.

Intoxication with organic mercury compounds derived from the fungicides or methylmercury was responsible for outbreaks of poisoning in Iraq (78), whereas ingestion of methylmercury-contaminated fish resulted in Minamata disease, an encephalopathy encountered along Minamata Bay in Japan. The neurologic picture of organic mercury poisoning in children is complex. Tingling and other sensory disturbances and progressive visual impairment, taking the form of constriction of visual fields, tunnel vision, or complete blindness, are almost invariable. Ataxia, tremor, impaired hearing, and mental deterioration also are encountered. A variety of involuntary movements are less common (79). Magnetic resonance imaging (MRI) shows atrophy of the ventral portion of the calcarine sulcus (80). Although neurologic degeneration was progressive in the Japanese epidemic, the more recently affected Iraqi children have had considerable functional recovery (78,81).

Methylmercury compounds also have been held responsible for congenital mercury poisoning. Affected infants show tremors, hypotonia, myoclonic jerks, and microcephaly (82,83). In clinically asymptomatic infants, *in utero* exposure to mercury does not appear to have any definite deleterious effects on neurodevelopment (84). Ethylmercury intoxication is less common and less severe than intoxication incurred from methylmercury. The neuropathology of organic mercury poisoning in children has been described by Takeuchi and coworkers (85). It consists of focal cerebral and cerebellar atrophy with the axonal retraction bulbs (torpedoes) on Purkinje cells resembling those seen in Menkes disease (see Chapter 1).

The diagnosis of mercury poisoning depends on the measurement of urinary mercury concentrations. Treatment is by oral administration of 2,3-dimercaptosuccinic acid (Succimer) (86). It is ineffective if not started promptly after exposure to mercury (86a).

Aluminum

Aluminum intoxication, usually caused by the ingestion of aluminum hydroxide, has been implicated in the pathogenesis of progressive dementia and seizures in children with chronic renal failure, whether or not they are undergoing maintenance dialysis. Aluminum intoxication is discussed more fully in Chapter 15.

Organic Toxins

Carbon Monoxide

Carbon monoxide poisoning is one of the major causes of death caused by toxins. In infants and small children the majority of cases results from faulty home heaters or, as in the Orient, the use of anthracite coal briquettes. The brain and the myocardium are most vulnerable to carbon monoxide. The principal effect of carbon monoxide is to interfere with tissue oxygenation by reducing the capacity of blood to transport oxygen and by shifting the blood oxyhemoglobin saturation curve, thus requiring blood oxygen tension to decrease to lower than normal values before a given amount of oxygen is released from hemoglobin. Carbon monoxide also reduces oxygen delivery to tissue by reducing cardiac output. In addition, carbon monoxide binds directly to iron-rich brain regions, notably the globus pallidus and the pars reticulata of the substantia nigra (87).

Neurologic symptoms of carbon monoxide toxicity include irritability, lethargy, and coma. In the Korean series of Kim and Coe, 14% of children presented with convulsions, in 13% there was neck stiffness, and 3% had blindness on admission. Computed tomographic scans showed diffuse cerebral edema and low-density areas in the basal ganglia, notably, the globus pallidus (88). On T2-weighted MRI, increased signal is seen in the basal ganglia (87). Chronic carbon monoxide poisoning can result from poorly ventilated heating systems and inadequately ventilated housing. Symptoms include hyperactivity, sleepiness, and headaches (89).

After apparent recovery, some 10% to 30% of patients, most of them of advanced age, who have had moderate to severe carbon monoxide poisoning develop delayed neurologic sequelae some 3 to 240 days after intoxication (90–92a). The sequelae include a variety of extrapyramidal symptoms, notably tremor, rigidity, and choreoathetosis. Additionally, Kim and Coe also encountered mental retardation, seizures, mutism, hemiparesis, and paraplegia (88). MRI in such patients shows a progressive demyelinating process (93). The underlying mechanism for the delayed neurologic symptoms requires further study. It is currently believed to involve carbon monoxide–mediated brain lipid peroxidation (92a,94).

The pros and cons for the treatment of carbon monoxide poisoning with hyperbaric oxygen are beyond the scope of this book. Suffice it to say that Weaver and colleagues have failed to show differences in outcome between patients who were treated with normobaric oxygen and those treated with hyperbaric oxygen (94a). The reader also is

referred to a paper by Rudge (95). The biological effects of carbon monoxide on pregnant mothers, fetuses, and newborn infants are reviewed by Ginsberg and Myers (96) and Longo (97).

Alcohol

Fetal Alcohol Syndrome

Alcohol is believed to affect the immature nervous system through chronic *in utero* exposure or through acute maternal intoxication.

In 1851, over 2000 years after Plutarch noted "one drunkard begets another" and Aristotle observed that "drunken women bring forth children like to themselves," Carpenter reviewed the then current data on alcohol use during pregnancy and concluded that offspring can experience mental and behavioral disabilities (98). More than 100 years later, French (99,100) and American (101) clinicians described a craniofacial and neurologic disorder with growth and psychomotor retardation called the *fetal alcohol syndrome* (FAS). Its frequency, as estimated by Clarren and Smith in 1978, is between 1 and 2 in 1,000 live-born babies, with partial expression of the syndrome, the fetal alcohol effects syndrome (FES), occurring in 3 to 5 in 1,000 live-born babies (101). A survey published in 1997 indicated that the combined rate of FAS and FES was at least 9.1 in 1,000 live births (102).

Data obtained from a variety of experimental models suggest that alcohol, or a metabolic product thereof, such as acetaldehyde, can adversely affect the developing brain through multiple mechanisms. These include direct effects such as a transient impairment in uterine blood flow, vasoconstriction of uterine vessels, and reduced fetal cerebral metabolic rate. In addition, alcohol is capable of affecting adversely DNA methylation, neurotransmitter receptors, signal transduction, trophic support of neurons, and membrane fluidization. The various potential mechanisms by which alcohol can damage the developing nervous system have been reviewed by West and colleagues (103) and Shibley and Pennington (104).

Even so, considerable debate surrounds the pathogenesis of FAS and FES. On the one hand, some researchers question whether there is a threshold amount of alcohol intake, beyond which fetal abnormalities can develop, and suggest that even the smallest amount of alcohol can be dangerous to the fetus. On the other hand, it is not known what role several other variables play in the production of FAS and FES. These variables include the type and quality of the alcoholic beverage consumed, particularly the presence of contaminants in illicitly procured alcohol, associated food and vitamin deficiencies, binge drinking, smoking during pregnancy, drug intake, low plasma zinc levels, and the stage of pregnancy when exposure occurred (105–107). Also not established is whether the same dysmorphology can occur in the absence of maternal alcohol intake. Lacking such data, it is unclear whether alcohol per se causes FAS and FES or whether high maternal alcohol intake is but a reflection of other environmental or genetic causes of mental retardation. An excellent review of the clinical application of the various animal models for *in utero* alcohol damage can be found in a 1984 Ciba Foundation Symposium (108) and a review by Dow and Riopelle (109).

Neuropathologic features of FAS include neuroglial and leptomeningeal heterotopias with aberrant neural and glial tissue incorporated within arachnoid and meninges (110). Lissencephaly, cerebellar dysplasia, and agenesis of the corpus callosum also have been described, and migration anomalies can involve the cerebellum and brainstem, as well as the cerebrum (111). Using material obtained for the most part during voluntary medical abortions, Konovalov and colleagues have shown that the proportion of fetuses showing these abnormalities in brain development increases with an increase in maternal ethanol intake (112), being lowest in women who were binge drinking during the first 3 months of pregnancy. They suggest that the teratogenic period for induction of the brain defects involves the initial 3 to 6 weeks of brain morphogenesis. These observations are at variance with those of Autti-Rämö and colleagues who found that the number of physical anomalies was significantly increased in infants exposed to alcohol throughout gestation, but not when heavy alcohol consumption, defined as in excess of 140 g per

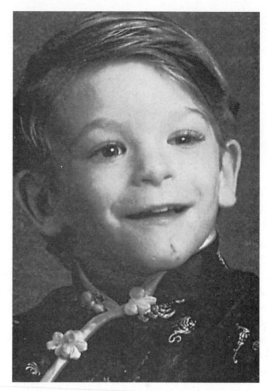

FIG. 9.1. Patient with fetal alcohol syndrome. This boy experienced intrauterine growth retardation and now shows mild mental retardation. His facies are typical, showing hypoplastic philtrum, thinning of upper lip, and flattening of the maxillary area. (Courtesy of Dr. William Torch, Neurodevelopmental and Neurodiagnostic Center, Reno, NV.)

week, was limited to the first or to the first and second trimesters (113).

The diagnosis of FAS is based entirely on history and the physical appearance of the child. In addition to confirmation of maternal alcohol abuse, the diagnostic criteria recommended by the Research Society on Alcoholism Fetal Alcohol Study Group require the following three: (a) the presence of prenatal or postnatal growth retardation; (b) CNS dysfunction such as developmental delay or intellectual impairment; and (c) at least two of the following: microcephaly, microphthalmia, short palpebral fissures, or all three, and hypoplastic philtrum with thin upper lip and flattening of the maxillary area (114) (Fig. 9.1). When a child demonstrates two of the three criteria, the condition is diagnosed with fetal alcohol effect (FAE). The use of this term has been challenged by Aase and colleagues on the basis of its imprecision, and that by labeling a child as having FAE, health workers presuppose that maternal alcohol abuse is the major or only cause of the child's problems (115).

Optic nerve hypoplasia is seen in up to one-half of children born to alcoholic mothers (116). Other ocular anomalies include microphthalmia, glaucoma, and cataracts (117). Less often, a sensorineural hearing loss and a variety of other minor physical anomalies occur (113). Outside the nervous system abnormalities of the heart (notably ventricular septal defects), joints (e.g., congenital dislocation of the hips and flexion-extension deformities), genitalia, or skeleton occur (118,119).

A considerable amount of work has been done to ascertain the long-term cognitive development of children diagnosed in infancy as having FAS or FAE. Two such studies can be cited as examples of the problems encountered in this endeavor. In the Finnish study of Autti-Rämö and colleagues, children who were subjected to heavy alcohol exposure throughout gestation had significantly lower scores on the Bayley Mental Scale and the Reynell Verbal Comprehension Test at 27 months of age. This study, however, failed to find any significant effect on intellectual development when heavy prenatal alcohol exposure was restricted to the first trimester. In this study, as in many others, social class and maternal education could have been confounding variables (120). In the German study of Spohr and coworkers, children were reexamined more than 10 years after their initial diagnosis (121). Many of the features of FAS and some of the minor physical anomalies had disappeared in the interval, so that it became difficult to diagnose FAS in a substantial proportion of children who initially had a mild expression of FAS. In severely affected children with FAS, the features of the condition tended to persist. In the series of Spohr and colleagues (121), 88% of FAS children were microcephalic at the first assessment at 3 years of age, and 65% at the second assessment at approximately 11 years of age. There was little improvement in IQ scores, and 69% of children had an IQ of 85 or less. It was noteworthy that not all children with

mild morphologic damage had normal intelligence and not all children with severe morphologic changes were mentally retarded. These findings are at variance with the observations of Mattsen and colleagues (122) who found that alcohol-exposed children displayed significant deficits in overall IQ measures even in the absence of any dysmorphic features.

Several other studies purport to demonstrate that even children whose IQs fall within the normal range have deficits in cognitive function, particularly in language development, and that school performance tends to deteriorate with time (121,123,124). It is quite likely that an adverse social environment contributes substantially to these features.

Acute Alcohol Poisoning

Acute alcohol intake by infants and young children initially induces a depression of the CNS, and if untreated, it causes marked hypoglycemia and convulsions several hours after ingestion (125,126). The mechanism for hypoglycemia is not completely understood. Wilson and coworkers suggest that ethanol inhibits hepatic gluconeogenesis because of an increase in the ratio of nicotinamide-adenine dinucleotide (reduced form) (NADH) to nicotinamide-adenine dinucleotide (NAD), and possibly also because it inhibits the carboxylation of pyruvate to oxaloacetate (127).

Theophylline (Aminophylline)

Theophylline, like other alkylxanthines, lowers the seizure threshold by antagonizing the anticonvulsant effect of endogenous adenosine (128). Neurologic symptoms can result from administration of a toxic dose of the drug, or from a therapeutic dose in children who have a lowered seizure threshold as a result of a preexisting seizure disorder or other previous brain injury or disease (129). Seizures are usually the most serious complication. These are often accompanied by cerebral vasoconstriction and ischemia. Ataxia, visual hallucinations, dyskinesias, and infantile spasms also have been reported as complications of theophylline toxicity (130–132). In premature infants, toxic effects include tachycardia, jitteriness, clonic posturing, and generalized seizures (133). Treatment of seizures involves the various anticonvulsants used for status epilepticus (see Chapter 13). Exchange transfusions also have been used in neonates given toxic dosages of theophylline.

Barbiturates

With the increased availability of other sedatives, the incidence of barbiturate intoxication in infants and children has diminished substantially since the 1980s.

Pharmacology

Barbiturates are general depressants. The mechanism of their action has been reviewed by Olsen and coworkers (134). In essence, toxic effects on the CNS result from the particular sensitivity of the reticular activating system to barbiturates. On a subcellular basis, barbiturates act on the γ-aminobutyric acid ($GABA_A$) receptor sites of postsynaptic neurons to increase the GABA-induced chloride current, thus potentiating the inhibitory effects of GABA.

The severity of intoxication induced by a given dose of barbiturate varies considerably. At comparable blood levels, slow-acting barbiturates are less toxic than rapid-acting thiobarbiturates. Other factors affecting the severity of clinical symptoms are the development of tolerance, as occurs in children treated with barbiturates for a convulsive disorder, and the rapidity with which the drug is metabolized by the liver.

Clinical Manifestations

Clinical symptoms of barbiturate intoxication are mainly those of CNS depression. A modified Glasgow Coma Scale, which scores both the level of consciousness and vital signs (respiratory rate, blood pressure, and hypothermia), has been suggested as a means of grading the severity of barbiturate intoxication (135). In severe intoxication, the child is comatose, although the deep tendon reflexes can persist and the plantar reflex is often positive. Barbiturates are respiratory depressants; they impair respiratory drive and the mechanisms responsible for rhythmic respiratory movements. Respiratory centers become insensitive to increased CO_2, and respiratory control becomes dependent on hypoxic drive, which, in turn, fails with progressively increasing barbiturate levels. As a consequence, respiration is affected early, and breathing becomes slow and shallow. Blood pressure decreases as a direct action of the drug on the myocardium and the depression of the medullary centers. A central antidiuretic action depresses urine formation. Hypoxia and pulmonary complications are common with severe barbiturate poisoning. Neuropathologic findings closely resemble those of fatal anoxia.

Diagnosis

The diagnosis of barbiturate intoxication in a child with severe CNS depression or coma rests on the history of drug ingestion or, in the absence of such a history, on the exclusion of other causes for coma and on the positive identification of the toxin.

The physical examination, which must be performed expeditiously, should be directed toward the exclusion of infectious, traumatic, metabolic, and vascular causes for the child's condition. Nuchal rigidity and focal neurologic signs make drug ingestion unlikely. Mitchell and colleagues (136) have stressed the frequency of miosis in children who are comatose owing to barbiturate intoxication and noted that miosis is usually absent in children admitted in coma as a consequence of head trauma or infection. The physician must always consider the possibility of nonaccidental barbiturate ingestion, which is an increasing form of child abuse (137).

A number of rapid urinary screening tests are available that produce characteristic color reactions in the presence of barbiturates or other toxins.

Treatment

Because barbiturate levels in brain correlate poorly with those in serum, serum barbiturate levels can only serve as a guide to assess the severity of intoxication. If the drug was ingested shortly before the child is examined, gastric lavage is done. When respirations are depressed, an airway is instituted and artificial respiration is used whenever necessary to maintain normal blood CO_2 and pH levels. Circulatory collapse, the chief cause of death in barbiturate intoxication, is prevented with plasma expanders or whole blood. Vasopressors are of relatively little value except in the initial management of severe hypotension (138). Forced diuresis with fluid loading and alkalinization by the intravenous administration of sodium bicarbonate facilitate urinary excretion of phenobarbital and other long-lasting barbiturates. Renal failure and hypothermia are other potentially serious complications of barbiturate intoxication (139).

In severe intoxication, or in children who because of renal or hepatic disease have impaired drug elimination, hemodialysis or peritoneal dialysis is the most effective means of removing the drug from the bloodstream (140). The effectiveness of peritoneal dialysis depends on the blood barbiturate level, which is usually high when long-acting barbiturates are ingested. Multiple doses of charcoal appear to be of little benefit. They decrease barbiturate serum half-life, but do not affect the clinical course (141).

Detoxification with hemoperfusion through charcoal coated with acrylic hydrocarbons also has been suggested. However, charcoal embolization to the CNS and pyrexia are significant complications of hemoperfusion; with the current mortality of barbiturate intoxication being less than 1%, it seems unwise to introduce another hazard into a child who will recover with simpler and less aggressive methods. The use of analeptics such as picrotoxin has been abandoned because they were found to induce cardiac arrhythmias and convulsions.

The presentation of benzodiazepine overdose is similar to that of barbiturate intoxication, and treatment is analogous, except that diuresis and forced alkalinization are unnecessary, because diazepines are metabolized by the liver. As a class, benzodiazepines are safer than barbiturates, and the mortality for intoxications is far smaller (139).

Phenothiazines

The neurotoxic actions of phenothiazines result from either an overdose or idiosyncratic adverse reactions to therapeutic dosages. The toxic responses include depression of consciousness, seizures, hypotension, loss of temperature control, and movement disorders. Movement disorders constitute the major adverse effects of therapeutic doses of phenothiazines. Although all phenothiazines can produce movement disorders, the extrapyramidal signs in children occur most commonly with prochlorperazine, haloperidol, thiaridazine, chlorpromazine, and clozapine (142).

Several kinds of movement disorders have been encountered. They can follow an acute ingestion or appear as side effects of chronic treatment. Younger children tend to have generalized manifestations, whereas adolescents tend to have signs localized to face and trunk (142). The most common are sudden episodes of opisthotonus accompanied by marked deviation of the eyes, and torticollis without loss of consciousness. Dystonic movements of the tongue, face, and neck muscles, drooling, trismus, ataxia, tremor, episodic rigidity, and oculogyric crises also are seen. Seizures are rare, but can be mimicked by violent dystonic movements.

A neuroleptic malignant syndrome has occasionally been encountered. The most common inciting drugs are haloperidol, phenothiazines, butyrophenones, and thioxanthines. The condition generally develops 3 to 9 days after initiation of neuroleptic treatment. It manifests by hyperthermia, muscular rigidity, extrapyramidal signs, opisthotonus, altered consciousness, and autonomic disturbances. Hyperthermia does not always have to be present (143). Serum creatine phosphokinase is elevated, and myoglobinuria is common. The condition lasts approximately 7 to 10 days (144). Drowsiness is common in patients who ingested toxic doses of phenothiazines, but rare when symptoms are caused by an idiosyncratic reaction to the drug. Persistence of the dyskinesias after withdrawal of the drug is relatively common in young adults, but rare in children (145). Other neurologic aspects of the movement disorder are considered in Chapter 2.

Extrapyramidal movements have been reported in newborns whose mothers received phenothiazines before delivery. The movement disorder is accompanied by hypertonia, tremor, and a poor suck reflex. It can persist for up to 12 months (146).

Diagnosis of phenothiazine intoxication depends on the history of drug ingestion. The most common appearance of the extrapyramidal disorder, namely as episodes of opisthotonus, trismus, and dystonic posturing, is distinctive. Paroxysmal choreoathetosis can present a similar picture, but its onset is gradual with a prolonged history of recurrent attacks. The presence of a positive urine ferric chloride test result (light pink to lilac) is common in chronic intoxication, but rare after acute drug ingestion.

Diphenylhydramine in a dose of 2 mg/kg, given intravenously over the course of 5 minutes, is an effective antidote for the extrapyramidal disorder appearing at therapeutic doses, and it often produces a dramatic response. Benztropine mesylate (0.5 mg/kg), given intravenously, or diazepam also is effective (142).

The neuroleptic malignant syndrome is treated by discontinuing the neuroleptic, reduction of hyperthermia by means of cooling blankets, and support of respiratory and cardiovascular status. The administration of dantrolene (0.5 mg/kg every 12 hours) or bromocriptine has been suggested, but controlled studies do not appear to show that either drug administered singly or in combination shortens the illness (147).

Antibacterial Agents

The increasing number of antibacterial agents used by clinicians for the treatment of various infectious diseases also has increased the incidence of neurologic complications associated with antibacterial therapy. The various clinical syndromes of neurotoxicity are shown in Table 9.4. They also have been reviewed by Thomas (148) and Wallace (149).

Encephalopathy/Seizures

The β-lactam antibiotics, notably penicillins, cephalosporins, and carbapenems, can manifest significant neurotoxicity. Studies on animal models have shown the toxic effect of penicillins to be caused by a dose-dependent inhibition of the GABA-gated chloride ion influx (148,149a).

The principal manifestations of β-lactam toxicity are seizures. The major risk factors for

TABLE 9.4. *Neurotoxicity of antibacterial therapy*

Syndrome	Drugs
Seizures, encephalopathy, organic brain syndrome	Cephalosporins
	Erythromycin
	Metronidazole
	Penicillins
	Rifampin
Cerebellar ataxia	Metronidazole
Pseudotumor cerebri	Nalidixic acid
	Nitrofurantoin
	Tetracyclines
	Trimethoprim-sulfamethoxazole
Aseptic meningitis	Trimethoprim-sulfamethoxazole
Myasthenic syndrome	Aminoglycosides
	Ampicillin
	Clindamycin
	Erythromycin
	Lincomycin
	Polymyxins
	Tetracycline
Optic neuritis	Chloramphenicol
	Ethambutol
	Isoniazid
Cochlear toxicity	Aminoglycosides
Vestibular toxicity	Aminoglycosides
	Erythromycin
	Tetracyclines
Peripheral neuropathy	Chloramphenicol
	Colistin
	Dapsone
	Ethionamide
	Isoniazid
	Metronidazole
	Nitrofurantoin

Adapted from Thomas RJ. Neurotoxicity of antibacterial therapy. *South Med J* 1994;9:869.

development of seizures are high-dose intravenous use of the antibiotic, impaired renal function, a preexisting or concurrent CNS disorder such as meningitis, and the concomitant use of drugs such as theophylline, which can lower the seizure threshold (149). In addition to seizures the β-lactams can cause hallucinations, and in the case of ceftazidime, absence status epilepticus (149).

Cochlear and Vestibular Damage

Several aminoglycoside antibiotics can induce damage to the eighth nerve. Gentamicin and tobramycin can damage both cochlear and vestibular components, whereas neomycin, kanamycin, and amikacin affect the auditory component predominantly. These complications are less common in children than in adults. Routine studies of brainstem auditory-evoked potentials during aminoglycoside therapy can detect high-frequency hearing loss as an early sign of ototoxicity (150). The development of ototoxicity is related to the dosage and duration of aminoglycoside therapy, the presence of impaired renal function, and probably a genetic predisposition to aminoglycoside susceptibility. Symptomatic hearing loss is seen initially as reduced high-frequency acuity, followed by impairment of lower frequency hearing, damage to the hair cells, and complete destruction of the organ of Corti with ultimate eighth nerve damage.

Neuromuscular Blockage

A myasthenic syndrome has been encountered in children treated with neomycin, ampicillin, gentamicin, and other aminoglycoside antibiotics. These drugs should therefore be used cautiously in children with neuromuscular disease, notably myasthenia gravis (151).

Pesticides

Organophosphates

Organophosphate insecticides are widely used on food crops throughout the world. These chemicals inhibit acetylcholinesterase and result in an accumulation of acetyl choline and overstimulation of the muscarinic postganglionic fibers of the parasympathetic nervous system. When ingested or inhaled, manifestations are of three types: acute, intermediate, and delayed. The acute syndrome represents a cholinergic crisis with headache, abdominal pain, irritability, sweating, miosis, and muscular twitching (152). After recovery, which generally occurs within 24 to 96 hours of the poisoning, an intermediate syndrome develops in many patients. This is characterized by profound muscular weakness, affecting predomi-

nantly the proximal and respiratory muscles, and often accompanied by cranial nerve palsies. Dystonia was seen in approximately 20% of Sri Lanka patients (153). Symptoms resolve within 1 to 5 weeks. A delayed polyneuropathy appears 2 to 3 weeks after the poisoning and often blends into the intermediate phase. It primarily affects the distal musculature, with recovery in 6 to 12 months. Controversy exists as to whether neurobehavioral effects persist after recovery (154).

Atropine has been recommended for treatment during the acute phase. For children younger than 12 years of age, the dose is 0.05 mg/kg, given intravenously. This is followed by a maintenance dosage of 0.02 to 0.05 mg/kg every 10 to 30 minutes until the cholinergic signs are no longer present or until pupils become dilated. Pralidoxime, given intravenously over the course of 15 to 30 minutes in a dose of 25 to 50 mg/kg, also has been recommended (155).

Organochlorines

Endrin is the most toxic of the organochlorine pesticides and has been responsible for several epidemics throughout the world. Symptoms are caused by CNS excitation. This results from suppression of the GABA-induced chloride current, and with it, suppression of the GABA-mediated synaptic inhibition (156). Symptoms occur within 12 hours of the poisoning. Convulsions are frequently the presenting symptom. Older children report headache, nausea, and muscle spasms just before the seizures (157). Phenobarbital or benzodiazepines are generally effective in controlling seizures, although recurrent convulsions are not unusual (158).

Lindane, another chlorinated hydrocarbon, has been used extensively in the form of Kwell for the treatment of scabies, and its accidental ingestion by toddlers is not unusual. If ingested in sufficient amounts, the substance can induce depression of consciousness, coma, and major motor seizures (159). The clinical picture of exposure to the various types of pesticides is reviewed by O'Malley (154).

Psychedelic Drugs

Fashions occur in psychedelic drugs, as they do in clothes. Currently, the use of 3,4-methylene-dioxymethamphetamine, also known as *ecstasy*, among college students and adolescents exceeds that of lysergic acid diethylamine and cocaine (160). Accidental poisoning with psychedelic drugs is uncommon in small children and is generally not life threatening.

Intoxication with phencyclidine is often produced by passive inhalation (161,162). The psychosis seen in older subjects is less common in small children than a depressed sensorium, hypotonia, dystonia or opisthotonus, and ataxia. Seizures as well as opisthotonus and a variety of ocular signs, notably horizontal or vertical nystagmus and miosis, can be encountered after phencyclidine or ecstasy ingestion (161,163). Treatment is symptomatic and observation of the intoxicated youngster usually suffices. A variety of barbiturates or phenothiazines can be used for sedation.

Hexachlorophene

Hexachlorophene, a chlorinated phenolic compound widely used as an antiseptic until 1972, when it became a prescription drug, has been shown to induce seizures when absorbed through burned or extensively excoriated skin. Significant amounts also are absorbed through the intact skin of small premature neonates (164).

Accidental ingestion of hexachlorophene by older children results in vomiting, hypotension, and a neurologic picture characterized by total blindness caused by deterioration of the optic nerves (165). Additionally, behavioral changes, convulsions, increased intracranial pressure, paralysis, and spastic paraparesis or paraplegia can occur (166).

Mepivacaine

In the past, the use of mepivacaine hydrochloride to induce paracervical or pudendal block in the course of labor resulted in accidental poisoning of the newborn by direct injection of the anesthetic. The clinical picture was reduced responsiveness, bradycardia, apnea, hypotonia, and seizures that commenced within 6 hours, usually between 1 and 3 hours of age. Mepivacaine intoxication is differentiated from perinatal asphyxia by the earlier onset of seizures and the abnormality of oculomotor reflexes, which in asphyxia tend to be preserved for the first few hours of life. The condition is self-limiting, and if asphyxia is prevented, infants return to normal by 18 hours of age (167).

Salicylate

A less widespread use of salicylates in this country has resulted in a significant reduction in the incidence of salicylate intoxication. Currently, most acute intoxications are the outcome of attempted suicide with aspirin or methylsalicylate (168). Both acute and chronic salicylate intoxication are associated with mental status depression whose severity is usually proportionate to the serum salicylate level (169). Additionally, a delayed encephalopathy owing to cerebral edema can develop. In some instances, this encephalopathy is associated with a rapid decrease in serum sodium concentrations, the consequence of inappropriate antidiuretic hormone secretion resulting from the action of salicylates on the brain (170). The administration of salicylates in a patient with an influenza virus or varicella infection can initiate Reye syndrome (see Chapter 6).

Eosinophilia-Myalgia Syndrome

Eosinophilia-myalgia syndrome is characterized by myalgia, eosinophilia, and a progressive neuropathy. Muscle biopsy demonstrates a perivascular eosinophilic infiltrate; sural nerve biopsy documents a demyelinating neuropathy with axonal degeneration (171). Involvement of the CNS includes seizures, dementia, and vascular infarctions (172). The condition is induced by consumption of tryptophan contaminated with 3-(phenylamino) alanine. This substance is chemically similar to 3-phenylamino-1,2-propanediol, an aniline derivative believed to be responsible for the contamination of rapeseed oil, which caused the toxic oil syndrome seen during 1981 in the central region of Spain (173). Cooking oil contaminated with polychlorinated biphenyls has been responsible for mass poisoning in Japan and central Taiwan. Neurologic symptoms include polyneuropathy. Children who were *in utero* when their mothers consumed contaminated oil were prone to severe developmental deficits (174).

Neonatal Drug Addiction

The increasing prevalence of drug abuse among women of child-bearing age has made relatively common the problem of neonates born to mothers addicted to cocaine, methamphetamine, heroin, or other opiates, or who receive methadone as part of a drug treatment program.

Cocaine

Four aspects of the effect of cocaine on the developing nervous system are considered: teratogenic effects, acute effects evident during the neonatal period, long-term effects on cognition, and accidental intoxication.

The most common teratogenic effect of cocaine is a reduction in head circumference. When cocaine-exposed infants are compared with control infants, head circumferences of the former group are significantly smaller. This observation in drug-exposed infants is probably significant, because it persists when birth weight and other confounding variables are controlled (175–177). Reports of other malformations are more anecdotal. These include disorders of midline prosencephalic development, septo-optic dysplasia, agenesis of the corpus callosum, and neuronal heterotopias (178). The mechanism for the teratogenic effects of cocaine is not clear.

The clinical picture of the drug-exposed neonate results from the effects of these drugs on intrauterine development and their postnatal withdrawal.

Cocaine is passed to the fetus through the maternal circulation during pregnancy and in breast milk. It acts as a sympathomimetic agent and impairs the reuptake of norepinephrine and epinephrine by presynaptic nerve endings, activating the adrenergic system and inducing vasoconstriction. Cocaine also impairs dopamine and serotonin reuptake. The vasoconstriction and reduced cerebral blood flow induced by cocaine probably are direct effects of the alkaloid and are not caused by an increase in catecholamines.

A neonate exposed *in utero* to cocaine can be born prematurely or be small for gestational age. As a rule, growth retardation is symmetric, as contrasted to the asymmetric growth retardation seen with maternal malnutrition (175). A number of physical and behavioral disturbances are common during the first few days of life. These include excessive jitteriness, tachycardia, tremors, irritability, poor feeding, an increased startle response, and abnormal sleep patterns, with excessive drowsiness after the hyperirritable stage (177,179,180). Seizures were observed in 81% of the neonates of Kramer and coworkers. They developed within 36 hours of birth (181). A transient dystonic reaction also has been reported (182). Cerebrospinal fluid (CSF) examination and neuroimaging study results are generally normal, although cerebral infarction has been encountered. The electroencephalogram (EEG) tends to be abnormal during the first few weeks of life, with multifocal bursts of spikes and sharp waves. Neurologic and electrical abnormalities are transient and usually do not continue beyond 3 weeks, although in the series of Kramer and colleagues, collected from Watts, California, one-half of the infants went on to develop epilepsy (181). The reason for persistence of seizures is unclear.

In utero exposure to cocaine has been implicated in several instances of cerebral infarction, usually in the distribution of the middle cerebral artery. Cerebral blood flow velocity is increased in the anterior cerebral artery for the first 2 days of life, an observation consistent with the presence of vasoconstriction (177). Although Dixon and Bejar have reported an abnormal cranial ultrasound in 41% of term cocaine-exposed newborns (183), the controlled study by King and coworkers found no difference in the incidence of neurosonographic abnormalities between cocaine-exposed infants and controls (177).

The effects of maternal drug addiction on the ultimate physical and cognitive development of offspring have not been clarified. The catch up in weight and length is analogous to that seen in small-for-date infants due to other causes. The effect of intrauterine cocaine exposure on head circumference becomes progressively less significant during the first and second years of postnatal life (176). When adequately controlled for socioeconomic status, there is also no significant impairment in early language development in children with *in utero* exposure to cocaine (184). In their review of the cognitive development of offspring of mothers with drug and alcohol abuse, Zuckerman and Bresnahan concluded that such infants are clearly at risk for developmental and behavioral problems, but that it is difficult to separate the biological vulnerability caused by prenatal drug exposure from the environmental vulnerability caused by an environment formed by drug use (106).

The clinical manifestations of accidental cocaine ingestion are a function of the age of the child when ingestion occurs. In the experience of Mott and colleagues, children younger than 7 years of age present with seizures, whereas in older children obtundation or delirium are the characteristic presenting symptoms (185).

Opiates

The effect of opiates on the fetus and on the newborn has been well studied. As a rule, symptoms are more severe than those resulting from exposure to cocaine. Approximately one-half of infants of addicted mothers weigh less than 2,500 g, and many of these are small for their gestational age. Additionally, 40% have a head circumference below the tenth percentile (186). Approximately two-thirds of infants born to heroin-addicted mothers develop symptoms (187). These symptoms generally become apparent during the first 48 hours of life. In order of frequency of occurrence, they are fist sucking, irritability, tremors, vomiting, high-pitched cry, sneezing, hypertonia, and abnormal sleep patterns (188,189). Seizures are relatively uncommon (187). The severity of the clinical course is related to the length of maternal addiction, the length of time from the last dose to birth, the magnitude of the drug doses taken, and the gestational age of the infant, with withdrawal symptoms being more severe in term infants (189). For reasons as yet undetermined, the incidence of intraventricular hemorrhage is less in neonates of opiate-dependent mothers than in infants of comparable weight born to nonaddicted mothers (190).

Untreated, the opiate withdrawal syndrome has a significant mortality. Administration of benzodiazepines is of considerable benefit. Clonidine, phenothiazines, barbiturates, methadone, and paregoric also have been recommended. Dosages and modes of administration of these drugs are reviewed by Yaster and coworkers (191).

Follow-up studies on infants of opiate- and methadone-addicted mothers indicate that the effects on growth parameters resolve by 1 to 2 years of age (192), and that antenatal exposure to illicit drugs does not increase infant mortality (193). Developmental scores and overall IQ are normal, but children have a higher incidence of behavioral abnormalities, notably temper tantrums and impulsivity, than children matched for socioeconomic status (194–196). As is the case for children of cocaine- and alcohol-addicted mothers, the developmental outcome is influenced more by the home environment than by exposure of the developing brain to toxin (196).

Kernicterus

The term *kernicterus*, originally coined by Schmorl in 1903 (197), has been used both pathologically and clinically. Pathologically, it indicates a canary yellow staining of circumscribed areas of the basal ganglia, brainstem, and cerebellum; clinically, it describes a syndrome consisting of athetosis, impaired vertical gaze, and auditory loss or imperception.

Up to 1990, kernicterus had nearly disappeared; its reemergence is probably the result of a shortened hospital stay for term neonates and a decreased concern about jaundice when it develops in breast-fed infants (198).

Pathology and Pathogenesis

On gross inspection, deposition of deep yellow pigment is noted in the meninges, choroid plexus, and numerous areas of the brain itself (199). The unique topography of neuronal damage in kernicterus is essentially the same in full-term and premature infants. Regions most commonly affected are the basal ganglia, particularly the globus pallidus, the subthalamic nucleus, the dentate nuclei, the cerebellar vermis, sectors H2 and H3 of the hippocampus, and the cranial nerve nuclei, notably the oculomotor, vestibular, and cochlear nuclei. The cerebral cortex is spared.

The microscopic alterations point to the cell membrane as the primary site of damage, with mitochondrial changes being secondary to disorganization of the cytoplasmic membranes.

Two distinct pathologic entities can be distinguished. In brains that are grossly stained yellow, the most frequently observed abnormality is a spongy degeneration and gliosis. In others, there is neuronal degeneration and deposition of the pigment within neurons, their processes, and the surrounding glial cells (200). Neurons can be in various stages of degeneration, the severity of degeneration being proportional to the age of the patient. A marked neuronal loss with demyelination and astrocytic replacement is observed in patients who die after the first month of kernicterus.

Although the exact pathogenesis of kernicterus in the term infant is far from clear, several factors acting in concert are involved. They include hyperbilirubinemia, reduced serum bilirubin-binding capacity, opening of the blood–brain barrier, and damaged or dead brain tissue.

The role of hyperbilirubinemia in the production of kernicterus has been known since the classic studies of Hsia and coworkers at Boston Children's Hospital (201). High bilirubin levels can be caused not only by Rh incompatibility but by several other conditions as well (202). The causes of neonatal hyperbilirubinemia and guidelines for treatment have been reviewed by Newman and Maisels (203) and Gourley (198).

Considerable evidence suggests that hyperbilirubinemia alone, even when extreme, is not sufficient for the production of kernicterus. Hyperbilirubinemia unaccompanied by isoimmunization or other adverse factors usually has no detrimental effect on motor and cognitive development or on hearing when these parameters are tested after the first year of life (204). At bilirubin levels of 30 mg/dL or higher, the likelihood of developing kernicterus is no greater than 50%. Thus, in a series of 105 full-term and 24 premature babies whose peak indirect bilirubin levels were between 20 and 30.8 mg/dL, only seven, two of them preterm, were found to have abnormal results on neurologic and psychological examination some 5 years later. Of these, one infant's jaundice was the result of Rh incompatibility. ABO incompatibility, sepsis, and unknown factors were responsible for jaundice in the remainder (205).

These observations, published in 1967, have since been amply verified from a number of centers (206). However, they must be qualified by the observation that kernicterus can develop in breast-fed infants in the absence of isoimmune or hemolytic disease (207). Kernicterus is extremely rare in adults, even when massive elevation of indirect serum bilirubin occurs. Patients with a congenital deficiency of glucuronyl transferase (the Crigler-Najjar I syndrome), whose indirect bilirubin levels typically range from 10 to 44 mg/dL, have been known to be free of neurologic symptoms for many years before developing a rapidly progressive extrapyramidal disorder, often after an infection (208). The clinical manifestations of Crigler-Najjar syndromes are reviewed by Labrune and colleagues (209) and Rubboli and colleagues (210). Most recently, the condition has been treated by infusion of hepatocytes (210a).

The most plausible current theory is that the clinical and pathologic picture of kernicterus results from antecedent or concomitant damage to the CNS with breakdown of the blood–brain barrier and uptake by brain of albumin-bound bilirubin (211). A number of factors, present singly or in concert, can act as noxious agents on the blood–brain barrier and nerve cells. Some of these, notably Rh hemolytic disease, ABO incompatibility, and hyperosmolarity, can do so by damaging the vascular endothelium of the brain, whereas prenatal and perinatal anoxia, sepsis, and acidosis can damage the nerve cell directly (212,213). Sepsis appears to be a particularly important factor. In the series of Pearlman and associates, two-thirds of infants who died of sepsis had kernicterus as evidenced by yellow discoloration of the susceptible nuclei and neuronal degeneration and necrosis in the stained lesions. In these infants, none of whom had any characteristic clinical abnormalities for kernicterus, neither acidosis nor the use of antibiotics known to displace bilirubin from albumin appeared to be responsible for the evolution of kernicterus (212).

The role of bilirubin-albumin binding in facilitating the entry of bilirubin into the brain is stressed by the observation that analbuminemic individuals do not develop kernicterus (214). In experimental animals, bilirubin deposited in brain is derived not only from the free fraction, but to a significant extent (30% to 60%) from the albumin-bound fraction. Whatever the source of the bilirubin, on theoretical grounds, free bilirubin is cytotoxic and induces an immediate and marked disturbance of brain energy metabolism. The exact mechanism by which bilirubin produces mitochondrial dysfunction is unknown. Several mechanisms have been proposed. Bilirubin binds to phospholipids and gangliosides of cellular membranes, and, as a consequence initiates a cascade of events. In experimental animals, these include interference with neuronal oxygen consumption and protein phosphorylation, and an alteration of the N-methyl-D-aspartate receptor (215,216). The role of drug-bilirubin interaction in the pathogenesis of kernicterus has been reviewed by Walker (217).

In premature infants, other factors in addition to an elevated serum bilirubin level are believed to be important in causing kernicterus. In the course of the 1980s and 1990s, the incidence of kernicterus in premature infants coming to autopsy, which up to then had been approximately 25%, has decreased significantly to approximately 4% for the period of 1983 to 1993 (218,219). The reasons for this decline are unclear. Jardine and Rogers have suggested that it is related to the discontinuation of benzyl alcohol, a bacteriostatic agent added to intravenous

fluids and medications (220). Other workers, however, have noted that the incidence of exposure to benzyl alcohol was no greater in infants who went on to develop kernicterus than in those who did not (221).

Clinical Manifestations

The jaundiced infant developing kernicterus becomes drowsy by the second to fifth day of life and begins to nurse poorly. The infant develops fever, has a monotonous cry, and loses the Moro reflex (222). Approximately 10% of infants who go on to develop kernicterus have no clinical manifestations during the neonatal period.

By 2 weeks of age, the infant usually has developed hypertonia, with opisthotonus, extensor spasms, and in approximately 10% of cases, clonic convulsions. Over the ensuing months, the infant becomes hypotonic, and by 4 years of age the syndrome characteristic of kernicterus has evolved. The striking constancy of neurologic symptoms in the older child with kernicterus is evident from Table 9.5 (223).

Athetosis is present almost invariably, often with dystonia, rigidity, and tremors. Gaze palsy can involve movements in all directions, but vertical gaze is by far the most commonly involved. Auditory imperception can take the form of a hearing loss, a receptive aphasia, or a combination of both. In a number of patients, the vestibular portion of the eighth nerve also is involved (198,205). Severe mental retardation is relatively uncommon in youngsters with kernicterus, although impaired hearing and gaze paralysis make psychometric testing extremely

TABLE 9.5. *Clinical picture of patients with kernicterus*

Number of children with severe neonatal jaundice due to Rh factor	248
Athetosis	93%
Gaze palsy	91%
Dental enamel dysplasia	83%
Auditory imperception	43%
Extrapyramidal rigidity	5%

From Perlstein MA. The clinical syndrome of kernicterus. In: American Academy for Cerebral Palsy. *Kernicterus and its importance in cerebral palsy.* Springfield, IL: Charles C Thomas, 1961;268. With permission.

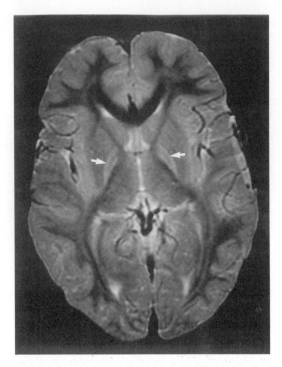

FIG. 9.2. Magnetic resonance imaging in kernicterus. T2-weighted images, 1.5T. The globus pallidus *(arrows)* is bilaterally demonstrated by both posteromedial and lateral outlines of high signal density. (Courtesy of Dr. Kenji Yokochi, Ohzora Hospital, Shizuoka, Japan.)

increased signal in the globus pallidus on T1-weighted images (198).

Diagnosis

The diagnosis of kernicterus in a term infant during the neonatal period rests on changes in body tone, abnormalities in eye movements, loss of the Moro reflex, and an abnormal cry, all in the presence of hyperbilirubinemia. The combination of extrapyramidal signs, ocular disturbances, and impaired hearing, although characteristic for kernicterus caused by isoimmunization, also can be seen in children who are only mildly jaundiced, but who have a history of prematurity and perinatal anoxia.

Treatment and Prognosis

The treatment of kernicterus rests on the prevention of severe hyperbilirubinemia. As pointed out by Maisels, it is known how, but not when, to treat hyperbilirubinemia. The role of exchange transfusions, multiple intrauterine transfusions, and phototherapy in the current treatment of isoimmunization and hyperbilirubinemia is discussed by Newman and Maisels (203) and Gourley (198). The use of metalloporphyrins for the prevention of neonatal jaundice has been reviewed by Gourley (198).

difficult. Of surviving children with kernicterus who could be tested, Byers and colleagues found 47% to have IQs between 90 and 110, and 27% between 70 and 90. The remainder (27%) had an IQ below 70 (224).

When brainstem auditory-evoked potentials are used to screen high-risk infants, one observes a correlation between maximum unbound bilirubin levels and abnormal central conduction times (225). It is becoming evident that any hearing loss in high-risk infants reflects the duration of hyperbilirubinemia and, more important, any associated hypoxia and respiratory acidosis (226,227).

MRI in children with kernicterus caused by Rh isoimmunization shows a symmetric increased signal in the globus pallidus on T2-weighted images (Fig. 9.2) (228). Some cases also show

Bacterial Toxins

The most potent nerve poisons known are produced by two anaerobic, spore-forming bacteria, *Clostridium botulinum* and *Clostridium tetani*.

Botulism

Botulism is induced by the ingestion of preserves and other canned goods in which *C. botulinum* has grown and produced toxin. The organism produces seven antigenically distinct protein toxins, of which A, B, and E are most commonly responsible for human disease.

The toxins produced by *C. botulinum* are lethal at the lowest dose per kilogram body weight of any of the known poisons. Calculated from data obtained in mice, the lethal dose for an adult is approximately 0.12 mg. Chemically, botulism toxin A, the most studied substance, is a simple polypeptide of known sequence with 33% homology to tetanus toxin. Its toxicity is lost with heat denaturation. Both botulinus and tetanus neurotoxins block the release of neurotransmitters. Whereas tetanus neurotoxin acts mainly on CNS synapses, the botulinum neurotoxins act peripherally on the terminal unmyelinated motor nerve fibrils blocking the release of acetylcholine. Three steps are involved: (a) irreversible binding of the toxin to the presynaptic nerve surface, (b) crossing of the toxin into the nerve terminal, probably by receptor-mediated endocytosis, and (c) disabling the release of acetylcholine by zinc-dependent proteolysis of three synaptic proteins (SNAP-25, VAMP, and syntaxin) involved in the exocytosis of neurotransmitters. A second, nonproteolytic inhibitory mechanism of action is believed to involve the activation of neuronal transglutaminases (229). The result is an interruption of transmission of the nerve impulse, producing a myasthenia-like syndrome (230).

Symptoms appear between 12 and 48 hours after ingestion of contaminated food. A prodromal period of nonspecific gastrointestinal symptoms is followed by the evolution of neurologic dysfunction (231). Initial symptoms include blurring of vision, impaired pupillary reaction to light, diplopia, and progressive weakness of the bulbar musculature. Paralysis of the major skeletal muscles follows, with death caused by respiratory arrest. In patients who do not die, convalescence is slow, and complete recovery of a totally paralyzed muscle can take as long as 1 year.

The clinical picture of botulism can be distinguished from various viral encephalitides by the early appearance in botulism of internal and external ophthalmoplegia, ptosis, and paralysis of the pupillary accommodation reflex. Electromyography (EMG) shows the motor unit action potentials to be brief and of small amplitude. Fibrillation potentials, consistent with functional denervation, are observed in approximately one-half of patients (232). Although the response to repetitive nerve stimulation is diagnostic for botulism, it may be normal in mild

cases, and incremental responses do not occur at slower rates of stimulation (5 Hz). In severe intoxication, transmitter release is blocked to such an extent that no increment occurs, even at rapid rates of stimulation (50 Hz) (233).

Infantile Botulism

This condition has its onset between ages 3 and 18 weeks and is characterized by hypotonia, hyporeflexia, and weakness of the cranial musculature. Infants often have an antecedent history of constipation and poor feeding, and a significantly large proportion (44%) has been fed honey (234).

Symptoms range from a mild disorder to one that resembles sudden infant death syndrome (SIDS). Bulbar signs predominate. These include a poor cry, poor sucking, an impaired pupillary light response, and external ophthalmoplegia. As the illness progresses, a flaccid paralysis develops. Autonomic dysfunction can be present; cardiovascular symptoms are absent, however, and the ECG remains normal (235). Almost all infants recover completely, with the illness lasting between 3 and 20 weeks. In 5% of infants, relapses occur 1 to 2 weeks after hospital discharge. The second bout of infantile botulism is just as severe or even more severe than the first attack (236).

The EMG results are similar to those seen in older individuals with botulism. It typically shows a pattern of brief duration, small-amplitude potentials with decremental response at low-frequency (3 to 10 Hz) repetitive stimulation, and an incremental (*staircase*) response at high-frequency (20 to 50 Hz) repetitive stimulation (237). The incremental response may not be seen in all muscles and is not as apparent at slower frequencies of nerve stimulation. Anticholinesterase medications should be withdrawn at least 8 hours before the study (237). When present, the finding of an incremental response to nerve stimulation is diagnostic, because the only other condition in which it is observed is Lambert-Eaton syndrome, an entity not seen in infants (238). The diagnosis can be confirmed by demonstrating the presence of toxin in serum before treatment (239).

Whereas botulism in older children and adults is generally, but not invariably, caused by the ingestion of preformed toxin, infant botulism results from the colonization of the gut with type A or type B spores of *C. botulinum*, and from the subsequent release of the toxin, which has been demonstrated in feces (240). Because spores of *C. botulinum* are ubiquitous and most individuals ingest *C. botulinum* without adverse effects, the cause for the illness is still obscure. A number of host factors, possibly constipation, immune deficiency, or unusual gut flora, also must be present to permit germination of the spores and production of the toxin within the gastrointestinal tract (241).

The diagnosis of infantile botulism is difficult to establish because the condition mimics septicemia, viral encephalitis, neonatal myasthenia gravis, and infectious polyneuritis. The predominance of bulbar symptoms in an infant who appears fairly aware of the surroundings should alert the clinician to the diagnosis and prompt the performance of an EMG.

In most cases, including all those of infant botulism, antitoxin administration is ineffective by the time botulism is diagnosed, and symptomatic therapy, including respiratory support and nasogastric feeding, must suffice. Recovery is slow. In the series of Schreiner and coworkers, the average duration of hospitalization in patients who required mechanical ventilation was 23 days (242). When treating with antibiotics, aminoglycosides that potentiate the paralysis must be avoided.

Tetanus

Tetanus is the result of an infection of wounded or damaged tissue by the spores of *Clostridium tetani*. Under anaerobic conditions, the spores germinate and the vegetative forms multiply to produce two toxins: a hemolysin and a neurotoxin.

The crystalline neurotoxin, tetanospasmin, is a 150,000-dalton protein, ranking second in potency only to botulism toxin. When tetanospasmin is treated with formalin, two molecules of protein polymerize to form toxoid, a nontoxic dimer with intact antigenicity that is used for immunizations.

Tetanus toxin enters the nervous system by binding to peripheral sensory, motor, and autonomic nerve terminals that are unprotected by a blood–brain barrier and traveling centrally by intra-axonal transport. The toxin binds to a highly specific protein receptor, and with lesser affinity to disialogangliosides and trisialogangliosides localized on the cell membrane (243). The toxin is then taken up by endocytosis and is transported retrograde via an intra-axonal transport system to the corresponding cell bodies, in the case of a peripheral injury, the alpha-motoneurons, at a rate of approximately 25 cm/day (244,245). When the toxin reaches the perikarya of motor neurons, it is passed transsynaptically to the surrounding presynaptic terminals, including the afferent fibers of the glycinergic inhibitors (246). The exact subcellular mechanism of action is similar to that of botulinum toxin in that it blocks exocytosis by proteolysis of synaptobrevin, one of the proteins involved in vesicle exocytosis (247).

The manifestations of tetanus result from the action of the toxin within the spinal cord and brainstem. The toxin blocks the release of GABA and glycine from the presynaptic terminals of the inhibitory polysynaptic circuits surrounding the motor neurons. Abolition of the inhibitory influence of afferent fibers on the motor neurons produces uncontrolled firing, which results in paroxysmal muscle spasms (248). At high toxin concentrations, excitatory transmission also is reduced, and the toxin prevents release of acetylcholine from the neuromuscular junction, thereby producing flaccid paralysis. Additionally, elevation of serum creatine phosphokinase and fluorescent binding techniques provide evidence that tetanospasmin produces direct injury to skeletal muscles.

Clinical Manifestations

Most commonly, symptoms appear approximately 1 week after injury. A number of authors have noted that the shorter the incubation period, the graver the infection. Trismus or stiffness of the neck and back is generally the earliest symptom. A characteristic retraction of the angles of the mouth has been termed *risus sardonicus* (Fig. 9.3). Rigidity becomes generalized, and tetanic spasms develop. These can be

Recovery from tetanus is slow. Approximately one-fourth of patients have major sleep disturbances for approximately 1 to 3 years. In approximately one-half, seizures, often accompanied by myoclonus, occur 1 to 2 months after apparent recovery and persist for 6 months to 1 year, with an average frequency of one major attack every 2 months (250).

Tetanus Neonatorum

Tetanus neonatorum is responsible for some 500,000 deaths a year, most of them in the developing countries, where umbilical cord sepsis and lack of maternal immunity contribute to its high incidence. In the United States, cases have been encountered in infants born to immigrant families (251).

The condition develops between the fourth and eighth day of life, with the more severe cases having a shorter incubation period. Irritability and trismus, with consequent inability to suck, are usually the earliest signs. As the disease progresses, infants develop opisthotonus and generalized tetanic spasms. These can be induced by stimulation, or in the more severe cases, appear spontaneously. In the most severe cases, the spasms become continuous and are accompanied by apneic episodes (252–254).

Treatment of neonatal tetanus is difficult even in technically more advanced countries. In their series of five patients, Adams and associates used nasotracheal intubation, mechanical ventilation, and neuromuscular blockade with pancuronium bromide to permit ventilatory control (255). Andersson has been successful with a relatively simple method of treatment. This consists of an initial intramuscular injection of diazepam (10 mg), followed by 5 to 10 mg of diazepam given by nasogastric tube four times daily, with additional diazepam administered rectally or intramuscularly as needed to maintain the infant free of spasms. Early nasogastric feedings are started to maintain the nutritional status of the infant. Diazepam is tapered when spasms and rigidity start to subside. This usually occurs after some 10 to 21 days (256). Metronidazole is preferred to penicillin or ampicillin, which like tetanus toxin are known antagonists of GABA (257). Einterz and Bates have reported on a similar regimen that they used in

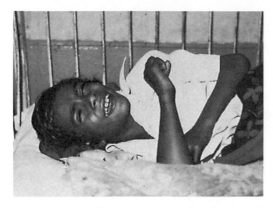

FIG. 9.3. Risus sardonicus in tetanus, causing an increased tone of all facial muscles, interfering with speech. Patient is a 6-year-old Pakistani boy after 7 days of therapy. (Courtesy of Dr. Muhammed Ibrahim Memon, Professor of Paediatric Medicine, Liaqut Medical College, Hyderabad, Pakistan.)

induced by various sensory stimuli or passive movements of the limbs, or they can occur spontaneously. Sudden respiratory failure, obstruction of the airway, and bronchopneumonia account for most deaths.

In some patients, muscular rigidity is initially localized to the area of the wound and only slowly extends to other muscles.

Tetanus owing to clostridial otitis media is distinctive in that trismus and risus sardonicus predominate over generalized spasms and rigidity.

Treatment of tetanus requires maintenance of an airway and adequate ventilation, administration of antitoxin as quickly as possible, debridement of the site of infection, treatment with an antibiotic such as penicillin to eradicate both vegetative and spore forms from the site of infection, and use of sedatives such as diazepam or phenobarbital. Patients who do not respond to any of these measures require neuromuscular blockade with curare-like agents. Despite these measures, the mortality of tetanus in children who demonstrate the full clinical picture is still high. In a 1987 series from Bombay, the overall mortality was 12%, and mortality in severe cases was 23%, with death being caused by unexpected cardiac arrest caused by arrhythmias, and to sudden hyperthermia and circulatory collapse (249).

Nigeria in a series of 237 cases of neonatal tetanus. They also have used phenobarbital (15 mg three times daily) via nasogastric tube (258). Other sedatives, including propanolol and paraldehyde, also have been recommended. Tetanus antiserum (30,000 to 40,000 U) is administered subcutaneously around the umbilicus, and 1,500 U are given intravenously, although Daud and colleagues believe that the mode of administering the antitoxin does not affect the outcome (259). Large amounts of intramuscular pyridoxine (100 mg/day) are said to lower mortality significantly (260). Even so, a series of some 200 cases of neonatal tetanus reported from developing countries indicates a mortality of at least 25%, and as recently as 1991, neonatal tetanus accounted for 30% to 70% of neonatal deaths in Africa (258). As is the case for older children and adults, the shorter the incubation period the more severe the disease, and the likelihood for survival increases when the incubation period is greater than 6 days.

Symptoms gradually abate after 25 to 45 days, and survivors appear neurologically and developmentally normal at 12 months of age.

Diphtheria

Although diphtheria is exceedingly rare in western countries as a result of widespread immunization programs, it still occurs with sufficient frequency in some of the developing countries to warrant mentioning its neurologic features (261). The clinical and pathologic features of diphtheria from the viewpoint of neurologists are reviewed in the classic publication by Miller Fisher and Adams (262).

Diphtheria results from an infection with *Corynebacterium diphtheriae*, which establishes itself on the mucous membranes of the throat or nasopharynx and can synthesize a potent, heat-labile toxin. This substance, a low-molecular-weight protein, interrupts the incorporation of amino acids into proteins (263). Once absorbed, the toxin is bound to membrane receptors and is transported intracellularly by endocytosis. The toxin does not cross the blood–brain barrier; its major effect is on the peripheral nervous system.

Neurologic symptoms are seen in 3% to 5% of children, with the incidence depending on the severity of the disease (261). The two types of symptoms are local paralyses and a polyneuropathy. Paralyses develop between the fifth and twelfth days of the illness and are marked by paralysis of the palate with a nasal voice, nasal regurgitation, and dysphagia. Hoarseness, numbness of the face, and ciliary paralysis with loss of accommodation ensue (262). Less often, the extraocular muscles are involved. Symptoms involving the other cranial nerves, such as deafness or loss of taste, have been noted on rare occasions. These deficits last 1 to 2 weeks, then gradually resolve.

A gradual evolution of a combined sensory and motor demyelinating, noninflammatory polyneuropathy, which affects mainly the lower extremities, can appear 5 to 8 weeks after the initial infection (262,264). The polyneuropathy progresses for 2 weeks, then resolves completely. The segmental demyelination responsible has a unique topography in that it is most marked in the anterior and posterior roots near the sensory ganglion. No inflammatory cells are evident (262).

Cardiac symptoms have been attributed to a toxin-induced myocarditis or to an involvement of the vagus nerve.

All these complications are preventable by early antitoxin therapy. Once symptoms have developed, treatment is nonspecific. Even so, most patients experience complete or functionally complete remission of symptoms.

Tick Paralysis

A progressive symmetric paralysis, associated with the bite of a wood or dog tick, is endemic in the Rocky Mountain and Appalachian regions of the United States. A similar condition also has been encountered in the Australian states of Victoria, Tasmania, and New South Wales, in Israel, and in South Africa (265,266). The disease also has been seen in one-humped Sudanese camels, llamas, and the red wolf (267). Symptoms are produced by a neurotoxin, secreted by the insect, that probably blocks depolarization in the terminal portions of the motor nerves and, in a manner as yet undelineated, also affects the large myelinated motor and sensory axons (268).

After a prodrome of a viral-like illness, the condition manifests by an unsteady gait, an ascending flaccid paralysis, and abnormalities of extraocular

TABLE 9.6. *Neurologic symptoms of animal venoms*

Animals	Symptoms	Action of venom	Reference
Coelentarata, jellyfish	Muscular weakness, respiratory paralysis	Unknown	Burnett et al. (276)
Mollusca, bivalve (infected by flagellate plankton, paralytic shellfish poisoning)	Ataxia, ascending paralysis, paresthesia	Binding to voltage-activated Na channel; blockade of nerve and muscle action potentials	Gessner et al. (277)
Mussels (contaminated)	Confusion, seizures, distal atrophy, alternating hemiparesis, ophthalmoplegia	Domoic acid, neuroexcitatory transmitter at glutamate receptor	Teitelbaum et al. (278)
Reptiles			
Crotalidae (rattlesnakes, water moccasins, copperheads)	Progressive paralysis	Direct action on central nervous system; inhibits neuromuscular transmission at motor end-plate, damages muscle	Holstegge et al. (279), Weber and White (280)
Elapidae (coral snakes, cobras)	Progressive paralysis, rapid onset	Competitive block of muscle nicotinic acetylcholine receptors	Watt et al. (281), Vijayaraghavan (282), Britt and Burkhart (283)
Arthropods			
Spiders, *Latrodectus* (black widow)	Local pain, abdominal rigidity, muscle spasms, convulsions	Massive exocytotic transmitter release followed by depletion and irreversible block	Moss and Binder (284), Ushkaryov (285), Davletov et al. (286), Woestman et al. (287)
Centruroides (scorpions)	Muscle spasms, convulsions	Several toxins depending on species; some act on Na channels, others on Ca-activated K channels	Berg and Tarantino (288), De Davila et al. (289)
Chordata			
Chondrichthyes (stingray)	Muscle spasms, convulsions	Unknown	Russell (290), Kizer et al. (291)
Osteichthyes (stonefish)	Local pain, paralysis, convulsions, slow recovery	Stonustoxin acts as cytolytic toxin liberates nitric oxide–synthase	Ghadessy et al. (292) Khoo, et al. (292a)
Puffer (ingestion of ovaries, liver)	Ataxia, paresthesias, muscular twitching, paralysis	Neuromuscular block, binds to voltage sensitive Na channel, blocks Na flux	Mills and Pasmore (293)
Ciguatera (reef fish)	Gastrointestinal symptoms, tingling of mouth, dizziness, ataxia, hallucinations, transient blurred vision or blindness, peripheral muscular weakness	Excitatory agent acts on Na channels	Cameron et al. (294), Williams et al. (295)

muscles. The paralysis can extend to involve the bulbar musculature. It is accompanied by areflexia and numbness or tingling of face and extremities. Fixed dilated pupils also have been observed.

Neurophysiologic studies disclose low-amplitude compound muscle action potentials with normal motor and sensory conduction velocities.

The early presence of impaired extraocular movements, and the fixed dilated pupils differentiate this condition from acute infectious polyneuritis. Infant botulism usually is seen in younger children and is not associated with ophthalmoplegia. Because scalp hair is one of the favorite sites for the tick, a thorough search for the insect should be conducted in children who have had a recent onset of a progressive weakness resembling infectious polyneuritis (269). After removal of the tick, recovery has been prompt in

TABLE 9.7. *Neurologic symptoms resulting from ingestion of plant toxins*

Plant	Symptoms	Toxin and action
Mushroom		
Amanita phalloides	Gastrointestinal symptoms, hepatic and renal dysfunction, hemorrhagic encephalopathy	Amatoxins inhibit RNA polymerase, phalloidin disrupts membranes (296–298)
Amanita muscaria	Dizziness, ataxia, convulsions	Mucimol activates γ-aminobutyric acid (296,297) receptors; ibotenic acid acts as glutamate receptor agonist
Inocybes	Perspiration, salivation, lacrimation, blurring of vision	Muscarine, a parasympathomimetic (296,297)
Psilocybes	Psychotropic effects	Psilocybin (296,297)
Gyromitra (brain fungus)	Gastrointestinal symptoms, renal and hepatic failure	Monomethyl hydrazine (296)
Chick-pea (*Lathyrus*)	Cramps, lower extremity weakness, sphincter dysfunction evolving into spastic paraparesis	β-*N*-oxalylamino-L-alanine (neuroexcitatory amion acid) (299,300)
Buckthorn	Flaccid quadriparesis, bulbar weakness	Segmental demyelination caused by at least four neurotoxins (301)
Nutmeg	Flushing, gastrointestinal symptoms, drowsiness or hyperactivity, hallucinations	Amino-derivatives of elemicin and myristicin (302)
Ricin (castor bean)	Hemorrhagic gastroenteritis, stupor, seizures	Ricin: ? proteolytic enzyme (303,304)
Jimsonweed (locoweed, thornapple)	Flushed face, dilated pupils, bizarre behavior, visual hallucinations, urinary retention	Atropine and scopolamine, anticholinergic action (305,306)
Pokeweed	Abdominal cramps, vomiting, diaphoresis, dizziness, lethargy, seizures	Phytolaccine (307)
Unripe akee nut	Jamaican vomiting sickness; symptoms similar to Reye syndrome (see Chapter 6)	Hypoglycin A, a cyclopropyl propionic acid (308,309)
Sugarcane (mildewed)	Impaired consciousness, seizures, delayed dystonia after recovery; computed tomography: bilateral hypodensities in putamen, globus pallidus	3-Nitropropionic acid (310)

the North American cases, but in the Australian cases there can be worsening of the paralysis over the subsequent 24 to 48 hours (266).

Removal of the tick arrests the progressive weakness. In the Australian experience of Grattan-Smith and colleagues, worsening of the paralysis occurred for 24 to 48 hours after tick removal (266). Full recovery can be expected, but often requires weeks to months.

Animal Venoms

Neurologic symptoms induced through the bite or sting of venomous animals usually are caused by impaired neuromuscular transmission and take the form of weakness or painful muscle spasms. In recent years considerable interest has focused on the molecular mechanisms of the various animal venoms, and their specific interactions with the various ion channels within the CNS and the neuromuscular junction. The chemistry and molecular biology of the various toxins are summarized by Adams and Swanson (270), the clinical picture by Russell (271), Southcott (272), and Campbell (273), and treatment by Auerbach (274). A review of the more toxic animals and pertinent references are presented in Table 9.6.

Plant Toxins

The neurologic symptoms of some of the more frequently encountered plant toxins are presented in Table 9.7. A complete and up-to-date review of the clinical presentation and management of plant toxins is given by Furbee and Wermuth (275).

NUTRITIONAL DISORDERS

Malnourished children constitute approximately 75% of the preschool population in developing countries. Grossly insufficient quantities of food, dietary imbalances, poor protein intake, lack of essential fatty acids and vitamins, climate, intercurrent bacterial or parasitic infections, and emotional deprivation all combine to predispose a child to nutritional diseases. Additionally, inadequate prenatal and perinatal care also can contribute to the final clinical picture.

Protein-Energy Malnutrition

Protein-energy malnutrition (also called protein-calorie malnutrition) refers to the severe clinical syndromes of marasmus and kwashiorkor, and to milder, often unappreciated cases of nutritional deficiencies. Kwashiorkor was first described in 1935 by Williams working in the Gold Coast, now Ghana (311). Kwashiorkor and marasmus are interrelated syndromes of malnutrition that in their most severe stages of development are distinct, with different causes and different metabolic pictures. Marasmus, primarily caused by caloric insufficiency, is of early onset and develops when infants are weaned before the end of their first year or when the available breast milk is reduced markedly. It is characterized by emaciation and growth failure (312,313). Kwashiorkor results from a diet containing adequate calories but insufficient protein. It is most common in children between 1 and 4 years of age, and frequently it is triggered by measles or various bacterial or parasitic infections (314). Whereas some workers have stressed the role of free radicals produced by bacterial or fungal toxins (aflatoxins) in the production of kwashiorkor (315,316), it is the view of most authorities that kwashiorkor is the result of multiple factors. These not only include dietary deficiencies and imbalances, but also multiple infections, parasitic infestations, dietary toxins, and maternal deprivation (317). Finally, it should be stressed that in many areas of the world symptoms of

kwashiorkor develop in a child who already has demonstrated retarded growth and mental development.

Clinical Manifestations

In mild to moderate forms of protein-energy malnutrition, a clinical distinction between marasmus and kwashiorkor is impossible. In certain areas of the world, diets giving rise to kwashiorkor also can be deficient in one or more vitamins, and signs of vitamin deficiency can accompany the more advanced stages. In West Africa, for instance, riboflavin deficiency is common; in Southeast Asia, thiamine deficiency can induce a mixed picture of protein-energy malnutrition and beriberi.

Certain changes in protein metabolism, notably a reduced serum albumin concentration, a reduced serum concentration of all essential amino acids except phenylalanine and histidine, and a normal or even higher than normal concentration of nonessential amino acids, are characteristic for kwashiorkor and can be used in making a biochemical diagnosis.

The clinical picture of kwashiorkor varies from one region of the world to another. The four basic symptoms and signs are edema, growth failure, behavioral changes, and muscle wasting. Other relatively common features include dyspigmentation of hair and skin, dermatitis, anemia, and hepatomegaly.

Neurologic Features

The effects of undernutrition on the immature nervous system have been the subject of intensive investigation. Neuropathologic studies reveal the brain of a malnourished infant to be small for the infant's chronologic age, and its number of neurons, degree of myelination, and total cerebral lipid content to be reduced (318,319). In interpreting these findings, one must note that in almost all instances these autopsies have been performed on children who died as a result of an infection in addition to protein and calorie deprivation.

Physiologic studies on children with severe protein-energy malnutrition conducted by Mehta, in collaboration with myself, indicated that the proportion of glucose undergoing aerobic oxidation by the brain is reduced, and that a significant proportion is converted to long-chain fatty acids (320).

Although these findings provide a biochemical basis for both the loss in myelination and the ultimate cognitive deficits of malnourished infants, the time during which the human brain is vulnerable to nutritional insults is still uncertain. Animal experiments indicate that a severe nutritional insult early in brain development can have a permanent adverse effect on cerebral structure and function. Periods of CNS growth spurt (in humans between 15 and 20 weeks' gestation, when neuronal multiplication is maximal, and between 30 weeks' gestation and the end of the first year of extrauterine life, when glial division occurs) are times when the brain is particularly vulnerable to experimental nutritional deficiency (321). As yet, these experimental data cannot be correlated with clinical experience.

Apathy is the most constant and earliest neurologic feature and is usual in children who weigh less than 40% of the expected amount (322). In the Indian series of Sachdeva and colleagues, 87% of children admitted for treatment of protein-energy malnutrition showed mental changes, 77% had muscle wasting, 70% weakness, and 40% hyporeflexia (323). More recent data from the Indian clinic of Chopra and his group are comparable (324). Most studies show that head circumference varies directly with nutritional status and is often below the third percentile for American children. It is less affected than height and weight. Hypotonia and reduced deep tendon reflexes are common; they are more marked in the lower extremities, particularly in the proximal musculature (325). "Soft" neurologic signs, notably impaired fine motor coordination, and the presence of choreoathetoid movements, are seen far more commonly in malnourished children than in control children with normal nutritional status.

The EEG has been studied by several groups. Generally, it demonstrates nonspecific abnormalities such as diffuse slowing. These are more commonly seen in malnourished than in control children (326). Nerve conduction times are significantly delayed in both the marasmic and the kwashiorkor forms of protein-energy malnutri-

tion, even in the absence of overt associated vitamin deficiencies. As a rule, the degree of delay correlates with the duration and the severity of the protein-energy malnutrition, and thus is more marked in marasmus (325). Approximately one-half of patients with the more severe forms of protein-energy malnutrition have segmental demyelination; when malnutrition is severe and long-standing, an arrest in myelination of peripheral nerves occurs, with a persistence of the small myelinated fibers and a relative lack of the large myelinated fibers (324).

Neuroimaging studies demonstrate widened cortical sulci, widened cerebellar folia, and enlarged ventricles. These abnormalities resolve quickly with nutritional rehabilitation, suggesting that they do not represent cerebral atrophy, but rather ventricular dilatation and enlargement of sulci as a consequence of a decrease in plasma proteins and reduced colloid osmotic pressure (327). It is of note that in the South African series of Gunston and coworkers, myelination was age appropriate even in children with severe kwashiorkor (327).

Psychological study results on malnourished infants show them to have cognitive inadequacies that result in delayed learning, particularly in reading and writing (328,329). Children who received supplementary feedings had higher verbal intelligence than their undernourished sibling controls, a difference that could not be accounted for by socioeconomic factors (330). However, other workers have found that the greatest postnatal influence on cognitive performance comes not from nutrition but from social stimulation (331). When children are subjected to either nutritional or social stimulation, the effect becomes evident within 18 months; it is almost immediate when both interventions are made available to them (Fig. 9.4) (332).

Treatment

The medical and social aspects of treatment of protein-energy malnutrition are reviewed by Jelliffe and Jelliffe (313). It is of note that with nutritional rehabilitation there is a rapid and striking increase in head circumference. This may become sufficiently marked to result in splitting

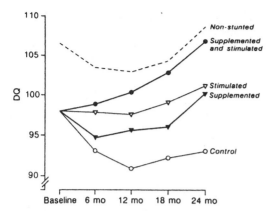

FIG. 9.4. Recovery from malnutrition in 129 Jamaican infants, aged 9 to 24 months, with stunted growth (length less than 2 standard deviations below the mean). The effect of nutritional supplementation is compared with that of psychosocial stimulation, combined nutritional and psychosocial interventions, and controls. A group of 32 nonstunted Jamaican infants served as reference. (DQ, developmental quotient.) (From Grantham-McGregor SM, et al. Nutritional supplementation, psychosocial stimulation, and mental development of stunted children: the Jamaican study. *Lancet* 1991; 338:15. With permission.)

of sutures and papilledema, suggesting the presence of pseudotumor cerebri.

Approximately one-fifth of children with kwashiorkor become drowsy in 3 to 4 days after being started on a normal diet. Although the condition is most often self-limited, it is occasionally accompanied by asterixis and can progress to coma with fatal outcome (333). The nature of this complication is unknown, but it is believed to reflect hepatic failure resulting from the ingestion of relatively large amounts of protein. Even more rarely, a transient syndrome marked by coarse tremors, parkinsonian rigidity, bradykinesia, and myoclonus has been observed in children with kwashiorkor 6 days to several weeks after starting the corrective high-protein diet (334). This condition is distinct from the infantile tremor syndrome.

Prognosis

Follow-up studies on children who experienced protein-energy malnutrition indicate that the younger the child at the time of the hospitalization for malnutrition, the less likely the child is to achieve intellectual parity (335,336).

Other studies, however, suggest that the cognitive delays of malnourished infants are reversible. Children whose nutrition was adequate during the first 2 years of life do not have a greater head circumference than their malnourished siblings at the same height. This finding suggests that malnutrition in early life has no apparent selective effect on head growth or, by inference, on brain size (337).

In contrast to data obtained from rats and other species, in humans there is no experimental support for a so-called critical period of intrauterine and early extrauterine brain development (i.e., a time when malnutrition induces irreversible damage). Whereas maternal undernutrition, particularly during the second half of gestation, results in reduced birth weights in one-half of infants, infants who are small for gestational age owing to maternal malnutrition have a better prognosis in terms of neurologic deficits than infants small for gestational age whose mothers were well nourished.

Summarizing sometimes contradictory data, one can conclude that malnutrition in isolation is not a lasting cause for permanently reduced mental competence or mental retardation (338). Rather, when intellectual inadequacy follows malnutrition in early life, it occurs not only as the result of protein-energy malnutrition, but because the infant's nervous system is inadequate from birth and interferes with its ability to feed and to interact emotionally with its mother (336).

Vitamin Deficiencies

The action of a vitamin in intermediary metabolism can be disturbed by its deficiency, by abnormally high vitamin requirements such as are seen in a variety of bacterial and parasitic infections, and by the inhibitory action of various antivitamin substances. Dietary factors antagonistic to the action of a vitamin include avidin (found in raw egg white), which is an antagonist to biotin, and the enzyme thiaminase (present in raw fish), which destroys dietary thiamine.

Although a deficiency in almost any of the vitamins can directly or indirectly affect the CNS, only components of the B complex group are known to be involved directly in brain function.

Deficiency of vitamin A can produce increased intracranial pressure, which can be reversed by dietary treatment. Chronic vitamin A intoxication also induces increased intracranial pressure, which is accompanied by craniotabes and cortical hyperostosis (339,340).

Vitamin E (tocopherol) deficiency is encountered in severe cases of cystic fibrosis and in other malabsorptive conditions. The syndrome of spinocerebellar degeneration and peripheral neuropathy occurring as a complication of tocopherol deficiency is described in the section on gastrointestinal diseases in Chapter 15.

The role of vitamin supplementation in preventing neural tube defects is covered in Chapter 4.

Thiamine Deficiency

The discovery of how thiamine participates in cerebral metabolism was an important part of the early history of neurochemistry and is reviewed by Peters (341) and Haas (342).

Thiamine functions in the form of pyrophosphate, which acts as a coenzyme for many enzyme systems. Generally speaking, thiamine pyrophosphate is involved in oxidative decarboxylation, nonoxidative decarboxylation, and various ketolases, notably the conversion of 5-carbon to 6-carbon sugars by means of the enzyme transketolase.

Pyruvate and α-ketoglutarate, whose decarboxylations are two integral steps of the Krebs cycle, exemplify enzymes responsible for oxidative decarboxylation. In thiamine deficiency, oxidation of pyruvate and α-ketoglutarate by the brain is reduced. As a consequence, cerebral oxygen and glucose consumption are lowered, and the concentrations of the two ketoacids (pyruvate and α-ketoglutarate) are increased in various tissues, including blood (343). When a thiamine-deficient individual is presented with a glucose load, the concentration of serum ketoacids increases to abnormal levels and remains elevated for several hours. At the same time, there is an increase in serum and CSF lactic and pyruvic acids.

Transketolase has been found to be more susceptible to thiamine deprivation than the ketoacid decarboxylases are, and the decrease in transketolase activity during induced thiamine deficiency is greater than the decrease of pyruvate decarboxylase activity (344). Dreyfus and Hauser postulated that failure in transketolase represents the basic biochemical lesion of thiamine deficiency, although the increase in transketolase activity with administration of thiamine was insufficient to account for the clinical improvement (345). In experimental studies, thiamine-deficient rats had a low glucose metabolic rate and limited glial proliferation in the vestibular nuclei. Both abnormalities were reversed by thiamine supplementation (346).

Thiamine deficiency is seen mainly in breast-fed infants, whose mothers, themselves, could have been thiamine deficient during pregnancy, and whose breast milk consequently contains inadequate amounts of thiamine. Thiamine deficiency occurs principally in Asia, where the milling of rice grain or the use of soda in the baking of bread excludes the vitamin from the diet. Not rare even now, the disease was one of the four principal causes of death in the Philippines as recently as 1960 (347), and extensive outbreaks of beriberi are still being reported from Africa (348). In the West, the condition is encountered in infants who are given unusual formulas, in critically ill infants on prolonged enteric feeding, and in children with malignancies, receiving intensive chemotherapy (349,350).

Two symptom complexes are seen: infantile beriberi and Wernicke-Korsakoff syndrome. Infantile beriberi appears suddenly, often after a bout of gastroenteritis, and is marked by weakness owing to acute peripheral neuritis, neck stiffness, and aphonia (voiceless cry) (351). Cardiac symptoms are not common in infants. The diagnosis can be established by the depressed thiamine concentrations in whole blood and CSF and by the low red cell ketolase activity (352). The experiences of Haridas in Malaya (351) and de Silva in Sri Lanka (312) illustrate the differential diagnosis and treatment of childhood thiamine deficiency in developing countries.

A neurologic picture resembling that seen in adults with Wernicke-Korsakoff syndrome is rare in children, but has been encountered in seriously ill patients receiving parenteral nutrition for a long time. More often, one sees a relatively nonspecific picture of lethargy, apneic spells, hypothermia, and deteriorating cardiovascular function (353,354). Generally, Wernicke-Korsakoff syndrome is clinically unsuspected and can develop rapidly in the absence of parenteral vitamin supplementation (355). In many instances, the diagnosis is made only on postmortem examination by noting the characteristic spongy changes in the mamillary bodies, hypothalamus, midbrain, and pons.

Infantile subacute necrotizing encephalopathy, a familial neurologic degenerative condition with pathologic changes reminiscent of Wernicke disease, has been termed pseudo-Wernicke syndrome, or, more recently, Leigh syndrome. It is accompanied by lactic acidosis and appears to be the consequence of a variety of enzymatic defects. This disease is more fully discussed in Chapter 1 in the section on mitochondrial disorders.

Pyridoxine Deficiency

Pyridoxine (vitamin B_6) in the form of its aldehyde derivative, pyridoxal-5-phosphate, is a coenzyme for numerous essential metabolic reactions within the nervous system. Both decarboxylation of glutamic acid to GABA, a neurotransmitter, and transamination of glutamic acid to α-ketoglutaric acid are impaired in animals receiving a pyridoxine-deficient diet. Several other amino acid decarboxylases, several transaminases, and serine hydroxymethyltransferase also are pyridoxine dependent. Pyridoxine also is involved in synaptogenesis, dendritic arborization, and in the maintenance of the normal neurotransmitter balance within the CNS.

In at least three conditions, a relative deficiency of pyridoxine is related to the appearance of seizures and potentially permanent neurologic deficits.

Dietary Pyridoxine Deficiency

Pyridoxine deficiency appears at 1 to 12 months of age in a significant proportion of infants whose intake of the vitamin is below 0.1 mg/day. Aside from seizures and hyperirritability, other symptoms of vitamin deficiency, notably anemia, can sometimes also be documented (356). Pyridoxine deficiency unaccompanied by other nutritional deficits is rarely encountered, even in the developing countries. A series of cases was seen, however, in the United States between 1952 and 1953 in a small percentage of infants fed a pyridoxine-deficient proprietary formula (357). More recently, prolonged seizures that were unresponsive to treatment with the usual anticonvulsant medications, but responded to pyridoxine (100 mg), were seen in an infant fed powdered goat's milk, a preparation devoid of pyridoxine and folic acid (358). Seizures owing to pyridoxine deficiency also are seen in infants who have been breastfed exclusively for longer than 6 months and in those who have had a jejunoileal bypass (359).

Pyridoxine Dependency

A familial pyridoxine dependency syndrome is marked by the evolution of seizures *in utero*, at birth, or at any time up to the end of the second year of life (360–362). The condition was first described by Hunt and colleagues (363) and is transmitted as an autosomal recessive trait. It is a relatively common entity, and one of the important causes for intractable seizures. Seizures are usually generalized or focal with secondary generalization, and are almost immediately arrested by the administration of intramuscular or intravenous pyridoxine (50 to 200 mg). Subsequently infants are often hypotonic and unresponsive (364). Microcephaly, if present, is corrected with pyridoxine treatment. Thus, pyridoxine dependency, like protein-energy malnutrition, is a rare cause of reversible microcephaly. The EEG usually shows a variety of paroxysmal discharges, including hypsarrhythmia and also normalizes promptly with pyridoxine administration. The dose of pyridoxine required to control seizures, to dramatically reverse the EEG abnormalities, and in older children to improve the IQ (2 to 50 mg/day) is many times the minimum daily requirement for the vitamin. MRI shows diffuse cortical atrophy, most marked in the frontal regions, and positron emission tomographic scan reveals a widespread cerebral hypometabolism (365).

CSF GABA levels are markedly reduced, and CSF glutamate levels are markedly elevated (364). Both levels return to normal with treatment. On autopsy, the GABA content of cerebral cortex has been found to be low, whereas the content of glutamic acid is elevated (366). No significant abnormalities in the activity of glutamic acid decarboxylase (GAD) have been demonstrated (367). Although a structural alteration in GAD with a diminished affinity of pyridoxine for the apoenzyme has been one plausible explanation for this disorder (368), knockout mice with selective elimination of both forms of GAD show an abnormal palate, but neither a seizure disorder nor any structural abnormalities of their cerebral cortex (369). Baumeister and coworkers, therefore, have suggested that glutamate, which has been shown to be elevated in CSF and cortex of pyridoxine-dependent subjects, hyperexcites the *N*-methyl-D-aspartate receptor inducing seizures and an encephalopathy (364).

The diagnosis of pyridoxine dependency rests on the presence of seizures that are intractable to the usual anticonvulsant medications, the prompt cessation of seizures with parenteral or oral pyridoxine administration, and, optimally, the recurrence of seizures after pyridoxine withdrawal.

Life-long continuous treatment with pyridoxine is necessary to prevent seizures and severe mental retardation. The dosage required for seizure control ranges between 0.2 and 30 mg/kg per day (369a). Larger amounts of pyridoxine have been given in some instances, but the vitamin can induce a reversible sensory neuropathy (370). The optimal dose of pyridoxine appears to vary between families, and regulation of pyridoxine dosage by aiming at normalization of CSF GABA and glutamine is probably indicated (371).

Hydrazine Toxicity

Treatment with isoniazide (INH), penicillamine, or other hydrazides capable of reacting with the aldehyde group of pyridoxal can induce symptoms of B_6 deficiency (372). With the increased prevalence of tuberculosis, and with INH being one of the first-line antituberculous drugs, the incidence of INH poisoning has increased, to the point where INH together with diphenhydramine and theophylline has become one of the three major causes for drug-induced seizures in the pediatric population (373,374). Dosages greater than 30 mg/kg can produce seizures. In addition, the characteristic clinical picture is that of a metabolic acidosis and coma (374). Seizures are often refractory to commonly used anticonvulsants, including intravenous benzodiazepines, and parenteral pyridoxine is necessary to control seizures (374).

Pellagra

Although pellagra is considered a multiple-deficiency disease, the main clinical manifestations—dermatitis, diarrhea, and diffuse cerebral disease—respond to therapy with nicotinic acid or tryptophan. Pellagra is endemic to areas where corn, a poor source of nicotinic acid, is the staple food, and where intake of meat, which provides tryptophan needed for the biosynthesis of nicotinic acid, also is low (375). Approximately one-half of the human minimum daily requirement of nicotinic acid is synthesized from tryptophan by micro-organisms, either in tissues or in the intestinal tract. Nicotinic acid is an integral component of two coenzymes involved in electron transfer, nicotinamide adenine dinucleotide and nicotinamide adenine dinucleotide phosphate. Both are essential for a variety of enzymatic reactions in carbohydrate and fatty acid metabolism.

Children who are mildly deficient in nicotinic acid are irritable or apathetic. With severe involvement, they become delirious or mentally obtunded, and they can show spasticity, coarse tremors of the face and hands, polyneuritis, and optic atrophy. In the experience of Malfait and colleagues, working in Malawi, dermatitis of the areas exposed to sunlight, particularly of the chest, arms, and neck (Casal's necklace), was seen in 80% of nicotinic acid–deficient subjects (376). Stomatitis was present in 60%, diarrhea in 20%, and mental disorders in 10%. Histologic examination of the brain shows degeneration of Betz cells of the motor cortex and, to a lesser extent, of the cerebellar Purkinje cells. In the spinal cord, degeneration of the posterior columns and the pyramidal and spinocerebellar tracts is seen. Demyelination of the peripheral nerves is common (377).

The experience of Spies and colleagues (378) in Alabama during the 1930s and the reviews by Still (379) and Lanska (380) provide the reader with an idea of the problems inherent in the differential diagnosis of pellagra and its therapy. Since then, the diagnosis of the condition is made by high-pressure liquid chromatography of serum nicotinamide metabolites (381). A pellagra-like skin rash also is seen in Hartnup disease and in some other genetic defects of tryptophan and kynurenine metabolism (see Chapter 1).

Subacute Combined Degeneration

Degeneration of the posterior and lateral columns of the spinal cord owing to deficiency of vitamin B_{12} (cobalamin) is rare in childhood. When seen, it can accompany one of the several forms of congenital pernicious anemia. The most likely form of subacute combined degeneration to be encountered in childhood is caused by a congenital defect of vitamin B_{12} absorption. This entity presents at 7 to 24 months of age with impaired mental development. Congenital intrinsic factor deficiency is less common. It, too, presents in this age group, with a similar neurologic picture (382). The condition can be associated with intestinal disease, regional ileitis, or celiac syndrome. Defective release of cobalamin from lysosomes, another genetic defect, is marked by developmental delay and a minimal vitamin B_{12}-responsive methylmalonic aciduria. Neither homocystinuria nor a megaloblastic anemia accompanies the condition. The various congenital disorders of cobalamin metabolism are covered in Chapter 1.

Many reports have described vitamin B_{12} deficiency in infants of mothers with undiagnosed pernicious anemia and in exclusively breast-fed infants whose mothers are vegans or vegetarians, thus excluding from the diet not only meat, but also eggs and dairy products (383,384). Megaloblastic anemia, always present with subacute combined degeneration in children, is accompanied by apathy, developmental regression, athetoid movements, and tremor (385,386). Alterations in sensorium can progress to coma (385,387). In older children, the presenting signs and symptoms of the condition are ataxia, spasticity, weakness of the lower extremities, loss of vibratory sensation, and mental retardation. Plasma homocysteine is increased, and plasma methionine is reduced. Excretion of methylmalonic acid and homocystine is increased (388).

Somatosensory-evoked potentials reveal the presence of CNS involvement even when overt clinical signs are absent (389). Vitamin B_{12} administration quickly corrects hematologic abnormalities. EEG and neuroimaging abnormalities also are reversible with treatment. However, cognitive and language development frequently remains delayed, particularly when neurologic symptoms appear during the first year of life (383,390). A combination tremor and myoclonus can appear after the initiation of treatment with cobalamin (386). In the experience of Pearson and colleagues, folic acid therapy often aggravates neurologic symptoms (391).

The pathogenesis of the neurologic deficits is still not understood. Hall has reviewed the role of vitamin B_{12} in normal nervous system function (392).

Infantile Tremor Syndrome

Infantile tremor syndrome is fairly common in India. It is seen in children between ages 6 months and 2 years with a history of developmental delay and severe malnutrition. Symptoms, which commence between May and July, include a tremor that can be generalized or confined to one or more extremities. The tremor is rapid, rhythmic, and coarse, and it disappears during sleep. It can be accompanied by myoclonic jerks, epilepsia partialis continua, or choreic movements. Affected children are pale and apathetic and have sparse, light-colored hair and prominent pigmentation over the knuckles. Despite treatment, the outcome is poor, and the majority is left with subnormal intelligence (393).

A number of deficiencies have been documented. These include a magnesium deficiency, and, more recently, a deficiency of vitamin B_{12}. In a series by Garewal and coworkers, concomitant malnutrition was documented in 82%, and an antecedent viral illness in 91% (394). The condition also was noted in infants of mothers who were strict vegetarians. Low serum B_{12} levels and a megaloblastic erythropoiesis could be demonstrated in 87%. In other series, magnesium deficiency with low CSF and urine magnesium levels was apparently well documented. The cause of this distinctive condition is still not clear, but tremors respond to supplementation with vitamin B_{12} or magnesium (393,394).

Tropical Myeloneuropathies

Several forms of progressive myeloneuropathies have been described in Third World countries, notably India and Africa. They fall into two clinical types with overlapping features: tropical spastic paraparesis and tropical ataxic neuropathy. Tropical spastic paraparesis is a slowly progressive spastic paraplegia that affects the pyramidal tracts and, to a lesser degree, the sensory systems, and is often accompanied by optic atrophy and a peripheral neuropathy. The condition is caused by the human T-cell lymphotropic virus 1 and is considered more extensively in Chapter 6.

Outbreaks of another form of acute spastic paraparesis, termed *konzo*, have been reported from a variety of areas in Africa, notably Tanzania, Mozambique, and Zaire, where cassava is the main staple crop. The condition affects boys predominantly, with its onset generally between 5 and 15 years of age. The onset is abrupt with difficulty in walking. This progresses over the course of 1 to 3 days to a complete and symmetric paraparesis with hyperreflexia and extensor plantar responses. In the majority of cases some degree of slow functional improvement occurs (395).

The cause for konzo is uncertain. High cyanide intake from the consumption of inadequately processed cassava has been proposed as one etiology. No antibodies to human T-cell lymphotropic virus 1 have been found.

Konzo is clinically similar to lathyrism, another acute form of spastic paraparesis seen in Ethiopia, India, and Bangladesh. This condition is caused by consumption of large amounts of the chick pea, *Lathyrus sativus*, which contains an excitatory amino acid, β-*N*-oxalylamino-L-alanine (396).

Tropical ataxic neuropathy (nonspastic paraparesis) differs from the various forms of tropical spastic paraparesis in the predominance of paresthesias in the lower extremities, the loss of proprioception and vibratory sensation, and the loss of deep tendon reflexes (397). Several exogenous factors have been proposed as causes for the condition. Ingestion of cassava beans and a consequent chronic cyanide toxicity plays an important role in some epidemics (398), but not in others (399). The role of the human T-cell lymphotropic virus 2 in the etiology of the condition has not been clarified.

A discussion of the amyotrophic lateral sclerosis-Parkinson disease-dementia complex seen in Guam and the other Mariana Islands and of the role of a plant excitant neurotoxin in causing this neurologic picture and those of the other toxic upper motor neuron diseases is outside the scope of this text. The reader is referred to reviews by Spencer and colleagues (400) and Ludolph and Spencer (300).

REFERENCES

1. Hestand HE, Teski DW. Diphenhydramine hydrochloride intoxication. *J Pediatr* 1977;90:1017–1018.
1a. Goetz CM, et al. Accidental childhood death from diphenhydramine overdosage. *Am J Emerg Med* 1990; 8:321–322.
2. Priest JH. Atropine response of eyes in mongolism. *Am J Dis Child* 1960;100:869–972.
3. Amitai Y, et al. Atropine poisoning in children during the Persian Gulf crisis. A national survey in Israel. *J Am Med Assoc* 1992;268:630–632.
4. Valdes-Dapena MA, Arey JB. Boric acid poisoning: three fatal cases with pancreatic inclusion and review of literature. *J Pediatr* 1962;61:531–546.
5. Cheng CT. Perak, Malaysia, mass poisoning. Tale of the nine emperor gods and rat tail noodles. *Am J Forensic Med Pathol* 1992;13:261–263.
6. von Muhlendahl KE, et al. Codeine intoxication in childhood. *Lancet* 1976;2:303–305.
7. Warden CR, Diekema DS, Robertson WO. Dystonic

reaction associated with dextromethorphan ingestion in a toddler. *Pediatr Emerg Care* 1997;13:214–215.

8. McCarron MM, Challoner KR, Thomson GA. Diphenoxylate-atropine (Lomotil) overdose in children: an update. *Pediatrics* 1991;87:694–700.

9. Robotham JL, Leitman PS. Acute iron poisoning. A review. *Am J Dis Child* 1980;134:875–879.

10. Mann KV, et al. Management of acute iron overdose. *Clin Pharm* 1989;8:428–440.

11. Martinez AJ, Boehm R, Hadfield MG. Acute hexachlorophene encephalopathy: cliniconeuropathological correlation. *Acta Neuropathol* 1974;28:93–103.

12. Martin-Bouyer G, et al. Outbreak of accidental hexachlorophene poisoning in France. *Lancet* 1982;1: 91–95.

13. Oakley CP Jr. The neurotoxicity of the halogenated hydroxyquinolines. *JAMA* 1983;225:395–397.

14. Selby G. Subacute myelo-optic neuropathy in Australia. *Lancet* 1972;1:123–125.

15. Shigematsu I, Yanagawa H. Data on clinoquinol and S.M.O.N. *Lancet* 1978;2:945.

16. Saraf KR, et al. Imipramine dose effects in children. *Psychopharmacologia* 1974;37:265–274.

17. Greene AS, Cromie WJ. Treatment of imipramine overdosage in children. *Urology* 1981;18:314–315.

18. Foreman HP, et al. Cerebral vasculitis and hemorrhage in an adolescent taking diet pills containing phenylpropanolamine: case report and review of the literature. *Pediatrics* 1989;83:737–741.

19. Parsons AC. Piperazine neurotoxicity: worm wobble. *Br Med J* 1971;4:792.

20. Lovejoy FH Jr, Mitchell AA, Goldman P. The management of propoxyphene poisoning. *J Pediatr* 1974; 85:98–100.

21. Espelin D, Done A. Amphetamine poisoning. Effectiveness of chlorpromazine. *N Engl J Med* 1968;278: 1361–1365.

22. Alldredge BK, Lowenstein DH, Simon RP. Seizures associated with recreational drug abuse. *Neurology* 1989;39:1037–1039.

23. Ellenhorn MJ, et al, eds. *Medical toxicology: diagnosis and treatment of human poisoning.* Baltimore: Williams & Wilkins, 1997.

24. Spencer PS, Schaumburg HH, eds. *Experimental and clinical neurotoxicology.* Baltimore: Williams & Wilkins, 1980.

25. Mack RB. Toxic encounters of the dangerous kind: Diphenoxylate (lomotil). *N C Med J* 1981;42:858.

26. Pearn J, et al. Accidental poisoning in childhood. Five year urban population study with 15 year analysis of fatality. *Br Med J* 1984;288:44–46.

27. Melis K, Bochener A. Acute poisoning in a children's hospital: an 8 year experience. *Acta Clin Belgica* 1990;13[Suppl.]:98–100.

28. Dana SL. *Lead Diseases, a treatise from the French of L. Tanquerel des Planches.* Lowell, MA: D. Bixby Co, 1848.

29. Blackfan KD. Lead poisoning in children with especial reference to lead as a cause of convulsions. *Am J Med Sci* 1917;153:877–887.

30. Holt LE. Lead poisoning in infancy. *Am J Dis Child* 1923;25:229–233.

31. Mahaffey KR. Exposure to lead in childhood—the importance of prevention. *N Engl J Med* 1992;327: 1308–1309.

32. Raghavan SRV, Gonick HC. Isolation of a low-molecular-weight lead-binding protein from human erythrocytes. *Proc Soc Exp Biol Med* 1977;155:164–167.

33. Rabinovitz MB, Wetherill GW, Kopple JD. Lead metabolism in the normal human. Stable isotope studies. *Science* 1973;182:725–727.

34. Klaassen CD. Heavy metals and heavy-metal antagonists. In: Hardman JG, Limbird LE, Molinoff PB, Ruddon RW, Gilman AG. eds. *Goodman and Gilman's the pharmacologic basis of therapeutics*, 9th ed. New York: Pergamon Press, 1996:1649–1654.

35. Landrigan PJ, Graef JW. Pediatric lead poisoning in 1987: the silent epidemic continues. *Pediatrics* 1987; 79:582–583.

36. Rogan WJ, Reigart JR, Gladen BC. Association of amino levulinate dehydratase levels and ferrochelatase inhibition in childhood lead exposure. *J Pediatr* 1986; 109:60–64.

37. Pocock SJ, Smith M, Baghurst P. Environmental lead and children's intelligence: a systematic review of the epidemiological evidence. *Brit Med J* 1994;309: 1189–1197.

38. American Academy of Pediatrics, Committee on Environmental Hazards. Statement on childhood lead poisoning. *Pediatrics* 1987;79:457–465.

39. Sassa S, Granick S, Kappas A. Effect of lead and genetic factors on heme biosynthesis in the human red cell. *Ann NY Acad Sci* 1975;244:419–440.

40. White JM, Harvey DR. Defective synthesis of γ and β globin chains in lead poisoning. *Nature* 1972;236:71–73.

41. Pentschew A. Morphology and morphogenesis of lead encephalopathy. *Acta Neuropathol* 1965;5:133–160.

42. Verity MA. Comparative observations on inorganic and organic lead neurotoxicity. *Environment Health Persp* 1990;89:43–48.

43. Winder C, Garten LL, Lewis PD. The morphological effects of lead on the developing central nervous system. *Neuropath Appl Neurobiol* 1983;9:87–108.

44. Behse F, Carlsen F. Histology and ultrastructure of alterations in neuropathy. *Muscle Nerve* 1978;1:368–374.

45. Thomas PK, Landon DN, King R. Diseases of the peripheral nerves. In: Graham DI, Lantos PL, eds. *Greenfields's neuropathology*, 6th ed, London: Edward Arnold, Ltd., 1997:417–419.

46. Blackman SS. Intranuclear inclusion bodies in the kidney and liver caused by lead poisoning. *Bull Johns Hopkins Hosp* 1936;58:384–403.

47. Freeman R. Chronic lead poisoning in children: a review of 90 children diagnosed in Sydney 1948–1967. 2. Clinical features and investigations. *Med J Aust* 1970;1:648–651.

48. Mellins RB, Jenkins CD. Epidemiologic and psychological study of lead poisoning in children. *JAMA* 1955;158:15–20.

49. Jenkins CD, Mellins RB. Lead poisoning in children. *Arch Neurol Psychiatry* 1957;77:70–78.

50. Mirando EH, Ranasinghe L. Lead encephalopathy in children: uncommon clinical aspects. *Med J Aust* 1970;2:966–968.

51. Anku VD, Harris JW. Peripheral neuropathy and lead poisoning in a child with sickle-cell anemia. *J Pediatr* 1974;85:337–340.

52. Park EA, Jackson D, Kajdi L. Shadows produced by lead in x-ray pictures of growing skeleton. *Am J Dis Child* 1931;41:485–499.

53. Smith M. The effects of low-level lead exposure on children. In: Smith MA, Grant LD, Sors AI, eds. *Lead exposure and child development: an international assessment.* London: Kluwer Academic Publishers, 1989:347.

54. Baghurst PA, et al. Environmental exposure to lead and children's intelligence at the age of seven years. The Port Pirie Cohort Study. *N Engl J Med* 1992; 327:1279–1284.

55. Committee on Environmental Health. Lead Poisoning: from screening to primary prevention. *Pediatrics* 1993;92:176–183.

56. Boeckx RL, Postl B, Coodin FJ. Gasoline sniffing and tetraethyl lead poisoning in children. *Pediatrics* 1977;60:140–145.

57. de la Burde B, Choat MS. Early asymptomatic lead exposure and development at school age. *J Pediatr* 1975;87:638–642.

58. Benson PF, Chisolm JJ Jr. A reliable qualitative urine coproporphyrin test for lead intoxication in young children. *J Pediatr* 1960;56:759–767.

59. Lockitch G, et al. Seizures in a 10-week-old infant: lead poisoning from an unexpected source. *Can Med Assoc J* 145:1991;1465–1468.

60. Committee on Drugs, American Academy of Pediatrics. Treatment guidelines for lead exposure in children. *Pediatrics* 1995;96:155–260.

61. Piomelli S, et al. Management of childhood lead poisoning. *J Pediatr* 1984;105:523–532.

62. Friedman JA, Weinberger HL. Six children with lead poisoning. *J Pediatr* 1988;112:799–804.

63. Jacob JM, Le Quesne PM. Toxic disorders. In: Adams JH, Duchen LW, eds. *Greenfield's neuropathology.* 5th ed. New York: Oxford University Press, 1992:881–987.

64. Yokoyama K, Araki S, Abe H. Distribution of nerve conduction velocities in acute thallium poisoning. *Muscle Nerve* 1990;13:117–120.

65. Chamberlain PH, et al. Thallium poisoning. *Pediatrics* 1958;22:1170–1182.

66. Cavanagh JB, et al. The effects of thallium salts, with particular reference to the nervous system changes. *Quart J Med* 1974;43:293–319.

67. Meggs WJ, et al. Thallium poisoning from maliciously contaminated food. *J Toxicol Clin Toxicol* 1994; 32:723–730.

68. Wainwright AP, et al. Clinical features and therapy of acute thallium poisoning. *Quart J Med* 1988;69: 939–944.

69. Kersjes MP, et al. An analysis of arsenic exposures referred to the Blodget Regional Poison Center. *Vet Hum Toxicol* 1987;29:75–78.

70. Russell DS. Changes in the central nervous system following arsphenamine medication. *J Pathol* 1937;45: 357–366.

71. Ohta M. Ultrastructure of sural nerve in a case of arsenic neuropathy. *Acta Neuropathol* 1970;16:233–242.

72. Gorby MS. Arsenic poisoning. *West J Med* 1988;49: 308–315.

73. Cullen NM, Wolf LR, St Clair D. Pediatric arsenic ingestion. *Am J Emerg Med* 1995;13:432–435.

74. Globus JH, Ginsburg SW. Pericapillary encephalorrhagia due to arsphenamine, so-called arsphenamine encephalitis. *Arch Neurol Psychiatr* 1933;30: 1226–1247.

75. Peterson RG, Rumack BH. D-penicillamine therapy of acute arsenic poisoning. *J Pediatr* 1977;91:661–666.

76. Cheek DB. Pink disease (infantile acrodynia). *J Pediatr* 1953;42:239–260.

77. Agocs MM, et al. Mercury exposure from interior latex paint. *N Engl J Med* 1990;323:1096–1101.

78. Amin-Zaki L, et al. Methylmercury poisoning in Iraqi children: clinical observation over 2 years. *Br Med J* 1978;1:613–616.

79. Elhassani SB. The many faces of methylmercury poisoning. *J Toxicol Clin Toxicol* 1983;19:875–906.

80. Korogi Y, et al. Representation of the visual field in the striate cortex: comparison of MR findings with visual field deficits in organic mercury poisoning. *Am J Neuroradiol* 1997;18:1127–1130.

81. Kurland LT, Faro SN, Siedler H. Minimata disease. *World Neurol* 1960;1:370–395.

82. Snyder RD. Congenital mercury poisoning. *N Engl J Med* 1971;284:1014–1016.

83. Marsh DO, et al. Fetal methylmercury poisoning: clinical and toxicological data on 29 cases. *Ann Neurol* 1980;7:348–353.

84. Myers GJ, et al. Summary of the Seychelles child development study on the relationship of fetal methylmercury exposure to neurodevelopment. *Neurotoxicology* 1995;16:711–716.

85. Takeuchi T, Eto N, Eto K. Neuropathology of childhood cases of methylmercury poisoning (Minimata Disease) with prolonged symptoms, with particular reference to the decortication syndrome. *Neurotoxicology* 1979; 1:120.

86. Aposhian HV. DMSA and DMPS—water soluble antidotes for heavy metal poisoning. *Annu Rev Pharmacol Toxicol* 1983;23:193–215.

86a. Nierenberg DW, et al. Delayed cerebellar disease and death after accidental exposure to dimethylmercury. *N Engl J Med* 1998;338:1672–1676.

87. Auer RN, Benevisti H. Hypoxia and related conditions. In Graham DI, Lantos PL, eds. *Greenfields's neuropathology*, 6th ed, London: Edward Arnold, Ltd., 1997:275–276.

88. Kim JK, Coe CJ. Clinical study on carbon monoxide intoxication in children. *Yonsie Med J* 1987;28: 266–273.

89. Khan K, Sharief N. Chronic carbon monoxide poisoning in children. *Acta Paediatr* 1995;84:742.

90. Garland H, Pearce J. Neurological complications of carbon monoxide poisoning. *Quart J Med* 1967; 36:445–455.

91. Zimmerman SS, Truxal B. Carbon monoxide poisoning. *Pediatrics* 1981;68:215–224.

92. Choi IS. Delayed neurologic sequelae in carbon monoxide intoxication. *Arch Neurol* 1983;40:433–435.

92a. Ernst A, Zibrak JD. Carbon monoxide poisoning. *N Engl J Med* 1998;339:1603–1608.

93. Murata T, et al. Serial proton magnetic resonance spectroscopy in a patient with the interval form of carbon monoxide poisoning. *J Neurol Neurosurg Psychiatr* 1995;58:100–103.

94. Thom SR. Carbon monoxide-mediated brain lipid peroxidation in the rat. *J Appl Physiol* 1990;68:997–1003.

94a. Weaver LK, et al. Carbon monoxide poisoning. *N Engl J Med* 1999;340:1290.

95. Rudge FW. Carbon monoxide poisoning in infants: treatment with hyperbaric oxygen. *South Med J* 1993;86:334–337.

96. Ginsberg MD, Myers RE. Fetal brain injury after maternal carbon monoxide intoxication. Clinical and neuropathologic aspects. *Neurology* 1976;26:15–23.

97. Longo LD. The biological effects of carbon monoxide on the pregnant woman, fetus and newborn infant. *Am J Obstet Gynecol* 1977;129:69–103.

98. Carpenter WV. *Use and abuse of alcoholic liquors.* Boston: Crosby & Nichols, 1851.

99. Heuyer C, et al. La descendance des alcooliques. *La Presse Med* 1957;29:657–658.

100. Lemoine P, Harousseau H, Borteyru J. Les enfants de parents alcooliques: anomalies observées. *Ouest Médicale* 1968;25:476–482.

101. Clarren SK, Smith DW. The fetal alcohol syndrome. *N Engl J Med* 1978;298:1063–1067.

102. Sampson PD, et al. Incidence of fetal alcohol syndrome and prevalence of alcohol-related neurodevelopmental disorder. *Teratology* 1997;56:317–326.

103. West JR, Chen WJ, Pantazis NJ. Fetal alcohol syndrome: the vulnerability of the developing brain and possible mechanisms of damage. *Metab Brain Dis* 1995;9:291–322.

104. Shibley IA, Pennington SN. Metabolic and mitotic changes associated with the fetal alcohol syndrome. *Alcohol Alcohol* 1997;32:423–434.

105. Forrest F, du V. Florey C. The relation between maternal alcohol consumption and child development: the epidemiological evidence. *J Publ Health Med* 1991; 13:247–255.

106. Zuckerman B, Bresnahan K. Developmental and behavioral consequences of prenatal drug and alcohol exposure. *Pediatr Clin North Am* 1991;38:1387–1406.

107. Day NL, Richardson GA. Prenatal alcohol exposure: a continuum of effects. *Semin Perinatol* 1991;15: 271–279.

108. Porter R, O'Connor M, Whelan J, eds. *Mechanisms of alcohol damage in utero.* London: Pitman, Ciba Foundation Symposium, 1984:103–123.

109. Dow KE, Riopelle RJ. Neurotoxicity of ethanol during prenatal development. *Clin Neuropharm* 1987; 10:330–341.

110. Wiesniewski K, et al. A clinical neuropathological study of the fetal alcohol syndrome. *Neuropediatrics* 1983;14:197–201.

111. Ferrer I, Galofre E. Dendritic spine anomalies in fetal alcohol syndrome. *Neuropediatrics* 1987;18:161–163.

112. Konovalov HV, et al. Disorders of brain development in the progeny of mothers who used alcohol during pregnancy. *Early Human Development* 1997;48: 153–166.

113. Autti-Rämö I, Gaily E, Granström M-L. Dysmorphic features in offspring of alcoholic mothers. *Arch Dis Child* 1992;67:712–716.

114. Sokol RJ, Clarren SK. Guidelines for use of terminology describing the impact of prenatal alcohol on the offspring. *Alcoholism* 1989;13:597–598.

115. Aase JM, Jones KL, Clarren SK. Do we need the term "FAE"? *Pediatrics* 1995;95:428–430.

116. Pinazo-Duran MD, et al. Optic nerve hypoplasia in fetal alcohol syndrome: an update. *Eur J Ophthalmol* 1997;7:262–270.

117. Strömland K, Hellström A. Fetal alcohol syndrome—an opthalmological and socioeducational prospective study. *Pediatrics* 1996;97:845–850.

118. Peiffer J, et al. Alcohol embryo- and fetopathy. *J Neurol Sci* 1979;41:125–137.

119. Nitowsky HM. Fetal alcohol syndrome and alcohol-related birth defects. *NY State J Med* 1982;82: 1214–1217.

120. Autti-Rämö I, et al. Mental development of 2-year-old children exposed to alcohol in utero. *J Pediatr* 1992;120:740–746.

121. Spohr H-L, Willms J, Steinhausen H-C. Prenatal alcohol exposure and long-term developmental consequences. *Lancet* 1993;341:907–910.

122. Mattsen SN, et al. Heavy prenatal alcohol exposure with or without physical features of fetal alcohol syndrome leads to IQ deficits. *J Pediatr* 1997;131:718–721.

123. Shaywitz SE, Caparulo B, Hodgson ES. Developmental language disability as a result of prenatal exposure to ethanol. *Pediatrics* 1981;68:850–855.

124. Larsson G, Bohlin A-B, Tunell R. Prospective study of children exposed to variable amounts of alcohol in utero. *Arch Dis Child* 1985;60:316–321.

125. Dickerman JD, Bishop W, Marks JF. Acute ethanol intoxication in a child. *Pediatrics* 1968;42:837–840.

126. Cummins LH. Hypoglycemia and convulsions in children following alcohol ingestion. *J Pediatr* 1961; 58:23–26.

127. Wilson NM, et al. Glucose turnover and metabolic and hormonal changes in ethanol induced hypoglycaemia. *Br Med J* 1981;282:849.

128. Young D, Dragunow M. Status epilepticus may be caused by loss of adenosine anticonvulsant mechanisms. *Neuroscience* 1994;58:245–261.

129. Bahls FH, Ma KK, Bird TD. Theophylline-associated seizures with "therapeutic" or low toxic serum concentrations: risk factors for serious outcome in adults. *Neurology* 1991;41:1309–1312.

130. Baker MD. Theophylline toxicity in children. *J Pediatr* 1986;109:538–542.

131. Pranzatelli MR, Albin RL, Cohen BH. Acute dyskinesias in young asthmatics treated with theophylline. *Pediatr Neurol* 1991;7:216–219.

132. Shields MD, et al. Infantile spasms associated with theophylline toxicity. *Acta Paediatr* 1995;84: 215–217.

133. Skopnik H, Bergt U, Heimann G. Neonatal theophylline intoxication: pharmacokinetics and clinical evaluation. *Eur J Pediatr* 1992;151:221–224.

134. Olsen RW, et al. Allosteric actions of central nervous system depressants including anesthetics on subtypes of the inhibitory γ-aminobutyric acid A receptor-chloride channel complex. *Ann NY Acad Sci* 1991;625: 145–154.

135. McCarron MM, et al. Short-acting barbiturate overdosage. Correlation of intoxication score with serum barbiturate concentration. *JAMA* 1982;248:55–61.

136. Mitchell AA, Lovejoy FH, Goldman P. Drug ingestions associated with miosis in comatose children. *J Pediatr* 1976;89:303–305.

137. Lorber J, Reckless JPD, Watson JBG. Nonaccidental poisoning: the elusive diagnosis. *Arch Dis Child* 1980;55:643–647.

138. Mann JB, Sandberg DH. Therapy of sedative overdosage. *Pediatr Clin North Am* 1970;17:617–628.

139. Bertino JS Jr, Reed MD. Barbiturate and nonbarbiturate sedative hypnotic intoxication in children. *Pediatr Clin North Am* 1986;33:703–722.

140. Lee HA. The role of peritoneal and haemodialysis treatment. In: Matthew H, ed. *Acute barbiturate poisoning.* Amsterdam: Excerpta Medica, 1971:205.

141. Pond SM, et al. Randomized study of the treatment of phenobarbital overdose with repeated doses of activated charcoal. *JAMA* 1984;251:3104–3108.

142. Knight ME, Roberts RJ. Phenothiazine and buty-rophenone intoxication in children. *Pediatr Clin North Am* 1986;33:299–309.

143. Lev R, Clark RF. Neuroleptic malignant syndrome presenting without fever: case report and review of the literature. *J Emerg Med* 1994;12:49–55.

144. Heiman-Patterson TD. Neuroleptic malignant syndrome and malignant hyperthermia. Important issues for the medical consultant. *Med Clin North Am* 1993; 77:477–492.

145. Shields WD, Bray PF. A danger of haloperidol therapy in children. *J Pediatr* 1976;88:301–303.

146. Guze BH, Guze PA. Psychotropic medication use during pregnancy. *West J Med* 1989;151:296–298.

147. Rosebush PI, Stewart T, Mazurek MF. The treatment of neuroleptic malignant syndrome. Are dantrolene and bromocriptine useful adjuncts to supportive care? *Br J Psychiatry* 1991;159:709–712.

148. Thomas RJ. Neurotoxicity of antibacterial therapy. *Southern Med J* 1994;87:869–874.

149. Wallace KL. Antibiotic-induced convulsions. *Crit Care Clin* 1997;13:741–762.

149a. Tsuda A, et al. Effect of penicillin on GABA-gated chloride ion influx. *Neurochem Res* 1994;19:1–4.

150. Fausti SA, et al. High frequency audiometric monitoring for early detection of aminoglycoside ototoxicity. *J Infect Dis* 1992;165:1026–1032.

151. Kaeser HE. Drug-induced myasthenic syndromes. *Acta Neurol Scand Suppl* 1984;100:39–47.

152. Zwiener RJ, Ginsberg CM. Organophosphate and carbamate poisoning in infants and children. *Pediatrics* 1988;81:121–126.

153. Senanayake N, Karalliede L. Neurotoxic effects of organophosphorus insecticides. An intermediate syndrome. *N Engl J Med* 1987;316:761–763.

154. O'Malley M. Clinical evaluation of pesticide exposure and poisonings. *Lancet* 1997;349:1161–1166.

155. Mortenson ML. Management of acute childhood poisoning caused by selected insecticides and herbicides. *Pediatr Clin North Am* 1986;33:421–445.

156. Narahashi T, et al. Sodium and GABA-activated channels as the targets of pyrethroids and cyclodienes. *Toxicol Lett* 1992;64–65:429–436.

157. Waller K, et al. Seizures after eating a snack food contaminated with the pesticide endrin. The tale of toxic taquitos. *West J Med* 1992;157:648–651.

158. Rowley DL, et al. Convulsions caused by endrin poisoning in Pakistan. Pediatrics 1987;79:928–934.

159. Aks SE, et al. Acute accidental lindane ingestion in toddlers. *Ann Emerg Med* 1995;26:647–651.

160. Schwartz RH, Miller NS. MDMA (ecstasy) and the rave: a review. *Pediatrics* 1997;100:705–708.

161. Kulberg A. Substance abuse: clinical identification and management. *Pediatr Clin North Am* 1986;33: 325–361.

162. Schwartz RH, Einhorn A. PCP intoxication in seven young children. *Pediatr Emerg Care* 1986;2:238–241.

163. Cooper AJ, Egleston CV. Accidental ingestion of ecstasy by a toddler: unusual cause for convulsion in a febrile child. *J Acid Emerg Med* 1997;14: 183–184.

164. Kimbrough RD. Review of recent evidence of toxic effects of hexachlorophene. *Pediatrics* 1973;51: 391–394.

165. Martinez AJ, Boehm R, Hadfield MG. Acute hexa-chlorophene encephalopathy: cliniconeuropathological correlation. *Acta Neuropathol* 1974;28:92–103.

166. Martin-Bouyer G, et al. Outbreak of accidental hexa-chlorophene poisoning in France. *Lancet* 1982;28: 93–103.

167. Hillman LS, Hillman RE, Dodson WE. Diagnosis, treatment and follow-up of neonatal mepivacaine intoxication secondary to paracervical and pudendal blocks during labor. *J Pediatr* 1979;95:472–477.

168. Chan TY. The risk of severe salicylate poisoning following the ingestion of topical medicaments or aspirin. *Postgrad Med J* 1996;72:109–112.

169. Done AK. Aspirin overdosage: incidence, diagnosis, and management. *Pediatrics* 1978;62[5 Pt 2 Suppl.]: 890–897.

170. Dove DJ, Jones T. Delayed coma associated with salicylate intoxication. *J Pediatr* 1982;100:493–496.

171. Heiman-Patterson TD, et al. Peripheral neuropathy associated with eosinophilia-myalgia syndrome. *Ann Neurol* 1990;28:522–528.

172. Tolander LM, et al. Neurologic complications of the tryptophan-associated eosinophilia-myalgia syndrome. *Arch Neurol* 1991;48:436–438.

173. Toxic Epidemic Study Group. Toxic epidemic syndrome, Spain 1981. *Lancet* 1982;2:697–702.

174. Tilson HA, Jacobson JL, Rogan WJ. Polychlorinated biphenyls and the developing nervous system: cross-species comparisons. *Neurotoxicol Teratol* 1990;12: 239–248.

175. Volpe JJ. Effect of cocaine use on the fetus. *N Engl J Med* 1992;327:399–407.

176. Chasnoff IJ, et al. Cocaine/polydrug use in pregnancy: two-year follow-up. *Pediatrics* 1992;89:284–289.

177. King TA, et al. Neurologic manifestations of in utero cocaine exposure in near-term and term infants. *Pediatrics* 1995;96:259–264.

178. Dominguez R, et al. Brain and ocular abnormalities in infants with in utero exposure to cocaine and other street drugs. *Am J Dis Child* 1991;145:688–695.

179. Oro AS, Dixon SD. Perinatal cocaine and methamphetamine exposure: maternal and neonatal correlates. *J Pediatr* 1987;111:571–578.

180. Doberczak TM, et al. Neonatal neurologic and electroencephalographic effects of intrauterine cocaine exposure. *J Pediatr* 1988;113:354–358.

181. Kramer LD, et al. Neonatal cocaine-related seizures. *J Child Neurol* 1990;5:60–64.

182. Beltran RS, Coker SR. Transient dystonia of infancy, a result of intrauterine cocaine exposure? *Pediatr Neurol* 1995;12:354–356.

183. Dixon SD, Bejar R. Echoencephalographic findings in neonates associated with maternal cocaine and methamphetamine use: incidence and clinical correlates. *J Pediatr* 1989;115:770–778.

184. Hurt H, et al. A prospective evaluation of early language development in children with in utero cocaine exposure and in control subjects. *J Pediatr* 1997;130:310–312.

185. Mott SH, Packer RJ, Soldin SJ. Neurologic manifestations of cocaine exposure in children. *Pediatrics* 1994;93:557–560.

186. Vargas GC, et al. Effect of maternal heroin addiction on 67 liveborn neonates. *Clin Pediatr* 1975;14:751–753.

187. Zelson C, Rubio E, Wasserman E. Neonatal narcotic addiction: 10-year observation. *Pediatrics* 1971;48: 178–189.

188. Schulman CA. Alterations of the sleep cycle in heroin addicted and "suspect" newborns. *Neuropädiatrie* 1969;1:89–100.

189. Ostrea EM, Chavez CJ, Strauss ME. A study of factors that influence the severity of neonatal narcotic withdrawal. *J Pediatr* 1976;88:642–645.

190. Cepeda EE, Lee MI, Mehdizadeh B. Decreased incidence of intraventricular hemorrhage in infants of opiate dependent mothers. *Scand Acta Paediatr* 1987;76:16–18.

191. Yaster M, et al. The management of opioid and benzodiazepine dependence in infants, children and adolescents. *Pediatrics* 1996;98:135–140.

192. Vance JC, et al. Infants born to narcotic dependent mothers: physical growth patterns in the first 12 months of life. *J Paediatr Child Health* 1997;33: 504–508.

193. Ostrea EM, et al. Mortality within the first 2 years in infants exposed to cocaine, opiate, or cannabinoid during gestation. *Pediatrics* 1997;100:79–83.

194. Kaltenbach K, Finnegan LP. Perinatal and developmental outcome of infants exposed to methadone in utero. *Neurotoxicol Teratol* 1987;9:311–313.

195. Wilson GS, et al. The development of preschool children of heroin-addicted mothers: a controlled study. *Pediatrics* 1979;63:135–141.

196. Orney A, et al. The developmental outcome of children born to heroin-dependent mothers, raised at home or adopted. *Child Abuse Negl* 1996;20: 385–396.

197. Schmorl G. Zur Kenntnis des Ikterus neonatorum insbesondere der dabei auftretenden Gehirnveränderungen. *Verh Dtsch Ges Pathol* 1903;6:109–115.

198. Gourley GR. Bilirubin metabolism and kernicterus. *Adv Pediatr* 1997;44:173–229.

199. Haymaker W, et al. Pathology of kernicterus and posticteric encephalopathy. In: American Academy for Cerebral Palsy. *Kernicterus and its importance in cerebral palsy.* Springfield, IL: Charles C Thomas, 1961:210–228.

200. Turkel SB, et al. A clinical pathologic reappraisal of kernicterus. *Pediatrics* 1982;69:267–272.

201. Hsia DYY, et al. Erythroblastosis fetalis VIII. Studies of serum bilirubin in relation to kernicterus. *N Engl J Med* 1952;247:668–671.

202. Gartner LM, et al. Kernicterus: high incidence in premature infants with low serum bilirubin concentrations. *Pediatrics* 1970;45:906–917.

203. Newman TB, Maisels MJ. Evaluation and treatment of jaundice in the term newborn: a kinder, gentler approach. *Pediatrics* 1992;89:809–818.

204. Rubin RA, Balow B, Fisch RO. Neonatal serum bilirubin levels related to cognitive development at ages 4 through 7 years. *J Pediatr* 1979;94:601–604.

205. Johnston WH, et al. Erythroblastosis fetalis and hyperbilirubinemia: a five-year follow-up with neurological, psychological and audiological evaluation. *Pediatrics* 1967;39:88–92.

206. Scheidt PC, et al. Intelligence at six years in relation to neonatal bilirubin level: follow-up of the National Institute of Child Health and Human Development clinical trial of phototherapy. *Pediatrics* 1991;87: 797–805.

207. Maisels MJ, Newman TB. Kernicterus in otherwise healthy, breast-fed term newborns. *Pediatrics* 1995;96:730–733.

208. Blumenschein SD, et al. Familial nonhemolytic jaundice with late onset of neurological damage. *Pediatrics* 1968;42:786–792.

209. Labrune PH, et al. Cerebellar symptoms as the presenting manifestations of bilirubin encephalopathy in children with Crigler-Najjar Type I disease. *Pediatrics* 1992;89:768–770.

210. Rubboli G, et al. A neurophysiological study in children and adolescents with Crigler-Najjar syndrome Type I. *Neuropediatrics* 1997;28:281–286.

210a. Fox IJ, et al. Treatment of the Crigler-Najjar syndrome Type I with hepatocyte transplantation. *N Engl J Med* 1998;338:1422–1426.

211. Watchko JF, Oski FA. Kernicterus in preterm newborns: Past, present, and future. *Pediatrics* 1992; 90:707–715.

212. Pearlman MA, et al. The association of kernicterus with bacterial infection in the newborn. *Pediatrics* 1980;65:26–29.

213. Bratlid D, Cashore WJ, Oh W. Effect of serum hyperosmolality on opening of blood–brain barrier for bilirubin in rat brain. *Pediatrics* 1983;71:909–912.

214. Levine RL, Fredericks WR, Rapoport SI. Entry of bilirubin into the brain due to opening of the blood–brain barrier. *Pediatrics* 1982;69:255–259.

215. Hansen TW, Mathiesen SB, Walaas SI. Modulation of the effect of bilirubin on protein phosphorylation by lysine-containing peptides. *Pediatr Res* 1997;42: 615–617.

216. Hoffman DJ, et al. The in vivo effect of bilirubin on the *N*-methyl-D-aspartate receptor/ion channel complex in the brains of newborn piglets. *Pediatr Res* 1996;40:804–808.

217. Walker PC. Neonatal bilirubin toxicity. A review of kernicterus and the implications of drug-induced bilirubin displacement. *Clin Pharmacokinet* 1987;13: 26–50.

218. Ahdab-Barmada M, Moossy J. The neuropathology of kernicterus in the premature neonate: diagnostic problems. *J Neuropath Exp Neurol* 1984;43:45–56.

219. Watchko JF, Classen D. Kernicterus in premature infants: current prevalence and relationship to NICHD Phototherapy Study Exchange Criteria. *Pediatrics* 1994;93:996–999.

220. Jardine DS, Rogers K. Relationship of benzyl alcohol to kernicterus, intraventricular hemorrhage, and mortality in preterm infants. *Pediatrics* 1989;83: 153–160.

221. Cronin CM, Brown DR, Ahdab-Barmada M. Risk factors associated with kernicterus in the newborn infant: importance of benzyl alcohol exposure. *Am J Perinatol* 1991;8:80–85.

222. Boreau T, Mensch-Dechene J, Roux-Doutheret F. Etude clinique de 34 cas d'ictere nucléaire par maladie hémolytique néonatale et de leur évolution. *Arch Fr Pediatr* 1964;21:43–85.

223. Perlstein MA. The clinical syndrome of kernicterus. In: American Academy for Cerebral Palsy. *Kernicterus and its importance in cerebral palsy.* Springfield, IL: Charles C Thomas, 1961:268–279.

224. Byers RK, Paine RS, Crothers B. Extrapyramidal cerebral palsy with hearing loss following erythroblastosis. *Pediatrics* 1955;15:248–254.

225. Nakamura H, et al. Auditory nerve and brainstem responses in newborn infants with hyperbilirubinemia. *Pediatrics* 1985;75:703–708.

226. Streletz L, et al. Brainstem auditory evoked potentials in fullterm and preterm newborns with hyperbilirubinemia and hypoxemia. *Neuropediatrics* 1986;17:66–71.

227. deVries LS, Laray S, Dubowitz LMS. Relationship of serum bilirubin to ototoxicity and deafness in high-risk low-birth-weight infants. *Pediatrics* 1985;76:351–354.

228. Yokochi K. Magnetic resonance imaging in children with kernicterus. *Acta Paediatr* 1995;84:937–939.

229. Tonello F, et al. Tetanus and botulism neurotoxins: a novel group of zinc-endopeptidases. *Adv Exp Med Biol* 1996;389:251–260.

230. Gutmann L, Pratt L. Pathophysiologic aspects of human botulism. *Arch Neurol* 1976;33:175–179.

231. Meyer KF. Food poisoning. *N Engl J Med* 1953;249: 843–852.

232. Oh SJ. Botulism: electrophysiological studies. *Ann Neurol* 1977;1:481–485.

233. Keesey JC. Electrodiagnostic approach to defects in neuromuscular transmission. *Muscle Nerve* 1989;12: 613–626.

234. Arnon SS. Infant botulism. *Annu Rev Med* 1980;31: 541–560.

235. Clay SA, et al. Acute infantile motor unit disorder. Infantile botulism? *Arch Neurol* 1977;34:236–243.

236. Glauser TA, Maguire HC, Sladsky JT. Relapse of infant botulism. *Ann Neurol* 1990;28:187–189.

237. Graf WD, et al. Electrodiagnosis reliability in the diagnosis of infant botulism. *J Pediatr* 1992;120: 745–749.

238. Cornblath DR, Sladky JT, Sumner A. Clinical electrophysiology of infantile botulism. *Muscle Nerve* 1983;6:448–452.

239. Krepler P, Piringer WA, Weingarten K. Botulismus bei Kindern. *Wien Klin Wochenschr* 1963;75: 541–547.

240. Arnon SS. Infant botulism: anticipating the second decade. *J Infect Dis* 1986;154:201–206.

241. Tardo C, Steele RW. Infant botulism. *Clin Pediatr* 1997;36:592–594.

242. Schreiner MS, Field E, Ruddy R. Infant botulism: a review of 12 years' experience at the Children's Hospital of Philadelphia. *Pediatrics* 1991;87:159–165.

243. Pierce EJ, et al. Characterization of tetanus toxin binding to rat brain membranes. Evidence for a high-affinity proteinase-sensitive receptor. *Biochem J* 1986;236:845–852.

244. Fishman PS, Carrigan DR. Motoneuron uptake from the circulation of the binding fragment of tetanus toxin. *Arch Neurol* 1988;45:558–561.

245. Price DL, Griffin JW. Immunocytochemical localization of tetanus toxin to synapses of spinal cord. *Neurosci Lett* 1981;23:149–155.

246. Schwab ME, Suda K, Thoenen N. Selective retrograde transsynaptic transfer of a protein, tetanus toxin, subsequent to retrograde axonal transport. *J Cell Biol* 1979;82:798–810.

247. Ahnert-Hilger G, Bigalke H. Molecular aspects of tetanus and botulinum neurotoxin poisoning. *Prog Neurobiol* 1995;46:83–96.

248. Bergey GK, Bigalke H, Nelson PG. Differential effects of tetanus toxin on inhibitory and excitatory synaptic transmission in mammalian spinal cord neurons in culture: a presynaptic locus of action for tetanus toxin. *J Neurophysiol* 1987;57:121–131.

249. Udwadia FE, et al. Tetanus and its complications: intensive care and management experience in 150 Indian patients. *Epidemiol Infect* 1987;99:675–684.

250. Illis LS, Taylor FM. Neurological and electroencephalographic sequelae of tetanus. *Lancet* 1971;1: 826–830.

251. Craig AS, et al. Neonatal tetanus in the United States: a sentinel event in the foreign-born. *Pediatr Infect Dis J* 1997;16:955–959.

252. Salimpour R. Cause of death in tetanus neonatorum. Study of 233 cases with 54 necropsies. *Arch Dis Child* 1977;52:587–594.

253. Tompkins AB. Tetanus in African children. *Arch Dis Child* 1959;34:398–405.

254. Pinheiro D. Tetanus of the newborn infant. *Pediatrics* 1964;34:32–37.

255. Adams JM, Kenny JD, Rudolph AJ. Modern management of tetanus neonatorum. *Pediatrics* 1979;64: 472–477.

256. Andersson R. High dose oral diazepam and early full alimentation in neonatal tetanus. *Tropical Doct* 1991;21:172–173.

257. Sanford JP. Tetanus—forgotten but not gone. *N Engl J Med* 1995;332:812–813.

258. Einterz EM, Bates ME. Caring for neonatal tetanus patients in a rural primary care setting in Nigeria: a review of 237 cases. *J Trop Pediatr* 1991;37:179–181.

259. Daud S, Mohammad T, Ahmad A. Tetanus neonatorum. *J Trop Pediatr* 1981;27:308–311.

260. Godel JC. Trial of pyridoxine therapy for tetanus neonatorum. *J Infect Dis* 982;145:547–549.

261. Singh M, et al. Diphtheria in Afghanistan—review of 155 cases. *J Trop Med Hyg* 1985;88:373–376.

262. Fisher CM, Adams RD. Diphtheritic polyneuritis—a pathological study. *J Neuropath Exp Neurol* 1956;15: 243–268.

263. London E. Diphtheria toxin: membrane interaction and membrane translocation. *Biochim Biophys Acta* 1992;1113:25–51.

264. Solders G, Nennesmo I, Persson A. Diphtheritic neuropathy, an analysis based on muscle and nerve biopsy and repeated neurophysiological and autonomic function tests. *J Neurol Neurosurg Psychiatry* 1989;52:876–880.

265. Tibballs J, Cooper SJ. Paralysis with Ixodes cornuatus envenomation. *Med J Aust* 1986;145:37–38.

266. Grattan-Smith PJ, et al. Clinical and neurophysiological features of tick paralysis. *Brain* 1997;120:1975–1987.

267. Beyer AB, Grossman M. Tick paralysis in a red wolf. *J Wildl Dis* 1997;33:900–902.

268. Kincaid JC. Tick bite paralysis. *Semin Neurol* 1990;10:32–34.

269. Mushatt DM, Hyslop NE Jr. Neurologic aspects of North American zoonoses. *Infect Dis Clin North Am* 1991;5:703–731.

270. Adams ME, Swanson G. Neurotoxins, 2nd ed. *Trends Neurosci* 1996;19 [Suppl.]:137.

271. Russell FE. *Snake venom poisoning*. Great Neck, NY: Scholium International, 1983.

272. Southcott RV. The neurologic effects of noxious marine creatures. In: Hornabrook RW, ed. *Topics on tropical neurology*. Philadelphia: FA Davis, 1975;165–258.

273. Campbell CH. The effects of snake venoms and their neurotoxins on the nervous system of man and animals. In: Hornabrook RW, ed. *Topics on tropical neurology*. Philadelphia: FA Davis, 1975:259–294.

274. Auerbach PS, ed. *Wilderness medicine: management of wilderness and environmental emergencies*, 3rd ed. St. Louis: Mosby, 1995.

275. Furbee B, Wermuth M. Life-threatening plant poisoning. *Crit Care Clinics* 1997;13:849–888.
276. Burnett JW. et al. Coelenterate venom research 1991–1995: clinical, chemical and immunological aspects. *Toxicon* 1996;34:1377–1383.
277. Gessner BD, Middaugh JP, Doucette GJ. Paralytic shellfish poisoning in Kodiak, Alaska. *West J Med* 1997;167:351–353.
278. Teitelbaum JS, et al. Neurologic sequelae of domoic acid intoxication due to the ingestion of contaminated mussels. *N Engl J Med* 1990;322:1781–1787.
279. Holstege CP, et al. Crotalid snake envenomation. *Crit Care Clin* 1997;13:888–921.
280. Weber RA, White RR. Crotalidae envenomation in children. *Ann Plast Surg* 1993;31:141–145.
281. Watt G, et al. Positive response to edrophonium in patients with neurotoxic envenoming by cobras (*Naja naja philippinensis*). A placebo-controlled study. *N Engl J Med* 1986;315:1444–1448.
282. Vijayaraghavan S, et al. Nicotinic receptors that bind α-bungarotoxin on neurons raise intracellular free Ca2+. *Neuron* 1992;8:353–362.
283. Britt A, Burkhart K. Naja naja cobra bite. *Am J Emerg Med* 1997;15:529–531.
284. Moss HS, Binder LS. A retrospective review of black widow spider envenomation. *Ann Emerg Med* 1987;16:188–192.
285. Ushkaryov YA, et al. Neurexins: Synaptic cell surface proteins related to the α-latrotoxin receptor and laminin. *Sciences* 1992;257:50–56.
286. Davletov BA, et al. High affinity binding of alpha-latrotoxin to recombinant neurexin I alpha. *J Biol Chem* 1995;270:23903–23905.
287. Woesstman R, Perkin R, Van Stralen D. The black widow: is she deadly to children? *Pediatr Emerg Care* 1996;12:360–364.
288. Berg RA, Tarantino MD. Envenomation by the scorpion centuroides exilicauda (*C. sculpturatus*): severe and unusual manifestations. *Pediatrics* 1991;87:930–933.
289. de Davila M, et al. Scorpion envenomation in Merida, Venezuela. *Toxicon* 1997;35:1459–1462.
290. Russell FE. Stingray injuries: a review and discussion of their treatment. *Am J Med Sci* 1953;226:611.
291. Kizer KW, McKinney HE, Auerbach PS. Scorpaenidae envenomation. A five year poison center experience. *JAMA* 1985;253:807–810.
292. Ghadessy FJ, et al. Stonustoxin is a novel lethal factor from stonefish (*Synanceja horrida*) venom. CDNA cloning and characterization. *J Biol Chem* 1996;271:25575–25581.
292a. Khoo HE, Chen D, Yuen R. Role of free thiol groups in the biological activities of stonustoxin, a lethal factor from stonefish (*Synanceja horrida*) verom. *Toxicon* 1998;36:469–476.
293. Mills AR, Pasmore R. Pelagic paralysis. *Lancet* 1988;1:161–164.
294. Cameron J, Flowers AE, Capra MF. Electrophysiological studies on ciguatera poisoning in man (Part II). *J Neurol Sci* 1991;101:93–97.
295. Williams RK, Palafox NA. Treatment of pediatric ciguatera fish poisoning. *Am J Dis Child* 1990;144:747–748.
296. DeWolfe FA. Neurologic aspects of mushroom intoxications. In: Vinken PJ, Bruyn GW, eds. *Intoxications of the nervous system, part I. handbook of clinical Neurology.* Vol. 36. Amsterdam: North-Holland, 1979:529–546.
297. McPartland JM, Vilgalys RJ, Cubeta MA. Mushroom poisoning. *Am Fam Phys* 1997;55:1797–1800, 1805–1809, 1811–1812.
298. Pond SM, et al. Amatoxin poisoning in Northern California, 1982–1983. *West J Med* 1986;145:204–209.
299. Spencer PS, et al. Lathyrism: evidence for role of the neuroexcitatory amino acid BOAA. *Lancet* 1986;2:1066–1067.
300. Ludolph AC, Spencer PS. Toxic models of upper motor neuron disease. *J Neurol Sci* 1996;139 [Suppl.]:53–59.
301. Villalobos R, Santos MA. Karwinskia palsy in childhood. *Acta Neuropediatr* 1996;2:154–159.
302. Mack RB. Toxic encounters of the dangerous kind. The nutmeg connection. *North Car Med J* 1982;43:439.
303. Mack RB. Toxic encounters of the dangerous kind. The baddest seed-ricin poisoning. *North Car Med J* 1982;43:584–589.
304. Lond JM, Roberts LM, Robertus JD. Ricin: structure, mode of action, and some current applications. *FASEB J* 1994;8:201–208.
305. Mack RB. Toxic encounters of the dangerous kind. "Loco" weed and the anticholinergic syndrome. *North Car Med J* 1982;43:650.
306. Savitt DL, Roberts JR, Siegel EG. Anisocoria from jimson weed. *JAMA* 1986;255:1439–1440.
307. Mack RB. Toxic encounters of the dangerous kind. Poke-weed. *North Car Med J* 1982;43:365.
308. Tanaka K. Jamaican vomiting sickness. In: Vinken PJ, Bruyn GW, eds. *Intoxications of the nervous system, part II. Handbook of clinical neurology,* Vol. 37. Amsterdam: North-Holland, 1979:511–539.
309. Trost LC, Lemasters JJ. The mitochondrial permeability transition: a new pathophysiological mechanism for Reye's syndrome and toxic liver injury. *J Pharmacol Exp Therap* 1996;278:1000–1005.
310. He F, et al. Delayed dystonia with striatal CT lucencies induced by a mycotoxin (3-nitropropionic acid). *Neurology* 1995;45:2178–2183.
311. Williams CD. Kwashiorkor—a nutritional disease of children associated with a maize diet. *Lancet* 1935;2:1151–1152.
312. DeSilva CC. Common nutritional disorders of childhood in the tropics. *Adv Pediatr* 1964;13:213–264.
313. Jelliffe DB, Jelliffe EFP. Protein-energy malnutrition. In: Strickland GT, ed. *Hunter's tropical medicine.* Philadelphia: WB Saunders, 1991:914–922.
314. Trowell HC, Davies JN, Dean RF. *Kwashiorkor.* London: Edward Arnold, Ltd., 1954.
315. Lenhartz H, et al. The clinical manifestation of the kwashiorkor syndrome is related to increased lipid peroxidation. *J Pediatr* 1998;132:879–881.
316. Hendrickse RG. Kwashiorkor: the hypothesis that incriminates aflatoxins. *Pediatrics* 1991;88:376–379.
317. Jelliffe DB, Jelliffe EFP. Causation of kwashiorkor: toward a multifactorial consensus. *Pediatrics* 1992;90:110–113.
318. Harper C, Butterworth R. Nutritional and metabolic disorders. In: Graham DI, Lantos PL, eds. *Greenfields's neuropathology,* 6th ed. London: Edward Arnold, Ltd., 1997:601–655.
319. Udani PM. Protein energy malnutrition (PEM), brain and various facets of child development. *Indian J Pediatr* 1992;59:165–186.

320. Mehta S, et al. Energy metabolism of brain in human protein-calorie malnutrition. *Pediatr Res* 1977;11: 290–293.

321. Dobbing J. Undernutrition and developing brain. *Am J Dis Child* 1970;120:411–415.

322. Udani PM. Neurological manifestations in kwashiorkor. *Indian J Child Health* 1960;9:103–112.

323. Sachdeva KK, Taori GM, Pereira SM. Neuromuscular status in protein-calorie malnutrition. Clinical, nerve conduction and electromyographic studies. *Neurology* 1971;21:801–805.

324. Chopra JS, et al. Effect of protein calorie malnutrition on peripheral nerves. A clinical, electrophysiological and histopathological study. *Brain* 1986;109:307–323.

325. Chopra JS, Sharma A. Protein energy malnutrition and the nervous system. *J Neurol Sci* 1992;110:820.

326. Agarwal KN, et al. Soft neurological signs and EEG pattern in rural malnourished children. *Acta Paediatr Scan* 1989;78:873–878.

327. Gunston, GD, et al. Reversible cerebral shrinkage in kwashiorkor: an MRI study. *Arch Dis Child* 1992;67: 1030–1032.

328. Cravioto J, DeLicardie ER, Birch HG. Nutrition, growth and neurointegrative development. An experimental and ecologic study. *Pediatrics* 1966;38:319–372.

329. Eichenwald HF, Fry PC. Nutrition and learning. *Science* 1969;163:644–648.

330. Evans D, et al. Intellectual development and nutrition. *J Pediatr* 1980;97:358–363.

331. Stein Z, Susser M. Early nutrition, fetal growth and mental function: observations in our species. In: Rassin DK, ed. *Current topics in nutrition and disease. Vol. 16. Basic and clinical aspects of nutrition and brain development.* New York: Alan R. Liss, 1987:323–338.

332. Grantham-McGregor SM, et al. Nutritional supplementation, psychosocial stimulation, and mental development of stunted children: the Jamaican study. *Lancet* 1991;338:15.

333. Balmer S, Howells G, Wharton B. The acute encephalopathy of kwashiorkor. *Dev Med Child Neurol* 1968;10:766–771.

334. Kahn E, Falcke HC. A syndrome simulating encephalitis affecting children recovering from malnutrition (kwashiorkor). *J Pediatr* 1956;49:37–45.

335. Cravioto J, Robles B. Evolution of adaptive and motor behavior during rehabilitation from kwashiorkor. *Am J Orthopyschiatry* 1965;35:449–464.

336. Birch HG, et al. Relation of kwashiorkor in early childhood and intelligence at school age. *Pediatr Res* 1971;5:579–585.

337. Graham GG, Adrianzen BT. Growth, inheritance and environment. *Pediatr Res* 1971;5:691–697.

338. Rosso P. Maternal nutrition and fetal growth: implications for subsequent mental competence. In: Rassin DK, ed. *Current topics in nutrition and brain development.* New York: Alan R. Liss, 1987:339–357.

339. Keating JP, Feigin RD. Increased intracranial pressure associated with probable vitamin A deficiency in cystic fibrosis. *Pediatrics* 1970;46:41–46.

340. Snodgrass SR. Vitamin neurotoxicity. *Mol Neurobiol* 1992;6:41–73.

341. Peters RA. Significance of thiamine in the metabolism and function of the brain. In: Elliott KA, Page IH, Quastel JH, eds. *Neurochemistry.* Springfield, IL: Charles C Thomas, 1962:267.

342. Haas RH. Thiamine and the brain. *Ann Rev Nutr* 1988;8:483–515.

343. Shimojyo S, Scheinberg P, Reinmuth O. Cerebral blood flow and metabolism in the Wernicke-Korsakoff syndrome. *J Clin Invest* 1967;46:849–854.

344. McCandless DW, Schenker S. Encephalopathy of thiamine deficiency: Studies of intracerebral mechanisms. *J Clin Invest* 1968;47:2268–2280.

345. Dreyfus PM, Hauser G. The effect of thiamine deficiency on the pyruvate decarboxylase system of the central nervous system. *Biochem Biophys Acta* 1965;104:78–84.

346. Sharp FR, Bolger E, Evans K. Thiamine deficiency limits glucose utilization and glial proliferation in brain lesions of symptomatic rats. *J Cereb Blood Flow Metab* 1982;2:203–207.

347. Valyasevi A. Infantile beriberi. In: Jelliffe DB, Sternfield JP, eds. *Diseases of children in the subtropics and tropics.* London: Edward Arnold, 1978:227–233.

348. Tang CM, et al. Outbreak of beriberi in The Gambia. *Lancet* 1989;2:206–207.

349. Hahn JS, et al. Wernicke encephalopathy and beriberi during total parenteral nutrition attributable to multivitamin infusion shortage. *Pediatrics* 1998;101:E10.

350. Seear M, et al. Thiamine, riboflavin, and pyridoxine deficiencies in a population of critically ill children. *J Pediatr* 1992;121:533–538.

351. Haridas L. Infantile beriberi in Singapore. *Arch Dis Child* 1947;22:23–33.

352. Wyatt DT, Noetzel MJ, Hillman RE. Infantile beriberi presenting as subacute necrotizing encephalomyelopathy. *J Pediatr* 1987;110:888–892.

353. Pihko M, Saarinen V, Paetau A. Wernicke encephalopathy: a preventable cause of death—report of two children with malignant disease. *Pediatr Neurol* 1989;5: 237–242.

354. Seear MD, Norman MG. Two cases of Wernicke's encephalopathy in children: an underdiagnosed complication of poor nutrition. *Ann Neurol* 1988;24: 85–87.

355. Barrett TG, et al. Potentially lethal thiamine deficiency complicating parenteral nutrition in children. *Lancet* 1993;341:901.

356. Bessey OA, Adam DJ, Hansen AE. Intake of vitamin B_6 and infantile convulsions. A first approximation of requirements of pyridoxine in infants. *Pediatrics* 1957;20:33–44.

357. Molony CJ, Parmelee AH. Convulsions in young infants as a result of pyridoxine (vitamin B_6) deficiency. *JAMA* 1954;154:405–406.

358. Johnson GM. Powdered goat's milk. *Clin Pediatr* 1982;21:494–495.

359. Heiskanen K, et al. Risk of low vitamin B_6 status in infants breast-fed exclusively beyond six months. *J Pediatr Gastroenterol Nutr* 1996;23:38–44.

360. Scriver CR, Hutchison JH. Vitamin B_6 deficiency syndrome in human infancy: biochemical and clinical observations. *Pediatrics* 1963;31:240–250.

361. Coker SB. Postneonatal vitamin B_6-dependent epilepsy. *Pediatrics* 1992;90:221–223.

362. Baxter P, et al. Pyridoxine-dependent seizures: demographic, clinical, MRI and psychometric features, and effect of dose on intelligence quotient. *Dev Med Child Neurol* 1996;38:998–1006.

363. Hunt AD, et al. Pyridoxine dependency: report of a

case of intractable convulsions in an infant controlled by pyridoxine. *Pediatrics* 1954;13:140–145.

364. Baumeister FAM, et al. Glutamate in pyridoxine-dependent epilepsy: neurotoxic glutamate concentration in the cerebrospinal fluid and its normalization by pyridoxine. *Pediatrics* 1994;94:318–321.

365. Shih JJ, Kornblum H, Shewmon DA. Global brain dysfunction in an infant with pyridoxine dependency: evaluation with EEG, evoked potentials, MRI and PET. *Neurology* 1996;47:824–826.

366. Kurlemann G, Menges EM, Palm DG. Low levels of GABA in CSF in vitamin B_6-dependent seizures. *Dev Med Child Neurol* 1991;33:749–750.

367. Lott IT, et al. Vitamin B_6-dependent seizures. Pathology and chemical findings in brain. *Neurology* 1978; 28:47–54.

368. Gordon N. Pyridoxine dependency: an update. *Dev Med Child Neurol* 1997;39:63–65.

369. Condie BG, et al. Cleft palate in mice with a targeted mutation in the gamma-aminobutyric acid-producing enzyme glutamic acid decarboxylase 67. *Proc Natl Acad Sci USA* 1997;94:11451–11455.

369a. Gospe SM. Current perspectives on pyridoxine-dependent seizures. *J Pediatr* 1998;132:919–923.

370. McLachlan RS, Brown WF. Pyridoxine dependent epilepsy with iatrogenic sensory neuronopathy. *Canad J Neurol Sci.* 1995;22:50–51.

371. Bankier A, Turner M, Hopkins I. Pyridoxine dependent seizures—a wider clinical spectrum. *Arch Dis Child* 1983;58:415–418.

372. Jaffe KA, Altman K, Merryman P. The antipyridoxine effect of penicillamine in man. *J Clin Invest* 1964;43: 1869–1873.

373. Olson KR, et al. Seizures associated with poisoning and drug overdose. *Am J Emerg Med* 1994;12:392–395.

374. Shah BR, et al. Acute isoniazide neurotoxicity in an urban hospital. *Pediatrics* 1995;95:700–704.

375. Spillane JD. *Nutritional disorders of the nervous system.* Edinburgh: E & S Livingstone, 1947.

376. Malfait P, et al. An outbreak of pellagra related to changes in dietary niacin among Mozambican refugees in Malawi. *Int J Epidemiol* 1993;22:504–511.

377. Meyer A. On parenchymatous systemic degeneration mainly in the central nervous system. *Brain* 1901;24: 47–115.

378. Spies TD, Walker AA, Wood AW. Pellagra in infancy and childhood. *JAMA* 1939;113:1481–1483.

379. Still CN. Nicotinic acid and nicotinamide deficiency: pellagra and related disorders of the nervous system. In: Vinken PJ, Bruyn GW, eds. *Handbook of clinical neurology.* Vol. 28. Amsterdam: North-Holland, 1977: 59–104.

380. Lanska DJ. Stages in the recognition of epidemic pellagra in the United States: 1865–1960. *Neurology* 1996;47:829–834.

381. Sauberlich HE. Newer laboratory methods for assessing nutrition of selected B complex vitamins. *Annu Rev Nutr* 1984;4:337–407.

382. Kapadia CR. Vitamin B_{12} in health and disease: part I—inherited disorders of function, absorption, and

transport. *Gastroenterologist* 1995;3:329–344.

383. Graham SM, Arvela OM, Wise GA. Long-term neurologic consequences of nutritional vitamin B_{12} deficiency in infants. *J Pediatr* 1992;121:710–714.

384. Kuhne T, Bubl R, Baumgartner R. Maternal vegan diet causing a serious infantile neurological disorder due to vitamin B_{12} deficiency. *Eur J Pediatr* 1991; 150:205–208.

385. Higginbottom MC, Sweetman L, Nyhan WL. A syndrome of methylmalonic aciduria, homocystinuria, megaloblastic anemia and neurologic abnormalities in a vitamin B_{12}-deficient breast-fed infant of a strict vegetarian. *N Engl J Med* 1978;299: 317–323.

386. Grattan-Smith PJ, et al. The neurological syndrome of infantile cobalamin deficiency: developmental regression and involuntary movements. *Movement Disorders* 1997;12:39–46.

387. Davis JR, Goldenring J, Lubin BH. Nutritional vitamin B_{12} deficiency in infants. *Am J Dis Child* 1981; 135:566–567.

388. McNicholl B, Egan B. Congenital pernicious anemia: effects of growth, brain, and absorption of B_{12}. *Pediatrics* 1968;42:149–156.

389. Zegers de Beyl D, et al. Somatosensory conduction in vitamin B_{12} deficiency. *Electroencephal Clin Neurophysiol* 1988;69:313–318.

390. von Schenck U, Bender-Gotze C, Koletzko B. Persistence of neurological damage induced by dietary vitamin B_{12} deficiency in infancy. *Arch Dis Child* 1997; 77:137–139.

391. Pearson HA, Vinson R, Smith RT. Pernicious anemia with neurologic involvement in childhood. *J Pediatr* 1964;65:334–339.

392. Hall CA. Function of vitamin B_{12} in the central nervous system as revealed by congenital defects. *Am J Hematol* 1990;34:121–127.

393. Sharda B, Bhandari B. Infantile tremor syndrome. *Indian Pediatr* 1987;24:415–421.

394. Garewal G, Narang A, Das KC. Infantile tremor syndrome: a vitamin B_{12} deficiency syndrome in infants. *J Trop Pediatr* 1988;34:174–178.

395. Howlett WP, et al. Konzo, an epidemic upper motor neuron disease studied in Tanzania. *Brain* 1990; 113:223–235.

396. Ludolph AC, et al. Studies on the aetiology and pathogenesis of motor neuron diseases. 1. Lathyrism: clinical findings in established cases. *Brain* 1987; 110:149–165.

397. Kazadi K, et al. Nonspastic paraparesis associated with HTLV-I. *Lancet* 1990;336:260.

398. Roman GC, Spencer PS, Schoenberg BS. Tropical myeloneuropathies. The hidden endemias. *Neurology* 1985;35:1158–1170.

399. Carton H, et al. Epidemic spastic paraparesis in Bandundu (Zaire). *J Neurol Neurosurg Psychiatr* 1986; 49:620–627.

400. Spencer PS, et al. Guam amyotrophic lateral sclerosis-Parkinson-dementia linked to a plant excitant neurotoxin. *Science* 1987;237:517–522.

Chapter 10

Tumors of the Nervous System

Bernard L. Maria and *John H. Menkes

*Department of Pediatrics, University of Florida College of Medicine, Gainesville, Florida 32610;
and *Departments of Neurology and Pediatrics, University of California, Los Angeles,
UCLA School of Medicine, and Department of Pediatric Neurology, Cedars-Sinai Medical Center,
Los Angeles, California 90048*

BRAIN TUMORS

Incidence

Tumors of the central nervous system (CNS) occur relatively frequently during the early years of life. They are the most common solid tumors of childhood and afflict approximately 1,500 patients every year in the United States (1,2). Reported incidence rates have varied from 2 to 5 per 100,000 children (3). Representing 20% of all malignancies, they are second only to leukemia in overall cancer incidence and account for a high proportion of deaths (4).

Although the incidence of leukemia has remained relatively stable, the incidence of brain tumors has increased approximately 2% per year in the past 20 years (5). A review of earlier studies on the incidence of intracranial space-occupying lesions indicates that the relative frequencies of pathologic varieties have changed Critchley, writing in 1925, found tuberculoma to be the most common intracranial tumor of childhood (6). Subsequent surveys by Bailey and associates (7) and Cuneo and Rand (8) stressed the preponderance of gliomas. Meningiomas and neurinomas were virtually absent, except in association with neurofibromatosis (9). Tuberculomas are now rare in the developed countries, but a series of 107 cases was reported from India as recently

as 1965 (10). From 1981 through 1993, the incidence of primitive neuroectodermal tumor/medulloblastoma (PNET/MB), the most common malignant posterior fossa tumor, has risen more than 4% per year (Table 10.1). This trend has not been fully explained, but improved detection through sensitive and specific neuroimaging technology, such as magnetic resonance imaging (MRI), may account for much of the increase (11). There is no conclusive data to show that toxic waste, air and water pollutants, irradiation, and electromagnetic fields in local environments are tumorigenic (11a). Furthermore, environmental influences ordinarily are e   xpected to be gender blind, and thus could not account for the 4% increase in PNET/MB, which elicits a male-to-female gender ratio of approximately 2.5:1.

Pediatric brain tumors include a spectrum of both glial and nonglial tumors that differ significantly in location and biologic behavior from that of adults (Table 10.2) (12,13). Subtentorial tumors constitute more than 50% of all intracranial space-occupying lesions in children; in adults, only 25% to 30% of tumors originate below the tentorium. In children younger than age 1 year, as in adults, supratentorial tumors are most frequent; in infancy these often arise from hamartomas or other congenital malformations (1).

TABLE 10.1. *Florida childhood cancer incidence 1981–1993, 0–14 years*

Tumor	Number of cancers	Annual % change
All	4,174	0.91
Leukemias	1,257	−0.31
Brain tumors	769	1.92
Glioma WM	214	3.36
Glioma WF	188	1.10
PNET	163	4.19
Neuroblastoma	293	3.25

PNET, primitive neuroectodermal tumor; WF, white female; WM, white male.

Table adapted from Roush SW, et al. The incidence of pediatric cancer in Florida, 1981 to 1986. *Cancer* 1992;69:2212–2219.

Pathogenesis

A discussion of the molecular origins of neoplasia within the nervous system is far beyond the scope of this text. Suffice it to say that the uncontrolled proliferation of a population of somatic cells is basically a genetic disorder, with multiple genetic abnormalities preceding the neoplastic transformation of normal tissue. Two distinct fundamental mechanisms appear to be operative. One is associated with the activation or overexpression of growth-promoting factors such as proto-oncogenes, and the other is the result of

TABLE 10.2. *Incidence of brain tumors in the pediatric population younger than 15 years of age versus all ages[a]*

Tumors	All ages (%)	Children (%)
Glioma	45	70
Astrocytoma	15	30
Glioblastoma	15	5
Oligodendroglioma	8	1
Medulloblastoma	4	20
Ependymoma	4	10
Meningioma	15	1
Neurinoma	6	<0.5
Pituitary adenoma	6	1
Metastases	5–20	<0.5
Craniopharyngioma	3	10

[a]Figures are estimates and are based on reports collected from the literature.

Table adapted from Tobias J, Hayward RD. Brain and spinal cord tumours in children. In: Thomas DGT, ed. *Neuro-oncology: primary malignant brain tumours.* Baltimore: The Johns Hopkins University Press, 1990:164–192.

loss or inactivation of genes that normally regulate or suppress cell growth, the tumor-suppressor genes. The mutation of the proto-oncogene to an oncogene has a dominant effect; only one of the cell's two gene copies needs to undergo the mutation. The inactivation of a tumor-suppressor gene is recessive, which means that both gene copies must be inactivated. Inactivation of tumor-suppressor genes is believed to be responsible for the development of tumors in neurofibromatosis and tuberous sclerosis (see Chapter 11).

The role of tumor viruses in CNS neoplasia of childhood is less clear. However, one-half of choroid plexus tumors and most ependymomas contain and express a segment of a gene related to the monkey polyoma virus (SV40). This virus, which is highly tumorigenic in rodents, could have an etiologic role in the development of some childhood neoplasms. It is also possible that certain human neoplasms provide a favorable microenvironment for viral replication in tissue that is latently infected with SV40 (14). From the data currently available, it is clear that the combination of accumulating events is distinct for each tumor type; what is still unknown is which molecular abnormality is the rate-limiting step that leads to neoplastic transformation.

Cytogenetic analysis of glial tumors has identified a variety of chromosomal abnormalities (Table 10.3) (15). These include extra copies of chromosome 7, loss of chromosomes 10, 17, or 22, and structural abnormalities of chromosome 9p and 19q. Loss of heterozygosity involving the short arm of chromosome 17 (17p) has been detected in astrocytomas. Deletions of the short arm of chromosome 17 (17p12-13.1) have been seen consistently in PNET/MB. Mutations of *p53*, a gene localized to the short arm of chromosome 17, have been found in a significant proportion of PNET/MB and oligodendrogliomas. The protein encoded by this gene, termed the "guardian of the genome," appears to function as a modulator of cell proliferation and repairs mutagenic alterations. Overexpression or amplification of the gene encoding for the epidermal growth factor receptor has been documented in some glioblastomas. This proto-oncogene is the normal cellular homologue of the viral oncogene v-*erbB*. The molecular biology of tumors has

TABLE 10.3. *Chromosomal and genetic alterations characteristic of specific types of brain tumors*

Tumor type	Chromosomal or LOH abnormality	Genetic alteration
Glioblastoma	+7	Unknown
	−9p	CDKN2A, CDKN2B
	−1-	Unknown
	−17p	p53 gene mutation
	Dmins	EGFR gene amplification and rearrangement
Oligodendroglioma	−1p	Unknown
	−19q	Unknown
Ependymoma	−22	?NF2 gene mutation
Medulloblastoma	−17p	Unknown
	Dmins	c-myc, N-myc gene amplification
Meningioma	−22	NF2 gene mutation
Schwannoma	−22	NF2 gene mutation

Dmins, double minute chromosomes; EGFR, epidermal growth factor receptor; LOH, loss of heterozygosity; NF2, neurofibromatosis 2.

From Bigner SH, et al. Brain tumors. In: Vogelstein B, Kintzler KW, eds. *The genetic basis of human cancer.* New York: McGraw-Hill, 1998:661–670. With permission of the authors.

been reviewed by Bigner and colleagues (15), Santarius and colleagues (16), and Ng and Lam (17). Complete and detailed reviews of newer developments in tumor cell culture, the effect of animal models on brain tumor research, and basic discoveries in neuro-oncology are also available elsewhere (18,19).

From a clinical point of view, the importance of genetic factors in the development of brain tumors is significant. Surveys of the incidence of tumors in relatives of brain tumor patients have demonstrated a higher incidence of CNS neoplasms and of leukemia, but no greater incidence of other malignancies (20). Craniopharyngiomas and some of the PNET/MBs are congenital and arise from an area of maldevelopment. Craniopharyngiomas arise from persistent remnants of the craniopharyngeal (Rathke's) pouch and PNET/MBs usually from primitive cell rests in the posterior medullary velum.

Postnatal factors, trauma in particular, have not proven significant in the development of brain tumors in children. In a few instances, irra-

diation has been implicated in the appearance of malignant mesodermal tumors at the radiation site. In one study, radiation for ringworm of the scalp was associated with an increased incidence of brain tumors occurring after an interval that ranged from 7 to 21 years (21).

Symptoms and Signs

Neurologic symptoms produced by brain tumors are general or local. General symptoms result from increased intracranial pressure, which results directly from progressive enlargement of the tumor within the limited volume of the cranial vault; local symptoms are due to the effects of the tumor on contiguous areas of the brain.

Pathophysiology

An intracranial mass produces cerebral compression by its intrinsic volume; by its encroachment on the ventricular system, obstructing the flow of cerebrospinal fluid (CSF) and producing ventricular dilatation; and particularly when malignant, by its ability to produce edema in white matter adjacent to the expanding mass.

As the tumor enlarges, the intracranial contents, primarily the ventricular spaces, are initially compressed. The duration of the initial asymptomatic period depends on the rate of tumor expansion and on whether the tumor's location causes it to compromise the circulation of CSF.

When the intracranial pressure approaches or equals the systemic arterial pressure, it causes the systemic arterial pressure to increase. Cushing noted that systemic hypertension was accompanied by bradycardia and slow irregular respirations (Cushing triad) (22,23). Compression of the venous channels, especially the large, draining venous sinuses, reduces cerebral blood flow. The resulting cerebral anoxia in turn produces vascular dilatation and a further increase in intracerebral volume and pressure (24).

A number of experiments have proven Cushing's contention that the pressure threshold for the induction of the vasopressor response is reached when intracranial pressure is at the level of systemic arterial pressure. Clinical experience, however, suggests that arterial hypertension first appears at lower pressures, particularly when a pressure differential exists above and below the tentorium. Under these instances, the pressure response can be triggered by local ischemia of the cerebral hemispheres or by distortion of the brainstem and subsequent medullary ischemia. With a further increase in intracranial pressure, the vasopressor mechanism fails, arterial pressure decreases, and cerebral blood flow is substantially reduced (25,26).

Pulmonary edema can accompany increased intracranial pressure (neurogenic pulmonary edema). Its pathogenesis is poorly understood; most likely, the edema is the direct result of an elevated pulmonary capillary pressure. Whether this elevation results from an increase in left atrial pressure (the consequence of left ventricular failure), as has been postulated for some years, or from a disturbance in hypothalamic function (with a consequent massive α-adrenergic discharge) has not been clarified (27). The rapid evolution of pulmonary edema after severe head trauma makes the latter alternative more attractive.

Increased intracranial pressure decreases cerebral blood flow when perfusion pressure (the difference between arterial pressure and intracranial pressure) decreases to approximately 40 mm Hg. At perfusion pressures below 40 mm Hg, cerebral blood flow decreases abruptly, and it eventually ceases completely (28). Additionally, asphyxia or shifts in the brainstem or in the cerebral hemispheres that arise from the mass effects of a tumor can affect cerebrovascular autoregulation and induce a decrease in cerebral blood flow at perfusion pressures higher than 40 mm Hg.

Aside from these circulatory disturbances, an expanding tumor produces a variety of mechanical deformations of the brain, especially in adults or in older children whose sutures cannot widen and whose cranium cannot enlarge in response to a prolonged increase in intracranial pressure.

Clinically, the most significant of these mechanical deformations are the various herniations, notably herniation of the cerebellar tonsils through the foramen magnum, a feature of infratentorial tumors, and herniation of the hippocampal gyrus, particularly the uncus, down through the tentorial opening (Fig. 10.1). This herniation is observed with supratentorial masses, especially ipsilateral temporal lobe tumors.

Both types of herniations can produce secondary brainstem dysfunction, most probably by circulatory impairment and edema.

Clinical signs of occipital lobe infarction from increased intracranial pressure are less frequent. This condition results from kinking of the posterior cerebral arteries as they become wedged against the rigid tentorial edge (29). Because arterial pressure usually exceeds intracranial pressure, even in the presence of a mass lesion, local or systemic circulatory disturbances contribute to the development of arterial insufficiency.

Impaired cranial nerve function commonly accompanies increased intracranial pressure (30). The abducens nerve can become compressed between the anteroinferior cerebellar artery and the pons, producing weakness or paralysis of the lateral rectus muscle. This cause of sixth nerve paralysis was originally suggested by Cushing (31) and Collier (32) as a "false localizing sign." Involvement of the oculomotor nerve can accompany uncal herniations. The oculomotor nerve, particularly its pupillomotor fibers, can be compressed by the posterior cerebral artery. Pressure on the nerve can produce transitory circulatory disturbances or actual grooving of the nerve with distal petechial hemorrhages from the vasa nervorum.

Clinical Manifestations

Increased intracranial pressure produces headaches, vomiting, impaired vision, and changes in consciousness, and, when sutures have not fused, an enlarging head.

Headache

Headache, a constant feature of increased intracranial pressure in adults, is less common in children, being noted in 70% of the series of Bailey and coworkers (7), and in approximately 50% of children younger than age 13 years (33). Headaches from brain tumors result from traction on the dura and blood vessels at the base of the brain. Pain may be generalized or localized and worsen with exertion. In children, the site of

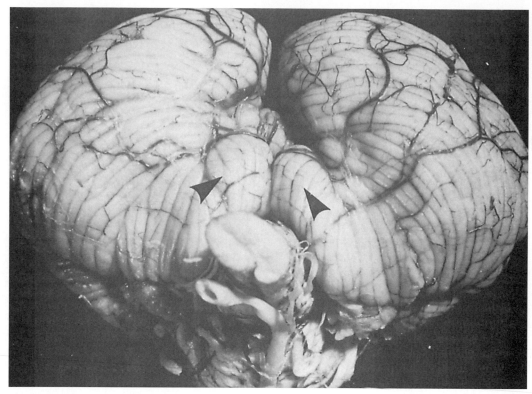

FIG. 10.1. Herniation of cerebellar tonsils. The view from the posterior aspect of the cerebellum demonstrates caudal displacement of the cerebellar tonsils resulting from increased intracranial pressure. The cone of herniated tonsillar tissue (*arrows*) impinges on the dorsal surface of the cervical spinal cord. (From Bell WE, McCormick WF. *Increased intracranial pressure in children*, 2nd ed. Philadelphia: Saunders, 1978. With permission.)

the pain, most commonly bifrontal, rarely assists in localizing the site of the tumor. Posterior fossa tumors, however, can produce irritation of the posterior roots of the upper cervical cord, resulting in pain in the back of the head and neck. Stiffness of the neck and a persistent head tilt, which can be adopted to avoid diplopia, also indicate a mass in the posterior fossa. Most commonly, the headache is transitory, occurring in the morning or awakening the child during the night. In children younger than 12 years of age, it can disappear temporarily with widening of the sutures, only to recur with further growth of the mass lesion. The majority of children who develop headache as a consequence of a brain tumor have had headache for less than 4 months (95%) or 2 months (85%) (34,35). Thus, if headache has been present for

4 months or longer and the neurologic and ophthalmologic examinations are normal, it is unlikely the child has a brain tumor.

Vomiting

Vomiting is one of the most constant signs of increased intracranial pressure in children. It occurred in 84% of patients in the series of Bailey and associates (7), and in 61% of children younger than 13 years of age in the 1975 series of Till (33). The reduced incidence of vomiting in the more recent series probably reflects an earlier referral. Vomiting can result from both increased intracranial pressure and from irritation of the brainstem by tumors of the posterior fossa. Contrary to general belief, vomiting in these patients is often not projectile and it can be

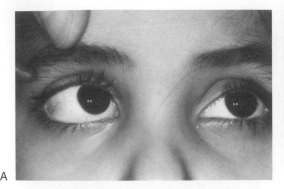

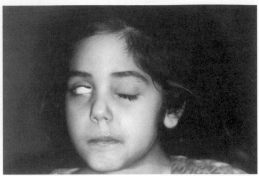

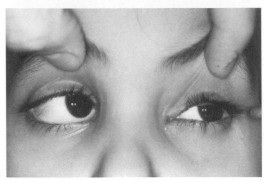

FIG. 10.2. Right-gaze palsy **(A)** caused by involvement of paramedian pontine reticular formation and of the abducens nucleus itself is present in this child with brainstem glioma. As compared with intact left gaze **(C)**, there is complete inability to move either eye to the right past the midline. Profound right peripheral facial paresis **(B)** is noted, with associated facial asymmetry and right orbicularis oculi weakness.

accompanied by nausea. Parents often note that vomiting relieves the headache. Like headaches, vomiting is most prominent in the morning and is unrelated to eating. Widening of the sutures can afford transitory relief.

Impaired Vision

Diplopia is usually the result of paralysis of one or both lateral recti muscles. Strabismus can be most striking at the end of a day and occasionally can fluctuate in parallel with the degree of increased intracranial pressure (Fig. 10.2).

Papilledema

Bailey and coworkers noted papilledema in 80% of children with brain tumors (7), whereas in the later series of Till it was absent in 45% of children younger than 13 years of age (33). Papilledema represents an abnormal elevation of the nerve head. Obliteration of the disk margins and absent pulsations of the central veins are the earliest and most important ophthalmoscopic findings. When increased intracranial pressure has developed acutely, vascular congestion with hemorrhages and exudates are also conspicuous (Fig. 10.3).

Papilledema should be distinguished from pseudopapilledema. Pseudopapilledema is a congenital anomaly associated with small anomalous disks, less commonly with drusen (hyaline bodies) buried below the surface of the disks and resulting in excessive glial proliferation at the disk margins. The nerve fibers appear raised, creating a blurred disk with or without vascular tortuosity. This anomaly can be transmitted as a dominant trait, and frequently it accompanies hyperopia or congenital malformations of the skull, such as brachycephaly. The clinical diagnosis of pseudopapilledema is often difficult and rests on the absence of physiologic cups, and the normal central emergence of vessels, and most important, the absence of other signs of increased intracranial pressure (36,36a). Although examination of the visual

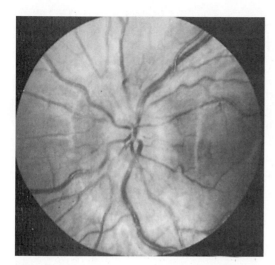

FIG. 10.3. Papilledema in 10-year-old girl with pseudotumor cerebri. The disc margins are elevated, and the retinal veins are tortuous and distended. (Courtesy of Dr. Robert Hepler, Department of Ophthalmology, University of California, Los Angeles, UCLA School of Medicine.)

fields demonstrates a normal blind spot, in contrast to the increased blind spot seen in true papilledema, this test is difficult to perform in young children.

Fluorescein fundus angiography has been advocated for distinguishing papilledema from pseudopapilledema. After the injection of fluorescein, the papilledematous optic disk discloses an increased capillary network, the presence of microaneurysms, and, most significantly, persistence of fluorescence at the disk margins or over the edematous disk area. Generally, these changes are not observed in pseudopapilledema (37).

In papilledema, visual symptoms usually are insignificant or limited to transient attacks of blurred vision. The concentric enlargement of the blind spot, detected when charting of visual fields is possible, is always asymptomatic.

Increased intracranial pressure is an important factor in the production of papilledema, but other causes can contribute. Papilledema can occur with normal intracranial pressure, as in infectious polyneuritis. Conversely, it sometimes fails to appear despite a prolonged increase in intracranial pressure.

The most favored hypothesis to explain the mechanism for papilledema is that the subarachnoid spaces surrounding the optic nerves, which are continuous with those inside the skull, allow a free transmission of intracranial pressure. When pressure is elevated, optic nerve tissue pressure increases. If communication between the ventricular and the perioptic spaces is blocked, as occurs in some patients with hydrocephalus, then papilledema does not develop, even after a long-standing elevation of intracranial pressure. The increased pressure within the optic nerve in turn interferes with axoplasmic flow and causes stasis at the optic nerve head. This produces axonal swelling and the clinical appearance of papilledema. Compression of vessels over the surface of the disk results in their dilatation and in the formation of microaneurysms and hemorrhages. Obstruction of venous and lymphatic drainage is probably secondary to the increase in optic nerve pressure, rather than being its cause (36a,38).

Although the presence of papilledema makes an intracranial mass highly probable, a number of other conditions must be excluded. In particular, choked optic disks also are encountered in pseudotumor cerebri, a condition characterized by increased intracranial pressure in the absence of a mass lesion.

Papilledema also can be found in the presence of subdural hematoma and in such systemic diseases as infectious polyneuritis, poliomyelitis, hypoparathyroidism, carbon dioxide retention, hypervitaminosis A, severe anemia, and lead poisoning.

Enlargement of the Head

Enlargement of the head is characteristic of a long-standing increase in intracranial pressure in infants and young children. In a series of brain tumors appearing during the first 2 years of life, an enlarging head was the most frequent presenting sign and was noted in 76% of infants (39). Enlargement of the head is not solely caused by brain tumors, but can occur in any child who has increased intracranial pressure and open sutures. Percussion of the head gives a high-pitched sound, termed *cracked pot* or *Macewen's sign.*

TABLE 10.4. *Location of tumors producing seizures in children*

Location	Number of cases
Temporal lobe	10
Frontal lobe	2
Parietal lobe	8
Entire hemisphere (diffuse or multiple tumors)	3
Other sites	5

Adapted from Low NL, Correll JW, Hammill JF. Tumors of the cerebral hemispheres in children. *Arch Neurol* 1965;13:547.

Seizures

Seizures are rarely an early indication of mass lesion; in one series they represented the initial symptom in approximately 15% of children with supratentorial lesions (40). Conversely, less than 1% of children with new onset seizures have a brain tumor as the etiology (41). Seizures become more frequent as the tumor grows and can be a late sign even in tumors of the posterior fossa. A complex partial seizure is the most common seizure type seen with intracranial masses, and the temporal lobe is the most common site for tumors producing seizures early in the course of illness (Table 10.4) (40).

Disturbances of Affect and Consciousness

Although mental disturbances or psychiatric disorders are fairly common with brain tumors in adults and indicate lesions of the frontal or temporal lobe, they are rarely observed in children. Children occasionally develop drowsiness, changes in personality, and irrational behavior, suggesting hypothalamic or thalamic involvement; changes in sleep patterns or in appetite are relatively common in frontal tumors. A progressive depression of consciousness resulting in drowsiness, stupor, and coma reflects increased intracranial pressure and compression of the reticular activating system. This compression can involve the reticular activating system in the upper brainstem when there is downward uncal or transtentorial herniation, or when, as a consequence of unilateral mass lesions, compression of the lower thalamus with horizontal displacement of the midbrain is seen (42).

Diagnosis

The diagnostic evaluation of the child suspected of harboring a brain tumor has undergone drastic changes since the 1970s. Classic texts, such as those by Bailey, Buchanan, and Bucy (7), published in 1939, bear witness to the early diagnostic difficulties presented by intracranial mass lesions. Formerly, initial evaluation involved the use of plain skull films and electroencephalography (EEG), followed by invasive procedures such as pneumoencephalography, ventriculography, and arteriography. This regimen has been superseded by various neuroimaging studies.

Diagnostic Neuroimaging

Advances in computer technology have helped establish more effective methods of identifying and characterizing pediatric brain tumors (10,43). The primary objective for any diagnostic MRI or computed tomographic (CT) study is to distinguish between normality and abnormality, and to determine the relevance of the findings on neuroimaging to the clinical situation. Establishing normality is typically more difficult than recognizing obvious pathology. Once a lesion is observed, the role of imaging shifts toward more specialized tasks, including interpreting the nature of the lesion, establishing the spatial relationship between the mass and eloquent areas of the brain, and staging the extent of disease.

In the initial evaluation of a child with a brain tumor, careful staging is particularly essential to appropriate treatment decisions. This process is critical, as the initial surgical resection may be the only time some tumors can be cured. Therefore, it is imperative that the full extent of the lesion is appreciated. Additionally, cytoreductive surgical intervention may not be warranted if evidence exists of distant spread. Several factors contribute to assisting the radiologist with the differential diagnosis of a particular tumor: the age of the patient (Table 10.5), the location of the tumor (Table 10.6), and the inherent imaging features (Tables 10.7 and 10.8).

Unlike in adults, many masses in children are not actually tumors, and a variety of pathologic lesions can mimic the picture of a brain tumor

TABLE 10.5. *Pediatric brain tumors and age at presentation*

Age	Benign masses	Malignant tumors
0–3 yr	Optic nerve and chiasm glioma, CPP, DIG, low-grade astrocytoma	Ependymoma, PNET/MB, CPC, teratoma, intermediate- and high-grade gliomas
4–12 yr	Migrational abnormalities, JPA, DNT, craniopharyngioma, cerebellar astrocytoma	High-grade gliomas, PNET/MB, ependymoma, BSG, ATT/RhT, germinoma
13–21 yr	Ganglioglioma, PXA, schwannoma, pituitary adenoma	High-grade gliomas, PNET/MB

ATT/RhT, atypical teratoid/rhabdoid tumor; BSG, brainstem glioma; CPC, choroid plexus carcinoma; CPP, choroid plexus papilloma; DIG, desmoplastic infantile ganglioglioma; DNT, dysembryoplastic neuroepithelial tumor; JPA, juvenile pilocytic astrocytoma; PNET/MB, primitive neuroectodermal tumor/medulloblastoma; PXA, pleomorphic xanthoastrocytoma.

Adapted from Quisling RG. Imaging for pediatric brain tumors. *Semin Pediatr Neurol* 1997;4:254–272.

TABLE 10.6. *Pediatric brain tumors and central nervous system location*

Intra-axial cerebrum	Low- and high-grade gliomas, CPP, CPC, DIG, DNT, PXA, PNETs (such as cerebral PNET or pineoplastoma)
Intra-axial cerebellum	JPA, PNET/MB, ependymoma, ATT/RhT
Intra-axial brainstem	Pilocytic or diffuse BSG, ganglioglioma, dorsally exophytic glioma, invasion by ependymomas, PNET/MB
Suprasellar region	Craniopharyngioma, optic pathway glioma, ectopic germ cell tumors, histiocytosis, lipodermoid, arachnoid cyst, adenoma dermoid/epidermoid, tuber cinereum hamartoma
Pineal region	Germ cell tumors, exophytic tectal glioma, exophytic vermic glioma, trilateral retinoblastoma, PNET, teratoma

ATT/RhT, atypical teratoid/rhabdoid tumor; BSG, brainstem glioma; CPC, choroid plexus carcinoma; CPP, choroid plexus papilloma; DIG, desmoplastic infantile ganglioglioma; DNT, dysembryoplastic neuroepithelial tumor; JPA, juvenile pilocytic astrocytoma; PNET/MB, primitive neuroectodermal tumor/medulloblastoma; PXA, pleomorphic xanthoastrocytoma.

Adapted from Quisling RG. Imaging for pediatric brain tumors. *Semin Pediatr Neurol* 1997;4:254–272.

on neuroimaging (Table 10.9). Some tumors are indolent, exhibiting virtually static biologic growth characteristics (44), whereas other mass lesions can display a mixture of both true tumor and cortical dysplastic features in the same region (45).

CT is used effectively for imaging the skull base, where the natural contrast of bone, air (paranasal sinuses), fat (nasopharyngeal/retrobulbar orbit), or CSF provides inherent contrast resolution. CT also is used whenever an imaging study is performed on an urgent basis. However, some tumors, especially those in the posterior fossa or temporal fossa, are best visualized with MRI and are occasionally missed by CT imaging (Fig. 10.4). This is particularly the case when the tumor is isodense and thus requires contrast infusion for its delineation (Fig. 10.5). In a brainstem glioma, for instance, sagittal scans demonstrate the rostrocaudal extent of the tumor (Fig. 10.6). Tumors involving the sella or the chiasmatic cistern are also more readily delineated by MRI than by CT, because interference from surrounding bone limits the accuracy of CT. In the experience of Sartor and coworkers, who compared the accuracy of CT scanning and MRI in delineating mass lesions in the sellar region, MRI was equivalent to CT scanning in 54% of cases, superior in 41%, and inferior in only 5% (46).

Because CT imaging concepts are similar to standard radiologic acquisitions, and CT is less

TABLE 10.7. *Magnetic resonance imaging features of benign tumors*

Little to no growth on serial imaging.
Epicenter in gray matter.
Unenhanced signal (in the solid portion) is similar in intensity to gray matter.
Cysts may be present but necrosis is absent.
Calcification (except in pineal region).
No contrast enhancement in DNTs.
Contrast enhancement in a mural nodule.
Tumor margins on T1 and T2 images correspond anatomically (T1/T2 concordance).

DNT, dysembryoplastic neuroepithelial tumor.

TABLE 10.8. *Magnetic resonance imaging features of malignant tumors*

Growth on serial imaging.
Evidence of tumor necrosis.
T1 and T2 spatial discordance.
Calcification in a pineal region tumor.
Malignant pattern of gadolinium enhancement:
  Subpial or subependymal enhancement suggesting tumor infiltration.
  Extension of a white matter centered mass through the gray matter cortical mantle.
Multicentricity or satellite lesions in the primary site or in more distant locations remote from the epicenter.
Distant spread in neuraxis. Such lesions can be shown by using a body coil and obtaining post contrast, sagittal, spin echo T1-weighted sequences followed by sagittal gradient using parameters that provide "white" CSF (a myelogram effect). Axial, post contrast, T1-weighted images are then obtained in the regions often involved by drop metastases, the cervical plexus and cauda equina regions. If any abnormality is observed on the sagittal images, then axial or coronal images would be obtained in these regions as well.

CNS, central nervous system; CSF, cerebrospinal fluid.
Note: Clinical history is important to the radiologist evaluating a CNS lesion and the probability that it is malignant. Patients with associated immune system dysfunction are at risk of having malignant tumors such as lymphoma. In addition, prior radiotherapy and chemotherapy increase the probability that a CNS lesion is malignant.

TABLE 10.9. *Pediatric brain tumor mimics*

Inflammatory	Tumefactive multiple sclerosis, myelin basic protein hypersensitivity, adrenoleukodystrophy
Infectious	Progressive multifocal leukoencephalopathy (papova virus), tuberculoma, cryptococcoma, neurocystercercosis, chronic empyema
Postsurgical	Reaction to shunt material, seroma, chronic hematoma
Postradiation	Radiation effect, radiation necrosis
Postchemotherapy	Progressive necrotizing leukoencephalopathy
Developmental	Cortical, subcortical, and periventricular heteropias, tuberous sclerosis
Dishistiogenesis	Neurofibromatosis, neurocutaneous melanosis
Vascular	Giant arterial or venous aneurysms (e.g., vein of Galen aneurysms), thrombosed vascular malformations, cavernous angioma, sequestered stroke

Adapted from Quisling RG. Imaging for pediatric brain tumors. *Semin Pediatr Neurol* 1997;4:254–272.

often required for neuroaxis tumor imaging, most of the following discussion focuses on MRI.

An understanding of the nature of a brain tumor and its location requires knowledge of T1, T2, and gadolinium-enhanced T1-weighted information (47). Unenhanced T1-weighted images can reveal areas of pathology that differ from normal brain by being either hyperintense or hypointense when compared with contiguous normal brain. Hyperintensity on T1-weighted images implies the presence of substances that naturally increase proton relaxation, such as methemoglobin (subacute residua of hemorrhage), melanin, dilute amounts of interstitial or intracellular calcification (postradiotherapy), and hyperconcentrated proteins (as might occur in a colloid-containing mass or hypercellular tumors). T1 hypointensity suggests changes related to either anisotropic effects (by structures containing either very large or rigidly

bound molecules, as seen in intratumoral desmoplasia or matrix calcification) or, alternatively, tissue containing unbound water (as seen in peritumoral edema, necrosis, or cyst formation) (48,49). T1 hypointensity reflects both extremes of hydrogen states: too tightly bound or too loosely bound compared with protons in adjacent brain parenchyma.

Information from T2-weighted sequences differs from T1-weighted data. In physical terms, T2 rate reflects the time required for the signal to degrade or to disappear from the image. It is a measure of loss of coherence of the magnetic vectors that had been refocused by the second radiofrequency pulse in spin echo sequences or by gradient applications in gradient echo imaging. Tissue with faster T2 rates disperses its signal faster than tissue with slower T2 rates, and hence exhibits less signal intensity on the image. Tissue in which the water molecules are bound within large complex molecules or within rigid tissue has faster T2 rates, and therefore destroys its signal more quickly (T2 hypointensity). Abnormal T2 hypointensity

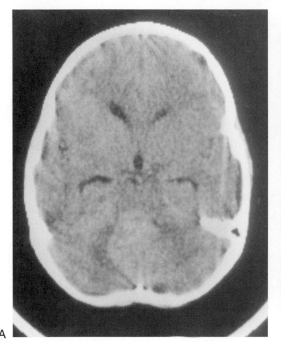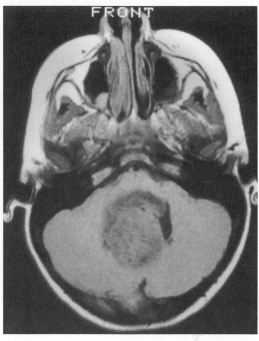

A B

FIG. 10.4. A: Computed tomographic scan of head shows ill-defined posterior fossa density that obliterates the fourth ventricle. **B:** Magnetic resonance imaging shows a well-defined midline posterior fossa tumor in the same patient. Magnetic resonance imaging is clearly superior to computed tomographic scanning in visualizing the tumor.

implies a more restricted bulk water pool. The latter occurs in fibrosis, ossification, and dehydrated tissues. Tissues that possess more unbound water molecules (such as CSF or vasogenic edema) have slower T2 rates and therefore exhibit a brighter signal. Abnormal T2 hyperintensity implies an increase in bulk tissue water.

For most intra-axial brain or spinal cord tumors, the T2-weighted sequences more accurately predict the extent of tumor infiltration. Although peritumoral tissue edema may not always contain tumor cells, the correlation is high. The zone of abnormality on standard spin echo T2-weighted images is a good measure of tumor infiltration.

Use of intravenously injected gadolinium (gadopentetate dimeglumine at 0.1 mmol/kg) or other paramagnetic compounds significantly improves the resolution of many brain tumors (45). T1-weighted, gadolinium-enhanced imaging is generally acquired in two orthogonal planes to ensure full appreciation of a tumor's

margins. The optimal planes of section, however, depend on the location of the tumor. Gadolinium enhancement arises whenever the capillary bed is expanded or vessels leak contrast through their walls. It assists in defining areas of edema and necrosis, cyst formation, spinal cord metastases, and extension of tumor to the leptomeninges or ependyma. High-grade tumors such as glioblastomas, ependymoblastomas, and PNET/MBs tend to enhance, whereas surrounding edema does not. Lack of enhancement increases the likelihood that the tumor is benign. MRI with gadolinium enhancement also is of considerable value in postoperative follow-up studies in distinguishing residual or recurrent tumor from edema, granulation tissue, and necrosis. As a rule, any structure that enhances with iodine on CT enhances on MRI with gadolinium; the reverse is not always the case.

Newer technologic developments are constantly unfolding (50,51). Some provide new information and some improve contrast

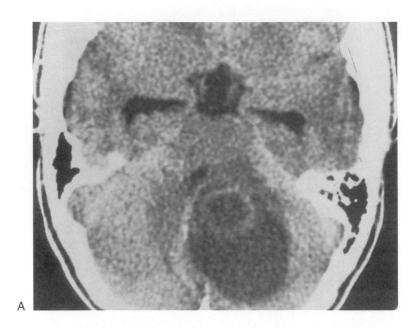

A

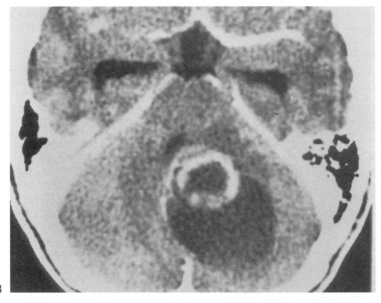

B

FIG. 10.5. Computed tomographic scans revealing cerebellar cystic astrocytoma in a 13-year-old boy. Computed tomographic scans before **(A)** and after **(B)** injection of iodinated contrast material show a large lesion predominantly involving the left cerebellar hemisphere, but extending to the vermis. The large, well-demarcated macrocyst contains proteinaceous fluid, which accounts for the high density of the cyst fluid compared with CSF in the suprasellar cistern, temporal horns, and third ventricle. **A:** A small fleck of calcium is noted medially within the wall of the macrocyst on the noncontrast computed tomography. An enhancing tumor nodule projects into the anterior portion of the macrocyst; some areas of the macrocyst wall are enhanced as well. (*Continued*)

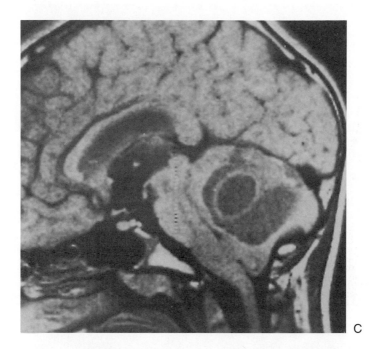

C

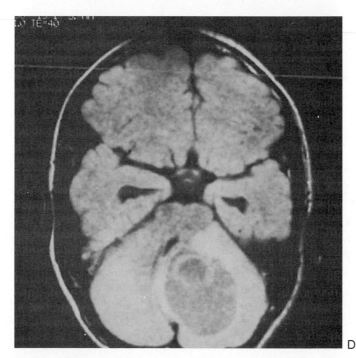

D

FIG. 10.5. *Continued.* T1-weighted magnetic resonance images in the sagittal **(C)** and axial **(D)** planes are shown also. These noncontrast magnetic resonance studies were done before gadolinium-diethylene-triaminepenta-acetic acid was approved for use in children. The magnetic resonance findings are concordant with the computed tomographic scan changes. If gadolinium-diethylenetriaminepenta-acetic acid could have been used, it probably would have enhanced abnormalities comparable with iodinated contrast on the computed tomographic scan. At surgery, a middle-grade astrocytoma was found. The macrocyst contained yellow fluid; small cysts and necrotic areas were found within the mural nodule. (Courtesy of Drs. Hervey D. Segall, Marvin D. Nelson, Jr., and Corey Raffel, Children's Hospital, Los Angeles.)

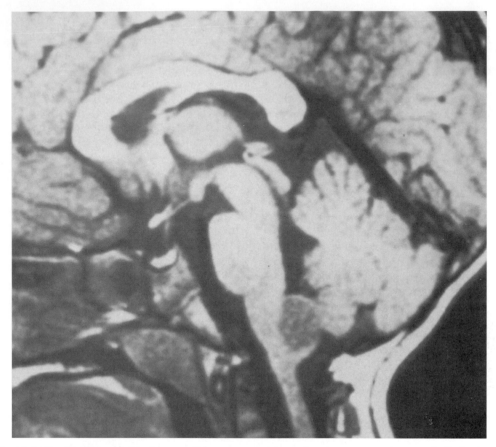

FIG. 10.6. Sagittal T1-weighted magnetic resonance scan showing a posterior exophytic brainstem glioma in a 6-year-old girl. The scan shows a rounded, sharply marginated, low-intensity tumor projecting posteriorly from the medulla. This was a grade II astrocytoma. (Courtesy of Dr. Hervey D. Segall, Department of Radiology, University of Southern California School of Medicine.)

resolution. Those currently receiving the most attention in the literature include fluid-attenuated inversion recovery (FLAIR) sequences, which are now preferred by many radiologists over standard T2 imaging, diffusion and perfusion imaging, and magnetization transfer techniques. The FLAIR sequence is especially useful in distinguishing pathologic tissue edema in locations where CSF abuts brain, especially along the cortical surface and within the depths of sulci. It has the disadvantage of taking longer to perform and thereby experiences interscan patient motion. This disadvantage has been obviated in part by using the fast scan techniques in conjunction with the FLAIR parameters to achieve scan times under 4 minutes. Other imaging techniques, including dif-

fusion imaging, perfusion imaging, and functional imaging (such as MR spectroscopy) are under development and may help characterize biologic behavior in the future (52,53).

Other Studies

Ancillary studies are often used to further delineate the nature and the extent of the tumor. MR arteriography, or conventional arteriography using digital subtraction techniques, helps delineate the blood supply to the mass lesion (54). Additionally, these procedures can indicate the degree of malignancy and exclude the presence of a vascular malformation (55).

The dangers attending lumbar puncture in the presence of increased intracranial pressure preclude its use as part of initial evaluation of a child with a suspected brain neoplasm. Because the presence and location of an intracranial abscess can readily be demonstrated by gadolinium-enhanced MRI, examination of the CSF is no longer used for this purpose. The appearance and composition of CSF in brain tumor patients were presented by Merritt in his classic study (56). Although CSF glucose level is almost always normal, it is reduced in some children with leukemic or lymphosarcomatous infiltration of the meninges and in meningeal carcinomatosis secondary to an ependymoma, a melanosarcoma, or a malignant tumor of the meninges (57).

Cytology can be performed on the CSF after centrifugation and can help determine whether the tumor has spread to the meninges or to the spinal subarachnoid space, as can occur in a PNET/MB (58).

The presence of malignant cells in the CSF indicates extensive seeding of the leptomeninges. False-positive results are rare. In the experience of Glass and associates, such results were encountered only in patients with lymphomas and were the consequence of mistakenly identifying lymphocytes as lymphoma cells (58). False-negative results are fairly common in all types of tumors, with the exception of acute lymphatic leukemia (58).

A less beneficial adjunct to the localization of an intracranial mass lesion is the EEG. Its greatest value lies in suggesting the presence of temporal lobe tumors in children with complex partial seizures. In such patients, the persistence of local slow-wave activity, overshadowing the spike and sharp-wave activity usually associated with seizures, points to a space-occupying lesion and calls for more definitive imaging studies.

Plain skull films can suggest an intracranial mass lesion if they show separation of sutures, erosion or enlargement of the sella turcica, or osteoporosis, especially thinning of the sphenoid ridge. Because the bones of the vault become more firmly joined, separation of sutures is rare in children older than 10 years of age and is practically nonexistent beyond age 20 years. In young children, sutures can spread after increased intracranial pressure lasting 10 days or even less, though suture separation takes longer to develop in older children (59). Radiographic evidence of calcification can be seen in 15% to 20% of intracranial tumors of childhood, mostly in the form of clusters of multiple specks. Approximately 50% of oligodendrogliomas, a rare tumor in childhood, develop radiologic signs of calcification (60). The most common tumor to produce suprasellar calcification is the craniopharyngioma, and it does so in approximately 70% to 80% of cases, usually along the superior aspect of the mass. In tuberous sclerosis, multiple calcifications varying in size from specks to up to 1 cm are usually located along the ventricular walls, less often within the cerebrum and the posterior fossa.

The use of ultrasound in the detection of intracranial tumors is limited to neonates and infants with an open fontanelle (61).

Positron emission tomography has considerable potential in delineating brain tumors. Primary brain tumors show good correlation between the uptake of labeled fluorodeoxyglucose (FDG) and the malignancy of the tumor as verified by its histology. Differences in uptake of FDG or labeled methionine also can assist in defining the site for a stereotactic biopsy. Additionally, the rate of FDG uptake after tumor irradiation generally allows one to differentiate between tumor recurrence, in which uptake is increased, and radiation necrosis, in which it is reduced (62). Corticosteroid therapy does not alter the positron emission tomographic scan. Thus, in the experience of Glantz and coworkers, 95% of patients with hypermetabolic abnormalities on the postoperative positron emission tomographic scan had recurrence of their tumor. Abscesses were, however, indistinguishable from recurrent tumors (63). The role of metabolic brain imaging as an adjunct to structural imaging is further discussed in the subsequent section dealing with radiotherapy.

MR spectroscopy has been used to determine the response of tumors to radiation or chemotherapy. This procedure is, however, still in its experimental stages (63a,63b).

Differential Diagnosis

Increased intracranial pressure is encountered not only in brain tumors, but also in various other mass lesions within the cranium. In infants, brain tumors cause increased intracranial pressure less commonly than hydrocephalus, intracranial hemorrhage, and infections do. Beyond 2 years of age, brain tumors become a progressively more frequent cause of increased intracranial pressure. Infections are encountered less often.

A brain abscess can act as a space-occupying lesion. It can arise from the direct spread of bacteria from an infected ear, mastoid, or paranasal sinus, or by hematogenous dissemination from a distant source. Brain abscesses are liable to occur in patients with congenital heart disease, particularly those who have a significant right-to-left shunt. The presence of increased intracranial pressure in patients with congenital heart disease should arouse immediate suspicion of a brain abscess. Only approximately 30% of these children have fever, so that its absence does not distinguish an abscess from a tumor. In most instances, MRI or CT scanning with contrast infusion is diagnostic of abscesses. This clinical entity is discussed more fully in Chapter 6.

In pseudotumor cerebri, intracranial pressure is elevated in the absence of a mass lesion. No localizing signs are present, the spinal fluid is normal, and imaging studies show the ventricular system to be normal or smaller than normal, but not displaced or distorted.

In the past, one of the differential diagnoses was lead encephalopathy. This was particularly the case when generalized convulsions coincided with a clinical picture of a posterior fossa tumor (see Chapter 9).

The clinical differentiation of hydrocephalus of nonneoplastic origin from midline brain tumors usually requires MRI. Like hydrocephalus, mass lesions can produce striking cranial enlargement during the early months of life, and a gradually expanding periaqueductal tumor, such as a fibrillary astrocytoma of the quadrigeminal plate, can produce aqueductal stenosis and ultimately complete obstruction. MRI demonstrates not only the distortion of the ventricular system that can accompany a brain tumor, but also any small mass that might have produced aqueductal obstruction (64). Normally, CSF flow through the aqueduct produces a signal void on T2-weighted images (i.e., an area of blackness); absence of the void indicates cessation of flow and partial or complete obstruction.

Severe herpes simplex encephalitis can simulate a rapidly expanding temporal lobe lesion because of the massive edema that accompanies the infection and because of its predilection for the temporal lobe. Additionally, a small proportion of children with cerebral degenerative diseases, notably disseminated acute encephalomyelitis (ADEM) and subacute sclerosing panencephalitis, can develop increased intracranial pressure and papilledema. When these signs are accompanied by predominantly unilateral signs, as they frequently are, the clinical diagnosis of brain tumor is unavoidable and is refuted only by neuroimaging studies that demonstrate white matter edema (65).

Treatment

Surgical extirpation remains the mainstay of treatment for pediatric brain tumors. The advent of the operating microscope, laser beam, and ultrasonographic methods have made it possible to increase the number of children having safe and complete tumor resections.

Most patients harboring a brain tumor rapidly improve with the administration of dexamethasone at a 0.1 to 0.5 mg/kg starting dose. This reduces increased intracranial pressure and allows the surgeon a much less explosive environment in which to radically resect the tumor. Then, if necessary, the child should be immediately transported to a brain tumor center. Other medications, such as phenytoin or fosphenytoin, can be used prophylactically in the perioperative period. The pediatric neurosurgeon is more than a technician in brain tumor surgery because the surgeon can provide vital information about extent of infiltration of the nervous system by direct observation of the brain tumor. Experience is the key to radical resection with low morbidity. The adaptation of the operating microscope to microneurosurgery has made it possible to extensively resect brain tumors in eloquent areas with minimal morbidity. The role of CT- and MRI-guided stereotactic biopsies in childhood brain tumors is appropriate and preferable to open biopsy in tumors involving the basal ganglia, thalamus, and midbrain. This simple, precise diagnostic test can provide an accurate diagnosis in approximately 95% of cases, with morbidity in the 2% to 5% range (66).

The most common error made during surgery is the discontinuation of a procedure when a tumor such as an astrocytoma, ependymoma, or PNET/MB is perceived to be emanating from the floor of the fourth ventricle (67). Commonly, these tumors involve the middle cerebellar peduncle adjacent to the fourth ventricle and should be totally resectable. Ependymoma can insinuate itself into an enlarged foramen of Luschka but the surgical attempt will be discontinued inappropriately when the surgeon perceives the lesion to be invading the brainstem.

Establishing the correct neuropathologic diagnosis of a pediatric brain tumor is critical in directing subsequent therapeutic efforts. Neuroimaging studies and perioperative frozen sections and touch preparations may be highly suggestive of a particular histologic type of tumor. However, a final diagnosis of surgically resected material often requires immunohistochemistry, flow cytometry, and electron microscopy. Therefore, it is best to wait 48 to 72 hours postoperatively for a final neuropathologic interpretation before discussing prognosis and any adjuvant treatment plans with the family.

Postsurgical Neuroimaging

The most important role of neuroimaging after surgery is to determine whether a mass has been completely resected and to assess the extent of any residual tumor. This information is most readily provided by serial imaging studies. Consequently, an immediate (24 to 48 hours) postoperative baseline study should be obtained. A variety of abnormalities can be observed. Postoperative edema can be present for days. Blood products can be seen for months. Tumor bed granulation tissue may be seen for years and can mimic residual tumor. MRI shows encephalomalacia, non-nodular contrast enhancement conforming to the encephalomalacia (granulation tissue), and hypodense susceptibility artifact in the same region as the enhancement on T2-weighted images. The reduced T2 signal is believed to be the result of microhemorrhages and hemosiderin deposition. Presence of nodular hyperintense abnormalities on T2-weighted sequences should raise the suspicion of residual neoplasia. Special attention to the depths of the middle fossa and to the cribriform plate is impor-

tant because subarachnoid space extends to these regions and may harbor metastatic tumor.

Another surgically related abnormality is dural thickening and enhancement associated with the presence of an indwelling ventricular-peritoneal shunt catheter. The dural changes may occur near the entrance of the shunt or in a more diffuse fashion overlying the surface of the brain. Benign dural thickening is not nodular and generally ranges from 1 to 3 mm. The ventricular-peritoneal shunt typically reduces the volume of the ipsilateral lateral ventricle more so than the contralateral side. The value of surveillance brain imaging varies by tumor type. The purpose of serial imaging is to document the response to treatment and make a diagnosis of recurrence or complications as soon as possible (68).

Radiotherapy

Radiotherapy can be used either as an adjuvant to surgery or for definitive therapy when complete resection is not feasible. Standard techniques of pediatric CNS radiotherapy, such as limited-field radiotherapy and craniospinal radiotherapy, have offered curative therapy for low-grade gliomas, PNET/MB, germinoma, and other tumor types. Advanced radiotherapy techniques, including conformal therapy, fractionated stereotactic radiotherapy, and stereotactic radiosurgery, are improving survival and reducing neurotoxicity. Many factors must be considered in deciding precisely how to safely use radiotherapy.

Within cells, the most abundant molecule is water. In addition, lipids, proteins, carbohydrates, and nucleotides are present. When ionizing radiation interacts with a cell, reactive species are created that damage cellular DNA (69). Tumor cells are particularly vulnerable to such damage because of aberrant cell cycle control mechanisms and because radiotherapy technique (multiple beams of radiation) delivers more radiation to the tumor site than to normal brain.

For each histologically defined pediatric brain tumor, there are critical radiation treatment parameters, such as total dose, time, and volume of tissue treated. Slow-growing focal tumors such as pilocytic and low-grade fibrillary astrocytomas may require limited-field radiation, whereas infiltrative tumors such as PNET/MB, germinoma, and atypical teratoid/ rhabdoid tumor require craniospinal radiation.

Another important factor in determining a treatment approach for pediatric brain tumors is whether radiation is used as a single modality, or in its more common role as a component of multimodal therapy. Timing of treatment and the dose delivered are affected by adjuvant chemotherapy, surgery, or both. Furthermore, patient age and tumor location in relationship to dose-limiting critical neural structures significantly influence the anticipated sequelae of treatment.

Modern brain imaging machines have made the use of stereotactic radiotherapy techniques possible and allowed for the delivery of large single doses of radiation to well-defined intracranial targets (70). In addition, radiation scatter is limited and thus, theoretically, should reduce late cognitive or endocrine effects from limited-field radiation of brain tumors. Advances in stereotactic treatment methods may soon supplant standard external-beam radiation, which has been used for decades (70).

In models of external-beam radiotherapy, treatment planning begins with construction of a face mask for reproducible position. Using this system along with standard relocation technologies such as laser beams, a patient can be repositioned daily with an accuracy of 3 to 9 mm (71). Stereotactic radiosurgery requires placement of a stereotactic head ring, which is attached to the patient's skull. Imaging in reference to the ring can then identify mathematical coordinates for each pixel in the CT or MRI images that directly corresponds to points in the patient positioned in the ring. Treatment planning identifies a coordinate at the center of a treatment plan, and data can be transferred to a treatment delivery machine with high accuracy (72). The technique uses the equivalent of hundreds of radiation beams delivered with circular fields via multiple arcs of treatment. This allows the radiation dose to be delivered accurately and to fall off optimally outside the treatment volume. Although a large single-dose treatment has radiobiologic disadvantages for more malignant tumors, the advantage of accu-

rate avoidance of normal tissue with steep dose gradients has made this a proven therapy for several entities, including arteriovenous malformations (see Chapter 12), ependymomas, acoustic schwannomas, metastases, and meningiomas (73,74).

Use of stereotactic radiosurgery in benign and malignant tumors in children has been less well defined than in adults, although interest in this technique is increasing. Further details of this procedure are provided by Bova and coworkers (75) and Flickinger and coworkers (76).

Immediate and Long-Term Effects of Radiation Therapy

As improved surgical and radiation techniques have lengthened survival of children with brain tumors, concern has grown about the quality of life in survivors and about the nature and extent of radiation-induced deficits.

Pathologic and experimental studies indicate that the major pathophysiology of radiation-induced brain damage results from damage to the vascular endothelium, tissue that is more radiosensitive than neurons. This results in obstruction of small and medium-sized blood vessels with ensuing thrombosis and infarction of deep white matter, but relative sparing of cortex and subcortical white matter. Large vessel injury is far less common (77). Additional or alternative mechanisms of brain injury have been proposed. These involve direct injury to glia and axons, and, less likely, an autoimmune vasculitis (78). Vasogenic edema is probably responsible for acute reactions that develop within a few weeks of radiation.

Neurologic symptoms can develop during radiation, or shortly thereafter, or have their onset after an interval of many months or years.

Acutely, craniospinal radiation may produce nausea and vomiting within 2 to 6 hours of treatment because the radiation beam exits through the stomach and bowel. In contrast, some children exhibit anticipatory nausea and vomiting that occurs before or within 2 hours of treatment. Symptoms are typically well controlled with antiemetics such as prochlorperazine, but occasionally require newer, more potent agents such as ondansetron.

Several weeks after the start of radiotherapy, patients lose hair and complain of skin soreness, erythema, and sore throat. These side effects begin to abate 1 to 2 weeks after therapy. Use of topical cream should be avoided unless the radiation oncologist is consulted, because many are oil-based and contain metal, which increases the surface radiation dose during therapy. After therapy is complete, aloe-based creams are recommended, and occasionally corticosteroid-based creams or newer matrix gels are used. Craniospinal radiation can cause thrombocytopenia, leukopenia, and anemia; thrombocytopenia delays completion of radiation treatment. Thus, complete blood counts should be obtained weekly during radiotherapy. If a delay is necessary, any limited-field external beam boost or fractionated stereotactic approaches may be used in the interim. These regionally limited treatments allow bone marrow recovery without placing the patient at risk for future tumor progression.

Acute radiation encephalopathy occurs in the course of treatment whenever large daily fraction doses are administered. The underlying pathology is that of cerebral edema caused by vascular damage and an ensuing increase in vessel wall permeability, which in turn produces perivascular edema, and in the most severe cases, microhemorrhage and thrombi. Cortical neurons disappear, and fibrillary gliosis extends from the cortical surface into the deeper layers of gray matter. Radiation injury to brain parenchyma results in intravascular and perivascular microcalcifications. These are most common at the junction of cortical gray and white matter and the basal ganglia (79).

The clinical picture varies. In general, it consists of lethargy, nausea and vomiting, seizures, and an exacerbation of preexisting neurologic deficits. MRI shows focal, multifocal, or diffusely increased signal in white matter on T2-weighted images (80). Lesions tend to start as small foci that progress with time. They are irreversible and do not correlate well with neurologic or developmental deficits (81). Acute radiation encephalopathy can be treated with corticosteroids, but it is preferable to prevent complications by administering low daily dosages, particularly in the rare instance in which radiotherapy is considered essential in infants and young children.

During therapy, some children are fatigued and do not make optimal effort in cognitive testing. Thus, it is best to complete radiation treatment before assessing cognition. Fatigue usually diminishes weeks to months after therapy, although many patients experience an early delayed response termed the *somnolence syndrome* in the 6 weeks to 3 months after radiotherapy.

The late effects of radiotherapy include impaired cognition, defective endocrine function, and the development of a second neoplasia.

A reduction of cognitive function is encountered in children irradiated for supratentorial and infratentorial tumors (69). Retrospective studies indicate that between 10% and 80% of surviving children who have undergone either local or whole-brain radiation therapy demonstrate a significant loss in full-scale IQ (79). Craniospinal radiation can be expected to lower IQ by 10 to 20 points (82). In addition, almost all children who have retained a normal IQ can be found to have some degree of attention and memory deficit (82). Visual perceptual skills, learning abilities, memory, and adaptive behavior are also adversely affected (83,84). These cognitive deficits are most evident in children younger than 7 years of age and appear to progress over the course of several years after completion of radiotherapy (85,86). Infants younger than 3 years of age have the worst prognosis in terms of intellectual development (87,88). Adjuvant chemotherapy, particularly intraventricular or intrathecal methotrexate, is believed to increase the risk for the development of dementia, as does a tumor localized to the cerebral hemispheres or the hypothalamus (82,89). Thus, the commonly used regimen of cranial irradiation and methotrexate can induce a necrotizing encephalopathy several months to years after completion of treatment. The incidence of necrotizing encephalopathy is dose related with respect to methotrexate and irradiation.

Neuroimaging studies in children with reduced cognition demonstrate white matter damage. On MRI, increased signal is seen in the periventricular white matter on T2-weighted images. The involved area has a scalloped appearance; often it extends to the gray-white matter junction (90). Zimmerman and colleagues have graded the white matter changes observed on MRI (91). There appears to be a direct relationship between the volume of brain irradiated and the development of white matter changes (92); the correlation between the severity of white matter involvement and the neurologic and cognitive deficits is not as good. This is particularly true for young children whose abnormalities on MRI tend to be less pronounced than those of older children (93).

Because of these sequelae, hyperfractionated approaches to treatment have been designed for treatment of the youngest children who must receive radiotherapy for tumor control. Careful attention to obtaining baseline studies before beginning radiotherapy is essential, as is recognition that the tumor itself plus surgery, chemotherapy, and psychosocial factors all contribute to function and coping.

A second important late effect of irradiation of the craniospinal axis is a disturbance in various growth and endocrine functions. This is seen in some 70% to 90% of patients (88,94). Although acutely not problematic, pituitary function can decline with time in 50% to 70% of patients, depending on the radiation dose and fractionation used. As a rule, the hypothalamus is more sensitive to radiation than the pituitary, and growth hormone secretion is affected first (79). An irreversible growth hormone deficiency becomes apparent 1 or more years after completion of irradiation and produces a gradual diminution of growth rate (95,96). In the series of Constine and coworkers, only 36% of children who received cranial irradiation, and 25% of children who received craniospinal irradiation, attained a height greater than the third percentile (94). Irradiation of the spine significantly affects the overall crown-rump height of a young patient. Furthermore, the musculature and size of the vertebral bodies and sternum may be affected by treatment. These growth anomalies yield a characteristic body habitus (69). In addition, cranial treatment in young children can affect skull growth. These growth anomalies are important to recognize because

musculoskeletal function and appearance are important determinants of self-esteem, coping, and social function in children and adolescents. Gonadotropin deficiency with delayed or precocious puberty also is encountered. Seventy percent of irradiated postpubertal girls had oligomenorrhea, and 30% of postpubertal boys had low testosterone levels. Symptoms of hypothyroidism were seen in 28%, and 62% had low total or free serum thyroxine levels (94). Diabetes insipidus owing to irradiation has not been reported (95).

Replacement of growth, thyroid, adrenal, and sex hormones should be overseen by an endocrinologist (97,98). No conclusive data show an increased risk of tumor recurrence with growth hormone replacement. As an extra precaution, however, it is common practice for endocrinologists to ensure there has been no residual tumor or evidence of tumor progression for at least 2 years before starting growth hormone therapy. In addition, many recommend more frequent brain imaging in the first year of growth hormone therapy.

An uncommon but devastating late effect is a second unrelated malignancy within or outside the CNS (99–101). It is estimated that one in six children who have had a brain tumor develop this complication years after radiation (102). A different type of cancer found within a radiation field at a significant interval after completion of treatment is considered a radiation-induced malignancy (101). In the series of Meadows and colleagues (99), 68% of tumors developed in radiation-exposed tissue. Tumors result not only from prior radiation, but also reflect a genetic predisposition to malignancies. These second cancers can be highly malignant and respond poorly to available therapies (99,103).

Children treated with high-dose radiation are also at a nine-fold increase in risk for developing second, unrelated CNS tumors. These appear at intervals of years to decades after irradiation and are often highly malignant (79).

Late radiation encephalopathy is a much less common complication. It develops several months to years after completion of treatment and is caused by brain necrosis or atrophy. The clinical picture is highlighted by headaches, seizures, and focal neurologic signs, notably hemiparesis. The course is slowly progressive. Imaging studies demonstrate low-density lesions within the brain. Symptomatic intraparenchymal hemorrhages outside the primary brain tumor site also have been recorded as a late complication (104). The exact cause of late radiation encephalopathy is unknown, but it is believed to result from a large total radiation dosage or large daily fractions (105).

Rarely, one observes a transitory episode of demyelination that appears some 2 to 3 months after completion of radiation and slowly resolves over the course of 6 to 8 weeks.

A late-onset myelopathy is another rare complication. Symptoms can be acute or chronically progressive. They range in severity from mild sensory signs, or lower motor neuron disease, to an acute paraplegia or quadriplegia (106). Cerebrovascular disease, manifested by strokes or transient ischemic attacks, can develop years to decades after completion of radiotherapy, particularly when radiotherapy is combined with chemotherapy. Damage to medium or large vessels, in particular, the carotid artery and its major branches, often can be documented (107). Recurrent attacks of migrainelike headaches lasting 2 to 24 hours and associated with focal symptoms such as aphasia or hemiparesis can represent a late complication of irradiation and chemotherapy (108). Children respond to propanolol or other antimigraine medications. Cerebral arteriography can trigger such an attack in these children.

In view of the high incidence of serious complications, there has been a trend toward delaying radiotherapy in patients younger than 3 years of age; prolonged postoperative chemotherapy is the preferred treatment. Such a regimen appears to be well tolerated, and its results compare favorably with those obtained in children treated with postoperative radiation and adjuvant chemotherapy. It appears, therefore, that postponement of radiation therapy is a feasible alternative for small children and infants (109).

Neuroimaging after Radiotherapy

Neuroimaging can disclose a variety of changes consequent to radiotherapy. Most commonly one sees mucositis within the paranasal sinuses and mastoid air cells and replacement of fat in marrow space. T2 hyperintensity may persist for months after stereotactic radiotherapy or radiosurgery. Standard-dose craniospinal radiotherapy produces few acute or subacute changes. Patients receiving whole-brain or craniospinal radiation may, after a period of several months, develop mild diffuse brain or spinal cord atrophy and chronic ischemic demyelination.

Radiation dosages that exceed neural tolerance produce radiation necrosis or progressive necrotizing leukoencephalopathy. The latter is usually seen when radiation therapy is used in conjunction with chemotherapy. The appearance of radiation necrosis on MRI and CT studies mimics residual or recurrent tumor (Fig. 10.7). Metabolic imaging tools such as FDG positron emission tomography, or thallium 201 single-photon emission CT (SPECT) can characterize metabolic activity within lesions (110–113). Neoplastic lesions have increased uptake of FDG and thallium, whereas radiation necrosis has decreased FDG metabolism as compared with normal surrounding brain; no thallium uptake occurs on SPECT imaging (113). Evidence exists that thallium is a more sensitive marker of viable tumor, whereas FDG provides information about metabolic activity in brain surrounding tumor (113). Despite these advances in metabolic characterization of lesions that arise after radiotherapy, biopsy is still the diagnostic gold standard.

Chemotherapy

One of the problems with traditional chemotherapy is that it is difficult to get drugs into tumors of the brain or spinal cord because such tumors have incompletely disrupted blood–brain barriers. Despite this limitation, clinical trials have shown safety and efficacy of chemotherapy in selected pediatric brain tumors, such as PNET/MB, germinoma, and pilocytic astrocytoma, and in infants with various malignant lesions. To overcome the blood–brain barrier, strategies have been designed to concentrate chemotherapy agents within brain tumors. One of the proposed strategies is to implant a pump

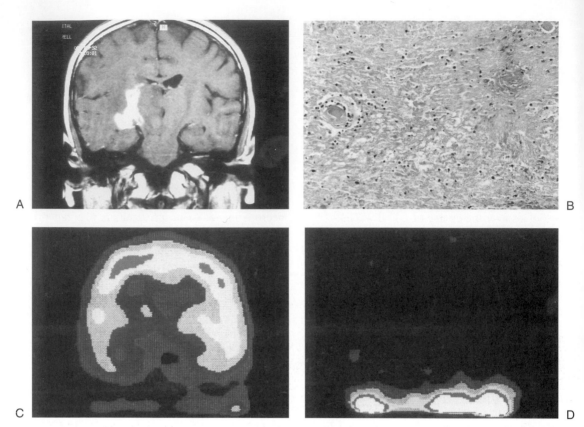

FIG. 10.7. T1-weighted coronal magnetic resonance imaging with gadolinium demonstrates deep white matter enhancing lesion in right hemisphere **(A)**. ^{99m}Tc HMPAO uptake **(B)** was decreased and ^{201}Tl uptake was absent **(D)**. Histologic preparation **(C)** reveals coagulative necrosis, consistent with radiation effect, and no evidence of tumor (hematoxylin and eosin, ×66). The patient was originally thought to have had a low-grade glioma and thus received radiotherapy. The patient is free of tumor more than 8 years from diagnosis.

that administers chemotherapy. The pump is a self-contained delivery system connected to the brain or spinal cord. Although pumps have the capacity to deliver drugs more uniformly than pills or injections and to bypass the blood–brain barrier, their overall effectiveness for managing brain tumors remains inconclusive (114).

Another approach is the use of polymer matrixes (plastic) to improve local therapy of malignant brain tumors. The new plastics enable the drugs to diffuse into the tumor bed in a continuous, uniform fashion. The plastic casings also protect unstable drugs from the body's own enzymes that may prematurely break them down. The pliability of plastics enables them to be molded into a variety of shapes and sizes that

can be surgically implanted or injected into precise locations in the body (114). Langer and colleagues demonstrated that polymer systems can be used to treat malignant adult brain tumors (114). Carmustine (BCNU)–containing polymer disks have been implanted to deliver tumor-killing doses of BCNU even after 4 weeks. Preliminary evidence suggests that implanting a BCNU polymer disk into the area where a tumor has been resected reduces the recurrence rate of such tumors (114,115). No studies have as yet tested pumps or polymer systems in malignant pediatric brain tumors.

Another option has been the use of chemotherapy in conjunction with drugs such as mannitol to disrupt the blood–brain barrier and thus permit better access of systemic chemotherapy to tumor cells. Preliminary experiments have shown that this approach results in a high incidence of seizures and other complications without demonstrating evidence of better tumor control. The approach has not been tested for safety or efficacy in children with malignant brain tumors.

It has become clear that chemotherapy increases disease-free survival in some children (37). As a consequence, by using chemotherapy, radiation can be delayed and neurotoxicity ameliorated in many infants (116). Chemotherapy can reduce the size of low-grade glioma, optic glioma, and oligodendroglioma (117). High-grade glioma and ependymoma, however, are relatively chemoresistant (118). It is important to recognize that the chemosensitivity of brain tumors varies greatly among tumor types and among patients with a particular histologic type.

Chemotherapeutic agents are toxic not only to malignant cells but also to normal ones (119). Because they are carried out by the blood circulation, they can affect any tissue in the body. Most drugs have preferential activity for rapidly proliferating cells such as hair follicles (alopecia), bone marrow (anemia, thrombocytopenia, granulocytopenia), intestinal mucosa, and gonads. In many cases, the effects are temporary when used in conventional doses. The spectrum of systemic side effects from chemotherapy is dependent on agent and dosage (120).

Almost all agents cause transient alopecia, which begins within a month of starting treatment and resolves when treatment is discontinued. Chemotherapy can affect all three hematologic cell lines. Anemia and thrombocytopenia may require transfusions. Weekly blood counts are indicated in most cases. Nausea and vomiting are common within 4 to 5 hours of administration and may persist for a few days. These symptoms are best controlled with the serotonin antagonist ondansetron. Stomatitis, glossitis, and proctitis occur with the beginning of neutropenia and disappear once the blood count recovers.

Vincristine frequently causes transient constipation and jaw pain (121). Virtually all patients develop hyporeflexia or areflexia. Less common side effects include foot drop, wrist drop, cranial nerve palsies, and vocal cord paralysis. Seizures with hyponatremia and inappropriate secretion of antidiuretic hormone can occur. Cisplatin can produce irreversible hearing loss in the high-frequency range. It also can cause severe hearing loss in the normal speech frequency range, especially if combined with radiotherapy. The dose-limiting toxicity of cisplatin is nephrotoxicity, and most patients ultimately have a permanent reduction of the glomerular filtration rate. More complete and detailed accounts of the systemic and neurotoxic complications of chemotherapy alone or in combination with radiotherapy are covered in Chapter 15 and are discussed in several excellent texts and reviews (122,123).

Neuroimaging after Chemotherapy

Chemotherapy can produce a variety of changes in the brain, ranging from mild atrophy to a destructive encephalopathy. The most severe complication of chemotherapy, usually seen in tandem with radiotherapy, is progressive necrotizing leukoencephalopathy (PNL) (124). PNL is characterized on MRI and CT as multicentric areas of contrast enhancement scattered randomly throughout cerebral white matter. The sites of the lesions do not necessarily correspond anatomically with the site of the primary tumor or the epicenter of radiotherapy. The findings may be more intense along the tract of an Ommaya reservoir catheter, presumably because of a higher concentration of chemotherapy from intraventricular injections. In time, the lesions calcify and their widespread presence is associated with diminished IQ, neurobehavioral disturbances, and neuroendocrine sequelae (Fig. 10.8).

Brain changes have been associated with the use of specific chemotherapeutic agents (e.g., cyclosporine) that have been given intravenously rather than intrathecally. These agents can infrequently produce a zone of infarction in deep capillary beds. For the most part, these have occurred in the parieto-occipital regions and produced vision loss. The mechanism is presumed to be related to a regional vasculopathy, platelet activation, and capillary zone infarction.

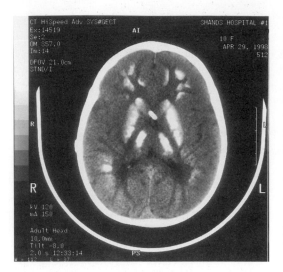

FIG. 10.8. Computed tomographic scan in axial plane shows widespread calcifications in both cerebral hemispheres resulting from radiotherapy and chemotherapy treatment.

Cutting-Edge Therapies

Several new therapeutic approaches, including the use of biologic therapies, are being evaluated in the laboratory and clinical trials. One of the more intellectually satisfying approaches is that of gene therapy. This modality offers hope for ultimately treating the root cause of the problem by replacing defective genes, amplifying the immune response to neoplasia, and sensitizing tumor cells to systemic therapies (suicide gene therapy).

Gene therapy involves the transfer of one or more genes and the sequences controlling their expression into target cell populations. Theoretically, gene therapy replaces defective genes, alters the immune response, and inserts drug-sensitizing genes. Currently, the most efficient delivery systems to transfer genes intracellularly are viral vectors such as adenovirus, adeno-associated virus, and retrovirus.

Insertion of the thymidine kinase gene from herpes virus into tumor cells can sensitize them to intravenous ganciclovir (125,126). A replication-incompetent retrovirus (murine leukemia virus) contained within vector-producer cells (fibroblast vector-producer cells) is used to deliver thymidine kinase gene from herpes virus. This gene therapy strategy is the most mature innovative approach and has been tested *in vitro*, in animals, and in a series of adult and pediatric clinical trials (126).

Pivotal to the thymidine kinase gene from herpes virus strategy is the *bystander effect*, which results in a larger number of tumor cells being killed than those that have been genetically altered. Immunocompetence and the presence of gap junctions between tumor cells are required experimentally to obtain the bystander effect. The various hurdles inherent to the strategy of gene therapy are reviewed by Maria and colleagues (125–127).

For the time being, however, surgery, radiotherapy, and chemotherapy continue to be the mainstays of pediatric brain tumor management, and despite the many promising approaches, the problem with treating deep or inaccessible tumors still remains.

SPECIFIC TUMOR TYPES

There have been many attempts to classify CNS tumors based not only on traditional morphology, but also on their biologic, immunopathologic, and genetic features. The most recently updated classification was published by the World Health Organization in 1993 and was based, whenever possible, on the histiogenesis of tumors and their biologic behavior (127a,128–130). Because the same type of tumor can produce totally different clinical pictures depending on its site, this chapter, for the greater part, adheres to a location-based classification.

Pediatric brain tumors include a spectrum of both glial and nonglial tumors that differ significantly in location and biologic behavior from those found in adults. Brain tumors in infants and children most often arise from central neuroepithelial tissue, whereas a significant number of adult tumors arise from CNS coverings (e.g., meningioma) or adjacent tissue (e.g., pituitary adenoma) or are metastases.

Tumors of the Posterior Fossa

Cerebellar Tumors

The cerebellum can be the site of various neoplastic processes, three of which are particularly common in children. These are the cerebellar pilocytic astrocytoma, a generally benign tumor arising from the cerebellar hemispheres or vermis, the PNET/MB, a malignant invasive tumor

TABLE 10.10. *Frequencies of common pediatric brain tumors in the infratentorial compartment*

Tumor	%
Medulloblastoma	32.4
(desmoplastic medulloblastoma)	5.4
Pilocytic astrocytoma	28.3
Ependymoma	12.0
Fibrillary astrocytoma	3.8
Astrocytoma, NOS	3.7
Protoplasmic astrocytoma	2.5
Anaplastic astrocytoma	2.4

NOS, not otherwise specified.
Adapted from Gilles FH. Pediatric brain tumors: classification. In: Morantz RA, Walsh JW, eds. *Brain tumors. A comprehensive text.* New York: Marcel Dekker Inc, 1994:109–134.

arising from the fetal cerebellar granular layer of the anterior and posterior medullary vela, and the ependymoma, which arises from the ependymal layer of the fourth ventricle (131). The incidence of the various neoplasms in the infratentorial compartment is shown in Table 10.10 (132).

Pathology

Astrocytomas. These tumors are derived from the astrocytic neuroglial cells and can arise from either the vermis or the lateral lobes of the cerebellum. They are almost always well circumscribed and tend to be cystic, with the neoplasm confined to a small intramural nodule (see Fig. 10.5). Occasionally, astrocytomas form a solid tumor mass involving the cerebellum, vermis, and their brainstem connections.

The microscopic appearance of cerebellar astrocytomas varies considerably even within the same tumor. On the basis of histologic characteristics, Gilles and his group distinguished two tumor types whose resectability and long-term survival can be predicted (132,133). The *pilocytic astrocytoma* represents a distinct subtype of glioma that is most common in children and is genetically and biologically distinct from the diffuse, infiltrating gliomas that affect both adults and children. It constitutes approximately two-thirds of all cerebellar astrocytomas and 28% of posterior fossa tumors (132). On gross inspection, the tumor arises most commonly from the cerebellum, where it frequently projects as a mural nodule into a macroscopically well-circumscribed fluid-filled cyst (Figs. 10.5 and 10.9A

and B). Solid (noncystic) variants also are encountered. Microscopically, the tumor is characterized by a "biphasic" pattern that consists of areas containing tightly packed, piloid ("hairlike") tumor cell processes alternating with areas having numerous microscopic cysts (Fig. 10.9C). The latter often coalesce to form larger cysts. Nonspecific changes of astrocytic cell processes such as eosinophilic granular bodies and Rosenthal fibers are also characteristic. The latter are intracytoplasmic, opaque, homogeneous, strongly eosinophilic beaded masses that stain deep purple with Mallory's phosphotungstic acid hematoxylin. Their presence indicates a degenerative change and they can be found in other tumors, notably in craniopharyngiomas. In an otherwise typical pilocytic astrocytoma, the presence of vascular proliferation or nuclear atypia does not correlate with aggressive behavior as it does in diffuse astrocytomas. Mitoses are rare. Although grossly circumscribed, these tumors may locally infiltrate adjacent tissues and may extend into the adjacent subarachnoid space. Neither of these features suggests a tendency for aggressive behavior. Anaplastic (malignant) pilocytic astrocytomas are rare (134). Although most pilocytic astrocytomas have normal karyotypes (135), deletions on the long arm of chromosome 17 have been reported (136). A *p53* mutation (exon 9, codon 324) was identified in one of seven pilocytic astrocytomas, but this was a silent mutation and its significance is uncertain (137).

Diffuse astrocytomas can occur anywhere in the CNS and are as common in the posterior fossa as in the supratentorial space (138). Diffuse astrocytomas constitute a spectrum of infiltrating astroglial tumors that display increasing grades of anaplasia and include the low-grade diffuse (fibrillary) astrocytoma, anaplastic (intermediate grade) astrocytoma, and glioblastoma multiforme (high grade). Collectively, these tumors account for 12.4% of pediatric infratentorial tumors (132). These intra-axial tumors are similar in histology and biological behavior to those affecting adults (131,138,139). Common pathologic features of this group are extensive infiltration of CNS tissue and a tendency of lower grade lesions to progress to higher grade lesions. Diffuse (fibrillary) astrocytomas tend to arise in white matter and often extensively invade adjacent gray matter struc-

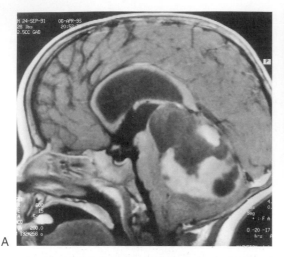

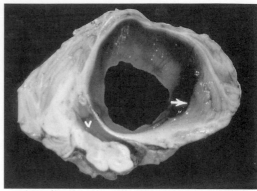

B

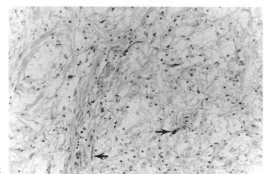

C

FIG. 10.9. Cerebellar pilocytic astrocytoma consisting of a large, well-circumscribed tumor that compresses the fourth ventricle (v) **(A and B)**. Arrow **(B)** indicates a mural nodule of solid tumor. **C:** The histologic section from the mural nodule of a pilocytic astrocytoma. The tumor contains abundant piloid (hairlike) processes and microscopic cysts. Arrows indicate Rosenthal fibers (hematoxylin and eosin, original magnification ×200).

tures. In contrast to the pilocytic astrocytoma, these tumors are difficult to eradicate by surgery alone because of poor demarcation between tumor and surrounding normal tissues, and a higher biologic propensity for regrowth.

Histologically malignant astrocytomas (anaplastic astrocytoma and glioblastoma multiforme) of childhood are infiltrative, biologically aggressive neoplasms (Figs. 10.10 and 10.11) (140). Microscopically, they are characterized by perivascular pseudorosette formation, necrosis, high cell density or mitotic figures, and calcifications, which usually are minute. In this type of glioma, microcyst formation is less common (occurring in 23% of cases).

Cytogenetic characteristics of pediatric malignant astrocytomas differ from those most commonly encountered in adults. Structural abnormalities in chromosomes 9, 13, 17, and double minutes were observed in malignant

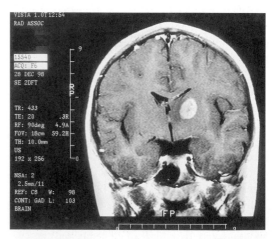

FIG. 10.10. Coronal magnetic resonance imaging with contrast shows inhomogenously enhancing left thalamic anaplastic astrocytoma in a 9-year-old child with a 3-month history of right hand tremor.

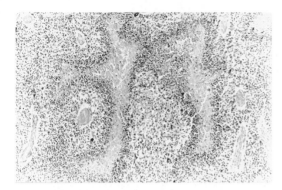

FIG. 10.11. Histologic section demonstrates increased cellularity and classic pseudopalisading necrosis of glioblastoma multiforme.

astrocytomas (anaplastic astrocytoma and glioblastoma) of childhood, whereas the most common chromosomal abnormalities in adult glioblastomas are losses of chromosomes 10 and 19q or gains in chromosome 7 (135). Furthermore, to date, the chromosomal abnormalities found in malignant astrocytomas of childhood are similar to those reported in a genetically distinct subset of glioblastomas that was found to arise in young adults (141).

Distinguishing between these various tumor types is difficult in many cases and changes from one type of tumor to another have been noted with tumor recurrence (142). Additionally, spinal seeding with astrocytomas that appear benign on histologic examination has been observed (143).

Calcification of cerebellar tumors is usually minute, but was seen in 26% of patients in Russell and Rubinstein's series (131).

Primitive Neuroectodermal Tumor/Medulloblastoma. The PNET/MB is the prototype of embryonal brain tumors and is among the most common malignant solid tumors of childhood. It accounts for 38% of pediatric infratentorial tumors (132). Unlike astrocytomas, MBs are derived from primitive neurons, the neuroblasts. Most of the laterally placed tumors arise from the fetal granular layer, a superficial layer of the cerebellar cortex present at birth, which disappears during the first year of life. The more numerous midline tumors are believed to arise from embryonal cell rests in the posterior medullary velum, the site of a germinal bud from which the exter-

nal granular layer is derived (144). In some instances, the origin of the tumor has been traced back to the thirteenth week of gestation, a period of active cerebellar histiogenesis (145).

Macroscopically, these tumors are soft, friable, and moderately well demarcated from the remainder of the cerebellum. In general, they infiltrate the floor or lateral wall of the fourth ventricle and extend into its cavity (Fig. 10.12). The tumor grows backward, occluding the foramen magnum and infiltrating the meninges. It can metastasize by way of the CSF into the subarachnoid space of the spinal canal, with spinal ("drop") metastasis characteristic. Less commonly, the tumor spreads over the cerebral convexity (Fig. 10.13). In the spinal canal the cord and cauda equina become coated with metastatic tumor deposits. The site most frequently involved is the lower end of the spinal cord.

Histologically, PNET/MBs are highly cellular and are composed of small to medium-sized cells with round to oval, often molded (carrot-shaped) hyperchromatic nuclei and poorly defined cell borders. Homer Wright rosettes (ring-like accumulations of tumor cell nuclei around a neurophil-containing or fibrillary core) are occasionally observed (Fig. 10.14). These tumors express a variety of neuronal/neuroendocrine markers, including synaptophysin (a 38-kd synaptic vesicle protein) and neurofilament proteins (146,147). Photoreceptor differentiation (retinal S-antigen and rhodopsin) is identified in 27% to 50% of these tumors (139,148). Glial fibrillary acidic protein (GFAP) has been reported in some 13% to 62% of PNET/MBs (149). One study found that patients with PNET/MBs that contained sheets or clumps of GFAP-immunoreactive neoplastic cells had a threefold increased risk of recurrence compared with those tumors without GFAP immunoreactivity. However, the prognostic value of immunohistochemical data has been controversial.

The most common molecular genetic abnormality identified to date in PNET/MB is loss of heterozygosity of chromosome 17p, which occurs in 30% to 50% of cases and seems to predict a poor prognosis (150,151). However, the PNET/MB-related locus on 17p appears to be

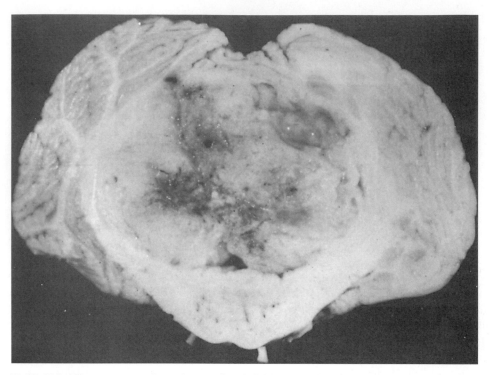

FIG. 10.12. Primitive neuroectodermal tumor/medulloblastoma invading the fourth ventricle and the midline cerebellum.

distinct from *p53* (152). Flow cytometric analyses have indicated a worse prognosis for DNA diploid tumors, whereas aneuploid tumors have a better prognosis (153,154).

The desmoplastic variant of PNET/MB is found in approximately 10% of PNET/MBs and tends to affect an older age group. In contrast to the classic midline form, it often arises laterally in a cerebellar hemisphere. The presence of reticulin-free "pale islands" is a characteristic histopathologic feature (155).

Ependymomas. Ependymomas account for 6% to 15% of brain tumors in children (156). Although these tumors can arise from any part of the ventricular system, the roof and the floor of the fourth ventricle are the most common sites of origin in childhood (Fig. 10.15A). Grossly, fourth ventricular ependymomas are exophytic growths that arise from the ventricular floor and fill the ventricle. Tumor may extend into the basal subarachnoid space through the foramina of Lushka or protrude into the cisterna magna. Ependymomas invade adjacent parenchymal structures but are less overtly infiltrative than high-grade astrocytomas. In appearance ependymomas are gray-tan, granular, and may contain cysts and areas of hemorrhage. Microscopically, the tumor is composed of a uniform population of cells with round to oval nuclei and fibrillary processes; the latter directed toward

FIG. 10.13. ▶ Primitive neuroectodermal tumor/medulloblastoma containing astrocytic elements. Sagittal **(A)** and axial **(B)** magnetic resonance images in this boy show a tumor within the fourth ventricle. It is of low signal intensity (darker than brain, but less dark than CSF) on the T1-weighted imaging **(A)**. The lesion appeared to arise from the roof of the fourth ventricle. Although the neoplasm compressed the posterior aspect of the pons and medulla, it seemed separable from the brainstem. This was confirmed at surgery. (Courtesy of Drs. Hervey D. Segall and J. Gordon McComb, Departments of Radiology and Neurosurgery, Children's Hospital, Los Angeles.)

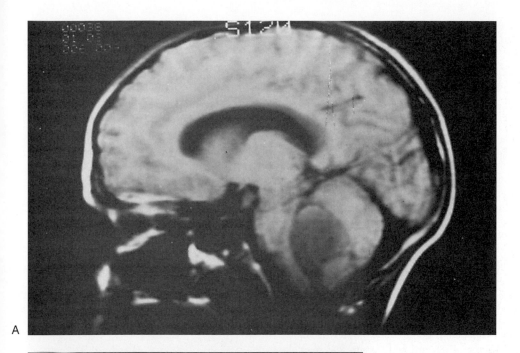

A

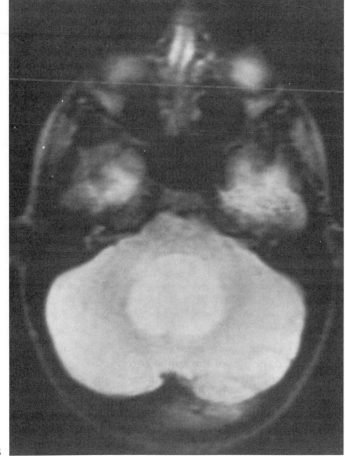

B

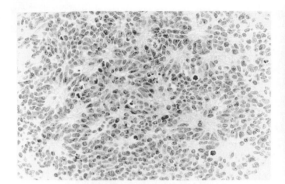

FIG. 10.14. Histology of primitive neuroectodermal tumor of the cerebellum (primitive neuroectodermal tumor/medulloblastoma) with several Homer Wright rosettes (hematoxylin and eosin, original magnification, ×1,000).

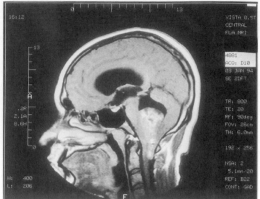

A

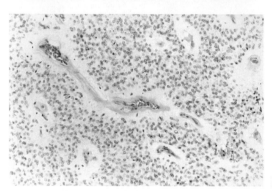

B

FIG. 10.15. A: Sagittal magnetic resonance imaging shows large contrast-enhancing ependymoma filling most of fourth ventricle. **B:** Histologic section of ependymoma shows a uniform population of cells with round to slightly oval nuclei and indistinct cell borders. Perivascular clear areas (*pseudorosettes*) represent tumor cell processes oriented perpendicular to intratumoral vessels (hematoxylin and eosin, original magnification, ×500).

abundant intratumoral blood vessels forming a distinct perivascular pseudorosette pattern (Fig. 10.15B). Better differentiated examples may contain tubular structures and canals. Although ependymal tumors with increased cellularity, pleomorphism, mitoses, and necrosis have been termed *anaplastic* or *malignant*, such histologic features have been less predictive of aggressive behavior than they are in diffuse astrocytomas (157). The association of a high number of mitoses and high cell density with incomplete pseudorosettes allows one to make the diagnosis of the anaplastic variant in supratentorial ependymomas (158). It is important to note that histologically benign ependymomas can hemorrhage and invade the brainstem (44). Paradoxically, the presence of calcifications in the tumor has a poor prognosis. Conversely, high cell density and nuclear polymorphism suggest a good prognosis (159).

Chromosomal abnormalities identified in ependymomas include monosomy and deletions of chromosome 22, trisomy of chromosome 7, loss of sex chromosomes, and structural rearrangements of chromosome 2 (139). In addition, chromosomes 9 and 11 may harbor genes involved in the pathogenesis of ependymoma. A germ-line mutation of the tumor-suppressor gene *p53* has been implicated in the pathogenesis of anaplastic ependymoma (160). A deletion of chromosome 1 has been identified

in the myxopapillary ependymoma, a distinct subtype that arises in the filum terminale.

Other Tumors. Other tumor types involving the cerebellum and its contiguous structures include undifferentiated sarcomas, some of which are of leptomeningeal origin, glioblastomas, and cerebellar hemangioblastoma, which is discussed in Chapter 11 under von Hippel–Lindau disease. Some of the uncommon CNS tumors are reviewed in Table 10.11.

Acoustic nerve tumors, which are common in adults, are rare in children; when seen they are usually bilateral and a manifestation of neurofibromatosis 2 (see Chapter 11).

TABLE 10.11. *Some less common central nervous system tumors of childhood*

Tumor	Most common site	Characteristics	Reference
Pleomorphic xanthoastrocytoma	Temporal lobe	Slow growing, may exhibit anaplastic features, can undergo malignant transformation	161–166
Ganglioglioma	Temporal lobe (38%), parietal lobe (30%), frontal lobe (18%), cerebellum, brainstem, spinal cord	Slow growing, benign, often cystic; associated with cortical dysplasia, neoplastic astroglial elements and ganglion cells	168–171
Desmoplastic infantile ganglioglioma	Supratentorial with frontoparietal predilection, often involves leptomeninges	Benign, partially cystic, extensive deposition of stromal collagen	172–174
Dysembryoplastic neuroepithelial tumor	Temporal lobe, caudate nucleus	Slow growing and benign, bundles of axons attached to oligodendroglial-like cells, cystic areas, adjacent cortical dysplasia	175–178
Medulloepithelioma	Supratentorial and infratentorial	Responds poorly to treatment; tumor cells and vesicular structures resembling embryonic neural tube	179
Atypical teratoid/ malignant rhabdoid tumors	Posterior fossa (65%), other areas of neuraxis	Highly malignant; histologically mixed with primitive neuroectodermal tumor and rhabdoid elements; prognosis worse than primitive neuroectodermal tumor/medulloblastoma	180–184
Dermoids and epidermoids	Extradural: scalp, skull; intradural: temporal lobe, posterior fossa, suprasellar region	Arise from trapped pouches of ectoderm; epidermoids have squamous epithelium, dermoids contain squamous epithelium, hair, sebaceous and sweat glands	185,186
Central neurocytoma	Supratentorial ventricular system	Generally benign, uniform round cells, with evidence of neuronal differentiation	187

Clinical Manifestations

The three tumors described previously are frequently indistinguishable clinically. Intracranial pressure is increased, and the cerebellum and its contiguous structures are involved.

In cerebellar tumors, the growing mass soon obstructs the ventricular system, making increased intracranial pressure a common presenting sign (Table 10.12). Early on, headaches are generally unlocalized or frontal; subsequently, they are suboccipital. When the tumor is unilateral, the child often holds the head tilted, with the head bent toward the more involved hemisphere while the chin points to the other side.

Vomiting is the most common presenting sign of cerebellar tumors. Usually it results from increased intracranial pressure, but at times it can be caused by direct pressure on the medullary vagal nuclei or the vomiting center.

The progressive evolution of cerebellar signs was described by Cushing in 1931 (188):

A child apparently healthy in all respects begins toward the end of the first decade, possibly after a fall or an attack of whooping cough, to have early morning headaches and vomiting. Nothing much is made of this by the family doctor, should he be called in, for the child subsequently feels perfectly well, has had breakfast, and wants to go out and play. This daily performance may continue for a considerable time, the child even going to school meanwhile. There may then be a remission of weeks or perhaps months and the episode be forgotten. On their reoccurrence, the symptoms are likely to be more pronounced and are apt to be ascribed to some gastrointestinal disturbance. This appears the more probable since the child finds that strain-

TABLE 10.12. *Presenting manifestations in patients 18 years of age or less with cerebellar tumors*

Initial signs or symptoms	Medulloblastoma	Astrocytoma
Vomiting	29	34
Headaches	10	38
Unsteadiness	22	15
Visual impairment	1	1
Strabismus	5	7
Enlarging head	0	1
Pain or stiffness of neck	1	3
Others (head tilt, malaise, dizziness, lumbar pain, hemiparesis)	8	4

From Cushing H. Experiences with the cerebellar astrocytomas. *Surg Gynecol Obstet* 1931;52:129. With permission.

ing at stool brings on a headache and there is a tendency to become constipated. What is more, a mild daily laxative usually serves completely to mask the symptoms.

This sort of thing continues off and on until it becomes evident that the child is a little clumsy at play and gets knocked over easily. Very possibly, before this, the periodic headache and vomiting will have ceased completely or at least have occurred at much longer intervals; and if parents are observant they may notice that the child's head in the interim has increased in size more rapidly than it should. This, however, is usually discounted for the child meanwhile has become free from complaints and in all respects appears alert and well.

Matters may run on in this way for an indefinite time, possibly with some increase in clumsiness of movement or in some instances with no noticeable change whatever until it suddenly becomes apparent, perhaps at school, that the child's sight is poor. To counteract this, glasses are usually prescribed; but even should an ophthalmoscope be resorted to, a child's retina is less easily examined than that of an adult and, because of the decompressive effects of the enlarging head, the optic papillae often show no measurable swelling and the fact of their being pale and with margins blurred may easily pass unrecognized.

Due to the insidious nature of the symptomatic onset, it is in this preamaurotic stage of the process that even today the victims of these midcerebellar astrocytomas . . . unfortunately continue to be admitted to hospital.

The length of time that a child with a cerebellar neoplasm is symptomatic before being hospitalized is a function of the malignancy of tumor and the readiness of the primary physician to request a consultation or perform imaging studies. In the experience of Park and coworkers, who in 1983 reported on a series of children with PNET/MB compiled between 1950 and 1980, the clinical history lasted less than 6 weeks in 51% of cases and less than 12 weeks in 76% of cases (189). By contrast, in the 1987 experience of Diebler and Dulac, the mean interval between the first signs of a cerebellar astrocytoma and diagnosis was approximately 4 months, and approximately 3 months for children with an ependymoma (190).

The most common cerebellar symptom is unsteadiness of gait, owing to involvement of the vermis. The child stands with the feet widely separated and quickly loses balance if the center of gravity is displaced. On attempting to walk, the child sways and staggers. Often, the impairment in gait is at its worst on awakening and lessens with prolonged activity. Disturbances of speech indicate more advanced involvement of the vermis. Speech is slow and monotonous, and syllables are uttered in a jerky, explosive manner.

Disorders of limb movement (dysmetria, adiadochokinesia or slowing and dissociation of rapid alternating movements, and intention tremor) and disorders of posture (hypotonia), both of which indicate involvement of the cerebellar hemispheres, are seen less commonly during the early stages of the process. Some tumors located exclusively along the midline, notably PNET/MBs arising from the vermis, can elicit no localizing symptoms. Hypotonia is more marked on the ipsilateral side. As a consequence, the child tends to stagger to the side of the lesion. The rebound phenomenon, the pendular deep tendon reflexes, and other evidence of postural instability are also more marked on the side of the lesion.

Nystagmus, although in general a classic sign of cerebellar disease, usually occurs late in chil-

TABLE 10.13. *Magnetic resonance characteristics
of specific histologic types of posterior fossa tumors*

	Hypointense on T1	Hyperintense on T2	Enhanced on T1	Cystic component
Medulloblastoma	42/42	0/42	20/22	0/42
Pilocytic astrocytoma	23/23	23/23	23/23	18/23
Malignant glioma	17/17	17/17	6/17	1/17
Fibrillary astrocytoma	8/8	8/8	4/8	0/8
Astrocytoma	7/7	7/7	5/7	1/7
Ganglioglioma	1/1	1/1	1/1	1/1
Ependymoma	8/10	6/10	9/10	0/10

Note: The signal intensity change is relative to that of normal gray matter. The numbers indicate the proportion of cases showing such change.
Adapted from Zimmerman RD, Bilaniuk LT, Rebsamen S. Magnetic resonance imaging of pediatric posterior fossa tumors. *Pediatr Neurosurg* 1992;18:58.

dren with posterior fossa tumors. When present, it is almost always bilateral and more noticeable with lateral than with vertical gaze. Although nystagmus is usually conjugate, the rapid phase is occasionally more evident in the direction of the predominantly involved hemisphere, with a slow drift back to the midline. The oscillations are slow (2 to 3 per second) and coarse.

Seizures are rare in cerebellar tumors, although Jackson, Holmes, and numerous other, older authors have described tonic cerebellar seizures with retraction of the head, arching of the back, flexion of the elbows, and rigid extension of the legs (191). These episodes are accompanied by disorders of respiration and can terminate fatally. They do not represent true seizures, but result from compression of the vermis or lower brainstem.

Diagnosis

The only distinguishing feature in the clinical course of the three major cerebellar tumors is the duration of symptoms before hospitalization. If symptoms have lasted more than 12 months, a benign cerebellar astrocytoma is most likely. With symptoms of more recent onset, clinical differentiation might not be possible. Although the CT scan was once considered a nearly flawless means of localizing a cerebellar tumor and was a guide to tumor type, MRI, particularly with gadolinium-diethylenethriaminepenta-acetic acid (DTPA) enhancement, provides an excellent and generally preferable diagnostic means.

An PNET/MB presents as a centrally located, generally uniformly homogeneous, dense tumor on precontrast scans, but after administration of contrast material shows homogeneous enhancement with sharp borders. The pilocytic astrocytoma presents as a uniform zone of low density with sharp borders; an enhanced tumor nodule is observed in the majority of instances. The diffuse astrocytoma has a low density on precontrast scans, but tends to become enhanced. Calcification within a mass located near the fourth ventricle should suggest the diagnosis of an ependymoma or, in children from Third World countries, a tuberculoma (192).

The MRI characteristics of the various posterior fossa tumors are shown in Table 10.13. Little difference is seen in unenhanced T1-weighted signal intensity between benign and malignant tumors (193,194). Most posterior fossa tumors enhance after the administration of gadolinium contrast so that presence or absence of enhancement provides no clue as to tumor type in posterior fossa neoplasms. On T2-weighted images the PNET/MB is isointense to gray matter, whereas all types of astrocytomas are hyperintense (195) (see Fig. 10.13). Generally, there is no clear demarcation between the tumor itself and any surrounding edema. The increased protein content of a cyst results in a high-intensity signal on T2-weighted images. This increased signal is usually readily differentiated from the tumor itself.

Some children with posterior fossa PNET/MBs show evidence of metastases. In the series of Park and associates (189), these were localized to the supratentorial region in 15% of patients with, most commonly, the frontal lobes being invaded. Clinically silent spinal cord metastases were detected in 19% of patients in a more recent series (196) (see Fig. 10.13). When symptomatic, the child complains of pain, spinal tenderness, urinary symptoms, and, in the most advanced stage, spinal cord compression and paraplegia. Systemic metastases, mainly to the skeleton, were seen in 10% of PNET/MBs.

Occasionally, tumors outside the posterior fossa induce signs simulating cerebellar involvement. A long-standing increase in intracranial pressure can result in ataxia and unsteadiness of gait. Frontal lobe tumors, rare in childhood, also can produce ataxia. In contrast to cerebellar ataxia, dysmetria and adiadochokinesia are absent in approximately 40% of patients with frontal lobe ataxia, and nystagmus is absent in approximately 65%. The ataxia is generally thought to arise from interruption of frontopontocerebellar fibers or interruption of afferent cerebellar fibers in the dentatorubrothalamocortical system (197). Craniopharyngiomas rarely can show predominantly cerebellar signs. Involuntary movements, consisting of rhythmic myoclonus of the face and arms, have been seen in an occasional child with a posterior fossa neoplasm (197). Although the diagnosis of posterior fossa masses with such unusual clinical features was difficult at one time, neuroimaging studies now readily localize the responsible lesion.

An unusual tumor of the cerebellum that produces prolonged and slowly progressive cerebellar signs was first described by Lhermitte and Duclos (198). The most striking feature of this condition is the replacement of the granular cell layer by a hamartomatous mass of pleiomorphic ganglion cells. Although the condition usually presents in adult life, it probably represents an abnormality in cell migration or a phakomatosis (199). Examination of tissue by immunohistochemistry shows that most of the abnormal neurons in the lesion are derived from granule cells, with a small subpopulation of cells demonstrating Purkinje cell–specific monoclonal and polyclonal antibodies (200). Lhermitte-Duclos disease is occasionally associated with Cowden disease, a rare autosomal dominant condition manifested by multiple hamartomas and other neoplasms (199,201). A mutation of the *PTEN/MMAC 1* gene, a tumor-suppres-

sor gene, has been found in some patients with Lhermitte-Duclos disease (202).

Treatment and Prognosis of Posterior Fossa Tumors

Astrocytomas. The treatment for pilocytic astrocytomas is gross total resection, whenever possible. Some surgeons prefer to place a shunt before performing surgery to diminish the volume of the excessively dilated ventricle. Evacuation of an associated cyst can relieve symptoms for long periods, but does not prevent ultimate refilling. After resection, patients should have an MRI and neurologic examination every 6 months for the first 2 years. With total tumor resection the outcome for the cystic variety of type A glioma is extremely good; in fact, in a series reported by Matson as early as 1956, the cure rate was 94% (203). With better surveillance, disease-free survival rates are equally good (204). If the resection is partial, as is often the case for midline supratentorial lesions, radiotherapy is recommended, and more frequent MRIs and neurologic examinations are indicated. In children younger than 3 years of age with partially resected or progressive supratentorial pilocytic astrocytomas, chemotherapy is recommended. As a rule, fibrillary astrocytomas are less responsive to chemotherapy than pilocytic astrocytomas.

Gross surgical excision of the diffuse astrocytoma is far more difficult. These tumors tend to arise in white matter and often extensively invade adjacent gray matter structures. In contrast to the pilocytic astrocytoma, there is a poor demarcation between tumor and surrounding normal tissues, and the tumor has a higher biologic propensity for regrowth. In the series of Schneider and colleagues total resection was achieved in only 37.5% (205). In children who underwent partial tumor resection followed by postoperative radiotherapy, the 5-year and 10-year survival rates were 70% and 63%, respectively (206).

It is as yet an unresolved question whether postoperative radiotherapy decreases the recurrence rate and improves survival of children with subtotally removed cerebellar astrocytomas. The difficulty of assessing the benefits of radiotherapy are because of the long survival of children in whom subtotal resection was the only therapy, and the lack of uniformity in radiation dosages and techniques. However, the adverse effects of radiation to the developing brain are clearly known, particularly when radiation is administered to children younger than age 3 years. It is, therefore, our recommendation that radiation therapy is best deferred in small children, even if tumor resection is incomplete, and that children be followed closely with imaging studies and not be irradiated unless tumor progression is documented (207). In all instances, MRI studies and neurologic examinations are required every 2 to 4 months in the first 2 years from diagnosis. Generally, a child can be considered cured of his or her neoplasm if the child remains free of any evident recurrence for a period equivalent to his or her age at diagnosis plus 9 months (Collins' law) (208). The effectiveness of chemotherapy on this tumor is still uncertain, and more studies are needed before specific agents and doses can be routinely recommended for treatment of diffuse astrocytomas in children.

Management of Primitive Neuroectodermal Tumor/Medulloblastoma. Management of PNET/ MB is a far more difficult task, but in the course of the past two decades, survival for children with this type of tumor has gradually improved (209). Advances in surgical technique, radiotherapy, and chemotherapy have culminated in 5-year progression-free survival rates as high as 85% (210). A number of studies have concluded that survival is improved with gross total resection, especially in patients with localized disease at the time of diagnosis (209,211,212). However, although 5-year survival rates have climbed to more than 50%, late recurrences have been reported, and late effects of therapy are common (213).

The decision of what treatment to recommend after surgery of PNET/MB is difficult because of conflicting results from clinical trials around the world. The value of chemotherapy, given before or after radiotherapy, is currently under investigation, with several ongoing study groups using different regimens. A current trend favors adjunct chemotherapy, which appears to be particularly beneficial in high-risk children, namely those with a tumor invading the fourth ventricle or infiltrating the brainstem, those younger than 4 years of age, and those who underwent a subtotal resection. Conversely, low-risk patients are those in whom more than 75% of the tumor is resected surgically, as confirmed by imaging studies, who have a negative spinal cord MRI study result and CSF cytology, have no evidence of CNS or extraneural metastases, and who are older than 2 years of age (214).

In the experience of Packer and colleagues, reported in 1991, chemotherapy did not improve 5-year disease-free survival of children with standard risk disease. However, there was a significant 5-year survival advantage from using chemotherapy in high-risk groups, as based on tumor size, degree of brainstem involvement, and evidence of CSF dissemination (210). Other studies also have reported a significantly better event-free survival in high-risk patients receiving chemotherapy (215). A randomized postoperative trial in which adjuvant postradiation chemotherapy (nitrogen mustard, vincristine, procarbazine, and prednisone) was tested against radiotherapy (216) showed that both groups had almost identical overall and event-free survival at 10 years postdiagnosis. (216).

Based on available information on surgery, radiotherapy, and chemotherapy, the following recommendations can be made. The goal should be to achieve a gross total resection of the PNET/MB, but the risks of surgical mortality and morbidity from removing brainstem components of the tumor probably outweigh the benefits of a complete excision. PNET/MB is often large in the area of the roof of the fourth ventricle and requires extensive suboccipital craniectomy and incision through the vermis for total microsurgical resection. Probably fewer benefits accrue from achieving a gross total surgical resection in patients with CSF dissemination of tumor. A critical aspect to defining the risk of tumor recurrence is determining the extent of invasion of the floor of the fourth ventricle by microscopic inspection of the ependymal lining. Postoperative craniospinal imaging and CSF cytology are required to determine if CSF and neuroaxis spread have occurred (217).

After near total resection, current therapy includes reduced-dose craniospinal radiotherapy followed by chemotherapy. It is well established that the entire neuroaxis must be treated with radiotherapy (218,219). If the resection is partial or the patient has other, aforementioned risk factors for tumor recurrence, standard dose craniospinal radiotherapy is recommended, followed by chemotherapy. It is premature to consider using low-dose radiotherapy until more information is available from ongoing clinical trials. Taken together, the results from the studies on chemotherapy in PNET/MB suggest that cisplatin, etoposide, vincristine, and cyclophosphamide produce the greatest survival benefit to patients with poor-risk disease. Optimal combinations of existing agents and doses, relation to radiotherapy, and new agents must be studied before they can be routinely recommended for high-risk patients. All children should have MRIs and neurologic examinations every 3 to 4 months in the first 2 years after diagnosis. Careful attention to growth, development, endocrine function, behavior, and cognition are pivotal in long-term follow-up.

Management of Ependymomas. Total surgical resection of ependymomas arising from the floor of the fourth ventricle is difficult and dangerous. In fact, improvement in survival statistics since 1980 is probably because of improved surgical technique and lower perioperative deaths (220). Evidence exists that patients undergoing a radical resection have twice the survival rate as those receiving a partial resection (221). Surgery should be followed by limited-field radiotherapy for low-grade ependymomas (222). For supratentorial anaplastic ependymomas, limited-field radiotherapy and chemotherapy are recommended (223,224). For posterior fossa anaplastic ependymomas, craniospinal radiotherapy and chemotherapy are recommended, although symptomatic spinal seeding is rare (225–227).

The only prospective randomized trial to evaluate the role of chemotherapy in ependymomas showed no improvement in outcome (228). Interestingly, infants with ependymomas showed a significant response to chemotherapy (109,229). In view of the observation that infants who received 2 years of chemotherapy have a lower 5-year survival than those who only receive 1 year of chemotherapy, Duffner and coworkers recommend that after maximal surgical resection, radiation therapy should not be delayed more than 1 year (230).

MRIs and neurologic examinations are required every 2 to 4 months in the first 2 years from diagnosis. As the 5-year survival for infants and children harboring an ependymoma is only 50%, it will be necessary to test the safety and efficacy of new radiotherapy strategies and chemotherapy agents (156,231,232).

A condition, termed *cerebellar mutism* has been encountered after resection of a posterior fossa tumor. It occurs within a few hours to up to 9 days after surgery and can last as long as 20 weeks (232a). The nature of the condition is poorly understood, and a transient oral apraxia or a loss of ability to initiate oral movements appear to be the most likely explanations (232b). Rarely, transient visual impairment accompanies the mutism (232c).

Brainstem Tumors

Tumors of the brainstem produce a clinical picture with a variable initial presentation but a uniformly fatal progression. They account for 10% of pediatric CNS neoplasms (233,234). Although nearly all brainstem gliomas are malignant by virtue of their location, morphologic studies show them to be a nonhomogeneous group, with a variety of appearances ranging from the benign, well-differentiated astrocytoma to the highly malignant glioblastoma.

Pathology

Most commonly, tumor of the brainstem arises from the pons and appears as a symmetric enlargement of the brainstem, bulging into the floor of the fourth ventricle, a pathologic feature termed "pontile hypertrophy" (Fig. 10.16). Approximately 80% of pediatric brainstem gliomas are diffusely infiltrating astrocytomas and, of these, approximately 50% are histologi-

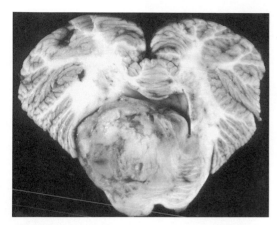

FIG. 10.16. Brainstem glioma diffusely expanding the pons and effacing normal structures.

cally malignant at presentation (234). Extensive infiltration of tumor along white matter tracts is typical. Characteristically, cells grow by insinuating themselves between preexisting structures, separating but not destroying them; hence, the relative paucity of signs in the earlier stages of tumor growth (Figs. 10.6 and 10.17).

Microscopic examination shows the glioma to be composed of elongated bipolar cells that resemble a fibrillary astrocytoma (233). Like astrocytomas of the cerebral hemispheres, but in contrast to cerebellar astrocytomas, brainstem tumors tend to show anaplasia, and certain areas, primarily those deep in the tumor, ultimately resemble glioblastoma multiforme. In their series of 21 tumors, Berger and coworkers found that all but one had the microscopic appearance of an anaplastic astrocytoma or a glioblastoma multiforme, and that frequently what appeared to be a benign tumor harbored highly malignant cells (235). Metastasis and invasion of the meninges are rare, but dissemination into the subarachnoid space of the spinal cord is well documented. Based on combined CT and morphologic studies, the Toronto group proposed the following classification (236):

Group I tumors arise from the floor of the fourth ventricle and grow exophytically into the fourth ventricle, with only limited brainstem infiltration. This type of a tumor constituted 22% of pediatric brainstem gliomas. Histologically, it generally is a grade I to II astrocytoma.

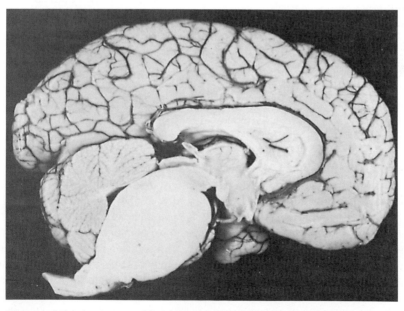

FIG. 10.17. Glioma of the brainstem. The tumor has diffusely infiltrated the brainstem, producing *hypertrophy*. Note the relative lack of dilatation of lateral ventricles. (Courtesy of Dr. P. Cancilla, Department of Pathology, University of California, Los Angeles, UCLA School of Medicine.)

Group II tumors, which constituted 51% of brainstem gliomas in the Toronto series, are intrinsic and diffusely infiltrative. Histologically, they are grade III astrocytomas or glioblastomas.

Group III tumors, which constituted 8% of brainstem gliomas, have a cystic component.

Group IV tumors, constituting 18% of the series, are focal tumors intrinsic to the brainstem, commonly located in the cervicomedullary area. They tend to be low-grade astrocytomas.

Von Deimling and colleagues and Louis and colleagues reported losses of portions of chromosome 17p, mutations of *p53*, and allelic losses of chromosome 10q in brainstem gliomas, a pattern similar to a subset of supratentorial glioblastomas that occurs in young adults (141,237).

Clinical Manifestations

Brainstem gliomas present with an insidious onset of symptoms and signs that have remained unchanged in the many series published since the 1930s (238) (Table 10.14). In contrast to the comparatively uniform evolution of the clinical picture in cerebellar tumors, the initial symptoms of a brainstem neoplasm are variable. The most commonly encountered brainstem tumor (group II, using the Toronto terminology) is characterized by the presence of four major features: cranial nerve palsies, pyramidal tract signs, cerebellar signs, and progression to advanced stages, usually without increase in intracranial pressure (236,239). In most patients, the period from onset of symptoms to diagnosis is less than 6 months, and it is usually under 2 months (240,241). Manifestations appear at 2 to 12 years of age, with peak incidence at 6 years. Vomiting and disturbances of gait are the most common presenting complaints. Less frequent is the gradual or rapid onset of a hemiparesis or evidence of cranial nerve involvement, especially facial weakness, strabismus, or difficulties in swallowing. The presence of a head tilt and changes in personality are other relatively common early signs (see Table 10.14) (239).

Vomiting, unaccompanied by headache, is caused not by increased intracranial pressure, but by direct infiltration of the medullary vomiting center. Impairment of gait is caused in part by involvement of the cerebellum or its pedun-

TABLE 10.14. *Incidence of neurologic signs and symptoms in children with brainstem tumors*

Sign/symptom	Incidence/number of patients
Gait disturbance	47/48
Squinting	25/48
Vomiting	22/48
Headache	21/48
Dysarthria	19/48
Facial weakness	15/48
Personality change	11/48
Dysphagia	10/48
Drowsiness	10/48
Head tilt	5/48
Hearing loss	4/48
Pyramidal tract signs	41/48
Cranial nerve involvement	
VII	64/78
IX and X	54/78
VI	48/78
V (sensory)	38/78
V (motor)	13/48
XII	13/48
VIII	12/78
Cerebellar signs	62/78
Nystagmus	
Horizontal	26/48
Vertical	14/14
Papilledema	24/78
Gaze paralysis	
Horizontal	22/48
Vertical	5/48
Hemisensory deficit	5/48

Adapted from Bray PF, Carter S, Taveras JM. Brainstem tumors in children. *Neurology* 1958;8:17; and Matson DD. *Neurosurgery of infancy and childhood.* Springfield, IL: Charles C Thomas, 1969.

cles, and in part by hemiparesis. Various neurologic signs found in affected children result from involvement of the major structures within the brainstem: the pyramidal tracts, nuclei of the various cranial nerves, and corticopontocerebellar fibers Corticospinal tracts are usually involved early. Patients develop a spastic hemiparesis, increased deep tendon reflexes, and an extensor plantar response.

The cranial nerves most commonly affected by the neoplasm are the seventh and the sixth. Because the nucleus of the facial nerve is involved, facial weakness is almost invariably of lower motor neuron type. Dysfunction of the ninth and tenth nerves leads to drooling, difficulty in swallowing, and often insidious loss of weight. Sixth nerve weakness often is associ-

TABLE 10.15. *Incidence of neurologic signs and symptoms in 16 patients with dorsally exophytic brainstem gliomas (group I)*

Sign/symptom	Number of patients
Hydrocephalus	12
Ataxia	11
Cranial nerve signs	8
Headache	6
Failure to thrive	5
Nystagmus	4
Long tract signs	1

Modified from Stroink AR, et al. Transependymal benign dorsally exophytic brainstem gliomas in childhood: diagnosis and treatment recommendations. *Neurosurgery* 1987;20:439.

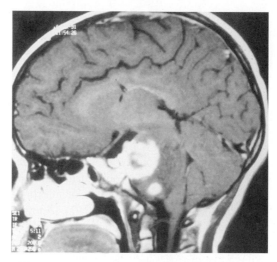

FIG. 10.18. Sagittal magnetic resonance imaging shows enlarged pons and contrast-enhancing malignant glioma with associated edema.

ated with horizontal conjugate gaze palsy. It is, therefore, caused by involvement of the brainstem, rather than being a false localizing sign resulting from increased intracranial pressure.

Functions of some of the other structures within the brainstem, notably the sensory pathways within the medial lemniscus, appear to be more resistant to tumor encroachment, and hemisensory deficits are rare. Infiltration of the reticular substances occasionally produces alterations in personality and changes in eating and sleeping patterns. In contrast to cerebellar tumors, impairment of consciousness is less common.

The progression of symptoms is relentless. As one cranial nerve after another becomes involved, patients become unable to swallow or speak, the extremities become completely paralyzed, and, finally, the patient has impairment of consciousness with deepening coma and respiratory or cardiac irregularities ending in death. The average survival time for the untreated patient is approximately 15 months from the date of the patient's first hospitalization (242).

Symptoms and signs of group I tumors differ from those of group II tumors in that hydrocephalus is seen in 75% of the patients, as compared with 16% of children with group II tumors. Hydrocephalus results from the tumor's extension into the fourth ventricle and its obstruction of CSF circulation. Cerebellar deficits are also more common than in group II tumors; long tract signs are rare (Table 10.15) (243).

Diagnosis

The diagnosis suggested by the clinical features of a brainstem neoplasm can be confirmed by imaging studies. MRI, which has the capability of imaging in any plane and provides sagittal views of the posterior fossa, is the preferred procedure for characterization of the neoplasm. Imaging typically shows a diffuse, infiltrative, variable-enhancing tumor that enlarges and distorts the brainstem (Fig. 10.18). The technique provides excellent visualization of exophytic tumors and delineation of intrinsic brainstem tumors, with sagittal views often clearly showing the rostrocaudal extent of the mass (see Fig. 10.6) (244). The neoplasm is almost always hypointense on T1-weighted images, and in the experience of Barkovich and colleagues, was always hyperintense on T2-weighted images (245). The presence or absence of gadolinium enhancement provides an indication as to the degree of malignancy of the tumor. As a rule, the greater the enhancement, the more malignant the tumor. MRI also indicates the presence and extent of tumor spread and allows visualization of areas of necrotic degeneration. Necrotic degeneration indicates a particularly poor prognosis, even if it appears after radiotherapy (246).

Several clinical entities should be considered in the differential diagnosis. These include a brain abscess, cysticercosis, tuberculoma, and a vascular malformation. The appearance of these lesions on MRI is often difficult to distinguish from a neoplasm, and serial studies or a biopsy of the lesion is sometimes necessary. In some instances, symptoms and signs of a brainstem glioma have receded spontaneously, leading to complete recovery. This condition has been termed *brainstem encephalitis*. It is probably identical to the Miller Fisher syndrome, a variant of infectious polyneuritis (see Chapter 7) (247). Another important condition in the differential diagnosis of brainstem glioma is the diffuse cerebellar astrocytoma that displaces and sometimes invades the brainstem. Such tumors may radiologically mimic intrinsic diffuse brainstem gliomas, but, in contrast, are amenable to near complete resections and may not require further therapy.

Treatment of Brainstem Gliomas

Treatment of brainstem gliomas depends on the tumor group. For group I tumors, Stroink and coworkers advocate subtotal resection, with radiotherapy being used only when tumor recurs (243). Generally, the morphologic appearance of the tumor correlates with survival time (248), and in the case of the diffuse brainstem gliomas, there is no evidence that microscopic examination of tissue obtained by stereotactic biopsy is a better predictor of clinical progression than neuroimaging (249). In addition, the presence of lower brainstem dysfunction is a contraindication to biopsy because patients will likely require tracheostomy postoperatively. Astrocytic tumors involving the midbrain have a much better prognosis than those involving the pons; medullary lesions have a somewhat better prognosis than pontine lesions.

Less common forms of brainstem glioma include focal, cystic, cervicomedullary, and tectal types (Toronto groups III and IV). In contrast to the diffuse type, these tumors tend to be well circumscribed and exophytic and display histologic and biologic characteristics of pilocytic astrocytomas (see Fig. 10.6). Such tumors may have a much more favorable prognosis than diffuse

brainstem gliomas and can be approached surgically with the intent to safely resect the lesions. However, morbidity is high, with the exception of lesions that are predominantly exophytic, and rare focal tumors that extend to the surface of the brainstem and can be shelled out without surgically incising normal brainstem tissue.

The principles of surgical excision of brainstem gliomas, whether exophytic or intrinsic, entail adequate exposure and visualization with an operating microscope. The concept is to excise the offending, noninfiltrating component of this lesion, which is best done with bipolar coagulation and suction. Use of ultrasonic aspirators and laser probes can aid in the early excision of these lesions, but once the tumor–brainstem interface is reached, careful tactile monitoring is required. The glial tumor in the cerebellum proper should be excised totally, and this entails staying in a plane of normal brain tissue surrounding the tumor. Again, this resection is best done with tactile feedback to the surgeon because visualization becomes confusing when tissue becomes charred and discolored using the laser. Focal pilocytic brainstem gliomas that have been excised can be followed conservatively with MRI every 3 to 4 months in the first 2 years. In the absence of clinical or radiographic recurrence, radiotherapy and chemotherapy should be deferred. Nonpilocytic focal brainstem gliomas or partially resected pilocytic brainstem gliomas should be treated with conformal or stereotactic radiotherapy. Progressive pilocytic lesions in infants should be treated with chemotherapy rather than radiotherapy. There have been no controlled clinical trials examining the benefits and risks of radiotherapy or chemotherapy in focal brainstem gliomas.

For group II tumors, a surgical approach is impossible, leaving radiotherapy and chemotherapy as principal treatments. The prognosis for these children is, to say the least, discouraging, regardless of the histology at the time of biopsy.

Radiation therapy produces transient clinical remissions in approximately 60% of this group, with initial improvement being noted some 3 to 6 weeks after the onset of treatment, most commonly as partial clearing of cranial nerve signs. Mean survival is between 6 and 12 months. Tumors that arise from the mesencephalon or those that extend into the cerebellopontine and prepontine cisterns fare a little better (236). The response to a second course of irradiation is usually poor (250,251).

Hyperfractionated radiotherapy, which entails the use of a large number of smaller fractions given in the same overall treatment time and allows a higher total dose to be directed at the tumor, is being used at the University of Florida and several other centers (252). Although the results are still difficult to interpret, they show a slight improvement in terms of 1- and 2-year survival (253).

Few studies have evaluated the efficacy of chemotherapy in brainstem gliomas backed by objective neuroimaging (254). A number of chemotherapeutic agents have been tried, notably BCNU, lomustine (CCNU), vincristine, cisplatin, carboplatin, and various alkylators. To date, when responses to chemotherapy do occur, they are of short duration, although exceptions have been encountered (233,255,256). For example, one study reported 80% partial response (four of five) to high-dose cyclophosphamide (257). This has not been corroborated by other investigators. One of us (B.M.) has treated six newly diagnosed children with diffuse brainstem gliomas with high-dose cyclophosphamide and thiotepa followed by bone marrow reinfusion. One patient had a partial response and one had minor response to chemotherapy (233,258). On recovery they were given hyperfractionated radiotherapy. The patient with a partial response to chemotherapy then achieved a complete response and is free of disease or late effects 8 years from diagnosis (258). Kretschmar and colleagues evaluated high-dose cyclophosphamide and cisplatin and radiotherapy before radiation in 32 pediatric patients (259). Of 32 patients, 3 had a partial response, 23 had stable disease, and 6 had progressive disease. Median survival was 9 months.

Neither brachytherapy, the implant of ^{125}I into the tumor, or immunotherapy, in the form of intraventricular interleukin-2 or interferon-β, have improved survival significantly (259a). The direct transfer by means of a retroviral vector of specific tumor-suppressor genes, of genes that encode a product toxic to tumors, or of genes whose products induce apoptosis in tumors, are new therapeutic approaches that are still experimental (259b,259c). It is clear that new treatment strategies are required to reduce the high mortality of diffuse brainstem gliomas.

Midline Tumors

A number of pathologically diverse tumors arising from the midline of the supratentorial region are grouped together because their initial clinical pictures share several features. These include the insidious development of increased intracranial pressure often caused by hydrocephalus, as well as by the bulk of the tumor, visual impairment, abnormalities of endocrine or metabolic function, and alterations of consciousness or personality.

Most common of these midline tumors are the craniopharyngioma (55% of midline lesions, and 5% to 6% of all pediatric intracranial tumors) and the glioma of the optic nerve (19% of midline lesions) (260). Other tumors, such as pinealomas, and various intraventricular neoplasms, such as colloid cysts of the third ventricle, papillomas of the choroid plexus, and ependymomas of the lateral or third ventricle, are much rarer (Table 10.16).

Craniopharyngioma

Pathology

The craniopharyngioma is located in the suprasellar region in 43% of patients, and in

TABLE 10.16. *Frequencies of common pediatric brain tumors in the suptratentorial compartment*

Tumor	Percent
Craniopharyngioma	14.9
Anaplastic astrocytoma	12.5
Pilocytic astrocytoma	12.2
Fibrillary astrocytoma	8.9
Unclassifiable or unknown	8.5
Germ cell tumors (including teratomas)	5.3
Ependymoma	5.0
Choroid plexus papilloma (including anaplastic varieties)	4.4

Adapted from Gilles FH. Pediatric brain tumors: classification. In: Morantz RA, Walsh JW, eds. *Brain tumors. A comprehensive text.* New York: Marcel Dekker;1994:109.

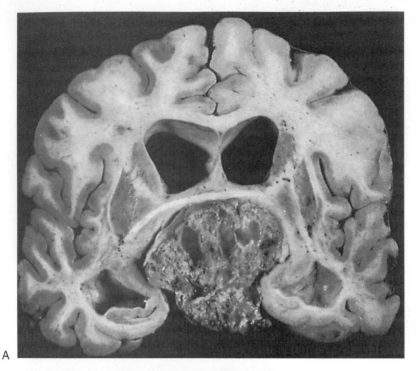

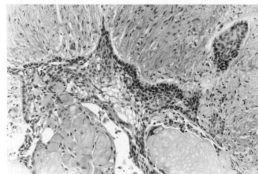

FIG. 10.19. A: Craniopharyngioma. Large tumor obstructing the third ventricle and causing hydrocephalus. (From Merritt HH. *A textbook of neurology*, 7th ed. Philadelphia: Lea & Febiger, 1984. With permission.) **B:** Note intraepithelial vacuolated areas (*stellate reticulum*) and islands of *wet* keratin (hematoxylin and eosin, original magnification ×500).

both intrasellar and suprasellar regions in 53%. Purely intrasellar craniopharyngiomas are rare in childhood. The tumor is believed to arise from small rests of squamous cells, normally encountered where the stalk joins with the pars distalis of the pituitary gland and is considered to represent remnants of the embryonal Rathke's pouch. If so, the tumor would be present at birth, but because of its slow growth, symptoms can be delayed for years to several decades. An adamantinomatous type usually is seen in children. Grossly, this neoplasm is char-

acterized by the presence of cysts containing viscous material, and calcifications. A *papillary* variant, lacking calcifications, occurs almost exclusively in adults (260a).

As the craniopharyngioma expands forward it begins to compress the optic chiasm. With downward expansion, the pituitary gland is compressed; with upward expansion, the third ventricle becomes distorted (Fig. 10.19A). Posterior expansion occurs into the posterior fossa, but rarely causes posterior fossa signs. Large tumors are partly or completely cystic and contain a cloudy brown fluid with a high concentration of cholesterol often seen as floating crystals.

Microscopically, the tumor's appearance can vary greatly. In some areas, the cysts are lined with stratified squamous epithelium with peripheral accumulation of tumor cells and more internally situated loose, degenerative-appearing epithelium called *stellate reticulum*. Plump deposits of so-called wet keratin that may undergo dystrophic calcification are typical (Fig. 10.19B). Deposition of lamellar bone also can occur. In other areas, the tumor consists of epithelial masses with poorly cellular connective tissue, resembling the enamel pulp of developing teeth, and termed *adamantinoma* because of its resemblance to a similar tumor arising from the jaw. Craniopharyngiomas are locally invasive and the adjacent brain tissue usually shows an exuberant reactive gliosis. The latter may contain large numbers of Rosenthal fibers that also can be seen in juvenile pilocytic astrocytomas (138).

On the basis of morphologic appearance and growth characteristics in tissue culture, Liszczak and colleagues distinguished two tumor types (261). In the majority of specimens, cells have the typical appearance and growth characteristics of epithelioid cells, with a smooth cell surface demonstrable by electron microscopy. Cells from atypical tumors contain cholesterol crystals and demonstrate some features characteristic of neoplastic transformation, with surface microvilli being evident on electron microscopy. Clinically, patients with atypical tumors tend to be younger and are more likely to experience early tumor recurrence.

Clinical Manifestations

In craniopharyngioma, as in many other midline neoplasms, the availability of imaging studies has facilitated diagnosis and, hence, significantly reduced the duration of symptoms before diagnosis. Whereas Northfield, compiling a series of patients in 1957 (262), recorded an interval of between 2 and 5 years between onset of symptoms and diagnosis, time before diagnosis is now shorter. As a consequence, treatment occurs sooner and increased intracranial pres-

TABLE 10.17. *Presenting signs and symptoms in children with craniopharyngiomas*

Sign/symptom	Percent of children	
	1968	1980
Increased intracranial pressure	65	24
Impaired vision or field defects	62	57
Endocrine abnormalities	41	53
Papilledema	41	9
Ataxia	9	0
Intracranial calcification	79	86
Erosion of sella	50	Large majority
Psychological symptoms	24	—

Adapted from Richmond IL, Wilson CB. Parasellar tumors in children. I. Clinical presentation, preoperative assessment, and differential diagnosis. *Childs Brain* 1980;7:73; and Bingas B, Wolter M. Das Kraniopharyngiom. *Fortschr Neurol Psychiatr* 1968;36:117.

sure is seen less frequently, and when present, it is less marked.

In approximately one-half of the younger patients, presenting symptoms are those of increased intracranial pressure, whereas in older children, visual complaints and endocrine abnormalities are common (Table 10.17) (263,264).

A variety of visual disturbances can be encountered, depending on the location of the tumor and the direction of its expansion. They include unilateral and bilateral optic atrophy and various field deficits. Unilateral or bilateral temporal field cuts are the most common disturbance, often commencing as field cuts in both upper bitemporal quadrants. Homonymous hemianopia (Fig. 10.20) and unilateral blindness are noted also (263). The hemianopia is the result of direct encroachment of the tumor on the optic chiasm or optic tracts. It should be noted that the craniopharyngioma is the intracranial tumor that causes the greatest loss of vision and the most extensive field cut even though the optic disks remain normal for a long time.

Disturbances in endocrine function result from either compression of the pituitary itself by a tumor both above and within the sella or hypothalamic involvement by a suprasellar tumor.

In the experience of Imura and coworkers, hypopituitarism was seen in 91% of patients with craniopharyngioma (265). Most had multiple hormone deficiencies. Delayed growth is the

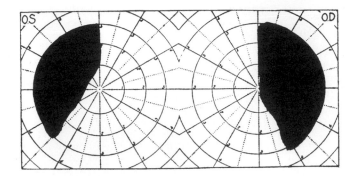

FIG. 10.20. Craniopharyngioma. Bitemporal hemianopia is almost complete. (OS, left eye; OD, right eye.) (Courtesy of Dr. Robert Hepler, Department of Ophthalmology, UCLA Center for the Health Sciences, Los Angeles.)

most common result of the endocrine disturbance, and growth hormone deficiency can be documented in more than one-half of affected children (263,266). A low gonadotropin level is found in approximately one-half of the pubertal patients. The failure of gonadotropic activity results in a reduced output of 17-ketosteroids and delayed or absent secondary sexual development. Abnormalities in follicle-stimulating hormone and luteinizing hormone output are seen in approximately one-third of patients, as are an elevation of prolactin and a reduction in thyroid-stimulating hormone (263,265).

Diabetes insipidus is a less common preoperative finding and is seen in 10% to 20% of children. Hypotension is seen occasionally and is sometimes related to hyponatremia owing to chronic adrenal insufficiency. A rare patient has oliguria with an inappropriate output of antidiuretic hormone. Precocious puberty was not seen in the series of Imura and coworkers. Nevertheless, the question of CNS lesions is frequently raised in patients with true precocious puberty. In boys, congenital or acquired disorders of the CNS can be implicated in 80% to 90% of these cases, whereas in girls, CNS lesions, most frequently a hypothalamic hamartoma, are responsible for 20% to 30% (267).

Disturbances of personality or dementia are not unusual and include periods of visual and olfactory hallucinations, abnormalities of sleep cycle, and dementia. These symptoms are believed to arise from hypothalamic involvement, although in some instances they can reflect a chronic increase of intracranial pressure. Seizures caused by impingement of the tumor on the medial aspect of the temporal lobe

are seen on occasion. Attacks of shivering or of falling without apparent loss of consciousness are somewhat rarer, but still characteristic.

A confusing finding is the occasional presence of cerebellar signs resulting from involvement of the red nucleus and its connections (268). Should cerebellar signs be accompanied by increased intracranial pressure, the erroneous clinical diagnosis of a posterior fossa tumor is almost inevitable, unless one keeps in mind that cerebellar signs occur late in the clinical course of a craniopharyngioma, but relatively early in posterior fossa tumors.

Diagnosis

The craniopharyngioma is characterized by a gradual development of increased intracranial pressure, visual disturbances, and endocrine dysfunction. Plain radiographs of the skull, at one time used as the initial diagnostic procedure, usually revealed eroded clinoid processes. Approximately 80% of children had curvilinear areas of suprasellar calcification. The tumor is readily demonstrable by imaging studies. CT scan reveals the cyst, with the increased density of its capsule, accompanied by calcifications (Fig. 10.21). Even though MRI does not reveal calcifications, sagittal views provide better information about the location, extent, and vascular relationships of the tumor. The size of the cyst and its proportions of keratin and cholesterol also can be determined. Cysts of Rathke's pouch are more likely to be hyperintense on T1-weighted images owing to the high cholesterol content of the cyst and the presence of methemoglobin (269). The signal on T2-weighted

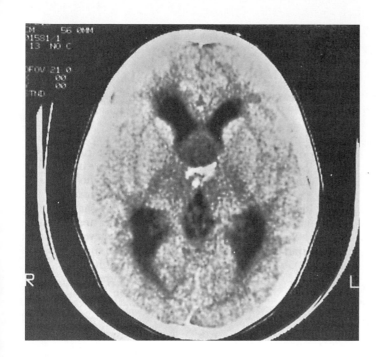

FIG. 10.21. Craniopharyngioma. Computed tomographic scan without contrast. The tumor consists of a cyst anteriorly and a calcified area posteriorly. The ventricular system, in particular the third ventricle, is somewhat enlarged. This 10-year-old boy had a 1-year history of growth failure and several months of intermittent headaches and vomiting. Papilledema and a field cut were seen on initial examination. The tumor could be only partially resected.

images is variable. When the optic tracts show increased signal on T2-weighted images, as is occasionally the case, and astrocytic gliosis is adjacent to the tumor as a result of an inflammatory response to the leaking contents of the cyst, the neoplasm can be misinterpreted as a glioma (270).

Other diagnostic studies are not helpful. The EEG either is normal or shows diffuse slowing. Of Russell and Pennybacker's patients, 75% had elevated spinal or ventricular fluid protein content (271).

Differential Diagnosis

Imaging studies readily differentiate between a craniopharyngioma and the various other commonly encountered space-occupying lesions in the sellar and suprasellar areas, notably optic glioma, chordoma, suprasellar arachnoid cyst, and the rare suprasellar meningioma. Even without their assistance, the clinical picture can provide important clues about the nature of the underlying neoplasm.

In an optic glioma, vision is lost early, and there is a high incidence of neurofibromatosis 1 (von Recklinghausen disease).

Chordomas are rare tumors in this region. They are believed to arise from notochord rest cells and in the majority of cases are located along the clivus (272). Those arising from the superior portion of the clivus can involve the chiasm and thus their clinical picture can mimic a craniopharyngioma. Chordomas that arise from the inferior portion of the clivus have a clinical picture suggesting a brainstem glioma with cranial nerve involvement and cerebellar deficits. In childhood, the course of these tumors is usually acute, and they tend to metastasize to the lungs (273,274).

Pinealomas, particularly those with extensions or implantations into the anterior portion of the third ventricle, can be mistaken clinically for suprasellar cysts. These tumors tend to compress the upper part of the mesencephalon and produce paralysis of upward gaze, impaired pupillary light reaction, and precocious puberty. At other times, the presenting symptom is increased intracranial pressure owing to meningeal invasion.

The most common presenting symptoms of chromophobe and eosinophilic adenomas include pituitary hypersecretion and failure of sexual maturation.

Suprasellar arachnoid cysts also present with midline tumor symptoms (275). In order of frequency, symptoms of these cysts include hydro-cephalus (87% of affected children), increased head size (57%), vision loss (30%), and ataxia (28%). Additionally, some children with this con-dition develop the *bobble-head* syndrome (276).

When tumors of the anterior third ventricle become symptomatic in infancy, they produce the diencephalic syndrome. The outstanding features of this condition, as first described by Russell (277), are emaciation in spite of normal food intake, hypoglycemia, hyperkinetic behav-ior, vomiting, a characteristic pale, elf-like facies, and exceptional alertness or euphoria. Visual impairment becomes evident during the later months of the illness. Imaging studies are diagnostic and reveal the tumor encroaching into the third ventricle. Tumors producing this syndrome are usually astrocytomas of the third ventricle or optic gliomas.

Treatment and Prognosis

With earlier diagnosis now possible, with a bet-ter understanding of preoperative, intraopera-tive, and postoperative hormonal and fluid requirements, and with the availability of micro-surgical techniques, total resection of the tumor as verified by postoperative neuroimaging can be achieved with minimal neurologic and endocrine damage in 70% to 90% of patients (278,279). Nevertheless, the respective roles of radical surgery and limited surgery with radio-therapy continue to be debated. In some series, the results of the two approaches are equivalent, or show long-term results of combined surgery and radiation to be better than results with total resection alone (280–282). At the UCLA Center for Health Sciences and at the University of Florida College of Medicine we favor radical surgery. As a rule, total removal is easier in chil-dren than in adults, because in adults chronic leakage of cyst fluid often results in the forma-tion of dense adhesions (278,283).

The neurosurgical approach differs for each case and depends on the location of the tumor. If total removal is impossible, as is the case when the tumor is large or when neighboring brain is invaded, surgery is limited to partial removal to avoid high morbidity and mortality. Under these circumstances tumor recurrence is likely. As a rule, complete tumor removal also is less likely the more marked the ventricular dilatation at the time of surgery (284). Because regrowth of the tumor is often delayed for many years, and because of the deleterious effects of radiotherapy on the developing brain, we believe that the sta-tus of the tumor should be followed with imaging studies, and that radiotherapy be delayed until necessary, even when tumor removal has been shown to be subtotal (285,286). Recurrences can be treated by another attempt at surgery or a com-bination of radiotherapy and surgery. In the expe-rience of Jose and coworkers, 72% of patients with recurrent tumor treated with combined radiotherapy and surgery experienced a 10-year progression-free survival (280). Brachytherapy with stereotactic installation of ^{32}P or yttrium 90 colloid into the cyst also has been advocated (287,288). It appears to be effective when more than 50% of the tumor bulk is cystic (289).

Vision does not improve, and endocrine dis-turbances are generally exacerbated after surgi-cal treatment (284). All children in the series of Lyen and Grant had hormonal deficiencies, most commonly (100% in Lyen and Grant's series) impaired growth hormone secretion (290). A defect in the output of gonadotropins is seen in 93%, and reduced adrenocorticotropic hormone (ACTH) and thyroid-stimulating hormone out-put also is observed in most affected children. Up to three-fourths of the children develop dia-betes insipidus, which is usually permanent and can be accompanied by an absent or impaired sense of thirst (284,291). Poor postoperative control of this condition can lead to cerebral vein thrombosis. Morbid postoperative obesity is common and interferes with social adaptation (292). In obese patients, there is MRI evidence of preoperative hypothalamic damage (292). As a rule, absence of calcification on neuroimaging is associated with a significantly better progres-sion-free survival (285). Postoperative endocrine therapy and its results are reviewed by Lyen and Grant (290) and de Vile and associates (284). It is of note that no significant difference in mor-bidity was seen after complete tumor excision without radiotherapy or subtotal excision with adjuvant irradiation (284). In the series of

Fahlbusch and colleagues, which comprised both children and adults, the 10-year recurrence-free survival rate was 83% after what was deemed total removal, and 50.5% after subtotal removal. Tumor recurrences occurred mostly within the first 5 years after surgery (292a). Without adequate hormone replacement, minor infections can lead to rapid deterioration or sudden death.

A variety of psychological deficits can be seen in subjects who have undergone surgical treatment of craniopharyngioma. These include visual perceptual dysfunction and frontal lobe deficits, notably a lack of inhibitory control and perseveration. The frontal lobe deficits can be caused by hypothalamic injury rather than direct trauma to the frontal lobes by surgery (293).

TUMORS OF THE OPTIC PATHWAY

Pathology

This heterogenous group of tumors represent 3% to 6% of pediatric brain tumors. Approximately one-third affect the optic nerve and the remainder involve the optic chiasm, hypothalamus, third ventricle, and optic tracts, singly or in combination. Tumors that arise from the optic nerve are histologically similar to the cerebellar pilocytic astrocytoma. They occur within or outside the orbit as a fusiform dilatation of the nerve. Neoplasms arising within the orbit tend to spread through the optic foramina and expand into the cranium in a dumbbell fashion. Tumors arising from the optic chiasm or hypothalamus can invade the third ventricle or grow inferiorly to compress the pituitary gland (294). On histologic examination, the neoplasm consists of oligodendroglia or astrocytes similar to the glial tumors arising from the cerebral hemispheres. Many optic nerve tumors are associated with neurofibromatosis. In this condition, the neoplasm is usually a glioma, less often a meningioma of the optic sheath (5).

Clinical Manifestations

A strong association exists between gliomas of the optic nerve and neurofibromatosis type 1; between 33% and 70% of patients with chias-

TABLE 10.18. *Symptoms and signs in 56 children with optic glioma*

Symptom/sign	Determined by patient history	Determined by physical examination
Diminished visual acuity	28	53
Exophthalmos	25	29
Nystagmus	8	14
Strabismus	6	17
Field cut	1	12
Disc change		
Pallor		36
Pallor and blurring		11
Blurring		8
Increased intracranial pressure	3	15
Enlarged head	1	4
Multiple café au lait spots		12
Hemiparesis		4

From Chutorian AM, et al. Optic gliomas in children. *Neurology* 1964;14:83. With permission.

mal gliomas have the clinical features of neurofibromatosis type 1 (295,296). Conversely, optic gliomas are the most common intracranial tumors in neurofibromatosis type 1.

The various signs and symptoms seen in patients with gliomas of the optic nerve are depicted in Table 10.18 (297). A more recent clinical series compiled in 1981 by Iraci and coworkers (298), indicates little difference in the initial clinical presentation as a consequence to the ready availability of the newer imaging techniques. In approximately one-half of patients, poor vision is the presenting symptom. In infancy, it can become evident as searching nystagmus or failure to fix on and follow objects. Deterioration of eyesight can progress so insidiously that children can have an apparent sudden loss of vision. Exophthalmos develops when the tumor grows anteriorly. Because exophthalmos is easily recognized, affected patients have a relatively shorter illness before hospitalization than those whose tumor expands posteriorly into the third ventricle.

Other ocular symptoms, such as strabismus, are less frequent presenting symptoms and are usually secondary to impaired vision. Increased intracranial pressure and endocrine abnormalities such as precocious puberty, diabetes insipidus, and growth retardation are uncommon early symptoms of

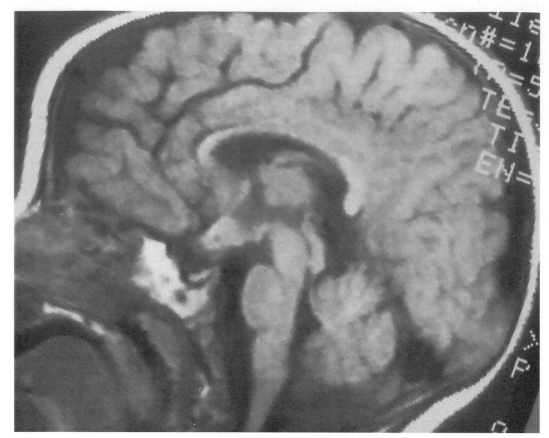

FIG. 10.22. Glioma of optic nerve and chiasm. Sagittal view on a T1-weighted magnetic resonance scan in a 6-month-old boy. A mass compresses and obliterates the optic and infundibular recesses of the anterior portion of the third ventricle. From there, the tumor extends anteroinferiorly. (Courtesy of Drs. Hervey D. Segall, William Kneeland, and William Bank, Children's Hospital, Los Angeles.)

optic gliomas. They indicate that the tumor has extended into the area surrounding the third ventricle and, therefore, are associated with a poor prognosis.

Almost all children with gliomas have abnormalities of the optic disks. These consist of primary optic atrophy, papilledema, or a mixture of the two abnormalities. These findings accompany a variety of visual field defects.

Diagnosis

Neuroimaging imaging studies readily detect gliomas of the optic nerve and delineate their extent (Fig. 10.22). An optic nerve sheath meningioma is distinguished by an increased signal on T1-weighted, gadolinium-enhanced images, with the hyperintensity sharply delineated from the optic nerve, which does not appear enlarged (299).

Treatment and Prognosis

Because the natural progression of this tumor is so variable, there is considerable controversy as to its best management (300). Some tumors remain static for years, and others progress rapidly. Consequently, no uniform management exists, and observation, chemotherapy, radiotherapy, and surgeries have been suggested by various authorities (301). We believe that the unilateral tumor confined to the optic nerve and producing a severely proptotic blind eye should be removed with the globe left in place. This allows the physician to monitor for tumor growth by either funduscopy or neuroimaging. The prognosis for patients with this type of tumor presentation is excellent, and the likelihood of posterior extension was only 5% in the series of Alvord and Lofton (302).

Treatment of bilateral tumor or a tumor that involves the optic chiasm and structures posterior to the chiasm is more uncertain (295). Tao and coworkers have demonstrated that radiotherapy can shrink the tumor and stabilize vision in 88% of patients, and provide a 10-year freedom from disease progression in 100% of 29 children (303). Even so, many clinicians, including ourselves, believe that the benefits of radiotherapy are difficult to prove (303). Using a regimen of 5,000 to 5,500 cGy given over the course of 6 to 8 weeks, Tenny and associates recorded a 50% survival over a mean follow-up period of 13 years (304). This figure, however, should be compared with a 64% survival of untreated patients with chiasmal gliomas followed by Imes and Hoyt for a median of 20 years (295), and a 10-year survival rate of 83% in untreated patients reported by Jenkin and colleagues (305). If treatment is decided on, children younger than age 5 years should receive chemotherapy in preference to radiotherapy (304).

The benefits of chemotherapy, however, are equally uncertain. Packer and coworkers using a combination of actinomycin-D and vincristine for patients with chiasmatic pilocytic astrocytomas induced significant tumor shrinkage (306). Petronio and colleagues used a five-drug regimen that included 6-thioguanine, procarbazine, dibromodulcitol, BCNU, and vincristine (307). Ten of 19 patients had a partial response and five had disease stabilization. Packer and colleagues treated 23 children with recurrent and 37 with newly diagnosed low-grade glioma using a 10-week induction cycle of carboplatin and vincristine, followed by maintenance treatment with the same drugs (308). Of newly diagnosed patients 62% had an objective response, and of children with recurrent disease, 52% of had an objective response. A similar partial response was seen by Chamberlain and colleagues who treated recurrent chiasmatic-hypo-

thalamic gliomas with 21-day courses of oral etoposide (309).

From these data we can conclude that chemotherapy can result in low-grade glioma shrinkage in more than one-half of patients treated (308) and should be used for tumors that are not surgically resectable and in young children (younger than age 3 years) for whom radiotherapy is contraindicated. In all cases, glioma of the optic chiasm or posterior structures should be treated only when its growth has been documented by neuroimaging studies or by progression of clinical symptoms, particularly deterioration of vision.

Optic gliomas associated with neurofibromatosis type 1 are no more aggressive than those unaccompanied by neurofibromatosis type 1, and from the wealth of conflicting follow-up studies, one gathers that the outlook for patients with optic gliomas and neurofibromatosis type 1 is no worse than for those without neurofibromatosis type 1 with respect to morbidity or mortality from the optic glioma. Patients with neurofibromatosis type 1, however, have an increased likelihood of succumbing to tumors arising from other sites in the body.

PINEAL TUMORS

Tumors of the pineal region account for 3% to 10% of all pediatric intracranial tumors (310,311). On histologic examination, at least four types of pineal tumors can be distinguished: (a) germ cell tumors, including germinomas, benign and malignant teratomas, and choriocarcinomas, which arise from the pineal body or structures immediately surrounding it; (b) pinealomas, which arise from the pineal parenchyma cells; (c) epidermoid cysts; and (d) gliomas. Russell and Sachs, Jooma and Kendall, and the Toronto Neurosurgical Group have observed the germinoma to be the most common, accounting for approximately one-half of pineal neoplasms (312–314). Germinomas are biphasic tumors consisting of a neoplastic component of large, glycogen-rich, germ cells with large nuclei and prominent nucleoli, and a nonneoplastic component of small mature lymphocytes. The germ cell component is immunoreactive for placental alkaline phophatase. Approximately 5% to 50% of germinomas con-

TABLE 10.19. *Eye signs in pineal tumors*

Sign	Percent
Dilated pupils	31
Impaired light reaction	50
Diplopia	25
Nystagmus	38
Limitation of upward gaze	31
Papilledema	56
Abducens palsy	25

From Posner M, Horrax G. Eye signs in pineal tumors. *J Neurosurg* 1946;3:15. With permission.

tain syncytiotrophoblastic tumor giant cells that elaborate β-human choriogonadotropic hormone. The presence of such cells in an otherwise typical germinoma does not indicate the presence of a choriocarcinoma element.

Other germ cell tumors, including the embryonal carcinoma, endodermal sinus tumor (yolk sac tumor), choriocarcinoma, and teratoma (mature and immature), are much less common than germinomas and tend to occur as mixed tumors rather than one particular type.

Primary tumors of the pineal parenchyma are rare and include the pineocytoma, pineoblastoma (PNET), intermediate, and mixed types. Details of the pathology and patient outcomes have been reported recently by Schild and colleagues (315). Pineal tumors should be distinguished from a benign pineal cyst. This lesion shows a rim of calcification and enhances with contrast. It is a relatively common, nonneoplastic entity that is usually asymptomatic and is often discovered serendipitously on MRI (316,317).

Clinical Manifestations

Germ cell tumors occur predominantly in male subjects. In the series of Hiraga and colleagues, 74% of patients presenting before 15 years of age were male; when presentation was after 15 years of age, 92% were male (318). Initial symptoms depend to some extent on the nature of the tumor. In the series of Kageyama and coworkers, the predominant symptoms of patients with a pineal germinoma include Parinaud's sign (paralysis of conjugate upward gaze) (76%), increased intracranial pressure (67%), Argyll Robertson pupil (46%), diplopia (32%),

diabetes insipidus (32%), and hypopituitarism (24%) (319). Increased intracranial pressure often arises acutely as a result of aqueductal obstruction or meningeal infiltration. The other neurologic signs, notably the limitation of conjugate upward gaze, impaired pupillary light reaction in the presence of an intact accommodative response (Argyll Robertson pupil), and central deafness, are caused by pressure on the corpora quadrigemina (Table 10.19) (320).

Cerebellar signs, resulting from transmitted pressure, were seen in 14% of the Japanese series of Kageyama (319). An abnormally calcified pineal body is seen in approximately 20% of patients with pinealoma, but precocious puberty is relatively uncommon; it was seen in only 3% and 14%, respectively, of the two Japanese series of Kageyama and colleagues and Hiraga and colleagues. It is far more common in boys harboring a malignant teratoma or in choriocarcinoma (313,318). Calcifications are common in more malignant tumors. Some 70% of patients with malignant teratomas have other signs of hypothalamic disturbance, including obesity, somnolence, polyphagia, and diabetes insipidus. The mechanism whereby pineal tumors produce precocious puberty is still unclear, and probably is not uniform.

A greater than chance association between bilateral retinoblastoma and a midline intracranial malignancy, most commonly a malignant pinealoma, has been reported (trilateral syndrome). In the series of Pesin and Shields, the retinoblastoma was diagnosed between 4 years before and 5 months after the diagnosis of the intracranial tumor (321).

Diagnosis

Increased intracranial pressure in the presence of pupillary abnormalities and impaired upward gaze in a male subject should always suggest a pineal tumor. Imaging studies are highly accurate in detecting and characterizing these tumors (322). The sagittal cut on MRI is optimal for visualizing the extent of the tumor, whereas CT scanning is generally superior to MRI for characterizing its histology, in that CT scanning is able to demonstrate the presence of calcifications, an indication of a benign or malignant teratoma (323). Normally, a calcified pineal body is rarely seen in a child younger than age 10 years. In the experience of Zimmerman, the youngest normal child with a calcified pineal body was 6 years old (322).

Increased secretion of β-human chorionic gonadotropins and α-fetoprotein has been noted in patients with pinealoma. Generally, their presence indicates a malignant teratoma rather than a germinoma (324).

Treatment and Prognosis

Despite the availability of human choriogonadotropic and α-fetoprotein markers and imaging studies, it is not always possible to differentiate preoperatively between germinomas, which are not amenable to total excision, and teratomas, which are amenable if benign (324). Tissue diagnosis, therefore, is important and the preferred treatment is definitive surgery for benign tumors (325).

No consensus exists on optimal therapy for germinomas (325). It is appropriate to offer a CT-guided biopsy and ventricular-peritoneal shunt followed by radiotherapy (low-dose craniospinal radiotherapy followed by conformal or stereotactic radiotherapy). The recommended approach has a low operative risk and a high cure rate. The alternative surgical approach is to perform a craniotomy and resect the tumor, but unlike PNET/MBs, there is no evidence that gross tumor resection produces a more favorable outcome in germinomas. The outcome is relatively good for germinomas, and 70% to 100% 5-year survival rates are commonly reported for localized tumors (317,325,326).

Other tumors, particularly the nongerminomatous germ cell tumors in the pineal region in which α-fetoprotein or human choriogonadotropic can be detected in serum or CSF, have a much lower 5-year survival rate than germinomas. Treatment for the more malignant germ cell tumors consists of debulking, followed by induction, multidrug chemotherapy, and focal radiotherapy using a protocol analogous to that used for PNET/MBs (325,327). Most patients harboring a pineal tumor do not

require ventricular-peritoneal shunting after CT biopsy and craniospinal radiotherapy. Edwards and associates, however, have suggested prophylactic spinal irradiation (325). Risk of systemic dissemination of tumor is small.

TUMORS OF LATERAL AND THIRD VENTRICLES

Intraventricular tumors are rare in children. The most common histologic types encountered are papillomas of the choroid plexus of the lateral ventricles, colloid cysts arising from the third ventricle, and ependymomas.

Choroid Plexus Papillomas

Choroid plexus papillomas are intraventricular tumors that arise as cauliflowerlike masses that histologically can resemble normal choroid plexus. These papillary neoplasms show increased cell density and low mitotic activity. Increased mitotic activity, lack of the papillary architecture, and evidence of invasion suggest a potential for local recurrence and aggressive behavior. Like ependymomas, choroid plexus carcinomas are most common in young children, usually the age of 3 years (328,329). The clinical picture is generally a progressive increase in intracranial pressure and hydrocephalus caused by increased CSF production and blockage of CSF flow. This is accompanied by ataxia and an organic mental syndrome.

Choroid plexus tumors can occur in various familial syndromes, including von Hippel–Lindau, Li-Fraumeni, and Aicardi's syndromes, but consistent abnormal genetic loci have not yet been identified (330,331). Although abnormal polyoma virus sequences have been associated with these tumors, a definitive role in pathogenesis remains uncertain.

Choroid plexus papillomas that are surgically resected may not require further therapy. The most common surgical approach is to first interrupt the vascular supply and then remove the tumor by a transventricular approach. Recurrent papillomas or more malignant carcinomas should be treated with chemotherapy followed by reoperation and limited-field radiotherapy (332). The most effective chemotherapy seems to be plat-inum-based regimens (e.g., cisplatin, bleomycin, vinblastine), as first suggested by Maria and colleagues (333).

Colloid Cysts of the Third Ventricle

Colloid cysts of the third ventricle constitute between 0.5% to 1.0% of brain tumors (334). Unlike choroid plexus papillomas, they do not show any predilection for early childhood; in the series of Mathiesen and coworkers only 8% of patients were younger than 15 years (334). On microscopic examination, the cyst is lined by cuboidal, pseudostratified, or columnar ciliated and mucous-secreting epithelial cells (335). Headache was the principal symptom in all children. In some instances, particularly when the cyst is located in the vicinity of the foramen of Monro, symptoms appear acutely or intermittently with paroxysmal attacks of headache and vomiting, terminated by a brief period of unconsciousness, with complete but transient recovery (336,337).

The diagnosis is readily made by imaging studies. Microsurgical removal of these tumors is currently preferred. Damage to the left fornix in the course of surgery can impair verbal memory, whereas bilateral fornix damage can induce amnesia (338).

Tumors of the Pituitary

Pituitary adenomas are uncommon in children; in the large pediatric series of Rorke and colleagues, they accounted for only 1.1% of all intracranial tumors with the majority occurring around or after puberty (44). They arise from the adenohypophysis and are histologically monomorphous and benign appearing. The most frequently encountered neoplasm is a prolactin-secreting adenoma (339). This tumor is more common in girls and manifests by amenorrhea, usually accompanied by galactorrhea. Headaches and visual disturbances are occasionally present. Some of the prolactin-secreting adenomas are invasive and extend into the suprasellar cisterns. ACTH-secreting tumors are next most common, producing the clinical picture of Cushing disease

(339). ACTH-secreting microadenomas might not be detected by imaging studies, even if MRI with gadolinium enhancement is used.

Microadenomas can be removed by transsphenoidal microsurgery. The procedure is preferable to irradiation, which induces pituitary-hypothalamic dysfunction. Macroadenomas cannot be cured surgically (340). Endocrinologic follow-up is critical to successful management of such patients.

TUMORS OF THE CEREBRAL HEMISPHERES

Tumors of the cerebral hemispheres are less frequent in children than in adults and account for approximately 40% of brain tumors (341). In children, it is often difficult to arrive at an early diagnosis, because increased intracranial pressure appears late, focal signs are difficult to elicit, and the relatively high incidence of idiopathic epilepsy in childhood makes the appearance of seizures less alarming than when their onset is at a later age. Before the advent of imaging studies, tumors of the cerebral hemispheres commonly grew to enormous sizes before diagnoses were made, and, not surprisingly, surgical therapy was often unsuccessful.

Pathology

Histologically, the most common types of tumors, accounting for 30% of neoplasms in the series of Gjerris (341), are the astrocytomas, in pure form or in conjunction with other cell types, such as oligodendrogliomas, and the malignant glioblastomas. The microscopic classification of childhood astrocytomas, used at University of California, Los Angeles, takes into account the cellularity of the neoplasm, its vascularity, nuclear detail, and the presence and amount of necrosis.

Four grades of *astrocytomas* are distinguished: Grade I, the most benign, has hypercellularity as its major feature. Grade I astrocytomas must be differentiated from astrocytosis. Grade II is marked by the presence of vascular proliferation and pleomorphism. Grade III demonstrates hyperchromatic nuclei and malignant cytologic features such as mitosis. As in adults, the histologically malignant astrocytomas (anaplastic astrocytoma and glioblastoma multiforme, grade IV gliomas) of childhood are infiltrative, biologically aggressive neoplasms characterized by a marked variation in cell size and areas of necrosis (see Figs. 10.10 and 10.11). Cytogenetic characteristics of pediatric malignant astrocytomas differ from those most commonly encountered in adults. Structural abnormalities in chromosomes 9, 13, 17, and double minutes were observed in malignant astrocytomas (anaplastic astrocytoma and glioblastoma) of childhood, whereas the most common chromosomal abnormalities in adult glioblastomas are losses of chromosomes 10 and 19q or gains in chromosome 7 (135). Furthermore, to date, the chromosomal abnormalities found in malignant astrocytomas of childhood are similar to those reported in a genetically distinct subset of glioblastomas that was found to arise in young adults (141).

Oligodendrogliomas are infiltrative glial neoplasms composed primarily of oligodendrocytes. They account for only approximately 2% of pediatric intracranial tumors (44). They arise most commonly in the frontal lobe, but may occur anywhere in the neuroaxis. These frequently calcified tumors are composed of a uniform population of round cells with clear perinuclear cytoplasm. Tumors are usually permeated by a delicate meshwork of angulated capillaries. Allelic deletions of chromosomes 1p and 19q appear to occur preferentially in oligodendrogliomas (342,343).

Less commonly encountered tumors of the cerebral hemispheres include epidermoid cysts, sarcomas, and ganglion cell tumors. The ganglion cell tumors include a spectrum of brain tumors that have in common a population of neoplastic or hamartomatous mature neurons, termed *ganglion cells*.

The *ganglioglioma* is the prototype of this group (344). Approximately 75% of gangliogliomas are in the temporal lobe. Less common locations include the brainstem, spinal cord, optic nerve and chiasm, pineal gland, and cerebellum. These slowly growing neoplasms are usually well circumscribed, often cystic, and

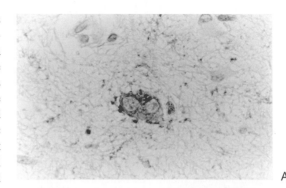

A

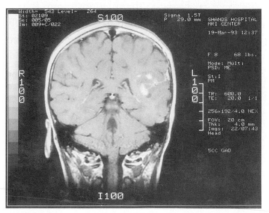

B

FIG. 10.23. **A:** Histology shows ganglioglioma with binucleate ganglion cells immunostained for synaptophysin. Unstained cells at upper right hand corner are of astrocytic lineage (original magnification ×1,200). **B:** Coronal magnetic resonance imaging with contrast shows ganglioglioma surrounding the left sylvian fissure.

may be associated with adjacent areas of cortical dysplasia (345,346). Gangliogliomas are composed of two histologic components: a neoplastic astroglial element that tends to be well differentiated (low grade) and a population of ganglion cells. The latter have features of mature neurons including large vesicular nuclei, prominent nucleoli, cytoplasmic Nissl substance, immunoreactivity for neuronal antigens such as neurofilament protein and synaptophysin, and little proliferative activity (345). Abnormal ganglion cells of a ganglioglioma tend to occur in clusters, have abnormally oriented cell processes, and may occasionally be binucleated (Fig. 10.23A) (347). Varying degrees of calcification, desmoplasia, lymphocytic infiltration, and pilocytic differentiation also may be observed. Although rare malignant degeneration has been described, surgical resection is the treatment of choice and is curative in many cases (347). No consistent genetic abnormalities have been reported.

In the temporal lobe, these tumors can be missed with CT scanning because they are often isodense with brain. MRI clearly shows gangliogliomas (Fig. 10.23B). In the brainstem, these tumors can be focal. In the area of the medulla, they can be found in the area postrema. Rarely, posterior fossa ganglioglioma can seed into the CSF and spread through the neuroaxis. Radiotherapy is often recommended postoperatively in posterior fossa gangliogliomas, although no clinical trials have been conducted.

Meningiomas are rare during childhood, and meningeal tumors are often highly malignant meningeal sarcomas (348,349). A number of children with a meningioma have clinical or pathologic evidence of neurofibromatosis or tuberous sclerosis. Metastatic tumors are rare in childhood. The only form that seeds into the CNS with any frequency is the neuroblastoma.

Clinical Manifestations

The clinical picture depends on the location of the tumor rather than on its histologic characteristics (40). Signs of increased intracranial pressure, headaches, and vomiting occur in approximately 50% of patients and are the initial complaints in approximately 25% of affected children. Seizures occur in approximately 50% of patients, most commonly in children with temporal lobe tumors. Many patients exhibit a combination of different seizure patterns; nearly 50% of seizure patients experience complex partial seizures, either alone or in combination with generalized seizures or have generalized seizures with a focal component. Absence attacks are rarely seen (Table 10.20).

Patients experiencing uncinate seizures (i.e., complex partial seizures with olfactory or gustatory hallucinations) are no more likely to harbor a temporal lobe glioma than those with other forms of complex partial epilepsy (350). A prolonged history of often intractable seizures can

TABLE 10.20. *Characteristics of seizures in 49 patients with tumors of the cerebral hemispheres*

	Percent
Seizure type	
Generalized	49
Generalized with focal components	25
Psychomotor	39
Focal	39
Petit mal	0
Other seizure forms	6
Duration of seizures before diagnosis of tumor	
<6 mo	39
6–12 mo	6
1–3 yr	18
3–5 yr	12
5–10 yr	20
>10 yr	2
Location of tumor producing seizures	
Temporal lobe	36
Frontal lobe	7
Parietal lobe	29
Other sites or diffuse	29

Adapted from Low NL, Correll JW, Hammill JF. Tumors of the cerebral hemispheres in children. *Arch Neurol* 1965;13:547.

precede demonstration of a tumor (see Chapter 13) (351,352). Children who experience seizures owing to an underlying tumor tend to be normal on neurologic examination and are of normal intelligence. Additionally, neurologic evaluation uncovers no other plausible cause for their seizures; however, the EEG demonstrates persistent focal slowing (352).

Other symptoms are related to the presence of hemiparesis. Hemisensory signs and aphasia are rare. Approximately 15% of patients show ataxia, usually as the outcome of involvement of the frontopontocerebellar pathways, but often clinically misinterpreted as being caused by a posterior fossa mass.

Supratentorial malignant tumors are relatively rare in early childhood; they occur predominantly in older children and adolescents. Most commonly, they represent a malignant degeneration of previously diagnosed low-grade astrocytomas appearing at the irradiated site, or occurring in patients who received prophylactic whole-brain radiation for acute lymphoblastic leukemia (99,103). Malignant gliomas are also more likely to develop in children with neurofibromatosis. Leptomeningeal spread is seen in approximately 30% of these tumors, usually in conjunction with tumor recurrence. An intratumoral hemorrhage occurred in 18% of children followed by Dropcho and coworkers at the Sloan-Kettering Cancer Center (353).

Diagnosis

Imaging studies, in particular MRI, confirm the clinical diagnosis of a cerebral hemisphere tumor. Calcifications within the tumor, which were found in 23% of children reported by Low and associates (40), are best demonstrated by CT scan. When CT scanning is performed with contrast material, it usually is definitive, although, on occasion, it fails to disclose a tumor that is subsequently discovered with MRI or on surgical resection of an epileptic focus. For this reason, MRI with gadolinium enhancement is the preferred study for youngsters with seizure disorders who are suspected as harboring a neoplasm.

For the initial diagnostic evaluation, EEG can help localize a structural lesion to some extent, particularly with tumors of the temporal lobe. The CSF can be under increased pressure with increased protein content.

Treatment and Prognosis

Low-grade gliomas have a relatively good prognosis, with 5-year survival ranging from 75% to 85% (354–356). Patients typically present with hemiparesis and seizures that can be managed with anticonvulsants after gross total resection. If seizures are a major component of the clinical course, then intraoperative corticography helps reduce the incidence of postoperative seizures (357). Intraoperative monitoring of evoked potentials is useful in reducing morbidity in these cortical and white matter resections. After a partial resection, limited-field radiotherapy is currently the standard of care. It is important that every effort be made to distinguish pilocytic astrocytoma from low-grade fibrillary astrocytoma, because pilocytic tumors are often curable by surgery alone.

Diffuse astrocytomas of the cerebral hemispheres, even when localized to the periphery of the cerebrum and appearing well circumscribed, infiltrate adjacent tissues so readily that complete surgical removal is often impossible. In the large series by Gjerris, collected in 1978 before MRI, 45% of tumors were believed to have been totally removed, yet less than one-half of these children were alive 15 years later (341). Frontal lobe tumors can be treated by lobectomy and, therefore, have a better prognosis. Intermediate- or high-grade astrocytic tumors are best treated with radical resection followed by limited-field radiotherapy and chemotherapy. Chemotherapy should be used first in children younger than 3 years of age so as to minimize the late effects of radiotherapy. Clinical trials show that radiotherapy can be averted altogether in some cases.

On the whole, chemotherapy has produced but modest improvement in survival of patients with anaplastic astrocytoma and has failed to make a significant difference in the outcome of children with glioblastoma multiforme. The best results are obtained when children are treated with a combination of radiotherapy followed by chemotherapy (358,359). In all series the most important prognostic factor for a given patient was the extent of tumor resection (360).

MRIs and neurologic examinations are required every 2 to 4 months in the first 2 years from diagnosis. More studies are needed before specific agents and doses can be routinely recommended for treatment of diffuse astrocytomas in children.

Low-grade oligodendrogliomas that have been totally resected may be followed conservatively without further therapy. If the resection is partial, then limited-field radiotherapy should be given. For anaplastic oligodendrogliomas, surgery should be followed by limited-field radiotherapy and chemotherapy. Because oligodendrogliomas are relatively rare in children, most of the information available on chemotherapy safety and efficacy comes from adult clinical trials. These have shown malignant oligodendrogliomas to be chemosensitive and responsive to nitrosourea-based therapy (361). MRIs and neurologic examinations are required every 2 to 4 months in the first 2 years from diagnosis. For patients who relapse, melphalan may be tried with strong consideration of consolidating responders with high-dose chemotherapy and stem cell rescue (361,362).

Brachytherapy is one of the newer therapeutic approaches designed to improve the poor prognosis of the more malignant hemisphere tumors. It involves the stereotactic implantation into the tumor of a source of high radioactivity, such as ^{125}I or yttrium 90 (259a,287,363). This therapeutic regimen can offer significantly prolonged survival times for children with highly anaplastic lesions, in particular those that have a significant cystic component. Stereotactic radiosurgery (gamma knife) is the precise delivery of a single fraction of radiation to an imaging-defined target. The technique has found little application for nonmetastatic malignant tumors, and lesions greater than 35 mm are poor candidates because with larger lesions there is an increase in radiation-related complications (364,364a). Clinical trials with cytokines and other angiogenesis inhibitors are in their preliminary stages (365). Most other new agents are disappointing, as is neutron therapy, and the disruption of the blood–tumor barrier by the administration of hyperosmolar mannitol. Locally directed immunotherapy, in the form of lymphokine-activated killer cells and interleukin-2 instilled into the glioma, results in cerebral edema and neurologic side effects (365).

BRAIN TUMORS IN CHILDREN YOUNGER THAN 3 YEARS OF AGE

The most common histologic types of tumors occurring in children younger than 3 years of age are ependymomas, PNET/MBs, choroid plexus papillocarcinomas, astrocytomas, and teratomas (366,367). Thus, most tumors are malignant and require multimodal therapy. The 5-year survival rate for young children with brain tumors is poor, and ranges from 20% to 40% (368,369). Late effects are common, with endocrinopathies in 70%, neurologic sequelae in 65%, and cognitive decline in 85% of infants (370). Radiotherapy has been implicated as a primary factor in the high incidence of mental retardation because of its effects on axonal growth, dendritic arborization, and synaptogenesis. Studies, therefore, have been initiated to determine the efficacy of postoperative chemotherapy in halting tumor progression in children younger than 3 years of age (371).

Clinical trials of postoperative chemotherapy in children younger than 3 years of age with malignant brain tumors at the MD Anderson Cancer Center, St. Jude Children's Hospital, and the Children's Hospital of Philadelphia provided preliminary data suggesting chemotherapy could effectively defer radiotherapy (372–374). Subsequent studies have confirmed that chemotherapy can be an effective substitute to radiotherapy in preventing progression of malignant brain tumors in a minority of children under age 3 years with malignant brain tumors. In the Children's Cancer Group "eight-drugs-in-1-day" treatment series, the 3-year progression-free survival was 22% for PNET/MBs, 0% for pineal PNETs, 55% for supratentorial nonpineal PNETs, and 26% for ependymomas (375).

These studies show that chemotherapy can be an effective substitute to radiotherapy in preventing progression of malignant brain tumors in the minority of children younger than 3 years of age with malignant brain tumors. More time, however, is needed to assess the late effects of such therapy in long-term survivors and to see whether radiotherapy is ultimately required to maintain tumor control. Because radiotherapy has such detrimental effects on cognition in young children, more effective treatment strategies are required that limit the use of radiotherapy.

High-Dose Chemotherapy

High-dose chemotherapy followed by reinfusion of autologous stem cells (harvested from the bone marrow or the peripheral blood) holds promise to further improve survival in children with malignant brain tumors and may produce sustained remissions in patients with selected tumor types who are at high risk for tumor progression (376,377). Effective use of autologous peripheral blood stem cells rather than bone marrow has enhanced hematologic recovery from high-dose therapy and has decreased the risk of life-threatening complications (378). Much more information about safety and efficacy is required, however, before high-dose chemotherapy can be routinely recommended in the treatment of malignant pediatric brain tumors.

SPINAL CORD TUMORS

In childhood, spinal cord neoplasms are less common than brain tumors. Although the exact prevalence of spinal tumors is uncertain owing to varying criteria used in published accounts, they represent approximately 10% to 20% of CNS tumors. An estimated 1 in 400 new patients referred to a child neurology center has a spinal cord tumor (379). Most series report an equal distribution across sexes (380,381) and in the series of Pascual-Castroviejo, most patients were younger than 7 years old (379–383). A comprehensive review of spinal cord tumors has been edited by Pascual-Castroviejo (384).

Pathology

Spinal cord tumors can arise anywhere along the neuraxis. They have been categorized as extradural extramedullary, intradural extramedullary, or intramedullary (Table 10.21). Extradural tumors were the most common (43%) among the 1,234 spinal tumors in a series reported by DiLorenzo and colleagues (380). In the extradural space, the most common tumors are neuroblastomas, sarcomas, and other primary tumors of bone (383). Benign tumors, such as neurofibromas, dermoid cysts, and teratomas, are usually extradural or intradural extramedullary. The two most common intramedullary tumors are low-grade astrocytomas followed by ependymomas and other gliomas (Fig. 10.24) (385,386). Rarely, primitive neuroectodermal tumors or malignant gliomas can arise from a child's spinal cord and seed the neuroaxis (387–389) (see Fig. 10.17). Intramedullary tumors occasionally are associated with a cystic cavity that does not communicate with the spinal subarachnoid space.

During the first 3 years of life, a variety of tumors are encountered. These include teratomas, lipomas, neuroblastomas, dermoids, and epidermoids (386). The most frequent benign histologic types, in decreasing order, are

TABLE 10.21. *Tumors of the spinal cord*

Intramedullary tumors	Intradural extramedullary tumors	Extradural tumors
Astrocytoma	Spinal teratoma	Peripheral nerve tumors
Ependymoma	Dermoid and epidermoid cyst	Neurofibroma
Medulloblastoma	Spinal neurenteric cyst	Lymphoma
Others	Intraspinal cyst	Osseous tumors
	Meningioma	
	Schwannoma (neurinoma)	
	Neurofibroma	
	Spinal hemangioma	
	Extraneural (lymphoma)	

Adapted from Escalona-Zapata J. Epidemiology of spinal cord tumors in children. In: Pascual-Castroviejo I, ed. *International review of child neurology series: spinal tumors in children and adolescents.* New York: Raven, 1990:11.

histiocytosis X, osteoid osteoma, and aneurysmal cyst (382).

Pathologic features have been reviewed by Escalona-Zapata (387) and cytogenetic studies reported by Chadduck and colleagues (390).

Clinical Manifestations

Clinical presentation of spinal cord tumors depends on the location of the lesion. Most tumors are slow growing, and it is not unusual for symptoms to exist for several months before diagnosis. Whereas intramedullary lesions usually produce symmetric weakness and atrophy of the affected segments, extramedullary tumors tend to affect nerve roots before the spinal cord and, therefore, begin with unilateral pain in a segmental distribution. This pain is often described as sharp "electric-like," radiating down a limb. It is accompanied by paresthesias and numbness (391). Valsalva maneuvers (coughing, sneezing, straining) frequently cause or exacerbate back pain in patients with extramedullary lesions. Extramedullary lesions must be large before they produce upper motor neuron weakness or a sensory level. When weakness does occur, it is typically unilateral. In both extramedullary and

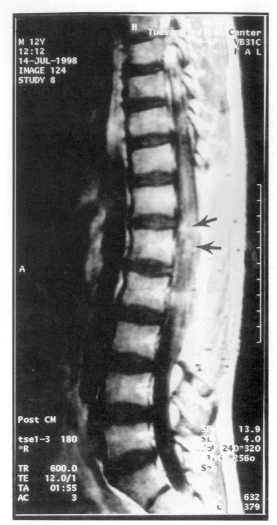

FIG. 10.24. Sagittal magnetic resonance imaging of spinal cord shows intramedullary ependymoma (*arrows*).

intramedullary tumors impaired gait and stiffness, and pain in the back or the legs is a common early complaint and can precede the onset of neurologic signs by a long time (392).

Intramedullary lesions produce bilateral weakness, spasticity, atrophy, a sensory level, sphincter disturbance, and hyperreflexia. In a study by Constantini and colleagues, the most common reasons for radiologic investigation in infants with intramedullary lesions were pain (42%), motor regression (36%), gait abnormali-

ties (27%), torticollis (27%), and progressive kyphoscoliosis (24%) (393).

On examination, two types of neurologic findings can be elicited: those that result from segmental spinal cord involvement, and those that result from interruption of ascending and descending tracts within the cord. Segmental weakness, atrophy, hyporeflexia, and sensory changes are caused by involvement of central gray matter or nerve roots. Spasticity, sensory deficits to a definable spinal cord level, and sphincteric involvement are caused by interruption of long tracts. Extramedullary tumors can cause Brown-Séquard syndrome [6% of patients in the series of Levy and coworkers (391)]. Classically, this syndrome follows hemisection of the spinal cord after trauma and includes homolateral weakness, spasticity, ataxia, and contralateral loss of pain and temperature sensation. Incomplete forms of this syndrome, however, are more common in patients with spinal cord tumors.

In infants and small children, an absolute loss of response to pinprick below a specific spinal level usually cannot be established. Diminished or absent sweating below the appropriate level, however, is frequently demonstrable on examination or by the iodine starch sweat test, particularly with intramedullary lesions (394). Somatosensory-evoked potentials can further delineate the sensory level of spinal cord tumors. Deep tendon reflexes below the level of the lesion are exceptionally brisk in tumors compressing the spinal cord, and an extensor plantar response occurs. Impaired bladder function is a late finding that dictates emergency surgery. Initial bladder symptoms are increased urgency followed by incontinence or retention of urine (395,396).

Nystagmus or papilledema can accompany spinal cord tumors. In some instances, the papilledema is caused by impaired CSF absorption, a consequence of the mucinous protein material that is formed by the degenerative changes within the tumor. Other factors also can operate in the production of papilledema; these include infiltration of the meninges by tumor, subarachnoid hemorrhage, and hydrocephalus, the last caused by Arnold-Chiari malformations (397,398). The unusual combination of papilledema and hydrocephalus should alert the clinician to an associated spinal cord tumor, particularly a teratoma.

Diagnosis

Spinal cord tumors are rare in childhood, so early recognition hinges on careful neurologic examination and localization of the offending lesion. Neurologic condition on admission, regardless of specific tumor type, is an important prognostic factor for functional recovery after therapy (399,400). Local spinal pain is a rare complaint in childhood; if present, a neurologic examination must be performed to evaluate neural function in tissue underlying the painful bony segment (401). The sudden onset of back pain is more likely caused by trauma or infection (e.g., empyema). The spine should be examined for point tenderness by gently percussing vertebral tips with a large soft rubber reflex hammer. Any scoliosis or limitation in flexion and extension of the pediatric spine is suspect for the presence of a spinal mass. Eeg-Olofsson and coworkers have noted that recurrent abdominal pain can be the first symptom of a thoracic intramedullary spinal cord tumor (402). Another finding that points to a spinal cord neoplasm is the presence of a painful scoliosis, with pain elicited or aggravated by physical effort, coughing, sneezing, or flexion of neck or back (403). The neurologic examination of motor and sensory function is intended to identify the likely diseased segment so that spinal imaging is directed to the epicenter of the neoplasm. Examination of the anus for gaping is important in evaluating medullary function.

MRI has replaced plain films, myelography, and CT as the preferred imaging study when spinal tumor is suspected (404). Faster imaging technologies have made motion artifacts uncommon, especially when a particular spinal segment is suspect. MRI is useful in separating neoplasms from edema or syrinx. Once the site and extent of the lesion are localized and defined by MRI with gadolinium enhancement, it is important to also image the cranium. Malignant pediatric brain tumors (e.g., PNET/MB, ependymoma) can present with gross spinal subarach-

noid metastasis before the appearance of symptoms pointing to a lesion above the foramen magnum. In addition, intramedullary spinal tumors may be associated with rostral extension of hydromyelia into the brainstem that can produce lower cranial nerve dysfunction. Rarely, as occurs in neurofibromatosis, a patient has spinal and intracranial tumors (e.g., schwannomas, meningiomas). Detailed aspects of imaging parameters (plane, slice thickness, weighting) best suited to viewing CNS tumors are reviewed by Quisling (405). As a rule, sagittal images are the most important plane for screening the spine.

Treatment and Prognosis

The treatment of spinal neoplasms depends on the involved segment (cervical, thoracic, lumbar, sacral), the location of the tumor (intradural versus extradural), tumor type (benign versus malignant), and tumor extent (localized versus infiltrative). Extramedullary tumors that can be totally removed surgically have an excellent prognosis. Even partial removal of a tumor is compatible with long periods of partial or complete symptomatic relief, particularly when surgery is followed by radiotherapy. Intramedullary tumors can sometimes be removed by microsurgical techniques (406). Because there is a higher incidence of incomplete excision of benign intramedullary tumors, treatment for this type of tumor is more controversial. The goal of therapy is to remove as much of the tumor as possible to improve neurologic function, and to reduce the risk of local recurrence and metastasis. For histologically benign extradural tumors (osteoid osteoma, aneurysmal bone cyst), intradural extramedullary tumors (dermoids, epidermoids, meningiomas, schwannomas), or intramedullary tumors (low-grade astrocytomas, lipomas), the prognosis is excellent after tumor removal by microsurgical techniques (Fig. 10.25). For intramedullary surgery, intraoperative spinal cord monitoring has a favorable effect on neurologic outcome (407). Surgical technique is reviewed in detail by Epstein (408) and Mottl and Koutecky (409).

Spinal column deformity after laminectomy can be a serious long-term problem for children in whom a curative tumor operation has been per-

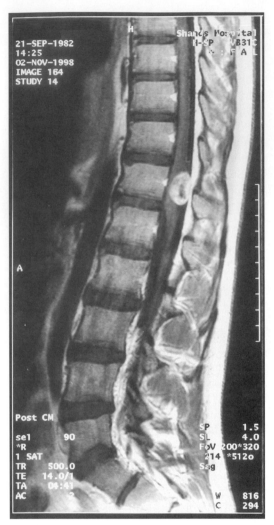

FIG. 10.25. Sagittal magnetic resonance imaging shows well-circumscribed spinal cord schwannoma.

formed. Radiotherapy has been associated with an excellent outcome in patients with intramedullary tumors (astrocytomas, ependymomas), but there have been no controlled studies testing the safety and efficacy of radiotherapy in children with intramedullary spinal cord tumors. Thus, most neuro-oncology centers favor surgery alone (408–410). In addition, radiotherapy increases the risk of spinal column deformity in the growing child (393). Other complications of irradiation of the spinal cord include an acute reaction, a transient postirradiation myelopathy, or an irreversible myelomalacia (411).

Postirradiation myelopathy appears several months after irradiation and is characterized by transient paresthesias and by sensations similar to electric shock in the extremities, precipitated by flexion of the cervical spine (Lhermitte's sign). Symptoms tend to resolve in the course of several months. Myelomalacia can result in a rapidly evolving paraplegia, the consequence of pathology in capillaries and small arteries (412). The time-dose relationship producing these complications has not been fully established, but, as in postirradiation encephalopathy, the complications have been encountered even after conservative doses, notably in infants and small children (413). Unusual complications of cord irradiation include amyotrophy, acute transverse myelitis, and slowly progressive myelopathy that advances to complete or incomplete transverse myelitis (411).

Radiotherapy and chemotherapy are targeted at malignant spinal tumors after surgery, but the prognosis is poor for malignant gliomas, neuroblastomas, and sarcomas (400). There is no evidence that the extent of surgical resection affects outcome in children with histologically malignant lesions. Every effort must be made to preserve neurologic function and to tailor radiotherapy and chemotherapy to the individual patient's age, pathology, tumor extent, and functional status.

PSEUDOTUMOR CEREBRI (IDIOPATHIC INTRACRANIAL HYPERTENSION, BENIGN INTRACRANIAL HYPERTENSION)

Pseudotumor cerebri (idiopathic intracranial hypertension, benign intracranial hypertension), in which increased intracranial pressure occurs in the absence of a space-occupying lesion, was first recognized by Quincke in 1893 (414).

Pathology and Pathophysiology

Pseudotumor cerebri is caused by various causes. Johnston and Paterson, who in 1974 compiled one of the largest reported series, found middle ear infection to be responsible for 24.3% of cases, nonspecific infections responsible for 13.9%, minor head injuries responsible for 4.4%, and withdrawal from corticosteroid therapy responsible for 1.2% (415). Pseudotumor cerebri also has been seen secondary to hypo- and hypervitaminosis A, and after the administration of isoretinoin for acne, nitrofurantoin for urinary tract infection, chlortetracycline, and tetracycline (416,417). It may follow varicella, as a consequence of transient protein S deficiency caused by the presence of an anti–protein S antibody (417a). Other, more unusual causes include profound iron deficiency anemia, hypoparathyroidism, Addison disease, disseminated lupus erythematosus, and carbon dioxide retention secondary to chronic lung disease (418). Some of these associations, however, may exist coincidentally. In children younger than 10 years of age, thrombosis of one or more of the dural sinuses, particularly the lateral sinus, as a sequel to otitis or mastoiditis, is probably still one of the most common abnormalities (419,420). The term *otitic hydrocephalus*, which has been used to designate this condition, is inappropriate because the ventricular system is always normal or even small. In older subjects, the cause of increased intracranial pressure is usually obscure. Endocrine disturbances also have been implicated in view of the relationship of pseudotumor cerebri to menarche, disorders of the menstrual cycle, obesity, and rapid discontinuation of prolonged corticosteroid therapy (421).

The pathophysiology for increased intracranial pressure is still unclear, and it is likely that more than one mechanism is at fault. Johnston and Paterson postulated that an increase in the volume of CSF is responsible (415). Because CSF formation in pseudotumor cerebri is diminished, there probably is increased resistance to its absorption, possibly at the level of the arachnoid villi. McComb points out that if this were indeed the case, there should be a progressive accumulation of CSF, with a new equilibrium established at a larger volume and at a higher pressure of CSF, which is not the case in pseudotumor cerebri (422). Anatomic examinations have revealed increased brain water content in some instances. MRI studies performed on obese young women with pseudotumor cerebri have confirmed the presence of increased white matter water. Additionally, the most severely

affected patients show areas of increased signal intensity on T2-weighted images, an indication of focal areas of edema (423).

Clinical Manifestations

Patients develop nonspecific signs of increased intracranial pressure, such as intermittent headaches, vomiting, blurred vision, and diplopia. In otitic hydrocephalus, these symptoms are often preceded by a partially treated otitis (424,425). Headaches tend to worsen at night, and in the child with migraine pseudotumor cerebri aggravates a typical migrainous attack. Papilledema is evident in the majority of cases; it was present in 82% in the series of Soler and colleagues (417). Visual impairment is usually slight, particularly in patients whose intracranial pressure has been elevated for only a short time. In contrast to patients with increased intracranial pressure secondary to mass lesions, the level of consciousness and intellectual functioning remains normal (425). A variety of cranial nerve palsies have been encountered. Most common is sixth nerve palsy, which is seen in up to one-half of children (426). An occasional patient has third, fourth, or hypoglossal nerve palsy (427).

Diagnosis

The diagnosis of pseudotumor cerebri is made after exclusion of other causes for increased intracranial pressure, particularly mass lesions localized to the midline or to the silent areas of the brain such as the frontal lobes. Generally, imaging studies reveal a ventricular system that is midline and normal or somewhat reduced in size (423,428).

The CSF is generally normal, although mild pleocytosis is not unusual. In a few instances, obstruction of the lateral sinus has been documented by carotid angiography or retrograde jugular venography.

Treatment and Prognosis

Although there are no randomized controlled studies and the natural course of the condition is unknown, treatment is directed toward maintaining the intracranial pressure within near normal limits to reduce the danger of permanent visual damage. Twice daily serial lumbar punctures have been used; in the experience of Soler and colleagues the increased CSF pressure resolved in 18% of children after one lumbar puncture. Acetazolamide was effective in 55% of the children who did not respond to the lumbar puncture (417). Some of the unresponsive children obtained symptomatic relief with 1 to 2 weeks of corticosteroid therapy. The remainder, some 23% in the series of Soler and colleagues, required surgery. Optic nerve sheath fenestration or lumboperitoneal shunts are the most commonly used procedures. Because of the significant incidence of shunt failures and other complications, optic nerve sheath fenestration is probably the procedure of choice (429). Corbett and Thompson believe that an asymptomatic patient with no visual field loss and normal visual acuity should not be treated, rather the patient should be followed by a neurologist and an ophthalmologist (430). We personally would prefer more frequent follow-up examinations than at intervals of 6 to 12 months as suggested by the authors. Indications for surgery are a loss of visual field or visual acuity or a severe headache that does not respond to medication or lumbar puncture. The various treatment methods have been reviewed by Baker and coworkers (431). Recurrences are rare: They were recorded in some 10% of subjects in Johnston and Paterson's series (415), and in only one patient in Grant's series of 79 patients (432). Some 10% of patients are left with visual defects that are permanent or require more than a year to resolve (415,433). These appear to be most common in women with systemic hypertension (434).

REFERENCES

1. Cohen ME, Duffner PK, eds. *Brain tumors in children. Principles of diagnosis and treatment.* New York: Raven Press, 1994.
2. Maria BL, ed. Teamwork in pediatric neuro-oncology. In: Bodensteiner JB, ed. *Seminars in pediatric neurology.* Philadelphia: WB Saunders Co, 1997:251–253.
3. Miltenburg D, Louw DF, Sutherland GR. Epidemiology of childhood brain tumors. *Can J Neurol Sci* 1996;23:118–122.
4. Pollack IF. Brain tumors in children. *N Engl J Med* 1994;331:1500–1507.
5. Roush SW, et al. Progress in childhood cancer care in Florida. 1970–1992. *J Fla Med Assoc* 1993;80:747–751.
6. Critchley M. Brain tumours in children: their general symptomatology. *Br J Child Dis* 1925;22:251–264.
7. Bailey P, Buchanan DN, Bucy PC. *Intracranial tumors of infancy and childhood.* Chicago: University of Chicago Press, 1939.
8. Cuneo HM, Rand CW. *Brain tumors of childhood.* Springfield, IL: Charles C Thomas, 1952.
9. Crouse SK, Berg BO. Intracranial meningiomas in childhood and adolescence. *Neurology* 1972;22: 135–141.
10. Dastur HM, Desai AD. Comparative study of brain tuberculomas and gliomas based on 107 case records of each. *Brain* 1965;88:375–396.
11. Roush SW, et al. The incidence of pediatric cancer in Florida, 1981 to 1986. *Cancer* 1992;69:2212–2219.
11a. Packer RJ. Brain tumors in children. *Arch Neurol* 1999;56:421–425.
12. Bleyer WA. The U.S. pediatric cancer clinical trials programmes: international implications and the way forward. *Eur J Cancer* 1997;33:1439–1447.
13. Tobias J, Hayward RD. Brain and spinal cord tumours in children. In: Thomas DGT, ed. *Neuro-oncology: primary malignant brain tumours.* Baltimore: The Johns Hopkins University Press, 1990: 164–192.
14. Huang H, et al. Identification in human brain tumors of DNA sequences specific for SV40 large T antigen. *Brain Pathol* 1999;9:33–44.
15. Bigner SH, et al. Brain tumors. In: Vogelstein B, Kintzler KW, eds. *The genetic basis of human cancer.* New York: McGraw-Hill, 1998:661–670.
16. Santarius T, et al. Molecular aspects of neuro-oncology. *Clin Neurol Neurosurg* 1997;99:184–195.
17. Ng HK, Lam PY. The molecular genetics of central nervous system tumors. *Pathology* 1998;30:196–202.
18. Muir DF. Translational research models in neuro-oncology. In: Bodensteiner JB, Maria BL, eds. *Seminars in pediatric neurology.* Philadelphia: WB Saunders, 1997:292–303.
19. Kornblith PL, Walker MD, eds. *Advances in neuro-oncology II.* Armack: Futura Publishing Co Inc, 1997.
20. Farwell J, Flannery JT. Cancer in relatives of children with central-nervous-system neoplasms. *N Engl J Med* 1984;311:749–753.
21. Modan B, et al. Radiation-induced head and neck tumors. *Lancet* 1974;1:277–279.
22. Cushing H. Concerning a definite regulatory mechanism of the vasomotor center which controls blood pressure during cerebral compression. *Bull Hopkins Hosp* 1901;12:290–292.
23. Cushing H. Some experimental and clinical observations concerning states of increased intracranial tension. *Am J Med Sci* 1902;124:375–400.
24. Marmarou A, Tabaddo RK. Intracranial pressure: physiology and pathophysiology. In: Cooper PR, ed. *Head injury,* 3rd ed. Baltimore: Williams & Wilkins, 1993:203–224.
25. Kety SS, Shenkin HA, Schmidt CF. The effects of increased intracranial pressure on cerebral circulatory function in man. *J Clin Invest* 1948;27:493–510.
26. Langfitt TW, Weinstein JD, Kassell NF. Cerebral vasomotor paralysis produced by intracranial hypertension. *Neurology* 1965;15:622–641.

27. Theodore J, Robin ED. Speculations on neurogenic pulmonary edema (NPE). *Annu Rev Resp Dis* 1976;113:405–411.

28. Miller JD. Disorders of cerebral blood flow and intracranial pressure after head injury. *Clin Neurosurg* 1982;29:162–173.

29. Lindenberg R. Compression of brain arteries as pathogenetic factor for tissue necroses and their areas of predilection. *J Neuropathol Exp Neurol* 1955;14: 223–243.

30. McNealy DE, Plum F. Brain stem dysfunction with supratentorial mass lesion. *Arch Neurol* 1962;7:10–32.

31. Cushing H. Strangulation of the nervi abducentes by lateral branches of the basilar artery in cases of brain tumour. With an explanation of some obscure palsies on the basis of arterial constriction. *Brain* 1910;33: 204–235.

32. Collier J. The false localizing signs of intracranial tumour. *Brain* 1904;27:490–508.

33. Till K. *Paediatric neurosurgery.* Oxford: Blackwell Scientific Publications, 1975.

34. Honig PJ, Charney EB. Children with brain tumor headaches. Distinguishing features. *Am J Dis Child* 1982;136:121–124.

35. The epidemiology of headache among children with brain tumor. Headache in children with brain tumors. The childhood brain tumor consortium. *J Neurooncol* 1991;10:31–46.

36. Savino PJ, Glaser JS. Pseudopapilledema versus papilledema. *Int Ophthalmol Clin* 1977;17:115–137.

36a. Sanders MD. Papilloedema: "the pendulum of progress." *Eye* 1997;11:267–294.

37. Anmarkrud N. The value of fluorescein fundus angiography in evaluating optic disc oedema. *Acta Ophthalmol* 1977;55:605–615.

38. Hayreh SS. Optic disc edema in raised intracranial pressure. V. Pathogenesis. *Arch Ophthalmol* 1977;95: 1553–1565.

39. Gordon GS, Wallae SJ, Neal JW. Intracranial tumours during the first two years of life: presenting features. *Arch Dis Child* 1995;73:345–347.

40. Low NL, Correll JW, Hammill JF. Tumors of the cerebral hemispheres in children. *Arch Neurol* 1965;13:547–554.

41. Burton LJ, et al. Headache etiology in a pediatric emergency department. *Pediatr Emerg Care* 1997;13:1–4.

42. Ropper AH. Lateral displacement of the brain and level of consciousness in patients with an acute hemispheral mass. *N Engl J Med* 1986;314:953–958.

43. Kuttesch JF. Advances and controversies in the management of childhood brain tumors. *Curr Opin Oncol* 1997;9:235–240.

44. Rorke LB. Pathology of brain tumors in infants and children. In: Tindall GT, Cooper PR, Barrow DL, eds. *The practice of neurosurgery.* Baltimore: Williams & Wilkins, 1996:733–754.

45. Tovi M, et al. Delineation of gliomas with magnetic resonance imaging using Gd-DTPA in comparison with computed tomography and positron emission tomography. *Acta Radiol* 1990;31:417–429.

46. Sartor K, et al. MR imaging in infra-, para-, and retrosellar mass lesions. *Neuroradiology* 1987;29:19–29.

47. Knopp MV, et al. Functional neuroimaging in the assessment of CNS neoplasms. *Eur Radiol* 1997; 7[Suppl 5]:209–215.

48. Brant-Zawadzki M, et al. Gd-DTPA in clinical MR of the brain: 1. Intraaxial lesions. *AJR Am J Roentgenol* 1986;147:1223–1230.

49. Dean B, et al. Gliomas: classification with MR imaging. *Radiology* 1990;174:411–415.

50. Kramer ED, et al. Staging and surveillance of children with central nervous system neoplasms: recommendations of the neurology and tumor imaging committees of the Children's Cancer Group. *Pediatr Neurosurg* 1994;20:254–263.

51. Rydberg JN, et al. Initial clinical experience in MR imaging of the brain with a fast fluid-attenuated inversion-recovery pulse sequence. *Radiology* 1994;193: 173–180.

52. Tsuchiya K, Mizutani Y, Hachiya J. Preliminary evaluation of fluid-attenuated inversion-recovery MR in the diagnosis of intracranial tumors. *AJR Am J Neuroradiol* 1996;17:1081–1086.

53. Kizu O, et al. Application of proton chemical shift imaging in monitoring of gamma knife radiosurgery on brain tumors. *Magn Reson Imaging* 1998;16:197–204.

54. Mistretta CA, Crummy AB, Strother CM. Digital angiography: a perspective. *Radiology* 1981;139: 273–276.

55. Brody AS. New perspectives in CT and MR imaging. *Neurol Clin* 1991;9:273–286.

56. Merritt HH. The cerebrospinal fluid in cases of tumors of the brain. *Arch Neurol Psychiatry* 1935;34: 1175–1187.

57. Berg L. Hypoglycorrhachia of noninfectious origin. Diffuse meningeal neoplasia. *Neurology* 1953;3: 811–824.

58. Glass JP, et al. Malignant cells in cerebrospinal fluid (CSF): the meaning of a positive CSF cytology. *Neurology* 1979;29:1369–1375.

59. Taveras JM, Wood EH. *Diagnostic neuroradiology*, 2nd ed. Baltimore: Williams & Wilkins, 1976:131.

60. Weir B, Elvidge AR. Oligodendrogliomas. An analysis of 63 cases. *J Neurosurg* 1968;29:500–505.

61. Babcock DS, Han BK. The accuracy of high resolution, real-time ultrasonography of the head in infancy. *Radiology* 1981;139:665–676.

62. Janus TJ, et al. Use of [18$_F$]fluorodeoxyglucose positron emission tomography in patients with primary malignant brain tumors. *Ann Neurol* 1993;33:540–548.

63. Glantz MJ, et al. Identification of early recurrence of primary central nervous system tumors by [18$_F$]fluorodeoxyglucose positron emission tomography. *Ann Neurol* 1991;29:347–355.

63a. Waldrop SM, et al. Treatment of brain tumors in children is associated with abnormal MR spectroscopic ratios in brain tissue remote from the tumor site. *AJNR Am J Neuroradiol* 1998;19:963–70.

63b. Koutcher JA, et al. Evaluation of chemotherapy and radiation enhancement and 31P NMR spectral changes induced by biochemical modulation *Cancer Invest* 1997;15:111–20.

64. Kemp SS, et al. Magnetic resonance imaging of the cerebral aqueduct. *Neuroradiology* 1987;29:430–436.

65. Kazner E, Lanksch W, Steinhoff H. Cranial computerized tomography in the diagnosis of brain disorders in infants and children. *Neuropaediatrie* 1976;7:136–174.

66. Mickle JP. Neurosurgery for pediatric brain tumors. *Semin Pediatr Neurol* 1997;4:273–281.

67. D'Angio GJ, et al. Key problems in the management of children with brain tumors. *Int J Radiat Oncol Biol Phys* 1990;18:805–810.
68. Steinbok P, et al. Value of postoperative surveillance imaging in the management of children with some common brain tumors. *J Neurosurg* 1996;84:726–732.
69. Buatti JM, et al. Radiotherapy for pediatric brain tumors. *Semin Pediatr Neurol* 1997;4:304–319.
70. Friedman WA, Bova FJ. Stereotactic radiosurgery. *Contemp Neurosurg* 1989;11:1–7.
71. Rabinowitz I, et al. Accuracy of radiation field alignment in clinical practice. *Int J Radiat Oncol Biol Phys* 1985;11:1857–1867.
72. Friedman WA, Bova FJ, Spiegelmann R. Linear accelerator radiosurgery at the University of Florida. *Neurosurg Clin N Am* 1992;3:141–166.
73. Auchter RM, et al. A multiinstitutional outcome and prognostic factor analysis of radiosurgery for resectable single brain metastasis. *Int J Radiat Oncol Biol Phys* 1996;35:27–35.
74. Lunsford LD. Contemporary management of meningiomas: radiation therapy as an adjuvant and radiosurgery as an alternative to surgical removal. *J Neurosurg* 1994;80:187–190.
75. Bova FJ, et al. The University of Florida frameless high-precision stereotactic radiotherapy system. *Int J Radiat Oncol Biol Phys* 1997;38:875–882.
76. Flickinger JC, Kondziolka D, Lunsford LD. Clinical applications of stereotactic radiosurgery. *Cancer Treat Res* 1998;93:283–297.
77. Benson PJ, Sung JH. Cerebral aneurysms following radiotherapy for medulloblastoma. *J Neurosurg* 1989;70:545–550.
78. Ball WS, Prenger EC, Ballard ET. Neurotoxicity of radio/chemotherapy in children: pathologic and MR correlation. *Am J Neuroradiol* 1992;13:761–776.
79. Duffner PK, Cohen ME. The long-term effects of central nervous system therapy on children with brain tumors. *Neurol Clin* 1991;9:479–495.
80. Curran WJ, et al. Magnetic resonance imaging of cranial radiation lesions. *Int J Radiat Oncol Biol Phys* 1987;13:1093–1098.
81. Kramer JH, et al. Absence of white matter changes on magnetic resonance imaging in children treated with CNS prophylactic therapy for leukemia. *Cancer* 1988;61:928–930.
82. Ellenberg L, et al. Factors affecting intellectual outcome in pediatric brain tumor patients. *Neurosurgery* 1987;21:638–644.
83. Glauser TA, Packer RJ. Cognitive deficits in long-term survivors of childhood brain tumors. *Child Nerv Syst* 1991;7:2–12.
84. Armstrong C, et al. Biphasic patterns of memory deficits following moderate-dose partial-brain irradiation: neuropsychologic outcome and proposed mechanisms. *J Clin Oncol* 1995;13:2263–2271.
85. Duffner PK, Cohen ME, Parker MS. Prospective intellectual testing in children with brain tumors. *Ann Neurol* 1988;23:575–579.
86. Radcliffe J, et al. Three- and four-year cognitive outcome in children with noncortical brain tumors treated with whole-brain-radiotherapy. *Ann Neurol* 1992;32:551–554.
87. Cohen BH, et al. Brain tumors in children under 2 years: treatment, survival and long-term prognosis. *Pediatr Neurosurg* 1993;19:171–179.
88. Suc E, et al. Brain tumours under the age of three. The price of survival. A retrospective study of 20 long-term survivors. *Acta Neurochir* 1990;106:93–98.
89. Jannoun L, Bloom HJG. Long-term psychological effects in children treated for intracranial tumors. *Int J Radiat Oncol Biol Phys* 1990;18:747–753.
90. Curnes JT, et al. MRI of radiation injury to the brain. *AJR Am J Roentgenol* 1986;147:119–124.
91. Zimmerman RD, et al. Periventricular hyperintensity as seen by magnetic resonance: prevalence and significance. *AJR Am J Neuroradiol* 1986;7:13–20.
92. Constine LS, et al. Adverse effects of brain irradiation correlated with MR and CT imaging. *Int J Radiat Oncol Biol Phys* 1988;15:319–330.
93. Tsuruda JS, Kortman KE, Bradley WG. Radiation effects on cerebral white matter: MR evaluations. *AJR Am J Neuroradiol* 1987;8:431–437.
94. Constine LS, et al. Hypothalamic-pituitary dysfunction after radiation for brain tumors. *N Engl J Med* 1993;328:87–94.
95. Rappaport R, Brauner R. Growth and endocrine disorders secondary to cranial irradiation. *Pediatr Res* 1989;25:561–567.
96. Cassady JR. Developmental toxicity: unique radiation toxicity in children which deserves study. *Radiat Oncol Invest* 1993;1:77–80.
97. Samaan NA, et al. Hypothalamic, pituitary and thyroid dysfunction after radiotherapy to the head and neck. *Int J Radiat Oncol Biol Phys* 1982;8:1857–1867.
98. Awwad S, Gregor A. Hormonal abnormalities in survivors of primary brain tumors. *Radiother Oncol* 1993;27:171–172.
99. Meadows AT, et al. Second malignant neoplasms in children: an update from the Late Effects Study Group. *J Clin Oncol* 1985;3:532–538.
100. Malone M, Lumley H, Erdohazi M. Astrocytoma as a second malignancy in patients with acute lymphoblastic leukemia. *Cancer* 1986;57:1979–1985.
101. Harrison MJ, et al. Radiation-induced meningiomas: experience at the Mount Sinai Hospital and review of the literature. *J Neurosurg* 1991;75:564–574.
102. Ater JL, et al. MOPP chemotherapy without irradiation as primary postsurgical therapy for brain tumors in infants and young children. *J Neurooncol* 1997;32:243–252.
103. Walter AW, et al. Secondary brain tumors in children treated for acute lymphoblastic leukemia at St. Jude Children's Research Hospital. *J Clin Oncol* 1998;16:3761–3767.
104. Allen JC, et al. Brain and spinal cord hemorrhage in long-term survivors of malignant pediatric brain tumors: a possible late effect of therapy. *Neurology* 1991;41:148–150.
105. Sheline GE. Irradiation injury of the human brain: a review of clinical experience. In: Gilbert HA, Kagan AR, eds. *Radiation damage to the nervous system.* New York: Raven Press, 1980:39.
106. Duffner PK, Cohen ME. Long-term consequences of CNS treatment for childhood cancer. Part II. Clinical consequences. *Pediatr Neurol* 1991;7:237–242.

107. Mitchell WG, et al. Stroke as a late sequela of cranial irradiation for childhood brain tumors. *J Child Neurol* 1991;6:128–133.
108. Shuper A, et al. "Complicated migraine-like episodes" in children following cranial irradiation and chemotherapy. *Neurology* 1995;45:1837–1840.
109. Duffner PK, et al. Postoperative chemotherapy and delayed radiation in children less than three years of age with malignant brain tumors. *N Engl J Med* 1993;328:1725–1731.
110. Maria BL, Drane WE, Quisling RG. Metabolic imaging in children with brain tumors. *Int Pediatr* 1993;8:233–238.
111. Maria BL, et al. ^{201}Thallium SPECT imaging in childhood brain tumors. *Pediatr Neurosurg* 1994;20:11–18.
112. Maria BL, et al. Correlation between gadolinium-DTPA contrast enhancement and thallium-201 chloride uptake in pediatric brainstem gliomas. *J Child Neurol* 1997;12:341–348.
113. Maria BL, et al. Comparative value of thallium and glucose SPECT imaging in childhood brain tumors. *Pediatr Neurol* 1998;19:351–357.
114. Langer LF, Brem H, Langer R. New technologies for fighting brain disease. *Technol Rev* 1991;94:62.
115. Mitchell MS. Combining chemotherapy with biological response modifiers in treatment of cancer. *J Natl Cancer Inst* 1988;80:1445–1450.
116. Kuhl J, et al. Primary chemotherapy after surgery and delayed irradiation in children under three years of age with medulloblastoma-pilot trial of the German pediatric brain tumor study group. *Med Pediatr Oncol* 1992;20:387.
117. Levin VA, ed. *Cancer in the nervous system*. New York: Churchill Livingstone Inc, 1996.
118. Lefkowitz I, et al. Adjuvant chemotherapy of childhood posterior fossa (PF) ependymoma: craniospinal radiation with or without CCNU, vincristine (VCR) and prednisone (P). *Proc Am Soc Clin Oncol* 1989;8:878.
119. Kolker JD, Weichselbaum RR. Radiobiology update. In: Kornblith PL, Walker MD, eds. *Advances in neuro-oncology II*. Armack: Futura Publishing Co Inc, 1997.
120. Maria BL. Brain tumors: current management in child neurology. Maria BL, ed. Hamilton, Ontario, Canada: BC Decker Inc, 1999:336–341.
121. Rowinski EK, Donehower RC. Vinca alkaloids and epipodophyllotoxins. In: Perry MC, ed. *The chemotherapy source book*. Baltimore: Williams & Wilkins: 1992:359–383.
122. Green DM, D'Angio GJ, eds. *Late effects of treatment for childhood cancer*. New York: Wiley-Liss Inc, 1992.
123. Perry MC, ed. *The chemotherapy source book*. Baltimore: Williams & Wilkins, 1996.
124. Maria BL, Dennis M, Obonsawin M. Severe permanent encephalopathy in acute lymphoblastic leukemia. *Can J Neurol Sci* 1993;20:199–205.
125. Maria BL, et al. Gene therapy for neurologic disease: benchtop discoveries to bedside applications. 1. The bench. *J Child Neurol* 1997;12:1–12.
126. Maria BL, et al. Gene therapy for neurologic disease: benchtop discoveries to bedside applications. 2. The bedside. *J Child Neurol* 1997;12:77–84.
127. Maria BL, Friedman T. Gene therapy in neuro-oncology: lessons learned from pioneering studies. In: Bodensteiner JB, Maria BL, eds. *Seminars in pediatric neurology*. Philadelphia: WB Saunders, 1997:333–339.
127a. Kleihues P, Burger PC, Scheithauer BW. The new WHO classification of brain tumours. *Brain Pathol* 1993;3:255–268.
128. Burger PC, Fuller GN. Pathology—trends and pitfalls in histologic diagnosis, immunopathology, and applications of oncogene research. *Neurol Clin* 1991;9:249–271.
129. Vagner-Capodano AM, et al. Cytogenic studies in 45 pediatric brain tumors. *Pediatr Hematol Oncol* 1992;9:223–235.
130. Bigner SH, et al. Chromosomal characteristics of childhood brain tumors. *Cancer Genet Cytogenet* 1997;97:125–134.
131. Russell DS, Rubinstein LJ, eds. *Pathology of tumours of the nervous system*, 5th ed. London: E. Arnold, 1989.
132. Gilles FH. Pediatric brain tumors: classification. In: Morantz RA, Walsh JW, eds. *Brain tumors. A comprehensive text*. New York: Marcel Dekker Inc, 1994:109–134.
133. Gilles FH, et al. Histologic features and observational variation in cerebellar gliomas in children. *Natl Cancer Inst Monogr* 1977;58:175–181.
134. Tomlinson FH, et al. The significance of atypia and histologic malignancy in pilocytic astrocytoma of the cerebellum: a clinicopathologic and flow cytometric study. *J Child Neurol* 1994;9:301–310.
135. Agamanolis DP, Malone JM. Chromosomal abnormalities in 47 pediatric brain tumors. *Cancer Genet Cytogenet* 1995;81:125–134.
136. von Deimling A, et al. Deletions on the long arm of chromosome 17 in pilocytic astrocytoma. *Acta Neuropathol (Berl)* 1993;86:81–85.
137. Patt S, et al. p53 gene mutations in human astrocytic brain tumors including pilocytic astrocytomas. *Hum Pathol* 1996;27:586–589.
138. Burger PC, Scheithauer BW. Tumors of the nervous system. In: *Atlas of tumor pathology, third series, fascicle 10*. Washington, DC: Armed Forces Institute of Pathology, 1994.
139. Lantos PL, Vandenberg SR, Kleihues P. Tumors of the nervous system. In: Graham DI, Lantos PL, eds. *Greenfield's neuropathology*, 6th ed. London: Arnold, 1997:583–879.
140. Maria BL, et al. Diffuse leptomeningeal seeding from a malignant spinal cord astrocytoma in a child with neurofibromatosis. *J Neurooncol* 1986;4:159–163.
141. von Deimling A, et al. Subsets of glioblastoma multiforme defined by molecular genetic analysis. *Brain Pathol* 1992;3:19–26.
142. Shapiro K, Katz M. The recurrent cerebellar astrocytoma. *Childs Brain* 1983;10:168–176.
143. Civitello LA, et al. Leptomeningeal dissemination of low-grade gliomas in childhood. *Neurology* 1988;38:562–566.
144. Rubinstein LJ. Cytogenesis and differentiation of primitive central neuroepithelial tumors. *J Neuropathol Exp Neurol* 1972;31:7–26.
145. Rorke LB. Origin and histogenesis of medulloblastoma. In: Zeltxer PM, Pochedly C, eds. *Medulloblastomas in children*. New York: Praeger, 1986:14–21.
146. Schwechheimer K, Wiedenmann B, Franke WW. Synaptophysin: a reliable marker for medulloblastomas. *Virchows Arch A Pathol Anat Histopathol* 1987;411:53–59.
147. Molenaar WM, Trojanowski JO. Biological markers of glial and primitive tumors. In: Salcman M, ed. *Neuro-*

biology of brain tumors: concepts in neurosurgery. Vol. 4. Baltimore: Williams & Wilkins, 1991:185–210.

148. Maraziotis J, et al. Neuron-associated class III beta-tubulin isotype, retinal S-antigen, synaptophysin and glial fibrillary acidic protein in human medulloblastomas: a clinicopathological analysis of 36 cases. *Acta Neuropathol* 1992;84:355–363.

149. Janss AJ, et al. Glial differentiation predicts poor clinical outcome in primitive neuroectodermal brain tumors. *Ann Neurol* 1996;39:481–489.

150. Cogen PH, et al. Involvement of multiple chromosome 17p loci in medulloblastoma tumorigenesis. *Am J Hum Genet* 1992;50:584–589.

151. Batra SK, et al. Prognostic implications of chromosome 17p deletions in human medulloblastomas. *J Neurooncol* 1995;24:39–45.

152. Biegel JA, et al. Evidence for a 17p tumor related locus distinct from p53 in pediatric primitive neuroectodermal tumors. *Cancer Res* 1992;52:3391–3395.

153. Gajjar AJ, et al. Relation of tumor-cell ploidy to survival in children with medulloblastoma. *J Clin Oncol* 1993;11:2211–2217.

154. del Charco JO, et al. Medulloblastoma: time-dose relationship based on a 30-year review. *Int J Radiat Oncol Biol Phys* 1998;42:147–154.

155. Katsetos CD, et al. Cerebellar desmoplastic medulloblastomas. A further immunohistochemical characterization of the reticulin-free pale islands. *Arch Pathol Lab Med* 1989;113:1019–1029.

156. Undjian S, Marinov M. Intracranial ependymomas in children. *Childs Nerv Syst* 1990;6:131–134.

157. Reyes-Mugica M, et al. Ependymomas in children: histologic and DNA-flow cytometric study. *Pediatr Pathol* 1994;14:453–466.

158. Schiffer D, et al. Histologic prognostic factors in ependymoma. *Childs Nerv Syst* 1991;7:177–182.

159. Rorke LB. Relationship of morphology of ependymoma in children to prognosis. *Prog Exp Tumor Res* 1987;30:170–174.

160. Tominaga T, et al. Anaplastic ependymomas: clinical features and tumour suppressor gene p53 analysis. *Acta Neurochir (Wien)* 1995;135:163–70.

161. Kepes JJ, Rubenstein LJ, Eng LF. Pleomorphic xanthoastrocytoma: a distinctive meningocerebral glioma of young subjects with relatively favorable prognosis: a study of 12 cases. *Cancer* 1979;44:1839–1852.

162. Kepes J. Pleomorphic xanthoastrocytoma: the birth of a diagnosis and a concept. *Brain Pathol* 1993;3:269–274.

163. Kordek R, et al. Pleomorphic xanthoastrocytoma with a gangliomatous component: an immunohistochemical and ultrastructural study. *Acta Neuropathol (Berl)* 1995;89:194–197.

164. Powell SZ, et al. Divergent differentiation in pleomorphic xanthoastrocytoma. Evidence for a neuronal element and possible relationship to ganglion cell tumors. *Am J Surg Pathol* 1996;20:80–85.

165. Paulus W et al. Molecular genetic alterations in pleomorphic xanthoastrocytoma. *Acta Neuropathol (Berl)* 1996;91:293–297.

166. Tonn JC, et al. Pleomorphic xanthoastrocytoma: report of six cases with special consideration of diagnostic and therapeutic pitfalls. *Surg Neurol* 1997;47:162–169.

167. Wisoff JH, et al. Neurosurgical management and influence of extent of resection on survival in pediatric high-grade astrocytomas: a report on CCG-945. *J Neurosurg* 1993;78:344A.

168. Wolf HK, et al. Ganglioglioma: a detailed histopathological and immunohistochemical analysis of 61 cases. *Acta Neuropathol (Berl)* 1994;88:166–173.

169. Miller DC, Lang FF, Epstein FJ. Central nervous system gangliogliomas. Part 1: Pathology. *J Neurosurg* 1993;79:859–866.

170. Jay V, et al. Malignant transformation in a ganglioglioma with anaplastic neuronal and astrocytic components. Report of a case with flow cytometric and cytogenetic analysis. *Cancer* 1994;73:2862–2868.

171. Johnson JH Jr, et al. Clinical outcome of pediatric gangliogliomas: ninety-nine cases over 20 years. *Pediatr Neurosurg* 1997;27:203–207.

172. Vandenberg SR. Desmoplastic infantile ganglioglioma and desmoplastic cerebral astrocytoma of infancy. *Brain Pathol* 1993;3:275–281.

173. Taratuto AL, et al. Superficial cerebral astrocytoma attached to dura. Report of six cases in infants. *Cancer* 1984;54:2505–2512.

174. Sperner J, et al. Clinical, radiological and histological findings in desmoplastic infantile ganglioglioma. *Child Nerv Syst* 1994;10:458–462.

175. Daumas-Duport, C, et al. Dysembryoplastic neuroepithelial tumor: a surgically curable tumor of young patients with intractable partial seizures. Report of thirty-nine cases. *Neurosurgery* 1988;23:545–556.

176. Daumas-Duport, C. Dysembryoplastic neuroepithelial tumors. *Brain Pathol* 1993;3:283–295.

177. Hirose T, et al. Dysembryoplastic neuroepithelial tumor (DNT): an immunohistochemical and ultrastructural study. *J Neuropathol Exp Neurol* 1994;53:184–195.

178. Cervera-Pierot P, et al. Dysembryoplastic neuroepithelial tumors located in the caudate nucleus area: report of four cases. *Neurosurgery* 1997;40:1065–1069.

179. Molloy PT, et al. Central nervous system medulloepithelioma: a series of eight cases including two arising in the pons. *J Neurosurg* 1996;84:430–436.

180. Rorke LB, Packer RJ, Biegel JA. Central nervous system atypical teratoid/rhabdoid tumors of infancy and childhood: definition of an entity. *J Neurosurg* 1996;85:56–65.

181. Rorke LB, Packer RJ, Biegel JA. Central nervous system atypical teratoid/rhabdoid tumors of infancy and childhood. *J Neurooncol* 1995;24:21–28.

182. Haas JE, et al. Ultrastructure of malignancy rhabdoid tumor of the kidney. A distinctive renal tumor of children. *Hum Pathol* 1981;12:646–657.

183. Biegel JA, et al. Molecular analysis of a partial deletion of 22q in a central nervous system rhabdoid tumor. *Genes Chromosomes Cancer* 1992;5:104–108.

184. Yachnis AT, et al. Characterization of a primary central nervous system atypical teratoid/rhabdoid tumor and derivative cell line: immunophenotype and neoplastic properties. *J Neuropathol Exp Neurol* 1998;57:961–971.

185. Smirniotopoulos JG, Chiechi MV. Teratomas, dermoids, and epidermoids of the head and neck. *Radiographics* 1995;15:1437–1455.

186. Gormley WB, et al. Craniocerebral epidermoid and dermoid tumours: a review of 32 cases. *Acta Neurochir* 1994;128:115–121.

187. Mackenzie IR. Central neurocytoma: histologic atypia, proliferation potential, and clinical outcome. *Cancer* 1999;85:1606–1610.

188. Cushing H. Experiences with the cerebellar astrocytomas. *Surg Gynecol Obstet* 1931;52:129–204.

189. Park TS, et al. Medulloblastoma: clinical presentation and management. Experience at the Hospital for Sick Children, Toronto, 1950–1980. *J Neurosurg* 1983;58: 543–552.

190. Diebler C, Dulac O. *Pediatric neurology and neuroradiology.* Berlin: Springer-Verlag, 1987:296.

191. Stewart TG, Holmes G. Symptomatology of cerebellar tumours: a study of forty cases. *Brain* 1904;27: 522–591.

192. Welchman JM. Computerized tomography of intracranial tuberculomata. *Clin Radiol* 1979;30: 567–573.

193. Komiyama M, et al. MR imaging: possibility of tissue characterization of brain tumors using T1 and T2 values. *Am J Neuroradiol* 1987;8:65–70.

194. Stack JP, et al. Gadolinium-DTPA as a contrast agent in magnetic resonance imaging of the brain. *Neuroradiology* 1988;30:145–154.

195. Zimmerman RD, Bilaniuk LT, Rebsamen S. Magnetic resonance imaging of pediatric posterior fossa tumors. *Pediatr Neurosurg* 1992;18:58–64.

196. O'Reilly G, Hayward RD, Harkness WF. Myelography in the assessment of children with medulloblastoma. *Br J Neurosurg* 1993;7:183–188.

197. Grant FC. Cerebellar symptoms produced by supratentorial tumors: further report. *Arch Neurol Psychiatry* 1928;20:292–308.

198. Lhermitte J, Duclos P. Sur un ganglioneurome diffus du cortex du cervelet. *Bull Assoc Franc Cancer* 1920;9:99107.

199. Padberg GW, et al. Lhermitte-Duclos disease and Cowden disease: a single phakomatosis. *Ann Neurol* 1991;29:517–523.

200. Hair LS, et al. Immunohistochemistry and proliferative activity in Lhermitte-Duclos disease. *Acta Neuropathol (Berl)* 1992;84:570–573.

201. Koch R, et al. Lhermitte-Duclos disease as a component of Cowden's syndrome. Case report and review of the literature. *J Neurosurg* 1999;90: 776–779.

202. Sutphen R et al. Severe Lhermitte-Duclos disease with unique germline mutation of PTEN. *Am J Med Genet* 1999;82:290–293.

203. Matson DD. Cerebellar astrocytomas in childhood. *Pediatrics* 1956;18:150–158.

204. Warnick RE, Edwards MS. Pediatric brain tumors. *Curr Probl Pediatr* 1991;21:129–173.

205. Schneider JH, Raffel C, McComb JG. Benign cerebellar astrocytomas of childhood. *Neurosurgery* 1992;30:58–63.

206. Bloom HJ, Glees J, Bell J. The treatment and long-term prognosis of children with intracranial tumors: a study of 610 cases, 1950 to 1981. *Int J Radiat Oncol Biol Phys* 1990;18:723–745.

207. Wallner KE, et al. Treatment results of juvenile pilocytic astrocytoma. *J Neurosurg* 1988;69: 171–176.

208. Collins VP, Loeffler RK, Tivey H. Observations on growth rates of human tumors. *AJR Am J Roentgenol* 1956;76:988–1000.

209. Packer RJ. Chemotherapy for medulloblastoma/primitive neuroectodermal tumors of the posterior fossa. *Ann Neurol* 1990;28:823–828.

210. Packer RJ, et al. Improved survival with the use of adjuvant chemotherapy in the treatment of medulloblastoma. *J Neurosurg* 1991;74:433–440.

211. Evans AE, et al. The treatment of medulloblastoma. Results of a prospective randomized trial of radiation therapy with and without CCNU, vincristine, and prednisone. *J Neurosurg* 1990;72:572–582.

212. Johnson DL, et al. Quality of long-term survival in young children with medulloblastoma. *J Neurosurg* 1994;80:1004–1010.

213. Duffner PK, et al. Second malignancies in young children with primary brain tumors following treatment with prolonged postoperative chemotherapy and delayed irradiation: a Pediatric Oncology Group study. *Ann Neurol* 1998;44:313–316.

214. Levin VA, et al. Treatment of medulloblastoma with procarbazine, hydroxyurea, and reduced radiation doses to whole brain and spine. *J Neurosurg* 1988;68: 383–387.

215. Tait DM, et al. Adjuvant chemotherapy for medulloblastoma: the first multicentre control trial of the international Society of Pediatric Oncology (SIOP 1). *Eur J Cancer* 1990;26:464–469.

216. Krischer JP, et al. Nitrogen mustard, vincristine, procarbazine, and prednisone as adjuvant chemotherapy in the treatment of medulloblastoma. *J Neurosurg* 1991:74;905-909.

217. Prayson RA, Fischler DF. Cerebrospinal fluid cytology. An 11-year experience with 5951 specimens. *Arch Pathol Lab Med* 1998;122:47-51.

218. Salazar OM. Primary malignant cerebellar astrocytomas in children: a signal for postoperative craniospinal irradiation. *Int J Radiat Oncol Biol Phys* 1981;7:1661–1665.

219. Keene DL, Hsu E, Ventureyra E. Brain tumors in childhood and adolescence. *Pediatr Neurol* 1999;20: 198–203.

220. Jayawickreme DP, Hayward RD, Harkness WF. Intracranial ependymomas in childhood: a report of 24 cases followed for 5 years. *Childs Nerv Syst* 1995;11:409–413.

221. Undjian S, Marinov M. Intracranial ependymomas in children. *Childs Nerv Syst* 1990;6:131–134.

222. Furie DM, Provenzale JM. Supratentorial ependymomas and subependymomas: CT and MR appearance. *J Comput Assist Tomogr* 1995;19:518–526.

223. Palma L, Celli P, Cantore G. Supratentorial ependymomas of the first two decades of life. Long-term follow-up of 20 cases (including two subependymomas). *Neurosurgery* 1993;32:169–175.

224. Ernestus RI, et al. Prognostic relevance of localization and grading in intracranial ependymomas of childhood. *Childs Nerv Syst* 1996;12:522–526.

225. Lyons MK, Kelly PJ. Posterior fossa ependymomas: report of 30 cases and review of the literature. *Neurosurgery* 1991;28:659–664.

226. Rousseau P, et al. Treatment of intracranial ependymomas of children: review of a 15-year experience. *Int J Radiat Oncol Biol Phys* 1994;28:381–386.

227. McLaughlin MP, et al. Ependymoma: results, prognostic factors, and treatment recommendations. *Int J Rad Oncol Biol Phys* 1998;40:845–850.

228. Lefkowitz I, et al. Adjuvant chemotherapy of childhood ependymomas with or without CCNU, vincristine, and prednisone. *Pediatr Neurosci* 1989;14:149.

229. Geyer JR, et al. Survival of infants with primitive neuroectodermal tumors or malignant ependymomas of the CNS treated with eight drugs in 1 day: a report from the children's cancer group. *J Clin Oncol* 1994;12:1607–1615.

230. Duffner PK, et al. Prognostic factors in infants and very young children with intracranial ependymomas. *Pediatr Neurosurg* 1998;28:215–222.

231. Chiu JK, et al. Intracranial ependymoma in children: analysis of prognostic factors. *J Neurooncol* 1992;13: 283–290.

232. Zorlu AF, et al. Intracranial ependymomas: treatment results and prognostic factors. *Radiat Med* 1994;12: 269–272.

232a. van Mourik M, et al. Complex orofacial movements and the disappearance of cerebellar mutism: report of five cases. *Dev Med Child Neurol* 1997;39:686–690.

232b. Dailey AT, McKhann GM, Berger MS. The pathophysiology of oral pharyngeal apraxia and mutism following posterior fossa tumor resection in children. *J Neurosurg* 1995;83:467–475.

232c. Liu GT, et al. Visual impairment associated with mutism after posterior fossa surgery in children. *Neurosurgery* 1998;42:253–256.

233. Maria BL, et al. Brainstem glioma: I. Pathology, clinical features, and therapy. *J Child Neurol* 1993;8:112–128.

234. Mantravardi RVP, et al. Brainstem glioma: an autopsy study of 25 cases. *Cancer* 1982;49:1294–1296.

235. Berger MS, et al. Pediatric brain stem tumors: radiographic, pathological and clinical correlations. *Neurosurgery* 1983;12:298–302.

236. Stroink AR, et al. Diagnosis and management of pediatric brain-stem gliomas. *J Neurosurg* 1986;65:745–750.

237. Louis DN, et al. Molecular genetics of pediatric brain stem gliomas. Application of PCR techniques to small and archival brain tumor specimens. *J Neuropathol Exp Neurol* 1993;52:507–515.

238. Louis DN, et al. Molecular genetics of pediatric brain stem gliomas. Application of PCR techniques to small and archival brain tumor specimens. *J Neuropathol Exp Neurol* 1993;52:507–515.

239. Bray PF, Carter S, Taveras JM. Brainstem tumors in children. *Neurology* 1958;8:17.

240. Flores LE, et al. Delay in the diagnosis of pediatric brain tumors. *Am J Dis Child* 1986;140:684–686.

241. Cohen ME, et al. Prognostic factors in brainstem gliomas. *Neurology* 1986;36:602–605.

242. Panitch HS, Berg BO. Brain stem tumors of childhood and adolescence. *Am J Dis Child* 1970;119: 465–472.

243. Stroink AR, et al. Transependymal benign dorsally exophytic brain stem gliomas in childhood: diagnosis and treatment recommendations. *Neurosurgery* 1987;20:439–444.

244. Packer RJL. Brainstem gliomas of childhood: Magnetic resonance imaging. *Neurology* 1985;35:397–401.

245. Barkovich AJ, et al. Brainstem gliomas: a classification based on magnetic resonance imaging. *Pediatr Neurosurg* 1990;16:73–83.

246. Nelson MD Jr, Soni D, Baram TZ. Necrosis in pontine gliomas: radiation induced or natural history? *Radiology* 1994;191:279–282.

247. Schain RJ, Wilson G. Brain stem encephalitis with radiographic evidence of medullary enlargement. *Neurology* 1971;21:537–539.

248. Albright AL, et al. Prognostic factors in pediatric brain-stem gliomas. *J Neurosurg* 1986;65:751–755.

249. Albright AL, et al. Magnetic resonance scans should replace biopsies for the diagnosis of diffuse brain stem gliomas: a report from the Children's Cancer Group. *Neurosurgery* 1993;33:1026–1029.

250. Edwards MS, Levin VA, Wilson CB. Chemotherapy of pediatric posterior fossa tumors. *Childs Brain* 1980;7:252–260.

251. Wilson CB. Diagnosis and treatment of childhood brain tumors. *Cancer* 1975;35:950–956.

252. Edwards MSB, et al. Hyperfractionated radiation therapy for brain-stem gliomas: A phase I–II trial. *J Neurosurg* 1989;70:691–700.

253. Freeman CR, et al. Hyperfractionated radiation therapy in brain stem tumors. *Cancer* 1991;68:474–481.

254. Finlay JL, et al. Randomized phase III trial in childhood high-grade astrocytoma comparing vincristine, lomustine, and prednisone with the eight-drugs-in-1-day regimen. *J Clin Oncol* 1995;13:112–123.

255. Zeltzer PM, et al. Prolonged response to carboplatin in an infant with brainstem glioma. *Cancer* 1991;67: 43–47.

256. Gaynon PS, et al. Carboplatin in childhood brain tumors. A Children's Cancer Study Group Phase II trial. *Cancer* 1990;66:2465–2469.

257. Allen JC, Helson L. High-dose cyclophosphamide chemotherapy for recurrent CNS tumors in children. *Am J Pediatr Hematol Oncol* 1990;112:297–300.

258. Kedar A, et al. High-dose chemotherapy with marrow reinfusion and hyperfractionated irradiation for children with brainstem glioma. *Proc Am Soc Clin Oncol* 1994;177:428–436.

259. Krestchmar CS, et al. Pre-irradiation chemotherapy and hyperfractionated radiation therapy 66 Gy for children with brain stem tumors: a phase II study of the Pediatric Oncology Group Protocol 8833. *Cancer* 1993;72:1404–1413.

259a. Chuba PJ, et al. Permanent I-125 brain stem implants in children. *Childs Nerv Syst* 1998;14:570–577.

259b. Culver KW, et al. In vivo gene transfer with retroviral vector-producer cells for treatment of experimental brain tumors. *Science* 1992;256:1550–1552.

259c. Fueyo J, et al. Targeting in gene therapy for gliomas. *Arch Neurol* 1999;56:445–448.

260. Richmond IL, Wilson CB. Parasellar tumors in children. I. Clinical presentation, preoperative assessment, and differential diagnosis. *Childs Brain* 1980;7:73–84.

260a. Crotty TB, et al. Papillary craniopharyngioma: a clinicopathological study of 48 cases. *J Neurosurg* 1995;83:206–214.

261. Liszczak T, et al. Morphological, biochemical, ultrastructural, tissue culture and clinical observations of typical and aggressive craniopharyngiomas. *Acta Neuropathol* 1978;43:191–203.

262. Northfield DWC. Rathke-pouch tumours. *Brain* 1957;80:293–312.

263. Epstein F, McCleary EL. Intrinsic brain-stem tumors of childhood. Surgical indications. *J Neurosurg* 1986;64:11–15.

264. Bingas B, Wolter M. Das Kraniopharyngiom. *Fortschr Neurol Psychiatr* 1968;36:117–195.
265. Imura H, Kato Y, Nakai Y. Endocrine aspects of tumors arising from suprasellar, third ventricular regions. *Prog Exp Tumor Res* 1987;30:313–324.
266. Newman CB, Levine LS, New MI. Endocrine function in children with intrasellar and suprasellar neoplasms. *Am J Dis Child* 1981;135:259–262.
267. Cacciari E, et al. How many cases of true precocious puberty are idiopathic? *J Pediatr* 1983;102:357–360.
268. Bailey P. Concerning the cerebellar symptoms produced by suprasellar tumors. *Arch Neurol Psychiatry* 1924;11:137–150.
269. Ito H, et al. Preoperative diagnosis of Rathke's cleft cyst. *Childs Nerv Syst* 1987;3:225–227.
270. Brummitt ML, Kline LB, Wilson ER. Craniopharyngioma: pitfalls in diagnosis. *J Clin Neuroophthalmol* 1992;12:77–81.
271. Russell RWR, Pennybacker JB. Craniopharyngioma in the elderly. *J Neurol Neurosurg Psychiatry* 1961;24:1–13.
272. Watkins L, et al. Skull base chordomas: a review of 38 patients, 1958–1988. *Br J Neurosurg* 1993;7:241–248.
273. Kaneko Y, et al. Chordoma in early childhood: a clinicopathological study. *Neurosurgery* 1991;29:442–446.
274. Matsumoto J, Towbin RB, Ball WS. Cranial chordomas in infancy and childhood: a report of two cases and review of the literature. *Pediatr Radiol* 1989;20:28–32.
275. Hoffman HJ, et al. Investigation and management of suprasellar arachnoid cysts. *J Neurosurg* 1982;57:597–602.
276. Nellhaus G. The bobble-head doll syndrome. A "tic" with a neuropathologic basis. *Pediatrics* 1967;40:250–253.
277. Russell A. A diencephalic syndrome of emaciation in infancy and childhood [Abstract]. *Arch Dis Child* 1951;26:2–74.
278. Shillito J. Treatment of craniopharyngioma. *Clin Neurosurg* 1986;33:533–546.
279. Yasargil MG, et al. Total removal of craniopharyngiomas. Approaches and long-term results in 144 patients. *J Neurosurg* 1990;73:3–11.
280. Jose CC, et al. Radiotherapy for the treatment of recurrent craniopharyngioma. *Clin Oncol (R Coll Radiol)* 1992;5:287–289.
281. Rajan B, et al. Craniopharyngioma—long-term results following limited surgery and radiotherapy. *Radiother Oncol* 1993;26:1–10.
282. Regine WF, Kramer S. Pediatric craniopharyngiomas: long-term results of combined treatment with surgery and radiation. *Int J Radiation Oncology Biol Phys* 1992;24:611–617.
283. Hoffman HJ. Craniopharyngiomas. *Can J Neurol Sci* 1985;12:348–352.
284. de Vile CJ, et al. Management of childhood craniopharyngioma: can the morbidity of radical surgery be predicted? *J Neurosurg* 1996;85:73–81.
285. Fisher PG, et al. Outcomes and failure patterns in childhood craniopharyngiomas. *Childs Nerv Syst* 1998;14:558–563.
286. Richmond IL, Wilson CB. Parasellar tumors in children. II. Surgical management, radiation therapy and follow-up. *Childs Brain* 1980;7:85–94.

287. Bernstein M, Laperriere NJ. A critical appraisal of brachytherapy for pediatric brain tumors. *Pediatr Neurosurg* 1990–91;16:213–218.
288. Van den Berge JH, et al. Intracavitary brachytherapy of cystic craniopharyngiomas. *J Neurosurg* 1992;77:545–550.
289. Backlund EO. Colloidal radioisotopes as part of a multi-modality treatment of craniopharyngiomas. *J Neurol Sci* 1989;33:95–97.
290. Lyen KR, Grant DB. Endocrine function, morbidity and mortality after surgery for craniopharyngioma. *Arch Dis Child* 1982;57:837–841.
291. Honegger J, Buchfelder M, Fahlbusch R. Surgical treatment of craniopharyngiomas: endocrinological results. *J Neurosurg* 1999;90:251–257.
292. de Vile CJ, et al. Obesity in childhood craniopharyngioma: relation to post-operative hypothalamic damage shown by magnetic resonance imaging. *J Clin Endocrin Metab* 1996;81:2734–2737.
292a. Fahlbusch R, et al. Surgical treatment of craniopharyngiomas: experience with 168 patients. *J Neurosurg* 1999;90:237–250.
293. Anderson CA, et al. Neurobehavioral outcome in pediatric craniopharyngioma. *Pediatr Neurosurg* 1997;26:255–260.
294. Martin P, Cushing H. Primary gliomas of chiasm and optic nerves in their intracranial portion. *Arch Ophthalmol* 1923;52:209–241.
295. Imes RK, Hoyt WF. Childhood chiasmal gliomas. Update on the fate of patients in the 1969 San Francisco study. *Prog Exp Tumor Res* 1987;30:108–112.
296. Listernick R, Charrow J. Neurofibromatosis type 1 in childhood. *J Pediatr* 1990;116:845–853.
297. Chutorian AM, et al. Optic gliomas in children. *Neurology* 1964;14:83–95.
298. Iraci G, et al. Gliomas of the optic nerve and chiasm: a clinical review. *Childs Brain* 1981;8:326–349.
299. Lindblom B, Truwit CL, Hoyt WF. Optic nerve sheath meningioma. Definition of intraorbital, intracanalicular, and intracranial components with magnetic resonance imaging. *Ophthalmology* 1992;99:560–566.
300. Dunn DW, Purvin V. Optic pathway gliomas in neurofibromatosis. *Dev Med Child Neurol* 1990;32:820–824.
301. Hoffman HJ, et al. Optic pathway/hypothalamic gliomas: a dilemma in management. *Pediatr Neurosurg* 1993;19:186–195.
302. Alvord EC, Lofton S. Gliomas of the optic nerve or chiasm. *J Neurosurg* 1988;68:85–98.
303. Tao ML, et al. Childhood optic chiasm gliomas: radiographic response following radiotherapy and long-term clinical outcome. *Int J Radiat Oncol Biol Phys* 1997;39:579–587.
304. Tenny RT, et al. The neurosurgical management of optic glioma. Results in 104 patients. *J Neurosurg* 1982;57:452–458.
305. Jenkin D, et al. Optic glioma in childhood. Resection, irradiation or surveillance? The University of Toronto experience [Abstract]. *Pediatic Neurosurg* 1990–91;16:1–27.
306. Packer RJ, et al. Treatment of chiasmatic/hypothalamic gliomas of childhood with chemotherapy: an update. *Ann Neurol* 1988;23:79–85.
307. Petronio J, et al. Management of chiasmal and hypothalamic gliomas of infancy and childhood with chemotherapy. *J Neurosurg* 1991;74:701–708.

308. Packer RJ, et al. Carboplatin and vincristine for recurrent and newly diagnosed low-grade gliomas of childhood. *J Clin Oncol* 1993;11:850–856.
309. Chamberlain MC, Grafe MR. Recurrent chiasmatic-hypothalamic glioma treated with oral etoposide. *J Clin Oncol* 1995;13:2072–2076.
310. Vaquero J, Ramiro J, Martínez R. Clinicopathological experience with pineocytomas: report of five surgically treated cases. *Neurosurgery* 1990;27:618–619.
311. Edwards MSB, Hudgins RJ, Wilson CB. Pineal region tumors in children. *J Neurosurg* 1988;68:689–696.
312. Russell WO, Sachs E. Pinealoma: a clinicopathologic study of seven cases with a review of the literature. *Arch Pathol* 1943;35:869–888.
313. Jooma R, Kendall BE. Diagnosis and management of pineal tumors. *J Neurosurg* 1983;58:654–665.
314. Hoffman HJ, et al. Experience with pineal region tumors in childhood. *Neurol Res* 1984;6:107–112.
315. Schild SE, et al. Pineal parenchymal tumors: clinical, pathologic, and therapeutic aspects. *Cancer* 1994;72:870–880.
316. Bodensteiner JB, et al. Incidental pineal cysts in a prospectively ascertain normal cohort. *Clin Pediatr* 1996;35:277–279.
317. Stein BM, Bruce JN. Surgical management of pineal region tumors. *Clin Neurosurg* 1992;39:509–532.
318. Hiraga S, et al. A study of 31 juvenile patients with primary intracranial germ cell tumor [Abstract]. *Pediatr Neurosurg* 1990–91;16:1–18.
319. Kageyama, N, et al. Intracranial germinal tumors. *Prog Exp Tumor Res* 1987;30:255–267.
320. Posner M, Horrax G. Eye signs in pineal tumors. *J Neurosurg* 1946;3:15–24.
321. Pesin SR, Shields JA. Seven cases of trilateral retinoblastoma. *Am J Ophthalmol* 1989;107:121–126.
322. Zimmerman RA. Computed tomography on pineal, parapineal and histologically related tumors. *Radiology* 1980;137:669–677.
323. Ganti SR, et al. CT of pineal region tumors. *Am J Neuroradiol* 1986;7:97–104.
324. Hoffman HJ. Pineal region tumors. *Prog Exp Tumor Res* 1987;30:281–288.
325. Edwards MSB, Hudgins RJ, Wilson CB. Pineal region tumors in children. *J Neurosurg* 1988;68:689–696.
326. Vaquero J, Ramiro J, Martínez R. Clinicopathological experience with pineocytomas: report of five surgically treated cases. *Neurosurgery* 1990;27:618–619.
327. Lapras C, et al. Direct surgery for pineal tumors: Occipital-transtentorial approach. *Prog Exp Tumor Res* 1987;30:268–280.
328. Packer RJ, et al. Choroid plexus carcinoma of childhood. *Cancer* 1992;69:580–585.
329. Pierga JY, et al. Carcinoma of the choroid plexus: a pediatric experience. *Med Pediatr Oncol* 1993;21:480–487.
330. Zwetsloot CP, Kros JM, Pay y Gueze HD. Familial occurrence of tumors of the choroid plexus. *J Med Genet* 1991;28:492–494.
331. Trifiletti RR, et al. Aicardi syndrome with multiple tumors: a case report with literature review. *Brain Dev* 1995;17:283–285.
332. Johnson DL. Management of choroid plexus tumors in children. *Pediatr Neurosci* 1989;15:195–206.
333. Maria BL, et al. Response of a recurrent choroid plexus tumor to combination chemotherapy. *J Neurooncol* 1985;3:259–262.
334. Mathiesen T, et al. Third ventricle colloid cysts: a consecutive 12-year series. *J Neurosurg* 1997;86:5–12.
335. Macaulay RJ, et al. Histological and ultrastructural analysis of six colloid cysts in children. *Acta Neuropathol* 1997;93:271–276.
336. Teng P, Papatheodorou C. Tumors of cerebral ventricles in children. *J Nerv Ment Dis* 1966;142:87–93.
337. Antunes JL, Louis KM, Ganti SR. Colloid cysts of the third ventricle. *Neurosurgery* 1980;7:450–455.
338. McMackin D, et al. Correlation of fornix damage with memory impairment in six cases of colloid cyst removal. *Acta Neurochir* 1995;13:12–18.
339. Styne DM, et al. Treatment of Cushing's disease in childhood and adolescence by transsphenoidal microadenomectomy. *N Engl J Med* 1984;310:889–893.
340. Kanter SL, et al. Pituitary adenomas in pediatric patients: are they more invasive? *Pediatr Neurosci* 1985;12:202–204.
341. Gjerris F. Clinical aspects and long-term prognosis in supratentorial tumors in infancy and childhood. *Acta Neurol Scand* 1978;57:445–470.
342. Reifenberger J, et al. Molecular genetic analysis of oligodendroglial tumors shows preferential allelic deletions on 19p and 1p. *Am J Pathol* 1994;145:1175–1190.
343. Kraus JA, et al. Shared allelic losses on chromosomes 1p and 19q suggest a common origin of oligodendroglioma and oligoastrocytoma. *J Neuropathol Exp Neurol* 1995;54:91–95.
344. Sutton LN, et al. Cerebral gangliogliomas of childhood. *Prog Exp Tumor Res* 1987;30:239–246.
345. Wolf HK, et al. Ganglioglioma: a detailed histopathological and immunohistochemical analysis of 61 cases. *Acta Neuropathol (Berl)* 1994;88:166–173.
346. Miller DC, Lang FF, Epstein FJ. Central nervous system gangliogliomas. Part 1. Pathology. *J Neurosurg* 1993;79:859–866.
347. Jay V, et al. Malignant transformation in a ganglioglioma with anaplastic neuronal and astrocytic components. Report of a case with flow cytometric and cytogenetic analysis. *Cancer* 1994;73:2862–2868.
348. Cooper M, Dohn DF. Intracranial meningiomas in childhood. *Cleve Clin Quart* 1974;41:197–204.
349. Merten DF, et al. Meningiomas of childhood and adolescence. *J Pediatr* 1974;84:696–700.
350. Howe JG, Gibson JD. Uncinate seizures and tumors, a myth reexamined. *Ann Neurol* 1982;12:2–27.
351. Page LK, Lombroso CT, Matson DD. Childhood epilepsy with late detection of cerebral glioma. *J Neurosurg* 1969;31:253–261.
352. Blume WT, Girvin JP, Kaufmann JCE. Childhood brain tumors presenting as chronic uncontrolled focal seizure disorders. *Ann Neurol* 1982;12:538–541.
353. Dropcho EJ, et al. Supratentorial malignant gliomas in childhood: a review of fifty cases. *Ann Neurol* 1987;22:355–364.
354. Laws ER Jr, et al. Neurosurgical management of low-grade astrocytoma of the cerebral hemispheres. *J Neurosurg* 1984;61:665–673.
355. Gajjar A, et al. Response of pediatric low grade gliomas to chemotherapy. *Pediatr Neurosurg* 1993;19:113–120.

356. North CA, et al. Low-grade cerebral astrocytomas. Survival and quality of life after radiation therapy. *Cancer* 1990;66:6–14.

357. Berger MS, Ojemann GA, Lettich E. Neurophysiological monitoring during astrocytoma surgery. *Neurosurg Clin N Am* 1990;1:65–80.

358. Mahaley MS Jr, et al. National survey of patterns of care for brain-tumor patients. *J Neurosurg* 1989;71:826–836.

359. Phuphanich S, et al. Supratentorial malignant gliomas of childhood. Results of treatment with radiation therapy and chemotherapy. *J Neurosurg* 1984;60:495–499.

360. Sposto R, et al. The effectiveness of chemotherapy for treatment of high grade astrocytoma in children: results of a randomized trial. *J Neurooncol* 1989;7:165–177.

361. Cairncross JG, Macdonald DR. Malignant oligodendroglioma: a chemosensitive tumor. *Proc ASCO* 1988;7:3–33.

362. Mahoney DH Jr, et al. High-dose melphalan and cyclophosphamide with autologous bone marrow rescue for recurrent/progressive malignant brain tumor in children: a pilot pediatric oncology group study. *J Clin Oncol* 1996;14:382–388.

363. Sneed PK, et al. Long-term follow-up after high-activity ^{125}I brachytherapy for pediatric brain tumors. *Pediatr Neurosurg* 1996;24:314–322.

364. Coffey RJ, Lunsford LD, Flickinger JC. The role of radiosurgery in the treatment of malignant brain tumors. *Neurosurg Clin N Am* 1992;3:231–244.

364a. Pollock BE, et al. The Mayo Clinic gamma knife experience: indications and initial results. *Mayo Clin Proc* 1999;74:5–13.

365. Fathallah-Shaykh H. New molecular strategies to cure brain tumors. *Arch Neurol* 1999;56:449–453.

366. Tomita T, McLone DG. Brain tumors during the first twenty-four months of life. *Neurosurgery* 1985;17:913–919.

367. Cohen BH, et al. Brain tumors in children under 2 years: treatment, survival and long-term prognosis. *Pediatr Neurosurg* 1993;19:171–179.

368. Deutsch M. Radiotherapy for primary brain tumors in very young children. *Cancer* 1982;50:2785–2789.

369. Jooma R, Kendall BE, Hayward RD. Intracranial tumors in neonates: a report of seventeen cases. *Surg Neurol* 1984;21:165–170.

370. Suc E, et al. Brain tumours under the age of three. The price of survival. A retrospective study of 20 long-term survivors. *Acta Neurochir (Wien)* 1990;106:93–98.

371. Strauss LC, et al. Efficacy of postoperative chemotherapy using cisplatin plus etoposide in young children with brain tumors. *Med Pediatr Oncol* 1991;19:16–21.

372. Tait DM, et al. Adjuvant chemotherapy for medulloblastoma: the first multicentre control trial of the International Society of Paediatric Oncology (SIOP I). *Eur J Cancer* 1990;26:464–469.

373. Krischer JP, et al. Nitrogen mustard, vincristine, procarbazine, and prednisone as adjuvant chemotherapy in the treatment of medulloblastoma. *J Neurosurg* 1991;74:905–909.

374. Kovnar EH, et al. Preirradiation cisplatin and etoposide in the treatment of high-risk medulloblastoma and other malignant embryonal tumors of the central nervous system: a phase II study. *J Clin Oncol* 1990;8:330–336.

375. Finlay J, et al. Randomized phase III trial in childhood high-grade astrocytomas comparing vincristine, lomustine and prednisone with eight-drug-in-one-day regimen. *J Clin Oncol* 1995;13:112–123.

376. Maria BL. High dose chemotherapy in the treatment of children with infiltrative brain tumors. *Int Pediatr* 1993;8:244–249.

377. Kedar A, et al. High-dose chemotherapy with marrow reinfusion and hyperfractionated irradiation for children with high-risk brain tumors. *Med Pediatr Oncol* 1994;23:428–436.

378. Shen V, et al. Collection and use of peripheral blood stem cells in young children with refractory solid tumors. *Bone Marrow Transplant* 1997;19:197–204.

379. Pascual-Castroviejo I. Epidemiology of spinal cord tumors in children. In: Pascual-Castroviejo I, eds. *International review of child neurology series: spinal tumors in children and adolescents*. New York: Raven Press, 1990:1–10.

380. Di Lorenzo N, Giuffre R, Fortuna A. Primary spinal neoplasms in childhood: analysis of 1234 published cases (including 56 personal cases) by pathology, sex, age and site. Differences from the situation in adults. *Neurochirurgia (Stuttg)* 1982;25:153–164.

381. Arseni C, Horvath L, Iliescu D. Intraspinal tumours in children. *Psychiatr Neurol Neurochir* 1967;70:123–133.

382. Stella G, et al. Benign tumors of the pediatric spine: statistical notes. *Chir Organi Mov* 1998;83:15–21.

383. Murovic J, Sundaresan N. Pediatric spinal axis tumors. *Neurosurg Clin N Am* 1992;3:947–958.

384. Pascual-Castroviejo I, ed. *Spinal tumors in children and adolescents*. New York: Raven Press, 1990.

385. Steinbok P, Cochrane DD, Poskitt K. Intramedullary spinal cord tumors in children. *Neurosurg Clin N Am* 1992;3:931–945.

386. O'Sullivan C, et al. Spinal cord tumors in children: long-term results of combined surgical and radiation treatment. *J Neurosurg* 1994;81:507–512.

387. Escalona-Zapata J. Epidemiology of spinal cord tumors in children. In: Pascual-Castroviejo I, eds. *International review of child neurology series: spinal tumors in children and adolescents*. New York: Raven Press, 1990:11–34.

388. Kwon OK, et al. Primary intramedullary spinal cord primitive neuroectodermal tumor with intracranial seeding in an infant. *Childs Nerv Syst* 1996;12:633–636.

389. Nam DH, et al. Intramedullary anaplastic oligodendroglioma in a child. *Childs Nerv Syst* 1998;14:127–130.

390. Chadduck WM, Frederick AB, Sawyer JR. Cytogenetic studies of pediatric brain and spinal cord tumors. *Pediatr Neurosurg* 1991–92;17:57–65.

391. Levy WJ, Bay J, Dohn D. Spinal cord meningioma. *J Neurosurg* 1982;57:804–812.

392. Richardson FL. A report of 16 tumors of the spinal cord: the importance of spinal rigidity as an early sign of disease. *J Pediatr* 1960;57:42–54.

393. Constantini S, et al. Intramedullary spinal cord tumors in children under the age of 3 years. *J Neurosurg* 1996;85:1036–1043.

394. Buchanan DN. Tumors of the spinal cord in infancy [Abstract]. *Arch Neurol Psychiatry* 1950;63:835.

395. Haft H, Ransohoff J, Carter S. Spinal cord tumors in children. *Pediatrics* 1959;23:1152–1159.

396. Ross AT, Bailey OT. Tumors arising within the spinal canal in children. *Neurology* 1953;3:922–930.
397. Oi S, Raimondi AJ. Hydrocephalus associated with intraspinal neoplasms in childhood. *Am J Dis Child* 1981;135:1122–1124.
398. Rifkinson-Mann S, Wisoff JH, Epstein F. The association of hydrocephalus with intramedullary spinal cord tumors: a series of 25 patients. *Neurosurgery* 1990;27:749–754.
399. Innocenzi G, et al. Intramedullary astrocytomas and ependymomas in the pediatric age group: a retrospective study. *Childs Nerv Syst* 1996;12:776–780.
400. Bouffet E, et al. Prognostic factors in pediatric spinal cord astrocytoma. *Cancer* 1998;83:2391–2399.
401. Robertson PL. Atypical presentations of spinal cord tumors in children. *J Child Neurol* 1992;7:360–363.
402. Eeg-Olofsson O, Carlsson E, Jeppson S. Recurrent abdominal pains as the first symptom of spinal cord tumor. *Acta Paediatr Scand* 1981;70:595–597.
403. Taylor LJ. Painful scoliosis: a need for further investigation. *BMJ* 1985;292:120–122.
404. Blaser S, Harwood-Nash D. Pediatric spinal neoplasms. *Top Magn Reson Imaging* 1993;5:190–202.
405. Quisling RG. Imaging for pediatric brain tumors. *Semin Pediatr Neurol* 1997;4:254–272.
406. Epstein FJ, Farmer JP, Schneider SJ. Intraoperative ultrasonography: an important surgical adjunct for intramedullary tumors. *J Neurosurg* 1991;74:729–733.
407. Kothbauer K, Deletis V, Epstein FJ. Intraoperative spinal cord monitoring for intramedullary surgery: an essential adjunct. *Pediatr Neurosurg* 1997;26: 247–254.
408. Epstein FJ. Surgical treatment of intramedullary spinal cord tumors of childhood. In: Pascual-Castroviejo I, eds. *International review of child neurology series: spinal tumors in children and adolescents*. New York: Raven Press, 1990:51–70.
409. Mottl H, Koutecky J. Treatment of spinal cord tumors in children. *Med Pediatr Oncol* 1997;29:293–295.
410. Goh KY, Velasquez L, Epstein FJ. Pediatric intramedullary spinal cord tumors: is surgery alone enough? *Pediatr Neurosurg* 1997;27:34–39.
411. Godwin-Austin RB, Howell DA, Worthington B. Observations in radiation myelopathy. *Brain* 1975;98:557–568.
412. DiChiro G, Herdt JR. Angiographic demonstration of spinal cord arterial occlusion in post-radiation myelomalacia. *Radiology* 1973;106:317–319.
413. Wara WM, et al. Radiation tolerance of the spinal cord. *Cancer* 1975;35:1558–1562.
414. Quincke H. Ueber Meningitis serosa. Volkmann's Sammlung klinischer Vorträge. N F 1893, Nr. 67. Cited in: Quincke H. Ueber Meningitis serosa und verwandte Zustände. *Deutsch Z Nervenheilk* 1897;9:149–168.
415. Johnston I, Paterson A. Benign intracranial hypertension. I. Diagnosis and prognosis. *Brain* 1974;97: 289–300.
416. Feldman MH, Schlezinger NS. Benign intracranial hypertension associated with hypervitaminosis A.

Arch Neurol 1970;22:1–7.
417. Soler D, et al. Diagnosis and management of benign intracranial hypertension. *Arch Dis Child* 1998;78: 89–94.
417a. Konrad D, Kuster H, Hunziker UA. Pseudotumour cerebri after varicella. *Eur J Pediatr* 1998;157: 904–906.
418. Walker AE, Adamkiewicz JJ. Pseudotumor cerebri associated with prolonged corticosteroid therapy: reports of four cases. *JAMA* 1964;188:779–784.
419. Gills JP, Kapp JP, Odom GL. Benign intracranial hypertension: pseudotumor cerebri from obstruction of dural sinuses. *Arch Ophthalmol* 1967;78:592–595.
420. Rush JA. Pseudotumor cerebri: clinical profile and visual outcome in 63 patients. *Mayo Clin Proc* 1980;55:541–546.
421. Greer M. Benign intracranial hypertension. IV. Menarche. *Neurology* 1964;14:569–573.
422. McComb JG. Recent research into the nature of cerebrospinal fluid formation and absorption. *J Neurosurg* 1983;59:369–383.
423. Moser FG, et al. MR imaging of pseudotumor cerebri. *Am J Radiol* 1988;4:903–909.
424. Foley J. Benign forms of intracranial hypertension—"toxic" and "otitic" hydrocephalus. *Brain* 1955;78: 1–41.
425. Greer M. Benign intracranial hypertension. I. Mastoiditis and lateral sinus obstruction. *Neurology* 1962;12:472–476.
426. Babikian P, Corbett J, Bell W. Idiopathic intracranial hypertension in children: the Iowa experience. *J Child Neurol* 1994;9:144–149.
427. Speer C, et al. Fourth cranial nerve palsy in pediatric patients with pseudotumor cerebri. *Am J Ophthalmol* 1999;127:236–237.
428. Jacobson DM, et al. Computed tomography ventricular size has no predictive value in diagnosing pseudotumor cerebri. *Neurology* 1990;40: 1454–1455.
429. Rosenberg ML, et al. Cerebrospinal fluid diversion procedures in pseudotumor cerebri. *Neurology* 1993;43:1071–1072.
430. Corbett JJ, Thompson HS. The rational management of idiopathic intracranial hypertension. *Arch Neurol* 1989;46:1049–1051.
431. Baker RS, Baumann RJ, Buncic JR. Idiopathic intracranial hypertension (pseudotumor cerebri) in pediatric patients. *Pediatr Neurol* 1989;5:5–11.
432. Grant DN. Benign intracranial hypertension. A review of 79 cases in infancy and childhood. *Arch Dis Child* 1971;46:651–655.
433. Guidetti B, Giuffre R, Gambacorta D. Follow-up study of 100 cases of pseudotumor cerebri. *Acta Neurochir* 1968;18:259–267.
434. Corbett JJ, et al. Visual loss in pseudotumor cerebri. Follow up of 57 patients from 5 to 41 years and a profile of 14 patients with permanent severe visual loss. *Arch Neurol* 1982;39:461–474.

Chapter 11

Neurocutaneous Syndromes

John H. Menkes and *Bernard L. Maria

*Departments of Neurology and Pediatrics, University of California, Los Angeles,
UCLA School of Medicine, and Department of Pediatric Neurology, Cedars-Sinai Medical Center, Los
Angeles, California 90048; and *Department of Pediatrics, University of Florida
College of Medicine, Gainesville, Florida 32610*

The neurocutaneous syndromes are marked by the conjoined abnormalities of skin and nervous system. The term *phakomatoses* (*phakomatosis* from φακοσ, Greek for *lentil*) is reserved for a group of diseases in which the subject is predisposed to tumors of the skin, nervous system, and other organs. The major entities included among the phakomatoses are the neurofibromatoses, tuberous sclerosis (TS), Sturge-Weber syndrome (SWS), von Hippel–Lindau disease, and ataxia-telangiectasia (AT).

Additionally, numerous other conditions exist, many of uncertain heredity and some extremely rare, in which abnormalities of skin are linked with those of the nervous system. These are detailed in a book edited by Gomez (1).

NEUROFIBROMATOSIS (VON RECKLINGHAUSEN DISEASE)

No longer considered to be a single disorder, neurofibromatosis has been divided into at least two genetically distinct forms. The common form, once known as *peripheral neurofibromatosis*, is called *neurofibromatosis 1* (NF1). The other, rarer form, once termed *central neurofibromatosis*, is now called *neurofibromatosis 2* (NF2). Additionally, several authorities distinguish segmental neurofibromatosis, in which the features of NF1 are confined to one part of the body, spinal neurofibromatosis, characterized by the late appearance of spinal cord tumors, and a condition marked by autosomal dominant café au lait spots.

Neurofibromatosis 1

NF1 is characterized by multiple tumors within the central and peripheral nervous systems, cutaneous pigmentation, and lesions of the vascular system and viscera. Additionally, a tendency exists for a variety of tissues to undergo malignant transformation. Although it was described initially in the eighteenth century, and more succinctly in 1849 by Smith (2), von Recklinghausen in 1882 first combined the various features of the condition and termed it *neurofibromatosis* (3). The disease occurs in approximately 1 in 3,000 live births and is transmitted as a dominant trait with variable expression but virtually complete penetrance by the age of 5 years (4). It is the most common single-gene defect to affect the nervous system. Approximately one-half of the cases appear to be sporadic, and the mutation rate has been estimated at 1 in 10,000 gametes per generation, one of the highest mutation rates in humans (5). Stephens and coworkers found that 93% of new mutations were in the paternally derived chromosome (6). For as yet unknown reasons, no parental age effect occurs. As determined by linkage analysis and translocation breakpoints, the gene for NF1 is located on the long arm of chromosome 17, near the centromere (q11.2). It has been cloned and consists of 59 exons that are spread out over 350 kb of genomic DNA and gives rise to several alternatively spliced transcripts (7). The gene encodes a cytoplasmic protein, named *neurofibromin*, which contains a large amino acid segment that is homologous to the functional domain of the *p21ras*-GTPase activating protein. This protein inactivates the tumor gene *p21ras* by stimulating its GTPase activity and converting the active form of *p21ras* into its inactive form. Inasmuch as the active form of *p21ras* is a specific growth regulator for astrocytes, the NF1 gene functions as a tumor-suppressor gene (8,9,9a). This is confirmed by the observation that loss of NF1 gene expression occurs in at least some neurofibroma, in neurosarcoma, and in leukemic cells derived from NF1 subjects (8,10,11). Neurofibromin also has been shown to be associated with cytoplasmic microtubules in the brain and is believed to be involved in signaling within the central nervous system (CNS).

The NF1 gene is large and is intrinsically hypermutable; more than 100 mutations have been described, and only rarely has the same mutation been identified in unrelated patients. Mutations include large deletions seen in 7.5% to 17% of patients (12,12a), frame shifts, stop mutations, and point mutations. The majority (60% to 70%) of mutations result in the formation of truncated and nonfunctioning neurofibromin. Somatic mosaicism is fairly common; its exact frequency has not been ascertained (12). NF1 gene expression is complex and is modulated posttranscriptionally by numerous alternative splicings and RNA editing (13). Some of the alternative transcripts lack tumor suppressor activity and are developmentally regulated. Their role in producing the clinical phenotype of NF1 is not understood (13,14).

It, therefore, comes as no surprise that there is much variability in the expression of NF1, even within the same family. Correlation between the genetic mutation and the clinical expression is poor. However, a significant proportion of subjects with severe manifestations including dysmorphic features have large deletions in the NF1 gene (15).

Pathology

The most striking neuropathologic feature is the presence of tumors along the major peripheral nerves, with the ulnar and radial nerves being involved most frequently. Neurofibromas are the most common tumor type, but schwannomas also can be seen. Tumors that are prone to develop within the CNS include primarily optic gliomas; pilocystic astrocytomas of the third ventricle, cerebellum, and spinal cord; and high-grade astrocytomas (16). Additionally, neurofibromatosis has been associated with a number of other neoplastic processes with a greater than random frequency (17). These include leukemia, Wilms tumor, neuroblastoma, and pheochromocytoma. A syndrome of multiple endocrine neoplasia characterized by bilateral pheochromocytomas, medullary thyroid carcinoma, and multiple neuromas and café au lait lesions has been delineated (18). Although generally benign, both central and peripheral neurofibromas can undergo malignant degeneration. This is particularly likely to occur with the plexiform neurofibroma, for which the risk for malignant transformation to neurofibrosarcoma has been estimated at 5% (19).

Clinical Manifestations

NF1 is a progressive disease process that can affect almost every organ. When many peripheral lesions are present, few lesions tend to be within the CNS. The reverse also is true (20).

The most common skin lesions are the café au lait spots. These are numerous light brown areas, usually located over the trunk, with smooth, well-defined borders and uniform pigmentation. They are seen in virtually every patient with NF1, and they result from an aggregation of neural crest-derived pigmented melanoblasts in the basal layer of the epidermis (4). They are present at birth and their number and size increase until puberty. According to Crowe and associates, at least six such lesions are necessary for a diagnosis of NF1 (21). Less frequent are diffuse freckling, freckling under the armpits, and large areas of faintly increased pigmentation (melanoderma). Although usually present before the onset of neurologic symptoms, these pigmentary abnormalities are not striking during infancy but intensify with age, particularly after puberty.

Various types of cutaneous tumors can be found (Fig. 11.1). The most characteristic for NF1 is the pedunculated molluscum fibrosum and the subcutaneous neurofibromas. The latter consist of an overgrowth of Schwann cells admixed with tortuous nerve fibers and perineural fibroblasts. They are located singly or in groups along nerve trunks. Generally, cutaneous tumors tend to enlarge slowly throughout life. Plexiform neuromas can occur in all affected tissues and lead to hypertrophy of one or more extremity, exophthalmos, or defects of the skull and orbit. Multiple nodules within the iris (iris hamartomas) (Fig. 11.2) were first described by Lisch (22). Lisch nodules are seen in almost all affected individuals aged 21 or more years, but only in one-half of children aged 5 to 6 years (23). Initially light colored, they become darker with time.

Short stature is common. It was seen in 31.5% of patients in the series of Huson and Rosser (4).

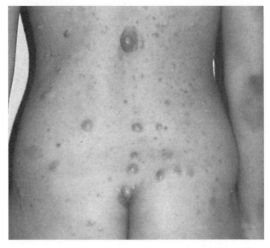

FIG. 11.1. Neurofibromatosis. Posterior view demonstrating various types of cutaneous tumors. These include the pedunculated molluscum fibrosum and subcutaneous neurofibromas. Note the area of hyperpigmentation of the right elbow and a typical café au lait lesion. (Courtesy of Dr. V. M. Riccardi, Neurofibromatosis Institute, La Crescenta, CA.)

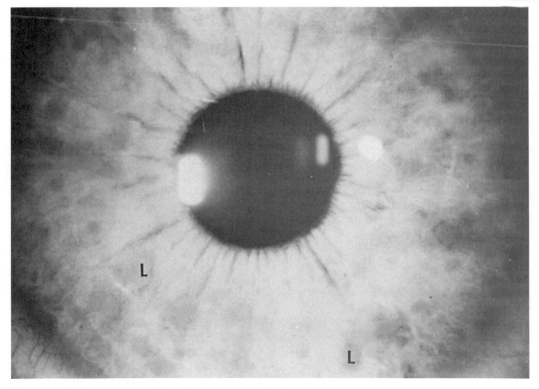

FIG. 11.2. Lisch nodules of iris (L). (Courtesy of Dr. Bronwyn Bateman, Department of Ophthalmology, University of Colorado School of Medicine, Denver.)

A large proportion of these children experiences growth hormone deficiency. The cause of this deficiency is not clear; in some instances it is probably the result of an intracranial tumor involving the hypothalamic region (23a). Various skeletal abnormalities have been described. Of these, low cervical or thoracic kyphoscoliosis is encountered most often. It was noted in 32% of children in the series of Holt, and its incidence increases with age (24). Less commonly, one observes scalloping of the posterior portion of the vertebral bodies. This scalloping is caused by a dural ectasia, the consequence of congenital weakness of the dura and the resulting pressure on the vertebral bodies. Anterior and lateral meningoceles, which are more common in adults, also result from the dural weakness. Bony rarefactions, the consequence of subperiosteal neurofibromas, can arise within the spine, the pelvis (particularly the iliac wings), or the skull. These rarefactions can induce pathologic fractures. Bony overgrowth, often with contiguous elephantiasis, is seen in approximately 10% of patients. Radiographic findings are reviewed by Holt (24) and Klatte and coworkers (25).

Hypertension can develop owing to the presence of a pheochromocytoma, which is seen in 1% to 4% of subjects. It also can be the result of renal artery stenosis, the most common of a variety of arterial abnormalities seen in neurofibromatosis (26,27). The microscopic picture of these arterial abnormalities is one of an intense subintimal proliferation of the spindle cells, which are believed to be of Schwann cell origin.

Neurologic manifestations can be grouped into five major categories (28,29).

Cognitive Disabilities

Although as many as 40% of children with neurofibromatosis have learning disabilities, only a small proportion are severely retarded (19,30). Thus, in the series of Ferner and colleagues only 8% of patients with NF1 had an IQ below 70 (31). All studies designed to investigate the cognitive deficits of NF1 subjects have shown a significant lowering in full-scale IQ when compared with unaffected siblings (31,32). As a rule, children tend to do better on verbal than on performance tasks and show deficits in visuospatial areas, attention, short-term memory, and reading (31,32). These deficits are believed to result from cortical heterotopias and other malformations of cerebral architecture such as glial nodules and other hamartomatous lesions (33), as well as from the presence of abnormal myelin. Malformations have been demonstrated by magnetic resonance imaging (MRI) as small focal areas of increased signal (*unidentified bright objects*) on T2-weighted scans in at least 43% of patients with neurofibromatosis (34). Areas of increased signal are located with particular frequency in the globus pallidus, brainstem, and cerebellum (35). Generally, they are asymptomatic and do not progress; rather, they tend to diminish or disappear over the years. In the experience of DiMario and Ramsby, lesions in the basal ganglia and cerebellum decrease in size and number over time, whereas lesions in the brainstem tended to increase in both number and size (36). Studies present conflicting data as to whether the number of abnormalities seen on MRI correlates with the severity of cognitive deficits (37,38). When lesions are seen in the brainstem they should not be confused with a neoplasm (33). Macrocephaly is common, and 16% of children in Riccardi's series and 45% of children in the series of Huson and Rosser had a head circumference at or above the 98th percentile (4,19,30). We have not seen a patient with neurofibromatosis and microcephaly.

Intracranial Tumors

Intracranial tumors can arise at any time of life, the optic pathway being the most common and the earliest site of involvement (39). In the series of Holt, optic pathway gliomas were found in 23% of children with neurofibromatosis (24). This compares with an incidence of 15% in the series of Huson and Rosser (4) and 19% in the series of Listernick and colleagues (40). The tumor is benign and histologically corresponds to a pilocystic astrocytoma. It is more common in girls, with a female to male ratio of 2:1 (40). Approximately one-half of patients who harbor optic pathway tumors develop signs or symptoms. The principal initial symptoms include proptosis and precocious puberty. The latter is seen in approximately 40%

of subjects and results from compression of the hypothalamus by the tumor. The presence of precocious puberty in a child with NF1, therefore, should always arouse the suspicion of an enlarging intracranial tumor.

Decreased visual acuity is rarely a presenting complaint in children even though it can be demonstrated by examination. The natural history of these optic pathway tumors in subjects with NF1 is not known and their growth rate differs considerably from one patient to the next. In the series of Listernick and colleagues (40) no tumor growth was seen as determined by MRI over a mean interval of 2.4 years. Only a small proportion of intraorbital tumors progress, whereas tumors that involve the optic chiasm are more likely to progress. The consensus statement from the NF1 Optic Pathway Glioma Task Force has concluded that MRI screening of children with NF1 for optic pathway gliomas has only limited value, and even though asymptomatic tumors are often found these only rarely progress. Serial visual acuity examinations in symptomatic children are preferable and less costly. Radiotherapy has been shown to halt tumor progression, but there has been concern that it could transform the tumor to a higher grade glioma (41).

Focal or generalized seizures can appear early in childhood and were seen in 7% of patients in the series of Huson and Rosser (4). Some of these patients had an electroencephalographic picture consistent with hypsarrhythmia. Because a significant proportion of patients with seizures and neurofibromatosis are ultimately found to have intracranial tumors, a child with cutaneous neurofibromatosis and seizures should be suspected of harboring a tumor and should receive imaging studies.

Tumors of the Peripheral Nerves

Tumors of the peripheral nerves can arise at any age and can involve any of the major nerves. Even though these tumors are occasionally painful, surgical removal must be weighed carefully against the possibility of the procedure producing considerable neurologic deficit. Malignant degeneration of neurofibromas occurs in less than 3% of children, but appears more frequently in adults (19).

Tumors also can arise within the autonomic nerve supply of various viscera. According to Kissel and Schmitt, the stomach, tongue, mediastinum, large intestines, and adrenal medulla are the most common sites (42).

Intraspinal Tumors

Intraspinal tumors are generally slower to develop than intracranial tumors and asymptomatic spinal cord tumors are commonly detected on routine neuroimaging studies. The youngest patient with a symptomatic intraspinal tumor in Canale's series was 20 years of age (28). Approximately one-half of intraspinal tumors are multiple, and occasionally, they are accompanied by malformations such as syringomyelia. Familial spinal neurofibromatosis is a variant of NF1. The condition is marked by the development of multiple spinal cord tumors during adult life (42–44).

Cerebrovascular Accidents

Cerebrovascular accidents are common and can be responsible for the abrupt evolution of neurologic signs. They result from cerebrovascular occlusive disease and most commonly affect the supraclinoid portion of the internal carotid artery or one of its major branches (45,46). More than one-half of the patients with occlusive disease of the internal carotid have the arteriographic picture of moyamoya disease (45,46).

The incidence of some of the neurologic manifestations encountered in NF1 and NF2 is presented in Table 11.1 (28).

Several conditions are related to NF1. Watson syndrome, characterized by dominantly transmitted pulmonary valve stenosis, café au lait spots, and low to normal intelligence, is believed to be allelic with NF1 (47). The concurrence of Noonan syndrome with NF1 may represent either a contiguous gene syndrome or the coincidental segregation of two autosomal dominant conditions (see Chapter 3).

Diagnosis

Despite the advances in understanding the molecular biology for NF1 and NF2, the diagnosis for both conditions is still largely based on clin-

TABLE 11.1. *Neurologic manifestations in 92 patients with neurofibromatosis (NF1 and NF2)*

Patients without neurologic manifestations	49
Patients with neurologic manifestations	43
Intracranial tumors	15
Optic glioma	5
Bilateral acoustic tumors	1
Multiple tumors	6
Intraspinal tumors	14
Multiple tumors	6
Associated with intracranial tumors	5
Peripheral nerve tumors	10
Seizures	11
Intracranial tumors	5
Mental retardation	9
Radicular pain	4

Modified from Canale D, Bebin Y, Knighton RS. Neurologic manifestations of von Recklinghausen's disease of the nervous system. *Confin Neurol* 1964;24:359.

ical criteria. The diagnostic criteria for NF1 are two or more of the following:

- Six or more café au lait macules whose greatest diameter is more than 5 mm in prepubertal patients and more than 15 mm in postpubertal patients
- Two or more neurofibromas of any type, or one or more plexiform neurofibroma
- Freckling in the axillary or inguinal region
- Optic glioma (tumor of the optic pathway)
- Two or more Lisch nodules (iris hamartomas)
- A distinctive osseous lesion such as sphenoid dysplasia or thinning of long bone cortex
- A first-degree relative with NF1 according to the previously mentioned criteria (48–50)

DNA testing for the diagnosis of NF1 is limited, because present techniques detect only approximately 70% of mutations (4). Although a solitary café au lait spot can occur in the normal population, the incidence of more than four such lesions in nonaffected persons is low, and, in the absence of other symptoms of neurofibromatosis, the lesions can indicate a partial penetrance of the disease (51). Conversely, some 75% of individuals with proven NF1 have six or more café au lait spots 1 cm or more at the largest diameter (21).

Both parents should be examined with particular attention to the presence of café au lait spots, subcutaneous neurofibromas, and Lisch nodules. Detection of Lisch nodules often requires slit-lamp examination by an ophthalmologist. If one parent has the stigmata of NF1, the condition in the offspring is not a new mutation, and a 50% chance exists for it to occur in each subsequent sibling. The risk for the patient's own potential offspring is the same. If neither parent has any abnormalities, a new mutation is presumed, and the recurrence risk for NF1 is no greater than in the general population. Prenatal diagnosis of the condition can be made by linkage analysis, if two or more family members are affected (50).

Treatment and Prognosis

Therapy is symptomatic. Most pediatric patients with NF1 should be seen in a multispecialist clinic at intervals of at least 6 months to 1 year to detect and manage the various potential complications. The necessity or value of routine cranial MRI scans is a matter of debate, because it is becoming apparent that the detection of asymptomatic lesions does not alter clinical management (50). Surgical removal of centrally located neoplasms is often life saving. When tumors are confined to peripheral nerves, the long-term prognosis is generally good. The prognosis for intracranial tumors depends on their location and whether they are single or multiple. In a follow-up study of patients with NF1 first reported in 1951, Sorensen and coworkers found that survival was limited by an incidence of neoplasms that was four times greater than seen in the normal population. Thus, 84% of patients developed a glioma, and second tumors were seen five to eight times more frequently than expected. Malignancies were encountered in one-third of the cohort, with female subjects having a higher incidence than male subjects. Second neoplasms were seen in 83% of patients with optic gliomas and in 43% of patients with other types of gliomas (52).

Neurofibromatosis 2

NF2 is genetically and clinically distinct from NF1. It is far less common, with an estimated incidence of 1 in 33,000 to 40,000, and it is characterized by the development of CNS tumors, notably bilateral vestibular schwannomas (49). The gene for NF2 has been mapped to the long arm of chromosome 22 (22q11) and has been cloned. Its gene product, merlin (schwannomin), shares significant homology with several actin-associated proteins (49a). Merlin is localized to the cell membrane and is believed to act as a membrane-cytoskeletal linker. It serves as a tumor suppressor by playing a role in the regulation of cell-cell adhesion, and in the reorganization of the actin cytoskeleton in response to growth factors, confluency, and changes in the shape of the cell (53,54). Merlin is absent from almost all schwannomas and from many meningiomas and ependymomas isolated from subjects with NF2. A large number of gene mutations have been documented. Some 90% of patients have gross truncations of merlin as a result of nonsense or frame-shift mutations (55). These patients tend to be younger at onset of symptoms and at diagnosis, and tend to harbor a large number of tumors (56).

Clinical Manifestations

In contrast to NF1, clinical manifestations and age of onset are similar within a given family, but differ considerably between families (57). The clinical manifestations of NF2 are highlighted by the presence of bilateral vestibular schwannomas (acoustic neuromas), which become manifest in more than 95% of genetically affected subjects (58). Generally, these tumors become symptomatic at puberty or thereafter. In addition, schwannomas occur in the other cranial nerves and the spinal and cutaneous nerves. Other tumors of the CNS seen in this condition include cranial and spinal meningiomas and multiple tumors of glial and meningeal origin. These tumors are readily detectable by imaging studies, with the acoustic neuromas appearing as a mass in the cerebellopontine angles or enlargement of the gasserian ganglia (34,59). As a rule, the mean age of onset of symptoms is in the second decade of life. In the series of Mautner and colleagues it was 17 years, with the age ranging from 2 to 36 years (59). In the same series, 44% of patients presented with deafness. Café au lait lesions were

present in only 43% and in this series as in others they rarely number more than six (60,61). Cataracts (posterior subcapsular or cortical) were seen in 81%, and seizures were presenting complaints in 8%. Peripheral nerve tumors were seen in 68%. These are predominantly schwannomas, but also can be neurofibromas (60). These appear as discrete, well-circumscribed slightly raised lesions with a roughened, slightly pigmented surface. Other skin lesions such as nodular tumors or neurofibromas also are less common than in NF1. According to Riccardi, acoustic neuromas and optic glioma never coexist in a patient (19).

Diagnosis

As is the case for NF1, the diagnosis of NF2 rests on clinical grounds. The criteria for NF2 are one or more of the following conditions:

- Bilateral eighth nerve masses (vestibular schwannomas) seen with imaging techniques
- A parent, sibling, or child with NF2 and either unilateral eighth nerve mass or any two of the following conditions: neurofibroma, meningioma, glioma, schwannoma, or juvenile posterior subcapsular lenticular opacity (48,60,62)

Patients with unilateral vestibular schwannomas and cataracts, or meningioma, glioma, or schwannoma are suspect for NF2, as are patients with multiple meningiomas plus unilateral vestibular schwannoma, cataracts, or glioma (60).

In 10% of cases of NF2 there is an identifiable mutation in merlin; for the remainder of patients, prenatal diagnosis requires a linkage study using DNA derived from at least two affected family members, if these are available.

Tuberous Sclerosis

Although the earliest report of a patient with TS is said to have been made by von Recklinghausen in 1863 (63), its first complete, albeit mainly pathologic, description is attributed to Bourneville, who, in 1880, was the first to call it TS (64). This is a protean disorder, chiefly manifested by mental deficiency, epilepsy, and skin lesions. It occurs with a frequency of 1 in 6,000 to 15,400 and is transmitted as an autosomal

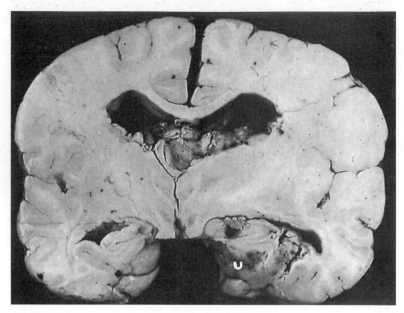

FIG. 11.3. Tuberous sclerosis. A large intraventricular tuber produces increased intracranial pressure, flattening of the gyri, and herniation of the right temporal uncus (U). (Courtesy of Dr. P. Cancilla, Department of Pathology, University of California, Los Angeles, UCLA School of Medicine.)

dominant gene (65,66). Approximately one-third of cases are familial, and the rest are new mutations.

TS is genetically heterogeneous, with loci on chromosome 9q34.3 (*TSC1*), and 16p13.3 (*TSC2*). Each locus accounts for approximately 50% of familial cases (67). The phenotypic expression of the two genetic defects appears to be similar if not identical. *TSC1* codes for hamartin, a 130-kd protein with no significant homology to any other known vertebrate protein (68). *TSC2* codes for tuberin, a 200-kd protein, which functions as a tumor-suppressor gene (69). It acts as a GTPase activator for *rap1*, which is an effective proliferation signal, expressed in several tissues, notably astrocytes. *Rap1* also is involved in morphogenesis and cell migration (69a). Tuberin is most abundant in cerebral gray matter and increases during prenatal and postnatal development (70). The protein also may be involved in neuronal differentiation (71). Hamartin and tuberin associate physically *in vivo*, and inactivation of either is believed to prevent the formation of a functional protein complex (72).

Mutations in the *TSC2* genes are more readily detected in sporadic than in familial cases (73). Penetrance is variable. No family with two or more affected offspring has been encountered in which one parent did not have adenoma sebaceum or some other skin lesion characteristic for TS (74). Conversely, the risk of having more than one affected child is low when both parents are clinically unaffected because under such circumstances the condition is probably a new mutation.

Pathology

Abnormalities can be found in the brain, eyes, skin, kidneys, bones, heart, and lungs. In the brain, three types of abnormalities occur: cortical tubers, subependymal nodules, and disorders of myelination. The most characteristic gross abnormality is the presence of tubers. These are numerous hard areas of gliotic tissue of varying size, after which this condition is named. Tubers can be located in the convolutions of any part of the cerebral hemispheres (Fig. 11.3). Less com-

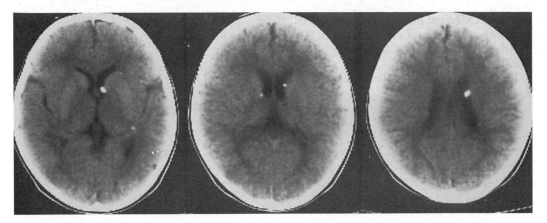

FIG. 11.4. Noncontrast computed tomographic scan of tuberous sclerosis, taken at several levels, shows typical calcified subependymal tubers at the margins of the lateral ventricles and projecting slightly into the ventricles. (Courtesy of Dr. Hervey D. Segall, Children's Hospital of Los Angeles.)

monly they are in the cerebellum, brainstem, or spinal cord. On histologic examination they are sclerotic areas that consist of an overgrowth of atypical giant astrocytes, and groups of large, bizarre, and frequently vacuolated "monster cells." Blood vessels in sclerotic regions show hyaline degeneration of their walls. In approximately one-half of subjects, calcium is deposited within the gliotic areas to an extent as to be visible on plain radiography of the skull or on computed tomographic (CT) scanning (Fig. 11.4). Subependymal nodules are found in the ventricular walls, particularly in the region of the foramen of Monro. They are multiple small, tumor-like nodules that project into the ventricles and that because of their appearance on pneumoencephalography were described as "candle drippings." Calcification of these nodules is common and increases with age. Subependymal giant cell astrocytomas arise from subependymal nodules, particularly in the area surrounding the foramen of Monro, and transitions between gliosis and astrocytomas are common. Their incidence in TS is approximately 10% to 15% (75). Although only rarely malignant, they often obstruct the foramen of Monro. It is of note that approximately one-half of high-grade and low-grade sporadic adult astrocytomas show reduced or absent expression of tuberin (75a). In the remainder, the majority have an increased expression of *rap1*.

Myelination usually is diminished in the gliotic areas within and surrounding the cortical tubers. In addition, islets occur consisting of heterotopic cells within white matter. These are distributed in a linear pattern that follows the normal migratory path of primitive neurons between the germinal layer of the ventricles and the cortical surface.

Tumors also can arise from various viscera. In the heart, the characteristic lesion is the rhabdomyoma. The incidence of these tumors in children with TS can be as high as 50%. Characteristically, they are multiple and well circumscribed. Rhabdomyomas cause as many as one-fourth of infants to die from circulatory failure during the first few days of life, well before developing other stigmata of TS. Between 50% and 80% of patients develop multiple renal tumors, which are usually benign and of mixed embryonal type. Lungs are rarely involved, but when lesions are present in the lungs they are usually cystic or fibrous. Other organs can be the seat of fibrocellular hamartomas (1). The pathologic features of the disease are extensively reviewed by Bender and Yunis (76).

Clinical Manifestations

Manifestations of TS vary considerably with respect to age of onset, severity, and rate of progression. The four main types of manifestations

TABLE 11.2. *Clinical picture in 71 patients with tuberous sclerosis*

Manifestation	43 Patients with mental retardation	26 Patients with average intelligence
Seizures	43	26
Major motor seizures	19	6
Minor seizures	6	5
Major and minor seizures	7	3
Seizure onset before 1 year of age	28	4
Seizure onset before 5 years of age	38	8
Adenoma sebaceum	37	22
Appearance of skin lesion before 2 years of age	17	9
Appearance of skin lesion after 9 years of age	2	3
Retinal tumors	21	13
Intracranial calcifications	20	15

From Lagos JC, Gomez MR. Tuberose sclerosis: reappraisal of a clinical entity. *Mayo Clin Proc* 1967;42:26. With permission.

are mental retardation, seizures, cutaneous lesions, and tumors in various organs including the brain. The frequency of the major signs and symptoms is given in Table 11.2 (77).

The degree of mental retardation varies widely, and for unknown reasons, a significant proportion of youngsters develops autistic features. Approximately one-third of patients diagnosed as having TS on the basis of other clinical manifestations maintain a normal intelligence. In others, language and perceptual development is slowed. Of retarded patients studied by Borberg, 15% developed normally for the first few years of life, showing the first signs of intellectual deterioration between 8 and 14 years of age (78). This deterioration can be the consequence of either frequent, uncontrolled seizures or the development of increased intracranial pressure caused by an obstruction at the foramen of Monro. In some series the number of tubers is greater in subjects with mental retardation than in those with normal intelligence, whereas in others there is no consistent relationship between intelligence and the number of tubers, and mental retardation reflects the early onset of seizures (75,79).

Seizures, the most common presenting complaint in all patients with TS, occur at some time in all patients who are retarded. Infantile spasms are the most common seizures during infancy (80). Between one-fourth and one-half of children presenting with this type of seizure ulti-

mately develop TS (81). Later, generalized convulsions or focal seizures can occur. Seizures can appear as early as the first week of life. The earlier the onset of seizures, the more likely the infant is to be mentally retarded (Table 11.2). Of 90 children whose seizures began before 1 year of age, only 8% were deemed to have average intelligence (82). Gomez and colleagues have postulated the presence of an epileptogenic factor, independent of cerebral TS, that facilitates the early onset of seizures, and, in turn, impairs normal CNS development (83). The severity of the seizures is unpredictable (84). As is discussed in Chapter 13, vigabatrin (150 mg/kg per day) is extremely effective in the management of infantile spasms caused by TS and is now considered to be the treatment of choice (85).

Autism or pervasive developmental disorder is a prominent feature of TS. In a series of TS patients from the University of California, Los Angeles, 28.5% satisfied the clinical features for autism, and a further 14.2% met the criteria for pervasive developmental disorder (86). In other series of patients with TS the incidence of autistic disorders was even higher (87). Bolton and Griffiths have commented on the association of autism with tubers within the temporal lobes (88). This challenging observation needs to be confirmed.

Adenoma sebaceum (angiofibroma) is the characteristic cutaneous lesion of TS (Fig. 11.5). These lesions consist of a red, papular rash over

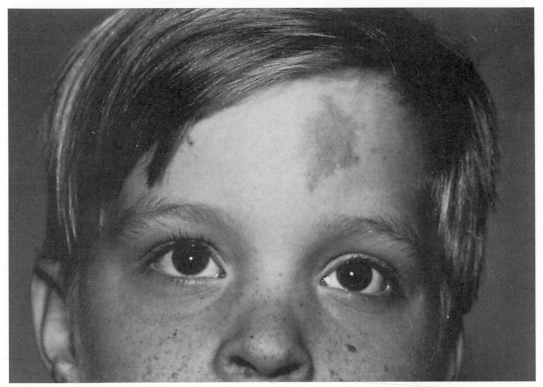

FIG. 11.5. Tuberous sclerosis. Characteristic fibrous plaque of the forehead and facial angiofibroma in a boy with an early stage of the condition. (From Gomez MR, ed. *Neurocutaneous diseases. A practical approach.* Boston: Butterworths, 1987. With permission.)

the nose, chin, cheeks, and malar region, appearing between ages 1 and 5 years. In the experience of Pampiglione and Moynahan, 12% of affected children developed this skin lesion by 1 year of age, and 40% by 3 years of age (89). Depigmented nevi, resembling vitiligo, in the form of oval areas with irregular margins (*ash leaf*) over the trunk and extremities are equally common. Generally, they appear earlier than the adenoma sebaceum. They can be noted at birth and are seen before 2 years of age in more than one-half of the subjects (89,90). They are more readily visualized when the skin is illuminated with ultraviolet light (Wood lamp). Depigmented nevi differ from vitiligo in that in vitiligo the melanocytes are absent, whereas in depigmented macules the melanocytes are normal, but the melanosomes are reduced and contain less melanin. Hypopigmented macules are seen in 0.8% of apparently healthy newborns (91).

Of the other cutaneous abnormalities, flattened fibromas are the most common. They appear in a variety of areas, including the trunk, gingivae, and periungual regions. In some infants, fibromas are found along the hairline or eyebrows. Another striking, but less common, lesion is the shagreen patch. This is an uneven thickening of skin, grayish green or light brown, raised above the surrounding surface, usually in the posterior lumbosacral region. Café au lait spots are seen in 7% to 16% of subjects. Their incidence is not much greater than in the general population and their presence in isolation should not prompt the diagnosis of neurofibromatosis. A significant percentage of subjects have patches of gray or white hair. Their presence can precede that of the depigmented nevi and thus can be the earliest clinical manifestation of TS (92). The abnormality is seen in 0.3% of apparently healthy newborns (91).

Intracranial tumors are less frequent in TS than in neurofibromatosis, but occurred in 15% of the series of Kapp and coworkers (93). Although the numerous intraventricular nodules are technically tumors, they usually do not grow to the extent of producing increased intracranial pressure. Tumors are found in the neighborhood of the foramen of Monro, arising from either the walls of the lateral ventricles or the anterior portion of the third ventricle. On the basis of their histology, they have been classified as giant cell astrocytomas.

The usual symptoms indicating the presence of an expanding mass in a patient with TS are headache, vomiting, and diminished vision. Papilledema is common, and occasionally lateralizing signs such as hemiparesis can develop. In as many as 50% of patients, tumors are detected in the retina, where they usually arise from the nerve head (94). Other common retinal anomalies are hyaline or cystic nodules (95). Further sites for neoplasms include the skin, lung, kidneys, bone, liver, and spleen (96,97). Patients require lifelong follow-up for early detection of potentially life-threatening conditions. The major causes of death include status epilepticus, renal disease, brain tumors, and lymphangiomyomatosis of the lung (98).

Diagnosis

As a rule, the diagnosis of TS is based on the characteristic skin lesions, seizures, and intellectual impairment or deterioration. In infants, the combination of depigmented areas of skin, infantile spasms, and delayed development is diagnostic. Griffiths and Martland suggest that the role of neuroimaging is to confirm the clinical suspicion of TS, evaluate the extent of the abnormality, look for associated but clinically unsuspected abnormalities, and follow the progression of the disease (99).

The CT scan is the simplest way to confirm the diagnosis of TS. It demonstrates multiple scattered calcium deposits varying in size up to several centimeters and located close to the wall of the lateral and third ventricles near the foramen of Monro (see Fig. 11.4). In the series of Kingsley and coworkers, only 5% of patients

with clinical features of TS had a normal CT scan result (75). Calcified masses within the cortex and white matter also are seen, as is cerebral cortical atrophy and ventricular dilatation, but the CT does not show cortical tubers unless they have become calcified (75). Whereas MRI is inferior to CT scanning for the detection of calcified lesions, it is preferable for the visualization of cortical tubers, the various white matter lesions, areas of heterotopias, and hamartomas. MRI also demonstrates islets of abnormal heterotopic giant cells that extend radially from the ependyma to the cortex. These are particularly common in the frontal lobes and the cerebellum (35,100). Cortical tubers can be found in 95% to 100% of patients with TS. They appear as thickened cortical gray matter that is hyperintense on T2-weighted images with indistinct gray-white differentiation. Fluid attenuated inversion recovery (FLAIR) sequences, which suppress the signal from cerebrospinal fluid (CSF), can be used to demonstrate smaller tubers (101). Subependymal nodules are hypointense on T1-weighted images. They are seen in approximately 95% of TS subjects, with the amount of calcification increasing with age. Gadolinium-enhanced MRI can be helpful in distinguishing a subependymal giant cell astrocytoma from a benign subependymal nodule (35,102) (Fig. 11.6). Hence, both CT and MRI studies are necessary for the complete evaluation of the child with TS, particularly for the detection of the heterotopias, which in our experience have proven to be troublesome seizure foci.

Equally diagnostic for TS are the cyst-like foci in the phalanges in approximately two-thirds of subjects. These are not seen at birth, but appear around puberty. A periungual or subungual fibroma (Koenen tumor), also characteristically appearing after puberty, is virtually diagnostic of TS, as are retinal hamartomas, which can be visualized in approximately one-half of patients (82).

Electroencephalography and the CSF are of relatively little diagnostic importance. Approximately one-third of children have hypsarrhythmia, which can persist in a modified form in patients up to 8 years of age (89). Focal and multifocal paroxysmal discharges also are seen.

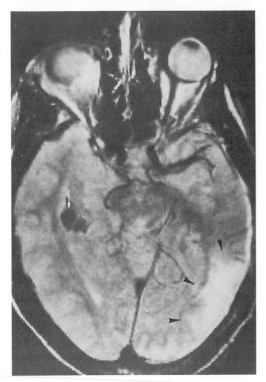

FIG. 11.6. Magnetic resonance imaging of tuberous sclerosis. A large cortical tuber is seen as a signal void corresponding to the calcification seen on computed tomographic scan. This area is surrounded by a fine hyperintense rim (*white arrow*). An area of high signal intensity with blurred margins corresponds to another large cortical tuber (*arrowheads*). (Courtesy of Dr. Nadine Martin, Départment de Neuroradiologie, Capital Beaujon, Clichy, France.)

Slow-wave abnormalities are often indicative of large intracerebral calcifications or masses.

The CSF protein content can be elevated, particularly in patients in whom intraventricular nodules have expanded, interfering with CSF circulation.

In numerous patients, incomplete forms of TS have been recognized by means of genetic surveys. These include isolated adenoma sebaceum, isolated retinal hamartomas, adenoma sebaceum with intracranial tumors but no seizures or intellectual deterioration, and visceral tumors without cerebral involvement (74,77,84). In the experience of Roach who used MRI to screen

apparently normal parents of children with TS, only 0.8% of the parents had typical MRI findings but a normal physical examination (103). Thus, a careful physical examination of parents is nearly as sensitive and much more cost effective than imaging studies. Incompletely affected individuals can have children with complete TS, a fact that should be kept in mind when offering genetic counseling. When both parents appear to be unaffected, the recurrence risk for a second child with TS has been calculated to be 1 in 22 after one affected offspring and one in three after two affected offspring (4).

The genetic diagnosis of TS has limited application. Two-thirds of the cases are sporadic, and a substantial fraction of even the most severe cases could be caused by mosaicism and missed by screening of leukocytes (103a). Genetic linkage testing has not been used routinely for the prenatal diagnosis of TS.

Treatment and Prognosis

No specific treatment is available. As stated elsewhere in this section, seizures are managed with anticonvulsant medications. In selected patients, resection of a single cortical epileptogenic tuber by stereotactic techniques or open craniotomy can result in a marked reduction of seizure frequency (104). Whether pertussis immunizations provoke the onset of infantile spasms in subjects with TS predisposed to such seizures is a matter of considerable controversy (104a). In view of studies that suggest as much and the observations of Gomez and associates that pertussis immunization can precede the onset of infantile spasms by less than 24 hours in infants with TS, pertussis immunization with whole cell vaccine is best withheld (83).

Resection of intraventricular tumors is reserved for children who develop ventricular obstruction. In view of the long survival of patients who do not receive radiation therapy for their mass lesions, we cannot draw any conclusions about its usefulness as an adjunct to surgery.

Whether patients should undergo periodic neuroimaging to detect the development of subependymal giant cell astrocytomas is a matter of debate (105). Whatever position a clinician wishes to take on this issue, regular neurologic examinations of the patient with TS are indicated. The management of cardiac rhabdomyomas and the various renal tumors that can develop in TS is outside the scope of this text.

Sturge-Weber Syndrome

SWS, as described by Sturge in 1879 (106) and Kalischer in 1897 (107), is a sporadic condition characterized by a port-wine vascular nevus on the upper part of the face, saltatory neurologic deterioration, and eventual neurodevelopmental delay. The hallmark intracranial vascular anomaly is a leptomeningeal angiomatosis that involves one or more lobes in one or both hemispheres (106). Although a port-wine stain on the face is a relatively common malformation, occurring in approximately 3 in 1,000 births, only 5% of infants affected with this type of a cutaneous lesion have SWS (108). Conversely, 13% of patients with cerebral manifestations of SWS do not have a facial nevus (109).

Pathogenesis and Pathology

In SWS, abnormalities of the skin, leptomeninges, choroid, and cortex can be traced to malformation of an embryonic vascular plexus, arising within the cephalic mesenchyme between the epidermis (neuroectoderm) and the telencephalic vesicle. Interference with the development of vascular drainage of these areas at approximately 5 to 8 weeks of gestation subsequently affects the face, eye, leptomeninges, and brain. Imaging findings in SWS can best be explained by the model of low-flow angiomatosis involving the leptomeninges (110). The angiomatosis is accompanied by poor superficial cortical venous drainage, with enlarged regional transmedullary veins developing as alternate pathways (Fig. 11.7). The ipsilateral choroid plexus may become engorged. Vascular stasis promotes chronic hypoxia of both cortex and underlying white matter. Ultimately, tissue loss and dystrophic calcification occur. Key radiologic features, therefore, are leptomeningeal enhancement of the angiomatosis, enlarged transmedullary veins, enlarged choroid plexus, white matter abnormalities, atrophy, and cortical calcifications.

Two structural aspects of SWS compromise cerebral blood flow. First, obstruction in the angiomatosis creates stasis, decreased venous return, and hypoxia. Under such conditions, neuronal metabolism suffers. Second, the lack of normal leptomeningeal vessels hinders neuroglial oxygenation, particularly at times of increased demand, such as when seizures occur. The resulting hypoxia is associated with several physiologic changes: abnormal drainage into the deep plexus and hypertrophy of the choroid plexus, increased capillary permeability, alterations in pH, calcium deposition, cerebral atrophy, and disruption of the blood–brain barrier (111–113). Poor venous drainage in one or both hemispheres is indicated by the presence of enlarged cortical vessels that extend beyond the borders of the leptomeningeal angiomatosis (114). The vascular compromise accounts for neurologic deterioration and eventual neurodevelopmental delay. The phenomenon of saltatory neurologic deterioration has been explained by the development of repeated thromboses, which are caused by microcirculatory stasis in the leptomeningeal angiomatosis. The stasis results in progressive, recurrent infarction that underlies loss of neurologic function.

On pathologic examination of the brain, the essential feature is a leptomeningeal angiomatosis with a predilection for the occipital or occipitoparietal region of one cerebral hemisphere (115). On microscopic examination the walls of these vessels are encrusted with iron and calcium deposits. Cortical calcifications usually are found in the degenerated cortex underneath the vascular malformations; in the less affected areas, calcifications are localized to the cortical tissue surrounding the walls of the smaller blood vessels. Calcification of microglia and neurons is a less common finding.

Clinical Manifestations

SWS is a progressive disease. The cutaneous port-wine nevus is present at birth and involves at least one eyelid or the supraorbital region of the face (112). It is initially pale red and gradually assumes the deep port-wine color. The angiomas also com-

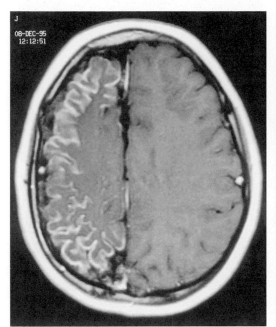

A

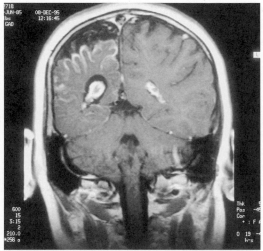

B

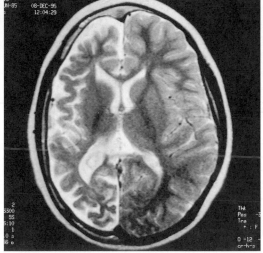

C

FIG. 11.7. Magnetic resonance imaging **(A)** in axial plane shows contrast-enhancing angiomatosis overlying the right cerebral hemisphere. Note hypertrophy of the choroid plexus in the coronal section **(B)**. Axial T2-weighted magnetic resonance imaging **(C)** shows widespread atrophy of the right hemisphere.

monly affect the mucous membranes of the pharynx and other viscera. An angioma of the choroid membrane of the eye is often associated with unilateral congenital glaucoma and buphthalmos. Bilateral facial nevi are not uncommon and were seen in 33% of patients in the series of Pascual-Castroviejo and colleagues (116). Approximately one-fourth of these patients had bilateral cerebral lesions on imaging studies.

Some 75% to 90% of affected patients develop focal or generalized seizures (117,118). These are usually the initial neurologic manifestation and frequently begin in the first year of life. Seizures can progressively become more refractory to medication and can be followed by transient or permanent hemiparesis. Hemiparesis, often with homonymous hemianopia, ultimately develops. In the Mayo Clinic series, some 67% of patients with a unilateral lesion and seizures were mentally handicapped (109). This is comparable with the data of Sujansky and Conradi who found that 71% of SWS subjects with seizures required special education (117), and that of Pascual-Castroviejo and colleagues, who found that the IQ of 70% of SWS subjects was less than 90 (116). By contrast, all patients without seizures were mentally normal (109,117). Glaucoma can be present at birth or develop over the years in up to 60% of patients (117). Less commonly, symptoms owing to hemangiomas involve the viscera. These include hematuria and gastrointestinal hemorrhages. Intracranial hemorrhages are rare.

Diagnosis

Most port-wine stains occur as an isolated anomaly. However, the coincidence of a facial vascular nevus and seizures should suggest SWS. Neuroimaging studies document the gradual but inexorable progression of the disease. This is particularly true for those children who develop seizures. MRI is presently the diagnostic modality of choice. In infants the unenhanced MRI can be normal, and the most reliable diagnostic features are leptomeningeal enhancement on MRI after gadolinium administration, enlarged transmedullary veins, and unilateral hypertrophy of the choroid plexus (see Fig. 11.7) (118–120). CT scan can reveal the localization and extent of intracranial calcifications (Fig. 11.8). Rarely present at birth, these become evident in nearly 90% of patients by the end of the second decade of life (109). Characteristically, calcifications are arranged in parallel lines ("railroad tracks") or serpentine convolutions that are most striking in the occipital and parieto-occipital areas (see Fig. 11.8). In older subjects MRI not only shows the pial angiomatosis, but also adjacent cerebral atrophy and enlargement of the lateral ventricles ipsilateral to the vascular nevus. Depending on the age when the study is performed, arteriography or MR arteriography can demonstrate abnormalities in approximately 50% of subjects. These include venous angiomas, thrombotic lesions, and other vascular anomalies (121,122). Functional cerebral imaging by means of a positron emission tomography (PET) or a single photon emission CT (SPECT) scan shows hypometabolism and hypoperfusion (Fig. 11.9) (123). The affected area is more extensive than the area of CT or MRI abnormalities (120). In infants who have not yet experienced a seizure, generally accelerated myelination and hyperperfusion of the affected region is seen (114,120,124).

The characteristic intracranial calcifications and seizures unaccompanied by a facial nevus also are seen in some patients with celiac disease (125). This condition is covered in Chapter 15.

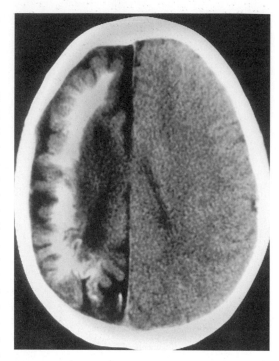

FIG. 11.8. Computed tomographic scan in axial plane shows widespread calcification in right hemisphere of the same patient in Figure 11.3.

Klippel-Trenaunay syndrome is a nonhereditary condition that shares a number of clinical features with SWS. In essence, it consists of cutaneous vascular nevi, which can appear at any site of the body and vary in size, venous varicosities, and hypertrophy of the bone and soft tissues (126,127). In some instances, the syndrome is associated with seizures, facial hemihypertrophy, and intracerebral calcifications (128) (see Chapter 12).

An association of large facial hemangiomas and abnormalities of the posterior fossa, notably the Dandy-Walker syndrome, posterior fossa arachnoid cyst, or cerebellar hypoplasia, has been recorded (129). There also is an autosomal dominant condition characterized by cerebral or cerebellar arteriovenous malformations, cutaneous vascular malformations, and seizures (130).

Treatment and Prognosis

Most patients with SWS have seizures; approximately one-third have glaucoma. As soon as the

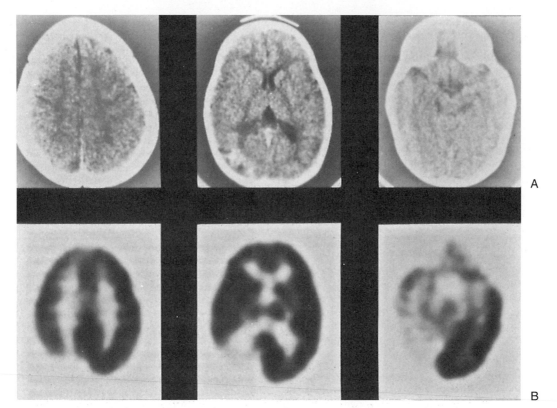

FIG. 11.9. Sturge-Weber disease. Computed tomographic scan and fluorodeoxyglucose positron emission tomography scans of a 13-month-old girl with bilateral capillary hemangiomas affecting all three divisions of the fifth cranial nerve. The hemangioma was more intense on the left, and there was left-sided glaucoma. Seizures began at 1 year of age, developmental milestones were normal, and no hemiparesis was seen. **A:** Computed tomographic scan showing early left occipital calcifications. **B:** Positron emission tomography scan indicating marked hypometabolism of occipital, temporal, and posterior parietal regions of the left hemisphere. (Courtesy of Dr. Harry Chugani, Division of Pediatric Neurology, Wayne State University, Detroit, MI.)

port-wine stain is noted, ophthalmologic consultation should be obtained, as aggressive medical and surgical management of glaucoma can preserve vision. Some children have rare complex partial seizures, but in the context of SWS, carbamazepine should be initiated after the first seizure. Effective seizure control may limit neurologic impairment and improve quality of life. More than 50% of patients have near complete control of seizures; an additional 39% have partial control (131). Despite general agreement that surgical resection (lobectomy, hemispherectomy) reduces seizure frequency, there is still debate about patient selection and the timing of surgery. Surgical guidelines have been developed for SWS patients (132). Hemispherectomy should be reserved for patients with clinically significant seizures who fail to respond to an adequate trial of antiepileptic drugs. However, there is no convincing data that early hemispherectomy halts neurodevelopmental deterioration in SWS, and surgery in SWS should be considered in the same way as it is for intractable epilepsy from other causes.

Anecdotal evidence associates aspirin therapy at 3 to 5 mg/kg per day with two-thirds fewer stroke-like episodes (132,133). The data are sufficiently compelling to propose a clinical trial, and it is reasonable to consider aspirin prophylaxis in children with transient neurologic deficits mimicking transient ischemic attacks. Because of the known association between aspirin and Reye syndrome, natural varicella, and influenza, the same precautions must be taken for SWS as those recommended by the American Heart Association for children with Kawasaki disease.

Increasing evidence suggests that SWS is associated with structurally diseased brain underlying and remote from the angiomatosis, defects in cerebral perfusion and metabolism, and dynamic changes in blood flow and glucose metabolism (133,134).

Von Hippel–Lindau Disease

The association of cerebellar hemangioblastomas with angiomas of the spinal cord, multiple congenital cysts of the pancreas, and kidney and renal carcinoma was first recorded by Lindau in 1926 (135), although retinal hemangiomas had already been described by Collins (136) and more definitively by von Hippel in 1904 (137). The condition is transmitted as a dominant trait with variable penetrance. Its prevalence is 1 in 40,000 to 50,000 (138). The von Hippel–Lindau (*VHL*) gene has been localized to the tip of the short arm of chromosome 3 (3p25-p26). It codes for two different tumor-suppressor proteins (139,140).

As a rule VHL disease does not present during the pediatric years. Symptoms are delayed until the second or third decade and can be referred to the eye with sudden intraocular hemorrhage, or to the posterior fossa with increased intracranial pressure or cerebellar signs (141). Of the gene carriers, 51% have retinal hemangiomatosis and 46% have CNS hemangioblastoma. Most commonly (52% of cases), the neoplasm is located in the cerebellum. It can be found in the spinal cord in 44% and in the brainstem in 18% of patients with CNS hemangioblastoma (142).

Associated with the retinal and cerebral lesions are a number of systemic lesions that tend to progress and become apparent during adult life. These include cysts in the pancreas (found in 72% of autopsied patients with VHL), kidneys (59% of autopsies), liver (17% of autop-

sies), epididymis (7% of autopsies), and various other organs. Additionally, VHL is associated with renal carcinoma (45% of autopsies) and pheochromocytomas (17% of autopsies). The high incidence of pheochromocytomas, which are often bilateral, appears to be limited to certain families in whom pheochromocytomas are usually the first expression of the disease, becoming manifest as early as 5 years of age (143).

A high CSF protein content is seen in the majority of subjects, and approximately 50% of patients with cerebellar tumors have polycythemia, the consequence of erythropoietin production by the tumor. MRI appears to be an excellent means for screening and follow-up examinations of affected family members in that it can detect neoplasms before the development of symptoms (144).

Ataxia-Telangiectasia

AT is characterized by slowly progressive cerebellar ataxia, choreoathetosis, telangiectasis of the skin and conjunctivae, and susceptibility to sinobronchopulmonary infections, lymphoreticular neoplasia, and other malignancies. It was described by Syllaba and Henner in 1926 (145), by Louis-Bar in 1941 (146), and more definitively in 1958 by Boder and Sedgwick (147), who presented the first clinical and neuropathologic delineation of the disease and named it AT.

Pathology and Pathogenesis

The gene for AT (*ATM, AT*, mutated) has been mapped to the long arm of chromosome 11 (11q23.3). It has been cloned and it codes for a large phosphoprotein, structurally similar to the signal transduction enzymes phosphatidyl inositol 3-kinases. These proteins are involved in the cellular responses to DNA damage, cell-cycle control, and maintaining telomere length (148,149). The ATM protein is localized in both the nucleus and cytoplasm. Screening for the gene has disclosed a large variety of mutations, most of which are unique for a given family, with nonconsanguinous patients being compound heterozygotes (148,150). The majority of mutations give rise to a truncated and nonfunctioning protein (150). As a result a number of biochemical and cellular abnormalities occur.

One basic lesion results in a marked increase in cellular sensitivity to ionizing radiation. This sensitivity is accompanied by a normal response to ultraviolet irradiation. Radiosensitivity of AT cells appears to result from an inability to recognize and respond to the presence of DNA damage by inhibition of DNA synthesis. In normal cells reduced DNA synthesis provides time for DNA repair before DNA synthesis is resumed at its preinjury rate. Although there is no defect in the ability to repair or remove strand breaks, fibroblasts derived from patients with AT contain increased amounts of topoisomerase II, an enzyme involved in inducing the transient breaks in double-stranded DNA (151).

Another feature of AT that arises from cellular sensitivity to ionizing radiation is the increased incidence of chromosomal breaks and rearrangements. Spontaneous intrachromosomal recombination rates are 30 to 200 times higher in fibroblasts derived from patients with AT than in normal cells (152). Translocations between chromosomes 7 and 14 are particularly frequent and can occur in the vicinity of the genes that code for the T-cell receptor and IgG genes (148).

Another basic characteristic of AT is a variety of immunologic abnormalities involving both the cellular and the humoral arms of the immune system (148). Low levels of serum and secretory IgA are found in 70% to 80% of patients (153). Additionally, low or borderline values for IgG_2 and IgG_4 are almost invariable (154). IgE is decreased or absent in 80% to 90% of patients, whereas IgM, IgG_1, and IgG_3 levels tend to be high (154). In most subjects, the deficiency of IgA and IgE results from impaired synthesis, although a high catabolic rate, the consequence of circulating anti-IgA antibodies, also has been noted (155). As a consequence of these humoral deficits, antibody response to various bacterial and viral antigens is deficient. Impaired cellular immunity is common in older children and is reflected in hypoplastic, embryonic-appearing tonsils, adenoids, and lymphoid tissue.

ATM protein is believed to also be involved in a complex system that prevents apoptosis after DNA damage. A defect in this system could be responsible for cell death within the nervous stem as well as within the thymus and the vascular endothelium (148,156).

Such a cell loss is the most striking finding on neuropathologic examination. This is most clearly seen in the cerebellar cortex where extensive loss of both Purkinje cells and internal granular cells occurs. Surviving Purkinje cells contain eosinophilic cytoplasmic inclusion bodies. Older patients show demyelination of the posterior columns and the dorsal spinocerebellar tracts (157,158). In some instances loss of anterior horn cells also occurs. Examination of peripheral nerves can reveal lipid inclusions in Schwann cells and a slight degree of axonal degeneration (158). Vascular malformations have been found inconsistently within the nervous system and the meninges (159).

Clinical Manifestations

AT is not a rare condition. Next to tumors of the posterior fossa, it is the most common cause for progressive ataxia in children younger than 10 years of age.

Cerebellar signs appear in infancy or early childhood. The telangiectases, which are characteristically located over the exposed areas, bulbar conjunctivae, bridge of the nose, ears, neck, and antecubital fossae, are first seen at between 3 and 10 years of age (Fig. 11.10) and become more marked with exposure to sunlight (160,161). Thinning and premature graying of the hair and loss of skin elasticity and subcutaneous fat also are prominent.

Approximately 85% of patients develop choreoathetosis, apraxia of eye movements, and nystagmus. Hypotonia, diminished reflexes, and generalized muscular weakness also have been observed and occur later. Imaging studies show cerebellar atrophy. Although normal initially, intelligence usually becomes impaired as the illness progresses, perhaps owing to diminished stimulation. Most patients experience recurrent sinopulmonary infections. Neoplastic disease is common. In particular, children with AT are 40 to 100 times more likely to develop lymphoma, leukemia, lymphosarcoma, and Hodgkin's disease

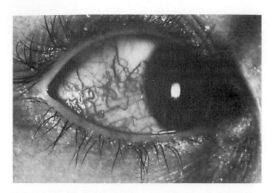

FIG. 11.10. Telangiectasia of the bulbar conjunctiva in a 12-year-old child with ataxia-telangiectasia. (From Boder E, Sedgwick RP. Ataxia-telangiectasia. In: Goldensohn ES, Appel S, eds. *Scientific approaches to clinical neurology.* Philadelphia: Lea & Febiger, 1977. With permission.)

than their peers (162). Other associated neoplasms include basal cell carcinoma, adenocarcinoma of the stomach, ovarian dysgerminoma, and a variety of brain tumors. In obligatory heterozygotes, the incidence of malignancies is increased threefold, with breast cancer being the most likely malignancy to be encountered in an AT heterozygote (163,164). Approximately one-half of patients develop an unusual form of diabetes in adolescence, characterized by hyperglycemia with only rare glycosuria, absence of ketosis, hypersecretion of insulin, and peripheral resistance to the action of insulin (165).

As expected from their *in vitro* fibroblast radiation sensitivity, children with AT are unusually sensitive to radiotherapy (166). It is unknown whether this radiosensitivity extends to the malignant cell lines derived from AT subjects.

Generally, the clinical course is downhill, although neurologic deterioration decelerates after adolescence. Death results from bronchopulmonary infection or malignancies.

Diagnosis

The diagnosis of AT is not difficult when the oculocutaneous lesions and the neurologic picture, particularly the oculomotor apraxia, are fully developed. In their absence, a young child

often presents with progressive cerebellar ataxia. Friedreich ataxia, the late infantile or juvenile neuronal ceroid lipofuscinoses, Refsum disease, and abetalipoproteinemia must all be considered.

Several laboratory tests assist in the diagnosis. The most constant abnormality is an elevated serum α-fetoprotein. Elevated α-fetoprotein levels are found in up to 95% of patients and precede by several years the appearance of telangiectases (167,168). An elevated carcinoembryonic antigen was also present in nearly all patients with AT. The characteristic defect in serum immunoglobulins, the demonstration of impaired delayed hypersensitivity responses, and the demonstration of spontaneous chromosome breaks also can assist in the diagnosis. Prenatal diagnosis of the disease by genotype analysis is now possible (169).

Milder forms of AT have been recognized. These patients have a later onset of neurologic symptoms, absence of telangiectatic lesions, less severe ataxia, and a longer life span (150). In these patients the ATM protein is present but in reduced amounts.

The Nijmegen breakage syndrome is an autosomal recessive disorder characterized by microcephaly, a bird-like facies, growth retardation, immune deficiency, an increased incidence of lymphoid cancers, and cellular sensitivity to ionizing radiation. The gene for this disorder differs from the AT gene; it has been localized to the long arm of chromosome 8 (170).

Treatment

No specific treatment prevents the neurologic progress of AT. Intercurrent sinopulmonary infections can be prevented by γ-globulin therapy or treated with antibiotics and postural drainage using a regimen similar to that used for cystic fibrosis.

Incontinentia Pigmenti and Hypomelanosis of Ito

Incontinentia pigmenti and hypomelanosis of Ito have considerable clinical similarity. Incontinentia pigmenti (Bloch-Sulzberger syndrome) is an X-linked disorder with lethality in male subjects.

TABLE 11.3. *Some neurocutaneous syndromes*

Condition	Signs and symptoms	Reference
Angiomatoses		
Wyburn-Mason syndrome	Facial nevus flammeus, telangiectases intracranial cirsoid aneurysm, racemose angioma of retina, seizure disorder, and variable degree of mental retardation	177,178
Cutaneomeningospinal angiomatosis (Cobb syndrome)	Vascular skin nevus at birth, angioma of spinal cord, neurologic symptoms appearing in childhood (see Chapter 12)	179
Riley-Smith syndrome	Macrocephaly, pseudopapilledema, multiple hemangiomas	180,181
Osler-Weber-Rendu disease	Telangiectases on tongue, face, mucous membranes, liver, and brain, epistaxes, intracranial hemorrhage, autosomal dominant hereditary pattern	Chapter 12
Gass syndrome	Cavernous hemangiomas of retina, intracranial cavernous hemangiomas, angiomatous hamartomas of skin	182
Linear nevus sebaceus	Yellow papules in linear patches (may be evident at birth), mental retardation, seizures, various developmental and vascular anomalies of CNS	183,184
Leopard syndrome	Lentigenes, electrocardiographic abnormalities, ocular hypertelorism, pulmonic stenosis, abnormal genitalia, retardation, sensorineural deafness, autosomal dominant gene	1,187
Xeroderma pigmentosum (De Sanctis-Cacchione syndrome)	Neurologic abnormalities (20%; 90% in Japan), microcephaly, mental deterioration, ataxia, choreoathetosis sensorineural hearing loss, peripheral neuropathy	188, Chapter 3
Kippel-Trenaunay syndrome	Capillary hemangioma, lymphedema, angioma of gut and bladder, hypertrophy of long bones, macrocephaly, intracranial and intraspinal angiomas	Chapter 12
Neurocutaneous melanosis	Multiple pigmented skin nevi present at birth, meningeal melanosis tending to become malignant, hydrocephalus, seizures	185,186

It is characterized by incontinence of melanin from the melanocytes in the basal layer of the epidermis into the superficial dermis. The skin lesions are erythematous and bullous at birth, crusting with residual pigmentation. They tend to follow a dermatome distribution. Neurologic symptoms are seen in up to 30% of patients (171). These include seizures, spasticity, microcephaly, and mental retardation (172). MRI discloses a variety of abnormalities. These include hypoplasia of the corpus callosum, neuronal heterotopias, and small or large vessel occlusion (173).

Hypomelanosis of Ito is characterized by hypopigmented lesions occurring in whorls and located on the trunk, head, or extremities, following a dermatome distribution. In the series of Pascual-Castroviejo and colleagues, mental retardation and seizures were found in 76% of subjects, macrocephaly in 23%, and hemihypertrophy in 20% (174). Some 10% of patients showed infantile spasms during the first year of life, and another 10% had autistic behavior. In addition, a variety of ophthalmologic abnormalities occur, notably microphthalmos and choroidal atrophy. Gray matter heterotopias, cerebellar atrophy, and intracranial arteriovenous malformations are occasionally seen on imaging studies (175). The disorder is probably heterogeneous, and in some instances the phenotype may result from the loss of pigmentation genes (176).

Some of the other less common neurocutaneous syndromes are presented in Table 11.3.

REFERENCES

1. Gomez MR, ed. *Neurocutaneous diseases. A practical approach.* Boston: Butterworths, 1987.
2. Smith RW. *A treatise on the pathology diagnosis and treatment of neuroma.* Dublin: Hodgis and Smith, 1849.
3. von Recklinghausen FD. *Ueber die multiplen Fibrome der Haut und ihre Beziehung zu den multiplen Neuromen.* Berlin: A. Hirschwald, 1882.
4. Huson SM, Rosser EM. The phakomatoses. In: Rimoin DL, Connor JM, Pyeritz RE, eds. *Principles and practice of medical genetics*, 3rd ed. New York: Churchill Livingstone, 1996:2269–2302.
5. Huson SM, et al. A genetic study of von Recklinghausen neurofibromatosis in Southeast Wales. I. Prevalence, fitness, mutation rate, and effect of parental transmission on severity. *J Med Genet* 1989; 26:704–711.
6. Stephens K, et al. Preferential mutation of the neurofibromatosis type 1 gene in paternally derived chromosomes. *Hum Genet* 1992;88:279–282.
7. Li Y, et al. Genomic organization of the neurofibromatosis 1 gene (NF1). *Genomics* 1995;25:9–18.
8. Legius E, et al. Somatic deletion of the neurofibromatosis type 1 gene in a neurofibrosarcoma supports a tumour suppressor gene hypothesis. *Nat Genet* 1993;3:122–126.
9. Brodeur GM. The NF1 gene in myelopoiesis and childhood myelodysplastic syndromes. *N Engl J Med* 1994;330:637–639.
9a. Gutmann DH. Recent insights into neurofibromatosis type 1: clear genetic progress. *Arch Neurol* 1998;55: 778–780.
10. Sawada S, et al. Identification of NF1 mutations in both alleles of a dermal neurofibroma. *Nature Genet* 1996;14:110–112.
11. Side L, et al. Homozygous inactivation of the NF1 gene in bone marrow cells from children with neurofibromatosis type 1 and malignant myeloid disorders. *N Engl J Med* 1997;336:1713–1720.
12. Rasmussen SA, et al. Constitutional and mosaic large NF1 gene deletions in neurofibromatosis type 1. *J Med Genet* 1998;35:468–471.
12a. Tonsgard JH, et al. Do NF1 deletions result in a characteristic phenotype? *Am J Med Genet* 1998;73:80–86.
13. Skuse GR, Cappione AJ. RNA processing and clinical variability in neurofibromatosis type I (NF1). *Hum Mol Genet* 1997;6:1707–1712.
14. Gutmann DH. Recent insights into neurofibromatosis type 1. *Arch Neurol* 1998;55:778–780.
15. Wu BL, Schneider GH, Korf BR. Deletion of the entire NF1 gene causing distinct manifestations in a family. *Am J Med Genet* 1997;69:98–101.
16. Pearce J. The central nervous system pathology in multiple neurofibromatosis. *Neurology* 1967;17:691–697.
17. Hope DG, Mulvihill JJ. Malignancy in neurofibromatosis. In: Riccardi VM, Mulvihill JJ, eds. *Advances in neurology. Neurofibromatosis (von Recklinghausen disease).* New York: Raven Press, 1981:33–55.
18. Schimke RM, et al. Syndrome of bilateral pheochromocytoma, medullary thyroid carcinoma and multiple neuromas. A possible regulatory defect in the differentiation of chromaffin tissue. *N Engl J Med* 1968;279:1–7.
19. Riccardi VM. *Neurofibromatosis: phenotype, natural history, and pathogenesis*, 2nd ed. Baltimore: Johns Hopkins University Press, 1992.
20. Huson SM, Hughes RAC, eds. *The neurofibromatoses: pathogenetic and clinical overview.* London: Chapman-Hall, 1994.
21. Crowe F, Scholl W, Neel J. *Clinical, pathological and genetic study of multiple neurofibromatosis.* Springfield, IL: Charles C Thomas, 1956.
22. Lisch K. Über Beteilung der Augen, insbesondere das Vorkommen von Irisknötchen bei der Neurofibromatose (Recklinghausen). *Z Augenheilk* 1937;93: 137–143.
23. Lubs ME, et al. Lisch nodules in neurofibromatosis type 1. *N Engl J Med* 1991;324:1264–1266.
23a. Howell SJ, et al. Growth hormone replacement and the risk of malignancy in children with neurofibromatosis. *J Pediatr* 1998;133:201–205.
24. Holt JF. Neurofibromatosis in children. *Am J Radiol* 1978;130:615–639.
25. Klatte EC, Franken EA, Smith JA. The radiographic spectrum in neurofibromatosis. *Semin Roentgenol* 1976;11:17–33.
26. Pellock JM, et al. Childhood hypertensive stroke with neurofibromatosis. *Neurology* 1980;30:656–659.
27. Zachos M, et al. Neurofibromatosis type 1 vasculopathy associated with lower limb hypoplasia. *Pediatrics* 1997;100:395–398.
28. Canale D, Bebin Y, Knighton RS. Neurologic manifestations of von Recklinghausen's disease of the nervous system. *Confin Neurol* 1964;24:359–403.
29. Michaux L, Feld M, eds. *Les phakomatoses cérébrales.* Paris: Droust, 1963.
30. Huson SM, Harper PS, Compston DAS. Von Recklinghausen neurofibromatosis: a clinical and population study in southeast Wales. *Brain* 1988;111: 1355–1381.
31. Ferner RE, Hughes RA, Weinman J. Intellectual impairment in neurofibromatosis 1. *J Neurol Sci* 1996;138:125–133.
32. Hofman KJ, et al. Neurofibromatosis type 1: the cognitive phenotype. *J Pediatr* 1994;124:S1–S8.
33. Duffner PK, et al. The significance of MRI abnormalities in children with neurofibromatosis. *Neurology* 1989;39:373–378.
34. Bognanno JR, et al. Cranial MR imaging in neurofibromatosis. *Am J Neuroradiol* 1988;9:461–468.
35. Truhan AP, Filipek PA. Magnetic resonance imaging. Its role in the neuroradiologic evaluation of neurofibromatosis, tuberous sclerosis, and Sturge–Weber syndrome. *Arch Dermatol* 1993;129:219–226.
36. DiMario FJ, Ramsby G. Magnetic resonance imaging lesion analysis in neurofibromatosis type 1. *Arch Neurol* 1998;55:500–505.
37. North K, et al. Specific learning disability in children with neurofibromatosis type 1: significance of MRI abnormalities. *Neurology* 1994;44:878–883.
38. Legius E, et al. Neurofibromatosis type 1 in childhood: correlation of MRI findings with intelligence. *J Neurol Neurosurg Psychiatry* 1995;59:638–640.
39. Rodriguez HA, Berthrong M. Multiple primary intracranial tumors in von Recklinghausen's neurofibromatosis. *Arch Neurol* 1966;14:467–475.
40. Listernick R, et al. Natural history of optic pathway tumors in children with neurofibromatosis type 1: a longitudinal study. *J Pediatr* 1994;125:63–66.

41. Listernick R, et al. Optic pathway gliomas in children with neurofibromatosis 1: consensus statement from the NF1 Optic Pathway Glioma Task Force. *Ann Neurol* 1997;41:143–149.

42. Kissel P, Schmitt J. Les formes viscerales des phakomatoses. In: Michaux L, Feld M, eds. *Les phakomatoses cérébrales.* Paris: Droust, 1963.

43. Ars E, et al. A clinical variant of neurofibromatosis type 1: familial spinal neurofibromatosis with a frameshift mutation in the NF1 gene. *Am J Hum Genet* 1998;62:834–841.

44. Poyhonen M, et al. Hereditary spinal neurofibromatosis: a rare form of NF1? *J Med Genet* 1997;34: 184–187.

45. Taboada D, et al. Occlusion of the cerebral arteries in Recklinghausen's disease. *Neuroradiology* 1979;18: 281–284.

46. Hilal SK, et al. Primary cerebral arterial occlusive disease in children. II. Neurocutaneous syndromes. *Radiology* 1971;99:87–93.

47. Riccardi VM. Genotype, malleotype, phenotype, and randomness: lessons from neurofibromatosis-1 (NF-1). *Am J Hum Genet* 1993;53:301–304.

48. Listernick R, Charrow J. Neurofibromatosis type 1 in childhood. *J Pediatr* 1990;116:845–853.

49. Evans DGR, et al. A genetic study of type 2 neurofibromatosis in the United Kingdom. I. Prevalence, mutation rate, fitness, and confirmation of maternal transmission effect on severity. *J Med Genet* 1992;29: 841–846.

49a. Gutmann DH, et al. Increased expression of the NF2 tumor suppressor gene product, merlin, impairs cell motility, adhesion and spreading. *Hum Mol Genet* 1999; 8:267–275.

50. Gutmann DH, et al. The diagnostic evaluation and multidisciplinary management of neurofibromatosis 1 and neurofibromatosis 2. *JAMA* 1997;278:51–57.

51. Whitehouse D. Diagnostic value of the café-au-lait spot in children. *Arch Dis Child* 1966;41:316–319.

52. Sorensen SA, Mulvihill JJ, Nielsen A. Long-term follow-up of von Recklinghausen neurofibromatosis: survival and malignant neoplasms. *N Engl J Med* 1986;314:1010–1015.

53. Shaw RJ, McCatchey AI, Jacks T. Regualtion of the neurofibromatosis type 2 tumor suppressor protein, merlin, by adhesion and growth arrest stimuli. *J Biol Chem* 1998;273:7757–7764.

54. Skoles DR, et al. Neurofibromatosis 2 tumour suppressor schwannomin interacts with beta II-spectrin. *Nat Genet* 1998;18:354–359.

55. MacColin M, et al. A point mutation associated with a severe phenotype of neurofibromatosis 2. *Ann Neurol* 1996;40:440–445.

56. Parry DM, et al. Germ-line mutations in the neurofibromatosis 2 gene: correlations with disease severity and retinal abnormalities. *Am J Hum Genet* 1996; 59:529–539.

57. Parry DM, et al. Neurofibromatosis 2 (NF2): clinical characteristics or 63 affected individuals and clinical evidence for heterogeneity. *Am J Med Genet* 1994;52: 450–461.

58. Wertelecki W, et al. Neurofibromatosis 2: clinical and DNA linkage studies of a large kindred. *N Engl J Med* 1988;319:278–283.

59. Mautner VF, et al. The neuroimaging and clinical spectrum of neurofibromatosis 2. *Neurosurgery* 1996; 38:880–885.

60. Mautner VF, et al. Skin abnormalities in neurofibromatosis 2. *Arch Dermatol* 1997;133:1539–1543.

61. Evans DG, et al. A clinical study of type 2 neurofibromatosis. *QJM* 1992;84:603–618.

62. Martuza RL, Eldridge R. Neurofibromatosis 2 (bilateral acoustic neurofibromatosis). *N Engl J Med* 1988; 318:684–688.

63. von Recklinghausen FD. Ein Herz von einen Neugeborenen welches mehrere theils nach aussen, theils nach den Höhlen prominierende Tumoren (Myomen) trug. *Verh Berl Ges Geburtsh* 1863;15:73.

64. Bourneville DM. Contributions a l'étude de l'idiotie. III. Sclerose tubereuse des circonvolutions cérébrales. *Arch Internat Neurol (Paris)* 1880;1:81–91.

65. Hunt A, Lindenbaum RH. Tuberous sclerosis: a new estimate of prevalence within the Oxford region. *J Med Genet* 1984;21:272–277.

66. Editorial. Progress in tuberous sclerosis. *Lancet* 1990;336:598–599.

67. Kwiatkowski DJ, et al. An index marker map of chromosome 9 provides strong evidence for positive interference. *Am J Hum Genet* 1993;53:1279–1288.

68. Van Slegtenhorst, M, et al. Identification of the tuberous sclerosis gene TSC1 on chromosome 9q34. *Science* 1997;277:805–808.

69. Jin F, et al. Suppression of tumorigenicity by the wild-type tuberous sclerosis 2 (Tsc2) gene and its C-terminal region. *Proc Natl Acad Sci U S A* 1996;93: 9154–9159.

69a. Asha H, et al. The rap1 GTPase functions as a regulator of morphogenesis in vivo. *EMBO J* 1999;18: 605–615.

70. Mizuguchi M, et al. Loss of tuberin from cerebral tissues with tuberous sclerosis and astrocytoma. *Ann Neurol* 1996;40: 941–944.

71. Soucek T, et al. A role of the tuberous sclerosis gene-2 product during neuronal differentiation. *Oncogene* 1998;16:2197–2204.

72. Van Slegtenhorst M, et al. Interaction between hamartin and tuberin, the TSC1 and TSC2 gene products. *Hum Mol Genet* 1998;7:1053–1057.

73. Au KS, et al. Germ-line mutational analysis of the TSC2 gene in 90 tuberous sclerosis patients. *Am J Hum Genet* 1998;62:286–294.

74. Bundy S, Evans K. Tuberous sclerosis: a genetic study. *J Neurol Neurosurg Psychiatry* 1969;32:591–603.

75. Kingsley DPE, Kendall BE, Fitz CR. Tuberous sclerosis: a clinicoradiological evaluation of 110 cases with particular reference to atypical presentation. *Neuroradiology* 1986;28:38–46.

75a. Wienecke R, et al. Reduced TSC2 RNA and protein in sporadic astrocytomas and ependymomas. *Ann Neurol* 1997;42:230–235.

76. Bender BL, Yunis EJ. The pathology of tuberous sclerosis. *Pathol Annu* 1982;17:339–382.

77. Lagos JC, Gomez MR. Tuberose sclerosis: reappraisal of a clinical entity. *Mayo Clin Proc* 1967;42:26–49.

78. Borberg A. Clinical and genetic investigation into tuberous sclerosis and Recklinghausen's neurofibromatosis: contribution to elucidation of interrelationship and eugenics of the syndromes. *Acta Psychiatr Neurol Scand* 1951;71[Suppl]:11–239.

79. Shepherd CW, Houser OW, Gomez MR. MR findings in tuberous sclerosis complex and correlation with seizure development and mental impairment. *Am J Neuroradiol* 1995;16:149–155.

80. Roth JC, Epstein CJ. Infantile spasms and hypopigmented macules: early manifestations of tuberous sclerosis. *Arch Neurol* 1971;25:547–551.
81. Della Rovere M, Hoare RD, Pampiglione G. Tuberose sclerosis in children: an EEG study. *Dev Med Child Neurol* 1964;6:149–157.
82. Gomez MR, ed. *Tuberous sclerosis*, 2nd ed. New York: Raven Press, 1988.
83. Gomez MR, et al. Tuberous sclerosis, early onset of seizures, and mental subnormality: study of discordant monozygous twins. *Neurology* 1982;32:604–611.
84. Critchley M, Earl CJ. Tuberose sclerosis and allied conditions. *Brain* 1932;55:311–346.
85. Chiron C, et al. Randomized trial comparing vigabatrin and hydrocortisone in infantile spasms due to tuberous sclerosis. *Epilepsy Res* 1997;26:389–395.
86. Gutierrez GC, Smalley SL, Tanguey PE. Autism in tuberous sclerosis complex. *J Autism Dev Disord* 1998;28:97–103.
87. Gillberg IC, Gillberg C, Ahlsén G. Autistic behaviour and attention deficits in tuberous sclerosis: a population-based study. *Dev Med Child Neurol* 1994;36: 50–56.
88. Bolton PF, Griffiths PD. Association of tuberous sclerosis of temporal lobes with autism and atypical autism. *Lancet* 1997;349:392–395.
89. Pampiglione G, Moynahan EJ. The tuberous sclerosis syndrome: clinical and EEG studies in 100 children. *J Neurol Neurosurg Psychiatry* 1976;39:666–673.
90. Gold AP, Freeman JM. Depigmented nevi: the earliest sign of tuberose sclerosis. *Pediatrics* 1965;35:1003–1005.
91. Alper JC, Holmes LB. The incidence and significance of birthmarks in a cohort of 4641 newborns. *Pediatr Dermatol* 1983;1:58–68.
92. McWilliam RC, Stephenson JBP. Depigmented hair. The earliest sign of tuberous sclerosis. *Arch Dis Child* 1978;53:961–963.
93. Kapp JP, Paulson GW, Odom GL. Brain tumors with tuberose sclerosis. *J Neurosurg* 1967;26:191–202.
94. McLean JM. Glial tumors of the retina. In relation to tuberous sclerosis. *Am J Ophthalmol* 1956;41:428–432.
95. Grover WD, Harley RD. Early recognition of tuberous sclerosis by funduscopic examination. *J Pediatr* 1969;75:991–995.
96. Dawson J. Pulmonary tuberose sclerosis and its relationship to other forms of the disease. *QJM* 1954;47:113–145.
97. Reed WB, Nickel WR, Campion G. Internal manifestations of tuberous sclerosis. *Arch Dermatol* 1963;87:715–728.
98. Shepherd CW, et al. Causes of death in patients with tuberous sclerosis. *Mayo Clin Proc* 1991;66:792–796.
99. Griffiths PD, Martland TR. Tuberous sclerosis complex: the role of neuroradiology. *Neuropediatrics* 1997;28:244–252.
100. Inoue Y, et al. CT and MR imaging of cerebral tuberous sclerosis. *Brain Dev* 1998;20:209–221.
101. Takanashi J, et al. MR evaluation of tuberous sclerosis: increased sensitivity with fluid-attenuated inversion recovery and relation to severity of seizures and mental retardation. *Am J Neuroradiol* 1995;16:1923–1928.
102. Martin N, et al. Gadolinium-DTPA enhanced MR imaging in tuberous sclerosis. *Neuroradiology* 1990;31:492–497.
103. Roach ES. Diagnosis and management of neurocutaneous syndromes. *Semin Neurol* 1988;8:83–96.
103a. Kwiatkowska J, et al. Mosaicism in tuberous sclerosis as a potential cause of the failure of molecular diagnosis. *N Engl J Med* 1999;340:703–707.
104. Bebin EM, Kelly PJ, Gomez MR. Surgical treatment for epilepsy in cerebral tuberous sclerosis. *Epilepsia* 1993;651–657.
104a. Goodman M, Lamm SH, Bellman MH. Temporal relationship modeling: DTP or DT immunizations and infantile spasms. *Vaccine* 1998;16:225–231.
105. Webb DW, Fryer AE, Osborne JP. Morbidity associated with tuberous sclerosis: a population study. *Dev Med Child Neurol* 1996;38:146–155.
106. Sturge WA. A case of partial epilepsy apparently due to a lesion of one of the vasomotor centres of the brain. *Trans Clin Soc Lond* 1879;12:162–167.
107. Kalischer S. Demonstration des Gehirns eines Kindes mit Teleangiectasie der linksseitgen Gesichts-Kopfhaut und Hirnoberfläche. *Berl Klin Wchnschr* 1897;34:10–59.
108. Tan OT, Sherwood K, Gilchrist BA. Treatment of children with port-wine stains using the flashlamp-pulsed tunable dye laser. *N Engl J Med* 1989;320:416–421.
109. Gomez MR, Bebin EM. Sturge-Weber Syndrome. In: Gomez MR, ed. *Neurocutaneous disease. A practical approach*. Boston: Butterworths, 1987:356–367.
110. Maria BL, Hoang KBN, Robertson RL, Barnes PD, Drane WE, Chugani HT. Imaging CNS pathology in Sturge-Weber syndrome. In: Bodensteiner JB, Roach SE. *Sturge-Weber syndrome*. Mt. Freedom, NJ: The Sturge-Weber Foundation, 1999.
111. Norman MG, Schoene WC. The ultrastructure of Sturge-Weber disease. *Acta Neuropathol (Berl)* 1977;37:199–205.
112. Alexander GL, Norman RM. The Sturge-Weber syndrome. Bristol: John Wright and Sons Ltd, 1960.
113. Sperner J, Schmauser I, Bittner R, et al. MR-imaging findings in children with Sturge-Weber syndrome. *Neuropediatrics* 1990;21:146–152.
114. Segall HD, Ahmadi J, McComb JG, Zee CS, Becker TS, Han JS. Computed tomographic observations pertinent to intracranial venous thrombotic and occlusive disease in childhood. State of the art, some new data, and hypothesis. *Radiology* 1982;143:441–449.
115. Wohlwill FJ, Yakovlev PI. Histopathology of meningo-facial angiomatosis (Sturge-Weber disease). *J Neuropathol Exp Neurol* 1957;16:341–364.
116. Pascual-Castroviejo I, et al. Sturge-Weber syndrome: study of 40 patients. *Pediatr Neurol* 1993;9:283–288.
117. Sujansky E, Conradi S. Outcome of Sturge-Weber syndrome in 52 adults. *Am J Med Genet* 1995;57:35–45.
118. Pinton F, et al. Early single photon emission computed tomography in Sturge-Weber syndrome. *J Neurol Neurosurg Psychiatry* 1997;63:616–621.
119. Griffiths P, et al. Choroid plexus size in young children with Sturge-Weber syndrome. *Am J Neuroradiol* 1996;17:175–180.
120. Benedikt RA, et al. Sturge-Weber syndrome: cranial MR imaging with Gd-DTPA. *Am J Neuroradiol* 1993;14:409–415.
121. Bentson JR, Wilson GH, Newton TH. Cerebral venous drainage pattern of the Sturge-Weber syndrome. *Radiology* 1971;101:111–118.
122. Vogl TJ, et al. MR and MR angiography of Sturge-Weber syndrome. *Am J Neuroradiol* 1993;14:417–425.
123. Chugani HT, Mazziotta JC, Phelps ME. Sturge-Weber syndrome: a study of cerebral glucose utiliza-

tion with positron emission tomography. *J Pediatr* 1989;114:244–253.

124. Adamsbaum C, et al. Accelerated myelination in early Sturge-Weber syndrome: MRI-SPECT correlations. *Pediatr Radiol* 1996;26:759–762.

125. Tiacci C, et al. Epilepsy with bilateral occipital calcifications: Sturge-Weber variant or a different encephalopathy? *Epilepsia* 1993;34:528–539.

126. Kramer W. Klippel-Trenaunay syndrome. In: Vinken PS, Bruyn GW, eds. *Handbook of clinical neurology*, Vol. 14. Amsterdam: North-Holland Publishing, 1968: 390–404.

127. Barek L, Ledor S, Ledor K. The Klippel-Trenaunay syndrome: a case report and review of the literature. *Mt Sinai J Med (NY)* 1982;49:66–70.

128. Heuser M. De l'entité nosologique des angiomatoses neurocutanées (Sturge-Weber et Klippel-Trénaunay). *Rev Neurol* 1971;124:213–228.

129. Reese V, et al. Association of facial hemangiomas with Dandy-Walker and other posterior fossa malformations. *J Pediatr* 1993;122:379–384.

130. Leblanc R, Melanson D, Wilkinson RD. Hereditary neurocutaneous angiomatosis. Report of four cases. *J Neurosurg* 1996;85:1135–1142.

131. Sujansky E, Conradi S. Sturge-Weber syndrome: age of onset of seizures and glaucoma and the prognosis for affected children. *J Child Neurol* 1995;10:49–58.

132. Roach ES, Riela AR, Chugani HT, Shinnar S, Bodensteiner JB, Freeman J. Sturge-Weber syndrome: recommendations for surgery. *J Child Neurol* 1994; 9:190–192.

133. Maria BL, Neufeld JA, Rosainz LC, et al. CNS structure and function in Sturge-Weber syndrome: evidence of neurologic and radiologic progression. *J Child Neurol* 1998;13:606–661.

134. Maria BL, Neufeld JA, Rosainz LC, et al. High prevalence of bihemispheric structural and functional defects in Sturge-Weber syndrome. *J Child Neurol* 1998;13:595–605.

135. Lindau A. Studien über Kleinhirncysten: Bau, Pathogenese und Beziehungen zur Angiomatosis retinae. *Acta Pathol Microbiol Scand* 1926;[Suppl 1]:1–128.

136. Collins ET. Intra-ocular growths. I. Two cases, brother and sister, with peculiar vascular new growth, probably primarily retinal, affecting both eyes. *Trans Ophthalmol Soc UK* 1894;14:141–149.

137. von Hippel, E. Ueber eine sehr seltene Erkrankung der Netzhaut. *Acta Ophthalmol* 1904;59:83–103.

138. Neumann HPH, et al. Central nervous system lesions in von Hippel–Lindau syndrome. *J Neurol Neurosurg Psychiatry* 1992;55:898–901.

139. Pause A, et al. The von Hippel–Lindau tumor suppressor gene is required for cell cycle exit upon serum withdrawal. *Proc Natl Acad Sci U S A* 1998;95: 993–998.

140. Schoenfeld A, Davidowitz EJ, Burk RD, A second major native Von Hippel–Lindau gene product initiated from an internal translation start site, functioning as a tumor suppressor. *Proc Natl Acad Sci U S A* 1998;95:8817–8822.

141. Maher ER, et al. Clinical features and natural history of von Hippel–Lindau disease. *QJM* 1990;77: 1151–1163.

142. Filling-Katz MR, et al. Central nervous system involvement in von Hippel–Lindau disease. *Neurology* 1991; 41:41–46.

143. Atuk NO, et al. Familial pheochromocytoma, hypercalcemia, and von Hippel–Lindau disease. *Medicine (Baltimore)* 1979;58:209–218.

144. Sato Y, et al. Hippel–Lindau disease: MR imaging. *Radiology* 1988;166:241–246.

145. Syllaba L, Henner K. Contribution à l'indépendance de l'athétose double idiopathique et congénitale. *Rev Neurol (Paris)* 1926;45:541–562.

146. Louis-Bar D. Sur un syndrome progressif comprenant des télangiectasies capillaires cutanées et conjonctivale symétriques à disposition naevoïde et des troubles cérébelleux. *Confin Neurol* 1941;4:32–42.

147. Boder E, Sedgwick RP. Ataxia-telangiectasia. A familial syndrome of progressive cerebellar ataxia, oculocutaneous telangiectasia and frequent pulmonary infection. *Pediatrics* 1958;21:526–554.

148. Lavin MF, Shiloh Y. The genetic defect in ataxiatelangiectasia. *Annu Rev Immunol* 1997;15:177–202.

149. Kastan M. Ataxia-telangiectasia—broad implications for a rare disorder. *N Engl J Med* 1995;333:662–663.

150. Gilad S, et al. Genotype-phenotype relationships in ataxia-telangiectasia and variants. *Am J Hum Genet* 1998;62:551–561.

151. Epstein RJ. Topoisomerases in human disease. *Lancet* 1988;1:521–524.

152. Meyn MS. High spontaneous intrachromosomal recombination rates in ataxia-telangiectasia. *Science* 1993;260:1327–1330.

153. McFarlin DE, Strober W, Waldmann TA. Ataxiatelangiectasia. *Medicine (Baltimore)* 1972;51: 281–314.

154. Oxelius VA, Berkel AI, Hanson LA. IgG2 deficiency in ataxia-telangiectasia. *N Engl J Med* 1982;306: 515–517.

155. Strober W, et al. Immunoglobulin metabolism in ataxia telangiectasia. *J Clin Invest* 1968;47:1905–1915.

156. Meyn MS. Ataxia-telangiectasia and cellular responses to DNA damage. *Cancer Res* 1995;55:5991–6001.

157. Solitare GB, Lopez VF. Louis-Bar's syndrome (ataxia-telangiectasia): neuropathologic observations. *Neurology* 1967;17:23–31.

158. De Leon GA, Grover WD, Huff DS. Neuropathologic changes in ataxia-telangiectasia. *Neurology* 1976;26: 947–951.

159. Agamanolis DP, Greenstein JL. Ataxia-telangiectasia. Report of a case with Lewy bodies and vascular abnormalities within cerebral tissue. *J Neuropathol Exp Neurol* 1979;38:475–488.

160. Reed WB, et al. Cutaneous manifestations of ataxiatelangiectasia. *JAMA* 1966;195:746–753.

161. Sedgwick RP, Boder E. Ataxia-telangiectasia. In: Vinken PJ, Bruyn GW, eds. *Handbook of clinical neurology*, Vol. 14. Amsterdam: North-Holland Publishing Co, 1972:267–339.

162. Toledano SR, Lange BJ. Ataxia-telangiectasia and acute lymphoblastic leukemia. *Cancer* 1980;45: 1675–1678.

163. Swift M, et al. Breast and other cancers in families with ataxia-telangiectasia. *N Engl J Med* 1987;316: 1289–1294.

164. Swift M, et al. Incidence of cancer in 161 families affected by ataxia-telangiectasia. *N Engl J Med* 1991;325:1831–1836.

165. Schalch DS, McFarlin DE, Barlow MH. An unusual form of diabetes mellitus in ataxia telangiectasia. *N Engl J Med* 1970;282:1396–1402.

166. Pritchard J, et al. The effects of radiation therapy for Hodgkin's disease in a child with ataxia telangiectasia. A clinical, biological and pathological study. *Cancer* 1982;50:877–886.

167. Boder E. Ataxia-telangiectasia. In: Gomez MR, ed. *Neurocutaneous diseases. A practical approach.* Boston: Butterworths, 1987:95–117.

168. Cabana MD, et al. Consequences of the delayed diagnosis of ataxia-telangiectasia. *Pediatrics* 1998;102: 98–100.

169. Gatti RA, et al. Prenatal genotyping of ataxia-telangiectasia. *Lancet* 1993;342:376.

170. Cerosaletti KM, et al. Fine localization of the Nijmegen breakage syndrome gene to 8q21: evidence for a common founder haplotype. *Am J Hum Genet* 1998;63: 125–134.

171. Landy SJ, Donnai D. Incontinentia pigmenti (Bloch-Sulzberger syndrome). *J Med Genet* 1993;30:53–59.

172. O'Doherty NJ, Norman RM. Incontinentia pigmenti (Bloch-Sulzberger syndrome) with cerebral malformation. *Dev Med Child Neurol* 1968;10:168–174.

173. Lee AG, et al. Intracranial assessment of incontinentia pigmenti using magnetic resonance imaging, angiography, and spectroscopic imaging. *Arch Pediatr Adolesc Med* 1995;149:573–580.

174. Pascual-Castroviejo I, et al. Hypomelanosis of Ito. A study of 76 infantile cases. *Brain Dev* 1998;20:36–43.

175. Pini G, Faulkner LB. Cerebellar involvement in hypomelanosis of Ito. *Neuropediatrics* 1995;26: 208–210.

176. Pellegrino JE, et al. Mosaic loss of 15q11q13 in a patient with hypomelanosis of Ito: is there a role for the P gene? *Hum Genet* 1995;96:485–489.

177. Wyburn-Mason R. Arteriovenous aneurysm of midbrain and retina, facial naevi, and mental changes. *Brain* 1943;66:163–209.

178. Patel U, Gupta SC. Wyburn-Mason syndrome: a case report and review of the literature. *Neuroradiology* 1990;31:544–546.

179. Kissel P, Dureux JB. Cobb syndrome. Cutaneo-meningospinal angiomatosis. In: Vinken PJ, Bruyn GW, eds. *Handbook of clinical neurology*, Vol. 14. Amsterdam: North-Holland Publishing Co, 1972: 429–445.

180. Riley HD, Smith WR. Macrocephaly, pseudopapilledema and multiple hemangiomata. A previously undescribed heredofamilial syndrome. *Pediatrics* 1960;26:293–300.

181. Arch EM, et al. Deletion of PTEN in a patient with Bannayan-Riley-Ruvalcaba syndrome suggests allelism with Cowden disease. *Am J Med Genet* 1997;71:489–493.

182. Gass JDM. Cavernous hemangioma of the retina. A neuro-oculo-cutaneous syndrome. *Am J Ophthalmol* 1971;71:799–814.

183. Pavone L, et al. Epidermal nevus syndrome: a neurologic variant with hemimegalencephaly, gyral malformations, mental retardation, seizures, and facial hemihypertrophy. *Neurology* 1991;41:266–271.

184. Prensky AL. Linear sebaceous nevus. In: Gomez MR, ed. *Neurocutaneous diseases*. Boston: Butterworths, 1987:335–344.

185. Fox H, et al. Neurocutaneous melanosis. *Arch Dis Child* 1964;39:508–516.

186. Demirci A, et al. MR of parenchymal neurocutaneous melanosis. *Am J Neuroradiol* 1995;16:603–606.

187. Coppin BD, Temple IK. Multiple lentigines syndrome (LEOPARD syndrome or progressive cardiomyopathic lentiginosis). *J Med Genet* 1997;34: 582–586.

188. Robbins JH, et al. Neurological disease in xeroderma pigmentosum. Documentation of a late onset type of the juvenile onset form. *Brain* 1991;114: 1335–1361.

Chapter 12

Cerebrovascular Disorders

John H. Menkes and *Harvey B. Sarnat

*Departments of Neurology and Pediatrics, University of California, Los Angeles,
UCLA School of Medicine, and Department of Pediatric Neurology, Cedars-Sinai Medical Center,
Los Angeles, California 90048; and *Departments of Pediatric Neurology and Neuropathology,
University of Washington School of Medicine, Children's Hospital and Regional Medical Center,
Seattle, Washington 98105*

This chapter discusses the various disorders caused by primary disease processes affecting the blood vessels of the central nervous system (CNS). It includes congenital anomalies of the cerebral arteries and veins and ischemic and hemorrhagic lesions resulting from disease processes affecting the cerebral vasculature. The cerebrovascular complications of infections, blood dyscrasias, trauma, and a variety of systemic diseases are discussed in other chapters.

Cerebrovascular disorders constitute a far smaller proportion of the neurologic diseases of childhood than of adulthood. Whereas cerebrovascular disease is the most common neurologic disorder of adults, a survey of the pediatric population of Rochester, Minnesota, disclosed an annual incidence rate of 2.52 cases of cerebrovascular disease per 100,000 (1). This figure compares with an incidence of 100 to 300 per 100,000 population per year in adults and of 110 cases of perinatal intracranial hemorrhage per 100,000 live-born babies (2). The distribution of the various forms of cerebrovascular disease in children younger than 15 years is depicted in Table 12.1. Occlusive vascular disease and CNS hemorrhages are approximately equally common, with cardiac abnormalities and arteriovenous malformations (AVMs) representing the most frequently documented causes.

According to classic neurology, cerebrovascular disease has three aspects: the basic patho-

logic process affecting the vessel, the pathologic changes induced in brain tissue by infarction or hemorrhage, and the neurologic picture caused by these changes (3).

CEREBRAL INFARCTION

Occlusive vascular diseases in childhood have various causes. Their relative incidences in the experience of Williams and coworkers is depicted in Table 12.2 (4). Many of the entities are discussed in other sections of this book and are therefore referred to only briefly in this chapter. The MELAS syndrome, a mitochondrial disorder marked by encephalopathy, lactic acidosis, and stroke-like episodes, is considered in the section on Mitochondrial Disorders in Chapter 1. Vascular occlusions resulting from vasculitic or rheumatic diseases are covered in Chapter 7. Vascular occlusions secondary to trauma, notably trauma to the internal carotid artery, are covered in Chapter 8. Thromboses associated with migraine are covered in Chapter 13. Thromboses owing to various inborn metabolic errors, notably homocystinuria and Fabry disease are covered in Chapter 1.

Cerebrovascular accidents have long been recognized as complications of cyanotic congenital heart disease. They are most common in infants younger than 2 years of age, particularly in those with severe cyanosis and hypoxia. Infec-

TABLE 12.1. *Cerebrovascular disease in 69 children younger than 15 years of age*

Occlusive vascular disease	38 patients (55%)
Preexisting heart disease	18
Unknown cause	13
Moyamoya disease	3
Other conditions	4
Central nervous system hemorrhage	31 patients (45%)
Arteriovenous malformations	13
Unknown	7
Aneurysms	6
Preexisting heart disease	1
Other conditions	4

From Schoenberg BS, Mellinger JF, Schoenberg DG. Cerebrovascular disease in infants and children: a study of incidence, clinical features, and survival. *Neurology* 1978;28:763. With permission.

TABLE 12.2. *Comparison of etiologies for cerebrovascular occlusive disease in age groups 1 to younger than 15 years of age and 15 to 18 years of age*

Subtype	Age 1 to less than 15 years, number (%)	Age 15 to 18 years, number (%)
Total number	81	11
Cardioembolic	11 (14)	3 (27)
Cyanotic heart disease	8	0
Valvular heart disease	1	0
Myoendocarditis	2	1
Patent foramen ovale/ atrial septal defect	0	2
Other	39 (48)	6 (55)
Prothrombotic, sickle cell	17	1
Prothrombotic, other	5	0
Dissection	0	3
Moyamoya	9	1
Vasculitis	3	1
Miscellaneous	5	0
Unknown	31 (38)	2 (18)

Adapted from Williams LS, et al. Subtypes of ischemic stroke in children and young adults. *Neurology* 1997; 49:1541.

tions, diarrhea, and dehydration are common precipitating factors. In most instances, infarctions occur in the distribution of the middle cerebral artery, and porencephalic cysts occasionally mark the area of tissue destruction (see Chapter 15). Mitral valve prolapse and cardiomyopathies also can be responsible.

Several genetic defects result in a predisposition to vascular thrombosis, the consequence of either increased deposition or decreased dissolution of fibrin. These conditions include several forms of antithrombin III deficiency and inherited defects of protein C and protein S. These three entities account for approximately 15% of families with inherited thrombophilia (5). Deficiencies of antithrombin III, a coagulant inhibitor, and defects in proteins C and S, and resistance to activated protein C caused by factor V Leiden increase the risk for venous thrombosis (6). Proteins C and S are naturally occurring anticoagulants, whose deficiencies are inherited as autosomal dominant traits. Cerebral arterial or venous thromboses have been seen in both homozygotes and heterozygotes for these two conditions. The heterozygotes can be asymptomatic or they can develop thromboses in the presence of other predisposing factors such as infection or dehydration (7,8). Resistance to activated protein C is the most common hereditary risk factor for venous thrombotic events in infants and children. Most commonly it is caused by a

point mutation in the gene for coagulation factor V, the factor V Leiden mutation (8a). Less often one encounters increased prothrombin and defects of heparin cofactor II and of plasminogen (9). In many instances, moderately elevated levels of homocysteine such as are seen in heterozygotes for homocystinuria, or homozygotes for a point mutation in the enzyme methylenetetrahydrofolate reductase interact with genetic defects in coagulation factors to increase exponentially the risk for arterial or venous thromboses (9a). Other acquired environmental insults also can contribute to the development of thrombosis in a predisposed, but otherwise asymptomatic, individual. A comprehensive review of the hypercoagulable states has been edited by Bertina (10).

Acquired protein S deficiency has been described in several disease states, notably in the nephrotic syndrome and in malignancies, such as leukemia (11). The condition is marked by a high incidence of thromboembolic events (12). Deficiencies in protein C or S appear to represent important risk factors for intracerebral occlusive disease in the pediatric population. In the experience of the Los Angeles Children's Hospital, the incidence of protein C and protein S deficiencies was 2% and 5% of all ischemic cerebrovascular accidents (13).

An association between the presence of antiphospholipid antibodies and thrombotic events has been well documented. Antiphospholipid antibodies include the lupus anticoagulants, which interrupt formation of the prothrombin activator complex and prolong the activated partial thromboplastin time, and the anticardiolipid antibodies whose presence induces a false-positive biological test for syphilis (14). Antiphospholipid antibodies occur in approximately 50% of children with systemic lupus erythematosus (15), but are also found in other autoimmune disorders and in individuals without any obvious underlying diseases (primary antiphospholipid antibody syndrome).

A number of cerebrovascular syndromes, including cerebrovascular occlusions, are the result of hemoglobinopathies, notably sickle cell disease (hemoglobin SS) and sickle cell hemoglobin C disease (hemoglobin SC). These conditions are considered in Chapter 15. Other syndromes involve an underlying phakomatosis (e.g., neurofibromatosis or tuberous sclerosis) or a neurocutaneous syndrome, entities covered in Chapter 11. The multitude of causes for occlusive vascular disease in the pediatric population is reviewed by Riela and Roach (16).

When one of the larger cerebral arteries becomes obstructed, the region affected includes both the cortex and underlying white matter. Classic neuropathology distinguishes between hemorrhagic and pale infarcts. In the hemorrhagic infarct, the region, which is usually gray matter, is congested and stippled with petechial hemorrhages. In a pale infarct, affected tissue, usually white matter, appears pale with considerable amounts of swelling. Microscopic examination reveals massive necrosis of all tissue elements, with the damage becoming progressively less severe toward the periphery of the infarct. The repair process is initiated by a polymorphonuclear infiltration, which, after 4 to 5 days, is replaced by mononuclear phagocytes. These ingest the various products of cellular and myelin disintegration. With time, cystic spaces replace the damaged parenchyma, and hypertrophic and hyperplastic astrocytes lay down a fiber network. The extent of tissue damage resulting from an infarction is extremely difficult to predict and depends in part on the availability of collateral flow.

In attempting to understand the pathophysiology of brain ischemia, one must distinguish between primary and secondary injury. Primary injury refers to the cellular damage caused directly by the insult, whereas secondary injury refers to the various derangements set into motion by the primary injury (17). A considerable amount of investigation has been directed toward understanding the nature of the secondary injury in the hope of preventing some of the damage induced by it. The processes of secondary injury are reviewed in Chapter 5 in connection with cell damage induced by perinatal asphyxia and in Chapter 15 in reference to postnatal anoxia and hypoglycemia.

Although the pathophysiologic consequences of an ischemic insult to the brain of an older infant or child are in many ways similar to the effects of asphyxia on the neonatal brain, several significant differences exist. These are outlined in Table 12.3.

TABLE 12.3. *Manifestations of cerebral ischemia*

	Global cerebral ischemia (asphyxia)	Focal cerebral ischemia (stroke)
Duration of insult	Short (5–15 min)	Long
Distribution of injury	Selectively vulnerable areas	Densely ischemic tissue surrounded by zone of less dense ischemia (penumbra zone)
Cell types affected	Neurons	All cells, including vasculature
Inflammatory component	Moderate	Strong
Development of irreversible injury	Rapid	Slow

Cerebral ischemia tends to be focal and prolonged, whereas asphyxia, being limited by the viability of brainstem centers, is briefer and tends to affect the entire brain, even though the response of the immature cerebral vasculature to asphyxia can produce secondary focal ischemia or hemorrhage. Tissue damage in cerebral ischemia is marked by the presence of a central core where ischemia is severe and infarction develops rapidly, and a marginally perfused area surrounding the core, termed the *penumbra*, which has the capacity to recover should perfusion be restored promptly. This contrasts with the picture of neuronal damage in asphyxia in which a selective vulnerability of neuronal populations occurs. Because the immature brain has more limited capabilities for repair, its cellular response to tissue destruction differs from the response of the older nervous system. On a biochemical level, the role of lactic acid in producing cell damage appears to be more important in the mature than in the neonatal brain, perhaps because the greater permeability of the immature blood–brain barrier to lactate prevents its local accumulation. The pathophysiology of brain ischemia is reviewed by Macdonald and Stoodley (18) and the cellular mechanisms of ischemic cell death by Kristiàn and Siesjö (19), by Sweeney and colleagues (20), and by Dirnagle and coworkers (20a).

Interruption of blood supply induces a rapid energy failure. This leads to a depletion of adenosine triphosphate (ATP) and consequently to the initiation of anaerobic glycolysis with accumulation of lactic acid and intracellular and extracellular acidosis. Lack of ATP also causes failure of active cellular pumps, which results in Na^+ and Cl^- influx and K^+ efflux. These ionic changes depolarize the cell membrane. As a consequence, there is an influx of calcium into the cell and an increased release of glutamate. As the major excitatory neurotransmitter, glutamate further increases intracellular calcium levels. The increase of intracellular calcium to nonphysiologic levels ultimately results in neuronal death by necrosis or apoptosis. The role of calcium-dependent proteases and phospholipases, free radicals, nitric oxide, cytokines, and stress genes in neuronal death is beyond the scope of this chapter. The mechanisms involved are discussed more fully in Chapters 5 and 15 and are summarized in Table 15.1.

A considerable degree of cellular damage, particularly in the area of the penumbra, does not immediately follow the interruption of the blood supply, but can be delayed for as long as several hours after the infarction. This delayed cellular death is probably related to events initiated by reperfusion of the partially infarcted tissue. The role of calcium in mediating delayed neuronal death is not fully understood. The various hypotheses have been reviewed by Kristiàn and Sjesjö (19), Sweeney and colleagues (20), and Dirnagle and coworkers (20a).

CEREBRAL HEMORRHAGE

The pathophysiology of intracerebral hemorrhage as seen in the full-term and premature newborn has been the subject of considerable attention among neonatologists and neonatal neurologists. It is discussed in Chapter 5.

In older age groups, intracerebral hemorrhage results from a defect in the wall of one of the blood vessels, either as a consequence of trauma (see Chapter 8) or because of various vascular malformations. Bleeding secondary to systemic hypertension, as well as the various blood dyscrasias, is discussed in Chapter 15.

Blood from a ruptured aneurysm or an AVM can enter the subarachnoid space or, after entering the overlying brain, it can dissect through the brain substance and pass into the ventricular system. Much less commonly, blood finds its way into the subdural spaces. A subarachnoid hemorrhage is accompanied by aseptic meningitis and an alteration of cerebrovascular reactivity. Although some of the brain damage results from actual tissue destruction by blood, the mere presence of blood in the subarachnoid space is responsible for a considerable proportion of the neurologic deficits that accompany bleeding into the subarachnoid spaces.

Both experimental and clinical data indicate that blood arising from a ruptured aneurysm and entering the subarachnoid space, particularly the basilar cisterns, induces a biphasic vasospasm whose severity is proportional to the amount of blood in the spinal fluid (21,22). The phenomenon is much less common when the hemorrhage results from an AVM or from trauma (23), and its role in producing neurologic deficits after a subarachnoid hemorrhage is less important in the child than in the adult. A summary of the pathophysiology is nevertheless indicated.

The first phase of vasospasm begins within minutes after the bleeding and lasts for approximately 1 hour. The second phase is of far longer duration. It occurs in less than one-half of adult patients and probably in an even lower proportion of the pediatric population, but it can produce devastating and frequently fatal neurologic symptoms. The spasm commences some 3 to 24 hours after bleeding, is maximal within 6 to 8 days, and can last for as long as several weeks (24). Clinical manifestations include headache, a change in sensorium, and the subsequent evolution of focal neurologic deficits.

Which of the components of blood is responsible for the vasospasm is still controversial. Horky and colleagues have postulated that ferrous iron, released from oxyhemoglobin, induces vasospasm either by generating free radicals and lipid peroxides or by binding the vasodilator nitric oxide (25). Probably no single substance or mechanical factor is involved, and certain substances released from the subarachnoid clot either are direct spasmogens or sensitize the blood vessels to other vasoactive compounds (26).

After a subarachnoid hemorrhage, an acute and persistent decrease in cerebral blood flow occurs, with the degree of cerebral blood flow reduction proportional to the amount of vasoconstriction. The resultant cerebral ischemia in part is responsible for the neurologic symptoms seen with a CNS hemorrhage (27). Additionally, increased intracranial pressure results from the blood that has entered the confined space of the cranial cavity. The combination of vasospasm and increased intracranial pressure is particularly ominous, as it reduces cerebral perfusion pressure and undoubtedly contributes to reduced cerebral blood flow (28). A poststenotic dilatation of the blood vessels in the marginally perfused cerebral tissue further complicates the condition. Another important contributory factor to infarction secondary to vasospasm is hypovolemia. This is accompanied by hyponatremia, which is caused by excessive renal sodium excretion, rather than being due to the syndrome of inappropriate antidiuretic hormone (SIADH). The atrial natriuretic factor and a digoxin-like factor are believed to be important in causing increased natriuresis (29).

Clinical and experimental evidence shows that the cerebral blood vessels become structurally abnormal during the second phase of vasoconstriction, with endothelial damage, subendothelial thickening, and smooth muscle necrosis producing the sustained vascular contraction (23). In addition, there is evidence for an impairment of endothelial-dependent vascular relaxation (30). This can be caused by decreased production of nitric oxide from the endothelial cells, and a decreased endothelial mRNA for nitric oxide synthase has been demonstrated in experimental animals (30). The combined effect of these factors complicates medical and surgical therapy and has a profound influence on the ultimate outcome of an intracranial hemorrhage (27).

OCCLUSIVE VASCULAR DISEASE

Glueck and associates have stressed the importance of familial lipid and lipoprotein abnormalities in children with occlusive vascular disease (31). In particular, low levels of high-density lipoproteins and high levels of triglycerides can predispose to occlusive vascular disease. Familial hypoalphalipoproteinemia, an autosomal dominant disorder, is associated with premature cerebrovascular accidents. Additionally, a high percentage of children with occlusive cerebrovascular disease have first-degree relatives with histories of coronary heart disease and cerebrovascular accidents (31). A significant association exists between nonhemorrhagic strokes or transient ischemic attacks and the presence of a patent foramen ovale. In the experience of Webster and coworkers, right-to-left shunting, as demonstrated by contrast echocardiography, could be demonstrated in 50% of stroke patients younger than age 40 years, as compared with only 15% of control subjects (32).

Arterial Thrombosis (Acute Hemiplegia)

In adult life, arterial occlusion is most frequently the consequence of arteriosclerosis of the cerebral vasculature. In childhood, arterial occlusion usually results from congenital dysplasia of the vessels, cerebral arteritis, trauma, or thromboembolic disease, the last usually in infants or children with congenital heart disease. The various causes for acute hemiplegia as published in 1970 are depicted in Table 12.4 (33). More recent series compiled from Finland (34) and France (35) have a somewhat similar distribution, except that in the Finnish series postmigrainous stroke hemiplegia accounted for 15% of acute hemiplegia.

The syndrome of acute hemiplegia was first described in the nineteenth century by a number of authors, including Freud (36), often under the term Marie-Strümpell encephalitis, a nomenclature designed to stress its supposed relationship to polioencephalitis. As defined by Ford and Schaffer (37), acute infantile hemiplegia is characterized by the sudden onset of hemiplegia in infancy or early childhood, usually before 6 years of age. The syndrome is not rare; Ford recalled observing some 200 patients with this condition at the Harriet Lane Home in Baltimore (38).

Pathology

In a large proportion of cases, the lesion causing acute hemiplegia can be delineated by cerebral arteriography or MR angiography (MRA) (1,33,39,40). On the basis of the arteriographic picture, Solomon and associates (33) and Hilal and associates (41) distinguished five categories.

1. Extracranial occlusions in the cervical portion of the internal carotid artery, generally

TABLE 12.4. *Causes for acute hemiplegia in 86 children*

Cause	Number of patients
Trauma	11
Central nervous system infections	11
Cardiac disease	10
Sickle cell anemia	5
Arteriovenous malformation	4
Documented occlusive vascular disease	16
Unknown origin	25
Miscellaneous	4

From Solomon GE, et al. Natural history of acute hemiplegia of childhood. *Brain* 1970;93:107. With permission of Oxford University Press.

the consequence of blunt trauma to the nasopharynx.
2. A marked and progressive stenosis or complete occlusion of the supraclinoid segment of the internal carotid artery and of its branches, notably the proximal portions of the middle and anterior cerebral arteries. Associated with this stenosis or occlusion is a prominent collateral network within the basal ganglia (Fig. 12.1). Additionally, extensive collaterals can exist between the meningeal branches of the external carotid artery and the leptomeningeal vessels on the cerebral surface. These abnormalities are usually bilateral and in many instances are progressive (42). This radiographic picture has been termed *moyamoya disease*.
3. Basal arterial occlusion, but without the presence of telangiectasia. Generally, the internal carotid artery is stenosed or completely occluded in its supraclinoid segment. The occlusion is believed to be caused by an arteritis, possibly as an aftermath of ear, throat, or sinus infections. This angiographic picture probably represents an early stage of moyamoya disease (43).
4. Stenosis at the origin of the internal carotid artery or occlusion of one or more branches of the distal portion of the middle cerebral artery (33,41). This picture is less common than that of moyamoya disease.
5. In the fifth group of children with acute hemiplegia, arteriography is normal. In the majority of this group, the hemiparesis follows multiple generalized or focal seizures (33,44). Norman has postulated that neuronal destruction resulting from the seizures and consequent hypotension and cerebral hypoperfusions results in tissue destruction occurring in a laminar distribution within the cerebral cortex and is responsible for the hemiparesis (45). Although in most cases of status epilepticus the neuronal loss is bilateral, in a number of instances cortical damage is almost exclusively unilateral, particularly when seizures are superimposed on a preexisting, but clinically inapparent, cerebral malformation or asphyxial birth injury.

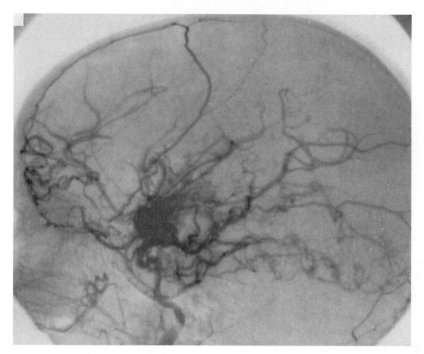

FIG. 12.1. Moyamoya disease in 3-year-old boy with acute right hemiplegia. The left cerebral angiogram demonstrates an obstruction of the internal carotid artery, probably at the origin of the posterior communicating artery. There is a net-like cluster of blood vessels in the area of the basal ganglia, probably arising from the lenticulostriate arteries. (Courtesy of Dr. Gabriel Wilson, Department of Radiology, University of California, Los Angeles, UCLA School of Medicine.)

Of the various types of vascular abnormalities resulting in arterial thrombosis, moyamoya disease has aroused the most attention. This condition was first described by Takeuchi in 1963 and more fully delineated by Suzuki (43). [*Moyamoya* is a Japanese term, first used by Kudo. It refers to something hazy, "just like a puff of cigarette smoke drifting in the air" (46).]

Moyamoya disease is not a single entity, but is best considered to be a syndrome. Takeuchi and associates (47) and Gadoth and Hirsch (48) distinguished two forms, primary and secondary (moyamoya syndrome). Primary moyamoya disease with a strong hereditary predisposition is fairly common among Japanese patients (0.1 in 100,000 per year), and 10% of Japanese cases are familial (43,49). One gene has been mapped to the short arm of chromosome 3 (3p24.2-p26) (49a). In the pediatric age group, girls are more frequently affected, with the peak age of onset being before 5 years (49). The initial symptoms include motor disturbances, mainly an alternating and generally nonprogressive hemiparesis, transient ischemic attacks, speech disturbances, and seizures (43). Mental deterioration is seen in approximately one-third of children, and involuntary movements appear in approximately 5%. Intracranial hemorrhage is unusual in children, but not in adults. Transient ischemic attacks are seen in some 20% of children. These are readily brought on by crying or hyperventilation; electroencephalograms (EEGs) taken during such events reveal a rapid and marked buildup and a rebuildup of slow waves 20 to 60 seconds after cessation of hyperventilation (49). Japanese workers have classified moyamoya disease into four types: the hemorrhagic type characterized by subarachnoid bleeding, the epileptic type by repeated seizures, the infarct type by permanent paresis, and the transient ischemic attack type marked by

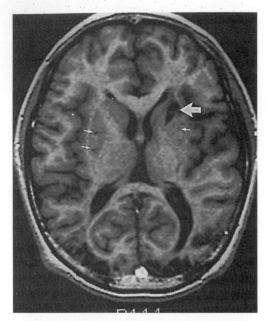

FIG. 12.2. Moyamoya disease. Axial T1-weighted magnetic resonance imaging in 13-year-old with moyamoya. An infarct is visible on the left, at the border between the caudate nucleus and the internal capsule (*arrow*). Prominent signal voids are seen in the basal ganglia (*small arrows*). (Courtesy of Dr. John Curran, Department of Radiology, UCLA Center for the Health Sciences, Los Angeles.)

recurrent transient ischemic attacks. The last type is the most common form seen in Japan.

Sequential arteriography or MRA indicates several stages of primary moyamoya disease. Initially, narrowing of the carotid fork is seen. This is followed by dilatation of the major cerebral arteries and the appearance of collateral circulation, the moyamoya vessels. Subsequently, the middle and anterior cerebral arteries disappear, with ultimate reduction and disappearance of the moyamoya vessels.

Magnetic resonance imaging (MRI) and MRA are equally informative and permit visualization of the stenotic internal carotid artery and the moyamoya vessels in the basal ganglia (37,46). In addition, the area or areas of infarction are demonstrable by MRI (Fig. 12.2), with the infarcted area being visualized as early as 2 to 3 hours after the vascular occlusion. Diffusion-weighted MRI can be used to evaluate

ischemic lesions within minutes after the onset of stroke (50,50a). This technique can be used also to demonstrate tissue, which is not irreversibly compromised.

Untreated, transient ischemic attacks tend to lessen over the years but intellectual deterioration and persistent motor deficits become progressively worse. Intellectual deterioration was noted in 65% of children who had moyamoya disease for longer than 5 years (51). Early onset of symptoms and hypertension were related to a poor prognosis, whereas the presence of seizures was not. Conversely, children with the transient ischemic attack form of moyamoya disease tend to do somewhat better in terms of mental status and activities of daily living (51a).

A variety of extracranial-intracranial bypass procedures have been proposed as treatment of moyamoya disease. These procedures produce direct, indirect, or combined anastomotic revascularization. Direct revascularization includes anastomosis of the superficial temporal artery or the occipital artery to the middle cerebral artery. Indirect bypasses, which are more or less effective, are placement of a dural graft, encephalo-duro-arteriosynangiosis (EDAS), and encephalo-arteriosynangiosis in which branches of the scalp arteries are used as donor arteries. Other indirect bypasses include encephalo-myo-synangiosis (EMS) in which a pedunculated temporalis muscle flap is placed over the temporoparietal lobe and omental transplantation. These procedures are often combined with direct or other indirect revascularization procedures. Indirect revascularization, technically less difficult, is used first in most Japanese centers, with direct anastomosis reserved for patients whose symptoms persist (43,52).

According to proponents of indirect revascularization, surgery for moyamoya disease results in the development of collaterals from the external carotid arterial system into the territory of the middle cerebral artery. This is associated with a decrease in the abnormal moyamoya vessels, and a significant improvement for children with transient ischemic attacks and involuntary movements (53). When mental handicap is relatively mild, improvement can be expected in the majority of instances (43). In the exclusively pediatric series of Hoffman, 70% of children treated by EDAS, sometimes supplemented by EMS, had an excellent outcome, 17% had a good outcome, but were left with a significant neurologic deficit (54). The various procedures and results are more fully described by Hoffman (54) and Kashiwagi and colleagues (55).

The cause for the underlying arterial occlusion and the circumstances conducive to the development of these extensive collaterals are obscure. Intimal fibrous thickening of the arterial walls of intracranial vessels are common (56), with similar changes in extracranial vessels. Suzuki has postulated an underlying autoimmune vasculitis as the etiology for primary moyamoya disease (43). More recently, mRNA levels for elastin were noted to be elevated, and Yamamoto and colleagues have suggested an abnormal regulation of extracellular matrix metabolism (57).

Secondary moyamoya disease (moyamoya syndrome) is caused by a variety of underlying conditions. In the series of patients seen at the Hospital for Sick Children, Toronto, neurofibromatosis 1 was by far the most common and accounted for 54% of children with moyamoya syndrome (54). Other causes reported in the literature include sickle cell disease (58), tuberous sclerosis (59), Down syndrome (60), congenital heart disease (61), Williams syndrome (61a), Schimke immuno-osseous dysplasia (61b), hypomelanosis of Ito (61c), and various CNS infections such as tuberculous meningitis (43), and varicella, which can induce a vasculitis. A rare association of AVMs in the cerebral hemisphere with moyamoya syndrome may be more than coincidental; the ischemia of the AVM may stimulate the neovascularity of moyamoya (57a).

Clinical Manifestations

Regardless of the angiographic findings, the clinical picture of arterial thrombosis unaccompanied by systemic diseases is fairly uniform. Little can be added to the description of acute hemiparesis given by Freud (36). The following is his description of an acute ischemic stroke:

> A child who has hitherto been well, and without hereditary predisposition, is suddenly taken ill at an age between a few months to 3

years. The etiology of the disease either remains unexplained or is attributed to a concurrent infection. The presenting symptoms may be either stormy, with fever, convulsions, and vomiting, or insignificant; they may last 1 day or up to several weeks. The disease cannot be diagnosed with certainty in this initial stage. A hemiparesis may appear at this point, or not until later. It spreads in the usual manner: first face, then arm, then leg. At first it is a flaccid paresis, but very soon it becomes spastic, with increased reflexes and contractures. Partial or complete aphasia appear commonly, but are usually transient; hemianopsia or paralyses of the ocular muscles are rare. The paresis may vanish, or else recur in bouts with increasing severity; most commonly it is permanent. Improvement is more likely in the leg than the arm; in such a case the child walks with circumduction of the affected hip. Improvement of the paresis is very commonly associated with posthemiplegic chorea together with a greater or lesser degree of residual spasticity. Growth atrophy of the affected limbs, which is often extensive, becomes apparent during the pubertal growth spurt. Impaired intelligence of varying degree is seldom absent. Epileptic seizures may make their appearance at a variable interval after the initial illness. These are at first unilateral; later they become generalized and severe. There is no time limit to the appearance of epileptic seizures.

As indicated by Freud's description, and confirmed in our experience and by the series of Ingram (62) and Lanska and colleagues (63), acute hemiplegia regardless of cause usually occurs before age 3 years. Nearly 90% of Ingram's patients were younger than age 3 years. In the series of Lanska and colleagues, 53% of children who experienced an acute presentation of a stroke did so prior to 3 years of age. Approximately 60% of Ingram's and 43% of Lanska's patients had unilateral or generalized seizures at the onset of hemiplegia or shortly thereafter. According to Hilal and coworkers (41), seizures tend to be more common when the angiographic picture demonstrates the moyamoya vessels. The duration of the convulsion varies; it can be as long as 24 hours. After the convulsion, neurologic function is lost or severely impaired. Headache is an important feature of basal arterial occlusion without telangiectasia. These observations probably reflect the changes in the clinical picture with the evolution of moyamoya syndrome. As Freud noted, involvement of the arm is almost always more extensive than of the leg. Crothers and Paine (64) and Aicardi and associates (65) found disturbances in sensation and hemianopia to be relatively common. They were seen in 11% each in the series of Lanska and coworkers. Atypical presentations, as with recurrent severe headache (hemiplegic migraine), or hemichorea have been noted (63,66).

Although Freud considered children who develop acute hemiplegia as having been "hitherto well," this actually is not the case, and only applied to 17% of children with acute hemiplegia in the series of Lanska and colleagues (63). The preponderance of children in the more recent series have had a history of congenital heart disease; some of these probably develop hemiplegia as a consequence of cerebral emboli. In a significant proportion, hemiplegia developed during uterine development, and became apparent to parents during the first year of life as a pathologic hand preference. The increased attention paid to an infant during an acute febrile illness frequently prompts recognition of a preexisting deficit. Earlier writers noted the high incidence of abnormal birth or gestation (62), but it is our experience and that of Lanska and colleagues that abnormalities during delivery or during the perinatal period are uncommon (see Chapter 5) (63). They were seen in only 25% of infants presenting with pathologic early hand preference, and in none of the older infants or children who presented with acute hemiplegia (63). Some 20% have had a history of prior convulsions. In most of these patients, single or multiple seizures initiate the hemiparesis (postconvulsive hemiparesis).

Diagnosis

The initial diagnostic evaluation of an acutely hemiparetic child should include an examina-tion of the cerebrospinal fluid (CSF) and an imaging study. The CSF is usually normal. A few patients have mild pleocytosis (less than 50 cells per μL) and an elevated protein. The EEG is of little assistance. It can reveal unilateral or predominantly unilateral slowing and decreased voltage over the affected side.

In an emergency setting, a CT scan is the preferred study. Starting within 4 to 6 hours of the infarction, the scan shows one or more nonhomogeneous lucent areas with indistinct margins. These generally enhance with contrast. An MRI study shows evidence of the infarct within 2 to 3 hours of the event. This study can be supplemented by MRA. Should CT and MRI results be negative despite a persistent hemiparesis, diffusion-weighted MRI, a technique that is becoming increasingly available, can be used to delineate the potentially infarcted area (50,50a). A mass effect resulting from edema becomes most prominent 48 hours after the infarction and can persist for a week or longer. A small number of scans show hemorrhage in the infarcted region. A few days after the event, gyral enhancement after the infusion of contrast material is apparent. Starting within a week of the infarction, the necrotic areas gradually become homogeneous with well-defined margins. In long-standing hemiplegias, neuroimaging demonstrates unilateral hemispheral atrophy with widening of sulci, narrowing of gyri, and dilatation of the ventricles (Fig. 12.3). Imaging studies performed on children who have had a long-standing infarct can sometimes disclose intracerebral calcification, an indication of a hemorrhagic component to the child's infarct. Alterations of the bony vault are seen also. This radiographic picture, referred to as the Dyke-Davidoff syndrome, can become evident as early as 9 months after the onset of the hemiparesis (33).

Cerebral arteriography or MRA are indicated for every child with an acute onset of hemiparesis to establish an anatomic diagnosis. In many institutions, MRA is valuable for initial screening, with cerebral arteriography continuing as the imaging gold standard. As a rule, angiography is more likely to reveal the cause of a cerebral hemorrhage, whereas MRA or MRI delineate nonhemorrhagic lesions (67). Compli-

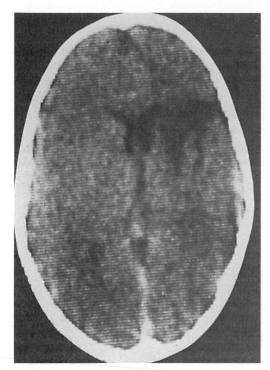

FIG. 12.3. Computed tomographic scan in acute hemiplegia. This child fell while running with a Popsicle stick in his mouth and sustained intraoral trauma to the internal carotid artery, which was shown to be completely occluded angiographically. The computed tomographic scan obtained at a later date shows cerebral infarction. The adjacent frontal horn dilatation and shift to the side of infarction indicates the presence of focal atrophy. (Courtesy of Drs. Hervey D. Segall, Forrest Johnson, and Philip Stanley, Children's Hospital, Los Angeles.)

cations from cerebral arteriography are rare, even when the procedure is carried out shortly after the onset of the hemiparesis.

Differential Diagnosis

Various conditions can produce sudden onset of hemiplegia in a child. In addition to the causes already discussed, hemiplegia of acute onset can result from periarteritis nodosa, bacterial or viral infections, including acquired immunodeficiency syndrome, trauma, cardiac abnormalities, sickle cell disease and other hemoglobinopathies, AVMs,

mitochondrial disorders (MELAS), demyelinating diseases, and homocystinuria.

Evaluation of the child who has experienced a cerebral thrombotic episode should involve screening for the presence of antiphospholipid antibodies, including the lupus anticoagulant and anticardiolipin antibody, screening for factor V Leiden, determination of antithrombin III levels, and measurement of protein C activity and total and free protein S antigen levels. Screening of serum for hyperlipidemia, urine for homocystine, and a cardiac evaluation, including echocardiography, also should be performed (8a, 68). An elevation in blood or CSF lactate is not indicative of a mitochondrial disorder, because cerebral ischemia of any cause can increase blood and CSF lactate levels.

Todd's paralysis must be considered in the differential diagnosis of acute hemiplegia. This entity is a transient paresis that follows a generalized focal or jacksonian seizure. Although in most cases the weakness clears in a few hours, apparently uncomplicated Todd's paralysis can persist for up to several days in some cases (see Chapter 13).

The sudden onset of hemiparesis is also characteristic of hemiplegic migraine. This relatively uncommon, often familial condition is characterized by the association of migraine and hemiplegia, with the hemiplegia usually occurring as an aura to the attack. Cerebral angiography during the prodromal stage either is normal or shows constriction of the internal carotid artery system (see Chapter 13). Stroke is a rare complication of migraine in adolescents. Whereas stroke is not associated with any particular arterial anomaly, antecedent migraine attacks tend to have been unusually severe (69).

Treatment and Prognosis

Treatment of acute cerebral thrombosis and consequent cerebral infarction is directed toward increasing cerebral perfusion and salvaging threatened tissue.

A variety of therapies have been advocated for the treatment of an acute cerebral infarction. Hemodilution using various volume expanders, calcium channel blockers, notably nimodipine, corticosteroids, and naloxone, an opiate antagonist, have all produced negative results in placebo-controlled trials. Anticoagulation using orally administered low-molecular-weight heparin, and thrombolysis using recombinant tissue plasminogen activator have been found to be effective in adult patients, the latter when given within 3 hours of the thrombotic event. The effectiveness of these therapeutic options in pediatric stroke patients still needs to be demonstrated (70). The risk of developing an intracranial hemorrhage as a result of thrombolytic therapy appears to be low in children (71). The clinical value of the various antagonists to the excitatory amino acid receptors has not yet been demonstrated (72). The effectiveness of various sodium-channel blockers, which may inhibit the release of glutamine from ischemic neurons, thus reducing postsynaptic excitotoxicity, as well as other forms of neuroprotection, has not been demonstrated for adult patients, and clinical benefits are even less certain in the pediatric population (72a).

The decision to use anticoagulants depends on the relative risks of recurrent stroke as compared with the likelihood of a postinfarction hemorrhage. As a rule, anticoagulants are used in children with gradually worsening strokes, recurrent emboli, and in the hypercoagulable state. Details of anticoagulation using heparin or low-molecular-weight heparin in pediatric patients are presented by Sutor and colleagues (73) and Massicotte and colleagues (74).

Increased intracranial pressure secondary to cerebral edema is a rare complication of cerebral infarction in the pediatric population. Corticosteroids should not be used routinely in such circumstances; they are ineffective in cytotoxic edema. Hypothermia and inhalations of 5% carbon dioxide or oxygen have been ineffective. Prophylactic anticonvulsants have no role in the treatment of children with thrombotic cerebral infarcts.

In children who have experienced an attack of acute hemiplegia, more than 50% of survivors have a residual hemiparesis or convulsions, but the frequency of residual motor deficits is quite variable and probably reflects the underlying cause of the hemiplegia (63,75). Generally, residua are more likely when hemiplegia results from a vascular occlusion rather than from a hem-

orrhagic episode (1). Seizures persist in approximately 75% of patients with postconvulsive hemiplegia, particularly in those whose illness began with multiple seizures (33,44). Complete recovery from the motor deficit and residual intellectual and behavioral abnormalities is less likely in this group than in patients whose hemiparesis was unaccompanied by seizures. When children with postconvulsive hemiplegia are excluded, the incidence of late seizures is much smaller (19% in the series of Lanska and coworkers) (63).

In many children, seizures continue for years and are intractable to anticonvulsants. Under these circumstances, hemispherectomy should be considered. The procedure and its indications and contraindications are discussed in Chapter 13.

A full discussion of the role of an organized rehabilitation program in the long-term treatment of the child with hemiplegia is outside the scope of this text. The reader is referred to a text by Molnar (76).

Cerebral Embolism

During the neonatal period, embolisms can arise from the placenta (see Chapter 5). In childhood, cerebral embolism usually is encountered within the framework of cardiac disease, specifically cyanotic congenital heart disease, bacterial endocarditis, or rheumatic valvular disease. Less often, a fat embolism can emanate from a fracture of a long bone (77–79) or occur after intravenous fat infusions (80). Air embolisms can be induced in the course of open heart surgery or various other thoracic surgical procedures (81). Additionally, they are encountered in underwater swimmers after prolonged breath holding and in scuba divers as a consequence of too rapid decompression (82). See Chapter 8, section on Neurologic Injury from Undersea Diving.

The clinical picture of cerebral embolism as a consequence of cardiac disease includes acute onset of a variety of neurologic symptoms, notably loss of consciousness, seizures, hemiparesis, aphasia, or hemianopia. Prodromal signs either are absent or are as relatively insignificant as headache or vomiting.

Fat embolism usually is seen within 48 hours after a fracture of the pelvis or the lower extremities; extremity fracture is often complicated by multiple transport maneuvers. Aside from the neurologic picture of altered consciousness, convulsions, and hemiparesis, patients almost invariably have tachypnea, fever, and a petechial rash over the upper chest, face, and axillae (78). Cerebral edema can complicate the neurologic picture. The MRI shows scattered, high-signal intensity lesions on T2-weighted images (83). Management involves administration of oxygen and corticosteroids. In the experience of Moore and associates, none of 17 patients had neurologic residua (78). Other workers have dissented on the effectiveness of corticosteroid therapy. Gossling and Pellegrini (77) and Batra (84) review the current concepts of the physiopathology of fat embolism.

Air embolism to the brain is marked by an abrupt loss of consciousness, with or without unilateral symptoms in the distribution of the carotid artery system. Less often, brainstem signs occur. Treatment consists of immediate recompression followed by administration of oxygen.

It is often difficult to determine whether an arterial filling defect as seen on arteriography or by MRA represents an embolus or a thrombus. Whenever there are multiple filling defects in multiple arterial branches, the diagnosis of thromboembolic disease is most likely (39).

Dural Sinus and Cerebral Vein Thrombosis

Once a common entity, considered "a dramatic and dangerous complication of many diseases" (85), thrombosis of the cerebral dural sinuses or veins has become relatively infrequent owing to the use of fluid therapy and antibiotics. At present, this clinical picture is seen in infants with severe, usually cyanotic, congenital heart disease, and the various other genetic or acquired conditions already cited, which are associated with a hypercoagulable state. In the 1992 series of Barron and coworkers, treatment with L-asparaginase was responsible for the hypercoagulable state in two-thirds of older children. The remainder was caused by antithrombin III or protein C deficiency (86).

Purulent venous thrombosis, once common, is relatively uncommon nowadays. In their classic studies of thrombosis of the dural venous sinuses (published in 1933 and 1937, respectively), Byers and Hass (87) and Bailey and

Hass (88) found 96% of cases of dural venous sinus thrombosis in children younger than 3 years of age. In approximately 50%, thrombosis was caused by a septic process arising from an adjacent focus: the mastoid, upper lip, or orbit. In approximately 5%, thrombosis followed a surgical procedure. In the 1992 series of Barron and colleagues, local infections were deemed responsible in 27% of older infants and children who experienced cerebral venous thrombosis (86). In infants with cyanotic congenital heart disease, the thrombus generally involves the dural sinus, most often the superior longitudinal (sagittal) sinus, and the tributary cerebral veins. In 31 infants whose thromboses were not the consequence of an infection, Bailey and Hass found involvement of the superior longitudinal sinus in 31, of the lateral sinus in 17, and of the superior cerebral veins in 15 (88). Several children had thromboses in more than one sinus.

The clinical picture is protean and nonspecific, and thrombosis must be considered whenever neurologic symptoms complicate a febrile illness in an infant with cyanotic congenital heart disease or some other debilitating condition (89). Most commonly, thrombosis induces changes in consciousness, focal or generalized seizures, focal motor deficits, and evidence of increased intracranial pressure in the form of papilledema or a full fontanel. Dilatation of the scalp veins and the caput medusae of Lermoyez (90), said to be a classic sign of superior sagittal sinus thrombosis, must be rare; it was found in none of Kalbag and Woolf's personal cases (85). In the series of Barron and colleagues, 60% of children presented with headache, 20% with seizures, 33% had an altered mental status, and 27% had cranial nerve palsies (86). Abnormalities in the CSF depend on when in the course of the illness the specimen is secured. Soon after thrombosis, the CSF is clear and under slightly increased pressure. Later, increased pressure is seen in approximately 50% of instances. The fluid can be xanthochromic or grossly bloody, and a striking increase of protein content can occur (88). Pleocytosis in the absence of an infection is not unusual.

The diagnosis of sinus or cortical vein thrombosis by neuroimaging studies is difficult and full of pitfalls, even in the most expert hands. Whenever cerebral angiography is used, the venous phase must be adequately visualized and venous subtraction films must be obtained. In most instances, the CT picture is nonspecific, with swelling or focal hypodensities. MRI is superior to CT scanning in that it can demonstrate sinus or venous thromboses not visualized on CT (91). In the experience of Zimmerman and Bilaniuk (39), MRI was diagnostic in 80% of infants and children. MRA with two- and three-dimensional time of flight techniques with and without gadolinium contrast material, a technique that demonstrates both fast and slow flow, also has been used for visualization of venous and dural sinus thrombosis (92). In the hands of Lee and colleagues and Wang (92,93), MRA and MR venography were superior to MRI in visualizing the intracranial vessels, and MR venography was the technique of choice for evaluating the dural sinuses and cerebral veins. Ozsvath and colleagues consider CT venography to be superior to MR venography in the identification of cerebral veins and dural sinuses (94).

Aside from maintaining an adequate state of hydration and performing the usual supportive measures, little can be done to help the infant or child with cerebral sinus or vein thrombosis once this process has begun (86). Heparin has been used in the hope that its early administration will prevent the spread of the thrombus. At present, no randomized study documents the effectiveness of heparin, and heparin is contraindicated when there is evidence of cortical vein thrombosis and thus a significant likelihood for cerebral hemorrhage (95,96).

The outcome depends on the age and the site of the thrombosis. Neonates generally have significant residua, whereas older infants or children have a 95% chance of escaping neurologic deficits. When the thrombosis affects the deep venous structures, including the internal cerebral vein and its tributaries, the vein of Galen, or the straight sinus, the outcome is generally poor. By contrast, patients with superficial cortical vein thrombosis have a fairly good prognosis (39,86).

Alternating Hemiplegia

Alternating hemiplegia is a rare but clinically distinct condition first described by Verret and Steele (97). It is characterized by repeated attacks of hemiplegia affecting either or both sides of the body, autonomic disturbances occurring independently from, or in conjunction with, the hemiplegia, oculomotor disturbances, notably nystagmus and extraocular palsies, and mental deterioration. Attacks usually begin before 18 months of age, are abrupt in onset, and last from minutes to days (98). The neurologic examination is generally normal between episodes, although some children demonstrate a variety of dyskinesias. Neuroimaging studies and neuropathologic examinations have been unremarkable. Between attacks the EEG is normal, but during an episode of hemiplegia the EEG frequently shows an increase in slow-wave components. During an attack, SPECT has demonstrated hypoperfusion of the hemisphere contralateral to the hemiparesis (99). This is often followed by hyperperfusion (100). Neuropathology is consistent with the results of recurrent attacks of hypoxia-ischemia, with extensive involvement of the hippocampus explaining the cognitive decline (101).

The pathophysiology of alternating hemiplegia is unknown. Vasospasm with cerebral hypoperfusion, such as is seen in attacks of complicated migraine or an atypical manifestation of epilepsy, are currently the most favored mechanisms. Often there is a family history of migraine, notably of hemiplegic migraine, or of alternating hemiplegia. Sleep, even for a brief period of a few minutes, frequently abolishes the hemiparesis and the infant or child awakens free of neurologic deficit. This feature heightens speculation that it is a form of migraine or a metabolic disturbance (101a). EEG monitoring during sleep cycles, with or without transient hemiparesis, fails to disclose paroxysmal activity or abnormal sleep stages. The long-term prognosis for children with alternating hemiplegia is guarded because most show evidence of developmental and intellectual decline. Seizures do not generally appear, early or late in the course of the disease.

Another hypothesis of the intermittent deficit with shifting laterality is that it is caused by a mitochondrial disorder, but efforts to demonstrate evidence of mitochondrial cytopathy by muscle biopsy have not yielded consistent or convincing evidence (101b,101c). Yet another theory of pathogenesis of alternating hemiplegia is that it is a channelopathy, of calcium channels in particular, analogous to hypokalemic periodic paralysis, but again the evidence is lacking (101a). It is not even certain whether alternating hemiplegia is a single disease entity or a syndrome of multiple etiologies.

In addition to the classic disorder, a dominant alternating hemiplegia has been described, as well as a condition in which there is alternating paroxysmal dystonia with hemiparesis, and alternating hemiplegia with livido reticularis. These extremely rare entities are reviewed by Andermann and colleagues (102).

Anticonvulsants and antimigraine agents are ineffective. Flunarizine, a calcium-channel blocker (5 mg/day for children less than 40 lbs body weight), has reduced the frequency of attacks in some children, but rarely abolishes them completely (103). In our experience the medication has been ineffective.

ARTERIAL DISSECTIONS

Dissections of the intracranial and cervical arteries are quite rare in childhood. They can occur spontaneously or as a result of an injury with sudden stretching of an artery, which leads to tearing of the intima. With a tear in the intima the force of the blood separates the intima from the media forming a dissecting hematoma, which progressively reduces the arterial lumen and can eventually occlude it. The most common sites for traumatic dissection are the cervical segments of the carotid arteries, the vertebral artery, and the proximal portions of the middle cerebral artery. Occasionally, multivessel dissection is seen (104). Traumatic cervical artery dissection can occur as a consequence of a blunt blow to the neck or from hyperextension of the neck. Injury also can be precipitated by the child falling while carrying an object in the mouth (Popsicle injury). The trauma frequently is minor, and the interval between trauma and the onset of symptoms can be as long as weeks or months. Recurrent dissection has been encountered in 8% (105). Spontaneous dissection of the internal carotid artery is encountered as a complication of Marfan syndrome and Ehlers-Danlos disease, type IV (106). In some patients there is a reduced production of type III colla-

gen (107). In many instances, however, no clear precipitating cause can be found (107a).

The clinical presentation is mainly with headache, transient ischemic attacks, hemiparesis, or seizures. When headache is present, it precedes the onset of ischemic symptoms by an interval, which in the experience of Schievink and colleagues ranged from less than 1 minute to 5 days (104). Spontaneous dissection of the intracranial arteries involves the supraclinoid portion of the internal carotid artery with additional involvement of the ipsilateral middle cerebral artery, or less often, the contralateral middle cerebral artery. Isolated involvement of the middle cerebral artery also has been noted. In most children there is an ischemic stroke. This can be preceded by headache and accompanied by seizures.

MRI and MRA are useful in the evaluation of arterial dissection, in that they can demonstrate complete or partial obstruction of the affected vessel. These studies are supplemented by conventional arteriography (108).

Anticoagulation therapy usually is recommended for adults, as there is a significant risk for intracranial hemorrhage. Because recovery is usually good or excellent, we recommend conservative management.

CENTRAL NERVOUS SYSTEM HEMORRHAGE

The most common cause of primary CNS hemorrhage in infants and children is vascular anomalies. The most important of these are the angiomas, which can be classified as arteriovenous, venous, cavernous, or capillary. In children, neurologic symptoms as a consequence of angiomas are approximately 10 times more common than symptomatic intracranial aneurysms or anomalies of the circle of Willis.

Streeter has reviewed the embryology of the cerebral vascular system (109). He defines five stages: (a) the formation of the primordial vascular plexus, (b) the formation of blood vessels, (c) stratification into superficial and deep components, (d) rearrangement of vessels with obliteration of some trunks and creation of others, and (e) differentiation into morphologically recognizable arteries, veins, and capillaries. Disturbance or arrest of vascular development accounts for all vascular malformations except aneurysms (110). The embryology of the cerebral vasculature is covered in greater detail in Chapter 4.

Angioma

Under the term *angiomas*, McCormick and colleagues include a variety of vascular malformations of the brain (111). These are true developmental malformations rather than vascular neoplasms, although some can proliferate and produce progressive destructive changes in the surrounding parenchyma. Malformations range from huge cavernous venous angiomas that often do not bleed to tiny subependymal cryptic angiomas that at times bleed massively and simultaneously obliterate themselves. Table 12.5 depicts the type, location, and relative frequencies of brain angiomas (111). Two-thirds of the lesions are in the cerebrum, with AVMs being the most common, constituting 56% of all vascular malformations of the brain (111).

Arteriovenous Malformation

Pathogenesis

AVMs result from the embryonic failure of capillary development between artery and vein. This malformation in turn produces an enlargement of the vessels and abnormal shunting of blood. On gross examination of the brain, the lesion has a "bag of worms" appearance, which is caused by the tangled mass of dilated veins, the frequently enlarged and tortuous arteries feeding these venous channels, and the interposed thickened, dilated, and hyalinized vessels. The malformation can extend from the cortical meningeal surface through the parenchyma to the ventricular cavity, and its size can vary from 1 mm to more than 10 cm. Calcifications within the walls of the vessel and the surrounding parenchyma are common, and some ossification can be present. Hemosiderin can be found in the gliotic parenchyma as a consequence of extravasated blood. The pathology of these lesions is reviewed by Rorke (112). In the pediatric series of Kondziolka and colleagues, 67% of malformations were in the cerebral hemispheres, 13% in the cerebellum, 11% in the brainstem, and 5% in the thalamus or basal ganglia (113). The distribution of lesions is similar for other series.

AVMs must be differentiated from the rarely encountered carotid-cavernous fistula, which almost always is traumatic in origin (see Chapter 8). Spontaneous carotid-cavernous fistulas have been reported, however, in patients with type IV Ehlers-Danlos syndrome (114,115).

Clinical Manifestations

Only one-half of AVMs are symptomatic. In our experience, small lesions are often deep and silent and bleed massively. Large lesions are characterized by seizures and focal neurologic signs and bleed less extensively. In most large studies of symptomatic AVMs, 10% become clinically manifest during the first decade, and up to 45% are evident by the second or third decade (116). These lesions are seen twice as frequently in male subjects. In the overwhelming majority, 79% in the series of Kondziolka and colleagues (113), intracranial hemorrhage is the initial presentation. In 23% of patients, the hemorrhage

TABLE 12.5. *Type, location, and frequency of brain angioma*

Type	Location			
	Cerebral	Cerebellar	Brainstem	Total
Telangiectasia	22	6	32	60
Cavernous angiomas	59	11	10	80
Venous angiomas	48	22	13	83
Arteriovenous malformations	217	52	18	287
Total	346	91	73	510

From McCormick WF, Hardman JF, Boulter TR. Vascular malformations ("angiomas") of the brain with special reference to those occurring in the posterior fossa. *J Neurosurg* 1968;28:241. With permission.

recurs from a few days to many years after the first event (117). A chronic seizure disorder, recurrent headache, and progressive neurologic deficits are less common presentations. Progressive neurologic deficits can result from the AVM acting as a space-occupying lesion, or, more commonly, are caused by arterial steal away from normal surrounding brain into a high-flow AVM or venous hypertension transmitted from the malformation into the surrounding brain (118). Rarely, the condition is familial, being transmitted as an autosomal dominant disorder accompanied by polycystic kidneys (119).

When a hemorrhage develops, it is generally parenchymal, but depending on the location of the AVM, blood can dissect into the subarachnoid space and the ventricular system. The most frequent clinical picture is that of a child who either has been completely asymptomatic or has experienced periodic migraine-like headaches, and who suddenly has a severe headache, vomiting, nuchal rigidity, and seizures (116,120,121). As a consequence of the massive bleeding, the patient can develop signs and symptoms of increased intracranial pressure with transtentorial or foramen magnum pressure cones. The mortality from a hemorrhage depends on the location of the AVM. In the series of Kondziolka and colleagues, it was 4.5% for cerebral AVMs, but 57% when the hemorrhage arose from a cerebellar malformation (113).

Less commonly (12% to 22% of children), an AVM presents with a focal or generalized seizure (113,121). Focal seizures can be simple partial, with or without generalization, and, less often, complex partial. Generalized tonic-clonic seizures are seen in some 20% of subjects (122). Control of seizures is relatively easy and, in the experience of Murphy, some 50% of patients were free of seizures for a minimum of 2 years (122). Other symptoms include progressive hemiparesis, behavioral abnormalities, and dementia. Intracranial bruits were found in only 25% of patients with AVMs reported by Kelly and coworkers (121). Rarely, an AVM can thrombose and produce ischemic focal neurologic deficits.

Relatively more common in the adult, AVMs in the posterior fossa become manifest before 20 years of age in less than 10% to 25% of cases

(113,123). Symptoms are those of a cerebellar or brainstem lesion. Because most AVMs in this region are small, usually less than 2 cm in diameter, intracranial bruits are rarely heard. A pontine angioma can mimic a similarly placed neoplasm by presenting with insidious and progressive brainstem deficits (123). Hydrocephalus can complicate this type of AVM (111).

A spinal cord syndrome owing to an AVM is rare in childhood. Symptomatic spinal cord AVMs are more frequent in the cervical region, whereas in adults they are more likely to be located in the thoracolumbar region. In the pediatric series of Aminoff and Edwards (124), 55% of children presented with a subarachnoid hemorrhage. Symptoms are marked by sudden severe pain at the site of the hemorrhage, which spreads to involve the entire back. Older children and adults often experience impairment of motor function, usually coming on after physical effort, and recurrent pain and paresthesias of girdle or root distribution. Sensory symptoms can present as fluctuating lower abdominal pain or sciatica and can last from several minutes to hours. Symptoms are produced by small hemorrhages, and stepwise progression of long tract signs below the lesion follows each attack. In 34%, a spinal cord AVM coexists with a cutaneous angioma in the same or an adjacent dermatome (125,126). The skin lesions include port-wine–stained angiomas (Cobb syndrome) (127) or telangiectasia (Osler-Weber-Rendu syndrome). An important clinical decision must be made in managing children with facial angiomas with respect to which patients to investigate for intracranial vascular lesions. Port-wine stains involving the cutaneous distribution of the ophthalmic branch of the trigeminal nerve are most likely to be associated with intracranial vascular malformations, especially if they are extensive; those involving two or more trigeminal branches nearly always have intracranial components (127a).

Osler-Weber-Rendu syndrome (OWRS) (hereditary hemorrhagic telangiectasia) consists of a group of autosomal dominant disorders, the gene for the most common of which is located on the long arm of chromosome 9 (9q33-q34). The gene encodes endoglin, a component of the transforming growth factor-β_1 receptor (TGF) complex (128). TGF inhibits growth of many cell types, including hematopoietic cells and lymphocytes. The clinical manifestations of OWRS involve vascular abnormalities of the nose, skin, gastrointestinal tract, lung, and brain. In the nose, telangiectases result in epistaxis, whereas in the lungs there are AVMs. In the experience of Putman and colleagues who systematically screened subjects with OWRS with MRI, 23% had abnormalities suggesting a vascular malformation. Follow-up angiography showed that all subjects had at least one AVM, and 39% had three or more AVMs (129,130). These lesions can result in subarachnoid hemorrhage, seizures, and if the AVM involves the spinal cord, paraparesis (125,130,131). Brain abscess can develop in the presence of pulmonary AVM and right-to-left shunt (132).

In the Klippel-Trenaunay syndrome, which occurs sporadically, a spinal cord AVM is associated with hypertrophy of one or more limbs or of the face, as well as with generally unilateral hemangiomas of the skin (see Chapter 11). Less often, a spinal cord AVM coexists with an AVM of the brain (126,133). Vertebral angiomas behave as extradural mass lesions, producing spinal cord and nerve root compression syndromes and deficits (134).

Should an AVM become symptomatic in infancy, its initial manifestations can be increased intracranial pressure and hydrocephalus. These result from the mass effect of the lesion itself, from an intracerebral hematoma, intraventricular hemorrhage, or dissection of a superficial cortical hemorrhage into the subdural space.

Diagnosis

When confronted by clinical evidence of a sudden intracranial hemorrhage, namely, severe headache, vomiting, and nuchal rigidity, the physician must consider the presence of an AVM or, less likely, an aneurysm. An intracranial bruit, which should always be listened for, is heard in a significant percentage of patients with AVMs. The incidence varies markedly from one series to the next and probably reflects the care with which the skull is auscultated. Unlike a benign bruit, it is accompanied by a thrill and has a much louder and harsher quality. Intracranial bruits are heard in a significant per-

centage of normal children (see Introduction) and in a variety of conditions characterized by increased cerebral blood flow. These include anemia, thyrotoxicosis, and meningitis. Bruits also accompany hydrocephalus, and some, not necessarily vascular, intracranial tumors.

Although plain skull radiography has revealed intracranial calcifications in up to 10% of children with AVMs (121), currently the initial diagnostic procedure of choice in the child who presents with an acute intracranial hemorrhage is a CT scan. If used, contrast enhancement identifies virtually all vascular lesions larger than 1.5 mm in diameter (135) and can even detect angiographically occult vascular malformations. The CT scan also can determine the presence and extent of hydrocephalus and a secondary intracerebral hematoma, and, hence, is immediately helpful in the surgical management of a pressure cone (136). Both MRI and MRA are invaluable for the more definitive evaluation of AVMs. MRI can show the presence and extent of any associated hematomas and the relationship of the angioma to the ventricular system, but does not obviate the need for angiography (39,137). Angiography remains the definitive diagnostic procedure and is invariably required before a nonemergency surgical procedure. When angiography is performed, bilateral carotid and vertebral studies are indicated, inasmuch as other vascular malformations can coexist with the malformation responsible for neurologic symptoms. Additionally, saccular aneurysms can coexist with AVMs in some 4% to 10% of patients (116, 117,121). In planning the angiographic procedure, one must remember that a small fraction of AVMs is supplied exclusively by the external carotid artery (138).

The CSF examination is of little value. In the patient who is deteriorating acutely as a consequence of an expanding hematoma or intraventricular dissection of blood, and who has signs of tentorial or foramen magnum herniation, it is contraindicated.

Spinal cord AVMs are difficult to document. CT has been of little help. When the malformation has a significant intramedullary component, MRI or MRA can identify the presence and the location of the malformation. When the AVM is localized to the dura of the spinal cord, the lesion cannot usually be demonstrated by these procedures (39). In such cases, a dilated epidural venous plexus can sometimes be demonstrated by an MRI of the spinal cord.

Treatment

Children with AVMs should be treated aggressively because of the risk of future catastrophic hemorrhage (138a). Surgical removal of an AVM is indicated if the operative risk is less than the risk determined by the natural history of the AVM. Spetzler and Martin have proposed a grading system for AVMs that takes into account the size of the malformation, whether venous drainage occurs through the cortical venous system or through deep veins such as the internal cerebral veins, and the location of the lesion with reference to areas whose injury results in a disabling neurologic deficit (139,140). In their experience, grade I and II AVMs, which constitute 26% of all AVMs, were removed without difficulty, with neither mortality nor major neurologic deficit. Grade IV and V AVMs, which constitute 38% of all AVMs, often require preoperative and intraoperative embolization and a multistaged surgical removal. Preoperative embolization changes a vascular lesion into an avascular tangle of thrombosed vessels, and thereby facilitates their surgical removal. Embolization alone has been tried, but the cure rate with this procedure has been between 8% and 16% (118). Complications from embolization include transient neurologic deficits, strokes, and hemorrhage.

Stereotactic radiosurgical treatment (Gamma knife) is a minimally invasive and effective alternative to surgical removal of an AVM. The effectiveness of this procedure depends in part on the size of the AVM; and the smaller the lesion, the higher the rate of obliteration. In children, most neurosurgeons opt for a definitive procedure designed to completely remove or obliterate the malformation (141).

The outcome depends on the size and location of the malformation. After surgery, 10% of patients with grade I and II AVMs were left with major, and 20% with minor, neurologic deficits. Complete surgical removal almost certainly prevents recurrence, whereas incomplete removal and ligation of feeding vessels does not. Incomplete obliteration by embolization also fails to provide protection from recurrent hemorrhage, even if follow-up angiography appears to show complete obliteration of the lesion (142).

Contrasted with this surgical experience are the data indicating that the mortality for the initial hemorrhage is greater in children than in adults, ranging between 7.1% and 13.3%. In children, a ruptured AVM has approximately a 2% to 4% risk of recurrence per year, whereas an unruptured AVM has a 32% risk of bleeding by 10 years of age, and 85% by 25 years of age (143). The latter values are significantly higher than those for adults (144). In particular, even trivial head trauma incurred during sports can result in rupture of an AVM (145). One must, therefore, conclude that surgery is indicated whenever an AVM is detected in children, even when there has been no antecedent hemorrhage (146).

The results of surgical resection when performed for seizure control are under dispute. In the experience of Murphy, the results were not good, and seizure control was not improved after resection of the AVM. In some cases, seizures started after surgery (122). By contrast, Kondziolka and coworkers found that excision of an AVM responsible for a chronic seizure disorder produced complete seizure control off anticonvulsants in 73% of children (113).

The current consensus is that the younger the child, the greater the indication for attempted resection of an accessible lesion because of the longer period the child is vulnerable to either rupture or gliosis and atrophy of the surrounding parenchyma. In inoperable lesions, stereotactic radiosurgery offers another therapeutic approach (141,147).

Vein of Galen Malformations

The great vein of Galen is a single midline vein lying in the subarachnoid space dorsal to the midbrain. It is formed by the union of the paired internal cerebral veins that course in the medial wall of the thalamus, the basal veins of Rosenthal, and the superior cerebellar vein. Joining the inferior sagittal sinus soon after its origin, the vein of Galen empties into the straight sinus. It drains the medial deep nuclei of the forebrain, the medial surfaces of the occipital and tempo-

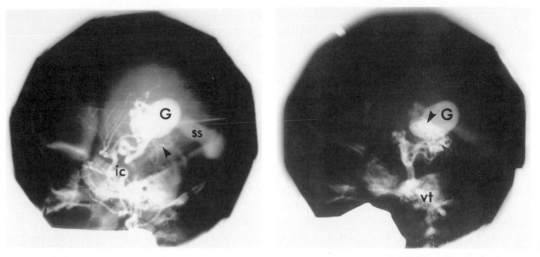

A

B

FIG. 12.4. Term neonate with vein of Galen malformation, presenting with high-output congestive heart failure and hydrocephalus. Left lateral views of arteriograms by selective catheterization and injection of the **(A)** left internal carotid (ic) and **(B)** left vertebral (vt) arteries. From both anterior (carotid) and posterior (vertebrobasilar) circulatory sources, while contrast material is still seen in these major vessels during the infusion, a large aneurysmal sac, representing the dilated vein of Galen (G), is seen filling with contrast and blood. Even the straight sinus (ss) is visualized at the same time, indicating a large component of arteriovenous fistulous shunt. In addition, aggregates of numerous smaller pathologic vessels (*arrowheads*) are seen, another component of this complex vascular malformation. The right carotid injection in this child (not shown) yielded similar results to the left carotid injection. The blood supply to this congenital vascular malformation was therefore from all three major vessels, both carotids and the basilar artery, making surgical treatment extremely difficult.

ral lobes, and the superior surface of the cerebellum. Malformations of the vein of Galen are complex and are sometimes called "aneurysms of the vein of Galen" because of the great dilatation caused by the arteriovenous fistula component, but this term is not entirely accurate because the angiomatous portion is equally important and creates an AVM (147a). Some malformations represent direct fistulas between the arteries and veins, others have an intervening vascular cluster or represent a venous malformation without arteriovenous shunting (Figs. 12.4 and 12.5) (39,148,149). Neuropathologic studies of the vein of Galen malformation show intimal thickening of the abnormal vascular channels, which could produce higher vascular resistance (149a).

Three distinct age-dependent presentations occur (150). Generally, the larger the arteriovenous shunt, the earlier the lesion becomes man-

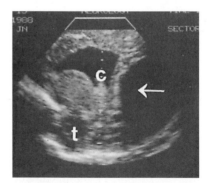

FIG. 12.5. Vascular malformation of the vein of Galen in a 3-day-old child. This full-term infant presented with a sudden change in level of consciousness, tachycardia, tachypnea, and cyanosis. There was a loud bruit over the cranium. Ultrasonography, sagittal view, demonstrates a massive malformation (*arrow*) that has pushed the choroid plexus (c) anteriorly. The right lateral ventricle and the temporal horn (t) are enlarged.

ifest clinically. Signs appearing during the neonatal period are primarily those of congestive heart failure (149–151). Shunting of a large volume of blood results in increased peripheral resistance and increased cardiac output. This produces high-output heart failure with cardiomegaly, a wide arterial pulse pressure, and a narrow arteriovenous oxygen difference (150). A loud, harsh, systolic or systolic-diastolic intracranial bruit, which is often heard without auscultation, is noted in a large proportion of neonates and in nearly every symptomatic infant.

When signs of a vein of Galen malformation appear during early infancy, initial manifestations take the form of hydrocephalus (42%), seizures (26%), or distention and tortuosity of scalp veins (26%) (149). Hydrocephalus is caused by aqueductal obstruction by the vein of Galen or by subarachnoid adhesions associated with intracranial hemorrhage. The older child with a malformation of the vein of Galen presents with an acute subarachnoid hemorrhage, focal seizures, or headaches. Because in this age group the arteriovenous flow is relatively small, intracranial bruits are rare (149). Cerebral atrophy and periventricular leukomalacia are not unusual and can be the result of a "steal phenomenon" (151).

Both MRI and MRA demonstrate the malformation. MRA is able to distinguish the high flow arterial feeding vessels from the low flow venous lesions. Conventional arteriography is performed as the initial component of the interventional procedure. In the neonate, the presence of a malformation of the vein of Galen can often be demonstrated by ultrasonography (see Fig. 12.5).

Surgical treatment of the malformation has had poor results, with only 10% of infants surviving ligation of the feeding vessels. One-half of these infants were neurologically impaired (152). The poor outcome is in part because the vascular lesion is fed by all major cerebral vessels, both carotids and the vertebrobasilar circulation (see Fig. 12.4). With the development of precise invasive radiologic procedures for controlled transarterial embolization of synthetic cyanoacrylate compounds, the vascular malformation may be reduced significantly in size in some children (152a). A minority of patients experience sponta-

neous thrombosis of the malformation in childhood without treatment (152a,152b), and rarely adults have thrombosis of the straight sinus as late as 64 years of age (152c).

At present, endovascular techniques with transarterial embolization of the malformation represent the primary treatment (153). Although infants who present during the neonatal period fare poorly, this procedure is more successful in older infants (154). Even though in many instances embolization does not produce a cure, it still allows the neonate to develop to an age when more definitive surgical treatment can be attempted (155). When hydrocephalus develops, as it does not infrequently, the complication is treated by placement of a ventriculoperitoneal shunt (153).

Venous Angioma

Venous angioma is the most common asymptomatic intracranial vascular malformation, being found in some 2.6% of individuals coming to autopsy (156).

Although the clinical presentation of venous angioma does not differ from that of AVMs, these lesions are pathologically distinct. The anomalous vein has a reduced amount of smooth muscle and elastic tissue. The lesion tends to be smaller than an AVM, although it can vary from 1 mm up to several centimeters in diameter. Ultimately, 15% to 20% calcify, and, occasionally, ossification and amyloid deposition occur (157). Because capillaries are interposed between artery and vein, bruits are seldom heard, and jugular blood is venous in its oxygen content. In the experience of Wyburn-Mason, venous angiomas are also the most common vascular malformation of the spinal cord (126). An association with facial nevi and hydrocephalus has been described (158). Because these malformations have a low risk of bleeding or causing symptoms, they are treated conservatively when discovered incidentally (144).

Cavernous Angioma

Cavernous angioma is frequently clinically silent, detected only incidentally by CT scan or

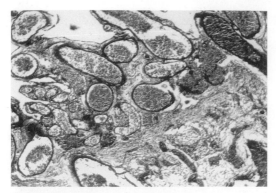

FIG. 12.6. Histopathologic section of a cavernous hemangioma within the brain parenchyma in the parietal lobe of a 7-year-old girl. Multiple closely clustered thin-walled vascular channels are seen that vary greatly in size but lack the muscular walls of arterioles, arteries, or veins. The lumina are filled with blood. Because of the large diameter and thin walls of these pathologic vessels, they are subject to rupture, causing intracerebral and subarachnoid hemorrhage (Verhoeff–van Gieson stain, ×250 original magnification).

MRI. Unlike the other vascular malformations, cavernous angiomas have a significant familial incidence, compatible with transmission as a dominant trait in some 5% of families (159,160a). One of at least three genes responsible for familial cavernous angioma (CCM1) has been mapped to the long arm of chromosome 7q11.2-21 (161). It encodes a protein which in an as yet unknown manner appears to regulate angiogenesis (161a). When families, including asymptomatic relatives, are investigated with MRI, penetrance approaches 100% (160).

Most cavernous angiomas in children occur in the cerebral hemispheres, and the long-term results of surgical resection are generally good (162). Surgery should be considered once the diagnosis is established to prevent catastrophic subsequent intracerebral hemorrhages. In the brainstem, once they become symptomatic, cavernous angiomas also may cause progressive morbidity from repeated hemorrhages and can even be fatal (163). After surgical resection, the vascular malformation may regrow and again become symptomatic, but complete excision is feasible, safe, and potentially curative in lesions located superficially and away from the floor of the fourth ventricle (163).

Cavernous angiomas usually do not become clinically apparent until adult life. Patients generally present with seizures, less commonly as vascular accidents or severe headache. The lesion is responsible for 12% of intracranial hemorrhages owing to vascular anomalies (164). Most of the cavernous angiomas are located in the cerebral hemispheres. Typically, they involve the rolandic area (Fig. 12.6). They can accompany similar lesions in the retina, liver, kidneys, or skin (159,165).

Capillary Angiomas and Telangiectasia

Though the terms *capillary angioma* and *telangiectasis* (plural, telangiectasia) are used interchangeably by some authors, there is an important distinction both pathologically and in biological behavior (147a). The neural tissue between the pathologic vessels in capillary angiomas is usually gliotic and contains no neurons; the cerebral parenchyma between vessels in telangiectasia is normal and includes normal neurons, a normal concentration of glial cells, and normal fibers, the ratios depending on the involved region of the brain. The vessels themselves are more constant in size and are morphologically consistent with capillaries in telangiectasia, whereas in angiomas the vessels are more variable in diameter and many are thin-walled, resembling the smaller vessels of cavernous angiomas (see Fig. 12.6). Unlike capillary angiomas, telangiectasia always remain asymptomatic and never cause intraparenchymal hemorrhage, result in neurologic deficits, or behave as neuronal irritants to cause seizures. The most common site of telangiectasia is in the basis pontis, where they are usually discovered in children or adults as an unsuspected, incidental finding at autopsy.

Much smaller than either AVMs or venous angiomas, capillary angiomas are usually found in the posterior fossa, particularly in the pons or medulla, occasionally in the cerebellum (111). This lesion, admixed with a venous angioma, constitutes the basic abnormality in Sturge-Weber syndrome (see Chapter 11). Capillary angiomas also can be found in the subependymal deep cortical region, where they tend to be solitary and often are discovered incidentally postmortem. Because of their location in the brainstem or subependymal region, they can be responsible for massive and catastrophic hemorrhage in these regions.

Aneurysms

Approximately 7% of the population develops an aneurysm 2 mm or larger by the time of death (157). Inasmuch as the vast majority of aneurysms are not congenital, but are acquired during life, the condition is rare in children (166). Although aneurysms are approximately one-tenth as frequent as AVMs, they have a greater tendency to rupture. Of patients younger than 20 years of age who have experienced a spontaneous subarachnoid hemorrhage, 40% have an aneurysm and 27% have an AVM. In the remaining 33% of patients, the bleeding is of unknown origin (167). In this series of Sedzimir and Robinson, only 10% of patients developed symptoms before 10 years of age (167).

From these data it is obvious that when a preadolescent patient develops a spontaneous intracranial hemorrhage, it is far more likely to be caused by an AVM than an aneurysm.

Aneurysms in childhood have no gender or racial predilection, and their rupture bears little relationship to systemic hypertension or physical activity. Whereas aneurysms are usually located on or adjacent to the circle of Willis in adults, in children 50% of aneurysms originate from the carotid bifurcation, 25% from the anterior cerebral artery, and 12.5% from the posterior cerebral artery (168). The majority of childhood aneurysms are of the giant type, and only 25% of them have the small, saccular shape typical for adults. Fusiform aneurysm of the basilar artery, which is not an uncommon form in adults with arteriosclerosis, is extremely unusual in children (169). Multiple aneurysms were only seen in 3% of children

(170). The pathology of these malformations is reviewed by Rorke (112).

Pathogenesis

In aneurysms appearing during childhood, the most common cause is a congenital weakness of the vascular media. Familial occurrence has been reported, and in 6% to 20% two or more cases of intracranial aneurysms are confirmed (171). In some families the transmission of the disorder is compatible with an autosomal dominant trait (172) and autosomal recessive in others (173). Among first-degree relatives of patients with an aneurysmal subarachnoid hemorrhage the risk of a ruptured intracranial aneurysm is four times higher than in the general population (174). In a cooperative screening study by MRA published in 1999, unruptured aneurysms were found in 4% of first-degree relatives. In 48%, aneurysms were less than 5 mm in diameter. In view of the substantial risks of prophylactic therapy, the risk of rupture must be weighed against the adverse psychological and functional risks of a diagnostic study and subsequent surgery (174a).

The association of aneurysms with neuroepithelial cysts, agenesis of the corpus callosum, and other cerebral malformations suggests that congenital factors operate in the formation of some aneurysms (175). In particular, a deficiency of type III collagen has been demonstrated to be responsible for the various vascular defects observed in the severe, autosomal recessive form of Ehlers-Danlos disease type IV (176), and for at least a significant proportion of patients diagnosed as having a congenital cerebral aneurysm (177). Aneurysms have also been reported in Pompe disease (glycogenosis type 2) and in various disorders of connective tissue, including the more benign autosomal dominant form of Marfan syndrome (178) and in pseudoxanthoma elasticum. In our opinion, this last association is so rare that it might be no more than coincidental.

In the 1973 series of Thompson and coworkers (179), only 9% of childhood aneurysms were mycotic. These usually were more peripheral and were most commonly encountered in children with congenital heart disease. A traumatic origin could be documented in 14%. In 12% of instances, intracranial aneurysms, usually of the saccular type, are associated with coarctation of the aorta, and in 4% with bilateral polycystic kidneys (180,181).

The larger the aneurysm, the more likely it is to rupture. This is particularly true for aneurysms larger than 1 cm in diameter, the size at which they tend to become symptomatic during childhood.

Clinical Manifestations

Sudden massive intracranial hemorrhage is by far the most common clinical manifestation in children. The ruptured aneurysm spills blood into the subarachnoid space, providing sudden severe headache, vomiting, meningeal irritation, and increased intracranial pressure. With progressive bleeding, focal neurologic deficits, seizures, impaired consciousness, and retinal hemorrhages can occur. Retinal hemorrhages can be flame shaped and localized near blood vessels, or ovoid and near or on the optic disc (174). They can dissect between retinal layers (subhyaloid hemorrhage). An intracerebral hematoma occurs in one-fourth to one-half of children and can produce a sudden increase in intracranial pressure. Other clinical manifestations, such as cranial nerve palsies and focal neurologic deficits consequent to embolization, are almost always confined to adults. In the experience of Patel and Richardson (180), 11 out of 58 youngsters with ruptured intracranial aneurysms had a prior history of headaches; in only one did these headaches take the form of classic migraine. A more recently conducted prospective study of patients presenting with acute serious headache and proven to have a subarachnoid hemorrhage did not uncover any minor, premonitory hemorrhages (182).

Diagnosis

Bruits are seldom heard in the unruptured aneurysm. Whenever the sudden onset of a severe headache associated with vomiting and photophobia implies a ruptured aneurysm, a CT scan is the first diagnostic procedure. If both the CT scan, performed within 12 hours of the onset of symptoms, and a subsequent CSF examination

are normal, angiography will probably not uncover an aneurysm (183). Aneurysms larger than 5 mm can be seen by MRI or MRA (170). MRI is superior to CT scanning for demonstrating the aneurysm and for delineating the various complications of an aneurysmal bleed, such as an intraventricular hemorrhage, a subdural hemorrhage (which is a relatively common complication in infants), an intracerebral hematoma, or acute hydrocephalus (184). When none of these study results are positive, digital subtraction cerebral angiography remains as the most definitive diagnostic procedure (185).

Treatment

A ruptured cerebral aneurysm has traditionally been treated by a neurosurgeon. Considerable controversy surrounds the clinical management of vasospasm resulting from the extravasated blood and the timing of the operation. The results of elective surgery are excellent in terms of morbidity and mortality, but mortality is high among patients awaiting elective aneurysm clipping. Because the mortality of early surgery is no longer as prohibitive as it was a decade or two ago, and because early surgery seems to prevent the delayed cerebral vasospasm, many authorities now opt for early surgery (174). Clipping of the aneurysm or endovascular therapy by insertion of a soft metallic coil, or a combination of the two procedures are the most commonly used approaches.

When an aneurysm is detected during an evaluation for headache or when it is encountered adventitiously, surgery is indicated if the aneurysm is greater than 1 cm in diameter. Such an aneurysm is likely to rupture, a generally fatal event (186). Aneurysms at the juncture of the internal carotid and posterior communicating arteries, and aneurysms within the vertebrobasilar system have a higher rate of rupture than other aneurysms (186a). Conversely, aneurysms smaller than 1 cm are not likely to subsequently rupture or to be responsible for neurologic symptoms.

Children appear to tolerate surgery better than adults, particularly when it is performed with the patient in a satisfactory state of alert-

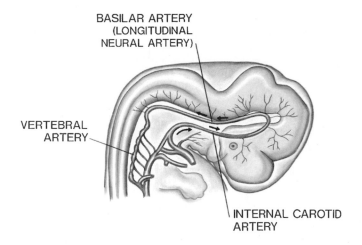

BASILAR ARTERY
(LONGITUDINAL
NEURAL ARTERY)

VERTEBRAL
ARTERY

INTERNAL CAROTID
ARTERY

A   **12mm. (6 WEEKS GESTATION)**

FIG. 12.7. A and B. Diagrams showing the changes in the posterior circulation of the developing human embryonic and fetal brain. The carotid arterial system develops sooner than does the verte-brobasilar system, and the anterior part of the circle of Willis also develops late. The basilar artery forms by the fusion of a pair of parallel adjacent vessels at the base of the embryonic brain, the paired longitudinal neural arteries, to create the single, midline vessel at the base of the brainstem, by approximately 6 weeks' gestation. Blood flow in the paired longitudinal neural arteries, and initially in the basilar artery, is rostrocaudal from the internal carotid arteries through a series of paired, tran-sitory embryonic arteries that connect the carotid and basilar arteries; these vessels are called the trigeminal, otic, and hypoglossal arteries, named for the nerves with which they are associated anatomically. The posterior communicating arteries of the circle of Willis are not yet formed. Because of the embryonic pontine and cervical flexures, the carotid and basilar arteries are oriented nearly parallel and in close proximity, unlike the adult, facilitating the development of the embryonic com-municating (i.e., trigeminal, otic, and hypoglossal) arteries; this relationship is best appreciated in the lateral view. The vertebral arteries form from a coalescence of paired plexuses of small, immature vessels, associated temporally with the formation of the vertebral neural arches, but they are not ready to provide complete blood flow into the basilar artery until approximately 8 weeks' gestation. At that time, a reversal of blood flow occurs in the basilar artery from rostrocaudal to caudorostral, the mature state. As this new direction of flow becomes established, the transient trigeminal, otic, and hypoglossal arteries progressively atrophy and disappear by approximately 9 weeks' gestation.

ness (168). Although operative mortality is low, many of the survivors are left with significant cognitive deficits, primarily because of a high incidence of cerebral infarction resulting from the delayed vasospasm.

The technology of endovascular treatment of intracranial aneurysms is changing rapidly. It is reviewed by McDougall and colleagues (187). For further discussion of the problem of intracra-nial aneurysms, which is primarily one of adult neurology and neurosurgery, the reader should consult various current neurosurgical texts.

**Vascular Malformations
Caused by Persistent or Anomalous
Fetal Cerebral Arteries**

The pattern of cerebrovascular circulation in the embryo and early fetus differs from the mature pattern because of the sequence of development of major cerebral arteries, which also results in changes in direction of blood flow in the basilar artery in particular. The changes in ontogenesis are illustrated in Figure 12.7 and are explained in the legend.

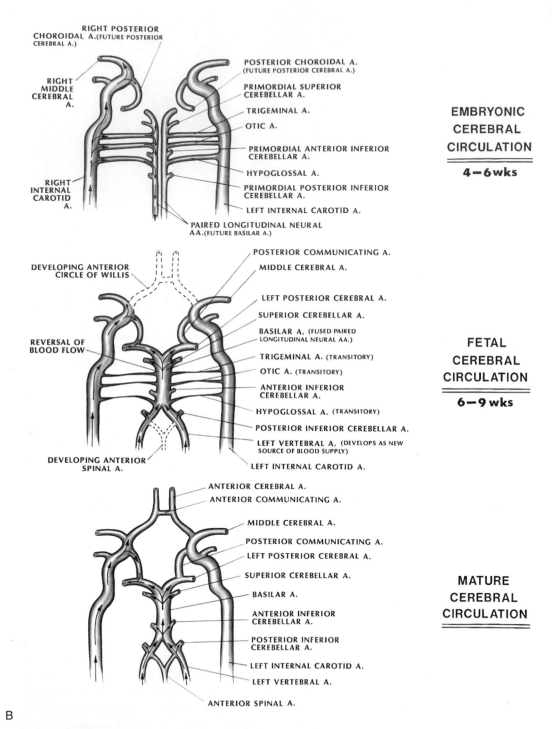

RIGHT POSTERIOR CHOROIDAL A.(FUTURE POSTERIOR CEREBRAL A.)

POSTERIOR CHOROIDAL A. (FUTURE POSTERIOR CEREBRAL A.)

RIGHT MIDDLE CEREBRAL A.

PRIMORDIAL SUPERIOR CEREBELLAR A.

TRIGEMINAL A.

OTIC A.

PRIMORDIAL ANTERIOR INFERIOR CEREBELLAR A.

HYPOGLOSSAL A.

RIGHT INTERNAL CAROTID A.

PRIMORDIAL POSTERIOR INFERIOR CEREBELLAR A.

LEFT INTERNAL CAROTID A.

PAIRED LONGITUDINAL NEURAL AA.(FUTURE BASILAR A.)

EMBRYONIC CEREBRAL CIRCULATION

4—6wks

POSTERIOR COMMUNICATING A.

MIDDLE CEREBRAL A.

DEVELOPING ANTERIOR CIRCLE OF WILLIS

LEFT POSTERIOR CEREBRAL A.

SUPERIOR CEREBELLAR A.

BASILAR A. (FUSED PAIRED LONGITUDINAL NEURAL AA.)

REVERSAL OF BLOOD FLOW

TRIGEMINAL A. (TRANSITORY)

OTIC A. (TRANSITORY)

ANTERIOR INFERIOR CEREBELLAR A.

HYPOGLOSSAL A. (TRANSITORY)

POSTERIOR INFERIOR CEREBELLAR A.

LEFT VERTEBRAL A. (DEVELOPS AS NEW SOURCE OF BLOOD SUPPLY)

DEVELOPING ANTERIOR SPINAL A.

LEFT INTERNAL CAROTID A.

FETAL CEREBRAL CIRCULATION

6—9 wks

ANTERIOR CEREBRAL A.

ANTERIOR COMMUNICATING A.

MIDDLE CEREBRAL A.

POSTERIOR COMMUNICATING A.

LEFT POSTERIOR CEREBRAL A.

SUPERIOR CEREBELLAR A.

BASILAR A.

ANTERIOR INFERIOR CEREBELLAR A.

POSTERIOR INFERIOR CEREBELLAR A.

LEFT INTERNAL CAROTID A.

LEFT VERTEBRAL A.

ANTERIOR SPINAL A.

MATURE CEREBRAL CIRCULATION

B

FIG. 12.7. Continued.

In addition to the maturational changes of major cerebral arteries, the microcirculation of the brain also undergoes an important developmental evolution (188,189). This evolution affects the vulnerability of the fetus and preterm infant to lesions seen rarely after 36 weeks' gestation, such as extensive white matter infarcts, periventricular leukomalacia, and germinal matrix hemorrhages. The penetrating vessels supplying the white matter of the cerebral mantle are mostly end-arterioles with few anastomoses, hence little collateral circulation, in the fetus and premature. The vascular channels of the germinal matrix are immature, thin-walled vessels rather than mature capillaries. Their thin endothelial cells are easily damaged by hypoxia and acidosis, and often rupture during reperfusion after an episode of transient systemic hypotension. These factors are discussed more extensively in Chapter 5.

Striatal arteries develop a muscularis wall at approximately 24 weeks' gestation, but most other cerebral vessels do not form a smooth muscular wall until the last few weeks of fetal life, and the muscularization of intracerebral arteries occurs in a centripetal direction (188).

An uncommon and usually clinically silent anomaly sometimes discovered in the course of cerebral angiography and at times by MRA is a persistence of one of the three major transitory embryonic arteries that communicates between the internal carotid arteries and the basilar artery before the vertebral arteries are established. The most rostral of this group of paired vessels, the trigeminal artery, is the most common (190–192) (Fig. 12.8), but persistence of the otic and hypoglossal arteries also occurs, either individually or conjointly (193–196). Persistence of paired embryonic vessels may be unilateral or bilateral. Many variants are seen: the trigeminal artery may form mainly an anastomosis between the internal carotid and the superior or inferior cerebellar arteries (197–201). Although usually occurring as anomalies in patients with otherwise normal brains, a persistent trigeminal artery occurs with greater frequency in holoprosencephaly (202). In other cases, it is reported in association with cerebellar malformations or hypoplasias (203).

Although not a cause of neurologic deficit or symptoms in themselves, these anomalies of

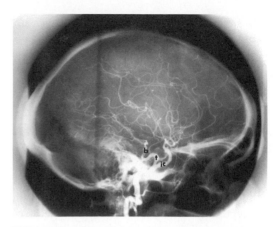

FIG. 12.8. Persistent embryonic trigeminal artery in a 46-year-old woman. Left lateral views of left internal carotid injection of cerebral angiogram by selective catheterization. A large trigeminal artery (t) appears as an aberrant communication between the internal carotid (ic) and basilar (b) arteries. Distal arterial blood flow is seen in both the anterior (middle and anterior cerebral) and posterior (posterior cerebral) circulations after carotid injection. After vertebral injection, only a small amount of flow was seen in the basilar artery and posterior cerebral circulation, and the right internal carotid injection showed a pattern similar to that shown by the left carotid injection, demonstrating that the carotid arteries supply nearly all of the blood to the brain in this anomalous condition, as in the embryo. This circulatory pattern was entirely asymptomatic, and the woman was neurologically normal; this arteriogram was performed because of an unrelated small anterior communicating aneurysm (not shown) causing a mild subarachnoid hemorrhage for the first time in her life.

persistent fetal cerebral arteries render such patients vulnerable to more extensive and often life-threatening infarction in the event of carotid artery thrombosis, because the carotid artery provides the main blood supply to posterior fossa structures and to the posterior cerebral artery territory, as well as to its normal distribution to the middle and anterior cerebral territories. Carotid occlusion is most commonly caused by trauma or infection in childhood and to atherosclerosis in older adults. In some patients, a persistent trigeminal artery coexists with a saccular aneurysm or with an angioma to produce deficits of cranial nerves III, V, IV, or

VI, and the associated vascular lesions may cause spontaneous subarachnoid hemorrhage (204,205). In rare cases, multifocal AVMs of the brain have been described with persistent fetal carotid-basilar anastomoses (196).

Agenesis of the carotid arteries is another developmental malformation that leads to either an aberrant blood supply of the internal carotid territories or to neurologic deficits resulting from poor development of supratentorial structures (205–208). Bilateral dissecting aneurysms of the internal carotid arteries might be a result of hypoplasia of these vessels, or at least of stenosis of the supraclinoid segment (107a). Various anomalous loops, kinks, or tortuosities in the internal carotid artery may occur during development and may cause neurologic symptoms secondary to ischemic atrophy of the involved hemisphere (209). Developmental dysplasias of the cerebrum are reported rarely in association with carotid agenesis, accompanied by facial hemangioma (210). True developmental agenesis of the carotid arteries, in contrast to acquired occlusions later in fetal or postnatal life, is generally associated with absence of the carotid canals at the base of the skull, which may be demonstrated radiographically or by CT scan (211).

Anomalies of the circle of Willis are extremely common, being encountered in nearly 50% of autopsy cases; however, these are probably of no clinical significance in children.

REFERENCES

1. Schoenberg BS, Mellinger JF, Schoenberg DG. Cerebrovascular disease in infants and children: a study of incidence, clinical features, and survival. *Neurology* 1978;28:763–768.
2. Schoenberg BS, Schoenberg DG. Spectrum of paediatric cerebrovascular disease. In: Rose FC, ed. *Clinical neuroepidemiology*. New York: State Mutual Books, 1980.
3. Editorial. A classification and outline of cerebrovascular diseases. *Neurology* 1958;8:409–434.
4. Williams LS, et al. Subtypes of ischemic stroke in children and young adults. *Neurology* 1997;49:1541–1545.
5. Zoller B, et al. Activated protein C resistance due to a common factor V gene mutation is a major risk factor for venous thrombosis. *Annu Rev Med* 1997;48:45–58.
6. Martinez HR, Rangel Guerra RA, Marfil LJ. Ischemic stroke due to deficiency of coagulation inhibitors. Report of 10 young adults. *Stroke* 1993;24:19–25.
7. Israels SJ, Seshia SS. Childhood stroke associated with protein C or S deficiency. *J Pediatr* 1987;111:562–564.
8. van Kuijck MAP, et al. Neurological complications in children with protein C deficiency. *Neuropediatrics* 1994;25:16–19.
8a. Lawson SE, et al. Congenital thrombophilia and throbosis: a study in a single centre. *Arch Dis Child* 1999;81:176–178.
9. Bauer KA. Hypercoagulability—a new cofactor in the protein C anticoagulant pathway. *N Engl J Med* 1994;330:566–567.
9a. Phillips MD. Interrelated risk factors for venous thromboembolism. *Circulation* 1997;95:1749–1751.
10. Bertina RM, ed. Hypercoagulable states. *Semin Hematol* 1997;34:167–264.
11. Packer RJ. Cerebral vascular accident related to cancer. In: Edwards MSB, Hoffman HJ, eds. *Cerebral vascular disease in children and adolescents*. Baltimore: Williams & Wilkins, 1989:429–440.
12. Kemkes-Matthes B. Acquired protein S deficiency. *Clin Investig* 1992;70:529–534.
13. Koh S, Chen LS. Protein C and S deficiency in children with ischemic cerebrovascular accident. *Pediatr Neurol* 1997;17:319–321.
14. Roddy SM, Giang DW. Antiphospholipid antibodies and stroke in an infant. *Pediatrics* 1991;87:933–935.
15. Shergy WJ, Kredich DW, Pisetsky DS. The relationship of anticardiolipin antibodies to disease manifestations in pediatric systemic lupus erythematosus. *J Rheumatol* 1988;10:41–51.
16. Riela AR, Roach ES. Etiology of stroke in children. *J Child Neurol* 1993;8:201–220.
17. Young W. The post-injury responses in trauma and ischemia: secondary injury or protective mechanisms? *CNS Trauma* 1987;4:27–51.
18. Macdonald RL, Stoodley M. Pathophysiology of cerebral ischemia. *Neurol Med Chir (Tokyo)* 1998;38:1–11.
19. Kristiàn T, Siesjö BK. Calcium in ischemic cell death. *Stroke* 1998;29:705–718.
20. Sweeney MI, et al. Cellular mechanisms involved in brain ischemia. *Can J Physiol Pharmacol* 1995;73:1525–1535.
20a. Dimagl U, Iadecola C, Moskowitz MA. Pathobiology of ischaemic stroke: an integrated view. *Trends Neurosci* 1999;22:391–397.
21. Seiler RB, et al. Cerebral vasospasm evaluated by transcranial ultrasound correlated with clinical grade and CT-visualized subarachnoid hemorrhage. *J Neurosurg* 1986;64:594–600.
22. Kiwak KJ, Heros RC. Cerebral vasospasm after subarachnoid hemorrhage. *Trends Neurosci* 1987;10:89–92.
23. Heros RC, Zervas NT, Varsos V. Cerebral vasospasm after subarachnoid hemorrhage: an update. *Ann Neurol* 1983;14:600–608.
24. Meyer CHA, et al. Progressive change in cerebral blood flow during the first three weeks after subarachnoid hemorrhage. *Neurosurgery* 1983;12:58–76.
25. Horky LL, et al. Role of ferrous iron chelator 2,2'-dipyridyl in preventing delayed vasospasm in a primate model of subarachnoid hemorrhage. *J Neurosurg* 1998;88:298–303.
26. Jakobsen M. Role of initial brain ischemia in subarachnoid hemorrhage following aneurysm rupture. A

pathophysiological survey. *Acta Neurol Scand Suppl* 1992;141:1–33.

27. Fisher CM, Roberson GH, Ojemann RG. Cerebral vasospasm with ruptured saccular aneurysm: the clinical manifestations. *Neurosurgery* 1977;1:245–248.

28. Bederson JB, et al. Acute vasoconstriction after subarachnoid hemorrhage. *Neurosurgery* 1998;42:352–360.

29. Wijdicks EFM, et al. Atrial natriuretic factor and salt wasting after aneurysmal subarachnoid hemorrhage. *Stroke* 1991;22:1519–1524.

30. Hino A, et al. Changes in endothelial nitric oxide synthase mRNA during vasospasm after subarachnoid hemorrhage in monkeys. *Neurosurgery* 1996;39:562–567.

31. Glueck CJ, et al. Pediatric victims of unexplained stroke and their families: familial lipid and lipoprotein abnormalities. *Pediatrics* 1982;69:308–316.

32. Webster M, et al. Patent foramen ovale in young stroke patients. *Lancet* 1988;2:11–12.

33. Solomon GE, et al. Natural history of acute hemiplegia of childhood. *Brain* 1970;93:107–120.

34. Riikonen R, Santavuori P. Hereditary and acquired risk factors for childhood stroke. *Neuropediatrics* 1994;25:227–233.

35. Giroud M, et al. Stroke in children under 16 years. Clinical and etiological difference with adults. *Acta Neurol Scand* 1997;96:401–406.

36. Freud S. Die Infantile Cerebrallähmung. In: Nothnagel H, ed. *Spezielle Pathologie und Therapie*, Vol. 9, Pt. 3. Vienna: Holder, 1897.

37. Ford FR, Schaffer AJ. The etiology of infantile acquired hemiplegia. *Arch Neurol Psychiatry* 1927;18:323–347.

38. Ford FR. *Diseases of the nervous system in infancy, childhood and adolescence*, 5th ed. Springfield, IL: Charles C Thomas, 1966.

39. Zimmerman RA, Bilaniuk LT. Pediatric brain, head and neck, and spine magnetic resonance angiography. *Magn Res Q* 1992;8:264–290.

40. Isler W, ed. *Acute hemiplegias and hemisyndromes in childhood. Clinics in developmental medicine*, Vols. 41–42. Philadelphia: JB Lippincott, 1971.

41. Hilal SK, et al. Primary cerebral arterial occlusive disease in children. Part I: Acute acquired hemiplegia. *Radiology* 1971;99:71–86.

42. Handa J, Handa H. Progressive cerebral arterial occlusive disease: analysis of 27 cases. *Neuroradiology* 1972;3:119–133.

43. Suzuki J. *Moyamoya disease*. Berlin: Springer-Verlag, 1986.

44. Aicardi J, Amsili J, Chevrie JJ. Acute hemiplegia in infancy and childhood. *Dev Med Child Neurol* 1969;11:162–173.

45. Norman RM. Neuropathological findings in acute hemiplegia in childhood with special reference to epilepsy as pathogenic factors. *Little Club Clin Dev Med* 1962;6:37–48.

46. Kudo T. Spontaneous occlusion of the circle of Willis. A disease apparently confined to Japanese. *Neurology* 1968;18:485–496.

47. Takeuchi K, et al. Factors influencing the development of moyamoya phenomenon. *Acta Neurochir* 1981;59:79–86.

48. Gadoth N, Hirsch M. Primary and acquired forms of moyamoya syndrome: a review and three case reports. *Isr J Med Sci* 1980;16:370–377.

49. Fukui M. Current state of study on moyamoya disease in Japan. *Surg Neurol* 1997;47:138–143.

49a. Ikeda H, et al. Mapping of a familial moyamoya disease gene to chromosome 3p24.2-p26. *Am J Hum Genet* 1999;64:533–537.

50. Connelly A, et al. Diffusion-weighted magnetic resonance imaging of compromised tissue in stroke. *Arch Dis Child* 1997;77:38–41.

50a. Zivin JA. Diffusion-weighted MRI for diagnosis and treatment of ischemic stroke. *Ann Neurol* 1997;41:567–568.

51. Kurokawa T, et al. Prognosis of occlusive disease of the Circle of Willis (Moyamoya disease) in children. *Pediatr Neurol* 1985;1:274–277.

51a. Imaizumi T, et al. Long-term outcomes of pediatric moyamoya disease monitored to adulthood. *Pediatr Neurol* 1998;18:321–325.

52. Miyamoto S, et al. Pitfalls in the surgical treatment of moyamoya disease. Operative techniques for refractory cases. *J Neurosurg* 1988;68:537–543.

53. Yamada Y, Matsushima Y, Suzuki S. Childhood moyamoya disease before and after encephalo-duro-arteriosynangiosis: an angiographic study. *Neuroradiology* 1992;34:318–322.

54. Hoffman HJ. Moyamoya disease and syndrome. *Clin Neurol Neurosurg* 1997;99[Suppl 2]:S39–S44.

55. Kashiwagi S, et al. Revascularization with split duro-encephalo-synangiosis in the pediatric Moyamoya disease—surgical result and clinical outcome. *Clin Neurol Neurosurg* 1997;99[Suppl 2]:S115–S117.

56. Hosoda Y, Ikeda K, Hirose S. Histopathological studies on spontaneous occlusion of the circle of Willis (cerebrovascular moyamoya disease). *Clin Neurol Neurosurg* 1997;99[Suppl 2]:S203–S208.

57. Yamamoto M, et al. Increase in elastin gene expression and protein synthesis in arterial smooth muscle cells derived from patients with Moyamoya disease. *Stroke* 1997;28:1733–1738.

57a. Lichtor T, Mullan S. Arteriovenous malformation in moyamoya syndrome. *J Neurosurg* 1987;67:603–608.

58. Seeler RA, et al. Moyamoya in children with sickle cell anemia and cerebrovascular occlusion. *J Pediatr* 1978;93:808–810.

59. Kramer HH, Karch D, Seibert H. Moyamoya-ähnliche cerebrovaskuläre Affektionen bei tuberoser Sklerose. *Monatsschr Kinderheilk* 1981;129:595–597.

60. Fukuyama Y, Osawa M, Kanai N. Moyamoya disease (syndrome) and the Down syndrome. *Brain Dev* 1992;14:254–256.

61. Lutterman J, et al. Moyamoya syndrome associated with congenital heart disease. *Pediatrics* 1998;101:57–60.

61a. Kaplan P, Levinson M, Kaplan BS. Cerebral artery stenoses in Williams syndrome cause strokes in childhood. *J Pediatr* 1995;126:943–945.

61b. Boerkoel CF, et al. Schimke immunoosseous dysplasia complicated by moyamoya phenomenon. *Am J Med Genet* 1998;78:118–122.

61c. Echenne BP, Leboucq N, Humbertclaude V. Ito hypomelanosis and moyamoya disease. *Pediatr Neurol* 1995;13:1691–1671.

62. Ingram TT. *Paediatric aspects of cerebral palsy*. Edinburgh, Scotland: ES Livingstone, 1964.

63. Lanska MJ, et al. Presentation, clinical course, and outcome of childhood stroke. *Pediatr Neurol* 1991;7: 333–341.

64. Crothers B, Paine RS. *The natural history of cerebral palsy*. Cambridge: Harvard University Press, 1959.

65. Aicardi J, Amsili J, Chevrie JJ. Acute hemiplegia in infancy and childhood. *Dev Med Child Neurol* 1969;11: 162–173.

66. Schoenberg BS, et al. Moyamoya disease presenting as a seizure disorder. A case report. *Arch Neurol* 1977;34: 511–512.

67. Roach ES, Riela AR. *Pediatric cerebrovascular disorders*. Mount Kisco, NY: Futura, 1988.

68. Sutor AH, Uhl M. Diagnosis of thromboembolic disease during infancy and childhood. *Semin Thromb Hemostasis* 1997;23:237–246.

69. Bogousslavsky J, et al. Migraine stroke. *Neurology* 1988;38:223–227.

70. Andrew M. Indications and drugs for anticoagulation therapy in children. *Thromb Res* 1996;81[Suppl 2]: S61–S73.

71. Zenz W, et al. Intracerebral hemorrhage during fibrinolytic therapy in children: a review of the literature of the last thirty years. *Semin Thromb Hemost* 1997; 23:321–332.

72. Lees KR. Cerestat and other NMDA antagonists in ischemic stroke. *Neurology* 1997;49[Suppl 4]: S66–S69.

72a. Lees KR. Does neuroprotection improve stroke outcome? *Lancet* 1998;351:1447–1448.

73. Sutor AH, et al. Heparin therapy in pediatric patients. *Semin Thromb Hemost* 1997;23:303–319.

74. Massicotte P, et al. Low-molecular-weight heparin in pediatric patients with thrombotic disease: a dose finding study. *J Pediatr* 1996;128:313–318.

75. Gold AP, Hammill JF, Carter S. Cerebrovascular diseases. In: Farmer TW, ed. *Pediatric neurology*, 3rd ed. Philadelphia: JB Lippincott, 1983.

76. Molnar GE, ed. *Pediatric rehabilitation*. Baltimore: Williams & Wilkins, 1992.

77. Gossling HR, Pellegrini VD. Fat embolism syndrome. A review of the pathophysiology and physiological basis of treatment. *Clin Orthop* 1982;165:68–82.

78. Moore P, James O, Saltos N. Fat embolism syndrome: incidence, significance and early features. *Austr NZ J Surg* 1981;51:546–551.

79. Robert JH, et al. Fat embolism syndrome. *Orthop Rev* 1993;22:567–571.

80. Barson AJ, Chistwick ML. Fat embolism in infancy after intravenous fat infusions. *Arch Dis Child* 1978;53: 218–223.

81. Stoney WS, et al. Air embolism and other accidents using pump oxygenators. *Ann Thorac Surg* 1979;29: 336–340.

82. Gillen HW. Symptomatology of cerebral gas embolism. *Neurology* 1968;18:507–512.

83. Satoh H, et al. Cerebral fat embolism studied by magnetic resonance imaging, transcranial Doppler sonography, and single photon emission computed tomography: case report. *J Trauma* 1997;43:345–348.

84. Batra P. The fat embolism syndrome. *J Thorac Imaging* 1987;2:12–17.

85. Kalbag RM, Woolf AL. *Cerebral venous thrombosis*. London: Oxford University Press, 1967.

86. Barron TF, et al. Cerebral venous thrombosis in neonates and children. *Pediatr Neurol* 1992;8:112–116.

87. Byers RK, Hass GM. Thrombosis of the dural venous sinuses in infancy and childhood. *Am J Dis Child* 1933;45:1161–1183.

88. Bailey OT, Hass GM. Dural sinus thrombosis in early life. I. The clinical manifestations and extent of brain injury in acute sinus thrombosis. *J Pediatr* 1937;11: 755–771.

89. Banker BQ. Cerebral vascular disease in infancy and childhood. I. Occlusive vascular disease. *J Neuropathol Exp Neurol* 1961;20:127–140.

90. Lermoyez M. Un signe de la thrombose du sinus longitudinal supérieur. *Ann Mal Oriel Larynx* 1897;23[Pt 2]:497–507.

91. Hanigan WC, et al. MRI of cerebral vein thrombosis in infancy: a case report. *Neurology* 1986;36:1354–1356.

92. Lee BC, Park TS, Kaufman BA. MR angiography in pediatric neurological disorders. *Pediatr Radiol* 1995;25:409–419.

93. Wang AM. MRA of venous sinus thrombosis. *Clin Neurosci* 1997;4:158–164.

94. Ozsvath RR, et al. Cerebral venography: comparison of CT and MR projection venography. *AJR Am J Roentgenol* 1997;169:1699–1707.

95. Bousser MG, et al. Cortical venous thrombosis: a review of 38 cases. *Stroke* 1985;16:199–213.

96. Southwick FS, Richardson EP Jr, Swartz MN. Septic thrombosis of the dural venous sinuses. *Medicine* 1986;65:82106.

97. Verret S, Steele JC. Alternating hemiplegia in childhood: a report of eight patients with complicated migraine beginning in infancy. *Pediatrics* 1971;47: 675–680.

98. Aicardi J, Bourgeois M, Goutières F. Alternating hemiplegia of childhood: clinical findings and diagnostic criteria. In: Andermann F, Aicardi J, Vigevano F, eds. *Alternating hemiplegia of childhood*. New York: Raven Press 1995:3–18.

99. Zupanc ML, Perlman SB, Rust RS. Single photon emission computed tomography studies in alternating hemiplegia of childhood. In: Andermann F, Aicardi J, Vigevano F, eds. *Alternating hemiplegia of childhood*. New York: Raven Press 1995:99–108.

100. Aminian A, Strashun A, Rose A. Alternating hemiplegia of childhood: studies of regional cerebral blood flow using 99mTc-hexamethylpropylene amine oxime single-photon emission computed tomography. *Ann Neurol* 1993;33:43–47.

101. Becker LE. Alternating hemiplegia of childhood: a neuropathologic review. In: Andermann F, Aicardi J, Vigevano F, eds. *Alternating hemiplegia of childhood*. New York: Raven Press 1995:57–66.

101a. Rho JM, Chugani HT. Alternating hemiplegia of childhood: insights into its pathophysiology. *J Child Neurol* 1998;13:39–45.

101b. Nevsimalová S, Dittrich J, Havlová M, et al. Alternating hemiplegia in childhood: a cross-sectional study. *Brain Dev* 1994;16:189–194.

101c. De Stefano N, Silver K, Andermann F, et al. Mitochondrial dysfunction in patients with alternating hemiplegia of childhood. In: Andermann F, Aicardi J, Vigevano F, eds. *Alternating hemiplegia of childhood*. New York: Raven Press 1995:115–124.

102. Andermann E, et al. Benign familial nocturnal alternating hemiplegia of childhood. *Neurology* 1994;44: 1812–1814.

103. Silver K, Andermann F. Alternating hemiplegia of childhood: a study of 10 patients and results of flunarizine treatment. *Neurology* 1993;43:36–41.

104. Schievink WI, Mokri B, Piepgras DG. Spontaneous dissections of cervicocephalic arteries in childhood and adolescence. *Neurology* 1994;44:1607–1612.

105. Schievink WI, Mokri B, O'Fallon M. Recurrent spontaneous cervical artery dissection. *N Engl J Med* 1994;330:393–397.

106. Schievink WI, et al. Cerebrovascular disease in Ehlers-Danlos syndrome type IV. *Stroke* 1990;21:626–632.

107. van den Berg JSP, et al. The role of type III collagen in spontaneous cervical artery dissections. *Ann Neurol* 1998;43:494–498.

107a. Adelman LS, Doe FD, Sarnat HB. Bilateral dissecting aneurysms of the internal carotid arteries. *Acta Neuropathol* 1974;29:93–97.

108. Mann CI, et al. Posttraumatic carotid artery dissection in children: evaluation with MR angiography. *AJR Am J Roentgenol* 1993;160:134–136.

109. Streeter GL. The developmental alterations in the vascular system of the brain of the human embryo. *Carnegie Inst Washington Contr Embryol* 1918;8:5–38.

110. Padget DH. The development of the cranial arteries in the human embryo. *Carnegie Inst Washington Contr Embryol* 1948;32:205–262.

111. McCormick WF, Hardman JF, Boulter TR. Vascular malformations ("angiomas") of the brain with special reference to those occurring in the posterior fossa. *J Neurosurg* 1968;28:241–251.

112. Rorke LB. Pathology of cerebral vascular disease in children. In: Edwards MSB, Hoffman HJ, eds. *Cerebral vascular disease in children and adolescents.* Baltimore: Williams & Wilkins, 1989:95–138.

113. Kondziolka D, et al. Arteriovenous malformations of the brain in children: a 40-year experience. *Can J Med Sci* 1992;19:40–45.

114. Schoolman A, Kepes JJ. Bilateral spontaneous carotid-cavernous fistulae in Ehlers-Danlos syndrome. *J Neurosurg* 1967;26:82–86.

115. Lach B, et al. Spontaneous carotid-cavernous fistula and multiple arterial dissections in type IV Ehlers-Danlos syndrome. Case report. *J Neurosurg* 1987;66: 462–467.

116. Paterson JH, McKissock WA. A clinical survey of intracranial angiomas with special reference to their mode of progression and surgical treatment. A report of 110 cases. *Brain* 1956;79:233–266.

117. Michelson WJ. Natural history and pathophysiology of arteriovenous malformations. *Clin Neurosurg* 1979;26:307–313.

118. Halbach VV, Higashida RT, Hieshima GB. Interventional neuroradiology. *Am J Radiol* 1989;153:467–476.

119. Proesmans W, et al. Autosomal dominant polycystic kidney disease in the neonatal period: association with a cerebral arteriovenous malformation. *Pediatrics* 1982;70:971–975.

120. Henderson WR, Gomez RD. Natural history of cerebral angiomas. *BMJ* 1967;4:571–574.

121. Kelly JJ, Mellinger JF, Sundt TM. Intracranial arteriovenous malformations in childhood. *Ann Neurol* 1978; 3:338–343.

122. Murphy MJ. Long-term follow-up of seizures associated with cerebral arteriovenous malformations. *Arch Neurol* 1985;42:477–479.

123. Zeller RS, Chutorian AM. Vascular malformations of the pons in children. *Neurology* 1975;25:776–780.

124. Aminoff MS, Edwards MSB. Spinal arteriovenous malformations. In: Edwards MSB, Hoffman HJ, eds. *Cerebral vascular disease in children and adolescents.* Baltimore: Williams & Wilkins, 1989;321–335.

125. Riché MC, et al. Arteriovenous malformations (AVM) of the spinal cord in children. Review of 38 cases. *Neuroradiology* 1982;22:171–180.

126. Wyburn-Mason R. *The vascular abnormalities and tumours of the spinal cord and its membranes.* London: Kimpton, 1943.

127. Kissel P, Dureux JB. Cobb syndrome: cutaneomeningospinal angiomatosis. In: Vinken PJ, Bruyn GW, eds. *Handbook of clinical neurology,* Vol. 14. New York: Elsevier, 1972:429–445.

127a. Pascual-Castroviejo I. The association of extracranial and intracranial vascular malformations in children. *Can J Neurol Sci* 1985;12:139–148.

128. Pece N, et al. Mutant endoglin in hereditary hemorrhagic telangiectasia type 1 is transiently expressed intracellularly and is not a dominant negative. *J Clin Invest* 1997;100:2568–2579.

129. Guttmacher AE, Marchuk DA, White RI. Hereditary hemorrhagic telangiectasia. *N Engl J Med* 1995;333: 918–924.

130. Putman CM, et al. Exceptional multiplicity of cerebral arteriovenous malformations associated with hereditary hemorrhagic telangiectasia (Osler-Weber-Rendu syndrome). *Am J Neuroradiol* 1996;17: 1733–1742.

131. Sobel D, Norman D. CNS manifestations of hereditary hemorrhagic telangiectasia. *Am J Neuroradiol* 1984;5:569–573.

132. Roman G, et al. Neurological manifestations of hereditary hemorrhagic telangiectasia (Rendu-Osler-Weber disease): report of 2 cases and review of the literature. *Ann Neurol* 1978;4:130–144.

133. Hoffman HJ, Mohr G, Kusunoki T. Multiple arteriovenous malformations of the spinal cord and brain in a child. Case report. *Childs Brain* 1976;2:317–324.

134. McAllister VL, Kendall BE, Bull JWD. Symptomatic vertebral haemangiomas. *Brain* 1975;98:71–80.

135. Bergström M, Riding M, Greitz T. The limitations of definition of blood vessels with computer intravenous angiography. *Neuroradiology* 1976;11:35–40.

136. Leblanc R, Ethier R, Little JR. Computerized tomography in arteriovenous malformations of the brain. *J Neurosurg* 1979;51:765–772.

137. Young IR, et al. NMR imaging in the diagnosis and management of intracranial angiomas. *Am J Neuroradiol* 1983;4:837–838.

138. Holla PS, et al. Radiographic features of vascular malformations. In: Smith RR, Haerer A, Russell WF, eds. *Vascular malformations and fistulas of the brain.* New York: Raven Press, 1982.

138a. Kondziolka D, Humphreys RP, Hoffmann HJ, et al. Arteriovenous malformations of the brain in children: a forty year experience. *Can J Neurol Sci* 1992;19:40–45.

139. Spetzler RF, Martin NA. A proposed grading system for arteriovenous malformations. *J Neurosurg* 1986;65: 476–483.

140. Hamilton MG, Spetzler RF. The prospective application of a grading system for arteriovenous malformations. *Neurosurgery* 1994;34:2–7.

141. Lunsford LD. Stereotactic radiosurgical procedures for arteriovenous malformations of the brain. *Mayo Clin Proc* 1995;70:305–307.

142. Fournier D, et al. Endovascular treatment of intracerebral arteriovenous malformations: experience in 49 cases. *J Neurosurg* 1991;75:228–233.

143. Celli P, et al. Cerebral arteriovenous malformations in children: clinical features and outcome of treatment in children and in adults. *Surg Neurol* 1984;22:43–49.

144. Wilkins RH. Natural history of intracranial vascular malformations: a review. *Neurosurgery* 1985;16:421–430.

145. Nishi T, et al. Ruptures of arteriovenous malformations in children associated with trivial head trauma. *Surg Neurol* 1987;28:451–457.

146. Brown RD, et al. The natural history of unruptured intracranial arteriovenous malformations. *J Neurosurg* 1988;68:352–357.

147. Loeffler JS, et al. Role of stereotactic radiosurgery with a linear accelerator in treatment of intracranial arteriovenous malformations and tumors in children. *Pediatrics* 1990;85:774–782.

147a. Challa VR, Moody DM, Brown WR. Vascular malformations of the central nervous system. *J Neuropathol Exp Neurol* 1995;54:609–621.

148. Litvak J, Yahr MD, Ransohoff J. Aneurysms of the great vein of Galen and midline cerebral arteriovenous anomalies. *J Neurosurg* 1960;17:945–954.

149. Gold AP, Ransohoff J, Carter S. Vein of Galen malformation. *Acta Neurol Scand* 1964;40[Suppl 11]:131.

149a. Yamashita Y, Nakamura Y, Okudera T, et al. Neuroradiological and pathological studies on neonatal aneurysmal dilation of the vein of Galen. *J Child Neurol* 1990;5:45–48.

150. Holden AM, et al. Congestive heart failure from intracranial arteriovenous fistula in infancy. Clinical and physiological considerations in eight patients. *Pediatrics* 1972;49:30–39.

151. Pasqualin A, et al. Midline giant arterio-venous malformations in infants. *Acta Neurochir* 1982;64:259–271.

152. Johnston IH, et al. Vein of Galen malformation: diagnosis and management. *Neurosurgery* 1987;20:747–758.

152a. Lasjaunias P, Garcia-Monaco R, Rodesch G, et al. Vein of Galen malformation. *Childs Nerv Syst* 1991;7:360–367.

152b. Gangemi M, Maiuri F, Donati PA, Iaconetta G. Spontaneous thrombosis of aneurysm of the vein of Galen. *Acta Neurol (Napoli)* 1988;10:113–118.

152c. Mayberg MR, Zimmerman C. Vein of Galen aneurysm associated with dural AVM and straight sinus thrombosis. *J Neurosurg* 1988;68:288–291.

153. Chisholm CA, et al. Aneurysm of the vein of Galen: prenatal diagnosis of perinatal management. *Am J Perinatol* 1996;13:503–506.

154. Borthne A, et al. Vein of Galen vascular malformations in infants: clinical, radiological and therapeutic aspect. *Eur Radiol* 1997;7:1252–1258.

155. Moriarty JL, Steinberg GK. Surgical obliteration for vein of Galen malformation: a case report. *Surg Neurol* 1995;44:365–369.

156. Sarwar M, McCormick WF. Intracerebral venous angioma: case report and review. *Arch Neurol* 1978;35:323–325.

157. McCormick WF. Vascular disorders of nervous tissue: anomalies, malformations and aneurysms. In: Bourne GH, ed. *The structure and function of nervous tissue.* New York: Academic Press, 1969.

158. Orr LS, et al. The syndrome of facial nevi, anomalous cerebral venous return and hydrocephalus. *Ann Neurol* 1978;3:316–318.

159. Dobyns WB, et al. Familial cavernous malformations of the central nervous system and retina. *Ann Neurol* 1987;21:578–583.

160. Rigamonti D, et al. Cerebral cavernous malformations: incidence and familial occurrence. *N Engl J Med* 1988;319:343–347.

160a. Labauge P, et al. Hereditary cerebral cavernous angiomas: clinical and genetic features in 57 French families. *Lancet* 1998;352:1892–1897.

161. Gil-Nagel A, Dubovsky J, Wilcox KJ, et al. Familial cerebral cavernous angioma: a gene localized to a 15-cM interval on chromosome 7q. *Ann Neurol* 1996;39:807–810.

161a. Laberge-le Couteulx S, et al. Truncating mutations in CCM1, encoding KRIT1. Cause hereditary cavernous angiomas. *Nature Genet* 1999;23:189–193.

162. Scott RM, Barnes P, Kupsky W, Adelman LS. Cavernous angiomas of the central nervous system in children. *J Neurosurg* 1992;76:38–46.

163. Zimmerman RS, Spetzler RF, Lee S, et al. Cavernous malformations of the brain stem. *J Neurosurg* 1991;75:32–39.

164. Ochiai C, Saito I, Sano K. Intracranial hemorrhage with cerebral vascular malformation. In: Smith RR, Haerer A, Russell WF, eds. *Vascular malformations and fistulas of the brain.* New York: Raven Press, 1982.

165. Russell DS, Rubinstein LJ. *The pathology of tumours of the nervous system,* 4th ed. London: E Arnold, 1977.

166. Storrs BB, et al. Intracranial aneurysms in the pediatric age-group. *Childs Brain* 1982;9:358–361.

167. Sedzimir CB, Robinson J. Intracranial hemorrhage in children and adolescents. *J Neurosurg* 1973;38:269–281.

168. Heiskanen O, Vilkki J. Intracranial arterial aneurysms in children and adolescents. *Acta Neurochir* 1981;59:55–63.

169. Read D, Esiri MM. Fusiform basilar artery aneurysm in a child. *Neurology* 1979;29:1045–1049.

170. Zimmerman RA, et al. MRI of cerebral aneurysm. *Acta Radiol* 1987;369:108–109.

171. Ronkainen A, et al. Familial intracranial aneurysm. *Lancet* 1997;349:380–384.

172. ter Berg HWM, Bijlsma JB, Willemse J. Familial occurrence of intracranial aneurysms in childhood: a case report and review of the literature. *Neuropediatrics* 1987;18:227–230.

173. Bromberg JEC, et al. Familial subarachnoid hemorrhage, distinctive features and patterns of inheritance. *Ann Neurol* 1995;38:929–934.

174. Schievink WI. Intracranial aneurysms. *N Engl J Med* 1997;336:28–40.

174a. The Magnetic Resonance Angiography in Relatives of Patients with Subarachnoid Hemorrhage Study Group. Risks and benefits of screening for intracranial aneurysms in first-degree relatives of patients with sporadic subarachnoid hrmorrhage. *N Engl J Med* 1999;341:1344–1350.

175. Shuanghoti S, Netsky MG, Switter DJ. Combined congenital vascular anomalies and neuroepithelial (colloid) cysts. *Neurology* 1978;28:552–555.

176. North KN, et al. Cerebrovascular complications in Ehlers-Danlos syndrome type IV. *Ann Neurol* 1995;38:960–964.

177. Hegedüs K. Some observations on reticular fibers in the media of the major cerebral arteries. A comparative study of patients without vascular diseases and those with ruptured berry aneurysms. *Surg Neurol* 1984;22:301–307.

178. Braunsdorf WE. Fusiform aneurysm of basilar artery and ectatic internal carotid arteries associated with glycogenosis type 2 (Pompe's disease). *Neurosurgery* 1987;21:748–749.

179. Thompson JR, Harwood-Nash DC, Fitz CR. Cerebral aneurysms in children. *Am J Roentgenol* 1973;118: 163–175.

180. Patel AN, Richardson AE. Ruptured intracranial aneurysm in the first two decades of life. A study of 58 patients. *J Neurosurg* 1971;35:571–576.

181. Chapman AB, et al. Intracranial aneurysms in autosomal dominant polycystic kidney disease. *N Engl J Med* 1992;327:916–920.

182. Linn FH, et al. Prospective study of sentinel headache in aneurysmal subarachnoid haemorrhage. *Lancet* 1994;344:590–593.

183. Editorial. Headaches and subarachnoid haemorrhage. *Lancet* 1988;1:80.

184. Jenkins A, et al. Magnetic resonance imaging of acute subarachnoid hemorrhage. *J Neurosurg* 1988;68: 731–763.

185. Weisberg LA. Computed tomography in aneurysmal subarachnoid hemorrhage. *Neurology* 1979;29: 802–808.

186. Wiebers DO, et al. The significance of unruptured intracranial saccular aneurysms. *J Neurosurg* 1987;66: 23–29.

186a. Caplan LR. Should intracranial aneurysms be treated before they rupture? *N Engl J Med* 1998;339: 1774–1775.

187. McDougall CG, et al. Endovascular treatment of basilar tip aneurysms using electrolytically detached coils. *J Neurosurg* 1996;84:393–399.

188. Kuban KCK, Gilles FH. Human telencephalic angiogenesis. *Ann Neurol* 1985;17:539–548.

189. Norman MG, O'Kusky JR. The growth and development of microvasculature in human cerebral cortex. *J Neuropathol Exp Neurol* 1986;45:222–232.

190. Morris ED, Moffat DB. Abnormal origin of the basilar artery from the cervical part of the internal carotid and its embryological significance. *Anat Rec* 1956;125:701–711.

191. Tibbs PA, Walsh JW, Minix WB. Persistent primitive trigeminal artery and ipsilateral acquired blepharoptosis. *Arch Neurol* 1981;38:323–324.

192. Saltzman G. Patent primitive trigeminal artery studied by cerebral angiography. *Acta Radiol* 1959;51: 329–336.

193. Bruetman ME, Fields WS. Persistent hypoglossal artery. *Arch Neurol* 1963;8:369–372.

194. Anderson RA, Sondheimer FK. Rare carotid-vertebrobasilar anastomoses with notes on the differentia-

tion between proatlantal and hypoglossal arteries. *Neuroradiology* 1976;11:113–118.

195. Khodadad G. Persistent hypoglossal artery in the fetus. *Acta Anat* 1977;99:477–481.

196. Garza-Mercado R, Cavazos E, Urrutia G. Persistent hypoglossal artery in combination with multifocal arteriovenous malformations of the brain: case report. *Neurosurgery* 1990;26:871–876.

197. Teal JS, Rumbaugh CL, Bergeron RT, et al. Persistent carotid-superior cerebellar artery anastomosis: a variant of persistent trigeminal artery. *Neuroradiology* 1972;103:335–341.

198. Chambers AA, Lukin R. Trigeminal artery connection to the posterior inferior cerebellar arteries. *Neuroradiology* 1975;9:121–123.

199. Chambers AA, Lukin R. Trigeminal artery connection to the posterior inferior cerebellar arteries. *Neuroradiology* 1975;9:121–123.

200. Haughton VM, Rosenbaum AE, Pearce J. Internal carotid artery origins of the inferior cerebellar arteries. *AJR Am J Roentgenol* 1978;130:1191–1192.

201. Siqueira M, Piske R, Ono M, Rarino R Jr. Cerebellar arteries originating from the internal carotid artery. *Am J Neuroradiol* 1993;14:1229–1235.

202. Zingesser LH, Schechter MM, Medina A. Angiographic and pneumoencephalographic features of holoprosencephaly. *AJR Am J Roentgenol* 1966;97: 5651–574.

203. Pascual-Castroviejo I, Tendero A, Martinez-Bermejo JM, et al. Persistence of the hypoglossal artery and partial agenesis of the cerebellum. *Neuropediatrics* 1975;6:184–189.

204. Wise BL, Palubinskas AJ. Persistent trigeminal artery (carotid-basilar anastomosis). *J Neurosurg* 1964;21: 199 206.

205. Turnbull I. Agenesis of the internal carotid artery. *Neurology* 1962;12:588–590.

206. Hussain SA, Araj JS, Forman JF, Rosenberg JC. Congenital absence of the internal carotid artery. *Arch Pathol* 1968;90:265–270.

207. Cali RL, Berg R, Rama K. Bilateral internal carotid artery agenesis: a case study and review of the literature. *Surgery* 1993;113:227–233.

208. Yokochi K, Iwase K. Bilateral internal carotid artery agenesis in a child with psychomotor developmental delay. *Pediatr Neurol* 1996;15:76–78.

209. Sarkari NBS, Holmes JM, Bickerstaff ER. Neurological manifestations associated with internal carotid loops and kinks in children. *J Neurol Neurosurg Psychiatry* 1970;33:194–200.

210. Pascual-Castroviejo, Viaño J, Pascual-Pascual SI, Martínez V. Facial haemangioma, ageneseis of the internal carotid artery and dysplasia of cerebral cortex: case report. *Neuroradiology* 1995;37:692–695.

211. Quint DJ, Silbergleit R, Young WC. Absence of the carotid canals at skull base CT. *Radiology* 1992; 182:477–481.

Chapter 13

Paroxysmal Disorders

John H. Menkes and *Raman Sankar

*Departments of Neurology and Pediatrics, University of California, Los Angeles, UCLA School
of Medicine, and Department of Pediatric Neurology, Cedars-Sinai Medical Center, Los Angeles,
California 90048; and *Departments of Neurology and Pediatrics, University of California, Los Angeles,
UCLA School of Medicine, Mattel Children's Hospital at UCLA, Los Angeles, California 90095*

This chapter discusses conditions manifested by sudden, recurrent, and potentially reversible alterations of brain function.

EPILEPSY

Epilepsy was known to the ancient Babylonians and was described by Hippocrates, who considered it a disease of the brain. Its history, related by Tempkin, spans that of medicine itself (1). Hughlings Jackson concisely defined epilepsy as "an occasional excessive and disordered discharge of nerve tissue" (2). More recently, epilepsy has been defined as recurrent convulsive or nonconvulsive seizures caused by partial or generalized epileptogenic discharges in the cerebrum.

The epilepsies represent a group of diseases for which recurrent seizures represent their principal manifestation.

Estimates of the incidence of epilepsy depend on whether a single convulsive or nonconvulsive episode and febrile seizures are included in the definition. According to Millichap, febrile seizures account for 2% of all childhood illnesses (3). More recent estimates of the prevalence of single and recurrent nonfebrile seizures in children younger than 10 years of age range from 5.2 to 8.1 per 1,000 (4,5). By age 40 years, the cumulative incidence is 1.7% to 1.9% (4,5).

Classification

The epilepsies have been designated as primary (idiopathic), secondary (symptomatic), or reactive (Table 13.1). The term *primary* implies that, with the present knowledge, no structural or biochemical cause for the recurrent seizures can be found. In general, the primary epilepsies are genetically transmitted, and they tend to have a better prognosis for seizure control. The term *secondary* (symptomatic) epilepsy indicates that the cause of the seizure can be discovered. Such seizures are the principal manifestation of many diseases. They occur in the course of many congenital or acquired conditions of the nervous system, or they can complicate systemic disease. The designation of an epileptic condition as cryptogenic implies that the underlying etiology is symptomatic, but not readily demonstrable by available diagnostic techniques (6). In the reactive epilepsies, seizures are the consequence of an abnormal reaction of an otherwise normal brain to physiologic stress or transient insult. A notable example is febrile seizures. Not all epilepsies can be categorized conveniently. Some are atypical, others are rare, and for a significant proportion data necessary for classification are inadequate or incomplete.

The characteristics for all epilepsies are recurrent convulsive or nonconvulsive seizures. The 1989

TABLE 13.1. *Scheme for organizing epileptic conditions*

	With generalized seizures	With partial (focal) seizures

Primary (idiopathic) epilepsies
  Without structural lesions;
    benign; genetic
	Absence (petit mal) epilepsy
	Juvenile absence epilepsy
	Many generalized tonic-clonic
	  seizures
	Juvenile myoclonic epilepsy
	Benign neonatal seizures
		Benign epilepsy with centrotemporal
		  spikes (rolandic epilepsy)
		Childhood epilepsy with occipital
		  spikes

Secondary (symptomatic) epilepsies
  With anatomic or known bio-
    chemical lesions
	Infantile spasms
	
	Lennox-Gastaut syndrome
		Temporal lobe (psychomotor)
		  epilepsy
		Epilepsies caused by gray matter
		  heterotopias, polymicrogyria
		Epilepsies caused by focal post-
		  asphyxial gliosis

Conditions with reactive seizures
  Abnormal reaction of an other-
    wise normal brain to physio-
    logic stress or transient
    epileptogenic insult
	Febrile seizures
	Most toxic- and metabolic-
	  induced seizures
	Many isolated tonic-clonic
	  seizures
	Early post-traumatic seizures
		Partial seizures occur when condi-
		  tions with reactive seizures are
		  superimposed on transient or pre-
		  existing nonepileptogenic brain
		  injury, as often seen with head
		  trauma, hypernatremia, hypo-
		  glycemia

Adapted from Engel J. *Seizures, epilepsies and the epileptic patient.* Philadelphia: FA Davis, 1989.

classification scheme of the International League Against Epilepsy (ILAE) elected a hierarchy of dichotomies in which the initial categorization is based on whether the epilepsy is localization-related or generalized (6). This distinction was, in fact, made by Hughlings Jackson more than 100 years ago (7) (Table 13.2). Localization-related epilepsies (partial or focal) seizures are classified into simple, complex, and secondarily generalized. Simple partial seizures involve preserved consciousness, whereas complex partial seizures are those with impaired consciousness. The prevalence of the various seizure types is presented in Table 13.3.

The descriptive classification of epileptic syndromes is extremely useful clinically. The so-called epileptic syndromes are distinctive in that they demonstrate characteristic age of onset, seizure types, electroencephalographic (EEG) features, and prognosis. This is particularly valuable in pediatric epileptology, because the immature brain often produces stereotypic epileptic behaviors that are a function of its stage of development, rather than etiology. Childhood syndromes can be considered as benign or catastrophic based on their responsiveness to treatment, the possibility of remission of seizures, and the long-term prognosis for normal cognitive development.

Etiology

Recurrent seizures are thought to result from a genetic predisposition, underlying neuropathologic changes, and chemicophysiologic alterations in the nerve cell and its connections. Each of these factors is considered in turn. Attributed causes for epilepsy in children and adolescents are presented in Table 13.4 (8).

Genetic Factors

Numerous studies suggest that the genetic susceptibility to seizures is normally distributed in the general population, and that there is a threshold above which the condition becomes clinically evident.

An interaction between one or more genes and various nongenetic events operates in several

TABLE 13.2. *Classification of epileptic seizures*

I. Partial (focal or local) seizures
  Simple partial seizures
    Seizures with motor signs
    Seizures with somatosensory or special
      sensory symptoms
    Seizures with autonomic symptoms or signs
    Seizures with psychic symptoms
  Complex partial (psychomotor) seizures
    Simple partial onset followed by impairment of
      consciousness
    Seizures with impairment of consciousness
      at outset
  Partial (focal) seizures evolving to secondarily
    generalized (tonic-clonic, grand mal) seizures
    Simple partial (focal) seizures evolving to
      generalized (grand mal) seizures
    Complex partial (psychomotor) seizures evolving
      to generalized (grand mal) seizures
    Simple partial (focal) seizures evolving to com-
      plex partial psychomotor seizures evolving
      to generalized seizures
II. Generalized seizures (convulsive and noncon-
    vulsive)
  Absence seizures
    Typical absences (petit mal attacks)
    Atypical absences (atypical petit mal attacks)
  Myoclonic seizures
  Clonic seizures
  Tonic seizures
  Tonic-clonic seizures (grand mal seizures)
  Atonic seizures (akinetic or astatic seizures)
III. Unclassified epileptic seizures

From Commission on Classification and Terminology of the International League Against Epilepsy. Proposal for revised clinical and electroencephalographic classification of epileptic seizures. *Epilepsia* 1981;22:489. With permission.

conditions accompanied by seizures. These include head trauma, brain tumors, and congenital hemiplegia (9,10). Genetic factors appear to be most significant in patients with the various primary epilepsies (11). In one study, Lennox and Lennox found a 70% concordance for monozygotic twins and 5.6% concordance for dizygotic twins for epilepsies without organic brain lesions (12). Metrakos and Metrakos found a 12% incidence of seizures among parents and siblings of children with absence seizures; 45% of siblings had an abnormal EEG. They proposed that this EEG abnormality is an expression of an autosomal dominant gene with nearly complete penetrance during childhood and low penetrance in infancy and adult life (13). Gerken and Doose, interpreting data derived from their

clinic, concluded that it was unlikely that a single autosomal dominant gene was responsible for the 3-Hz spike and wave trait and suggested a polygenic inheritance with neurophysiologic and genetic heterogeneity (14).

In families with centrotemporal spikes or sharp-wave discharges and rolandic seizures, EEG abnormalities are transmitted in a dominant manner with age-dependent penetrance (11). Only 12% of relatives with EEG abnormalities, however, develop clinically apparent seizures. A significant genetic predisposition also occurs in juvenile myoclonic epilepsy, in photosensitive seizures, and in the various other primary generalized epilepsies. In seizures with secondary generalization, the genetic factors, although demonstrable through controlled twin studies, are not as striking as in the primary generalized epilepsies. However, even in absence epilepsy, in which the genetic factor is most prominent, the overall risk of developing seizures is only 8% for siblings of affected subjects, and 2% in as yet unaffected siblings older than 6 years of age (15). For offspring of subjects with absence seizures, the risk for EEG abnormalities is 64%, and for seizures 6.7% (16). When promazine is used to activate the EEG, 73.5% of 7- to 14-year-old siblings of subjects with idiopathic absence seizures develop an abnormal EEG (17).

In the previous edition of this book, we mentioned the localization of genes for juvenile myoclonic epilepsy, benign neonatal convulsions, and Unverricht-Lundberg myoclonic epilepsy. The pace of activity in this area has accelerated considerably, and in addition to linkage studies and localization, cloning of several specific genes has been accomplished. The first epilepsy gene to be cloned was that believed to be responsible for autosomal dominant nocturnal frontal lobe epilepsy (18). It has been mapped to chromosome 20q13.2-13.3 and encodes the nicotinic acetylcholine receptor alpha-4 subunit (CHRNA 4). The same authors later reported a different mutation in the same gene for a different pedigree with this syndrome (19). Another gene for this condition has been mapped to chromosome 15q24, whereas in some families linkage studies have excluded both of these genes (20). The discovery of muta-

TABLE 13.3. *Prevalence rates per 1,000 of specific seizure types in children aged newborn to 9 years*

Seizure type	Ohtahara et al. (1981)[a]	Cowen et al. (1989)	Kurland (1959)
All types	8.21 (n = 2,378)	5.24 (n = 626)	5.79 (n = 29)
Generalized	2.57	2.22	—
Primary generalized	1.99	1.29	—
Grand mal	1.82	1.18	3.20
Petit mal	0.11	0.06	1.20
Myoclonus	0.07	0.05	—
Secondary generalized	0.58	0.94	—
Lennox-Gastaut syndrome	0.29	0.13	—
Infantile spasms (West syndrome)	0.14	0.19	—
Others	0.14	0.61	—
Partial	3.60	1.17	—
With elementary symptomatology	0.71	0.43	0.60
With complex symptomatology	0.21	0.30	0.40
Secondarily generalized	2.68	0.43	—
Mixed	0.12	0.02	—
Unclassified	1.92	1.82	0.40

[a]n, total number of prevalent cases in children aged 0 to 9 years. Includes single and recurrent afebrile seizures. From Cowen LD, et al. Prevalence of the epilepsies in children and adolescents. *Epilepsia* 1989;30:94. With permission.

tions in this gene was perplexing to many, because this receptor has not been considered to be involved in the modulation of neuronal excitability relevant to seizure disorders.

The finding that benign familial neonatal convulsions are attributable to mutations of voltage-gated potassium channels, KCNQ2 (21,22) and KCNQ3 (23) is more in tune with our understanding of the mechanisms of excitability. Altered K^+-channel function could impair neuronal repolarization and thus contribute toward increased excitability. The

TABLE 13.4. *Attributed causes for epilepsy in children and adolescents by sex: prevalent cases, 1983*

Cause	Male		Female		Total	
	Number	Percent	Number	Percent	Number	Percent
Idiopathic	428	68	375	70	803	69
Congenital	17	3	19	4	36	3
CNS malformation	9	1	11	2	20	2
MH, DD	5	<1	6	1	11	1
Phacomatoses	3	<1	1	<1	4	<1
Other	—	—	1	<1	1	<1
CNS infection	19	3	14	3	33	3
Toxic/metabolic	15	2	11	2	26	2
CNS neoplasm	2	<1	1	<1	3	<1
Perinatal	45	7	36	7	81	7
Birth trauma	9	1	1	<1	10	1
Asphyxia/hypoxia	17	3	21	4	38	3
Other perinatal	9	1	2	<1	11	1
Multiple perinatal	10	2	12	2	22	2
Traumatic	23	4	20	4	43	4
Other and multiple	77	12	57	11	134	12
Total	626	100	533	100	1,159	100

CNS, central nervous system; DD, developmental delay (includes the diagnoses of mental retardation, psychomotor retardation, failure to thrive, and developmental delay); MH, motor handicap (includes the diagnoses of cerebral palsy, monoplegia, diplegia, hemiplegia, and quadriplegia). From Cowen LD, et al. Prevalence of the epilepsies in children and adolescents. *Epilepsia* 1989;30:94. With permission.

extremely transient nature of this disorder suggests that compensatory changes probably take place in other genes controlling excitatory or inhibitory ion channels.

One of us (R.S.) has reviewed these developments (23a). Many other epilepsy syndromes appear to be genetically heterogeneous based on different linkages found from the study of different pedigrees.

Neuropathologic Factors

Seizures can occur in patients with almost any pathologic process that affects the brain. Two types of abnormalities are seen: those that are responsible for recurrent seizures, and those that are the consequence of recurrent seizures.

Gowers stated more than 100 years ago that seizures begat seizures (24). The question whether lesions produce seizures or seizures produce lesions has been extensively investigated.

Lesions Responsible for Recurrent Seizures

A variety of morphologic changes can cause recurrent seizures. They range from the most obvious, such as some of the major developmental anomalies (see Chapter 4) or postasphyxial changes (see Chapter 5), to minor dysgenetic lesions such as the gray matter heterotopias (see Chapter 4). Although morphologic alterations would not be expected to be found in the primary epilepsies, sometimes they are (25). Mutations in the gene *filamin 1* have been reported to be responsible for the aberrance in migration that results in periventricular heterotopia (26). A number of authors have called attention to minor developmental anomalies in the molecular layer of the cerebral cortex and in the cerebellar cortex, some of which are clearly the result of disturbed cell migration (27). Malformations, notably gray matter heterotopias, *cryptic tubers*, or angiomas arising within the temporal lobe, can cause recurrent seizures. Such lesions also can be found in other areas of the brain (28,29). The genetic basis of some of the dramatic cerebral malformations associated with severe epilepsies of early childhood, such as the double cortex syndrome or band heterotopia are also beginning to be understood (30,31) (see Chapter 4). Mutations in the gene *doublecortin* that resides in the X chromosome (Xq22) result in severe lissencephaly in boys that is often lethal, whereas the migrational anomaly seen in girls with such mutations appears to be the double cortex syndrome.

Altered neuronal migration that results in granule cell disorganization in the dentate gyrus has been seen in tissue resected from patients with temporal lobe epilepsy (32). Although initially this was thought to be a congenital lesion, provocative data from Parent and colleagues demonstrates that, even in mature animals, status epilepticus can result in neurogenesis in the dentate gyrus, and that the nascent granule cells may migrate aberrantly. The data suggest that aberrant synapse formation by these cells could contribute to abnormal excitability (33).

The role of infectious processes in the pathogenesis of epilepsy has received relatively little attention since Aguilar and Rasmussen established that some epileptic patients with focal seizures, slowly progressive intellectual deterioration, and cerebral atrophy demonstrate a pathologic picture consistent with a viral encephalitis (34). Attempts at viral isolation have been unsuccessful in these cases. Nevertheless, it is likely that not only focal epilepsy, but also other forms of seizure disorders, particularly disorders beginning in early childhood in previously healthy children (such as epileptogenic encephalopathy) are caused by a smoldering viral disease within the brain (35,36) (see Chapter 6).

Lesions Secondary to Recurrent Seizures

Among the lesions considered to be secondary to recurrent seizures are those that result from the physical trauma that often attends seizures, and those that result from hypoxia, vascular alterations, or the action of the excitatory neurotransmitters.

Meldrum and colleagues (37) explored the possibility that the seizure itself, rather than systemic changes, was responsible for brain damage. They showed that brain damage occurred in the absence of systemic abnormalities in paralyzed, ventilated, adolescent baboons that were subjected to prolonged, bicuculline-induced seizures. Although the neurochemical changes attending cell death owing to prolonged seizures are similar to those seen in ischemia and hypoglycemia, significant differences in the time course and anatomic distribution of brain damage occur (see Table 15.1).

Under clinical conditions, damage results from a combination of the increased metabolic demands that accompany excessive neuronal activity and the reduced circulation and substrate supply induced by the combination of hyperthermia, hypoglycemia, hypotension, and hypoxia. Cell death under these conditions occurs through a process that resembles cell death in asphyxia, namely through the release of excitotoxins that increase intracellular calcium in the course of prolonged seizures. A more extensive discussion can be found in Chapter 5.

Several areas of the brain, especially the hippocampus, appear to be particularly vulnerable to recurrent and prolonged seizures. Anatomic manifestations of cell damage to the hippocampus include loss of interneurons in the hilus, pyramidal cell loss within the Sommer's sector (prosubiculum and subfield CA1 of Ammon's horn), and subfield CA3, with consequential glial scarring and atrophy (38,39). Using Golgi techniques to study the hippocampus and dentate nucleus, Scheibel and associates have observed loss of dendritic spines and deformation of the dendritic shaft (40). This selective hippocampal vulnerability has been postulated to result from a high density of excitatory receptors on nerve cells in Sommer's sector (41). Other factors also could be operative. Using *in situ* hybridization techniques, Sommer and coworkers showed unique developmental patterns in the mRNA expression of the Glu R-1, -2, and -3 glutamate receptor subunits in CA1, CA3, and the dentate gyrus. Differences in receptor structure could result in differences in receptor function and differences with maturation in resistance of the hippocampus to epileptic damage (42). The protective role of calbindin, a calcium-binding protein, from glutamate-induced neurotoxicity also could account for the selective nerve cell loss (43).

Within the gray matter of the cerebral hemispheres, neuronal cell loss is most likely to occur in laminae 3 and 4, where the thalamocortical afferents terminate. Damage also occurs in the pars reticularis of the substantia nigra, globus pallidus, and thalamus. In animal models, the substantia nigra has been demonstrated to play an important role in the propagation of seizures, and damage to this structure could conceivably contribute to increased propensity for seizures (44). The caudate nucleus appears to be spared (45).

There had been some controversy as to the effect of seizures on the immature brain. One of us (R.S.) has reviewed the arguments for both sides in this controversial issue (46). Some types of experimental seizures fail to produce histologic lesions (46). This observation gave rise to the argument that the immature brain is not vulnerable to seizure-induced damage. This argument runs contrary to the observations on surgically resected tissue from epileptic children which show structural alterations that can be attributed to seizures (47,48). More recent work has shown that the effect of seizures on the developing brain is age- and model-specific, and also that seizures may be associated with the induction of apoptosis in specific cell populations (49,50). Even neonatal animals seem to be vulnerable to seizure-induced brain alterations.

Brief but recurrent seizures induced by pentylenetetrazol have been shown to contribute to morphologic and functional alterations in neonatal rat pups (51–53). The question whether brief but recurrent seizures also have the potential to induce brain damage cannot be answered with assurance in humans. In terms of clinical practice, patients with recurrent seizures are invariably treated with antiepileptic drugs, which on their own can affect development (54); the natural history of the condition without treatment is, therefore, impossible to study. Autopsy material does not permit an easy distinction of the pathology that caused the frequent seizures from the effect of the seizures themselves.

The studies of Shewmon and Erwin are more directly applicable to the clinical problem. These workers have demonstrated that interictal spikes, when followed by prominent inhibitory after potentials, can transiently disrupt cortical function. Thus, frequent interictal spikes could interfere with modality-specific learning (55).

TABLE 13.5. *Possible etiologic factors for complex partial seizures*

Factor	Mesial temporal sclerosis, 47[a] cases	Small tumors, 21 (24) cases	Miscellaneous lesions, 10 (13) cases	Equivocal lesions, 22 cases	Totals, 100 cases
Positive family history	6	0	2 (4)	0	8
Difficult or precipitate birth	7	4	3	7	21
Infantile convulsions	13	1	1	1	16
Difficult/precipitate birth and infantile convulsions	6	1	0	0	7
Head injury	5	6	3 (5)	5	19
Other factors[b]	11	1 (2)	4	4	20
None of above factors	5	10	2	7	—

[a]The figures without parentheses refer to pure cases of each subgroup, and those with parentheses refer to cases with a dual pathology, including mesial temporal sclerosis.

[b]For example, meningitis, mastoid disease, febrile illnesses in infancy without convulsions.

Modified from Falconer MA, Serafetinides EA, Corsellis JAN. Etiology and pathogenesis of temporal lobe epilepsy. *Arch Neurol* 1964;10:233.

Presumably, recurrent electrical discharges could influence activity-dependent plasticity of the developing brain.

Mesial Temporal Sclerosis (Ammon's Horn Sclerosis, Hippocampal Sclerosis)

The damage seen in the hippocampus obtained by surgical resection in chronic temporal lobe epilepsy differs from that seen in postmortem specimens after status epilepticus (56,57). In contrast to the selective damage seen after status epilepticus, the hippocampus of subjects with chronic temporal lobe epilepsy shows more widespread damage throughout the CA1, CA2, and CA3 subfields, as well as the dentate granule cells (56). Hippocampal cell loss ranges from mild and random to almost complete. Although initially the changes have a bilateral distribution, with time, one hemisphere becomes more affected (58). This pathologic abnormality has been designated as mesial temporal sclerosis (MTS) or hippocampal sclerosis. It was seen in 47% of resected temporal lobes in the series of Falconer and associates (Table 13.5) (59), and in 64% of a more recent series compiled by Engel and associates (60). Cell loss and gliosis in the amygdala also has been observed and can occur in the absence of significant hippocampal changes (61). In more severe cases, nerve cell loss and gliosis involves not only the entire hippocampus, but

also the uncus, amygdala, and adjacent cortex (Fig. 13.1). Atrophic changes in the cerebellum or the thalamus are not uncommon.

The cause or causes of MTS are still under debate. When seizures arise outside the hippocampus and are propagated into the hippocampus, hippocampal cell densities are normal in the majority of cases. Therefore, it would appear that MTS initiates temporal lobe seizures, rather than the converse (62). MTS has been seen as early as 1 year of age, and combined morphologic and electrophysiologic studies suggest that the seizure focus is generated in part when abnormal, recurrent, monosynaptic excitatory synapses are formed after damage to normal intrahippocampal synapses (63). A detailed analysis of the epileptogenic potential of the lesions produced by intrahippocampal or systemic kainic acid or by ischemia led Franck to conclude that hippocampal sclerosis and seizures are both symptoms of an underlying pathology, and that although MTS may be produced by seizures, the development of epilepsy as a syndrome does not depend on cell loss or plasticity in the hippocampus (64). However, the anatomic features of MTS may become incorporated into, and sustain, an epileptic focus.

Vascular, metabolic, or immunologic factors, acting singly or in concert, can be responsible (65,66). Epidemiologic studies have been used to ascertain risk factors for this condition. Febrile convulsions were seen in 20% of subjects, as com-

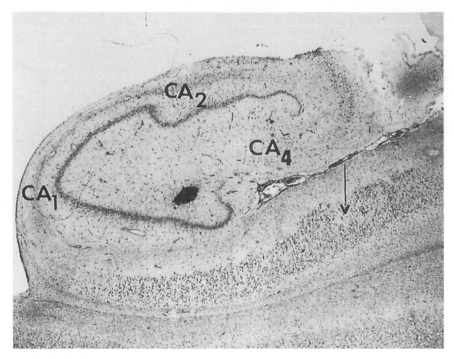

FIG. 13.1. Mesial temporal sclerosis in 23-year-old man. Onset of complex partial seizures began at age 6 years with a frequency of up to seven per day. A few major motor seizures occurred each year. Cross-section of the cornu Ammonis shows the extent of injury of the pyramidal cell layer. Neurons of areas CA_4, CA_2, and CA_1 are markedly reduced in number. There are also focal areas of cell loss in the subiculum (*arrow*) (Gridley stain, ×10). (Courtesy of the late Dr. W. Jann Brown, Department of Pathology, University of California, Los Angeles, UCLA School of Medicine.)

pared with 2% of controls. The majority experienced at least one complicated febrile seizure. An increased incidence of head trauma and neonatal convulsions also could be documented. Additionally, there was a significant association with maternal seizures (67). In a significant population of patients, the brain, after a lifetime of recurrent epileptic attacks, shows neither gross nor microscopic abnormalities. This observation reflects the current limitation of morphologic studies in furthering our understanding of the epilepsies.

Basic Mechanisms of Epileptogenesis

We must notice what the normal function of nerve tissue is. Its function is to store up and expend force.
—H. Jackson, 1873 (68)

It should be stated at the outset that modulation of transmitter effects, of voltage-gated channels, and of cell electrical properties involves processes that occur continually during normal brain function. This plasticity is the basis of the cortex to learn from experience. It seems that the same plastic mechanisms are involved in epileptogenicity. One extreme result of such plasticity is the hyperexcitability and hypersynchrony that characterize epileptiform activities. The risk of epileptiform activity is the price that has to be paid for a nervous system that is so adaptive (69).

Each clinical form of epilepsy is generated by a different set of mechanisms. In general, there is greater understanding presently of generators of focal epileptiform activity than generalized epileptiform activities. Cellular aspects of epileptogenesis are reviewed by Dichter and Ayala (70), and by Lothman and Collins (71).

Neurophysiology and Neurochemistry

From a neurophysiologic point of view, an epileptic seizure has been defined as an alteration of central nervous system (CNS) function resulting from spontaneous electrical discharge in a diseased neuronal population of cortical gray matter or the brainstem.

Epileptogenesis requires a set of epileptogenic neurons, the presence of disinhibition, and circuitry to permit multicellular synchronization.

Partial Epilepsies

An epileptic neuron has, among other characteristics, an increased electric excitability and the ability to sustain an autonomous paroxysmal discharge that can be influenced from the outside by synaptic activity. Intracellular recordings within an epileptic focus reveal that during the time when an interictal discharge is recorded on the scalp EEG, a compact population of neurons displays a stereotyped abnormality called paroxysmal depolarization shift (PDS). A PDS is characterized by a sudden, large, and sustained (approximately 30 mV for 70 to 150 msec) depolarization that is synchronized in many neurons. Multiple, high-frequency action potentials are superimposed on the PDS. The PDS and the EEG spike can occur spontaneously or can be triggered by afferent stimuli. The PDS is followed by a hyperpolarization of 10 to 20 mV below the resting potential that lasts 700 msec or longer. During this period the focus is refractory to afferent stimulation.

The large and lasting depolarization that characterizes a PDS is attributed to the triggering of voltage-gated calcium channels by the incoming action potential. This depolarizing calcium conductance is mediated by a subtype of excitatory amino acid receptor, which is characterized by its high affinity to *N*-methyl-D-aspartate (NMDA). The calcium channel is regulated by magnesium through a voltage-dependent block that can be removed by the initial sodium influx triggered by the action potential. The rise in intracellular calcium in turn triggers the opening of a specific type of potassium channel that initiates the hyperpolarization phase.

Another requirement for epileptogenesis is the spread of localized epileptic discharges to induce a clinical seizure during which thousands of neurons fire synchronously for prolonged periods.

Several experimental systems have been used to study how localized discharges are able to spread. In a nonepileptic brain, an area of neuronal hyperpolarization, the inhibitory surround, surrounds the region of synchronous paroxysmal discharges. This inhibitory surround limits the duration of the interictal discharge, determines its frequency, and prevents its progression into a full-blown seizure. Neurons can become hyperpolarized by several processes that can differ from one set of neurons to another.

When the interictal spike discharge is to be followed by a seizure, the hyperpolarization potentials of a population of neurons become progressively smaller and ultimately disappear, to be replaced by depolarization.

The mechanisms responsible for this transition from interictal to ictal period probably involve nonsynaptic processes such as electrical field effects (ephaptic interactions) and electrotonic coupling via gap junctions (72). Changes in the extracellular environment, such as K^+ and Ca^{2+} concentrations, also can affect the excitability of neuronal populations (73,74).

The observation that normal neurons can become epileptogenic by repeated stimulation, a process termed *kindling*, has provided a model for the study of the development of complex partial epilepsy (75,76). Kindling refers to a process by which brief trains of subconvulsive electrical stimuli are repeatedly delivered at appropriate intervals to a susceptible area of the brain. Initially, these stimuli produce afterdischarges, which become progressively more prolonged until they give rise to limbic and clonic motor seizures. When stimulations are continued for even longer periods, spontaneous seizures appear. Once established, the effects of kindling are permanent. Kindling also can be achieved by chemical stimulation of the cortex.

During kindling, the mossy fiber pathway (efferent from the granule cells of the dentate gyrus) undergoes reorganization of its synaptic connections (77). The resulting recurrent excita-

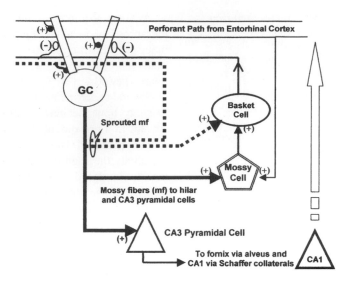

FIG. 13.2. Hippocampal circuitry and seizure-induced circuit reorganization. Granule cells (GC) receive their major input via the perforant path. The perforant path also stimulates hilar interneurons (such as mossy cells and basket cells) to provide feed-forward inhibition of the granule cells. Granule cell axons, the mossy fibers, make synaptic contact with CA3 pyramidal cells. Mossy fiber collaterals innervate the hilar interneurons such as the mossy cell shown in the diagram. Mossy cells are excitatory to GABAergic basket cells, which provide feedback inhibition to the granule cell. Sprouting of mossy fibers (in response to seizure-induced loss of CA3 pyramidal cells and hilar mossy cells) can result in enhanced excitation by forming autapses (an axon sprout synapsing with the dendrites of the same cell) and can augment synchronization by stimulating neighboring granule cells (not shown), thus contributing to epileptogenicity. It also has been suggested that the sprouted mossy fibers may restore inhibition lost after seizure-induced death of hilar mossy cells by direct stimulation of deafferented (dormant) basket cells.

tory connections have been implicated in the progressive development of hypersynchronous discharge. Such synaptic reorganization associated with loss of pyramidal cells in the CA3 subfield has been demonstrated in human epileptic tissue (78–80). Sloviter has suggested that the recurrent mossy fiber terminals include synapses on inhibitory interneurons (81).

Using his perforant path stimulation model of status epilepticus, Sloviter has studied the development of mossy fiber sprouting, chronic epilepsy, and time-dependent alterations in dentate inhibition. He suggested that the recurrent mossy fiber terminals include synapses on inhibitory interneurons (81,82). In his conceptualization, the hilar basket cells [inhibitory, γ-aminobutyric acid (GABA)-ergic] are deafferented by the loss of another group of cells, the mossy cells (excitatory, glutamatergic), which normally receive mossy fiber input, and drive the inhibitory basket cells (Fig.

13.2); hence the term *dormant basket cell hypothesis* for this concept. Mossy fiber sprouting compensates for the loss of drive to the basket cells. GABAergic cells, indeed, appear to be preserved in human epileptic tissue (83) and also in animal models (82), thus supporting this concept. Data derived by the study of slices from resected hippocampi suggest that the decrease in granule cell inhibition cannot be solely explained by a decrease in excitatory input onto inhibitory interneurons and may reflect changes at the interneuron-granule cells synapse or in the number of specific inhibitory interneurons (84).

Studies have compared the expression of excitatory amino acid receptor subunits and glutamic acid dehydrogenase (GAD) (presynaptic marker for GABA terminals) to the extent of mossy fiber sprouting in tissue from patients who underwent surgery. Patients' granule cell KA2 and GluR5 mRNA levels were increased in association with aberrant fascia dentata mossy fiber sprouting; however, increased glutamic acid dehydrogenase immunoreactivity also was present in such tissue (85,86).

The preceding discussions pertain to the structural plasticity that may be associated with focal epileptogenesis. There is also evidence for functional plasticity of synapses. Excitatory synapses show robust enhancement when they undergo repetitive high-frequency activation (87). This includes facilitation during the course of sustained stimulation and long-term potentiation that lasts hours to days after such a burst of activity in excitatory synapses. In contrast, similar repetitive high-frequency driving diminishes the efficacy of inhibitory (GABAergic) synapses (88,89).

Three factors determine whether a focal seizure will become generalized. The first is the excitability of the epileptic neurons, the second is the ease with which an electric discharge can be propagated from the focus, and the third is the threshold of the brainstem centers for disseminating an electric discharge. The last is believed to reflect in part a genetic predisposition, and in part the frequency with which the brainstem centers are activated by the primary epileptic focus.

Current concepts propose that a secondarily generalized tonic-clonic seizure results from the axonal propagation of the cortical ictal discharge to the contralateral cortex, and to subcortical structures via intrahemispheric and interhemispheric association pathways. The substantia nigra, in particular, appears to be involved, at least in the control of experimental seizures (90).

Once neuronal excitation derived from the epileptic cortical focus spreads to involve the brainstem, particularly the midbrain and the pontine reticular formation, a generalized seizure develops almost instantly. These areas are responsible for the dissemination of epileptic potentials (91,92). With the subcortical neurons involved by the epileptic discharge, a positive excitatory feedback circuit is established between the cortex and the subcortical neurons, inducing discharges at a rate of 10 to 40 Hz. This circuit is responsible for the tonic phase of the focal motor seizure. As inhibitory neurons are recruited, a negative inhibitory feedback circuit develops, which periodically interrupts the excitatory activity and produces the clonic phase of the seizure. When the negative feedback wins

ascendancy, the seizure subsides, leaving the neuronal membrane in a far greater hyperpolarized state than before the onset of the seizure.

Considerable evidence suggests that postictal (Todd's) paralysis, a common sequel to a focal seizure, is caused by persistence of the active inhibitory state, rather than by metabolic exhaustion of epileptic neurons (93).

The various areas of the cortex differ in their potential for secondary generalization. A number of areas including the temporal, frontal, and prefrontal cortex have particularly strong corticofugal projections to the centrencephalic system, and focal lesions within them readily induce a generalized seizure discharge (94,95). By contrast, the potential for secondary generalization is low in the motor strip. Additionally, small cortical lesions are more likely to induce a focally restricted seizure, whereas multiple or diffuse cortical lesions are more likely to result in a generalized seizure.

Primary Generalized Epilepsies

The pathophysiology of the primary generalized epilepsies is less well understood, and much of the experimental data is based on animal models that might not be applicable to the human epilepsies. In the 1940s, Penfield introduced the concept of centrencephalic epilepsy. This idea was that a generalized spike and wave discharge, such as occurs in absence epilepsy, originates in the rostral brainstem structures and the diencephalon, with the thalamus being responsible for the sudden generalized cortical discharge (96).

Gloor and Fariello postulate that in the primary generalized epilepsies the cortex is in a diffusely hyperexcitable state, perhaps as a result of the discharge of a group of excitatory neurons. As a result, an epileptic discharge can be triggered by excitation of the brainstem and the midline thalamic reticular system induced by thalamocortical input (97). Engel suggests that the firing of a small group of excitatory neurons stimulates a set of inhibitory neurons that have connections throughout the cortex. A second burst of properly timed excitatory impulses then produces a synchronized discharge over a wide area of the cortex (98). Thus the spike-wave discharges arise from the rhythmic, reverberatory interactions between interconnected thalamic and cortical neurons.

The oscillations in the thalamocortical circuits rely in part on the intrinsic membrane properties of the involved thalamic neurons. These neurons undergo slow, calcium-dependent depolarizations, attributed to the so-called T-channel (99). These low-threshold calcium currents provide the pacemaker quality to these cells that forms the basis of the thalamocortical reverberations. These spike-wave paroxysms are abolished by substances such as trimethadione or ethosuximide, which have a specific effect of abolishing calcium currents associated with the T-channel (99).

Clinically, such a discharge produces grand mal or absence epilepsy. In the latter condition, quick excitation of a neuronal inhibitory system prevents a prolonged clinical seizure and the development of the tonic-clonic components. These seizures can occur without known cerebral injury or disease, and, as indicated previously, they have a high rate of genetic transmission.

Views on the propagation of cortical electrical discharges have been considerably modified in the last few years, and the importance of the cortex in the production of both primary and secondarily generalized seizures has become increasingly evident from implanted or surface electrodes and from ictal and interictal PET scanning. These techniques have shown also the marked discrepancies between the scalp EEG and the actual seizure focus in approximately one-third of patients with refractory seizures (100,101).

Excitatory and Inhibitory Neurotransmitters

Excitatory neurotransmitters can play a role in the development of seizure discharges. Glutamate and aspartate are the major excitatory neurotransmitters found in the mammalian brain (102). Focal application of glutamate to hippocampal slices induces a calcium ion current and depolarizes the neuron. Another excitatory neurotransmitter system, the cholinergic system, has been successfully manipulated to produce experimental limbic seizures (103). Although the development of antiepileptic drugs based on their action at excitatory amino acid receptors is an active area of current research, presently available antimuscarinic agents are not likely to be useful as anticonvulsants because of their widespread central and peripheral sites of action.

Nicotinic receptors have not been thought to be important in the mechanisms underlying seizures. The recent finding of an association between autosomal dominant nocturnal frontal lobe epilepsy and mutations in the gene for a nicotinic cholinergic receptor subunit (CHRNA4) was thus surprising to investigators (19,20).

GABA has been shown to have inhibitory postsynaptic activity and is one of the principal inhibitory neurotransmitters in the mammalian brain. The role of inhibitory GABA-releasing neurons in producing hyperpolarization has been well established, and temporary disinhibition might predispose a normal neuronal population to epileptiform activity. The GABA receptor has been found in all areas of the brain (104). This receptor is coupled to the chloride channel (chloride ionophore), so that GABA binding to its receptor results in a rapid opening of the chloride channel, with an ensuing increase in the postsynaptic membrane conductance to chloride. Increased chloride ion permeability stabilizes the cell near its resting membrane potential and reduces its response to excitatory inputs. Modulation of the GABA receptor-chloride ionophore complex mediates the actions of benzodiazepines and barbiturates, as well as the convulsant effect of picrotoxin and its analogues (105). Interactions at the GABA receptor-chloride ionophore complex also underlie some of the mechanisms of action of felbamate and topiramate. These substances all have receptor sites on the GABA receptor complex. The receptor protein has been isolated and purified, and the genes coding for its two subunits have been cloned (106,107). The physiology and pharmacology of the receptor assembly depend on the subunit composition (107–109). No genetic diseases resulting from a defect in these genes have been demonstrated as yet.

Convulsions can be induced by substances that block the biosynthesis of GABA. Allylglycine, an inhibitor of glutamic acid decarboxylase, the enzyme promoting conversion of glutamic acid to GABA, is a potent epileptogenic compound (66). Inhibition of GABA binding to its receptor by bicuculline and inhibition of the postsynaptic GABA-chloride conductance responses by picrotoxin also induces convulsions. When GABAergic inhibition is progressively blocked with picrotoxin, stimulation of one neuron excites more and more neurons until neuronal behavior begins to resemble a seizure. Conversely, a number of compounds that elevate nerve-terminal GABA concentrations are potential anticonvulsants (110). These include such inhibitors of GABA transaminase as γ-vinyl-GABA (vigabatrin) and valproate. It is unclear, however, whether the anticonvulsant effects of valproate are indeed related to its elevation of brain GABA because this effect is seen only at supratherapeutic levels.

Magnetic resonance (MR) spectroscopy has provided evidence that gabapentin and topiramate also measurably increase brain concentrations of GABA even though they do not inhibit GABA transaminase (111,112). Extracellular (presumably also synaptic) concentration of GABA is increased by the nipecotic acid derivative, tiagabine (113).

Pyridoxine functions as a coenzyme for glutamic acid decarboxylase. Consequently, an increased glutamic acid to GABA ratio is expected in pyridoxine deficiency, a state marked by prolonged seizures. In pyridoxine dependency, an autosomal recessive disorder also characterized by seizures, the GABA content of brain is reduced, and brain glutamic acid concentration is elevated (114). Even though skin fibroblasts show reduced activity of pyridoxal-dependent glutamic acid decarboxylase, no abnormality in the two genes coding for glutamic acid decarboxylase, the biosynthetic enzyme for GABA, has been documented (115).

This relatively simple model for the epileptogenicity of insufficient inhibition and excessive excitation may, however, not hold true. Strong inhibition can predispose to hypersynchronization, and in petit mal seizures hyperfunction of GABAergic inhibitory pathways is evident (116). Brainstem and diencephalic influences, which normally induce slow-wave sleep, also increase cortical neuronal synchronization and raise the potential for epileptogenicity. In some of the experimental epilepsies, notably the reflex epilepsy of Mongolian gerbils, the number of GABAergic neurons is increased (117).

A role for other inhibitory neurotransmitters, notably the opioid peptides, in the production of interictal inhibition, and a role for postictal

depression have been suggested from various animal models (118). At low dosages, morphine and other opioids have anticonvulsant activity that is reversed by naloxone, whereas at higher dosages they act as convulsants, producing a petit mal–like seizure disorder. The relevance of these observations to human petit mal is uncertain, although positron emission tomography (PET) has revealed increased opiate receptor binding in the temporal cortex in patients with complex partial seizures (119).

Adenosine is another potent inhibitor of cortical neurons, acting primarily by depressing spontaneous neuronal firing or synaptic transmission through its inhibition of the presynaptic release of excitatory neurotransmitters. In a rat model of limbic status epilepticus, an adenosine A1 receptor agonist antagonized the development of status (120). Evidence from *in vivo* microdialysis experiences, performed intraoperatively on humans, suggests that adenosine may be a potential mediator of seizure arrest and postictal refractoriness (121). The clinical use of adenosine and of adenosine analogues has not been investigated extensively (122), and there is evidence that systemically administered adenosine analogues do not cross the blood–brain barrier (123). Moreover, the widespread effects of adenosine in the brain may not permit the development of a highly specific anticonvulsant with minimal CNS side effects.

Catecholamines and Indolamines

Adrenergic neurotransmitters are believed to play a significant role in the regulation of cortical excitability; consequently, a number of laboratories have searched for abnormalities in this system. Brain norepinephrine levels are low in several species of epileptic animals, and a decrease in brain norepinephrine concentration increases their seizure susceptibility. Conversely, an increase in brain norepinephrine levels decreases seizure severity (124). The lesioning of noradrenergic projections from the locus ceruleus lowers the threshold for forebrain and brainstem seizures (125). On the other hand, an increase in tyrosine hydroxylase has been found in human epileptic cortex, and the density of α_1-adrenoreceptor binding sites is reduced (126). It is not clear whether these findings in human tissue have relevance to epileptogenesis or merely reflect the effect of chronic epilepsy.

The serotonergic system also influences the expression of seizures. In view of the recent popularity of highly selective serotonin-uptake antagonists as antidepressants, it is of interest that fluoxetine (Prozac) appears to have anticonvulsant effects (127–129). Experiments have suggested that the antiepileptic action of fluoxetine on CA1 neurons is caused by an enhancement of endogenous serotonin that in turn seems mediated by 5-hydroxytryptamine-1A (5-HT1$_A$) receptor (130,131). Interestingly, in a genetic rat model of absence epilepsy, a 5-HT1$_A$ agonist increased spike waves in a dose-dependent manner (132). Genetically altered mice lacking the gene for 5-HT2$_C$ receptor seem to exhibit spontaneous seizures while the wild type background could be made to mimic such behavior by the administration of a specific 5-HT2$_C$ antagonist (133).

Biochemical Alterations Induced by Seizures

During a brief seizure, the brain undergoes several biochemical alterations. Cerebral oxygen and glucose consumption increase strikingly, but with maintenance of adequate ventilation, the increase in cerebral blood flow is sufficient to meet the increased metabolic requirements of the brain.

These studies, derived from experimental animals, have been confirmed in the epileptic human by PET. Autoradiography using labeled 2-deoxyglucose as a substrate provides excellent information on the local cerebral glucose metabolism. Using this technique, cerebral metabolism is generally found to be increased in the area of the epileptic focus during a seizure. In some instances, the area of increased metabolic activity extends to adjacent tissue and into areas of neuronal projection (134). In absence seizures, a marked and diffuse increase in cerebral metabolic rate occurs (135). The hypermetabolism probably reflects the enhanced excitatory and inhibitory neuronal activity during a seizure.

By contrast, the interictal metabolic picture reveals areas of hypometabolism (100,136). These observations, important to the localiza-

tion of epileptic foci, are discussed in a subsequent section of this chapter.

When a generalized seizure lasts 30 minutes or longer, it is usually accompanied by apnea. Apnea induces hypoxia and carbon dioxide retention. As a result of the energy demands of the convulsing muscles, the subject becomes hypoxic and hyperpyrexic (137). Oxygen tension within the brain decreases, a shift toward anaerobic metabolism occurs, and lactic acid accumulates (138). MR spectroscopy performed on rabbits subjected to status epilepticus corroborates these data. Phosphocreatine levels decrease, inorganic phosphorus levels increase, lactate increases, and intracellular pH decreases within 30 minutes of the onset of seizures (139). The increase in cerebral lactate after prolonged seizures results from activation of phosphofructokinase, which is a primary regulatory enzyme for cerebral glycolysis (139).

Clinical Manifestations

To facilitate presentation of the clinical manifestations of seizures, which vary even in a given patient, each of the common epilepsies is discussed. A miscellaneous group of less common epilepsies is then covered, with literature references for more extensive reading. Finally, the discussion turns to febrile seizures and the problem of seizures during the neonatal period.

Epilepsies Characterized by Generalized Tonic-Clonic (Grand Mal) Seizures

A generalized tonic-clonic seizure, occurring as a manifestation of primary generalized epilepsy, occurring as a secondary generalization of a partial epilepsy, or alternating with other seizure forms is the most common epileptic manifestation of childhood (see Table 13.3) (140). These conditions do not represent a homogeneous group, but are seen in a variety of clinical settings.

The seizure can be primary generalized or secondarily generalized. A primary generalized seizure can occur without warning, whereas a secondarily generalized seizure can be preceded by an aura. Occasionally, the child might be irritable or might manifest unusual behavior for several hours before the seizure. In localizing the epileptic focus, the aura offers the most important clinical clue, more reliable at times than the EEG. The examining physician should always try to elicit its history. The most common epileptic aura is a sensation of dizziness or an unusual feeling of ascending abdominal discomfort. These sensations have been attributed to a discharge in the area of visceral sensory representation, but offer less evidence for the site of the epileptic focus than do focal sensory symptoms (141).

In the classic form of an attack, the aura, if present, can be followed by rolling up of the eyes and loss of consciousness. A generalized tonic contraction of the entire body musculature occurs, and the child can utter a piercing, peculiar cry, after which he or she becomes apneic and cyanotic. With the onset of the clonic phase of the convulsion, the trunk and extremities undergo rhythmic contraction and relaxation. As the attack ends, the rate of clonic movements slows, and finally the movements cease abruptly. The duration of a seizure varies from a few seconds to half an hour or more. A series of attacks at intervals too brief to allow the child to regain consciousness between attacks is known as status epilepticus. Because status epilepticus is one of the few neurologic conditions requiring emergency treatment, it will be referred to again in the section on treatment.

After the seizure, the child can remain semiconscious and then confused for several hours. When examined soon after an attack, he or she is poorly coordinated, with mild impairment of fine movements. Truncal ataxia, increased deep tendon reflexes, clonus, and extensor plantar responses can be present. Occasionally, the child appears blind and speechless. Postictally, he or she may vomit or complain of severe headache.

The major motor attack has numerous variations. Occasionally, particularly when drug therapy has been partly effective in controlling a secondarily generalized seizure, a typical aura occurs but is not followed by a seizure. In other patients, either the tonic or the clonic phase is too brief to be noted. Attacks can occur at any time of the day or night, although their frequency is somewhat greater shortly before or after the child falls asleep or awakens. Approximately one-fourth of patients experience nocturnal seizures; the remainder experience diurnal or mixed seizures. Generally, patients who for 1 year or more have experienced seizures only during sleep are unlikely to have attacks at other times of the day. In some girls, seizures occur a few days before or shortly after their menstrual period.

A generalized tonic-clonic seizure or other epileptic manifestations can be precipitated by infection and fever, fatigue, emotional disturbances, hyperventilation and alkalosis, and drugs.

Fever can induce a seizure not only in children experiencing febrile seizures, but also in patients who previously had recurrent epileptic attacks unassociated with fever. In some children, dehydration and ketosis accompanying an acute infectious illness decrease seizure frequency.

In a few children, excessive fatigue or lack of sleep appears to precede a seizure, but probably does not represent an important precipitating factor. Considerable clinical evidence indicates that epileptic children have fewer seizures when engaged in regular strenuous physical activity. Although fatigue seems to have little effect on the EEG, sleep deprivation can activate the EEG of epileptic patients and can precipitate seizures (142).

Parents often believe that emotional disturbances precipitate seizures in epileptic children. No evidence supports this idea, however, and there is no justification for parents' failing to set limits to the behavior of their epileptic child.

Hyperventilation and alkalosis induce absence attacks in approximately 90% of patients subject to them, but are less effective in precipitating other seizure forms.

A variety of drugs can induce single seizures or status epilepticus. In the experience of Messing and coworkers, isoniazid and psychotropic medications accounted for approximately one-half of cases (143). Other drugs implicated in bringing on seizures include cocaine (144), theophylline, and penicillin. Isoniazid (INH) antagonizes glutamic acid decarboxylase by binding with its cofactor, pyridoxal phosphate, thus interfering with the biosynthesis of GABA. Demonstrable decreases in brain GABA levels result from INH administration. An increasing number of patients has presented with status epilepticus and encephalopathy attributable to INH overdoses (144,145). In these cases, immediate administration of pyridoxal (vitamin B_6) is crucial. Theophylline acts as an adenosine antagonist, whereas penicillin acts as a GABA antagonist and interferes with benzodiazepine binding in the brain (122). For INH and theophylline, the convulsive effects tend to be dose related (143). Various anticonvulsants, notably phenytoin, when given in toxic amounts, increase seizure frequency. Trimethadione, which was formerly used in the treatment of absence epilepsy, occasionally precipitated a grand mal seizure within 1 to 2 days of first being administered. The sudden withdrawal of anticonvulsant medication, particularly barbiturates and benzodiazepines, is the most common cause for status epilepticus. Finally, adolescent patients should be warned against excessive alcohol consumption.

Spontaneous variations in the frequency of attacks are common and must be taken into account when judging the effectiveness of anticonvulsant medication. In the experience of van Donselaar and colleagues, who studied untreated tonic-clonic seizures in children younger than 16 years of age, 42% showed a decelerating pattern, and ultimately became seizure free even in the absence of anticonvulsant treatment. An accelerating pattern of seizure frequency was seen in only 20% of children with four or more untreated seizures (146). Some children have seizures during early childhood, then remain asymptomatic until puberty, when their attacks recur for 4 to 7 years.

Epilepsies with Typical Absence (Petit Mal) Seizures

Typical absence seizures are most commonly identified with absence (petit mal) epilepsy. In its pure form, an absence (petit mal) attack was defined by Gowers as a "transient loss of consciousness without conspicuous convulsions" (24).

The onset of seizures is usually abrupt, and the child suddenly develops an estimated 20 or more attacks each day. The characteristic attack is a brief arrest of consciousness, usually lasting 5 to 10 seconds, appearing without warning or aura. There can be a slight loss of body tone, causing the child to drop objects from his or her hand, but this loss is rarely profound enough to induce a fall. Minor movements occur in approximately 70% of patients; these are usu-

ally lip-smacking or twitching of the eyelids or face, often at the three per second frequency of the EEG abnormality (Fig. 13.3). Urinary incontinence is rare (147). The seizure terminates abruptly, and the patient is often unaware of the lapse of consciousness. The occurrence and duration of a lapse can be determined by reciting to the child a series of numbers during the attack and asking the child to repeat them when consciousness appears to have returned. Attacks first appear during childhood; in 64% of instances, they begin between 5 and 9 years of age. They are more common in girls; Dalby's series had 99 female and 62 male subjects (148).

When attacks are frequent, the child's intellectual processes are slowed and, often, the first indication is a deterioration in schoolwork and behavior (149). Responsiveness to auditory stimuli is impaired in the majority of patients in 0.1 to 0.4 seconds after the onset of a generalized spike-wave paroxysm, but it recovers in 2 to 3 seconds after the cessation of the attack. Extrapolations from spike-wave discharges associated with focal epilepsies have implicated the slow-wave component of the spike-wave complex in the interrupted cognitive function (55). Even brief and clinically undetectable attacks can impair intellectual performance.

Some absence attacks are more complex, and their appearance can be difficult to differentiate from complex partial seizures. They involve brief behavioral automatisms or, less commonly, prolonged symmetric myoclonic movements of the head or extremities (myoclonic petit mal). In the series of Sato and coworkers, some 40% of patients with typical absence seizures also experienced a grand mal attack, either before or after the onset of their absence attack (150). This figure is probably high and perhaps reflects the patterns of referral to a university center.

On a clinical basis, absence attacks must be distinguished from brief complex partial seizures; the latter are often preceded by an aura and followed by postictal depression. Additionally, brief complex partial seizures tend to be less frequent and clustered. Routine EEG studies in most instances clarify the situation. In a child with typical absence attacks, the EEG demonstrates a 3-Hz spike-wave discharge, which occasionally slows as the seizure pro-

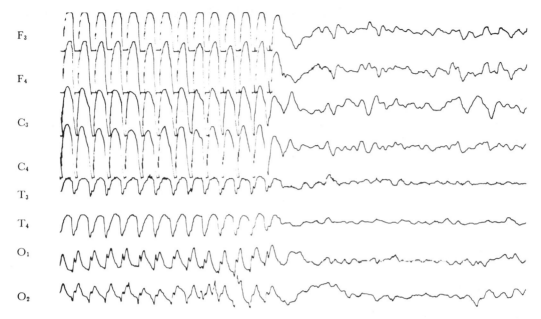

FIG. 13.3. Three-hertz (three per second) spike-wave discharges in an 11-year-old girl with frequent absence (petit mal) attacks. In this instance, a clinically evident seizure lasting 19 seconds was induced by hyperventilation. (F_3, left frontal; F_4, right frontal; C_3, left central; C_4, right central; T_3, left temporal; T_4, right temporal; O_1, left occipital; O_2, right occipital.)

gresses. The interictal EEG is normal in approximately one-half of patients, and the background EEG frequency is generally age appropriate (151). Approximately 10% of children with clinical and EEG features of typical absence attacks have a focal onset to their EEG seizures and demonstrate focal cortical lesions (152).

Typical absence seizures also should be differentiated from atypical absence attacks, which are associated with the Lennox-Gastaut syndrome (atypical petit mal, petit mal variant). This relatively common seizure type is associated with a variety of CNS insults, and the majority of affected children have a significant developmental delay. Unlike typical absence attacks, the frequency of atypical attacks is cyclic, in that seizure-free periods alternate with days or weeks of a high seizure frequency. The EEG shows complexes occurring at 1.5 to 2.5 Hz, or multiple spike and wave discharges. Diffuse slowing of background activity was seen in 85% of children in the series of Holmes and coworkers (151).

Absence attacks are a common prelude to juvenile absence epilepsy. Its characteristic features consist of typical absence attacks, seen in

approximately one-third of patients, and commencing later than those of typical childhood absence epilepsy. Brief myoclonic jerks that generally occur on awakening usually develop around 15 years of age (i.e., several years after the appearance of absence attacks), and tonic-clonic seizures follow some months thereafter. Attacks tend to occur much less frequently than they do in absence seizures, usually once a day or less (152). Intelligence is normal. The interictal EEG in juvenile absence epilepsy demonstrates discharges not only at 3 Hz, but also at 4 to 6 Hz (153). The background activity is usually normal. Photosensitivity is seen in approximately one-third of patients (154).

Experimental studies designed to clarify the mechanism for absence seizures have already been reviewed (97,98,155).

Epilepsies with Complex Partial Seizures (Psychomotor Seizures, Temporal Lobe Seizures)

Complex partial seizures have been defined as seizures that arise from a limited area of one cerebral hemisphere and produce a period of impaired consciousness that varies from mild to profound. Although these seizures are most characteristically associated with lesions of the temporal lobe and have been called temporal lobe seizures, they also can be associated with lesions of the frontal (156) or occipital lobes (157). As the terminology indicates, they are focal seizures.

The epilepsies characterized by this seizure type are heterogeneous. Pathologic alterations seen within the surgically resected temporal lobe have been summarized in Table 13.5 (158).

The most common abnormality is MTS (Ammon's horn sclerosis or hippocampal sclerosis). In the series of Harvey and colleagues, it was seen in 21% of children aged 15 years or younger, with new onset temporal lobe epilepsy (159). The association of this characteristic lesion with both epileptogenicity and seizure-related damage has been discussed in the Neuropathologic Factors section previously in this chapter. Less commonly, 13% of cases in the series of Harvey and colleagues (159), a variety of tumors in the epileptogenic cortex can occur. These include hamartomas, which occasionally undergo malignant transformation, small gliomatous nodules, hemangiomas, and lesions suggestive of tuberous sclerosis (160,161). In early childhood, however, tumors are the most common etiology for complex partial seizures. Thus, in the series of Wyllie and colleagues, comprising children younger than 12 years of age who underwent temporal lobectomy, tumors were seen in 64%, as compared with MTS, seen in 29%. It is of note that 75% of children with MTS in the series of Wyllie and coworkers had a history of previous febrile convulsions (162). When bilateral MTS develops early in life, usually after prolonged seizures or status epilepticus, the clinical picture is marked by loss of language, or failure of language development, and impaired social and adaptive learning (163).

In a significant proportion of patients with complex partial seizures, focal abnormalities are found outside the hippocampus, in the limbic portion of the frontal lobes, in the lateral temporal lobe, and in nonlimbic areas outside the temporal lobe (164). In these instances, the ictal discharge probably spreads from the focus to involve the temporal lobe.

TABLE 13.6. *Clinical manifestations of complex partial seizures in childhood*

Seizure manifestation	Number of patients with manifestations (total 25)		
	Age 1–6	Age 7–16	Total
Aura	6	10	16
Altered consciousness	12	13	25
Change in position of body or limbs	10	11	21
Integrated but confused activity	8	11	19
Staring or dazed expression	10	8	18
Epigastric sensation, nausea, vomiting	9	5	14
Oral movements, drooling	8	5	13
Muttering, mumbling, hissing	5	5	10
Walking, wandering	4	6	10
Pallor or flushing	5	4	9
Rubbing or fumbling	4	5	9
Speech (usually irrelevant or incoherent)	3	5	8
Affective disturbance (fear, anger)	5	3	8
Stiffening of body or limbs	5	3	8
Falling	4	3	7
Aggressive activity	4	3	7
Dreamy state	2	3	5
Forced thinking or ideational blocking	1	4	5
Searching or orienting movements	1	3	4
Abdominal pain	3	1	4
Incontinence (urinary)	2	1	3
Perceptual disturbance (visual, auditory)	0	3	3

Modified from Glaser GH, Dixon MS. Psychomotor seizures in childhood: a clinical study. *Neurology* 1956; 6:646.

Even though seizures start before 10 years of age in approximately 75% of children (67), typical complex partial seizures are rarely seen until 10 years of age. Rather, children who later develop complex partial attacks can have an antecedent history of convulsive seizures associated with chewing, lip-smacking, or other oral automatisms (165). Additionally, they can experience a variety of behavior disorders, enuresis, nightmares, and sleepwalking (166).

Seizure manifestations in older children are presented in Table 13.6. The aura can consist of a variety of subjective phenomena. In children, Glaser and Dixon have found intense anxiety usually associated with visceral sensations to be the most common antecedent to complex partial seizures (167). Wyllie and colleagues have noted that a large proportion of children complain of a "funny" or bad taste (162). An epigastric "rising" sensation is also common. Olfactory hallucinations (uncinate fits) are usually described as unpleasant but unidentifiable odors. Their association with temporal lobe tumors is a matter of some dispute. In Daly's series, almost 40% of 55 patients who experienced this aura were found to have neoplasms (168). Similarly, in the series of Acharya and colleagues 73% of patients with such an aura harbored a tumor (169). By contrast, Howe and Gibson found a tumor incidence of only 8.1% in their series of 37 patients, which is comparable with the 9.1% overall incidence of gliomas in patients with temporal lobe seizures (170).

Hallucinatory experiences, most commonly a feeling of déjà vu, an adventitious sense of familiarity, and visual hallucinations, have been reported by children with complex partial seizures (171). According to Mullan and Penfield, they occur more frequently when the focus is in the nondominant temporal lobe (172).

Paroxysmal emotional states, particularly fear, are not rare in children and are commonly reported by parents. Rage reactions or temper tantrums are unusual auras of a complex partial seizure, and purposeful aggressive acts are uncommon in the course of seizure. A detailed history of the aura can assist in localizing the seizure focus, but does not help in lateralizing it. Whereas experiential auras, such as fear and déjà vu, almost invariably originate from the temporal lobes, notably the neocortex (164), cephalic auras, such as a sensation of dizziness or lightheadedness are of less localizing value and can emanate from either frontal or temporal areas. Viscerosensory auras were found to accompany a temporal lobe focus in 76% of subjects, and somatosensory auras accompanied a parieto-occipital focus in 62% (173).

On the basis of the initial seizure manifestations, Delgado-Escueta and associates have divided complex partial seizures into two types (174). In the more common form, type I, the seizure originates from the temporal lobe. Patients briefly stop all activity after their aura.

They stand still, stare, or turn pale. Shortly thereafter, minor motor acts are initiated. Prolonged postictal confusion is common in these patients. In type II, seizures originate from outside the temporal lobe, most commonly from the frontal lobe. In this type automatisms initiate the attack. Commonly, these involve chewing and smacking movements, purposeless fumbling or patting of the hands, and picking at clothes. Postictal confusion is brief in this group of patients. Drop attacks as part of temporal lobe seizures are unusual in childhood (175).

The final part of the seizure generally involves more complex motor acts. The child might move about the room, begin to undress, and occasionally utter stereotyped or nonsensical phrases. In the majority of cases, these automatisms usually do not last longer than 5 minutes, although reliable observers have recorded prolonged complex partial seizures. Complex partial status epilepticus (psychomotor status) is extremely rare, and to our knowledge it has never initiated complex partial epilepsy (176,177). In children, the condition manifests by impaired consciousness with intermittent staring and wandering eye movements and intermittent automatisms, such as picking at clothes. At other times, it can result in a prolonged period of amnesia. The condition should be differentiated from absence status or hysterical amnesia. Depth electrode studies suggest that the seizure focus is more commonly within the frontal lobes (178). A variety of electrocardiographic abnormalities can accompany complex partial seizures. These can be responsible for some of the sudden deaths seen in inadequately treated epileptic patients (179).

Following the seizure, the patient experiences postictal confusion, drowsiness, or clouding of consciousness. When fully recovered, the child has complete amnesia for the entire attack.

As with major motor seizures, the frequency of complex partial seizures varies, but in contrast to typical absence attacks, more than three to four attacks a day is uncommon (167).

The possibility of complex partial seizures is often raised in a child with behavior problems who has an abnormal EEG result. Aird and Yamamoto examined this question and found that approximately one-half of children with behavior problems have an abnormal EEG result. Of all patients studied, 27% had EEG foci primarily involving the temporal lobe (180). Although some authors vigorously dispute this predilection to behavior disturbances (181), others support it and have found behavior disturbances to be three times as common in this as in the other types of epilepsy (182). Additionally, symptoms suggesting complex partial seizures are highly prevalent among violent juveniles (183). Several further studies have confirmed these observations. In a series published in 1980, the incidence of abnormal behavior was 36% (184). The cause of the seizures, their duration, and the presence of associated grand mal attacks do not seem to affect the likelihood of psychiatric disturbances. However, boys whose seizure focus is located in the dominant hemisphere and whose seizures commence between 5 and 10 years of age appear to be particularly vulnerable (182). In most instances, the psychiatric illness commences during adolescence; its manifestation before 12 years of age is unusual.

The basis for these psychiatric phenomena has undergone considerable speculation. The most attractive hypothesis states that recurrent complex partial seizures kindle a limbic dopamine system, whose paroxysmal activity does not produce seizures but does produce serious behavior disturbances (185). The role of limbic kindling in the genesis of psychiatric illness is outside the scope of this text. Adamec and Stark-Adamec and Weiss and Post review this subject (186,187).

Epilepsies Characterized by Simple Partial Seizures (Focal Seizures, Partial Seizures with Elementary Symptoms)

Focal seizures are characterized by the development of localized motor or sensory symptoms without impairment of consciousness. In a large proportion of children, these seizures spread to other parts of the body, ultimately becoming generalized with loss of consciousness. On rare occasions, progression follows an orderly sequence, a phenomenon known as the *jacksonian march*. This type of a seizure is generally considered to be symptomatic of a structural cortical lesion.

Perhaps the most common focal attack observed in children is the versive seizure (188). Most often, this consists of turning the eyes, or the eyes and head, away from the side of the focus. In some patients, the upper extremity on the side toward which the head turns is abducted and extended, and the fingers are clenched. Thus, the child appears to look at his closed fist.

The patient may be aware of this movement or may simultaneously lose consciousness. By means of combined telemetry and EEG monitoring, the cortical areas of discharge responsible for this form of seizure have been found to be either the contralateral temporal lobe or the contralateral frontal lobe, anterior to the rolandic gyrus. Patients whose seizure starts with versive movements and who retain awareness of them tend to have a frontal lobe seizure focus. Patients whose seizure starts with staring and automatisms tend to have a temporal lobe focus (174,189,190). EEG changes, as recorded on scalp electrodes, are seen in only approximately one-third of patients during telemetry-verified attacks of a variety of simple partial seizures. Therefore, the presence of an unaltered EEG does not speak against the diagnosis (191).

Focal motor seizures are particularly common in hemiplegic children. The epileptic movements are usually clonic and begin in the hemiplegic hand, and are often heralded by localized sensory symptoms. The clonic movements spread over the entire affected side, ultimately becoming generalized in many cases. Postictal weakness (Todd's paralysis) commonly follows this kind of seizure and can last for several hours or for a day or more.

Whereas adults have a high positive correlation between Todd's paralysis and a structural cortical lesion, children do not, and often attacks of alternating left- and right-sided focal seizures with postictal paralyses are the initial events in a child with apparently idiopathic epilepsy. This observation probably reflects a smaller and less readily detectable focus in the pediatric population.

A heterogeneous group of conditions are characterized by focal (simple partial) seizures. In approximately one-half of patients, one can document an underlying structural lesion. These lesions include developmental malformations, notably gray matter heterotopias and localized pachygyria, gliosis resulting from asphyxial damage or perinatal and postnatal physical trauma, and a variety of space-occupying lesions. In the remainder of patients with simple partial seizures, no obvious etiology can be demonstrated. Several clinically distinct types of these idiopathic focal epilepsies have been recognized. They are characterized by the absence of anatomic or functional focal lesions and by a benign course with normal intellectual development and spontaneous cure. Aside from febrile seizures and a family history of seizures for approximately one-third of children, no obvious antecedents exist. The frequency of these conditions is difficult to ascertain. Roger and Bureau believe they constitute some 60% of partial epilepsies seen in school-aged children (192).

The most common and most clearly delineated of the idiopathic focal epilepsies is midtemporal epilepsy (sylvian epilepsy, rolandic epilepsy, benign childhood epilepsy with centrotemporal spikes). In the experience of Loiseau and coworkers, it represented 10.7% of children seen in a specialized private practice (193). A high incidence of similar seizures occurs in first-degree relatives, and an autosomal dominant form of rolandic epilepsy has been reported (194). In approximately 75% of children this type of a seizure commences between ages 5 and 10 years. Seizures are infrequent, in the majority of cases occurring less than three or four times a year, and are generally brief. Most characteristically, attacks commence with a somatosensory aura, usually referred to the tongue, cheek, or gums, and less often to the abdomen. As a result of motor interference, speech is arrested, the child salivates, and tonic or tonic-clonic movements involve the face. Consciousness is preserved in some 60% of children. Because approximately three-fourths of the attacks occur during sleep, a good patient history is difficult to obtain. The interictal EEG shows midtemporal spikes, probably a reflection of discharges arising from the rolandic cortex (195,196). In contrast to other seizures having a temporal spike focus, the prognosis in this condition is excellent (197); most children

respond well to anticonvulsant therapy. In the experience of Lombroso, almost 50% were seizure free within 3 years of their first attack, and in more than 30% the EEG reverted to normal as well (195). Beaussart and Faou share this optimism. In their series of 334 cases, no patient had seizures after age 13 years, even when anticonvulsants had been withdrawn (198).

Infantile epilepsy with an occipital focus (199) is much less common. The age of onset is variable; in the experience of Beaumanoir, it ranged between 15 months and 17 years (199). Attacks are initiated by hemianopia, phosphenes (white or colored luminous spots), or visual hallucinations. Amaurosis or nonvisual symptoms follow. The latter include unilateral convulsions, automatisms, or generalized tonic-clonic seizures. Aphasia is not unusual. The interictal EEG demonstrates nearly continuous unilateral or bilateral high-voltage spike-wave discharges from the occipital or posterior temporal regions. This is generally suppressed by eye opening. The prognosis is excellent with or without anticonvulsant therapy, and all children in Beaumanoir's series were seizure free with a normal EEG by 9 to 13 years of age (199). This condition has been reviewed by Sveinbjornsdottir and Duncan (200).

The European epileptologists also distinguish a focal epilepsy with midtemporal spikes and affective symptoms. Seizures commence with a sensation of fear or terror and proceed with chewing and swallowing movements and speech arrest. Consciousness is depressed. Unlike complex partial seizures, seizures cease with therapy, and no evidence for a focal lesion can be found on clinical examination or by imaging studies (191).

Lennox-Gastaut Syndrome (Myoclonic-Astatic Petit Mal)

The epileptic syndromes considered in this section share an early onset, an EEG picture characterized by spike-wave forms other than the regular 3 Hz, and poor prognosis, in terms of both seizure control and ultimate intellectual development. Livingston and associates have used the term *minor motor seizures* to designate the epilepsies described in this section (201). This term has been abandoned in recent years; not only is there nothing minor about these seizures, but the term is overly broad and encompasses a variety of seizures with limited expression, regardless of their etiology and EEG features.

Types of Seizures

Based on the different clinical manifestations of the epileptic attacks, at least four seizure types can be distinguished: atonic (astatic or akinetic) seizures, brief tonic seizures, atypical petit mal seizures, and myoclonic seizures (202).

Atonic (Akinetic) Seizures. Atonic seizures are characterized by a sudden, momentary loss of posture or muscle tone. In the infant who is able to sit but cannot yet stand, atonic spells consist of a sudden dropping forward of the head and neck, the *salaam seizure*, such as is seen as part of infantile spasms. In older children, the loss of postural tone precipitates the child violently to the ground. Consciousness is lost only momentarily, but the force of the fall commonly produces injuries of the face and head. Atonic spells recur frequently during the course of a day and are particularly common during the morning hours and shortly after the child awakens.

Tonic Seizures. Tonic seizures are characterized by a brief generalized increase in muscle tone. These seizures are frequent during non–rapid eye movement (REM) sleep and generally are the most common form of seizure in the Lennox-Gastaut syndrome, and also the type most resistant to anticonvulsant therapy (203).

Atypical Petit Mal Seizures. Atypical petit mal seizures are characterized by absence seizures that, unlike true petit mal, tend to occur in cycles and can disappear for periods of several days (204). These seizures can occur by themselves or can be accompanied by grand mal or complex partial seizures.

Myoclonic Seizures. The term *myoclonic seizure* includes a variety of seizures characterized by myoclonus, that is, single or repetitive contractures of a muscle or a group of muscles. For therapeutic and prognostic purposes,

myoclonus has been classified into two forms: epileptic and nonepileptic (205). Myoclonic seizures account for approximately 7% of the epilepsies that have an onset during the first 3 years of life (206). In primary generalized epileptic myoclonus, the myoclonic jerks consist of small, random, recurring twitches, most evident in the fingers and hands. They synchronously involve muscles on both sides of the body. An EEG abnormality, originating most commonly from the frontal leads, precedes the myoclonus, suggesting that a hyperexcitable cortex responds to a subcortical input with the paroxysm. This form of myoclonus usually is seen with chronic epileptic disorders. In the series of Wilkins and associates, it was part of the Lennox-Gastaut syndrome in more than one-half of the subjects (207).

Myoclonic seizures also are seen as a nonspecific symptom in several forms of viral encephalitis, metabolic disturbances such as uremia, and progressive cerebral degenerative diseases such as the various lysosomal storage diseases, some of the leukodystrophies, Menkes disease, and Unverricht-Lundberg disease (see Chapter 1).

Several types of nonepileptic myoclonus have been recognized. Cortical reflex myoclonus is believed to result from hyperexcitability of a small region of the sensory portion of the sensorimotor cortex. The muscular contractions are irregular and are precipitated or aggravated by sensory stimuli, most commonly by light, noise, or tapping on the face or chest. Postural changes intensify the contractions. The movements disappear in sleep. The EEG is clearly abnormal, and a paroxysm precedes both the spontaneous and the reflex-induced myoclonic jerks. Giant somatosensory-evoked potentials are characteristic for this type of myoclonus (208).

In reticular reflex myoclonus, the myoclonic jerks affect the entire body, with the flexor muscles being more involved than the extensors. The seizures are believed to be the result of hyperexcitability of the caudal brainstem reticular formation, possibly the nucleus reticularis gigantocellularis (205). An EEG spike usually follows the first electromyographic evidence of myoclonus. Another nonepileptic form of myoclonus is considered to be of spinal cord or brainstem origin. The muscular contractions are rhythmic and are unaffected by sensory stimuli. They persist during sleep. The EEG can be normal or abnormal, and response to anticonvulsant medication is poor.

Nonepileptic myoclonus is also encountered in the context of involuntary movements in some of the disorders of the extrapyramidal system. It is seen in normal individuals while falling asleep. Rarely, frequent but nonprogressive myoclonic movements occur unaccompanied by other types of epileptic attacks or intellectual subnormality. This condition is termed *paramyoclonus multiplex* or *essential myoclonus*. It is probably transmitted by an autosomal dominant gene, and is considered to be related to the various dystonias covered in Chapter 2 (209). Closely related to this condition is the exaggerated startle response (hyperekplexia), which is transmitted by a gene mapped to chromosome 5q33-35 and coding for the glycine receptor α-1 subunit (210). This condition is covered more extensively in Chapter 2. In hyperekplexia patients exhibit momentary muscular stiffness and loss of voluntary postural control without loss of consciousness. Other features of this condition include transient hypertonia during infancy, nocturnal jerking of the legs, insecure gait, and low average intelligence. No other epileptic phenomena occur, although the EEG can have paroxysmal features. Minor, quantitatively less severe forms of this condition also have been observed. The condition should be distinguished from startle epilepsy, a type of reflex epilepsy (211). Treatment with clonazepam appears to be beneficial (212).

Causes

The causes for the Lennox-Gastaut syndrome are multiple. In the experience of Lennox and Davis, compiled in 1950, 50% of patients had a history of perinatal cerebral injury, another 20% might have had an attack of encephalitis or meningitis, and 13% had major complications of gestation (213). Currently, complications of gestation appear to be the most significant cause, with perinatal asphyxia, infections, and genetic factors following in order of importance.

Onset of the Lennox-Gastaut syndrome seizures ranges from age 6 months to approximately age 16 years. In some two-thirds of instances, the onset is between 2 and 14 years of age (214). In some patients, 6% of Kruse's series, the Lennox-Gastaut syndrome follows infantile spasms (214). In approximately one-half of the children, one or more major motor attacks, with or without fever, precede the illness. Brett delineated a group of children who experience a sudden onset of major seizures that, after a seizure-free interval of approximately 1 week, are followed by the Lennox-Gastaut syndrome and progressive intellectual deterioration (36). This entity, termed *epileptogenic encephalopathy* by Brett, is not rare. Its cause is unknown, but in view of the occasional cerebrospinal fluid (CSF) pleocytosis, it might be infectious. Atonic, myoclonic, or atypical absence seizures can continue throughout the patient's lifetime. In three-fourths of patients, generalized tonic-clonic or focal seizures also can appear.

Lennox-Gastaut syndrome correlates with an EEG result that Lennox and Davis termed the *petit mal variant* (Fig. 13.4) (213). It is an asymmetric, sometimes lateralized, slow (2.0 to 2.5 Hz) polyspike-wave discharge (atypical spike-wave discharge), which, in contrast to the 3-Hz synchronous discharge of petit mal, is less likely to be provoked by hyperventilation.

Mental development of the child with Lennox-Gastaut syndrome is usually slow. In part this reflects the underlying brain disease, and in part it is the result of the frequency of seizures. Characteristically, the earlier motor milestones are attained at the expected age, but subsequent evaluations reveal subnormal intelligence in a large proportion of affected children. In the series of Blume and associates, 35% of patients attained an IQ of 75 or above, and only 10% scored above 100 on psychometric testing (215). In the experience of Chevrie and Aicardi, the incidence of retardation was even higher (203).

Infantile Spasms (West Syndrome)

Infantile spasms most commonly develop between 3 and 8 months of age, with only 8% of cases first being encountered in infants older

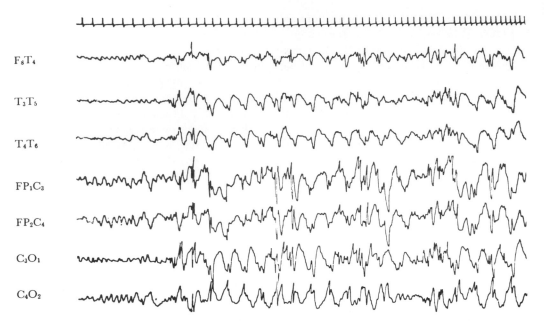

FIG. 13.4. Atypical polyspike-wave discharge. Photically (5 Hz) induced myoclonic seizure in a 14-year-old girl. The electroencephalogram shows 3-Hz multiple spike-wave discharges. (F_8T_4, right frontotemporal; T_3T_5, left frontotemporal; T_4T_6, right temporal; FP_1C_3, left frontopolar-central; FP_2C_4, right frontopolar-central; C_3O_1, left central-occipital; C_4O_2, right central-occipital. Top lead is photostimulator.)

than 2 years of age. It occurs somewhat more frequently in male infants. Attacks are characterized by a series of sudden muscular contractions by which the head is flexed, the arms are extended, and the legs are drawn up. A cry or giggling can precede or follow the seizure, and the infant can flush or can turn pale or cyanotic.

Other clinical presentations of infantile spasms occur less commonly. They include head nodding and extensor spasms characterized by extension rather than flexion of arms, legs, and trunk. Rarely, the attacks are concluded by a brief clonic seizure.

Lightning attacks (Blitzkrämpfe) (216) are a variant involving a single, momentary, shock-like contraction of the entire body (217).

Clusters of seizures recur frequently, particularly on waking, and some children have 50 to 100 each day. In Jeavons and Bower's series of 112 children, mental development was normal up to the onset of seizures in 52% and was definitely or probably delayed in the remainder (218). More recent series have had a higher incidence of

delayed mental development before the onset of seizures. In 66% of patients, the EEG has the characteristics of hypsarrhythmia, namely diffuse dysrhythmia with high-voltage slow waves and multiple spike-wave discharges (Fig. 13.5) (218). This unique electrical pattern becomes apparent after 3 to 4 months of age. In some infants, it is most evident in non-REM sleep. During REM sleep and immediately after arousal from REM or non-REM sleep, the EEG can be normal for up to several minutes (219). The discharges tend to favor the posterior areas of the brain. This contrasts with the paroxysmal discharges in Lennox-Gastaut syndrome, which are most evident anteriorly. The significance of this finding is not clear, particularly because many children with infantile spasms progress to Lennox-Gastaut syndrome. To our knowledge there has not been a systematic study of EEG maturation in infantile spasms.

Hypsarrhythmia persists for some years, then is superseded by a variety of other paroxysmal abnormalities. These include focal discharges, most commonly arising from the temporal

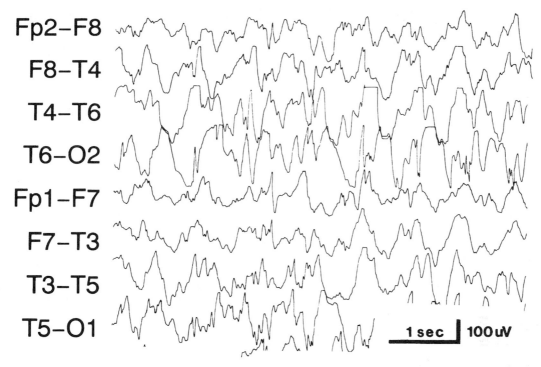

Fp2–F8

F8–T4

T4–T6

T6–O2

Fp1–F7

F7–T3

T3–T5

T5–O1

1 sec | 100 uV

FIG. 13.5. Hypsarrhythmia in a 6-month-old girl with infantile spasms. The record is characterized by mountainous slow waves, multifocal spikes, and sharp waves. (Fp2–F8, right frontopolar-frontal; F8–T4, right frontotemporal; T4–T6, right temporal; T6–O2, right temporal-occipital; Fp1–F7, left frontopolar-frontal; F7–T3, left frontotemporal; T3–T5, left temporal; T5–O1, left temporal-occipital.)

areas, multifocal spike discharges, and an atypical spike-wave pattern.

Attacks are often associated with a discharge of multiple spike-wave or polyspikes. Sudden suppression of electric activity begins with an attack and persists briefly after its completion.

Although infantile spasms are considered as a generalized epilepsy, the neuroanatomic substrates responsible for them are poorly understood. A marked decrease in REM sleep has led to the proposal that the basic abnormality is at the pontile level in proximity to centers regulating sleep cycles (220). This hypothesis is supported by the finding on interictal PET scan of hypermetabolism of the brainstem. Additionally, hypermetabolism of the lenticular nucleus occurs, which suggested to Chugani and coworkers a neuronal circuitry involving cortex, lenticular nucleus, and brainstem in the generation of infantile spasms (221).

Infantile spasms are classified as cryptogenic or symptomatic. Cryptogenic spasms, a minority of the cases of infantile spasms [less than 15% in the series of Riikonen (222)], occur in infants with normal birth and development until the onset of seizures, in whom no obvious cause for the convulsions can be demonstrated. A variety of prenatal and perinatal insults are responsible for the majority of cases in the symptomatic group. Abnormalities of gestation, manifested by a history of maternal infection and prematurity, are particularly common. Perinatal asphyxia or traumatic birth injuries are seen less often. Neonatal seizures are a common precursor, and symptomatic neonatal hypoglycemia is encountered in some 18% of infants (222). In the remainder of the infants, tuberous sclerosis is the major etiologic factor, with intracerebral calcifications detectable by CT scanning in up to 25%. Infantile spasms also are seen in neurofibromatosis, agenesis of the corpus callosum, and metabolic diseases such as phenylketonuria maple syrup urine disease and pyridoxine dependency (222a). In a small group of infants, spasms begin shortly after pertussis immunization with the whole cell vaccine. Whether this association is fortuitous, as suggested by Bellman and coworkers (223), or whether pertussis vaccine indeed represents a rare cause for infantile spasms has not been resolved.

As might be expected, a variety of neuropathologic findings have been reported. These include structural malformations of cortical gray matter. The most commonly observed abnormality observed in surgically resected specimens is a hamartomatous proliferation of multipotential neuroectodermal cells (224). Other alterations include focal cortical dysplasia, ulegyria, lissencephaly, unilateral megalencephaly, and pachygyria (225). Focal areas of cortical microdysgenesis are encountered commonly. These are not readily detectable by magnetic resonance imaging (MRI) during the first few months of life, but can be visualized indirectly in subsequent studies by a focal delay in maturation of subcortical white matter. This can only be visualized by repeated imaging studies (226). Cytomegalovirus infection (227) and spongy degeneration of gray and white matter are less common (228). In most children, the outlook for normal intellectual development is poor, even though in approximately 50%, infantile spasms have ceased by 3 years of age or are replaced by the Lennox-Gastaut syndrome or by major motor attacks (229). According to Jeavons and Bower, none of the patients whose development was already retarded when infantile spasms began had a subsequent normal intellectual development, whereas 29% of infants believed to have developed normally up to the onset of seizures were found to be neurologically intact and intellectually in the normal or low-normal range when their infantile spasms disappeared (218). More recent series, such as those of Riikonen (222) and Gaily and coworkers (229a), present comparable results. The latter workers observed 67% of infants with cryptogenic infantile spasms to have normal intelligence when tested between the ages of 4 and 6 years. Specific cognitive deficits were found in 42% of children in this group. Riikonen found that in children whose infantile spasms are attributed to tuberose sclerosis, the long-term prognosis is worse than in other symptomatic or cryptogenic cases of infantile spasms (230). By contrast, the prognosis is relatively good when infantile spasms accompany neurofibromatosis (231).

It is not clear whether in the idiopathic cases early adrenocorticotropic hormone (ACTH) therapy affects mental development. Lerman and Kivity suggest that optimal results are obtained when treatment is initiated within a month after the onset of seizures and when high doses are given for a prolonged period (232). In the experience of these workers, complete recovery (i.e., neither seizures nor mental retardation) was seen in some 60% of children who had early therapy. The more recent series of Glaze and coworkers does not have a sufficient number of cryptogenic cases to determine the benefit of early therapy. Certainly, early ACTH therapy does not alter the uniformly poor outcome of symptomatic infantile spasms (233). In this respect, it is of interest that the relapse after ACTH treatment is much higher in patients with tuberose sclerosis than in other forms of symptomatic infantile spasms (230). Even when treatment does not improve mental functioning, it can have a beneficial effect on seizure control and on the EEG in over one-half of the cases.

Many regimens for ACTH treatment have been proposed. As a rule, at higher ACTH doses a greater proportion of remissions occurs, but also a higher incidence of major adverse reactions. One convenient treatment schedule follows: ACTH is given intramuscularly in a daily dose of 80 to 120 U. This dose is maintained until spasms and the hypsarrhythmia disappear. If a response is noted, the dose is changed to 40 to 80 U every other day, and then gradually reduced to half that dose. This is maintained for approximately 3 more months. Thereafter, the dosage is reduced further by 10 U at 2-month intervals until the drug is completely withdrawn or the minimal dosage for seizure control is reached. One of us (JHM) has recommended a starting dose of 40 U, which is increased at weekly increments to 60 U and 80 U if there has not been any response. A prospective study has indicated that there is no difference in the effectiveness of high-dose and low-dose regimens with respect to seizure control and normalization of the EEG (234). Whether this is also true in terms of ultimate cognitive abilities is not known. Side reactions to ACTH include hypertension, which can become apparent at a dosage of 80 U/day, gastroenteritis, sepsis, osteoporosis, and unexplained CNS hemorrhage. The incidence of these complications varies considerably and probably reflects the different treatment schedules. In some series, it can be as high as 37% (235), whereas others have not shown any serious morbidity (236). One interesting concomitant to ACTH therapy is an enlargement of the cerebral ventricular system, which is disclosed by serial neuroimaging studies. This enlargement, which is occasionally permanent, is believed to reflect loss of water, owing to altered CSF absorption (237).

The mechanism by which ACTH controls infantile spasms is a matter of some debate. Baram and colleagues have shown that in infantile spasms CSF levels of ACTH and cortisol are reduced and have postulated that there is an increased synthesis of corticotropin-releasing hormone (CRH), which in infant rats has been shown to induce seizures originating from the amygdala. They suggest that ACTH desensitizes the CRH receptors and thus induces a negative feedback on CRH release (238). ACTH could also modulate second messenger systems or increase the expression of several genes and thus accelerate myelination, in this manner shortening a vulnerable, hyperexcitable period (239). In that respect, it is significant that several studies, as well as our own experience, indicate that ACTH is a potent anticonvulsant for Lennox-Gastaut syndrome (236,240).

In a prospective, randomized study, high-dose ACTH (150 U/m^2 per day) was more effective than prednisone by both clinical and EEG criteria (241). Prats and coworkers have suggested treating infantile spasms with extremely high doses of sodium valproate (100 to 300 mg/kg per day). According to their protocol, the anticonvulsant is given for 21 days or until the EEG resolves. Then the medication is reduced to 25 to 50 mg/kg per day (242). Although their results require confirmation, the outcome of children treated with valproate appears to be as good or better than those treated with ACTH both in terms of seizure control and normal intellectual development.

Chiron and coworkers have used vigabatrin with considerable success in the treatment of infantile spasms associated with tuberose sclerosis (243). In a retrospective study, vigabatrin was found to be as effective as ACTH in controlling seizures and offering a good developmental outcome. Side effects were less frequent in vigabatrin-treated children than in those who received ACTH (244). Appleton recommends starting at 25 to 50 mg/kg per day and increasing the dosage to a maximum of 80 to 120 mg/kg per day. In their group of children, making up 81% of symptomatic infantile spasms, 81% experienced total cessation of spasms. On follow-up 2 years later, 67% had remained seizure free (245). Currently, vigabatrin has become the first-line drug for the treatment of infantile spasms, particularly when these occur in a setting of tuberose sclerosis (246,246a).

As ominous as infantile spasms are in terms of ultimate mental development, Lombroso and Fejerman were able to distinguish a benign form (247). In this condition, myoclonic attacks are accompanied by normal intellectual development and a normal EEG, in contrast to infantile spasms in which the EEG is abnormal at the onset of seizures or becomes abnormal within a few months, as is the case in young infants. In the benign form of the condition, myoclonus ceases before 2 years of age, and no other seizures supervene.

Attacks characterized by shuddering and resembling myoclonic seizures can occur in monosodium glutamate poisoning and also can be noted as a prelude to familial (essential) tremor (see Chapter 2).

A syndrome of infantile spasms, mental retardation, chorioretinitis, colobomas of the retina, and agenesis of the corpus callosum limited to female subjects was first described by Aicardi and coworkers (Aicardi syndrome) (see Chapter 4) (248–250).

Juvenile Absence Epilepsy

Typical absence epilepsy should be distinguished from juvenile absence epilepsy. This is a genetically heterogeneous condition, transmitted as a dominant trait. Several genes have been implicated in this condition. One of the candidate genes encoding the GABA receptor (*GABABR1*) has been mapped to chromosome 6p21.3, close to the location of the gene for some patients with juvenile absence epilepsy (251).

Juvenile absence epilepsy has a prevalence of 0.5 to 1.0 per 1,000 and represents some 4% of the primary generalized epilepsies (154).

Symptoms usually become apparent in adolescence, with age of onset between 12 and 18 years (154). Seizures are characterized by sudden myoclonic jerks of shoulders and arms that usually appear shortly after awakening. A large majority of patients also experience grand mal attacks. As a rule, myoclonic jerks precede grand mal seizures. Up to one-third of patients also experience absence attacks, which tend to precede the onset of myoclonic jerks (154). Intelligence remains normal. The interictal EEG is characteristic, in that it demonstrates 4- to 6-Hz polyspike and wave complexes, with photosensitivity in approximately 30% (252). Valproic acid is effective in up to 90% of subjects, but has to be continued for the remainder of the patient's life, because withdrawal of anticonvulsants results in seizure recurrence in some 90% of patients, even after many years of complete control (250,253).

Miscellaneous Seizure Forms

A number of epileptic conditions are manifested by unusual seizure forms. These are seen too rarely to warrant more than a brief description. The following types deserve mention.

Abdominal Seizures

Paroxysmal attacks of abdominal pain can occur as an aura for a major motor attack or can be the only manifestation of a seizure. The abdominal pain is usually periumbilical, radiating to the epigastrium. In the majority of cases it lasts 5 to 10 minutes, but it can persist for 24 to 36 hours. It is usually associated with disturbed awareness (254).

The pediatrician often sees a child who has recurrent bouts of paroxysmal abdominal pain accompanied by vomiting and in whom the usual gastrointestinal evaluation result has been normal. Only a small proportion of these children has abdominal epilepsy. A more common cause of this complaint is childhood migraine. A history of pain and vomiting is common in small children who subsequently develop the usual clinical picture of migraine. The diagnosis of abdominal epilepsy rests on the presence of other epileptic manifestations, usually complex partial seizures, an abnormal EEG pattern during or between attacks, and, less convincingly, a favorable response to anticonvulsants, usually carbamazepine, valproate, or phenytoin (255).

Epilepsia Partialis Continua

Epilepsia partialis continua, a variant of a simple partial (focal) seizure, is characterized by clonic movements, usually localized to the face or upper extremities, that persist over long periods either continuously or with only brief interruptions. Consciousness is not impaired, but postictal weakness is usually evident. We have seen several children with this condition who had an underlying chronic encephalitis of the kind described by Aguilar and Rasmussen (34) and Rasmussen and McCann (256). Rasmussen syndrome was the most common cause for epilepsia partialis continua in the series of Thomas and coworkers (257). This condition, and its relationship to immune disorders and a variety of infectious agents, and its treatment is considered in Chapter 6. Various space-occupying lesions, including tumor, abscess, and cerebral cysticercosis, are less frequent causes for epilepsia partialis continua. Epilepsia partialis continua also has been encountered in various metabolic disorders, notably nonketotic hyperglycinemia (see Chapter 1).

Nonconvulsive Status Epilepticus Absence Status (Generalized Nonconvulsive Status Epilepticus, Petit Mal Status)

Two types of nonconvulsive status epilepticus have been recognized: a generalized form, also termed *absence status* or *petit mal status*, and a partial type, termed *complex partial status epilepticus* (258).

Absence status is the more common form of nonconvulsive status epilepticus. It is characterized by a prolonged state of clouded mental

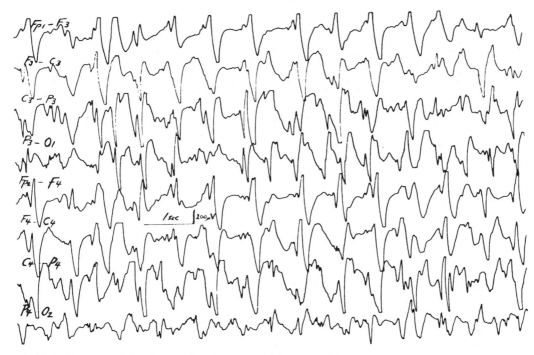

FIG. 13.6. Absence status (generalized nonconvulsive status) in a 26-month-old girl with mild retardation and 14-day history of drowsiness. Note the enormously high voltage of the spike and sharp waves. (C, central; F, frontal; O, occipital; P, parietal.) (Marker indicates 200 μV.) (Courtesy of Dr. E. Niedermeyer, Johns Hopkins Hospital, Baltimore, MD.)

activity usually accompanied by an EEG picture of atypical, slow spike-wave complexes and polyspike discharges. Untreated, the condition can last from several hours to 2 years (259). Absence status almost always occurs in children with preexisting organic cerebral lesions, a history of intellectual retardation, and a variety of other seizure forms (Fig. 13.6) (260). Approximately one-fourth of children with Lennox-Gastaut syndrome enter absence status one or more times during their lifetime (214).

Farran and coworkers have suggested that absence status is seen in patients with cerebellar anomalies and a consequent defect in the inhibitory system mediated by the Purkinje cells (261). The PET scan obtained during an attack fails to confirm this supposition in that it demonstrates only diffuse hypometabolism of fluorodeoxyglucose (262).

Complex partial status epilepticus is characterized by altered mentation, with impaired or absent language function, and a variable degree of responsiveness. The EEG during an attack shows various abnormalities, ranging from focal temporal spike and wave discharges to rhythmic slowing.

Benzodiazepines (lorazepam or diazepam) or valproate are the best drugs for treatment of both forms of nonconvulsive status, followed by institution or resumption of long-term anticonvulsant therapy (262a).

Landau-Kleffner Syndrome

Landau-Kleffner syndrome, which has attracted considerable attention in recent years, is marked by an acquired aphasia in children who have had normal language and motor development (263). Symptoms develop between 4 and 7 years of age. A variety of seizures accompany this condition in approximately 80% of cases. They can be rare and can disappear completely before adolescence. The EEG abnormalities are diagnostic. They include bilateral independent tem-

TABLE 13.7. *Unusual seizure forms*

Seizure type	Characteristics	Reference
Gelastic	Paroxysmal laughter associated with transitory loss of consciousness	Gascon and Lombroso (838)
Reflex	Seizures evoked by a number of specific sensory stimuli:	
	Light	Jeavons and Harding (839)
	Language	Geschwind and Sherwin (840)
	Sound	Forster (271)
	Music	Critchley (841)
	Somatosensory stimulus (e.g., tapping, brushing teeth)	Forster (271), Calderon-Gonzalez et al. (842)
	Decision making (e.g., chess)	Ingvar and Nyman (843)
	Reading	Critchley (844)
Running	Episodic alteration of awareness associated with running; running may occur in an ictal twilight state, postictally, as a preconvulsive phenomenon, and possibly as an attack of paroxysmal compulsive behavior	Strauss (845)

poral or temporoparietal spikes, or spike and wave discharges, and in a large proportion of children, a continuous spike and wave discharge during as much as 90% of the sleeping state (264). Neuroimaging study results are normal. The aphasia frequently fluctuates in severity, but as a rule, the earlier the onset of symptoms, the worse the prognosis in terms of language function (265). Other aspects of higher cortical function are preserved. Although in the initial report the condition was seen in two brothers, the etiology remains totally unknown.

Valproate, ethosuximide, and the benzodiazepines can improve the condition; phenobarbital and carbamazepine are generally ineffective. ACTH or corticosteroids also can be partially effective (266). Other therapeutic approaches include the use of intravenous immunoglobulins, which can be effective in some patients (267), and multiple subpial transections (268). As a rule, the EEG abnormalities regress with time, leaving the child with a severe receptive and expressive aphasia.

Landau-Kleffner syndrome has much in common with a condition in which subclinical electrical status epilepticus occurs during slow-wave sleep (ESES) (269,270). In the former, there is an isolated disturbance of language function, whereas in the latter, other cognitive functions are also affected. The clinical course and response to anticonvulsants is similar for the two conditions, and many workers consider ESES to be a variant of the Landau-Kleffner syndrome or to represent a clinical continuum (264,270).

Other Seizures

Rarer seizure forms are summarized in Table 13.7. The most likely of these to be encountered are the reflex seizures. This term denotes seizures that are repeatedly initiated by clearly defined stimuli. Reflex epilepsies account for some 5% of all epilepsies, with visually induced reflex (photogenic) epilepsy being the most common form, constituting 53% of Forster's series (271). Visual reflex epilepsy includes television epilepsy and video game epilepsy, and most cases of epilepsy in which the child induces his or her own seizures by looking at a light source and rapidly moving the hand back and forth in front of the eyes "fanning" (272,273). Other patients, not included in the group of reflex epileptic patients, can have both photogenic and nonphotogenic seizures or, even more commonly, can show only a photoconvulsive response on the EEG (274).

The mechanism for reflex seizures is unclear. The most attractive theory is that the attacks are caused by hyperexcitability of the sensory cortex, perhaps combined with a lack of cortical inhibition for a certain type of afferent input.

Treatment consists of avoiding the specific stimulus that induces seizures and administering anticonvulsants, preferably valproate or clonazepam. It is of note that the frequency of the TV or video game screen is important in provoking a seizure, with a 100-Hz screen being significantly safer than a 50-Hz screen. In addition, the distance of the child from the screen is also important, in that 1 m is safer than 50 cm (273).

Diagnosis

The diagnostic process in a child with epileptic seizures has two phases: the ascertainment of the type of seizure and its focus, if any, and an attempt to understand the cause for the attacks.

A thorough history, taken not only from the parent but also from the child, is crucial for arriving at a diagnosis. Usually, the physician is not able to witness an attack, and hospitalizing the child in the hope of recording a seizure is financially prohibitive, although in some instances it ultimately may be necessary.

Differential Diagnosis

The diagnosis of a generalized tonic-clonic seizure is usually made without much difficulty, although psychogenic seizures (hysteric seizures) also should be kept in mind despite their current relative rarity (275). The best discussion of the differential diagnosis between the two conditions is by Gowers, who emphasized the following points (24):

1. In the hysteric convulsion, the aura is absent or consists of palpitation, malaise, or a choking sensation.
2. During a hysteric attack, consciousness is impaired rather than lost.
3. The movements accompanying a hysteric seizure are somewhat coordinated, but lack the definite sequence of a true tonic-clonic seizure. Tonic spasms are long and severe, often associated with opisthotonus or brief and irregular clonic movements.
4. Micturition and tongue biting are rarely seen in a hysteric attack.

5. The hysteric attack terminates suddenly, and the patient often resumes his or her former activities.

To these criteria, distinguishing hysteric seizures, proposed more than 100 years ago, can now be added the absence of abnormalities on EEG or video-telemetry EEG recordings during a hysteric attack (275,276).

Childhood hysteria can be encountered as early as 6 years of age. Although it is still more common in girls, in children younger than 10 years of age, the sexes are affected equally (277).

Lazare has listed several psychological criteria for the diagnosis of a conversion symptom, such as a hysterical seizure (278):

1. A disorder of somatization (i.e., long-standing psychosomatic symptoms affecting several organ systems)
2. An associated psychopathology (e.g., depression, personality disorder, schizophrenia)
3. A model for the symptom, based on the patient's own previous illness, or on that of an important figure in the patient's life

Less important criteria for the diagnosis of a conversion reaction are emotional stress before the onset of symptoms, a disturbed sexuality (i.e., a history of seduction or incest), and the patient's being the youngest child. These considerations do not always allow a definite diagnosis, and it is important to remember that casual evaluation can lead to an erroneous diagnosis.

Grand mal attacks also should be differentiated from syncope. Syncope is rare in childhood, being more common in adolescence, particularly in girls. The attacks usually occur in the upright position and are preceded by fatigue or emotional stress. Syncopal attacks are occasionally terminated by a brief generalized tonic or tonic-clonic convulsion, probably the result of cerebral anoxia. An EEG recording during a syncopal attack, if available, shows diffuse electric slowing rather than seizure activity (279).

Another condition requiring differentiation from grand mal attacks is breath-holding. Breath-holding spells are limited to children younger than age 6 years. They are precipitated by crying in response to emotional upsets. The attack is

TABLE 13.8. *Episodic disorders*
that mimic seizures

Benign neonatal sleep myoclonus (282,830)
Normal but excessive motor activity during active
   (rapid eye movement) sleep in infants
Jitteriness of newborns (including drug withdrawal in
   maternal addiction)
Breath-holding spells (802)
Gastroesophageal reflux (Sandifer syndrome) (846)
Sleep disorders, including pavor nocturnus, sleep
   mycoclonus, and narcolepsy
Familial essential myoclonus (209)
Familial paroxysmal hypnogenic dystonia
Familial paroxysmal dyskinesias
Abnormal startle reaction (hyperekplexia)
Infantile shuddering attacks (see Chapter 2)
Nocturnal paroxysmal dystonia (848)
Transient paroxysmal dystonia of infancy (847)
Migraine and syncope
Habit spasms, tics, Gilles de la Tourette syndrome
Pseudoseizures
Benign paroxysmal vertigo of childhood (see Chapter 6)

From Tharp BR. An overview of pediatric seizure disorders and epileptic syndromes. *Epilepsia* 1987;28[Suppl 1]:S36. With permission.

usually brief and accompanied by intense cyanosis or pallor. The child can be limp or opisthotonic. A short clonic convulsion induced by cerebral anoxia can terminate the spell.

Tharp has listed a variety of other disorders that mimic seizures (Table 13.8) (280).

A few comments with respect to some of the more commonly encountered diagnostic problems follow.

The differentiation between a prolonged absence seizure with motor accompaniments and a brief complex partial seizure should take the following items into account: that a complex partial seizure lasts longer and includes a greater variety of movements; that absence attacks do not have an aura, occur far more frequently than psychomotor seizure, and can often be elicited by hyperventilation; that the patient with a complex partial seizure has partial clouding of consciousness for a brief period after the seizure has ended; and that the interictal EEG abnormalities in absence epilepsy are generally diagnostic.

Pavor nocturnus (night terror) should be distinguished from nocturnal complex partial seizures or major motor seizures. Pavor nocturnus is a paroxysmal sleep disturbance occurring during arousal from slow-wave sleep. The child appears agitated or leaves bed crying and in apparent ter-

ror. Heart rate and respiratory rate are increased. The episode is brief, often lasting less than a minute, and the child returns to sleep. Generally, efforts to rouse the child fail, and the child has no recollection of the attack. The EEG during pavor nocturnus is normal (281), and children generally outgrow this condition.

Myoclonic seizures of the body or extremities commonly occur when a child drops off to sleep and can be unusually violent in a few families. The syndrome of severe nocturnal myoclonus, although benign and not amenable to drug therapy, must be differentiated from a true nocturnal epileptic seizure (282).

Tics are usually distinguished from myoclonic seizures because the patient is able to control tics voluntarily, they consist of the same movement each time, and they occur in patients who manifest other evidence of psychological disturbance and are aggravated by emotional strain.

Spasmus nutans (see Chapter 7) is often confused with epileptic seizures, particularly salaam seizures. Unlike in salaam seizures, children with spasmus nutans do not lose consciousness during an attack, and intellectual development remains normal. Vertical or horizontal nystagmus affecting one or both eyes is a common feature of spasmus nutans. Head thrusts and blinking observed in congenital ocular motor apraxia have been mistaken for the seizure manifestations of Lennox-Gastaut syndrome (283).

Patient History

Because the diagnosis of a seizure disorder relies to a great extent on the history furnished to the physician, an intentionally falsified history leads to the erroneous diagnosis of epilepsy. Over the last few years, we have seen an increasing number of children with Munchausen disease by proxy who have been brought in with a history of a seizure disorder or recurrent apnea (284). *Fictitious epilepsy*, the term used by Meadow, is a not at all rare form of child abuse and can lead to years of unwarranted invalidism (285). Its diagnosis is difficult but should be considered when, in addition to epilepsy, the youngster suffers from other disorders equally difficult to document. These include diarrhea and food allergies, hematuria and hematemesis, and

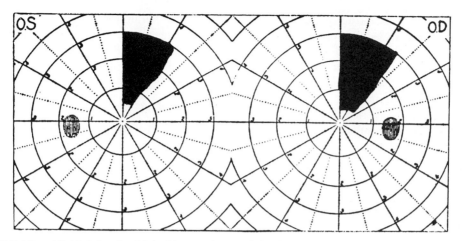

FIG. 13.7. Visual field defect in child with complex partial seizures and temporal lobe tumor. The child has a superior quadrantal hemianopia with sparing of the macula. (OD, right eye; OS, left eye.) (Courtesy of Dr. R. Hepler, Department of Ophthalmology, University of California, Los Angeles, UCLA School of Medicine.)

apneic episodes. Additionally, the patient often has an inexplicable mixture of overdosing and undertreatment, as verified by blood anticonvulsant levels. When fictitious epilepsy is suspected, verification of the history from individuals outside the family (e.g., teachers) and observation in the hospital are indicated.

Physical Examination

The physical examination in a patient with a seizure disorder can be abnormal when the patient has underlying cerebral pathology (Fig. 13.7). A small fraction of children with long-standing seizure disorders unaccompanied by neurologic abnormalities harbor a cerebral tumor. Although imaging studies, especially MRI, disclose the neoplasm, it is impractical and far too costly to subject every child who has experienced a seizure to imaging studies. What makes the diagnosis even more difficult is the fact that in most of the children with an underlying tumor, neither the type of seizure nor the initial EEG suggests a focal disorder; even a CT scan performed as part of an initial evaluation can be normal. Page and associates compiled the clinical features that they consider indicative of a cerebral tumor in children with a seizure disorder (Table 13.9) (286). The physician must keep in mind that the physical examination also can be abnormal when the patient is examined shortly after a seizure, and when cerebral dysfunction results from recurrent seizures or is the consequence of anticonvulsant medication.

TABLE 13.9. *Warning signs of cerebral neoplasms in 23 children with long-standing seizure disorder and brain tumor*

	Time before diagnosis of tumor	
Parameter	6–24 mo	Less than 6 mo
Deterioration of behavior and school performance	9	3
Slow wave focus on electroencephalography	8	11
Seizure pattern changed or increased in frequency	8	5
Abnormalities on plain skull film	3	9
Specific neurologic signs	1	13
Signs reflecting increased intracranial pressure	0	12

Modified from Page LK, Lombroso CT, Matson DD. Childhood epilepsy with late detection of cerebral glioma. *J Neurosurg* 1969;31:253.

Following a severe seizure, the patient can be confused and transient neurologic signs, including intention tremor, incoordination, weakness of one or more extremities, and pathologic exaggeration of reflexes, are common. When convulsions recur at brief intervals, these signs can persist for prolonged periods.

Cerebral damage can result from recurrent seizures. Usually this damage takes the form of intellectual deterioration and emotional disturbance. The incidence of these complications is treated in the section on Prognosis.

A number of anticonvulsants can induce neurologic abnormalities (Table 13.10).

Laboratory Tests

Laboratory studies are directed toward uncovering the cause of the seizures. Various diagnostic procedures are customarily performed on patients with seizures who lack a history or neurologic findings that point to a diagnosis.

Blood Chemistries

Serum glucose and calcium levels are obtained for all infants with seizures and for older children whose histories raise the possibility of a metabolic disturbance (see Chapter 15). In neonates, an evaluation of renal function is indicated also. Serum electrolyte disturbances are rare in patients with recurrent seizures. In children with seizures owing to hypernatremia, the history usually suggests a fluid imbalance.

Electroencephalography

The EEG can be useful in determining the type of seizure the patient experiences. It differentiates between absence and complex partial seizures, and between absence attacks and atypical petit mal. Occasionally, it can assist in establishing a diagnosis when the history is inadequate or not diagnostic. The EEG must be interpreted in conjunction with the patient's history. A normal EEG, seen in approximately one-half of epileptic patients, does not exclude the diagnosis of epilepsy, nor does an abnormal EEG necessarily establish it. King and colleagues have found that it is easier to differentiate between a primary generalized and a secondarily generalized seizure disorder if the initial EEG is performed within 24 hours of the seizure. They also recommend that should the initial EEG be normal, a second, sleep-deprived EEG should be performed (287).

Electric abnormalities can be seen during an overt attack as well as between seizures. Generalized tonic-clonic seizures arising from subcortical excitation can be recorded on the EEG, but the abnormalities are usually obscured by move-

TABLE 13.10. *Neurologic complications of commonly used antiepileptic drugs*

Drug	Most common neurologic complications
Phenobarbital	Hyperkinetic behavior, drowsiness
Methylphenobarbital	Hyperkinetic behavior, drowsiness
Primidone	Drowsiness, ataxia, dizziness, dysarthria, diplopia, nystagmus, personality changes
Phenytoin	Nystagmus on vertical and horizontal gaze, truncal ataxia, intention tremor, dysarthria, aggravation of seizures, permanent cerebellar degeneration, personality disturbances
Ethosuximide	Headache, dizziness, hiccups, personality disturbances
Diazepam	Drowsiness, ataxia, hallucinations, blurred vision, diplopia, headaches, slurred speech, tremors, extrapyramidal movements
Clonazepam	Ataxia, drowsiness, dysarthria, irritability, belligerence, and other behavior disturbances
Carbamazepine	Diplopia, disturbed coordination, drowsiness, headaches, visual hallucinations, peripheral neuritis or paresthesias, extrapyramidal movements
Valproic acid	Ataxia, tremor (dose-related), asterixis, drowsiness, or stupor (when given in conjunction with phenobarbital)
Vigabatrin	Dyskinesias, visual field defects
Topiramate	Dizziness, ataxia, somnolence, psychomotor slowing, impaired memory
Lamotrigine	Dizziness, ataxia, somnolence, diplopia, blurred vision
Gabapentin	Somnolence, dizziness, ataxia
Felbamate	Insomnia, somnolence, mononeuritis, choreoathetosis

ment artifacts. One exception is the major seizure with a focal cortical origin. In this condition, random focal spiking or spike-wave discharges that had already been seen during the interseizure period increase in frequency and amplitude and spread both contiguously and via subcortical centers. Generalization can occur within a fraction of a second after the onset of the focal seizure; less commonly, it develops slowly over as long as 20 seconds. Following the seizure, electric activity is depressed. Recovery starts with slow waves, normal cortical activity first appearing contralateral to the epileptic focus, then ipsilateral, and finally over the focus itself.

Less commonly, the ictal tracing is marked by suppression of electrical activity, or low-voltage fast activity, an indication of disinhibition.

The EEG during an absence attack shows bilateral high-voltage synchronous alternating spike-wave complexes, most commonly 3 Hz (see Fig. 13.3). As the discharge continues, the frequency of the spike-wave complexes tends to slow down.

In most patients with complex partial seizures, the EEG patterns accompanying the seizure are slow, rhythmic, and usually bilaterally synchronous, 4- to 6-Hz discharges, most prominent in the frontal and temporal areas, but becoming generalized as the seizure progresses. At the conclusion of the attack, the EEG is featureless, and recovery of normal activity is delayed for many minutes.

The interseizure record in patients with major motor attacks can be normal or can demonstrate a number of nonspecific abnormalities, including disorganization, spike discharges, loss of α-rhythm or loss of the highest expected frequency activity for the child's age, and, occasionally, continuous or intermittent focal slowing. This last finding, particularly when it is continuous, should always raise the possibility of an underlying tumor or other structural lesion and indicates the need for imaging studies.

In the patient with absence (petit mal) epilepsy, the interseizure EEG record is almost always abnormal, with isolated or grouped symmetric 3-Hz spike-wave discharges, often most prominent in the frontal leads. The discharge frequency can be increased by hyperventilation.

In complex partial seizures, the interseizure tracing is normal or shows nonspecific abnormalities or spike foci, which usually arise from the anterior portions of the temporal lobes (Fig. 13.8). Often, the seizure focus is apparent only during the transition between wakefulness and sleep, and a combined wake and sleep tracing should always be obtained from children suspected of having complex partial seizures. In approximately 80% of children with this condition, three serial wake and sleep recordings uncover an abnormality. In a number of patients, secondary spike foci can be recorded from the opposite temporal lobe. It is rare to find focal temporal spike discharges in children younger than 8 years of age, even in those with a classic clinical picture of complex partial seizures.

Atypical spike-wave discharges (i.e., spike-wave discharges at a frequency less than 2.5 Hz) and polyspike-wave discharges are common in children with Lennox-Gastaut syndrome. They indicate a poor prognosis in terms of seizure control and normal intellectual function. The high positive correlation between hypsarrhythmia and infantile spasms has already been discussed.

With EEG maturation, the EEG in patients with seizure disorders can undergo significant changes. Focal spike activity tends to migrate from the occipital to the midtemporal and ultimately to the anterior temporal leads (288). In patients with 3-Hz generalized spike-wave discharges, an improvement in clinical status can be associated with the disappearance of the abnormal EEG pattern, which is often replaced by a wandering spike focus (289). In patients with focal seizure discharges, mirror spike activity can appear. In some, this second focus is suppressed by anticonvulsants; in others, it becomes the only active focus (289).

For further information on the clinical aspects of EEG, the reader is referred to one of the several standard EEG texts.

Lumbar Puncture

Lumbar puncture is not performed routinely in patients with seizure disorders. Because a significant proportion of infants with bacterial or

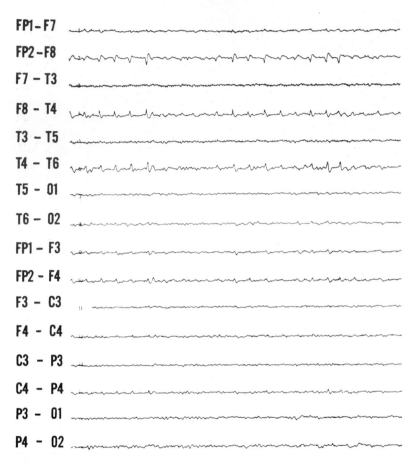

FIG. 13.8. Right anterior temporal spike discharge in patient with complex partial seizures. (C, central; F, frontal; FP, frontopolar; O, occipital; P, parietal; T, temporal.) (Courtesy of Dr. Gregory Walsh, Department of Neurology, University of California, Los Angeles, UCLA School of Medicine.)

tuberculous meningitis have a febrile seizure as their initial symptom (see Chapter 6), we believe a lumbar puncture is indicated in patients who have experienced their first febrile seizure and in all infants having their first seizure.

Although the CSF is by definition normal in the majority of patients with idiopathic epilepsy, minor abnormalities were found in the classic study of Lennox and Merritt (290). In 4% of their patients, pleocytosis was slight (5 to 10 cells/μL), and in 10%, protein content was increased (45 to 85 mg/dL). Both abnormalities were believed to be related to the presence of small areas of cerebral contusion that resulted from a fall attending

the seizure. They had disappeared when the spinal tap was repeated several weeks later. More recent studies are consistent with these observations (291,292). However, we suspect that abnormalities in cell count and protein level reflect the cerebral edema, disturbed autoregulation, and the breakdown of the blood–brain barrier that attend a prolonged seizure and that have been documented by MRI (293).

Imaging Studies

MRI, CT scans, and, to a lesser extent, PET scans are the procedures currently used in the evaluation of a child with a seizure disorder. These studies are particularly important when surgical treatment is contemplated. Skull radiography is no longer part of a seizure workup.

An imaging study is indicated for the child with recurrent seizures under several circumstances: in the presence of an abnormal neurologic examination, including dysmorphic features, or skin lesions suggestive of a phakomatosis (64%); in the presence of focal EEG abnormalities, particularly focal slowing (63%); with a history of neonatal seizures (100%); and with a history compatible with simple partial or complex partial seizures (52% and 30%, respectively). The numbers in parentheses represent percentage of positive CT scan results seen by Yang and coworkers in their series of seizure patients (294); the percentages of positive combined CT and MRI studies would undoubtedly be higher.

Whether imaging studies also are indicated for children who by history and examination do not fulfill these criteria is a matter of individual judgment. Children whose neurologic examination and EEG are normal have a low yield of positive scan results, as do children with primary generalized seizures [5% and 8%, respectively, in the series of Yang and coworkers (294)]. In confirmation of this experience, King and coworkers found no MRI abnormalities in any of their patients with EEG-confirmed primary generalized seizures (287).

Several studies have compared CT scans and MRI for their respective advantages and disadvantages in evaluating a seizure patient. Although the two procedures occasionally provide complementary information, MRI is the preferred initial screening procedure. Unlike CT scanning, MRI detects congenital malformations of the cortex, gray matter heterotopias, and a large proportion of arteriovenous malformations, some of which can be angiographically occult. MRI is also an excellent screening test for detecting neoplasms, particularly when it is used with gadolinium enhancement. On the other hand, CT scans are more sensitive for small foci of calcification.

The joint use of EEG and imaging studies has been applied most successfully in the evaluation of patients with focal seizure disorders. MRI is

effective in detecting underlying abnormalities in the cortical architecture of children with simple partial epilepsies (287,295) (Fig. 13.9). In young children with intractable partial epilepsies, malformations of the cortex are detectable on MRI. These abnormalities are most common in the central cortical area, particularly in the region of the operculum. The complexity of cortical gyration makes difficult the detection of subtle abnormalities, and when MRI is correlated with pathologic examination of brain tissue resected from epileptic seizure foci, only approximately one-half of the malformations were detected before surgery by MRI (296). MRI results are abnormal in most patients with severe mesial temporal sclerosis, and in a large proportion of subjects with pathologically proven mild to moderate sclerosis (297,298). These abnormalities are best demonstrated with T2-weighted images. Additionally, MRI can detect small epileptogenic lesions in the temporal lobe, notably hamartomas and low-grade gliomas (299,300).

Transient abnormalities at the site of an actively discharging epileptic focus can be visualized by MRI, particularly on T2-weighted images (301). These abnormalities can reflect hyperemia or can be caused by a shift of water from the extracellular compartment into dendrites or glia (302). Similar changes also can be visualized on CT scans. The abnormalities take from 1 to 48 hours to develop and can resolve within 1 week or as late as 12 weeks (303). Additionally, some drugs, notably digoxin and heparin, can increase the signal intensity on MRI (304).

In contrast to CT scanning and MRI, PET scanning provides three-dimensional functional images of the brain. Although in most centers PET scanning is still a research study, this procedure has become part of the diagnostic evaluation of a youngster with focal seizures or with intractable generalized seizures, and assists in the surgical treatment of intractable epilepsies. Fluorodeoxyglucose, which measures glucose metabolism, is the most commonly used tracer. The interictal PET scan demonstrates focal areas of hypometabolism corresponding to the site of the epileptic focus as determined by EEG, and to focal changes on MRI (305) (Fig. 13.10). During a seizure, this area of hypometabolism becomes

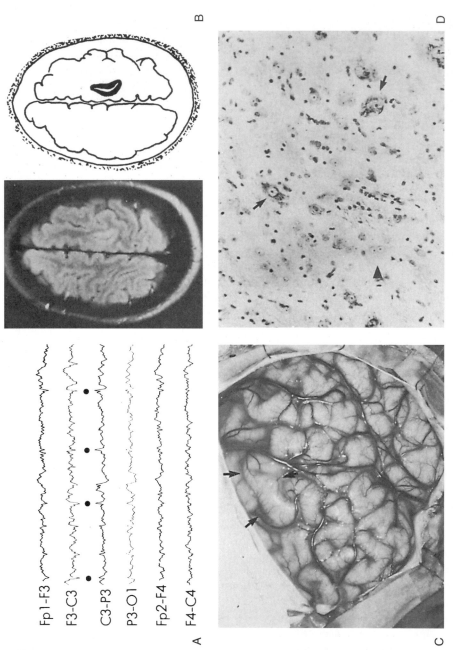

FIG. 13.9. An 18-year-old girl with onset at 6 years of age of focal myoclonus involving right arm and shoulder and right hemiparesis. **A:** Representative section of electroencephalogram showing frequent sharp waves with phase reversals over the left central region (C3). (C, central; F, frontal; O, occipital; P, parietal.) **B:** Magnetic resonance imaging showing left hemiatrophy and an area of slightly increased signal corresponding to the abnormal gyrus (see adjacent diagram). **C:** Left cerebral hemisphere at operation. Note enlarged gyrus (*black arrows*). **D:** Microscopic section at junction of cortex and white matter showing disruption of cortical lamination with abnormally large dysplastic neurons (*arrows*) and large astrocytes (*arrowhead*) (Luxol fast blue, ×130). (Courtesy of Drs. R. Kuzniecky and F. Andermann, Department of Neurology, McGill University, Montreal, Canada.)

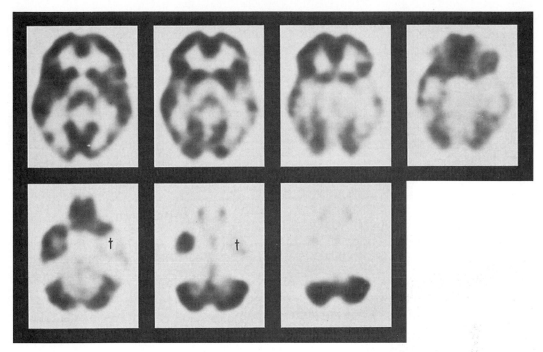

FIG. 13.10. Positron emission tomography using labeled fluorodeoxyglucose. Interictal scan in a patient with complex partial seizures since age 5 years. There is a zone of relative hypometabolism in the left temporal lobe (t). The electroencephalogram on this patient showed a left mesial temporal spike focus. Computed tomographic scans showed possible enlargement of the left temporal horn, but angiographic and pneumoencephalographic studies were normal. Pathologic examination following left temporal lobectomy revealed a mesial temporal lobe sclerosis. (From Engel J, Crandall PH, Rausch R. The partial epilepsies. In: Rosenberg RN, et al., eds. *The clinical neurosciences*, Vol. 2. *Neurology/neurosurgery*. New York: Churchill Livingstone, 1983. With permission.)

hypermetabolic. When the seizure is generalized, such as in children with absence attacks, hypermetabolism is generalized (306). Focal areas of hypometabolism have been found in children with infantile spasms and in the Lennox-Gastaut syndrome (262). The relative value of localizing a seizure focus by means of EEG, MRI, and PET has been a matter of some debate. Most centers, including ours, consider a PET to be more likely to detect a focal temporal abnormality than structural imaging studies, and we have seen a number of patients with PET abnormalities in whom MRI had been normal (307). The experiences of Won and colleagues with respect to the comparative ability of MRI, interictal PET, and ictal single photon emission CT (SPECT) show that PET was the best study to correctly localize the epileptic focus. SPECT and MRI were equally useful

(308). In our experience and that of Theodore and colleagues, the anatomic distribution of neuronal cell loss correlates poorly with the degree and the spatial extent of PET hypometabolism (309). The advantages and drawbacks of SPECT in the localization of epileptic foci are considered in the Introduction.

In the majority of instances, abnormal imaging studies do not influence treatment of the child with a seizure disorder. For the physician who must practice defensive medicine under the legal sword of Damocles, these logical guidelines are, however, of little help.

Cerebral Angiography

Cerebral angiography, requiring hospitalization, is hardly ever indicated, except to determine the vascular anatomy as part of the preoperative evaluation before removal of a seizure focus.

Magnetoencephalography

In contrast to EEG, which records the electrical potentials, magnetoencephalography records the magnetic fields generated by the brain. Although these fields are extremely small, the magnetic fields generated by epileptiform discharges can be localized three-dimensionally, particularly when the focus is in the more superficial areas of the cortex. At this time, the procedure is primarily a research tool and does not yet offer any significant advantages over other diagnostic studies (310,311).

Telemetry and Other Tests to Determine Focal or Generalized Cerebral Dysfunction

A number of tests can be used to localize an epileptogenic focus in patients whose seizures have remained intractable with standard medical therapy or in whom the epileptic nature of recurrent episodes has not been clarified. Several techniques have been used for long-term EEG monitoring. The most commonly employed is a combined EEG telemetry and video monitoring (312). For this procedure, the child is admitted to the hospital and is continuously monitored until enough ictal events have been recorded to determine the epileptic nature of the attacks, the epileptic seizure type, and the site of onset. Because the monitoring system is portable, the child is free to move around the ward and can engage in usual ward activities (313). Prolonged (8- to 10-hour) EEG recordings in the laboratory are somewhat simpler, but require considerable cooperation by the patient. An ambulatory cassette recorder allows the child to remain at home or attend school, while the parent or teacher keeps a log of the activities. We have found the ambulatory technique useful to determine whether or not recurrent episodes are epileptic but of lesser value in the localization of the seizure focus.

Sphenoidal electrodes have been used to localize epileptic discharges generated by mesial temporal sclerosis in patients with complex partial seizures. Although electrodes are fairly easily placed in the cooperative adult, their use in children requires analgesia and sedation. Once in place, the electrodes are generally well tolerated. Other procedures used to localize an epileptic discharge and select patients for surgical ablation include thiopental activation intended to evoke focal attenuation of barbiturate-induced fast activity (314), the use of methohexital to distinguish between primary and secondary epileptic foci (315), and the pharmacologic ablation of a hemisphere with intracarotid amobarbital.

The activation of focal epileptiform discharges with pentylenetetrazol is no longer done in most institutions.

Metabolic Screening Studies and Cytogenetics

Metabolic screening studies and cytogenetics are performed when seizures are coupled with mental retardation of indiscernible cause or are associated with periods of prolonged impairment of consciousness. Generally, screening of plasma amino acids and other metabolites is combined with determination of urine organic acids, blood ammonia levels, and blood and CSF lactate and pyruvate levels. Several cytogenetic abnormalities are coupled with a seizure disorder. These are reviewed in Chapter 3.

Treatment

Clinical Aspects of Treatment

The objective in the treatment of the epileptic patient is complete control of seizures, or at least a reduction in their frequency to the point at which they no longer interfere with physical and social well-being. Two aspects of therapy are discussed: who to treat and how to treat.

Candidates

Although all authorities agree that all patients with recurrent seizures should be treated as soon as the diagnosis is established, considerable controversy surrounds the optimal method of dealing with certain groups of patients.

Febrile Seizures

The treatment of febrile seizures is discussed in the section on Specific Seizure Types.

Isolated Tonic-Clonic (Grand Mal) Seizure

We believe that treatment of this type of seizure is optional and depends on the risk for recurrence and a variety of social factors, notably patient and family anxiety, and compliance.

Several studies have attempted to assess the recurrence risk after a first seizure. Generally, the risk is a function of the type of seizure and the time interval between the first seizure and the patient's visit to the doctor. Recurrence rates for a generalized tonic-clonic seizure have ranged from 24% to 71%. Hauser and associates reported a recurrence risk of 24% for idiopathic, mainly generalized tonic-clonic seizures. Patients who had experienced two or more seizures by the time they were first diagnosed were excluded from the study (316). When patients are seen within 1 day of their first tonic-clonic seizure, the recurrence risk is much greater. In the experience of Elwes and coworkers, the cumulative probability of recurrence in untreated children and adults was 20% by 1 month, 32% by 3 months, 46% by 6 months, 62% by 1 year, and 71% by 3 to 4 years (317). These statistics are consistent with a recurrence risk of 84% obtained in a demographic survey in Kent, England (5). Recurrence is most likely in children with neurologic or developmental abnormalities, complex partial seizures, and a paroxysmal EEG (318,319). Recurrence was also more likely for children whose seizures were idiopathic, and for those who had a parent or sibling with nonfebrile seizures (316,320). A history of an antecedent febrile seizure or the age when the initial seizure was experienced does not affect the likelihood of recurrence (319,320).

In children, one-half of the observed recurrences were encountered during the first 6 months of follow-up (320). An overall incidence of 48.3% for recurrences of childhood generalized motor seizures was obtained in a prospective study of both treated and untreated subjects (320).

In view of these relatively optimistic experiences, and a 30% incidence of significant side reactions to anticonvulsant therapy, we are reluctant to treat the youngster who has suffered a first isolated idiopathic grand mal seizure and whose neurologic examination and EEG are normal, except on insistence of the family. Other authorities are of a similar opinion, but consensus suggests that if two or more tonic-clonic seizures occur in a period of less than 1 year, treatment is indicated.

Breath-Holding Spells

We have found antiepileptic drugs to be of no value in preventing recurrence of attacks. Our experience is shared by Stephenson who recommends a trial of atropine for breath-holding spells, and for resistant reflex anoxic seizures (321).

Syncopal Attacks

Anticonvulsant therapy is of little use in preventing either the attack or the clonic seizure that can terminate it.

One or More Episodes the Epileptic Nature of Which Cannot Be Established with Certainty

Three options are open for the management of one or more episodes the epileptic nature of which cannot be established with certainty. One can defer therapy until the clinical picture becomes clear. If the patient probably experienced a seizure equivalent, one can institute a clinical trial with carbamazepine, which is relatively more effective in seizure equivalents than most other anticonvulsants. If the episodes are sufficiently frequent, inpatient telemetry or outpatient ambulatory cassette EEG monitoring are invaluable (313,322).

Drugs

Principles

Once treatment has been decided on, several therapeutic principles should be kept in mind.

1. The selection of the preferred drug is based on the type of seizure and on the potential toxicity of the drug.
2. Treatment should begin with one drug, its dosage being increased until seizures are

TABLE 13.11. *Which anticonvulsants should be monitored?*

Drug	Therapeutic levels[a] μmol/L (μg/mL)	Value rating[b]	Comments
Phenytoin	40–80 (10–20)	*****	Monitoring essential for good therapy. Accurate dosing difficult without serum levels, because of saturable metabolism. Low therapeutic ratio, disguised toxicity and frequency of drug interactions add weight to the case of routine monitoring.
Carbamazepine	20–40 (5–10)	***	Monitoring useful. Clinical symptoms (especially eye symptoms) are often helpful in determining dose limit, but water intoxication and increase in fit frequency may be caused by high serum level. Standardization of sampling time advisable.
Ethosuximide	350–750 (50–100)	***	Monitoring in children is less acceptable, but can be helpful as a guide to correct dose.
Phenobarbital	70–180 (15–40)	**	Tolerance develops and therefore therapeutic range difficult to define.
Primidone (unchanged)		*	Phenobarbitone is major metabolite; therefore, this should be monitored if indicated. Occasional measurement of primidone useful in slow metabolizers.
Valproic acid	350–700 (50–100)	*	Timed specimens essential. Little evidence that management is improved by monitoring. Possibility of *hit and run* effect.
Clonazepam		*	Sedation is usually dose limiting; serum levels unhelpful because of development of receptor tolerance.

[a]Evidence for these ranges is, in some cases, inadequate.
[b]The greater the number of asterisks, the greater the value of monitoring.
From Richens A. *Textbook of epilepsy*, 4th ed. Edinburgh: Churchill, 1993. With permission.

controlled or the child develops toxicity. If the drug does not control seizures, it is discontinued gradually while a second drug is instituted and its dosage is increased.

This concept of monotherapy (i.e., the preferential use of a single anticonvulsant in the treatment of seizures) has gained considerable support from a number of clinical studies. These have documented various disadvantages of polytherapy (323,324). First, chronic toxicity is directly related to the number of drugs consumed by the child. Even though none of them may be present in toxic level, their effect, particularly on sensorium and intellectual performance, is cumulative. Second, drug interactions might not only enhance toxicity, but might lead to loss of seizure control. Third, polytherapy can aggravate seizures in a significant proportion of patients. Finally, polytherapy makes it difficult to identify the cause of an adverse reaction.

In the experience of Reynolds and Shorvon (323), the conversion of polyther-apy to monotherapy is associated with improved seizure control and intellectual performance. One of us (J.H.M.) had made comparable observations many years before (325). In approximately one-fourth of patients, a single anticonvulsant, however, does not control seizures, and two drugs are required.

3. Alterations in drug dosage should be made gradually, usually not more frequently than once every 5 to 7 days.

4. The chance of controlling epilepsy with a lesser known drug when first-line medications have failed is small. Conversely, the chances of inducing perplexing side reactions with a new or rarely used drug are great.

5. Once seizures are controlled, the medication should be continued for a long time.

6. The value of anticonvulsant blood levels is considerable for patients receiving phenobarbital, phenytoin, carbamazepine, and ethosuximide (Table 13.11). Plasma levels of these drugs should be monitored frequently, particularly in patients whose seizures are

not responding to therapy or who develop evidence of drug intoxication. Although some anticonvulsants show a good correlation between blood levels and efficacy as well as signs of intoxication, the relationship between drug dosage and blood levels is variable, particularly in the case of valproate, clonazepam, and phenytoin, and there is no correlation between valproate toxicity and serum levels (326). The correlation between dose and blood levels is highly variable for gabapentin because of a saturable transporter needed for absorption that results in decreased bioavailability with increasing dosage. Insufficient data exist to correlate drug levels with clinical efficacy for most of the newer antiepileptic drugs. Therapeutic blood levels for the more commonly employed anticonvulsants are listed in Table 13.11 (327–330). In their clinical interpretation, the physician should remember Kutt's statement that there are "as many therapeutic plasma levels as there are patients" (331). Whether drug levels should be determined routinely in seizure-free patients is a matter of some debate (332,333). Despite evidence that epileptic drug monitoring does not improve the overall degree of seizure control, we believe that the metabolic changes in a growing youngster who is receiving one of the readily monitored anticonvulsants dictate obtaining levels at regular intervals.

7. Routine hematologic and hepatic evaluations have been suggested on the assumption that the serious hematologic and hepatic abnormalities, which occasionally develop in patients receiving anticonvulsants, are preceded by an asymptomatic phase that can be detected by laboratory examinations. This is not the case, and we believe that there is little value in routine blood counts and liver function tests. Wyllie and Wyllie have pointed out that if every patient receiving anticonvulsants were to be monitored as suggested by the *Physicians' Desk Reference*, the annual costs of epileptic therapy would be astronomic (334).

8. Anticonvulsant medication should be withdrawn gradually. Sudden withdrawal of medication, particularly barbiturates, is one of the most common causes of status epilepticus.

Cellular Mechanisms and Animal Models

The history of modern pharmacologic treatment of the epilepsies can be said to start in the middle of the nineteenth century when bromides were tried with some success for the control of convulsions. This approach predates the treatises on epilepsy by John Hughlings Jackson (2,68) and William Gowers (24). Bromides were first used by Sir Charles Locock in treating eclamptic seizures and catamenial seizures.

Phenobarbital was adopted in 1912 after Hauptmann observed its ability to suppress seizures when he used it to sedate a ward of noisy psychiatric and epileptic patients during the night. Introduction of more specific anticonvulsants for clinical application followed the availability of the first animal seizure model, the maximal electroshock (MES) model (335). The history and principles of the development of anticonvulsants has been reviewed by one of us (R.S.) (336).

As newer antiepileptic drugs with a variety of different mechanisms of action become available, it becomes important to categorize these agents in a manner consistent with preclinical and clinical pharmacology. Preclinical pharmacology involves an understanding of the cellular mechanisms of action, usually at the level of membrane ion channels. This information is correlated with the expression of seizures in animal models. Finally, the action of antiepileptic drugs at cellular and experimental levels must be correlated with their action in the epileptic patient. The principal molecular actions of the major anticonvulsants are presented in Table 13.12.

It is beyond the scope of this text to detail the large number of animal models that have been developed to study the various types of epilepsy; these have been reviewed by Fisher (337). Two models important in the development of antiepileptic drugs are the MES model, which is highly predictive of antiepileptic drug activity against tonic-clonic seizures, and the pentylenetetrazol or metrazol (MET) model, which is useful in the development of compounds with activity against absence seizures. The proto-

TABLE 13.12. *Principal molecular actions of clinically important anticonvulsants*

	PHT CBZ	BZD	PB	ESM	VPA	AZM	FBM	GBP
Inhibits voltage-gated sodium channels	+				+		+	
Inhibits sodium currents through non-NMDA receptors								
Inhibits calcium currents through NMDA receptors							+	
Inhibits low-threshold T-type voltage-gated calcium channels				+	+?			
Enhances GABA$_A$-receptor mediated chloride currents		+	+				+	
Inhibits presynaptic GABA reuptake								
Increases brain GABA by inhibiting GABA transaminase					+			
Increases brain GABA through unknown mechanisms								+
Inhibits brain carbonic anhydrase activity						+		
Novel actions not yet clearly defined					+			+

AZM, acetazolamide; BZD, benzodiazepines; CBZ, carbamazepine; ESM, ethosuximide; FBM, felbamate; GABA, γ-aminobutyric acid; GBP, gabapentin; NMDA, *N*-methyl-D-aspartate; PB, phenobarbital; PHT, phenytoin; VPA, valproic acid.

typical compounds active in the MES model are phenytoin and carbamazepine. The compound in current use that typifies activity in the MET model is ethosuximide. In our discussion we categorize antiepileptic drugs according to their activity in the MES and MET animal models.

On a cellular level, the activity of antiepileptic drugs results from their action on cellular (neuronal) excitability, in particular, their effects on various ion channels, either directly or through a neurotransmitter system. These aspects are covered by Rho and Sankar in a current and comprehensive review (338).

Several antiepileptic drugs, classically phenytoin and carbamazepine, reduce sustained, high-frequency, repetitive firing (SRF) of cortical neurons in a use-dependent manner. This effect is attributable to the antagonism of Na$^+$ anductance in voltage-gated channels. Both phenytoin and carbamazepine are active in the MES model

and inactive in the MET animal model. They protect humans against tonic-clonic seizures, but can exacerbate absence seizures. Use-dependent blockade of voltage-dependent sodium channels is demonstrated also by valproic acid, felbamate, lamotrigine, and topiramate.

Trimethadione and ethosuximide possess the specific ability to block low-threshold T-type calcium currents exhibited by rhythmically firing thalamic neurons. This action of trimethadione and ethosuximide is attributed to their activity against MET-induced spike and wave epilepsy in animal models, and may explain their activity against absence epilepsy. The newer anticonvulsant zonisamide has activity against both voltage-gated sodium channels and T-calcium channels.

Barbiturates and benzodiazepines function by enhancing GABA-mediated chloride currents, and thus hyperpolarize the neuronal membrane.

They bind to different sites on the GABA-receptor, chloride ionophore complex, and enhance the action of GABA. Benzodiazepines increase the frequency of channel openings, whereas barbiturates enhance the duration of an individual channel opening. Both felbamate and topiramate have the ability to enhance GABA-mediated Cl^- currents. The kinetics of felbamate action resemble that of barbiturates (339), whereas the kinetics of topiramate-induced Cl^- channel openings resemble that of benzodiazepines (340). The activity of topiramate at this site is not antagonized by the benzodiazepine antagonist flumazenil, suggesting that this is a novel site on this receptor-ionophore complex. All such compounds tend to have some activity in both MES and MET models and tend to be active against a wide variety of human epilepsies.

Other ways exist to influence GABAergic activity than by direct binding to the GABA receptor. Tiagabine functions by antagonizing the reuptake of GABA, whereas vigabatrin, an investigational agent in the United States, functions by inhibiting GABA transaminase, the enzyme that inactivates GABA by converting it to succinic semialdehyde. The anticonvulsant effect of valproic acid is still unexplained and at therapeutic dosages its action on GABAergic systems is probably not significant.

Several new anticonvulsants that act on the excitatory amino acid receptors and their associated ion channels are being developed, but to date few have made it into clinical practice. Two antiepileptic drugs in current use have activity against excitatory amino acid sites. At least one mechanism of action of felbamate has been shown to involve a dose-dependent antagonism of ligand-gated calcium currents mediated by glutamate at the NMDA receptor (341). Topiramate, on the other hand, shows activity against Na^+ currents triggered by the binding of glutamate to non-NMDA receptors, such as the kainate- or AMPA-sensitive sites, in addition to its antagonism of voltage-gated Na^+ channels.

Underlining the limited knowledge of antiepileptic drug action is the fact that gabapentin, an antiepileptic drug, has activity in both MES and MET models, but does not function by any of the previously described mechanisms.

A more extensive review of antiepileptic drug action has been prepared by Rho and Sankar (338).

Selection of Anticonvulsant

Which drug to use to treat a patient with a seizure disorder depends on the type of seizure or epilepsy syndrome. Preferred drugs are presented in Table 13.13. Often the choice of drug depends not only on the seizure history of the patient, but also on the personal preference of the physician. We therefore have presented in this table the individual preferences of the two coauthors. At the time of the first visit of a patient with recurrent seizures, we have made it a practice to outline in the chart the proposed course of therapy and the drugs we intend to use in order of preference.

Phenobarbital. Phenobarbital is an effective anticonvulsant in the treatment of generalized tonic-clonic (grand mal) and simple partial (focal) seizures. The therapeutic dosage of phenobarbital varies from patient to patient. Therefore, we prefer to start at approximately 4 to 5 mg/kg per day, given in two divided doses. The drug is absorbed slowly from the gastrointestinal tract, and under clinical conditions (4 mg/kg body weight), 95% of the maximum serum level is reached in 2 to 3 weeks (see Table 13.11) (342). Svensmark and Buchthal have shown that in most patients with major motor seizures controlled by phenobarbital, the drug was effective at serum levels of 10 to 15 μg/mL. These levels were achieved by an oral dose of 2 to 3 mg/kg in children weighing 10 to 20 kg and approximately 2 mg/kg in larger children (343). Figure 13.11 shows the ratio of phenobarbital levels to dosage in several age groups and the effect exerted by the concurrent intake of valproate sodium (344). The maximum variation in serum concentration with one daily dose of phenobarbital is between 7% and 14%. Therefore, in most cases, two daily doses of the anticonvulsant suffice for seizure control.

Toxic levels of phenobarbital vary between individuals, but generally, no permanent sedation is seen with levels below 35 μg/mL. There is considerable variability in the extent of tolerance that develops with prolonged use of the drug. Of

TABLE 13.13. *Some drugs used in the control of epileptic disorders[a]*

Primary generalized tonic-clonic		Absence	Complex partial		Lennox-Gastaut		Simple partial		Infantile spasms
J.M.	*R.S.*	*J.M., R.S.*	*J.M.*	*R.S.*	*J.M.*	*R.S.*	*J.M.*	*R.S.*	*J.M., R.S.*
CBZ	VPA	ESM	CBZ	CBZ	VPA	TPM	CBZ	CBZ	VGB
VPA	TPM	VPA	VPA	GBP	LMT	VPA	VPA	GBP	ACTH
PB	LMT	LMT	PHY	TPM	TPM	LMT	TPM	VPA	B₆[b]
PHY	CBZ	AZM	PMD	VPA	FBM	FBM	PHY	TPM	NTZ
PMD	PB		PB	LMT	KGD	KGD[c]	PMD	LMT	VPA
TPM	PHY		VGB	PHY	ACTH		VGB	PHY	OZP
	PMD			PMD					
				TIA					

ACTH, adrenocorticotropic hormone; AZM, acetazolamide; B₆, pyridoxine; CBZ, carbamazepine; CZP, clonazepam; ESM, ethosuximide; FBM, felbamate, GBP, gabapentin; KGD, ketogenic diet; LMT, lamotrigine; NTZ, nitrazepam; PB, phenobarbital; PHY, phenytoin; PMD, primidone; TIA, tiagabine; TPM, topiramate; VGB, vigabatrin; VPA, valproic acid.

[a]In this table drugs have been arranged in order of personal preference of each of the two authors. Anticonvulsants that have been found less effective have not been listed. Careful evaluation of patients should be undertaken to identify those with a surgically remediable syndrome before embarking on exhaustive trials with more than two of the listed antiepileptic drugs.

[b]Even though pyridoxine deficiency and dependency are rare, there is a noteworthy fraction of infants who benefit from pyridoxine therapy.

[c]The ketogenic diet and vagus nerve stimulation are often worth trying in patients who are not candidates for resective surgery. They can be considered after the failure of more than two antiepileptic drugs and in subjects who are sensitive to the side effects of most antiepileptic drugs.

ingested phenobarbital, 30% is excreted unchanged in the urine; the rest is oxidized in the liver by para-hydroxylation to form para-hydroxyphenobarbital. In some instances, the administration of phenobarbital induces an elevation of transaminase activity. As confirmed by electron microscopy on liver biopsies, this elevation is the consequence of enzyme induction, rather than cellular damage (345).

The major side reactions encountered with phenobarbital are drowsiness and hyperactivity; however, the long-term effect of phenobarbital and the other anticonvulsants on intellectual performance is a matter of much debate. As documented by PET scanning, performed before and after withdrawal of therapeutic doses, phenobarbital produces a significant (37%) reduction in local glucose cerebral metabolism (346). Some authors have found that the drug induces a major depressive disorder (347), disturbances in sleep, fussiness, and impaired concentration, whereas others, confirming an initial impairment in cognitive functions, show that these side effects disappear after the first year of therapy (348,349). Whereas Thompson and Trimble showed that

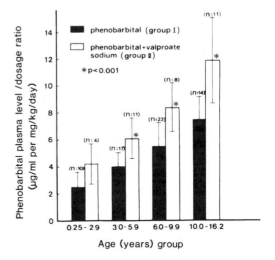

FIG. 13.11. Plasma concentration to dosage ratios in children of various age groups receiving phenobarbital alone and in combination with valproate sodium (mean dosage, 22 mg/kg per day). Each value represents the mean plus or minus standard deviation. The number in parentheses indicates the number of patients in each group. (From Suganuma T, et al. The effect of concurrent administration of valproate sodium on phenobarbital plasma concentration/dosage in pediatric patients. *J Pediatr* 1981;99:314. With permission.)

substitution of carbamazepine for phenobarbital or phenytoin resulted in improved memory, concentration, and mental and motor speed (350), Mitchell and coworkers found that when phenobarbital levels were in the middle of the therapeutic range, there was little dose-dependent effect on reaction time, attention, and impulsivity (351). Farwell and colleagues in a double-blind, counter-balanced, crossover study of children receiving phenobarbital for prevention of febrile convulsions found that children receiving phenobarbital performed significantly poorer than patients receiving placebo in measurements of cognitive function and behavior (352). These observations are supported by a study of de Silva and colleagues, who found that 60% of children receiving phenobarbital for the treatment of generalized tonic-clonic or partial seizures developed side effects leading to drug withdrawal. This was in contrast to 4% to 9% of unacceptable side effects for phenytoin, carbamazepine, or sodium valproate (353).

Methylphenobarbital. Methylphenobarbital has been used in the place of phenobarbital because it was believed to have fewer side effects. Because methylphenobarbital is demethylated to phenobarbital in the liver, we would not expect it to have any advantages over phenobarbital in terms of seizure control.

Primidone. Primidone is an effective anticonvulsant for generalized tonic-clonic, simple partial seizures and complex partial seizures. Unlike phenobarbitol, primidone, by itself, has no effect on postsynaptic GABA responses on Cl⁻ currents. It behaves much like phenytoin in abolishing sustained, repetitive firing in cultured neurons, presumably antagonizing Na⁺ currents.

In children, primidone is started at low levels, generally 25 mg per day, given in two divided doses. The daily dose is gradually increased until the average effective dose (150 to 500 mg per day given in three divided doses) is reached. This procedure is intended to circumvent the marked sedation that often occurs when the drug is started at the higher levels. Toxic symptoms are caused by primidone itself and appear when only primidone is detectable in serum. Generally, prior exposure to phenobarbital makes the subject less likely to develop primidone toxicity (354). Primidone is converted into two active metabolites, phenobarbital and phenylethylmalonamide. Hence, monitoring of blood levels can be used only to determine compliance.

Phenytoin. Phenytoin is as effective as phenobarbital and carbamazepine in controlling tonic-clonic seizures. It has lost considerable favor as a long-term anticonvulsant for use in pediatric practice because of the wide variability in its absorption, the effect of other anticonvulsants and even mild intercurrent illnesses on its rate of metabolism, and the relatively high incidence of side reactions (355).

Depending on the size of the child, the average effective dose of phenytoin is 5 to 10 mg/kg per day. The drug is slowly absorbed from the gastrointestinal tract, and at a dose of 4 to 6 mg/kg per day, equilibrium levels in the blood are established between 7 and 10 days after initiation of therapy (see Table 13.11) (356). The daily fluctuations in serum concentrations in children who weigh less than 30 kg are sufficiently large to require the drug to be administered at approximately 8-hour intervals (354,357). Phenytoin is metabolized in the liver, mainly by the P450 mixed oxidase system, which hydroxylates the drug at the para-position (358). The concurrent administration of phenobarbital has little effect on phenytoin blood levels, and the small alterations that do occur are unpredictable (359). Phenytoin produces a number of untoward reactions; in many instances, these are related to overdosage and can be relieved by reducing the drug intake.

Clinically effective phenytoin levels range from 10 to 20 µg/mL. Nystagmus at lateral gaze appears with blood levels of 15 to 30 µg/mL, ataxia appears at above 30 µg/mL, and lethargy or aggravation of seizures appears at levels of 40 µg/mL or higher (360). Irreversible degeneration of the cerebellar Purkinje cells can occur after chronic intoxication or severe acute intoxication (361), and cerebellar atrophy has been demonstrable by imaging studies. Because seizures can be controlled at an average blood level of 18 µg/mL, reduction of dosage in patients with toxic levels usually has no adverse effects on the frequency of convulsions (356).

The rate of phenytoin metabolism varies considerably and appears to be under polygenetic control. A small proportion of patients has a defect in the para-hydroxylation of phenytoin and develop toxic symptoms at the usual daily dosages (362). Low phenytoin tolerance also is seen in patients with liver disease and in those receiving chemotherapeutic drugs against tuberculosis. Small infants eliminate only 1% to 20% of the drug in a 24-hour period and often develop toxic side effects (357).

One of the major drawbacks of phenytoin therapy is a long and worrisome list of common side reactions.

Approximately 2% to 5% of patients receiving phenytoin develop fever, a morbilliform rash, and lymphadenopathy within 2 weeks of the start of therapy. Blood levels at the time of the reaction are in the therapeutic range, and symptoms clear after the medication is discontinued (363). Although some authorities believe that phenytoin can be restarted, we have been hesitant to do so because the drug is known to induce a variety of severe hypersensitivity reactions, including antinuclear antibodies, a lupus-like disease, and Stevens-Johnson syndrome (364). In a multinational case control study, the risk for Stevens-Johnson syndrome and for toxic epidermal necrolysis was significantly increased during the first 8 weeks of phenytoin therapy. Carbamazepine, phenobarbital, and lamotrigine also increased the risk for these dermatologic complications (365).

Antinuclear antibodies have been detected not only in patients receiving phenytoin, but also in those receiving phenobarbital or ethosuximide exclusively. Although the presence of antinuclear antibodies in asymptomatic children has aroused considerable concern, it is not an indication for discontinuation of anticonvulsants (see Chapter 7). The incidence of malignant lymphomas and Hodgkin's disease in patients receiving long-term therapy with phenytoin or other hydantoins is 4 to 10 times greater than expected, a finding suggesting that phenytoin-induced lymphadenopathy is not necessarily benign (366).

According to Kapur and associates, 93% of patients with phenytoin levels between 10 and 20 µg/mL develop gum hyperplasia, and 75% of patients develop hirsutism (367). Gum hyperplasia can be reduced by strict oral hygiene, daily gum massage, and repeated excision of hyperplastic tissue. Coarsening of facial features, and increased skin pigmentation are other, relatively common, adverse effects of phenytoin therapy. Patients on prolonged phenytoin therapy can develop megaloblastic anemia and lowered serum folate concentrations, which respond to folic acid therapy (368). The mechanism by which the drug alters folate metabolism is still uncertain, and Weber and associates have suggested that megaloblastic anemia seen in the course of phenytoin therapy reflects inadequate food composition or intake (369). Although prolonged folate deficiency can induce an organic brain syndrome in the absence of subacute combined degeneration of the cord, folate therapy has no effect on the behavior or mental function of chronic epileptic patients (370). Plasma biotin levels of patients on long-term anticonvulsant therapy are reduced, but what role, if any, biotin deficiency plays in the cerebellar deficits of some patients on long-term phenytoin therapy is still unclear (371). Reduced plasma vitamin E levels are commonly noted in seizure patients and have prompted the addition of vitamin E (400 IU/day) to the anticonvulsant regimen with apparent improvement in seizure control (372).

A disturbed vitamin D metabolism resulting in hypocalcemic rickets, decreased serum calcium and phosphorus, and increased alkaline phosphatase is seen in some ambulatory, noninstitutionalized patients after long-term therapy with phenytoin, primidone, or phenobarbital (373). Anticonvulsants have been shown to accelerate the conversion of the vitamin D sterols to polar compounds other than the active vitamin D metabolites such as 25-hydroxycholecalciferol. This observation suggests that children who are on long-term anticonvulsant therapy should be maintained on vitamin D supplementation and should be encouraged to participate in outdoor activities and to receive adequate exposure to sunlight (374).

Peripheral neuropathy also can result from prolonged anticonvulsant therapy. Deep tendon reflexes are lost in approximately one-half of patients receiving phenytoin for longer than 15 years (375).

Several reports have called attention to the occurrence of hyperglycemia in persons receiving phenytoin. In short-term experiments, the drug impairs glucose-induced insulin release, but this effect is temporary, and in clinical practice, hyperglycemia has been encountered only at drug levels that produce signs of neurotoxicity (376).

Phenytoin encephalopathy is generally seen with toxic blood levels, but has rarely been reported as an idiosyncratic reaction at therapeutic levels. Mentally retarded subjects are particularly vulnerable to this syndrome (377).

The teratogenic effect of phenytoin and other anticonvulsants has attracted considerable attention. As delineated by Hanson and Smith (378), the fetal hydantoin syndrome is characterized by intrauterine and postnatal growth deficiency, mental retardation, hypoplasia of the distal phalanges with small nails, ocular hypertelorism, a low and broad nasal bridge, and a bowed upper lip. Early work suggested that 11% of phenytoin-exposed fetuses developed this syndrome and that there was a significant incidence (7.1%) of major congenital malformations in children of women who received not only phenytoin, but other anticonvulsants as well (379). This incidence was somewhat higher than the incidence of malformations in epileptic women who were not taking anticonvulsants (1.8%). Shapiro and associates noted, however, that malformations are also higher in offspring of epileptic fathers (4.5%). They suggested that a genetic transmission of malformations is at work (380). More recent studies on offspring of mothers who were receiving mainly phenytoin monotherapy and whose blood levels were carefully monitored and maintained in the low therapeutic range, found a 1% to 2% risk of serious developmental anomalies, a value slightly greater than the risk in the general population (381). The observation that infants who developed fetal hydantoin syndrome have low amniocyte epoxide hydrolase activity needs to be confirmed, but could open up a means for assessing the risk for the syndrome (382,383). The suggestion that mutations in the gene for microsomal epoxide hydrolase are responsible for anticonvulsant teratogenicity or hypersensitivity reactions has not been confirmed. (484) No association between maternal epileptic seizures during pregnancy and minor malformations in the offspring was found in several other studies. It is the present consensus that not only phenytoin, but other hydantoins, as well as phenobarbital, valproate, and carbamazepine, increase the incidence of fetal malformations, particularly when combinations of anticonvulsants are being used (384,385).

Mephenytoin. Mephenytoin, which is chemically related to phenytoin, was once used in the treatment of generalized tonic-clonic and complex partial seizures. Unlike phenytoin, it did not appear to cause hirsutism, gingival hyperplasia, or many of the cerebellar deficits associated with the use of phenytoin (386).

Carbamazepine. Carbamazepine is an iminostilbene, chemically unrelated to any of the other major anticonvulsants. It appears to function by antagonizing sodium currents in a manner similar to phenytoin (387).

Children with complex partial and tonic-clonic seizures are most likely to benefit from the drug (388). The starting dosage in children aged 6 to 12 years is 10 to 25 mg/kg per day, and maximum dosage for effective seizure control in that age range is approximately 600 to 800 mg per day. The suggested starting dosage for children younger than 6 years of age is 10 mg/kg per day. Although optimal therapeutic levels are generally stated to be between 4 and 12 µg/mL (389), carbamazepine-plasma protein binding and the conversion of carbamazepine to a pharmacologically active 10,11-epoxide, which cannot readily be assayed, complicate the interpretation of serum concentrations in children (390). Ratios of carbamazepine to its epoxide range from 4 to 1 in children receiving carbamazepine monotherapy to 3 to 1 in those receiving other anticonvulsants as well (388). The ratio between the epoxide and carbamazepine tends to decrease with increasing age (391). The ratio between the dosage of carbamazepine and the blood concentration is linear for any given child, but the ratio varies considerably among children. On the average, dosage increments of 2 mg/kg increase carbamazepine concentration by 1 µg/mL (388). The drug is given two to four times daily. Two sustained release preparations, Tegretol-XR and Carbatrol, are available in the United States. The latter is a sprinkle preparation. Oxcarbazepine, a keto-substituted analogue, has a pharmacologic spectrum and potency similar to that of carbamazepine, but a lower incidence of side reactions (392). Its release in the United States is expected in the near future.

Clearance of carbamazepine increases for the first month after initiation of therapy as a consequence of induction of the metabolic enzymes. When carbamazepine is used in conjunction with another drug, notably valproic acid, protein binding is decreased, with an ensuing increase in unbound carbamazepine and toxicity at lower blood levels (388).

Diplopia is the most common side reaction encountered in patients receiving carbamazepine. It can disappear spontaneously or after reduction of drug dosage. Lesser and coworkers, however, found no clear relationship between such toxic side effects and either free or total plasma carbamazepine levels (324). Transient drowsiness, incoordination, and vertigo can be seen with initiation of therapy or when the dosage is increased too rapidly (393).

Other side reactions include a variety of rashes, hyponatremia, hepatic dysfunction, and leukopenia (394). Rashes are undoubtedly the most common and were encountered in 5% of children in the series of Pellock (393). Hyponatremia is believed to result from an antidiuretic effect of carbamazepine or an excessive release of antidiuretic hormone. It is usually mild and reversible with fluid restriction (395). A stable, nonprogressive leukopenia is not rare. In the series of Pellock, a leukopenia of less than 4,000 per μL was seen in 12.7% of children; only 2.3% had counts below 3,000. These cases of leukopenia were not progressive and therefore did not require discontinuation of the drug; blood counts reversed spontaneously in 75% of children. In some of these patients, a minor viral illness can induce the decrease in the number of white cells. The experiences of Camfield and coworkers have been similar. In their series, 9% of children on carbamazepine also had an elevated aspartate aminotransferase level (396). Isolated cases of rash followed by acute hepatic failure during the first few weeks of carbamazepine therapy have been reported, as have a few instances of systemic lupus erythematosus (397).

Administration of therapeutic doses of carbamazepine to children with atypical absence and other minor motor seizures can aggravate the seizure disorder or induce absence status; less often a continuous, nonepileptic myoclonus is seen (398,399). Less commonly encountered side reactions include dystonic movements. The concurrent administration of other drugs can induce carbamazepine neurotoxicity by inhibiting its metabolism. These drugs include calcium channel blockers such as diltiazem and verapamil, propoxyphene hydrochloride, isoniazid, and erythromycin (400).

Despite the various potential side reactions, carbamazepine has the advantage over phenobarbital or phenytoin in that it improves cognitive functions and makes patients feel brighter and more alert (351,401). Additionally, behavior was thought to be improved in 15% of children in Pellock's series (393). The experience of Forsythe and his group differs from these studies, in that patients receiving carbamazepine monotherapy demonstrated impairment in recent recall and slowed information processing at therapeutic drug levels (402).

Generic substitution for carbamazepine raises problems in patients in whom the therapeutic to toxic window is narrow, because of the reduced shelf-life of some products, and a relatively large range in bioavailability of the various generic preparations. These concerns have been reviewed by Nuwer and colleagues (403).

Ethosuximide. The most effective drug for the treatment of absence (petit mal) seizures is ethosuximide. In experimental models, the drug blocks pentylenetetrazol-induced seizures. Starting doses for children are 250 mg twice daily or 20 mg/kg per day. Optimal therapeutic plasma levels are between 40 and 100 μg/mL (329). We use ethosuximide by itself in the treatment of absence attacks unless the patient has had a history of other seizure types, in which case valproate monotherapy or combined phenobarbital and ethosuximide therapy can be used.

Phenytoin, which increases the frequency of absence attacks, should not be used in the patient with combined major and absence seizures. Side effects of ethosuximide are generally minor. They include gastrointestinal upsets, usually during the first few days of drug therapy, skin rashes, headaches, and, occasionally, hematologic abnormalities, principally a reversible leukopenia (329).

Trimethadione. Until the introduction of etho-suximide in 1958, trimethadione had been the drug of choice in the treatment of absence attacks. Like ethosuximide, it blocks pentylene-tetrazol seizures. Its tendency to predispose patients to major motor seizures and the induction of bone marrow depression in approximately 5% of patients made it inferior to ethosuximide.

Valproic Acid. Since its introduction into clinical practice in the 1970s, valproic acid, either as its sodium or magnesium salt or as a free acid, has proven highly effective, not only for minor motor seizures, but also for tonic-clonic absence, simple partial, and complex partial seizures (404).

The exact mechanism of drug action is unknown and the drug probably acts through a combination of several mechanisms (405). Valproic acid increases GABA synthesis and release, and reduces the release of the epileptogenic amino acid γ-hydroxybutyric acid. It also is believed to potentiate the postsynaptic GABA inhibitory effect, block spike generation, and inhibit the excitatory neuronal pathways (406,407). It may also inhibit GABA-transaminase and succinic semialdehyde dehydrogenase activities, and thus elevate GABA concentrations in CSF and within the brain. There is, however, considerable doubt whether increased GABA concentrations are important for anticonvulsant action because valproic acid demonstrates an antiepileptic effect before brain GABA levels increase.

Starting dosages for children are 15 to 20 mg/kg per day given two to three times a day, with the dose increased at weekly intervals to an amount that provides seizure control, usually in the range of 20 to 70 mg/kg per day. Serum valproic acid levels and anticonvulsant action are poorly correlated. Even though several authorities consider 50 to 100 µg/mL to represent optimal drug levels, we have found that fasting valproic acid levels are not reproducible and only monitor valproic acid concentrations to verify compliance. Bourgeois (408) and a *Lancet* editorial (409) have taken the same position.

The dose-serum concentration relationship is complex, in part because of the short half-life of valproic acid, and in part because of its high degree of plasma protein binding. At low plasma valproic acid levels, protein binding is 90% to 95%, but with increasing dosages, the proportion of valproic acid bound to protein decreases progressively, and, as a consequence, the total serum concentration of valproic acid does not increase in proportion to the dose (328). The concentration of valproate in brain tissue resected from patients with chronic epilepsy is extremely low. In part, the low concentrations reflect the fact that valproate is not bound to lipids; in part, they can be accounted for by gliosis in the surgical specimens (410).

Although the plasma half-life is short (i.e., 6 to 15 hours when valproic acid is administered alone, and even less when valproic acid is given in combination with other anticonvulsants), the practice of administering the drug in two to four daily doses might not be required; once-daily administration of enteric-coated valproic acid appears to provide equally good seizure control (411). Absorption of valproate sprinkles is slower, but as complete as the syrup. Because there is less fluctuation in the serum levels, this preparation of valproate can be given every 12 hours (412).

With the widespread use of valproic acid, numerous side reactions have been encountered. The most common of these are a variety of gastrointestinal upsets (404). In part, these can be reduced by taking the medication after meals, by a gradual increase in dosage, or by the use of an enteric-coated preparation. Increased appetite is another common side reaction, seen in 11% of patients receiving enteric-coated valproic acid in the Collaborative Study Group (413). We have noted that significant weight gain is encountered in the patients who respond best to the drug. Thinning of hair is encountered less often (1% of patients in the Collaborative Study Group).

The effects of valproic acid on liver function have generated serious concern (414). Dose-related elevations of liver enzymes are seen in up to 44% of patients receiving valproic acid as the sole anticonvulsant. Usually, these abnormalities are transient or resolve with dosage reduction. Far more serious is a Reye syndrome–like hepatic failure usually encountered during the first 3 months of therapy. This complication is unrelated to valproic acid dosage, and its incidence is highest (1 in 543) in children younger than 2 years of age receiving polytherapy (414). Infants with mental retardation and those with medical conditions other than epilepsy are particularly prone to fatal hepatic failure. Children younger than 2 years of age who were on monotherapy had an incidence of 1 in 8,213, whereas those older than 2 years of age on monotherapy had an incidence of 1 in 45,000 (415). Only one case of a child older than 10 years of age and receiving monotherapy has been reported (414).

The cause for valproic acid–induced acute hepatic failure is still unclear, although an unsaturated metabolite of valproic acid, 2-n-propyl-4-pentenoic acid, is believed to be indirectly responsible. This substance inhibits hepatic cytochrome P450, inhibits fatty acid β-oxidation, and induces hepatic microvesicular steatosis, the characteristic cellular abnormality in valproic acid–induced liver injury. Liver microsomes from phenobarbital-treated rats catalyzed the desaturation of valproic acid to 2-n-propyl-4-pentenoic acid, implying that patients who concurrently receive valproic acid and phenobarbital are at particular risk for hepatic failure (416). Inasmuch as 2-n-propyl-4-pentenoic acid is seen in approximately 10% of children on valproic acid, its presence cannot be used to predict fatal hepatotoxicity (417). In any case, there is no continuum between those patients who show an elevation in serum liver enzymes and those who develop hepatic failure. Thus, routine monitoring of liver function does not prevent hepatic failure (418). It also should be pointed out that valproate hepatotoxicity should be distinguished from the syndrome of progressive cerebral degeneration, which is associated with liver disease (see Chapter 2) (419). Adverse effects of valproic acid are not limited to the liver, and microvesicular lipid droplets also are seen between myofibrils near mitochondria (420).

Hyperammonemia is a common accompaniment of valproic acid therapy. Laub encountered fasting ammonia levels between 33 and 143 µg/mL in otherwise asymptomatic patients receiving therapeutic dosages of valproic acid. Following protein load, ammonia levels rose even further (58 to 426 µg/mL). There is no correlation between elevated ammonia levels and hepatic failure, and finding high blood ammonia should not prompt discontinuation of valproic acid therapy (421).

Sedation owing to valproic acid is seen in some 10% of patients (413). When it occurs, it is self-limiting and is often attributable to other, concurrently administered anticonvulsants. Episodes of stupor also have been encountered. These are almost invariably seen in children being treated for complex partial seizures with valproic acid, either exclusively or in combination with other anticonvulsants (422). Whether hyperammonemia has a role in the development of stupor is unclear (423). What has been amply demonstrated, however, is that valproic acid elevates serum levels of a variety of other anticonvulsants, notably phenobarbital (424), ethosuximide (425), primidone, and carbamazepine. Valproic acid lowers total phenytoin concentrations, but by displacing phenytoin from its plasma binding sites, it increases the proportion of free phenytoin; thus, toxicity is encountered at lower phenytoin levels (426). The combination of valproic acid and clonazepam has strong hypnotic effects, and, in some instances, it induces absence status. These complex anticonvulsant drug interactions once more underline the advisability of monotherapy.

Tremor and asterixis have been encountered in patients receiving valproic acid (404). We, and others, have seen that in most instances tremor develops only at doses greater than 40 to 50 mg/kg per day and is reduced or cleared by lowering the dosage (427). Some of these children have a family history of essential tremor. Asterixis is rare and is associated with polytherapy (428). A decrease in platelet count, which is often transient, is also dose related. It appears to have an autoimmune basis, and in general is not sufficiently severe to require reduction or withdrawal of valproic acid. The thrombocytopenia can be aggravated with infections and at such times can result in bruising or minor bleeding phenomena (429). In a large proportion of children receiving valproic acid, one observes a reduction in factor VIII/von Willebrand factor complex. This results in a prolonged bleeding time, but aside from nosebleeds, or mild bleeding from the gums or skin, this defect is generally asymptomatic. It is unrelated to the dosage of valproic acid, or whether the child is on monotherapy or polytherapy (430). Many epilepsy centers discontinue valproic acid before surgical procedures. Ward and coworkers, however, have shown that surgical blood loss in the course of temporal lobectomy was no greater in patients receiving valproate than in those who were not (431).

Much rarer side reactions to valproic acid therapy include hyperglycinemia (432) and pancreatitis (433). Hyperglycinemia is believed to be caused by inhibition of the glycine cleavage system by valproic acid, valproyl-CoA, or both (432). Pancreatitis manifests by epigastric pain, nausea, and vomiting. It is unrelated to dosage, but is more commonly encountered in patients who are on polytherapy. In most instances this complication develops during the first few months of therapy. In the series of Asconape, an asymptomatic elevation of serum amylase levels was seen in 11% of patients receiving valproate (434). Edema of face and limbs has been encountered in children receiving valproate for more than a year. The reason for this complication is not clear (435).

A variety of endocrine disorders has been described. These include centripetal obesity and menstrual disorders. In women who have been on long-term valproate therapy, obesity, polycystic ovaries, and hyperandrogenism are a frequent occurrence (436).

Valproic acid therapy lowers serum free carnitine levels, although the exact mechanism is still unclear. Valproic acid, a C8 fatty acid, forms carnitine esters that are readily excreted in urine. Additionally, valproic acid reduces hepatic β-oxidation of fatty acids, which are then excreted as acylated carnitine. Although low carnitine levels have been seen in children with Reye syndrome, carnitine therapy does not prevent hepatic dysfunction (437,438). There is no correlation between valproic acid dosage and carnitine levels or between carnitine and ammonia levels. Because children with low carnitine levels are asymptomatic, dietary carnitine supplementation is not indicated (438), and in a double-blind, placebo-controlled study, the administration of carnitine in children receiving valproate monotherapy or polytherapy was no more effective than placebo in relieving non-specific symptoms such as hypotonia and lethargy (439).

In approximately 1% to 2% of pregnancies, maternal intake of valproic acid has resulted in the development of neural tube defects in offspring (440). A syndrome of facial anomalies similar to that seen in offspring of mothers receiving hydantoin therapy also has been reported. Determinations of α-fetoprotein levels on pregnant women receiving valproic acid are indicated (see Chapter 4).

Despite these side reactions, valproic acid is an excellent anticonvulsant, not only because it provides better seizure control, but because it does so without sedating the child. Nevertheless, patients on this drug should be seen by a physician at 2- to 3-month intervals, and routine blood studies, particularly platelet counts, should be obtained at every visit. Whether liver function tests are needed is more problematic.

Benzodiazepine Anticonvulsants. Several agents are used in the treatment of epilepsy. In experimental models, all of them have been shown to enhance the GABA-mediated chloride currents.

Clonazepam. In our experience, clonazepam is an effective anticonvulsant for most types of minor motor seizures. It is instituted in gradually increasing dosages beginning at 0.05 mg/kg per day in three or four divided doses, and increased by 0.05 mg/kg every fifth to seventh day until seizures are controlled or until a dose of 0.25 mg/kg is reached. Thereafter, the dose is increased more slowly to 0.5 mg/kg if needed or until side effects are encountered. Side effects include ataxia, drowsiness, dysarthria, irritability or belligerence, and excessive weight gain (441,442). Emotional disturbances that occur commonly with this drug are often aggravated when it is combined with barbiturates or other benzodiazepines (443). Although seizure control is exceedingly good when clonazepam is first initiated, the drug's effectiveness is lost within a few weeks or months in approximately one-third to one-half of subjects. Olsen suggested that the receptor-chloride channel complex is directly involved in the development of tolerance, or that an endogenous benzodiazepine antagonist is produced (105). Clonazepam is most effective in akinetic seizures and atypical petit mal. It is ineffective in infantile spasms.

Nitrazepam. Nitrazepam, a benzodiazepine, which differs from clonazepam by its lack of a chlorine atom, is an effective anticonvulsant for most minor motor seizures (444). Because elevated hepatic enzymes are seen in approximately one-half of patients, its use has been restricted in the United States. The drug is readily available in Europe and Latin America, however. Nitrazepam induces cricopharyngeal incoordination with impaired swallowing and aspiration. Its use has been coupled with sudden death probably caused by aspiration in infants who were on dosages higher than 0.8 mg/kg per day and who had intractable epilepsy (445,445a).

Clorazepate. Clorazepate appears to be another potentially useful benzodiazepine for the treatment of various seizure disorders. Clorazepate is a prodrug. It is converted to *N*-desmethyldiazepam, a long-acting metabolite, whose half-life has been estimated to be between 30 and 150 hours (446). Its usefulness as an adjunctive agent in a variety of seizure types has been reported and the data has been summarized by Ko and colleagues (447). In our service at UCLA, we have used it as a well-tolerated adjunct in refractory patients, and as monotherapy in treating transient seizure problems in organ transplant recipients to avoid pharmacokinetic interactions of antiepileptic drugs with drugs used to prevent rejection of transplanted organs. The latter use is being replaced with gabapentin.

Midazolam. The use of midazolam for the treatment of acute seizures and status epilepticus is increasing (448,449). Compared with barbiturates, which are mitochondrial toxins at high doses, the use of midazolam in the induction of coma is likely to result in much less cardiac toxicity that necessitates the use of pressors and inotropes to support the patient. O'Regan and colleagues have described the intranasal use of midazolam to treat acute seizures successfully in the emergency department (450). Chamberlain and associates found that intramuscular use of midazolam achieved a more rapid cessation of seizures in an emergency room setting than diazepam administered after placement of intravenous access (451).

Diazepam and Lorazepam. Diazepam and lorazepam are used mainly for the treatment of status epilepticus and febrile convulsions. They are discussed under these sections. We have had no experience with other benzodiazepines, notably clobazam, which is being used extensively in Europe and Canada. In the experience of the Canadian Study Group, clobazam is as effective as carbamazepine or phenytoin for the treatment of partial and some generalized childhood epilepsies, with no greater adverse cognitive effects than are encountered with carbamazepine (452,453).

Acetazolamide. Acetazolamide has been viewed favorably as an anticonvulsant in the treatment of refractory childhood seizures, including absence seizures, menstruation-related generalized seizures, and complex partial seizures, by a group of epileptologists, notably Millichap (454). In menstruation-related generalized seizures, we start the drug approximately 5 days before the expected menses and continue it until its end.

Felbamate. Felbamate is effective in both the MET and MES animal models. It also inhibits NMDA currents and facilitates GABA currents. Up to 1994, the drug had been used widely as an add-on anticonvulsant or as monotherapy for both refractory partial onset seizures and the Lennox-Gastaut syndrome (455,456). The drug was started at 15 mg/kg per day in three to four divided doses, with the dose increased by 15 mg/kg per day at weekly intervals to 45 mg/kg per day or higher (up to 200 mg/kg per day) should there be no clinical response and no adverse reactions. Valproate, phenytoin, and carbamazepine epoxide steady-state plasma concentrations increase with the addition of felbamate; therefore, when felbamate is used as adjunctive therapy, the present antiepileptic drug dosage is reduced by approximately 20%, and plasma levels of the other anticonvulsant should be verified during the initial stages of felbamate treatment. Several cases of a sometimes irreversible aplastic anemia, some in patients on felbamate monotherapy, have been reported. The incidence of this complication in approximately 1 in 10,000 patients is far higher than background incidence of aplastic anemia. Thompson and colleagues have suggested that some patients may have an increased propensity to form a reactive metabolite, 3-carbamoyl-2-phenylpropionaldehyde, which is readily transformed to atropaldehyde, a compound proposed to play a role in the development of toxicity during felbamate therapy (457). As a consequence of this toxicity, the use of felbamate has been restricted to patients who absolutely require this drug for seizure control. Other, less severe reactions seen in children include rash, insomnia, and loss of appetite. The American Academy of Neurology has recommended the use of felbamate for patients with the Lennox-Gastaut syndrome who are older than 4 years of age, and who have been unresponsive to primary antiepileptic drugs. The drug is recommended also for intractable partial seizures in patients older than age 18 years who have failed standard antiepileptic drug therapy. The drug may be continued in those patients who have been receiving it for more than 18 months. The use of felbamate is optional in children with intractable partial epilepsy, primary generalized epilepsy unresponsive to primary anticonvulsants, children younger than 4 years of age with Lennox-Gastaut syndrome, and in those patients who experience unacceptable sedative or cognitive side effects with traditional antiepileptic drugs (458).

Gabapentin. Although designed as a GABA agonist, the mode of action of this anticonvulsant, a structural analogue of GABA, is still uncertain. Significant elevations in brain GABA levels as measured by MR spectroscopy have been demonstrated in epileptic patients treated with gabapentin (459). The drug is effective for secondarily generalized tonic-clonic seizures and complex partial seizures (460). It is usually given to adults in dosages of 2,400 to 3,600 mg per day, but much higher dosages appear to be well tolerated. To date, reported side effects include somnolence, fatigue, dizziness, and weight gain (461). Several reports on the efficacy of gabapentin monotherapy for partial and secondarily generalized seizures have appeared in the recent literature (462–464). The advantages of gabapentin are that it is not bound by plasma albumin, does not undergo hepatic metabolism, or induce cytochrome P450 isoen-

zymes. Therefore, it can be added to other regimens without concerns about pharmacokinetic interactions. It is also devoid of problems with hypersensitivity reactions and bone marrow toxicity. It has demonstrated minimal cognitive effects in a placebo-controlled study of refractory epileptic patients (464a).

Based on experience with animal models (465), gabapentin should not be used in primary generalized spike-wave epilepsies. This is confirmed by its lack of efficacy in absence seizures (466), and its exacerbation of symptomatic generalized epilepsy of the Lennox-Gastaut type (467).

Lamotrigine. Lamotrigine resembles phenytoin and carbamazepine in animal models, being most effective in the MES model (468). The drug reduces sustained repetitive firing in cultured neurons (469) and prolongs the inactivation of voltage-gated sodium channels (470). Lamotrigine appears to have activity against generalized seizures (471). Its efficacy against partial seizures has been demonstrated in a monotherapy trial in which this antiepileptic drug appeared to be well tolerated (472).

Lamotrigine also has been shown to be useful in the Lennox-Gastaut syndrome (473,474), juvenile myoclonic epilepsy (475), and typical and atypical absence seizures (476).

When lamotrigine is used as monotherapy, optimal doses range between 3 and 6 mg/kg per day, with the starting dose approximately one-fourth of that amount. When lamotrigine is given to a child who is already receiving valproate, a starting dose of 0.1 to 0.2 mg/kg per day is recommended, with the dosage being built up slowly to a maximum of 5 mg/kg. Because valproate inhibits lamotrigine metabolism, higher doses produce severe toxicity (477,478). This is particularly evident in children receiving both lamotrigine and valproate. When lamotrigine is added to carbamazepine, phenytoin, or phenobarbital, drugs that induce hepatic enzymes, the half-life of lamotrigine is decreased, and higher lamotrigine dosages are required (479).

The most commonly encountered side effect is a variety of rashes, including severe reactions such as Stevens-Johnson syndrome or toxic epidermal necrolysis (480). The estimated incidence of these severe reactions in children of between 1 in 50 to 100 has resulted in the manufacturer and the U.S. Food and Drug Administration suggesting that lamotrigine not be used as first-line therapy of seizures in children. The incidence in adults of such reactions appears to be in the same order of magnitude as with phenytoin and carbamazepine. Schlienger and colleagues also found that 74% of the patients who had a severe skin reaction to lamotrigine (Stevens-Johnson syndrome or toxic epidermal necrolysis) were also co-medicated with valproic acid (480). A slow titration rate, beginning at 25 mg every other day, has been proposed as a means to minimize the chance of developing a rash. Buchanan suggests that patients on lamotrigine monotherapy be started on 12.5 mg per day, with the dosage increased by 12.5 mg every 2 weeks. Patients who are on a combination of valproate and lamotrigine should be started on a dosage of 12.5 mg every 3 days for 2 weeks, then increased to 12.5 mg every 2 days for 2 weeks, then 12.5 mg per day, with further dosage increases every 2 weeks (481). Less commonly encountered side reactions include a syndrome of multiorgan dysfunction and disseminated intravascular coagulation after a flu-like illness in children who received a combination of lamotrigine and valproate (482). No controlled studies on the cognitive side effects of the drugs are as yet available, but the drug does not appear to have any long-term effects in healthy adults (483).

Topiramate. Topiramate, a fructose derivative, has demonstrated potent anticonvulsant activity in several animal models, with the exception of those involving seizures induced by chemoconvulsants (484). Its mechanisms of action include activity against both voltage-gated and ligand-gated (at AMPA-Kainate subtypes of glutamate receptors)· Na$^+$ channels as well as enhancement of GABA-mediated Cl$^-$ currents (338). In addition, topiramate also seems to elevate brain GABA levels (485,486) and acts as a weak carbonic anhydrase inhibitor.

Topiramate has been demonstrated to be effective against partial seizures, generalized seizures, as well as the drop attacks and major motor seizures in the Lennox-Gastaut syndrome (487–490). The major side effect of the drug is its adverse action on cognitive function, with subjects performing worse on tests of verbal memory and psychomotor speed. In addition, adult subjects have reported difficulties with expressive speech, memory, and slowed thinking (483). These studies are consistent with clinical observations from many centers including our own.

Vigabatrin. Vigabatrin (γ-vinyl GABA), an irreversible inhibitor of GABA transaminase, was first licensed as an antiepileptic agent in Britain and the Republic of Ireland in 1989 (491). It binds irreversibly to GABA transaminase (GABA-T), the enzyme that breaks down GABA. This action increases the brain levels of GABA, increasing inhibition in the brain and thereby decreasing the likelihood of seizures.

Vigabatrin has been approved for treatment in nearly 50 countries worldwide but its approval in the United States has stalled because of concerns about toxicity to the visual system. These concerns include reports of severe, persistent visual field defects noted in association with treatment with vigabatrin (492–494).

Interestingly, development of vigabatrin in the United States had previously been delayed for several years because of concerns about white matter toxicity (intramyelinic edema) encountered in experimental animals, then resumed when such toxicity could not be demonstrated in humans.

The clinical efficacy of vigabatrin in partial seizures has been documented in several studies, summarized by one of us (R.S.) (491). The most promising effect of the drug is in infantile spasms, especially its unique and extraordinary efficacy in the subset whose spasms are caused by tuberous sclerosis (495–499). Its dramatic efficacy in this subpopulation, when compared with the poor responses of these patients to ACTH (230), mandates a separate risk to benefit analysis of this medication in pediatric patients (500). Vigabatrin is not effective in children with Lennox-Gastaut syndrome (501).

The recommended starting dose is 40 mg/kg per day, which is increased to 80 to 100 mg/kg per day, as required. In infantile spasms, dosages of more than 100 mg/kg per day have been used with some effect (243). Side effects include drowsiness, agitation and confusion, and a variety of dyskinesias such as akathisia, hyperkinesia, and forced laughter (502).

Other Anticonvulsants. Older anticonvulsants, notably phenacemide, paramethadione, and methsuximide, are rarely used in the treatment of seizures. Calcium channel antagonists have anticonvulsant activity in experimental seizure models, and preliminary clinical trials using flunarizine for complex partial and generalized tonic-clonic seizures suggest that these drugs have a significant anticonvulsant activity in the human as well (503).

Ketogenic Diet

Although the value of fasting in the treatment of seizures has been recognized since biblical times, the ketogenic diet, which attempts to reproduce the ketosis and acidosis of starvation, was introduced only in 1921 (504). Despite the development of a variety of new and effective anticonvulsants in this country and abroad, it remains an attractive alternate means for the treatment of Lennox-Gastaut syndrome and other intractable seizures (505). The diet involves restricting protein and carbohydrate intake and supplying 80% of caloric intake through fats. The mechanism by which this regimen controls convulsions is still unknown. It is independent of respiratory or metabolic acidosis and of the accumulation of ketone bodies. Starvation induces the activity of D-3-hydroxybutyrate dehydrogenase and allows the brain to metabolize ketone bodies. It is still unclear if the benefits of the diet in seizure disorders stem primarily from the switch in cerebral metabolism involving the use of β-hydroxybutyrate instead of glucose as an energy substrate. The metabolic and endocrine aspects of this diet have been reviewed in detail by one of us (R.S.) (506).

The diet is most effective in children with minor motor seizures between 2 and 5 years of age. Older children do not respond as well because they fail to maintain an adequate degree of ketosis. We reserve the ketogenic diet for children who have been unable to tolerate anticonvulsant drugs because of multiple allergies.

Details of the induction and maintenance of the diet are presented by Livingston (507). Medium-chain triglycerides as a substitute for a ketogenic diet have been advocated by Huttenlocher and associates (508). We have had relatively little experience with this regimen, but it appears to be as effective as the ketogenic diet and is better tolerated by some children.

The increasing popularity of the diet in the 1990s prompted a multicenter study to evaluate its effectiveness (509). This study found that 10% of the patients became free of seizures on the diet. One-half the patients received considerable benefit from the diet, whereas the other one-half had dropped out of the diet by the end of the year, either because of lack of efficacy or adverse effects. There have been concerns among clinicians as how to best screen patients for safety with this diet. To state that physicians should avoid placing a child with seizures on the diet if the child also demonstrates hypotonia and developmental delay, with metabolic acidosis and abnormalities of organic or amino acids, is too general to provide adequate guidance. A child with such a presentation could have pyruvate dehydrogenase deficiency, and hence may stand to benefit significantly from the ketogenic diet. On the other hand, a child with a primary or acquired carnitine deficiency or a defect in the β-oxidation of fatty acids sustains significant morbidity if fasted or placed on the diet. If a patient has undergone a muscle biopsy earlier in the workup for hypotonia and weakness, a biopsy showing a few ragged-red fibers may not be a contraindication to the diet, but the appearance of a lipid myopathy is. Increased serum pyruvate and lactate along with alaninuria may not be a problem, but increased dicarboxylic acid excretion points at a potential for trouble. We, therefore, suggest that in the presence of an abnormal pattern of urinary organic acids the type of dicarboxylic aciduria be determined, before the child is started on a ketogenic diet. We should point out that dicarboxylic aciduria and carnitine deficiency can occur in a patient who is on both valproic acid and the ketogenic diet. In addition, children who present with a history of seizures and intermittent encephalopathy in the course of minor infections should be carefully evaluated for the nature of the metabolic abnormality before considering the ketogenic diet.

We agree with Demeritte and colleagues (510) that organic acid screening be done before and after the initiation of the ketogenic diet. However, we do not recommend that patients on the diet be supplemented routinely with carnitine. Rather, we agree with recommendations from a roundtable discussion on the role of L-carnitine supplementation in children with epilepsy that suggests that carnitine supplementation be reserved for children with demonstrable carnitine deficiency (511). Even though most centers offering the ketogenic diet have patients who are also on valproate, one study has hinted at the added risk for complications in such patients (512).

Anticonvulsants in Children with Systemic Disease

Phenobarbital can be administered in the presence of severe hepatic disease. Even though hepatic hydroxylation of the drug is impaired, with consequent doubling of its half-life, increased elimination of unchanged phenobarbital reduces the importance of hepatic metabolism.

Carbamazepine levels are altered in hepatic disease. Metabolism of the drug is reduced significantly, reducing its clearance. This effect is counteracted by reduced plasma binding and increased free carbamazepine. Generally, however, levels tend to increase and must be monitored carefully, keeping in mind that the free carbamazepine fraction is higher than normal.

No modification of clearance or bioavailability of carbamazepine has been observed in renal failure. In cardiac failure, carbamazepine absorption, which is normally erratic, is reduced. However, the drug is metabolized more slowly than usual, thus reducing its clearance. Carbamazepine can cause increased sodium and water retention, which may aggravate cardiac symptoms.

In cirrhosis and renal disease, the free fraction of valproic acid increases two- to threefold. The intrinsic metabolism of the drug is reduced, however, so that the actual clearance remains essentially normal.

The metabolism of the benzodiazepines is unaffected by renal or hepatic disease. Among the newer agents, gabapentin, topiramate, and lamotrigine offer the benefits of not having significant systemic toxicity, protein binding, or hepatic induction. This permits the use of these agents in children with renal or hepatic disease, including those who are transplant recipients maintained on immunosuppressants with brittle pharmacokinetic properties.

Summary

In summarizing medical therapy for seizure disorders, we would like to point out several common errors.

The physician fails to diagnose correctly the type of seizure experienced by the child. This failure is almost always because an inadequate history was obtained. Misinterpretation of EEGs also contributes to the failure to diagnose the seizure syndrome.

Anticonvulsants are not given in sufficiently high dosage. No drug should be abandoned unless the physician is certain that it has no beneficial effects and unless toxic symptoms are verified.

Another error results from the physician placing too much reliance on newer anticonvulsants in the hope that one of them will *turn off* seizures. Frequent changes in medication and altering the dosage of more than one drug at the same time should be avoided.

Finally, the tendency for polytherapy to increase seizure frequency has been insufficiently appreciated. Many years ago, one of us (J.H.M.) found that complete discontinuation of anticonvulsant medication can produce significant, and sometimes permanent, improvement in approximately one-third of patients with Lennox-Gastaut syndrome, and we believe that periodic withdrawal or reduction of anticonvulsants is indicated in such patients whose seizures remain under poor control (325).

Surgical Procedures

When epilepsy is intractable to medical treatment, surgical resection of the tissue responsible for the epilepsy should be considered. Only some 5% to 10% of all cases of epilepsy, approximately 10,000 new cases annually, turn out to have a medically intractable condition. Approximately one-third of these, some 3,000 new patients per year, will ultimately become candidates for currently available surgical procedures (513). The traditional criteria for choosing a suitable candidate, developed largely from centers concentrating on temporal lobectomies and extratemporal cortical resections for partial seizures, have stressed the need for precise localization of the epileptic focus (514). There are also commonly accepted criteria regarding what constitutes medical intractability, what is an acceptable deficit, and the minimal IQ below which a patient is not a suitable candidate (514). The present indications and criteria for surgical interventions have been reviewed by Duchowny and colleagues (514a).

Many of these criteria have been modified significantly to accommodate the distinctive aspects of the developing brain. This is reflected in the criteria set forth in the most current edition of Engel's treatise on epilepsy surgery, which differ from those set up in 1987 (515). The background and rationale for these revised criteria have been described by Shewmon and associates (516).

Shewmon and coworkers have shown that the presence of bilaterally independent, multifocal, interictal epileptiform discharges in a young child does not necessarily indicate widespread epileptogenicity (517), and thus is not a contraindication to focal resection (516). They also point out that the iatrogenic introduction of significant new neurologic deficits, such as hemiparesis and hemianopsia, is acceptable in some conditions. In conditions such as Rasmussen syndrome or Sturge-Weber disease, the underlying disease can eventually lead to the same deficit; but early intervention may eliminate the frequent interruptions to the developmental processes of the *good* cortex by the *nociferous* cortex, and also takes advantage of the plasticity of the *good* cortex when it is at its maximum. Considerations of development and plasticity also affect the determination of what seizure disorder is intractable, and what is the best timing for surgery. Furthermore, mental retardation

or developmental delay is common in children who benefit substantially from resective surgery and thus is not a contraindication.

Shewmon and coworkers also have pointed out the complexities involved in the localization of a seizure focus (516,517). Ictal epileptiform abnormalities are sometimes not clearly lateralized; in childhood epileptic syndromes such as West syndrome, the ictal EEG tends to be generalized even when a lateralized zone of cortical abnormality exists. However, the nonepileptiform abnormalities, such as focal bursts of slowing or asymmetry in the generation of beta rhythms in response to barbiturates, or asymmetry of sleep spindles can suggest the presence of an underlying lateralized zone of cortical abnormality.

Neuroimaging aspects of presurgical evaluation of candidates have been reviewed (518,519), and the special considerations for presurgical noninvasive and semi-invasive neurophysiologic tests are outlined by Duchowny and colleagues (520). In neuroimaging infants with cortical microdysplasias, the timing of the MRI is of crucial importance because of the progression of myelination affecting the MR signal characteristics. One of us (R.S.) has demonstrated that even microscopic cortical abnormalities may become discernible by changes in the maturation of the adjacent white matter (226). Thus, an infant with West syndrome with a normal MRI at the age of 4 to 6 months may have to be reimaged several months later if the clinical course warrants considering surgical treatment.

Use of newer ligands such as the benzodiazepine receptor ligand ^{11}C-flumazenil have not significantly improved the utility of PET scanning compared with traditional interictal metabolic mapping with PET using ^{18}F-fluorodeoxyglucose (521).

In "nonlesional" (normal MRI) neocortical epilepsies in older children and adults, interictal SPECT and PET are usually not helpful in localization. In these cases ictal SPECT is of considerable value. The regional blood flow data determined by interictal SPECT can be combined with either ictal or postictal studies to generate a subtraction SPECT. The co-registration of subtraction data with the MRI significantly enhances the sensitivity and specificity of localization (522,523).

Anterior Temporal Lobectomy

The most commonly used surgical procedure, anterior temporal lobectomy, is offered to patients with medically intractable complex partial seizures. Surgery consists of the removal of the anterior portion of the temporal lobe, usually 4 to 5 cm of the dominant lobe or 6 to 7 cm when the epileptic focus is on the nondominant side. In this procedure, the amygdala, anterior hippocampus, and anterior temporal neocortex are removed. When surgery is performed on the dominant temporal lobe, care is taken to avoid the areas for language function. The earlier the surgery, the greater the plasticity for language development. Children younger than 10 years of age can transfer their language to the side contralateral to the resected side, if the resection involves the language dominant side. In many centers, a total temporal lobe resection is performed. This includes the amygdala and 1 to 2 cm of the hippocampus (524). Generally, cure or significant improvement in seizure control is better with the more extensive surgery. Anticonvulsants are continued for at least 2 years after surgery.

For a patient to be a suitable candidate for anterior temporal lobectomy, EEG must demonstrate a consistent ictal onset in one temporal lobe. Additionally, lateralization of language dominance should be confirmed by the Wada test, the intracarotid injection of amobarbital sodium (Amytal). This test also ascertains whether the contralateral temporal lobe will support memory. Within the near future, functional MRI will undoubtedly supplant the invasive procedures currently required to localize language function (525). The EEG focus is confirmed by imaging studies, including the demonstration of hypometabolism by a PET scan, if such is readily available. In recent years, quantitative volumetric studies of the hippocampal formation using MRI have begun to approach the diagnostic accuracy established by PET (526–529). The usefulness of ictal SPECT in the presurgical evaluation of patients with temporal lobe epilepsy has been favorably compared with the sensitivity and specificity of interictal PET (530,531). Should these studies leave doubt about a temporal lobe focus, or should they suggest multiple foci, chronic recordings from stereotactically implanted depth electrodes are desirable. These can localize the site of the earliest ictal discharge with greater accuracy than is possible with scalp recordings, and complement localization derived from the PET scan (136). In some patients, recording with depth electrodes shows nonlateralized EEG epileptiform activity to arise from a single, surgically accessible focus (532). Lesser and coworkers have presented an algorithm, used at the Johns Hopkins Epilepsy Center, for evaluation and treatment of patients with intractable complex partial seizures (533).

Anterior temporal lobectomy is most effective in children with mesial temporal lobe sclerosis or a hamartoma of the temporal lobe. In the experience of Delgado-Escueta and Walsh, the outcome of anterior temporal lobectomy is excellent for seizure control when paroxysmal discharges arise from within the hippocampus or amygdala (534). Conversely, when the epileptic focus is outside the hippocampus or amygdala, response to this type of surgery is not as good (535). These results have been challenged by other workers and need to be confirmed. A consensus, however, suggests that the longer seizure control remains complete, the less likely is a recurrence. Improvement in the behavior disorder that often accompanies complex partial seizures usually parallels seizure control, but can take considerable time to become apparent. Results with children suggest that performing a temporal lobectomy at an earlier age leads to a better outcome than when the procedure is done during adult years (536). Postoperatively there appears to be a decrease in immediate and delayed verbal memory scores in preadolescent children. This is particularly evident in those who performed above the median preoperatively (537). Immediate verbal memory was more affected in those children who had a left temporal lobectomy.

Limited Temporal Resections

More restricted resections such as selective amygdalohippocampectomy (538) or selective lateral neocortical resections sparing the amygdala and the hippocampus (539) are performed in few centers and the indications for these procedures are not standardized. Hence, it is difficult to compare the outcome from these procedures with that from the standard anterior lobectomy. Even after the standard procedure, some patients with good seizure control continue to experience auras, suggesting that widely distributed areas extending beyond the resected regions may harbor epileptogenicity.

Extratemporal Neocortical Resections

Children with intractable simple partial seizures whose epileptic focus as determined by EEG and imaging studies is localized to the lateral convexity of the brain also can be suitable candidates for surgical resection of the affected area (540).

When partial seizures arise from a focus outside the limbic system or the temporal neocortex, the definition of the area of resection has to consider a possible overlap of the epileptogenic areas with areas of eloquent cortex such as the primary motor and somatosensory and language areas. To do so often requires invasive monitoring with subdural grids or strips to define the focus or foci, and stimulation studies to define and map eloquent areas. Both procedures require general anesthesia, and neither can be used in children for motor or language mapping. Alternate means of mapping the epileptogenic area include depth electrodes and intraoperative electrocorticography. In a series published in 1992, the risks of hemorrhage or infection from MRI-guided depth electrodes were less than 1% (541). Results from the Montreal Neurological Institute suggest that the outcome of frontal resections is not nearly as good as that of central, parietal, or occipital resections, probably because the epileptogenic area cannot be resected completely without sacrificing eloquent cortex (542). The percentage of patients who became completely free of seizures subsequent to surgery was 26% in frontal resections, as compared with 34% in central, parietal, and occipital resections. These

figures contrast with a 70% seizure-free rate after temporal lobectomies (542,543).

Section of Corpus Callosum

A small proportion of children with medically intractable complex partial seizures of frontal lobe origin and primary or secondary generalized tonic-clonic, atonic, clonic, or myoclonic seizures are suitable candidates for section of the corpus callosum (544,545). EEG in such cases generally demonstrates generalized or multifocal discharges arising from one or both hemispheres. The effectiveness of the procedure is based on interruption of the spread of epileptic discharges from one hemisphere to the other (546). Transection of the anterior two-thirds of the corpus callosum and complete transection have been used, with the latter procedure generally being more effective (547).

Complete transection of the corpus callosum and the anterior and hippocampal commissures produces an unusual cerebral disconnection syndrome. Patients experience difficulties performing tasks in which the sensory inflow is restricted to one hemisphere, and in which the response involves the hand for which the cortical representation is in the opposite hemisphere. Transient mutism also is encountered after surgery (524,548).

Children who improve the most as a result of this procedure are those with atypical absence, atonic (akinetic), and tonic-clonic seizures (549). Children with tonic seizures are least likely to be improved. At UCLA, the number of callosotomy procedures has decreased in recent years because of the reemergence of the ketogenic diet and the availability of vagus nerve stimulation.

Hemispherectomy

Hemispherectomy also has been used in the treatment of intractable seizures and developmental delay in children with lateralized zones of cortical abnormality. This can result from cortical dysplasias resulting from the various migrational disorders covered in Chapter 4, vascular infarcts, or the Sturge-Weber syndrome (see Chapter 11). Total hemispherectomy, in reality a hemicortectomy, spares the basal ganglia and thalamus. Functional hemispherectomy is a subtotal hemispherectomy involving resection of the central cortex and the temporal lobe with complete disconnection of the remaining abnormal cortex. The latter procedure was developed to avoid CNS hemosiderosis. This progressive and ultimately fatal syndrome of hydrocephalus and CNS hemosiderosis was seen in as many as one-third of patients after many seizure-free years. It was believed to result from a lack of adequate support for the remaining hemispheres and from consequent bouts of small bleeds into the intracranial cavity (550). However, in cases where there is no hemiparesis and the frontal lobe appears free of epileptiform discharges, a parieto-temporo-occipital resection that spares motor function can be performed.

Our own approach had been to drain the surgical cavity externally when the CSF is highly proteinaceous, and internalize a shunt when the CSF clears. This appears to minimize the possibility of pseudomembrane formation and to reduce the vulnerability to hemorrhagic complications as long-term sequelae of anatomic hemispherectomies. Rasmussen introduced the concept of the functional hemispherectomy, in which the central cortex and the temporal lobe are removed, leaving behind a frontal remnant and a parieto-occipital remnant, with a complete callosal resection and disconnection of the descending tracts (551). Our experience at UCLA suggests that seizure recurrence caused by incomplete disconnection is not an uncommon sequelae of the functional hemispherectomies. Our present approach at UCLA is the peri-insular hemispherotomy, a modified version of functional hemispherectomy introduced by Villemure and Mascott (552).

In the series of Tinuper and coworkers from the Montreal Neurological Institute, seizures remained totally controlled over an average follow-up period of 7 years in 78% of patients (550). Additionally, IQ improved significantly in the majority of patients without worsening of the hemiparesis. Preoperative unilateral hypometabolism, as disclosed on the PET scan, correlates with good surgical results (552a). Chugani and coworkers believe that the degree of functional recovery is greater if the procedure is performed

early in life than if it is delayed (552a). In his 1996 analysis of the data, Peacock reported that seizure control in the 50 patients who underwent hemispherectomy at UCLA with more than 1 year follow-up was 90% or better reduction in seizure frequency in 44 of 50 (88%). Motor function of the preoperatively hemiparetic extremities was improved or unchanged postoperatively in 38 of 50 (76%) of the patients (553). In a more recent analysis of the UCLA experience, Mathern and associates found that seizure relief and antiepileptic drug usage after resective surgery for symptomatic cortical dysplasia and noncortical dysplasia etiologies was comparable with complex partial temporal lobe epilepsy cases up to 2 years postsurgery (554). Furthermore, at 5 years postsurgery patients with cortical dysplasia had outcomes better than presurgery, but worse than temporal lobe epilepsy cases. Similar results have been reported from the Cleveland Clinic (555).

Vagal Nerve Stimulation

Intermittent stimulation of the vagus nerve using a neurocybernetic prosthesis is an approach to achieving seizure control that has been approved in the United States, Canada, and several European Union countries. The mechanism of action of vagal nerve stimulation is poorly understood. The vagus nerve consists of approximately 80% afferent fibers, and these fibers terminate in the nucleus of the solitary tract. Axons from this nucleus project to a number of cortical and subcortical structures including the amygdala, hippocampus, hypothalamus, thalamus, and the insular cortex.

Even though acute changes in neurotransmitter metabolites have been demonstrated in the CSF (556), the gradual increase in efficacy of chronic stimulation suggests some plastic changes in circuitry. Indeed, Henry and associates have shown that the increases in acute blood flow in the thalamus correlate with chronic efficacy of vagal nerve stimulation in reducing seizure frequency (557).

The programmable pulse generator (neurocybernetic prosthesis) is implanted in the patient's chest on the upper left side. The signals are conveyed to the vagus nerve by leads that terminate in helical, bipolar stimulating electrodes. Stimulation parameters are adjusted noninvasively via a radio frequency programming wand from a PC-compatible computer. The adjustable stimulation parameters include signal frequency (typically set at 30 Hz), signal pulse width (typically 500 μs), signal on time (typically 30 s), signal off time (typically 5 minutes), and the output current that is gradually increased over several visits in increments of 0.25 mA in the range of 0.25 to 4.0 mA. In our practice most children who receive benefit with the device do so between 1.5 and 3.0 mA. Those who have an aura can activate the device by a handheld magnet, if they perceive the aura between stimulations in the duty cycle to attempt aborting the seizure.

Clinical efficacy has been demonstrated in adults (558–560), as well as in children (561). Experience thus far suggests that partial as well as idiopathic and symptomatic generalized epilepsies are responsive. Efficacy is seen within 6 months after implantation and seems to improve up to 18 months. This method is especially valuable for children who remain refractory to available medical therapy or exhibit severe adverse reactions to antiepileptic drugs and whose epilepsies are not amenable to resective surgical therapy.

Treatment of Status Epilepticus (Convulsive Status Epilepticus)

A patient is said to be in status epilepticus when seizures occur so frequently that over the course of 30 or more minutes he or she has not recovered from the coma produced by one attack before the next attack supervenes. Status epilepticus is one of the few true emergencies in the practice of pediatric neurology. Consensus states that the more prolonged the status, the worse the outcome.

As has been reviewed elsewhere in this chapter, experimental studies indicate that convulsions lasting longer than 20 to 30 minutes can induce brain damage. Several systemic factors, acting singly or in concert, are believed to be responsible. During the initial stages of status (i.e., for the first 30 minutes or so) cardiac output

increases. Tachycardia and systemic hypertension lead to a two- to threefold increase in cerebral blood flow, with a marked increase in cerebral oxygen consumption. During this period plasma glucose and glucose uptake by the brain is increased. In due time, the brain requirements for oxygen outstrip its supply, and when status lasts longer than 30 to 60 minutes, decompensation sets in (562–564). From that time on, cerebral autoregulation breaks down, cardiac output decreases, and there is arterial hypotension and reduced cerebral perfusion. With increased oxygen demands and inadequate oxygen delivery to the brain, cellular metabolism energy fails, and with mitochondrial damage, the organ reverts to anaerobic metabolism with consequent cellular acidosis, increased CSF lactate, and cerebral edema. Ultimately, there is respiratory failure and hyperthermia (562).

Additionally, prolonged and abnormal electrical discharges, by themselves, can cause neuronal damage. The mechanism by which this occurs has not been fully substantiated, but involves enhanced glutaminergic excitatory transmission that leads to excessive depolarization of neurons and increased intracellular calcium and sodium. These ion changes initiate a cascade of events that lead to cell death (565). This subject is also reviewed in Chapters 5 and 15.

Status epilepticus is not part of the natural history of the epilepsies, but rather is a complication induced by changes in medication or intercurrent infections. Its incidence has increased with the advent of the newer anticonvulsant drugs, and in a study published in 1989, 3.7% of epileptic patients experienced one or more bouts of status epilepticus (566). In children, 85% of status epilepticus develops during the first 5 years of life and 25% during the first year of life (563).

Status epilepticus also can occur as an isolated phenomenon, particularly in children experiencing viral encephalitis or brain abscess or can occur after an open head injury, especially of the frontal lobes. It can be the initial epileptic attack in patients with secondary (symptomatic) epilepsy or can appear in the course of chronic primary (idiopathic) epilepsy. Maytal and coworkers (566) analyzed the causes of status epilepticus in children. In their series, approximately one-fourth of cases occurred without an obvious precipitating cause in patients who had a prior CNS insult. One-fourth were precipitated by fever and thus represented febrile convulsions, and one-fourth were caused by an acute neurologic insult, such as meningitis, trauma, and anoxia or were due to withdrawal of anticonvulsants. In approximately one-fourth, the precipitant for status was unknown.

Four sequential aspects to the management of the patient in status should be followed. They are (a) maintenance of vital functions, (b) institution of drug therapy to control convulsions, (c) diagnosis of the cause for the condition, and (d) prevention of further convulsions (567).

The physician who treats a child in status should act promptly to maintain an adequate airway, prevent aspiration of mucus, and secure the child from injury induced by the violence of the convulsions. Hyperthermia and hypotension should be corrected.

Several modes of therapy have been used, each with its advantages and disadvantages. We currently favor the use of lorazepam as the first-line anticonvulsant. The drug is highly lipid soluble and penetrates rapidly into the brain. Lorazepam is administered as an intravenous bolus at a dosage of 0.1 mg/kg, up to a maximum of 4 mg, or 0.06 mg/kg for children older than 13 years of age (568). The drug is administered over the course of 3 or more minutes. Should seizures continue for more than 10 minutes, the initial dose is repeated (569). In most children with generalized or focal status epilepticus, seizures stop within 5 minutes of the administration of lorazepam. The principal side effect is respiratory depression, which can require assisted ventilation. Unlike with diazepam, the likelihood of this complication is not increased by concurrent or antecedent administration of barbiturates. The serum half-life of lorazepam is approximately 15.7 hours (568), and sequential doses of lorazepam are often necessary; in the Los Angeles Children's Hospital series, sequential doses were used in 30% of cases (568). The effectiveness of lorazepam diminishes with successive doses.

Diazepam is another effective agent in the treatment of status epilepticus. Like lorazepam

it is highly lipid soluble and as judged from concurrent EEGs the drug enters the brain in 1.0 to 9.5 minutes (570). It is highly protein bound, and its redistribution within the body limits its duration of action within the brain to less than 30 minutes. This contrasts with an 8- to 12-hour duration of CNS action of lorazepam (571). Diazepam is administered intravenously at a dosage of 0.3 to 0.5 mg/kg, up to a maximum of 20 mg, and at a rate of 1 to 2 mg per minute (569). In one-third of patients, seizures stop within 3 minutes after diazepam is injected, and in the majority, within 5 minutes (572). From the range of suggested dosages and from clinical experience, it is apparent that the amount required for seizure control varies considerably among individuals. The principal advantages of diazepam are its rapid effectiveness, its margin of safety, and its ability to control seizures of cortical, as well as centrencephalic origin (573). The principal side effects of diazepam are respiratory depression and hypotension. They are most likely to occur in patients receiving a combination of drugs, particularly diazepam and phenobarbital (574).

Rectal diazepam (0.5 mg/kg for children aged 2 to 5 years, 0.3 mg/kg for children aged 6 years or older) is administered by means of a rubber tube inserted 4 to 5 cm beyond the anus. It appears to be a simple and safe means of controlling prolonged major motor seizures (575,576).

The use of intravenous phenytoin in the treatment of status epilepticus has been advocated by several groups (564,577). Phenytoin enters the brain more rapidly than phenobarbital, but not as rapidly as diazepam. Once phenytoin has controlled seizures, immediate recurrence is unlikely. The major drawback to phenytoin is its delivery into the circulation. For intravenous use, phenytoin should be mixed only in normal saline or half-normal saline; it is poorly soluble in dextrose 5% in water, and precipitates when mixed. Because of the likelihood of precipitation in nonalkaline saline solutions, phenytoin should not be diluted more than 100 mg/100 mL. A suitable volume is approximately 50 mL, and an in-line filter should be used. Phenytoin is given as an initial intravenous bolus of 10 mg/kg. To prevent cardiovascular toxicity, the drug is given at a rate of less than 1 mg/kg per minute (569,571). A second bolus of 5 mg/kg is given an hour later. This is followed by an intravenous maintenance dose of 10 mg/kg per 24 hours. Shorvon and Richard and coworkers recommend a somewhat higher loading dose (15 mg/kg), with subsequent intravenous doses adjusted according to blood levels obtained at 2 and 8 hours (564,578). The former group recommends changing to oral maintenance phenytoin at 28 hours. We prefer the use of carbamazepine or phenobarbital for maintenance after status, particularly in infants and small children.

The main advantages of phenytoin are a half-life of 24 or more hours and lack of significant CNS depression. For this reason the drug is usually preferred for patients with status following a head injury, in whom preservation of consciousness is desirable. The anticonvulsant should not be administered intramuscularly, because it is absorbed too slowly to result in effective anticonvulsant serum and tissue levels (579).

Fosphenytoin, a disodium phosphate ester of phenytoin, has found wide acceptance for the treatment of status and in many centers has replaced phenytoin. The drug is completely water soluble and is rapidly and completely converted to phenytoin. It can be administered both intravenously at a dosage of 10 to 20 mg/kg, or intramuscularly (577,580). Holmes and Riviello recommend its use in children whose status has lasted longer than 10 minutes (581). Evrard and colleagues recommend prompt combined treatment with a benzodiazepine such as lorazepam, which has GABAergic action and counteracts the excitatory effect of released glutamate, with phenytoin in the form of fosphenytoin, which antagonizes the release of excitatory amino acids, and believe that these two drugs have a synergistic effect (582).

Another means of controlling status epilepticus is by the use of sodium phenobarbital. The initial dose of 15 mg/kg is administered intravenously at a rate of 2 mg/kg per minute intramuscularly, or even subcutaneously. Because the drug requires 15 minutes to penetrate the blood–brain barrier regardless of its mode of administration, the rate at which seizures are controlled is slower than with lorazepam or diazepam, and it is now reserved for those children whose seizures have failed to respond to a benzodiazepine within 15 to 40 minutes after its administration (581).

If phenobarbital is to be used as a backup to a benzodiazepine, the child must be intubated. Aside from its slow rate of action, the disadvantages of phenobarbital are the depression of consciousness and respiration when the drug is used in dosages required for the control of status epilepticus (583).

Refractory seizures are seizures that have continued for 60 minutes or longer despite adequate anticonvulsant therapy. They frequently develop in the presence of acute CNS injury, or a neurodegenerative disease. When brain edema is suspected, as is the case when status follows a head injury, corticosteroids or other antiedematous agents should be given. In addition, one may have to resort to midazolam or pentobarbital. Midazolam, an injectable benzodiazepine, is given in a bolus dose of 0.2 mg/kg, followed by an infusion of 1 to 5 µg/kg per minute (584). Pentobarbital is given in a loading dose of 5 to 15 mg/kg, followed by a maintenance infusion of 1 to 5 mg/kg per hour (581), with the dosages of pentobarbital being adjusted to maintain an EEG burst suppression pattern (585). Although monitoring the electrical activity of the brain whenever a patient is in status is always desirable, this measure becomes mandatory in the patient with refractory status (569,581).

Other drugs that have been used for the treatment of status epilepticus include intravenous valproate (10 to 20 mg/kg) and lidocaine (586,587). Clinical experience with long-term use of lidocaine is limited, however.

Whatever the means for treating status, the physician must keep in mind that the intravenous route is the preferred way to administer anticonvulsants; that the most common mistake is to give repeated, yet insufficient, doses of anticonvulsants; and that he or she should avoid using more than one anticonvulsant drug.

Following termination of status, the patient is maintained on parenteral anticonvulsant therapy, until the patient has regained consciousness. Oral medication is then resumed. With successive doses the effectiveness of lorazepam and diazepam is progressively reduced, and these agents cannot be used for long-term seizure control.

With prompt and appropriate therapy, mortality owing to status has fallen to essentially nil. However, a significant percentage of patients can die as a consequence of the condition that precipitated status. In the 1989 series of Maytal and coworkers, no deaths occurred in 137 children with unprovoked or febrile status (566). In the series of Phillips and Shanahan, also published in 1989, only 1% of patients died (588). With current therapy, the incidence of residua is low and is essentially nil when status results from a febrile seizure. Although some 9% of children are left with new motor or cognitive deficits, these usually are the consequence of the underlying neurologic condition that caused status. In terms of outcome, the duration of status is less important than its etiology (566). The clinician who cares for children who have experienced an episode of status should keep in mind that such children have a 4% to 6% likelihood of experiencing one or more additional episodes of status, and that children who have had more than one episode of status have approximately a one in three risk of further episodes (589).

Prognosis

The outcome of medical therapy for epilepsy depends on the type of seizure and its natural course (590). Generally, spontaneous remission or control of seizures by anticonvulsants is greatest in children with idiopathic seizures and age of onset between 2 and 12 years (591). Clinically, such children have normal intellect, no abnormalities on neurologic examination, and no focal lesions on imaging studies. In the experience of Camfield and coworkers who studied children with generalized tonic-clonic, partial, and partial with secondarily generalized seizures, 83% were successfully treated with a single anticonvulsant. Treatment was more likely to be successful in children with generalized tonic-clonic seizures, and treatment failures were more likely in children with complex partial seizures. Of the 17% of children who did not respond to the first anticonvulsant, 42% ulti-

mately became free of seizures and were in remission at the end of 4 or more years (592). As in most other studies, the success of anticonvulsant treatment for children with neurologic deficits was significantly less than in the remainder of the study group.

Between 25% and 83% of children younger than 16 years of age who have had a single nonfebrile seizure experience a recurrence, with the median time to recurrence 5.7 months. In the series of Shinnar and colleagues, 88% of recurrences occurred within 2 years, and only 3% recurred after 5 years (593). The lower recurrence figures are derived from prospective studies (594), whereas the higher figures are derived from retrospective studies (595). As many as 70% of the group with recurrent seizures have only a small number of further attacks before going into remission, which in approximately 90% is permanent (596). In 30% seizures continued. These chronic cases constitute the mainstay of a pediatric neurologist's practice. With successful treatment of children in this group, some 30% enter a long remission, whereas 70% continue to experience occasional seizures despite adequate therapy and compliance. Generally, the longer the period between the onset of seizures and their control, the less likely the chance for significant remissions. The remission rate is 60% if seizures do not come under control within a year of their onset. This contrasts with a remission rate of 10% if seizures remain uncontrolled for more than 4 years, and 5% for those who continue to experience seizures for 10 or more years after their diagnosis (597). However, even in medically intractable seizures, frequency of attacks tend to diminish over the years, especially in those who maintain a normal IQ (598).

Some clinical features can be singled out for prognostic significance.

Remissions occurred in 13% of neurologically intact children with grand mal epilepsy who had experienced fewer than 20 such seizures (599) and in 75% to 80% of children with childhood absence (petit mal) epilepsy (600). In our experience, it is the rare child with normal intelligence whose seizures are not completely or nearly completely controlled with adequate medical supervision and good compliance. Despite good seizure control, the social outcome is not as favorable. In part, this is because of associated learning disorders, and in part, the consequence of a chronic illness (601).

Adverse prognostic factors include partial or mixed seizures, an abnormal neurologic examination, mental retardation, and inadequate seizure control during the early years of the disorder (602). Complete remission is least likely in children with minor motor attacks.

A particularly favorable prognosis is seen in the following seizures:

Sylvian seizures (i.e., attacks in which the EEG demonstrates a centrotemporal spike discharge) and the other benign partial epilepsies of childhood (603)

Partial seizures on falling asleep or waking, absences, or brief atonic and myoclonic seizures in which the EEG demonstrates continuous, generalized spike-wave paroxysmal activity during sleep

Benign myoclonic seizures

Nocturnal myoclonus

Absence seizures also have a favorable prognosis. In a follow up performed 15 years after seizure onset, 65% of patients were in remission, and 18% were taking anticonvulsants. Of the latter group 38% were seizure free. Seventeen percent were not taking anticonvulsants and continued to experience seizures. Of the total cohort, 15% had progressed to juvenile myoclonic epilepsy. The factors that predicted treatment failure included the presence of cognitive problems, development of nonconvulsive status, the appearance of tonic-clonic seizures after the onset of anticonvulsant therapy, an abnormal EEG background, and a history of generalized seizures in first-degree relatives (604).

Of patients with complex partial seizures, 84% experienced complete seizure control at the end of the first year (592); 61% were in remission at the end of 4 or more years; 35% experienced sporadic seizures, and 4% had intractable epilepsy. Favorable predictive signs in complex partial seizures are good intelligence, a family history of seizures, and a right temporal seizure focus. According to Lindsay and colleagues, unfavorable factors include early onset of

seizures, frequent grand mal seizures, an associated hyperkinetic syndrome, and attacks of rage during childhood (605).

Approximately one-third of patients with nocturnal tonic-clonic seizures ultimately can be expected to experience daytime attacks as well (606). Although there are no controlled studies that determine whether early and effective anticonvulsant therapy influences the chances for a spontaneous remission, Reynolds and other members of his group, including Shorvon, believe that epilepsy must be treated early and effectively to preclude the evolution of a chronic epileptic condition (596,607). We agree with their position.

Aside from dying from unrelated disorders, epileptic patients can die in status epilepticus as a consequence of their underlying brain disease (e.g., tumor or a CNS degenerative disorder), accidentally as a result of a seizure, and, most perplexing, without any apparent cause. Patients in the last group usually experience tonic-clonic seizures that before death appeared to have been relatively well controlled. Approximately one-half die in their sleep and less than 10% have therapeutic anticonvulsant blood levels at the time of death (608). The most likely explanation for their demise is that it is a seizure-related event, possibly neurogenic pulmonary edema (609,610).

Although older studies suggested that intellectual deterioration was relatively common in subjects whose seizures were secondary to cerebral injury or malformation, there are few modern data to support or refute this observation. A prospective study, reported in 1986, did not find a difference between IQs of neurologically normal seizure patients and their normal siblings, and it failed to demonstrate deterioration of IQ as a consequence of seizures (611). The data of Huttenlocher and Hapke, published in 1990, confirm these observations (598).

Despite these optimistic data, without doubt a significant percentage of patients with recurrent seizures, some 15% in the experience of Trimble, deteriorate intellectually over time (612). Examination of patients in Trimble's group revealed that they had significantly higher serum levels of phenytoin and primidone, and lower folic acid levels than the group who did not experience deterioration. When seizure frequency was factored out, these findings still persisted with respect to phenytoin and folic acid. Other studies also have implicated anticonvulsant therapy, particularly polytherapy, in intellectual deterioration. Addy concluded that an association between poor cognitive function and phenobarbital or phenytoin intake has been reported too often to continue considering them as first-line anticonvulsants for the pediatric population (613). Trimble and his group have demonstrated that phenobarbital and phenytoin, given singly or jointly, impair immediate and delayed memory, and interfere with performance on visual and auditory scanning tasks (612). Eliminating polytherapy or changing the anticonvulsant to carbamazepine tended to improve cognitive function within 3 months. Even with therapeutic anticonvulsant levels of drugs such as phenobarbital, children experience subtle cognitive effects (614). Carbamazepine or valproic acid probably produce less striking cognitive impairment than phenobarbital.

Behavior disturbances are common in epileptic children. In part, they stem from the deleterious effects of a chronic illness, but frequently they, too, are induced by drug therapy and disappear spontaneously once the anticonvulsant is withdrawn (615). Additionally, it is likely that children with complex partial seizures are particularly prone to disordered behavior. Abnormal behavior or psychoses also can be part of the ictal phenomenon, as in some patients with absence status, or they can follow a seizure (616).

In view of the adverse effects of long-term anticonvulsant therapy, medication should be withdrawn as soon as feasible. There has been considerable controversy about when drugs should be discontinued after prolonged seizure control. Several studies have attempted to answer this question and have found that recurrence risks are similar after seizure-free intervals of 2, 3, or 4 years (591,617,618).

Holowach and coworkers discontinued anticonvulsants after 4 years of seizure control and encountered a relapse rate of 28%, which increased by another 4% when the follow-up was extended to 15 years (619). More than one-half of recurrences were seen during the first year after anticonvulsant withdrawal and 85% occurred by 5 years after withdrawal. Other studies have come up with similar recurrence rates, even though in some studies drug withdrawal was started after a 2-year seizure-free interval (599,620). Neither the sex of the patient nor the age when drugs are withdrawn affect the relapse rate. Children with neurologic dysfunction or an abnormal neurologic examination have a higher incidence of recurrence. The relapse rate was highest in children with juvenile myoclonic epilepsy and complex partial seizures and lowest in benign rolandic epilepsy and absence seizures (620). These results probably reflect the relatively high proportion of patients with idiopathic epilepsy in the last two groups. In the experience of some workers, the age of seizure onset also influences the likelihood of relapse. The prognosis is poorest for those with onset younger than 2 years of age, less so for those with seizure onset at age 12 years or older, and best for those with onset between 2 and 12 years of age (591). Children with seizure onset after 12 years of age had a higher risk for recurrence (618). By contrast, Gherpelli and colleagues noted that the age of seizure onset did not influence the likelihood for recurrence after anticonvulsant withdrawal, but found that in their series the greater the number of seizures experienced by the patient before control, the greater the likelihood for relapse (621).

Whether the EEG can predict a relapse is still unresolved. Whereas Thurston and coworkers (619) did not consider EEG findings to be an important predictor of seizure recurrence, Shinnar and coworkers, Tennison and coworkers, and Peters and colleagues did (618,620,622). In the experience of Shinnar and coworkers, EEG slowing, but not epileptiform features, signaled an increased risk for relapse (620). Tennison and coworkers and Peters and colleagues found that the presence of paroxysmal EEG discharges was predictive for recurrence (618,622). As a rule, the EEG is more predictive for relapse in children with idiopathic epilepsy than in those with epilepsy secondary to a known CNS abnormality (617). In all studies, risk of recurrence has been highest during the first few months after withdrawal, with 50% or more of recurrences occurring within 6 months after withdrawal was initiated (617,619). Callaghan and coworkers found that the factors predictive for relapse are the same as in an adult population (623). The rate of anticonvulsant withdrawal does not appear to influence the frequency of relapse, although withdrawal over the course of less than a month is inadvisable, and abrupt withdrawal is known to initiate status epilepticus (622).

Based on these studies, we consider withdrawal of anticonvulsants after approximately 2 years of seizure control. Generally, we withdraw medication over 2 to 3 months. When the child has been on polytherapy, one drug is completely stopped before the other is tapered.

The social problems incurred by an epileptic child in terms of his or her relationship to family and peers are so considerable that they are beyond the scope of this book. The reader is referred to books by O'Donohoe (140) and the chapter by Craig and Oxley in the volume by Laidlaw and colleagues (624) for a more extensive discussion.

In our opinion epileptic children should participate in all normal activities, including sports. Children should be permitted to swim with a friend in a supervised pool. The hyperventilation incurred in the more strenuous athletics is accompanied by a buildup of carbon dioxide, and therefore should not induce seizures. The more hazardous contact sports, such as high school football, are best avoided, however, as they should be for nonepileptic youngsters, and swimming should be done under competent adult supervision (624,626). Kemp and Sibert, who reviewed drowning accidents in epileptic children, found that no child who participated in supervised swimming drowned (625). Most states and countries restrict an epileptic patient from driving a car. Considering the likelihood that a youngster who has been seizure free for 2 or more years will continue to be seizure free, we have no hesitation in recommending such a patient for a driver's license. When it comes to withdrawing medication in such a youngster, we are reluctant to do so, for fear that seizure recurrence will result in loss of the license. The dilemma between maintaining anticonvulsants for longer than necessary and inducing a serious social inconvenience requires an individualized decision.

Specific Seizure Types

Febrile Seizures

The term *febrile seizure* is used to designate seizures associated with fever, but it excludes those caused by infections of the CNS. By definition, a minimum body temperature of 37.8° to 38.5° C or 100.1° to 101.4° F is required for a seizure to be considered febrile. Febrile seizures represent one of the most common neurologic disorders of childhood. In 1924, Patrick and Levy found an incidence of 4.2% of febrile seizures in an unselected group of children attending Well Baby Clinics (627). Several other subsequent studies have shown an incidence between 2% and 4% (628–630). The condition is somewhat more common in male subjects.

Etiology and Clinical Manifestations

The cause for febrile seizures is still unknown. Certainly, genetic factors play an important role. In the series of Berg and colleagues (630), 24% of children with febrile seizures had a first-degree relative with febrile seizures; only 20% had no family history of febrile seizures. The mode of inheritance has not been established, but an autosomal dominant or a polygenic transmission appears to be the most likely (628). From clinical and genetic studies it has become evident that the genes for febrile seizures differ from those causing afebrile seizures. At least four autosomal dominant genes for febrile seizures have been mapped by genetic linkage studies. These have been localized to chromosome 19p13.3, 19q, 8q13-21 (631,632), and 2q23-34 (632a). The gene defect localized to chromosome 19p is a mutation in the sodium channel beta1 subunit SCN1B (632b).

In the prospective study of Berg and colleagues, only 4% of children with febrile seizures had a first-degree relative with afebrile seizures (630). Berg also pointed out that if febrile seizures were a manifestation of epilepsy, the risk for a second febrile seizure would equal the risk for a second afebrile seizure. In actuality the risk for the former was 34% as compared with a risk of 2% to 3% for afebrile seizures. Additionally, the factors that predict recurrent febrile seizures, namely young age and a family history of febrile seizures, do not predict occurrence of subsequent afebrile seizures (633).

In most patients, the height of body temperature appears to be an important factor in triggering the seizures, and Millichap has postulated a convulsive threshold beyond which the seizure is precipitated (3,634). Although the rate at which body temperature increases has been frequently cited as a contributing factor in the development of seizures, EEG data obtained on children with artificially induced fever indicate that this is not the case (635). What appears clear, however, is that in a significant proportion of infants a febrile seizure occurs at the same time or shortly after fever is recognized. In the series of Berg and colleagues, 44% of infants had experienced less than 1 hour of fever at the time of their febrile convulsion; only 13% had fever of more than 24 hours' duration (630). Other authors concur with this observation. In the experience of Autret and colleagues, a febrile seizure was the first manifestation of an illness in 42% of infants treated for febrile seizures (636). Another risk factor is a history of febrile convulsions in a first-degree relative (634).

Aside from human herpesvirus 6 infections and roseola (exanthema subitum), which are responsible for some one-third of first-time febrile seizures (629,637), epidemic diseases are a relatively infrequent cause of febrile seizures. More commonly, a convulsion accompanies an upper respiratory infection or severe gastroenteritis, particularly when caused by *Shigella* (638,639). In none of the infectious illnesses has there been evidence for direct involvement of the brain by the organisms. From these data, the best conclusion is that febrile seizures occur when, as a result of genetic predisposition, the immature neuronal membrane is particularly susceptible to temperature elevations and responds by breaking down.

The first febrile seizure occurs between 6 months and 3 years of age in 93% of affected children (3). Generally, patients with febrile seizures are considered to consist of two distinct groups: the majority (96.9%) has an entity Liv-

ingston designated as a simple febrile seizure (507). The remainder (3.1%) had complex febrile seizures. These are defined as seizures of greater than 30 minutes' duration, seizures repeated within the same day, or having focal features.

Diagnosis

In the child who has just experienced a first febrile seizure, the clinician is frequently called on to make a decision with respect to obtaining a lumbar puncture, neuroimaging studies, and a subsequent EEG.

Whether the infant who has just experienced his or her first febrile seizure should undergo a lumbar puncture has been a matter of some debate. Despite Lorber and Sunderland's advocacy for a selective lumbar puncture (640), we believe that the diagnostic skills required to ascertain whether an infant is more ill than his or her physical signs suggest are so considerable that it is best to err on the side of safety and perform the tap. This is particularly so for infants younger than 2 months of age, and the study of Green and coworkers documenting the low incidence of occult meningitis in children between the ages of 2 months and 15 years does little to alter our stance (641).

We do not believe that the neurologically healthy child who has experienced his or her first febrile seizure should undergo neuroimaging studies. Freeman and Vining concur with our position (642).

The EEG is of little value in predicting recurrence of febrile seizures or the evolution of afebrile seizures. In the Bulgarian series of Sofijanov and colleagues, the EEG, taken 7 to 20 days after a febrile seizure, was normal or nonspecifically abnormal in 78% of children (643). A paroxysmal abnormality was found in 20%, with a generalized or focal fast spike and wave discharge being the most commonly observed paroxysmal abnormality. Stores found a far lower incidence of paroxysmal discharges (1.4% to 3.0%). Their presence was of no predictive value, and he believes that the procedure made more trouble than it was worth (644). Freeman and Vining also consider an EEG to be unnecessary after a first febrile seizure (642). We, too, believe that the EEG only rarely contributes to the management of infants with febrile seizures, but find that, in general, the medically sophisticated population in Southern California expects or even demands this procedure.

Treatment

Treatment of the febrile seizure consists of controlling the convulsion with anticonvulsants in dosages analogous to those recommended for the treatment of status epilepticus, reduction of body temperature by conductive or evaporative cooling of the patient, and treatment of the acute infection responsible for the fever.

There is considerable controversy as to the management of a child who has experienced his or her first febrile seizure. The evidence is overwhelming that antipyretics do not prevent recurrence of febrile seizure (645). Neither phenobarbital nor oral diazepam (0.2 mg/kg) administered at the time of illness have been effective when given singly or in combination (646,647). Somewhat better results have been obtained with higher doses of diazepam (0.33 mg/kg).

Current consensus, however, proposes that patients who have one or more of the risk factors cited in the section on prognosis should be considered for treatment with continuous prophylactic medication (648). The effectiveness of continuous prophylactic phenobarbital is controversial. Wolf found that febrile seizures could be prevented by maintaining phenobarbital levels at 15 µg/mL or more; two more recent studies suggest that prophylactic treatment with phenobarbital does not lessen the risk for recurrence (352,646,649). However, in both series, drug levels were either unavailable or subtherapeutic in a large proportion of children who had seizure recurrence. Behavior disorders are common in children on long-term phenobarbital, particularly in those who have had an antecedent history of behavior disturbances (646). Additionally, the IQ of children receiving prophylactic phenobarbital is significantly lower than that of controls (352).

Administration of rectal diazepam at the onset of a febrile illness provides an alternative to phenobarbital treatment. This approach appears to reduce significantly the risk for a sub-

sequent febrile seizure, but does not prolong the time between the first febrile seizure and the next breakthrough (650). Administration of rectal phenobarbital at the onset of a febrile illness is ineffective (651). Neither phenytoin (652) nor carbamazepine (653) are effective in preventing recurrences. Although in some series valproic acid (30 mg/kg per day) appeared to prevent subsequent febrile seizures (654,655), this has not been confirmed (649).

Continuous prophylactic anticonvulsant therapy has been considered for children without risk factors. However, with only a 30% likelihood of a recurrence of the first febrile seizure, and no evidence that treatment of febrile seizures prevents subsequent afebrile (i.e., epileptic) seizures or has an adverse effect on intellect, the only rationale for treating febrile seizures in such children is to allay family anxiety. When treatment has been elected for children who are developmentally delayed or who have an abnormal neurologic examination, phenobarbital is given for approximately 1 to 2 years, monitoring blood levels. Should we encounter side effects, we change to oral or rectal diazepam (0.5 mg/kg per day) to be given at the onset of subsequent fevers.

Prognosis

Three aspects of prognosis are usually of concern to the family and to the physician: the likelihood of further febrile convulsions, the likelihood of subsequent afebrile seizures, and the likelihood that a prolonged febrile seizure will induce permanent neurologic or intellectual damage.

Most studies predict that approximately one-third of infants who experience a febrile seizure will experience one or more further febrile seizures. The risk for recurrence is greatest in the first 6 to 12 months after the initial seizure, and the likelihood for recurrence is enhanced in infants who convulse at temperatures below 40° C. A family history for either febrile or afebrile seizures makes a recurrence more likely, as does an initial febrile seizure at an early age, the last factor simply by increasing the length of time during which the child is susceptible to further febrile convulsions (656). The duration of the initial seizure does not influence the likelihood of a recurrent febrile seizure (656).

Five risk factors predispose the child with febrile seizures to subsequent epilepsy (639, 657–660). In order of importance they are antecedent neurologic or developmental abnormalities, epilepsy in a first-degree relative, complex febrile seizures, onset of febrile seizures before 1 year of age, and multiple recurrences of febrile seizures (661). The importance of prior neurologic deficits in increasing the likelihood for subsequent afebrile seizures has been stressed by Maytal and Shinnar who noted that a complex febrile seizure does not increase the risk for subsequent afebrile seizures in an infant who is neurologically normal (662). Other studies, including the British cohort study of Verity and colleagues, have come to similar conclusions (663).

In the collaborative study conducted under the auspices of the National Institutes of Health, the incidence of epilepsy by 7 years of age was 1.1% in children with febrile seizures who did not have any of the previously mentioned risk factors. This compared with an incidence of 0.5% in the general population. In the Mayo Clinic study by Annegers and coworkers, the cumulative risk for subsequent epilepsy in children with febrile seizures was 2.4% (660). In children whose neurologic status before their first febrile seizure was not normal, and whose first febrile seizure was severe, the incidence of epilepsy rose to 9.2% (657). A similar greater risk of afebrile seizures is seen in children with focal, prolonged, or repeated febrile seizures, being 50% when all these factors were combined (660). Probably a preexisting brain abnormality predisposes to both complex febrile seizures and subsequent afebrile seizures.

Afebrile seizures after febrile seizures are usually major motor and tend to appear within 1 year after the first febrile seizures (Table 13.14) (657,658,660,664).

Autopsy studies performed on the rare infant who died after a prolonged febrile seizure reveal anoxic changes affecting the hippocampus, neocortex, thalamus, and cerebellum. It is not clear whether these alterations represent precursors to mesial temporal sclerosis, which is a common pathologic finding in patients with complex partial seizures (158). MRI studies are commensu-

TABLE 13.14. *Time of appearance of spontaneous nonfebrile seizures in relation to onset of febrile seizures in 313 patients with both types of seizures*

Time of appearance of nonfebrile seizures	Patients with febrile seizures	
	Number	Percent
Before febrile seizures	20	6.4
Close to febrile seizures	21	6.7
Years after febrile seizures		
1 mo to 1 yr	147	46.9
1–4	54	17.3
5–9	47	15.1
10–14	14	4.5
15–35	10	3.1

Modified from Lennox WG. Significance of febrile convulsions. *Pediatrics* 1953;11:341.

rate with pathologic examination. In adults with temporal lobe epilepsy who provided a history of prolonged febrile seizures, neuroimaging uncovered a higher incidence of atrophy of the amygdala and mesial temporal sclerosis than in patients with temporal lobe seizures who had not experienced prolonged febrile convulsions (665). Fernández and coworkers suggest that in familial febrile convulsions a subtle preexisting malformation of the hippocampus, possibly a migrational disturbance, is a prerequisite for the development of hippocampal sclerosis after febrile convulsions (666). Although at least one-third of patients with complex partial seizures have a retrospective history of febrile seizures, prospective studies, which might not have been carried out long enough, show an incidence of complex partial seizures in only 4.3% of children who develop epilepsy after febrile seizures (658).

Although intuitively one would expect that prolonged febrile seizures are detrimental to ultimate intellectual function, the IQs of children who were developmentally normal before their first seizure and who did not have any subsequent afebrile seizures were no lower than the IQs of their asymptomatic siblings, regardless of the duration of the first febrile seizure (667,668). These observations are confirmed by more recent studies published in 1998 (669). Complications of febrile seizures are extremely rare: death occurs in 0.08% and persistent hemiplegia is unusual (639,657,670). Subsequent mental retardation was noted in only 1% of 400 children with febrile seizures; in none did the febrile seizure last longer than 5 minutes, and one-half of the mentally retarded children already had a history of delayed milestones before their first febrile seizure (651).

Neonatal Seizures

Because seizures occur with relatively high frequency during the neonatal period and present special problems for diagnosis and treatment, they are considered separately.

Etiology

The incidence rate of seizures during the neonatal period ranges between 2.0 and 2.8 in 1,000 live births for term neonates. It is 13.5 in 1,000 live births for infants weighing less than 2,500 g, and 57.5 in 1,000 for infants weighing less than 1,500 g (671,672). The various causes for seizures during the newborn period and their relative frequency as determined by autopsy are presented in Table 13.15 (673). Currently, the most common identifiable causes are hypoxic-ischemic encephalopathy and infections, especially sepsis and bacterial meningitis (see Chapter 6). In the study of Ronen and coworkers, prenatal, perinatal, and postnatal hypoxic ischemic encephalopathy accounted for 40% of neonatal seizures, and infections for 20% of neonatal seizures (672). Physical trauma, resulting in intracerebral and intraventricular hemorrhage, is less common. Developmental anomalies of the brain are probably more common than would appear from the data of Mizrahi (673) and the autopsy series of Volpe (674) because a large proportion of infants with these anomalies do not die from them, and others who have a poor Apgar score are frequently included in the group with hypoxic-ischemic encephalopathy.

Characteristically, seizures owing to perinatal asphyxia and its complications start within the first 24 hours of life. According to Volpe, 60% of asphyxiated infants who experience a seizure have their first seizure within 12 hours of birth (674). Neonatal seizures owing to developmental

TABLE 13.15. *Etiology of neonatal seizures (1971 and 1986)*

Etiology	Percent (1986)	Percent (1971)
Hypoxic-ischemic encephalopathy	46	36
Infection	17	4
Intracerebral hemorrhage	7	
Intraventricular hemorrhage	6	
Infarction	6	
Hypoglycemia	5	5
Congenital anomaly of CNS	4	6
Inborn errors of metabolism	4	
Subarachnoid hemorrhage	2	
Unknown	2	23
Hypocalcemia	0	31

Modified from Mizrahi EM. Neonatal seizures: problems in diagnosis and classification. *Epilepsia* 1987;28 [Suppl]:S46.

defects also start in the first 3 days of life; the age when seizures start, therefore, will not assist in diagnosing their etiology, or in the case of a perinatal asphyxial insult, its timing (675).

Hypoglycemic seizures are relatively common during the neonatal period, but as shown in Table 13.15, hypocalcemic seizures have become extremely rare over the last three decades. In the series of Ronen and colleagues, published in 1999, seizures caused by hypocalcemia or hypomagnesemia accounted for 5.6% of neonatal seizures (672). Hypoglycemic seizures are more common in small-for-gestational-age infants and offspring of diabetic mothers, and generally they appear during the second day of life. In the majority of these children, hypoglycemia is preceded by perinatal asphyxia or other causes for perinatal stress (672). A more extensive discussion of these seizures can be found in Chapter 15. Seizures are common in newborn infants who have infections of various types, the most important being sepsis and bacterial meningitis. These conditions are covered in Chapter 6.

The narcotic withdrawal syndrome in newborn infants of mothers who are narcotics addicts has been recognized with increased frequency in recent years. Although seizures are uncommon among these infants, they have been observed in the most severely affected. Seizures are most likely to be encountered in infants born to mothers taking barbiturates, particularly the short-acting type, in neonates passively addicted to alcohol, and in infants born to methadone-addicted mothers (676). Signs of neonatal withdrawal usually appear during the first or second day of life, but can be delayed for up to several days.

In exceptional instances, inborn errors of metabolism are responsible for neonatal seizures (see Chapter 1).

Clinical Manifestations

Only a small fraction of neonates experience classic tonic-clonic convulsions (677). Rather, neonatal seizures are difficult to recognize, and their appearance reflects the immature nervous system of the newborn infant and its inability to propagate epileptic discharges. Volpe delineated these various seizure types in order of decreasing frequency: subtle, tonic, multifocal clonic, focal clonic, and generalized focal or multifocal myoclonic seizures (674,678). In the EEG-monitored series of Scher and colleagues, subtle seizures were also the most common and accounted for 71% of seizures seen in term infants, and 68% of seizures seen in preterm infants (675). Other workers have encountered a much lower incidence of subtle seizures (672,679). It is possible that because of their unimpressive clinical appearance subtle seizures are frequently overlooked. Subtle seizures (or motor automatisms) are characterized by rhythmic eye movement, chewing, or unusual rowing, swimming, or pedaling movements of arms and legs. Tonic seizures can be generalized or focal. Generalized tonic seizures are more common and are marked by sustained hyperextension of the upper and lower extremities or of the trunk and neck. Focal or multifocal clonic movements of the extremities are usually at one to three jerks per second. They can be distinguished from tremor or jitteriness, which is observed in approximately one-half of healthy neonates, by the fact that in the latter condition, the rate of rhythmic movements is faster, usually five to six per second. The movements in jitteriness are of equal amplitude around a fixed axis and can be stopped by restraining or repositioning the limb (680). Other seizure forms include symmetric posturing of limbs or trunk, and atonic attacks

characterized by arrest of movement with the infant becoming limp and unresponsive. In the experience of Mizrahi and Kellaway, apnea was never seen as the sole seizure manifestation (677). In the series of Ronen and colleagues, apneic seizures were more frequently seen in infants of less than 38 weeks' gestation (672).

When seizures are correlated with simultaneously recorded EEG, it becomes evident that not all seizure types are accompanied by cortical seizure activity and that not all electrocortical seizures are clinically manifest (electroclinical disassociation) (677,681). In particular, motor automatisms and generalized tonic seizures can occur without associated EEG seizure activity, implying that these movements originate from subcortical gray matter or that they represent brainstem-release phenomena. Mizrahi and Kellaway favor the latter alternative and argue against treatment of these phenomena with anticonvulsants for fear of further depression of the higher centers (677).

Although these various seizure forms cannot yet be related to gestational age or to etiology, seizures without corresponding EEG abnormalities are more likely to be seen after hypoxic-ischemic encephalopathy and are a poor prognostic sign. In a significant proportion of nonparalyzed term infants, EEG seizures occur in the absence of obvious clinical findings. In the series of Connell and coworkers, clinical seizures accompanied EEG seizures in only 47% of term infants; in approximately two-thirds of these, the clinical evidence for seizures was not at all obvious (679). As many as 70% of preterm infants do not show any clinical evidence for seizures despite a concurrent paroxysmal EEG (679).

Treatment

The primary concern of the physician treating the neonate with seizures is the immediate identification of those causes that are amenable to specific treatment. Therefore, appropriate studies must be performed to exclude sepsis, meningitis, hypoglycemia, hyponatremia, hypocalcemia, and hypomagnesemia. Intramuscular pyridoxine (25 to 50 mg) also should be given as a therapeutic trial to exclude pyridoxine dependency (682).

When the underlying cause for seizures cannot be treated specifically, the physician must be content with symptomatic therapy. Phenobarbital is the anticonvulsant most commonly used during the neonatal period. The drug is administered in an intramuscular or intravenous loading dose of 15 to 20 mg/kg, with the intravenous dose being given over the course of 15 minutes. Loading doses of up to 30 mg/kg are well tolerated (683). Peak concentrations are reached within 1 to 6 hours, and maintenance dosages of 3 to 4 mg/kg per day are initiated once the blood barbiturate level falls below 15 to 20 μg/mL. Because the drug has a half-life of more than 6 days in the neonate, this usually does not occur until 5 to 7 days of age (683–685). These drug schedules apply irrespective of the gestational age of the infant. Nevertheless, for optimal seizure control, daily or twice daily barbiturate levels must be secured, with optimal levels being between 16 and 40 μg/mL (678,681).

We have not had much success controlling neonatal seizures using oral or parenteral phenytoin. Painter and coworkers have found intravenous phenytoin to be equally effective as phenobarbital in controlling seizures (686). In our experience, the relation between drug dosage and serum levels is unpredictable, and toxic reactions are common, probably because of the immaturity of the hepatic hydroxylating system responsible for phenytoin detoxification. The drug is administered orally or parenterally in dosages of 5 to 15 mg/kg per day (687). The experience with fosphenytoin has been similar in that therapeutic serum phenytoin levels are difficult to maintain (688).

Diazepam given intravenously (0.5 mg/kg) also has been suggested as an anticonvulsant in the newborn infant, although it is no better than phenobarbital for the treatment of neonatal seizures (674). Also, its short half-life (18 hours in term infants) makes it a poor drug for maintenance (681).

Intravenous lidocaine has been used by European physicians. Hellström-Westas and colleagues suggest a bolus of 1.5 to 2.2 mg/kg, and a continuous infusion of 4.7 to 6.3 mg/kg per hour for 24 hours. The drawbacks of this medication include the development of acidosis and bradycardia, and the propensity of lidocaine to induce seizures when given for longer than 24 hours (689). We have had no experience with either anticonvulsant in neonates; rather, we have found that if seizures are not controlled by phenobarbital, they are usually poorly controlled by other drugs. The ultimate prognosis for intellectual development in such infants, most of whom have congenital cerebral malformations or severe hypoxic ischemic encephalopathy, is poor.

Infants with electrocortical paroxysmal discharges but no apparent clinical seizures present a therapeutic dilemma. Although considerable experimental evidence suggests that uncontrolled seizures have a deleterious effect on the developing brain, so does chronic administration of phenobarbital (51). Not wishing to treat an EEG abnormality, we prefer to delay the use of anticonvulsants under such circumstances until clinical evidence for seizures exists. Volpe is of the same opinion (674,678). On the other hand, PET and nuclear MR (NMR) studies suggest that seizures documented by EEG exacerbate the brain damage produced by the underlying insult (690).

Prognosis

As a rule, the prognosis for neonatal seizures depends on the underlying cause. Follow-up studies on infants with neonatal seizures are summarized in Table 13.16. In this series from Pittsburgh, compiled by Bergman and coworkers, 47% of infants were normal at 1 to 5 years of age, and 24.7% died (691). Infants with seizures caused by perinatal asphyxia or malformations of the CNS have a fair prognosis for survival, but not for normal intellectual development and freedom from subsequent seizures (692). In a series of neonates with EEG-confirmed seizures, 70% of infants who survived perinatal asphyxia experienced epilepsy, developmental delay, or cerebral palsy (690). In the relatively current experience of Volpe (674), 50% of infants with neonatal seizures had normal development, whereas only 10% of infants whose seizures were the result of intraventricular hemorrhage, and none of those with congenital anomalies of the brain, escaped intellectual deficits (674). It should be noted that every patient who experienced a chronic seizure

TABLE 13.16. *Outcome of 131 infants with neonatal seizures*

Cause	Number of patients	Death or severe or moderate impairment	Normal or mild impairment
Hypoxia-ischemia, intracranial hemorrhage, or both[a]	77	41	34
≤31 wk[b]	28	16	11
32–36 wk	14	10	4
≥37 wk[b]	35	15	19
16			
Infection, bacterial or viral[c]	16	7	9
Metabolic			
Hypoglycemia	7	2	5
Hypocalcemia	2	0	2
Hyperbilirubinemia	1	1	0
Transient hyperammonemia	1	1	0
Brain malformations/genetic syndromes	5	5	0
Trauma	4	0	4
Narcotic withdrawal	2	0	3
Unknown	16	4	12
Total	**131**	**61**	**68**

From Bergman L, et al. Outcome in neonates with convulsions treated in an intensive care unit. *Ann Neurol* 1983;14:642. With permission.

[a]Outcome unknown for two patients with hypoxic-ischemic seizures.
[b]Gestational age.
[c]Twelve meningitis and four sepsis.

disorder secondary to hypoxic-ischemic encephalopathy also had cerebral palsy or mental retardation (690). The incidence of permanent neurologic sequelae is similar in other studies, although results from the Collaborative Project are somewhat more optimistic in that 70% of 7-year-old children who had experienced seizures during the neonatal period were neurologically and intellectually intact (693). The differences in outcomes could reflect the inclusion of hypocalcemic seizures in the Collaborative Project. When neonatal seizures recur in later life, they usually do so before the third year, and preventive therapy with phenobarbital appears to be ineffectual. Infantile spasms or minor motor seizures are particularly common and were seen in approximately one-half of children who experienced a recurrence of their neonatal seizures (694).

The clinical appearance of the child can provide important prognostic clues. Prolonged and repetitive seizures are associated with a bad outcome, either in terms of mortality or significant neurologic residua. A persistently abnormal neurologic examination, in particular abnormalities of eye movements, suggests a poor prognosis, as does the presence of subtle seizures. The interictal EEG is also of considerable prognostic help. The presence of burst-suppression patterns, low voltage background, or multifocal sharp waves are particularly ominous findings; only 12% of infants showing multifocal sharp waves achieved normal development (695).

The outlook is better for the infant who is seizure free at discharge. In the experience of Painter and coworkers (696), only 6% of neonates who had experienced a seizure but were free of seizures at the time of hospital discharge had a recurrence. Bad prognostic factors are a 5-minute Apgar score of less than 7, seizures lasting more than 30 minutes, and the need for prolonged resuscitation (697).

Considerable controversy exists, but little data, regarding how long anticonvulsants should be given to an infant who has experienced neonatal seizures. Although experimental data derived from rats suggest an adverse effect of phenobarbital on the developing nervous system, the applicability of these results to the human, whose brain is more mature at birth, has not been demonstrated unequivocally.

We maintain adequate phenobarbital blood levels for the first 3 months of life. Thereafter, in the presence of normal development, continued freedom from seizures, and a normal EEG, we allow the infant to outgrow the phenobarbital dosage, so that when blood levels drop below 15 µg/mL, the drug can be discontinued.

A syndrome of infantile epileptic encephalopathy was first described by Ohtahara and colleagues (698). The condition is marked by severe and recurrent seizures, mainly tonic spasms or partial motor seizures and a striking and persistent burst-suppression EEG. With maturation, many of these infants develop West syndrome and then Lennox-Gastaut syndrome (699). The outcome is poor in terms of intellectual development and seizure control.

A syndrome, termed *benign idiopathic neonatal seizures* is characterized by the onset of seizures during the latter part of the first week of life. In the experience of Volpe (674), 5% of term infants fell into this group. The seizures are generally multifocal clonic and last less than 24 hours (700). Their cause is as yet unexplained, and almost all infants become seizure free with normal intellectual development.

Another rare and genetically heterogeneous condition, termed *benign familial neonatal convulsions*, is characterized by the occurrence of focal or generalized clonic seizures during the second or third day of life (701,702). The interictal EEG is normal, and seizures usually stop by 6 months of age. The condition is transmitted as a dominant trait. One gene has been mapped to the long arm of chromosome 20q13.3 and codes for a voltage-gated potassium channel, KCNQ2. (703). A second gene has been mapped to chromosome 8q24 and codes for another potassium channel gene, KCNQ3 (704).

MIGRAINE AND OTHER TYPES OF CHRONIC HEADACHE

Migraine is the most common of the paroxysmal disorders to affect the brain. The term designates a chronic recurrent headache, often familial and unilateral, and often preceded by visual disturbances and accompanied by nausea or vomiting.

Pathophysiology and Genetics

The pathogenesis of migraine is still a matter of uncertainty. Many theories have been proposed. Each answer some aspect of the clinical picture, but none completely accounts for the complexity of symptoms and their evolution. The classic vascular theory of migraine pathophysiology holds that an attack has two phases. The prodromal phase is characterized by vasospasm that induces cerebral ischemia and the various transient focal symptoms that initiate the attack. The second phase, characterized by extracranial and intracranial vasodilation, is responsible for the pulsating headache, which is generally felt in the distribution of the trigeminal nerve and the upper cervical roots (705). The vascular theory has been supplemented by a neuronal theory of migraine. This proposes that classical migraine (i.e., migraine preceded by an aura or other focal symptoms) is related to a paroxysmal depolarization of cortical neurons. During the initial phase of the attack a cortical spreading depression is elicited at the occipital pole of the brain. The term *cortical spreading depression* is used to describe a depression of spontaneous EEG and other cortical electrical activities spreading across the cerebral cortical surface in the wake of a variety of noxious stimuli (706). The cortical spreading depression moves anteriorly in the course of the attack at a rate of approximately 2 mm/minute. At the wave front, transient ionic changes cause neurons and glia to depolarize with ensuing neuronal silence. Associated with these changes there are dramatic alterations in the ion distribution between intracellular and extracellular departments. These changes are believed to trigger the migraine aura and to induce a 20% to 25% reduction in cerebral blood flow. Cerebral ischemia is probably the result of arteriolar vasoconstriction, and in most instances is not of primary importance in the induction of the migraine aura or of focal neurologic symptoms. Generally, oligemia in the posterior part of the brain is the most characteristic alteration of regional cerebral blood flow in attacks of classical migraine (707). Cerebral blood flow in the areas of the brain not affected by cortical spreading depression remains normal. Regional blood flow in the brainstem is increased, however, with maximal increase in the region corresponding to the dorsal raphe nucleus and the locus caeruleus (707a). The course followed by the spreading oligemia is independent of vascular patterns and appears to be related to neuronal cytoarchitecture (708). As a rule, the cortical spreading depression stops at the central sulcus. Ventral propagation of the cortical spreading depression to the pain-sensitive meningeal trigeminal fibers that innervate the intracranial and dural blood vessels is believed to induce the headache, although some experimental evidence suggests the contrary (709). A number of vasoactive substances are released. These include vasoactive intestinal peptide, substance P, and calcitonin gene-related peptides. The role of these substances in the evolution of the headache is not clear (708,710). The factors that induce the onset of cortical spreading depression are multiple and are also not well clarified. No doubt, they are both exogenous and endogenous. In part, they include any disturbance of K^+ homeostasis, genetic predisposition, stress, and dietary factors, and the antidromic release of vasoactive peptides from the trigeminovascular system (708,711).

In migraine without an antecedent aura (common migraine) there are, however, no consistent changes in cerebral blood flow (712), and the mechanisms other than cortical spreading depression that are responsible for this form of migraine are poorly understood. They could involve extracranial and intracranial arterial dilatation (713).

In addition to the vascular changes seen in classical migraine, there are a variety of abnormalities in the metabolism and concentrations of neurotransmitters, notably serotonin and its metabolites. At the onset of an attack serotonin is released from platelets, and during an attack there is a transient reduction in serotonin turnover (713,714) and there appears to be an enhancement in serotonin turnover between attacks (714a). This observation corresponds to the finding obtained by PET of an increased serotonin synthesis capacity in all brain regions in patients having migraine without aura (714a). Of the various serotonin receptors 5-HT1, 5-HT2, and 5-HT_3 are involved in the pathophysiology of migraine. 5-HT1 receptors are inhibitory. The postsynaptic 5-HT1_B receptor is located on intracranial blood vessels, whereas the presynaptic receptor, 5-HT1_D is located on the trigeminal nerve ending. Most of the drugs used for the acute treatment of migraine are $5\text{-HT1}_B/5$-

$HT1_D$ agonists, whereas medications such as propanolol and methysergide are antagonists to the excitatory 5-HT2 receptors (715).

A number of substances can initiate an attack of migraine. These include prostaglandin E_1, tyramine, and phenylethylamine. Tyramine and phenylethylamine can be found in a variety of foods, notably cheese and chocolate, and are responsible for consistently initiating migraine attacks in a significant proportion of adults. In children, however, these amines are of lesser import (716). Considerable evidence suggests that the brain is not the only organ affected during an attack of migraine; alterations in renal functions, particularly polyuria and increased histidine excretion, have been demonstrated.

The familial transmission of migraine has been known for many centuries. Although in the past the condition was considered to be transmitted as an autosomal disorder, current genetic data do not support this pattern. Almost all genetic studies have been confounded by the high prevalence of migraine in the general population, which facilitates a chance familial occurrence. In addition, inclusion of a family history of migraine as a diagnostic criterion, differences in migraine case definition, and variation in case ascertainment (referral to a clinic versus a population survey) all have hindered valid genetic studies. However, over the last few years several studies have shed light on the genetics of the disorder. Twin studies have supported a strong genetic component in the etiology of migraine, with a significantly higher concordance rate among monozygotic twins compared with dizygotic twins (717,718,718a). Subjects with classical migraine are more likely to have first-degree relatives with classical migraine than with common migraine, and vice versa. From data such as these it has become evident that migraine with aura (classical migraine) and migraine without aura (common migraine) are genetically distinct entities (719). Although some authors have postulated an autosomal recessive model with reduced penetrance, it is more likely that both migraine entities have a multifactorial inheritance, and that there is no evidence for any specific mendelian transmission (720,721). In any case, the frequency of migraine indicates that in the future, multiple genes will almost certainly be implicated.

Clinical Manifestations

An excellent review of the clinical presentations and treatment of migraine can be found in the monograph by Barlow (722).

Migraine is relatively common in children. A survey published in 1997, of 3- to 11-year-old children in British general practice using a questionnaire and a structured interview disclosed that depending on the diagnostic criteria 3.7% to 4.9% of children experienced migraine. Of these 1.5% had migraine with aura (723).

Migraine begins surprisingly early in life. Initial complaints are paroxysmal, recurrent abdominal pain, restlessness, head banging, or sudden alterations in personality. A history of motion sickness or car sickness can be elicited in approximately two-thirds of patients (724). Because these symptoms are nonspecific, the diagnosis of migraine is generally not made until the child is old enough to relate the symptoms. Approximately one out of five patients has the first attack before age 5 years (725). Boys are affected almost twice as often as girls (726).

Headaches are characteristically paroxysmal and are separated by symptom-free intervals. Commonly, an attack begins in the early morning hours, often awakening the child. In the classic form of migraine, many attacks of headache are preceded by an aura. In children the most common symptoms involve nausea, vomiting, abdominal pain, and disturbances of vision. Some of the older children describe scintillating scotomata moving across one or both visual fields, and in adults visual symptoms are the most common manifestation of the aura (727). Vision is blurred, and the child can have a transient hemianopsia or even complete blindness in one eye (amaurosis fugax). Both can terminate with the onset of contralateral headache or can last for several days unaccompanied by head pain (728). A family history of the disorder can be elicited in over one-half of the patients and was found in 72% in the data compiled by Prensky (726).

Other symptoms preceding the headache include numbness and tingling in one arm or over the entire side, hemiplegia, aphasia, or apraxia (729). In most instances, symptoms appearing during the pre-headache phase are completely reversible, but in some children, function returns slowly, and an occasional case of persistent hemianopsia or hemiparesis has been reported (730,731).

In some older subjects, headaches begin over one eye and spread to involve the entire hemicranium. Attacks occur from 2 to 10 times a day and last on the average for 45 minutes. They may occur during sleep and awaken the patient. The pain is extremely severe and throbbing and is accompanied by nasal congestion, tearing, conjunctival injection, and photophobia (732). Ptosis is seen in approximately one-half of children, and there often is perspiration over the face and body. These attacks are frequently episodic, with periods of 1 to 3 months during which headaches are frequent, followed by periods of remission lasting several months to years. In the series of Maytal, boys were affected six times more frequently, and the frequency and duration of attacks increased at puberty (733).

In younger children, migraine headache is bifrontal or poorly localized and is almost invariably accompanied by pallor, nausea, and vomiting (722). Occasionally, vomiting can be sufficiently intense and prolonged to induce acidosis and mimic cyclic vomiting. The relationship between migraine and cyclic vomiting is not clear. Some patients with cyclic vomiting have a strong family history of migraine, and a significant proportion develop migraine in adult life (734,735). An attack of migraine lasts anywhere from half an hour to several days. Most commonly, the headache appears in the morning and ends as the child goes to sleep in the late afternoon or evening.

In a significant proportion of children, focal neurologic symptoms present during an attack persist beyond the headache phase. These cases are designated as complicated migraine.

Occasionally, unilateral ptosis or complete third nerve palsy accompanies the migraine, a condition termed *ophthalmoplegic migraine* (736). In this form of migraine, headache is usually localized to the forehead. In the initial attacks, the paralysis lasts for only a few hours. With repeated bouts it can persist for weeks or months or can even become permanent. The cause for the ophthalmoplegia is unknown.

Vascular anomalies are frequently considered in the differential diagnosis of ophthalmoplegic migraine and should be excluded by imaging studies. When nonionic contrasts are used in children, high-resolution digital angiography is not accompanied by a statistically significant increased risk.

Atypical attacks of migraine occur more commonly in childhood than in adult life. Vertigo is not unusual (737). It can precede headache or persist beyond the onset of the headache. In other instances, recurrent paroxysms of vertigo are replaced after a few years by typical migraine headaches.

A syndrome of basilar artery migraine has been observed (738). Vertigo, tinnitus, ataxia, dysarthria, and diplopia can precede the onset of headache and are believed to result from brainstem ischemia. The first attack can occur in children ranging in age from infancy to adolescence. Although symptoms clear after an hour to several hours, residua after multiple attacks have been reported (739).

Periods of confusion have been encountered in association with migraine headaches (740). The duration of the confusion can last from several hours to up to 1 week (741). In some instances, a period of confusion is triggered by a relatively minor head injury. This leads to an obvious but false diagnosis of an epidural or subdural hematoma (742). In our experience, attacks tend to recur as frequently as once a month, but are ultimately replaced by typical migraine (743). Other types of headache syndromes, some not at all uncommon, are summarized in Table 13.17.

Children with migraine often show a characteristic personality. They are meticulous, compulsive, and unusually mature for their age, striving to excel at school and to please the family at home. Additionally, they have considerable difficulty in expressing anger or rage (744).

Diagnosis

The differential diagnosis of headache in a child is a common task for the clinician. In the series of children younger than age 7 years evaluated for headaches, Chu and Shinnar found that 75% were experiencing migraine. Common migraine was the most frequent form, and only 17% of children could relate the presence of an aura (745). In 72 patients from the Winnipeg pediatric neurologic outpatient service, which handled referrals up to 18 years of age, common migraine (migraine without aura) was also the most frequently seen form of headache and accounted for 61% of patients (746). Migraine with aura accounted for 15% of children, tension headaches for 3% of children, and mixed migraine and tension-type headaches were seen in 15%. There was only one patient with sinus headaches.

In evaluating a child with headaches, the physician should first determine how many different types of headaches are experienced by the child, and then obtain their description, one by one. A headache diary can be used to assist in the diagnosis of headaches (747). Such a diary also helps determine the relative frequency of migrainous and nonmigrainous headaches. For each of the types of headache it is important to determine whether they are intermittent, progressive, or static, their duration, whether they are triggered by any specific foods or activities, the quality of the pain, and their location (748). It is also necessary to determine what the child does during an attack. Typically, children with migraine headaches cease activities and prefer to lie down.

From their temporal patterns, Rothner distinguishes four categories of headaches in older children: acute, paroxysmal and recurrent, chronic and progressive, and chronic and nonprogressive (749). He separates acute headaches into those in which the pain is generalized and those in which it is localized. Although the causes for acute generalized headache are multiple, ranging from the first attack of migraine to a subarachnoid hemorrhage, thorough physical and neurologic examinations and some basic laboratory studies provide a diagnosis in almost every instance. Acute localized headaches can be caused by head trauma; 12% of children seen by Chu and Shinnar had post-traumatic headaches (745). In the Winnipeg series, post-traumatic headaches accounted for only 3% of patients (746). Other causes include sinusitis, glaucoma, optic neuritis, and a variety of atypi-

TABLE 13.17. *Less common headache syndromes in children and adolescents*

Syndrome	Symptoms	References
Occipital neuralgia	Unilateral or bilateral pain in posterior part of head, infrequent to continuous.	Rothner (732)
Temporal mandibular joint dysfunction	Dull, aching unilateral pain below ear, frequently aggravated by chewing.	Belfer ML, Kaban LB. (750)
Exertional headaches	Headaches precipitated by coughing, sneezing, laughing, or sports. Pain is generalized and lasts from 15 minutes to 12 hours.	Symonds C. Cough headache. *Brain* 1956;79:557
Hemicrania continua	Steady, severe headache over frontal area, unaccompanied by nausea. Good response to indomethacin.	Rothner (732)
Ice cream headache	Cold-induced, severe but of short duration.	Raskin NH, Knittle SC. Ice cream headache and orthostatic symptoms in patients with migraine. *Headache* 1976;16:222
Ice pick headache	Single or repeated episodes of brief, sharp, jabbing pain over orbit, temple, or parietal area.	Raskin NH, Schwartz RK. Icepick-like pain. *Neurology* 1980;30:203

cal facial pains, some of which are caused by temporomandibular joint dysfunction. These conditions are more likely to occur in adults (750) (see Table 13.17).

The diagnosis of migraine rests on the periodicity of the paroxysmal headaches and their initiation by stress. The diagnostic criteria for migraine that have been established for adults by the International Headache Society have been modified for children. They are summarized in Table 13.18 (751). In the experience of Maytal and coworkers the International Headache Society criteria are satisfactory for the diagnosis of pediatric migraine with aura (classical migraine), but when applied to children suffering from migraine without aura (common migraine) these criteria have a high specificity, but a poor sensitivity when the clinical diagnosis is used as a gold standard (752). A number of clinical diagnostic criteria have been delineated (753): an aura, generally visual, is seen in 10% to 50% of children (725); gastrointestinal symptoms, mainly nausea and vomiting, but also anorexia and abdominal pain in 70% to 100%; a positive family history in 44% to 87%; unilateral headaches (less common in children than in adults) in 25% to 66%; and a history of motion sickness in 45% to 65%.

EEG abnormalities, which are not unusual in the child with migraine headaches, were found in 27% of Holguin and Fenichel's series (725), in 20% of patients in the series of Chu and Shinnar (745), and in 23% of the series of Friedman and Pampiglione (754). In the experience of Kramer and colleagues, epileptiform EEG abnormalities were encountered in 11% in both migraine and tension headaches (755). We too have encountered an occasional patient whose EEG is definitely abnormal. In such instances, one must consider the possibility that the headache represents a true epileptic equivalent, an aura of a major motor seizure, or a postictal state of a clinically inapparent seizure (756). We have treated a few of these patients with anticonvulsants, notably carbamazepine or phenytoin, and, contrary to the observations of Friedman and Pampiglione, have occasionally found them to be beneficial (754). Even though the history of migraine headache might be convincing, the possibility of an underlying space-occupying lesion should not be forgotten. We have seen several children in whom the appearance of a malignant posterior fossa tumor aggravated long-standing migraine. Paroxysmal headaches also can be caused by intraventricular tumors, such as a colloid cyst of the third ventricle (see Chapter 10) (757).

The question whether neuroimaging should be part of the workup for a child presenting with recurrent headache has been a matter of considerable concern. In the series of Chu and Shinnar

TABLE 13.18. *International Headache Society criteria for pediatric migraine*

With aura
A. At least two attacks fulfilling B
B. At least three or more of the following:
   1. One or more fully reversible aura symptoms indicating focal cerebral cortical, brainstem dysfunction, or both.
   2. At least one aura symptom develops gradually over more than 4 minutes or two or more symptoms occur in succession.
      Aura symptoms include homonymous visual disturbance, unilateral paresthesias and/or numbness, unilateral weakness, aphasias or unclassifiable speech disturbance.
   3. No aura symptom lasts more than 60 minutes. If more than one aura symptom is present, accepted duration is proportionally increased.
   4. Headache follows aura with a free interval of less than 60 minutes. It also may begin before or simultaneously with the aura.
C. At least one of the following:
   1. History, physical, and neurologic examinations do not suggest any other disorder
   2. History, physical, and neurologic examinations do suggest another disorder, but it is ruled out by appropriate investigations
Without aura
A. At least five attacks fulfilling B through D
B. Headache attack lasting 2 to 48 hours
C. Headache has at least two of the following:
   1. Unilateral location
   2. Pulsating quality
   3. Moderate to severe intensity
   4. Aggravation by routine physical activity
D. During headache at least one of the following:
   1. Nausea, vomiting, or both
   2. Photophobia, phonophobia, or both

Adapted from Seshia SS, et al. International Headache Society criteria and childhood headache. *Dev Med Child Neurol* 1994;36:419–428.

(745), some 30% of 104 children younger than the age of 7 years who presented with headache underwent imaging. In only one instance, a child with Chiari I malformation, did these studies uncover a previously unknown finding. In the series of Maytal and coworkers neuroimaging studies disclosed cerebral abnormalities in 3% of pediatric headache patients. All abnormalities were deemed to be unrelated to the presenting complaint (758). In older children and adolescents, the incidence of abnormal findings in the face of a normal neurologic examination is even lower. It is, therefore, our policy to defer neuroimaging, unless there is excessive parental concern. McAbee and coworkers, who have studied the value of MRI in children with migraine, concur (759). On the other hand, chronic headaches that are steadily or intermittently progressive or occur in children younger than 7 years of age should prompt a thorough diagnostic investigation. In such children, the presumptive diagnosis is increased intracranial pressure owing to tumors or other space-occupying lesions. The question of how to go about finding the rare youngster in whom headache is the first and only sign of an intracerebral tumor has been addressed by several groups, most recently by Straussberg and Amir, who recommend performing imaging studies on youngsters younger than 4 years of age in whom headache is accompanied by vomiting, even when the neurologic examination is normal (760). Battistella and colleagues found that headache was the first symptom in 27% of children with brain tumors, and the only presenting symptom in 10%. The authors noted that headache associated with brain tumors had a high incidence of projectile vomiting, nocturnal or morning onset, and a lack of triggering factors. Also of note was that rest or sleep failed to relieve the pain and that nausea, photophobia, and phonophobia infrequently accompanied headaches associated with brain tumors (761).

On rare occasion attacks of migraine accompanied by temporary unilateral sensory symptoms, aphasia, or motor deficits are associated with a CSF lymphocytic pleocytosis, and an aseptic inflammation of the leptomeningeal vasculature (762).

Chronic nonprogressive headaches are almost invariably functional. Generally, they are not seen in children younger than 10 years of age. In some, they are a manifestation of anxiety and tension; other affected children have an underlying history of depression (763). Psychological and psychoeducational tests are often useful in this group (764). Ramadan, however, points out that prolonged, tension type, or migraine-like headaches can be seen in 15% to 75% of patients with Chiari I malformation (765). Hyperventilation syndrome, another cause for chronic nonprogressive headache (766), can be accompanied by giddiness, paresthesias, brief loss of consciousness, and blurring of vision. Hyperventilation syndrome is diagnosed by inducing the symptoms by brief, voluntary hyperventilation. The condition must be differentiated from absence seizures (767).

Treatment

The treatment of migraine is symptomatic or prophylactic. The patient and the patient's parents should be informed of the child's lifelong predisposition to headaches and of the essentially benign nature of the condition. Generally, attacks should be treated only if they are frequent or severe enough to interfere with the child's activities. When attacks occur infrequently, as is usually the case in children, pharmacologic treatment is abortive; preventive treatment is used less commonly.

The acute attack of migraine is treated by bedrest in a dark room and the administration of analgesics. Acetylsalicylic acid is usually of little help except in mild attacks. In the experience of Hämäläinen and coworkers acetaminophen (15 mg/kg) is effective for moderate or severe attacks (768). Other medications used for severe attacks include naproxen (Aleve), ibuprofen (Motrin, Advil), butalbital (Fiorinal), phenacetin, or caffeine singly or in combination (722,769).

For most older children, another drug of choice for intermittent therapy is ergotamine tartrate, a medication that induces strong arterial vasoconstriction. It is given orally at the beginning of an attack, usually in the form of Cafergot, a proprietary preparation containing ergotamine tartrate (1 mg) and caffeine (100 mg) per tablet. If necessary, it is followed by a second tablet after 30 minutes. Ergotamine is contraindicated for patients who develop hemianopsia or hemiparesis during the constrictive phase of an attack. Because smaller children rarely inform their parents approximately the onset of the headache, the usefulness of Cafergot is somewhat limited (722).

Sumatriptan, a selective 5-HT1 receptor agonist, has been effective in the treatment of a migraine attack in adults. The drug induces vasoconstriction of the large basal intracranial arteries and thereby increases the blood flow velocity in the middle cerebral artery and the internal carotid artery. As yet, no evidence exists that its effectiveness is related to this phenomenon (770). Several other triptans also have been used to be effective in the acute treatment of migraine in adults. These include zolmitriptan, naratriptan, and rizatriptan. However, in a placebo-controlled crossover study on a pediatric population, sumatriptan was found to be no better than ibuprofen (771).

Propranolol has been advocated as a preventive for childhood migraine. In children who weigh less than 35 kg, the maximum dosage is 20 mg three times daily; in those weighing more than 35 kg, it is 40 mg three times daily. Although this drug is a fairly good prophylactic, many children complain of difficulty in falling asleep (772). Flunarizine, a calcium-channel blocker, given in doses of 5 mg per day, also has been used with some effect as a preventive in children with common and classical migraine (773,774). No data on the effectiveness of other calcium-channel blockers in children are available, and the rationale for their effectiveness is still unknown (775).

Divalproex (Depakote) also has been used as a migraine preventive in children and adults (776). At present, it is our favorite preventive medication, and we give it in dosages of 15 to 20 mg/kg per day. In a single-blind, placebo-controlled study performed on adults it was as effective as propanolol in the prophylaxis of migraine without aura (777).

Methysergide (Sansert), a 5-HT2 antagonist, is rarely used in children because of its propensity to induce thrombophlebitis (778). The use of tricyclics or monoamine oxidase inhibitors such as phenelzine (Nardil) has not been fully explored in a pediatric population.

Food allergies are commonly believed to trigger attacks. A double-blind study suggests that some foods, notably cow's milk, eggs, chocolate, oranges, wheat, benzoic acid, cheese, tomatoes, and rye, can provoke attacks, and that their exclusion results in improvement in the majority of children (779).

A number of other activities and measures have been proposed to relieve migraine. These include yoga, karate, and biofeedback. Despite many examples of dramatic effectiveness, none of these techniques can be shown to work consistently. The effectiveness of any form of intervention in a disease that exhibits as much periodicity as migraine does can be evaluated only through long-term studies.

The outlook for the patient with migraine headaches is excellent, and in most instances the condition does not interfere with schoolwork. In approximately two-thirds of children, attacks persist throughout life, although many patients are intermittently free of them for long periods or their headaches are at least partly relieved by medication or a less stressful family and school environment (716,780).

Familial Hemiplegic Migraine

In some families, transient attacks of hemiplegia followed by contralateral headache are transmitted as an autosomal dominant trait (781,782). Attacks generally start with numbness of the hand, accompanied by a homonymous hemianopsia, and spreading to involve the face, tongue, and the remainder of the body. Aphasia and weakness are common. Migraine-like headache can precede or follow the neurologic symptoms. Full neurologic recovery can take 24 hours or longer. In a large proportion of patients, attacks are triggered by relatively minor head injuries (783). In approximately 20% of patients, familial hemiplegic migraine is accompanied by progressive cerebellar ataxia (784).

The elucidation of the molecular genetics of this condition represents one of the major recent advances in the understanding of the pathophysiology of migraine. Familial hemiplegic migraine is a heterogenic condition, and to date two genes have been implicated. In approximately one-half of the families with familial hemiplegic migraine the condition has been mapped to chromosome 19p13 and codes for a brain-specific P/Q type calcium channel alpha$_1$-subunit gene (CACNL1A4) (784). This condition is allelic with episodic ataxia type 2, and all cases of familial hemiplegic migraine with progressive ataxia map to this site (see Chapter 2). A number of mutations in the gene have been documented; a considerable proportion of mutation carriers are asymptomatic

(785). A second locus has been mapped to the long arm of chromosome 1, and the mutation may affect a potassium channel or another calcium channel gene (783). In some families both loci have been excluded, an observation that underlines the heterogeneity of the condition (786).

Cyclic Vomiting

Although in most instances cyclic vomiting is not a paroxysmal disorder, it is considered here because of its relationship to migraine. Gee characterized the condition as producing fits of vomiting that recur after intervals of uncertain lengths and continue for a few hours or several days (787). Cyclic vomiting is neither uncommon nor benign. Its incidence can be as high as 10% of unselected school children, with peak occurrence between ages 6 and 11 years (734). Attacks start as early as 1 year of age; in 82%, the first attack occurs before age 6 years (788). Aside from vomiting, symptoms include headache (seen in 36% of children in the series of Hoyt and Stickler) (788), fever (43%), and abdominal pain (18%). Hypertension also can be present. Curiously, there appears to be a high incidence of prematurely gray hair in affected children and their mothers (735). The EEG is more likely to be abnormal than in the general population, but there is no evidence that the condition represents a seizure equivalent or that it responds to anticonvulsants (789).

In 64% of children, attacks last 4 days or less; in 11%, they last longer than 1 week (788). A variety of medications have been suggested, but none are convincingly effective. Thus, treatment is directed toward maintaining fluid and electrolyte balance. Because a variety of emotional stresses are believed to trigger attacks, psychotherapy is considered an important therapeutic adjunct (790).

Important in understanding the nature of the condition is the widespread observation that children with cyclic vomiting become adults with migraine and have a positive family history of migraine (734,735). In the series of Hammond, 75% of adults who experienced cyclic vomiting during childhood suffered from migraine. Approximately two-thirds still have recurrent bouts of vomiting (734). A high percentage of children In this group respond favorably to antimigraine therapy, notably sumatriptan (791).

Cyclic vomiting must be distinguished from several other entities. Most commonly, recurrent vomiting occurs in severely retarded youngsters. In many instances, this vomiting is the consequence of gastroesophageal reflux (792). Symptoms can respond to small feedings and antacid therapy. The effectiveness of postprandial upright positioning is a matter of dispute. In some instances, even fundal plication is ineffective. Other neurologic conditions inducing recurrent vomiting include dysautonomia, the various disorders of urea cycle and organic acid metabolism, notably dicarboxylic aciduria (scc Chapter 1), mitochondrial DNA mutations, and abdominal epilepsy (793,794). Additionally, functional disorders are common in children older than 5 years of age. Less often, one encounters thc irritable bowel syndrome, lactose intolerance, inflammatory bowel disease, and *Giardia* infections. In infants, intussusception, constipation, and urinary tract infections must be excluded.

SYNCOPE

Syncope or fainting is characterizcd by transient loss of consciousness resulting from inadequate cerebral perfusion and from anoxia. Four major causes can be distinguished: (a) vasovagal, (b) reflex, (c) decreased venous return, and (d) cardiac.

In the first three entities, syncope results from a sudden decrease in blood pressure in a child who is upright. In vasovagal syncope, which accounts for approximately 75% of instances, it is the result of pain or some obvious emotional upset. In reflex syncope, the event is precipitated by hyperventilation, violent coughing, hot baths, or micturition (795). Syncope resulting from Valsalva maneuver is probably the consequence of reduced venous return. Adolescents subject to postural hypotension can faint when maintaining an upright posture for long periods.

Cardiac syncope is seen in children with cardiac asystole (Stokes-Adams syndrome), parox-

ysmal changes in cardiac rhythm, obstruction to left ventricular outflow, or anemia. Syncopal attacks caused by a prolonged QT interval have a familial incidence and occasionally present with a seizure. Attacks are frequently induced by exercise or excitement (796). Two distinct clinical conditions marked by a prolonged QT interval have been described. The Romano-Ward syndrome is transmitted as an autosomal dominant trait. Four genes have been found responsible. They involve the cardiac potassium and the cardiac sodium channels. In the Jervell-Lange-Nielsen syndrome, an autosomal recessive condition, caused by a homozygous mutation of a cardiac potassium channel gene, prolongation of the QT interval is accompanied by congenital deafness (797,798). Syncope preceded by dyspnea can be seen in systemic mastocytosis. Because skin involvement is not invariable, this condition must be kept in mind under such circumstances (799).

Syncope is rare in childhood, but more common during adolescence, particularly in girls. Fainting spells consist of an initial period during which the patient experiences a number of premonitory symptoms including restlessness, pallor, sweating, and reduction in vision. These are followed by loss of consciousness. In two-thirds of the patients followed by Livingston for recurrent syncope, unconsciousness lasted less than 5 minutes; in the remainder, it persisted for 5 to 30 minutes (507). Approximately 40% of syncopal attacks are accompanied by a convulsion. Usually this is a tonic spasm followed by confusion lasting several minutes. Less often, there are clonic movements or a tonic-clonic convulsion. Subjects who experience convulsive syncope have a normal EEG and a negative family history for seizure disorders. Their blood pressure and heart rate during an attack do not differ significantly from subjects who experience uncomplicated syncope, and the cause of this phenomenon is unknown (800).

The differentiation between syncope and epilepsy is difficult and has already been discussed. In many cases, electrocardiographic monitoring and echocardiography are more valuable than EEG in arriving at a diagnosis. A tilt-table test is probably of limited value in the usual clinical setting (801). In general, the longer the period of unconsciousness, the greater the likelihood of an epileptic equivalent. In such patients, anticonvulsant therapy is often beneficial in reducing the frequency of attacks. Finally, syncope can precipitate a convulsion in an epileptic individual.

BREATH-HOLDING SPELLS

It is common for a small child to hold his or her breath when crying. These episodes, termed *breath-holding spells*, are readily recognized and follow a distinct clinical pattern.

In a typical attack, the child who has been frightened or frustrated begins to cry and ceases breathing. Usually the breath is held in expiration, and after a few seconds the infant becomes cyanotic to varying degrees. Consciousness is lost, the infant becomes limp and can experience a few clonic convulsions of the extremities. Lombroso and Lerman found breath-holding spells in 4.6% of infants, with the majority of spells (76%) beginning in infants between 6 and 18 months of age (802). In a large number, the first attack was observed during the neonatal period. The frequency of attacks varies considerably. Approximately 10% of patients experience two or more attacks a day, and another 20% experience an average of one spell a day. A family history of breath-holding spells can be elicited in a significant number of first-degree relatives. In the series of DiMario and Sarfarazi, 27% of parents and 21% of siblings had current or prior breath-holding spells. These authors suggest that the condition is transmitted as an autosomal dominant with reduced penetrance (803).

With increasing age, spells become less common; in almost all instances they finally disappear by age 5 to 6 years. Lombroso and Lerman believe that infants with breath-holding spells can be divided into two well-defined groups of approximately equal size: one group in which spells are conspicuously cyanotic and another in which they are characterized by pallor (802). The latter group is particularly sensitive to vagal stimulation as elicited by ocular compression, which induces a prolonged asystole and an occasional seizure. Gauk and coworkers demon-

strated a rapid decrease in arterial oxygen saturation as measured by ear oximetry, probably the result of oxygen use (804).

As indicated previously, a breath-holding spell accompanied by a seizure can be differentiated from an epileptic convulsion (apneic seizure) in that an obvious precipitating factor, which has induced the child to cry, can always be elicited in the breath-holding spell. Cyanosis generally follows the onset of convulsions in an epileptic attack, but it precedes breath-holding spells (805). Finally, the interictal EEG is invariably normal in patients with breath-holding spells. Apneic seizures, which represent true epileptic attacks probably arising from the limbic system, can occur during both the waking and sleeping state. They are generally seen in neurologically damaged infants and are accompanied by EEG abnormalities. Treatment with anticonvulsants can be effective in apneic seizures.

In the experience of Daoud and colleagues iron therapy significantly reduced the frequency of breath-holding spells, even though not all children who responded were iron deficient and not all iron-deficient children responded (806). Drug therapy for breath-holding spells is neither indicated nor effective, although atropine is said to be helpful in the pallid type of breath-holding spell. Donma, however, has found piracetam, a cyclic derivative of GABA, to be extremely effective in the control of breath-holding spells (807). These observations have not been confirmed. Basically, breath-holding spells are triggered by a disciplinary conflict between parent and child, with the child using the attacks or the threat of an attack to assert him- or herself and to express anger. Proper family counseling and assurance to parents that the attacks do not represent any danger to the child are often effective in stopping them (805).

Although breath-holding spells disappear spontaneously in every case, many patients become prone to syncope and develop behavior disturbances, particularly temper tantrums. The incidence of true epilepsy in children with breath-holding spells, however, is no greater than is found in the general population.

One of the most difficult problems confronting the clinician is the patient with paroxysmal episodes of aggressive and explosive behavior, a condition commonly termed *episodic dyscontrol*. In a significant proportion of cases, the first attack follows a head injury; in other instances, a history of temper tantrums, learning disabilities, and isolated seizures are seen. The neurologic aspects of this entity are reviewed more extensively by Rickler (808).

NARCOLEPSY

Narcolepsy is characterized by paroxysmal attacks of irrepressible sleep. The somnolence is occasionally associated with transient loss of muscular tone or cataplexy. Narcolepsy has a familial incidence and is transmitted by a dominant gene with incomplete penetrance. Of white people with narcolepsy, 97% are tissue type HLA-DR2 positive (809,810). Whether this observation implies that the gene for narcolepsy is linked to the HLA genes is still obscure, as is the role played in the disease by immune factors (811).

Pathogenesis

Narcolepsy was first described by Westphal in 1877 (812); its neurophysiologic basis has been found to represent abnormal recurrent episodes of REM sleep. Healthy subjects always go into non-REM sleep first, changing to REM sleep after a variable period, averaging 140 minutes in children 19 to 45 months of age (813). By contrast, the sleep attack of most typical narcoleptic subjects shows an appearance of REM sleep within 5 minutes. The cataplectic attack often associated with narcolepsy has been explained as resulting from the intrusion into wakefulness of the motor inhibitory process that is an essential part of normal REM periods; whenever cataplexy is not interrupted it goes on into REM sleep.

There is a strong genetic predisposition to narcolepsy, and almost 100% of patients with narcolepsy and cataplexy have first-degree relatives similarly affected (814). Because monozygotic twins have a significant rate of discordance, the condition is believed to be multifactorial.

The pathogenesis of narcolepsy is still obscure (815,816). Some evidence suggests that the pontile reticular formation is involved in REM sleep, and both REM-on cells (i.e., cells that fire selectively during REM sleep) and REM-off cells are located in this region. Most of the REM-on cells are cholinergic or cholinoceptive, whereas REM-off cells are noradrenergic or serotonergic (816,817). It has been suggested that in narcolepsy the monoamine-dependent inhibition of REM sleep is defective. Using D1- and D2-specific ligands, no abnormalities in striatal receptor binding, however, have been documented by PET (818).

Clinical Manifestations

Narcolepsy is common, with a prevalence of just under 0.1% (819). It first appears during the late second or third decade of life, although spells can develop as early as 2 to 3 years of age (820,821). In preschool children, unexpected, abrupt falls are the most common initial complaint; in older children these are accompanied by repetitive falling asleep in class, difficulty waking in the morning, and abnormal behavior in school, notably hyperactivity and an attention deficit disorder (821). Attacks of sleep usually occur while the child is at rest. Although the patient can resist them, he or she can do so only briefly. If not disturbed, sleep lasts from a few minutes to half an hour, after which the patient awakens and is completely alert. Narcoleptic sleep is usually shallow, and the patient can easily be aroused.

Cataplexy is associated with narcolepsy in approximately 75% of children. In general, the history indicates that during an emotional reaction, particularly laughter, anger, or surprise, the child loses all muscular tone and falls to the ground, but retains consciousness. The attack is short and rarely lasts more than a minute.

Some children experience both narcolepsy and cataplexy on separate occasions; others experience somnolence as a result of excitement, and if sleep occurs, they undergo a cataplectic attack. The condition persists throughout adult life, the frequency of attacks varying over the years without showing a definite trend toward improvement or worsening.

A narcoleptic attack is distinguished from a true seizure in that the patient is easily aroused and once awake does not show postictal confusion, which is a common sequel to an epileptic attack. Narcolepsy is unrelated to the Kleine-Levin syndrome of recurrent somnolence and morbid hunger, which is occasionally encountered in adolescence (822,823), and to the excessive somnolence of the patient with obesity and carbon dioxide retention (pickwickian syndrome) (824).

Diagnosis

The diagnosis of narcolepsy is based on the clinical history, HLA typing, and polysomnographic recordings during night sleep (814,821,825). These characteristically demonstrate a diminished latency for the onset of REM sleep. In older children, a multiple sleep latency test can be obtained. This is a standardized test in which children are asked to fall asleep in bed in a dark and comfortable room. Daytime sleep attacks also demonstrate a sleep-onset REM period (819). Additionally, HLA typing of white or Asian patients must demonstrate DQw6. Most narcoleptic patients also express DRw15. Even in black narcoleptics, the incidence of these HLA types is markedly higher than in the general black population (810). It has been shown that some children who present with hyperactivity and attention deficit disorders or with various learning disabilities experience underlying narcolepsy or other sleep disorders, but how commonly this occurs has not been determined (826).

Treatment

Methylphenidate or dextroamphetamine are the preferred drugs to combat sleep attacks. Modafinil, a psychostimulant, which has been introduced into this country, is believed to be equally effective (826a). Pemoline is generally used in younger children. Monoamine inhibitors suppress REM sleep for extended periods. Their adverse effects, including insomnia, hypotension, and alterations in personality, limit their usefulness (827). A child with narcolepsy tolerates large doses of these drugs (40 to 60 mg methylphenidate per day), but the drugs rarely give complete relief, although 50% of patients report a reduction in frequency and severity of attacks.

Cataplexy does not respond to these drugs. Imipramine, clomipramine, and fluoxetine inhibit REM sleep and are effective in treating cataplexy (814,815,828). Frequent brief daytime naps should be encouraged and reduce the dose of stimulants required to keep the child awake. Teachers and family should be made to understand that narcolepsy is a chronic physical illness, and that sleep attacks cannot be controlled by the child.

PARASOMNIAS

The term *parasomnia* refers to a variety of motor and autonomic disturbances in sleep that are relatively common in childhood. They include infantile myoclonic jerks, bruxism, head banging, sleepwalking, enuresis, and night terrors (814,829).

Infantile myoclonic jerks are seen during stage 1 and 2 of non-REM sleep. They consist of rhythmic jerks of the limbs that can be severe enough to interfere with sleep. The condition tends to be familial and subsides within the first 2 years, although in some families it persists throughout life. Attacks are not stimulus sensitive, and because the EEG during an attack is normal, telemetry readily distinguishes infantile myoclonic jerks from a nocturnal myoclonic seizure (830). The condition also should be distinguished from benign myoclonic epilepsy of infancy, which is seen also in healthy infants. Benign myoclonic epilepsy attacks have their onset between 6 months and 3 years; they are brief and involve the upper extremities and the head (831). Unlike sleep myoclonus, this condition can appear throughout the day; the EEG taken during an attack always shows bursts of generalized spike-wave and polyspike-wave discharges. Photic stimulation can provoke a myoclonic seizure (832).

Bruxism and head banging also occur before sleep or during stages 1 and 2 of non-REM sleep. These phenomena are relatively common in infants and young children, with the incidence of head banging in healthy infants being as high as 15% (833). Both entities are more common in blind, mentally retarded, or autistic infants. Onset of head banging is generally in the latter half of the first year of life, and in most healthy infants the condition is transient, disappearing in a few months or, at the latest, before 4 years of age. The most plausible cause for head banging is that the condition is stress related, and that infants experience a need for motor release. Treatment for head banging is usually unnecessary, and head injury does not occur; when it does, child abuse should be suspected. If excessive, both head banging and bruxism can require the bedtime use of chloral hydrate or benzodiazepines. When the condition persists, psychiatric evaluation should be considered.

Some 15% of healthy children sleepwalk. This phenomenon generally occurs during stages 3 and 4 of non-REM sleep. In some, sleepwalking alternates with episodes during which the child sits up in bed and performs semipurposive movements. If awakened, the child is transiently confused. Attacks last from a few seconds to a few minutes, rarely up to an hour (834). An EEG taken during the episode shows it to commence with paroxysmal bursts of slow-wave activity and to continue with a mixture of wake and sleep activity. Sleepwalking tends to be familial, and it occurs more frequently during periods of stress (835).

A discussion of night terrors and the various other sleep disorders is outside the scope of this text. The interested reader is referred to reviews by Vgontzas and Kales (814), Broughton (819,836) and Ferriss (837) and to a book by Sheldon and coworkers (834).

REFERENCES

1. Tempkin O. *The falling sickness*, 2nd ed. Baltimore: The Johns Hopkins University Press, 1971.
2. Jackson JG. On convulsive seizures. *BMJ* 1890;1: 703–707, 765–771, 821–827.
3. Millichap JG. *Febrile convulsions.* New York: Macmillan, 1968.
4. Baumann RJ. Classification and population studies of epilepsy. In: Anderson VA, et al., eds. *Genetic basis of the epilepsies.* New York: Raven Press, 1982:11–20.
5. Goodridge DMG, Shorvon SD. Epileptic seizures in a population of 6000. I. Demography, diagnosis and classification, and role of the hospital services. *BMJ* 1983;287:641–645.
6. Commission on Classification and Terminology of the International League Against Epilepsy. Proposal for revised classification of epilepsies and epileptic syndromes. *Epilepsia* 1989;30:389–399.
7. Hughlings-Jackson J. On right- or left-sided spasm at the onset of epileptic paroxysms, and on crude sensation warnings, and elaborate mental states. *Brain* 1880;3:192–206.
8. Cowan LD, et al. Prevalence of the epilepsies in children and adolescents. *Epilepsia* 1989;30:94–106.
9. Andermann E. Multifactorial inheritance of generalized and focal epilepsy. In: Anderson VE, et al., eds. *Genetic basis of the epilepsies.* New York: Raven Press, 1982:355–374.
10. Hauser WA, Hesdorffer DC. *Epilepsy: frequency, causes and consequences.* New York:Demos Publications, 1990.
11. Blandfort M, Tsuboi T, Vogel F. Genetic counseling in the epilepsies. I. Genetic risks. *Hum Genet* 1987; 76:303–331.
12. Lennox WG, Lennox MA. *Epilepsy and related disorders.* Boston: Little, Brown and Company, 1960.
13. Metrakos K, Metrakos JD. Genetics of convulsive disorders. II. Genetic and electroencephalographic studies in centrencephalic epilepsy. *Neurology* 1961;11: 474–483.
14. Gerken H, Doose H. On the genetics of EEG-anomalies in childhood. III. Spike and waves. *Neuropädiatrie* 1973;4:88–97.
15. Metrakos JD, Metrakos K. Childhood epilepsy of subcortical ("centrencephalic") origin. *Clin Pediatr* 1966;5:537–542.
16. Tsuboi T. Seizures of childhood. A population-based and clinic-based study. *Acta Neurol Scand* 1986;74 [Suppl 110]:12–37.
17. Degen R, Degen H-E, Roth C. Some genetic aspects of idiopathic and symptomatic absence seizures: waking and sleep EEG in siblings. *Epilepsia* 1990;31: 784–794.
18. Steinlein OK, et al. A missense mutation in the neuronal nicotinic acetylcholine receptor alpha 4 subunit is associated with autosomal dominant nocturnal frontal lobe epilepsy. *Nat Genet* 1995;11: 201–203.
19. Steinlein OK, et al. An insertion mutation of the CHRNA4 gene in a family with autosomal dominant nocturnal frontal lobe epilepsy. *Hum Mol Genet* 1997;6:943–947.
20. Steinlein OK. New insights into the molecular and genetic mechanisms underlying idiopathic epilepsies. *Clin Genet* 1998;54:169–175.
21. Biervert C, et al. A potassium channel mutation in neonatal human epilepsy. *Science* 1998;279:403–406.
22. Singh NA, et al. A novel potassium channel gene, KCNQ2, is mutated in an inherited epilepsy of newborns [see comments]. *Nat Genet* 1998;18:25–29.
23. Charlier C, et al. A pore mutation in a novel KQT-like potassium channel gene in an idiopathic epilepsy family [see comments]. *Nat Genet* 1998;18:53–55.
23a. Giza C, Sankar R. Pathogenesis of the developmental epilepsies. *Curr Opin Pediatr* 1998;10:567–574.
24. Gowers WR. *Epilepsy and other chronic convulsive diseases: their causes, symptoms, and treatment.* London: William Wood and Co, 1885.
25. Giza CC, et al. Periventricular nodular heterotopia

and childhood absence epilepsy. *Pediatr Neurol* 1999;20:315–318.

26. Fox JW, et al. Mutations in filamin 1 prevent migration of cerebral cortical neurons in human periventricular heterotopia. *Neuron* 1998;21:1315–1325.

27. Meencke HJ, Janz D. Neuropathological findings in primary generalized epilepsy: a study of eight cases. *Epilepsia* 1984;25:8–21.

28. Corsellis JA, Falconer MA. "Cryptic tubers" as a cause of focal epilepsy [Abstract]. *J Neurol Neurosurg Psychiatry* 1971;34:104–105.

29. Pollen DA, Trachtenberg MC. Neuroglia: gliosis and focal epilepsy. *Science* 1970;167:1252–1253.

30. Gleeson JG, et al. Doublecortin, a brain-specific gene mutated in human X-linked lissencephaly and double cortex syndrome, encodes a putative signaling protein. *Cell* 1998;92:63–72.

31. Gleeson JG, et al. Characterization of mutations in the gene doublecortin in patients with double cortex syndrome [see comments]. *Ann Neurol* 1999;45:146–153.

32. Houser CR. Granule cell dispersion in the dentate gyrus of humans with temporal lobe epilepsy. *Brain Res* 1990;535:195–204.

33. Parent JM, et al. Dentate granule cell neurogenesis is increased by seizures and contributes to aberrant network reorganization in the adult rat hippocampus. *J Neurosci* 1997;17:3727–3738.

34. Aguilar NJ, Rasmussen T. Role of encephalitis in pathogenesis of epilepsy. *Arch Neurol* 1960;2:663–676.

35. Gupta PC, Roy S, Tandon PN. Progressive epilepsy due to chronic persistent encephalitis: report of four cases. *J Neurol Sci* 1974;22:105–120.

36. Brett EM. On a peculiar mode of onset of epilepsy in childhood: epileptogenic encephalopathy. *J Neurol Sci* 1967;4:315–338.

37. Meldrum BS, Vigouroux RA, Brierley JB. Systemic factors and epileptic brain damage: prolonged seizures in paralyzed, artificially ventilated baboons. *Arch Neurol* 1973;29:82–87.

38. Corsellis JAN, Bruton CJ. Neuropathology of status epilepticus in humans. *Adv Neurol* 1983;34:129–139.

39. Wasterlain CG, et al. Pathophysiological mechanisms of brain damage from status epilepticus. *Epilepsia* 1993;34[Suppl 1]:S37–53.

40. Scheibel ME, Crandall PH, Scheibel AB. The hippocampus-dentate complex in temporal lobe epilepsy. A Golgi study. *Epilepsia* 1974;15:55–80.

41. Greenamyre JT, et al. Autoradiographic characterization of *N*-methyl-*D*-aspartate, quisqualate- and kainate-sensitive glutamate binding sites. *J Pharmacol Exp Ther* 1985;233:254–263.

42. Sommer B, et al. Flip and flop: a cell-specific functional switch in glutamate-operated channels of the CNS. *Science* 1990;249:1580–1584.

43. Goodman JH, et al. Calbindin-D28k immunoreactivity and selective vulnerability to ischemia in the dentate gyrus of the developing rat. *Brain Res* 1993;606:309–314.

44. Iadarola MJ, Gale K. Substantia nigra: site of anticonvulsant activity mediated by gamma-aminobutyric acid. *Science* 1982;218:1237–1240.

45. Auer RN, Siesjö BK. Biological differences between ischemia, hypoglycemia, and epilepsy. *Ann Neurol* 1988;24:699–707.

46. Sankar R, Wasterlain, CG, Sperber EF. Seizure-induced changes in the immature brain. In: Schwartzkroin PA, et al., eds. *Brain development and epilepsy.* Oxford: Oxford University Press, 1995:268–288.

47. Represa A, et al. Hippocampal plasticity in childhood epilepsy. *Neurosci Lett* 1989;99:351–355.

48. Mathern GW, et al. Children with severe epilepsy: evidence of hippocampal neuron losses and aberrant mossy fiber sprouting during postnatal granule cell migration and differentiation. *Dev Brain Res* 1994;78:70–80.

49. Sankar R, et al. Patterns of status epilepticus-induced neuronal injury during development and long-term consequences. *J Neurosci* 1998;18:8382–8393.

50. Sankar R, Shin DH, Wasterlain CG. Serum neuron-specific enolase is a marker for neuronal damage following status epilepticus in the rat. *Epilepsy Res* 1997;28:129–136.

51. Holmes GL, Ben-Ari Y. Seizures in the developing brain: perhaps not so benign after all. *Neuron* 1998;21:1231–1234.

52. Holmes GL, et al. Consequences of neonatal seizures in the rat: morphological and behavioral effects. *Ann Neurol* 1998;44:845–857.

53. Holmes GL, et al. Mossy fiber sprouting after recurrent seizures during early development in rats. *J Comp Neurol* 1999;404:537–553.

54. Holmes GL. The long-term effect of seizures on the developing brain: clinical and laboratory issues. *Brain Dev* 1991;13:393–409.

55. Shewmon DA, Erwin RJ. Focal spike-induced cerebral dysfunction is related to the after-coming slow wave. *Ann Neurol* 1988;23:131–137.

56. Meldrum BS. Excitotoxicity and epileptic brain damage. *Epilepsy Res* 1991;10:55–61.

57. DeGiorgio CM, et al. Hippocampal pyramidal cell loss in human status epilepticus. *Epilepsia* 1992:33:23–27.

58. Bruton C. *The neuropathology of temporal lobe epilepsy.* New York: Oxford University Press, 1988.

59. Falconer MA, Serafetinides EA, Corsellis JAN. Etiology and pathogenesis of temporal lobe epilepsy. *Arch Neurol* 1964;10:233–248.

60. Engel J, et al. Pathological findings underlying focal temporal lobe hypometabolism in partial epilepsy. *Ann Neurol* 1982;12:518–528.

61. Hudson LP, et al. Amygdaloid sclerosis in temporal lobe epilepsy. *Ann Neurol* 1993;33:622–631.

62. Babb TL, et al. Temporal lobe volumetric cell densities in temporal lobe epilepsy. *Epilepsia* 1984;25:729–740.

63. Babb TL, et al. Glutamate decarboxylase-immunoreactive neurons are preserved in human epileptic hippocampus. *J Neurosci* 1989;9:2562–2574.

64. Franck JE. Cell death, plasticity, and epilepsy. In: Schwartzkroin PA, ed. *Epilepsy: models, mechanisms, and concepts.* Cambridge: Cambridge University Press, 1993:281–303.

65. Engel J. Epileptic brain damage: how much excitement can a limbic neuron take? *Trends Neurosci* 1983;6:356–357.

66. Meldrum BS, Horton RW, Brierley JB. Epileptic brain damage in adolescent baboons following seizures induced by allylglycine. *Brain* 1974;97:407–418.

67. Rocca WA, et al. Risk factors for complex partial

seizures: a population-based case-control study. *Ann Neurol* 1987;21:22–31.

68. Taylor J. *Selected writings of John Hughlings Jackson.* Vol. 1. London: Hodder & Stoughton, 1931.

69. Schwartzkroin PA. "Normal" brain mechanisms that support epileptiform activities. In: Schwartzkroin PA, ed. *Epilepsy: models, mechanisms, and concepts.* Cambridge: Cambridge University Press, 1993:358–370.

70. Dichter MA, Ayala GF. Cellular mechanisms of epilepsy: a status report. *Science* 1987;237:157–164.

71. Lothman EW, Collins RC. Seizures and epilepsy. In: Pearlman AL, Collins RC, eds. *Neurobiology of disease.* Oxford: Oxford University Press, 1990:593–617.

72. Dudek FE, Snow RW, Taylor CP. Role of electrical interactions in synchronization of epileptiform bursts. *Adv Neurol* 1986;44:593–617.

73. Heinemann U. Changes in the neuronal micro-environment and epileptiform activity. In: Wieser HG, Speckman EJ, Engel J, eds. *Current problems in epilepsy 3: the epileptic focus.* London: John Libbey & Co, Ltd, 1987:27–44.

74. Prince DA, Schwartzkroin PA. Non-synaptic mechanisms in epileptogenesis. In: Chalozonitis N, Boiusson M, eds. *Abnormal neuronal discharges.* New York: Raven Press, 1978:1–12.

75. Goddard GV, McIntyre DC, Leech CK. A permanent change in brain function resulting from daily electrical stimulation. *Exp Neurol* 1969;25:295–330.

76. McNamara J. Kindling: an animal model of complex partial epilepsy. *Ann Neurol* 1984;16[Suppl]:S72–S76.

77. Sutula T, et al. Synaptic reorganization in the hippocampus induced by abnormal functional activity. *Science* 1988;239:1147–1150.

78. Sutula T, et al. Mossy fiber synaptic reorganization in the epileptic human temporal lobe. *Ann Neurol* 1989;26:321–330.

79. Houser CR, et al. Altered patterns of dynorphin immunoreactivity suggest mossy fiber reorganization in human temporal lobe epilepsy. *J Neurosci* 1990;276–282.

80. Babb TL, et al. Synaptic reorganization by mossy fibers in human epileptic fascia dentata. *Neuroscience* 1991;42:351–363.

81. Sloviter RS. Possible functional consequence of synaptic reorganization in the dentate gyrus of kainic acid–treated rats. *Neurosci Lett* 1992;137:91–96.

82. Sloviter RS. Permanently altered hippocampal structure, excitability, and inhibition after experimental status epilepticus in the rat: the "dormant basket cell" hypothesis and its possible relevance to temporal lobe epilepsy. *Hippocampus* 1991;1:41–66.

83. Babb TL, et al. Glutamate decarboxylase immunoreactive neurons are preserved in human epileptic hippocampus. *J Neurosci* 1989;9:2562–2574.

84. Williamson A, Patrylo PR, Spencer DD. Decrease in inhibition in dentate granule cells from patients with medial temporal lobe epilepsy. *Ann Neurol* 1999;45:92–93.

85. Mathern GW, et al. Altered hippocampal kainate-receptor mRNA levels in temporal lobe epilepsy patients. *Neurobiol Dis* 1998;5:151–176.

86. Mathern GW, et al. Hippocampal GABA and glutamate transporter immunoreactivity in patients with temporal lobe epilepsy. *Neurology* 1999;52:453–472.

87. Zucker RS. Frequency dependent changes in excitatory synaptic efficacy. In: Dichter MA, ed. *Mechanisms of epileptogenesis—the transition to seizure.* New York: Plenum Publishing, 1988:163–168.

88. Dichter MA. Modulation of inhibition and the transition to seizures. In: Dichter MA, ed. *Mechanisms of epileptogenesis—the transition to seizure.* New York: Plenum Publishing, 1988:169–182.

89. Kapur J, Stringer JL, Lothman LW. Evidence that repetitive seizures in the hippocampus cause a lasting reduction of GABAergic inhibition. *J Neurophysiol* 1989;61:417–426.

90. Gale K. Progression and generalization of seizure discharge: anatomical and neurochemical substrates. *Epilepsia* 1988;29[Suppl 2]:S15–S34.

91. Burnham WM. Core mechanisms in generalized convulsions. *Fed Proc* 1985;44:2442–2445.

92. Browning RA. Role of the brain-stem reticular formation in tonic-clonic seizures: lesion and pharmacological studies. *Fed Proc* 1985;44:2425–2431.

93. Efron R. Post-epileptic paralysis: theoretical critique and report of a case. *Brain* 1961;84:381–394.

94. Niedermeyer E, Laws ER Jr, Walker AE. Depth EEG findings in epileptics with generalized spike-wave complexes. *Arch Neurol* 1969;21:51–58.

95. Goldring S. The role of prefrontal cortex in grand mal convulsion. *Arch Neurol* 1972;26:109–119.

96. Penfield W. Epileptic automatism and the centrencephalic integrating system. *Assoc Res Nerv Ment Dis* 1952;30:513–528.

97. Gloor P, Fariello RG. Generalized epilepsy: some of its cellular mechanisms differ from those of focal epilepsy. *Trends Neurosci* 1988;11:63–68.

98. Engel, J. *Seizures, epilepsy and the epileptic patient.* Philadelphia: FA Davis Co, 1989.

99. Coulter DA, Haguenard JR, Prince DA. Characterization of ethosuximide reduction of low-threshold calcium currents in thalamic neurons. *Ann Neurol* 1989;25:582–593.

100. Engel J, et al. Interictal cerebral glucose metabolism in partial epilepsy and its relation to EEG changes. *Ann Neurol* 1982;12:510–517.

101. Spenser S, et al. The localizing value of depth electroencephalography in 32 patients with refractory epilepsy. *Ann Neurol* 1982;12:248–253.

102. Cotman CW, Iverson LL. Excitatory amino acids in the brain-focus on NMDA receptors. *Trends Neurosci* 1987;10:263–265.

103. Turski WA, et al. Limbic seizures produced by pilocarpine in rats: a behavioral, electroencephalographic, and neuropathological study. *Behav Brain Res* 1983;9:315–335.

104. Olsen RW, et al. Benzodiazepine/barbiturate/GABA receptor-chloride ionophore complex in a genetic model for generalized epilepsy. *Adv Neurol* 1986;44:365–378.

105. Olsen RW. GABA-drug interactions. *Prog Drug Res* 1987;31:223–341.

106. Schofield PR, et al. Sequence and functional expression of the GABAA receptor shows a ligand-gated receptor super-family. *Nature* 1987;328:221–227.

107. Pritchett DB, et al. Importance of a novel GABAA receptor subunit for benzodiazepine pharmacology. *Nature* 1989;338:582–584.

108. Sigel E, et al. The effect of subunit composition of rat

brain GABAA receptors on channel function. *Neuron* 1990;5:703–711.

109. Macdonald RL, et al. Regulation of GABAA receptor channels by anticonvulsant and convulsant drugs and by phosphorylation. *Epilepsy Res Suppl* 1992; 265–277.

110. Gale K, Iadarola MJ. Seizure protection and increased nerve-terminal GABA: delayed effects of GABA transaminase inhibition. *Science* 1980;208: 288–291.

111. Petroff OA, et al. Human brain GABA and homo-carnosine increased after starting topiramate. *Neurology* 1998;50[Suppl 4]:A312.

112. Petroff OAC, et al. Topiramate increases brain GABA, homocarnosine, and pyrrolidinone in patients with epilepsy. *Neurology* 1999;52:473–478.

113. During M, et al. The effect of tiagabine hydrochloride on extracellular GABA levels in the human hippocampus. *Epilepsia* 1992;33[Suppl 3]:83.

114. Lott IT, et al. Vitamin B6-dependent seizures: pathology and chemical findings in brain. *Neurology* 1978; 28:47–54.

115. Gospe SM, Olin KL, Keen CL. Reduced GABA synthesis in pyridoxine-dependent seizures. *Lancet* 1994;343:1133–1134.

116. Fromm GH. Role of inhibitory mechanisms in staring spells. *J Clin Neurophysiol* 1986;3:297–311.

117. Peterson GM, Ribak CE, Oertel WH. A regional increase in the number of hippocampal GABAergic neurons and terminals in the seizure-sensitive gerbil. *Brain Res* 1985;340:384–389.

118. Engel J Jr, et al. Do altered opioid mechanisms play a role in human epilepsy? In: Fariello RF, et al., eds. *Neurotransmitters in seizures and epilepsy.* New York: Raven Press, 1984:263–274.

119. Frost JJ, et al. μ-opiate receptors measured by positron emission tomography are increased in temporal lobe epilepsy. *Ann Neurol* 1988;23:231–237.

120. Handforth A, Treiman DM. Effect of an adenosine antagonist and an adenosine agonist on status entry and severity in a model of limbic status epilepticus. *Epilepsy Res* 1994;18:29–42.

121. During MJ, Spencer DD. Adenosine: a potential mediator of seizure arrest and postictal refractoriness. *Ann Neurol* 1992;32:618–624.

122. Dragunow M. Purinergic mechanisms in epilepsy. *Progr Neurobiol* 1988;31:85–108.

123. Chin JH. Adenosine receptors in brain: neuromodulation and role in epilepsy. *Ann Neurol* 1989;26: 695–698.

124. Jobe PC, Laird HE. Neurotransmitter abnormalities as determinants of seizure susceptibility and intensity in the genetic models of epilepsy. *Biochem Pharmacol* 1981;30:3137–3144.

125. Mishra PK, et al. Role of norepinephrine in forebrain and brainstem seizures. Chemical lesioning of locus ceruleus with DSP4. *Exp Neurol* 1994;125: 58–64.

126. Brière R, et al. α–1 adrenoreceptors are decreased in human epileptic foci. *Ann Neurol* 1986;19:26–30.

127. Prendiville S, Gale K. Anticonvulsant effect of fluoxetine on focally evoked limbic motor seizures in rats. *Epilepsia* 1993;34:381–384.

128. Leander JD. Fluoxetine, a selective serotonin-uptake inhibitor, enhances the anticonvulsant effects of phenytoin, carbamazepine, and ameltolide (LY201116). *Epilepsia* 1992;33:573–576.

129. Favale E, et al. Anticonvulsant effect of fluoxetine in humans. *Neurology* 1995;45:1926–1927.

130. Salgado-Commissariat D, Alkadhi KA. Serotonin inhibits epileptiform discharge by activation of 5-HT1A receptors in CA1 pyramidal neurons. *Neuropharmacology* 1997;36:1705–1712.

131. Lu KT, Gean PW. Endogenous serotonin inhibits epileptiform activity in rat hippocampal CA1 neurons via 5-hydroxytryptamine 1A receptor activation. *Neuroscience* 1998;86:729–737.

132. Gerber K, et al. The 5-HT$_{1A}$ agonist 8-OH-DPAT increases the number of spike-wave discharges in a genetic rat model of absence epilepsy. *Brain Res* 1998;807:243–245.

133. Applegate CD, Tecott LH. Global increases in seizure susceptibility in mice lacking 5-HT2C receptors: a behavioral analysis. *Exp Neurol* 1998;154:522–530.

134. Engel J, et al. Local cerebral metabolism during partial seizures. *Neurology* 1983;33:400–413.

135. Engel J, Kuhl DE, Phelps ME. Patterns of human local cerebral glucose metabolism during epileptic seizures. *Science* 1982;218:64–66.

136. Engel J, et al. Comparative localization of epileptic foci in partial epilepsy by PCT and EEG. *Ann Neurol* 1982;12:529–537.

137. Meldrum BS, Horton RW. Physiology of status epilepticus in primates. *Arch Neurol* 1973;28:19.

138. Beresford HR, Posner JB, Plum F. Changes in brain lactate during induced cerebral seizures. *Arch Neurol* 1969;20:243–248.

139. Petroff OAC, et al. Combined ^{1}H and ^{31}P nuclear magnetic resonance spectroscopic studies of bicuculline-induced seizures in vivo. *Ann Neurol* 1986;20:185–193.

140. O'Donohoe NV. *Epilepsies of childhood*, 3rd ed. Oxford: Butterworth–Heinemann, 1994.

141. Van Buren JM. The abdominal aura. A study of abdominal sensations occurring in epilepsy and produced by depth stimulation. *Electroencephalogr Clin Neurophysiol* 1963;15:119.

142. Mattson RH, Pratt KL, Calverley JR. Electroencephalograms of epileptics following sleep deprivation. *Arch Neurol* 1965;13:310–315.

143. Messing RO, Closson RG, Simon RP. Drug-induced seizures: a 10-year experience. *Neurology* 1984;34: 1582–1586.

144. Olson KR, et al. Seizures associated with poisoning and drug overdose. *Am J Emerg Med* 1993;11: 565–568.

145. Blanchard PD, et al. Isoniazid overdose in the Cambodian population of Olmstead County, Minnesota. *JAMA* 1986;256:3131–3133.

146. Van Donselaar CA, et al. Clinical course of untreated tonic-clonic seizures in childhood: prospective hospital based study. *Brit Med J* 1997; 314:401–404.

147. Gastaut H, Roger J, Favel F. La miction au cours des absences petit mal. Le petit mal enuretique. *Rev Neurol* 1960;103:53–58.

148. Dalby MA. Epilepsy and 3 per second spike and wave rhythms. *Acta Neurol Scand* 1969;40[Suppl]:3.

149. Lennox WG. The petit mal epilepsies: their treatment with Tridione. *JAMA* 1945;129:1069–1074.

150. Sato S, Dreifuss FE, Penry JK. Prognostic factors in absence seizures. *Neurology* 1976;26:788–796.

151. Holmes GL, McKeever M, Adamson M. Absence seizures in children: clinical and electroencephalographic features. *Ann Neurol* 1987;21:268–273.

152. Berkovic SF, et al. Concepts of absence epilepsies: discrete syndromes or biological continuum? *Neurology* 1987;37:993–1000.

153. Janz D. Epilepsy with impulsive petit mal (juvenile myoclonic epilepsy). *Acta Neurol Scand* 1985;72: 449–459.

154. Delgado-Escueta AV, Serratosa JM, Medina MT. Juvenile myoclonic epilepsy. In: Wyllie E, ed. *The treatment of epilepsy: principles and practice,* 2nd ed. Baltimore: Williams & Wilkins, 1996:484–501.

155. Prevett MC, et al. Demonstration of thalamic activation during typical absence seizures using H_2 ^{15} O and PET. *Neurology* 1995;45:1396–1402.

156. Williamson PD, et al. Complex partial seizures of frontal lobe origin. *Ann Neurol* 1985;18:497–504.

157. Williamson PD, et al. Occipital lobe epilepsy: clinical characteristics, seizure spread patterns and results of surgery. *Ann Neurol* 1992;31:3–13.

158. Falconer MA, Serafitinides EA, Corsellis JAN. Etiology and pathogenesis of temporal lobe epilepsy. *Arch Neurol* 1964;10:233–248.

159. Harvey AS, et al. Temporal lobe epilepsy in childhood. Clinical, EEG, and neuroimaging findings and syndrome classification in a cohort with new-onset seizures. *Neurology* 1997;49:960–968.

160. Cavanagh JB. On certain small tumours encountered in the temporal lobe. *Brain* 1958;81:389–405.

161. Malamud N. The epileptogenic focus in temporal lobe epilepsy from a pathological standpoint. *Arch Neurol* 1966;14:190–195.

162. Wyllie E, et al. Temporal lobe epilepsy in early childhood. *Epilepsia* 1993;34:859–868.

163. DeLong GR, Heinz ER. The clinical syndrome of early-life bilateral hippocampal sclerosis. *Ann Neurol* 1997;42:11–17.

164. Pacia SV, et al. Clinical features of neocortical temporal lobe epilepsy. *Ann Neurol* 1996;40:724–730.

165. Yamamoto N, et al. Complex partial seizures in children: ictal manifestations and their relation to clinical course. *Neurology* 1987;37:1379–1382.

166. Aird RB, Venturini AM, Spielman PM. Antecedents of temporal lobe epilepsy. *Arch Neurol* 1967;16:67–73.

167. Glaser GH, Dixon MS. Psychomotor seizures in childhood: a clinical study. *Neurology* 1956;6:646–655.

168. Daly DD. Uncinate fits. *Neurology* 1958;8:250–260.

169. Acharya V, Acharya J. Lüders H. Olfactory epileptic auras. *Neurology* 1998;51:56–61.

170. Howe JG, Gibson JD. Uncinate seizures and tumors, a myth reexamined. *Ann Neurol* 1982;12:227.

171. Penfield W, Perot P. The brain's record of auditory and visual experience. A final summary and discussion. *Brain* 1963;86:595–616.

172. Mullan S, Penfield W. Illusions of comparative interpretation and emotion; production by epileptic discharge and by electrical stimulation in the temporal cortex. *Arch Neurol Psychiatry* 1959;81:269–284.

173. Palmini A, Gloor P. The localizing values of auras in partial seizures: a prospective and retrospective study. *Neurology* 1992;42:801–809.

174. Escueta AVD, Enrile BF, Treiman DM. Complex partial seizures on closed-circuit television and EEG: a study of 691 attacks in 79 patients. *Ann Neurol* 1982;11:292–300.

175. Gambardella A, et al. Late-onset drop attacks in temporal lobe epilepsy: a reevaluation of the concept of temporal lobe syncope. *Neurology* 1994;44:1074–1078.

176. Markand ON, Wheeler GL, Pollack SL. Complex partial status epilepticus (psychomotor status). *Neurology* 1978;28:189–196.

177. McBride MC, Dooling EC, Oppenheimer EY. Complex partial status epilepticus in young children. *Ann Neurol* 1981;9:526–530.

178. Williamson PD, et al. Complex partial status epilepticus: a depth-electrode study. *Ann Neurol* 1985;18:647–654.

179. Blumhardt LD, Smith PE, Owen L. Electrocardiographic accompaniments of temporal lobe epileptic seizures. *Lancet* 1986;1:1051–1056.

180. Aird RB, Yamamoto T. Behavior disorders of childhood. *Electroenceph Clin Neurophysiol* 1966;21:148–156.

181. Stevens JR, Hermann BP. Temporal lobe epilepsy, psychopathology, and violence: the state of the evidence. *Neurology* 1981;31:1127–1132.

182. Rutter M, Graham P, Yule W. A neuro-psychiatric study in childhood. Rutter M, Graham P, Yule W. *Clinics in developmental medicine.* London: Butterworth–Heinemann, 1970:35–36.

183. Pincus JH. Can violence be a manifestation of epilepsy? *Neurology* 1980;30:304–307.

184. Pritchard PB, Lombroso CT, McIntyre M. Psychological complications of temporal lobe epilepsy. *Neurology* 1980;30:227–232.

185. Stevens JR, Livermore A. Kindling in the mesolimbic dopamine system: animal model of psychosis. *Neurology* 1978;28:36–46.

186. Adamec RE, Stark-Adamec C. Limbic kindling and animal behavior–implications for human psychopathology associated with complex partial seizures. *Biol Psychiatry* 1983;18:269–293.

187. Weiss SR, Post RM. Kindling: separate vs. shared mechanisms in affective disorders and epilepsy. *Neuropsychobiology* 1998;38:167–180.

188. Ochs R, et al. Does head-turning during a seizure have lateralizing or localizing significance? *Neurology* 1984;34:884–890.

189. Wyllie E, et al. The lateralizing significance of versive head and eye movements during epileptic seizures. *Neurology* 1986;36:606–611.

190. McLachlan RS. The significance of head and eye turning in seizures. *Neurology* 1987;37:1617–1619.

191. Devinsky O, et al. Clinical and electroencephalographic features of simple partial seizures. *Neurology* 1988;38:1347–1352.

192. Roger J, Bureau M. Les épilepsies partielles idiopathiques de l'enfant (épilepsies partielles bénignes or primaries). *Rev Neurol* 1987;143:381–391.

193. Loiseau P, Duché B, Loiseau J. Classification of epilepsies and epileptic syndromes in two different samples of patients. *Epilepsia* 1991;32:303–309.

194. Scheffer IE, et al. Autosomal dominant rolandic epilepsy and speech dyspraxia: a new syndrome with anticipation. *Ann Neurol* 1995;38:633–642.

195. Lombroso CT. Sylvian seizures and midtemporal spike foci in children. *Arch Neurol* 1967;17:52–59.

196. Loiseau P, Beaussart M. The seizures of benign childhood epilepsy with Rolandic paroxysmal discharges. *Epilepsia* 1973;14:381–389.

197. Loiseau P, et al. Long-term prognosis in two forms of childhood epilepsy: typical absence seizures and

epilepsy with Rolandic (Centrotemporal) EEG foci. *Ann Neurol* 1983;13:642–648.

198. Beaussart M, Faou R. Evolution of epilepsy with Rolandic paroxysmal foci: a study of 324 cases. *Epilepsia* 1978;19:337–342.

199. Beaumanoir A. Infantile epilepsy with occipital focus and good prognosis. *Eur Neurol* 1983;22:43–52.

200. Sveinbjornsdottir S, Duncan JS. Parietal and occipital lobe epilepsy: a review. *Epilepsia* 1993;34:493–521.

201. Livingston S, Eisner V, Pauli L. Minor motor epilepsy: diagnosis, treatment and prognosis. *Pediatrics* 1958;21:916–928.

202. Menkes JH. Diagnosis and treatment of minor motor seizures. *Pediatr Clin North Am* 1976;23:435–442.

203. Chevrie JJ, Aicardi J. Childhood epileptic encephalopathy with slow spike-wave. A statistical study of 80 cases. *Epilepsia* 1972;13:259–271.

204. Janz D. *Die epilepsien*. Stuttgart: Georg Thieme Verlag, 1969.

205. Hallett M. The pathophysiology of myoclonus. *Trends Neurosci* 1987;10:69–73.

206. Hurst DL. Epidemiology of myoclonic epilepsy of infancy. *Epilepsia* 1990;31:397–400.

207. Wilkins D, Hallett M, Erba G. Primary generalised epileptic myoclonus: a frequent manifestation of minipolymyoclonus of central origin. *J Neurol Neurosurg Psychiatry* 1985;48:506–516.

208. Rothwell JC, Obeso JA, Marsden CD. On the significance of giant somatosensory evoked potentials in cortical myoclonus. *J Neurol Neurosurg Psychiatry* 1984;47:33–42.

209. Muller U, Steinberger D, Nemeth AH. Clinical and molecular genetics of primary dystonias. *Neurogenetics* 1998;1:165–177.

210. Vergouwe MN, et al. Hyperekplexia phenotype due to compound heterozygosity for GLAR1 gene mutations. *Ann Neurol* 1999;46:634–638.

211. Aguglia U, Tinuper P, Gastaut H. Startle-induced epileptic seizures. *Epilepsia* 1984;25:712–720.

212. Andermann F, et al. Startle disease or hyperekplexia. Further delineation of the syndrome. *Brain* 1980;103:985–997.

213. Lennox WG, Davis JP. Clinical correlates of fast and slow spike-wave electroencephalogram. *Pediatrics* 1950;5:626–644.

214. Kruse R. *Das myoklonisch-astatische Petit Mal.* Berlin: Springer-Verlag, 1968.

215. Blume WT, David RB, Gomez MR. Generalized sharp and slow wave complexes—associated clinical features and long-term follow-up. *Brain* 1973;96:289–306.

216. Asal B, Moro E. Über bösartige Nickkrämpfe in frühen Kindesalter. *Jahrb Kinderheilk* 1924;107:1–17.

217. Druckman RD, Chao D. Massive spasms in infancy and childhood. *Epilepsia* 1955;4:61–72.

218. Jeavons PM, Bower BD. *Infantile spasms*. London: The Spastics Society Medical Education and Information Unit in association with Butterworth–Heinemann, 1964:12.

219. Hrachovy RA, Frost JD, Kellaway P. Hypsarrhythmia: variations on the theme. *Epilepsia* 1984;25:317–325.

220. Hrachovy RA, Frost JD Jr, Kellaway P. Sleep characteristics in infantile spasms. *Neurology* 1981;31:688–694.

221. Chugani HT, et al. Infantile spasms: II. Lenticular nuclei and brain stem activation on positron emission tomography. *Ann Neurol* 1992;31:212–219.

222. Riikonen R. A long-term follow-up study of 214 children with the syndrome of infantile spasms. *Neuropediatrics* 1982;13:14–23.

222a. Baxter P. Epidemiology of pyridoxine dependent and pyridoxine response seizures in the U.K. *Arch Dis Child* 1999;81:431–433.

223. Bellman MH, Ross EM, Miller DL. Infantile spasms and pertussis immunization. *Lancet* 1983;1:1031–1034.

224. Vinters HV, et al. Morphologic substrates of infantile spasms: studies based on surgically resected cerebral tissue. *Child's Nerv Syst* 1992;8:8–17.

225. Jellinger K. Neuropathologic aspects of hypsarrhythmia. *Neuropädiatrie* 1970;1:277–294.

226. Sankar R, et al. Microscopic cortical dysplasia in infantile spasms: evolution of white matter abnormalities. *Am J Neuroradiol* 1995;16:1265–1272.

227. Midulla M, et al. Infantile spasms and cytomegalovirus infection. *Lancet* 1976;2:377.

228. Poser C, Low NL. Autopsy findings in three cases of hypsarrhythmia (infantile spasms with mental retardation). *Acta Paediatr Scand* 1960;49:695–706.

229. Jeavons PM, Harper JR, Bower BD. Long-term prognosis in infantile spasms: a follow-up report on 112 cases. *Dev Med Child Neurol* 1970;12:413–421.

229a. Gaily E, et al. Cognitive deficits after cryptogenic infantile spasms with benign seizure evolution. *Dev Med Child Neurol* 1999;41:660–664.

230. Riikonen R, Simell O. Tuberous sclerosis and infantile spasms. *Dev Med Child Neurol* 1990;32:203–209.

231. Workshop on infantile spasms. *Epilepsia* 1992;33:195.

232. Lerman P, Kivity S. The efficacy of corticotropin in primary infantile spasms. *J Pediatr* 1982;101:294–296.

233. Glaze DG, et al. Prospective study of outcome of infants with infantile spasms treated during controlled studies of ACTH and prednisone. *J Pediatr* 1988;112:389–396.

234. Hrachovy RA, Frost JD, Glaze DG. High-dose, long-duration versus low-dose, short-duration corticotropin therapy for infantile spasms. *J Pediatr* 1994;124:803–806.

235. Riikonen R, Donner MA. ACTH therapy in infantile spasms: side effects. *Arch Dis Child* 1980;55:664–672.

236. Snead OC, Benton JW, Myers GJ. ACTH and prednisone in childhood seizure disorders. *Neurology* 1983;33:966–970.

237. Carollo C, et al. CT and ACTH treatment in infantile spasms. *Childs Brain* 1982;9:347–353.

238. Baram T, et al. Cerebrospinal fluid corticotropin and cortisol are reduced in infantile spasms. *Pediatr Neurol* 1995;13:108–113.

239. Baram TZ. Pathophysiology of massive infantile spasms: perspective on the putative role of the brain adrenal axis. *Ann Neurol* 1993;33:231–236.

240. Charuvanji A, et al. ACTH treatment in intractable seizures of childhood. *Brain Dev* 1992;14:102–106.

241. Baram TZ, et al. High-dose corticotropin (ACTH) versus prednisone for infantile spasms: a prospective, randomized, blinded study. *Pediatrics* 1996;97:375–379.

242. Prats JM, et al. Infantile spasms treated with high doses of sodium valproate: initial response and follow-up. *Dev Med Child Neurol* 1991;33:617–625.

243. Chiron C, et al. Therapeutic trial of vigabatrin in refractory infantile spasms. *J Child Neurol* 1991;2 [Suppl]:S52–S59.

244. Cossette P, Riviello JJ, Carmant L. ACTH versus vigabatrin in infantile spasms: a retrospective study. *Neurology* 1999;52:1691–1694.

245. Appleton RF. A simple, effective and well-tolerated treatment regime for West syndrome. *Dev Med Child Neurol* 1995;37:185–187.

246. Wohlrab G, Boltshauser E, Schmitt B. Vigabatrin as a first-line drug in West syndrome: clinical and electroencephalographic outcome. *Neuropediatrics* 1998; 29:133–136.

246a. Vigevano F, Cilio MR. Vigabatrin versus ACTH as first-line treatment for infantile spasms: a randomized, prospective study. *Epilepsia* 1997;38:1270–1274.

247. Lombroso CT, Fejerman N. Benign myoclonus of early infancy. *Ann Neurol* 1977;1:138–143.

248. Aicardi J, Lefebvre J, Lerique-Koechlin A. A new syndrome: spasm in flexion, callosal agenesis, ocular abnormalities. *Electroencephalogr Clin Neurophysiol* 1965;19:609–610.[Abstract]

249. Dennis J, Bower BD. The Aicardi syndrome. *Dev Med Child Neurol* 1972;14:382–390.

250. Goutieres F, et al. Aicardi-Goutieres syndrome: an update and results of interferon-alpha studies. *Ann Neurol* 1998;44:900–907.

251. Sander T, et al. Refined mapping of the epilepsy susceptibility locus EJM1 on chromosome 6. *Neurology* 1997;49:842–847.

252. Wolf P, Goosses R. Relation of photosensitivity to epileptic syndromes. *J Neurol Neurosurg Psychiatry* 1986;49:1386–1391.

253. Grünewald RA, Chroni E, Panayiotopoulos CP. Delayed diagnosis of juvenile myoclonic epilepsy. *J Neurol Neurosurg Psychiatry* 1992;55:497–499.

254. Douglas EF, White PT. Abdominal epilepsy—a reappraisal. *J Pediatr* 1971;78:59–67.

255. Schäffler L, Karbowski K. Rezidivierende paroxysmale abdominale Schmerzen zerebraler Genese. *Schweiz Med Wschr* 1981;111:1352–1360.

256. Rasmussen T, McCann W. Clinical studies of patients with focal epilepsy due to "chronic encephalitis." *Trans Am Neurol Assoc* 1968;93:89–94.

257. Thomas JE, Reagan TJ, Klass DW. Epilepsia partialis continua. A review of 32 cases. *Arch Neurol* 1977;34:266–275.

258. Cascino GD. Nonconvulsive status epilepticus in adults and children. *Epilepsia* 1993;34[Suppl 1]:S21–S28.

259. Brett EM. Minor epileptic status. *J Neurol Sci* 1966;3:52–75.

260. Niedermeyer E, Khalifeh R. Petit mal status ("spike-wave stupor"). An electro-clinical appraisal. *Epilepsia* 1965;6:250–262.

261. Farran RD, McIntyre HB, Itabashi HH. Pathogenesis of spike-wave status: a clinical-pathological study implicating cerebellar disturbance. *Bull Los Angeles Neurol Soc* 1975;40:153–159.

262. Chugani HT, et al. The Lennox-Gastaut syndrome: metabolic subtypes determined by 2-deoxy-2-[^{18}F]fluoro-D-glucose positron emission tomography. *Ann Neurol* 1987;21:413.

262a. Kaplan PW. Intravenous valproate treatment of generalized nonconvulsive status epilepticus. *Clin Electroencephalogr* 1999;30:1–4.

263. Landau WM, Kleffner FR. Syndrome of acquired aphasia with convulsive disorder in children. *Neurology* 1957;7:523–530.

264. Hirsch E, et al. Landau-Kleffner syndrome: a clinical and EEG study of five cases. *Epilepsia* 1990;31:756–767.

265. Paquier PF, Van Dongen HR, Loonen MCB. The Landau-Kleffner syndrome or "acquired aphasia with convulsive disorder." Long-term follow-up of six children and a review of the recent literature. *Arch Neurol* 1992;49:354–359.

266. Marescaux C, et al. Landau-Kleffner syndrome: a pharmacologic study of five cases. *Epilepsia* 1990;31: 768–777.

267. Lagae LG, et al. Successful use of intravenous immunoglobulin in Landau-Kleffner syndrome. *Pediatr Neurol* 1998;18:165–168.

268. Grote CL, Van Slyke P, Hoeppner JA. Language outcome following multiple subpial transection for Landau-Kleffner syndrome. *Brain* 1999;122:561–566.

269. Jayakar PB, Seshia SS. Electrical status epilepticus during slow-wave sleep: a review. *J Clin Neurophysiol* 1991;7:299–311.

270. Rossi PG, et al. Landau-Kleffner syndrome (LKS): long-term follow-up and links with electrical status epilepticus during sleep (ESPS). *Brain Dev* 1999; 21:90–98.

271. Forster FM. *Reflex epilepsy, behavioral therapy and conditioned reflexes*. Springfield, IL: Charles C Thomas Publisher, 1977.

272. Darby CE, et al. The self-induction of epileptic seizures by eye closure. *Epilepsia* 1980;21:31–42.

273. Badinand-Hubert N, et al. Epilepsies and video games: results of a multicentric study. *Electroencephalogr Clin Neurophysiol* 1998;107:422–427.

274. Newmark ME, Penry JK. *Photosensitivity and epilepsy: a review*. New York: Raven Press, 1979.

275. Wyllie E, et al. Psychogenic seizures in children and adolescents: outcome after diagnosis by ictal video and electroencephalographic recording. *Pediatrics* 1990;85:480–484.

276. Williams DT, Spiegel H, Mostofsky DI. Neurogenic and hysterical seizures in children and adolescents: differential diagnostic and therapeutic considerations. *Am J Psychiatry* 1978;135:82–86.

277. Schneider S, Rice DR. Neurologic manifestations of childhood hysteria. *J Pediatr* 1979;94:153–156.

278. Lazare A. Conversion symptoms. *N Engl J Med* 1981;305:745–748.

279. Gastaut H, Fischer-Williams M. Electroencephalographic study of syncope: its differentiation from epilepsy. *Lancet* 1957;2:1018–1025.

280. Tharp BR. An overview of pediatric seizure disorders and epileptic syndromes. *Epilepsia* 1987;28[Suppl. 1]: S36–S45.

281. Tassinari CA, et al. Pavor nocturnus of non-epileptic nature in epileptic children. *Electroencephalogr Clin Neurophysiol* 1972;33:603–607.

282. Symonds CP. Nocturnal myoclonus. *J Neurol Neurosurg Psychiatry* 1953;16:166–171.

283. Altrocchi PH, Menkes JH. Congenital ocular motor apraxia. *Brain* 1960;83:579–588.

284. Mitchell I, et al. Apnea and factitious illness (Münchausen syndrome) by proxy. *Pediatrics* 1993;92: 810–814.

285. Meadow R. Fictitious epilepsy. *Lancet* 1984;2:25–28.

286. Page LK, Lombroso CT, Matson DD. Childhood epilepsy with late detection of cerebral glioma. *J Neurosurg* 1969;31:253–261.

287. King MA, et al. Epileptology of the first-seizure presentation: a clinical, electroencephalographic, and magnetic resonance imaging study of 300 consecutive patients. *Lancet* 1998;352:1007–1011.

288. Gibbs EL, Gillen HW, Gibbs FA. Disappearance and migration of epileptic foci in children. *Am J Dis Child* 1954;88:596–603.

289. Strobos RJ, Kavallinis GP. Changes in repeat electroencephalograms in epileptics. *Neurology* 1968;18:622–633.

290. Lennox WG, Merritt HH. Cerebrospinal fluid in "essential" epilepsy. *J Neurol Psychopathol* 1936;17:97–106.

291. Edwards R, Schmidley JW, Simon RP. How often does a CSF pleocytosis follow generalized convulsions? *Ann Neurol* 1983;13:460–462.

292. Barry E, Hauser WA. Pleocytosis after status epilepticus. *Arch Neurol* 1994;51:190–193.

293. Yaffe K, et al. Reversible MRI abnormalities following seizures. *Neurology* 1995;45:104–108.

294. Yang PJ, et al. Computed tomography and childhood seizure disorders. *Neurology* 1979;29:1084–1088.

295. Kuzniecky R, et al. Focal cortical myoclonus and Rolandic cortical dysplasia: clarification by magnetic resonance imaging. *Ann Neurol* 1988;23:317–325.

296. Kuzniecky R, et al. Magnetic resonance imaging in childhood intractable partial epilepsies: pathologic correlations. *Neurology* 1993;43:681–687.

297. Kuzniecky R, et al. Magnetic resonance imaging in temporal lobe epilepsy: pathological correlations. *Ann Neurol* 1987;22:341–347.

298. Williamson PD, et al. Characteristics of medial temporal lobe epilepsy: I. Interictal and ictal scalp electroencephalography, neuropsychological testing, neuroimaging, surgical results, and pathology. *Ann Neurol* 1993;34:781–787.

299. Theodore WH, et al. Pathology of temporal lobe foci: correlation with CT, MRI and PET. *Neurology* 1990;40:797–803.

300. Kuzniecky R, et al. Cortical dysplasia in temporal lobe epilepsy: magnetic resonance imaging correlations. *Ann Neurol* 1991;29:293–298.

301. Kramer RE, et al. Transient focal abnormalities of neuroimaging studies during focal status epilepticus. *Epilepsia* 1987;28:528–532.

302. McLachlan RS, Karlik SJ, Myles V. Nuclear magnetic resonance relaxometry in a penicillin model of focal epilepsy. *Epilepsia* 1988;29:396–400.

303. Sammaritano M, et al. Prolonged focal cerebral edema associated with partial status epilepticus. *Epilepsia* 1985;26:334–339.

304. Karlik SJ. Common pharmaceuticals alter tissue proton NMR relaxation properties. *Magn Reson Imaging Med* 1986;3:181–193.

305. Abou-Khalil BW, et al. Positron emission tomography studies of cerebral glucose metabolism in chronic partial epilepsy. *Ann Neurol* 1987;22:480–486.

306. Engel J, et al. Local cerebral metabolic rate for glucose during petit mal absences. *Ann Neurol* 1985;17:121–128.

307. Olson DM, et al. Electrocorticographic confirmation of focal positron emission tomographic abnormalities in children with intractable epilepsy. *Epilepsia* 1990;31:731–739.

308. Won HJ, et al. Comparison of MR imaging with PET and ictal SPECT in 118 patients with intractable epilepsy. *Am J Neuroradiol* 1999;20:593–599.

309. Theodore WH, et al. Temporal lobectomy for uncontrolled seizures: the role of positron emission tomography. *Ann Neurol* 1992;32:789–794.

310. Sutherling WW, et al. The magnetic field of epileptic spikes agrees with intracranial localizations in complex partial epilepsy. *Neurology* 1988;38:778–786.

311. Wheless JW, et al. A comparison of magnetoencephalography, MRI and V-EEG in patients evaluated for epilepsy surgery. *Epilepsia* 1999;40:931–941.

312. Scott CA, et al. Presurgical evaluation of patients with epilepsy and normal MRI: role of scalp video-EEG telemetry. *J Neurol Neurosurg Psychiatry* 1999;66:69–71.

313. Gotman J, Ives JR, Gloor P, eds. Long-term monitoring in epilepsy. *Electroenceph Clin Neurophysiol* 1985;[Suppl 37].

314. Engel J, Driver MV, Falconer MA. Electrophysiological correlates of pathology and surgical results in temporal lobe epilepsy. *Brain* 1975;98:129–156.

315. Morrell F, et al. Diagnostic value of the methohexital suppression test for differentiating independent secondary foci. *Neurology* 1984;34[Suppl 1]:124.

316. Hauser WA, et al. Seizure recurrence after a first unprovoked seizure. *N Engl J Med* 1982;307:522–528.

317. Elwes RDC, Chesterman P, Reynolds EH. Prognosis after a first untreated tonic-clonic seizure. *Lancet* 1985;2:752–753.

318. Shinnar S, et al. The risk of recurrence following a first unprovoked seizure in childhood: a prospective study. *Pediatrics* 1990;85:1076–1085.

319. Camfield PR, et al. Epilepsy after a first unprovoked seizure in childhood. *Neurology* 1985;35:1657–1660.

320. Hirtz DG, Ellenberg JH, Nelson KB. The risk of recurrence of nonfebrile seizures in children. *Neurology* 1984;34:637–641.

321. Stephenson JBP. *Fits and faints. Clinics in developmental medicine*. Oxford: MacKeith Press, 1990:109.

322. Ebersole JS, Leroy RF. Evaluation of ambulatory cassette EEG monitoring. III. Diagnostic accuracy compared to intensive inpatient EEG monitoring. *Neurology* 1983;33:853–860.

323. Reynolds EH, Shorvon SD. Monotherapy or polytherapy for epilepsy? *Epilepsia* 1981;22:110.

324. Lesser RP, et al. High-dose monotherapy in treatment of intractable seizures. *Neurology* 1984;34:707–711.

325. Hanson RA, Menkes JH. Iatrogenic perpetuation of epilepsy. *Trans Am Neurol Assoc* 1972;97:290–291.

326. Choonara IA, Rane A. Therapeutic drug monitoring of anticonvulsants: state of the art. *Clin Pharmacokinet* 1990;18:318–328.

327. Curless RG, Walson PD, Carter DE. Phenytoin kinetics in children. *Neurology* 1976;26:715–720.

328. Laidlaw J, Richens A, Chadwick D. *A textbook of epilepsy*, 4th ed. Edinburgh: Churchill Livingstone, 1993.

329. Browne TR, et al. Ethosuximide in the treatment of absence (petit mal) seizures. *Neurology* 1975;25:515–524.

330. Bourgeois BFD. Phenobarbital and primidone. In: Wyllie E, ed. *The treatment of epilepsy: principles and practice*, 2nd ed. Baltimore: Williams & Wilkins, 1996:845–855.

331. Kutt H. Relation of plasma concentration to seizure control. In: Woodbury DM, et al., eds. *Antiepileptic drugs*, 2nd ed. New York: Raven Press, 1982:241–246.

332. Chadwick DW. Overuse of monitoring of blood con-

centrations of antiepileptic drugs. *BMJ* 1987;294:723–724.

333. Pellock JM, Willmore LJ. A rational guide to routine blood monitoring in patients receiving antiepileptic drugs. *Neurology* 1991;41:961–964.

334. Wyllie E, Wyllie R. Routine laboratory monitoring for serious adverse effects of antiepileptic medications: the controversy. *Epilepsia* 1991;32[Suppl 5]: S74–S79.

335. Merritt HH, Putnam TJ. A new series of anticonvulsant drugs tested by experiments on animals. *Arch Neurol Psychiatry* 1938;38:1003–1015.

336. Sankar R, Weaver DF. Basic principles of medicinal chemistry. In: Engel J Jr, Pedley TA, eds. *Epilepsy: a comprehensive textbook*. Philadelphia: Lippincott–Raven Publishers, 1998:1393–1403.

337. Fisher RS. Animal models of the epilepsies. *Brain Res Rev* 1989;14:245–278.

338. Rho JM, Sankar R. The pharmacologic basis of antiepileptic drug action. *Epilepsia* 1999;40:1471–1483.

339. Rho JM, et al. Mechanism of action of the anticonvulsant felbamate: opposing effects on N-methyl-D-aspartate and γ-aminobutyric acid receptors. *Ann Neurol* 1994;35:229–234.

340. White HS, Brown SD, Woodhead JH, et al. Topiramate enhances GABA-mediated chloride flux and GABA-evoked chloride currents in murine brain neurons and increases seizure threshold. *Epilepsy Res* 1997;28:167–179.

341. Rho JM, Donevan SD, Rogawski MA. Mechanism of action of the anticonvulsant felbamate: opposing effects on N-methyl-D-aspartate and γ-aminobutyric acid A receptors. *Ann Neurol* 1994;35:229–234.

342. Buchthal F, Svensmark O, Simonsen H. Relation of EEG and seizures to phenobarbital in serum. *Arch Neurol* 1968;19:567–572.

343. Svensmark O, Buchthal F. Diphenylhydantoin and phenobarbital. Serum levels in children. *Am J Dis Child* 1964;108:82–87.

344. Suganuma T, et al. The effect of concurrent administration of valproate sodium on phenobarbital plasma concentration/dosage ratio in pediatric patients. *J Pediatr* 1981;99:314–317.

345. Aiges HW, et al. The effects of phenobarbital and diphenylhydantoin on liver function and morphology. *J Pediatr* 1980;97:22–26.

346. Theodore WH, et al. Barbiturates reduce human cerebral glucose metabolism. *Neurology* 1986;36:60–64.

347. Brent DA, et al. Phenobarbital treatment and major depressive disorder in children with epilepsy: a naturalistic follow-up. *Pediatrics* 1990;85:1086–1091.

348. Camfield CS, et al. Side effects of phenobarbitone in toddlers: behavioral and cognitive aspects. *J Pediatr* 1979;95:361–365.

349. Hellstrom B, Barlach-Christoffersen M. Influence of phenobarbital on the psychomotor development and behaviour in preschool children with convulsions. *Neuropädiatrie* 1980;11:151–160.

350. Thompson PJ, Trimble MR. Anticonvulsant drugs and cognitive functions. *Epilepsia* 1982;23:531–544.

351. Mitchell WG, et al. Effects of antiepileptic drugs on reaction time, attention and impulsivity in children. *Pediatrics* 1993;91:101–105.

352. Farwell JR, et al. Phenobarbital for febrile seizures—effects on intelligence and on seizure recurrence. *N Engl J Med* 1990;322:364–369.

353. De Silva M, et al. Randomized comparative monotherapy trial of phenobarbitone, phenytoin, carbamazepine or sodium valproate for newly diagnosed childhood epilepsy. *Lancet* 1996;347:709–713.

354. Gallagher BB, et al. Primidone, diphenylhydantoin and phenobarbital. Aspects of acute and chronic toxicity. *Neurology* 1973;23:145–149.

355. Dodson WE. Nonlinear kinetics of phenytoin in children. *Neurology* 1982;32:42–48.

356. Buchthal F, Svensmark O. Aspects of the pharmacology of phenytoin (Dilantin) and phenobarbital relevant to their dosage in the treatment of epilepsy. *Epilepsia* 1960;1:373–384.

357. Buchthal F, Svensmark O. Serum concentrations of diphenylhydantoin (phenytoin) and phenobarbital and their relation to therapeutic and toxic effects. *Psychiatr Neurol Neurochir* 1971;74:117–136.

358. Browne TR, Change T. Phenytoin: biotransformation. In: Levy R, et al., eds. *Antiepileptic drugs*, 3rd ed. New York: Raven Press, 1989:197–214.

359. Kutt H, et al. The effect of phenobarbital on plasma diphenylhydantoin level and metabolism in man and in rat liver microsomes. *Neurology* 1969;19:611–616.

360. Kutt H, McDowell F. Management of epilepsy with diphenylhydantoin sodium. Dosage regulation for problem patients. *JAMA* 1968;203:969–972.

361. Kokenge R, Kutt H, McDowell F. Neurological sequelae following Dilantin overdose in a patient and in experimental animals. *Neurology* 1965;15:823–829.

362. Kutt H, et al. Insufficient parahydroxylation as a cause of diphenylhydantoin toxicity. *Neurology* 1964;14:542–548.

363. Dawson KP. Severe cutaneous reactions to phenytoin. *Arch Dis Child* 1973;48:239–240.

364. Beernink DH, Miller JJ. Anticonvulsant-induced antinuclear antibodies and lupus-like disease in children. *J Pediatr* 1973;82:113–117.

365. Rzany B, et al. Risk of Stevens-Johnson syndrome and toxic epidermal necrolysis during first weeks of antiepileptic therapy: a control study. *Lancet* 1999;353:2190–2194.

366. Li FP, et al. Malignant lymphoma after diphenylhydantoin (dilantin) therapy. *Cancer* 1975;36:1359–1362.

367. Kapur RN, et al. Diphenylhydantoin-induced gingival hyperplasia: its relationship to dose and serum level. *Dev Med Child Neurol* 1973;15:483–487.

368. Reynolds EH. Folate metabolism and anticonvulsant therapy. *Proc R Soc Med* 1974;67–68.

369. Weber TH, et al. Long-term use of phenytoin: effects on whole blood and red cell folate and haematological parameters. *Scand J Haematol* 1977;18:81–85.

370. Reynolds EH. Anticonvulsants, folic acid, and epilepsy. *Lancet* 1973;1:1376–1378.

371. Krause K-H, et al. Biotin status of epileptics. *Ann NY Acad Sci* 1985;447:297–313.

372. Ogunmekan AO, Hwang PA. A randomized, double-blind, placebo-controlled, clinical trial of D-alpha-tocopheryl acetate (Vitamin E) as add-on therapy, for epilepsy in children. *Epilepsia* 1989;30:84–89.

373. Crosley CJ, Chee C, Berman PH. Rickets associated with long-term anticonvulsant therapy in a pediatric outpatient population. *Pediatrics* 1975;56:52–57.

374. Morijiri Y, Sato T. Factors causing rickets in institu-

tionalized handicapped children on anticonvulsant therapy. *Arch Dis Child* 1981;56:446–449.

375. Lovelace RE, Horwitz SJ. Peripheral neuropathy in long-term diphenylhydantoin therapy. *Arch Neurol* 1968;18:69–77.

376. Kutt H, Solomon GE. Phenytoin: relevant side effects. *Adv Neurol* 1980;27:435–445.

377. Ambrosetto G, et al. Phenytoin encephalopathy as probably idiosyncratic reaction. Case report. *Epilepsia* 1977;18:405–408.

378. Hanson JW, Smith DW. The fetal hydantoin syndrome. *J Pediatr* 1975;87:285–290.

379. Annegers JF, et al. Do anticonvulsants have a teratogenic effect? *Arch Neurol* 1974;31:364–373.

380. Shapiro S, et al. Anticonvulsants and parental epilepsy in the development of birth defects. *Lancet* 1976;1:272–275.

381. Gaily E, et al. Minor anomalies in offspring of epileptic mothers. *J Pediatr* 1988;112:520–529.

382. Buehler BA, et al. Prenatal prediction of risk of the fetal hydantoin syndrome. *N Engl J Med* 1990;322: 1567–1572.

383. Lindhout D. Pharmacogenetics and drug interactions: role in antiepileptic-drug-induced teratogenesis. *Neurology* 1992;42 [Suppl 5]:43–47.

383a. Green VJ, et al. Genetic analysis of microsomal epoxide hydrolase in patients with carbamazepine hypersensitivity. *Biochem Pharmacol* 1995;50:1353–1359.

384. Delgado-Escueta AV, Janz D. Consensus guidelines: preconception counseling, management, and care of the pregnant woman with epilepsy. *Neurology* 1992;42[Suppl. 5]:149–160.

385. Meadow SR. Anticonvulsant drugs in pregnancy. *Arch Dis Child* 1991;66:62–65.

386. Troupin AS, et al. Clinical pharmacology of mephenytoin and ethotoin. *Ann Neurol* 1979;6:410–414.

387. Reckziegel G, et al. Carbamazepine effects on Na$^+$ currents in human dentate granule cells from epileptogenic tissue. *Epilepsia* 1999;40:401–407.

388. Dodson WE. Carbamazepine efficacy and utilization in children. *Epilepsia* 1987;28[Suppl 3]:S17–S24.

389. Troupin A, et al. Carbamazepine—a double-blind comparison with phenytoin. *Neurology* 1977;27:511–519.

390. Westenberg HG, et al. Kinetics of carbamazepine and carbamazepine epoxide, determined by use of plasma and saliva. *Clin Pharmacol Ther* 1978;23:320–328.

391. Bertilsson L, Tomson T. Clinical pharmacokinetics and pharmacological effects of carbamazepine and carbamazepine-10,11-epoxide. An update. *Clin Pharmacokinet* 1986;11:177–198.

392. Dam M, et al. A double-blind study comparing oxcarbazepine and carbamazepine in patients with newly diagnosed previously untreated epilepsy. *Epilepsy Res* 1989;3:70–76.

393. Pellock JM. Carbamazepine side effects in children and adults. *Epilepsia* 1987; 28[Suppl 3]:S64–S70.

394. Perucca E, et al. Water intoxication in epileptic patients receiving carbamazepine. *J Neurol Neurosurg Psychiatry* 1978;41:713–718.

395. Van Amelsvoort T, et al. Hyponatremia associated with carbamazepine and oxcarbazepine therapy: a review. *Epilepsia* 1994;35:181–188.

396. Camfield C, et al. Asymptomatic children with epilepsy: little benefit from screening for anticonvulsant-induced liver, blood, or renal damage. *Neurology* 1986;36: 838–841.

397. Hadzic N, et al. Acute liver failure induced by carbamazepine. *Arch Dis Child* 1990;65:315–317.

398. Snead OC, Hosey LC. Exacerbation of seizures in children by carbamazepine. *N Engl J Med* 1985;313: 916–921.

399. Aguglia U, Zappia M, Quattrone A. Carbamazepine-induced nonepileptic myoclonus in a child with benign epilepsy. *Epilepsia* 1987;28:515–518.

400. Macphee GJ, et al. Verapamil potentiates carbamazepine neurotoxicity: a clinically important inhibitory interaction. *Lancet* 1986;1:700–703.

401. Dodrill CB, Troupin AS. Psychotropic effects of carbamazepine in epilepsy: a double blind comparison with phenytoin. *Neurology* 1977;27:1023–1028.

402. Forsythe I, et al. Cognitive impairment in new cases of epilepsy randomly assigned to carbamazepine, phenytoin and sodium valproate. *Dev Med Child Neurol* 1991;33:524–534.

403. Nuwer MR, et al. Generic substitutions for antiepileptic drugs. *Neurology* 1990;40:1647–1651.

404. Dean JC. Valproate. In: Wyllie E, ed. *The treatment of epilepsy: principles and practice*, 2nd ed. Baltimore: Williams & Wilkins, 1996:824–832.

405. Loscher W. Valproate: a reappraisal of its pharmacodynamic properties and mechanisms of action. *Prog Neurobiol* 1999;58:31–59.

406. Buchhalter JR, Dichter MA. Effects of valproic acid in cultured mammalian neurons. *Neurology* 1986;36: 259–262.

407. Johnston D. Valproic acid: update on its mechanisms of action. *Epilepsia* 1984;25[Suppl 1]:S1–S4.

408. Bourgeois BFD. Valproate. Clinical use. In: Levy R, et al., eds. *Antiepileptic drugs*. New York: Raven Press, 1989;633–642.

409. Editorial. Sodium valproate. *Lancet* 1988;2:1229–1232.

410. Shen DD, et al. Low and variable presence of valproic acid in human brain. *Neurology* 1992;42: 582–585.

411. Covanis A, Jeavons PM. Once-daily sodium valproate in the treatment of epilepsy. *Dev Med Child Neurol* 1980;22:202–204.

412. Cloyd JC, et al. Comparison of sprinkle versus syrup formulations of valproate for bioavailability, tolerance, and preference. *J Pediatr* 1992;120:634–638.

413. Collaborative Study Group, Bourgeois B, et al. Monotherapy with valproate in primary generalized epilepsies. *Epilepsia* 1987;28[Suppl 2]:S8–S11.

414. Bryant AE, Dreifuss FE. Valproic acid hepatic fatalities. III. U.S. experience since 1986. *Neurology* 1996;48:465–469.

415. Dreifuss FE, et al. Valproic acid hepatic fatalities. II. U.S. experience since 1984. *Neurology* 1989;39: 201–207.

416. Rettie AE, et al. Cytochrome P-450-catalyzed formation of delta-4-VPA, a toxic metabolite of valproic acid. *Science* 1987;235:890–893.

417. Tennison MB, et al. Valproate metabolites and hepatotoxicity in an epileptic population. *Epilepsia* 1988;29:543–547.

418. Jeavons PM. Sodium valproate and acute hepatic failure. *Dev Med Child Neurol* 1980;22:547–548.

419. Lenn NJ, et al. Fatal hepatocerebral syndrome in siblings discordant for exposure to valproate. *Epilepsia* 1990;31:578–583.

420. Melegh B, Trombitás K. Valproate treatment induces lipid globule accumulation with ultrastructural abnor-

malities of mitochondria in skeletal muscle. *Neuropediatrics* 1997;28:257–261.

421. Laub MC. Nutritional influence on serum ammonia in young patients receiving sodium valproate. *Epilepsia* 1986;27:55–59.

422. Marescaux C, et al. Stuporous episodes during treatment with sodium valproate: report of seven cases. *Epilepsia* 1982;23:297–305.

423. Coulter DL, Allen RJ. Secondary hyperammonaemia: a possible mechanism for valproate encephalopathy. *Lancet* 1980;1:1310–1311.

424. Bruni J, et al. Valproic acid and plasma levels of phenobarbital. *Neurology* 1980;30:94–97.

425. Mattson RH, Cramer JA. Valproic acid and ethosuximide interaction. *Ann Neurol* 1980;7:583–584.

426. Patsalos PN, Lascelles PT. Effect of sodium valproate on plasma protein binding of diphenylhydantoin. *J Neurol Neurosurg Psychiatry* 1977;40:570–574.

427. Hyman NM, Dennis PD, Sinclair KG. Tremor due to sodium valproate. *Neurology* 1979;29:1177–1180.

428. Bodensteiner JB, Morris HH, Golden GS. Asterixis associated with sodium valproate. *Neurology* 1981;31:194–195.

429. Barr RD, et al. Valproic acid and immune thrombocytopenia. *Arch Dis Child* 1982;57:681–684.

430. Kreuz W, et al. Valproate therapy induces von Willebrand disease type I. *Epilepsia* 1992;33:178–184.

431. Ward M, et al. Preoperative valproate administration does not increase blood loss during temporal lobectomy. *Epilepsia* 1996;37:98–101.

432. Mortensen PB, Kolvraa S, Christensen E. Inhibition of the glycine cleavage system: hyperglycinemia and hyperglycinuria caused by valproic acid. *Epilepsia* 1980;21:563–569.

433. Parker PH, et al. Recurrent pancreatitis induced by valproic acid. A case report and review of the literature. *Gastroenterology* 1981;80:826–828.

434. Asconape JJ, et al. Valproate-associated pancreatitis. *Epilepsia* 1993;34:177–183.

435. Ettinger A, Moshe S, Shinnar S. Edema associated with long-term valproate therapy. *Epilepsia* 1990;31: 211–213.

436. Isojärvi JIT, et al. Obesity and endocrine disorders in women taking valproate for epilepsy. *Ann Neurol* 1996;39:579–584.

437. Murphy JV, Groover RV, Hodge C. Hepatotoxic effects in a child receiving valproate and carnitine. *J Pediatr* 1993;123:318–320.

438. Laub MC, et al. Serum carnitine during valproic acid therapy. *Epilepsia* 1986;27:559–562.

439. Freeman JM, et al. Does carnitine administration improve the symptoms attributed to anticonvulsant medications? A double-blinded, crossover study. *Pediatrics* 1994;93:893–895.

440. Lindhout D, Omtzigt JG, Cornel MC. Spectrum of neural-tube defects in 34 infants prenatally exposed to antiepileptic drugs. *Neurology* 1992; 42 [4 Suppl 5]:111–118.

441. Hansen RA, Menkes JH. A new anticonvulsant in the management of minor motor seizures. *Dev Med Child Neurol* 1972;14:3–14.

442. Farrell K. Benzodiazepines in the treatment of children with epilepsy. *Epilepsia* 1986; 27[Suppl 1]:S45–S51.

443. Martin D, Hirt HR. Clinical experience with clonazepam (Rivotril) in the treatment of epilepsies in infancy and childhood. *Neuropädiatrie* 1973;4:245–266.

444. Markham CH. The treatment of myoclonic seizures of infancy and childhood with LA-1. *Pediatrics* 1964;34:511–518.

445. Murphy JV, et al. Deaths in young children receiving nitrazepam. *J Pediatr* 1987;111:145–147.

445a. Rintahaka PJ, et al. Incidence of death in patients with intractable epilepsy during nitrazepam treatment. *Epilepsia* 1999;40:492–496.

446. Wretlind M, et al. Disposition of three benzodiazepines after single oral administration in man. *Acta Pharmacol Toxicol* 1977;40:28–39.

447. Ko DY, et al. Benzodiazepines. In: Engel J Jr, Pedley TA, eds. *Epilepsy: a comprehensive textbook.* Philadelphia: Lippincott-Raven, 1998:1475–1489.

448. Kumar A, Bleck TP. Intravenous midazolam for the treatment of refractory status epilepticus. *Crit Care Med* 1992;20:483–488.

449. Parent JM, Lowenstein DH. Treatment of refractory generalized status epilepticus with continuous infusion of midazolam. *Neurology* 1994;44:1837–1840.

450. O'Regan ME, et al. Nasal rather than rectal benzodiazepines in the management of acute childhood seizures? *Dev Med Child Neurol* 1996;38:1037–1045.

451. Chamberlain JM, et al. A prospective, randomized study comparing intramuscular midazolam with intravenous diazepam for the treatment of seizures in children. *Pediatr Emerg Care* 1997;13:92–94.

452. Clobazam has equivalent efficacy to carbamazepine and phenytoin as monotherapy for childhood epilepsy. Canadian Study Group for Childhood Epilepsy. *Epilepsia* 1998;39:952–959.

453. Bawden HN, et al. The cognitive and behavioural effects of clobazam and standard monotherapy are comparable. Canadian Study Group for Childhood Epilepsy. *Epilepsy Res* 1999; 33:133–143.

454. Millichap JG. Acetazolamide in treatment of epilepsy [Letter]. *Neurology* 1991;41:764.

455. The Felbamate Study Group in Lennox-Gastaut Syndrome. Efficacy of felbamate in childhood epileptic encephalopathy (Lennox-Gastaut syndrome). *N Engl J Med* 1993;328:29–33.

456. Faught E, et al. Felbamate monotherapy for partial-onset seizures: an active-control trial. *Neurology* 1993;43:688–692.

457. Thompson CD, et al. Quantification in patient urine samples of felbamate and three metabolites: acid carbamate and two mercapturic acids. *Epilepsia* 1999;40:769–776.

458. French J, et al. Practice advisory: the use of felbamate in the treatment of patients with intractable epilepsy. *Neurology* 1999;52:1540–1545.

459. Petroff OA, et al. The effect of gabapentin on brain gamma-aminobutyric acid in patients with epilepsy. *Ann Neurol* 1996;39:95–99.

460. The U.S. Gabapentin Study Group Number 5. Gabapentin as add-on therapy in refractory partial epilepsy: a double-blind, placebo controlled, parallel group study. *Neurology* 1993;43:2292–2298.

461. UK Gabapentin Study Group. Gabapentin in partial epilepsy. *Lancet* 1990;335:1114–1117.

462. Bergey GK, et al. Gabapentin monotherapy: I. An 8-day, double-blind, dose-controlled, multicenter study in hospitalized patients with refractory complex partial or secondarily generalized seizures. The U.S. Gabapentin Study Group 88/89. *Neurology* 1997;49: 739–745.

463. Beydoun A, et al. Gabapentin monotherapy: II. A 26-week, double-blind, dose-controlled, multicenter study of conversion from polytherapy in outpatients with refractory complex partial or secondarily generalized seizures. The U.S. Gabapentin Study Group 82/83. *Neurology* 1997;49:746–752.

464. Chadwick DW, et al. A double-blind trial of gabapentin monotherapy for newly diagnosed partial seizures. International Gabapentin Monotherapy Study Group 945-77. *Neurology* 1998;51: 1282–1288.

464a. Leach JP, et al. Gabapentin and cognition: a double-blind, dose-ranging, placebo controlled study in refractory epilepsy. *J Neurol Neurosurg Psychiatry* 1997;62:372–376.

465. Hosford DA, Wang Y. Utility of the lethargic (lh/lh) mouse model of absence seizures in predicting the effects of lamotrigine, vigabatrin, tiagabine, gabapentin, and topiramate against human absence seizures. *Epilepsia* 1997;38:408–414.

466. Trudeau V, et al. Gabapentin in naive childhood absence epilepsy: results from two double-blind, placebo-controlled, multicenter studies. *J Child Neurol* 1996;11:470–475.

467. Vossler DG. Exacerbation of seizures in Lennox-Gastaut syndrome by gabapentin. *Neurology* 1996;46: 852–853.

468. Miller AA, et al. Pharmacological studies on lamotrigine, a novel potential antiepileptic drug: I. Anticonvulsant profile in mice and rats. *Epilepsia* 1986;27:483–489.

469. Cheung H, et al. An in vitro investigation of the action of lamotrigine on neuronal-activated sodium channels. *Epilepsy Res* 1992;13:107–112.

470. Lang DG, et al. Lamotrigine, phenytoin and carbamazepine interactions on the sodium current in N4TG1 Neuroblastoma cells. *J Pharmacol Exp Ther* 1993;266:820–835.

471. Beran RG, et al. Double-blind, placebo-controlled, crossover study of lamotrigine in treatment-resistant generalised epilepsy. *Epilepsia* 1998;39:1329–1333.

472. Gilliam F, et al. An active-control trial of lamotrigine monotherapy for partial seizures. *Neurology* 1998;51:1018–1025.

473. Dulac O, Kaminska A. Use of lamotrigine in Lennox-Gastaut and related epilepsy syndromes. *J Child Neurol* 1997;12[Suppl 1]:S23–S28.

474. Motte J, et al. Lamotrigine for generalized seizures associated with the Lennox-Gastaut syndrome. Lamictal Lennox-Gastaut Study Group. *New Engl J Med* 1997;337:1807–1812.

475. Buchanan N. The use of lamotrigine in juvenile myoclonic epilepsy. *Seizure* 1996;5:149–151.

476. Besag FMC, et al. Lamotrigine for the treatment of epilepsy in childhood. *J Pediatr* 1995;127:991–997.

477. Battino D, et al. Lamotrigine in resistant childhood epilepsy. *Neuropediatrics* 1993;24:332–336.

478. Yuen AWC, et al. Sodium valproate acutely inhibits lamotrigine metabolism. *Br J Clin Pharmacol* 1992;33:511–513.

479. Gram L. Potential antiepileptic drugs. Lamotrigine. In: Levy R, et al., eds. *Antiepileptic drugs.* New York: Raven Press, 1989:947–953.

480. Schlienger RG, et al. Lamotrigine-induced severe cutaneous adverse reactions. *Epilepsia* 1998;39[Suppl 7]; S22–S26.

481. Buchanan N. Lamotrigine: clinical experience in 200 patients with epilepsy with follow-up to four years. *Seizure* 1996;5:209–214.

482. Chattergoon DS, et al. Multiorgan dysfunction and disseminated intravascular coagulation in children receiving lamotrigine and valproic acid. *Neurology* 1997;49:1442–1444.

483. Martin R, et al. Cognitive effects of topiramate, gabapentin, and lamotrigine in healthy young adults. *Neurology* 1999;52:321–327.

484. Kramer LD, Reife RA. Topiramate. In: Engel J Jr, Pedley TA, eds. *Epilepsy: a comprehensive textbook.* Philadelphia: Lippincott–Raven Publishers, 1998: 1593–1598.

485. Kuzniecky R, et al. Topiramate increases cerebral GABA in healthy humans. *Neurology* 1998;51:627–629.

486. Petroff OAC, et al. Topiramate increases brain GABA, homocarnosine, and pyrrolidinone in patients with epilepsy. *Neurology* 1999;52:473–478.

487. Sachdeo RC, et al. Topiramate monotherapy for partial onset seizures. *Epilepsia* 1997;38:294–300.

488. Biton V, et al. A randomized, placebo-controlled study of topiramate in primary generalized tonic-clonic seizures. Topiramate YTC Study Group. *Neurology* 1999;52:1330–1337.

489. Elterman RD, et al. A double-blind, randomized trial of topiramate as adjunctive therapy for partial-onset seizures in children. Topiramate YP Study Group. *Neurology* 1999;52:1338–1344.

490. Sachdeo RC, et al. A double-blind, randomized trial of topiramate in Lennox-Gastaut syndrome. Topiramate YL Study Group. *Neurology* 1999;52:1882–1887.

491. Sankar R, Derdiarian AT. Vigabatrin. *CNS Drug Reviews* 1998;4:260–274.

492. Eke T, Talbot JF, Lawden MC. Severe persistent visual field constriction associated with vigabatrin. *Brit Med J* 1997;314:180–181.

493. Krauss GL, Johnson MA, Miller NR. Vigabatrin-associated retinal cone system dysfunction: electroretinogram and ophthalmologic findings. *Neurology* 1998;50:614–618.

494. Kälviäinen, et al. GABAergic Antiepileptic Drug Vigabatrin Causes Concentric Visual Field Defects. *Neurology* 1999;53:922–926.

495. Chiron C, et al. Therapeutic trial of vigabatrin in refractory infantile spasms. *J Child Neurol* 1991;2[Suppl]:S52–S59.

496. Aicardi J, et al. Vigabatrin as initial therapy for infantile spasms: a European retrospective survey. Sabril Investigator and Peer Review Groups. *Epilepsia* 1996;37:638–642.

497. Vigevano F, Cilio MR. Vigabatrin versus ACTH as first-line treatment for infantile spasms: a randomized, prospective study. *Epilepsia* 1997;38:1270–1274.

498. Chiron C, et al. Randomized trial comparing vigabatrin and hydrocortisone in infantile spasms due to tuberous sclerosis. *Epilepsy Res* 1997;26:389–395.

499. Hancock E, Osborne JP. Vigabatrin in the treatment of infantile spasms in tuberous sclerosis: literature review. *J Child Neurol* 1999;14:71–74.

500. Sankar R, Wasterlain CG. Is the devil we know the lesser of two evils? Vigabatrin and visual fields. [Editorial]. *Neurology* 1999;52:1537–1538.

501. Gibbs JM, Appleton RE, Rosenbloom L. Vigabatrin in intractable childhood epilepsy: a retrospective study. *Pediatr Neurol* 1992;8:338–340.

502. Jongsma MJ, et al. Reversible motor disturbances induced by vigabatrin. *Lancet* 1991;338:893.
503. Greenberg DA. Calcium channels and calcium channel antagonists. *Ann Neurol* 1987;21:317–330.
504. Wilder RM. The effects of ketonuria on the course of epilepsy. *Mayo Clin Proc* 1921;2:307–308.
505. Kinsman SL, et al. Efficacy of the ketogenic diet for intractable seizure disorders: review of 58 cases. *Epilepsia* 1992;33:1132–1136.
506. Sankar R, Sotero de Menezes M. Metabolic and endocrine aspects of the ketogenic diet. *Epilepsy Research* 1999;37:191–201.
507. Livingston S. *Comprehensive management of epilepsy in infancy, childhood, and adolescence.* Springfield, IL: Charles C Thomas Publisher, 1972.
508. Huttenlocher PR, Wilbourn AJ, Signore JM. Medium-chain triglycerides as a therapy for intractable childhood epilepsy. *Neurology* 1971;21:1097–1103.
509. Vining EP, et al. A multicenter study of the efficacy of the ketogenic diet. *Arch Neurol* 1998;55:1433–1437.
510. Demeritte EL, Ventimiglia J, Coyne M, Nigro MA. Organic acid disorders and the ketogenic diet. *Ann Neurol* 1996;40:305.
511. De Vivo DC, et al. L-carnitine supplementation in childhood epilepsy: current perspectives. *Epilepsia* 1998;39:1216–1225.
512. Ballaban-Gil K, et al. Complications of the ketogenic diet. *Epilepsia* 1998;39:744–748.
513. Hauser WA, Hesdorffer DC. The natural history of seizures. In: Wyllie E, ed. *The treatment of epilepsy: principles and practice*, 2nd ed. Baltimore: Williams & Wilkins, 1996:173–178.
514. Andermann F. Identification of candidates for surgical treatment of epilepsy. In: Engel J Jr, ed. *Surgical treatment of the epilepsies*. New York: Raven Press, 1987:51–70.
514a. Duchowny MS, et al. Indications and criteria for surgical intervention. In: Engel J Jr, Pedley TA, eds: *Epilepsy: a comprehensive textbook*, Philadelphia: Lippincott–Raven Publishers, 1998:1677–1685.
515. Shewmon DA, Engel J Jr. Overview: who should be considered a surgical candidate? In: Engel J Jr, ed. *Surgical treatment of the epilepsies,* 2nd ed. New York: Raven Press, 1993:23–34.
516. Shewmon DA, et al. Contrasts between pediatric and adult epilepsy surgery: rationale and strategy for focal resection. *J Epilepsy* 1990;3[Suppl]:141–155.
517. Shewmon DA, et al. Selective carotid amytal suppression of independent multifocal spikes in children [Abstract]. *Epilepsia* 1990:31:653.
518. Sankar R, Chugani HT. Strategies for diagnosis and treatment of childhood epilepsy. *Curr Opin Neurol Neurosurg* 1993;6:398–402.
519. Chugani HT, et al. Surgery for intractable infantile spasms: neuroimaging perspectives. *Epilepsia* 1993;34:764–771.
520. Duchowny MS, et al. Special considerations for preoperative evaluation in childhood. In: Engel J Jr, ed. *Surgical Treatment of the Epilepsies,* 2nd ed. New York: Raven Press, 1993:415–428.
521. Debets RM, et al. Is ^{11}C-flumazenil PET superior to 18_FDG PET and 123_I-iomazenil SPECT in presurgical evaluation of temporal lobe epilepsy? *J Neurol Neurosurg and Psychiatry* 1997;62:141–150.
522. O'Brien TJ, et al. Subtraction ictal SPECT co-registered to MRI improves clinical usefulness of SPECT in localizing the surgical seizure focus. *Neurology* 1998;50:445–454.
523. O'Brien TJ, et al. Subtraction SPECT co-registered to MRI improves postictal SPECT localization of seizure foci. *Neurology* 1999;52:137–146.
524. Brey R, Laxer KD. Type I/II complex partial seizures: no correlation with surgical outcome. *Epilepsia* 1985;26:657–660.
525. Souweidane MM, et al. Brain mapping in sedated infants and young children with passive-functional magnetic resonance imaging. *Pediatr Neurosurg* 1999;30:86–92.
526. Jack CR, Sharbrough FW, Twomey CK. Temporal lobe seizures: lateralization with MR volume measurements of hippocampal formation. *Radiology* 1990;175;423–429.
527. Lencz T, et al. Quantitative magnetic resonance in temporal lobe epilepsy: relationship to neuropathology and neuropsychological function. *Ann Neurol* 1992;31:629–637.
528. Bernasconi N, et al. Entorhinal cortex in temporal lobe epilepsy. *Neurology* 1999;52:1870–1876.
529. Lawson JA, et al. ILAE-defined epilepsy syndromes in children: correlation with quantitative MRI. *Epilepsia* 1998;39:1345–1349.
530. Ho SS, et al. Comparison of ictal SPECT and interictal PET in the presurgical evaluation of temporal lobe epilepsy. *Ann Neurol* 1995;37:738–745.
531. Markand ON, et al. Comparative study of interictal PET and ictal SPECT in complex partial seizures. *Acta Neurol Scand* 1997;95:129–136.
532. So N, et al. Depth electrode investigations in patients with bitemporal epileptiform abnormalities. *Ann Neurol* 1989;25:423–431.
533. Lesser RP, Fisher RS, Kaplan P. The evaluation of patients with intractable complex partial seizures. *Electroencephalogr Clin Neurophysiol* 1989;73:381–388.
534. Delgado-Escueta AV, Walsh GO. Type I complex partial seizures of hippocampal origin. Excellent results of anterior temporal lobectomy. *Neurology* 1985;35:143–154.
535. Walsh GO, Delgado-Escueta AV. Type II complex partial seizures: poor results of anterior temporal lobectomy. *Neurology* 1984;34:113.
536. Shields WD, Duchowny MS, Holmes GL. Surgically remediable syndromes of infancy and early childhood. In: Engel J Jr, ed. *Surgical treatment of the epilepsies*, 2nd ed. New York: Raven Press, 1993:35–48.
537. Szabo CA, et al. Neuropsychological effect of temporal lobe resection in preadolescent children with epilepsy. *Epilepsia* 1998;39:814–819.
538. Yasargil MG, et al. Selective amygdalohippocampectomy. Operative anatomy and surgical treatment. *Adv Tech Stand Neurosurg* 1985;12:93–123.
539. Keogan M, et al. Temporal neocorticectomy in the management of intractable epilepsy: long-term outcome and predictive factors. *Epilepsia* 1992;33:852–861.
540. Peacock WJ, et al. Special consideration for epilepsy surgery in childhood. In: Engel J Jr, ed. *Surgical treatment of the epilepsies*, 2nd ed. New York: Raven Press, 1993:541–548.

541. Pillay PK, Barnett G, Awad I. MRI-guided stereotactic placement of depth electrodes in temporal lobe epilepsy. *Br J Neurosurg* 1992;6:47–53.
542. Rasmussen T. Surgery for epilepsy arising in regions other than the temporal and frontal lobes. In: Purpura DP, et al., eds. *Neurosurgical Management of Epilepsies. Adv Neurol* 1975;8:207–226.
543. Olivier A. Surgery of extratemporal epilepsy. In: Wyllie E, ed. *The treatment of epilepsy: principles and practice*, 2nd ed. Baltimore: Williams & Wilkins, 1997:1060–1073.
544. Wyllie E. Corpus callosotomy for intractable generalized epilepsy. *J Pediatr* 1988;113:255–261.
545. Spencer SS. Corpus callosum section and other disconnection procedures for medically intractable epilepsy. *Epilepsia* 1988;29[Suppl 2]:S85–S99.
546. Blume WT. Corpus callosum section for seizure control: rationale and review of experimental and clinical data. *Cleve Clin Q* 1984;51:319–332.
547. Black MP, Holmes G, Lombroso C. Corpus callosum section for intractable epilepsy in children. *Pediatr Neurosurg* 1992;18:298–304.
548. Gazzaniga MS, Bogen JE, Sperry RW. Observations on visual perception after disconnexion of the cerebral hemisphere in man. *Brain* 1965;88:221–236.
549. Gates JR, et al. Corpus callosum section in children: seizure responses. *J Epilepsy* 1990;3[Suppl]:271–278.
550. Tinuper P, et al. Functional hemispherectomy for treatment of epilepsy associated with hemiplegia: rationale, indications, results, and comparison with callosotomy. *Ann Neurol* 1988;24:27–34.
551. Rasmussen T. Hemispherectomy for seizures revisited. *Can J Neurosci* 1983;10:71–78.
552. Villemure JG, Mascott C. Hemispherotomy: the peri-insular approach. Technical aspects. *Epilepsia* 1993;34[Suppl 6]:48.
552a. Chugani HT, et al. Surgical treatment of intractable neonatal-onset seizures: the role of positron emission tomography. *Neurology* 1988;38:1178–1188.
553. Peacock WJ, et al. Hemispherectomy for intractable seizures in children: a report of 58 cases. *Child's Nerv Syst* 1986;12:376–384.
554. Mathern GW, et al. Post-operative seizure control and anti-epileptic drug usage in pediatric epilepsy surgery patients: the UCLA experience, 1986–1997. *Epilepsia*, 2000, (in press).
555. Wyllie E, et al. Seizure outcome after epilepsy surgery in children and adolescents. *Ann Neurol* 1998;44:740–748.
556. Hammond EJ, et al. Neurochemical effects of vagus nerve stimulation in humans. *Brain Res* 1992;583:300–303.
557. Henry TR, et al. Acute blood flow changes and efficacy of vagus nerve stimulation in partial epilepsy. *Neurology* 1999;52:1166–1173.
558. Uthman B, et al. Treatment of epilepsy by stimulation of the vagus nerve. *Neurology* 1993;43:1338–1345.
559. Ben-Menachem E, et al. Vagus nerve stimulation for treatment of partial seizures: 1. A controlled study of effect on seizures. *Epilepsia* 1994;35:616–626.
560. Handforth A, et al. Vagus nerve stimulation therapy for partial-onset seizures. A randomized active control trial. *Neurology* 1998;51:48–55.
561. Murphy JV. Left vagal nerve stimulation in children with medically refractory epilepsy. The Pediatric VNS Study Group. *J Pediatr* 1999;134:563–566.
562. Lothman E. The biochemical basis and pathophysiology of status epilepticus. *Neurology* 1990;40[Suppl 2]:13–23.
563. Brown JK, Hussain IHM. Staus epilepticus: I. Pathogenesis. *Dev Med Child Neurol* 1991;33:317.
564. Shorvon S. Tonic clonic status epilepticus. *J Neurol Neurosurg Psychiatry* 1993; 56:125–134.
565. Holmes GL. Epilepsy in the developing brain: lessons from the laboratory and clinic. *Epilepsia* 1997;38: 12–30.
566. Maytal J, et al. Low morbidity and mortality of status epilepticus in children. *Pediatrics* 1989;83:323–331.
567. Payne TA, Black TP. Status epilepticus. *Crit Care Clin* 1997;13:17–38.
568. Crawford TO, Mitchell WG, Snodgrass SR. Lorazepam in childhood status epilepticus and serial seizures: effectiveness and tachyphylaxis. *Neurology* 1987;37:190–195.
569. Brown JK, Hussain IHM. Status epilepticus: II. Treatment. *Dev Med Child Neurol* 1991;33:97–109.
570. Franzoni E, Carboni C, Lambertini A. Rectal diazepam: a clinical and EEG study after a single dose in children. *Epilepsia* 1981;24:35–41.
571. Leppik IE. Status epilepticus. In: Wyllie E, ed. *The treatment of epilepsy: principles and practice*. Philadelphia: Lea & Febiger, 1993:678–685.
572. Delgado-Escueta AV, et al. Management of status epilepticus. *N Engl J Med* 1982;306:1337–1340.
573. Lombroso CT. Treatment of status epilepticus with diazepam. *Neurology* 1966;16:629–634.
574. Bell DS. Dangers of treatment of status epilepticus with diazepam. *BMJ* 1969;1:159–161.
575. Kriel RL. Home use of rectal diazepam for cluster and prolonged seizures. Efficacy, adverse reactions, quality of life, and cost analysis. *Pediatr Neurol* 1991;7:13–17.
576. Dreifuss FE, et al. A comparison of rectal diazepam gel and placebo for acute repetitive seizures. *N Engl J Med* 1998;338:1869–1875.
577. Runge JW, Allen FH. Emergency treatment of status epilepticus. *Neurology* 1996;46[Suppl 1]:S20–S23.
578. Richard MO, et al. Phenytoin monitoring in status epilepticus in infant and children. *Epilepsia* 1993;34:144–150.
579. Wilensky AJ, Lowden JA. Inadequate serum levels after intramuscular administration of diphenylhydantoin. *Neurology* 1973;23:318–324.
580. Pellock JM. Fosphenytoin use in children. *Neurology* 1996;46[Suppl 1]:S14–S16.
581. Holmes GL, Riviello JJ. Midazolam and pentobarbital for refractory status epilepticus. *Pediatr Neurol* 1999;20:259–264.
582. Evrard P, et al. Management of status epilepticus in the pediatric age group. In: Treiman DM, Wasterlain CG, eds. *Status epilepticus: mechanisms and management*. New York: Lippincott Williams & Wilkins (in press).
583. Shaner DM, et al. Treatment of status epilepticus: a prospective comparison of diazepam and phenytoin versus phenobarbital and optional phenytoin. *Neurology* 1988;38:202–207.
584. Koul RL, et al. Continuous midazolam infusion as treatment of status epilepticus. *Arch Dis Child* 1997;76:445–448.
585. Van Ness PC. Pentobarbital and EEG burst suppression in treatment of status epilepticus refractory to

benzodiazepines and phenytoin. *Epilepsia* 1990;31: 61–67.

586. Mitchell WG. Status epilepticus and acute repetitive seizures in children, adolescents, and young adults: etiology, outcome, and treatment. *Epilepsia* 1996;37 [Suppl 1]:S74–S80.

587. Kobayashi K, et al. Successful management of intractable epilepsy with intravenous lidocaine and lidocaine tapes. *Pediatr Neurol* 1999;21:476–480.

588. Phillips SA, Shanahan RJ. Etiology and mortality of status epilepticus in children. A recent update. *Arch Neurol* 1989;46:74–76.

589. Berg AT, et al. Status epilepticus in children with newly diagnosed epilepsy. *Ann Neurol* 1999;45:618–623.

590. Rodin EA. *The prognosis of patients with epilepsy.* Springfield, IL: Charles C Thomas Publisher, 1968.

591. Shinnar S, et al. Discontinuing antiepileptic drugs in children with epilepsy after a seizure free period: effect of age on outcome. *Epilepsia* 1991;32[Suppl. 3]: 69–70.

592. Camfield PR, et al. If a first antiepileptic drug fails to control a child with epilepsy, what are the chances of success with the next drug? *J Pediatr* 1997;131: 821–824.

593. Shinnar S, et al. The risk of seizure recurrence after a first unprovoked afebrile seizure in childhood: an extended follow-up. *Pediatrics* 1996;98:216–225.

594. Hauser WA, et al. Seizure recurrence after a first unprovoked seizure: an extended follow-up. *Neurology* 1990;40:1163–1170.

595. Sander JW, et al. National General Practice Study of Epilepsy: newly diagnosed epileptic seizures in a general population. *Lancet* 1990;336:1267–1271.

596. Shorvon SD. The temporal aspects of prognosis in epilepsy. *J Neurol Neurosurg Psychiatry* 1984;47: 1157–1165.

597. Annegers JF, Hauser WA, Elveback LR. Remission of seizures and relapse in patients with epilepsy. *Epilepsia* 1979;20:729–737.

598. Huttenlocher PR, Hapke RJ. A follow-up study of intractible seizures in childhood. *Ann Neurol* 1990;28:699–705.

599. Emerson R, et al. Stopping medication in children with epilepsy. *N Engl J Med* 1981;304:1125–1129.

600. Sato S, et al. Long-term follow-up of absence seizures. *Neurology* 1983;33:1590–1595.

601. Camfield C, et al. Biologic facts as predictors of social outcome of epilepsy in intellectually normal children: a population-based study. *J Pediatr* 1993;122: 869–873.

602. Reynolds EH, Elwes RD, Shorvon SD. Why does epilepsy become intractable? Prevention of chronic epilepsy. *Lancet* 1983;2:952–954.

603. Aicardi J. *Epilepsy in Children*, 2nd ed. New York: Raven Press, 1994.

604. Wirrell EC, et al. Long-term prognosis of typical childhood absence epilepsy. Remission or progression to juvenile myoclonic epilepsy. *Neurology* 1996;47:912–918.

605. Lindsay J, Ounsted C, Richards P. Long-term outcome in children with temporal lobe seizures. I. Social outcome and childhood factors. *Dev Med Child Neurol* 1979;21:285–298.

606. Gibberd FB, Bateson MC. Sleep epilepsy: its pattern and prognosis. *BMJ* 1974;2:403–405.

607. Reynolds EH. Early treatment and prognosis of epilepsy. *Epilepsia* 1987;28:97–106.

608. Terrence CF, Wisotzkey HM, Perper JA. Unexpected, unexplained death in epileptic patients. *Neurology* 1975;25:594–598.

609. Terrence CF, Rao GR, Perper JA. Neurogenic pulmonary edema in unexpected, unexplained death of epileptic patients. *Ann Neurol* 1981;9:458–464.

610. Nilsson L, et al. Risk factors for sudden unexplained death in epilepsy: a case-controlled study. *Lancet* 1999;353:888–893.

611. Ellenberg JH, Hirtz DG, Nelson KB. Do seizures in children cause intellectual deterioration? *N Engl J Med* 1986;314:1085–1088.

612. Trimble MR. Cognitive hazards of seizure disorders. *Epilepsia* 1988;29[Suppl 1]:S19–S24.

613. Addy DP. Cognitive function in children with epilepsy. *Dev Med Child Neurol* 1987;29:394–397.

614. Vining EPG, et al. Psychologic and behavioral effects of antiepileptic drugs in children: a double-blind comparison between phenobarbital and valproic acid. *Pediatrics* 1987;80:165–174.

615. Trimble MR, Reynolds EH. Anticonvulsant drugs and mental symptoms: a review. *Psychol Med* 1976;6: 169–178.

616. Goldensohn ES, Gold AP. Prolonged behavioral disturbances as ictal phenomena. *Neurology* 1960;10:19.

617. Gross-Tsur V, Shinnar S. Discontinuing antiepileptic drug treatment. In: Wyllie E, ed. *The treatment of epilepsy: principles and practice*, 2nd ed. Baltimore: Williams & Wilkins, 1997:799–807.

618. Peters ACB, et al. Randomized prospective study of early discontinuation of antiepileptic drugs in children with epilepsy. *Neurology* 1998;50:724–730.

619. Holowach-Thurston JH, et al. Prognosis in childhood epilepsy: additional follow-up of 148 children 15 to 23 years after withdrawal of anticonvulsant therapy. *N Engl J Med* 1982;306:831–836.

620. Shinnar S, et al. Discontinuing antiepileptic drugs in children with epilepsy: a prospective study. *Ann Neurol* 1994;35:534–535.

621. Gherpelli JLD, et al. Discontinuing medication in epileptic children: a study of risk factors related to recurrence. *Epilepsia* 1992;33:681–686.

622. Tennison M, et al. Discontinuing antiepileptic drugs in children. A comparison of a six-week and a nine-month taper period. *N Engl J Med* 1994;330:1407–1410.

623. Callaghan N, Garret A, Goggin T. Withdrawal of anticonvulsant drugs in patients free of seizures for two years: a prospective study. *N Engl J Med* 1988;318: 942–946.

624. Craig A, Oxley J. Emotional and psychiatric aspects of epilepsy. In: Laidlaw J, Richens A, Chadwick D, eds. *A textbook of epilepsy*, 3rd ed. Oxford: Butterworth–Heinemann, 1994:186–200.

625. Kemp AM, Sibert JR. Epilepsy in children and the risk of drowning. *Arch Dis Child* 1993;68: 684–685.

626. O'Donohoe NV. What should the child with epilepsy be allowed to do? *Arch Dis Child* 1983;58:934–937.

627. Patrick HT, Levy DM. Early convulsions in epileptics and in others. *JAMA* 1924;82:375–381.

628. Wallace SJ. *The child with febrile seizures.* London: John Wright, 1988.

629. Vanden-Berg BJ, Yerushalmy J. Studies on convulsive disorders in young children. I. Incidence of febrile and nonfebrile convulsions by age and other factors. *Pediatr Res* 1969;3:298–304.

630. Berg AT, et al. A prospective study of recurrent febrile seizures. *N Engl J Med* 1992;327:1122–1127.
631. Johnson EW, et al. Evidence for a novel gene for familial febrile convulsions, FEB2, linked to chromosome 19p in an extended family from the Midwest. *Hum Mol Genet* 1998;7:63–67.
632. Wallace RH, et al. Suggestion of a major gene for familial febrile convulsions mapping to 8q13-21. *J Med Genet* 1996;33:308–312.
632a. Peiffer A, et al. A locus for febrile seizures (FEB3) maps to chromosome 2q23-24. *Ann Neurol* 1999;46: 671–678.
632b. Wallace RH, et al. Febrile seizures and generalized epilepsy associated with a mutation in the Na+ channel beta1 subunit gene SCN1B. *Nature Genet* 1998;19:366–370.
633. Berg AT. Febrile seizures and epilepsy: the contribution of epidemiology. *Paediatr Perinat Epidemiol* 1992;6:145–152.
634. Berg AT, et al. Risk factors for a first febrile seizure: a matched case-control study. *Epilepsia* 1995;36: 334–341.
635. Baird HW III, Garfunkel JM. Electroencephalographic changes in children with artificially induced hyperthermia. *J Pediatr* 1956;48:28–33.
636. Autret E, et al. Double-blind, randomized trial of diazepam versus placebo for prevention of recurrence of febrile seizures. *J Pediatr* 1990;117:490–494.
637. Hall CB, et al. Human herpesvirus-6 infections in children. A prospective study of complications and reactivation. *N Engl J Med* 1994;331:432–438.
638. Fischler E. Convulsions as a complication of shigellosis in children. *Helv Paediatr Acta* 1962;17:389–394.
639. Lennox-Buchthal MA. Febrile convulsions. A reappraisal. *Electroencephalogr Clin Neurophysiol* 1973; [Suppl 32].
640. Lorber J, Sunderland R. Lumbar puncture in children with convulsions associated with fever. *Lancet* 1980;1:785–786.
641. Green SM, et al. Can seizures be the sole manifestation of meningitis in febrile children? *Pediatrics* 1993;92:527–534.
642. Freeman JM, Vining EPG. Decision making and the child with febrile seizures. *Pediatr Rev* 1992;13: 298–310.
643. Sofijanov N, et al. Febrile seizures: clinical characteristics and initial EEG. *Epilepsia* 1992;33:52–57.
644. Stores G. When does the EEG contribute to the management of febrile seizures? *Arch Dis Child* 1991;66: 554–557.
645. Camfield PR, et al. Prevention of recurrent febrile seizures. *J Pediatr* 1995;126:929–930.
646. Wolf SM, et al. The value of phenobarbital in the child who has had a single febrile seizure: a controlled prospective study. *Pediatrics* 1977;59:378–385.
647. Uhari M, et al. Effect of acetaminophen and low intermittent doses of diazepam on prevention of recurrences of febrile seizures. *J Pediatr* 1995;126:991–995.
648. Fishman MA. Febrile seizures: the treatment controversy. *J Pediatr* 1979;94:177–184.
649. McKinlay I, Newton R. Intention to treat febrile convulsions with rectal diazepam, valproate or phenobarbitone. *Dev Med Child Neurol* 1989;31:617–625.
650. Rosman NP, et al. A controlled trial of diazepam administered during febrile illnesses to prevent recurrence of febrile seizures. *N Engl J Med* 1993;329:79–84.

651. Wolf SM, Forsythe A. Epilepsy and mental retardation following febrile seizures in childhood. *Acta Paediatr Scand* 1989;78:291–295.
652. Hirtz DG, et al. Survey on the management of febrile seizures. *Am J Dis Child* 1986;140:909–914.
653. Camfield PR, Camfield CS, Tibbles AR. Carbamazepine does not prevent febrile seizures in phenobarbital failures. *Neurology* 1982;32:288–289.
654. Wallace SJ, Smith JA. Successful prophylaxis against febrile convulsions with valproic acid or phenobarbitone. *BMJ* 1980;280:353–354.
655. Mamelle N, et al. Prevention of recurrent febrile convulsions—a randomized therapeutic assay: sodium valproate, phenobarbital, and placebo. *Neuropediatrics* 1984;15:37–42.
656. Offringa M, et al. Risk factors for seizure recurrence in children with febrile seizures: a pooled analysis of individual patient data from five studies. *J Pediatr* 1994;124:574–584.
657. Nelson KB, Ellenberg JH. Predictors of epilepsy in children who have experienced febrile seizures. *N Engl J Med* 1976;295:1029–1033.
658. Tsuboi T, Endo S. Febrile convulsions followed by nonfebrile convulsions. A clinical, electroencephalographic and follow-up study. *Neuropädiatrie* 1977;8:209–223.
659. Nelson KB, Ellenberg JH. Prognosis in children with febrile seizures. *Pediatrics* 1978;61:720–727.
660. Annegers JF, et al. Factors prognostic of unprovoked seizures after febrile convulsions. *N Engl J Med* 1987;316:493–498.
661. Berg AT, Shinnar S. Unprovoked seizures in children with febrile seizures: short-term outcome. *Neurology* 1996;47:562–568.
662. Maytal J, Shinnar S. Febrile status epilepticus. *Pediatrics* 1990;86:611–617.
663. Verity CM, Ross EM, Golding J. Outcome of childhood status epilepticus and lengthy febrile convulsions: findings of national cohort study. *Brit Med J* 1993;307:225–228.
664. Lennox WG. Significance of febrile convulsions. *Pediatrics* 1953;11:341–357.
665. Cendes F, et al. Early childhood prolonged febrile convulsions, atrophy and sclerosis of mesial structures, and temporal lobe epilepsy; an MRI volumetric study. *Neurology* 1993;43:1083–1087.
666. Fernández G, et al. Hippocampal malformation as a cause of familial febrile convulsions and subsequent hippocampal sclerosis. *Neurology* 1998;50:909–917.
667. Ellenberg JH, Nelson KB. Febrile seizures and later intellectual performance. *Arch Neurol* 1978;35:17–21.
668. Verity CM, Butler NR, Golding J. Febrile convulsions in a national cohort followed up from birth. II. Medical history and intellectual ability at 5 years of age. *BMJ* 1985;290:1311–1315.
669. Verity CM, Greenwood R, Golding J. Long-term intellectual and behavioral outcomes of children with febrile convulsions. *N Engl J Med* 1998;338:1723–1728.
670. Wolf SM. Controversies in the treatment of febrile convulsions. *Neurology* 1979;29:287–290.
671. Lanska MJ, et al. A population-based study of neonatal seizures in Fayette County, Kentucky. *Neurology* 1995;45:724–732.
672. Ronen GM, Penney S, Andrews W. The epidemiology of clinical neonatal seizures in Newfoundland: a population-based study. *J Pediatr* 1999;143:71–75.

673. Mizrahi EM. Neonatal seizures: problems in diagnosis and classification. *Epilepsia* 1987;28[Suppl 1]:S46–S55.

674. Volpe JJ. *Neurology of the newborn*, 3rd ed. Philadelphia: WB Saunders, 1995:172–207.

675. Scher MS, et al. Electrographic seizures in preterm and full-term neonates: clinical correlates, associated brain lesions, and risk for neurologic sequelae. *Pediatrics* 1993;91:128–134.

676. Herzlinger RA, Kandall SR, Vaughan HG. Neonatal seizures associated with narcotic withdrawal. *J Pediatr* 1977;91:638–641.

677. Mizrahi EM, Kellaway P. Characterization and classification of neonatal seizures. *Neurology* 1987;37:1837–1844.

678. Volpe JJ. Neonatal seizures: current concepts and revised classification. *Pediatrics* 1989;84:422–428.

679. Connell J, et al. Continuous EEG monitoring of neonatal seizures: diagnostic and prognostic considerations. *Arch Dis Child* 1989;64:452–458.

680. Parker S, et al. Jitteriness in full-term neonates: prevalence and correlates. *Pediatrics* 1990;85:17–23.

681. Scher MS. Neonatal seizures. In: Wyllie E, ed. *The treatment of epilepsy: principles and practice*, 2nd ed. Baltimore: Williams & Wilkins, 1996:600–621.

682. Waldinger C, Berg RB. Signs of pyridoxine dependency manifest at birth in siblings. *Pediatrics* 1963;32:161–168.

683. Donn SM, Grasela TH, Goldstein CW. Safety of a higher loading dose of phenobarbital in the term newborn. *Pediatrics* 1985;75:1061–1064.

684. Painter MJ, et al. Phenobarbital and diphenylhydantoin levels in neonates with seizures. *J Pediatr* 1978;92:315–319.

685. Lockman LA, et al. Phenobarbital dosage for control of neonatal seizures. *Neurology* 1979;29:1445–1449.

686. Painter MJ, et al. Phenobarbital compared with phenytoin for the treatment of neonatal seizures. *N Engl J Med* 1999;341:485–489.

687. Bourgeois BFD, Dodson WE. Phenytoin elimination in newborns. *Neurology* 1983;33:173–178.

688. Takeoka M, et al. Fosphenytoin in infants. *J Child Neurol* 1998;13:537–540.

689. Hellström-Westas L, et al. Lidocaine for treatment of severe seizures in newborn infants. II. Blood concentrations of lidocaine and metabolites during intravenous infusion. *Acta Paediatr Scand* 1992;81:35–39.

690. Legido A, Clancy RR, Berman PH. Neurologic outcome after electroencephalographically proven neonatal seizures. *Pediatrics* 1991;88:583–596.

691. Bergman I, et al. Outcome in neonates with convulsions treated in an intensive care unit. *Ann Neurol* 1983;14:642–647.

692. Dennis J. Neonatal convulsions: aetiology, late neonatal status and long-term outcome. *Dev Med Child Neurol* 1978;20:143–158.

693. Holden KR, Mellits ED, Freeman JM. Neonatal seizures. I. Correlation of prenatal and perinatal events with outcomes. *Pediatrics* 1982;70:165–176.

694. Clancy RR, Legido A. Postnatal epilepsy after EEG-confirmed neonatal seizures. *Epilepsia* 1991;32:69–76.

695. Rose AL, Lombroso CT. Neonatal seizure states: a study of clinical, pathological and electroencephalographic features in 137 full-term babies with long-term follow-up. *Pediatrics* 1970;45:404–425.

696. Painter MJ, Bergman I, Crumrine P. Neonatal seizures. *Pediatr Clin North Am* 1986;33:91–109.

697. Mellits ED, Holden KR, Freeman JM. Neonatal seizures. II. A multivariate analysis of factors associated with outcome. *Pediatrics* 1982;70:177–185.

698. Ohtahara S, et al. Early-infantile epileptic encephalopathy with suppression-bursts. In: Roger J, et al., eds. *Epileptic syndromes in infancy, childhood and adolescence*, 2nd ed. London, John Libbey 1992:25–34.

699. Watanabe K, et al. Epilepsies of neonatal onset: seizure type and evolution. *Dev Med Child Neurol* 1999;41:318–322.

700. Pryor DS, Don N, Macourt DC. Fifth day fits: a syndrome of neonatal convulsions. *Arch Dis Child* 1981;56:753–758.

701. Quattlebaum TG. Benign familial convulsions in the neonatal period and early infancy. *J Pediatr* 1979;95:257–259.

702. Alfonso I, et al. Bilateral tonic-clonic epileptic seizures in non-benign familial neonatal convulsions. *Pediatr Neurol* 1997;16:249–251.

703. Singh NA, et al. A novel potassium channel gene, KCNQ2, is mutated in an inherited epilepsy of newborns. *Nat Genet* 1998;18:25–29.

704. Charlier C, et al. A pore mutation in a novel KQT-like potassium channel gene in an idiopathic epilepsy family. *Nat Genet* 1998;18:53–55.

705. Dalessio DJ. *Wolff's headache and other head pain*. New York: Oxford University Press, 1980.

706. Bures J, Buresova O, Krivanek J. *The mechanism and applications of Leao's spreading depression of electroencephalographic activity*. New York: Academic Press, 1974.

707. Oleson J, Edvinsson L. Migraine: a research field matured for the basic neurosciences. *Trends Neurosci* 1991;14:3–5.

707a. Weiller C, et al. Brain stem activation in spontaneous human migraine attacks. *Nature Med* 1995;1:658–660.

708. Lauritzen M. Pathophysiology of the migraine aura. The spreading depression therapy. *Brain* 1994;117:199–210.

709. Ingvardsen BK, et al. Possible mechanism of c-fos expression in trigeminal nucleus caudalis following cortical spreading depression. *Pain* 1997;72:407–415.

710. Goadsby PJ, Edvinsson L. The trigeminovascular system and migraine: studies characterizing cerebrovascular and neuropeptide changes seen in humans and cats. *Ann Neurol* 1993;33:48–53.

711. Lance JW. Current concepts of migraine pathogenesis. *Neurology* 1993;43[Suppl. 3]:S11–S15.

712. Ferrari MD, et al. Cerebral blood flow during migraine attacks without aura and effect of sumatriptan. *Arch Neurol* 1995;52:135–139.

713. Woods RP, Iacoboni M, Mazziotta JC. Bilateral spreading cerebral hypoperfusion during spontaneous migraine headache. *N Engl J Med* 1994;331:1689–1692.

714. Ferrari MD, et al. Serotonin metabolism in migraine. *Neurology* 1989;39:1239–1242.

714a. Chugani DC, et al. Increased brain serotonin synthesis in migraine. *Neurology* 1999;53:1473–1479.

715. Peroutka SJ. Antimigraine drug interactions with serotonin receptor subtypes in human brain. *Ann Neurol* 1988;23:500–504.

716. Congden PJ, Forsythe WI. Migraine in childhood: a study of 300 children. *Dev Med Child Neurol* 1979;21:209–216.

717. Larsson B, Bille B, Pederson N. Genetic influence in headaches: a Swedish twin study. *Headache* 1995;35: 513–519.

718. Ulrich V, et al. The inheritance of migraine with aura estimated by means of structural equation modelling. *J Med Genet* 1999;36:225–227.

718a. Gervil M, et al. Migraine without aura: a population-based twin study. *Ann Neurol* 1999;46:606–611.

719. Russell MB, Olesen J. Migrainous disorder and its relation to migraine without aura and migraine with aura. A genetic epidemiological study. *Cephalalgia* 1996;16:431–435.

720. Russell MB, Iselius L, Olesen J. Inheritance of migraine investigated by complex segregation analysis. *Hum Genet* 1995;96:726–730.

721. Ulrich V, et al. Analysis of 31 families with an apparently autosomal-dominant transmission of migraine with aura in the nuclear family. *Am J Med Genet* 1997;74:395–397.

722. Barlow CF. *Headaches and migraine in childhood. Clinics in developmental medicine.* Oxford: Blackwell Science, 1984:91.

723. Mortimer MJ, Kay J, Jaron A. Epidemiology of headache and childhood migraine in an urban general practice using ad hoc, Vahlquist and HIS criteria. *Dev Med Child Neurol* 1992;34:1095–1101.

724. Baloh RW. Neurotology of migraine. *Headache* 1997;37:615–621.

725. Holguin J, Fenichel G. Migraine. *J Pediatr* 1967;70: 290–297.

726. Prensky AL. Migraine and migrainous variants in pediatric patients. *Pediatr Clin North Am* 1976;23: 461–471.

727. Russell MB, Olesen J. A nosographic analysis of the migraine aura in a general population. *Brain* 1996; 119:355–361.

728. Hachinski VC, Porchawka J, Steele JC. Visual symptoms in the migraine syndrome. *Neurology* 1973;23: 570–579.

729. Rossi LN, Mumenthaler M, Vassella F. Complicated migraine (migraine accompagnée) in children. *Neuropädiatrie* 1980;11:27–35.

730. Kupersmith MJ, Warren FA, Hass WK. The non-benign aspects of migraine. *Neuro-ophthalmology* 1987;7:1–10.

731. Editorial. Migraine-related stroke in childhood. *Lancet* 1991;337:825–826.

732. Rothner AD. Miscellaneous headache syndromes in children and adolescents. *Semin Pediatr Neurol* 1995;2:159–164.

733. Maytal J. Childhood onset of cluster headaches. *Headache* 1992;275–279.

734. Hammond J. The late sequelae of recurrent vomiting of childhood. *Dev Med Child Neurol* 1974;16:15–22.

735. Smith CH. Recurrent vomiting in children. Its etiology and treatment. *J Pediatr* 1937;10:719–742.

736. Kuzemko JA, Young W. Ophthalmoplegic migraine. A case report. *Dev Med Child Neurol* 1967;9:427–429.

737. Eviatar L, Eviatar A. Vertigo in children. Differential diagnosis and treatment. *Pediatrics* 1977;59: 833–838.

738. Camfield PR, Metrakos K, Andermann F. Basilar migraine, seizures, and severe epileptiform EEG abnormalities: a benign syndrome in adolescents. *Neurology* 1978;28:584–588.

739. Golden GS, French JH. Basilar artery migraine in young children. *Pediatrics* 1975;56:722–726.

740. Gascon, G, Barlow, C. Juvenile migraine presenting as an acute confusional state. *Pediatrics* 1970;45:628–635.

741. Lee CH, Lance CW. Migraine stupor. *Headache* 1977;17:32–38.

742. Haas DC, Pineda GS, Lourie H. Juvenile head trauma syndromes and their relationship to migraine. *Arch Neurol* 1975;32:727–730.

743. Ehyai A, Fenichel GM. The natural history of acute confusional migraine. *Arch Neurol* 1978;35:368–369.

744. Menkes MM. Personality characteristics and family roles of children with migraine. *Pediatrics* 1974;53: 560–564.

745. Chu ML, Shinnar S. Headaches in children younger than 7 years of age. *Arch Neurol* 1992;49:79–82.

746. Seshia SS, et al. International headache society criteria and childhood headache. *Dev Med Child Neurol* 1994;36:419–428.

747. Metsähonkala L, Sillanpää M, Tuominen J. Headache diary in the diagnosis of childhood migraine. *Headache* 1997;37:240–244.

748. Rothner AD. The evaluation of headaches in children and adolescents. *Semin Pediatr Neurol* 1995;2: 109–118.

749. Rothner AD. Headaches in children: a review. *Headache* 1983;18:169–175.

750. Belfer ML, Kaban LB. Temporomandibular joint dysfunction with facial pain in children. *Pediatrics* 1982;69:564–567.

751. Winner P, et al. Classification of pediatric migraine: proposed revisions to the IHS criteria. *Headache* 1995;35:407–410.

752. Maytal J, et al. Pediatric migraine and the International Headache Society (IHS) criteria. *Neurology* 1997;48:602–607.

753. Barabas G, Matthews WS, Ferrari M. Childhood migraine and motion sickness. *Pediatrics* 1983;72: 188–190.

754. Friedman E, Pampiglione G. Recurrent headache in children (a clinical and electroencephalographic study). *Arch de Neurobiol* 1974;37[Suppl]:115–176.

755. Kramer U, et al. The value of EEG in children with chronic headache. *Brain Dev* 1994;16:304–306.

756. Schon F, Blau JN. Postepileptic headache and migraine. *J Neurol Neurosurg Psychiatry* 1987;50: 1148–1152.

757. Young WB, Silberstein SD. Paroxysmal headache caused by colloid cyst of the third ventricle: case report and review of the literature. *Headache* 1997;37:15–20.

758. Maytal J, et al. The value of brain imaging in children with headaches. *Pediatrics* 1995;96:413–416.

759. McAbee GN, et al. Value of MRI in pediatric migraine. *Headache* 1993;33:143–144.

760. Straussberg R, Amir J. Headaches in children younger than 7 years: are they really benign? *Arch Neurol* 1993;50:130–131.

761. Battistella PA, et al. Headache and brain tumors: different features versus primary forms in juvenile patients. *Headache Q* 1998;9:245–248.

762. Gomez-Aranda F, et al. Pseudomigraine with temporary neurological symptoms and lymphocytic pleocytosis. A report of 50 cases. *Brain* 1997;120: 1105–1113.

763. Ling W, Oftedal G, Weinberg W. Depressive illness in childhood presenting as severe headache. *Am J Dis Child* 1970;120:122–124.
764. Harrison RH. Psychological testing in headache: a review. *Headache* 1975;14:177–185.
765. Ramadan NM. Unusual causes of headaches. *Neurology* 1997;48:1494–1499.
766. Herman SP, Stickler GB, Lucas AR. Hyperventilation syndrome in children and adolescents: long-term follow-up. *Pediatrics* 1981;67:183–187.
767. Perkin GD, Joseph R. Neurological manifestations of the hyperventilation syndrome. *J Roy Soc Med* 1986; 79:448–450.
768. Hämäläinen ML, et al. Ibuprofen or acetaminophen for the acute treatment of migraine in children. A double-blind, randomized, placebo-controlled, crossover study. *Neurology* 1997;48:103–107.
769. Capobianco DJ, Cheshire WP, Campbell JK. An overview of the diagnosis and pharmacologic treatment of migraine. *Mayo Clin Proc* 1996;71: 1055–1066.
770. Caekebeke JFV, et al. Antimigraine drug sumatriptan increases blood flow velocity in large cerebral arteries during migraine attacks. *Neurology* 1992;42: 1522–1526.
771. Hämäläinen ML, Koppu K, Santavuori P. Sumatriptan for migraine attacks in children: a randomized placebo-controlled study. Do children with migraine respond to oral sumatriptan differently from adults? *Neurology* 1997;48:1100–1103.
772. Ludvigsson J. Propranolol used in prophylaxis of migraine in children. *Acta Neurol Scand* 1974;50: 109–115.
773. Andersson KE, Vinge E. β-adrenoreceptor blockers and calcium antagonists in the prophylaxis and treatment of migraine. *Drugs* 1990;39:355–373.
774. Sorge F, et al. Flunarizine in prophylaxis of childhood migraine: a double-blind, placebo-controlled study. *Cephalalgia* 1987;7[Suppl 6]:385–386.
775. Igarashi M, May WN, Golden GS. Pharmacologic treatment of childhood migraine. *J Pediatr* 1992;120: 652–657.
776. Mathew NT, et al. Migraine prophylaxis with divalproex. *Arch Neurol* 1995;52:281–286.
777. Kaniecki RG. A comparison of divalproex with propanolol and placebo for the prophylaxis of migraine without aura. *Arch Neurol* 1997;54: 1141–1145.
778. Fenichel GM, Battiata S. Thrombophlebitis secondary to methysergide maleate therapy. *J Pediatr* 1966;68:632–634.
779. Egger J, et al. Is migraine a food allergy? *Lancet* 1983;2:865–869.
780. Hinrichs WL, Keith HM. Migraine in childhood: a follow-up report. *Mayo Clin Proc* 1965;40:593–596.
781. Glista GG, Mellinger JF, Rooke ED. Familial hemiplegic migraine. *Mayo Clin Proc* 1975;50:307–311.
782. O'Hare JA, Feely MJ, Callaghan N. Clinical aspects of familial hemiplegic migraine in two families. *Irish Med J* 1981;74:291–295.
783. Gardner K, et al. A new locus for hemiplegic migraine maps to chromosome 1q31. *Neurology* 1997;49: 1231–1238.
784. Ophoff RA, et al. Familial hemiplegic migraine and episodic ataxia type 2 are caused by mutations in the Ca (2+) channel gene CACNL1A4. *Cell* 1996;87:543–552.
785. Denier C, et al. High prevalence of CACNA1A truncations and broader clinical spectrum in episodic ataxia type 2. *Neurology* 1999;52: 1816–1821.
786. Ducros A, et al. Mapping of a second locus for familial hemiplegic migraine to 1q21-q23 and evidence of further heterogeneity. *Ann Neurol* 1997;42: 885–890.
787. Gee S. On fitful or recurrent vomiting. *St. Bartholomew's Hospital Reports* 1882;18:1–6.
788. Hoyt CS, Stickler GB. A study of 44 children with the syndrome of recurrent (cyclic) vomiting. *Pediatrics* 1960;25:775–780.
789. MacKeith RCM, Pampiglione G. The recurrent syndrome in children. Clinical and EEG observations in 52 cases [Abstract]. *Electroenceph Clin Neurophys* 1956;8:161.
790. Reinhart JB, Evans SL, McFadden DL. Cyclic vomiting in children: seen through the psychiatrist's eye. *Pediatrics* 1977;59:371–377.
791. Li UK, et al. Is cyclic vomiting syndrome related to migraine? *J Pediatr* 1999;134:567 572.
792. Sondheimer JM, Morris BA. Gastroesophageal reflux among severely retarded children. *J Pediatr* 1979; 94:710–714.
793. Li BUK, et al. Heterogeneity of diagnoses presenting as cyclic vomiting. *Pediatrics* 1998;102:583–587.
794. Boles RG, et al. Cyclic vomiting and mitochondrial DNA mutations. *Lancet* 1997;350:1299–1300.
795. Katz RM. Cough syncope in children with asthma. *J Pediatr* 1970;77:48–51.
796. Garson A. Medicolegal problems in the management of cardiac arrhythmias in children. *Pediatrics* 1987;79:84–88.
797. Gospe SM, Choy M. Hereditary long Q-T syndrome presenting as epilepsy: electroencephalography laboratory diagnosis. *Ann Neurol* 1989;25:514–516.
798. Splawski I, et al. Molecular basis of the long-QT syndrome associated with deafness. *N Engl J Med* 1997; 336:1562–1567.
799. Travis WD, et al. Systemic mast cell disease. Analysis of 58 cases and literature review. *Medicine* 1988;67:345–368.
800. Lin JTY, et al. Convulsive syncope in blood donors. *Ann Neurol* 1982;11:525–528.
801. Lerman-Sagie T, et al. Head-up tilt for the evaluation of syncope of unknown origin in children. *J Pediatr* 1991;118:676–679.
802. Lombroso CT, Lerman P. Breathholding spells (cyanotic and pallid infantile syncope). *Pediatrics* 1967;39:565–581.
803. DiMario FJ, Sarfarazi M. Family pedigree analysis of children with severe breath-holding spells. *J Pediatr* 1997;130:647–651.
804. Gauk EW, Kidd L, Prichard JS. Mechanism of seizures associated with breath-holding spells. *N Engl J Med* 1963;268:1436–1441.
805. Livingston S. Breath-holding spells in children: differentiation from epileptic attacks. *J Am Med Assoc* 1970;212:2231–2235.
806. Daoud AS, et al. Effectiveness of iron therapy on breath-holding spells. *J Pediatr* 1997;130:547–550.
807. Donma MM. Clinical efficacy of piracetam in treatment of breath-holding spells. *Pediatr Neurol* 1998; 18:41–45.

808. Rickler KB. Episodic dyscontrol. In: Benson DF, Blumer D, eds. *Psychiatric aspects of neurologic disease.* New York: Grune & Stratton, 1982:49–73.
809. Billiard M, Seignalet J. Extraordinary association between HLA-DR2 and narcolepsy. *Lancet* 1985;1: 226–227.
810. Neely S, et al. HLA antigens in narcolepsy. *Neurology* 1987;37:1858–1860.
811. Langdon N, et al. Immune factors in narcolepsy. *Sleep* 1986;9:143–148.
812. Westphal C. Zwei Krankheitsfälle. II. Eigenthümliche mit Einschlafen verbundene Anfälle. *Arch Psychiat Nervenkr* 1877;7:631–635.
813. Ornitz EM, et al. The EEG and rapid eye movements during REM sleep in normal and autistic children. *Electroencephalogr Clin Neurophysiol* 1969;26:167–175.
814. Vgontzas AN, Kales A. Sleep and its disorders. *Ann Rev Med* 1999;50:387–400.
815. Guilleminault C, et al. Investigations into the neurologic basis of narcolepsy. *Neurology* 1998;50 [2 Suppl 1]:S8–S15.
816. Hishikawa Y, Shimizu T. Physiology of REM sleep, cataplexy, and sleep paralysis. *Adv Neurol* 1995;67: 245–271.
817. Aldrich MS. The neurobiology of narcolepsy. *Trends Neurosci* 1991;14:235–239.
818. MacFarlane JG, et al. Dopamine D2 receptors quantified in vivo in human narcolepsy. *Biol Psychiatry* 1997;41:305–310.
819. Broughton RJ. Polysomnography: principles and applications in sleep and arousal disorders. In: Niedermeyer E, Lopes da Silva F, eds. *Electroencephalography*, 3rd ed. Baltimore: Williams & Wilkins, 1993: 765–802.
820. Yoss RE, Daly DD. Narcolepsy in children. *Pediatrics* 1960;25:1025–1033.
821. Guilleminault C, Pelayo R. Narcolepsy in prepubertal children. *Ann Neurol* 1997;43:135–142.
822. Critchley M. Periodic hypersomnia and megaphagia in adolescent males. *Brain* 1962;85:627–656.
823. Orlosky MJ. The Kleine-Levin syndrome: a review. *Psychosomatics* 1982;23:609–621.
824. Ward WA Jr, Kelsey WM. The Pickwickian syndrome: a review of the literature and report of a case. *J Pediatr* 1962;61:745–750.
825. Kotagal S, Hartse KM, Walsh JK. Characteristics of narcolepsy in children. *Pediatrics* 1990;85: 205–209.
826. Chervin RD, et al. Symptoms of sleep disorders, inattention, and hyperactivity in children. *Sleep* 1997;20: 1185–1192.
826a. Beusterien KM, et al. Health-related quality of life effects of modafinil for treatment of narcolepsy. *Sleep* 1999;22:757–765.
827. Mitler MM, et al. Treatment of narcolepsy: objective studies on methylphenidate, pemoline, and protriptyline. *Sleep* 1986;9:260–264.
828. Shapiro WR. Treatment of cataplexy with clomipramine. *Arch Neurol* 1975;32:653–656.
829. Parkes JD. The parasomnias. *Lancet* 1986;2: 1021–1025.
830. Resnick TJ, et al. Benign neonatal sleep myoclonus: relationship to sleep states. *Arch Neurol* 1986;43: 266–268.
831. Dravet C. Les épilepsies myocloniques bénignes du nourisson. *Epilepsies* 1990;2:95–101.
832. Dravet C, Bureau M, Roger J. Benign myoclonic epilepsy in infants. In: Roger J, et al., eds. *Epileptic syndromes in infancy, childhood and adolescence.* London: John Libbey, 1985:23–29.
833. Leung KC, Robson WM. Head banging. *J Singapore Paediat Soc* 1990;32:14–17.
834. Sheldon SH, Spire J-P, Levy HB. *Pediatric sleep medicine.* Philadelphia: WB Saunders, 1992.
835. Kales A, et al. Hereditary factors in sleepwalking and night terrors. *Br J Psychiatry* 1980;137:111–118.
836. Broughton R. Childhood sleep walking, sleep terrors, and enuresis nocturna: their pathophysiology and differentiation from nocturnal epileptic seizures. *Sleep* 1978. Basel: S. Karger 1980:103–111.
837. Ferriss G. Sleep disorders. *Neurol Clin* 1984;2:51–69.
838. Gascon GG, Lombroso CT. Epileptic (gelastic) laughter. *Epilepsia* 1971;12:63–76.
839. Jeavons PM, Harding GF. *Photosensitive epilepsy.* Spastics Int Med Publ. London: William Heinemann Medical Books, Ltd, 1975.
840. Geschwind N, Sherwin I. Language-induced epilepsy. *Arch Neurol* 1967;16:25–31.
841. Critchley MacD. Musicogenic epilepsy. *Brain* 1937; 60:13–27.
842. Calderon-Gonzalez R, Hopkins I, McLean WT. Tap seizures. A form of sensory precipitation epilepsy. *JAMA* 1966;198:521–523.
843. Ingvar DH, Nyman GE. Epilepsia arithmetices. A new psychological mechanism in a case of epilepsy. *Neurology* 1962;12:282–287.
844. Critchley MacD, Cobb W, Sears TA. On reading epilepsy. *Epilepsia* 1959;1:403–417.
845. Strauss H. Paroxysmal compulsive running and the concept of epilepsia cursiva. *Neurology* 1960;10: 341–344.
846. Menkes JH, Ament ME. Neurologic disorders of gastroesophageal function. *Adv Neurol* 1988;49: 409–416.
847. Angelini L, et al. Transient paroxysmal dystonia in infancy. *Neuropediatrics* 1988;19:171–174.

Chapter 14

Diseases of the Motor Unit

John H. Menkes and *Harvey B. Sarnat

*Departments of Neurology and Pediatrics, University of California, Los Angeles, UCLA School of
Medicine, and Department of Pediatric Neurology, Cedars-Sinai Medical Center, Los Angeles,
California 90048; and *Departments of Pediatric Neurology and Neuropathology, University of
Washington School of Medicine, and Children's Hospital and Regional Medical Center, Seattle, Washington 98105*

But this form of myopathy, this pseudo-hypertrophic paralysis which was described by Duchenne (of Boulogne), that great worker in neuro-nosography, is so different in its clinical characters from the progressive spinal amyotrophies that they have rarely been confused clinically. Pseudo-hypertrophic paralysis is a disease of early youth. It is scarcely ever met with after twenty years of age. It is noticed that the child becomes clumsy in his walk, that he is more easily fatigued than the other children of his age; for it is always, quoting from Duchenne's description, in the lower extremities where it commences. Then the upper extremities may be attacked in their turn; but, whatever be the degree of the affection, the hands are generally absolved. Finally the muscles attacked, or at least a great number of them, present an augmentation of volume, an enormous increase in size, giving to the limb, or a segment of the limb, Herculean proportions. Anatomically this hypertrophy is characterized by lesions of the interstitial tissue, such as does not exist in the same degree in spinal amyotrophies. Moreover, and this is a peculiarity which is not found in Duchenne-Aran disease, heredity plays a great part in the development of pseudo-hypertrophic paralysis of the muscles. It often happens that several children are attacked in one family, and that some of their relatives may present the same affection.

J. M. Charcot, *Clinical Lectures on Diseases of the Nervous System*, 1889.

The *motor unit* consists of the motor neuron, its axon, the neuromuscular junction, and muscle fibers this single motor neuron innervates. The size of the motor unit varies greatly: Finely tuned small muscles, such as the extraocular muscles or the stapedius, have a 1:1 ratio, whereas large muscles not requiring such refined control, such as the glutei or quadriceps femoris, have a ratio of 1:200 or more. This chapter discusses disorders of the motor unit, or neuromuscular disorders, and excludes suprasegmental disorders of cerebral origin, such as spasticity, ataxia, and dyskinesias, that are not primary disturbances of the motor unit even though they may profoundly affect muscular function.

Neuromuscular disorders have a limited clinical expression with considerable overlap of symptoms and signs, hence their definitive diagnosis depends in part on the proper application of laboratory techniques. The procedures used most are serum myogenic enzymes, imaging of muscle, electromyography (EMG), electrophysiologic measurement of motor and sensory nerve conduction velocities, and muscle biopsy.

The latter procedure involves histochemistry, immunocytochemistry, biochemistry, and electron microscopy. Advances in genetics now provide molecular genetic markers for many specific diseases that may be diagnosed from a blood sample. Examples include many muscular dystrophies, spinal muscular atrophy (SMA), and several metabolic myopathies. The clinician must decide which of these procedures provides the needed information in the least invasive manner. At times, two procedures are complementary rather than competitive: nerve conduction velocity and nerve biopsy provide different information. At other times, one procedure confirms another: a blood polymerase chain reaction for Duchenne dystrophy is nondiagnostic in approximately one-third of cases, but the more precise dystrophin immunoreactivity of the muscle biopsy is diagnostic in all cases. Several excellent texts and review chapters deal with disorders of muscle: Engel and Franzini-Armstrong (1), Brooke (2), Dubowitz (3), Swash (4), and Sarnat (5). The best current monograph on pediatric disorders of peripheral nerve is by Ouvrier and colleagues (6).

LABORATORY INVESTIGATION OF NEUROMUSCULAR DISEASE

Muscle Enzymes

Degenerating or necrotic myofibers release several enzymes into the serum because of loss of integrity of the sarcolemmal membrane. These provide useful markers in blood for a few neuromuscular diseases, but not for those in which no degenerative changes occur or the process is so mild that renal clearance can compensate.

The gold standard of muscle enzymes is creatine kinase (CK), previously known as creatine phosphokinase. This enzyme of striated muscle is shared by only two other organs: cardiac muscle and central nervous system (CNS), and not by liver, pancreas, or other viscera. If elevated, isoenzymes may be measured in blood to separate the source: the MM band is striated muscle, MB band is heart, and BB is brain or spinal cord. The upper range of normal serum CK in childhood is approximately 180 IU/L, and the CK usually must be approximately three times

normal to be considered significant. Strenuous physical activity always results in a transient increase in serum CK, as shown in studies of athletes, so that the enzyme should be measured after a period of relative rest. It also is elevated after traumatic injury of muscle, hence it should not be measured for at least a week after muscle biopsy or EMG. It is transiently elevated in neonates because of minor contusions of muscle during labor and delivery, but is not elevated in infants delivered by cesarean section unless they have suffered prolonged labor and arrested descent within the maternal pelvis.

The serum CK may be mildly elevated (in the hundreds) in some neuromuscular disorders (e.g., SMA, limb-girdle muscular dystrophy), greatly elevated (in the thousands) in others (e.g., Duchenne and Becker muscular dystrophy, rhabdomyolysis), and remains normal in most (e.g., the congenital myopathies; mitochondrial cytopathies). In some myopathies it is variable from normal to high (e.g., polymyositis, dermatomyositis), depending on the activity of the inflammation and necrosis. The serum CK is, therefore, not a screening test for neuromuscular diseases, but a normal CK level always excludes Duchenne muscular dystrophy, even in the presymptomatic neonate.

Other *muscle enzymes* are not as specific as CK and may be misleading. The first such serum enzyme discovered was aldolase, but this enzyme is expressed in many tissues including in red blood cells where it is present in high concentrations. An elevated aldolase out of proportion to CK in the same sample is usually an artifact caused by hemolysis. The transaminases (e.g., aspartate aminotransferase, alanine aminotransferase), often regarded as *liver enzymes,* are also present in muscle, and some children with myopathy have undergone unnecessary liver biopsy for unexplained high liver enzymes because CK was not also measured. Enzymes other than CK rarely contribute to the diagnosis if CK is available.

Imaging of Muscle

In recent years, ultrasonography, computed tomography, and magnetic resonance imaging

(MRI) have been applied to muscle in various neuromuscular diseases and indeed may be helpful at times in diagnosing fatty or fibrous connective tissue replacement of muscle and distinguishing edematous or mostly dystrophic myofibers from normal muscle. The most useful of these methods is ultrasound. It is probably the simplest, least invasive, and least expensive (7). Plain roentgenography of the extremities may provide useful information about the ratio of the *muscle cylinder* and subcutaneous fat pad and about intramuscular calcifications, but ultrasonography should be reserved for soft tissues, not for bone as in the usual radiographs of the extremities.

Cardiac Evaluation

In some myopathies, cardiomyopathy may be present as well as involvement of striated muscle (e.g., Duchenne muscular dystrophy; Emery-Dreifuss muscular dystrophy; some cases of nemaline rod myopathy) or there may be a disturbance in the Purkinje conduction system (e.g., myotonic muscular dystrophy). Electrocardiography, roentgenography of the chest, and echocardiography may be indicated in selected cases. In muscular dystrophies in which cardiac involvement to some degree is almost universal at some stage in the disease, early consultation with a pediatric cardiologist should be requested even if the patient is asymptomatic, as a baseline for anticipated future problems.

Molecular Genetic Markers

Several molecular genetic DNA markers in blood now provide definitive diagnoses in specific diseases such as SMA and some cases of Duchenne dystrophy, and may obviate the need for more invasive diagnostic tests such as muscle biopsy. Muscle dystrophin is characterized and quantitated by means of the Western blot test or quantitated by immunohistochemistry or enzyme-linked immunosorbent assay (ELISA) (8). The polymerase chain reaction (PCR) blood test for Duchenne dystrophy is falsely normal, however, in approximately one-third of cases, but the more specific immunocytochemistry of anti-

bodies against various portions of the dystrophin molecule is diagnostic in all cases, but must be performed on frozen sections of muscle biopsy tissue. The ratio of myofibers expressing or not expressing dystrophin shown by specific antibodies to the rod domain, N-terminus, and C-terminus of the dystrophin molecule distinguishes Duchenne from Becker dystrophies and also detects the female carrier state and mildly affected girls. Immunocytochemical markers in the muscle biopsy for merosin (congenital muscular dystrophy), the family of sarcoglycans (limb-girdle muscular dystrophy), dystroglycans, and others are now available as well. Genetic markers for many other diseases undoubtedly will become commercially available in the next few years. These markers have an additional importance in prenatal diagnosis and for the detection of carrier states.

Electrophysiologic Studies

Motor and sensory nerve conduction velocities (NCV) are valuable diagnostic studies of children with neuropathies. They also help distinguish motor neuron disease from peripheral neuropathy, and axonal degeneration from primary demyelination. NCV can be measured in the facial nerve and the phrenic nerve as well as those of the extremities. NCV usually can be performed with surface electrodes on the skin, without the use of needles, and hence are less frightening to the child and are not painful.

EMG requires needle insertion into muscle and is less useful in pediatric conditions than in those of adults. EMG may provide useful information in distinguishing myopathy from neuropathy, but does not generally distinguish the exact type of myopathy, hence it is not an alternative to the more specific muscle biopsy in most cases. EMG has the advantage of being able to sample several muscles at one examination, to compare distal and proximal muscles, upper and lower extremities and axial muscles, and any presence of left and right asymmetries. In myopathies, the EMG characteristically shows a shortened mean duration and lower amplitude of the motor unit action potentials. A unique pattern is found in myotonic conditions. In contrast to

TABLE 14.1. *Histochemical reactions for muscle biopsies*

Stain	Indication
Hematoxylin and eosin	General survey
Modified Gomori trichrome	Intermyofibrillar network; Z-bands and nemaline rods
Nicotinamide-adenine dinucleotide (reduced form) dehydrogenase	Mitochondrial respiratory complex I
Succinate dehydrogenase	Mitochondrial respiratory complex II
Cytochrome-c oxidase	Mitochondrial respiratory complex IV
Myofibrillar (calcium-mediated) ATPase; pre-incubation at pH 4.3, 4.7, and 10.2 (or 9.8)	Fiber types and subtypes
Heavy-chain myosin	Fiber types (applicable to paraffin sections)
Acid phosphatase	Lysosomal enzyme
Alkaline phosphatase	Lysosomal enzyme
Periodic acid–Schiff	Glycogen and polysaccharides
Oil red O	Neutral lipids
Acridine orange fluorochrome	Nucleic acids, regenerating and denervated myofibers
Acetylcholinesterase	Nerve terminals

myopathies, neuropathic patterns are characterized by spontaneous activity at rest and motor unit action potentials of increased duration and amplitude.

EMG with repetitive nerve stimulation (i.e., evoked potential EMG) is a highly specific diagnostic test for myasthenia and is an example of one condition in which EMG is more definitive than the muscle biopsy. Other specialized EMG studies, such as macro-EMG and single-fiber EMG recording are available in some centers, but are not generally used for clinical diagnosis.

Muscle Biopsy

A muscle biopsy has become the most essential diagnostic procedure in evaluating a child with neuromuscular disease. It is a simple procedure generally performed in day-surgery under local anesthesia with a regional nerve block and does not require a general anesthetic. Needle biopsy has become popular in some centers, including the Cedars-Sinai Medical Center and UCLA. It can be performed percutaneously and has the advantage that repeated biopsies can be performed if necessary (8a). However, an open biopsy usually provides a better quality specimen for pathology and any biochemical studies.

The first decision is the choice of muscle to undergo biopsy. The muscle selected should be affected clinically, but not to such an advanced degree that all muscle tissue has degenerated

beyond recognition. Additionally, the muscle should not have been subjected to EMG study in the previous 4 to 6 weeks. Because all muscles do not normally have the same ratio of fiber types, this is an additional consideration. The deltoid, for example, normally expresses a 60 to 80% predominance of type I fibers, which at times can complicate interpretation of neurogenic changes. The muscle most studied and generally suitable for the diagnosis of most generalized neuromuscular diseases is the vastus lateralis (i.e., quadriceps femoris), a large proximal muscle not in the region of large blood vessels or major nerves.

The muscle sample is divided, and portions are used for routine examination, histochemistry, electron microscopy, and biochemical or enzymatic studies. For routine histologic examination, a portion of the specimen can be fixed in 10% buffered formalin and embedded in paraffin. For histochemical and most histologic studies, the tissue is frozen in liquid nitrogen and then stored at $-70°$ C. A separate piece of the biopsy should be frozen directly and preserved for possible biochemical studies.

The histochemical reactions generally used, together with their indications, are shown in Table 14.1. Histochemical studies have shown that muscle fibers in human skeletal muscle can be differentiated into two types: type I fibers, which are rich in oxidative enzymes but poor in ATPase and phosphorylase, and type 2 fibers, poor in oxidative enzymes but rich in ATPase and phosphorylase. Type 2 fibers have been subdivided into 2A, 2B, and 2C, according to the intensity of ATPase staining at pH 4.35 and 4.63. Type 2C fibers are seen in normal immature, but not adult, muscle. Normal muscle presents a mosaic of both types 1 and 2 fibers. A fuller discussion of histochemical techniques, the histochemistry of developing muscles, and the histologic changes in neurogenic muscular atrophies is presented by Dubowitz (3), Sarnat (5), and Engel and Franzini-Armstrong (1).

Immunocytochemistry has become important in muscle biopsy diagnosis only in the past few years. Frozen sections are required for all of the sarcolemmal region protein, such as dystrophin, spectrin, merosin, and the sarcoglycans (9). Intermediate filament proteins such as vimentin and desmin are important in some congenital myopathies and can be demonstrated both in frozen and paraffin sections. Heavy-chain myosin immunocytochemistry is the first technique to reliably distinguish fiber types in paraffin sections. Other special purpose immunocytochemical methods include antibodies against actin, tropomyosin, and for marking T and B lymphocytes to help distinguish different types of inflammatory myopathies.

Electron microscopy is needed only in selected cases. However, tissue submitted for electron microscopy can be used to prepare 1-μ epoxy resin-embedded sections that are suitable for examination in the light microscope after staining with toluidine blue. These thin sections are valuable to confirm the presence of inclusions, such as those seen in a variety of storage diseases, and other details. Thinner sections for electron microscopy usually are stained with uranyl acetate and lead citrate.

Biochemical Studies

In metabolic myopathies, particularly in the glycogenoses and lipid storage myopathies, quantitative assays may be performed on frozen muscle biopsy tissue for specific enzymatic activities, such as acid maltase, myophosphorylase, brancher and debrancher enzymes, phosphofructokinase, and carnitine palmitoyl-transferase.

Total muscle glycogen and fat and muscle carnitine content also may be measured. These tests are expensive and not routine; they are requested only if the clinical suspicion is strong and especially if the muscle biopsy histochemistry and ultrastructure support the diagnosis.

The increased awareness of mitochondrial diseases and the large number of different deletions and point mutations involving mtDNA have resulted in a much larger number of muscle biopsies now being performed with the specific question of ruling out a mitochondrial cytopathy. Quantitative analysis of each of the mitochondrial respiratory chain enzymes and of mtDNA can be performed on freshly frozen muscle biopsy tissue if there is sufficiently strong clinical or histochemical and ultrastructural evidence. A few mitochondrial cytopathies fail to exhibit morphologic or histochemical changes, so that normal routine biopsy results do not definitively exclude mitochondrial disease, but these cases are a small minority of the mitochondrial cytopathies. Frozen tissue remaining on the block after cutting frozen sections is not suitable for the quantitative analysis of mitochondrial respiratory complexes because the isopentane used to preserve the histologic detail and prevent ice crystal artifacts during the freezing process in liquid nitrogen interferes with the determination of complexes I through III and gives falsely low values. A portion of the muscle biopsy should be freshly frozen directly for possible later biochemical study.

DISEASES OF THE MOTOR NEURON

In children, the most common entity affecting the motor neuron in the brainstem and spinal cord is the SMAs. Poliomyelitis, once seen in epidemic proportions, is a rarity in Western countries. Other neurotropic agents including other enteroviruses that, like poliomyelitis, produce transient or permanent paralysis are considered in Chapter 6. A flaccid paralysis resembling poliomyelitis has been seen in some children who are recovering from an acute episode of asthma (Hopkins syndrome) (see Chapter 15). A familial degenerative disease resembling the adult form of amyotrophic lateral sclerosis is encountered rarely in pediatric practice. It is characterized by degeneration of the pyramidal tracts and the motor cells of the spinal cord and brainstem (10). Involvement of the motor neurons as part of generalized storage diseases is observed in some hereditary metabolic diseases such as GM₁ gangliosidosis, Hurler syndrome, infantile Gaucher disease, glycogenosis type II (Pompe), and neuronal ceroid-lipofuscinosis. These entities are considered under their appropriate sections in Chapter 1.

Spinal Muscular Atrophies

The SMAs are a group of relatively common diseases occurring in infancy or early childhood, transmitted by an autosomal recessive gene and manifested by widespread muscular denervation and atrophy. Carrier frequency has been estimated to fall between 1 in 50 to 80, and the disease has an overall incidence of 1 in 10,000 to 25,000, making it the second most common hereditary neuromuscular disease after Duchenne dystrophy. Three forms of SMA have been recognized. These are the infantile, acute form (SMA type 1 or Werdnig-Hoffmann disease), the intermediate form (SMA type 2), and the juvenile form (SMA type 3 or Kugelberg-Welander disease). Approximately one-fourth of cases of SMA fall into the type 1 variety, approximately one-half into type 2, and the remainder into type 3 (2). All three forms are caused by mutations in a gene, the telomeric survival motor neuron gene (*SMN1*) (11). Two copies of the gene are normally present, a telomeric copy, *SMN1*, and a centromeric copy, *SMN2*. The two genes have greater than 99% homology, and their exons differ in but two nucleotides (12). They encode identical proteins.

Pathologic Anatomy and Pathogenesis

Both Guido Werdnig, an Austrian neurologist from the University of Graz (13), and Johan Hoffmann, a German neurologist (14), in their original descriptions of the infantile form of the disease, pointed to the conspicuous loss of anterior horn cells along the entire length of the spinal cord. Some of the residual motor neurons are in the process of degenerating or are being phagocytized by microglial cells. Motor neurons in the brainstem, notably in the hypoglossal nucleus, are affected also. Some authors describe suprasegmental lesions, including loss of large pyramidal cells from layers 5 and 6 of the motor cortex. These findings must be interpreted in light of the severe agonal anoxia that is commonly encountered. In general, the absence of upper motor neuron involvement is an important clinical feature that distinguishes SMAs from degenerative motor neuron diseases such as amyotrophic lateral sclerosis.

Up to 95% of patients experiencing the various forms of SMA have a homozygous deletion or absence of exons 7 and 8 for both copies of the *SMN1* gene. Subjects who do not have detectable deletions have microdeletions or point mutations in the gene (15). In some patients with SMA types 2 and 3, *SMN1* is not deleted; rather it is replaced by *SMN2* (16). Two other genes have been mapped to the SMA critical region. Homozygous deletions of neuronal apoptosis inhibitory protein gene (*NAIP*) are seen in up to 69% of patients with SMA type 1. By contrast, only some 12 to 18% of patients with SMA types 2 and 3 are deleted for this gene (16a). A third gene in this region, shown to encode a subunit of the basal transcription factor (*TFIIH*) is deleted in approximately 15% of all types of SMA (16a). *NAIP* and *TFIIH* as well as a multicopy microsatellite marker in close proximity to *SMN1* have been proposed as SMA-modifying genes (16b,16c).

The genetic basis for the phenotypic variability of SMA is unclear. Milder forms of SMA appear to have more than two copies of *SMN2*, and in at least one asymptomatic subject with homozygous deletion of the *SMN1* gene, there were four copies of the *SMN2* gene (17).

The SMN protein is widely expressed in brain and a variety of non-CNS tissues (17a). The reason for the effect of gene mutation on the spinal motor neurons is still unclear. The most attractive hypothesis is that SMN protein has an antiapoptotic effect (17b). It therefore appears that SMA is a primary disorder of apoptosis, with the condition representing a physiologic process that becomes pathologic because of continued degeneration of motor neurons in late fetal life and postnatally (18).

Prominent glial proliferation often occurs in the proximal portion of the anterior spinal roots, an abnormality initiated in fetal life, and which was thought to induce secondary neuronal degeneration (19). In some instances, the glial bundles also are demonstrated in the posterior roots, accompanied by shrinkage of the dorsal root ganglion cells (20). An inconstant finding in SMA is loss of myelin from the posterior columns of thoracic and lumbar segments and in the corticospinal tracts (21). These phenomena are now believed to be secondary reactive changes. Removal of the peripheral target of the anterior horn cells accentuates the normal process of motor neuron apoptosis (22–24), but there is no evidence that the primary disorder in this disease is in the muscle target or that there is a distal-to-proximal *dying-back* axonal degeneration in the nerve.

There is selective loss of the large motor neurons, but a striking preservation of several types of motor neurons, notably some of the cervical cord (25) and those innervating extraocular muscles. This histologic contrast is expressed clinically as preservation of normal eye movements even in late stages of the disease. Some genes that program the differentiation and maintenance of motor neurons are expressed in all motor neurons, whereas others are expressed only in certain motor neurons and may provide a protective effect on oculomotor neurons by the principle of genetic redundancy (see Chapter 4 on neuroembryology).

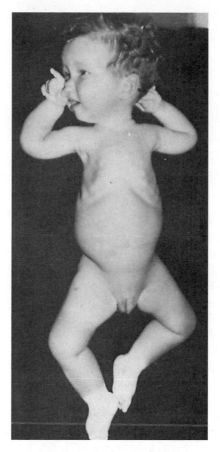

FIG. 14.1. A 1-year-old infant with severe spinal muscular atrophy showing intercostal recession and diaphragmatic breathing. Note frog-leg posture, ability to flex elbows and move hands, and normal facial expression. (Courtesy of Professor Victor Dubowitz, Royal Postgraduate Medical School, London.)

Clinical Manifestations

The clinical picture is marked by reduction of muscle power and spontaneous movement (26). Muscle weakness is symmetric and is more extensive in the proximal part of the limbs, and what little movement is left to the child is found in the small muscles of the hands and feet. At the same time, the affected muscles undergo atrophy, although this is concealed by the subcutaneous fat normally seen at this age. Muscles of the trunk, neck, and thorax are affected equally, although the diaphragm generally is spared until the late stages of the disease (27) (Fig. 14.1). Cardiac and smooth muscles are usually spared as well. With progression of the disease, involvement of bulbar musculature becomes more prominent, and atrophy and fasciculation of the tongue are noted. Deep tendon reflexes are nearly always markedly reduced or absent. There is no sensory loss, intellectual retardation, or sphincter disturbance.

TABLE 14.2. *Age of first clinical manifestations in infantile muscular atrophy*

Age	Percent of cases
Newborn	37
0–1 month	10
1–3 months	12
3–6 months	6
6–9 months	12
9–12 months	9
More than 1 year	8

Modified from Brandt S. *Werdnig-Hoffmann's progressive muscular atrophy.* Copenhagen: Ejnar Munksgaard, 1950.

The age at which the first clinical manifestations become apparent is presented in Table 14.2. It is evident from this table that there are at least two populations, one with onset of symptoms before 6 months of age, SMA type 1, and another with its onset after 6 months of age, SMA types 2 and 3.

In SMA type 1 (infantile SMA, Werdnig-Hoffmann disease), the onset is acute and the disease progresses rapidly. Infants who were already severely hypotonic at birth rarely survive the first year of life, whereas those whose weakness appears postnatally tend to deteriorate more slowly (28,29). Some infants can even experience transient improvement. This improvement is partly caused by a true stationary period in the disease, such as was already noted by Hoffmann in one of his earliest patients. Maturation of partially paralyzed muscles also can give the impression of improvement. In most instances, however, the disease is fatal by 3 years of age, with death generally resulting from a respiratory infection.

Children who experience SMA type 2 [29% in Brandt's series (26), 47% in the more recent series (2)] develop normally for the first 6 months of life, but by 18 months of age experience an arrest of their motor milestones. These children generally lack bulbar symptoms and their disease has a less malignant course (29). One unusual feature of this form of SMA is the presence of a tremor that affects the upper extremities (30) and can even be recorded on the electrocardiogram as a tremor of the baseline (31). Serum CK activity is elevated to approximately five times normal in approximately one-half of these patients, but is never in the thousands of units as in muscular dystrophy; hypertrophy of the gastrocnemius is not unusual (32).

SMA type 3, a milder form of SMA consistent with survival into adult life, was first described by Wohlfart and coworkers (33) and by Kugelberg and Welander (34). Muscular weakness develops after 18 months of age, and in some patients does not manifest until adult life. Adult onset SMA has been termed SMA type 4. It is characterized by involvement of the predominantly proximal muscles and thus bears close clinical resemblance to the muscular dystrophies. Unlike SMA types 1 and 2, impaired joint mobility is relatively common. The condition is differentiated from Duchenne muscular dystrophy by a less striking elevation in muscle enzymes, and from the other types of muscular dystrophies by the alterations seen on muscle biopsy (see Muscle Biopsy, later in this chapter). In some families, SMA types 1 and 2, or types 2 and 3, coexist. This observation represents a genetic puzzle, because haplotype analysis has shown that this variability cannot be accounted for by different alleles at the SMA locus (35).

In some families, a condition that clinically resembles Kugelberg-Welander disease is transmitted in an autosomal dominant manner (36). X-linked pedigrees also have been reported. Hexosaminidase A deficiency can resemble Kugelberg-Welander disease, but patients demonstrate mental deterioration (37).

Diagnosis

Genetic Studies

The definitive diagnosis may now be made by the marker in blood of the *SMN* gene, that usually shows deletions of exons 7 and 8 (15). Thus, in the series of van der Steege and colleagues, the *SMN1* gene, as determined by polymerase chain reaction, was homozygously absent or interrupted in 98.6% of SMA patients (37a). Muscle biopsy, which until only recently had been the diagnostic standard, can therefore be avoided in most patients except for the small fraction whose molecular genetic test results are negative or uninformative.

Biochemical Studies

The study of serum enzymes is important in the differential diagnosis of motor neuron disease. Serum CK is often normal in SMA type 1, but may be elevated in the hundreds, but never in the thousands. It usually is normal or only slightly elevated in the other types. The excretion of amino acids and creatine is generally normal during the early stages of the illness. None of these features are definitively diagnostic of SMA.

Neurophysiologic Studies

EMG findings help confirm the clinical diagnosis of motor neuron disease. Characteristically, the denervated muscles contract spontaneously, involving single muscle fibers (fibrillation) or entire motor units (fasciculation) (38). The finding most specific for the disease and not observed in any other condition marked by muscular denervation is the presence of spontaneous, rhythmic muscle activity at a frequency of 5 to 15 per second, which can be activated by voluntary effort. This abnormality can be recorded in approximately 75% of patients irrespective of age or severity of disease (39). In addition, the residual motor unit potentials are polyphasic and increased in amplitude and duration. With increased muscular effort, little increase occurs in the frequency of discharge and recruitment is impaired. Conduction velocity in the motor nerves is decreased in the more severely affected children (40). This is because of the preferential involvement of the largest motor neurons, which also have the most myelinated and fastest conducting axons.

Muscle Biopsy

Chemical analyses for glycogen, lipids, glycolytic enzymes, and mitochondrial enzymes are performed, with the selection of assays dictated by the clinical presentation.

In the SMAs, a biopsy shows the classic features of denervation atrophy (Fig. 14.2), but

perinatal denervation shows unique features not seen in neurogenic atrophy of mature muscle. Large patches of small, atrophic fibers of both histochemical types are present, and both scattered and grouped muscle fibers of exclusively type I also are present. The normal mosaic or *chessboard* pattern is lost. This uniformity of fiber type reflects an ongoing compensatory reinnervation (3). Electron microscopy adds little specific diagnostic information. The myofilaments are loosened, and mitochondria are diminished in number and show atrophic cristae. Muscle biopsies showing the perinatal pattern of denervation-reinnervation nearly always signify SMA, but are not definitively diagnostic because rare perinatal polyneuropathies may yield a similar picture.

Differential Diagnosis

The presenting signs of the infant with SMA type 1 (Werdnig-Hoffmann disease) are poor muscle tone and a marked delay in motor development. Because a variety of well-defined diseases present the picture of the floppy infant (Table 14.3), differential diagnosis on purely clinical grounds can be difficult. Unlike Walton writing in 1957, (41), we have found the most common cause for diminished muscle tone in a

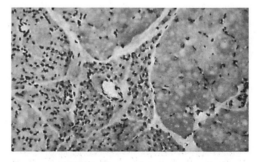

FIG. 14.2. Transverse section of muscle from a patient with Werdnig-Hoffmann disease. Note the relative preservation of muscle fibers in the right side of the field and atrophy of fibers on the left (hematoxylin and eosin, ×20). (Courtesy of Dr. P. Cancilla, Department of Pathology, University of California, Los Angeles, UCLA School of Medicine.)

TABLE 14.3. *Diagnosis of 107 cases of floppy infant*[a]

Diagnosis	Number of cases
Infantile muscular atrophy	67
Congenital muscular dystrophy	3
Polymyositis	1
Myasthenia gravis	1
Scurvy	2
Cerebral disease (atonic cerebral palsy)	14
"Benign congenital hypotonia"	17

[a]Complete recovery in eight patients.
Modified from Walton JH. The limp child. *J Neurol Neurosurg Psychiatry* 1957;20:144.

small infant to be *atonic cerebral palsy*, often secondary to cerebellar hypoplasia. Hypotonia also may result from major abnormalities of the cerebrum, both developmental malformations and disorders acquired in the perinatal period. Invariably, affected infants have considerable intellectual retardation. Spontaneous movements are present, and the tendon reflexes are easily elicited. Often when the infant is lifted by the trunk, the legs promptly become rigid, and a striking accentuation of the extensor thrust reflex is seen. Although some of these children remain hypotonic, others develop dyskinesias or a clear-cut hypertonia within 1 to 3 years. A more extensive discussion of this condition is found in Chapter 5.

Amyotonia congenita, now an obsolete term, was a clinical syndrome reported briefly in a single case by Oppenheim in 1900 (42). It represents a number of unrelated disease processes. It is important to differentiate these entities, now collectively termed *congenital myopathies* (benign congenital hypotonias), from the usually fatal SMA type 1. The term *congenital myopathy* is used to describe floppy infants with a marked delay in motor development. Some of these children recover completely, whereas others can be considered to have a stationary or, at worst, a slowly progressive muscular disorder. In these infants, the muscles are soft and flabby, and a remarkable range of passive movement is possible. Deep tendon reflexes are elicitable, and spontaneous movements are more prominent than in SMA type 1. Respiratory muscles are involved only slightly, and intellectual

development is usually normal. Histochemical and electron microscopic studies of muscle biopsies have delineated numerous distinct entities (see Congenital Myopathies, later in this chapter).

A relatively common clinical problem is that of a floppy infant with delayed gross motor milestones, notably delayed walking, but with normal or nearly normal fine motor development and speech and no demonstrable muscular disorder. This heterogeneous entity, termed *congenital laxity of ligaments* by the late Dr. Frank Ford (43), has more recently been designated *dissociated motor development* (44) or *benign maturation delay* (45).

In a series of such infants reported by Lundberg, 52% achieved normal development between 17 months and 6 years of age (44). A further 24% continued to have delayed motor milestones without any apparent cause. Ultimately 15% were found to have mild mental retardation. The remaining infants experienced various neuromuscular disorders, notably congenital deafness with hypoactive labyrinths and macrocephaly (45,46). Muscle biopsy revealed fiber size disproportion and showed a predominance of type 1 fibers, which persisted despite clinical improvement (45). Dissociated motor development should be distinguished from the less common Ehlers-Danlos syndromes, which are characterized by marked hyperelasticity of skin.

The syndrome of congenital fiber type disproportion (Table 14.4) is part of a broader spectrum of muscle dysmaturation. Both type 1 and type 2 fibers can be affected, with hypotrophic fibers, increased variability in fiber size, or a combination of both. Many infants who demonstrate dysmaturation of muscle, particularly when type 2 fibers are affected, also have significant developmental retardation (47).

Rarer causes for infantile hypotonia include various forms of congenital or neonatal myasthenia gravis, some of which can be diagnosed by the striking improvement in muscle strength after administration of an anticholinesterase drug. For diagnostic purposes, a slowly metabolized drug, such as neostigmine, is more suitable for infants than edrophonium chloride, whose effectiveness is often too fleeting to allow correct

TABLE 14.4. *Some congenital myopathies*

Myopathy	Characteristic clinical features	Muscle biopsy abnormalities	Reference
Nemaline	Dominant or recessive sporadic transmission; associated skeletal dysmorphism; respiratory problems	Rodlike expansions of Z-band	Shy et al. (325)
Central core disease	Dominant or sporadic transmission; associated congenital dislocation of hips	Central area of fiber devoid of mitochondria; myofibril disruption variable; defect in muscle ryanodine receptor	Shuaib et al. (340), Lynch et al. (440)
Myotubular (centronuclear)	Ptosis; weak external ocular muscles; usually sex-linked	Most fibers with one or more central nuclei	Spiro et al. (346), Kioschis et al. (436)
Multicore (minicore) disease	Nonprogressive proximal weakness; neck muscle weakness	Multiple small areas of severe filament disruption devoid of mitochondrial enzymes	Heffner et al. (422)
Congenital fiber disproportion type	Variable clinical picture; muscle contractures; congenital dislocation of hips	Type 1 fibers smaller than type 2; increased variability in fiber diameter; also seen in Krabbe leukodystrophy, fetal alcohol syndrome, Pompe disease, myotonic dystrophy, result of abnormal suprasegmental influence on fetal motor unit (e.g., cerebellar hypoplasia)	Dubowitz (31), Cavanagh et al. (423), Dchkhargani et al. (321), Sarnat (324)
Fingerprint	Tremors; mental retardation	Subsarcolemmal inclusions resembling fingerprints; also found in myotonic dystrophy; dermatomyositis	Engel et al. (424)
Sarcotubular	None	Dilated and fragmented sarcotubules in type 2 fibers	Jerusalem et al. (425)
Zebra body	None	Unique bodies on electron microscopy	Lake and Wilson (426)
Reducing body	None	Inclusions rich in sulfhydryl groups and RNA	Brooke and Neville (427)
Trilaminar	Rigidity of muscle tone gradually disappearing with age; increased serum creatine kinase	Distinctive three-zone fibers by histochemistry and electron microscopy	Ringel et al. (428)
Tubular aggregate	Cramps; muscle pain; proximal limb weakness; autosomal dominant	Tubular aggregates in subsarcolemmal region	Rohkamm et al. (429)
Cytoplasmic body	Progressive proximal muscle weakness; autosomal dominant or recessive	Inclusions in subsarcolemmal region	Goebel et al. (430), Mitrani-Rosenbaum et al. (437)
Cylindrical spiral	Cramps; percussion myotonia; autosomal dominant	Cylindric spirals	Bove et al. (431)
Myopathy with excessive autophagy	Early onset; affects proximal muscles; slow progression, marked creatine kinase elevation; sex-linked	Increased number of autophagic vacuoles	Kalimo et al. (432)
Polysaccharide storage myopathy	Proximal myopathy; no demonstrable abnormality of glycogen pathway	Branched-chain polysaccharides and mucoprotein storage	Thompson et al. (433)
Desmin storage myopathy	Congenital proximal myopathy; cardiomyopathy starting at any age; autosomal dominant distal myopathy	Intrasarcoplasmic accumulation of electron-dense granulofilamentous material, staining for desmin, an intermediate filament protein	Horowitz (434), Goldfarb et al. (438)

sequential assessment of muscle strength. Muscular dystrophy is only rarely seen in a small infant, but in no other condition is a significant elevation in serum enzymes, particularly in CK, common. In the absence of a family history of a dystrophic process, the diagnosis depends mainly on a muscle biopsy.

Finally, infantile botulism (see Chapter 9), Down syndrome, transection of the spinal cord, congenital polyneuritis, muscular hypotonia owing to Marfan syndrome or Prader-Willi syndrome, various chronic illnesses, malnutrition, or metabolic disorders (e.g., organic acidurias and mitochondrial disorders) also must be considered in the differential diagnosis of the hypotonic child.

Several rare conditions are transmitted as autosomal recessive traits in which amyotrophy of the limbs and of the bulbar musculature are combined with progressive pyramidal tract symptoms. In one of these disorders pseudobulbar palsy combines with progressive paraplegia, with symptoms appearing during the first decade of life. In another form, progressive fasciculations and atrophy of the hands, bulbar palsy, and spastic paraplegia appear during the second decade of life. EMG is consistent with denervation and the motor nerve conduction velocities are normal, but in contrast to the SMAs, the deep tendon reflexes are exaggerated (48).

Treatment

Treatment is purely symptomatic and is of no value in altering the course of infantile SMA type 1. In the forms with slower progression, treatment should be directed at maintaining joint mobility and avoiding contractures. The child should be fitted with a lightweight support for the spine to prevent kyphoscoliosis. If at all possible, the youngster should be encouraged to walk with braces. Active exercise can help strengthen still functioning muscles (2,31). Dysphagia may be a late complication in some patients, and aspiration is a risk.

Arthrogryposis

This entity refers to multiple congenital and nonprogressive contractures of the joints, which are fixed in flexion or, less commonly, in extension, accompanied by diminution and wasting of skeletal muscle. Other congenital malformations, particularly clubfoot and cerebral maldevelopment, are often part of the syndrome (49).

Arthrogryposis appears to have several causes, all involving impaired fetal mobility (50). In one group of infants (25% of an English series) (51), the neuromuscular apparatus was normal, and arthrogryposis was caused by external mechanical factors. Such factors include a malformed uterus (e.g., bicornuate uterus), the treatment of maternal tetanus with muscle relaxants, or oligohydramnios (e.g., Potter syndrome). In the remainder of infants, arthrogryposis results from a neuromuscular or a combined cerebral and neuromuscular disorder (50,51). The most common of these disorders is one in which the large anterior horn cells are markedly reduced, the muscle fibers are small and often hyalinized, and the EMG abnormalities are consistent with denervation (52). In contrast to the SMAs, no gliosis occurs, and the small neurons in the ventral horn of the spinal cord are preserved or even increased in number (53). In the experience of Quinn and colleagues, neurogenic arthrogryposis constituted 30% of cases (54). In other cases of arthrogryposis, the changes are compatible with congenital muscular dystrophy (55), congenital myotonic dystrophy (56), fibrosis of the anterior spinal roots, or evidence of embryonic denervation and maturation arrest of muscle (56). Such cases constituted 60% of subjects with arthrogryposis who came to autopsy (54).

Wynne-Davies and associates suggest that the incidence of arthrogryposis has increased considerably over the last few decades (51). Even though both autosomal dominant and autosomal recessive transmission have been postulated, when familial cases caused by a faulty fetal environment are discounted, there is little evidence for a genetic transmission. Rather, a viral or toxic etiology is more likely in the large majority of cases. In at least one instance maternal antibodies against the fetal form of the acetylcholine receptor were demonstrated (56a).

Arthrogryposis is marked by multiple and severe flexion and extension contractures of all extremities, notably the hips, elbows, and fingers. Skin creases are absent, and approximately one-fourth of affected infants have contractures of the temporomandibular joint. These contractures produce the typical round face and micrognathia (57). In one variant, amyoplasia, the shoulders are internally rotated, the elbows are extended, the wrists are flexed, and the hands clenched. In the lower extremities, the knees are generally flexed, and the feet are maintained in an equinovarus position. Some 10% to 30% of patients have various superimposed developmental malformations of the CNS (50).

In Pena-Shokeir syndrome I, a hetcrogeneous condition, arthrogryposis is accompanied by facial anomalies, pulmonary hypoplasia, intrauterine growth retardation, and a variety of cerebral malformations. There is a paucity of motor neurons and muscular atrophy (58). Pena-Shokeir syndrome type II manifests by arthrogryposis not associated with deficiency of motor neurons, but is accompanied by microcephaly, ocular defects, and a variety of skeletal abnormalities (59). Several other malformation syndromes, some with chromosomal disorders, can be accompanied by arthrogryposis. These are listed in review articles by Hageman and coworkers (50) and Hall (60).

Hall and coworkers (60,61), and Staheli and coworkers (62) distinguish several conditions termed *distal arthrogryposis*, which, in contrast to the proximal arthrogryposes, tend to be genetically transmitted and are marked by congenital contractures of hands and feet. The hand of such infants is characteristically tightly fisted with tight adduction of the thumb and medial overlapping of the fingers, similar to the position of the hand in the trisomy 18 syndrome (see Chapter 3). In some families, distal arthrogryposis is dominantly inherited, and in others it appears sporadically. A condition termed *distal arthrogryposis type II* also can have involvement of the proximal limb joints and associated congenital anomalies. In a significant proportion of families, arthrogryposis type II is dominantly inherited (61). Generally, patients with distal arthrogryposis have a better prognosis in terms of limb function than those with mainly proximal joint involvement.

The reduced fetal movements of arthrogryposis permit an *in utero* diagnosis by ultrasonography and, if necessary, by fetoscopy (63).

Treatment of arthrogryposis should commence immediately after birth, with passive motion exercises, braces, and casts. Subsequently, surgery is usually necessary, particularly for contractions of the lower extremities and hips. These procedures are contraindicated in the presence of considerable weakness and amyoplasia. Generally, functional improvement of extension contractures is better than that of flexion contractures, and arthrogryposis secondary to maternal factors has a better outlook than that owing to neuromuscular disorders (60,64). In selected cases, a muscle biopsy may be indicated to rule out myopathies, such as congenital muscular dystrophy, often associated with multiple congenital contractures.

DISEASES OF THE AXON

Disorders at this level of the motor unit result from genetic, infectious, postinfectious, traumatic, or toxic processes, and are, therefore, best discussed under their respective headings (see Chapters 2, 6, 7, 8, and 9, respectively).

In the differential diagnosis of muscular weakness, a polyneuritic process should always be considered. Although, supposedly, the presence of sensory loss in the affected area would easily distinguish polyneuritis from other disorders of the motor unit, an isolated motor neuropathy is far from rare. Commonly, motor weakness can overshadow sensory disturbances, the latter being particularly difficult to demonstrate in infants.

In general, the polyneuritides have a rapid onset, a feature they share only with the inflammatory muscular disorders: polymyositis and dermatomyositis. The site of muscular involvement is often a clue to the cause of the weakness; whereas the SMAs and the muscular dystrophies involve the proximal musculature preferentially, the polyneuritides usually affect the distal musculature. Ascending paralysis such as was originally described by Landry, Guillain, and Barré (see Chapter 7) is uncommon in infants. As a result of the predilection of the polyneuritides for the distal musculature, ankle reflexes are lost early in the illness; in the muscular dystrophies, they are retained.

The distinction between infectious polyneuritis and the hereditary motor and sensory neuropathies rests on the slower evolution of the neuropathies, their frequent association with skeletal deformities or cerebellar involvement, and the presence of a similar neuropathic condition in other members of the immediate family. In approximately two-thirds of children with infectious polyneuritis, the spinal fluid is abnormal. A classic picture of albuminocytologic dissociation, namely an elevated protein level in the absence of a cellular response, is common during the first 2 to 8 weeks of the illness. Motor nerve conduction times are usually slowed, although they can be normal during the initial phases of infectious polyneuritis. Although slowed motor conduction time, when present, is characteristic of infectious polyneuritis, it also can be seen with severe atrophy in anterior horn cell disease (poliomyelitis and the infantile SMA). In approximately one-half of the patients, the sensory nerve conduction times are also delayed. The histologic changes in affected muscle are rarely significant during the acute phase of infectious polyneuritis, whereas in chronic polyneuritis, the main abnormality is a widespread muscular atrophy.

DISEASES OF THE NEUROMUSCULAR JUNCTION

Myasthenia Gravis

Myasthenia gravis, a chronic disease characterized by unusual fatigability of voluntary muscles, was first described by Willis in 1672 (65). Three forms of myasthenia gravis are seen in childhood: juvenile myasthenia gravis, congenital myasthenia gravis, and transient neonatal myasthenia gravis. Aside from age of onset, there is no difference in terms of pathology and pathogenesis between juvenile myasthenia gravis and adult onset myasthenia gravis.

Pathologic Anatomy

The microscopic changes can be minute, even in severely affected muscles. On electron microscopy, the nerve terminals are small, and the cleft between the nerve and the subneural apparatus is widened. Additionally, the area reactive for acetylcholinesterase is reduced, but with no abnormality in the number or size of synaptic vesicles. In 70% to 80% of patients, there are pathologic changes in the thymus. Usually, these consist of lymphoid hyperplasia. Although thymomas occur in approximately 10% of all patients with myasthenia, they are extremely rare in childhood. Myocardial abnormalities have been found in approximately one-half of autopsied patients.

Pathogenesis

The functional lesion in juvenile myasthenia gravis is located at the neuromuscular junction and is the consequence of an antibody-mediated autoimmune reaction against the postsynaptic acetylcholine receptors in skeletal muscle (66). By contrast, the autoimmune response in Eaton-Lambert syndrome, a myasthenic syndrome seen in adults harboring a malignancy (most commonly a small cell carcinoma of the bronchus), is directed against the voltage-sensitive calcium channels on the presynaptic membrane.

Antibodies to the acetylcholine receptor protein have been demonstrated in the serum of all patients with generalized juvenile myasthenia gravis (67), and the electrophysiologic features of the disease can be reproduced in animals by repeated injections of IgG derived from myasthenic subjects or by antibodies against the acetylcholine receptors (68). Several lines of evidence indicate that antibody production against acetylcholine receptors is T-cell dependent. Serum antibodies against acetylcholine receptors are usually absent in congenital myasthenia gravis (but not in the maternally transmitted neonatal form) and in many cases limited to extraocular muscle involvement.

By means of the snake venom (bungarotoxin, which binds specifically to the acetylcholine receptor), these receptors have been localized to the postsynaptic folds. Myasthenic subjects show a 70% to 90% reduction in the number of functional acetylcholine receptors (69). The gross destruction of the acetylcholine receptor area, seen in subjects with long-standing myasthenia gravis, is probably the consequence of a cellular immune reaction. Three possible processes are a complement-mediated lysis of the postsynaptic membrane, an IgG-induced accelerated rate of degradation by endocytosis of cross-linked acetylcholine receptors, or an antibody-mediated blockage of the active site of the receptors (69).

The factors that induce and sustain an autoimmune reaction against the acetylcholine receptors are still unknown, although there are some hints about the nature of the process. Administration of penicillamine to patients with rheumatoid arthritis can induce myasthenia that is reversible within a few months after withdrawal of the medication. Whereas this observation suggests an alteration of the acetylcholine receptor because of exogenous factors, Lindstrom and coworkers believe that patients with myasthenia gravis respond to some endogenous source of native acetylcholine receptor, rather than to a bacterial or viral coat protein that would not have the identical autoantibody specifications (66).

The initial antiacetylcholine receptor sensitization probably occurs in the thymus. Extracts of thymic tissue have been found to contain acetylcholine receptors that are localized to myoid cells present in that tissue (70), and thymocytes of myasthenic patients produce acetylcholine receptor antibodies (71). These antibodies in most instances are specific for the embryonic acetyl choline receptor (72). Whereas an environmental factor might initiate an immune response against the acetylcholine receptors in the thymus of genetically predisposed subjects, examination by immunofluorescence of thymus derived from patients with myasthenia gravis does not show these cells to be the foci of immunologic stimulation (73). Alternatively, a possibly viral-induced derangement of function or communication between the various types of cells that regulate the intensity and duration of an immune reaction (immune regulation) might be responsible for the breakdown in tolerance to acetylcholine receptor protein.

What appears most likely at present is that autoimmune myasthenia gravis is a heterogeneous group of diseases, distinguishable by their clinical features, notably the age at onset of the illness, and by their human leukocyte antigen types, with each entity having a different pathogenetic mechanism. Thus, in some 10% to 15% of adult myasthenic patients, antibodies against acetylcholine receptor cannot be detected, and evidence suggests that in these subjects antibodies are directed to other parts of the end-plate, rather than to the acetylcholine receptor (74). The immunopathology has been reviewed by Hoedemaekers and colleagues (75) and Whitney and McNamara (76).

Juvenile myasthenia gravis, like adult myasthenia gravis, appears to result from T-cell initiated antibodies directed against end-plate acetylcholine receptor protein. Neonatal myasthenia is caused by the transfer of maternal acetylcholine receptor antibodies across the placenta. Maternal acetylcholine receptor antibodies are found in all infants of myasthenic mothers, whether infants are symptomatic or not, and myasthenic symptoms in an infant are not proportional to the amount of antibodies transferred to it from the mother (77,78). Rather, neonatal myasthenia appears to correlate with persistence of antibodies, possibly as a consequence of antibody synthesis by the myasthenic infant.

Clinical Manifestations

> Before noon, the stores of the spirit which influenced the muscle being almost spent, they are scarcely able to move hand and foot. . . . [T]his person for some time speaks freely and readily enough, but after long, hasty or laborious speaking, presently she becomes mute as a fish and cannot bring forth a word.

—T. Willis (65)

In the child, myasthenia gravis can take one of several forms (79,80).

Neonatal myasthenia is a transient disease seen in approximately one in seven infants born to mothers with myasthenia gravis. Symptoms usually appear during the first 24 hours, or, at the latest, by the third day of life. All affected infants have a paresis of the lower bulbar muscles, causing a weak cry and difficulty in sucking or swallowing. Generalized hypotonia is found in approximately one-half of the infants. Antibody titers against the acetylcholine receptor are elevated in the mother and infant. Symptoms respond promptly to anticholinesterase medication, and, even if untreated, the illness usually lasts less than 5 weeks.

Congenital myasthenia gravis designates children with myasthenia born to mothers without the disease (81,82). Generally, antibodies against the acetylcholine receptor protein are undetectable. Several syndromes have been recognized. These are outlined in Table 14.5 (82,83). Engel and coworkers and Misulis and Fenichel have divided these into presynaptic, synaptic, and postsynaptic defects (82,84). Presynaptic defects include at least two autosomal recessive conditions caused by defects in acetylcholine resynthesis and mobilization (82,85,86). Postsynaptic defects include several forms associated with a defect in the gene that codes for the collagen-like tail of acetylcholine esterase (87), and at least 56 mutations in one of the five genes coding for the adult or fetal subunits of the acetylcholine receptor (82). These entities are depicted in Table 14.5. The most common of these are at least 11 mutations that result in an autosomal dominant condition, which is the consequence of an abnormally prolonged open-time of the acetylcholine-ion channels, the *slow channel syndrome* (82,88,88a). Less common are the various mutations that cause the *fast channel syndrome*. In these mutations the postsynaptic response to acetylcholine is markedly diminished, although the number of acetylcholine receptors per end-plate is normal (89). Other defects in the genes coding for the acetylcholine receptor impair the receptor ligand-binding affinity (89a), and in another group of patients presenting with a familial, congenital myasthenic syndrome, the number of receptors is reduced, and end-plate structure is distorted (90–92). In the experience of Vincent and coworkers, who studied a European and Asian patient population, the most common form of congenital myasthenia, accounting for 40% of patients, is one in which the end-plate appears abnormal and the number of acetylcholine receptors is reduced (93).

The clinical picture of congenital myasthenia also is heterogeneous. In approximately one-half of children, symptoms commence before 2 years of age, and more than one sibling can be affected (80,86). In many instances, fetal movements are reduced, and neonates can have feeding difficulties, ptosis, limitation of eye movements, and a weak cry. The initial symptoms in congenital myasthenia gravis are not as severe as in the neonatal variety, and the diagnosis is, therefore, more difficult. A few patients with congenital myasthenia have spontaneous remissions, but the course of the disease is usually protracted, with mild symptoms that are refractory to both medical and surgical therapy (thymectomy).

Myasthenia can also begin during childhood (juvenile myasthenia). In this form, girls are

TABLE 14.5. *Myasthenic conditions of infancy and childhood*

Condition	Characteristic clinical features or reference
Juvenile myasthenia	Girls more commonly affected; AChR antibodies
Neonatal myasthenia	Transient; affects infants of myasthenic mothers
Congenital myasthenia	
Presynaptic	
Familial infantile myasthenia (defect in ACh resynthesis/packaging)	Mora et al. (102)
Paucity of synaptic vesicles	Walls et al. (228)
Postsynaptic	
Slow channel syndrome	Dominant, worsened by pyridostigmine; Gomex et al. (88), Engel et al. (88a)
Fast channel syndrome	Ohno et al. (89)
Recessive mutations of AChR subunits	Engel et al. (82)
End-plate AChE deficiency	Ohno et al. (87)

TABLE 14.6. *Symptoms and signs in 35 patients with juvenile myasthenia gravis*

Symptom or sign	Number of patients
Ptosis	32
Diplopia	30
Facial weakness	29
Dysphonia	29
Weakness of arms	29
Weakness of legs	29
Chewing weakness	22
External ophthalmoplegia	18
Respiratory difficulties	12

Adapted from Millichap JG, Dodge PR. Diagnosis and treatment of myasthenia gravis in infancy, childhood and adolescence. *Neurology* 1960;10:1007.

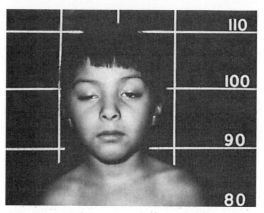

FIG. 14.3. Girl with myasthenia gravis. She has bilateral ptosis, more marked on the right, and the typical myasthenic facies. (Courtesy of Dr. Christian Herrmann, Jr., Department of Neurology, University of California, Los Angeles, UCLA School of Medicine.)

affected two to six times as frequently as boys. The onset of juvenile myasthenia can be insidious, although at times it is rapid and often a sequel to an acute febrile illness. Generally, muscles innervated by the cranial nerves are affected first, with bilateral ptosis the most common presenting sign (Table 14.6 and Fig. 14.3). It was seen in 81% of children in the series of Afifi and Bell and was unilateral in 33% (67). Generalized weakness and dysphagia are less common presenting symptoms. The clinical course is highly variable. Approximately one-half of the patients experience one or more remissions, usually during the early years of the illness. In others, symptoms progress to a certain point and then become stationary. In approximately 26% of cases, myasthenia is restricted to the extraocular musculature (67).

The characteristic feature of all forms of juvenile myasthenia gravis is the variability in muscular strength, with increasing weakness of the affected muscles with repeated contractions (Fig. 14.4). The child is usually at his or her best in the morning and becomes progressively weaker during the day, although partial or complete recovery can follow a nap. In approximately 10% to 20% of untreated cases, weakness becomes irreversible, and muscle wasting, particularly of the shoulder girdle and the extraocular muscles, becomes apparent. Despite hypotonia, the tendon jerks are normal or even exaggerated, but they can disappear after repeated elicitation.

Other autoimmune diseases are sometimes associated with juvenile myasthenia gravis. The most common of these are rheumatoid arthritis, juvenile diabetes mellitus, and thyroid disease, usually thyrotoxicosis (94). For reasons as yet unexplained, seizures are seen in as many as 12.5% of patients (95). Malignancies were seen in 5% of the Mayo Clinic pediatric series (96).

Myasthenia also can be seen in association with collagen vascular disease, notably systemic lupus

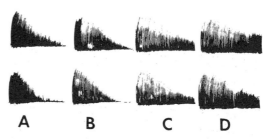

A   B   C   D

FIG. 14.4. Muscle ergograph in a patient with myasthenia gravis. **A:** Resting state. **B:** After intravenous atropine (0.4 mg). **C:** After intravenous Tensilon (2.0 mg). **D:** After intravenous edrophonium chloride (8.0 mg). Note the progressive decrease in amplitude in A and B, partly or completely corrected by edrophonium chloride. (Courtesy of Dr. C. Herrmann, Jr., Department of Neurology, University of California, Los Angeles, UCLA School of Medicine.)

erythematosus. Dobkin and Verity described a syndrome transmitted through an autosomal recessive gene and characterized by cardiomyopathy, excessive muscle fatigability with a predilection for the proximal musculature, and improvement with anticholinesterase drugs (97). Muscle biopsy revealed hypoplasia of type 1 muscle fibers and tubular aggregates of types 1 and 2 fibers.

The Eaton-Lambert myasthenic syndrome is rarely encountered in children. It has been observed after the administration of antibiotics (most frequently neomycin), in conjunction with surgery (98,99), and in acute leukemia (100).

Although most myasthenic syndromes are expressions of autoimmune disease, hereditary myasthenic syndromes also are known and transmitted as autosomal recessive and autosomal dominant traits (82,101). Congenital myasthenia gravis (see previous discussion) is in this category of genetically determined myasthenia.

Diagnosis

The diagnosis of myasthenia gravis is based on a history of abnormal fatigability of voluntary muscles and evidence of a prompt improvement of muscle weakness with anticholinesterase drugs. It is supported by a history of remissions and exacerbations and by the absence of any concurrent illness that might contribute to the muscular weakness.

For diagnostic purposes, the most widely used drug is edrophonium chloride (Tensilon). Approximately 5 mg is given intravenously to a 3- to 5-year-old child. Within 1 minute after the injection, a transient improvement in muscle strength is observed, usually lasting 4 to 5 minutes. Positive responses are diagnostically reliable. In some infants, a positive response can be obscured by the response to the injection, in which case a longer-acting anticholinesterase drug, neostigmine, should be used. After intramuscular injection of 0.5 to 1.5 mg of neostigmine, muscle strength begins to improve in 10 to 15 minutes and reaches its peak by 30 minutes. Both tests are nearly 100% reliable in generalized myasthenia, and in ocular myasthenia, which progresses to generalized myasthenia. In the series of Afifi and Bell, edrophonium gave positive test results in all cases of ocular myas-

thenia; neostigmine was positive only in 67% of cases (67). A number of conditions can give a false-positive result. These include drug-induced myasthenia gravis, botulism, brainstem gliomas, and Guillain-Barré syndrome (102). A confirmatory test, therefore, is required.

The presence of acetylcholine receptor antibodies in serum is the simplest diagnostic test in juvenile myasthenia, although false-negative results are not unusual, particularly in children whose symptoms are limited to the extraocular muscles. In the series of Afifi and Bell, acetylcholine receptor antibodies were found in 63% of cases (67). A similar incidence of positive serology has been reported in other series. When acetylcholine receptor antibodies are absent, it is necessary to consider one of the congenital myasthenic syndromes. This is not an academic exercise, because in juvenile myasthenia gravis therapy is not only supportive, but also directed against the immune-mediated response. Andrews and coworkers suggest that the rapid response to plasmapheresis frequently seen in children with juvenile myasthenia gravis can be used to distinguish this condition from congenital myasthenia gravis (103). It should be noted that antibody levels do not parallel disease severity.

Rapid stimulation of the distal (ulnar) or proximal (spinal, axillary, or facial) motor nerves produces a characteristic decrement in the amplitude of successive action potentials recorded from surface muscle electrodes and in the amplitudes of the mechanical excursions (see Fig. 14.4). This test is positive in some 80% of pediatric cases, but is usually negative in ocular myasthenia (104). Patients suspected of having myasthenia gravis on the basis of their clinical picture, but who have a normal EMG study, should undergo single-fiber EMG (105,106). The results of this study generally complement the results of the assay for acetylcholine receptor antibodies. One exception is congenital myasthenia gravis, in which single-fiber EMG is frequently positive; another exception is in children with the mild, predominantly ocular form of the disease (106).

In addition to penicillamine, a number of other drugs can induce or unmask myasthenia. These include β-adrenergic blockers, carnitine, aminoglycoside antibiotics, lithium carbonate, magnesium salts, trimethadione, and phenytoin (107).

Treatment

Treatment of the patient with juvenile myasthenia is generally lifelong, extending into all areas of activity. The three approaches to therapy are symptomatic, immunologic, and surgical. Treatment of the congenital myasthenias is solely symptomatic (108).

When juvenile myasthenia is mild or is restricted to the ocular musculature, treatment is generally symptomatic (i.e., using anticholinesterase drugs). At the University of California, Los Angeles, UCLA School of Medicine, pyridostigmine bromide (Mestinon) is the preferred drug. It is administered at a starting dosage of 15 mg two to three times a day (in tablet or syrup form) for a child 3 to 8 years old.

In the remaining patients, treatment should be immunologic. Mann and coworkers suggest a course of oral prednisone, starting out at high dosages (1 mg/kg per day) and tapering when improvement is sustained or when side effects require reduction of the dosages (109). Sarnat and associates have advocated a starting dosage of 2 mg/kg given every other day (110). Cholinesterase inhibitors are used as needed while the patient is receiving corticosteroids. Exacerbation of myasthenia gravis can be seen during the early days of corticosteroid therapy, usually toward the end of the first week, and can last approximately a week. Improvement is noted within approximately 2 weeks and becomes maximal in approximately 3 months. Plasmapheresis lowers the level of antibodies against the acetylcholine receptor protein. Dau recommends this procedure to stabilize patients whose course worsens markedly during initiation of prednisone therapy and as primary therapy in combination with immunosuppressive drugs such as azathioprine (111). Plasmapheresis also has been used to treat patients who remain unresponsive to other forms of therapy, to improve respiratory function before thymectomy, and to hasten remission after thymectomy. Improvement, often dramatic, is seen within 1 to 3 days after the start of the course. Immunosuppression with cyclosporine has been disappointing (112)

and is not used at our institutions. Intravenous immune globulin has been used in conjunction with other modes of therapy, particularly corticosteroids and plasmapheresis, in rapidly deteriorating patients with bulbar symptoms (113). There is little difference between the efficacy of three plasma exchanges and intravenous immune globulin (0.4 mg/kg per day for 3 or 5 consecutive days), although as a rule, intravenous gammaglobulin is better tolerated (113a). Intravenous immune globulin is ineffective in neonatal myasthenia gravis (114).

After establishment of maximal improvement, children should be considered for thymectomy (113,115,116). In general, the procedure is now indicated if symptoms recur after withdrawal of corticosteroids after 1 year of therapy or if corticosteroids fail to benefit the patient significantly. The best results from thymectomy may be predicted in children who have high titers of circulating antiacetylcholine receptor antibodies and who are symptomatic for less than 2 years. However, a long history of juvenile myasthenia gravis is not a contraindication to thymectomy; for both girls and boys, good operative results are possible. In the UCLA experience, the procedure is of considerable benefit when performed as early as the third year of life. The maximum benefit of thymectomy may be delayed for weeks or even several months, so that absence of an immediate and dramatic postoperative improvement should not be discouraging.

Proceeding according to this treatment schedule, Mann and associates found that up to 90% of patients have significant improvement or complete remission of their myasthenic symptoms, and that in some, corticosteroids and anticholinesterase drugs can even be tapered and discontinued (109).

In myasthenic children, the remission rate after thymectomy is 60% (117). This figure compares with a remission rate of 29% in children who did not undergo a thymectomy (117). In the series of Rodriguez and coworkers, the remission rate was higher in children who underwent thymectomy within 12 months of the onset of symptoms. It was also higher in patients who had experienced bulbar symptoms before surgery, in those having involvement of extremities, but neither ocular nor generalized weakness, and in those whose myasthenic symptoms presented between ages 12 and 16 years (96).

Patients with congenital forms of myasthenia can respond to anticholinesterases. When such treatment is unsatisfactory, Palace and colleagues have used 3,4-diaminopyridine. This substance blocks potassium conductance and increases the release of acetylcholine from the nerve terminal (117a).

Toxic Disorders

The toxins of *Clostridium tetani* and *C. botulinum* and the venom of cobras and of arachnoideae such as the black widow spider affect the neuromuscular junction. These toxins are reviewed by Swift (118) and are more extensively considered under their respective headings in Chapter 9.

DISEASES OF MUSCLE

Muscular Dystrophies

The muscular dystrophies are a group of diseases that are distinguished from other neuromuscular disorders by four obligatory criteria: (a) primary myopathies, not neurogenic; (b) genetically determined; (c) progressive diseases, some slowly progressive and compatible with normal longevity and others more rapidly progressive and leading to early death; and (d) myofiber degeneration at some stage in the disease (5).

An excellent review on the history of the terminology in muscular dystrophy was provided by Dubowitz (119). The name *muscular dystrophy*, meaning a growth disorder of muscle, was entrenched by Gowers in his "Clinical lecture on pseudohypertrophic muscular paralysis," a series of essays in *The Lancet* in 1879 (120).

From a clinical point of view there are at least six major forms of muscular dystrophy: Duchenne (Aran-Duchenne) muscular dystrophy, Becker muscular dystrophy (now known to be merely a mild form of Duchenne dystrophy with the same genetic defect), Emery-Dreifuss (humeroperoneal) muscular dystrophy, the congenital muscular dystrophies, facioscapulohumeral (Landouzy-Déjèrine) muscular dystrophy, and the limb-girdle

dystrophies. The characteristic clinical features of each entity are presented in Table 14.7 (121–123).

Pathologic Anatomy

Despite differences in the clinical picture, the same pathologic findings are shared by all muscular dystrophies. The earliest stages of the disease show a dilated sarcoplasmic reticulum, with an irregular orientation of the triads (124). As the illness progresses, there are repeated episodes of necrosis and regeneration of muscle cells. This process is probably initiated by a breakdown of the muscle cell membrane, and electron microscopy may reveal the absence of the plasma membrane around all or part of the circumference of the muscle fibers (125). Small losses of membrane can be repaired, but generally, regeneration is inadequate. As a consequence of the membrane defect, an influx of calcium ions can occur, activating the endogenous proteases and inducing lysis of the Z disc of the myofibril, which is probably the initial step in muscle breakdown. Subsequently, the number of muscle cells is reduced and variability in fiber size is increased. Sarcolemmal nuclei are swollen and increased in number, a regenerative reaction to the injury of muscle fibers. Over the years, this reaction becomes more extreme, and muscle fibers appear enlarged, forked, hyalinized, or atrophied. With further progression of the disease, large accumulations of collagen and fat cells are seen between muscle fibers, and these cells are partly responsible for the muscular hypertrophy (Fig. 14.5) (31).

Neither heart nor smooth muscle is spared, and there is myocardial degeneration with fatty infiltration and fibrosis of the myocardial fibers.

When muscular dystrophy is associated with mental retardation, brain sections can be normal or can disclose various developmental anomalies of the cortex, such as pachygyria, heterotopia, and disorders of cortical architecture (126).

Pathogenesis

The elucidation of the gene defect in Duchenne and Becker muscular dystrophy represents one of the most important triumphs of molecular

TABLE 14.7. Clinical features of muscular dystrophies

Type	Inheritance	Age at onset	Initial distribution	Pseudo-hypertrophy	Progression	Contractures	Cardiac involvement	IQ
Duchenne	Sex-linked recessive	Childhood (2–5 yr)	Pelvic girdle	>80%	Rapid	Common	50–80%	Often reduced
Becker	Sex-linked recessive	Childhood	Pelvic girdle	90%	Slow	Common, but mild	Rare (approximately 15%)	Normal
Emery-Dreifuss	Sex-linked	5–15 yr	Upper arms, peroneal muscles	None	Slow	Elbows, posterior cervical muscles	Common, severe	Normal
Congenital	Autosomal recessive	Birth	Proximal muscles	None	Slow, unpredictable	Common	Rare	Normal (except in Fukuyama variant)
Facioscapulo-humeral	Autosomal dominant	Childhood to adulthood	Face, shoulder girdle	Uncommon	Slow, with abortive forms	Rare	Rare	Normal
Limb-girdle	Usually autosomal recessive	10–20 yr	Shoulder or pelvic girdle	<30%	Variable	Late in disease	Rare	Normal
Distal	Autosomal recessive	12–30 yr	Gastrocnemius	None	Slow	None	None	Normal

After Rowland (121), Ringel et al. (122), Hopkins et al. (123), and Barohn et al. (211).

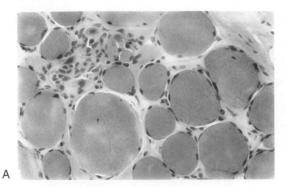
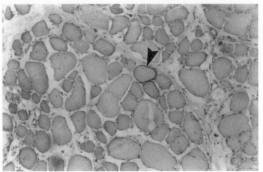

A   B

FIG. 14.5. Muscle biopsy of a 5-year-old boy with Duchenne muscular dystrophy. **A:** Myofibers are extremely variable in size with both hypertrophic and atrophic forms. They have an abnormally rounded rather than the normal polygonal contour in transverse section because of the proliferation of endomysial collagen that forms rigid sleeves around each fiber. A few fibers have internal nuclei. A zone of degenerating myofibers infiltrated by phagocytic cells is seen in the upper left of the figure. **B:** Immunocytochemistry shows absence of dystrophin at the sarcolemma of all myofibers, large and small, except for one (*arrowhead*) called a *revertant fiber* that expresses this protein as in normal fibers (**A**, hematoxylin and eosin, ×400; **B**, dystrophin, rod domain, ×250).

biology in the area of neurology. Inasmuch as it provides an example of strategies for positional cloning, we propose to review it in some detail.

Although the gene for Duchenne muscular dystrophy has long been known to be located on the X chromosome, the site was more precisely located to the small arm of the chromosome (Xp21) by cytogenetic studies on girls with Duchenne muscular dystrophy and X/autosomal translocations (127). A microscopically visible deletion at the same point was seen in a male subject with Duchenne muscular dystrophy, chronic granulomatous disease, and retinitis pigmentosa (128). Using an ingenious technique in which excess amounts of the defective genome were hybridized with DNA derived from a patient with an XXXY karyotype and in which the unmatched DNA was isolated, Kunkel and his group were able to prepare seven clones that were absent from the patient's genomic DNA, but present in normal individuals (129). One of these deletion-specific clones, pERT 87, was found to be tightly linked to the Duchenne muscular dystrophy gene and recognized deletions in a significant proportion of Duchenne muscular dystrophy patients (130,131).

Using the pERT 87 clone as a starting point, several other cloned fragments from the Xp21 region were isolated, a restriction enzyme map of the region involved in the Duchenne muscular dystrophy phenotype was drawn (132), and a small human cDNA transcript spanning the region of the pERT 87 locus was isolated (133). Subsequently, a much larger human Duchenne muscular dystrophy cDNA corresponding to the complete muscle transcript was isolated and sequenced. By means of this cDNA, deletion mutations have been found in some 65% of boys with Duchenne muscular dystrophy (134). In other instances, there have been point mutations or duplications of portions of the gene (135). Approximately 40% of all deletions start in the same region of the DNA (*hot spots*) (136,137).

Using portions of the coding sequence of the cDNA, Hoffman and coworkers produced a polyclonal antiserum that was directed against the protein product of the normal gene (138). The gene, which is 10 times larger than any other gene characterized to date, consists of approximately 2 million base pairs and produces dystrophin, a protein with a molecular weight of 427,000. Dystrophin is a low-abundance protein and constitutes but 0.002% of

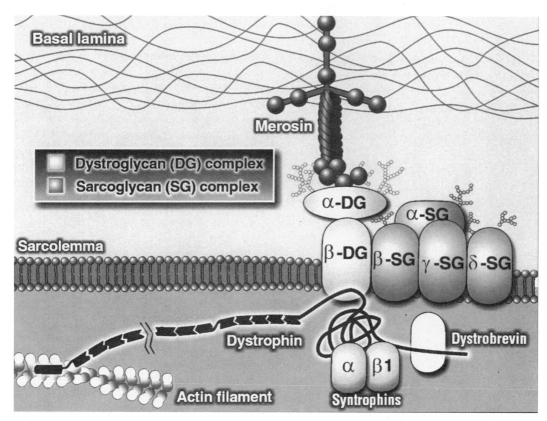

FIG. 14.6. The dystrophin-glycoprotein complex. Dystrophin contacts F-actin in the cytoplasm of the cell, and the dystrophin-glycoprotein complex forms a bridge across the membrane to the merosin subunit of laminin in the extracellular matrix. (Courtesy of R. G. Worton, The Ottawa Hospital, Research Institute, Ottawa.)

total muscle protein. It is a cytoskeletal protein, with a globular amino domain, a central rod-like domain, and a globular carboxy domain. It is localized to the inner surface of the sarcolemma, aggregating as a homotetramer that is associated with actin at its amino terminus and with a glycoprotein complex at its carboxy terminus. The dystrophin-glycoprotein complex, by which the membrane cytoskeleton is linked to extracellular glycoproteins, consists of several dystrophin-associated glycoproteins and dystrophin-associated proteins (Fig. 14.6). The membrane complex is markedly reduced in Duchenne muscular dystrophy. Its synthesis is normal, but in the absence of dystrophin, the glycoproteins become unstable and are degraded (139).

Dystrophin is present not only in muscle, but in a variety of other cell types (140). Although *in situ* hybridization demonstrates some expression of the gene in affected muscle (141), the complete dystrophin molecule is absent, or is present in less than 3% of normal levels in more than 90% of patients with classic Duchenne muscular dystrophy. It is present in reduced amounts, or in normal amounts but with an abnormal molecular configuration in boys with Becker muscular dystrophy (142). The phenotype of Duchenne and Becker muscular dystrophies does not always correlate with the size of the deletion in the dystrophin gene; some cases of undetectable dystrophin are paradoxically associated with only mild clinical manifestations (143). Rather, the effect of the deletion on dystrophin synthesis is important. If the deletion breaks up the codon triplet, and thereby shifts the reading frame, a premature stop codon is quickly generated, and dystrophin synthesis comes to a halt, leaving a small, truncated protein molecule without its carboxy terminal, which is rapidly degraded. If the deletion removes a triplet codon in its entirety, the reading frame is maintained, resulting in the synthesis of a dystrophin molecule with a shortened rod domain, but intact carboxy and amino domains. This is what occurs in Becker dystrophy (144). Good reviews of the genetic variations of the dystrophin gene and its protein transcription products are provided by Miller and Wessel (145), Mendell and colleagues (146), Ikezawa and colleagues (147), and Nigro and colleagues (148).

Dystrophin is associated with other proteins at the sarcolemmal region, which also may be defective; these include α- and β-dystroglycans (148–151) and utrophin. Utrophin is an autosomal homologue of dystrophin, being coded by a gene that has been mapped to the long arm of chromosome 6 (6q24). Like dystrophin it is a large protein that is found at the neuromuscular synapse and the myotendinous junction and is also expressed in several other tissues, notably lungs and intestines (151a).

Dystrophin is also expressed in smooth muscle and in brain, although the level of expression in brain is lower, and the structure of brain messenger RNA for dystrophin differs from that of muscle (152,153). This difference is because cortical dystrophin is transcribed from a promoter that is at least 90 kb upstream from the muscle promoter. Other, markedly truncated dystrophins can be found in normal brain and peripheral nerve. In particular, a 140-kD protein (Dp140) is found throughout the CNS (154,154a).

How the membrane defect results in the dystrophic process is not completely clear. It is likely that dystrophin stabilizes the muscle membrane during repeated cycles of muscle contraction. Lacking dystrophin, the normal interaction between sarcolemma and extracellular matrix is lost and, as a consequence, osmotic fragility of muscle fibers become increased (139). Possibly significant in the pathogenesis of the dystrophic process are the low potassium and high intrafiber sodium and calcium concentrations seen in dystrophic muscle (155). These electrolyte changes can reflect ionic leakage through the abnormal membrane of dystrophic fibers. Whether membrane leakage is also responsible for the elevation in serum CK activity is open to speculation. An incompletely explained finding is the presence in Duchenne muscular dystrophy of an occasional dystrophin-positive muscle fiber (see Fig. 14.5B). This could reflect the presence in muscle of an mRNA in which the reading frame has been restored by an as yet unknown mechanism (156).

Clinical Manifestations

Duchenne Muscular Dystrophy (Aran-Duchenne)

Transmitted in a sex-linked recessive manner, this disease was first described in 1868 by Duchenne (157), and more definitively in 1879 by Gowers (120,158). It is a relatively common condition with a prevalence of 1 in 25,000. Clinically, it is the most clearly defined of the muscular dystrophies. The disease becomes apparent in early childhood (121). The course is so gradual that initial symptoms are often overlooked. At first, these are often confined to difficulty in climbing stairs, in arising from the floor, or in performing other activities that involve the pelvic muscles. An early indication of pelvic weakness is the manner by which patients arise from the floor, by progressively "climbing up their thighs" (Gowers' sign) (158). Lordosis commonly appears with progression of the disease, and the child "straddles as he stands and waddles as he walks." Muscular wasting and a progressive and early enfeeblement of deep tendon reflexes accompany the advance of the disease. Subsequent to the initial stages, muscular involvement is invariably symmetric. In contrast to the generalized atrophy, there is striking pseudohypertrophy of the calves, and, less commonly, of the deltoids and infraspinati (Fig. 14.7). Contractures are common and occur chiefly at the hamstrings.

Enlargement of the heart, persistent tachycardia, and myocardial failure are seen in 50%

to 80% of patients at some time during the disease, and are reflected in significant electrocardiographic abnormalities. These result from metabolic abnormalities within a relatively circumscribed area of the posterolateral left ventricular wall (159).

Symptoms of smooth muscle dysfunction are frequently overlooked. Gastric hypomotility can result in sudden episodes of vomiting, abdominal pain, and distention (160). In a small number of patients, a history of diarrhea, malabsorption, or megacolon can be elicited, and there can be a disturbance in motor function of the esophagus. These clinical findings correspond to pathologic changes in smooth muscle, most characteristically a fatty infiltration of the myofibers, necrosis of the muscle fibers, and degenerative changes in the nuclei (160,161). Constipation, fecal retention, and distention of the bowel may result not only from smooth muscle involvement, but also from weakness of the striated rectus abdominus muscles, that do not provide for a sufficient increase in intra-abdominal pressure during defecation to assist in the peristaltic emptying of the rectum.

A number of children with muscular dystrophy have defective intellectual development (162). Significant abnormalities in cortical architecture, suggestive of prenatal maldevelopment, have been found in some, but not all, pathologic studies (126,163). The mean IQ of children is approximately 85, and its range appears to follow a normal (gaussian) distribution curve (31). Retardation is nonprogressive, and its severity is unrelated to the severity of muscular weakness. It is accompanied by cerebral atrophy as demonstrated by neuroimaging studies (164). Deletions in the exon 45 to 52 region in particular have in increased incidence of cognitive impairment. Lidov and colleagues postulate that such deletions affect the expression of the 140-kD isoform, which is important for CNS function and is localized to the postsynaptic regions of cortex (154a). It is of note that in mentally retarded patients with Becker dystrophy the deletion affects the Dp140 regulatory region (165).

Duchenne muscular dystrophy is but one of several muscle diseases in which the CNS is

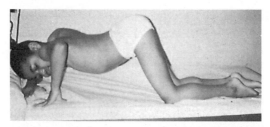

FIG. 14.7. Boy with Duchenne muscular dystrophy. The atrophy of the proximal musculature and the pseudohypertrophy of the gastrocnemius become particularly evident when the patient attempts to rise from the prone position.

also involved, usually in the form of mental retardation. These various conditions are listed in Table 14.8.

The course of the illness is steadily downhill. Death usually occurs in adolescence and results from secondary infections or intractable congestive heart failure.

The female carrier for muscular dystrophy is usually asymptomatic, but occasionally demonstrates pseudohypertrophy and mild weakness of the pelvic musculature. All gradations from apparent complete normality to a marked but focal dystrophy can be seen on biopsy (166). Both dystrophin-positive and dystrophin-negative fibers can be seen, a finding that supports the view, postulated by the Lyon hypothesis, that in the dystrophin-negative cells the paternal X chromosome, on which the muscular dystrophy gene is located, is active.

Becker Muscular Dystrophy

The incidence of Becker muscular dystrophy in the United Kingdom is 1 in 18,450 births, as compared with an incidence of 1 in 5,618 births for Duchenne muscular dystrophy. Because of the earlier demise of patients with Duchenne muscular dystrophy, the prevalence of the two diseases is about the same (167).

Symptoms begin somewhat later than in Duchenne muscular dystrophy, often after 8 years of age, and the ability to walk is retained beyond age 16 years (see Table 14.7). Pseudohypertrophy

TABLE 14.8. *Muscle diseases with central nervous system involvement*

Condition	Central nervous system signs and symptoms	Reference
Duchenne muscular dystrophy	Mental retardation	Dubowitz (31)
Myotonic dystrophy	Mental retardation	Harper (230)
Fascioscapulohumoral muscular dystrophy	Sensorineural hearing loss	Taylor et al. (202)
Centronuclear myopathy	Seizures, occasional mental retardation	Serratrice et al. (418)
Mitochondrial cytopathies	Protean CNS involvement	Ricci (419); Chapter 1
Glycerol kinase deficiency	Spasticity, mental retardation	Guggenheim et al. (420)
Systemic carnitine deficiency	Recurrent acute encephalopathy	Treem et al. (395)
Glycogenosis type II (Pompe disease)	Dementia, seizures	Chapter 1
Debre-Sémélaigné syndrome	Cretinism	Spiro et al. (355); Chapter 15
De Lange syndrome	Mental retardation, extrapyramidal signs	De Lange (352)
Congenital muscular dystrophies		Van der Knaap et al. (421), Tomé (441)[a]
Walker-Warburg syndrome	Severe mental retardation, macrocephaly, various eye abnormalities, diffuse agyric cortex, hypoplasia cerebellar vermis, abnormal white matter	Dobyns et al. (435)
Muscle-eye-brain disease	Mental retardation, microcephaly, eye abnormalities, cortical dysplasia less severe than in Walker-Warburg syndrome	Laverda et al. (439)
Fukuyama disease	Severe mental retardation, seizures, no eye abnormalities	Fukuyama et al. (174)
Merosin-deficient congenital muscular dystrophy	Mild mental retardation, seizures, diffuse white matter changes	Philpot et al. (186)

[a]Tomé (441) provides a classification of the congenital muscular dystrophies that is based on the merosin status in muscle biopsies.

is less likely to be present and the ankle reflexes are often lost. A diagnostic feature of this form of muscular dystrophy is the presence of pes cavus in 60% of subjects (122). Cardiac involvement is rare, and children have normal intelligence. Serum CK levels are markedly elevated. As has already been indicated, Becker muscular dystrophy results from a defect in the amount and structure of dystrophin.

A syndrome of X-linked myalgia and cramps with onset in early childhood, and elevated serum CK levels is accompanied by normal amounts of muscle dystrophin that is truncated at the amino end of the molecule. The relatively mild symptoms in this condition contrast with the severe symptoms that result from deletions at the carboxy end of the dystrophin protein (168,169).

Emery-Dreifuss Muscular Dystrophy

Emery-Dreifuss muscular dystrophy, a rare myopathy, appears between ages 5 and 15 years. Inheritance is usually X-linked, but autosomal dominant pedigrees have been encountered. The gene responsible for the X-linked form has been localized to the distal portion of the long arm (170). It encodes a single membrane spanning protein named *emerin*, which has been localized to the inner nuclear membrane. This protein is believed to stabilize the nuclear membrane against the mechanical stresses which develop during muscle contraction (170a). Weakness is diffuse or is maximal in biceps, triceps, and the peroneal muscles (171). Flexion contractures of the elbows, posterior cervical muscles, and Achilles tendons are prominent early in the course of the disease. The weakness progresses slowly, but all patients have severe and potentially fatal cardiac arrhythmias that can precede any apparent skeletal muscle weakness (see Table 14.7) (123,171). CK levels are only moderately elevated. Arrhythmias also can be seen in otherwise asymptomatic female carriers (172). Some girls with an Emery-Dreifuss phenotype but no apparent chromosomal abnormality might represent sporadic cases of the dominant form of the disease.

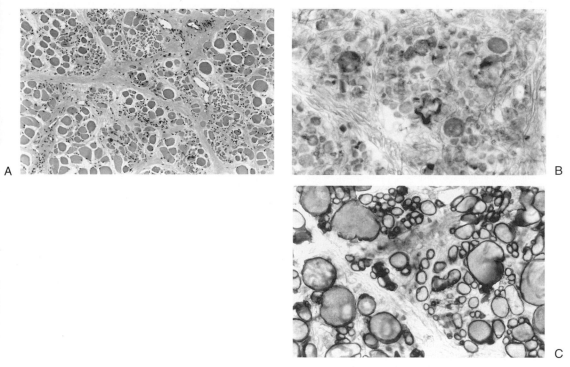

FIG. 14.8. Muscle biopsy of a 12-month-old girl with merosin-deficient congenital muscular dystrophy. **A:** Both perimysial (between fascicles) and endomysial (within fascicles) collagen is greatly increased and myofibers vary greatly in diameter and have a rounded contour, but few fibers show frank necrosis or degeneration. Compare with Fig. 14.5A. **B:** Immunocytochemistry for merosin shows lack of expression at the sarcolemmal region of myofibers of all sizes. **C:** Immunocytochemistry for α-sarcoglycan (adhalen) shows normal expression of this protein at the sarcolemma of both large and small myofibers. Normal merosin staining should appear similar (**A**, hematoxylin and eosin, ×100; **B**, merosin, ×250; **C**, α-sarcoglycan, ×400).

Congenital Muscular Dystrophy

This group of disorders is characterized by the presence at birth of a proximal muscular weakness, which progresses slowly and is accompanied by pathologic muscular changes that are consistent with muscular dystrophy (173). The congenital muscular dystrophies are among the less common causes of the floppy infant syndrome. Most appear to be transmitted as an autosomal recessive trait.

In one variant, first described by Fukuyama, severe mental retardation and seizures accompany muscular weakness (174). Although rare outside of Japan, this condition is second in frequency only to Duchenne muscular dystrophy in

that country. It is transmitted as an autosomal recessive disorder and is associated with a deficiency of one of the dystrophin-associated glycoproteins, which normally is expressed in both muscle and brain (173,175). One gene for this condition is localized to the long arm of chromosome 9 (9q31-33) (176). Muscle weakness is present from birth on, with contractures appearing early. In addition to generalized limb and trunk weakness, facial muscles are involved. CK levels are generally elevated and can reach 10 to 50 times normal after 6 months of age. Neuroimaging is often spectacular, with a massive decrease in the density of white matter in approximately one-third of infants (177). The electroencephalogram can show paroxysmal

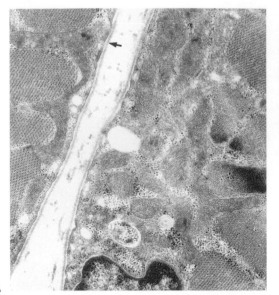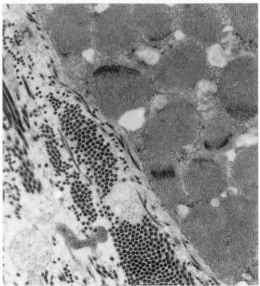

A   B

FIG. 14.9. Electron micrographs of sarcolemmal region of **(A)** normal myofibers and **(B)** myofibers in merosin-deficient congenital muscular dystrophy, the biopsy shown in Figure 14.2. **A:** The sarcolemma is normally a well-defined plasma membrane of the myofiber; external to it is a thin gray line corresponding to the basal lamina or basement membrane (*arrow*). **B:** In merosin deficiency, the basal lamina is absent or discontinuous and the sarcolemma is less distinct than normal. Collagen is seen between myofibers (**A** and **B**, Uranyl acetate and lead citrate, ×16,000).

discharges, and the visual-evoked potentials also can be abnormal. An inflammatory cell infiltration of muscle can be quite striking and has led some authors to postulate that congenital muscular dystrophy is the consequence of an intrauterine infection (176). Within the brain there is micropolygyria and hypoplasia of myelin. The condition is progressive and is generally fatal by the end of the first decade.

The other congenital muscular dystrophies may be divided into two groups, one with deficiency of merosin in muscle and the other in which merosin is normally expressed. Merosin, the α_2 chain or M-chain of laminin, is an extracellular matrix protein that attaches the sarcolemma (i.e., the plasma membrane of the muscle fiber) to the basal lamina or basement membrane. It is generally associated with the LAMA2 locus on 6q22, but some cases with merosin deficiency are not linked to this region (178). When merosin is absent, the basal lamina cannot form or disappear (Figs. 14.8 and 14.9), and the sarcolemma then degenerates secondarily, resulting in the eventual necrosis of the myofiber (179–183). The pathogenesis of the disease in the presence of merosin is less well understood, and the genotype and phenotype correlations in congenital muscular dystrophies are not always predictable (184–186). Infants with merosin deficiency usually have a poorer prognosis than those in whom merosin is present. Clinically the former group manifest with a greater generalized weakness and dysphagia, and often require a gastrostomy to prevent recurrent aspiration. Some infants also have apneic spells or respiratory insufficiency. CNS involvement, expressed as mental retardation, motor deficits, and cerebral cortical dysplasia, does not correlate well with the presence or absence of merosin or with the severity of the myopathy (187). A reduced expression of merosin also is associated with Fukuyama muscular dystrophy and muscle-eye-brain disease (188,189,189a). Patients with muscle-eye-brain disease present with congenital hypotonia, myopia, and mental retardation. Merosin expression is normal in Walker-Warburg syndrome (189a).

Merosin can be demonstrated by immunocytochemistry in frozen sections of the muscle biopsy, but also is present in skin and can be detected by skin biopsy. However, correlative studies of muscle and cutaneous merosin expression have not been documented sufficiently for the diagnosis to depend solely on skin biopsy. Merosin also is strongly expressed in Schwann cells, so that peripheral nerve is immunoreactive for merosin both in muscle and skin biopsies. This is in contrast to dystrophin, sarcoglycans, and other sarcolemmal region proteins. When merosin is absent from myofibers, it also is not expressed in Schwann cells.

One of the prominent histopathologic features of the congenital muscular dystrophies, with or without merosin deficiency, is a striking proliferation of endomysial collagen, evident even at birth, although the clinical progression of the disease may be slower than the neonatal muscle biopsy might have predicted. The number of frankly necrotic myofibers at any stage in the disease is never as great as in Duchenne dystrophy.

Another variant of congenital muscular dystrophy, Ullrich disease, is an autosomal recessive condition characterized by a nonprogressive or slowly advancing congenital muscle weakness, striking congenital contractures of the proximal joints, hyperextensibility of the distal joints, and normal intelligence (190–192). Hyperhidrosis and posterior protrusion of the calcaneus can be characteristic for this entity (192).

In the Walker-Warburg syndrome, congenital muscular dystrophy (189) is accompanied by type II lissencephaly (see Chapter 4), Dandy-Walker cyst, and cerebellar and retinal malformations. The condition is transmitted as an autosomal recessive trait (193).

In most of the other congenital muscular dystrophies, no cerebral involvement occurs, serum CK levels are mildly to moderately elevated, and the diagnosis depends on the muscle biopsy (194,195).

Facioscapulohumeral Muscular Dystrophy

As implied by its name, facioscapulohumeral muscular dystrophy (FSHD) is a group of diseases affects the muscles of the face, shoulder, and upper arm. The classic form of the condition,

described in 1885 by Landouzy and Déjèrine, is transmitted as an autosomal dominant trait with a frequency of 1 in 20,000 (196,196a). Initial symptoms tend to appear at a somewhat later age than in the Duchenne form, with penetrance being approximately 50% by age 14 years (197). The gene for this condition has been localized to the subtelomeric portion of the long arm of chromosome 4 (4q35), and deletions of integral copies of 3.3.kb units from a tandem repeat located near the gene have been associated with the clinical expression of the disease. Deletion of these units which are not transcribed is believed to induce repression of a more centromerically located gene (196a). Although a second gene for FSHD is thought to be located on the long arm of chromosome 10 (197a), in the experience of Wiljemenga et al., there was little genetic heterogeneity (198). This is somewhat surprising in view of the marked heterogeneity of clinical manifestations. The genetic phenomenon of *anticipation* often is demonstrated in families with this disease, a grandparent being only mildly involved from early adult life, a parent being more severely involved since late childhood or adolescence, and the infant or young child showing severe involvement since birth.

Pathologically, FSHD is a heterogeneous group, with a similar clinical picture being caused by muscular dystrophy, neurogenic muscular atrophy, polymyositis, myasthenia gravis, myotubular myopathy, nemaline myopathy, or Möbius syndrome (infantile FSHD) (199). A lymphocytic inflammatory myopathy is not unusual, particularly in children with a rapidly progressive course (199), but it is not an autoimmune disorder and does not respond to treatment with corticosteroids.

Initial symptoms usually include wasting of the shoulder girdle, prominent winging of the scapulae, and in many, but not all, families, development of myopathic facies. The lips cannot be pursed, and they protrude in what has been termed a *tapir's mouth*. The relative weakness of the zygomatic muscles results in an equally characteristic transverse smile. Muscular hypertrophy, contractures, and skeletal deformities are rare. Involvement tends to be symmetric, but asymmetric weakness is more common in this form than in any of the other dystrophies.

TABLE 14.9. *Protein defects in muscular dystrophies*

Protein	Gene mapping	Disease
Dystrophin	Xp21	Duchenne MD, Becker MD
α-Sarcoglycan (adhalin)	17q12-q21	Autosomal recessive limb-girdle MD
β-Sarcoglycan	4q12	Autosomal recessive limb-girdle MD
γ-Sarcoglycan	13q12	Severe, autosomal recessive, Duchenne-like Tunisian MD
Merosin (α_2 laminin)	6q22-q23	Congenital MD
Calpain-3	15q15	Autosomal recessive; usually mild limb-girdle MD, but considerable range in severity
Unknown	2p	Relatively mild, autosomal recessive MD (Myoshi myopathy)
Unknown	5q	Autosomal dominant
Unknown	1	MD associated with cardiomyopathy

MD, muscular dystrophy.
Adapted from Worton R. Muscular dystrophies: diseases of the dystrophin-glycoprotein complex. *Science* 1995;270:755; and Bushby K. Muscular dystrophy and allied disorders: research strategies. *Trans Biochem Soc* 1996;24:489.

Although cardiac involvement has been encountered, it occurs rarely. Progression of FSHD is sufficiently slow, and interrupted by periods of seeming remission, to allow a normal life span for a fairly large proportion of patients. When sought using fluorescence angiography, retinal vascular anomalies are not unusual, and in one study were encountered in 75% of subjects, including some who lacked muscular symptoms (200). FSHD also may be accompanied by Coats disease (congenital retinal dysgenesis with telangiectasia and retinal detachment) (201) or sensorineural hearing loss (202).

Several other variants have been recognized. These include Erb muscular dystrophy (scapulohumeral muscular dystrophy) and scapuloperoneal dystrophy. In some subjects with the latter condition, sometimes known as Davidenkow syndrome, autopsy studies have disclosed evidence for both progressive neurogenic and myopathic forms. The condition is linked to chromosome 12, and onset of symptoms is usually during the third decade of life (202a). In many instances, electrophysiologic and nerve biopsy document a motor neuropathy (203).

Limb-Girdle Muscular Dystrophy

These dystrophies comprise a number of distinct clinical conditions, which are summarized in Table 14.9. Transmission usually occurs in an autosomal recessive manner (*LGMD2*), but families in which the condition is transmitted in

a dominant manner have been well documented (*LGMD1*) (204). At least six different gene loci for the latter form have been described. Symptoms appear during the second or third decade, with muscles of either the shoulder or the pelvic girdle being affected initially. The rate of progression is highly variable, but generally, the course is far more benign than that of Duchenne muscular dystrophy. Approximately 30% of patients develop pseudohypertrophy, usually of the gastrocnemius, less commonly of the lateral vasti and deltoids. Using cDNA probes for the dystrophin gene, at least some of these patients have been found to have Becker muscular dystrophy (205). Cardiac involvement is rare, and intelligence is unaffected.

In many cases of recessively transmitted limb-girdle syndrome a deficiency of one of four sarcoglycans occurs (205a,205b). The first entity to be described was called *adhalen* as an anglicized version of the Arabic word for *muscle*, because it was first reported in Tunisian families with consanguinity. Adhalen is now termed α-sarcoglycan (206). Other limb-girdle dystrophies are caused by defects in β-, γ-, or δ-sarcoglycan (207–209). In the series of Duggan and colleagues, mutations in the α-sarcoglycan gene were the most common, with mutations in the β-sarcoglycan gene the next most frequent (207). Immunocytochemical antibodies are now commercially available to demonstrate each of these sarcoglycans in frozen sections of muscle biopsy (see Fig. 14.9). Adhalen, or α-sarcoglycan, generally is secondarily deficient when any of the other sarcoglycans are not normally expressed, so that deficiency of α-sarcoglycan alone does not prove that this defect is primary, but does provide a convenient screen for deficiency of any of the other sarcoglycans. Secondary deficiency of α-sarcoglycan also accompanies dystrophin deficiency in some cases of Duchenne muscular dystrophy. The genotype-phenotype correlation of the sarcoglycanopathies demonstrates that the pure α-form is the least severe with the slowest rate of progression. The condition is sometimes not expressed until adolescence or adult life. The other sarcoglycanopathies are associated with a more severe clinical course that begins in the prepubertal years (208,209).

One well-described type of autosomal recessive limb-girdle dystrophy (LGMD) is caused by a defect in the gene that codes for calpain-3 (209a). Calpain-3 is a muscle-specific calcium-activated neutral protease whose deficiency is associated with a mild form of LGMD with onset of symptoms at approximately 10 years of age and unaccompanied by cardiomyopathy or mental retardation (209a).

Another variant of LGMD that appears in childhood is accompanied by thrombocytopenia and is transmitted as an autosomal dominant disorder (210).

Muscular dystrophies that affect the distal musculature predominantly generally occur most commonly in the adult years. One form, with its onset in young adulthood, is transmitted as an autosomal recessive trait and progresses slowly (211). Another form is characterized by the presence of rimmed vacuoles within muscle (212), whereas another type has its onset in infancy (213). All these entities are rare, and Brooke has pointed out that myotonic dystrophy is the most common myopathy to affect the distal musculature in early life (2).

Diagnosis

Even though a fully developed case of muscular dystrophy can be readily diagnosed on clinical grounds (namely, by the proximal distribution of the involved muscles, the presence of pseudohypertrophy, and the absence of deep tendon reflexes at the proximal musculature), a com-

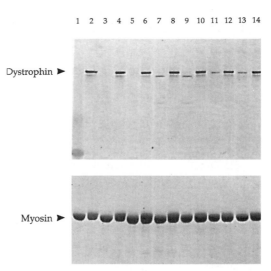

FIG. 14.10. Western blot on muscle biopsies from patients with muscular dystrophies. The dystrophin assay is run with two different antibodies: antibody corresponding to amino acids 1991–3112, and a carboxyl terminus antibody corresponding to amino acids 3669–3685. Lanes 3, 5: Patient with Duchenne muscular dystrophy; dystrophin levels are virtually absent. Lanes 7, 9: Patient with mild to moderate Becker muscular dystrophy. Dystrophin is present in reduced amounts at an abnormal location. Lanes 11, 13: Patient with severe Becker muscular dystrophy. Marked reduction of dystrophin, which is in its normal location. Lane 1 shows molecular weight markers; even numbered lanes are control biopsies. (Courtesy of Genica Pharmaceuticals Corporation, Worcester, MA.)

plete investigation, including serum CK levels and a muscle biopsy, is the first step toward arriving at a diagnosis.

A qualitatively altered dystrophin is consistent with the diagnosis of Becker muscular dystrophy; absent dystrophin indicates the diagnosis of Duchenne muscular dystrophy (Fig. 14.10). Abnormal immunohistochemistry for dystrophin in a girl indicates a carrier state. Normal dystrophin points to another form of muscular dystrophy, such as the limb-girdle or Emery-Dreifuss types (214).

Muscle tissue (100 mg maintained at –70° C) suffices for quantitation of dystrophin and determination of molecular weight by Western blotting. For ELISA analysis, much smaller amounts (5 mg of tissue) suffice. Neither the site of the muscle biopsy nor the age of the patient is important in the evaluation of dystrophin (142). The anatomic appearance of the muscle biopsy and the elevation of muscle enzymes are less specific diagnostic parameters.

Because the early stages of the dystrophic process are accompanied by a marked outflow of muscle enzymes into the circulation, the serum level of many soluble enzymes normally present in muscle tissue is increased. These include aspartate aminotransferase, alanine aminotransferase, lactic dehydrogenase, aldolase, and CK. Of these enzymes, an elevation of CK MM isozyme is the most sensitive and specific for the presence of a dystrophic process (215).

In the early stages of Duchenne muscular dystrophy, and even before clinical signs appear, serum CK levels are strikingly increased. Neither liver disease nor hemolysis of blood samples changes the serum activity of this enzyme, so that this abnormality is fairly specific for a dystrophic process. With progression of the disease, enzyme levels decrease. Dystrophies other than the Duchenne form, with the exception of the Fukuyama type of congenital muscular dystrophy, show less striking enzyme abnormalities, and clinically typical cases of LGMD with normal serum enzymes are not rare.

DNA markers derived from within the dystrophin gene locus have been used in the prenatal diagnosis of Duchenne muscular dystrophy using amniocytes or chorionic villus cells. Despite the large number of intragenic DNA polymorphisms available, the diagnosis is still fraught with errors. For one, the large size of the gene permits crossovers within it (216). Furthermore, in the two-thirds of cases in which no previous family history of the disease is seen, linkage analysis is inadequate (217). Finally, deletion mutants are detectable only in some 65% of cases. For these reasons, other diagnostic means must be used (218). These include sonographically guided fetal muscle biopsy for dystrophin analysis by immunofluorescence, or measuring dystrophin by immunocytochemical analysis on amniocytes in which

myogenesis was induced by infecting them with a retrovirus containing a gene that induces myogenesis (219).

In carriers of Duchenne or Becker muscular dystrophy, serum CK levels are elevated. This elevation is most striking younger than 16 years of age, and at that age, carrier detection, using the mean value of three or more separate CK estimations, is close to 100%. When mothers who are obligate carriers for Duchenne muscular dystrophy are screened by means of CK levels, the detection rate is approximately 70%. This discrepancy appears to be a function of the decrease in CK levels with age (220). The information obtained from the DNA probes can be correlated with the CK test data or immunohistochemistry for dystrophin on muscle biopsy to provide genetic information with 98% to 99% reliability (214).

Treatment

At present, no treatment is effective for any of the muscular dystrophies. The anecdotal effectiveness of courses of vitamin E, anabolic steroids, and combinations of amino acids has not withstood controlled trial. The interesting observation that boys with growth hormone deficiency have a milder form of Duchenne muscular dystrophy has led to a randomized, double-blind controlled trial using mazindol, a growth hormone inhibitor. This did not show any slowing of the progression of muscular weakness (221). A significant proportion of patients with FSHD, when treated with corticosteroids, experience dramatic, but often transient, clinical improvement that is coupled with a striking decrease in previously elevated serum CK levels (222). Long-term treatment with corticosteroids, however, may actually make the patient weaker by the added weight of additional subcutaneous adipose tissue that the weakened muscles must overcome, and because of other complications of chronic corticosteroid therapy in any patient.

Other potential therapeutic approaches include gene replacement, myoblast transplantation, or replacement of dystrophin by other, dystrophin-related proteins. The promises and problems inherent in these various approaches have been reviewed (223–225). To date, myoblast transfer has been the only therapeutic approach that has been used clinically. Although there have been few adverse effects, less than 1% of the donor cells survived to express dystrophin (226). The reason for poor survival is unclear; it does not appear to be caused by immune rejection (225,226).

As stated by Brooke (2), "incurable and untreatable are not synonymous." A treatment program for the child with muscular dystrophy not only offers a positive attitude and hope to family and child, but keeps the child as active as possible until such time, not too distant now, when molecular biology will offer a more definitive approach. In the early stages of the illness, passive stretching of affected muscles and the application of night splints can delay contractures. Children are encouraged to take as much exercise as they desire. Physiotherapy can be helpful in preventing contractures of the ankles and hips in particular, but once the contractures appear, therapy alone cannot reverse them. Because of progressive fibrosis of muscle, contractures often appear despite conscientious physiotherapy. If physiotherapy is too rigorous, it may actually accelerate the rate of degeneration of the fragile myofibers with abnormal sarcolemmal membranes, reflected as a further increase in serum CK, so that this therapy must be titrated to be forceful enough to prevent contractures without being excessive, causing further damage to the muscle.

While the child is still walking, major surgery is inadvisable. In the more advanced case, bracing is preferable to use of a wheelchair, because the latter promotes curvature of the spine. Body jackets tend to delay these deformities. Orthopedic measures, particularly those followed by prolonged bedrest, seem to hasten the downhill process and should be resorted to only when absolutely necessary.

A small proportion of children with mild or clinically inapparent muscle disease develop anesthesia-induced malignant hyperpyrexia, also known as malignant hyperthermia (227,228). To prevent this complication, local or spinal anesthesia should be used for all procedures, or dantrolene sodium may be administered for several hours before the anesthetic, which effectively blocks this complication. If general anesthesia is unavoidable, thiopental sodium is the preferred agent, and body temperature should be monitored throughout surgery.

Myotonic Disorders

A number of genetically distinct conditions share the clinical feature of myotonia of the voluntary muscles. In some, the myotonic phenomenon is the most evident aspect of the disease; in others, it is overshadowed by other symptoms. Although in the past the myotonias were believed to represent various expressions of the same genetic disorder, it is now apparent that they have different underlying biochemical defects and can be classified as *channelopathies* of the sarcolemma, related to either sodium or chloride channels.

From a clinical point of view, the myotonias can be divided into nondystrophic and dystrophic types. The nondystrophic myotonias are further divided into myotonia congenita, paramyotonia congenita, hyperkalemic periodic paralysis, and the various syndromes of continuous motor discharges (Table 14.10).

Myotonia is characterized by a failure of voluntary muscle to relax after contraction ceases and by a slow, tonic response to mechanical and electric stimulation. This phenomenon is most readily observed in the muscles of the hand, face, and tongue. Patients are unable to relax their grasp, and percussion of the thenar eminence can produce a dimple lasting several seconds. Repetitive movements lessen myotonia; exposure to cold aggravates it. It is useful to ask the patient if the condition is aggravated or improved on entering a warm bath or shower or a cold swimming pool.

The defects of sodium and chloride channels may be distinguished by a careful history and physical examination. In sodium channel disorders, the patient finds it increasingly difficult to relax muscle contractions with continued exercise; in chloride channel disorders, by contrast, exercise improves the myotonia or abolishes it temporarily,

TABLE 14.10. *Genetic classification of the myotonias*

Type of disease	Locus
Sodium channel diseases	Chromosome 17q23.1-q25.3
Hyperkalemic periodic paralysis (with or without myotonia)	(SCN4A gene)
Paramyotonia congenita	
Potassium-sensitive myotonia congenita (also known as myotonia fluctuans)	
Protein kinase-related disease	Chromosome 19q13.3
Myotonic dystrophy	
Chloride channel diseases	Chromosome 7q32(CLCN1)
Thomsen (autosomal dominant) myotonia congenita	
Becker (autosomal recessive) myotonia congenita	
Myotonia lesion	
Unknown	Unknown
Chondrodystrophic myotonia (autosomal dominant; also known as Schwartz-Jampel syndrome)	
Hyperkalemic periodic paralysis with dysrhythmias (Andersen syndrome)	

From Ptacek LJ, Johnson KJ, Griggs RC. Genetics and physiology of the myotonic muscle disorders. *N Engl J Med* 1993;328:482. With permission.

so that patients learn to do warm-up exercises before undertaking physical tasks. Moxley has written an excellent review of the myotonic disorders in children and adults that includes clinical, physiologic, and molecular genetic aspects (229).

Myotonic Dystrophy

Not a rare disease (incidence at birth is 13.5 in 100,000), myotonic dystrophy is transmitted as an autosomal dominant trait and is marked by the association of myotonia with a dystrophic process of muscle and multisystem involvement (230). The disorder is caused by a CTG trinucleotide expansion in the 3' untranslated region of *DM*, the gene that encodes a myotonic dystrophy protein kinase.

Although the disease usually appears in late adolescence or early adult life, it can manifest at birth (congenital myotonic dystrophy) or during the first decade (juvenile myotonic dystrophy). These congenital and juvenile forms of myotonic dystrophy constitute approximately 20% of all myotonic cases. As a rule, the disease shows an earlier onset and increasing severity of clinical manifestations in successive generations, a phenomenon termed *anticipation* (231).

In some patients, myotonia is severe and generalized, and dystrophic features are absent or develop late in life. In others, muscular atrophy

and weakness are the prominent abnormalities, with myotonia difficult to elicit or completely absent on physical examination and recognized only on EMG studies. Sometimes both clinical variants occur in the same family (232,233).

The distribution of muscular atrophy is characteristic for the disease. The face, sternocleidomastoids, and girdle musculature are the initial sites of atrophy. The wasted, weakened sternocleidomastoids and the facial atrophy marked by shrinkage of the masseter and temporal muscles produce a *hatchet face* appearance, which is distinctive even in a small child (Fig. 14.11). An inability to relax a smile, the *Cheshire cat smile*, is also characteristic (234). Myotonic dystrophy differs from most primary myopathies in that distal rather than proximal involvement predominates. This pattern is not caused by an accompanying neuropathy.

Smooth muscles, particularly those of the pharynx, esophagus, and gastrointestinal tract, are also involved, and myotonia of the anal sphincter has been described (235). The involved neonate and young infant may have loss of peristalsis because of the smooth muscle involvement, leading to chronic obstipation, fecal retention, and distention of the bowel (236). Conduction velocities are slowed in several motor nerves, and biopsy reveals a preferential loss of the larger myelinated fibers. The

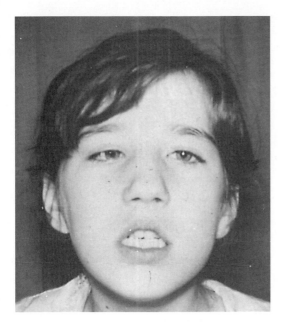

FIG. 14.11. An 11-year-old girl with myotonic dystrophy. Note the distinctive snarling appearance of the face. Her presenting symptoms were impaired speech and mild mental dullness. Because of the atrophy of the neck muscles, the profile can have a "hatchet face" appearance.

cause of the polyneuropathy is still unknown; it is not the result of entrapment or secondary to muscle disease (230). Electrocardiographic abnormalities were seen in 86% of Harper's patients. These include cardiac conduction defects, mainly a prolonged PR interval (70%), and arrhythmias, mainly atrial flutter seen in 15% (230). Myotonic dystrophy is accompanied by excessive daytime sleepiness and is a common cause of this symptom in childhood.

Posterior cortical cataracts can regularly be demonstrated in the adult with myotonic dystrophy and can even occur in the absence of either myotonia or dystrophy in the guise of senile or presenile cataracts. In juvenile myotonic dystrophy, cataracts usually are not seen until after 10 years of age, but occasionally neonates with symptomatic disease at birth have congenital cataracts in one or both eyes. The incidence in children with myotonic dystrophy is less than 30%, even when a careful slit-lamp examination

is performed. Pigmentary retinal degeneration is relatively common; an abnormal ERG can predate muscular symptoms. Mental retardation is seen in 80% of patients with myotonic dystrophy and occurs almost invariably in congenital myotonic dystrophy. In some instances, developmental delay is apparent before the onset of muscular symptoms.

Endocrine abnormalities such as frontal baldness, loss of body hair, and testicular atrophy are not seen in the affected child (237). Between 6.5% and 20.0% of patients ultimately develop an unusual insulin-resistant form of diabetes mellitus, which occasionally occurs before adolescence (238,239). Various immunologic abnormalities have been documented. Most consistent is an increased catabolism of IgG, which results in low serum concentrations of the immunoglobulin in approximately one-third of subjects, including some who have not yet developed muscle weakness (240,241).

The congenital form of myotonic dystrophy is almost invariably transmitted by an affected mother. In the DNA of infants, the number of CTG repeats ranges from 500 to 2,700, and the intergenerational expansion of the repeat depends on the sex of the transmitting parent (242). With maternal transmission of the myotonic dystrophy gene there is marked expansion of the repeat, whereas with paternal transmission there is reduced amplification or even contraction (243,244).

In congenital myotonic dystrophy, the disease expresses itself by a weak suck, delayed speech, retarded motor development, and generalized hypotonia especially involving the neck muscles. Infants are prone to perinatal asphyxia. Facial diplegia is evident in 87% of infants, delayed motor development in 87%, and mental retardation in 68% (230). Approximately one-half of mothers who carry an offspring with congenital myotonic dystrophy have polyhydramnios, sometimes sufficiently severe to require amniocentesis (236). Arthrogryposis can be noted at birth (56). Clinical myotonia is invariably absent before 1 year of age and is present in only 12% of 1- to 5-year-old children (230). MRI studies often reflect the perinatal asphyxial insults sustained by the infants (245).

The clinical course in the fully developed case of congenital myotonic dystrophy is one of gradual debilitation. Respiratory insufficiency, dysphagia and aspiration, and poor gastrointestinal motility may present life-threatening presentations in the neonatal period (236). Infants who survive the first year of life appear to improve over the course of the subsequent few years, only to deteriorate gradually with increasing muscular weakness, the appearance of myotonia, and the various other features of the adult form of the disease. Most significantly, these features include diabetes mellitus (239), cardiac involvement that usually takes the form of conduction defects, and ultimately, congestive heart failure (230) or sudden death as a consequence of tachyarrhythmias or bradyarrhythmias (246).

Diagnosis

In a typical case of myotonic dystrophy affecting an older child, the facial appearance is striking, myotonic phenomena can be elicited, and the family history is often helpful. In the small child or infant, the diagnosis is less obvious, and myotonic phenomena are detected neither clinically nor, in most instances, by EMG (247). Myotonia is never manifest in infancy and usually does not become evident, either clinically or by EMG, until 4 to 5 years of age. Rather, the characteristic aspects of the disease are facial diplegia and generalized hypotonia. Clinical and EMG examinations of the mother invariably show subclinical or overt signs of myotonic dystrophy (248).

Serum enzymes are usually normal. On EMG, prolonged trains of high-frequency discharges arising from single fibers or groups of muscle fibers occur in response to electrode insertion or movement. Amplified, their sound is highly characteristic, like that of a dive-bomber. Neuroimaging studies show ventricular enlargement, and in some instances hypoplasia of the corpus callosum, and abnormal myelination (247a).

Myotonia occasionally is observed in hyperkalemic periodic paralysis, polyneuritis, and polymyositis. A slowing in muscular contraction and relaxation, resembling myotonia, also can be seen in hypothyroidism.

A DNA probe that is specific for more than 96% of patients is available for the diagnosis of myotonic dystrophy and obviates the need for linkage analyses (249). Muscle biopsy is generally not required because it is not definitively diagnostic, though characteristic changes such as large numbers of centronuclear fibers and selective type I fiber atrophy in children and many stages of arrested maturation in neonates are strongly suggestive of the diagnosis.

Treatment

When myotonic dystrophy occurs in childhood, myotonia is rarely severe enough to warrant intensive treatment, and there is no evidence that improvement of the myotonia affects the dystrophic process. Procaine amine, quinine, corticosteroids, antihistamines, and calcium channel blockers such as nifedipine can be of benefit in children with myotonia caused by myotonic dystrophy or myotonia congenita (250,251). The side effects of these drugs at times are more disturbing than the myotonia. Medications that work at the sodium channel, such as carbamazepine, phenytoin, and especially mexiletine are often helpful in minimizing myotonia, but if the patient has predominantly weakness rather than myotonia, they are ineffective.

Pathologic Anatomy

Microscopic examination of muscle obtained from subjects with the adult form of myotonic dystrophy reveals nonspecific alterations in the appearance of the muscle fibers resembling that seen in other muscular dystrophies as a necrotizing myopathy, but usually with little or no connective tissue proliferation. The number of centronuclear fibers often is excessive. A characteristic finding shared only by a few other myopathies is selective type I myofibers atrophy, a feature shared with Emery-Dreifuss dystrophy but not seen in Duchenne, limb-girdle, or FSHD. Another of the histologic characteristics of the disease is a reorientation of peripheral myofibrils from a longitudinal disposition to one ringing the muscle fiber. The significance of this abnormality is uncertain; it is usually seen in long-standing myotonic dystrophy, and never in the congenital or early forms of the disorder. It also occurs in hypothyroidism, limb-girdle, and facioscapulo-humeral dystrophy, and also can be the result of trauma to muscle. None of the ultrastructural features of myotonic muscle are specific (252). The sarcolemmal membrane and basal lamina (basement membrane) are well preserved. Immunocytochemical expression of sarcolemma-associated proteins such as dystrophin, merosin, and the sarcoglycans is normal.

In neonatal myotonic dystrophy, the muscle fibers present an apparent maturational arrest. They are arrested in maturation in various stages of development within the same fascicles: myoblasts, myotubes, incomplete histochemical differentiation into type 1 and type 2 fibers, and persistent expression of excessive fetal intermediate filament proteins such as desmin and vimentin (253,254). The ultrastructure in the congenital disease shows additional features not seen at the light microscopic level: persistent fetal orientation of triads parallel to the long axis of the myofibril and lack of registry of Z-bands of adjacent myofibrils, features that normally mature at approximately 30-weeks' gestation. In some cases of congenital myotonic dystrophy, congenital muscle fiber-type disproportion (see Congenital Myopathies, later in this chapter) is the dominant pattern of the muscle biopsy.

Pathogenesis

DM, the gene for myotonic dystrophy, is located on the long arm of chromosome 19 (19q13.3) and codes for myotonin-protein kinase, a cyclic AMP-dependent protein kinase. Protein kinases modulate the activities of a variety of target proteins by phosphorylating some of their serine residues. In 1992, several groups who independently studied patients with myotonic dystrophy demonstrated an expansion on the 3' untranslated region of *DM* of a cytosinethymineguanine (CTG) trinucleotide repeat (255,256). The CTG sequence is repeated between 5 and 35 times in DNA derived from healthy subjects, but between 40 and 1,500 times in DNA derived from patients with myotonic dystrophy (242), and 1,500 to 2,500 times in DNA derived from subjects with

congenital myotonic dystrophy (243,244) (see Fig. 3.5). Rare families with the characteristic picture of myotonic dystrophy, but no triplet expansion, have been encountered (257). With transmission of the gene to subsequent generations, the length of the CTG repeat tends to increase. This is especially the case when the gene is transmitted by an affected mother. Concomitant with this increase there is a worsening of clinical symptoms in subsequent generations. When an affected father transmits the gene, on rare occasions, a contraction of the expanded repeat occurs into the normal range (258).

The mechanism that causes the CTG triplet expansion is still unknown. The expanded CTG repeats that occur outside the coding region are believed to create a gain-of-function mutation by increasing the size of the mRNA. This disrupts the activity of a CUG-binding protein, a nuclear ribonucleoprotein involved in the splicing of various genes. This protein accumulates in tissues obtained from patients with myotonic dystrophy (258a). Because patients have reduced reproductive ability, the gene pool needs to be replenished. This appears to happen by preferential transmission to offsprings of alleles with greater than 19 CTG repeats (259).

Molecular biology has started to unravel the physiologic defects that underlie the various myotonic disorders (see Table 14.10). The myotonic disorders result from an abnormality of muscle membrane excitability. Two major subgroups have been recognized. In one, the mutations involve the skeletal muscle chloride channel (*CLCN1*), and in the other they affect the gene that codes for the α-subunit of the skeletal muscle voltage-gated sodium channel (*SCN4A*) (260).

Three clinical entities are caused by a disorder of *CLCN1*. These are myotonia congenita (Thompsen disease), Becker generalized myotonia, and myotonia levior (260,261). In both dominant and recessive forms of myotonia congenita, muscle membrane chloride conductance is abnormal in that the rate of repolarization after an action potential is excessively slow (262).

To date, some 20 mutations in the gene coding for *SCN4A* have been recognized (260,263). The mutations result in a number of phenotypes, of which hyperkalemic periodic paralysis and paramyotonia congenita are the most common (264,265). The presence of genetic defects altering sodium channel function is consistent with the long-standing clinical observation that in both these diseases inactivation of sodium channels in muscle is abnormal (266).

Myotonia Congenita
(Thomsen Disease and Becker Disease)

Myotonia congenita (Thomsen disease and Becker disease) was first described in 1876 by Thomsen, an English physician, in himself and his own son (267). It is a rare disease, with the highest prevalence being in northern Finland, where it occurs in 7.3 per 100,000 (267a). In myotonia congenita, myotonia and muscle stiffness are first observed in infancy. Occasional choking episodes are not uncommon, as is prolonged closure of eyes after sneezing. Myotonia improves with exercise, and, in most instances, becomes less evident with increasing age. Muscular hypertrophy of the upper and lower extremities are commonly seen in later years (267a). Thomsen disease is transmitted as a dominant disorder; a recessive form of myotonia congenita also is recognized and is known as Becker disease (not to be confused with the Becker form of dystrophinopathy related to Duchenne muscular dystrophy) (268). These two patterns of inheritance are different diseases, not only in the mendelian pattern of inheritance, but because of different mutations within the same voltage-gated chloride channel gene (*CLCN1*) at the 7q32 locus (269). The dominant form is more benign. Myotonia levior is an even milder entity with later onset of myotonia than is seen in myotonia congenita and absence of muscle hypertrophy (261). In some families myotonia congenita is accompanied by hyperkalemic periodic paralysis, but this is yet another disease caused by a defect in the sodium rather than the chloride channels; this disorder is best classified as a form of paramyotonia congenita (see following discussion) (see Table 14.10).

The serum CK is normal or mildly elevated in the various forms of myotonia congenita. The muscle biopsy is normal or shows minimal, nonspecific alterations, such as excessive variation in myofiber diameter and poor differentiation of type II fiber subtypes with ATPase stains, but there is no myofiber degeneration, hence unlike myotonic dystrophy, Thomsen and Becker diseases are not muscular dystrophies. The EMG discloses myotonic discharges.

Paramyotonia Congenita (Eulenburg Disease)

In paramyotonia congenita, a dominantly inherited disorder, myotonia is usually recognized during infancy. It is brought on or aggravated by exposure to cold and worsens with continued exercise (270). Many individuals also experience prolonged periods of weakness and develop muscular wasting (271). In some, weakness accompanies an increase in serum potassium, a feature that overlaps with hyperkalemic periodic paralysis (272). The condition is caused by a mutation in the α-subunit of the skeletal muscle voltage-gated sodium channel (*SCN4A*) (260).

Rippling muscle disease is a clinically unique condition, which appears during the first or second decade of life. It is characterized by muscular stiffness and myalgia apparent after a period of rest. Symptoms abate with exercise. Generalized muscle hypertrophy occurs, especially in the calves, and grip myotonia. Tapping a muscle causes a peculiar rolling contraction across the muscle group that is unaccompanied by myotonic EMG discharges. One gene for this entity has been mapped to chromosome 1q41, but considerable genetic heterogeneity exists (272a).

Hyperkalemic Periodic Paralysis

Atypical cases of periodic paralysis had been recognized for several years before Gamstorp's classic description of this condition (273). In her subjects, attacks started in early childhood, did not respond to potassium, and were unaccompanied by an electrolyte imbalance.

Attacks often begin in infancy, and in 90% of cases, the disease becomes established by 10 years of age. The condition affects both sexes equally and is transmitted by an autosomal dominant gene with a strong penetrance. The gene has been mapped to the long arm of chromosome 17 (17q23.1-q25.3) and codes for a subunit of the sodium channel (SCN4A). Attacks occur approximately once per week and are precipitated by rest after physical exertion or the administration of potassium. Weakness first affects the pelvic musculature, but at times can become generalized. Average attacks last approximately 1 hour. During this time, the plasma potassium levels are usually higher than normal. Additionally, plasma phosphate levels tend to decrease, and patients respond to exercise with decreases in blood glucose and associated ketosis (274). Between attacks, muscle strength returns to normal, although a slowly progressive myopathy can develop in some families (275).

Hyperkalemic attacks can occur with myotonia or paramyotonia (cold-induced myotonia and weakness). The course of the paralytic attacks is similar in these conditions, and the disease also is transmitted in an autosomal dominant manner (276,277). When myotonia is present, it commonly affects the eyelids and produces a staring appearance. Percussion myotonia is noted occasionally, and in some families, potassium-induced paralysis and myotonia are jointly transmitted as a dominant disorder. Families in which hyperkalemic paralysis with paramyotonia coexist have been reported (278). These represent yet another mutation of the gene that codes for *SCN4A*.

Because hyperkalemia is not invariable, the diagnosis of hyperkalemic periodic paralysis is best established by inducing an attack through the careful oral administration of potassium (25 mg/kg), with concomitant monitoring by electrocardiography.

Treatment

Most attacks are mild and brief and do not require treatment. The administration of acetazolamide (125 mg/day for an 8-year-old child) has been successful in preventing attacks or reducing their severity (279). Inhalations of albuterol, a β-adrenergic stimulant, also have been found to be effective in the treatment of paralytic episodes (280).

Syndromes of Continuous Motor Neuron Discharges

Several rarely encountered conditions are characterized by continuous motor neuron discharges.

Schwartz-Jampel Syndrome (Chondrodystrophic Myotonia)

Schwartz-Jampel syndrome (chondrodystrophic myotonia) (281) is an autosomal recessive disorder marked by clinical and EMG myotonia and muscular atrophy. The condition has been mapped to the short arm of chromosome 1 (1p34-p36). However, there is considerable clinical and genetic heterogeneity. Giedion and coworkers have recognized three subtypes: 1A, apparent in childhood and marked by moderate bony dysplasia; 1B, which is apparent at birth with more striking bony changes; and type 2, which is manifest at birth and has increased mortality (282). Type 1A corresponds to the original patients of Schwartz and Jampel (282a). In all forms continuous motor neuron discharges involving the facial musculature produce blepharophimosis, a puckered mouth, and a characteristic pinched facies. Growth is retarded, and there is progressive limitation of joint movements in hips, wrists, fingers, and toes. Vertebral anomalies and deformities of chest and hips are almost always present. Mental development is generally normal (283). Myotonic EMG abnormalities have been observed in both parents. It is not known whether these EMG abnormalities reflect a dominant transmission of the disease or the partial expressivity of the heterozygote (284). Procainamide hydrochloride produces considerable relief from the myotonia and the painful muscle spasms.

This condition should be distinguished from the Van Dyke–Hansen syndrome, in which continuous motor neuron discharges are accompanied by episodic ataxia (285).

Isaacs Syndrome

Isaacs syndrome is characterized by the appearance at any time of life of muscle stiffness and cramps, impaired muscular relaxation, and widespread myokymia or fasciculations (286). The condition can be sporadic or can be inherited in an autosomal dominant manner (272). The motor neuron discharge is believed to arise from the peripheral motor axon because it is unaffected by peripheral nerve block and persists during sleep. Curare abolishes the abnormal discharges. EMG of the fully relaxed muscle discloses continuous discharges of normal motor unit potentials. Motor and sensory nerve conduction times are usually normal, although some of the familial cases have an associated peripheral neuropathy (287). The condition is nonprogressive and occasionally can improve. Relatively small amounts of phenytoin or carbamazepine decrease the abnormal muscle activity (288,289).

Isaacs syndrome is distinct from the stiff-man syndromes, one form of which is dominantly inherited and characterized by muscular symptoms at birth (stiff-baby syndrome or hyperekplexia) (290) (see Chapter 2). The other form is sporadic and usually appears in adult life or, rarely, in adolescence (291). In both forms, the motor unit discharges disappear with sleep and are relieved with diazepam, a drug that is ineffective in Isaacs syndrome. Because a peripheral nerve block abolishes the rigidity, Layzer believes that the abnormal motor unit discharges arise as a result of a defect in a descending spinal pathway that originates within the brainstem and inhibits muscle tone and exteroceptive spinal reflexes (292). This inhibition is enhanced by γ-aminobutyric acid and diminished by noradrenergic input. Solimena and coworkers have demonstrated autoantibodies against glutamic acid decarboxylase, the enzyme responsible for γ-aminobutyric acid synthesis within neurons, in patients with this syndrome (293).

Another condition to be considered in a child demonstrating continuous motor unit activity is malignant hyperthermia. Usually, this condition follows the administration of halothane or succinylcholine. It, too, is marked by generalized hypertonia, rigidity, and muscle fasciculation. Hyperthermia may not always be present, particularly in infants. The CK levels are markedly elevated, and a metabolic acidosis is usually demonstrable. Muscle biopsy in the acute stage or shortly thereafter shows a severe necrotizing myopathy. Malignant hyperthermia is, therefore, really acute rhabdomyolysis. Children with Duchenne muscular dystrophy, myotonic dystrophy, and especially central core disease (see Central Core Disease, later in this chapter) are particularly prone to this condition. Treatment is

with dantrolene (7 mg/kg), more effective if given before the anesthetic is administered (294).

Dermatomyositis

The idiopathic inflammatory myopathies can be classified into three groups: dermatomyositis, polymyositis, and inclusion body myositis (295). In children, dermatomyositis is the most common of these conditions; inclusion body myositis is seen almost exclusively in late adult life (296,297).

Dermatomyositis is a systemic disease that involves many organs and is primarily characterized by low-grade fever, fatigue, anorexia, a typical skin rash, muscular weakness, and pain.

Pathologic Anatomy

The primary site of involvement in childhood dermatomyositis is the intramuscular microvasculature. As a consequence, the most striking anatomic abnormalities are found in the blood vessels of the muscles, fat, nerves, connective tissue, and gastrointestinal tract. Here, the endothelial cells undergo degeneration and regeneration, with inclusion-like reticulotubular aggregates within their cytoplasm; these structures probably are clusters of duplicated sarcoplasmic reticulum. Other changes include a markedly decreased number of pinocytotic vesicles in the endothelial cytoplasm, hyperplasia of the intima, and multiple vascular occlusions. These alterations produce areas of muscle infarction, which are often accompanied by denervation atrophy secondary to occlusion of the nutrient vessels to the peripheral nerves.

A characteristic feature of dermatomyositis is the presence of several layers of atrophic fibers at the periphery of fascicles, with relative preservation of myofibers in the centers of fascicles. This condition is known as *perifascicular atrophy*. Most of the atrophic fibers at the periphery of fascicles are regenerating and only a few scattered degenerating fibers are demonstrated. This abnormality is seen in some 90% of children with dermatomyositis, but not in polymyositis. Degeneration of muscle fibers is disproportionately sparse in childhood dermato-myositis, in contrast to polymyositis of adults and children (296,298). Another distinguishing feature in the muscle biopsy is the absence of lymphocytes infiltrating and phagocytosing myofibers in dermatomyositis, whereas this is a typical histopathologic feature in polymyositis. Perifascicular atrophy is characteristic, but not necessarily diagnostic of dermatomyositis because it also occurs in other chronic small vessel ischemic diseases, such as in adults with diabetes mellitus and claudication of the legs.

Pathogenesis

The basic process that leads to dermatomyositis is an antibody or immune complex-mediated immune response against a vascular-endothelial component (299). The inflammatory cell in der-matomyositis is predominantly the B lympho-cyte, and the immune reaction is mediated by circulating antibodies against endothelial cells, by contrast with the aggressive T cells of polymyositis that cause a cell-mediated immune reaction. Kissel and coworkers believe that the first pathologic event is complement activation in the microvasculature and have demonstrated a membrane attack complex in the walls of recently damaged muscle (300). A variety of cytokines and chemokines, notably interleukin-1_α and 1_β, and tumor growth factor-β are impor-tant in the mediation of the inflammatory response (301). This process is followed by ischemic muscle fiber damage and by a cellular inflammatory response. We do not know what process or processes activate the complement cascade. The importance of genetic factors in the evolution of dermatomyositis is underlined by the 72% incidence of HLA-B8 tissue type in white children with dermatomyositis. This com-pares with its incidence of 21% in control sub-jects (302). The role of infectious agents in the evolution of the disease is less certain. The best evidence to date for their involvement is the demonstration of hybridization of coxsack-ievirus B-specific cDNA to a viral genomic RNA in skeletal muscle of several patients with acute dermatomyositis (303). Additionally, a

TABLE 14.11. *Clinical data on 34 children with dermatomyositis*

Symptom	Number of patients
Weakness	32
Facial skin lesions	31
Fever	29
Contractures	29
Weakness of bulbar musculature	17
Death	10
Subcutaneous calcifications	8

After Wedgewood RJ, Cook C, Cohen J. Dermato-myositis: report of 26 cases in children with a discussion of endocrine therapy in 13. *Pediatrics* 1953;12:447; and Banker BQ. Dermatomyositis of childhood. *J Neuropathol Exp Neurol* 1975;34:46.

large proportion of children with dermato-myositis develop high antibody titers against coxsackievirus B, suggesting cross-reactivity between components of an infectious agent and muscle or vascular endothelium, and formation of immune complexes that damage both tissues (304). Enteroviruses and toxoplasmosis also have been considered causative agents.

Clinical Manifestations

The onset of the disease can be insidious or acute and preceded by an infection. The most common early symptoms are weakness and easy fatigabil-ity (Table 14.11) (305). Typical skin changes, often at onset, include an erythematous, scaly, and occasionally violaceous discoloration of the upper eyelids. Subsequently, the skin of the peri-orbital region, malar areas, and extensor surfaces of the joints, particularly the knuckles, elbows, and knees, also can become affected. The rash tends to spare the phalanges, in contrast to that seen in systemic lupus erythematosus in which the phalanges are involved, and the knuckles are spared. Less commonly, the rash involves the neck and the upper chest. It is exacerbated by sunlight. At times, the skin becomes edematous.

Muscle weakness usually is generalized but always is most marked proximally. Weakness of the flexor muscles of the neck is observed in approximately one-half of children. Involve-ment of the bulbar musculature is an unfavorable prognostic sign; in the series of Wedge-wood and coworkers, reported in 1953, 75% of children with this sign died from the disease (305). Early flexion contractures at the ankles produce a tiptoe gait. The deep tendon reflexes are diminished or abolished.

The course of the disease is extremely variable. In some children, particularly those whose illness has an acute onset, the weakness advances rapidly over a period of several months and, with involvement of the bulbar musculature, terminates fatally. Perforation of the gastrointestinal tract is a frequent cause of death. In other children, the disease does not progress, but leaves the patient crippled by irreversible weakness, contractures, and subcutaneous calcium deposits.

Diagnosis

The diagnosis of dermatomyositis rests on (a) symmetric limb-girdle weakness, (b) muscle biopsy evidence of myositis and muscle necrosis, (c) increased levels of muscle enzymes in serum, (d) EMG changes of myositis, and (e) the presence of skin lesions (306,307). The appearance of cutaneous lesions may precede or follow the onset of myopathic weakness.

Routine laboratory studies are of little diagnostic help. In the active stage, the erythrocyte sedimentation rate is elevated, and the peripheral white cell count can be abnormal. Systemic lupus erythematosus cells are not demonstrated in peripheral blood, and the antistreptolysin titer is normal. The antinuclear antibody titer is occasionally positive, and the serum gamma-globulins are increased in approximately one-half of patients. Serum enzymes can be normal or slightly elevated. EMG examination can reveal myopathic action potentials exclusively, a combination of fibrillation potentials within resting muscles and myopathic action potentials, or repetitive high-frequency discharges evoked by mechanical stimulation of muscle (308). MRI of muscle can be used to follow disease involvement. Involved muscles have increased signal on T2-weighted images and normal T1-weighted images. Perimuscular edema and inflammatory changes of subcuta-neous fat are seen also (309). The muscle biopsy is usually diagnostic.

Differential Diagnosis

The muscle weakness seen in dermatomyositis must be distinguished from that associated with muscular dystrophy and polymyositis. In muscular dystrophy, as in dermatomyositis, muscle weakness involves the proximal muscles of the shoulder and pelvic girdle. However, bulbar signs, in particular swallowing difficulties, are extremely rare in muscular dystrophy. The onset of weakness is far more gradual in muscular dystrophy and contractures develop in its later stages. Finally, in childhood dermatomyositis, it is rare to see as striking an elevation in serum CK levels as occurs in the early phases of muscular dystrophy. Polymyositis is rare in childhood and lacks the dermal and vascular features of dermatomyositis (310). Instead, one observes widespread degeneration of muscle fibers and regenerative activity (Fig. 14.12). Inclusion body myositis is a disease of adult life. A somewhat similar pathologic picture, featuring inflammatory cell infiltrates but lacking the extensive vasculitis of dermatomyositis, is seen in a number of collagen vascular diseases, including rheumatic fever, rheumatoid arthritis, systemic lupus erythematosus, and mixed connective tissue disease (see Chapter 7). An inflammatory, corticosteroid-responsive myopathy, distinguished from dermatomyositis by the absence of vascular changes on muscle biopsy, is seen in infancy (311). This condition could be related if not identical to the Fukuyama type of congenital muscular dystrophy, in which inflammatory changes are fairly common. The eosinophilic myositis that resulted from toxic products in a tryptophan preparation is discussed in Chapter 9.

Treatment

Untreated, dermatomyositis has a poor prognosis. In the majority of affected children, however, the disease probably becomes quiescent after approximately 2 years, and treatment, therefore, is intended to carry the child through this period. The effectiveness of corticosteroid therapy in

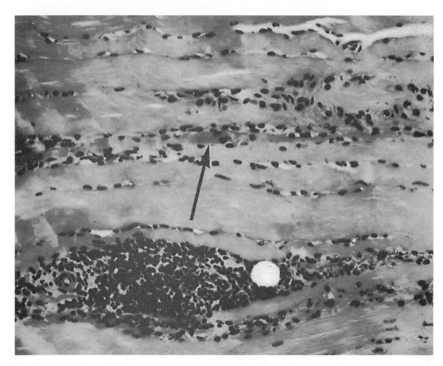

FIG. 14.12. Polymyositis. Inflammatory and degenerative changes in muscle in long-standing polymyositis. The arrow indicates a basophilic-staining muscle fiber. (From Merritt HH. *Textbook of neurology*, 5th ed. Philadelphia: Lea & Febiger, 1973. With permission.)

altering the course of dermatomyositis is still under dispute. However, most clinical centers, including our own, advocate instituting a regimen of prednisone (1.5 to 2.5 mg/kg per day for severe cases and 1.0 to 1.5 mg/kg per day for relatively mild cases). Dubowitz and his group, however, favor a starting dosage of 1 mg/kg per day for all patients. In their experience, and the experience of others, there are fewer relapses and less morbidity (31,307,308,312). This dosage is continued until remission has begun, as evidenced by a decrease in serum enzyme levels and by improvement in strength. It is then tapered and changed to alternate-day therapy at a level just sufficient to suppress symptoms. In many instances, corticosteroid therapy can be discontinued in 3 to 6 months.

When the disease is life-threatening or when symptoms are not controlled with prednisone alone, immunosuppressive therapy is indicated (313,314). This can take the form of biweekly injections of methotrexate (2 to 3 mg/kg per dose),

daily azathioprine (50 to 125 mg/day), or cyclosporine (2.5 to 7.5 mg/kg per day) (315). Later infertility is a risk with these drugs, in girls more than in boys. High-dose intravenous immune globulins have been used successfully. This management is indicated when there has been a relapse on previously effective therapy, when weakness persists despite high corticosteroid doses, or when corticosteroids cannot be reduced without precipitating a relapse. A dosage of 1 to 2 g/kg gammaglobulins, given in divided amounts over the course of 3 to 5 days, is generally recommended for initial therapy (316). Side reactions include headache, fever, and gastrointestinal upset. Plasmapheresis also has been used, but appears to be more effective in polymyositis.

In the experience of Spencer and coworkers, the course of the disease, when treated as indicated in this discussion, was chronic and continuous in 44% of children, chronic and polycyclic in 31%, and monocyclic in 25% (307). Although other series have not been as optimistic, these workers found that 78% of their patients were ultimately well and no longer taking medications.

Despite all current available therapy, the mortality in a series published in 1982 was still 10% (306).

Polymyositis

Although not rare in adults, particularly during the fifth and sixth decades, polymyositis is uncommon in children. It is a chronic inflammatory process of muscles leading to the insidious onset of weakness, without the constitutional symptoms and skin changes that accompany dermatomyositis. In contrast to dermatomyositis, polymyositis is a cell-mediated disease. Polymyositis can begin as early as the second year of life and usually first affects the pelvic musculature. Muscles are abnormally firm and occasionally painful. As the disease progresses, the weakness spreads to the upper limbs and the face. The clinical picture resembles that of muscular dystrophy and, from a clinical viewpoint, it is only the somewhat more rapid onset of muscle weakness and the arrest or retrogression of symptoms that suggest the diagnosis.

On microscopic examination, the affected muscles exhibit primary degeneration of muscle fibers, a considerable amount of regenerative activity, and round cell infiltration, especially around blood vessels (310) (see Fig. 14.12). In addition to perivascular cuffing by lymphocytes, there is often a true intramuscular vasculitis, with lymphocytes infiltrating the muscular wall of the vessel, endothelial swelling and proliferation, and occlusion of the lumen. The cause of the condition is obscure, but the presence of antibodies to myosin in some 90% of polymyositis patients suggests a virus-induced autoimmune process.

The course of the disease is generally downhill and, unlike in adult patients, treatment of children with corticosteroids does not seem to alter the outlook (317).

Other Inflammatory Diseases of Muscle

Rheumatic fever, rheumatoid arthritis, and the collagen vascular diseases can all be associated with an interstitial polymyositis, which is characterized by focal round cell infiltrates but lacks the vasculitis seen in dermatomyositis. Eosinophilic fasciitis may involve perivascular infiltrates within muscle of both lymphocytes and eosinophils.

A number of chronic infections, notably tuberculosis and sarcoidosis, can produce myositis. Among the types of myositis caused by parasitic infections, trichinosis is the most common entity (see Chapter 6). Also, the presenting symptom of toxoplasmosis can be polymyositis.

A relatively common entity that is best grouped with the inflammatory myopathies is myalgia cruris epidemica (318). This condition is characterized by transient severe pain and weakness affecting mainly the gastrocnemius and beginning 1 to 2 days after an upper respiratory infection. As indicated by its name, the condition occurs epidemically, most commonly in association with influenza. Muscle biopsy reveals a polymorphonuclear and mononuclear infiltrate and muscle cell necrosis. EMG studies indicate that the myositis extends beyond the clinically affected calf muscles.

Myositis also can accompany various virus infections, with symptoms usually limited to muscular aches and pains (319). In epidemic pleurodynia, however, muscles of the chest, back, and shoulders are notably painful. The myositis that accompanies human immunodeficiency virus infection is considered in Chapter 6. In some instances, accompanying cerebrospinal fluid pleocytosis indicates meningeal involvement. Pleurodynia is usually caused by a variety of coxsackievirus B. Myositis is also a feature of various parasitic diseases and of tropical polymyositis. A myopathy also is seen subsequent to treatment with penicillamine and zidovudine. Endomysial inflammation is seen in some of the muscular dystrophies, notably in FSHD, glycogen storage disease type II, and for approximately 1 month after the insertion of needle electrodes for EMG.

Congenital Myopathies

The term *congenital myopathy* encompasses a group of diseases of muscle present at birth and showing a nonprogressive course. The diagnosis of these diseases has, until recently, been confirmed only by muscle biopsy, but the elucidation of the genetic defect in some of these entities now provides DNA markers in blood. The muscle biopsy shows distinctive structural, histochemical, or both kinds of changes in each congenital myopathy, but none are necrotizing myopathies or muscular dystrophies. Nearly all the congenital myopathies are genetically determined but some, such as congenital muscle fiber-type disproportion, are syndromes that may be associated with systemic metabolic disease or may represent aberrant developmental defects of muscle maturation.

The ambiguous term "benign congenital hypotonia" previously denoted an infant with hypotonia and mild, nonprogressive weakness who either improved with maturation or at least held his own. Oppenheim's poorly described patients with amyotonia congenita, a now obsolete term, would probably belong to this group (42), along with a number of new and pathologically well-defined muscular disorders (see Table 14.4). Benign congenital hypotonia now is used only as a convenient wastebasket term to describe an infant or child with generalized hypotonia without major weakness and in whom the muscle biopsy, EMG, and all other laboratory study results are normal. It is not a diagnosis of a disease.

Congenital Muscle Fiber-Type Disproportion

Congenital muscle fiber-type disproportion (CMFTD) is defined only by muscle biopsy and requires three principal obligatory criteria: (a) disproportion in the ratio of types I and II myofibers, with 80% or more predominance of type I fibers (type II predominance is not CMFTD); (b) type I fibers that are uniformly smaller than normal from birth, whereas type II fibers are of normal diameter or mildly hypertrophic to compensate; and (c) no myofiber degeneration or regeneration (320). Other minor criteria include that the hypoplastic type I fibers retain their normal polygonal contour in transverse section and are not angular as are atrophic fibers. In some cases, an excessive number of central nuclei are found in myofibers.

In cases not associated with other congenital myopathies or with systemic or neuromuscular

metabolic diseases, the serum CK in CMFTD is invariably normal and the EMG also is normal or shows minimal nonspecific myopathic features. No molecular genetic marker exists to date. The diagnosis can be suspected from clinical features, but confirmation requires muscle biopsy with histochemistry. The incidence is unknown, but it may be the most common of the congenital myopathies.

Pure CMFTD occurs in some families and appears to follow an autosomal recessive inheritance. An autosomal dominant trait is suspected in other rare families, but is less certain. The clinical features are similar to those of nemaline rod myopathy (see following Nemaline Myopathy section), and include dolichocephaly, high palate, a generalized small mass of axial, appendicular and facial muscles, and occasionally scoliosis. Pharyngeal, respiratory, and extraocular muscles are not generally involved to the extent of causing clinically detectable deficits. Congenital contractures occasionally occur and respond well to gentle physiotherapy. Congenital subluxation of the hips is a rare complication. If central nuclei occur in myofibers as well as the CMFTD pattern, the clinical myopathic features, particularly generalized weakness, are more severe and ptosis and incomplete external ophthalmoplegia are often associated.

CMFTD also is seen as a syndrome or component of other diseases. Among neuromuscular and metabolic diseases, it is a regular part of globoid cell (Krabbe) leukodystrophy early in the course before the neuropathy produces changes of denervation-reinnervation (321,322). It is a reliable feature in the muscle biopsy of patients with nemaline rod disease (see following discussion) and is one of the patterns seen in the congenital form of myotonic dystrophy. CMFTD also is reported in some cases of glycogenoses II and III, multiple sulfatase deficiency, congenital hypothyroidism, fetal alcohol syndrome, rigid spine syndrome, minicore myopathy, and oculocerebrorenal disease of Lowe.

One of the most common nongenetic and nonneuromuscular etiologies of CMFTD is cerebellar hypoplasia and brainstem dysgeneses (323,324). Abnormal bulbospinal impulses that descend to influence the motor neuron during

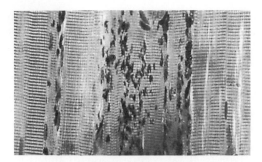

FIG. 14.13. Nemaline myopathy. Longitudinal section of muscle fibers showing rod-shaped structures occurring singly or in aggregates, the latter tending to a palisadelike arrangement (trichrome stain, ×30). (Courtesy of Dr. P. Cancilla, Department of Pathology, University of California Los Angeles, UCLA School of Medicine.)

the histochemical stage of muscle maturation (20- to 28-weeks' gestation) apparently cause distortions in the suprasegmental innervation of the fetal motor unit that alters the ratio of fiber types and the differential growth of each type of fiber (320). Generalized muscular hypotonia is a constant clinical feature of cerebellar hypoplasia as well (see Chapter 5). Should CMFTD be reported in the muscle biopsy during the course of investigation for hypotonia and mild weakness and is unexplained, particularly if the child does not have the typical facies and body habitus of the pure myopathic CMFTD, an MRI of the brain is indicated with special attention to structures in the posterior fossa.

Nemaline Myopathy

First described in 1963 independently by Shy and coworkers (325) and Conen and coworkers (326), nemaline myopathy is another common congenital myopathy. Two forms of this condition are now well defined. One is transmitted as an autosomal dominant condition with variable penetrance, whereas the other is transmitted as an autosomal recessive trait (327). The gene for the autosomal dominant condition has been localized to the long arm of chromosome 1 at the 1q21-q23 locus (328), and the gene for the autosomal recessive form is on the long arm of chromosome 2 at 2q21.2-q22 (329). The two

genetic entities are indistinguishable by clinical history or muscle biopsy.

Three clinical pictures have been recognized: a severe and almost always fatal neonatal form, which presents with hypotonia, weakness, and respiratory impairment; a milder form that also presents in the neonatal period, infancy, or early childhood and is either stationary or slowly progressive; and an adult onset form. The last form can have a benign course or at times progress rapidly (330). Children have a dysmorphic appearance, and deformities of the palate, spine, and feet have been observed. A cardiomyopathy has also been noted.

Aggregates of thread-like, intracytoplasmic rods are present in most muscle fibers (Fig. 14.13) (331). In frozen sections, they may be demonstrated by the modified Gomori trichrome stain, in which they appear red against the green of the myofibrillar proteins, and in paraffin sections they may be stained with phosphotungstic acid-hematoxylin or with the Luna-Parker acid fuscin stain. In electron microscopy these rods are found to represent an excessive accumulation of Z-band material with the same geometric periodicity as the Z-band and often seen arising from Z-bands between sarcomeres. In rare cases, intranuclear rods also are demonstrated, but how they form and become localized to sarcolemmal nuclei is unclear (332).

Chemical studies on the rod material suggest that it consists of several protein components, of which sarcomeric α-actinin is the most clearly defined, being present in increased amounts (333,334). The gene in the autosomal dominant form of nemaline myopathy, *TPM3*, transcribes for tropomyosin-3, whereas the gene for the autosomal recessive disease produces a large protein called *nebulin* (335). Both gene products are incorporated into the Z-band of the sarcomeres. Increased amounts of other normal components of the Z-band, such as actin and α-actinin, are probably secondary reactive changes.

An additional constant feature in the muscle biopsy is the presence of congenital muscle fiber-type disproportion (see previous discussion), particularly in infants. As the child grows older, and particularly in late childhood, adolescence and early adult life, a slow but gradual conversion of more of the remaining type II myofibers to type I occurs, until the muscle may contain a uniform population of small type I myofibers. This histochemical conversion is not necessarily associated with clinical progression of the disease, but some cases do appear to show increased weakness (336).

The presence of nemaline bodies is not diagnostic of nemaline myopathy, because it also may occur as a nonspecific finding. Nemaline bodies have been seen in skeletal muscle after experimental tenotomy and in a variety of human disease entities, including polymyositis, other autoimmune vascular disease, and in human immunodeficiency virus infection (337). An adult onset nemaline rod myopathy is sporadic and not related to either of the two genetic forms found in children.

Central Core Disease

Central core disease, transmitted as an autosomal dominant trait, is characterized by mild and nonprogressive muscle weakness that is either proximal or generalized and is of early onset. The basic defect in this condition is located in the gene for the ryanodine receptor. This gene codes for a tetramer receptor to a calcium channel found in the membrane of muscle sarcoplasmic reticulum. This nonvoltage-gated channel, which is characterized by its ability to bind ryanodine, a plant alkaloid, plays an important role in excitation-contraction coupling and calcium transport (338,339). Central core disease is often associated with muscle contractures around the knees and hips and with various skeletal defects, including congenital dislocation of the hips and patella, kyphoscoliosis, and pes cavus. There is high incidence of cardiac abnormalities, and virtually all subjects are susceptible to malignant hypothermia (340). This observation has been explained by the finding that malignant hyperthermia, like central core disease, results from a mutation in the same ryanodine receptor gene (341). The serum CK is generally normal when the patient is not experiencing malignant hyperthermic rhabdomyolysis.

When muscle is stained with trichrome, the central areas of affected muscle fibers stain blue, whereas peripheral fibers appear red. With histochemical stains specific for the mitochondrial oxidative enzymes, the central area stains less intensively than the periphery of the fiber, and there is a type I fiber predominance, often so extensive that only a few scattered type II fibers remain or none are found in the biopsy (342). Brooke has observed that the severity of the changes in muscle is unrelated to the clinical weakness (2).

Because of the close clinical and genetic association with malignant hyperthermia, patients with central core disease who require a general anesthetic should be pretreated with dantrolene sodium before surgery as a precaution.

Minicore (Multicore) Myopathy

Minicore (multicore) myopathy is distinct from central core disease (343). It manifests shortly after birth with a rather benign nonprogressive generalized hypotonia, but in adolescence approximately 10% of patients develop a rigid spine and progressive kyphoscoliosis. The Swash-Schwartz variant of familial multicore disease is marked by a myopathy that also includes external ophthalmoplegia (344). Hypertrophic cardiomyopathy is reported rarely. Other inconstant complications include endocrinopathies, small stature, and severe mental retardation, but most patients are intellectually normal.

The diagnosis is confirmed by muscle biopsy, which shows multiple cores within myofibers with defects in histochemical enzymatic activities in the cores. CMFTD is reported in a few infants. Poor registry of Z-bands, disarray of myofilaments, and cores of amorphous granular material are seen ultrastructurally. The disorder appears to be genetically heterogeneous.

Myotubular (Centronuclear) Myopathy

A group of disorders characterized by rows of central nuclei in most myofibers have been termed *myotubular myopathies* because of their similarity to the architecture of the normal human fetal myotube at 8- to 15-weeks' gestation. However, few other features support the hypothesis of true maturational arrest (345).

The most common form of centronuclear myopathy is transmitted as an autosomal dominant condition with variable penetrance. Children affected with this disorder show a slowly progressive weakness of the limb girdles and neck muscles, with acute fluctuations coinciding with respiratory illnesses (346). Although there is considerable clinical heterogeneity, ptosis and weakness of the extraocular muscles appear to be characteristic for most cases (347).

A more severe, X-linked recessive disease is well defined, in which hypotonia, diffuse weakness, inability to swallow, and respiratory failure appear during the neonatal period (348). The muscle biopsy is diagnostic and shows many abnormal features, but usually good histochemical differentiation is seen, although sometimes there is a predominance of type I fibers and registry of Z-bands, features that develop much later than the myotubular stage (343). The central nuclei in rows within the myofibers are always spaced with two to four nuclear diameters between them, unlike fetal myotubes, and the condensation of chromatin is that of the term neonate, not the fetus. Mothers, who are obligate carriers, can show mild muscle weakness and have minor changes in their muscle biopsy.

Infantile Myofibrillar Myopathy

Infantile myofibrillar myopathy is characterized clinically by mainly dysphagia in early infancy disproportionately severe in relation to the mild generalized weakness, although respiratory muscle insufficiency sometimes occurs. Gastrostomy often is required, but patients gradually improve and the gastrostomy can be removed by 3 to 4 years of age when the child is able to swallow adequately. Mild axial weakness may persist, with a mild Gowers' sign and a mild hip-waddle gait. Intelligence and neurologic development proceed normally.

The muscle biopsy is diagnostic. It shows ultrastructural changes of two or three disorganized sarcomeres with normal sarcomeres on either side of the same myofibril, and some severely atrophic fibers with disrupted myofilaments and fragmented Z-bands. Alterations in

cristae are demonstrated in some mitochondria. Massive type I fiber predominance and desmin accumulation are shown by light microscopy. In some families, mitochondrial defects in complex III, associated with 7.5-kb deletions of mtDNA are demonstrated, but other families do not show mitochondrial defects (349).

Mitochondrial Diseases (Mitochondrial Cytopathies)

Although muscle dysfunction is a prime feature in the majority of mitochondrial disorders, their discussion has been relegated to the chapter dealing with metabolic disorders of the nervous system (see Chapter 1).

Other Congenital Myopathies

A number of other rare congenital myopathies have now been recognized on the basis of their distinctive intramuscular structures. Their clinical and pathologic features are summarized in Table 14.4. Although these diseases were formerly termed *benign congenital hypotonias*, it is becoming clear that some are hardly benign, and that respiratory or bulbar musculature weakness can prove fatal at an early age.

Congenital Absence of Specific Muscles and Segmental and Generalized Amyoplasia

Unilateral or bilateral congenital absence of muscle is more frequently observed in the pectoral group than elsewhere. Absence of the abdominal musculature is commonly associated with defects of the urinary tract and hydronephrosis (350). The palmaris longus muscle of the volar forearm is congenitally absent in approximately 30% of normal individuals and is asymptomatic, compensated in function by the flexor carpi ulnaris and flexor carpi radialis.

Segmental amyoplasia is absence of muscles derived from defective somites in a segmental distribution. The most common segmental amyoplasia is associated with sacral agenesis. In this condition absent or defective myotomes belong to the same embryonic somites that fail to give rise to the sclerotomes that form the vertebral bodies at those same levels; dysplasia of the spinal cord occurs because of lack of induction by the notochord. Because all other components of muscle, such as the connective tissue, blood vessels, nerves, and tendons are derived from the lateral mesoderm or from the neural crest, and the myotomes form only the myofibers themselves, the other components are present, but the myofibers are replaced by fat. Sacral agenesis is most commonly associated with maternal diabetes mellitus, and *rumpless chicks* are experimentally produced by injecting insulin into incubating eggs. In the autosomal dominant form of sacral agenesis, the defective *Sonic hedgehog* is the same gene that has a mutation in a common form of holoprosencephaly, at the other end of the neural tube (see Chapter 4).

Generalized amyoplasia is not compatible with life and is probably caused by defective myogenic gene expression, as occurs in a mouse model. There are four genes using basic helix-loop-helix transcription factors recognized as critical in myogenesis; these proto-oncogenes are known as myogenic factor 5 (*myf5*), *myogenin*, which promotes the fusion of myoblasts to form myotubes, *herculin* (also known as *mrf4* or *myf6*) and *MyoD1*. *MyoD1* and *myf5* may compensate for each other if either is defective, but loss of both gene expressions cannot be compensated, nor can loss of *myogenin* or *herculin* alone (5,351).

Muscular Hypertrophy and Pseudohypertrophy

Hypertrophy of muscle is a physiologic process, such as work hypertrophy, the muscular enlargement induced by exercise. Pseudohypertrophy differs from hypertrophy because the enlargement of muscles is caused by a pathologic process.

Congenital muscular hypertrophy can be associated with several different conditions. Generalized pseudohypertrophy occurs in myotonia congenita (see previous discussion), and restricted pseudohypertrophy of the calves, tongue, and forearms occurs in Duchenne and Becker muscular dystrophies (see previous discussion). Pseudohypertrophy of muscle also may occur paradoxically in denervation, although neurogenic atrophy is the usual response. It sometimes occurs in hereditary sensory motor neuropathies.

In 1934, de Lange reported three children with generalized muscular enlargement, severe mental retardation, and widespread porencephaly (352). In some instances, the hypertrophy diminished as the children matured, but all patients remained severely mentally defective.

Hypothyroidism (Debre-Sémélaigne syndrome) (353,354) and myotonic dystrophy are other rare causes of congenital muscular pseudohypertrophy. In muscular pseudohypertrophy associated with hypothyroidism, type I muscle fibers are atrophied and oxidative enzyme activity is abnormal, with a collection of glycogen in the subsarcolemmal areas (355). Finally, in Beckwith-Wiedemann syndrome, generalized or unilateral muscle hypertrophy is associated with generalized or unilateral macroglossia. Additional features include omphalocele, facial nevus flammeus, neonatal hypoglycemia with pancreatic hyperplasia, gigantism with increased bone age, and mild microcephaly. This condition is covered in Chapter 3.

Periodic Paralysis

Hypokalemic Periodic Paralysis

The clinical picture of acute transient paralysis of the musculature of the trunk and extremities with complete freedom from symptoms between attacks was noted first by Shakhnovitch in 1882 (356) and by Westphal in 1885 (357). This condition is distinct from hyperkalemic periodic paralysis, considered in this chapter in conjunction with the myotonic disorders.

Pathogenesis

The disease is the consequence of mutations in the gene that encodes the muscle dihydropyridine-sensitive calcium channel α_1-subunit (*CACNL1A3*). The gene has been mapped to chromosome 1q32, but there is genetic heterogeneity. The gene encodes a dihydropyridine receptor that functions as a voltage-gated calcium channel (358).

The importance of potassium and sodium metabolism in the clinical manifestations of the disease is well documented. Severe attacks are usually preceded by sodium retention in the body. During an attack, the plasma potassium decreases as weakness develops. Symptoms usually become evident at a serum potassium concentration of 3 mEq/L and are marked at between 2.5 and 2.0 mEq/L. Because healthy subjects do not develop significant muscle weakness when, as a result of electrolyte imbalance, their serum potassium drops to 2.5 mEq/L, it is unlikely that weakness results directly from a potassium deficiency. More likely, the converse actually takes place, for weakened muscle has a higher potassium concentration than the same muscle sampled between attacks.

It appears likely that muscle weakness results from an abnormal ratio between sodium and potassium conductances. Muscle sodium content is considerably elevated between attacks and remains unchanged or only slightly reduced with the development of paralysis. These findings suggest that potassium shifts into the muscle before or along with the onset of paralysis (359).

A muscle biopsy performed during a paralytic attack reveals marked vacuolization of the sarcoplasm (360). This abnormality is caused by an enormous dilatation of the endoplasmic reticulum and disappears once normal muscle function is regained.

Clinical Manifestations

Hypokalemic periodic paralysis is quite rare. In Finland its current prevalence is 0.4 in 100,000 (361). It is transmitted as an autosomal dominant trait with 100% penetrance in male subjects and markedly reduced penetrance in female subjects. In 88% of cases, attacks first occur between the ages of 7 and 21 years. They can vary from slight transient weakness to almost complete paralysis (362). Most attacks last 6 to 24 hours and affect primarily the lower limbs. Bulbar and respiratory muscles are the last to become paralyzed, and death during an attack can occur in as many as

10% of patients. The most consistent factors predisposing to an attack are prolonged rest after vigorous exercise, a heavy carbohydrate meal, the administration of insulin, and exposure to cold. Administration of adrenocorticotropic hormone and a number of mineralocorticoid compounds, notably 2-methyl-9-α-fluorohydrocortisone, also induce paralysis.

During an attack, the subject has a flaccid paralysis that is most complete in the proximal musculature, a loss of deep tendon reflexes, and absent electric and mechanical excitability. Between attacks, patients are free of symptoms. Permanent wasting and proximal and distal muscle weakness can develop, however, even in patients who experience only rare attacks (363).

Treatment

Paralytic attacks are best treated by the oral administration of potassium. Prophylactically, a low carbohydrate diet and administration of supplemental potassium at bedtime is advisable. A low sodium intake and administration of diuretics, notably acetazolamide, also have been effective in preventing attacks or at least in reducing their frequency. Spironolactone, an aldosterone antagonist given in dosages of 100 to 200 mg/day, also appears to be of benefit. None of these drugs, however, prevents the development of progressive muscular atrophy.

Normokalemic Periodic Paralysis

Periodic attacks of severe weakness, commencing in early childhood and lasting up to several weeks, are the characteristic features of a third, extremely rare type of periodic paralysis, normokalemic paralysis, transmitted as an autosomal dominant. Large amounts of sodium (460 mEq/24 hours for the average adult) can relieve the weakness in this condition, and attacks can occasionally be prevented by the prolonged administration of acetazolamide (364).

Differential Diagnosis

When a child experiences recurrent attacks of muscular weakness, a number of conditions should be considered. Hypokalemic periodic paralysis is diagnosed by the family history, a clinical response to potassium, and concurrent hypokalemia. In the absence of a family history, recurrent paralytic attacks can be caused by a sporadic form of the disease. In some sporadic cases of hypokalemic periodic paralysis, observed mainly in young male adults of Asian background, thyrotoxicosis appears to be a major predisposing factor (365). Renal tubular acidosis, ingestion of licorice extract (366), or barium poisoning incurred by ingestion of table salt contaminated with barium chloride or flour contaminated with barium carbonate also must be considered when muscle weakness is accompanied by hypokalemia (367,368). In barium poisoning, muscle weakness results from an interruption of the passive efflux of intracellular potassium, with a consequent net increase in muscle cell potassium (368). Periodic attacks of muscle weakness are seen also in primary hyperaldosteronism. The striking alkalosis, hypernatremia, and hypokalemia that accompany the attacks aid diagnosis.

Hyperkalemic periodic paralysis is distinguished by the early onset of brief but frequent attacks and their induction through the administration of potassium. In normokalemic periodic paralysis, attacks are more severe and of longer duration, but sometimes are induced also by potassium.

In myasthenia gravis, weakness almost always affects the bulbar as well as the skeletal musculature, and deep tendon reflexes can be preserved during an attack. A clear-cut improvement in muscle strength after the administration of anticholinesterases confirms the diagnosis. Recurrent muscle weakness is seen also in myopathies associated with abnormal mitochondria and in polyneuropathies, particularly those accompanying intermittent acute porphyria. It is a prominent feature of paroxysmal myoglobinuria and muscle phosphorylase deficiency. Accidental or intentional ipecac ingestion can induce a reversible proximal myopathy (369,370).

Anderson syndrome is an autosomal dominant condition that is distinct from hypokalemic periodic paralysis. It is marked by periodic weakness, ventricular arrhythmias, short stature, and dis-

tinctive facial features, notably low-set ears, hypertelorism, and mandibular hypoplasia. A prolonged QT interval is seen in approximately 80% of subjects. Attacks of paralysis can be initiated by an oral potassium challenge but the shifts in serum potassium are inconsistent and hyperkalemia, normokalemia, or hypokalemia have been documented (371).

Muscle Phosphorylase Deficiency (Glycogenosis Type V, McArdle Disease)

This condition, described by McArdle in 1951 (372), was the first inheritable myopathy for which the enzymatic abnormality, an absence of muscle phosphorylase activity, was recognized. Clinical onset is in childhood, with painful muscle cramps and weakness after exertion and episodes of myoglobulinuria. In a typical case, when the forearm muscle is exercised with its arterial circulation occluded, the flexor muscles go into contracture within a minute and remain in this state for an hour or longer after circulation is restored (373). In contrast to normal muscle, there is no increase in venous lactate.

A severe neonatal form of myophosphorylase usually results in neonatal death from respiratory muscle failure and severe generalized weakness. Muscle biopsy shows an excess of glycogen and only scattered myofibers that express phosphorylase.

The disease is transmitted as an autosomal recessive disorder with a predilection for male subjects. The gene has been localized to the long arm of chromosome 11 (374). There is considerable genetic heterogeneity occurs, with at least 12 allelic variants and a high incidence of compound heterozygotes having been described (375). Several clinical variants have been reported including an infantile form, presenting with progressive muscular weakness (376).

Muscle biopsy shows an increased concentration of glycogen, and enzymatic studies reveal the specific defect in muscle phosphorylase activity. In some 85% of cases, immunologically reactive enzyme protein is undetectable. Some of the patients with biochemically inactive enzyme protein appear to have a defect in the enzyme-activating system, specifically in the cyclic

AMP-dependent muscle phosphorylase b kinase. This autosomal recessive condition has been designated as glycogenosis type VIII (377,378).

Muscle phosphorylase deficiency was the first neuromuscular disorder diagnosed by nuclear MR spectroscopy. By means of this technique it can be shown that with exercise, intramuscular pH does not decrease, but the concentration of phosphocreatine decreases excessively. There is no depletion of adenosine triphosphate (379). Erythrocyte and liver phosphorylase, enzymes that are chemically different, are present in normal amounts.

The sequence of biochemical events leading to contractures and myoglobinuria is still unclear. There is some evidence that premature fatigue results from impaired excitation-contraction coupling caused by an accumulation of adenosine diphosphate (380). Because glycogenolysis is interrupted, energy for ordinary muscular effort must be derived from the oxidation of glucose or fatty acids.

Congenital Defect of Phosphofructokinase (Glycogenosis Type VII)

Congenital defect of phosphofructokinase (glycogenosis type VII) is transmitted as an autosomal recessive trait with an increased incidence in male subjects. Subjects with a congenital defect of muscle phosphofructokinase tend to have a long history of easy fatigability and of weakness or stiffness induced by exertion (381). In addition, decreased insulin secretion occurs in response to glucose (382). An infantile form, presenting with congenital weakness and respiratory insufficiency, has been recognized also (383). CK levels are usually elevated and, as occurs in muscle phosphorylase deficiency, there is no increase in venous lactate with ischemic exercise. A mild hemolytic anemia is often present. In erythrocytes, enzyme activity is reduced by some 50%, but it is normal in leukocytes. Two subunits of phosphofructokinase M (muscle type) and L (liver type) have been recognized, with the muscle type subunit being inactive in this disease. The gene for phosphofructokinase has been mapped to chromosome 12q13.3, and numerous mutations have been described, with the disease being most frequent in the Ashkenazi Jewish population. Because the enzyme defect precludes glucose utilization in these individuals, energy for muscle contraction must be derived from fatty acid oxidation or, conceivably, from enhancement of the usually unimportant hexose monophosphate shunt.

Although many other defects of muscle carbohydrate metabolism are theoretically possible, the only well-documented ones at this time are caused by defects in phosphoglycerate mutase deficiency and aldolase A. Patients with phosphoglyceromutase deficiency have a lifelong history of muscle pains, cramps, and weakness after exercise (384). The enzyme defect also can result in hemolytic anemia, seizures, and mental retardation (380). Subjects with aldolase A deficiency present with unexplained episodes of jaundice and anemia, accompanied by a marked elevation in CK and microcephaly. Muscle biopsy discloses lipid accumulation and distorted and vacuolated mitochondrial cristae (385).

Myoadenylate deaminase deficiency appears to be a relatively common autosomal recessive entity that can be asymptomatic or can present with exertional myalgia during the first or second decade of life (386).

Defects of Mitochondrial Transport (Lipid Storage Myopathies)

Since their first description by Engel and coworkers in 1970 on the basis of a pathologic picture of lipid droplets within type 1 fibers (387), a number of distinct biochemical entities have been recognized, all sharing a defect in the use of long-chain fatty acids by skeletal muscle.

Carnitine (L-3-hydroxy-4-trimethylammonium butyrate) is present in large amounts in skeletal muscle, where it stimulates mitochondrial oxidation of the coenzyme A derivatives of long-chain fatty acids (acyl-CoA), notably palmitate, by facilitating their transport from cytoplasm into the inner mitochondrial compartment (Fig. 14.14). The transfer of palmitoyl acyl-CoA is accomplished by its transesterification to form a long-chain fatty acylcarnitine. This reaction is catalyzed by carnitine palmitoyl transferase I, an enzyme located on the outer surface of the inner

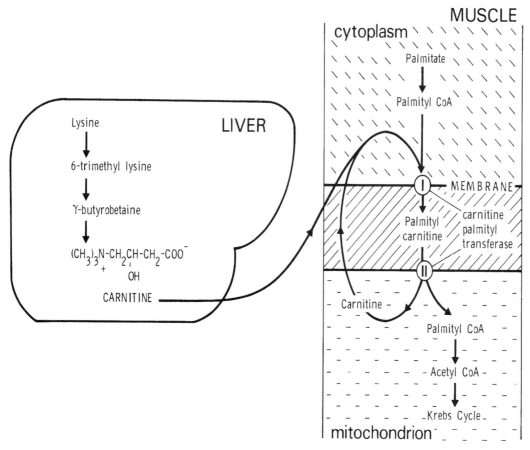

FIG. 14.14. Muscle carnitine metabolism. Not shown in this figure is a carnitine transporter that carries carnitine to the inner aspect of the outer mitochondrial membrane where carnitine palmityl transferase I (CPT I) catalyses its reaction with palmityl-CoA to form palmitylcarnitine. After the formation of palmitylcarnitine, a translocase carries the acylcarnitine to the inner aspect of the inner mitochondrial membrane where CPT II converts palmitylcarnitine to free carnitine and palmityl-CoA.

mitochondrial membrane. Carnitine is supplied for this reaction by a carnitine transporter. A translocase then carries the acylcarnitine across the barrier of the inner mitochondrial membrane. There the acylcarnitine complex is cleaved by a second carnitine palmitoyl transferase (II) to form acyl-CoA, which then enters the β-oxidation pathway (388).

Carnitine occurs naturally in food, notably in meat and fish, but the amounts ingested in a normal diet are insufficient to meet body requirements. Carnitine is also synthesized in several tissues, including liver, according to the pathway outlined in Figure 14.14. Aside from functioning in the transport of fatty acids into

mitochondria, carnitine is used to detoxify the acyl-CoA compounds. Large amounts of acyl-CoA derivatives, such as are seen in the various organic acidurias (see Chapter 1), can inhibit a variety of enzymes, notably the pyruvate dehydrogenase complex and glutamate dehydrogenase, which in turn aggravates the basic enzymatic defect and sets into motion a vicious circle. When the amount of carnitine is insufficient to buffer the toxic acyl-CoA compounds, a carnitine deficiency is said to exist (389).

Most workers distinguish between a primary and a secondary carnitine deficiency, with secondary deficiency being encountered far more commonly. In fact, doubt exists whether primary carnitine deficiency actually exists, or whether it reflects an underlying, as yet undiscovered metabolic defect reducing the concentration of free carnitine. Several infants who initially were thought to have a primary systemic carnitine deficiency were subsequently found to have a defect in medium-chain acyl-CoA dehydrogenase, another infant was found to have a defect in short-chain acyl-CoA dehydrogenase, and another patient with muscle carnitine deficiency was shown to have a defect in short-chain acyl-CoA dehydrogenase that for unknown reasons was restricted to muscle (390,391).

Normal total plasma carnitine concentrations run between 40 and 60 μmol/L, with between 70% and 90% of carnitine in the free (unesterified) state (391,392). Patients with secondary carnitine deficiency generally have a high ratio of plasma acylcarnitine (esterified carnitine) to free carnitine. The causes for secondary carnitine deficiency are multitudinous (393). Aside from its presence in the various acyl-CoA dehydrogenase deficiencies and the organic acidemias, it is seen in disorders of mitochondrial function, in several other inborn errors of metabolism, including maple syrup urine disease, in infants having an inadequate dietary intake, in Reye syndrome, in renal failure, and in patients receiving valproate or salicylates (389).

The primary carnitine deficiencies have been divided into systemic and muscle forms, a distinction that will likely turn out to be artificial. Systemic forms have low levels of carnitine in plasma, liver, and muscle, whereas muscle forms have low carnitine levels in muscle only.

The most clearly defined primary carnitine deficiency syndrome is an autosomal recessive disorder characterized by a defect in intracellular uptake of carnitine (394). This condition probably encompasses some of the previously reported cases of muscle carnitine deficiency. The clinical picture is highlighted by a progressive cardiomyopathy and weakness that develops in late infancy or early childhood. This was the clinical presentation in 70% of cases compiled by Stanley and coworkers (394). In 45%, the initial manifestation was an episode of hypoglycemic coma. Rarely, the presentation resem-

bles a sudden infant death syndrome-like episode (395). Plasma and muscle carnitine levels are markedly reduced and a defect in carnitine uptake has been shown in fibroblasts and leukocytes. The renal transport system for carnitine is believed to be impaired also, resulting in defective renal conservation of carnitine. Skeletal muscle contains lipid inclusions that are mainly seen in type 1 fibers. Electron microscopy shows the mitochondria to appear abnormal, with increased number and size, and intramitochondrial inclusions (396). There is an associated metabolic acidosis, probably secondary to an accumulation of lactic acid, and urinary organic acids are normal or show only slight elevations of medium-chain dicarboxylic acids.

The defect in this condition has been localized to a gene, mapped to chromosome 5q31, which codes for a plasmalemmal sodium ion-dependent, high-affinity carnitine transporter (397,398).

Response to treatment with oral carnitine (50 mg/kg per day L-carnitine) corrects the clinical signs of myopathy, although skeletal muscle carnitine levels remain markedly reduced.

Carnitine Palmitoyl Transferase Deficiencies

Cases with documented carnitine palmitoyl transferase II deficiency are more common than those with carnitine palmitoyl transferase I deficiency of which there are only a few adequately documented cases. In these, children present with recurrent Reye syndrome–like episodes, marked by nonketotic hypoglycemic coma, mild hyperammonemia, renal tubular acidosis, and elevated plasma free fatty acids (399). Treatment with medium-chain triglycerides that are transported into mitochondria without the need of the carnitine palmitoyl transferase system has been effective. The gene for carnitine palmitoyl transferase I deficiency has been mapped to chromosome 11q, whereas the gene for carnitine palmitoyl transferase II deficiency has been mapped to chromosome 1p32.

Carnitine palmitoyl transferase II deficiency has two modes of presentation. In older children or adults the disorder is characterized by exercise intolerance and attacks of rhabdomyolysis with myoglobinuria precipitated by fasting, cold stress, prolonged, but not necessarily strenuous, physical activity, or high fat intake (400,401). In newborns, carnitine palmitoyl transferase II deficiency is a generally lethal disease, marked by hypoglycemia, cardiac arrhythmia, or severe myopathy (402–404). Serum and muscle carnitine levels are generally reduced, and palmitoyl transferase activity is decreased in muscle and in various other tissues, including liver and fibroblasts (405). Although there is some lipid accumulation in muscle, this disorder is not a lipid myopathy in that there is little or no lipid storage in muscle (406). Probably, this enzymatic defect precludes the use of fatty acids required to maintain muscle energy when glycogen stores are depleted by prolonged exercise. A high carbohydrate intake before exercise usually prevents symptoms, and treatment with medium-chain triglycerides appears also to be effective.

Another disorder in mitochondrial oxidation of fatty acids affects the carnitine-acylcarnitine translocase. Symptoms develop in infancy and are marked by seizures, apnea, and bradycardia. Generalized muscle weakness becomes apparent in survivors (407). Dietary supplementation with carnitine appears to be ineffective in this condition.

Lipid Myopathy with Normal Carnitine Levels

In several instances, the pathologic picture of lipid inclusions within type 1 muscle fibers has been unaccompanied by any discernible disorder in the metabolism of fatty acids (408,409). The clinical picture of these conditions is variable; most patients have a congenital, nonprogressive myopathy. Because most of the clinical descriptions lack currently available biochemical and enzymatic studies, their nature is unclear. One form, Dorfman-Chanarin disease, is characterized by ichthyosis, cardiomyopathy, and neutral lipid storage in muscles, hepatocytes, granulocytes, and the gastrointestinal endothelium. It is accompanied by impaired oxidation of long-chain fatty acids (410). The various lipid storage myopathies have been reviewed by Di Donato (396).

Myoglobinuria

Myoglobinuria is a rare syndrome with a variety of causes, both hereditary and sporadic (31, 411,412).

Its causes include disorders resulting from defective energy production (e.g., exertional myoglobinuria), myoglobinuria accompanying convulsions, and the various hereditary enzymatic defects already discussed, notably muscle phosphorylase deficiency, phosphofructokinase deficiency, or deficient carnitine palmitoyl transferase activity (412). These conditions are reviewed by Tein and coworkers (413). Exercise-induced myoglobinuria and progressive muscular weakness also can be caused by a mutation in the mitochondrial DNA coding for cytochrome b, and myoglobinuria precipitated by febrile illness can be transmitted as a dominant trait (414,415).

Sporadic myoglobinuria also can be caused by hypoxia, as occurs in carbon monoxide poisoning, by a primary muscle injury, such as accompanies trauma or burns, or after an infectious illness, notably viral illnesses with myalgic prodromes. Additionally, myoglobinuria can be encountered subsequent to exposure to a variety of toxins and medications (e.g., alcohol, barbiturates, amphotericin B, clozapine, colchicine, cyclohexanone, and licorice). It also can follow insect bites and envenomation (416) (see Chapter 9).

Patients characteristically have severe muscle pain and weakness accompanied by the passage of brown urine. Serum enzymes are strikingly elevated, and blood creatine kinase values of 50,000 units or higher have been reported. Occasionally, acute renal tubular necrosis accompanies the attack.

The presence of myoglobin is suggested by a positive benzidine test in an erythrocyte-free urine. The pigment is identified by acrylamide gel electrophoresis or immunodiffusion techniques or, more simply, albeit less specifically, by dipsticks such as Hemoccult (416).

In evaluating a child, often an adolescent, with muscle pain and easy fatigability, a creatine kinase determination and an erythrocyte sedimentation test are the two most helpful screening tests (417). In the experience of Mills and Edwards, a specific diagnosis could be made in almost every patient with an elevated creatine kinase or erythrocyte sedimentation rate (417). An enzymatic defect, the most common cause, was seen in 15% of patients. In half of these, a mitochondrial myopathy was diagnosed by muscle biopsy. The remaining patients had muscle phosphorylase deficiency or, less often, muscle phosphofructokinase deficiency. Of the nonmetabolic cases with muscle pain, inflammatory and endocrine myopathies and a neurogenic disorder were the major diagnostic categories. Most of the undiagnosed patients were found to be depressed.

REFERENCES

1. Engel AG, Franzini-Armstrong C. *Myology: basic and clinical*, 2nd ed. New York: McGraw–Hill, 1994.
2. Brooke MH. *A clinician's view of neuromuscular diseases*, 2nd ed. Baltimore: Williams & Wilkins, 1986.
3. Dubowitz V. *Muscle biopsy. A practical approach*, 2nd ed. London: Baillière Tindall, 1985.
4. Swash M. *Neuromuscular diseases. A practical approach to diagnosis and management*, 3rd ed. Berlin: Springer-Verlag, 1997.
5. Sarnat HB. Neuromuscular disorders. In: Behrman RE, Kliegman RM, Arvin AM, eds. *Nelson textbook of pediatrics*, 16th ed. Philadelphia: WB Saunders, 1999:1867–1893.
6. Ouvrier RA, McLeod JG, Pollard JD. *Peripheral neuropathy in childhood*, 2nd ed. London, UK: MacKeith Press, 1999.
7. Zuberi SM, Matta N, Nawaz S. Muscle ultrasound in the assessment of suspected neuromuscular disease in childhood. *Neuromusc Disord* 1999;9:203–207.
8. Byers TJ, et al. ELISA quantitation of dystrophin for the diagnosis of Duchenne and Becker muscular dystrophies. *Neurology* 1992;42:570–576.
8a. Fukuyama Y, et al. Percutaneous needle muscle biopsy in the diagnosis of neuromuscular disorders in children. Histological, histochemical and electron microscopic studies. *Brain Dev* 1981;3:277–287.
9. Voit T, et al. Preserved merosin M-chain (or laminin-α2) expression in skeletal muscle distinguishes Walker-Warburg syndrome from Fukuyama muscular dystrophy and merosin-deficient congenital muscular dystrophy. *Neuropediatrics* 1995;26:148–155.
10. Refsum S, Skillicorn SA. Amyotrophic familial spastic paraplegia. *Neurology* 1954;4:40–47.
11. Lefebvre S, et al. Identification and characterization of a spinal muscular atrophy-determining gene. *Cell* 1995;80:155–165.
12. Monani UR, et al. A single nucleotide difference that alters splicing patterns distinguishes the SMA gene SMN1 from the copy gene SMN2. *Hum Mol Genet* 1999;8:1177–1183.
13. Werdnig G. Zwei frühinfantile hereditäre Fälle von progressiver Muskelatrophie unter dem Bilde der Dystrophie, aber auf neurotischer Grundlage. *Arch Psychiat Nervenkr* 1891;22:437–481.

14. Hoffmann J. Über chronische spinale Muskelatrophie im Kindesalter auf familiärer Basis. *Dtsch Z Nervenheilk* 1893;3:427–470.
15. Biros I, Forrest S. Spinal muscular atrophy: untangling the knot? *J Med Genet* 1999;36:1–8.
16. Burghes AHM. When is a deletion not a deletion? When it is converted. *Am J Hum Genet* 1997;61:9–15.
16a. Roy N, et al. Refined physical map of the spinal muscular atrophy gene (SMA) region at 5 q13 based on YAC and cosmid contiguous arrays. *Genomics* 1995; 26:451–460.
16b. Lorson CL, et al. A single nucleotide in the SMN gene regulates splicing and is responsible for spinal muscular atrophy. *Proc Natl Acad Sci U S A* 1999;96: 6307–6311.
16c. Scharf JM, et al. Identification of a candidate modifying gene for spinal muscular atrophy by comparative genomics. *Nat Genet* 1998;20:83–86.
17. McAndrew PE, et al. Identification of proximal spinal muscular atrophy carriers and patients by analysis of SMNT and SMNC gene copy number. *Am J Hum Genet* 1997;60:1411–1422.
17a. Battaglia G, et al. Expression of the SMN gene, the spinal muscular atrophy determining gene, in the mammalian central nervous system. *Hum Mol Genet* 1997;6:1961–1971.
17b. Iwahashi H, et al. Synergistic anti-apoptotic activity between Bcl-2 and SMN implicated in spinal muscular atrophy. *Nature* 1997;390:413–417.
18. Sarnat HB. Research strategies in spinal muscular atrophy. In: Gamstorp I, Sarnat HB, eds. *Progressive spinal muscular atrophies*. New York: Raven Press, 1984:225–233.
19. Chou SM, Nonaka I. Werdnig-Hoffmann disease: proposal of a pathogenetic mechanism. *Acta Neuropathol* 1978;41:45–54.
20. Probst A, et al. Sensory ganglion neuropathy in infantile spinal muscular atrophy. Light and electron microscopic findings in two cases. *Neuropediatrics* 1981;12: 215–231.
21. Kumagai T, Hashizume Y. Morphological and morphometric studies on the spinal cord lesion in Werdnig-Hoffmann disease. *Brain Dev* 1982;4:87–96.
22. Lowrie MB, Vrbovà G. Dependence of postnatal motoneurones on their targets: review and hypothesis. *Trends Neurosci* 1992;15:80–84.
23. Fidzianska A, Goebel HH, Warlo I. Acute infantile spinal muscular atrophy. Muscle apoptosis as a proposed pathogenetic mechanism. *Brain* 1990;113:433–445.
24. Altman J. Programmed cell death: the paths to suicide. *Trends Neurosci* 1992;15:278–280.
25. Kuzuhara S, Chou SM. Preservation of the phrenic motoneurons in Werdnig-Hoffmann disease. *Ann Neurol* 1981;9:506–510.
26. Brandt S. *Werdnig-Hoffmann's progressive muscular atrophy*. Copenhagen: Ejnar Munksgaard, 1950.
27. Mellins RB, et al. Respiratory distress as the initial manifestation of Werdnig-Hoffmann disease. *Pediatrics* 1974;53:33–40.
28. Pearce J, Harriman DG. Chronic spinal muscular atrophy. *J Neurol Neurosurg Psychiatry* 1966;29:509–520.
29. Dubowitz V. Infantile muscular atrophy: a prospective study with particular reference to a slowly progressive variety. *Brain* 1964;87:707–718.
30. Moosa A, Dubowitz V. Spinal muscular atrophy in childhood. Two clues to clinical diagnosis. *Arch Dis Child* 1973;48:386–388.

31. Dubowitz V. *Muscle disorders in childhood*, 2nd ed. Philadelphia: WB Saunders, 1995.
32. Van Wijngaarden GK, Bethlem J. Benign infantile spinal muscular atrophy. A prospective study. *Brain* 1973;96:163–170.
33. Wohlfart G, Fex J, Eliasson S. Hereditary proximal spinal muscular atrophy—a clinical entity simulating progressive muscular dystrophy. *Acta Psychiatr Neurol Scand* 1955;30:395–406.
34. Kugelberg E, Welander L. Heredofamilial juvenile muscular atrophy simulating muscular dystrophy. *Arch Neurol Psychiatry* 1956;75:500–509.
35. Müller B. Proximal spinal muscular atrophy (SMA) Types II and III in the same sibship are not caused by different alleles at the SMA locus. *Am J Hum Genet* 1992;50:892–895.
36. Tsukagoshi H, et al. Kugelberg-Welander syndrome with dominant inheritance. *Arch Neurol* 1966;14: 378–381.
37. Dale AJ, Engel AG, Rudd NL. Familial hexosaminidase A deficiency with Kugelberg-Welander phenotype and mental changes. *Ann Neurol* 1983;14:109.
37a. van der Steege G, et al. PCR-based DNA test to confirm clinical diagnosis of autosomal recessive spinal muscular atrophy. *Lancet* 1995;345:985–986.
38. Denny-Brown D, Pennybacker JB. Fibrillation and fasciculation in voluntary muscle. *Brain* 1938;61:311–338.
39. Buchthal F, Olsen PZ. Electromyography and muscle biopsy in infantile spinal muscular atrophy. *Brain* 1970;93:15–30.
40. Moosa A, Dubowitz V. Motor nerve conduction velocity in spinal muscular atrophy of childhood. *Arch Dis Child* 1976;51:974–977.
41. Walton JH. The limp child. *J Neurol Neurosurg Psychiatry* 1957;20:144–154.
42. Oppenheim H. Über allgemeine und localisierte Atonie der Muskulatur (Myatonia) im frühen Kindesalter. *Monatsschr Psychiatr Neurol* 1900;8:232–233.
43. Ford FR. Congenital laxity of ligaments. In: *Diseases of the nervous system in infancy, childhood and adolescence*, 5th ed. Springfield, IL: Charles C Thomas, 1966: 1219–1221.
44. Lundberg A. Dissociated motor development—developmental patterns, clinical characteristics, causal factors and outcome, with special reference to later walking children. *Neuropaediatrie* 1979;10:161–182.
45. Iannaccone ST, et al. Type 1 fiber size disproportion: morphometric data from 37 children with myopathic, neuropathic, or idiopathic hypotonia. *Pediatr Pathol* 1987;7:395–419.
46. Rapin I. Hypoactive labyrinths and motor development. *Clin Pediatr* 1974;13:922–923, 926–929, 934–937.
47. Verity MA, Gao YH. Dysmaturation myopathy: correlation with minimal neuropathy in sural nerve biopsies. *J Child Neurol* 1988;3:276–291.
48. Ben Hamida M, Hentati F, Ben Hamida C. Hereditary motor system diseases (chronic juvenile amyotrophic lateral sclerosis). Conditions combining a bilateral pyramidal syndrome with limb and bulbar amyotrophy. *Brain* 1990;113:347–363.
49. Peña CE, et al. Arthrogryposis multiplex congenita: report of two cases of a radicular type with familial incidence. *Neurology* 1968;18:926–930.
50. Hageman G, et al. The pathogenesis of fetal hypokinesia. A neurological study of 75 cases of congenital contractures with emphasis on cerebral lesions. *Neuropediatrics* 1987;18:22–33.
51. Wynne-Davies R, Williams PF, O'Connor JCB. The 1960 epidemic of arthrogryposis multiplex congenita. *J Bone Joint Surg* 1981;63B:76–82.
52. Strehl E, Vanasse M, Brochu P. EMG and needle muscle biopsy in arthrogryposis multiplex congenita. *Neuropediatrics* 1985;16:225–227.
53. Clarren SK, Hall JG. Neuropathologic findings in the spinal cords of 10 infants with arthrogryposis. *J Neurol Sci* 1983;58:89–102.
54. Quinn CM, Wigglesworth JS, Heckmatt J. Lethal arthrogryposis multiplex congenita: a pathological study of 21 cases. *Histopathology* 1991;19:155–162.
55. Pearson CM, Fowler WG Jr. Hereditary nonprogressive muscular dystrophy inducing arthrogryposis syndrome. *Brain* 1963;86:75–88.
56. Dyken PR, Harper PS. Congenital dystrophica myotonica. *Neurology* 1973;24:465–473.
56a. Vincent A, et al. Arthrogryposis multiplex congenita with maternal autoantibodies specific for a fetal antigen. *Lancet* 1995;346:24–25.
57. Hageman G, Willemse J. Arthrogryposis multiplex congenita. Review with comment. *Neuropediatrics* 1983; 14:6–11.
58. Hageman G, et al. The heterogeneity of the Pena-Shokeir syndrome. *Neuropediatrics* 1987;18:45–50.
59. Pena SDJ, Shokeir MHK. Autosomal recessive cerebro-oculo-facio-skeletal (COFS) syndrome. *Clin Genet* 1974;5:285–293.
60. Hall JG. Arthrogryposis and the other neuromuscular and motor neuron disorders. In: Hoffman HJ, Epstein F, eds. *Disorders of the developing nervous system.* Boston: Blackwell Scientific Publications, 1986:289–300.
61. Hall JG, Reed SD, Greene G. The distal arthrogryposes: delineation of new entities—review and nosologic discussion. *Am J Med Genet* 1982;11:185–239.
62. Staheli LT, et al. *Arthrogryposis: a text atlas.* Cambridge, UK: Cambridge University Press, 1998.
63. Miskin M, et al. Arthrogryposis multiplex congenita: prenatal assessment with diagnostic ultrasound and fetoscopy. *J Pediatr* 1979;95:463–464.
64. Williams P. The management of arthrogryposis. *Orthop Clin North Am* 1978;9:67–88.
65. Willis T. De Anima Brutorum Quae Hominis Vitalis ac Sensitiva Est, Exercitationes Duae. Altera pathologica morbos qui ipsam, & sedem eius primariam, nempe cerebrum & nervosum genus afficiunt, explicat, eorumque therapeias instituit. Oxford: E theatro Sheldoniano. Impensis Ric. Davis, 1672;565.
66. Lindstrom J, Shelton D, Fujii Y. Myasthenia gravis. *Adv Immunol* 1988;42:233–284.
67. Afifi AK, Bell WE. Tests for juvenile myasthenia gravis: comparative diagnostic yield and prediction of outcome. *J Child Neurol* 1993;8:403–411.
68. Protti MP, et al. Myasthenia gravis: recognition of a human autoantigen at the molecular level. *Immunol Today* 1993;14:363–368.
69. Engel AG, Arahata K. The membrane attack complex of complement at the endplate in myasthenia gravis. *Ann N Y Acad Sci* 1987;505:326–332.
70. Drachman DB, et al. Functional activities of autoantibodies to acetylcholine receptors and the clinical severity of myasthenia gravis. *N Engl J Med* 1982;307: 769–775.
71. Fujii Y, et al. Antibody to acetylcholine receptor in myasthenia gravis: production by lymphocytes from thymus or thymoma. *Neurology* 1984;34:1182–1186.

72. Manfredi AA, et al. T helper cell recognition of muscle acetylcholine receptor in myasthenia gravis. Epitopes on the gamma and delta subunits. *J Clin Invest* 1993;92:1055–1067.

73. Schluep M, et al. Acetylcholine receptors in human thymic myoid cells in situ: an immunohistological study. *Ann Neurol* 1987;22:212–222.

74. Mossman S, Vincent A, Newsom-Davis J. Myasthenia gravis without acetylcholine-receptor antibody: a distinct disease entity. *Lancet* 1986;1:116–119.

75. Hoedemaekers AC, van Breda Vriesman PJ, De Baets MH. Myasthenia gravis as a prototype autoimmune receptor disease. *Immunol Res* 1997;16:341–354.

76. Whitney KD, McNamara JO. Autoimmunity and neurological disease: antibody modulation of synaptic transmission. *Annu Rev Neurosci* 1999;22:175–195.

77. Keesey J, et al. Anti-acetylcholine receptor antibody in neonatal myasthenia gravis [Letter]. *N Engl J Med* 1977;296:55.

78. Lefvert AK, Osterman PO. Newborn infants to myasthenic mothers: a clinical study and an investigation of acetylcholine receptor antibodies in 17 children. *Neurology* 1983;13:133–138.

79. Millichap JG, Dodge PR. Diagnosis and treatment of myasthenia gravis in infancy, childhood and adolescence. *Neurology* 1960;10:1007–1014.

80. Fenichel GM. Clinical syndromes of myasthenia in infancy and childhood. A review. *Arch Neurol* 1978;35:97–103.

81. Greer M, Schotland M. Myasthenia gravis in the newborn. *Pediatrics* 1960;26:101–108.

82. Engel AG, Ohno K, Sine SM. Congenital myasthenic syndromes: recent advances. *Arch Neurol* 1999;56: 163–167.

83. Engel AG. The investigation of congenital myasthenic syndromes. *Ann NY Acad Sci* 1993;681:425–434.

84. Misulis KE, Fenichel GM. Genetic forms of myasthenia gravis. *Pediatr Neurol* 1989;5:205–210.

85. Mora M, Lambert EH, Engel AG. Synaptic vesicle abnormality in familial infantile myasthenia. *Neurology* 1987;37:206–214.

86. Albers JW, et al. Abnormal neuromuscular transmission in an infantile myasthenic syndrome. *Ann Neurol* 1984;16:28–34.

87. Ohno K, et al. Human endplate acetylcholinesterase deficiency caused by mutations in the collagen-like tail subunit (ColQ) of the asymmetric enzyme. *Proc Natl Acad Sci U S A* 1998;95:9654–9659.

88. Gomez CM, et al. A beta-subunit mutation in the acetylcholine receptor gate causes severe slow-channel syndrome. *Ann Neurol* 1996;39:712–723.

88a. Engel AG, et al. A newly recognized congenital myasthenic syndrome attributed to a prolonged open time of the acetylcholine-induced ion channel. *Ann Neurol* 1982;11:553–569.

89. Ohno K, et al. Congenital myasthenic syndrome caused by decreased agonist binding affinity due to a mutation in the acetylcholine receptor epsilon subunit. *Neuron* 1996;17:157–170.

89a. Uchitel O, et al. Congenital myasthenic syndrome attributed to an abnormal interaction of acetylcholine with its receptor. *Ann NY Acad Sci* 1993;681:487–495.

90. Vincent A, et al. Congenital myasthenia: end-plate acetylcholine receptors and electrophysiology in five cases. *Muscle Nerve* 1981;4:306–318.

91. Engel AG, et al. Newly recognized congenital myasthenic syndromes: I. Congenital paucity of synaptic vesicles and reduced quantal release. II. High conductance fast-channel syndrome. III. Abnormal acetylcholine receptor (AChR) interaction with acetylcholine. IV. AChR deficiency and short channel open time. *Prog Brain Res* 1990;84:125–137.

92. Engel AG, et al. Congenital myasthenic syndromes. I. Deficiency and short open-time of the acetylcholine receptor. *Muscle Nerve* 1993;16:1284–1292.

93. Vincent A, et al. Clinical and experimental observations in patients with congenital myasthenic syndromes. *Ann NY Acad Sci* 1993;681:451–460.

94. Schlezinger NS, Corin MS. Myasthenia gravis associated with hyperthyroidism in childhood. *Neurology* 1968;18:1217–1222.

95. Snead OC, et al. Juvenile myasthenia gravis. *Neurology* 1980;30:732–739.

96. Rodriguez M, et al. Myasthenia gravis in children. Long-term follow-up. *Ann Neurol* 1983;13:504–510.

97. Dobkin BH, Verity MA. Familial neuromuscular disease with type I fiber hypoplasia, tubular aggregates, cardiomyopathy, and myasthenic features. *Neurology* 1978;28:1135–1140.

98. McQuillen MP, Cantor HE, O'Rourke JR. Myasthenic syndrome associated with antibiotics. *Arch Neurol* 1968;18:402–415.

99. Pittinger C, Adamson R. Antibiotic blockade of neuromuscular function. *Ann Rev Pharmacol* 1972;12: 169–184.

100. Shapira Y, et al. A myasthenic syndrome in childhood leukemia. *Dev Med Child Neurol* 1974;16:668–671.

101. Middleton LT, et al. Inherited myasthenic syndromes. *Acta Myologica (Napoli)* 1998;2:47–53.

102. Oh SJ, Cho HK. Edrophonium responsiveness not necessarily diagnostic of myasthenia gravis. *Muscle Nerve* 1990;13:187–191.

103. Andrews PI, Massey JM, Sanders DB. Acetylcholine receptor antibodies in juvenile myasthenia gravis. *Neurology* 1993;43:977–998.

104. Vial C, et al. Myasthenia gravis in childhood and infancy. Usefulness of electrophysiologic studies. *Arch Neurol* 1991;48:847–849.

105. Keesey JC. AAEE minimonograph 33: electrodiagnostic approach to defects of neuromuscular transmission. *Muscle Nerve* 1989;12:613–626.

106. Kelly JJ, et al. The laboratory diagnosis of mild myasthenia gravis. *Ann Neurol* 1982;12:238–242.

107. Kaeser HE. Drug-induced myasthenic syndromes. *Acta Neurol Scand Suppl* 1984;100:39–47.

108. Keesey J. Myasthenia gravis. In: Raker RE, ed. *Conn's current therapy.* Philadelphia: WB Saunders, 1992: 902–908.

109. Mann JD, Johns TR, Campa JF. Long-term administration of corticosteroids in myasthenia gravis. *Neurology* 1976;26:729–740.

110. Sarnat HB, McGarry JD, Lewis JE. Effective treatment of infantile myasthenia gravis by combined prednisone and thymectomy. *Neurology* 1977;27:550–553.

111. Dau PC. Plasmapheresis therapy in myasthenia gravis. *Muscle Nerve* 1980;3:468–482.

112. Tindall RSA, et al. Preliminary results of a double-blind, randomized, placebo-controlled trial of cyclosporine in myasthenia gravis. *N Engl J Med* 1987;316:719–724.

113. Herrmann DN, Carney PR, Wald JJ. Juvenile myasthenia gravis: treatment with immune globulin and thymectomy. *Pediatr Neurol* 1998;18:63–66.

113a. Gajdos P, et al. Clinical trial of plasma exchange and high-dose intravenous immunoglobulin in myasthenia gravis. *Ann Neurol* 1997;41:789–796.

114. Tagher RJ, Baumann R, Desai N. Failure of intravenously administered immunoglobulin in the treatment of neonatal myasthenia gravis. *J Pediatr* 1999; 134:233–235.

115. Youssef S. Thymectomy for myasthenia gravis in children. *J Pediatr Surg* 1983;18:537–541.

116. Fonkelsrud EW, Herrmann C, Mulder DG. Thymectomy for myasthenia gravis in children. *J Pediatr Surg* 1970;5:157–165.

117. Palace J, Wiles CM, Newsom-Davis J. 3,4-diaminopyridine in the treatment of congenital (hereditary) myasthenia. *J Neurol Neurosurg Psychiatr* 1991;54:1069–1072.

117a. Lindner A, Schalke B, Toyka KV. Outcome in juvenile-onset myasthenia gravis: a retrospective study with long-term follow-up of 79 patients *J Neurol* 1997;244: 515–529.

118. Swift TR. Disorders of neuromuscular transmission other than myasthenia gravis. *Muscle Nerve* 1981;4:334–353.

119. Dubowitz V. What's in a name? Muscular dystrophy revisited. *Eur J Paediatr Neurol* 1998;2:273–284.

120. Gowers WR. Clinical lecture on pseudohypertrophic muscular paralysis. *Lancet* 1879;2:1,37,73,113.

121. Rowland LP. Muscular dystrophies, polymyositis and other myopathies. *J Chronic Dis* 1958;8:510–535.

122. Ringel SP, Carroll JE, Schold SC. The spectrum of mild X-linked recessive muscular dystrophy. *Arch Neurol* 1977;34:408–416.

123. Hopkins LC, Jackson JA, Elsas LJ. Emery-Dreifuss humeroperoneal muscular dystrophy: an X-linked myopathy with unusual contractures and bradycardia. *Ann Neurol* 1981;10:230–237.

124. Watkins SC, Cullen MJ. A qualitative and quantitative study of the ultrastructure of regenerating muscle fiber in Duchenne muscular dystrophy and polymyositis. *J Neurol Sci* 1987;82:181–192.

125. Carpenter S, Karpati G. Duchenne muscular dystrophy. Plasma membrane loss initiates muscle cell necrosis unless it is repaired. *Brain* 1979;102:147–161.

126. Rosman NP. The cerebral defect and myopathy in Duchenne muscular dystrophy. A comparative clinicopathologic study. *Neurology* 1970;20:329–335.

127. Zatz M, et al. Translocation (X^6) in a female with Duchenne muscular dystrophy, implications for the localisation of the DMD locus. *J Med Genet* 1981;18: 442–447.

128. Francke U, et al. Minor Xp21 chromosome deletion in a male associated with expression of Duchenne muscular dystrophy, chronic granulomatous disease, retinitis pigmentosa and McLeod syndrome. *Am J Hum Genet* 1985;37:250–267.

129. Kunkel LM, et al. Specific cloning of DNA fragments absent from the DNA of a male patient with an X-chromosome deletion. *Proc Natl Acad Sci U S A* 1985;82: 4778–4782.

130. Monaco AP, et al. Detection of deletions spanning the Duchenne muscular dystrophy locus using a tightly linked DNA segment. *Nature* 1985;316:842–845.

131. Kunkel LM, et al. Analysis of deletions in DNA of patients with Becker and Duchenne muscular dystrophy. *Nature* 1986;322:73–77.

132. van Ommen GJB, et al. A physical map of 4 million bp around the Duchenne muscular dystrophy gene on the human X chromosome. *Cell* 1986;47:499–504.

133. Monaco AP, et al. Isolation of candidate cDNAs for portions of the Duchenne muscular dystrophy gene. *Nature* 1986;323:646–650.

134. Koenig M, et al. Complete cloning of the Duchenne muscular dystrophy (DMD) cDNA and preliminary genomic organization of the DMD gene in normal and affected individuals. *Cell* 1987;50:509–517.

135. Roberts RG, Bobrow M, Bentley DR. Point mutations in the dystrophin gene. *Proc Natl Acad Sci U S A* 1992;89:2331–2335.

136. Forrest SM, et al. Preferential deletions of exons in Duchenne and Becker muscular dystrophies. *Nature* 1987;329:638–640.

137. Medori R, Brooke MH, Waterston RH. Genetic abnormalities in Duchenne and Becker dystrophies: clinical correlations. *Neurology* 1989;39:461–465.

138. Hoffman EP, Brown RJ, Kunkel LM. Dystrophin: the protein product of the Duchenne muscular dystrophy locus. *Cell* 1987;51:919–928.

139. Ibraghimov-Beskrovnaya O, et al. Primary structure of dystrophin-associated glycoproteins linking dystrophin to the extracellular matrix. *Nature* 1992;355:696–702.

140. Zubrzykcka-Gaarn EE, et al. The Duchenne muscular dystrophy gene product is localized in sarcolemma of human skeletal muscle. *Nature* 1988;333:466–469.

141. Scott MO, et al. Duchenne muscular dystrophy gene expression in normal and diseased human muscle. *Science* 1988;239:1418–1420.

142. Hoffman EP, et al. Characterization of dystrophin in muscle-biopsy specimens from patients with Duchenne's or Becker's muscular dystrophy. *N Engl J Med* 1988;318:1363 1368.

143. Blake DJ, Tinsley JM, Davies KE. Utrophin: a structural and functional comparison to dystrophin. *Brain Pathol* 1996;6:37–47.

144. England SB, et al. Very mild muscular dystrophy associated with the deletion of 40% of dystrophin. *Nature* 1990;343:180–182.

145. Miller G, Wessel HB. Diagnosis of dystrophinopathies: review for the clinician. *Pediatr Neurol* 1993;9:3–9.

146. Mendell JR, Sahenk Z, Prior TW. The childhood muscular dystrophies: diseases sharing a common pathogenesis of membrane instability. *J Child Neurol* 1995;10:150–159.

147. Ikezawa M, et al. Dystrophin gene analysis on 130 patients with Duchenne muscular dystrophy with a special reference to muscle mRNA analysis. *Brain Dev* 1998;20:165–168.

148. Nigro V, et al. Gene redundancies in the dystrophin-associated protein complex. *Acta Myologica (Napoli)* 1998;2:29–31.

149. Hattori N, et al. Undetectable dystrophin can still result in a relatively benign phenotype of dystrophinopathy. *Neuromusc Disord* 1999;9:220–226.

150. Salih MAM, et al. Muscular dystrophy associated with beta-dystroglycan deficiency. *Ann Neurol* 1996;40:925–928.

151. Brown RH Jr. Dystrophin-associated proteins and the muscular dystrophies: a glossary. *Brain Pathol* 1996; 6:19–24.

151a. Wilson J, et al. Up71 and Up140, two novel transcripts of utrophin that are homologues of short forms of dystrophin. *Hum Mol Genet* 1999;8:1271–1278.

152. Nudel U, et al. Duchenne muscular dystrophy gene product is not identical in muscle and brain. *Nature* 1989;337:76–78.

153. Lidov HGW. Dystrophin in the nervous system. *Brain Pathol* 1996;6:63–77.
154. Ahn AH, Kunkel LM. The structural and functional diversity of dystrophin. *Nat Genet* 1993;3:283–291.
154a. Lidov HGW, Selig S, Kunkel LM. Dp140: a novel 140 kDa CNS transcript from the dystrophin locus. *Hum Mol Genet* 1995;4:329–335.
155. Bodensteiner JB, Engel AG. Intracellular calcium accumulation in Duchenne dystrophy and other myopathies: a study of 567,000 muscle fibers in 114 biopsies. *Neurology* 1978;28:438–446.
156. Nicholson LVB, et al. Functional significance of dystrophin positive fibres in Duchenne muscular dystrophy. *Arch Dis Child* 1993;68:632–636.
157. Duchenne G. *De la paralysis musculaire pseudohypertrophique ou paralysis myo-sclerotique*. Paris: P. Asselin, 1868.
158. Gowers WR. *Pseudo-hypertrophic muscular paralysis*. London: J & A Churchill, 1879.
159. Perloff JK. Cardiac rhythm and conduction in Duchenne's muscular dystrophy: a prospective study of 20 patients. *J Am Coll Cardiol* 1984;3:1263–1268.
160. Barohn RJ, et al. Gastric hypomotility in Duchenne's muscular dystrophy. *N Engl J Med* 1988;319:15–18.
161. Huvos AG, Prudzanski W. Smooth muscle involvement in primary muscle disease. II. Progressive muscular dystrophy. *Arch Pathol* 1967;83:234–240.
162. Rosman NP, Kakulas BA. Mental deficiency associated with muscular dystrophy: a neuropathological study. *Brain* 1966;89:769–788.
163. Dubowitz V, Crome L. The central nervous system in Duchenne muscular dystrophy. *Brain* 1969;92:805–808.
164. Yoshioka M, et al. Central nervous system involvement in progressive muscular dystrophy. *Arch Dis Child* 1980;55:589–594.
165. Bardoni A, et al. Absence of brain Dp140 isoform and cognitive impairment in Becker muscular dystrophy. *Lancet* 1999;353:897–898.
166. Pearce GW, Pearce JM, Walton JN. The Duchenne type muscular dystrophy: histopathologic studies of the carrier state. *Brain* 1966;89:109–120.
167. Bushby KMD, Thambyayah M, Gardner-Medwin D. Prevalence and incidence of Becker muscular dystrophy. *Lancet* 1991;337:1022–1024.
168. Gospe SM, et al. Familial X-linked myalgia and cramps: a non-progressive myopathy associated with a deletion in the dystrophin gene. *Neurology* 1989;39:1277–1280.
169. Doriguzzi C, et al. Exercise intolerance and recurrent myoglobinuria as the only manifestation of Xp21 Becker type muscular dystrophy. *J Neurol* 1993;240:269–271.
170. Yates JR, et al. Emery-Dreifuss muscular dystrophy: linkage to markers in distal Xq28. *J Med Genet* 1993;30:108–111.
170a. Farley EA, Kendrick-Jones J, Ellis JA. The Emery-Dreifuss muscular dystrophy phenotype arises from aberrant targeting and binding of emerin at the inner nuclear membrane. *J Cell Sci* 1999;112:2571–2582.
171. Emery AEH, Dreifuss FE. Unusual type of benign X-linked muscular dystrophy. *J Neurol Neurosurg Psychiatry* 1966;29:338–342.
172. Dickey RP, Ziter FA, Smith RA. Emery-Dreifuss muscular dystrophy. *J Pediatr* 1984;104:555–559.
173. Matsumura K, Nonaka I, Campbell KP. Abnormal expression of dystrophin-associated proteins in Fukuyama-type congenital muscular dystrophy. *Lancet* 1993;341:521–523.
174. Fukuyama Y, Osawa M, Suzuki H. Congenital progressive muscular dystrophy of the Fukuyama type—clinical, genetic and pathological considerations. *Brain Dev* 1981;3:129.
175. Kinoshita M, et al. A case of congenital polymyositis—a possible pathogenesis of "Fukuyama type congenital muscular dystrophy." *Clin Neurol (Tokyo)* 1980;11:911–916.
176. Toda T, et al. Localization of a gene for Fukuyama type congenital muscular dystrophy to chromosome 9q-31-33. *Nat Genet* 1993;5:283–286.
177. Barkovich AJ. Neuroimaging manifestations and classification of congenital muscular dystrophies. *Am J Neuroradiol* 1998;19:1389–1396.
178. Muntoni F, et al. An early onset muscular dystrophy with diaphragmatic involvement, early respiratory failure and secondary α2 laminin deficiency unlinked to the LAMA2 locus on 6q22. *Eur J Paediatr Neurol* 1998;1:19–26.
179. Osari S, et al. Basement membrane abnormality in merosin-negative congenital muscular dystrophy. *Acta Neuropathol* 1996;91:332–336.
180. Fardeau M, et al. Dystrophie musculaire congénitale avec déficience en mérosine. *Rev Neurol (Paris)* 1996;152:11–19.
181. North KN, et al. Congenital muscular dystrophy associated with merosin deficiency. *J Child Neurol* 1996;11:291–295.
182. Tsao C-Y, et al. Congenital muscular dystrophy with complete laminin-alpha2-deficiency, cortical dysplasia, and cerebral white-matter changes in children. *J Child Neurol* 1998;13:253–256.
183. Castro-Gago M, et al. Distrofia cerebromuscular tipo occidental y distrofia muscular congénita deficiente en merosina: dos denominaciones para una misma entidad. *Rev Neurol (Barcelona)* 1998;157:459–462.
184. Pegoraro E, et al. Laminin alpha2 muscular dystrophy. Genotype/phenotype studies of 22 patients. *Neurology* 1998;51:101–110.
185. Cohn RD, et al. Laminin alpha2 chain-deficient congenital muscular dystrophy. Variable epitope expression in severe and mild cases. *Neurology* 1998;51: 94–101.
186. Philpot J, et al. Clinical phenotype in congenital muscular dystrophy: correlation with expression of merosin in skeletal muscle. *Neuromusc Disord* 1995;5:301–305.
187. Brett FM, et al. Merosin-deficient congenital muscular dystrophy and cortical dysplasia. *Eur J Paediatr Neurol* 1998;2:77–82.
188. Yamamoto T, et al. Localization of laminin subunits in the central nervous system in Fukuyama congenital muscular dystrophy: an immunohistochemical investigation. *Acta Neuropathol* 1997;94:173–179.
189. Voit T, et al. Preserved merosin M-chain (or laminin-alpha2) expression in skeletal muscle distinguishes Walker-Warburg syndrome from Fukuyama muscular dystrophy and merosin-deficient congenital muscular dystrophy. *Neuropediatrics* 1995;26:148–155.
189a. Haltia M, et al. Muscle-eye-brain disease: a neuropathological study. *Ann Neurol* 1997;41:173–180.
190. Ullrich O. Kongenitale, atonisch-sklerotische Muskeldystrophie; ein weiterer Typus der heredodegenerativen Erkrankungen des neuromuskulären Systems. *Z Ges Neurol Psychiatrie* 1930;126:171–201.

191. Nonaka I, et al. A clinical and histological study of Ullrich's disease (congenital atonic-sclerotic muscular dystrophy). *Neuropediatrics* 1981;12:197–208.

192. Furukawa T, Toyokura Y. Congenital, hypotonic-sclerotic muscular dystrophy. *J Med Genet* 1977;14:426–429.

193. Dobyns WB, et al. Diagnostic criteria for Walker-Warburg syndrome. *Am J Med Genet* 1989;32:195–210.

194. Donner M, Rapola J, Somer H. Congenital muscular dystrophy: a clinico-pathological and follow-up study of 15 patients. *Neuropaediatrie* 1975;6:239–258.

195. Pihko H, et al. CNS in congenital muscular dystrophy without mental retardation. *Neuropediatrics* 1992;23:116–122.

196. Landouzy L, Dejerine J. De la myopathie atrophique progressive. *Rev Med Franc* 1885;5:811–817, 253–366; 6:977–1027.

196a. Tupler R, et al. Profound misregulation of muscle-specific gene expression in fascioscapulohumeral muscular dystrophy. *Proc Natl Acad Sci USA* 1999;96:12650–12654.

197. Lunt PW, Harper PS. Genetic counselling in facioscapulohumeral muscular dystrophy. *J Med Genet* 1991;28:655–664.

197a. Fitzsimmons RB. Fascioscapulohumeral muscular dystrophy. *Curr Opin Neurol* 1999;12:501–511.

198. Wijmenga C, et al. Mapping of facioscapulohumeral muscular dystrophy gene to chromosome 4q35-qter by multipoint linkage analysis and in situ hybridization. *Genomics* 1991;9:570–575.

199. Rothstein TL, Carlson CB, Sumi SM. Polymyositis with facioscapulohumeral distribution. *Arch Neurol* 1971;25:313–319.

200. Fitzsimons RB, Gurwin EB, Bird AC. Retinal vascular abnormalities in facioscapulohumeral muscular dystrophy. *Brain* 1987;110:631–648.

201. Wulff JD, Lin JT, Kepes JJ. Inflammatory facioscapulohumeral muscular dystrophy and Coats syndrome. *Ann Neurol* 1982;12:398–401.

202. Taylor DA, et al. Facioscapulohumeral dystrophy associated with hearing loss and Coats syndrome. *Ann Neurol* 1982;12:395–398.

202a. Wilhelmsen KC, et al. Chromosome 12-linked autosomal dominant scapuloperoneal muscular dystrophy. *Ann Neurol* 1996;39:507–520.

203. Ronin GM, et al. Hereditary motor sensory neuropathy type I presenting as scapuloperoneal atrophy (Davidenkow syndrome). Electrophysiological and pathological studies. *Can J Neurol Sci* 1986;13:264–266.

204. Mohire MD, et al. Early-onset benign autosomal dominant limb-girdle myopathy with contractures (Bethlem myopathy). *Neurology* 1988;38:573–580.

205. Norman A, et al. Distinction of Becker from limb-girdle muscular dystrophy by means of dystrophin cDNA probes. *Lancet* 1989;1:466–468.

205a. Worton R. Muscular dystrophies: diseases of the dystrophin-glycoprotein complex. *Science* 1995;270:755–756.

205b. Bushby K. Muscular dystrophy and allied disorders: research strategies. *Trans Biochem Soc* 1996;24:489–496.

206. Ljunggren A, et al. Primary adhalin deficiency as a cause of muscular dystrophy in patients with normal dystrophin. *Ann Neurol* 1995;38:367–372.

207. Duggan DJ, et al. Mutations in the sarcoglycan genes in patients with myopathy. *New Engl J Med* 1997;336:618–624.

208. Politano L, Nigro V, Passamano L, et al. Clinical and genetic findings in sarcoglycanopathies. *Acta Myologica (Napoli)* 1998;2:33–40.

209. Angelini C, Fanin M, Freda MP, et al. The clinical spectrum of sarcoglycanopathies. *Neurology* 1999;52:176–179.

209a. Topaloglu H, et al. Calpain-3 deficiency causes a mild muscular dystrophy in childhood. *Neuropediatrics* 1997;28:213–216.

210. Mahon M, et al. Familial myopathy associated with thrombocytopenia: a clinical and histomorphometric study. *J Neurol Sci* 1988;88:55–67.

211. Barohn RJ, Miller RG, Griggs RC. Autosomal recessive distal dystrophy. *Neurology* 1991;1365–1370.

212. Nonaka I, et al. Autosomal recessive distal muscular dystrophy: a comparative study with distal myopathy with rimmed vacuole formation. *Ann Neurol* 1985;17:51–59.

213. Magee KR, DeJong RN. Hereditary distal myopathy with onset in infancy. *Arch Neurol* 1965;13:387–390.

214. Beggs AH, Kunkel LM. Improved diagnosis of Duchenne/Becker muscular dystrophy. *J Clin Invest* 1990;85:613–619.

215. Nanji AA. Serum creatine kinase isoenzymes: a review. *Muscle Nerve* 1983;6:83–90.

216. Darras BT, Harper JF, Francke U. Prenatal diagnosis and detection of carriers with DNA probes in Duchenne's muscular dystrophy. *N Engl J Med* 1987;316:985–992.

217. Cole CG, et al. Prenatal testing for Duchenne and Becker muscular dystrophy. *Lancet* 1988;1:262–266.

218. Kuller JA, et al. Prenatal diagnosis of Duchenne muscular dystrophy by fetal muscle biopsy. *Hum Genet* 1992;90:34–40.

219. Sancho S, et al. Analysis of dystrophin expression after activation of myogenesis in amniocytes, chorionic-villus cells, and fibroblasts. A new method for diagnosing Duchenne's muscular dystrophy. *N Engl J Med* 1993;329:915–920.

220. Nicholson GA, et al. Carrier detection in Duchenne muscular dystrophy: assessment of the effect of age on detection-rate with serum-creatine-kinase activity. *Lancet* 1979;1:692–694.

221. Griggs RC, et al. Randomized, double-blind trial of mazindol in Duchenne dystrophy. *Muscle Nerve* 1990;13:1169–1173.

222. Munsat TL. Inflammatory myopathy with facioscapulohumeral distribution. *Neurology* 1972;22:335–347.

223. Howell JM. Is there a future for gene therapy? *Neuromuscul Disord* 1999;9:102–107.

224. Fassati A, Murphy S, Dickson G. Gene therapy of Duchenne muscular dystrophy. *Adv Genet* 1997;35:117–153.

225. Qu Z, et al. Development of approaches to improve cell survival in myoblast transfer therapy. *J Cell Biol* 1998;142:1257–1267.

226. Gussoni E, Blau HM, Kunkel LM. The fate of individual myoblasts after transplantation into muscles of DMD patients. *Nat Med* 1997;3:970–977.

227. King JO, Denborough MA. Anesthetic-induced malignant hyperpyrexia in children. *J Pediatr* 1973;83:37–40.

228. Walls TJ, et al. Congenital myasthenic syndrome associated with paucity of synaptic vesicles and reduced quantal release. *Ann N Y Acad Sci* 1993;681:461–468.
229. Moxley RT III. Myotonic disorders in childhood: diagnosis and treatment. *J Child Neurol* 1997;12:116–129.
230. Harper PS. *Myotonic dystrophy*, 2nd ed. London: WB Saunders, 1989.
231. Harper PS, et al. Anticipation in myotonic dystrophy: new light on an old problem. *Am J Hum Genet* 1992; 51:10–16.
232. Calderon R. Myotonic dystrophy: a neglected cause for mental retardation. *J Pediatr* 1966;68:423–431.
233. Pruzanski W. Variants of myotonic dystrophy in preadolescent life. *Brain* 1966;89:563–568.
234. Edwards JH. Sign of the Cheshire cat. *Lancet* 1987; 2:581.
235. Camilleri M. Disorders of gastrointestinal motility in neurologic diseases. *Mayo Clin Proc* 1990;65: 825–846.
236. Sarnat HB, O'Connor T, Byrne PA. Clinical effects of myotonic dystrophy on pregnancy and the neonate. *Arch Neurol* 1976;33:459–465.
237. Dodge PR, et al. Myotonic dystrophy in infancy and childhood. *Pediatrics* 1965;35:319.
238. Stuart CA, et al. Insulin resistance in patients with myotonic dystrophy. *Neurology* 1983;33:679–685.
239. Walsh JC, et al. Abnormalities of insulin secretion in dystrophia myotonica. *Brain* 1970;93:731–742.
240. Wochner RD, et al. Accelerated breakdown of immunoglobulin G (IgG) in myotonic dystrophy: a hereditary error of immunoglobulin catabolism. *J Clin Invest* 1966;45:321–329.
241. Bundey S. Clinical evidence for heterogeneity in myotonic dystrophy. *J Med Genet* 1982;19:341–348.
242. Lavedan C, et al. Myotonic dystrophy: size- and sex-dependent dynamics of CTG meiotic instability, and somatic mosaicism. *Am J Hum Genet* 1993;52: 875–883.
243. Mulley JC, et al. Explanation for exclusive maternal origin for congenital form of myotonic dystrophy. *Lancet* 1993;341:236–237.
244. Hofmann-Radvanyi H, et al. Myotonic dystrophy: absence of CTG enlarged transcript in congenital forms, and low expression of the normal allele. *Hum Mol Genet* 1993;2:1263–1266.
245. Tanabe Y, et al. Neuroradiological findings in children with myotonic dystrophy. *Acta Paediatr Scand* 1992;81:613–617.
246. Moorman JR, et al. Cardiac involvement in myotonic muscular dystrophy. *Medicine* 1985;64:371–378.
247. Dubowitz V. *The floppy infant*. London: William Heinemann Medical Books, 1980.
247a. Martinello F, et al. Clinical and neuroimaging study of central nervous system in congenital myotonic dystrophy. *J Neurol* 1999;246:186–192.
248. Koh THHG. Do you shake hands with mothers of floppy babies? *BMJ* 1984;289:485.
249. Shelbourne P, et al. Direct diagnosis of myotonic dystrophy with a disease-specific DNA marker. *N Engl J Med* 1993;328:471–475.
250. Grant R, et al. Nifedipine in the treatment of myotonia in myotonic dystrophy. *J Neurol Neurosurg Psychiatry* 1987;50:199–206.
251. Hughes EF, Wilson J. Response to treatment with antihistamines in a family with myotonia congenita. *Lancet* 1991;337:25–27.
252. Schotland DL. An electron microscopic investigation of myotonic dystrophy. *J Neuropathol Exp Neurol* 1970; 29:241–253.
253. Sarnat HB, Silbert SW. Maturational arrest of fetal muscle in neonatal myotonic dystrophy. *Arch Neurol* 1976;33:466–474.
254. Sarnat HB. Vimentin and desmin in maturing skeletal muscle and developmental myopathies. *Neurology* 1992;42:1616–1624.
255. Aslanidis C, et al. Cloning of the essential myotonic dystrophy region and mapping of the putative defect. *Nature* 1992;355:548–551.
256. Brook JD, et al. Molecular basis of myotonic dystrophy: expansion of a trinucleotide (CTG) repeat at the 3' end of a transcript encoding a protein kinase family member. *Cell* 1992;68:799–808.
257. Thornton CA, Griggs RC, Moxley RT. Myotonic dystrophy without trinucleotide repeat expansion. *Ann Neurol* 1994;35:269–272.
258. Brunner HG, et al. Brief report: reverse mutation in myotonic dystrophy. *N Engl J Med* 1993;328:476–480.
258a. Phillips AV, Timchenko LT, Cooper TA. Disruption of splicing regulated by a CUG-binding protein in myotonic dystrophy. *Science* 1998;280:737–744.
259. Carey N, et al. Meiotic drive at the myotonic dystrophy locus? *Nat Genet* 1994;6:117–118.
260. Ackerman MJ, Clapham DJ. Ion channels—basic science and clinical disease. *N Engl J Med* 1997;336: 1575–1586.
261. Lehmann-Horn F, et al. Myotonia levior is a chloride channel disorder. *Hum Mol Genet* 1995;4:1397–1402.
262. Koch MC, et al. The skeletal muscle chloride channel in dominant and recessive human myotonia. *Science* 1992;257:797–800.
263. Rosenfeld J, Sloan-Brown K, George AL. A novel muscle sodium channel mutation causes painful congenital myotonia. *Ann Neurol* 1997;42:811–814.
264. Ptacek LJ, Johnson KJ, Griggs RC. Genetics and physiology of the myotonic muscle disorders. *N Engl J Med* 1993;328:482–489.
265. Wang J, et al. Molecular genetic and genetic correlations in sodium channelopathies: lack of founder effect and evidence for a second gene. *Am J Hum Genet* 1993;52:1074–1084.
266. Cannon SC, Brown RH, Corey DP. A sodium channel defect in hyperkalemic periodic paralysis: potassium-induced failure of inactivation. *Neuron* 1991; 6:619–626.
267. Thomsen J. Tonische Krämpfe in willkürlich beweglichen Muskeln in Folge von ererbter psychischer Disposition: Ataxia muscularis? *Arch Psychiat Nervenkr* 1876;6:702–718.
267a. Papponen H, et al. Founder mutations and the high prevalence of myotonia congenita in northern Finland. *Neurology* 1999;53:297–302.
268. Becker PE. Neues zur Genetik und Klassifikation der Muskeldystrophien. *Humangenetik* 1972;17:1–22.
269. Moxley RT III. Myotonic disorders in childhood: diagnosis and treatment. *J Child Neurol* 1997;12:116–129.
270. Johnson T, Friis ML. Paramyotonia congenita (von Eulenberg) in Denmark. *Acta Neurol Scand* 1980;61: 78–87.
271. Lundberg PO, Stalberg E, Thule B. Paralysis periodica paramyotonica: a clinical and neurophysiological study. *J Neurol Sci* 1974;21:309–321.

272. Auger RG, et al. Hereditary form of sustained muscle activity of peripheral nerve origin causing generalized myokymia and muscle stiffness. *Ann Neurol* 1984;15:13–21.

272a. Stephan DA, et al. A rippling muscle disease gene is localized to 1 q41: evidence for multiple genes. *Neurology* 1994;44:1915–1920.

273. Gamstorp I. Adynamia episodica hereditaria. *Acta Paediatr Scand* 1956;[Suppl]108:11–26.

274. Hoskins B, Vroom FQ, Jarrell MA. Hyperkalemic periodic paralysis. Effects of potassium, exercise, glucose and acetazolamide on blood chemistry. *Arch Neurol* 1975;32:519–523.

275. Bradley WG, et al. Progressive myopathy in hyperkalemic periodic paralysis. *Arch Neurol* 1990;47:1013–1017.

276. Gamstorp I. Adynamia episodica hereditaria, and myotonia. *Acta Neurol Scand* 1963;39:41–58.

277. Ricker K, Rohkamm R, Bohlen R. Adynamia episodica and paralysis periodica paramyotonia. *Neurology* 1986;36:682–686.

278. Layzer RB, Lovelace RE, Rowland LP. Hyperkalemic periodic paralysis. *Arch Neurol* 1967;16:455–472.

279. McArdle B. Adynamia episodica hereditaria and its treatment. *Brain* 1962;85:121–148.

280. Wang P, Clausen T. Treatment of attacks in hyperkalemic familial periodic paralysis by inhalation of salbutamol. *Lancet* 1976;1:221–223.

281. Huttenlocher PR, et al. Osteo-chondro-muscular dystrophy. *Pediatrics* 1969;44:945–958.

282. Giedion A, et al. Heterogeneity in Schwartz-Jampel chondrodystrophic myotonia. *Eur J Pediatr* 1997;156:214–223.

282a. Schwartz O, Jampel RS. Congenital blepharophimosis associated with a unique generalized myopathy. *Arch Ophthalmol* 1962;68:52–57.

283. Aberfeld DC, Hinterbuchner LP, Schneider M. Myotonia, dwarfism, diffuse bone disease and unusual ocular and facial abnormalities (a new syndrome). *Brain* 1965;88:313–322.

284. Ferrannini E, et al. Schwartz-Jampel syndrome with autosomal-dominant inheritance. *Europ Neurol* 1982;21:137–146.

285. Hansen PA, Martinez LB, Cassidy R. Contractures, continuous muscle discharges, and titubation. *Ann Neurol* 1977;1:120–124.

286. Isaacs H. Continuous muscle fibre activity in an Indian male with additional evidence of terminal motor fibre abnormality. *J Neurol Neurosurg Psychiatry* 1967;30:126–133.

287. Lazaro RP, Rollinson RD, Fenichel GM. Familial cramps and muscle pain. *Arch Neurol* 1981;38:22–24.

288. Lutschg I, et al. The syndrome of "continuous muscle fiber activity." *Arch Neurol* 1978;35:198–205.

289. Ashizawa T, et al. A dominantly inherited syndrome with continuous motor neuron discharges. *Ann Neurol* 1983;13:285–290.

290. Lingam S, Wilson J, Hart EW. Hereditary stiff-baby syndrome. *Am J Dis Child* 1981;135:909–911.

291. Daras M, Spiro AJ. "Stiff-man syndrome" in an adolescent. *Pediatrics* 1981;67:725–726.

292. Layzer RB. Stiff-man syndrome—an autoimmune disease? *N Engl J Med* 1988;318:1060–1062.

293. Solimena M, et al. Autoantibodies to GABA-ergic neurons and pancreatic β cells in stiff-man syndrome. *N Engl J Med* 1990;322:1555–1560.

294. Nelson TE, Flewellen EH. The malignant hyperthermia syndrome. *N Engl J Med* 1983;309:416–418.

295. Dalakas MC. Polymyositis, dermatomyositis, and inclusion-body myositis. *N Engl J Med* 1991;325:1487–1498.

296. Banker BQ. Dermatomyositis of childhood. *J Neuropathol Exp Neurol* 1975;34:46–75.

297. Riggs JE, et al. Childhood onset inclusion body myositis mimicking limb-girdle muscular dystrophy. *J Child Neurol* 1989;4:283–285.

298. Carpenter S, et al. The childhood type of dermatomyositis. *Neurology* 1976;26:952–962.

299. Hohlfeld R, et al. Cellular immune mechanisms in inflammatory myopathies. *Curr Opin Rheumatol* 1997;9:520–526.

300. Kissel JT, et al. The relationship of complement-mediated microvasculopathy to the histologic features and clinical duration of disease in dermatomyositis. *Arch Neurol* 1991;48:26–30.

301. Lundberg IE, Nyberg P. New developments in the role of cytokines and chemokines in inflammatory myopathies. *Curr Opin Rheumatol* 1998;10:521–529.

302. Pachman LM, Cooke N. Juvenile dermatomyositis: a clinical and immunologic study. *J Pediatr* 1980;96:226–234.

303. Bowles NE, et al. Dermatomyositis, polymyositis, and Coxsackie-B-virus infection. *Lancet* 1987;2:1004–1007.

304. Whitaker JN. Inflammatory myopathy: a review of etiologic and pathogenetic factors. *Muscle Nerve* 1982;5:573–592.

305. Wedgewood RJ, Cook C, Cohen J. Dermatomyositis: report of 26 cases in children with a discussion of endocrine therapy in 13. *Pediatrics* 1953;12:447–466.

306. Malleson P. Juvenile dermatomyositis: a review. *J Roy Soc Med* 1982;75:33–37.

307. Spencer CH, et al. Course of treated juvenile dermatomyositis. *J Pediatr* 1984;105:399–408.

308. Bohan A, et al. A computer-assisted analysis of 153 patients with polymyositis and dermatomyositis. *Medicine* 1977;56:255–286.

309. Hernandez RJ, et al. MR findings in children with dermatomyositis: musculoskeletal findings and correlation with clinical and laboratory findings. *Am J Roentgenol* 1993;161:359–366.

310. Carpenter S, Karpati G. The major inflammatory myopathies of unknown cause. *Pathol Ann* 1981;16:205–237.

311. Thompson CE. Infantile myositis. *Dev Med Child Neurol* 1982;24:307–313.

312. Miller G, Heckmatt JZ, Dubowitz V. Drug treatment of juvenile dermatomyositis. *Arch Dis Child* 1983;58:445–450.

313. Jacobs JC. Methotrexate and azathioprine treatment of childhood dermatomyositis. *Pediatrics* 1977;59:212–218.

314. Wallace DJ, Metzger AL, White KK. Combination immunosuppressive treatment of steroid-resistant dermatomyositis/polymyositis. *Arthritis Rheum* 1985;28:590–592.

315. Heckmatt J, et al. Cyclosporin in juvenile dermatomyositis. *Lancet* 1989;1:1063–1066.

316. Sussman GL, Pruzanski W. Treatment of inflammatory myopathy with intravenous gamma globulin. *Curr Opin Rheumatol* 1995;7:510–515.
317. Bohan A, Peter JB. Polymyositis and dermatomyositis. *N Engl J Med* 1975;292:344–347,403–407.
318. Lundberg A. Myalgia cruris epidemica. *Acta Paediatr Scand* 1957;46:18–31.
319. Ruff RL, Secrist D. Viral studies in benign acute childhood myositis. *Arch Neurol* 1982;39:261–263.
320. Sarnat HB. *Congenital muscle fiber-type disproportion.* Neurobase (computer textbook), 1999.
321. Dehkhargani F, et al. Congenital muscle fiber-type disproportion in Krabbe's leukodystrophy. *Arch Neurol* 1981;38:585–589.
322. Marjanovic B, et al. Association of Krabbe leukodystrophy and congenital muscle fiber type disproportion. *Pediatr Neurol* 1996;15:79–82.
323. Sarnat HB. Le cerveau influence-t-il le développement musculaire du foetus humain? Mise en évidence de 21 cas. *Can J Neurol Sci* 1985;12:111–120.
324. Sarnat HB. Cerebral dysgeneses and their influence on fetal muscle development. *Brain Dev* 1986;8:495–499.
325. Shy GM, et al. Nemaline myopathy: a new congenital myopathy. *Brain* 1963;86:793–810.
326. Conen PE, Murphy EG, Donohue WL. Light and electron microscopic studies of "myogranules" in a child with hypotonia and muscle weakness. *Can Med Assoc J* 1963;9:618–625.
327. Wallgren-Pettersson C, et al. Genetics of congenital nemaline myopathy: a study of 10 families. *J Med Genet* 1990;27:480–487.
328. Laing NG, et al. A mutation in the alpha tropomyosin gene TPM3 associated with autosomal dominant nemaline myopathy NEM1. *Nat Genet* 1995;9:75–79.
329. Wallgren-Pettersson C, et al. A gene for autosomal recessive nemaline myopathy assigned to chromosome 2q by linkage analysis. *Neuromuscul Disord* 1995;5: 441–443.
330. Martinez BA, Lake BD. Childhood nemaline myopathy: a review of clinical presentation in relation to prognosis. *Dev Med Child Neurol* 1987;29:815–820.
331. Rifai Z, et al. Intranuclear rods in severe congenital nemaline myopathy. *Neurology* 1993;43:2372–2377.
332. Goebel HH, Warlo I. Nemaline myopathy with intranuclear rods: intranuclear rod myopathy. *J Child Neurol* 1997;7:13–19.
333. Jennekens FGI, et al. Congenital nemaline myopathy. I. Defective organization of alpha-actinin is restricted to muscle. *Muscle Nerve* 1983;6:61–68.
334. Stuhlfauth I, et al. Congenital nemaline myopathy: II. Quantitative changes in alpha-actinin and myosin in skeletal muscle. *Muscle Nerve* 1983;6:69–74.
335. Pelin K, et al. Mutations in the nebulin gene associated with autosomal recessive nemaline myopathy. *Proc Natl Acad Sci U S A* 1999;96:2305–2310.
336. Wallgren-Pettersson C, Rapola J, Donner M. Pathology of congenital nemaline myopathy. A follow-up study. *J Neurol Sci* 1988;83:243–257.
337. Feinberg DM, Spiro AJ, Weidenheim KM. Distinct light microscopic changes in human immunodeficiency virus-associated nemaline myopathy. *Neurology* 1998;50:529–531.
338. Zhang Y, et al. A mutation in the human ryanodine receptor gene associated with central core disease. *Nat Genet* 1993;5:46–50.
339. Berridge MJ. Inositol trisphosphate and calcium signalling. *Nature* 1993;361:315–325.
340. Shuaib A, Paasuke RT, Brownell KW. Central core disease: clinical features in 13 patients. *Medicine* 1987;66:389–396.
341. Quane KA, et al. Mutations in the ryanodine receptor gene in central core disease and malignant hyperthermia. *Nat Genet* 1993;5:51–55.
342. Shy GM, Magee KR. A new congenital non-progressive myopathy. *Brain* 1956;79:610–621.
343. Panegyres PK, Kakulas BA. The natural history of minicore-multicore myopathy. *Muscle Nerve* 1991; 14:411–415.
344. Swash M, Schwartz MS. Familial multicore disease with focal loss of cross-striations and ophthalmoplegia. *J Neurol Sci* 1981;52:1–10.
345. Sarnat HB. Myotubular myopathy: arrest of morphogenesis of myofibres associated with persistence of fetal vimentin and desmin. Four cases compared with fetal and neonatal muscle. *Can J Neurol Sci* 1990;17: 109–123.
346. Spiro AJ, Shy GM, Gonatas NK. Myotubular myopathy. *Arch Neurol* 1966;14:1–14.
347. Campbell MJ, Rebeiz JJ, Walton JN. Myotubular, centronuclear or peri-centronuclear myopathy? *J Neurol Sci* 1969;8:425–443.
348. Barth PG, van Wijngaarden GK, Bethlen J. X-linked myotubular myopathy with fatal neonatal asphyxia. *Neurology* 1975;25:531–536.
349. Sarnat HB, Flores-Dinorin L, Marín-García J. Infantile myofibrillar myopathy: a new mitochondrial myopathy. *Neurology* 2000 (*in press*).
350. Dodge PR. Congenital neuromuscular disorders. *Res Publ Assoc Res Nerv Ment Dis* 1958;38:479–533.
351. Iannaccone ST. Myogenes and myotubes. *J Child Neurol* 1992;7:180–187.
352. DeLange C. Congenital hypertrophy of the muscles, extrapyramidal motor disturbances and mental deficiency. *Am J Dis Child* 1934;48:243–268.
353. Wilson J, Walton JN. Some muscular manifestations of hypothyroidism. *J Neurol Neurosurg Psychiatry* 1959;22:320–324.
354. Debré R, Sémélaigne G. Syndrome of diffuse muscular hypertrophy in infants causing athletic appearance. *Am J Dis Child* 1935;50:1351–1361.
355. Spiro AJ, et al. Cretinism with muscular hypertrophy (Kocher-Debré-Sémélaigne syndrome). Histochemical and ultrastructural study of skeletal muscle. *Arch Neurol* 1970;23:340–349.
356. Shakhnovitch. On a case of intermittent paraplegia [Abstract]. *London Med Rec* 1894;12:130.
357. Westphal C. Über einen merkwürdigen Fall von periodischer Lähmung aller vier Extremitäten, mit gleichzeitigen Erlöschen der electrischen Erregbarkeit während der Lähmung. *Berl Klin Wochenschr* 1885;31: 489–511.
358. Greenberg DA. Calcium channels in neurological disease. *Ann Neurol* 1997;42:275–282.
359. Layzer RB. Periodic paralysis and the sodium-potassium pump. *Ann Neurol* 1982;11:547–552.
360. Ionasescu V, et al. Hypokalemic periodic paralysis. Low activity of sarcoplasmic reticulum and muscle ribosomes during an induced attack. *J Neurol Sci* 1974;21:419–429.
361. Kantola IM, Tarssanen LT. Familial hypokalaemic periodic paralysis in Finland. *J Neurol Neurosurg Psychiatry* 1992;55:322–324.
362. Dyken M, Zeman W, Rusche T. Hypokalemic periodic paralysis: children with permanent myopathic weakness. *Neurology* 1969;19:691–699.

363. Links TP, et al. Permanent muscle weakness in familial hypokalaemic periodic paralysis. Clinical, radiological and pathological aspects. *Brain* 1990;113:1873–1889.

364. Meyers KR, et al. Periodic muscle weakness, normokalemia, and tubular aggregates. *Neurology* 1972;22:269–279.

365. Kelly DE, et al. Thyrotoxic periodic paralysis. Report of 10 cases and review of electromyographic findings. *Arch Intern Med* 1989;149:2597–2600.

366. Conn JW, Rovner DR, Cohen EL. Licorice-induced pseudoaldosteronism. Hypertension, hypokalemia, aldosteronopenia, and suppressed plasma renin activity. *JAMA* 1968;205:492–496.

367. Johnson CH, VanTassell VJ. Acute barium poisoning with respiratory failure and rhabdomyolysis. *Ann Emerg Med* 1991;20:1138–1142.

368. Stedwell RE, Allen KM, Binder LS. Hypokalemic paralyses: a review of the etiologies, pathophysiology, presentation, and therapy. *Am J Emerg Med* 1992;10:143–148.

369. Carraccio C, Blotny K, Ringer R. Sudden onset of profound weakness in a toddler. *J Pediatr* 1993; 122:663–667.

370. Mateer JE, et al. Reversible ipecac myopathy. *Arch Neurol* 1985;42:188–190.

371. Sansone V, et al. Anderson's syndrome: a distinct periodic paralysis. *Ann Neurol* 1997;42:305–312.

372. McArdle B. Myopathy due to a defect in muscle glycogen breakdown. *Clin Sci* 1951;10:13–33.

373. Rowland LP, et al. The clinical diagnosis of McArdle's disease. Identification of another family with deficiency of muscle phosphorylase. *Neurology* 1966;16:93–100.

374. Lebo RV, et al. High-resolution chromosome sorting and DNA spot-blot analysis assign McArdle's syndrome to chromosome 11. *Science* 1984;225:57–59.

375. Tsujino S, et al. Three new mutations in patients with myophosphorylase deficiency (McArdle disease). *Am J Hum Genet* 1994;54:44–52.

376. DiMauro S, Hartlage PL. Fatal myopathic form of muscle phosphorylase deficiency. *Neurology* 1978;28:1124–1129.

377. Ohtani Y, et al. Infantile glycogen storage myopathy in a girl with phosphorylase kinase deficiency. *Neurology* 1982;32:833–838.

378. van der Berg IET, Berger R. Phosphorylase b kinase deficiency in man: a review. *J Inherit Metab Dis* 1990;13:442–451.

379. Argov Z, Bank WJ. Phosphorus magnetic resonance spectroscopy (^{31}P MRS) in neuromuscular disorders. *Ann Neurol* 1991;30:90–97.

380. DiMauro S, Servidei S. Disorders of carbohydrate metabolism: glycogen storage diseases. In: Rosenberg RN, et al., eds. *The molecular and genetic basis of neurological disease*, 2nd ed. Boston: Butterworth–Heinemann, 1997:1067–1098.

381. Layzer RB, Rowland LP, Ranney HM. Muscle phosphofructo-kinase deficiency. *Arch Neurol* 1967;17:512–523.

382. Ristow M, et al. Deficiency of phosphofructo–1–kinase/muscle subtype in humans impairs insulin secretion and causes insulin resistance. *J Clin Invest* 1997;100:2833–2841.

383. Servidei S, et al. Fatal infantile form of muscle phosphofructo-kinase deficiency. *Neurology* 1986;36:1465–1470.

384. DiMauro S, et al. Muscle phosphoglycerate mutase deficiency. *Neurology* 1982;32:584–591.

385. Kreuder J, et al. Brief report: inherited metabolic myopathy and hemolysis due to a mutation in aldolase A. *N Engl J Med* 1996;334:1100–1104.

386. Verzijl HTFM, et al. Genetic characteristics of myoadenylate deaminase deficiency. *Ann Neurol* 1998;44:140–143.

387. Engel WK, et al. A skeletal muscle disorder associated with intermittent symptoms and a possible defect of lipid metabolism. *N Engl J Med* 1970;282:697–704.

388. Murthy MS, Pande SV. Characterization of a solubilized malonyl-CoA-sensitive carnitine palmitoyltransferase from the mitochondrial outer membrane as a protein distinct from the malonyl-CoA-insensitive carnitine palmitoyltransferase of the inner membrane. *Biochem J* 1990;268:599–604.

389. Stumpf DA, Parker WD, Angelini C. Carnitine deficiency, organic acidemias, and Reye's syndrome. *Neurology* 1985;35:1041–1045.

390. Turnbull DM, et al. Short-chain acyl CoA dehydrogenase deficiency associated with a lipid-storage myopathy and secondary carnitine deficiency. *N Engl J Med* 1984;311:1232–1236.

391. Coates PM, et al. Genetic deficiency of short-chain acyl-coenzyme A dehydrogenase in cultured fibroblasts from a patient with muscle carnitine deficiency and severe skeletal muscle weakness. *J Clin Invest* 1988;81:171–175.

392. Winter SC, et al. Plasma carnitine deficiency. Clinical observations in 51 pediatric patients. *Am J Dis Child* 1987;141:660–665.

393. Breningstall GN. Carnitine deficiency syndromes. *Pediatr Neurol* 1990;6:75–81.

394. Stanley CA, et al. Chronic cardiomyopathy and weakness or acute coma in children with a defect in carnitine uptake. *Ann Neurol* 1991;30:709–716.

395. Treem WR, et al. Primary carnitine deficiency due to a failure of carnitine transport in kidney, muscle, and fibroblasts. *N Engl J Med* 1988;319:1331–1336.

396. Di Donato S. Disorders of lipid metabolism affecting skeletal muscle: carnitine deficiency syndromes, defects in the catabolic pathway, and Chanarin disease. In: Engel AG, Franzini-Armstrong C, eds. *Myology*, 2nd ed. New York: McGraw-Hill, 1994;1587–1609.

397. Shoji Y, et al. Evidence for linkage of human primary systemic carnitine deficiency with D5S436: a novel gene locus on chromosome 5 q. *Am J Hum Genet* 1998;63:101–108.

398. Lamhonway AM, Tein I. Carnitine uptake defect: frameshift mutations in the human plasmalemmal carnitine transporter gene. *Biochem Biophys Res Commun* 1998;252:396–401.

399. Falik-Borenstein ZC, et al. Brief report: renal tubular acidosis in carnitine palmitoyltransferase type 1 deficiency. *N Engl J Med* 1992;327:24–27.

400. Kelly KJ, et al. Fatal rhabdomyolysis following influenza infection in a girl with familial carnitine palmityl transferase deficiency. *Pediatrics* 1989;84:312–316.

401. Vladutin G.D. Biochemical and molecular correlations in carnitine palmitoyltransferase II deficiency. *Muscle Nerve* 1999;22:949–951.

402. Hug G, Bove KE, Soukup S. Lethal neonatal multiorgan deficiency of carnitine palmitoyl transferase II. *N Engl J Med* 1991;325:1862–1864.

403. Demaugre F, et al. Infantile form of carnitine palmitoyltransferase II deficiency with hepatomuscular

symptoms and sudden death: physiopathological approach to carnitine palmitoyltransferase II deficiencies. *J Clin Invest* 1991;87:859–864.

404. Land JM, et al. Neonatal carnitine palmitoyltransferase-2 deficiency: a case presenting with myopathy. *Neuromuscul Disord* 1995;5:129–137.

405. Meola G, et al. Recessive carnitine palmityl transferase deficiency: biochemical studies in tissue cultures and platelets. *J Neurol* 1987;235:74–79.

406. Zierz S. Carnitine palmitoyl transferase deficiency. In: Engel AG, Franzini-Armstrong C, eds. *Myology*, 2nd ed. New York: McGraw–Hill, 1994;1577–1586.

407. Stanley CA, et al. Brief report: a deficiency of carnitine-acylcarnitine translocase in the inner mitochondrial membrane. *N Engl J Med* 1992;327:19–23.

408. Jerusalem F, Spiess H, Baumgartner G. Lipid storage myopathy with normal carnitine levels. *J Neurol Sci* 1975;24:273–283.

409. Sengers RC, et al. Cardiomyopathy and short stature associated with mitochondrial and/or lipid storage myopathy of skeletal muscle. *Neuropaediatrie* 1976;7:196–208.

410. Williams ML, et al. Ichthyosis and neutral lipid storage disease. *Am J Med Genet* 1985;20:711–726.

411. Tonin P, et al. Metabolic causes of myoglobinuria. *Ann Neurol* 1990;27:181–185.

412. Herman J, Nadler HL. Recurrent myoglobinuria and muscle carnitine palmitoyl transferase deficiency. *J Pediatr* 1977;91:247–250.

413. Tein I, DiMauro S, DeVivo DC. Recurrent childhood myoglobinuria. *Adv Pediatr* 1990;37:77–156.

414. Martin-Du Pan RC, et al. Mitochondrial anomalies in a Swiss family with autosomal dominant myoglobinuria. *Am J Med Genet* 1997;69:365–369.

415. Andreu AL, et al. A nonsense mutation (G15059A) in the cytochrome b gene in a patient with exercise intolerance and myoglobinuria. *Ann Neurol* 1999;45:127–130.

416. Knochel JP. Rhabdomyolysis and myoglobinuria. *Annu Rev Med* 1982;33:435–443.

417. Mills KR, Edwards RHT. Investigative strategies for muscle pain. *J Neurol Sci* 1983;58:73.

418. Serratrice G, et al. Centronuclear myopathy. Possible central nervous system origin. *Muscle Nerve* 1978;1:62–69.

419. Ricci E, et al. Disorders associated with depletion of mitochondrial DNA. *Brain Pathol* 1992;2:141–147.

420. Guggenheim MA, et al. Glycerol kinase deficiency with neuromuscular, skeletal and adrenal abnormalities. *Ann Neurol* 1980;7:441–449.

421. Van der Knaap MS, et al. Magnetic resonance imaging in classification of congenital muscular dystrophies with brain abnormalities. *Ann Neurol* 1997;42:50–59.

422. Heffner R, et al. Multicore disease in twins. *J Neurol Neurosurg Psychiatry* 1976;39:602–606.

423. Cavanagh NPC, Lake BD, McMeniman P. Congenital fiber type disproportion myopathy: a histologic diagnosis with an uncertain clinical outlook. *Arch Dis Child* 1979;54:735–743.

424. Engel AG, Angelini C, Gomez MR. Fingerprint body myopathy. *Mayo Clin Proc* 1972;47:377–388.

425. Jerusalem F, Engel AG, Gomez MR. Sarcotubular myopathy. *Neurology* 1973;23:897–906.

426. Lake BD, Wilson J. Zebra body myopathy: clinical, histochemical and ultrastructural studies. *J Neurol Sci* 1975;24:437–446.

427. Brooke MH, Neville HE. Reducing body myopathy. *Neurology* 1972;22:829–840.

428. Ringel S, et al. A new congenital neuromuscular disease with trilaminar muscle fibers. *Neurology* 1978;28:282–289.

429. Rohkamm R, et al. A dominantly inherited myopathy with excessive tubular aggregates. *Neurology* 1983;33:331–336.

430. Goebel HH, Schloon H, Lenard HG. Congenital myopathy with cytoplasmic bodies. *Neuropediatrics* 1981;12:166–180.

431. Bove KE, et al. Cylindrical spirals in a familial neuromuscular disorder. *Ann Neurol* 1980;7:550–556.

432. Kalimo H, et al. X-linked myopathy with excessive autophagy: a new hereditary muscle disease. *Ann Neurol* 1988;23:258–265.

433. Thompson AJ, et al. Polysaccharide storage myopathy. *Muscle Nerve* 1988;11:349–355.

434. Horowitz SH, Schmalbruch H. Autosomal dominant distal myopathy with desmin storage: a clinicopathologic and electrophysiologic study of a large kinship. *Muscle Nerve* 1994;17:151–160.

435. Dobyns WB, et al. Diagnostic criteria for Walker-Warburg syndrome. *Am J Med Genet* 1989;32:195–210.

436. Kioschis P, et al. Genomic organization of a 225-kb region in Xq28 containing the gene for X-linked myotubular myopathy (MTM1) and a related gene (MTMR1). *Genomics* 1998;54:256–266.

437. Mitrani-Rosenbaum S, et al. Hereditary inclusion body myopathy maps to chromosome 9p1-q1. *Hum Mol Genet* 1996;5:159–163.

438. Goldfarb LG, et al. Missense mutations in desmin associated with familial cardiac and skeletal myopathy. *Nat Genet* 1998;19:402–403.

439. Laverda AM, et al. Congenital muscular dystrophy, brain and eye abnormalities: one or more clinical entities? *Child Nerv Syst* 1993;9:84–87.

440. Lynch PJ, et al. A mutation in the transmembrane/luminal domain of the ryanodine receptor is associated with abnormal Ca2+ release channel function and severe central core disease. *Proc Natl Acad Sci U S A* 1999;96:4164–4169.

441. Tomé FMS. The saga of congenital muscular dystrophy. *Neuropediatrics* 1999;30:55–65.

Chapter 15

Neurologic Manifestations of Systemic Disease

John H. Menkes, *Burton W. Fink, †Carole G. H. Hurvitz,
‡Carol B. Hyman, §Stanley C. Jordan, and ‖Frederick Watanabe

*Departments of Neurology and Pediatrics, University of California, Los Angeles, UCLA School of Medicine, and Department of Pediatric Neurology, Cedars-Sinai Medical Center, Los Angeles, California 90048; *Department of Pediatrics, University of California, Los Angeles, UCLA School of Medicine, Los Angeles, California 90048; †Department of Pediatrics,University of California, Los Angeles, Center for the Health Sciences, and Department of Pediatric Hematology and Oncology, Cedars-Sinai Medical Center, Los Angeles, California 90048; ‡Department of Pediatrics, University of Southern California School of Medicine, and Children's Hospital of Los Angeles, Cedars-Sinai Medical Center, Los Angeles, California 90048; §Department of Pediatrics, University of California, Los Angeles, UCLA School of Medicine, and Department of Pediatric Nephrology and Transplant Immunology, Cedars-Sinai Medical Center, Los Angeles, California 90048; and ‖Department of Pediatrics, University of California, Los Angeles, UCLA School of Medicine, and Center for Liver Diseases and Transplantation, Cedars-Sinai Medical Center, Los Angeles, California 90048*

METABOLIC ENCEPHALOPATHIES

Extracerebral diseases can interfere with normal brain function by impairing the necessary supply of oxygen and glucose or by disturbing the ionic environment of neurons, glia, and cell processes.

Hypoxia and Hypoglycemia

Pathophysiology

Hypoxia-ischemia, hypoglycemia, and status epilepticus induce energy failure with consequent brain damage (1–3). The significant differences in the time course and distribution of brain damage that result from these three insults are depicted in Table 15.1. Primary events involve the release of glutamate and other excitatory amino acids and an increase in free cytosolic calcium concentration. Secondary (*downstream*) events include activation of calcium-dependent protein kinases and phosphorylases and hydrolysis of phospholipids with accumulation of diacylglycerides. The role of nitric oxide synthase, and free radical–mediated cell damage, and the altered expression of growth factors, heat shock, and stress proteins in cell death resulting from energy failure, have been reviewed by Siesjö (4), Choi (5), and Massa (6) (Fig. 15.1).

Cerebral function requires an adequate supply of oxygen and glucose. In adults, glucose is the only substrate oxidized by the brain, although under nonphysiologic conditions such as starvation, structural proteins and lipids can be used as well. The brain of an infant or younger child can oxidize substrates other than glucose, notably ketone bodies, and possibly glycerol and fatty acids (7,8). Glucose is supplied to the brain by the bloodstream and enters neurons and glia by facilitative transport. Six isoforms of facilitated glucose transporters (GLUT) have been cloned and are expressed in brain. Quantitatively GLUT1 and GLUT3 are the most important glucose transporters in brain. GLUT1 is expressed in the blood–brain barrier, whereas GLUT3 is the principal neuronal glucose transporter (9).

TABLE 15.1. *Neurobiological differences among ischemia, hypoglycemia, and epilepsy*

	Ischemia	Hypoglycemia[a]	Epilepsy
Energy level (% normal)	0–5	25	99
Predominant excitotoxin	Glutamate	Aspartate	Unknown
Lactic acidosis	Variable (depending on blood glucose)	Absent	Mildly elevated unless cerebral O_2 supply reduced
Duration of insult required to produce neuronal necrosis	2–10 min	10–20 min	45–120 min
Timing of neuronal death	2–4 d	1–8 hr postinsult	1–2 hr postinsult
Distribution of neuronal necrosis	Pan-necrosis	Selective neuronal necrosis	Selective neuronal necrosis and pan-necrosis
Location of brain damage			
Cerebral cortex	Middle laminae	Superficial laminae	Laminae 3 and 4
Hippocampus	CA 4, CA 1 pyramidal cells	Medial CA 1 cells dentate crest	CA 4 and CA 1
Basal ganglia, thalamus, midbrain	Thalamic reticular nucleus, caudate	Caudate	Caudate spared; globus pallidus, pars reticulata of substantia nigra

[a]We should emphasize that the studies on hypoglycemia were performed on adult animals, and that the times noted to neuronal necrosis and neuronal death refer to times after an isoelectric electroencephalogram. The relevance of these studies to newborn animals or the neonate is unknown.

Adapted from Auer RN, Siesjö BK. Biological differences between ischemia, hypoglycemia, and epilepsy. *Ann Neurol* 1988:24:699.

Compared with its rate of use, the glucose reserve of the brain, which is in the form of glycogen, is minute, and increased energy demands, as occur during a seizure, necessitate an increased rate of glucose transport across the blood–brain barrier.

Approximately 85% of glucose used by the adult brain is oxidized to CO_2 either through the Krebs tricarboxylic acid cycle, or after conversion to α-amino acids, mainly glutamic and aspartic acids. For these reactions, a constant oxygen supply (3.3 mL/100 g tissue per minute) is required. Glycolysis to lactate accounts for only approximately 10% of glucose used by the adult brain. The brain of newborn infants has a lower cerebral oxygen consumption and converts a considerably greater proportion of glucose to lactate and pyruvate (7). Values for cerebral metabolic rates for oxygen range from 0.4 to 1.3 mL/100 g per minute in term infants without neurologic injury, and 0.06 to 0.54 mL/100 g per minute in apparently normal preterm infants of 26 to 32 weeks' gestation (10). These values reflect the increased glycolytic ability of the immature brain and its reduced energy demands, in part a consequence of its reduced synaptic density. Reduced energy demands also explain to some degree the relative resistance of the newborn brain to hypoglycemic and hypoxic damage. See Chapter 5 for a more extensive discussion of perinatal asphyxia.

There is no constant relationship between blood glucose levels and the severity of neurologic symptoms, because the neurologic symptoms also reflect glucose levels within the brain, tissue energy requirements, and the ability of brain to draw on anaerobic glycolysis and other substrates for its metabolic needs (8).

The quantity of oxygen used by the brain is a function of the cerebral blood flow and the concentration difference for oxygen between arterial and cerebral venous blood. The principles involved in the measurement and calculation of brain oxygen consumption are discussed by Kety (11).

Neurologic symptoms can result from a reduction in arteriovenous oxygen difference. Such a reduction is seen in cyanotic congenital heart disease. According to Tyler and Clark,

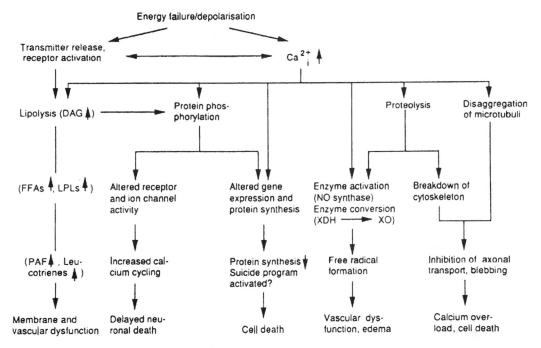

FIG. 15.1. Schematic diagram illustrating events resulting from energy failure. (DAG, diacylglycerides; FFA, free fatty acids; LPL, lysophospholipids; PAF, platelet activating factor; NO, nitric oxide; XDH, XO, xanthine oxidase, reduced and oxidized forms.) (From Siesjö BK. A new perspective on ischemic brain damage? *Prog Brain Res* 1993;96:1. With permission of the author.)

cerebral disturbances are encountered when the arterial oxygen saturation is 60% or less, although considerable individual differences occur in the degree to which the brain is susceptible to oxygen deprivation (12).

Cerebral anoxia also can result from reduced cerebral blood flow. The rate of cerebral blood flow depends on two factors: the pressure head (the difference between the arterial and venous pressure) and the resistance to blood flow through the cerebral vasculature. In aortic stenosis and in breath-holding spells, reduction of cerebral blood flow can induce neurologic symptoms, particularly syncope and seizures.

Several factors determine the extent and permanence of central nervous system (CNS) damage resulting from cerebral anoxia. These include the age of the subject, body temperature, extent and duration of anoxia, and intracellular pH. Siesjö and Plum (13) and more recently by Auer and Siesjö (14) have reviewed the patho-

physiology of anoxic brain damage beyond the neonatal period.

Brain regions containing a high density of excitatory amino acid (e.g., glutamate) receptors are the most vulnerable to hypoxic-ischemic insult, a finding that can at least partially account for patterns of hypoxic brain injury. This topic is more extensively covered in Chapter 5. The fact that damage from these insults can be attenuated by pharmacologic blockage of excitatory neurotransmission with receptor antagonists has triggered the search for similar agents suitable for clinical use (5). At present none are in general use in clinical situations.

Pathologic Anatomy

Bakay and Lee (15) and Auer and Siesjö (14) have described the basic pathologic alterations in the hypoxic brain. Structural damage can be limited to neurons or, if the hypoxia is more severe, it also involves glia and nerve fibers. The microscopic changes in neurons subjected to energy failure have been delineated by Auer and Beneviste (16). As a rule, associated glial cell damage is proportional to neuronal damage. In gray matter, astrocytes swell as a result of cellular overhydration, whereas in white matter, the intercellular space enlarges because of extracellular edema and alterations in the walls of the cerebral capillaries. Areas most sensitive to hypoxia, as occurs after sudden cardiac arrest, are the middle cortical layers of the occipital and parietal lobes, the hippocampus, amygdala, caudate nucleus, putamen, anterior and dorsomedial nuclei of the thalamus, and cerebellar Purkinje cells (17). Brainstem nuclei are more likely to be involved in infants than in older children.

When hypoxia is accompanied by hypotension, the ischemic lesions are concentrated along the arterial boundary zones of the cerebral cortex and cerebellum. With a prolonged insult, ischemic lesions tend to become generalized.

In hypoglycemia, there is selective neuronal necrosis of the superficial cortical layers, the hippocampus, and dentate gyrus. The cerebral cortical lesions are most conspicuous in the insular and the parieto-occipital cortices (18). The thalamus and nonneuronal elements are spared unless hypoglycemia is severe and prolonged (19–21). Damage to Purkinje cells is less than occurs after hypoxia (16,22). Infarction or hemorrhage are usually absent, even after a severe hypoglycemic insult (1). As occurs in hypoxia, the accumulation of excitatory neurotransmitters plays an important pathogenetic role in neuronal damage and death (1). The predominant release of aspartate into extracellular fluid in response to hypoglycemia contrasts with the release of glutamate in hypoxia and may account for the differences in the distribution of neuronal damage. The presence of acidosis, as occurs in hypercapnia, aggravates hypoglycemic neuronal damage, as does concurrent hypoxia (22,23).

Clinical Manifestations

Hypoxia

A number of clinical features are shared by all metabolic encephalopathies (24). The earliest symptom is a gradual impairment of consciousness. In infants, this can take the form of irritability, loss of appetite, and diminished alertness. Periods of hyperpnea can progress to Cheyne-Stokes respiration, a pattern of periodic breathing in which hyperpnea regularly alternates with apnea. The eyes move randomly, but ultimately, as the coma deepens, they come to rest in the forward position.

When anoxia occurs acutely, consciousness is lost within seconds. In cyanotic congenital heart disease, anoxia can take the form of brief syncopal attacks, often after crying, exertion, or eating, and most frequently occurring during the second year of life. Usually, at the onset of the attack, the child cries, then becomes deeply cyanotic and gasps for breath. Generalized seizures can terminate the more severe cyanotic episodes.

Should oxygen supply be restored immediately, recovery is quick, but when anoxia lasts longer than 1 to 2 minutes, neurologic signs persist transiently or permanently. These include impaired consciousness and decerebrate or decorticate rigidity. The prognosis for survival is relatively good for patients who after their anoxic episode exhibit intact brainstem function as manifested by normal vestibular responses, normal respiration, intact doll's eye movements, and pupillary light reactions (24).

The longer the duration of coma, the less likely the outlook for full recovery. In the series of Bell and Hodgson, which included all age groups, 17.5% of patients comatose for longer than 24 hours could be discharged from the hospital, but 70% of these subjects experienced significant and permanent neurologic impairment (25). There is fairly good evidence that some children who survive a major hypoxic episode without apparent neurologic residua are left with permanent visuoperceptual deficits (26).

The electroencephalogram (EEG) is of assistance in predicting the outcome of coma after cardiorespiratory arrest. A phasic tracing early in the recovery period indicates a good prognosis, whereas a flat EEG is never associated with full recovery except in cases of drug ingestion (27). Bilateral loss of cortical responses after median nerve stimulation on the somatosensory-evoked potential (SSEP) test is one of the best prognosticators for a poor outcome. Initial preservation of the cortical potentials does however not necessarily imply a good recovery (28,29). This is particularly true for small infants and serial SSEPs are indicated to ascertain whether they continue to remain intact (30). In term neonates the positive predictive value of an abnormal SSEP is also excellent, but in premature infants a normal response after stimulation of the median nerve had a poor predictive value with respect to normal outcome (30,31).

Near Drowning

In near drowning, the length of coma has even more significant prognostic implications than after cardiorespiratory arrest, and, as a rule, there is an all or nothing outcome, with few children experiencing mild degrees of neurologic damage. None of the patients still comatose in 15 to 30 minutes after their rescue survived without major neurologic residua, and 60% of subjects in this group died. In a Hawaiian series, all children who ultimately survived intact made spontaneous respiratory efforts within 5 minutes of rescue, and the majority of those did so within 2 minutes (32). The experiences from several other centers are similar in that all children who still required cardiopulmonary resuscitation on arrival at the hospital experienced permanent severe anoxic encephalopathy. Interestingly, the presence of convulsions does not indicate a bad prognosis although their persistence beyond 12 hours does. Fields concurs with that observation and lists the following factors that predict poor outcome: (a) submersion for more than 5 minutes; (b) serum pH below 7.0 at time of admission to the emergency room; (c) the need for cardiopulmonary resuscitation in the emergency room; (d) a delay before the first postresuscitation gasp; and (e) poor initial neurologic evaluation on resuscitation (33). Immersion

in cold or icy water appears to give a better chance for survival (34).

SSEPs and an EEG obtained during the second 24 hours after the accident have been used as additional prognostic indicators (35).

Numerous treatment regimens, many of unproved benefit, have been used for cerebral salvage. These include induced hypothermia, barbiturate coma, and intracranial pressure monitoring to control cytotoxic cerebral edema. None of these have been effective in improving the ultimate outcome (34,36). The neurologist attending a near-drowning victim should keep in mind that hypoglycemia and hyperglycemia can cause further neurologic damage. Hyperthermia should be avoided and seizures controlled, with phenytoin being the preferred anticonvulsant.

A postanoxic dystonic syndrome has been recognized in children. It appears 1 week to 36 months after the anoxic insult, and tends to worsen for several years. Dysarthria and dysphagia are common. Neuroimaging studies reveal putaminal lesions in the majority of such cases. Treatment is generally ineffectual. The pathophysiologic mechanism underlying this condition and the reason for its progression are totally unknown (37).

The persistent vegetative state (PVS) after near drowning is being seen with increasing frequency owing to the resuscitative facilities of most emergency rooms. According to data compiled in California and reported in 1994, survival of children in PVS is dependent on their age. Median survival of infants younger than 1 year of age was 2.6 years; of infants between 1 and 2 years, 4.2 years; and children between 2 and 6 years, 5.2 years (38). The same group of workers, reporting in 1999, found that in the mid-1990s the mortality rate for infants in PVS was only one-third of those in the early 1980s. A smaller decrease in mortality rates was recorded for children ages 2 to 10 years (38a). In the experience of Heindl and Laub 55% of children who are in PVS as a result of an anoxic event became conscious within 19 months of the injury. The quality of life was fairly good for those who recovered from PVS; 9% recovered completely, and another 52%

became independent in everyday life (39). After 9 months, less than 5% of children were able to recover from PVS (39). In the study of Ashwal and coworkers (38), children in PVS survive somewhat longer in institutions than at home; other studies have shown converse results (40). A more extensive consideration of the PVS can be found in Chapter 8.

Hypoglycemia

The neonate does not show any specific symptoms of hypoglycemia. Table 15.2 outlines the clinical picture of symptomatic hypoglycemia in term neonates, as recorded from a Scandinavian nursery (41).

Transient hypoglycemia has been observed in a relatively significant proportion of infants with intrauterine growth retardation, perinatal asphyxia, or other forms of perinatal stress (42,43), and in neonates born to mothers with diabetes or toxemia (44). The incidence of neonatal hypoglycemia is difficult to ascertain because of the different criteria used to define hypoglycemia and because of the varieties of feeding routines used in nurseries. Normal plasma glucose values during the first week of life have been published (45). With hypoglycemia defined as glucose levels of 20 mg/dL or less, the condition was identified in 5.7% of cases at the University of Illinois Hospital Nursery (46). The incidence is higher in low-birth-weight infants.

Symptoms of hypoglycemia may appear as early as 1 hour after birth, particularly in infants who are small for gestational age, but generally they are delayed until 3 to 24 hours. In approximately 25%, hypoglycemia does not become symptomatic until after 24 hours (41). An inconstant relationship exists between blood glucose levels and hypoglycemic symptoms. Some infants with blood sugar levels between 20 and 30 mg/dL develop hypoglycemic symptoms, whereas others whose levels fall below 20 mg/dL can remain asymptomatic (47). Evoked potentials have provided evidence for the critical value at which hypoglycemia affects the brain. SSEPs and brainstem auditory-evoked potentials become abnormal in term infants when their blood sugar falls below 41.5 and 45.0 mg/dL, respectively (48). Visual-evoked

TABLE 15.2. *Symptoms of neonatal hypoglycemia in 44 newborn patients[a]*

Principal symptoms	Number of infants
Tremors	33
Apnea, cyanosis, tachypnea	22
Convulsions	13
Lethargy	9
No symptoms or symptoms masked by another condition	7

[a]Hypoglycemia was considered to be significant if the blood sugar was 20 mg/dL or less on at least two separate occasions.
From Raivio KO. Neonatal hypoglycemia. *Acta Pediatr Scand* 1968;57:540. With permission.

responses remain normal at these levels. A rapid compensatory increase in cerebral blood flow resulting from recruitment of previously unperfused capillaries mediated by an increase in plasma epinephrine levels occurs at or below blood glucose values of 30 mg/dL (49–51). Magnetic resonance imaging (MRI) studies can show patchy hyperintensities in the occipital periventricular white matter. These lesions tend to resolve with prompt therapy (51a). From the point of view of a neurologist it therefore seems prudent that any blood glucose value of 45 mg/dL or less should be emergently corrected and followed closely to ensure normoglycemia.

The clinical management of hypoglycemia in the neonates is beyond the scope of this text. The reader is referred to a flow diagram by Cornblath and Schwartz (52).

It is difficult to know what the outlook is in terms of neurologic and cognitive deficits for neonates who develop symptomatic hypoglycemia. This is because of limitations of current definitions for neonatal hypoglycemia, our inability to determine at what glucose level hypoglycemia becomes symptomatic, and on the various other risk factors, which complicate the clinical course of hypoglycemic infants and confound every study on neurodevelopmental outcome (53). From a multitude of data derived from neonates without other major risk factors, who had severe hypoglycemia as a consequence of nesidioblastosis, it is clear that a significantly low plasma glucose level that persists over a prolonged period of time can indeed result in major brain damage. The risks of asymptomatic neonatal hypoglycemia are even more undefined, because low-birth-weight and stressed infants, the group with the highest incidence of hypoglycemia, are also subject to a variety of other prenatal and perinatal risks, notably hypoxic ischemic encephalopathy (54).

When older infants and children develop symptomatic hypoglycemia, the condition presents with autonomic symptoms, which accompany a progressive impairment of neurologic function. The serum glucose level at which symptoms appear varies, but any child with a blood glucose level of 46 mg/dL or less is suspect for hypoglycemia (55). Autonomic symptoms are mainly caused by increased adrenaline secretion. They include anxiety, palpitations, pallor, sweating, irritability, and tremors (55). During the initial stages, impaired neurologic function is manifested by dizziness, headache, blurred vision, somnolence, and slowed intellectual activity. Transient cortical blindness is seen only rarely (56). In fact, if permanent blindness accompanies hypoglycemia, one must consider the diagnosis of congenital optic nerve hypoplasia associated with hypopituitarism (see Chapter 4) (57). If hypoglycemia is prolonged, subcortical and diencephalic centers become inoperative. The brainstem, the area most resistant to hypoglycemia, is the last to be affected.

Almost all children develop generalized or focal seizures during a severe hypoglycemic episode. With even more prolonged involvement, tonic extensor spasms and shallow respirations develop. The response to intravenous glucose is immediate in patients who have not progressed to brainstem involvement. In children who have experienced prolonged unconsciousness or repeated hypoglycemic attacks the prognosis for complete recovery is poor and approximately one-half of the patients remain mentally retarded (58).

Not uncommonly, the clinician encounters a child whose first seizure occurred in the setting of suspected hypoglycemia, but who continues to experience seizures in the absence of hypoglycemia. Although prolonged hypoglycemia can indeed induce hippocampal damage and thus set up a seizure focus, we believe that isolated hippocampal damage is quite rare, and that, in the majority of such cases, both initial and sub-

sequent seizures are unrelated to hypoglycemia. Transient hemiparesis or aphasia has been seen in diabetic children, often in association with documented hypoglycemia. The cause of these focal deficits is unclear, but they could reflect focal seizures followed by Todd's paralysis (59).

Brain Death

The Ad Hoc Committee on Brain Death from the Children's Hospital, Boston, has defined brain death:

> Brain death has occurred when cerebral and brainstem functions are irreversibly absent. Absent cerebral function is recognized clinically as the lack of receptivity and responsivity, that is, no autonomic or somatic response to any sort of external stimulation, mediated through the brainstem. Absent brainstem function is recognized clinically when pupillary and respiratory reflexes are irreversibly absent. . . . Particularly in children, peripheral nervous activity, including spinal cord reflexes, may persist after brain death; however, decorticate or decerebrate posturing is inconsistent with brain death (60).

Recommendations made by a special task force appointed to set guidelines for determining brain death have been published (61). Although it is generally recognized that particular caution should be exerted when diagnosing brain death in small children, the task force further emphasized this age distinction by recommending different brain death criteria for infants between 7 days and 2 months of age, between 2 months and 1 year, and older than 1 year. The period of observation before declaration of brain death in the youngest group should be such that two examinations and EEGs to document electrocerebral silence are performed, separated by at least 48 hours. In the group from 2 months to 1 year of age, the interval between the two examinations and EEGs can be reduced to 24 hours. Furthermore, a repeat examination and EEG are not necessary in this group if radionuclide angiography demonstrates absent cerebral blood flow (62). In children older than 1 year, the task force recommended the period of observation be a minimum of 12 hours, unless corroborating tests added further support to the diagnosis of brain death. When the extent and reversibility of brain damage are difficult to assess because of the type of insult (e.g., hypoxic-ischemic encephalopathy), the observation period should be extended to at least 24 hours.

Some authorities have challenged these recommendations and a survey of pediatric intensive care units shows substantial variability even within the same pediatric intensive care unit with respect to criteria used by clinicians for the diagnosis of brain death (63). In a clinical and neuropathologic study of brain death, Fackler and coworkers found no support for employing distinct brain death criteria for infants between 2 months and 1 year of age (64). Other investigators question the validity of relying on the EEG to confirm brain death, because EEG activity is occasionally seen after brain death (65). Conversely, phenobarbital levels above 25 to 35 μL can suppress EEG activity in neonates (66). The brainstem-auditory evoked response cannot be used as a confirmatory laboratory criterion of brain death. Its absence is not predictive of brain death and persistence of peak I has occasionally been seen in brain dead infants (67). Although complete absence of cerebral blood flow is considered irrefutable evidence of brain death, cerebral blood flow is extremely low in normal term or preterm newborns (10).

We believe that as more sophisticated imaging techniques such as xenon-enhanced computed tomography (CT), single photon emission computed tomography (SPECT) (68), and positron emission tomography (PET) (69) are applied to the clinical evaluation of brain death in children, the criteria for making this diagnosis will become refined and perhaps simplified.

An important aspect in diagnosing brain death is the documentation of apnea. During this procedure, it is vital to prevent hypoxemia. Administration of 100% oxygen for 10 minutes is recommended before withdrawal of respiratory support. A catheter should be inserted into the endotracheal or tracheostomy tube, and oxygen be continued at 6 L/minute during the test. The arterial pCO_2 level should be allowed to increase to 60 mm Hg. Patients who are hypothermic or receiving medications that suppress respiration cannot be reliably tested using this procedure (70). When diabetes insipidus is seen, it reflects midbrain death (71).

Disorders of Acid–Base Balance

Pathology

Both pH and ionic concentrations within the CNS are controlled by the blood–brain barrier, which renders the brain relatively resistant to alterations in the electrolyte composition of serum. In disorders of acid–base balance, the blood pH correlates poorly with the presence or severity of neurologic symptoms. This is because cerebrospinal fluid (CSF) pH tends to fluctuate less than arterial pH, even with wide shifts in serum hydrogen ion concentrations. Resistance to shifts of systemic pH is most pronounced in metabolic acidosis, less evident in metabolic and respiratory alkalosis, and least effective in respiratory acidosis. Homeostatic factors maintaining the pH of CSF include alterations in cerebral blood flow, active transport of H^+ and HCO_3^-, and carbon dioxide removal. These factors are reviewed by Plum and Siesö (72). In respiratory acidosis, the pH of CSF deviates from normal as much as or more than arterial pH. This deviation often obscures the severity of acid–base disturbance and suggests measurements of CSF pH in encephalopathies associated with ion imbalance are preferable to those of blood pH.

Clinical Manifestations

The neurologic picture of acid–base disorders is nonspecific. Children become progressively more obtunded, finally delirious, and comatose. Seizures are rare. Often, the patient's clinical condition does not correlate well with either blood or CSF pH, although in patients with respiratory acidosis, neurologic symptoms are invariably present when the pH of CSF decreases below 7.25.

Disorders of Electrolyte Metabolism

Sodium and Potassium

Disturbances of serum electrolytes can induce changes in the ionic composition of the intracellular and extracellular compartments of the brain. These changes can have major effects on the excitability of the neural membrane and on the processing and transmission of neuronal signals. The membrane potential depends in part on the ratio of intracellular and extracellular sodium and potassium concentrations. Major shifts in serum sodium concentrations disrupt cerebral function as a result of altered osmolality of the cellular compartments. A normal potassium level is essential for the maintenance of the membrane potential. In contrast to the ease with which fluctuations in serum sodium concentration affect intracerebral sodium, the concentration of extracellular potassium within the brain, as reflected by CSF levels, varies little, even with such major shifts as those induced by intravenous infusions of potassium or by the administration of corticosteroids. It is, therefore, uncertain what role potassium plays in the evolution of cerebral symptoms commonly associated with hyperkalemia or hypokalemia. The effect of potassium on muscular function is reviewed in Chapter 14. The reader is also referred to a review by Katzman and Pappius (73) for a full discussion of the pathogenesis of cerebral symptoms in electrolyte disorders and to a review by Strange on disorders of osmotic balance (74).

TABLE 15.3. *Clinic conditions producing abnormalities of sodium concentration*

Hyponatremia
  Administration of salt-poor solutions in the presence of impaired function, acute overload of solute-free water in infants
  Water retention (congestive heart failure, hepatic cirrhosis)
  Depletion of intracellular solutes (diuretics, protein energy malnutrition, cystic fibrosis, adrenogenital syndrome)
  Postoperative hyponatremia, associated with non-osmotic release of antidiuretic hormone
  Inappropriate secretion of antidiuretic hormone in diseases involving the central and peripheral nervous systems (anatomic isolation of supraoptic nucleus of hypothalamus resulting in released firing of osmoreceptors)
  Encephalitis, meningitis, polyneuritis, diffuse cerebral damage in infancy, cerebral infarction, supratentorial and infratentorial brain tumors, subarachnoid hemorrhage
Hypernatremia
  Limited water intake
  Excessive evaporative losses (hyperpnea, increased environmental temperature)
  Excessive excretory losses (diarrhea, diabetes insipidus)
  Salt loading (often accompanied by excessive water loss)
  Sodium retention (hyperaldosteronism and Cushing syndrome)

Hyponatremia

Low-sodium syndromes can result from an increase in body water with retention of a normal sodium store or can occur after reduction of sodium stores. The clinical conditions associated with hyponatremia are outlined in Table 15.3.

In the experience of Arieff and colleagues, the most common cause for symptomatic hyponatremia in the pediatric population was administration of hypotonic fluids combined with extensive extrarenal loss of electrolyte-containing fluids (75). Oral water intoxication from increased intake of tap water during the summer months also induces symptomatic hyponatremia (76). Neurologic symptoms of hyponatremia include headache, nausea, incoordination, delirium, and, ultimately, generalized or focal seizures with apnea and opisthotonus

(77,78). On autopsy, cerebral edema and transtentorial herniation are seen (75,76).

Generally, severe neurologic symptoms with permanent residua do not develop at sodium levels above 130 mEq/L, unless plasma sodium has decreased rapidly. Some have advocated rapid correction of hyponatremia in a patient with neurologic symptoms using urea in conjunction with salt supplements and water restriction (79). A too rapid correction of hyponatremia has been thought to play a role in the development of central pontine myelinolysis (80), a frequently fatal disorder characterized clinically by confusion, cranial nerve dysfunction, and, in larger lesions, a "locked in" syndrome and quadriparesis. Pathologically, central pontine myelinolysis is characterized by symmetric destruction of myelin at the center of the pons. The pontile demyelination can be visualized by MRI (81).

According to Brunner and colleagues, central pontine myelinolysis is more likely to develop when the initial sodium level is less than 105 mEq/L, when hyponatremia has developed acutely, and when sodium levels are corrected too rapidly (82). Other investigators have challenged the concept that this condition is related to the rate of correction of hyponatremia, and the optimal rate for correcting hyponatremia is still controversial (83). According to Keating and colleagues, an optimal rate of correction is 2 to 3 mEq/L per hour (76).

Hypernatremia

Increased concentration of sodium in body fluids elevates fluid osmolality and induces severe cerebral manifestations. Major causes for hypernatremia are outlined in Table 15.3.

Luttrell and Finberg have delineated the factors responsible for neurologic symptoms. These are subdural hematomas, venous and capillary congestion, and hemorrhages, the last produced by shrinkage of the brain during dehydration (84).

Neurologic symptoms can also occur in the absence of any structural alteration and are probably the direct result of hyperosmolality. Symptoms are caused by cerebral edema, which is particularly likely to occur with rapid rehydration and is caused by an elevated content of chloride and potassium in the brain (85,86).

Hypernatremia is generally seen in infants younger than 6 months of age. All have clear evidence of dehydration. Patients have varying degrees of impaired consciousness and hyperpyrexia. Approximately one-third experience generalized convulsions and spasticity. Focal neurologic abnormalities, notably hemiparesis, are seen in approximately 10% of patients. Finberg found subdural hematomas in many of his hypernatremic infants (87). In some, neurologic symptoms, notably seizures, do not appear until 24 to 48 hours after the start of fluid therapy. These symptoms have been ascribed to cerebral edema and a lowered convulsive threshold developing with rehydration of the brain (85).

The mortality of children who develop neurologic symptoms with hypernatremia ranges from 10% to 20%. Approximately one-third of survivors have permanent sequels, notably seizures, spasticity, and mental retardation (88).

Chloride

Hypochloremia

A syndrome marked by anorexia, lethargy, failure to thrive, muscular weakness, and hypokalemic metabolic alkalosis was seen in infants who ingested a chloride-deficient formula for the preceding 1 or more months (89,90). Serum chloride as low as 61 mEq/L and arterial pH values as high as 7.74 were recorded (89). Usually, urinary chlorides were completely absent. Impaired growth of head circumference was documented in the majority of cases. Rehydration and chloride supplementation reversed all symptoms and resulted in a marked acceleration of motor milestones and in complete or partial recovery of the decelerated skull growth. Developmental testing in some of these children at 9 to 10 years of age indicated that children who had received this formula had significantly lower scores on the Wechsler Intelligence Scale for Children (WISC) and significantly higher risks for receptive and expressive language disorders (91). We have recognized a clinical picture of an expressive language delay, coupled with visuomotor deficits and an attention deficit disorder that often assumes the overfocused pattern (see Chapter 16). When the defect is more severe, the language and visuomotor problems can expand to a picture of generalized mental retardation, and the attention disorder can exhibit autistic features (92). A similar condition has been seen in nursing infants whose mothers' milk was for unknown reasons deficient in chloride (93).

Calcium

Calcium is the major extracellular divalent cation. Both high and low serum calcium levels are associated with neurologic symptoms. Total calcium in serum is found in three forms: protein bound, and therefore nondiffusible (30% to 55% of total); chelated (i.e., diffusible but nonionized; 15% of total); and ionized (remaining percentage). Generally, the appearance of neurologic symptoms cor-

TABLE 15.4. *Conditions producing hypocalcemia, hypomagnesemia, and neurologic symptoms*

Condition	Symptoms	Reference
Premature and critically ill term infants	Onset in first 48 hours of life, generalized neuromuscular hyperexcitability, convulsions, spontaneous attacks of apnea and cyanosis, hollow or squeaky cry, hyperactivity alternating with immobility	Craig and Buchanan (94), Nelson et al. (95), Cardenas-Rivero et al. (96)
Transient neonatal hypoparathyroidism, decreased urinary excretion of phosphate (neonatal tetany)	Seen mainly in bottle-fed infants; appears at 5–8 days of age; convulsions and generalized neuromuscular hyperexcitability	Cockburn et al. (97), Bainbridge et al. (98)
Maternal hyperparathyroidism	Major motor convulsions, refractory to anticonvulsants; appears in second week of life	Hartenstein and Gardner (99)
Vitamin D deficiency	Convulsions, laryngospasm, carpopedal spasm, muscular hypotonia; appears at 3–12 months of age	Eliot and Park (100), Gessner (101)
Hypoparathyroidism	Cataracts, photophobia, increased density of bones, ridging of teeth and nails, tetany and convulsions, increased intracranial pressure, mental deterioration, extrapyramidal disorder, calcification of basal ganglia	Simpson (102)
Pseudohypoparathyroidism	Obesity, dysmorphic appearance, round facies, stubby short hands and fingers, tetany and convulsions (88%), mental retardation (60%), syndrome unaltered by parathormone	Mallette (103), Cohen and Donnell (104)
Renal disease	Tetany, muscle cramps, fasciculations associated with moderate to severe acidosis, elevated serum potassium to calcium ratio, often unresponsive to calcium or magnesium administration	Tyler (105)
Hypomagnesemic tetany of infancy	Recurrent convulsions, appears first month of life, impaired magnesium absorption across gastrointestinal tract, transient hypoparathyroidism	Tsang (117)
DiGeorge syndrome	Cardiovascular defects, hypoplasia of parathyroids and thymus, seizures	Chapter 3

relates well with levels of ionized calcium of 2.5 mg/dL or less. The concentration of CSF calcium is normally approximately one-half that of serum calcium and represents the result of a secretory process, rather than the movement of diffusible and ionized calcium from the serum. Changes in the CSF concentration are relatively small, although large alterations in serum calcium values overcome homeostatic mechanisms (73).

Hypocalcemia

The clinical picture of hypocalcemia and its causes varies with the age of the affected child.

Some of the syndromes that produce hypocalcemia are outlined in Table 15.4.

Hypocalcemia was one of the more common causes of seizures during the neonatal period. The condition can be defined as a level of serum calcium below 7 mg/dL or of ionized calcium below 3.5 mg/dL. It is commonly seen in the preterm neonate or in the stressed term neonate (106). Two forms of neonatal hypocalcemia are encountered. One occurs during the first 2 days of life in premature and critically ill term infants. It is also seen in infants who have suffered perinatal asphyxia and in infants of mothers with insulin-dependent diabetes. As many as 50% of very-low-birth-weight infants have serum calcium levels below 7 mg/dL (107). The exact mechanism of this form of hypocalcemia is still obscure. Impaired vitamin D metabolism also has been excluded as a pathogenetic factor. Increased levels of calcitonin have been suggested as an etiologic factor in the hypocalcemia of prematurity, but not in that seen in infants of diabetic mothers (108). Decreased end-organ responsiveness, decreased calcium intake and absorption, and respiratory alkalosis are also believed to play a role (107). Less often, maternal hyperparathyroidism, congenital absence of the parathyroid glands, or disturbed renal function induce neonatal hypocalcemia (see Table 15.4). The second form of neonatal hypocalcemia is the classic neonatal tetany (late hypocalcemia), whose mechanism was first elucidated by Bakwin in 1937 (109). It occurs between the fifth and tenth days of life and results in part from intake of cow's milk, which induces an increased phosphate load. In this form of hypocalcemia, hyperphosphatemia and hypomagnesemia are commonly present (97). Additionally, low circulating parathyroid hormone levels are seen. With the widespread use of low-phosphate milk formulas this condition has virtually disappeared. In the series of Lynch and Rust, congenital heart disease was seen in 47% of infants with hypocalcemic seizures, and prematurity in 13%. Maternal hyperparathyroidism, idiopathic hypoparathyroidism, and DiGeorge syndrome were other causes. In 20% of infants there was no obvious cause for the seizures (110).

Neonatal hypomagnesemia has been recorded in association with hypocalcemia resulting from maternal hyperparathyroidism (106). It can also be the result of a selective malabsorption of magnesium (108) (see Table 15.4).

Hypocalcemic seizures can be focal, multifocal, or generalized. In the series of Lynch and Rust, multifocal clonic seizures were the most common. True tonic seizures or tonic-clonic (grand mal) attacks are unusual, and the latter seizure type was not encountered by Lynch and Rust (110). In the interictal period, infants generally are alert, and seizures without apparent loss of consciousness are not uncommon (97). Jitters were encountered in 35% of hypocalcemic infants in the 1971 series of Cockburn and coworkers (97), and in 27% of infants in the series of Lynch and Rust (110). An increased extensor tone is relatively common, as are increased deep tendon reflexes and ankle clonus. In contrast to neonates suffering from seizures owing to nonmetabolic causes, persistent focal neurologic deficits are not observed. The classic signs of tetany seen in the older child are usually absent. Carpopedal spasm was rare, stridor owing to laryngospasm, and Chvostek's sign (a brief contraction of the facial muscles elicited by tapping the face over the seventh nerve) was not noted in any of the hypocalcemic infants reported by Keen (111).

The EEG is frequently abnormal. It can demonstrate electroencephalo-graphic seizures (110).

The treatment of seizures caused by neonatal tetany consists primarily of the administration of calcium salts (see the section on neonatal seizures in Chapter 13). The long-term outlook of infants who have experienced seizures owing to late hypocalcemia is generally good and in the absence of subsequent neurologic insults the majority develop normally (97,110,111). Calcium deposition in necrotic areas of brains of stressed neonates has been related to the transient elevations of ionic calcium after parenteral administration of calcium gluconate (112).

In older infants and in children, neurologic symptoms of hypocalcemia include tetany and seizures. Tetany is characterized by episodes of muscular spasms and paresthesias mainly involving the distal portion of the peripheral nerves. Episodes appear abruptly and are precipitated by hyperventilation or ischemia. No alteration of consciousness occurs. Carpopedal spasm and laryngospasm are the two most frequent examples of tonic muscular spasms. Chvostek's sign is not diagnostic of tetany, because it is seen in healthy infants. Seizures can occur in the absence of tetany and are occasionally focal. Headaches and extrapyramidal signs are less common and are confined to older children or adults with hypoparathyroidism (113). In this condition, CT scans can show symmetric bilateral punctate calcifications of the basal ganglia, although only 50% show an association between this finding and the occurrence of extrapyramidal signs (113).

Pseudohypoparathyroidism is characterized by obesity, moon-shaped facies, mental retardation, cataracts, short, stumpy digits, enamel defects, and impaired taste and olfaction. Calcifications of the basal ganglia are seen in approximately one-third of instances. The condition is seen more commonly in females and is caused by an inability of renal tubules to respond to parathormone (103).

In neonates undergoing gastrostomy for various reasons, vitamin D malabsorption can lead to hypocalcemic seizures. This condition is treated by parenteral administration of vitamin D (114). Tetanic seizures also can result from sodium phosphate enemas (115).

Hypercalcemia

Aside from hyperparathyroidism, which is rare, hypercalcemia of childhood takes two forms: mild hypercalcemia and the hypercalcemia elfin-facies syndrome (Williams syndrome) (see Chapter 3). Patients with mild idiopathic hypercalcemia usually show a sudden failure to thrive between 3 and 7 months of age. The condition is probably the result of excess vitamin D intake and is reversible with restriction of calcium and vitamin D intake.

Williams syndrome is covered in Chapter 3. Neonatal hypercalcemia also is seen in the presence of subcutaneous fat necrosis and blue diaper syndrome. The latter is a rare familial disease in which hypercalcemia is associated with a defect in the intestinal transport of tryptophan. The blue diaper results from the oxidation of indican, a tryptophan derivative (116). Neurologic symptoms are generally absent, although optic nerve hypoplasia has accompanied this condition.

Magnesium

Since the 1970s, it has become apparent that a number of symptomatic infants with combined hypocalcemia and hypomagnesemia respond only to the administration of magnesium (117). This condition, termed *congenital hypomagnesemia*, is marked by recurrent tetany or convulsions, which commence during the first few weeks of life and respond to administration of magnesium but not calcium. Blood magnesium

levels can be as low as 0.04 mmol/L, as contrasted with mean normal levels of 0.8 mmol/L, with hypomagnesemia being defined as levels below 0.65 mmol/L (118). Although boys are overrepresented in reported cases, this condition is now believed to be transmitted as an autosomal recessive disorder (119), and in one extended Bedouin family it has been mapped to the long arm of chromosome 9 (9q) (120). The condition is caused by a selective defect in magnesium absorption in the small intestine (121). This is believed to result from a defect in a receptor or ion channel (120). Symptomatic hypocalcemia also occurs and is believed to be secondary to impaired synthesis or secretion of parathyroid hormone, or end-organ unresponsiveness to parathormone as a result of diminished activity of magnesium-dependent enzymes. When treated early and consistently, the outcome is good in terms of neurodevelopment, but untreated children can die or experience permanent brain damage (119). Congenital hypomagnesemia is distinct from primary familial hypomagnesemia, whose gene has been mapped to the long arm of chromosome 3 (122).

Hypomagnesemia also is seen in infants of diabetic mothers and in small-for-date infants. It has been described in conjunction with maternal hypoparathyroidism, neonatal hepatic disease, and increased loss of magnesium, as might occur after repeated exchange transfusions.

In older infants or children, low plasma magnesium levels are encountered in malabsorption syndromes, prolonged diarrhea, rickets, protein energy malnutrition or other forms of chronic malnourishment, and hypoparathyroidism (117,123).

Diagnosis of the Metabolic Encephalopathies

In most instances, the differential diagnosis of the metabolic encephalopathies rests on the clinical history and on laboratory examinations. The clinical and EEG pictures tend to be nonspecific and usually reflect dulling of consciousness and a diffuse cerebral disorder. The examining physician, therefore, must go through the differential diagnosis of impaired consciousness in an infant or child.

A history obtained quickly but competently is the first requirement for the differential diagnosis of coma. The physician must determine if loss of consciousness occurred without warning or was preceded by other symptoms, such as an upper respiratory infection, gastrointestinal disturbances, headaches, or unsteady gait. If the onset of unconsciousness was sudden, one has to consider acute poisoning, trauma, postictal stupor, or, less likely, an intracranial or subarachnoid hemorrhage. Trauma and acute subdural and extradural hemorrhages secondary to trauma are unlikely in the absence of external injuries and retinal hemorrhages and in the presence of a normal CT scan, whereas a normal CSF virtually excludes a subarachnoid hemorrhage. Focal neurologic signs are the rule in an intracerebral hemorrhage. Poisoning is often difficult to exclude, particularly in a toddler, and warrants gastric lavage and blood screening for toxins in all undiagnosed cases of coma. Making a diagnosis of postictal stupor is difficult after an unobserved convulsive attack unless one can elicit a history of a seizure disorder. Obstruction of the ventricular system by an intraventricular tumor, and hemorrhage arising from a hemangiomatous malformation within the brainstem are rare causes for sudden loss of consciousness.

When loss of consciousness is preceded by an illness, the diagnosis of metabolic encephalopathy, acute meningitis, encephalitis, or increased intracranial pressure must be considered. Examination of the eye grounds for papilledema, neuroimaging studies, blood chemistries, and a lumbar puncture are required to distinguish among the various entities. It is hazardous to arrive at a diagnosis of encephalitis in a patient who has normal CSF. Rather, one must consider other conditions. Acute toxic encephalopathy and Reye syndrome are two entities, which are now relatively uncommon. They were characterized by vomiting, seizures, and prolonged loss of consciousness. Because they have been postulated to have a viral cause, they are considered in Chapter 6.

NEUROLOGIC COMPLICATIONS OF PULMONARY DISEASE

In the past, neurologic problems in children with lung disease were encountered relatively infrequently, but with the recent advent of improved management for both acute and chronic pulmonary disease, and hence prolonged survival, such disorders are being recognized increasingly.

Extracorporeal membrane oxygenation (ECMO) is being used in most medical centers to treat neonates with uncontrollable respiratory failure (124). This invasive, technically complicated procedure is designed to functionally bypass the lungs. It requires systemic anticoagulation and generally necessitates ligation of the right common carotid artery, the right internal jugular vein, or both. Even though there is a compensatory response anatomically mediated through the circle of Willis, approximately one-fourth of infants demonstrate focal parenchymal lesions on postECMO MRI (125). As a rule, these are right-sided ischemic lesions, and contralateral hemorrhagic lesions consistent with hyperperfusion of the left cerebral hemisphere. In the experience of Mendoza and her group, 83% of ischemic lesions involved the right side and 70% of the hemorrhagic lesions occurred solely or predominantly on the side opposite the carotid ligation (126). These abnormalities are demonstrable on head ultrasound studies performed during the course of ECMO (127). Additionally, there is a significant incidence of left hemiparesis and left focal seizures. These deficits, seen during the neonatal period, however do not always translate into focal functional disabilities in later life. The neurodevelopmental outcome of infants who had been placed on ECMO has been surveyed in several centers. Most studies record a handicap rate of approximately 20% to 30% (128,129). The underlying diagnosis necessitating ECMO is in part a predictor of the outcome. Children who required ECMO because of meconium aspiration have higher developmental indices than those whose underlying diagnosis was sepsis (129), whereas children who develop bronchopulmonary dysplasia after ECMO fare less well (130). Serial plasma lactate concentrations obtained during the procedure may help predict the developmental outcome (131), as may the degree of abnormality seen on neuroimaging (132). The major causes of handicap are spastic quadriparesis, seizures, impaired cognitive functioning, and language delay (128). Additionally, approximately 20% of children have abnormal hearing, most commonly a sensorineural hearing loss (133,134). This figure, obtained by testing brainstem auditory-evoked potentials on ECMO-treated infants at the time of hospital discharge, may be falsely low, and at least in some infants hearing loss appears to have a delayed onset and to be progressive (135). The sensorineural hearing loss seen in children postECMO treatment parallels an incidence of 37% of generally bilateral sensorineural hearing loss in children with persistent fetal circulation who are not treated with ECMO. Although prolonged hyperventilation has been implicated in this deficit, other factors are probably operative (136,137).

Theophylline is commonly used in the nursery for the treatment of apnea and in older children for asthma and other pulmonary conditions. The major neurologic complication of theophylline therapy is the appearance of seizures, which are seen in all age groups, and are generally accompanied by elevated theophylline levels, although seizures have been observed at levels of 21 to 23 μg/mL (138,139). Seizures can be focal or generalized. When they are focal, one should suspect an underlying focal cerebral lesion. Theophylline-induced seizures are often difficult to control with anticonvulsants, and in some instances a toxic encephalopathy and permanent brain damage can ensue (140). Seizures are best avoided by careful monitoring of serum theophylline levels, and it would appear wise not to use the medication for the treatment of reactive airway disease in children who have an abnormally low seizure threshold.

In the past, a progressive degenerative disease of the CNS was seen in premature infants with bronchopulmonary dysplasia or other forms of severe and chronic lung disease who were receiving ventilatory support. This condition involved the cerebral cortex, brainstem, or basal ganglia (141). With improved control of the respirator variables, which affect mechanical ventilation, this entity is no longer encountered.

A distinctive neuromuscular syndrome has been encountered in children who had been on prolonged ventilatory support and nondepolarizing neuromuscular blocking agents. The condition is more common in the adult population and has been termed *critical illness neuromuscular disease* (142). Several overlapping syndromes are subsumed under that term. Some patients suffer from an axonal motor neuropathy, whereas in others a defect at the neuromuscular junction or a myopathy can be documented by electrophysiologic studies or biopsy (143). The clinical picture is similar and is highlighted by an inability of most such patients to be weaned from a respirator. Neurologic examination discloses a quadriparesis with absent or reduced reflexes, a neuropathic or myopathic electromyography result (EMG), and normal or only slightly elevated creatine kinase levels. Nerve conduction studies on patients with the axonal polyneuropathy show a mild slowing of motor velocity, and a muscle biopsy shows grouped atrophy. In critical illness myopathy there is a type II muscle fiber atrophy (144). The cause or causes for the clinical picture are obscure (145). Intravenous immune globulin has been suggested, but even without treatment affected children improve over the course of ensuing weeks or months.

The neurologic picture in chronic pulmonary disease (e.g., in advanced cystic fibrosis) results from hypoxia combined with carbon dioxide retention, and, to a lesser degree, from chronic respiratory acidosis. Children develop progressively deepening lethargy that, often with the onset of a respiratory infection, progresses to coma. Approximately 14% show papilledema, the consequence of increased intracranial pressure owing to chronic carbon dioxide retention, which induces dilatation of the cerebral vasculature (146). Seizures are rare. With evolution of the encephalopathy, asterixis and multifocal myoclonus become prominent. Asterixis consists of sudden flapping movements of the palms at the wrists (*liver flap*), most easily elicited when the arms are outstretched and the hands dorsiflexed.

During coughing paroxysms, such as are seen in cystic fibrosis, the most common neurologic complaints are lightheadedness and headache. Visual disturbances, paresthesias, tremor, and speech disturbances are occasionally encountered (147). All symptoms are reversible.

NEUROLOGIC COMPLICATIONS OF GASTROINTESTINAL AND HEPATIC DISEASE

Hepatic Encephalopathy

When the liver is damaged by acute or chronic disease, a characteristic set of neuropsychiatric symptoms develops termed *hepatic encephalopathy* (HE). The etiology of HE is still debated, but it is probably the consequence of systemic shunting of gut-derived constituents, caused by the impaired extraction by the failing liver (148,149).

Pathology and Pathogenesis

The morphologic changes in the brain are dominated by astrocytic alterations. The principal microscopic abnormalities include enlargement and increase in the number of protoplasmic astrocytes. These cells (Alzheimer II cells) are astrocytes with an enlarged, pale nucleus, and a marked diminution in glial fibrillary acidic protein. They are found throughout the cerebral cortex, basal ganglia, brainstem nuclei, and Purkinje layer of the cerebellum. They are most prominent in the chronic forms of liver disease and in patients dying after prolonged periods of coma (150). Neuronal changes are generally not seen. Less often, central pontine myelinolysis has been noted in children with hepatic failure (151).

According to current consensus HE is multifactorial (152,152a). The two most important factors in its pathogenesis are increased plasma and brain concentrations of ammonia and increased GABAergic neurotransmission.

Ammonia has been known to be neurotoxic for several decades. When astrocyte cultures are exposed to ammonia, they are transformed to Alzheimer II cells. From a neurophysiologic point of view, ammonia enhances neuronal inhibition, either by acting directly on the $GABA_A$ receptor complex and increasing selectively the binding of agonist ligands, or by promoting astrocytic synthesis of substances that activate the $GABA_A$ receptor complex (152).

However, approximately 10% of patients with HE have normal or only moderately elevated blood ammonia levels (153), and electrophysiologic experiments have shown that at the ammonia concentrations seen in hepatic failure, (0.5 to 2 mM), ammonia blocks the formation of hyperpolarizing inhibitory postsynaptic potentials, thus impairing postsynaptic inhibitory processes and increasing excitatory neurotransmission (154). These effects contrast with the clinical picture of hepatic coma, making it evident that hyperammonemia is not solely responsible for HE.

Increased GABA-mediated neurotransmission contributes significantly to the manifestations of HE. Primarily studied in chronic liver disease, GABAergic transmission is probably also affected in acute HE. Several mechanisms have been proposed. These include an increased availability of GABA in synaptic clefts, the result of ammonia-induced abnormalities in glial function, leading to decreased GABA reuptake, increased levels of benzodiazepine receptor agonists (155), loss of presynaptic feedback inhibition of GABA release caused by a decrease in the number of $GABA_B$ receptors, or increased transfer of GABA from blood to brain (154). Studies in both animal models and humans with HE have demonstrated transient improvement in mental status after administration of flumazenil, a benzodiazepine antagonist (156). The exact mechanism for improvement is unclear; it has been suggested that several, mostly unidentified endogenous or food-derived benzodiazepine-like substances act as ligands for the receptor (157).

Additional metabolic disturbances may contribute to the evolution of HE. High levels of ammonia can increase glutamine synthesis. Although glutamine itself is not neurotoxic, its metabolite alpha-ketoglutarate is. Furthermore, the increased synthesis of glutamine depletes the available amounts of alpha-ketoglutarate, reducing the concentration of high-energy phosphates, and slowing the reactions in the Krebs tricarboxylic acid cycle. Decreased oxygen consumption and glucose metabolism are probably secondary to HE rather than causative (152).

Evidence for the synergistic role of other neurotoxins such as mercaptans, short-chain fatty acids, and phenols, and the generation of false neurotransmitters such as octopamine is currently less strong (152). Additionally, liver

TABLE 15.5. *Signs and symptoms of hepatic encephalopathy*

Stage	Mental status/behavior	Motor/reflexes
I	Mild confusion Anxiety Irritability, agitation Altered sleep pattern Reduced attention Depression	Fine postural tremor Slowed coordination
II	Drowsiness, lethargy Gross personality change Disorientation (especially time) Poor recall Inappropriate behavior	Asterixis Dysarthria Suck and grasp reflexes Paratonia Ataxia
III	Delirium, profound confusion Paranoia Disorientation (time, place) Incomprehensible speech Somnolent but arousable	Hyperreflexia Seizures, myoclonus Hyperventilation Babinski sign Hypothermia Incontinence
IV	Coma	Decerebrate posturing Brisk oculocephalic reflexes

failure induces profound multisystem disturbances, which, in turn, can further impair neurologic function (158).

Clinical Manifestations

HE can occur in two forms: acutely, as in fulminant hepatic failure, and as a chronic, progressive encephalopathy. In children, acute hepatic failure is primarily responsible for clinically important HE. The most common predisposing causes are acute infectious hepatitis, ingestion of drugs (e.g., valproic acid, acetaminophen, isoniazid, halothane) or toxins (e.g., mushroom poisoning) (159), or Wilson disease (160). In infancy, galactosemia, fructosemia, or tyrosinemia can present as fulminant hepatic failure (see Chapter 1). In the past, Reye syndrome and hemorrhagic shock syndrome presented with fulminant liver failure (see Chapter 6).

The onset of the encephalopathy usually coincides with a deterioration of the general clinical condition. The principal signs and symptoms of hepatic coma are related to disorders of consciousness. The stages of HE are outlined in Table 15.5. It is of the utmost importance that the first signs of encephalopathy are recognized. Because the first evidence of encephalopathy

can be outbursts of violent agitation or uncharacteristic behavior, the early stage of HE is frequently misdiagnosed. The progression from stage I to stage IV can be exceedingly rapid. Hyperventilation can develop during stages II and III and can lead to alkalosis, low serum pCO_2, and a further deterioration of mental status. A fine tremor and more characteristically coarse flapping movements, termed *asterixis*, can be present in stages I and II, respectively, whereas decorticate and decerebrate postural responses accompany stage IV of HE. Choreic movements, a fluctuating rigidity of the limbs, dystonia, and periods of noisy delirium are particularly frequent in children (161).

Cerebral edema is a prominent part of the clinical picture of acute HE and is the principal cause of death, with brainstem herniation found in up to 80% of patients dying in fulminant hepatic failure (162). The cause of cerebral edema is unknown, and it is believed to be both vasogenic and cytotoxic, with the latter being more important. In vasogenic edema, there is a toxin-induced breakdown of the blood–brain barrier, with leakage of serum proteins through the capillary endothelium into the brain parenchyma. The cytotoxic aspects of cerebral edema result from an impaired cellular osmoregulation, which results in intracellular accumulation of fluids, mainly within astrocytes (163).

Although severe liver disease is a prerequisite for the appearance of HE, ascites, jaundice, edema, or hepatomegaly do not invariably accompany the neurologic involvement. In fact, frequently, as irreversible liver failure supervenes, previously elevated serum transaminase levels decrease rapidly, the coagulopathy worsens, the initially enlarged liver shrinks, and the total bilirubin climbs while the conjugated portion decreases.

In a majority of patients, the EEG shows paroxysmal and diffuse bursts of high-voltage slow-wave activity, a pattern that is not specific for HE but is highly indicative of one of the metabolic encephalopathies. Triphasic waves, characteristic for HE, are common in adults but rare in children. Clinical or EEG evidence of seizures is associated with a poor outcome (164).

Treatment and Prognosis

The advent of successful liver transplantation has revolutionized the management, treatment, and prognosis of children with liver failure and HE (165). Liver transplantation now offers a success rate of between 55% and 89% (166). Therefore, the child with HE requires meticulous medical management until either the liver resumes adequate function or a replacement organ is found. Management of the precipitating event, dietary protein restriction, avoidance of constipation, and alteration of the intestinal flora are the major aspects of the therapeutic regimen (167). The therapeutic value of flumazenil, a benzodiazepine antagonist, appears to be minimal in the pediatric population (168). Response to flunazenil is transient; the medication may precipitate an anaphylactic reaction. For a comprehensive discussion of the therapy of hepatic failure, the interested reader is referred to reviews by Jalan (149), Sherlock (153), and Devictor (169).

The neurologist involved in the treatment of the child in HE should consider that neurologic symptoms can result from six complications: hypoglycemia, sepsis, intracranial bleeding as a consequence of a coagulopathy, renal failure

(seen in approximately one-half of patients with hepatic failure), electrolyte disturbances (notably hyponatremia, hypokalemia, and hypocalcemia), and cerebral edema. Because cerebral edema mainly occurs on a cytotoxic basis, corticosteroids have no role in the management. The best course of management is by fluid restriction and assisted hyperventilation. Minimizing stimulation (lights, sound, endotracheal suctioning) avoids sharp increases in intracranial pressure that may become sustained and recalcitrant to therapeutic measures. Short-acting narcotics (fentanyl) can be administered to further blunt intracranial pressure increase from stimulation. The judicious use of osmotic diuretics, such as mannitol, is recommended (153). Hypothermia and barbiturate coma have been advocated, but should only be used if intracranial pressure is monitored. Extradural or subdural monitoring devices are increasingly used for children in stages III or IV (169). These allow management of intracranial pressure and permit documentation of cerebral hypoperfusion and the rapid fluctuations of intracranial pressure encountered during the transplant procedure (170). Placement requires an experienced neurosurgeon and may call for simultaneous administration of fresh frozen plasma. In the experience of Blei and coworkers, a potentially fatal hemorrhage was the most common complication of cerebral pressure monitoring in fulminant hepatic failure (171).

Liver transplantation is the definitive treatment in patients with acute or chronic hepatic failure, and in several major centers, including our own, results have been encouraging both in terms of survival rate and posttransplant complications. The decision on which patients to transplant and when surgery is to be done is beyond the scope of this text. Suffice it to say that the mortality of patients in stage IV HE is 63% to 80%. In particular, patients who have developed cerebral edema fare badly and are not suitable candidates for liver transplant (172). In the experience of the Children's Hospital of Pittsburgh, 70% of children who developed cerebral edema as demonstrated by CT scan died, and 15% were left with severe to profound neurologic deficits. The remainder was left with moderate deficits that prevented them from an independent lifestyle (172). Sustained increases in intracranial pressure resulting in diminished cerebral perfusion pressure (less than 40 torr for more than 2 hours) is generally accepted as a contraindication to liver transplantation (173). In addition, the cause of hepatic failure and a variety of other prognostic indicators must be considered (174). In particular, the longer the interval between the onset of jaundice and the development of HE, the worse the outcome (175). As a rule, somatosensory-evoked potentials are superior to EEG in terms of prognosis, and a lack of a thalamocortical potential presages a poor outcome (176).

Neurologic Complications of Liver Transplantation

Neurologic complications of liver transplantation occur in 30% to 60% of patients. They can be categorized into problems related to the underlying disease, problems related to the transplant procedure, side effects of immunosuppressive drugs, and neurologic complications arising from immunosuppression (177).

In the pediatric age group infectious complications resulting from immunosuppression are the most common. These may take the form of acute meningitis, subacute chronic meningitis, a meningoencephalitis, or a brain abscess. Conti and Rubin provide a timetable for the occurrence of infections in the transplant patient (178). Opportunistic infections of the CNS during the first month after transplantation are rare. Between 1 and 6 months after transplantation, the risk for CNS infections is the greatest. The organisms responsible for these infections differ from those causing infections in the immunocompetent child. Organisms include herpesvirus, cytomegalovirus, *Listeria monocytogenes*, *Aspergillus*, and *Nocardia* (178). At 6 months posttransplant, patients are at risk for cryptococcal meningitis and cytomegalovirus. The most common organism to cause acute meningitis in the immunocompromised child is *Listeria monocytogenes*. *Cryptococcus*, *Listeria*, and *Mycobacterium tuberculosis* can be responsible for subacute infections. Abscess is most commonly caused by *Aspergillus*, *Nocardia*, and toxoplasmosis.

Neurologic symptoms can also result from the use of immunosuppressive agents. Cyclosporine induces neurologic symptoms in some 10% to 25% of patients (179). The most common neurologic symptom is tremor. This can be caused by sympathetic activation, a leukoencephalopathy, or can be a part of generalized cerebellar dysfunction (180). Less often, one can observe seizures. In some patients these appear to be related to metabolic derangements, notably hypomagnesemia. Seizures are more likely to occur with the intravenous form of cyclosporine (Sandimmune) than with the oral form of the drug. The neurologic consultant is often asked whether to start anticonvulsant therapy and which anticonvulsant is most appropriate. By inducing the hepatic P450 system most anticonvulsants interfere with the metabolism of immunosuppressive agents, thus increasing their required dosage. Benzodiazepines, gabapentin, and valproate are the drugs of choice in that they tend to have a lesser effect on cyclosporine metabolism (177).

Other serious complications include cerebellar symptoms, mental confusion, polyneuropathy, a motor spinal cord syndrome, thromboembolic phenomena, visual hallucinations, and transient cortical blindness. Neuroimaging studies disclose diffuse white matter abnormalities and the EEG reveals diffuse slowing. The CSF is generally normal (181,182). An encephalopathy, characterized by confusion, cortical blindness, quadriparesis, seizures, intracranial hemorrhage, and coma, also has been encountered (182–184). It is often reversed after discontinuation or reduction of the immune suppressant and has been linked to low serum cholesterol levels in that hypocholesterolemia upregulates the low-density lipoprotein receptor, which increases intracellular transport of cyclosporine (185,186). A dose-dependent myopathy has been encountered some 5 to 25 months after initiation of cyclosporine therapy (187). In a small proportion of patients cyclosporine induces a hemolytic uremic syndrome or thrombotic thrombocytopenic purpura with ensuing neurologic symptoms (188,189).

Tacrolimus is a potent new immunosuppressant, which is used increasingly in children. The spectrum and incidence of neurotoxicity is similar to that of cyclosporine. A severe postural tremor and, less frequently, mutism and speech apraxia and seizures are the most common manifestations (190,191). Headaches are also commonly seen, especially early after transplantation, a time when immunosuppression is highest. OKT3 is a monoclonal murine IgG immunoglobulin used for short courses in severe acute organ rejection. This agent can induce a sterile CSF pleocytosis. Symptoms include fever, headache, photophobia, meningism, cerebral edema, and transient hemiparesis. They are reversed by cessation of OKT3 treatment (192,193).

At dosages required for immune suppression, corticosteroids may induce mental status changes, a steroid myopathy, cerebrovascular changes owing to hypertension, and pseudotumor cerebri, which can develop after corticosteroid withdrawal. Neurologic complications of the other immunosuppressive agents are covered by Walker and Brochstein (179). A primary CNS lymphoma is seen in some 2% of organ transplant patients.

The clinical picture of these various complications most often takes the form of an encephalopathy, characterized by changes in mental status. This picture was encountered in 50% of children in the University of Pittsburgh hepatic transplant series of Martinez and coworkers (194). The most important causes were infections, intracranial bleeds, and metabolic abnormalities. Seizures were seen less often (33% of children), and focal neurologic deficits occurred in 13%. Parkinsonian symptoms of bradykinesia and hypokinesia, cog-wheel rigidity, and resting tremor have been noted after bone marrow transplantation (195). In the series of Martinez and colleagues, the most common pathologic findings in children dying after having undergone a liver transplantation were cerebral edema, a variety of ischemic and hemorrhagic vascular lesions, and infections, mainly caused by cytomegalovirus, aspergillosis, and candidiasis (194). A liver transplant series reported from the University of California, Los Angeles, UCLA School of Medicine shows similar neuropathologic sequelae (196). Aspergillosis of the CNS is a particularly common infection in immunocompromised children. In the University of California, Los Angeles, UCLA School of Medicine series, 1.1% of adult

and pediatric patients had disseminated aspergillosis with multiple brain abscesses. Solitary or multiple subcortical infarctions of the cerebral hemispheres or cerebellum and meningeal involvement are other common features of aspergillosis. The diagnosis could not be made during the lifetime in more than one-half of the cases, and blood culture results are generally negative (197). Central pontine myelinolysis and focal pontine leukoencephalopathy also have been encountered. Central pontine myelinolysis is most commonly seen in liver transplant recipients, but it has also been seen after renal transplant (198,199). Focal pontine leukoencephalopathy refers to a pathologic picture of multiple microscopic foci of vacuolization, necrosis, calcification, and axonal injury of the pontocerebellar or corticospinal tracts of the basis pontis (196). Neither of these conditions was diagnosed during the lifetime of the patient (199). In most instances, clinicopathologic correlation is difficult and the factors that lead to one or the other neuropathologic abnormality are obscured by the multiplicity of complications that befall transplant patients before their demise.

The neurologic consequences of the transplant procedure are related to the major fluid and electrolyte shifts that can occur during the course of the operation. All these factors contribute to the neurologic mortality associated with liver failure. Intracranial hemorrhage secondary to coagulopathy and severe ischemic injury secondary to hypoperfusion are uncommon but devastating consequences. Patients with fulminant hepatic failure can continue to experience encephalopathy and life-threatening cerebral edema for several days after the transplant. Intraoperative intracranial pressure may increase secondary to the stress of surgery, supine operating position, or fluid shifts. Rapid shifts in sodium concentrations in the perioperative period have been associated with the development of central pontine myelinolysis (194).

Children who are long-term survivors of liver transplantation after chronic hepatic failure are at greater risk for intellectual and neuropsychological deficits than are children with other chronic illnesses. Whether this is an effect on cognitive functioning of the pretransplant hepatic disease or the posttransplant immune suppressant therapy remains to be established (200).

Vitamin E Deficiency States

The recognition that vitamin E deficiency is associated with a number of neurologic manifestations points to the important role played by vitamin E in normal neurologic function (201). Generally, vitamin E deficiency induces a spinocerebellar degeneration, resembling that seen in spinocerebellar (Friedreich's) ataxia. This picture is seen in a variety of conditions marked by chronic malabsorption (202). Thus, children with chronic cholestatic liver disease can develop a syndrome characterized by areflexia, gait disturbance, decreased proprioception and vibratory sensation, and gaze paresis (203). Dystonia is seen less commonly (162). Nerve conduction velocities and nerve action potential amplitudes are decreased (204). In most instances, serum vitamin E levels have been low. In one series, 80% of children older than 5 years of age with chronic cholestasis and vitamin E deficiency developed clinically significant neurologic abnormalities, with areflexia being the earliest sign (205). A similar clinical picture is encountered in abetalipoproteinemia. Here, too, vitamin E levels can be strikingly reduced (see Chapter 1). A normal serum vitamin E level does not exclude a deficiency in the vitamin, because hyperlipidemia can produce a false elevation in serum vitamin E levels. The ratio of vitamin E to total serum lipids (cholesterol, triglycerides, and phospholipids) is considered a better indicator of vitamin E deficiency (206).

A rare autosomal recessive disorder is caused by mutations in the gene for the alpha-tocopherol transfer protein. This protein incorporates alpha-tocopherol into lipoprotein particles during their assembly in liver cells. The defect results in a decrease in serum vitamin E levels (207). Several allelic variants have been recognized. In some the clinical picture resembles that of spinocerebellar ataxia with peripheral neuropathy; in others ataxia is accompanied by retinitis pigmentosa. The age of onset can be as early as the first decade, and the disease is relentlessly progressive. Vitamin E in large doses (400 to 1,200 IU) can stabilize or improve neurologic symptoms (208,209). The neuropathologic picture of vitamin E deficiency regardless of cause resembles that previously described for vitamin E deficiency in rats and monkeys. It includes a loss of large diameter myelinated sensory axons in the spinal cord and peripheral nerves, with spheroid formation. These findings are most pronounced in the posterior columns (210,211). The tocopherol content of biopsied peripheral nerve is reduced in vitamin E–deficient patients with peripheral neuropathy. In some cases, chemical changes precede anatomic evidence for peripheral nerve degeneration (212). Ultrastructural evidence of electron-dense accumulations in muscle fibers also has been reported (213,214).

Inflammatory bowel disease (Crohn's disease) is usually unaccompanied by neurologic complications unless an associated vitamin E deficiency exists. Prolonged use of metronizadole (Flagyl) for the treatment of the condition can result in a clinical or subclinical sensory polyneuropathy or a combined sensory-motor polyneuropathy.

When subjects with inflammatory bowel disease undergo MRI studies, a large proportion demonstrate increased signal in white matter. These changes are unaccompanied by neurologic symptoms and their clinical significance, if any, is still uncertain (215).

The association of celiac disease with a seizure disorder, notably with complex partial seizures, and bilateral occipital or fronto-occipital calcifications has been encountered with some frequency in Europe and Latin America (216). In many instances the distribution of the calcifications resembles that seen in Sturge-Weber disease. Folate deficiency has been documented in some patients, whereas in others there has been nephrogenic diabetes insipidus. The nature of this condition is unknown. Seizures are treated with anticonvulsants and a gluten-free diet (217).

Whipple Disease

Whipple disease, with or without nervous system involvement, although usually a disease of middle-aged men, has been encountered in children (218). Adults can have one of three patterns of CNS involvement. The most common pattern consists of myoclonus, ataxia, and ocular abnormalities with progressive dementia. The second pattern is hypothalamic dysfunction, notably sleeping and waking disturbances, and polydipsia. Additionally, there are abnormalities of gaze and dementia. In the third pattern, no clinically evident neurologic deficits are seen, but at autopsy, periodic acid–Schiff-positive material is stored in the brain (219). The diagnosis and treatment of Whipple disease is beyond the scope of this text.

NEUROLOGIC COMPLICATIONS OF RENAL DISEASE

Uremia

Pathology

The pathogenesis of cerebral symptoms in uremia is still unknown and it is generally accepted that several toxins are responsible. Urea is the most studied of these. It has been known for some time that the severity of cerebral symptoms correlates poorly with levels of serum urea, and hemodialysis sometimes reverses symptoms without lowering blood urea (220). Creatinine, p-cresol, the guanidines, and parathormone may each be responsible for some aspect of the various neurologic symptoms encountered in uremia, notably the peripheral neuropathy and the myopathy (221,222). Cerebral blood flow studies have shown a defect in oxygen use. In part, this defect might be caused by nonspecific increases in brain permeability and disordered membrane function, which could allow toxic products, possibly a variety of organic acids, to enter the brain. These acids could alter the function of the sodium-potassium ion pump. Disorders in blood and CSF electrolytes can aggravate the clinical picture, as can bouts of acute hypertensive encephalopathy (223). The neurologic symptoms in uremia have been reviewed by Fraser and Arieff (224).

Clinical Manifestations

The principal neurologic symptoms of uremia are abnormalities in mental status, tremor, myoclonus, asterixis, convulsions, and muscle cramps (105,225). Peripheral nerve involvement is common in patients with uremia. Most frequently, it takes the form of a polyneuropathy. This can be a symptomatic mixed motor and sensory neuropathy, or it can be subclinical, detected only by nerve conduction studies. In one report, 76% of uremic children had a significantly reduced peroneal motor nerve conduction velocity without any clinical evidence of neuropathy (226). When symptoms develop, they begin with sensory abnormalities in the lower extremities. The condition can progress slowly to total flaccid quadriplegia. Nerve biopsy can reveal primarily an axonal neuropathy, progressive axonal neuropathy with secondary demyelination, or predominantly demyelinating neuropathy (227). Less commonly, patients develop a mononeuropathy, cranial nerve palsies, and choreoathetosis. Restless legs syndrome is seen in a large proportion of uremic patients (228). Signs of hypocalcemia and hypomagnesemia are often present. On rare occasions, one can encounter a primary myopathy (229).

In hypertensive encephalopathy, such as occurs with acute glomerulonephritis, patients develop symptoms and signs of increased intracranial pressure, with headache, vomiting, disturbance of vision, and papilledema. Seizures and transient focal cerebral syndromes, including hemiparesis and cortical blindness, are also common.

As a rule, developmental quotients of children who develop chronic renal failure before 1 year of age are more affected than those of children who go into uremia after 3 years of age (230). In the experience of McGraw and Haka-Ikse, more than 50% of patients with chronic renal failure present since infancy had significant developmental delay (231). This is accompanied by a significant reduction in the head circumference.

Neuroimaging studies of the brain of patients with end-stage uremia reveal a high incidence of cerebral atrophy, suggesting an adverse effect of uremia on brain development (232). MRI of patients with cortical blindness demonstrates increased signals in occipital white matter and cortex on T2-weighted images. These tend to resolve over the ensuing weeks (233).

Treatment and Prognosis

Treatment of uremia involves correction of electrolyte disturbance and maintenance of normal plasma composition. These have been greatly assisted by the use of dialysis. In some instances, neurologic symptoms can become aggravated after peritoneal dialysis or hemodialysis. Some workers have suggested that urea in the brain does not equilibrate freely with urea in blood, so that water enters the brain along an osmotic gradient. This is generally referred to as the dialysis-dysequilibrium syndrome. Gradual changes in blood electrolytes and earlier dialysis prevent some neurologic complications. In general, motor symptoms tend to improve once blood urea levels are lowered, whereas sensory symptoms tend to remain fixed. The sensory neuropathy does, however, respond dramatically to renal transplant (234). The correction of anemia by means of recombinant erythropoietin improves intellectual function (235).

Successful renal transplantation is associated with acceleration in head growth and improved intellectual functioning. Improvement can continue for more than 1 year after the transplant (236,237). Nevertheless, prospective studies of children with moderate to severe congenital renal disease indicate that both cognitive and motor developmental delay is common. This delay reflects, in part, a toxic effect of uremia on brain growth and maturation, and, in part, chronic malnutrition, the various metabolic disturbances, and also an antecedent brain malformation. In the series of Bock and coworkers, approximately one-half of infants with congenital renal disease maintained normal development. In the remainder, development was delayed or deteriorated. Neither the cause for the renal disease, nor its severity influenced the neurologic or cognitive status (238).

Treatment of convulsions in uremic patients depends on the cause of the seizures. Seizures accompanying the dysequilibrium states are usually self-limiting and often can be prevented by close supervision of dialysis. Chronic seizures are best treated with phenobarbital or phenytoin, with recognition that serum protein binding, particularly for phenytoin, is reduced in uremia. As a result, both therapeutic and toxic effects of the drug are encountered at lower serum levels than of patients with normal renal function. Nevertheless, anticonvulsant activity can usually be achieved with the usual doses, because the free fraction of phenytoin remains unchanged (239). No modification of carbamazepine clearance or bioavailability has been observed. In renal failure, the free fraction of valproate increases two- to threefold. However, the intrinsic metabolism of the drug is reduced so that the actual clearance remains normal. The metabolism of the various benzodiazepines is unaffected. Both phenytoin and phenobarbital are known to hasten the metabolism of corticosteroids and the immunosuppressant drugs cyclosporine and FK506. This causes ineffective immunosuppression in renal transplant recipients and reduced cadaver allograft survival (240). Hence, Wassner and coworkers have suggested that anticonvulsants not be administered to patients right after transplant unless absolutely essential, and if they are given, corticosteroid dosage should be increased accordingly (240). Alternatively, a benzodiazepine can be used. The various drug interactions are considered by Cutler (241). (See Chapter 13 for a discussion of anticonvulsant therapy of patients with renal failure.)

Complications of Treatment of Chronic Uremia

As a consequence of the various methods of therapy currently available for what at one time was considered an irreversible renal disease, various neurologic complications have been encountered.

Generally, neurologic complications are seen more frequently after hemodialysis than after peritoneal dialysis (242). Restlessness, headache, nausea, and vomiting are relatively common after more extreme adjustments of urea levels or acidosis. Seizures followed by impaired consciousness were seen in some 8% of patients subjected to dialysis before 1965, but are now less common (242). These symptoms have been attributed to the osmotic gradient established when, as a consequence of the blood–brain barrier urea is removed more rapidly from the blood than from the brain. Headaches also can be caused by impaired vascular regulation by the damaged kidneys, because bilateral nephrectomy resulted in complete relief of headaches in 70% of subjects despite continued dialysis (243).

Cerebral hemorrhages and central retinal vein occlusion are less common complications of hemodialysis (244).

With repeated dialyses, a variety of syndromes are encountered that have been attributed to a deficiency of vitamins or other nutritional factors. These include a peripheral sensorimotor neuropathy (burning feet or restless legs syndrome) (242), central pontine myelinolysis (151), Wernicke encephalopathy (245), and leg cramps. Restless legs syndrome and leg cramps respond to vitamin supplementation; in particular, leg cramps respond to vitamin E or quinine (246).

Dialysis dementia is characterized by rapidly progressive speech disturbance, myoclonus, asterixis, seizures, and personality changes. Impaired bulbar function, weakness, and diffuse EEG abnormalities also can be seen (247). Untreated, the condition usually terminates in death within a few years (248). Though initially reported only in patients on chronic dialysis, the syndrome is now known to occur in patients with chronic renal failure who have never undergone dialysis (249).

The role of aluminum in causing dialysis dementia is well established (250). The metal enters the body not only through dialysis fluid, but also orally, in the form of various aluminum resins taken by many uremic patients (251), and even through some infant formulas (252,253). Furthermore, citrates promote aluminum absorption, and the elevated parathormone levels, often found in uremic individuals, promote entry of aluminum into the body and brain (254). Discontinuation of aluminum gel (255), chelation of aluminum by deferoxamine (256), and parathyroidectomy (257) have all been reported to reverse dialysis dementia.

A progressive encephalopathy with a clinical picture similar to dialysis dementia has been recognized in children who developed chronic renal insufficiency before 1 year of age and who have not been dialyzed. It is characterized by developmental delay, the evolution of microcephaly, seizures, hypotonia, and involuntary movements, including chorea and tremor (258,259). Various causes have been suggested for this clinical picture, including the oral inges-

tion of aluminum in the form of aluminum hydroxide, chronic malnutrition, and the neurotoxic effects of chronic renal failure during a vulnerable period of brain growth.

Another syndrome that is clinically indistinguishable from dialysis dementia is occasionally seen in uremic patients who develop acute hypercalcemia. It is easily reversed by normalizing calcium levels (260).

The neurologic complications attending renal homotransplants are mainly the result of immunosuppressive therapy. Like the complications after hepatic transplants, considered earlier in this chapter, they include a variety of infections, notably fungal infections resulting from *Aspergillus* or *Candida* (261) and viral infections with cytomegalovirus and herpes simplex (262). In an autopsy study on renal transplant patients, 58% of subjects who succumbed to infection died of bacterial infection, 27% of fungal infection and 6% of viral infection (263). The clinical picture of these secondary infections is highlighted by disturbances of behavior and seizures. Fungal infections, in particular, are seen in children who have been on prolonged immunosuppressive therapy, and their appearance is unrelated to preexisting treatment with antibiotics. It is often difficult to establish an antemortem diagnosis. Imaging studies should be performed before lumbar puncture, which can be dangerous in the presence of a large brain abscess.

The neurologic complications of cyclosporine therapy are similar to those encountered after hepatic transplants, but appear to be less frequent (264). Side effects of FK506 and OKT3 are covered in the section on liver transplantation.

Symptomatic hypoglycemia can develop in infants or children a few months to several years after transplantation. The etiology is probably multifactorial, but in the series of Wells and coworkers, almost all affected patients were receiving propranolol when they developed hypoglycemia. In such cases, propranolol should be discontinued and frequent feedings initiated (265).

Approximately 6% of renal homograft recipients, followed for up to 8 years, have developed neoplasms. The majority of these neoplasms has involved the CNS and includes reticulum cell sarcomas, lymphomas, and less commonly, Hodgkin disease (266–268).

Hemolytic Uremic Syndrome

Hemolytic uremic syndrome, a heterogeneous group of disorders, shares the following features: microangiopathy, hemolytic anemia, and thrombocytopenia. Because it now appears that the classic or primary hemolytic uremic syndrome, seen in infants or young children, is in part the consequence of endothelial damage resulting from an infection, principally with the verotoxin-producing *Escherichia coli*, 0157:H7, hemolytic uremic syndrome is considered in Chapter 6. Secondary hemolytic uremic syndrome, resulting from a variety of drugs, notably cyclosporine, is seen mainly in adults.

NEUROLOGIC COMPLICATIONS OF CARDIAC DISEASE

In addition to the neurologic effects of hypoxia, cerebral complications can be encountered in a significant proportion of children with congenital or acquired heart disease. Such complications can be classified into those that occur as a consequence of the anatomic abnormality, and those that are at risk to develop after the treatment of such congenital or acquired abnormalities.

Congenital Heart Disease

Left-to-Right Shunts

Patients with uncomplicated atrial septal defects, ventricular septal defects, or patent ductus arteriosus are, in the main, not at risk for neurologic complications. This is based on the basic physiology of a left-to-right shunt in which the pulmonary circuit serves as a buffer against insult to the brain. However, should patients with such lesions not be operated on and develop pulmonary vascular disease, the Eisenmenger's complex, a shunt reversal can develop, with consequent direct communication between the right side of the heart and the

systemic circulation. This flow reversal puts the patient at risk for a cerebral embolus.

Cerebral embolization also can occur as a consequence of bacterial endocarditis. Currently, most cases of bacterial endocarditis are caused by congenital heart disease, notably ventricular septal defect and patent ductus arteriosus. Bacterial endocarditis has not been reported in a secundum atrial septal defect. Because the vegetations in a ventricular septal defect tend to occur on the right ventricular side, neurologic accidents secondary to this form of a congenital heart disease are rare. In the patient with a patent ductus arteriosus, vegetations also can occur on the pulmonary artery side but with a potential extension into the aorta. Children with unrepaired atrial septal defects are at risk for paradoxical emboli. In this defect the right and left atrial pressures are generally equal. However, when intrathoracic pressures increase, the usual left-to-right shunt can then be reversed into a shunt from the right atrium to the left atrium. This exposes the patient to the possibility of an emboli, septic or otherwise, being routed to the brain with potential neurologic sequelae (269,270).

On the whole, with the widespread prophylactic use of antibiotics for dental surgery and for the treatment of bacterial infections, and with progressively earlier surgical correction of most cardiac malformations, bacterial endocarditis is rarely seen (270).

The clinical picture of cerebral embolization can be a sudden disturbance of consciousness, hemiparesis, seizures, or aphasia. Most patients show hematuria, the result of embolization to the kidneys. Rarely, cerebral embolization is the first sign of bacterial endocarditis or secondary to the presence of immune complex.

The diagnosis of the cerebral embolization rests on the demonstration of sepsis by means of repeated blood cultures. Large intracardiac vegetations can be detected by echocardiography. Diffusion-weighted MRI and conventional MRI can demonstrate increased signal consistent with cerebral ischemia resulting from embolization. Treatment consists of parenteral antibacterial therapy against the invading organism, most commonly α- or γ-streptococcus or staphylococcus (270).

OBSTRUCTIVE LESIONS

In the obstructive lesions category, we consider the complications of aortic stenosis, pulmonary stenosis, and coarctation of the aorta. Each of these three lesions can be responsible for bacterial endocarditis and subsequent cerebral vascular or peripheral embolization, although the incidence of that process in pulmonary stenosis is extremely low.

Unique to aortic stenosis is the potential for an acutely decreasing cardiac output with reduced coronary artery flow leading to an arrhythmia such as ventricular tachycardia or fibrillation. Such an event in turn leads to diminished cerebral blood flow and the risk of seizures resulting from cerebral hypoxia.

Coarctation of the Aorta

The association of coarctation of the aorta with intracranial arterial aneurysms is well documented. Although intracranial arterial aneurysms are seen in only a small percentage of children with coarctation, they account for approximately one-fourth of aneurysms in childhood (271). Like arterial aneurysms in general, these are located around the circle of Willis and its major branches, particularly the anterior communicating artery. Arterial aneurysms are more fully discussed in Chapter 12.

A rare complication of surgery for repair of the coarctation is spinal cord damage. The nature of the repair requires occlusion proximally and distally to the site of the coarctation. Generally, children with fewer collateral vessels and the longest period of aortic occlusion are more disposed to this complication. Other factors, including the degree of compromise to the circulation of the spinal cord and variations in the anatomy of the blood supply to the spinal cord, play important roles (272,273).

Spinal cord damage can result in residua ranging from mild weakness to complete paraplegia, with transection usually at the midthoracic level. Somatosensory-evoked potentials (SSEP) after posterior tibial nerve stimulation can be monitored during surgery to detect spinal cord ischemia (274).

Cyanotic Congenital Heart Disease

Cyanotic congenital heart disease includes the traditional *five T's*, namely, transposition of the great arteries, tetralogy of Fallot, truncus arteriosus, tricuspid atresia, and total anomalous pulmonary venous connection. Generally speaking, each of these lesions allows a connection between systemic venous blood passing into the heart and the cerebral circulation without the lungs acting as an intervening filter. As such, any peripheral infection could cause a neurologic event such as a brain abscess or a cerebral vascular accident.

Unique to the patient with tetralogy of Fallot is the additional risk of an acute hypoxic episode, known as "TET" spells. These result from a sudden increase in the infundibular stenosis, which then increases the flow of hypooxygenated blood from the right ventricle through the ventricular septal defect to the aorta and into the cerebral circulation. Attacks occur most frequently between 6 months and 3 years of age and are precipitated by crying, dehydration, and fever. Many attacks occur shortly after the child wakes up. In approximately one-half of the children, severe cyanotic attacks are followed by a generalized convulsion (275). The EEG during such an attack shows high-voltage slow-wave activity, but no spike discharges (276). These spells may be transient and short-lived. However, frequent spells lead to repeated cerebral insults and have the potential for permanent diminished cerebral function.

Brain abscesses are seen in older children, usually those older than 2 years of age. Early repair of most types of cyanotic cardiac lesions has reduced the incidence of brain abscess. Those with a residual right-to-left shunt remain at risk for this complication, however. The risk of brain abscess is proportional to the degree of cyanosis (277). The diagnosis and treatment of brain abscesses in children with cyanotic heart disease are discussed more extensively in Chapter 6.

Any patient with inoperable cyanotic heart disease is at risk for progressive hemoconcentration with a potential increase in hematocrit to the high 60s or low 70s. This results in a small but recognizable risk of a cerebral vascular accident secondary to either embolic phenomenon or intrinsic vascular occlusion. The majority of cerebral infarcts in such children are caused by vascular occlusions, most often in the distribution of the middle cerebral artery. Venous thrombi are more common than arterial occlusions (278,279). Dehydration, fever, and iron deficiency anemia also play a role in the evolution of cerebrovascular accidents in nonsurgical patients (280) (see Chapter 12).

A cerebrovascular accident is marked by a sudden onset of hemiplegia or aphasia. Seizures can accompany the acute episode; in some 10% of children, they can follow the cerebrovascular accident after a latent period of 6 months to 5 years. Approximately 20% of children, particularly those who incur a cerebrovascular accident during the early years of life, are left mentally retarded (281).

The differential diagnosis of hemiplegia and seizures in a child with cyanotic congenital heart disease is discussed in the section on brain abscess (see Chapter 6). We should point out that in cyanotic children, funduscopy is of little help in ascertaining the presence of increased intracranial pressure. Retinal changes consisting of dilated and tortuous veins and blurring of the disc margins can be observed in the majority of these children. This retinopathy is related to decreased oxygen tension and secondary polycythemia, rather than to retention of carbon dioxide or increased venous pressure (282).

Prolonged hypoxemia with pO_2 levels less than 25 torr in a patient with as yet unoperated cyanotic heart disease can lead to acidosis and potential cerebral vascular deficiencies. The symptoms may be seizures and, on a long-term basis, diminution in intellectual capability.

Additionally, a variety of developmental CNS anomalies can accompany many types of congenital heart disease. In a survey of children scheduled to undergo open heart surgery, preoperative neurologic evaluation found neurologic

TABLE 15.6. *Incidence of neurologic abnormalities in various types of congenital heart disease*[a]

Congenital heart disease	Incidence of neurologic abnormalities (%)
Transposition of the great arteries	2.3
Patent ductus arteriosus	11.0
Ventricular septal defects	8.6
Atrial septal defects	11.0
Tetralogy of Fallot	8.7
Coarctation of aorta	5.4
Aortic stenosis	0–5.0
Truncus arteriosus	5.4
Hypoplastic left-sided heart syndrome	29.0

[a]The high incidence of neurologic abnormalities in atrial septal defects and patent ductus arteriosus could reflect the fact that it was the central nervous system anomalies (e.g., postrubella syndrome) rather than the congenital heart disease that brought the child to the physician's attention.

Adapted from Greenwood RD, et al. Extracardiac abnormalities in infants with congenital heart disease. *Pediatrics* 1975;55:485; and Glauser TA, et al. Congenital brain anomalies associated with the hypoplastic left heart syndrome. *Pediatrics* 1990;85:984.

and neurobehavioral abnormalities in more than one-half of the group. One-third of subjects were microcephalic, and 44% were hypotonic (282a). The incidence of the neurologic abnormalities in the various major types of congenital heart disease is outlined in Table 15.6. Malformations of the CNS are seen in approximately 7% of children with congenital heart disease (283) (Table 15.6). In the original study, published in 1975, the highest incidence of CNS anomalies was seen in children with patent ductus arteriosus and atrial septal defects. In part, this may have reflected the fact that it was the CNS anomalies, rather than what in most instances was a mild cardiac defect, that brought the children to their doctors' attention. A high incidence of CNS anomalies is seen also in patients with the hypoplastic left-sided heart syndrome (284). A significant proportion of infants who have both congenital heart disease and a CNS malformation have chromosomal anomalies such as Down syndrome or a well-established syndrome such as congenital rubella, Cornelia de Lange, or Rubinstein-Taybi.

Acquired Heart Disease

Cardiomyopathy

This diagnosis applies to patients whose hearts are uncommonly dilated (dilated cardiomyopathy) or demonstrate an abnormal hypertrophy, generally of the ventricular septum itself. The latter condition has been termed asymmetric septal hypertrophy, hypertrophic cardiomyopathy, or idiopathic hypertrophic subaortic stenosis. Dilated cardiomyopathy can be the aftermath of acute myocarditis or may be idiopathic. In the presence of a chronically dilated heart, there can be stasis and clot formation, and the potential for emboli into the systemic circuit and the subsequent risk of a cerebral vascular accident. Hypertrophic cardiomyopathy can cause subtle or acute decrease in left ventricular output, decreased coronary blood flow, ventricular arrhythmia, syncope, and the potential of hypoxic brain damage.

Rheumatic Fever

Once a relatively common condition, rheumatic fever has gone through a phase of near nonrecognition, followed by a resurgence in the 1980s, and more recently a quiescence. The principal neurologic complications of acute rheumatic fever and rheumatic heart disease are Sydenham chorea (see Chapter 7) and cerebral embolization secondary to bacterial endocarditis or cardiac arrhythmias.

Arrhythmias

It is well known that ventricular arrhythmias may develop during the postoperative period in patients who have undergone open heart surgery in which the ventricle has been involved in the repair, such as tetralogy of Fallot, truncus arteriosus, or ventricular septal defect. The neurologist must remember that ventricular tachycardia can progress to fibrillation and to cardiac arrest with cerebral hypoxia.

The same sequence of events can occur in the patient with ventricular ectopy unrelated to surgery. Clinically, the presenting symptom is one of syncope. The differential diagnosis

between cardiac and primary neurologic causes for syncope is considered in Chapter 13.

Neurologic complications caused by hypertension, whether due to renal disease or to essential hypertension, are discussed more fully in a text on adult neurology. The interested reader is referred to a review by Wright and Mathews on hypertensive encephalopathy in a pediatric population (285). The condition is rare and generally develops in association with renal disease. As a rule, the percentage increase over base blood pressure rather than the actual magnitude of the level determines the development of neurologic symptoms. The most common presenting symptoms are focal or generalized seizures, headaches, and impaired vision. In the series of Wright and Mathews, papilledema was seen in approximately one-third of children whose discs were examined (285). Imaging studies are nonspecific or can demonstrate white matter hypodensity on CT, whereas MRI can show focal cortical and white matter increased signal on T2-weighted images. A reduction of the hypertension by 20% to 25% is usually adequate to improve or reverse neurologic symptoms within 24 to 48 hours.

The association of hypertension with lower motor neuron facial nerve palsy has been noted by several clinicians (286). The association of hypertension with pheochromocytoma and neurofibromatosis or pheochromocytoma with von Hippel–Lindau disease is also well recognized (see Chapter 11). Other neurologic conditions in which hypertension is not uncommon include familial dysautonomia, Guillain-Barré syndrome, increased intracranial pressure, and various viral diseases that can affect the brainstem, classically poliomyelitis.

A reversible syndrome of headache, altered mental status, seizures, and loss of vision due to cortical blindness is associated with hypertension, particularly with a rapid increase in blood pressure. It can occur in the setting of severe renal disease or in association with chemotherapy or immunosuppressant therapy (287,288). MRI demonstrates hypointense T1 and hyperintense T2 signal involving gray and white matter mainly in the posterior regions (Fig. 15.2) (289). The condition has been termed *occipital parietal encephalopathy*. Its pathophysiology is similar to that of hypertensive encephalopathy in that the condition results when systemic blood pressure exceeds the autoregulatory capacity of the cerebral vasculature, with consequent breakdown of the blood–brain barrier and transudation of fluid into the brain. It is believed that the relative lack of sympathetic innervation of the posterior circulation may predispose the parietal occipital region to vasodilation and breakdown of the blood–brain barrier (290). The condition is reversible on lowering the blood pressure or discontinuation of immune suppressants.

Systemic hypertension is seen in the neonate, most commonly in association with bronchopulmonary dysplasia, and can result in cerebrovascular accidents (291). Sudden reduction of the hypertension, such as follows the use of captopril, has resulted in seizures or the development of an intracranial hemorrhage, in which case the neurologic status improves concurrent with an increase in systolic blood pressure (292).

Congestive heart failure in neonates has been observed secondary to large cerebral arteriovenous malformations (see Chapter 12). Although arteriovenous malformations are readily delineated by neuroimaging studies, their clinical recognition is often difficult. Audible bruits over the cranium can be heard in many of these patients, but also are heard in approximately 15% of healthy infants younger than 1 year of age. Cutaneous abnormalities around the head and neck and dilated neck veins are perhaps more reliable indications of the diagnosis.

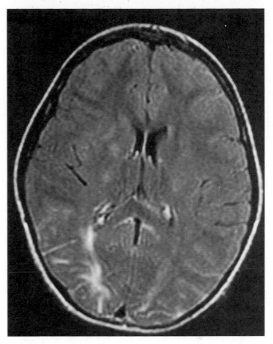

FIG. 15.2. Occipital parietal encephalopathy. This T1-weighted axial magnetic resonance image demonstrates increased signal in the right occipital parietal region. The patient was a 9-year-old girl with chronic renal disease on home peritoneal dialysis. She developed status epilepticus after apparent fluid overload. On admission, her blood pressure was 195/140. She had hypotonia in the right upper extremity, and hypertonia in the other extremities. There was no papilledema. (Courtesy of Dr. Franklin G. Moser, Department of Radiology, Cedars-Sinai Medical Center, Los Angeles.)

NEUROLOGIC SEQUELAE AFTER INTERVENTION TECHNIQUES

Cardiac Catheterization

Cardiac catheterization, originally primarily a diagnostic tool, now serves as both an avenue for diagnosis and treatment. Common to both purposes is the introduction of sheaths, catheters, balloons, and devices into arteries and veins. As a result, a significant risk exists of vessel compromise or occlusion and clot formation with emboli and air emboli. Further, the implanting of devices into the patent ductus arteriosus, atrial septum, and other vessels presents a nidus for thrombus, clots, and emboli. Neurologic complications rarely attend cardiac catheterization. In children, thromboembolic complications predominate and appear most commonly when the procedure is performed in the first few months of life.

Neurologic Complications of Cardiac Surgery

Since the 1960s we have witnessed improved diagnostic techniques and an increased aggressiveness in the surgical approach to the management of the child with heart disease. As a result, the incidence of neurologic complications attending cardiac surgery has become better defined. Also, improved survival of more serious types of heart disease has been accompanied by a more noticeable number of children with neurologic defects (293).

The basic technique of open heart surgery initially isolated the heart for surgical repair and, at the same time, protected the other organs. Research demonstrated that lowering body temperatures permitted a longer time of perfusion with continued protection of the organs. Shortly thereafter, the technique of profound hypothermia with circulatory arrest was developed. With this technique, the patient's body temperature is decreased to 15° to 17° C. The blood volume is stored in the oxygenator compartment of the heart-lung system. Experimental work suggests that a window of safety for this technique is 1 hour (294–296).

After repair, the blood is returned to the patient, the patient gradually rewarmed, and the surgical procedure completed. The parameters of this technique, in addition to standard open heart surgical techniques, expose the patient to hypoxic-ischemic encephalopathy. Vanucci and colleagues have pointed out that this can be a sequel to inadequate blood flow to vital regions of the brain. The various causes include prolonged cardiac arrest beyond the perceived safety margin, intraoperative or postoperative systemic hypoxia and hypotension, and cerebral vascular occlusive insults secondary to thrombi or embolization (297).

Clinically, one may see seizures in the immediate postoperative period. Rappaport and coworkers, in a selected group of patients with transposition of the great arteries, spoke to the recognition of seizures and the potential risk of long-term neurologic and developmental sequelae (298). Although studying a different subset of patients, Uzark and colleagues reported on a group of patients with single ventricle undergoing the Fontan procedure with no deficiency in intellectual development, but for some deficits in visual motor integration (299). These patients, however, did not require circulatory arrest and were cyanotic before the onset of surgical intervention.

Actual figures on the incidence of neurologic complication after cardiac surgery vary, depending on the care and detail of the neurologic evaluation and on the period during which the series was collected. Currently, they range between 5% and 25%. Sotaniemi, reporting in 1980 on 100 consecutive patients who underwent open heart surgery, found a 37% incidence of postoperative cerebral disorders. In his experience, the incidence of cerebral complications was proportional to the duration of cardiac bypass (300). It must be pointed out, however, that many factors, such as cross clamp time, complete or partial circulatory arrest, blood gas manipulation, and brain hypothermia, affect the supply and demand of oxygen in cerebral tissue. Thus, conclusions as to the cause of these complications must be drawn carefully and related specifically to the techniques used at a specific institution at a specific time.

Ferry divided the neurologic complications into acute and chronic forms (301). In the pediatric population the most prominent of the acute complications are focal and generalized seizures, intracranial hemorrhage, and spinal cord infarction (302).

Neuropathologic changes, when present, have been attributed to impaired cerebral blood flow, hypoxia or hypotension, reduced microvascular perfusion consequent to gas, microparticulate, or platelet embolization, a nonpulsatile blood flow, and the altered rheologic states of cardiopulmonary bypass and hypothermia (303).

Several factors are responsible for impaired cerebral blood flow. Hypotensive episodes can be related to the surgical procedure. Additionally, considerable evidence suggests that hypothermia, when used with cardiopulmonary bypass, produces a marked reduction in cerebral blood flow (304). Additionally, during deep hypothermia there si a loss of cerebrovascular autoregulation. The reduction in cerebral blood flow is not immediately reversible postoperatively, and brain oxygenation remains impaired for some time after rewarming (305).

During the immediate postoperative period, major neurologic deficits include alterations of consciousness, behavioral changes, and defects in intellectual function, particularly in recent memory and in those modalities that pertain to perception and synthesis of visual patterns. Additionally, we and several other groups have observed a curious dyskinesia, which is frequently localized to the orofacial region and can be accompanied by developmental delay (306,307). In the large series of Medlock and coworkers, involuntary movements were seen in 1.2%; in other series, the incidence ranged from 1.1% to 18.0% (307). On neuropathologic examination, there is marked neuronal loss and gliosis in the globus pallidus, chiefly in the lateral segment (308). The cause for the dyskinesia is unknown. In the majority of children the involuntary movements improve in the course of several days to 3 weeks and ultimately clear completely.

When intraoperative hypoxic or hypotensive brain damage has been extensive, patients do not recover consciousness postoperatively. They often experience focal or generalized seizures. On examination they are in extensor rigidity with papilledema and fixed, dilated pupils. Focal signs can be evident, even though autopsy reveals widespread anoxic changes throughout both hemispheres. Symptoms of cerebral emboli include hemiplegia, visual field defects, and seizures. These deficits are not likely to resolve spontaneously, and permanent residua are not unusual (302). As many patients undergo surgical repair in the early neonatal period or in infancy, signs of cerebral compromise are even more difficult to detect.

As is the case after renal or hepatic transplantation, neurologic sequelae of heart transplantation can be divided into perioperative and late complications.

The perioperative complications are those encountered with cardiopulmonary bypass surgery and hypothermia and have already been cited. Late complications are related to chronic immunosuppressants and include opportunistic intracranial infection and, less commonly, lymphoproliferative disorders, and the complications that attend the use of cyclosporine and other immunosuppressive agents (309,310).

Chronic Complications

Evidence exists that prolonged hypoxia adversely affects the developing nervous system. Chronic hypoxia in children with cyanotic congenital heart disease is associated with motor dysfunction, poor attention span, and low academic achievement (311). In the experience of Bellinger and colleagues, the incidence of developmental sequelae is greater the longer the duration of circulatory arrest (312). Neurocognitive abnormalities occur less frequently in children operated on before 14 months of age, as compared with those who undergo surgery later. Newburger and associates also found that the age at which major cardiac surgery is performed correlates inversely with cognitive function (313). These data suggest that postponement of repair in a child with cyanotic congenital heart disease is associated with progressive impairment of cognitive abilities.

Attacks of syncope occasionally occur in unrepaired patients with tetralogy of Fallot, or after placement of a Blalock-Taussig shunt. This condition, called the *subclavian steal syndrome*, is caused by obstruction in the proximal portion of the vertebral artery and consequent siphoning off of blood from the vertebral-basilar system into the subclavian and subsequently the pulmonary artery. This shunt can be demonstrated by arteriography (314).

Injuries to the brachial plexus can result from traction in the course of surgery. A postoperative polyneuropathy has been rarely encountered, but is mainly seen in adults. This complication may be related to the duration of induced hypothermia. Unilateral or, more rarely, bilateral phrenic nerve injury with ensuing diaphragmatic paralysis and respiratory insufficiency is an uncommon complication of cardiac surgery. Approximately one-half of the children require diaphragmatic plication (315).

NEUROLOGIC COMPLICATIONS OF HEMATOLOGIC DISEASES

Anemia

Neurologic symptoms accompanying anemia usually result from cerebral hypoxia. They include irritability, listlessness, and impaired intellectual function. The relationship between the various red blood cell disorders and cerebrovascular accidents has been reviewed by Grotta (316).

The effects on neurodevelopmental outcome of chronic iron deficiency anemia experienced during the first 2 years of life have been a matter of some debate. In the Chilean experience of Walter and colleagues, developmental test performance, particularly on language items, was impaired in children whose hemoglobin values had been below 10.5 g for more than 3 months. Correction of the iron deficiency failed to improve the performance scores (317). Similar results have been obtained from other parts of the world (318). Like the effects of lead, these results are confounded by a variety of environmental, particularly socioeconomic factors (318). Some of these aspects are covered in Chapter 16.

Congenital Aplastic Anemia (Fanconi's Anemia)

This autosomal recessive syndrome probably represents several genetically distinct entities whose molecular biology is incompletely delineated. The syndrome is characterized by the inadequate proliferation or differentiation of hematopoietic stem cells. Clinically, it is marked by association of pancytopenia and bone marrow hypoplasia with a variety of congenital anomalies (319). These include skeletal defects, growth retardation, microcephaly, microphthalmus, ptosis, facial weakness, strabismus, deafness, and malformations of ears, kidneys, and heart (320). Generalized hyperpigmentation, and café-au-lait spots are seen in 51% and 23% of children, respectively. Both types of skin lesions can be present also. Approximately 20% of children with Fanconi's anemia develop malignancies (321).

Hereditary Hemoglobinopathies

Sickle Cell Disease

Sickle cell disease results from a genetic, structural abnormality of hemoglobin that is found predominantly in individuals of African ancestry but also may be found in individuals of Mediterranean, Indian, and mideastern descent. In the United States it occurs mainly in blacks (approximately 1 in 600) and in Hispanics of Caribbean or South American origins. Sickle cell in the homozygous state (SS) or in combination with another hemoglobin disorder may result in significant morbidity and mortality. Because neurologic problems are among the most frequent and devastating complications and in many instances can be prevented, present-day management is directed toward their prevention (322,323).

Serious neurologic problems occur primarily in patients with SS or S Beta^0 thalassemia (at least 29%) and less frequently in those with SC disease (approximately 5%) or S Beta$^+$ thalassemia (322,324–326). At least 25% of children with sickle cell have evidence of sickle-related neurovascular disease during the first decade of life and some are younger than 2 years of age at diagnosis (327,328). MRI was found to be positive for prior infarctions in 10% of patients aged 1 to 4 years with no history of CNS symptoms (328). Findings of the Cooperative Study of Sickle Cell Disease suggest that neurovasculopathy is present by 6 years of age in most children who will be affected (324,329). The magnitude of CNS-related problems is much greater than the incidence of overt stroke, reported to be 5.5% to 12.0% (324,329). When a group of 312 children with sickle cell disease, with and without a history of CNS symptoms, were screened with brain MRI, 13% with no prior history of CNS problems were shown to have brain abnormalities (silent stroke) (329). Another group of children without prior stroke was studied, beginning at 12 months of age, by age appropriate neurologic and neuropsychological test procedures, and those with positive findings had a high incidence of abnormalities identified by MRI, MR angiography or transcranial Doppler ultrasonography (TCD) (330). The addition of positron emission tomography and single photon emission CT to anatomic imaging identified an even greater number with neuronal damage (331,332).

Sickle hemoglobin causes neurovasculopathy by changing the shape and rheology of the red cell (333). Sickle red cells are more adherent to the endothelium than normal red cells even when the hemoglobin is oxygenated.

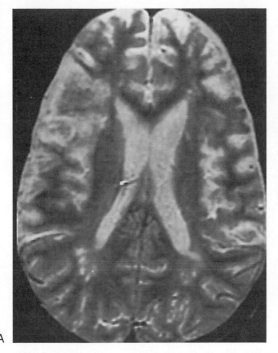
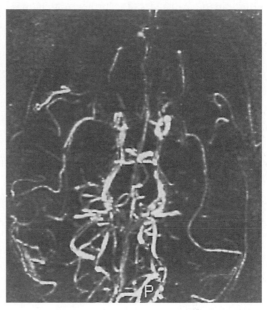

A   B

FIG. 15.3 **A:** Sickle cell disease. This T2-weighted axial magnetic resonance image (2,000/80/1) demonstrates extensive patchy hyperintensity bilaterally in the distribution of the middle cerebral artery. The lesions are consistent with the clinical history of repeated episodes of stroke in this 9-year-old girl. (Courtesy of Dr. John Curran, Department of Radiology, UCLA Center for the Health Sciences, Los Angeles.) **B:** Magnetic resonance angiography in the same child demonstrates a severe loss of arterial supply in the middle cerebral artery distribution bilaterally. (Courtesy of Dr. John Curran, Department of Radiology, UCLA Center for the Health Sciences, Los Angeles.)

When it is deoxygenated, the process is markedly enhanced and the red cells become rigid and sickle in shape. There is evidence that under intra-arterial pressure the jet stream of blood containing sickle cells is sufficient to cause endothelial damage and start thrombosis (334). Intimal proliferation occurs, narrowing the vascular lumen (334). Blood flow, which is more rapid than normal because of the anemia, is even more rapid through the narrower lumen, bombarding the distal endothelium with sickle cells at an increasingly higher rate (334). The reason the young child is especially susceptible to CNS damage from sickling may be that the higher oxygen requirement of the child's brain necessitates a much higher blood flow than is required by the older child or adult (335).

Neuropathologic findings include widespread narrowing of the major cerebral arteries, smaller vessels, and distal microvasculature as a result of endothelial proliferation. This is sometimes accompanied by focal dilatation, thrombosis, neovascularization, and hemorrhage (327,334,335). Most infarcts are located in the major arterial border zones, confirming that the primary pathogenic mechanism is large vessel disease with distal hypoperfusion, and that distal small vessel disease accounts for only a minority of symptoms of cerebral ischemia (Fig. 15.3A) (336,337). Occlusion or segmental narrowing of the larger arteries or veins can be demonstrated by MRI and MR angiography (Fig 15.3B) (338). Both large and small vessel disease usually occur in combination (334). Neovascularization may present a pattern of moyamoya (335,339). Cerebral infarction is the most frequent complication and occurs most often in children (340,341), whereas intracranial hemorrhage affects more adults than children. Both processes can occur simultaneously (324,334). Intracranial hemorrhage in children is usually subarachnoid and has a higher mortality than infarction (340). Hemorrhage may result from an aneurysm in the circle of Willis and be amenable to surgery (341). In a neuropathologic study, infarcts were found in 50% of autopsied brains and were most extensive in the distal perfusion areas of the internal carotid arteries, particularly in the boundary zone between the anterior and middle cerebral artery boundary zone (342). For patients with a history of overt stroke, lesions were typically in the cortex and deep white matter, whereas in patients with silent stroke they were confined to the deep white matter (329). The most common areas of infarction and ischemia were frontal lobe (78%), parietal lobe (51%), and temporal lobe (15%). Lesions in the occipital lobe, cerebellum, and brainstem were uncommon. Among patients with lesions of infarction and ischemia, both hemispheres were affected in 60%, and 20% each had an affected right or left hemisphere. Generalized, focal, or both kinds of atrophy were present in 30 (14%) of SS patients and 5 (5%) of SC patients. Twenty of these also had lesions of infarction and ischemia (329).

Neurologic problems may be acute or chronic. The acute problems are emergencies and require immediate diagnosis and treatment. They include bacterial meningitis, the consequences of increased susceptibility to infection, overt stroke, or transient focal signs or symptoms of neurologic deficit. Stroke is the most frequent and can occur as an isolated event or in combination with a sickle cell crisis, especially after a transient ischemic attack or acute chest syndrome, infection, transfusion, or other systemic illness. Findings include changes in sensorium, focal seizures, aphasia, hemiparesis, transient weakness or inability to move an extremity, paresthesia of an extremity, ataxia, and homonymous hemianopia. Spinal cord infarction, mononeuropathies, and multiple cranial neuropathies also have been reported (343). These findings can be irreversible or transient, but those that are transient may be caused by vasospasm and in most instances precede an overt clinical stroke (324). Chronic neurologic symptoms include headaches and the residua of prior infarcts or brain hypoperfusion such as seizures and a variety of cognitive deficits including short attention span, delayed speech development, behavior and school learning problems. Cognitive deficits occur more frequently in children with sickle cell than in their siblings or in other healthy children (326). Imaging studies have confirmed that many of the children with cognitive deficits had experienced silent strokes (326,329,330,341). Seizures can result from an acute infarction or be part of a chronic process often in association with other neurologic abnormalities. Severe headaches can occur with intracranial hemorrhage, be related to increased cerebral blood flow, or be unrelated to sickle cell disease (322,344).

Diagnostic procedures include a careful history of prior events as well as of the acute problem, neurologic examination, and neural imaging studies. Bacterial meningitis needs to be considered. Neurologic examination may fail to elicit subtle evidence of frontal or temporal lobe disease or extension of a previous infarction (345). Transcranial Doppler ultrasonography (TCD) can identify large vessel stenosis and has been found to be useful as a screening procedure to identify those children who are at high risk for future infarction, including those with no prior history of CNS disease (323,329,330). A flow velocity of 200 cm/second or greater in the internal carotid or middle cerebral artery is considered to be positive. In a controlled trial of 130 children identified as high risk by TCD there was a 92% decrease in the incidence of first stroke in those treated with transfusion compared with the observation group (346).

Imaging studies using gadolinium as contrast medium appear to be safe and can identify both large and small vessel disease, areas of ischemia and infarction, and atrophy (see Fig. 15.3A and B). Angiography using high-viscosity radiopaque dyes is contraindicated, however, because of a 5% risk of inducing infarction (328,333). After a stroke the MRI becomes positive within 2 to 4 hours in 90% of patients (347). Positron emission tomography (PET) and single photon emission CT (SPECT) may identify lesions not found by the other techniques and can be useful in monitoring the effectiveness of therapy (332). The EEG can reveal slow-wave foci. Hyperventilation, normally a routine part of an EEG procedure, can trigger a neurologic deficit in children with sickle cell by inducing cerebral arteriolar constriction and consequent cerebral edema (348). Unfortunately, no single test identifies all patients with CNS pathology.

Clinical stroke, whether the symptoms persist or are transient, must be treated with immediate transfusion, preferably exchange transfusion, using blood phenotypically matched at least for Kell and Rh subgroups, if available. Untreated, there is a greater than 65% likelihood of recurrent cerebral infarctions, with progressively more extensive clinical deficits occurring within the next 36 months (324). The patient should remain on transfusion therapy to suppress the hemoglobin S level to less than 20% because with levels of 30% or greater there is a significant recurrence rate (347,349). In some instances, the moyamoya syndrome can be reversed or improved by transfusion. Although red cell transfusion is the only effective therapy at present, in the future it may be replaced by anti-sickling agents, some of which are under development (350,351). Hydroxyurea has not been shown to be effective in preventing stroke, and neurologic complications have occurred after bone marrow transplant.

For unknown reasons children with sickle cell disease have an increased risk of developing lead neuropathy when exposed to the metal (352).

Sickle Cell Trait

There have been case reports of cerebral vascular occlusive events in sickle cell trait, but convincing evidence of an etiologic role for the hemoglobinopathy is lacking (353,354).

Congenital Hemolytic Anemia

Several forms of congenital hemolytic anemia have been associated with neurologic deficits, most commonly developmental retardation. In all of these forms, an enzymatic defect affects red cell glycolysis. Muscle glycolysis also can be defective. In the most common of these disorders (pyruvate kinase deficiency), neurologic

symptoms result from kernicterus as a consequence of severe neonatal jaundice. Deficiency of erythrocyte phosphoglycerate kinase, an X-linked disorder, causes hemolytic anemia of variable severity and is accompanied by a slowly progressive extrapyramidal disease characterized by a resting tremor, dystonic posturing of the extremities, and hyperlordosis (355). When the enzyme defect affects both red cells and muscle, patients also can present with recurrent myoglobinuria, mental retardation, and a seizure disorder. In some no apparent hemolytic anemia is seen (356). Triosephosphate isomerase deficiency also is accompanied by a progressive neurologic disorder with onset in infancy (357). Symptoms and signs are variable. They include dystonia, tremor, and involvement of the spinal motor neurons and pyramidal tract. Intellectual development is usually normal (358). In other families the clinical picture is one of chronic hemolytic anemia, myopathy, and mental retardation (359). Muscle biopsy can show abnormalities in mitochondrial structure (360).

Thalassemia

In thalassemia, neurologic symptoms are rare, but one-third of patients, homozygous for β-thalassemia, have myalgia, a myopathy with weakness and wasting of the proximal muscles in the lower extremities, hyporeflexia, and a myopathic EMG pattern (361). On muscle biopsy a moderate variation in fiber size is seen, with fiber atrophy and preponderance of type 1 fibers (362). Because in many such children serum vitamin E levels are low, treatment with the vitamin should be considered. High-dose deferoxamine, used for iron chelation in patients with thalassemia and congenital hypoplastic anemia, can lead to visual and auditory neurotoxicity characterized by decreased visual acuity, loss of color vision, deafness, and abnormal visual and auditory-evoked potentials. Partial or complete recovery can be seen after discontinuation of the drug (363).

Occasionally, one encounters spinal cord compression as a consequence of extramedullary hematopoiesis. Neuroimaging studies demon-

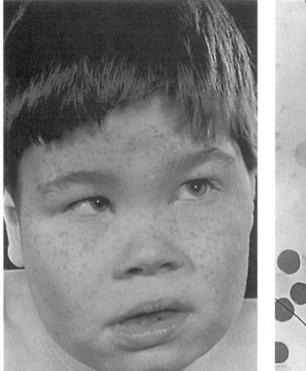

A

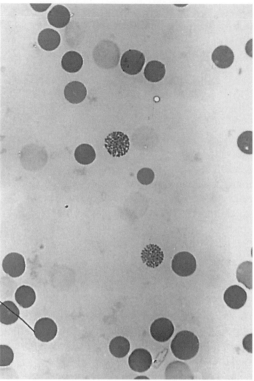

B

FIG. 15.4 A: Eight-year-old boy with hemoglobin H disease. He has hypotonia, seizures, and severe mental retardation. Appearance is marked by microcephaly, relative hypertelorism, depressed nasal bridge, a pouting lower lip, and a small triangular nose with anteverted nares. **B:** Blood smear stained with 1% brilliant cresyl blue, showing hemoglobin H inclusions. (Courtesy of Drs. Richard Gibbons and Douglas R. Higgs, MRC Molecular Haematology Unit, John Radcliffe Hospital, Oxford, England.)

strate an extradural block. Localized irradiation is recommended for this complication (364).

The association of mental retardation and α-thalassemia was first reported by Weatherall and coworkers (365). Two distinct syndromes have been recognized. In one group extensive deletions of the short arm of chromosome 16 could be detected. These subjects exhibit mild to moderate mental retardation accompanied by a variety of dysmorphic features. The other group is an X-linked condition in whom mental retardation is more severe. In these children the clinical features have been striking. They include microcephaly, hypertelorism, midface hypoplasia with a pouting lower lip, and hypotonia (Fig. 15.4A). Anemia is usually not severe, and this syndrome can best be diagnosed by demonstrating the presence of hemoglobin H in red cells. All affected cases have been male, and the condition is believed to be transmitted as an X-linked trait (366). We suspect that this entity is not at all rare, but the anemia is frequently not marked and hemoglobin H is not invariably detected by electrophoresis and requires special staining techniques. For this purpose, fresh venous blood is incubated for at least 4 hours or preferably overnight at room temperature, with an equal volume of 1% brilliant cresyl blue in 0.9% saline. Inclusions are seen in 0.8% to 40.0% of cells (Fig. 15.4B) (367). Hemoglobin H disease has a relatively high prevalence in Asians; it is seen sporadically in Mediterranean populations.

Optimally, severely retarded male subjects in these ethnic groups should be screened for the presence of hemoglobin H.

Neonatal Polycythemia

Polycythemia, as defined by a venous hematocrit of more than 65% during the first week of life, and hyperviscosity occur in 1% to 4% of newborns and up to 40% of affected infants have long-term neurologic and developmental sequelae.

Neurologic symptoms from neonatal polycythemia are generally thought to result from reduced cerebral blood flow caused by increased blood viscosity. This in turn leads to cerebral hypoxia and ischemia. Roscnkrantz and coworkers have postulated that the elevation of arterial oxygen content in infants with polycythemia compensates for the reduced cerebral blood flow and allows for normal oxygen delivery to the brain. On the basis of animal experiments they suggest that the decreased plasma glucose fraction of blood in polycythemic animals results in a reduced glucose delivery to the brain and consequently a reduction in glucose metabolism (368). These experimental studies are supported by clinical data that show that polycythemic infants with concurrent hypoglycemia tend to experience more neurologic and developmental deficits than normoglycemic infants (369).

The most frequently encountered signs and symptoms of neonatal polycythemia are headache, paresthesias, vertigo, tinnitus, seizures, and visual disturbances. Intracranial hemorrhage is seen on rare occasions (370). We also have seen thrombotic cerebrovascular accidents in neonates with unrecognized or poorly treated polycythemia. In one prospective study, 38% of newborns with polycythemia and the neonatal hyperviscosity syndrome had evidence of motor and neurologic abnormalities at 1 to 3 years of age. As has already been cited, in the experience of Black and coworkers the presence of hypoglycemia posed an additional risk and raised this figure to 55% (371). Peripheral neuropathy has been noted also. It probably is not an unusual complication, but can only be detected by electrodiagnostic studies (372). Controlled studies show that partial exchange transfusions reverse many of the physiologic abnormalities and improve most symptoms, but do not improve the long-term neurologic and developmental outcome (373). The relatively poorer outcome of polycythemic infants could in part reflect the high incidence of antecedent fetal disorders in this group.

Coagulation Disorders

Intracranial hemorrhage is the leading cause of death in hemophilia owing to factor VIII deficiency (374). Up to 10% of subjects experience an intracranial hemorrhage; in approximately one-half, trauma is documented. Also in approximately one-half, the site of bleeding is within the subdural or epidural spaces. Subgaleal bleeding is the most common hemorrhagic complication in vaginally delivered hemophilic infants. The majority of infants with subgaleal hemorrhage were delivered by vacuum extraction (375). After head trauma, neurologic symptoms tend to develop after a symptom-free interval that can last several hours to 4 or more days, attesting to the importance of indolent bleeding in the hemophiliac child. A CT scan should therefore be performed; in most instances it discloses the site and extent of the bleeding (376). Martinowitz and coworkers advise immediate replacement of missing factor and evacuation of any clot, if no improvement occurs within a few hours (374). The rationale behind surgery is that an intracranial hemorrhage activates the fibrinolytic system, promoting the breakdown of the clot and subsequent rebleeding. These authors also recommend antifibrinolytic therapy with tranexamic acid (0.1 to 0.15 g/kg per day). Whenever a lumbar puncture is indicated, it should be deferred until factor VIII replacement therapy has been completed to avoid epidural or subarachnoid bleeding (377). Although CNS bleeding caused by coagulation defects is rare in the newborn period, coagulation studies should be obtained in any infant who has experienced an intracranial hemorrhage (378). A spinal extradural hematoma is a less common neurologic complication of hemophilia (379).

Patients with factor IX (plasma thromboplastin antecedent) deficiency have a clinical picture essentially identical to that of factor VIII deficiency. Intracranial hemorrhages occur rarely but apparently spontaneously in this condition, as well as in factor VII deficiency and in the von Willebrand diseases (380,381). The neurologic complications of acquired immunodeficiency syndrome seen in some hemophiliac children are covered in Chapter 6.

Thrombocytopenic Purpuras

In young children, idiopathic thrombocytopenic purpura occurs as an acute, self-limiting disorder. Less often it is a chronic disease with remissions and exacerbations. Intracranial hemorrhages are rare in both entities. In patients with the chronic form, learning disorders and behavioral problems are common, and significant EEG abnormalities are seen in approximately 50% of cases. Minute, multiple capillary bleeding is believed to account for these findings (382). Generally, the febrile thrombocytopenic child is at a significant risk for intracranial hemorrhage.

Neurologic complications occur in 1% to 8% of patients with Schönlein-Henoch purpura, usually as a result of hypertension, vasculitis, or renal involvement (383). The most frequently seen neurologic manifestations are headaches and mental status changes (384). Other complications include seizures and focal neurologic deficits, notably hemiparesis, aphasia, chorea, ataxia, and cortical blindness. Peripheral nervous system involvement, manifested by a mononeuropathy (385), and polyradiculoneuropathy can be encountered also (384).

Neonatal Alloimmune Thrombocytopenia

Neonatal alloimmune thrombocytopenia is caused by infants having platelet antigen that differs from that of their mothers' and alloimmunization occurs during pregnancy inducing a transient severe thrombocytopenia. CNS hemorrhages develop in 10% to 15% of infants (386). The thrombocytopenia is transient, but maternal platelet transfusion or intravenous IgG improves the platelet count. Subsequent pregnancies of a mother who has had one infant with this condition are at high risk for thrombocytopenia, and the likelihood of intracranial bleeding increases in later pregnancies.

Thrombotic Thrombocytopenic Purpura

In thrombotic thrombocytopenic purpura, a rare and occasionally familial condition usually confined to adult life, platelet aggregation in the microvasculature results in intracapillary and intra-arteriolar thrombi that are widespread throughout the brain. Rarely thrombosis can involve the middle cerebral artery or other large arteries (387). The thromboses result in cerebral ischemia and a variety of neurologic symptoms. These have been reviewed by Lawlor and coworkers (388). The condition responds promptly to plasma exchange (388). Thrombotic thrombocytopenic purpura is related to hemolytic uremic syndrome, an entity in which platelet aggregation occurs in the microvasculature. Hemolytic uremic syndrome is covered in Chapter 6.

Hemorrhagic Disease of the Newborn

Hemorrhagic disease of the newborn can result in intracerebral and subarachnoid hemorrhage or in the evolution of a subdural hematoma (389). The condition is most often encountered in fully breast-fed infants who failed to receive prophylactic vitamin K after birth (390). Early and late forms of the condition have been described. In the early form of the disease, onset of bleeding occurs during the first day of life. Infants usually present with gastrointestinal bleeding (391). The peak age for the late form is 4 weeks. In the German series of Sutor and colleagues, 58% of infants had intracranial hemorrhage (392). Mothers who are receiving anticonvulsant medications are particularly prone to bearing offspring with symptomatic hemorrhagic disease (393).

Intracranial hemorrhage is commonly seen in the framework of the hemorrhagic disease that accompanies disseminated intravascular coagulation, a condition that complicates a variety of serious illnesses in the newborn.

NEUROLOGIC COMPLICATIONS OF NEOPLASTIC DISEASE

This section deals only with neoplastic disease that arises outside the nervous system. Primary tumors of the nervous system are discussed in Chapter 10.

Leukemia

With the advent of effective antileukemic chemotherapy and, hence, longer patient survival, neurologic complications in acute leukemia have become more common, and their diagnosis and treatment have become major medical problems. Neurologic complications are of two kinds: those attending the disease and those resulting from the therapy used to control the disease.

Central Nervous System Leukemia

Some controversy exists as to what constitutes CNS leukemia. The Children's Cancer Group (CCG) considers the diagnosis of CNS leukemia to be established when the CSF cell count is greater than 5 and lymphoblast cells are found on microscopic examination or on cytospin counts (394).

Pathology

Neurologic complications result from leukemic infiltrations of the meninges, brain, and cranial or peripheral nerves or from intracranial hemorrhage and infections. In one neuropathologic study, published in 1978, CNS lesions were found in 93% of children who died from leukemia (395). The present incidence of CNS lesions is undoubtedly much lower. The most common lesion in the 1978 study was cerebral atrophy, seen in 65%, followed in frequency by leptomeningeal infiltrations and various forms of hemorrhage.

Meningeal leukemia (CNS leukemia) is seen in all types of acute leukemia and can occur at any stage of the disease. It is generally thought that CNS leukemia results from the entrance into the CNS of leukemic cells from the blood as a consequence of petechial hemorrhages and a failure of systemically administered chemotherapeutics to cross the blood–brain barrier. Leukemic

TABLE 15.7. *Presenting symptoms and signs in 50 episodes of central nervous system leukemia occurring in 29 patients*

Neurologic symptoms or signs	Episodes (%)
Vomiting	80
Headache	70
Papilledema	70
Increased appetite and weight gain	26
Cranial nerve palsies	16
Seizures	8
Visual disturbance	4
Ataxia	4

From Hardisty RM, Norman PM. Meningeal leukemia. *Arch Dis Child* 1967;42:441. With permission.

cells are first seen in the walls of the superficial arachnoid veins. Cells then extend into the deeper arachnoid vessels, from there into the CSF, and finally they penetrate the vessel walls and invade brain parenchyma. The pathology of CNS leukemia and the neurologic complications of therapy have been reviewed by Price (396).

Clinical Manifestations

At the time when leukemia is first diagnosed, approximately 4% to 5% of children have CNS involvement (397). More frequently, CNS involvement occurs in the late stages of the disease and is frequently present at relapse. Presenting symptoms and signs of CNS leukemia are shown in Table 15.7. These include signs of increased intracranial pressure with vomiting, headache, and papilledema. Seizures are less frequent. Although nuchal rigidity was not noted by Hardisty and Norman (398), we have found it on numerous occasions. Cranial nerve palsies are relatively common and result from leukemic infiltration of the basilar meninges. Nerves most commonly affected are the facial, abducens, and auditory. In the series of Ingram and coworkers facial nerve palsy was seen in over 90% of children who developed cranial nerve palsies as a part of the first CNS relapse (399). Increased appetite and sudden weight gain, an indication of hypothalamic infiltration, have also been noted (398). Rarely, epidural spinal cord compression is seen at the time of diagnosis (400). This complication can be treated effectively with systemic chemotherapy and local radiation. The hyperleukocytosis that occurs in chronic myelogenous leukemia and is occasionally encountered in acute lymphoblastic leukemia can induce a leukostatic syndrome. Neurologic signs include papilledema, hearing loss, impaired vestibular function, and a variety of focal neurologic deficits. Symptoms respond promptly when the leukocyte level is lowered (401).

CNS relapse after complete remission occurs in 6% to 8% of children with acute lymphoblastic leukemia. With the more recent treatment protocols, 64.5% of children with acute lymphoblastic leukemia who experienced CNS relapse were in apparently complete hematologic remission. Of these children, only 29% had neurologic signs and symptoms, and the diagnosis was made by examination of the CSF (397).

Diagnosis

The CSF cell count is generally increased. The sugar content is reduced in approximately 60% of cases, and the protein content is increased in approximately 50% of children who present with CNS symptoms (402). CT scans of the skull often show splitting of the sutures. MRI studies can demonstrate meningeal enhancement, particularly after the infusion of gadolinium (402a).

Prophylaxis and Treatment

Because leukemic cells are sequestered in the CNS even in the absence of overt clinical or CSF manifestations of CNS leukemia, CNS treatment is delivered as an early part of intervention (403). The optimal treatment for CNS leukemia is still under debate. CNS leukemia is usually sensitive to chemotherapy and there has been a trend to use intensive intrathecal chemotherapy and individualized systemic therapy with blood level monitoring of chemotherapeutic agents (404). Such a regimen prevents overt CNS leukemic manifestations in some 90% of cases and in part has contributed to the dramatic increase in long-term survival (405).

The presence of CNS leukemia at the time of diagnosis is an ominous prognostic sign, even though with intensive therapy most of these children go into temporary remission. The ultimate outlook for children who experience a CNS relapse after their initial remission is not good, even when the diagnosis is made by routine lumbar puncture in an asymptomatic patient (406). Treatment requires intensive systemic chemotherapy using multiple agents, intrathecal therapy, and craniospinal irradiation. Using such a protocol on a series of 20 children, Ribeiro and his group managed to achieve a second complete remission in all, with a 5-year second complete remission rate of 70% (407). The CCG has reported a 48% 5-year remission rate after CNS relapse (408). It is evident that the ideal therapy has yet to be devised.

Both acute and long-term complications of CNS prophylaxis are encountered when a combination of intrathecal therapy and cranial irradiation is used.

Neurologic complications seen in the course of intracranial irradiation include headache and, on rare occasion, seizures. These side effects have become uncommon with the lower radiation doses currently in use. On MRI a transient, diffusely increased signal is seen on T2-weighted images. This finding probably reflects vasogenic edema (409). A transient episode of somnolence of fever has been seen 6 to 8 days after cranial irradiation. This condition clears spontaneously. It may be a predictor of later neuropsychological deficits (410).

A subacute leukoencephalopathy is seen as a late effect of therapy, particularly after the combination of intrathecal methotrexate and CNS irradiation (411,412). The condition is caused by a polyoma virus (the JC virus), which is normally acquired at an early age, and becomes reactivated to cause a lytic infection of oligodendroglia that induce demyelination. The clinical picture is one of a rapid evolution of dementia, spasticity, and ataxia developing in the course of several days to weeks. Focal neurologic signs, including hemiparesis and blindness, also can be noted. Seizures and changes in consciousness are not uncommon (413). The condition can be fatal or can gradually resolve, with partial recovery of neurologic function. A polymerase chain reaction assay on CSF has been used to detect the presence of viral DNA (414).

Delayed effects appear several months to years after CNS prophylaxis and are marked focal neurologic signs, notably seizures of hemiparesis. Although clinical and neuroimaging correlates are poor, MRI shows progressive focal, multifocal, or diffusely increased signal in white matter (415). Additionally, CT scans reveal a calcifying microangiopathy (416). Changes are frequently bilateral and are most pronounced in the putamen and internal capsule, but also can affect the cerebral and cerebellar cortex (417). The cortical calcifications can resemble the "railroad tracks" of Sturge-Weber syndrome. They are most likely to be seen in children who received prophylactic irradiation before 5 years of age.

On rare occasions, one encounters isolated optic atrophy as a consequence of the combined use of cranial irradiation and chemotherapy (418). In addition, a large proportion of children develops secondary malignancies with a sevenfold increase in all second malignancies, and a 22-fold increase in the incidence of brain tumors over the general population (419).

Long-term follow-up of leukemic children has uncovered deficits in such areas as overall intellectual functioning, academic achievement, attention, concentration, and short-term memory (420). These deficits are more severe after cranial irradiation than after intrathecal or systemic methotrexate and are particularly evident in children treated before 3 to 5 years of age. They can progress over time (421–424). Intensive intrathecal and systemic chemotherapy also has the potential to lead to long-term neuropsychological deficits. The mechanism for the cognitive deficits is not clear.

In apparently asymptomatic children who have undergone treatment for leukemia, the incidence of neuroimaging abnormalities can be as high as 75%. Most commonly, there is cerebral atrophy. MRI studies can show increased white matter signal on T2-weighted images (425). On positron emission tomography cerebral white matter glucose metabolism is reduced in subjects who had been treated with a combination of cranial irradiation and intrathecal chemotherapy, but was normal in those who had received intrathecal therapy alone. Metabolic rates in cortical and subcortical gray matter are reduced, regardless of the mode of therapy (426). Radiation injury to the

brain is more extensively covered in Chapter 10.

The use of immunosuppressants in the treatment of leukemia predisposes the child to a variety of infectious agents that can invade the CNS. Of the various viral encephalitides, herpes zoster, cytomegalovirus, and herpes simplex are the most common (402). Atypical subacute sclerosing panencephalitis also has been encountered with or without antecedent measles (427). Other infections of the CNS can be caused by a variety of organisms: *Staphylococcus aureus*, *Pseudomonas*, *Escherichia coli*, and a variety of fungi, most commonly, *Candida* and *Cryptococcus*.

More recently, with CNS leukemia on the wane because of preventive therapy, other destructive lesions have been found in the brains of leukemic children who come to autopsy (395,428). As has already been noted, progressive multifocal encephalopathy, a condition that is not rare in immunocompromised individuals or in adults who experience malignant tumors, has been seen in children with acute leukemia. Central pontine myelinolysis, another disorder more familiar to the nonpediatric neurologist, also has been described in childhood leukemia (429).

CNS involvement also occurs in acute nonlymphoblastic leukemia, a heterogeneous group of malignancies that accounts for some 20% of childhood leukemia and that is commonly accompanied by chromosome abnormalities (430). CNS involvement at diagnosis is more common in acute nonlymphoblastic leukemia than in acute lymphoblastic leukemia. At the time of diagnosis some 5% to 15% have abnormal CSF. Neurologic symptoms at time of diagnosis are rare and are mainly seen in infants. CNS prophylaxis appears to have little effect on the incidence of CNS relapse, and the overall prognosis is not as good as for acute lymphoblastic leukemia (431).

Neurologic Complications from Antineoplastic Agents

A number of neurologic disorders results from the agents used in the treatment of leukemia. These are reviewed by Allen (432) and Pizzo and colleagues (433).

Vincristine is used widely to induce the initial remission. Its neurologic side effects mainly are a dose-dependent peripheral neuropathy, with the drug's initial effect being on the muscle spindle (434). The Achilles tendon reflexes are depressed or lost in almost all patients. Less often, paroxysmal abdominal pain, weakness of the distal musculature of the lower extremities, and paresthesias in a stocking-glove distribution occur. Cranial nerve involvement, usually optic neuritis, ptosis, ophthalmoplegia, and facial palsy, has been noted less often, and almost always in association with peripheral muscle weakness and atrophy. Autonomic disturbances, including constipation, paralytic ileus, bladder atony, and orthostatic hypotension, also have been encountered. The isolated appearance of cranial nerve signs in a leukemic child who has been treated with vincristine should suggest meningeal infiltration rather than a side effect of vincristine therapy. It is an indication to perform a diagnostic lumbar puncture (435). Another common side effect is jaw pain, seen with the first dose of vincristine. The CSF is normal in vincristine neuropathy (435,436). Motor and sensory nerve conduction times are usually normal, even when the neuropathy is severe (437). Vincristine neuropathy is largely reversible on discontinuation of the drug. Less often, an episode of seizures and coma accompanies or follows a course of vincristine therapy (438). The inadvertent intrathecal administration of vincristine results in an ascending and generally fatal myeloencephalopathy (439). Early irrigation of CSF and treatment with glutamic acid occasionally arrests the process (440,441).

Intrathecal methotrexate can induce at least two distinct neurologic disorders (442). Most common is a chemical arachnoiditis with fever, headaches, back pain, and nuchal rigidity. A more serious complication is the development of a transient or persistent paraparesis or paraplegia (443).

L-asparaginase, an enzyme used in induction therapy for acute leukemia, has been associated with a variety of adverse reactions affecting the nervous system (444). The most serious of these complications, seen in 1% to 2% of children, are intracranial thromboses and hemorrhagic infarcts, which result in headache, obtundation, focal seizures, and hemiparesis (445,446). Symptoms occur a few weeks after L-asparaginase initiation and are believed to result from the enzyme's causing deficiencies of antithrombin, plasminogen, and fibrinogen, with a subsequent disruption of plasma hemostasis. Because thrombosis of the cerebral veins or dural sinuses is common under these circumstances, MRI or angiography is required to establish the diagnosis. Administration of fibrinogen, or fresh frozen plasma is the usual treatment. For unclear reasons, the risk of recurrence with further L-asparaginase therapy is low (447). An acute brain syndrome has been encountered also (444).

A number of other antineoplastic agents can induce neurologic complications in children with neoplastic disease.

Cisplatin, a drug used against neuroblastoma, osteosarcoma, and other tumors, can produce a high-frequency hearing loss, particularly in young children (448). As deduced from animal studies, damage is the result of destruction of hair cells in the organ of Corti (449). A sensory peripheral neuropathy also has been attributed to cisplatin (450).

On rare occasions, the use of cytosine arabinoside is associated with paraplegia, blindness, and a peripheral neuropathy (451). With high-dose arabinoside, the incidence of CNS toxicity increases. Complications include cerebellar signs, seizures, and a leukoencephalopathy. Symptoms usually become apparent within 24 hours after the last treatment, and in some instances are irreversible (452). Postmortem examination on some of these patients has disclosed evidence of cerebellar degeneration, characterized by a depletion of Purkinje cells (453).

Fluorouracil, a pyrimidine analogue that interferes with DNA synthesis, can cause cerebellar injury with ensuing dysfunction of gait and coordination. These symptoms are reversible with discontinuation of the drug (451).

In patients receiving phenytoin and undergoing a combined chemotherapeutic treatment program, particularly those who receive methotrexate, serum phenytoin levels can decrease, thereby lowering the seizure threshold. The exact cause of this interaction is unknown, but is believed to involve increased phenytoin clearance (454).

Bone marrow transplantation is being performed increasingly for leukemia, as well as for aplastic anemia and a variety of inborn errors of metabolism (455). The complications are similar to those encountered after other organ transplants.

In a series published in 1984, 59% of children receiving bone marrow transplants developed neurologic complications, notably cerebrovascular accidents and CNS infections (meningitis or meningoencephalitis). Herpes zoster infections were seen in 23% (456). Aspergillosis, *Listeria monocytogenes*, and cytomegalovirus also can be encountered. Cerebrovascular complications are usually the consequence of endocarditis (457). Rare neuromuscular complications of chronic graft-versus-host disease after bone marrow transplantation include myasthenia gravis (458) and an inflammatory myopathy (459). The side effects of immune suppressant therapy are covered in the section on hepatic transplants.

The long-term effects of chemotherapy and total body irradiation before bone marrow transplantation have been studied extensively. Generally, the younger the child and the greater the dose of irradiation, the more likely a developmental delay. In addition, there are delayed growth and endocrine abnormalities.

Lymphoma and Hodgkin Disease

Primary CNS lymphoma is rare in children, and the neurologic complications of lymphomas generally result from an infiltration of the CNS and meninges. Symptoms and signs of increased intracranial pressure are present. A peripheral neuropathy also has been encountered (460). When present, CNS involvement often presages a fatal outcome (461). CNS involvement at diagnosis is encountered in approximately 20% of children with Burkitt lymphoma and develops despite prophylactic therapy (462). Paraplegia resulting from spinal cord compression, cranial neuropathies, and meningeal infiltration are the most common abnormalities. With intensive multidrug chemotherapy the prognosis for 5-year survival has improved considerably (463).

Neurologic complications of Hodgkin disease are relatively unusual in childhood. They can take the form of infiltrations along the floor of the cranial cavity and the overlying meninges with an extension to the cranial nerves. Intracranial granulomas are rare (464). Progressive multifocal encephalopathy, an acute disseminated demyelination, can also be encountered in Hodgkin disease and lymphosarcoma.

NEUROLOGIC COMPLICATIONS OF ENDOCRINE DISORDERS

Thyroid Gland

Pathology

The brain and thyroid act on each other reciprocally. The anterior hypothalamus controls the thyrotropic function of the pituitary by regulating thyroid-stimulating hormone secretion, which in turn is under feedback control by blood thyroxine or T_3 concentrations. Thyroid hormone regulates the various processes, which are part of the final stage of brain differentiation. These include dendritic arborization, axonal growth, synaptogenesis, neuronal migration, and myelination. A review of the role of thyroid hormone in brain development and of the molecular basis of the various actions of thyroid hormone in the developing brain is far beyond the scope of this book. The interested reader is referred to reviews by Dussault and Ruel (465), Bernal and Nunez (466), Oppenheimer and Schwartz (467), and Burrow and colleagues (468).

In essence, thyroid hormones act almost ubiquitously, but the brain's responsiveness to them is maximal during the last stages of development and maturation. During this period thyroid hormones interact with specific receptors to alter genomic activity and affect synthesis of a variety of brain-specific proteins. In the human fetus, thyroxine is synthesized after 10 to 14 weeks' gestation. Because maternal thyroxine is unable to cross the placenta to any significant degree, an inability of the fetus to initiate or maintain thyroid synthesis can affect brain development during the latter part of gestation (469). Therefore, the degree of thyroid deficiency suffered by the athyrotic fetus influences the extent of intellectual retardation.

Structural abnormalities in the brain of hypothyroid individuals often incorporate characteristics of the immature organ. Both cerebrum and cerebellum partake of the developmental delay. As a consequence of increased neuronal cell death and defective oligodendrocyte differentiation, cortical neurons are smaller and fewer, axons and dendrites are hypoplastic, and myelination is retarded.

Hypothyroidism

Clinical Manifestations

The clinical picture of hypothyroidism depends on the degree of thyroid insuffi-

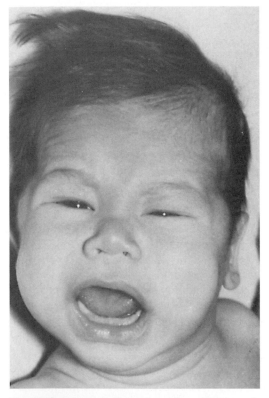

FIG. 15.5. Congenital hypothyroidism. Five-month-old child presenting with developmental delay and hypotonia. Note the immature facies and coarse hair. Additionally, the anterior fontanelle was enlarged, the posterior fontanelle was still patent, and there was a hoarse cry and an umbilical hernia. A history of diminished motor activity was elicited also.

ciency and the time of its onset. With respect to neurologic symptoms, five clinical forms can be distinguished: (a) neonatal nongoitrous hypothyroidism, (b) congenital goitrous hypothyroidism, (c) goitrous hypothyroidism with deafness (Pendred syndrome), (d) endemic cretinism, and (e) congenital thyroid deficiency with muscular hypertrophy (Kocher-Debré-Sémélaigne syndrome).

In neonatal nongoitrous hypothyroidism, the thyroid gland is absent or too small to keep the patient euthyroid. At birth, symptoms of hypothyroidism are difficult to detect. Affected infants tend to have a prolonged gestation and a birth weight greater than 4 kg. They also tend to have prolonged neonatal jaundice, abdominal distention, a large posterior fontanelle, mottling of the skin, and decreased motor activity. Osseous development is often retarded, and an umbilical hernia is present in approximately one-half of affected infants (470). Sensorineural hearing loss is present in at least 10% of these infants (471). Auditory brainstem-evoked responses can indicate a delayed wave I (472). The cause of the hearing loss is believed to result from developmental abnormalities of the cochlea.

Symptoms become more clear-cut by the second month of life. By then, infants are more obviously placid, with diminished spontaneous movements, generalized hypotonia, and a husky, grunting cry. The head appears large with coarse, lusterless hair and widely open sutures and fontanelle (Fig. 15.5). Motor and intellectual development is delayed. One-third of patients are spastic, uncoordinated, and experience cerebellar ataxia (473). The EEG also reflects delayed development of the brain (474).

When hypothyroidism develops after 3 years of age, intelligence is not irreversibly damaged. Impaired memory, poor school performance, and generalized slowing of movement and speech are prominent. The muscles are weak and pseudohypertrophic. A significant reduction in the speed of muscular contraction and relaxation can be demonstrated by EMG and can be visible on neurologic examination.

At least nine major defects in the biosynthesis, storage, secretion, delivery, and use of thyroid hormone have been delineated. These entities are transmitted as autosomal recessive traits and are responsible for congenital goitrous hypothyroidism. The association of sensorineural deafness with goitrous hypothyroidism, Pendred syndrome, is transmitted as an autosomal recessive disorder (475,476). The condition accounts for an estimated 7.5% of childhood deafness.

Endemic cretinism is by far the most prevalent form of hypothyroidism, affecting some 800 million people, mainly in Third World countries (477). It results from dietary iodine deficiency, which induces maternal hypothyroidism and deficient transfer of thyroid hormone across the placenta with ensuing fetal hypothyroidism. The neurologic picture includes a small head circumference, mental retardation, pyramidal tract signs, extrapyramidal deficits, notably focal or generalized dystonia, and a characteristic gait. The gait, which resembles that of parkinsonian patients, is marked by slow turning and reduced arm swing. Stance is broad based with flexion of hips and knees and knock-knees. Deafness, resulting from cochlear damage, is seen in as many as 90% of children with endemic cretinism, and in some areas of the world can be the sole neurologic abnormality (477,478).

The CT scan discloses calcifications of the basal ganglia in 30% of subjects, principally those with severe and long-standing hypothyroidism. MRI demonstrates widening of the sylvian fissures, a nonspecific developmental abnormality, and hyperintensity of the globus pallidus and substantia nigra on T1-weighted images (479). The selective vulnerability of these areas to thyroid deficiency has been postulated to reflect the density of T_3 receptors (480).

Supplementation of the maternal diet with iodine before the third trimester of pregnancy improves neurologic and psychological development in offspring. Treatment with iodine during the first two trimesters of pregnancy prevents the development of neurologic symptoms. Treatment during the third trimester is ineffective. These observations confirm experimental work showing the importance of thyroid hormone in neural differentiation and synaptogenesis (481).

Kocher, in 1892 (482), and Debré and Sémélaigne, in 1935 (483), described infants with an unusual combination of diffuse muscular hypertrophy and congenital thyroid deficiency. The muscular hypertrophy is unexplained, for neither fiber enlargement nor an infiltrative process has been found with light or electron microscopy (484,485).

Transient hypothyroxinemia is common in premature infants and is believed to reflect hypothalamic-pituitary immaturity. In the study of Reuss and colleagues preterm infants whose blood thyroxine concentrations were more than 2.6 standard deviations below the mean were at increased risk for cerebral palsy and developmental delay (486).

Diagnosis

The diagnosis of congenital hypothyroidism is often considered in a child with developmental retardation. The infantile facies, protuberant abdomen, and dry hair and skin evoke the suspicion of the condition (487). The diagnosis can be confirmed by documenting retarded osseous development, delayed growth, and infantile bodily proportions. More specific are the determination of serum T_4 and T_3 concentrations and an elevated thyroid-stimulating hormone level.

Treatment and Prognosis

Synthetic levothyroxine (Synthroid) is the accepted treatment of hypothyroidism. When treatment is started within the first weeks of life, somatic growth and head circumference is normal (488), but the prognosis for mental function is less clear-cut.

A meta-analysis of published data has concluded that in all studies there was a trend toward lower IQ and poorer motor skills in infants with congenital hypothyroidism as compared with controls (489). The most important independent risk factor for eventual outcome was the severity of congenital hypothyroidism at the time of diagnosis as defined by the initial T_4 level and skeletal maturation. Age at start of treatment, dose of T_4 and plasma T_4 during treatment was less important in determining eventual cognitive development. It should be noted, however, that in the studies included for analysis the mean age specified for the start of treatment ranged from 16 to 32 days (489). Children with congenital hypothyroidism who remain hypothyroid for the first 3 months of life frequently suffer residual cerebellar deficits and speech defects (490,491). One curious complication of excessive thyroid therapy for cretinism is the development of craniosynostosis (492).

Hyperthyroidism

Clinical Manifestations

The association of hyperthyroidism with neuromuscular disease is much more frequent in adults than in children. The condition is more common in girls than in boys; a quoted gender ratio is 6:1. Neuromuscular disorders seen in the course of hyperthyroidism include exophthalmic ophthalmoplegia, thyrotoxic myopathy, myasthenia gravis, and periodic paralysis (493). Cerebral symptoms begin insidiously and at first are nonspecific. The child is irritable, nervous, and unable to concentrate, has a short attention span, and does poorly in school. Exophthalmos is the most characteristic sign. It can be unilateral early in the disease, and when severe is accompanied by papilledema and central scotomata. The chorea of hyperthyroidism can be continuous or paroxysmal (494) and can be related to hypersensitivity of brain dopamine receptors in this condition (495). Tremor and increased deep tendon reflexes are seen in the more toxic children, and seizures, usually generalized, are encountered in a small proportion of children (496). Presentation in status epilepticus and coma also has been encountered (497). In some instances, previously diagnosed epilepsy can become more difficult to control. Cranial nerve palsies are rarely seen in childhood hyperthyroidism. Thyrotoxicosis is occasionally associated with myasthenia gravis or with familial periodic paralysis (see Chapter 14).

Congenital hyperthyroidism is rare. Most commonly it is seen in offspring of hyperthyroid mothers. Although usually transient, the condition can persist for several years. Affected infants can develop craniosynostosis, and long-term follow-up shows that a high proportion of infants with long-standing neonatal Graves disease has residual hyperactivity and major visuomotor deficits (498).

A gain of function mutation in the thyrotropin receptor gene also leads to congenital hyperthyroidism (499). This condition is probably responsible for the majority of infants with congenital hyperthyroidism whose mothers do not have Graves disease.

Diagnosis

In thyrotoxic children, the thyroid gland is nearly always enlarged. Radioactive iodine uptake is increased, and the concentrations of serum T_4 and T_3 are elevated. Measurement of the proportion of free to bound T_4 confirms the diagnosis.

Thyroiditis, which can simulate thyrotoxicosis, is suggested by the presence of a symptomatic goiter in an euthyroid child. The clinical manifestations of thyroiditis can vary from symptoms suggesting hyperthyroidism to symptoms of hypothyroidism.

Treatment

Thyrotoxicosis is treated with propylthiouracil or methimazole. Details of treatment are beyond the scope of this text. Once thyroid function returns to normal, neuromuscular and most other neurologic symptoms remit.

Parathyroid Gland

The neurologic symptoms of hypoparathyroidism and hyperparathyroidism are the direct or indirect result of disordered calcium metabolism and are, therefore, considered in the section dealing with the disturbances of electrolyte metabolism.

Adrenal Gland

Neurologic symptoms accompanying disorders of the adrenal gland are usually the result of disturbed serum electrolytes and osmolarity. They are referred to in another portion of this chapter. Adrenoleukodystrophy is discussed in Chapter 2. The association of catatonia, vertigo, chorea, and papilledema with Addison disease also has been recorded (500).

A syndrome of adrenal insufficiency, absent tears, and achalasia with addisonian skin pigmentation and hypoglycemia goes under the name of Allgrave syndrome. Symptoms usually develop before 5 years of age and include achalasia, mental retardation, microcephaly, optic atrophy, nerve deafness, ataxia, and increased muscle tone (501).

Pituitary Gland

Neurologic symptoms associated with disorders of pituitary function can result from direct involvement of the perisellar and hypothalamic regions by a mass originating from the pituitary gland or neighboring structures (see Chapter 10). Less commonly, the neurologic picture evolves in conjunction with direct trauma or a destructive lesion affecting this area, such as occurs with histiocytosis X, sarcoidosis, and other granulomatous diseases.

MRI is preferable to CT scans for detecting small masses in these regions. Using MRI, girls with precocious puberty having its onset before 2 years of age were found to harbor a lesion suggestive of a hypothalamic hamartoma. When precocious puberty had a later onset the MRI was normal (502).

MRI is employed also in the evaluation of patients with growth hormone deficiency. In a series of Agyropoulou and colleagues, approximately one-half of these children showed an interruption of the pituitary stalk. The significance of this finding is not clear, but interruption of the pituitary stalk can result from head injury, a prenatal developmental defect, or a perinatal insult (503,504). The incidence of these abnormalities is even higher when there are multiple pituitary deficiencies (502).

Neurologic complications of other pituitary disorders are rare, although a hypertrophic neuropathy is a distinct complication of acromegaly (505).

The Laurence-Moon-Bardet-Biedl syndrome is a clinically and genetically heterogeneous autosomal disorder. As first described by Laurence and Moon, the condition is characterized by mental retardation, spinocerebellar ataxia, retinitis pigmentosa, progressive spastic paraparesis, and hypogonadism (506). Patients subsequently described by Bardet and Biedl suffered from mental retardation, retinitis pigmentosa, hypogonadism, obesity, and polydactyly (507). In the series of Green and coworkers, retinal dystrophy and renal abnormalities were present in all patients, obesity was seen in 96%, polydactyly in 58%, and mental retardation in 41% (508). The

condition is common in Arabs, and aminoaciduria and end-stage renal failure is seen in a significant proportion of patients. Visual failure is progressive (509). Although pituitary dysfunction has been held responsible for the hypogonadism, recent immunocytologic and histologic studies have failed to show any pituitary abnormalities (510). At least four genetic loci are associated with this condition. The genes for this condition in European families studied by Bruford and colleagues were linked to chromosomes 11, 15, and 16 (511). In Arab families, the gene for the Bardet-Biedl syndrome has been localized to the long arm of chromosome 16 (16q21). However, in another pedigree all three of these loci were excluded, an indication of the genetic heterogeneity of the Bardet-Biedl syndrome (511,512). The Bardet-Biedl syndrome should be distinguished from the Alström syndrome, an autosomal recessive condition in which retinitis pigmentosa, hypogonadism, and obesity are accompanied by a sensorineural hearing loss (513).

Polydactyly also is seen as part of the various orofaciodigital syndromes. These entities are frequently accompanied by a variety of brain defects. These include agenesis of the corpus callosum, hydrocephalus, heterotopic gray matter, and various congenital anomalies of the posterior fossa, notably agenesis or hypoplasia of the cerebellar vermis, or Dandy-Walker syndrome (514).

A syndrome of cerebral gigantism (Sotos syndrome), first described by Sotos in 1964 (515), does not appear to be rare. Patients are generally mentally retarded and their facies are unusual, with frontal bossing, hypertelorism, macrocrania, and prognathism. Birth weights are commonly above the 90th percentile, and for the first 4 to 5 years, children experience a growth spurt that subsequently subsides. Convulsions and sexual precocity are occasionally present. Most cases are sporadic, but transmission as a dominant trait has been reported in several families. In addition to mental retardation, which is found in more than 80% of cases, perceptual handicaps are common in subjects with apparently normal IQs (516). Abnormalities of cortical architecture have been documented on autopsy and by MRI studies (517). Plasma growth hormone levels are normal and the cause for this syndrome is unknown (518). Sotos syndrome has been associated with fragile X syndrome (519).

Hypopituitarism can be seen in septo-optic dysplasia (De Morsier syndrome), a condition characterized by optic nerve hypoplasia and absence of the septum pellucidum (see Chapter 4). It also can be associated with a number of neurologic abnormalities, notably seizures, nystagmus, and varying degrees of mental retardation (see Chapter 4).

Growth failure is commonly seen in children who are severely retarded or who have other forms of serious and long-standing brain dysfunction. In the series of Castells and associates (520), the IQs of all children so affected were below 60, and the majority had severe microcephaly and a retarded bone age. In view of an impaired growth hormone response to a variety of stimuli, hypothalamic function appears to be faulty in at least some of these patients.

Several conditions in which delayed growth accompanies mental retardation have been described. Many of these are also associated with other neurologic features and with chromosomal disorders (see Chapter 3 for a more extensive discussion).

Diabetes

Of the neurologic complications of diabetes in children, the most common is peripheral neuropathy. The mechanism for this disorder has been reviewed by Winegrad (521). This condition is usually asymptomatic, although careful neurologic examination of diabetic patients can reveal slight distal weakness in the lower extremities, wasting of the interossei muscles, and diminished deep tendon reflexes. Conduction velocity in the peroneal nerve is abnormally slow in 11% of diabetic children between 8 and 15 years of age, even in the absence of clinical signs for peripheral neuropathy (522). Somatosensory-evoked potentials to bilateral peroneal nerve stimulation are also abnormal in a significant percentage of neurologically asymptomatic juvenile diabetic patients, suggesting an additional defect in spinal afferent transmission (523). The presence of a neuropathy correlates with the duration of the diabetes and is more commonly seen in children

whose disease has been under poor control (522,524). This view is confirmed by a more recent study, which indicates that duration of diabetes, patient age, and diabetic control each significantly and independently influence the prevalence of delayed motor conduction in diabetic patients aged 6 to 23 years (525). Moreover, the presence of retinopathy in these patients correlates closely with the conduction velocity.

Although polyradiculopathy is a complication primarily of adult diabetics, in rare instances it can be seen in juvenile diabetics (526). Pain, dysesthesia, and weakness are the primary complaints. Clinical and EMG evidence point to involvement of multiple nerve roots or proximal segmental nerves.

Involvement of the cranial nerves and cerebrovascular disease are not encountered in diabetic children, although some authors believe that acute and transient hemiparesis may be a complication of juvenile insulin-dependent diabetes (527). We have not observed involvement of the cranial nerves or cerebral vascular disease in diabetic children.

When diabetes has its onset before 5 years of age and especially when it is complicated by episodes of severe hypoglycemia resulting in seizures, the condition is associated with a mild impairment of psychomotor efficiency, attention, and verbal skills (527a). When diabetes develops after 5 years of age, hypoglycemia does not appear to affect cognitive function (528).

Neurologic symptoms are seen in diabetic coma, in the course of treatment of diabetic ketoacidosis, and in hyperosmolar nonketotic diabetic coma. The cause of neurologic impairment in diabetic ketoacidosis is not well understood. For some time, it has been known that under these circumstances cerebral oxygen uptake is reduced by 40% (529), and that cerebral blood flow is decreased, but the role of the various metabolic abnormalities present in diabetic coma in causing these changes has not been completely clarified.

It is unlikely that accumulation of ketone bodies is solely responsible, as the CSF concentrations of β-hydroxybutyrate and acetoacetate vary widely when obtundation first becomes apparent (530). In severely acidotic patients

CSF pH is normal or even elevated. Hyperosmolality per se also does not correlate well with the patient's state of alertness. It appears, therefore, that a multitude of factors, including brain intracellular pH, impaired oxygen use, hyperosmolality, and disseminated intravascular coagulation inducing localized areas of cerebral hyperperfusion act jointly to cause the depression of sensorium.

A number of deaths from irreversible cerebral edema have occurred in the course of apparently adequate treatment of diabetic ketoacidosis (531). In the experience of Bello and Sotos, the incidence of this complication was 0.7% of children presenting in diabetic ketoacidosis. Patients who experience this complication are younger and more likely to have new onset diabetes. They have had a longer duration of ketoacidosis and a higher serum glucose level than those who do not develop cerebral edema (532).

The pathophysiology that leads to this complication is not entirely clear. Duck and colleagues have proposed that a rapid reduction of blood hyperosmolality with treatment and a slower change in the cerebral hyperosmolality owing to the presence of substances termed *idiogenic osmoles* can result in the entrance of water into the brain and consequent cerebral edema (533). Van der Meulen and coworkers hypothesized that cell swelling during treatment of diabetic ketoacidosis results from conditions favoring the activation of the sodium-potassium exchanger, a plasma-membrane transport system that regulates cytoplasmic pH. Apparently, weak organic acids, such as ketoacids and free fatty acids, present in cytoplasm, are known to activate the exchanger, which, in the presence of extracellular sodium, leads to cell swelling (534). Neither the use of bicarbonate nor the rate of decline of glucose, or excessive secretion of antidiuretic hormone, or the rate of fluid administration are responsible for the development of cerebral edema. Rather, it could represent vasogenic edema, the result of damage to the capillary endothelium and an increased reactivity of the immature cerebral vasculature (531).

Prediction and diagnosis of this complication is difficult, because characteristic clinical or biochemical features are lacking and neuroimaging studies indicate that subclinical cerebral edema is fairly common during therapy of diabetic ketoacidosis in the pediatric age group (535). Rather, the patient's failure to recover consciousness, despite adequate treatment with insulin and fluids, suggests the presence of cerebral edema. The presence of high blood sugar levels and hyperpyrexia should alert the clinician to the imminence of cerebral edema. Duck and Wyatt suggest that excessive secretion of vasopressin exacerbates brain swelling and recommend limiting the rate of fluid administration (536). Dexamethasone has been used in treatment of cerebral edema, but in our experience, it is usually given too late to be effective. Mannitol, administered as soon as cerebral edema is diagnosed, might be more beneficial (537). In any case, early intervention is effective, even though the incidence of death or neurologic handicap is quite high even with the most expert care.

Nonketotic hyperosmolal diabetic coma is rare in children. Neurologic symptoms are believed to result from brain swelling (538). In addition to impaired consciousness, patients can develop hemiparesis and generalized or focal seizures. This condition has been treated successfully with low-dose insulin infusion while intracranial pressure is monitored (539).

The neurologic complications of hypoglycemia are discussed at another point in this chapter.

A familial syndrome of juvenile diabetes mellitus and optic atrophy has been reported sporadically since 1938. The condition is transmitted as a recessive trait and is marked by early onset of diabetes, subsequent evolution of optic atrophy, a sensorineural hearing loss, ataxia, peripheral neuropathy, and anosmia (Wolfram syndrome) (540).

REFERENCES

1. Auer RN. Progress review: hypoglycemic brain damage. *Stroke* 1986;17:699–708.
2. Choi DW. Excitotoxic cell death. *J Neurobiol* 1992;23:1261–1276.

3. Nakanishi S. Molecular diversity of glutamate receptors and implications for brain function. *Science* 1992;258: 597–603.
4. Siesjö BK. A new perspective on ischemic brain damage? *Prog Brain Res* 1993;96:1–9.
5. Choi D. Antagonizing excitotoxicity: a therapeutic strategy for stroke? *Mt Sinai J Med* 1998;65:133–138.
6. Massa SM, Swanson RA, Sharp FR. The stress gene response in brain. *Cerebrovasc Brain Metab Rev* 1996; 8:95–158.
7. Kraus H, Schlenker S, Schwedesky D. Developmental changes of cerebral ketone body utilization in human infants: Hoppe-Seyler's. *Z Physiol Chem* 1974;355: 164–170.
8. Levitsky LL, Paton JB, Fisher DE. Cerebral utilization of alternative substrates to glucose: an explanation for asymptomatic neonatal hypoglycemia. *Pediatr Res* 1973;7:418.
9. Vanucci SJ, Maher F, Simpson IA. Glucose transporter proteins in brain: delivery of glucose to neurons and glia. *Glia* 1997;21:2–21.
10. Altman DI, et al. Cerebral metabolism in newborns. *Pediatrics* 1993;92:99–104.
11. Kety SS. Blood flow and metabolism of the human brain in health and disease. In: Elliott KA, Page IH, Quastel JH, eds. *Neurochemistry*. Springfield, IL: Charles C Thomas Publisher, 1962.
12. Tyler HR, Clark DB. Loss of consciousness and convulsions with congenital heart disease. *Arch Neurol Psychiatr* 1958;79:506–510.
13. Siesjö BK, Plum F. Pathophysiology of anoxic brain damage. In: Gaull GE, ed. *Biology of brain dysfunction*. Vol. I. New York: Plenum Press, 1973: 319–372.
14. Auer RN, Siesjö BK. Biological differences between ischemia, hypoglycemia, and epilepsy. *Ann Neurol* 1988;24:699–707.
15. Bakay L, Lee JC. The effect of acute hypoxia and hypercapnia on the ultrastructure of the central nervous system. *Brain* 1968;91:697–706.
16. Auer R, Beneviste H. Hypoxia and related conditions. In: Graham DI, Lantos PL, eds. *Greenfield's neuropathology*. Vol. 1. 6th ed. New York: Oxford University Press, 1997:263–314.
17. Brierley JB, et al. Neocortical death after cardiac arrest. *Lancet* 1971;2:650–655.
18. Fujioka M, et al. Specific changes in human brain after hypoglycemic injury. *Stroke* 1997;28:584–587.
19. Banker BQ. The neuropathological effects of anoxia and hypoglycemia in the newborn. *Dev Med Child Neurol* 1967;9:544–550.
20. Auer RN, et al. Neuropathologic findings in three cases of profound hypoglycemia. *Clin Neuropathol* 1989;8:63–68.
21. Auer RN, Siesjö BK. Hypoglycemia: brain neurochemistry and neuropathology. *Baillière Clin Endocrinol Metab* 1993;7:611–625.
22. Kristián T, Gidö G, Siesjö BK. The influence of acidosis on hypoglycemic brain damage. *J Cereb Blood Flow Metab* 1995;15:78–87.
23. Bachelard H, et al. Studies on metabolic regulation using NMR spectroscopy. *Dev Neurosci* 1993;15: 207–215.
24. Plum F, Posner JB. *Diagnosis of stupor and coma*. 3rd ed. Philadelphia: FA Davis Co, 1980.
25. Bell JA, Hodgson HJ. Coma after cardiac arrest. *Brain* 1974;97:361–372.
26. Bell TS, Ellenberg L, McComb JC. Neuropsychological outcome after severe pediatric near-drowning. *Neurosurgery* 1985;17:604–608.
27. Pampiglione G, et al. Transitory ischemia/anoxia in young children and the prediction of quality of survival. *Ann N Y Acad Sci* 1978;315:281–292.
28. Frank LM, Furgiuele TL, Etheridge JE. Prediction of chronic vegetative state in children using evoked potentials. *Neurology* 1985;35:931–934.
29. Pohlman-Eder B, et al. How reliable is the predictive value of SEP (somato sensory evoked potentials) patterns in severe brain damage with special regard to the bilateral loss of cortical responses? *Intensive Care Med* 1997;23:301–308.
30. Majnemer A, Rosenblatt B. Evoked potentials as predictors of outcome in neonatal intensive care unit survivors: review of the literature. *Pediatr Neurol* 1996; 14:189–195.
31. Pierrat V, Eken P, de Vries LS. The predictive value of cranial ultrasound and of somatosensory evoked potentials after nerve stimulation for adverse neurological outcome in preterm infants. *Dev Med Child Neurol* 1997;39:398–403.
32. Fandel I, Bancalari E. Near-drowning in children: clinical aspects. *Pediatrics* 1976;58:573–579.
33. Fields AI. Near-drowning in the pediatric population. *Crit Care Clin* 1992;8:113–129.
34. DeNicola LK, et al. Submersion injuries in children and adults. *Crit Care Clin* 1997;13:477–502.
35. Kruus S, et al. The prognosis of near-drowned children. *Acta Paediatr Scand* 1979;68:315–322.
36. Biggart MJ, Bohn DJ. Effect of hypothermia and cardiac arrest on outcome of near-drowning accidents in children. *J Pediatr* 1990;117:179–183.
37. Bhatt MH, Obeso JA, Marsden CD. Time course of postanoxic akinetic-rigid and dystonic syndromes. *Neurology* 1993;43:314–317.
38. Ashwal S, Eyman RK, Call TL. Life expectancy of children in a persistent vegetative state. *Pediatr Neurol* 1994;10:27–33.
38a. Strauss DJ, Shavelle RM, Ashwal S. Life expectancy and median survival time in the permanent vegatative state. *Pediatr Neurol* 1999;21:626–631.
39. Heindl UT, Laub MC. Outcome of persistent vegetative state following hypoxia or traumatic brain injury in children and adolescents. *Neuropediatrics* 1996;27: 94–100.
40. Wintermute GJ. Childhood drowning and near-drowning in the United States. *Am J Dis Child* 1990;144:663–669.
41. Raivio KO. Neonatal hypoglycemia. *Acta Paediatr Scand* 1968;57:540–546.
42. Lubchenco LO, Bard H. Incidence of hypoglycemia in newborn infants classified by birth weight and gestational age. *Pediatrics* 1971;47:831–838.
43. Gutberlet RL, Cornblath M. Neonatal hypoglycemia revisited, 1975. *Pediatrics* 1976;58:10–17.
44. Lubchenco LO. *The high risk infant*. Philadelphia: WB Saunders, 1976.
45. Srinivasan G, et al. Plasma glucose values in normal neonates: a new look. *J Pediatr* 1986;109:114–117.
46. Pildes R, et al. The incidence of neonatal hypoglycemia: a completed survey. *J Pediatr* 1967;70:76–80.

47. Guthrie R, van Leeuwen GV. The frequency of asymptomatic hypoglycemia in high risk newborn infants. *Pediatrics* 1970;46:933–936.

48. Koh THHG, et al. Neural dysfunction during hypoglycemia. *Arch Dis Child* 1988;63:1353–1358.

49. Skov L, Pryds O. Capillary recruitment for preservation of cerebral glucose influx in hypoglycemic, preterm newborns: evidence for a glucose sensor? *Pediatrics* 1992;90:193–195.

50. Pryds O, Greisen G, Friis-Hansen B. Compensatory increase of CBF in preterm infants during hypoglycemia. *Acta Paediatr Scand* 1988;77:632–637.

51. Pryds O, Chirstensen NJ, Friis-Hansen B. Increased cerebral blood flow and plasma epinephrine in hypoglycemic, preterm neonates. *Pediatrics* 1990;85:172–176.

51a. Kinnala A, et al. Cerebral magnetic resonance imaging and ultrasonography findings after neonatal hypoglycemia. *Pediatrics* 1999;103:724–729.

52. Cornblath M, Schwartz R. Hypoglycemia in the neonate. *J Pediatr Endocrinol* 1993;6:113–129.

53. Cornblath M, et al. Hypoglycemia in infancy: the need for a rational definition. *Pediatrics* 1990;85:834–837.

54. Haworth JC. Neonatal hypoglycemia: how much does it damage the brain? *Pediatrics* 1974;54:3–4.

55. Gregory JW, Aynsley-Green A. Hypoglycemia in the infant and child. *Ballière Clin Endocrinol Metab* 1993;7:683–704.

56. Garty BZ, Dinari G, Nitzan M. Transient acute cortical blindness associated with hypoglycemia. *Pediatr Neurol* 1987;3:169–170.

57. Costello JM, Gluckman PD. Neonatal hypopituitarism: a neurological perspective. *Dev Med Child Neurol* 1988;30:190–199.

58. Haworth JC, Coodin FJ. Idiopathic spontaneous hypoglycemia in children: report of seven cases and review of the literature. *Pediatrics* 1960;25:748–765.

59. Wayne EA, et al. Focal neurologic deficits associated with hypoglycemia in children with diabetes. *J Pediatr* 1990;117:575–577.

60. Ad Hoc Committee on Brain Death, The Children's Hospital Boston. Determination of brain death. *J Pediatr* 1987;110:15–19.

61. Task Force for the Determination of Brain Death in Children. Guidelines for the determination of brain death in children. *Neurology* 1987;37:1077–1078.

62. Schwartz JA, Baxter J, Brill DR. Diagnosis of brain death in children by radionuclide cerebral imaging. *Pediatrics* 1984;73:14–18.

63. Mejia RA, Pollack MM. Variability in brain death determination practices in children. *JAMA* 1995;274:550–553.

64. Fackler JC, Troncoso JC, Gioia FR. Age-specific characteristics of brain death in children. *Am J Dis Child* 1988;142:999–1003.

65. Grigg MM, et al. Electroencephalographic activity after brain death. *Arch Neurol* 1987;44:948–954.

66. Ashwal S, Schneider S. Brain death in the newborn. *Pediatrics* 1989;84:429–437.

67. Ashwal S. Brain death in early infancy. *J Heart Lung Transplant* 1993;12:S176–S178.

68. Darby JM, et al. Xenon-enhanced computed tomography in brain death. *Arch Neurol* 1987;44:551–554.

69. Spudis EV. The persistent vegetative state—1990. *J Neurol Sci* 1991;102:128–136.

70. Rowland TW, Donnelly JH, Jackson AH. Apnea documentation for determination of brain death in children. *Pediatrics* 1984;74:505–508.

71. Outwater KM, Rockoff MA. Diabetes insipidus accompanying brain death in children. *Neurology* 1984;34:1243–1246.

72. Plum F, Siesjö BK. Recent advances in CSF physiology. *Anesthesiology* 1975;42:708–730.

73. Katzman R, Pappius H. *Brain electrolytes and fluid metabolism.* Baltimore: Williams & Wilkins, 1973.

74. Strange K. Regulation of solute and water balance and cell volume in the central nervous system. *J Am Soc Nephrol* 1992;3:12–27.

75. Arieff AI, Ayus JC, Fraser CL. Hyponatremia and death or permanent brain damage in healthy children. *BMJ* 1992;304:1218–1222.

76. Keating JP, Schears GJ, Dodge PR. Oral water intoxication in infants. An American epidemic. *Am J Dis Child* 1991;145:985–990.

77. Mangos JA, Lobeck CC. Studies of sustained hyponatremia due to central nervous system infection. *Pediatrics* 1964;34:503–510.

78. Editorial. Excess water administration and hyponatremic convulsions in infancy. *Lancet* 1992;339:153–155.

79. Decaux G, et al. Hyponatremia in the syndrome of inappropriate secretion of antidiuretic hormone: rapid correction with urea, sodium chloride, and water restriction therapy. *JAMA* 1982;247:471–474.

80. Laureno R. Central pontine myelinolysis following rapid correction of hyponatremia. *Ann Neurol* 1983;13:232–242.

81. Brunner JE, et al. Central pontine myelinolysis after rapid correction of hyponatremia: a magnetic resonance imaging study. *Ann Neurol* 1988;23:389–391.

82. Brunner JE, et al. Central pontine myelinolysis and pontine lesions after rapid correction of hyponatremia: a prospective magnetic resonance study. *Ann Neurol* 1990;27:61–66.

83. Arieff AI, Ayus JC. Treatment of symptomatic hyponatremia: neither haste nor waste. *Crit Care Med* 1991;19:748–751.

84. Luttrell CN, Finberg L. Hemorrhagic encephalopathy induced by hypernatremia. *Arch Neurol Psychiatr* 1959;81:424–432.

85. Hogan GR, et al. Pathogenesis of seizures occurring during restoration of plasma tonicity to normal in animals previously chronically hypernatremic. *Pediatrics* 1969;43:54–64.

86. Swanson PD. Neurological manifestations of hypernatremia. In: Vinken PJ, Bruyn GW, eds. *Handbook of clinical neurology.* Vol 28. New York: Elsevier Science, 1977:443–461.

87. Finberg L. Pathogenesis of lesions in the nervous system in hypernatremic states. I. Clinical observation of infants. *Pediatrics* 1959;23:40–45.

88. Morris-Jones PH, Houston IB, Evans RC. Prognosis of the neurologic complications of acute hypernatremia. *Lancet* 1967;2:1385–1389.

89. Grossman H, et al. The dietary chloride deficiency syndrome. *Pediatrics* 1980;66:366–374.

90. Rodriguez-Soriano J, et al. Biochemical features of dietary chloride deficiency syndrome: a comparative study of 30 cases. *J Pediatr* 1983;103:209–214.

91. Malloy MH. The follow-up of infants exposed to

chloride-deficient formulas. *Adv Pediatr* 1993;40: 141–158.

92. Kaleita TA, Kinsbourne M, Menkes JH. A neurobe-havioral syndrome after failure to thrive on chloride-deficient formula. *Dev Med Child Neurol* 1991;33: 626–635.

93. Hill ID, Bowie MD. Chloride deficiency syndrome due to chloride-deficient breast milk. *Arch Dis Child* 1983;58:224–226.

94. Craig WS, Buchanan MF. Hypocalcemic tetany developing within 36 hours of birth. *Arch Dis Child* 1958;33:505–511.

95. Nelson NA, Finnstrom O, Larsson L. Plasma ionized calcium, phosphate and magnesium in preterm and small for gestational age infants. *Acta Paediatr Scand* 1989;78:351–357.

96. Cardenas-Rivero N, et al. Hypocalcemia in critically ill children. *J Pediatr* 1989;114:946–951.

97. Cockburn F, et al. Neonatal convulsions associated with primary disturbance of calcium, phosphorus and magnesium metabolism. *Arch Dis Child* 1973;48: 99–108.

98. Bainbridge R, et al. Transient congenital hyper-parathyroidism: how transient is it? *J Pediatr* 1988; 111:866–868.

99. Hartenstein H, Gardner LI. Tetany of the newborn associated with maternal parathyroid adenoma. *N Engl J Med* 1966;274:266–268.

100. Eliot MM, Park EA. Rickets. In: McQuarrie I, ed. *Brenneman's practice of pediatrics*. Vol. 1. Hagers-town, MD: WF Prior, 1949.

101. Gessner BD, et al. Nutritional rickets among breast-fed black and Alaska native children. *Alaska Med* 1997;39:72–74.

102. Simpson JA. Neurologic manifestation of idiopathic hypoparathyroidism. *Brain* 1952;75:76–90.

103. Mallette LE. Pseudohypoparathyroidism. *Curr Ther Endocrinol Metab* 1997;6:577–581.

104. Cohen ML, Donnell GN. Pseudohypoparathyroidism and hypothyroidism: case report and review of the lit-erature. *J Pediatr* 1960;56:369–382.

105. Tyler RH. Neurologic disorders in renal failure. *Am J Med* 1968;44:734–748.

106. Mizrahi A, London RD, Gribetz D. Neonatal hypocal-cemia: its causes and treatment. *N Engl J Med* 1968; 278:1163–1165.

107. Koo WWK, Tsang RC. Calcium and magnesium homeostasis. In: Avery GB, Fletcher MA, MacDonald MG, eds. *Neonatology: pathophysiology and man-agement of the newborn*, 4th ed. Philadelphia: JB Lip-pincott Co, 1994:585–604.

108. Venkataraman PS, et al. Pathogenesis of early neona-tal hypercalcemia: studies of serum calcitonin, gastrin, and plasma glucagon. *J Pediatr* 1987;110:599–603.

109. Bakwin H. Pathogenesis of tetany of the newborn. *Am J Dis Child* 1937;54:1211–1226.

110. Lynch BJ, Rust RS. Natural history and outcome of neonatal hypocalcemic and hypomagnesemic seizures. *Pediatr Neurol* 1994;11:23–27.

111. Keen JH. Significance of hypocalcemia in neonatal convulsions. *Arch Dis Child* 1969;44:356–361.

112. Changaris DG, et al. Brain calcification in severely stressed neonates receiving parenteral calcium. *J Pediatr* 1984;104:941–946.

113. Muenter MD, Whisnant JP. Basal ganglia calcifica-tion, hypoparathyroidism, and extrapyramidal motor manifestations. *Neurology* 1968;18:1075–1083.

114. Taitz LS, Wales JKH, Spitz L. Hypocalcaemic seizures following gastrectomy. *Eur J Pediatr* 1983;141:36–38.

115. Edmondson S, Almquist TD. Iatrogenic hypocal-cemic tetany. *Ann Emerg Med* 1990;19:938–940.

116. Libit SA, Ulstrom RA, Doeden D. Fecal pseudo-monas aeruginosa as a cause of the blue diaper syn-drome. *J Pediatr* 1972;81:546–547.

117. Tsang RC. Neonatal magnesium disturbances—a review. *Am J Dis Child* 1972;124:282–293.

118. Maggioni A, Orzalesi M, Mimouni FB. Intravenous correction of neonatal hypomagnesemia: effect on ionized magnesium. *J Pedatr* 1998;132:652–655.

119. Shalev H, et al. Clinical presentation and outcome in primary familial hypomagnesaemia. *Arch Dis Child* 1998;78:127–130.

120. Walder RY, et al. Familial hypomagnesemia maps to chromosome 9q, not to the X chromosome: genetic linkage mapping and analysis of a balanced transloca-tion breakpoint. *Hum Mol Genet* 1997;6:1491–1497.

121. Milla PJ, et al. Studies in primary hypomagnesaemia: evidence for defective carrier-mediated small intesti-nal transport of magnesium. *Gut* 1997;20:1028–1033.

122. Shalev H, et al. Clinical presentation and outcome in primary familial hypomagnesaema. *Arch Dis Child* 1998;78:127–130.

123. Salet J, Fournet JP. Les hypomagnesemies de l'enfant (en dehors de la periode neo-natale). *Ann Pediatr* (Paris) 1971;18:39–45.

124. Kanto WP. A decade of experience with neonatal extracorporeal membrane oxygenation. *J Pediatr* 1994;124:335–347.

125. Lago P, et al. MRI, MRA, and neurodevelopmental outcome following neonatal ECMO. *Pediatr Neurol* 1995;12:294–304.

126. Mendoza JC, Shearer LL, Cook LN. Lateralization of brain lesions following extracorporeal membrane oxygenation. *Pediatrics* 1991;88:1004–1009.

127. Lazar EL, et al. Neuroimaging of brain injury in neonates treated with extracorporeal membrane oxy-genation: lessons learned from serial examinations. *J Pediatr Surg* 1994;29:186–190.

128. Schumacher RE, et al. Follow-up of infants treated with extracorporeal membrane oxygenation for new-born respiratory failure. *Pediatrics* 1991;87:451–457.

129. Robertson CM, et al. Neurodevelopmental outcome after neonatal extracorporeal membrane oxygenation. *Can Med Assoc J* 1995;152:1981–1988.

130. Kornhauser MS, et al. Adverse neurodevelopmental outcome after extracorporeal membrane oxygenation among neonates with bronchopulmonary dysplasia. *J Pediatr* 1998;132:307–311.

131. Cheung PY, Robertson CM, Finer NN. Plasma lactate as a predictor of early childhood neurodevelopmental outcome of neonates with severe hypoxaemia requir-ing extracorporeal membrane oxygenation. *Arch Dis Child Fetal Neonatal Ed* 1996;74:F47–F50.

132. Glass P, et al. Severity of brain injury following neona-tal extracorporeal membrane oxygenation and outcome at age 5 years. *Dev Med Child Neurol* 1997;39: 441–448.

133. Hofkosh D, et al. Ten years of extracorporeal mem-brane oxygenation: neurodevelopmental outcome. *Pediatrics* 1991;87:549–555.

134. Glass P, Miller M, Short B. Morbidity for survivors of extracorporeal membrane oxygenation: neurodevelopmental outcome at 1 year of age. *Pediatrics* 1989;83:72–78.

135. Desai S, et al. Sensitivity and specificity of the neonatal brain-stem auditory evoked potential for hearing and language deficits in survivors of extracorporeal membrane oxygenation. *J Pediatr* 1997;131:233–239.

136. Hendricks-Muñoz KD, Walton JP. Hearing loss in infants with persistent fetal circulation. *Pediatrics* 1988;81:650–658.

137. Walton JP, Hendricks-Muñoz K. Profile and stability of sensorineural hearing loss in persistent pulmonary hypertension. *J Speech Hear Res* 1991;34:1362–1370.

138. Gal P, et al. Theophylline-induced seizures in accidentally overdosed neonates. *Pediatrics* 1980;65:547–549.

139. Richards W, Church JA, Brent DK. Theophylline-associated seizures in children. *Ann Allergy* 1985;54:276–279.

140. Bigler ED. Theophylline neurotoxicity resulting in diffuse brain damage. *Dev Med Child Neurol* 1991;33:179–181.

141. Perlman JM, Volpe JJ. Movement disorder of premature infants with severe bronchopulmonary dysplasia: a new syndrome. *Pediatrics* 1989;84:215–218.

142. Sheth RD, et al. Critical illness neuromuscular disease in children manifested as ventilatory dependence. *J Pediatr* 1995;126:259–261.

143. Lacomis D, Petrella JT, Giuliani MJ. Causes of neuromuscular weakness in the intensive care unit: a study of ninety-two patients. *Muscle Nerve* 1998;21:610–617.

144. Gutmann L, et al. Acute type II myofiber atrophy in critical illness. *Neurology* 1996;46:819–821.

145. Rich MM, et al. Muscle is electrically inexcitable in acute quadriplegic myopathy. *Neurology* 1996;46:731–736.

146. Austen FK, Carmichael NW, Adams RD. Neurologic manifestations of chronic pulmonary insufficiency. *N Engl J Med* 1957;257:579–590.

147. Stern RC, Horwitz SJ, Doershuk CF. Neurologic symptoms during coughing paroxysms in cystic fibrosis. *J Pediatr* 1988;112:909–912.

148. Fraser CL, Arieff AI. Hepatic encephalopathy. *N Engl J Med* 1985;313:865–873.

149. Jalan R, Hayes PC. Hepatic encephalopathy and ascites. *Lancet* 1997;350:1309–1315.

150. Adams RD, Foley JM. The neurological disorder associated with liver disease. *Assoc Res Nerv Ment Dis Proc* 1953;32:198–237.

151. Valsamis MP, Peress NS, Wright LD. Central pontine myelinolysis in childhood. *Arch Neurol* 1971;25:307–312.

152. Jones EA, Weissenborn K. Neurology and the liver. *J Neurol Neurosurg Psychiatry* 1997;63:279–293.

152a. Blei AT, Butterworth RF. Hepatic encephalopathy. *Semin Liver Dis* 1996;16:233–239.

153. Sherlock S. Fulminant hepatic failure. *Adv Intern Med* 1993;38:245–267.

154. Jones EA, Basile AS. Does ammonia contribute to increased GABA-ergic neurotransmission in liver failure? *Metab Brain Dis* 1998;13:351–360.

155. Jones EA, Basile AS. The involvement of ammonia with the mechanisms that enhance GABA-ergic neurotransmission in hepatic failure. *Adv Exp Med Biol* 1997;420:75–83.

156. Mullen KD, Basile AS. Benzodiazepine-receptor antagonists and hepatic encephalopathy: where do we stand? *Gastroenterology* 1993;105:937–940.

157. Mullen KD, et al. Could an endogenous benzodiazepine ligand contribute to hepatic encephalopathy? *Lancet* 1988;1:457–459.

158. Butterworth RF, Pomier Layrargues G. Benzodiazepine receptors and hepatic encephalopathy. *Hepatology* 1990;11:499–501.

159. Riegler JL, Lake JR. Fulminant hepatic failure. *Med Clin North Am* 1993;77:1057–1083.

160. Klein AS, et al. Amanita poisoning: treatment and the role of liver transplantation. *Am J Med* 1989;86:187–193.

161. Walia BN, et al. Fulminant hepatic failure and acute intravascular haemolysis as presenting manifestations of Wilson's disease in young children. *J Gastroenterol Hepatol* 1992;7:370–373.

162. Danks DM. Copper-induced dystonia secondary to cholestatic liver disease. *Lancet* 1990;335:410.

163. Lidofsky SD, et al. Intracranial pressure monitoring and liver transplantation for fulminant hepatic failure. *Hepatology* 1992;16:1–7.

164. Blei AT. Cerebral edema and intracranial hypertension in acute liver failure: distinct aspects of the same problem. *Hepatology* 1991;13:376–379.

165. Navelet Y, et al. Insuffisance hepato-cellulaire aigue grave de l'enfant: aspects EEG prognostiques. *Neurophysiol Clin* 1990;20:237–245.

166. Schafer DF, Shaw BMJ. Fulminant hepatic failure and orthoptic liver transplantation. *Semin Liver Dis* 1989;9:189–194.

167. Lidofsky SD. Liver transplantation for fulminant hepatic failure. *Gastroenterol Clin North Am* 1993;22:257–269.

168. Devictor D, et al. Flumazenil in the treatment of hepatic encephalopathy in children with fulminant liver failure. *Intensive Care Med* 1995;21:253–256.

169. Devictor D, et al. Management of fulminant hepatic failure in children—an analysis of 56 cases. *Crit Care Med* 1993;21[Suppl 9]:S348–S349.

170. Munoz SJ, et al. Factors associated with severe intracranial hypertension in candidates for emergency liver transplantation. *Transplantation* 1993;55:1071–1074.

171. Blei AT, et al. Complications of intrapressure monitoring in fulminant hepatic failure. *Lancet* 1993;341:157–158.

172. Alper G, et al. Outcome of children with cerebral edema caused by fulminant hepatic failure. *Pediatr Neurol* 1998;18:299–304.

173. Hoofnagle JH, et al. Fulminant hepatic failure: summary of a workshop. *Hepatology* 1995;21:240–252.

174. O'Grady JG, et al. Early indicators of prognosis in fulminant hepatic failure. *Gastroenterology* 1989;97:439–445.

175. Rivera-Penera T, et al. Delayed encephalopathy in fulminant hepatic failure in the pediatric population and the role of liver transplantation. *J Pediatr Gastroenterol Nutr* 1997;24:128–134.

176. Kullmann F, et al. Subclinical hepatic encephalopathy: the diagnostic value of evoked potentials. *J Hepatol* 1995;22:101–110.

177. Patchell R. Neurological complications of organ transplantation. *Ann Neurol* 1994;36:688–703.

178. Conti DJ, Rubin RH. Infection of the central nervous system in organ transplant recipients. *Neurol Clin* 1988;6:241–260.

179. Walker RW, Brochstein JA. Neurologic complications of immunosuppressive agents. *Neurol Clin* 1988;6:261–278.

180. Scherrer U, et al. Cyclosporine-induced sympathetic activation and hypertension after heart transplantation. *N Engl J Med* 1990;323:693–699.

181. Rubin AM, Kang H. Cerebral blindness and encephalopathy with cyclosporin A toxicity. *Neurology* 1987;37:1072–1076.

182. Stein DP, et al. Neurological complications following liver transplantation. *Ann Neurol* 1992;31:644–649.

183. Krom RAF, et al. The first 100 liver transplantations at the Mayo Clinic. *Mayo Clin Proc* 1989;64:84–94.

184. Adams DH, et al. Neurological complications following liver transplantation. *Lancet* 1987;1:949–951.

185. de Groen PC, et al. Central nervous system toxicity after liver transplantation. The role of cyclosporin and cholesterol. *N Engl J Med* 1987;317:861–866.

186. Wijdicks EFM, Wiesner RH, Krom RAF. Neurotoxicity in liver transplant recipients with cyclosporine immunosuppression. *Neurology* 1995;45:1962–1964.

187. Arrelano F, Krupp P. Muscular disorder associated with cyclosporin. *Lancet* 1991;337:915.

188. Oursler DP, Holley KE, Wagoner RD. Hemolytic uremic syndrome after bone marrow transplantation without total body irradiation. *Am J Nephrol* 1993;13:167–170.

189. van Buren D, et al. De novo hemolytic uremic syndrome in renal transplant recipients immunosuppressed with cyclosporine. *Surgery* 1985;96:54–62.

190. Eidelman BH, et al. Neurologic complications of FK 506. *Transplant Proc* 1991;23:3175–3178.

191. Wijdicks EFM, et al. FK506-induced neurotoxicity in liver transplantation. *Ann Neurol* 1994;35:498–501.

192. Osterman JD, et al. Transient hemiparesis associated with monoclonal CD3 antibody (OKT3) therapy. *Pediatr Neurol* 1993;9:482–484.

193. Strominger MB, Liu GT, Schatz NJ. Optic disk swelling and abducens palsies associated with OKT3. *Am J Ophthalmol* 1995;119:664–665.

194. Martinez AJ, Estol C, Faris AA. Neurologic complications of liver transplantation. *Neurol Clin* 1988;6:327–348.

195. Mott SH, et al. Encephalopathy with parkinsonian features in children following bone marrow transplantations and high-dose amphotericin B. *Ann Neurol* 1995;37:810–814.

196. Ferreiro GA, et al. Neuropathologic findings after liver transplantation. *Acta Neuropathol* 1992;84:1–14.

197. Walsh TJ, Hier DB, Caplan LR. Aspergillosis of the central nervous system: clinicopathological analysis of 17 patients. *Ann Neurol* 1985;18:574–582.

198. Hall WA, Martinez AJ. Neuropathology of pediatric liver transplantation. *Pediatric Neurosci* 1989;15:269–275.

199. Estol CJ, et al. Central pontine myelinolysis after liver transplantation. *Neurology* 1989;39:493–498.

200. Stewart SM, et al. Neuropsychological outcome of pediatric liver transplantation. *Pediatrics* 1991;87:367–376.

201. Muller DPR, Lloyd JK, Wolff OH. Vitamin E and neurological function. *Lancet* 1983;1:225–228.

202. Perlmutter DH, et al. Intramuscular vitamin E repletion in children with chronic cholestasis. *Am J Dis Child* 1987;141:170–174.

203. Rosenblum JL, et al. A progressive neurologic syndrome in children with chronic liver disease. *N Engl J Med* 1981;304:503–508.

204. Cynamon HA, et al. Effect of vitamin E deficiency on neurologic function in patients with cystic fibrosis. *J Pediatr* 1988;113:637–640.

205. Guggenheim MA, et al. Vitamin E deficiency and neurologic disease in children with cholestasis: a prospective study. *J Pediatr* 1983;102:577–579.

206. Sokol RJ, et al. Vitamin E deficiency with normal serum vitamin E concentrations in children with chronic cholestasis. *N Engl J Med* 1984;310:1209–1212.

207. Cavalier L, et al. Ataxia with isolated vitamin E deficiency: heterogeneity of mutations and phenotypic variability in a large number of families. *Am J Hum Genet* 1998;62:301–310.

208. Stumpf DA. Friedreich's disease: V. variant form with vitamin E deficiency and normal fat absorption. *Neurology* 1987;37:168–174.

209. Hentati A, et al. Human α-tocopherol transfer protein: gene structure and mutations in familial vitamin E deficiency. *Ann Neurol* 1996;39:295–300.

210. Perlmutter DH, et al. Intramuscular vitamin E repletion in children with chronic cholestasis. *Am J Dis Child* 1987;141:170–174.

211. Larnaout A, et al. Friedrich's ataxia with isolated vitamin E deficiency: a neuropathological study of a Tunisian patient. *Acta Neuropathol* 1997;93:633–637.

212. Traber MG, et al. Lack of tocopherol in peripheral nerves of vitamin E-deficient patients with peripheral neuropathy. *N Engl J Med* 1987;317:262–265.

213. Werlin SL, et al. Neuromuscular dysfunction and ultrastructural pathology in children with chronic cholestasis and vitamin E deficiency. *Ann Neurol* 1983;13:291–296.

214. Neville HE, et al. Ultrastructural and histochemical abnormalities of skeletal muscle in patients with chronic vitamin E deficiency. *Neurology* 1983;33:483–488.

215. Geisler A, et al. Focal white-matter lesions in brain of patients with inflammatory bowel disease. *Lancet* 1995;345:897–898.

216. Nunes ML, et al. Early onset bilateral calcifications and epilepsy. *Pediatr Neurol* 1995;13:80–82.

217. Ferroir JP, et al. Epilepsie, calcifications cérébrales et maladie coeliaque. *Rev Neurol* (Paris) 1997;153:354–356.

218. Barakat AY, Bitar J, Nassar VH. Whipple's disease in a seven-year-old child: report of a case. *Am J Proctol* 1973;24:312–315.

219. Schmitt BP, et al. Encephalopathy complicating Whipple's disease: failure to respond to antibiotics. *Ann Intern Med* 1981;94:51–52.

220. Ringoir S. An update on uremic toxins. *Kidney Int* 1997;52[Suppl 62]:S2–S4.

221. Avram MM, Feinfeld DA, Huatuco AH. Search for the uremic toxin: decreased motor-nerve conduction velocity and elevated parathyroid hormone in uremia. *N Engl J Med* 1978;298:1000–1003.

222. Lazaro RP, Kirshner HS. Proximal muscle weakness in uremia: case reports and review of the literature. *Arch Neurol* 1980;37:555–558.

223. Raskin NH, Fishman RA. Neurologic disorders in renal failure. *N Engl J Med* 1976;294:143–148, 204–210.
224. Fraser CL, Arieff AI. Nervous system complications in uremia. *Ann Intern Med* 1988;109:143–153.
225. Lockwood AH. Neurologic complications of renal disease. *Neurol Clin* 1989;7:617–627.
226. Mentser MI, et al. Peripheral motor nerve conduction velocities in children undergoing chronic hemodialysis. *Nephron* 1978;22:337–341.
227. Said G, et al. Different patterns of uremic polyneuropathy: clinicopathologic study. *Neurology* 1983;33:567–574.
228. Pirzada NA, Morgenlander JC. Peripheral neuropathy in patients with chronic renal failure. A treatable source of discomfort and disability. *Postgrad Med* 1997:249–261.
229. Berretta JS, Holbrook CT, Haller JS. Chronic renal failure presenting as proximal muscle weakness in a child. *J Child Neurol* 1986;1:50–52.
230. Crittenden M, et al. Intellectual development of children with renal insufficiency and end stage renal disease. *Int J Pediatr Nephrol* 1985;6:265–280.
231. McGraw ME, Haka-Ikse K. Neurologic-developmental sequelae of chronic renal failure in infancy. *J Pediatr* 1985;106:579–582.
232. Passer JA. Cerebral atrophy in end-stage uremia. *Proc Dialysis Transplant Forum* 1977;7:91–94.
233. Hauser RA, Lacey DM, Knight MR. Hypertensive encephalopathy. Magnetic resonance imaging demonstration of reversible cortical and white matter lesions. *Arch Neurol* 1988;45:1078–1083.
234. Ibrahim MM, et al. Effect of renal transplantation on uraemic neuropathy. *Lancet* 1974;2:739–742.
235. Temple RM, Deary IJ, Winney RJ. Recombinant erythropoietin improves cognitive function in patients maintained on chronic ambulatory peritoneal dialysis. *Nephrology. Dialysis. Transplantation.* 1995;10:1733–1738.
236. Davis ID, Chang P-N, Nevins TE. Successful renal transplantation accelerates development in young uremic children. *Pediatrics* 1990;86:594–600.
237. So SKS, et al. Growth and development of infants after renal transplantation. *J Pediatr* 1987;110:343–350.
238. Bock GH, et al. Disturbances of brain maturation and neurodevelopment during chronic renal failure in infancy. *J Pediatr* 1989;114:231–238.
239. Dodson WE, et al. Management of seizure disorders: selected aspects. *J Pediatr* 1974;89:527–540.
240. Wassner SJ, et al. Allograft survival in patients receiving anticonvulsant medications. *Clin Nephrol* 1977;8:293–297.
241. Cutler RE. Cyclosporine drug interactions. *Dialysis & Transplantation* 1988;17:139–151.
242. Tyler HR. Neurological complications of dialysis, transplantation and other forms of treatment in chronic uremia. *Neurology* 1965;15:1081–1088.
243. Graham JR, Bana D, Yap A. Headache, hypertension and renal disease. *Res Clin Stud Headache* 1978;6:147–154.
244. Barton CH, Vaziri ND. Central retinal vein occlusion associated with hemodialysis. *Am J Med Sci* 1979;277:39–47.
245. Lopez RI, Collins GH. Wernicke's encephalopathy. *Arch Neurol* 1968;18:248–259.
246. Roca AO, et al. Dialysis leg cramps. Efficacy of quinine versus vitamin E. *ASAIO J* 1992;38:M481–M485.
247. Hughes JR, Schreeder MT. EEG in dialysis encephalopathy. *Neurology* 1980;30:1148–1154.
248. Alfrey AC, et al. Syndrome of dyspraxia and multifocal seizures associated with chronic hemodialysis. *Trans Am Soc Artif Int Organs* 1972;18:257–261,266–267.
249. Foley CM, et al. Encephalopathy in infants and children with chronic renal disease. *Arch Neurol* 1981;38:656–658.
250. Geary DF, et al. Encephalopathy in children with chronic renal failure. *J Pediatr* 1980;96:41–44.
251. Andreoli SP, Bergstein JM, Sherrard DJ. Aluminum intoxication from aluminum-containing phosphate binders in children with azotemia not undergoing dialysis. *N Engl J Med* 1984;310:1079–1084.
252. Freundlich M, et al. Infant formula as a cause of aluminum toxicity in neonatal uraemia. *Lancet* 1985;2:527–529.
253. Andreoli SP. Aluminium levels in children with chronic renal failure who consume low-phosphorus infant formula. *J Pediatr* 1990;116:282–285.
254. Mayor GH, et al. Parathyroid hormone-mediated aluminum deposition and egress in the rat. *Kidney Int* 1980;17:40–44.
255. Masselot JP, et al. Reversible dialysis encephalopathy: role for aluminum-containing gels [Letter]. *Lancet* 1978;2:1386–1387.
256. Ackrill P, et al. Successful removal of aluminum from a patient with dialysis encephalopathy [Letter]. *Lancet* 1980;2:692–693.
257. Ball JH, Butkus DE, Madison DS. Effect of subtotal parathyroidectomy on dialysis dementia. *Nephron* 1977;18:151–155.
258. Rotundo A, et al. Progressive encephalopathy in children with chronic renal insufficiency in infancy. *Kidney Int* 1982;21:486–491.
259. Trompeter RS, et al. Neurologic complications of renal failure. *Am J Kidney Dis* 1986;7:318–328.
260. Rivera-Vazquez AB, et al. Acute hypercalcemia in hemodialysis patients: distinction from dialysis dementia. *Nephron* 1980;25:243–246.
261. Rifkind D, et al. Systemic fungal infections complicating renal transplantations and immunosuppressive therapy. *Am J Med* 1967;43:28–38.
262. Schneck SA. Neuropathological features of human organ transplantation. I. Probable cytomegalovirus infection. *J Neuropathol Exp Neurol* 1965;24:415–429.
263. Reis MA, Costa RS, Ferraz AS. Causes of death in renal transplant recipients: a study of 102 autopsies from 1968 to 1991. *J R Soc Med* 1995;88:24–27.
264. Grimm PC, Ettenger R. Pediatric renal transplantation. *Adv Pediatr* 1992;39:441–493.
265. Wells TG, Ulstrom RA, Nevins TE. Hypoglycemia in pediatric renal allograft recipients. *J Pediatr* 1988;113:1002–1007.
266. Schneck SA, Penn I. Central neoplasms associated with renal transplantation. *Arch Neurol* 1970;22:226–233.
267. Penn I. Tumor incidence in human allograft recipients. *Transplant Proc* 1979;11:1047–1151.
268. Gayal RK, McEvoy L, Wilson DB. Hodgkin disease after renal transplantation in childhood. *J Pediatr Hematol Oncol* 1996;18:392–395.

269. Johnson DH, Rosenthal A, Nadas AS. A 40-year review of bacterial endocarditis in infancy and childhood. *Circulation* 1975;51:581–588.
270. Lerner PI. Neurologic complications of infective endocarditis. *Med Clin N Am* 1985;69:385–398.
271. Matson DD. Intracranial arterial aneurysms in childhood. *J Neurosurg* 1965;23:578–583.
272. Schuster SR, Gross RE. Surgery for coarctation of the aorta. A review of 500 cases. *J Thorac Cardiovasc Surg* 1962;43:54–70.
273. Albert ML, Greer WE, Kantrowitz W. Paraplegia secondary to hypotension and cardiac arrest in a patient who has had previous thoracic surgery. *Neurology* 1969;19:915–918.
274. Guerit JM, et al. The usefulness of the spinal and subcortical components of the posterior tibial nerve SEP's for spinal cord monitoring during aortic coarctation repair. *Electroencephalogr Clin Neurophysiol* 1997;104:115–121.
275. Tyler HR, Clark DB. Incidence of neurological complications in congenital heart disease. *Arch Neurol Psychiatry* 1957;77:17–22.
276. Kalyanaraman K, et al. The electroencephalogram in congenital heart disease. *Arch Neurol* 1968;18:98–106.
277. Fischbein CA, et al. Risk factors for brain abscess in patients with congenital heart disease. *Am J Cardiol* 1974;34:97–102.
278. Tyler HR, Clark DB. Cerebrovascular accidents in patients with congenital heart disease. *Arch Neurol Psychiatr* 1957;77:483–489.
279. Berthrong M, Sabiston DC Jr. Cerebral lesions in congenital heart disease. *Bull Hopkins Hosp* 1951;89:384–406.
280. Martelle RR, Linde LM. Cerebrovascular accidents with tetralogy of Fallot. *Am J Dis Child* 1961;101:206–209.
281. Cotrill CM, Kaplan S. Cerebral vascular accidents in cyanotic congenital heart disease. *Am J Dis Child* 1973;125:484–487.
282. Peterson RA, Rosenthal A. Retinopathy and papilledema in cyanotic congenital heart disease. *Pediatrics* 1972;49:243–249.
282a. Limperopoulos C, et al. Neurologic status of newborns with congenital heart defects before open heart surgery. *Pediatrics* 1999;103:402–408.
283. Greenwood RD, et al. Extracardiac abnormalities in infants with congenital heart disease. *Pediatrics* 1975;55:485–492.
284. Glauser TA, et al. Congenital brain anomalies associated with the hypoplastic left heart syndrome. *Pediatrics* 1990; 85:984–990.
285. Wright RR, Mathews KD. Hypertensive encephalopathy in childhood. *J Child Neurol* 1996;11:193–196.
286. Lloyd AV, Jewitt DE, Still JD. Facial paralysis in children with hypertension. *Arch Dis Child* 1966;41:292–294.
287. Hinchey J, et al. A reversible posterior leukoencephalopathy syndrome. *N Engl J Med* 1996;334:494–500.
288. Pavlakis SG, et al. Occipital-parietal encephalopathy: a new name for an old syndrome. *Pediatr Neurol* 1997;16:145–148.
289. Jones BV, Egelhoff JC, Patterson RJ. Hypertensive encephalopathy in children. *Am J Neuroradiol* 1997; 18:101–106.
290. Sheth RD, et al. Parietal occipital edema in hypertensive encephalopathy: a pathogenetic mechanism. *Eur Neurol* 1996;36:25–28.
291. Abman SH, et al. Systemic hypertension in infants with bronchopulmonary dysplasia. *J Pediatr* 1984;104:928–931.
292. Perlman JM, Volpe JJ. Neurologic complications of captopril treatment of neonatal hypertension. *Pediatrics* 1989;83:47–52.
293. Bellinger D, et al. Cognitive development of children following early repair of transposition of the great arteries using deep hypothermic circulatory arrest. *Pediatrics* 1991;87:701–707.
294. Treasure T, et al. The effect of hypothermic circulatory arrest time on cerebral function, morphology and biochemistry. An experimental study. *J Thorac Cardiovasc Surg* 1983;86:761–770.
295. Wells FC, et al. Duration of circulatory arrest does influence the psychological development of children after cardiac operation in early life. *J Thorac Cardiovasc Surg* 1983;86:823–831.
296. Blackwood M, et al. Developmental outcome in children undergoing surgery with profound hypothermia. *Anesthesiology* 1986;85:437–440.
297. Vanucci R, et al. Diagnosis and management of neurologic complications in infants and children. In: *Complications in cardiothoracic surgery*. St. Louis: Mosby Year Book, 1991:68.
298. Rappaport L, et al. Relation of seizures after cardiac surgery in early infancy to neurodevelopmental outcome. Boston Circulatory Arrest Study Group. *Circulation* 1998;97:773–779.
299. Uzark K, et al. Neurodevelopmental outcomes in children with Fontan repair of functional single ventricle. *Pediatrics* 1998;101:630–633.
300. Sotaniemi KA. Brain damage and neurological outcome after open-heart surgery. *J Neurol Neurosurg Psychiatry* 1980;43:127–135.
301. Ferry PC. Neurologic sequelae of open-heart surgery in children. An "irritating question." *Am J Dis Child* 1990;144:369–373.
302. Puntis JW, Green SH. Ischaemic spinal cord injury after cardiac surgery. *Arch Dis Child* 1985;60:517–520.
303. Moody DM, et al. Brain microemboli during cardiac surgery or aortography. *Ann Neurol* 1990;28:477–486.
304. Greeley WJ, et al. Effects of cardiopulmonary bypass on cerebral blood flow in neonates, infants and children. *Circulation* 1989;80:1209–1215.
305. Greeley WJ, et al. The effect of deep hypothermia and circulatory arrest on cerebral blood flow and metabolism. *Ann Thorac Surg* 1993;56:1464–1466.
306. Huntley DT, Al-Mateen M, Menkes JH. Unusual dyskinesia complicating cardiopulmonary bypass surgery. *Dev Med Child Neurol* 1993;35:631–641.
307. Medlock MD, et al. A 10-year experience with post-pump chorea. *Ann Neurol* 1993;34:820–826.
308. Kupsky WJ, Drozd MA, Barlow CF. Selective injury of the globus pallidus in children with post-cardiac surgery choreic syndrome. *Dev Med Child Neurol* 1995;37:135–144.
309. Montero CG, Martinez AJ. Neuropathology of heart transplantation: 23 cases. *Neurology* 1986;36:1149–1154.
310. Hall WA, et al. Central nervous system infections in heart and heart-lung transplant recipients. *Arch Neurol* 1989;46:173–177.

311. O'Dougherty M, et al. Cerebral dysfunction after chronic hypoxia in children. *Neurology* 1985;35:42–46.
312. Bellinger DC, et al. Developmental and neurologic status of children after heart surgery with hypothermic circulatory arrest or low-flow cardiopulmonary bypass. *N Engl J Med* 1995;332:549–555.
313. Newburger JW, et al. Cognitive function and age at repair of transposition of the great arteries in children. *N Engl J Med* 1984;310:1495–1499.
314. Kurlan R, Krall RL, Deweese JA. Vertebrobasilar ischemia after total repair of tetralogy of Fallot. Significance of subclavian steal created by Blalock-Taussig anastomosis. *Stroke* 1984;15:359–362.
315. Tonz M, et al. Clinical implications of phrenic nerve injury after pediatric cardiac surgery. *J Pediatr Surg* 1996;31:1265–1267.
316. Grotta JC, et al. Red blood cell disorders and stroke. *Stroke* 1986;17:811–817.
317. Walter T, et al. Iron deficiency anemia: adverse effects on infant psychomotor development. *Pediatrics* 1989;84:7–17.
318. Wasserman G, et al. Independent effects of lead exposure and iron deficiency anemia on developmental outcome at age 2 years. *J Pediatr* 1992;121:695–703.
319. Alter BP. Fanconi's anaemia and its variability. *Br J Haematol* 1993;85:9–14.
320. Minagi H, Steinbach HL. Roentgen appearance of anomalies associated with hypoplastic anemias of childhood: Fanconi's anemia and congenital hypoplastic anemia (erythrogenesis imperfecta). *AJR Am J Roentgenol* 1966; 97:100–109.
321. Alter BP, Young NS. The bone marrow failure syndromes. In: Nathan DG, Orkin SH, eds. *Hematology of infancy and childhood*. Philadelphia: WB Saunders, 1998:259–273.
322. Adams JJ. Neurologic complications. In: Embury SH, Hebbel RP, Mohandas N, ed. *Sickle cell disease*. New York: Raven Press, 1994:599–621
323. Adams R, McKie V, Nichols F. The use of transcranial ultrasonography to predict stroke in sickle cell disease. *N Engl J Med* 1992;326:605–610.
324. Powars D, Wilson B, Imbus C. The natural history of stroke in sickle cell disease. *Am J of Medicine* 1978;65:461–471.
325. Portnoy BA, Herion JC. Neurological manifestations in sickle cell disease. *Ann Intern Med* 1972;76:643–652.
326. Armstrong FD, Thompson RJ, Wang W. Cognitive functioning and brain magnetic resonance imaging in children with sickle cell disease. *Pediatrics* 1996;97:864–870.
327. Powars D. Natural history of disease: the first two decades. In: Embury SH, Hebbel RP, Mohandas N, eds. *Sickle cell disease*. New York: Raven Press, 1994:395–412.
328. Wang W, Langston J, Steen G. Silent infarction of the central nervous system [CNS] occurs in very young children with sickle cell anemia: an MRI/MRA study. *J Pediatr Hematol Oncol* 1996;18:461–463.
329. Moser FG, Miller ST, Bello JA. The spectrum of brain MR abnormalities in sickle-cell disease: a report from the cooperative study of sickle cell disease. *Am J Neuroradiol* 1996;17:965–972.
330. Groncy P, Softley T, Queralt J. Proceedings of the American Society of Pediatric Hematology/Oncology at Alexandria, VA. September, 1995.
331. Ohene-Frempong K, Weiner SJ, Sleeper LA. Cerebrovascular accidents in sickle cell disease: rates and risk factors. *Blood* 1998;91:288–294.
332. Powars DR, et al. Cerebral vasculopathy in sickle cell anemia: diagnostic contribution of positron emission tomography *Blood* 1999;93:71–79.
333. Huttenlocher PR, Moohr JW, Johns L. Cerebral blood flow in sickle cell cerebrovascular disease. *Pediatrics* 1984;73:615–621.
334. Koshy M, Thomas C, Goodwin J. Vascular lesions in the central nervous system in sickle cell disease [neuropathology]. *J Am Acad Min Phys* 1990;1:71–78.
335. Powars D, Adams RJ, Nichols FT. Delayed intracranial hemorrhage following cerebral infarction in sickle cell anemia. *J Am Assoc Minority Physicians* 1990;1:79–82.
336. Adams RJ, et al. Cerebral infarction in sickle cell anemia: mechanics based on CT and MRI. *Neurology* 1988;38:1012–1017.
337. Greer M, Schotland D. Abnormal hemoglobin as a cause of neurologic disease. *Neurology* 1962;12:114–123.
338. Witnitzer M, et al. Diagnosis of cerebrovascular disease in sickle cell anemia by magnetic resonance angiography. *J Pediatr* 1990;117:551–555.
339. Van Hoff J, Ritchey AK, Shaywitz BA. Intracranial hemorrhage in children with sickle cell disease. *AJDC* 1985;139:1120–1123.
340. Sarnaik SA, Lusher JM. Neurologic complications of sickle cell anemia. *Am J Pediatr Hematol Oncol* 1982;4:386–394.
341. Powars D. Sickle cell anemia and major organ failure. *Hemoglobin* 1990;14:573–598.
342. Rothman SM, Fulling KH, Nelson JS. Sickle cell anemia and cerebrovascular occlusion. *J Pediatr* 1978;93:808–810.
343. Asher SW. Multiple cranial neuropathies, trigeminal neuralgia, and vascular headache in sickle cell disease, a possible common mechanism. *Neurology* 1980;30:210–211.
344. Pavlakis SG, et al. Neurologic complications of sickle cell disease. *Adv Pediatr* 1989;36:247–276.
345. Wasserman AL, Wilimas JA, Fairclough DL. Subtle neuropsychological deficits in children with sickle cell disease. *Am J Pediatr Hematol Oncol* 1991;13:14–20.
346. Adams RJ, McKie VC, Hsu L. Prevention of a first stroke by transfusions in children with sickle cell anemia and abnormal results on transcranial doppler ultrasonography. *N Engl J Med* 1998;339:5–11.
347. Pavlakis SG, et al. Brain infarction in sickle cell anemia: magnetic resonance imaging correlates. *Ann Neurol* 1988;23:125.
348. Allen JP, et al. Neurologic impairment induced by hyperventilation in children with sickle cell anemia. *Pediatrics* 1976;58:124–126.
349. Groncy P, Softley T, Bradley W. Proceedings of the American Society of Pediatric Hematology/Oncology at San Francisco, CA; February, 1997.
350. Brugnara C. Cation homeostasis. In: Embury SH, Hebbel RP, Mohandas N, eds. *Sickle cell disease*. New York: Raven Press, 1994:608–612.

351. Niihara Y, Zerez CR, Akiyama DS. Increased red cell glutamine availability in sickle cell anemia: demonstration of increased active transport, affinity, and increased glutamate level in intact red cells. *J Lab Clin Med* 1997;130:83–90.
352. Erenberg G, Rinsler SS, Fish BG. Lead neuropathy and sickle cell disease. *Pediatrics* 1974;54:438–441.
353. Greenberg J, Massey EW. Cerebral infarction in sickle cell trait. *Ann Neurol* 1985;18:354–355.
354. Feldenzer JA, Bueche MJ, Venes JL. Superior sagittal sinus thrombosis with infarction in sickle cell trait. *Stroke* 1987;18:656–660.
355. Konrad PN, et al. Erythrocyte and leukocyte phosphoglycerate kinase deficiency with neurologic disease. *J Pediatr* 1973;82:456–460.
356. Sugie H, et al. Recurrent myoglobinuria in a child with mental retardation: phosphoglycerate kinase deficiency. *J Child Neurol* 1989;4:95–99.
357. Valentine WN, et al. Hereditary hemolytic anemia with triosephosphate isomerase deficiency. Studies in kindreds with coexistent sickle cell trait and erythrocyte glucose-6- phosphate dehydrogenase deficiency. *Am J Med* 1966;41:27–41.
358. Poll-The BT, et al. Neurological findings in triosephosphate isomerase deficiency. *Ann Neurol* 1985;17:439–443.
359. Eber SW, et al. Triosephosphate isomerase deficiency: haemolytic anaemia, myopathy with altered mitochondria and mental retardation due to a new variant with accelerated enzyme catabolism and diminished specific activity. *Eur J Pediatr* 1991;150:761–766.
360. Bardosi A, et al. Myopathy with altered mitochondria due to a triosephosphate isomerase (TPI) deficiency. *Acta Neuropathol* 1990;79:387–394.
361. Logothetis J, et al. Thalassemia major (homozygous β-thalassemia). *Neurology* 1972;22:294–304.
362. Shapira Y, et al. Myopathological findings in thalassemia major. *Eur Neurol* 1990;30:324–327.
363. Olivieri NF, et al. Visual and auditory neurotoxicity in patients receiving subcutaneous deferoxamine infusions. *N Engl J Med* 1986;314:869–873.
364. Issaragrisil S, Piankijagum A, Wasi P. Spinal cord compression in thalassemia: report of 12 cases and recommendations for treatment. *Arch Intern Med* 1981;141:1033–1036.
365. Weatherall DJ, et al. Hemoglobin H disease and mental retardation: a new syndrome or a remarkable coincidence? *N Engl J Med* 1981;305:607–612.
366. Gibbons RJ, et al. Clinical and hematological aspects of the X-linked alpha-thalassemia/mental retardation syndrome (ATR-X). *Am J Med Genet* 1995;55:288–299.
367. Gibbons RJ, et al. A newly defined X-linked mental retardation syndrome associated with a-thalassemia. *J Med Genet* 1991;28:729–733.
368. Rosenkrantz TS, et al. Cerebral metabolism in the newborn lamb with polycythemia. *Pediatr Res* 1988;23:329–333.
369. Black VD, et al. Developmental and neurologic sequelae of neonatal hyperviscosity syndrome. *Pediatrics* 1982;69:426–431.
370. Wiswell TE, Cornish JD, Northam RS. Neonatal polycythemia: frequency of clinical manifestations and other associated findings. *Pediatrics* 1986;78:26–30.
371. Black VD, et al. Developmental and neurologic sequelae of neonatal hyperviscosity syndrome. *Pediatrics* 1982;69:426–431.
372. Yiannikas C, McLeod JG, Walsh JC. Peripheral neuropathy associated with polycythemia vera. *Neurology* 1983;33:139–143.
373. Werner EJ. Neonatal polycythemia and hyperviscosity. *Clin Perinatol* 1995;22:693–710.
374. Martinowitz U, Heim M, Tadmor R. Intracranial hemorrhage in patients with hemophilia. *Neurosurgery* 1986;18:538–541.
375. Ljung R, et al. Normal vaginal delivery is to be recommended for haemophilial carrier gravidae. *Acta Paediatrica* 1994;83:609–611.
376. Kinney TR, et al. Computerized tomography in the management of intracranial bleeding in hemophilia. *J Pediatr* 1977;91:31–35.
377. Olsen ER. Intracranial surgery in hemophiliacs. *Arch Neurol* 1969;21:401–412.
378. Joffe G, Buchanan GR. Intracranial hemorrhage in newborn and young infants with hemophilia. *J Pediatr* 1988;113:333–336.
379. Hutt PJ, et al. Spinal extradural hematoma in an infant with hemophilia A: an unusual presentation of a rare complication. *J Pediatr* 1996;128:704–706.
380. Smith CH, Miller DR, Baehner RL, Miller LP. *Blood diseases of infancy and childhood: in the tradition of C.H. Smith*. St. Louis: CV Mosby, 1989.
381. Davies-Jones GAB, Preston FE, Timperly WR. *Neurological complications in clinical haematology*. Oxford: Blackwell Science, 1980.
382. Matoth Y, Zaizov R, Frankel JJ. Minimal cerebral dysfunction in children with chronic thrombocytopenia. *Pediatrics* 1971;47:698–706.
383. Lewis IC, Philpott MG. Neurological complications in the Schonlein-Henoch syndrome. *Arch Dis Child* 1956;31:369–371.
384. Belman AL, et al. Neurologic manifestations of Schoenlein-Henoch purpura: report of three cases and review of the literature. *Pediatrics* 1985;75:687–692.
385. Ritter FJ, Seay AR, Lahey ME. Peripheral mononeuropathy complicating anaphylactoid purpura. *J Pediatr* 1983;103:77–78.
386. Uhrynowska M, Maslanka K, Zupanska B. Neonatal thrombocytopenia: incidence, serological and clinical observations. *Am J Perinatol* 1997;14:415–418.
387. Kelly PJ, et al. Middle cerebral artery main stem thrombosis in two siblings with familial thrombotic thrombocytopenic purpura. *Neurology* 1998;80:1157–1160.
388. Lawlor ER, et al. Thrombotic thrombocytopenic purpura: a treatable cause of childhood encephalopathy. *J Pediatr* 1997;130:313–316.
389. McNinch AW, Orme RL, Tripp JH. Haemorrhagic disease of the newborn returns. *Lancet* 1983;1:1089–1090.
390. Choau WT, Chou ML, Eitzman DV. Intracranial hemorrhage and vitamin K deficiency in early infancy. *J Pediatr* 1984;105:880–884.
391. Lulseged S. Haemorrhagic disease of the newborn: a review of 127 cases. *Ann Trop Paediatr* 1993;13:331–336.
392. Sutor AH, Dagres N, Niederhoff H. Late form of vitamin K deficiency bleeding in Germany. *Klin Padiatr* 1995;207:89–97.
393. Yerby MS. Risks of pregnancy in women with epilepsy. *Epilepsia* 1992;33[Suppl 1]:S23–S26.

394. Smith M, et al. Uniform approach to risk classification and treatment assignment for children with acute lymphoblastic leukemia. *J Clin Oncol* 1996; 14:4–6.
395. Crosley CJ, et al. Central nervous system lesions in childhood leukemia. *Neurology* 1978;28:678–685.
396. Price RA. The pathology of CNS leukemia. In: Mastrangelo R, Poplack DG, Riccardi R, eds. *CNS leukemia: prevention and treatment.* Boston: Martinus Nijhoff, 1983:1–10.
397. Gelber RD, et al. Central nervous system treatment in childhood acute lymphoblastic leukemia. *Cancer* 1993;72:261–270.
398. Hardisty RM, Norman PM. Meningeal leukemia. *Arch Dis Child* 1967;42:441–447.
399. Ingram LC. Cranial nerve palsy in childhood acute lymphoblastic leukemia. *Cancer* 1991;67:2262–2268.
400. Kataoka A, et al. Epidural spinal cord compression as an initial symptom in childhood acute lymphoblastic leukemia: rapid decompression by local irradiation and systemic chemotherapy. *Pediatr Hematol Oncol* 1995;12:179–184.
401. Maurer HS, et al. The effect of initial management of hyperleukocytosis on early complications and outcome of children with acute lymphoblastic leukemia. *J Clin Oncol* 1988;6:1425–1432.
402. Pierce MI. Neurologic complications in acute leukemia in children. *Pediatr Clin North Am* 1962;9: 425–442.
402a. Schumacher M, Orszagh M. Imaging techniques in neoplastic meningiosis. *J Neurooncol* 1998;38:111–120.
403. Pinkel D, Woo S. Prevention and treatment of meningeal leukemia in children. *Blood* 1994;84: 355–366.
404. Evans WE, et al. Conventional compared with individualized chemotherapy for childhood acute lymphoblastic leukemia. *N Engl J Med* 1998;338: 499–505.
405. Steinherz PG. Radiotherapy vs. intrathecal chemotherapy for CNS prophylaxis in childhood ALL. *Oncology* 1989;3:47–53.
406. Hustu HO, et al. Prevention of central nervous system leukemia by irradiation. *Cancer* 1973;32:585–597.
407. Ribeiro JC, et al. An intensive re-treatment protocol for children with isolated CNS relapse of acute lymphoblastic leukemia. *J Clin Oncol* 1995;13: 333–338.
408. Gaynon PS, et al. Survival after relapse in childhood acute lymphoblastic leukemia: impact of site and time to first relapse—the Children's Cancer Group Experience. *Cancer* 1998;82:1387–1395.
409. Wilson DA, et al. Transient white matter changes on MR images in children undergoing chemotherapy for acute lymphocytic leukemia: correlation with neuropsychologic deficiencies. *Radiology* 1991;180: 205–209.
410. Ch'ien LT, et al. Long-term neurological implications of somnolence syndrome in children with acute lymphocytic leukemia. *Ann Neurol* 1980;8:273–277.
411. Peylan-Ramu N, et al. Abnormal CT scans in asymptomatic children after prophylactic cranial irradiation and intrathecal chemotherapy. *N Engl J Med* 1978;298:815–818.
412. DeVivo DC, et al. Leukoencephalopathy in childhood leukemia. *Neurology* 1977;27:609–613.
413. Ochs JJ, et al. Seizures in childhood lymphoblastic leukaemia patients. *Lancet* 1984;2:1422–1424.
414. Hammarin A-L, et al. Analysis of PCR as a tool for detection of JC virus DNA in cerebrospinal fluid for diagnosis of progressive multifocal leukoencephalopathy. *J Clin Microbiol* 1996;34:2929–2932.
415. Curran WJ, et al. Magnetic resonance imaging of cranial radiation lesions. *Int J Radiat Oncol Biol Phys* 1987;13:1093–1098.
416. Chen CY, et al. Childhood leukemia: central nervous system abnormalities during and after treatment. *Am J Neuroradiol* 1996;17:295–310.
417. Price RA, Birdwell DA. The central nervous system in childhood leukemia. III. Mineralizing microangiopathy and dystrophic calcification. *Cancer* 1978;42:717–728.
418. Fishman ML, et al. Optic atrophy following prophylactic chemotherapy and cranial radiation for acute lymphocytic leukemia. *Am J Ophthalmol* 1976;82: 571–576.
419. Neglia JP, et al. Second neoplasms after acute lymphoblastic leukemia in childhood. *N Engl J Med* 1991;325:1330–1336.
420. Stehbens JA, et al. CNS prophylaxis of childhood leukemia: what are the long-term neurological, neuropsychological, and behavioral effects? *Neuropsychol Rev* 1991;2:147–177.
421. Jannoun L. Are cognitive and education development affected by age at which prophylactic therapy is given in acute lymphoblastic leukaemia? *Arch Dis Child* 1983;58:953–958.
422. Crist W, et al. Clinical and biologic features predict a poor prognosis in acute lymphoid leukemias in infants: a Pediatric Oncology Group study. *Blood* 1986;67: 135–140.
423. Butler RW, et al. Neuropsychologic effects of cranial irradiation, intrathecal methotrexate, and systemic methotrexate in childhood cancer. *J Clin Oncol* 1994;12:2621–2629.
424. Hill JM, et al. A comparative study of the long-term psychosocial functioning of childhood acute lymphoblastic leukemia survivors treated by intrathecal methotrexate with or without cranial radiation. *Cancer* 1998;82:208–218.
425. Kramer JH, et al. Absence of white matter changes on magnetic resonance imaging in children treated with CNS prophylaxis therapy for leukemia. *Cancer* 1988;61:928–930.
426. Phillips PC, et al. Abnormal cerebral glucose metabolism in long-term survivors of childhood acute lymphocytic leukemia. *Ann Neurol* 1991;29:263–271.
427. Sluga E, Budka H, Pichler E. Slow virus "Enzephalitis" nach Masern bei zytostatisch behandelter Leukämie im Kindesalter. *Wien Klin Wochenschr* 1975;87:248–251.
428. Price RA, Jamieson PA. The central nervous system in childhood leukemia. II. Subacute leukoencephalopathy. *Cancer* 1975;35:306–318.
429. Mellor D. Encephalitis and encephalopathy in childhood leukemia. *Dev Med Child Neurol* 1976;18: 90–94.
430. Mrózek K, et al. Clinical significance of cytogenetics in acute myeloid leukemia. *Semin Oncol* 1997:17–34.
431. Steuber CP, et al. A comparison of induction and maintenance therapy for acute nonlymphocytic leukemia in childhood: results of a Pediatric Oncology Group study. *J Clin Oncol* 1991;9:247–258.

432. Allen JC. The effects of cancer therapy on the nervous system. *J Pediatr* 1978;93:903–909.
433. Pizzo PA, Poplack DG, Bleyer WA. Neurotoxicities of current leukemia therapy. *Am J Pediatr Hematol Oncol* 1979;1:127–140.
434. Rosenthal S, Kaufman S. Vincristine neurotoxicity. *Ann Intern Med* 1974;80:733–737.
435. Sandler SG, Tobin W, Henderson ES. Vincristine induced neuropathy. *Neurology* 1969;19:367–374.
436. Evans AE. Cerebrospinal fluid of leukemic children without central nervous system manifestations. *Pediatrics* 1963;31:1024–1027.
437. Casey EB, et al. Vincristine neuropathy—clinical and electrophysiological observations. *Brain* 1973;96: 69–86.
438. Martin J, Mainwaring D. Coma and convulsions associated with vincristine therapy. *BMJ* 1973;4: 782–783.
439. Bain PG, et al. Intrathecal vincristine: a fatal chemotherapeutic error with devastating central nervous system effects. *J Neurol* 1991;238:230–234.
440. Dyke RW. Treatment of inadvertent intrathecal injection of vincristine. *N Engl J Med* 1989;321: 1270–1271.
441. Michelagnoli MP, et al. Potential salvage therapy for inadvertent intrathecal administration of vincristine. *Br J Haematol* 1997;99:364–367.
442. Duttera MJ, et al. Irradiation, methotrexate toxicity, and the treatment of meningeal leukemia. *Lancet* 1973; 2:703–707.
443. Robain O, et al. Necrotizing leukoencephalopathy complicating treatment of childhood leukaemia. *J Neurol Neurosurg Psychiatr* 1984;47:65–72.
444. Cairo MS. Adverse reactions of L-asparaginase. *Am J Pediatr Hematol Oncol* 1982;4:335–339.
445. Cairo MS. Intracranial hemorrhage and focal seizures secondary to use of L-asparaginase during induction of ALL. *J Pediatr* 1980;97:829–833.
446. Priest JR, et al. A syndrome of thrombosis and hemorrhage complicating L-asparaginase therapy for childhood acute lymphoblastic leukemia. *J Pediatr* 1982; 100:984–989.
447. Feinberg WM, Swenson MR. Cerebrovascular complications of L-asparaginase therapy. *Neurology* 1988;38:127–133.
448. McHaney VA, et al. Hearing loss in children receiving cisplatin chemotherapy. *J Pediatr* 1983;102: 314–317.
449. Weatherly RA, et al. Cis-platinum ototoxicity in children. *Laryngoscope* 1991;101:917–924.
450. Roelofs RI, et al. Peripheral sensory neuropathy and cisplatin chemotherapy. *Neurology* 1984;34:934–938.
451. Goldberg ID, Bloomer WD, Dawson DM. Nervous system toxic effects of cancer therapy. *JAMA* 1982;247:1437–1441.
452. Baker WJ, Royer GI, Weiss RB. Cytarabine and neurologic toxicity. *J Clin Oncol* 1991;9:679–693.
453. Winkelman MD, Hines JD. Cerebellar degeneration caused by high-dose cytosine arabinoside: a clinicopathological study. *Ann Neurol* 1983;14:520–527.
454. Jarosinski PF, et al. Altered phenytoin clearance during intensive chemotherapy for acute lymphoblastic leukemia. *J Pediatr* 1988;112:996–999.
455. Kadota RP. Bone marrow transplantation for diseases of childhood. *Mayo Clin Proc* 1984;59:171–184.
456. Wiznitzer M, et al. Neurological complications of bone marrow transplantation in childhood. *Ann Neurol* 1984;16:569–576.
457. Patchell RA, et al. Neurologic complications of bone marrow transplantation. *Neurology* 1985;35: 300–306.
458. Bolger GB, et al. Myasthenia gravis after allogeneic bone marrow transplantation: relationship to chronic graft-versus-host disease. *Neurology* 1986;36: 1087–1091.
459. Urbano-Marquez A, et al. Inflammatory myopathy associated with chronic graft-versus-host disease. *Neurology* 1986;36:1091–1093.
460. Woodman R, Shin K, Pineo G. Primary non-Hodgkins lymphoma of the brain. *Medicine* 1985; 64:425–430.
461. Murphy SB. Childhood non-Hodgkin's lymphoma. *N Engl J Med* 1979;299:1446–1448.
462. Ziegler JL, et al. Central nervous system involvement in Burkitt's lymphoma. *Blood* 1970;36:718–728.
463. Mazza JJ, et al. Aggressive chemotherapy in the treatment of Burkitt's and non-Burkitt's undifferentiated lymphoma. *Leuk Lymphoma* 1995;18:289–296.
464. Sohn D, Valensi Q, Miller SP. Neurologic manifestations of Hodgkin's disease. *Arch Neurol* 1967;17: 429–436.
465. Dussault J, Ruel J. Thyroid hormones and brain development. *Annu Rev Physiol* 1987;49:321–334.
466. Bernal J, Nunez J. Thyroid hormones and brain development. *Eur J Endocrinol* 1995;133:390–398.
467. Oppenheimer JH, Schwartz HL. Molecular basis of thyroid hormone-dependent brain development. *Endocr Rev* 1997;18:462–475.
468. Burrow GN, Fisher DA, Larsen PR. Maternal and fetal thyroid function. *N Engl J Med* 1994;331:1072–1078.
469. Fisher DA. Thyroid function in the fetus. In: Fisher DA, Burrow GN, eds. *Perinatal thyroid physiology and disease.* New York: Raven Press, 1975:21.
470. Smith DW, et al. Congenital hypothyroidism: signs and symptoms in newborn period. *J Pediatr* 1975;87: 958–962.
471. Vanderschueren-Lodeweyckx M, et al. Sensorineural hearing loss in sporadic congenital hypothyroidism. *Arch Dis Child* 1983;58:419–422.
472. Laureau E, et al. Somatosensory evoked potentials and auditory brain-stem responses in congenital hypothyroidism. II. A cross-sectional study in childhood. Correlations with hormonal levels and developmental quotients. *Electroenceph Clin Neurophysiol* 1987;67:521–530.
473. Wilkins L. The effects of thyroid deficiency upon the development of the brain. *Assoc Res Nerv Ment Dis Proc* 1962;39:150–155.
474. Schultz MA, et al. Development of electroencephalographic sleep phenomena in hypothyroid infants. *Electroencephalogr Clin Neurophysiol* 1968;25: 351–358.
475. Batsakis JG, Nishiyama RH. Deafness with sporadic goiter: Pendred's syndrome. *Arch Otolaryngol* (Chicago) 1962;76:401–407.
476. Reardon W, Trembath RC. Pendred syndrome. *J Med Genet* 1996;33:1037–1040.
477. Halpern J-P, et al. The neurology of endemic cretinism. A study of two endemias. *Brain* 1991;114: 825–841.

478. Wang YY, Yang SH. Improvement in hearing among otherwise normal school children in iodine-deficient areas of Guizhou, China, following use of iodized salt. *Lancet* 1985;2:518–520.

479. Ma T, et al. Magnetic resonance imaging of brain and the neuromotor disorder in endemic cretinism. *Ann Neurol* 1993;34:91–94.

480. Weinberger C, et al. A neural thyroid hormone receptor gene. In: DeLong GR, Robbins J, Condliffe PG, eds. *Iodine and the brain*. New York: Plenum, 1989:29–38.

481. Xue-Yi C, et al. Timing of vulnerability of the brain to iodine deficiency in endemic cretinism. *N Engl J Med* 1994;331:1739–1744.

482. Kocher T. Zur Verhütung des Cretinismus und cretinoider Zustände nach neuen Forschungen. *Dtsch Z Chir* 1892;34:556–626.

483. Debré R, Sémélaigne G. Syndrome of diffuse muscular hypertrophy in infants causing an athletic appearance. Its connection with congenital myxedema. *Am J Dis Child* 1935;50:1351–1361.

484. Cross HE, et al. Familial agoitrous cretinism accompanied by muscular hypertrophy. *Pediatrics* 1963;41: 413–420.

485. Spiro AJ, et al. Cretinism with muscular hypertrophy (Kocher-Debré-Sémélaigne syndrome): histochemical and ultrastructural study of skeletal muscle. *Arch Neurol* 1970;23:340–349.

486. Reuss ML, et al. The relation of transient hypothyroxinemia in preterm infants to neurologic development at two years of age. *N Engl J Med* 1996; 334: 821–827.

487. Andersen HS. Studies in hypothyroidism in children. *Acta Paediatr* 1961;[Suppl]:125.

488. Aronson R, et al. Growth in children with congenital hypothyroidism detected by neonatal screening. *J Pediatr* 1990;116:33–37.

489. Derksen-Lubsen G, Verkerk PH. Neuropsychologic development in early treated congenital hypothyroidism: analysis of literature data. *Pediatr Res* 1996; 39:561–566.

490. Wiebel J. Cerebellar-ataxic syndrome in children and adolescents with hypothyroidism under treatment. *Acta Paediatr Scand* 1976;65:201–205.

491. MacFaul R, et al. Neurological abnormalities in patients treated for hypothyroidism from early life. *Arch Dis Child* 1978;53:611–619.

492. Penfold JL, Simpson DA. Premature craniosynostosis: a complication of thyroid replacement therapy. *J Pediatr* 1975;86:360–363.

493. Mosier HD. Hyperthyroidism. In: Gardner LI, ed. *Endocrine and genetic diseases of childhood and adolescence*, 2nd ed. Philadelphia: WB Saunders, 1975.

494. Fishbeck KH, Layzer RB. Paroxysmal choreoathetosis associated with thyrotoxicosis. *Ann Neurol* 1979; 6:453–454.

495. Klawans HL Jr, Shenker DM. Observations on the dopaminergic nature of hyperthyroid chorea. *J Neurol Transm* 1972;33:73–81.

496. Jabbari B, Huott AD. Seizures in thyrotoxicosis. *Epilepsia* 1980;21:91–96.

497. Radetti G, et al. Thyrotoxicosis presenting with seizures and coma in two children. *Am J Dis Child* 1993;147:925–927.

498. Hollingsworth DR, Mabry CC. Congenital Graves' disease: four familial cases with long-term follow-up and perspective. *Am J Dis Child* 1976;130:148–155.

499. Kopp P, et al. Congenital hyperthyroidism caused by a mutation in the thyrotropin-receptor gene. *N Engl J Med* 1995;332:150–154.

500. Jefferson A. A clinical correlation between encephalopathy and papilledema in Addison's disease. *J Neurol Neurosurg Psychiatry* 1956;19:21–27.

501. Grant DB, et al. Neurological and adrenal dysfunction in the adrenal insufficiency/alacrima/achalasia (3A) syndrome. *Arch Dis Child* 1993;68:779–782.

502. Cacciari E, et al. Endocrine function and morphological findings in patients with disorders of the hypothalo-pituitary area: a study with magnetic resonance. *Arch Dis Child* 1990;65: 1199–1202.

503. Argyropoulou M, et al. Magnetic resonance imaging in the diagnosis of growth hormone deficiency. *J Pediatr* 1992;120:886–891.

504. Rappaport R. Magnetic resonance imaging in pituitary disease. *Growth Genetics & Hormones* 1995:11:1–5.

505. Stewart BM. The hypertrophic neuropathy of acromegaly. *Arch Neurol* 1966;14:107–110.

506. Laurence JZ, Moon RC. Four cases of retinitis pigmentosa occurring in the same family and accompanied by general imperfection of development. *Ophthal Rev* 1866;2:32–41.

507. Farag TI, et al. Bardet-Biedl and Laurence-Moon syndromes in a mixed Arab population. *Clin Genet* 1988;33:78–82.

508. Green JS, et al. The cardinal manifestations of Bardet-Biedl syndrome, a form of Laurence-Moon-Biedl syndrome. *N Engl J Med* 1989;321:1002–1009.

509. Jacobson SG, Borruat FX, Apathy PP. Patterns of rod and cone dysfunction in Bardet-Biedl syndrome. *Am J Ophthalmol* 1990;109:676–688.

510. Whitaker MD, et al. The pituitary gland in the Laurence-Moon syndrome. *Mayo Clin Proc* 1987; 62:216–222.

511. Bruford EA, et al. Linkage mapping in 29 Bardet-Biedl syndrome families confirms loci in chromosomal regions 11q13, 15q22.3-q23, and 16q21. *Genomics* 1997;41:93–99.

512. Kwitek-Black AE, et al. Linkage of Bardet-Biedl syndrome to chromosome 16q and evidence for non-allelic genetic heterogeneity. *Nat Genet* 1993;5:392–396.

513. Goldstein JL, Fialkow PJ. The Alstrom syndrome: report of three cases with further delineation of the clinical, pathophysiological, and genetic aspects of the disorder. *Medicine* 1973;52:53–71.

514. Leão MJ, Ribeiro-Silva ML. Orofaciodigital syndrome type I in a patient with severe CNS defects. *Pediatr Neurol* 1995;13:247–251.

515. Sotos JF, et al. Cerebral gigantism in childhood: a syndrome of excessively rapid growth with acromegalic features and a nonprogressive neurologic disorder. *N Engl J Med* 1964;271:109–116.

516. Dodge PR, Holmes SJ, Sotos JF. Cerebral gigantism. *Dev Med Child Neurol* 1983;25:248–252.

517. Milunsky A, Cowie VA, Donoghue EC. Cerebral gigantism in childhood. A report of two cases and a review of the literature. *Pediatrics* 1967;40:395–402.

518. Cole TRP, Hughes HE. Sotos syndrome. *J Med Genet* 1990;27:571–576.

519. Beener FA, Veenema H, de Pater JM, Cerebral gigantism (Sotos syndrome) in two patients with fra(X) chromosomes. *Am J Med Genet* 1986;23:221–226.

520. Castells S, Reddy CM, Hashemi S. Metabolic

responses to human growth hormone in children with cerebral dwarfism. *J Pediatr* 1976;89:958–960.

521. Winegrad AI. Does a common mechanism induce the diverse complications of diabetes? *Diabetes* 1987;36:396–406.

522. Eeg-Olofsson O, Petersen I. Childhood diabetic neuropathy. *Acta Paediat Scand* 1966;53:163–176.

523. Cracco J, Castells S, Mark E. Spinal somatosensory evoked potentials in juvenile diabetes. *Ann Neurol* 1984;15:55–58.

524. Solders G, et al. Nerve conduction and autonomic nerve function in diabetic children. A 10-year follow-up study. *Acta Paediatr* 1997;86:361–366.

525. Hoffman WH, Hart ZH, Frank RN. Correlates of delayed motor nerve conduction and retinopathy in juvenile-onset diabetes mellitus. *J Pediatr* 1983;102:351–356.

526. Bastron JA, Thomas JE. Diabetic polyradiculopathy: clinical and electromyographic findings in 105 patients. *Mayo Clin Proc* 1981;56:725–732.

527. MacDonald JT, Brown DR. Acute hemiparesis in juvenile insulin-dependent diabetes mellitus (JIDDM). *Neurology* 1979;29:893–896.

527a. Rovet JF, Ehrlich RM. The effect of hypoglycemic seizures on cognitive function in children with diabetes: a 7-year prospective study. *J Pediatr* 1999;134:503–506.

528. Bjørgass, M, et al. Cognitive function in type 1 diabetic children with and without episodes of severe hypoglycemia. *Acta Paediatr* 1997;86:148–153.

529. Kety SS, et al. The blood flow and oxygen consumption of the human brain in diabetic acidosis and coma. *J Clin Invest* 1948;27:500–510.

530. Ohman JL, et al. The cerebrospinal fluid in diabetic ketoacidosis. *N Engl J Med* 1971;284:283–290.

531. Rosenbloom AL. Intracerebral crises during treatment of diabetic ketoacidosis. *Diabetes Care* 1990;13:22–33.

532. Bello FA, Sotos JF. Cerebral oedema in diabetic ketoacidosis in children. *Lancet* 1990;336:64.

533. Duck SC, et al. Cerebral edema complicating therapy for diabetic ketoacidosis. *Diabetes* 1976;25:111–115.

534. Van der Meulen JA, Klip A, Grinstein S. Possible mechanism for cerebral oedema in diabetic ketoacidosis. *Lancet* 1987;2:306–308.

535. Krane EJ, et al. Subclinical brain swelling in children during treatment of diabetic ketoacidosis. *N Engl J Med* 1985;312:1147–1151.

536. Duck SC, Wyatt DT. Factors associated with brain herniation in the treatment of diabetic ketoacidosis. *J Pediatr* 1988;113:10–14.

537. Franklin B, Liu J, Ginsberg-Fellner F. Cerebral edema and ophthalmoplegia reversed by mannitol in a new case of insulin-dependent diabetes mellitus. *Pediatrics* 1982;69:87–90.

538. Joosten R, et al. Hyperglycemic nonketotic diabetic coma. *Eur J Pediatr* 1981;137:233–236.

539. Vernon DD, Postellon DC. Nonketotic hyperosmolal diabetic coma in a child: management with low-dose insulin infusion and intracranial pressure monitoring. *Pediatrics* 1986;77:770–772.

540. Cremers CW, Wijdeveld PG, Pinckers AJ. Juvenile diabetes mellitus, optic atrophy, hearing loss, atonia of the urinary tract and bladder, and other abnormalities (Wolfram syndrome). *Acta Paediatr Scand* 1977;264[Suppl]:3–16.

Chapter 16

Disorders of Mental Development

Marcel Kinsbourne and *William D. Graf

*Department of Cognitive Studies, Tufts University, Medford, Massachusetts 02155;
and °Departments of Pediatrics and Neurology, University of Washington School of Medicine,
and Children's Hospital and Regional Medical Center, Seattle, Washington 98105*

A developmental disability is an abnormality of the central nervous system (CNS), manifest during the developmental period, which results in significant lifelong impairment in any combination of physical, cognitive, sensory, speech and language, and neuropsychological functions. This chapter considers the nature, diagnosis, and management of those developmental disorders and disabilities that implicate higher cortical function.

The developmental period begins with embryonic gastrulation and the formation of the neuroectoderm and continues until approximately 5 years of age. A disorder of mental development is an impairment in the acquisition of one or more complex skills that is not caused by an acquired brain lesion, sensory or motor impairment, or lack of opportunity to learn.

NATURE OF DEVELOPMENTAL DISORDERS

The most distinctive aspect of postnatal neurologic maturation in humans is the gradual acquisition of an extensive repertoire of cognitive skills. The newborn is devoid of cerebrally controlled behavior patterns, to the point that in the first 6 weeks of life it is hard to distinguish the behavior of a normal from an anencephalic infant. Different brain regions assume control over specific aspects of function in a pre- dictable sequence and timing: brainstem before cerebrum, and sensorimotor before association cortex.

The bulk of the variance in IQ in the general population reflects genetic diversity (1). There is normally a high correlation between an individual's performance on various mental tests, a phenomenon that has given rise to the construct of *g*, or general intelligence. But many adverse biological, genetic, environmental, and gene-environment interaction (ecogenetic) influences can reduce the rate of intellectual development. Development may be globally delayed, resulting in mental retardation. In other cases it is decreased only for some components of intelligence. This results in "scatter" between normal scores on some tests, and low scores on tests that are sensitive to the cognitive processes that are developing abnormally slowly. This "discrepancy" profile is typical of learning disabilities. Any cognitive skill may be selectively impaired, but it is the impairments that have a social effect that attract attention. Those selective cognitive deficits that result in delayed language development, abnormal play, and social skills commonly become apparent during the second and third years of life. Selective deficits in attention, concentration, and learning that leave a child lacking readiness for instruction in academic areas may not be recognized until the preschool or grade school period. Such disorders are usually diagnosed on functional and behavioral criteria, when biological validation of the diagnosis is not feasible.

Most true developmental disorders reach an end-point of persisting deficits, although signs and symptoms may change with age. There may be gradual improvement (e.g., compensation, reorganization, and maturation in a child, possibly because of structured special education) or worsening (e.g., the increasing effect of an intractable seizure disorder, or the gradual deceleration of development that is typical in Down syndrome). Some deficits take the form of developmental immaturity, in which the child's function is quantitatively insufficient for the chronologic age but qualitatively normal for a child of a younger age. In others, such as autism, qualitatively abnormal behavior is apparent in the first 3 years of life. The lag in the emergence of the impaired cognitive or behavioral function often does not resolve over time, and the child reaches a plateau at a lower than normal end-point of cognitive maturity. This occurs because the damaged area had not yet assumed control over behavior at the time of the injury.

NEURODEVELOPMENTAL LAG

As the normal brain matures, different areas assume control over specific aspects of behavior in a predictable sequence and with predictable timing. The normal cognitive and language developmental milestones are presented in Table 16.1. When an area is damaged after the skill has been acquired, its control over the skill is impaired, and an acquired deficit results. In neurodevelopmental lag, the effects of an early lesion or maldevelopment become apparent many months or years later, as persistence of immature behavior patterns and slower than normal emergence of skills. The newborn is innately equipped with a limited behavioral repertoire of synergisms (root, suck, startle, and so froth) that serve to satisfy vital needs or attract care taking. These coordinated movement patterns occur spontaneously or appear as reflexive responses to stim-

TABLE 16.1. *Typical cognitive and language developmental milestones of infancy and childhood*

Age	Early cognitive milestones	Early language milestones
From birth	Interest in faces; begins to make eye contact	Phonologic discrimination
Few mo	A social smile should develop before 6 weeks of age Laughing out loud is a reliable milestone that should occur around 4 months of age	Responsive vocalization, turn-taking, cooing (vowels)
6–8 mo	Grabbing for objects, exploring surroundings	Babbling consonants/vowels,syllables, dada, baba
10–12 mo	Pointing to indicate wanted object; comprehension of words	2–3 words with meaning; imitation of animals
18–22 mo	Should follow simple commands, indicate body parts, ask for objects by pointing, and imitate actions	Vocabulary spurt; jargonizing develops interspersed with intelligent words; receptive language and understanding are more developed than speech
	Onlooker behavior, nonsocial activity, and solitary independent play	By 2 years: word combinations/many single words; expansion of comprehension
Around 2 yr	Limited social participation; parallel play	2-word utterances; mostly intelligible to family; comprehend many sentences
By 3 yr	Beginning social play (the child talks about play, borrows/lends toys, controls who may play in the group)	Speaks in grammatical sentences (with some errors); mostly intelligible to strangers (still makes phonologic errors)
Thereafter	Cooperative play; acts out make-believe themes	Phonology by school age; vocabulary increases life-long

ulation. They gradually disappear according to a well-delineated schedule in the course of infancy or childhood. A miscellany of neurologic disorders that give rise to neurodevelopmental lag may cause synergisms to persist. They then become apparent as "soft signs" on the neurologic examination. Soft signs are signs that would have been normal in a younger child. They are of two kinds, both relative to expectation for the child's age: (a) unwanted movements (e.g., persistent asymmetric tonic neck response, unwanted associated and mirror movements); and (b) imperfect execution, such as slowness in speeded sequential activities such as finger tapping or finger-thumb sequencing, or in alternating movements, such as pronation-supination or flexion-extension at the ankle (dysdiadochokinesis). Dyspraxia, or clumsiness, in the absence of long tract signs, is diagnostically nonspecific. The overall trend of motor development is toward increasingly precise control over an ever widening repertoire of discrete movement combinations, whereas sensory development tends toward a finer, more exact differentiation between various stimuli (2).

In developmentally delayed children, just as in healthy children, development proceeds along the same lines, although at a slower rate, depending on the severity of the neurologic lesion. Thus, with increasing age and neurologic maturation, scores on quantitative scales for soft signs decline, regardless of diagnosis (3). Considerable consistency in neuromotor developmental status has been demonstrated over periods as long as 10 years (4). Signs of sensorimotor immaturity are often lower-level analogues to later emerging cognitive immaturity, behavior problems, and attention deficits. Thus, early signs of developmental delay indicate a high risk of long-term functional developmental disabilities, depending on the distribution and severity of the underlying cause, but they do not provide an adequate basis for prognosis, although an association between persisting mirror movements and aggressive psychopathology (both disinhibitory phenomena?) has been documented (5).

In the past, sensorimotor and cognitive immaturities were bracketed together as "minimal brain dysfunction" (MBD) (6). This construct was intended to counteract the now virtually extinct tendency to ascribe developmental delays to intrapsychic problems. These miscellaneous neurocognitive immaturities do not necessarily coincide with or affect specific academic skills, and they cannot be used to arrive at any conclusion about mental development or the nature of a cognitive deficit. Nor do the antecedents of minimal brain dysfunction differ qualitatively from those of major brain dysfunctions such as cerebral palsy or mental retardation, which also are end results of a host of different neuropathologies. Whether minor or major developmental impairments occur, or other deficits, depends on the distribution and severity of the insult, rather than its cause.

CLASSIFICATION OF DEVELOPMENTAL DISORDERS AND DISABILITIES

All disorders of cognitive development should be classified on both an etiologic and descriptive and functional basis. However, regardless of the clinician's skill, many patients with developmental disorders remain without a conclusive etiologic diagnosis. Provided that the diagnostic evaluation is reasonably complete, the medical record should then describe the developmental disorder as "of uncertain etiology." This characterization urges the diagnostic process to continue with each subsequent clinic or office visit and acknowledges that "the best test in neurology is the test of time."

In the absence of a precise medical diagnosis, it is preferable to describe the characteristics of the abnormal developmental process rather than to record inferences such as "cerebral dysfunction," "organicity," or "static encephalopathy." When evaluating a developmentally delayed child, it is invaluable to record qualitative and quantitative descriptions of the mental status, including use of language, play skills, visual and auditory recognition, reasoning, orientation to spatial relationships, impulse control, and the ability to sustain attention. Most neurodevelopmental disorders that result in mild disability affect quality of life but do not curtail longevity. Beyond the diagnostic evaluation, children with most developmental disorders only require the customary standard of medical care treatments throughout their lives. The need for additional specific medical interventions for certain neurologic disorders (e.g., diets for metabolic disorders or epilepsy, pharmacologic treatment for severe behavioral problems), or for nonmedical therapy programs, must be continually reevaluated for evidence of cost-effectiveness on long-term outcome.

PRACTICAL APPROACHES TO NEURODEVELOPMENTAL DISORDERS

Two fundamental practice models in clinical medicine are the medical model and the rehabilitation model (Fig. 16.1). In the evaluation and management of children with disorders of neurologic development, the practice of both models should coincide; however, it may be helpful to maintain the individual perspectives of these models in discussions with parents and caretakers. These perspectives are particularly important for neurologic disorders for which there are no specific treatments.

Medical Model

Developmental disorders have a wide variety of causes and their severity is determined by the timing, duration, and intensity of the genetic error, biological insult, or environmental influence. Few children with developmental disorders have a specific, identifiable genetic or biological etiology. A thorough search for diagnostic clues is nonetheless important. In addition to the family history with a three-generation pedigree, information is required from the prenatal, perinatal, and early postnatal periods. The physician should inquire into the development of motor skills, comprehension of speech, emergence of words and formed, intelligible sentences, and quality of social play skills. The physical examination includes measuring head circumference, body size and growth, assessing vision and hearing, ocular funduscopy, and searching for facial, skeletal, somatic, and dermatoglyphic anomalies and asymmetries, visceromegaly, neurocutaneous lesions and depigmentations, and other

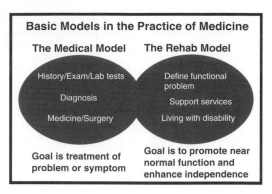

FIG. 16.1. The practice of the medical model and the rehabilitation model should coincide.

signs of chronic illness. Hand preference and pencil grip are observed, as well as the presence of abnormal postures and involuntary movements. The various clinical clues in the evaluation of developmental disorders are presented in Table 16.2. A useful semiquantified neurodevelopmental examination is the Physical and Neurologic Examination for Subtle Signs (7). It evaluates the child's ability to walk in various ways, balance and hop, and the time the child takes to move tongue, fingers, hands, and feet in various ways 20 times.

The mental status examination assesses the child's orientation, relatedness to, and interest in the examiner, caregiver, siblings, peers, and other people in the child's environment; the quality of reciprocal social exchange in verbal and nonverbal communication (e.g., eye contact, gestures, facial expression); ability to engage in reciprocal imaginative play with representational toys; presence of perseverative, stereotypic, and ritualistic behavior; and presence of problematic behaviors, such as attention difficulties, overactivity, aggression, and self-injury.

The laboratory evaluation of choice for developmental disorders continues to change as understanding of the human genome leads to improved syndrome delineation and advances in cytogenetic, molecular, and neuroimaging techniques become clinically available. A routine protocol cannot replace the detailed assessment of the individual patient or clinical judgment. The incidence of identifiable meta-

TABLE 16.2. *Clinical clues in the determination of developmental disorders and their etiology*

Clinical clue	Etiologic category	Examples
Family member with known condition, mental retardation, other developmental disabilities, multiple miscarriages	Genetic	Mendelian dominant, recessive, X-linked; some mitochondrial disorders; cytogenetic/chromosomal anomalies
Facial dysmorphism, severe central nervous system malformation	Genetic or acquired during embryogenesis	CHARGE syndrome, anencephaly, holoprosencephaly, septo-optic dysplasia
Evidence of neuroblast migrational disorder, hydrocephalus, congenital microcephaly	Genetic or acquired during the fetal period	Lissencephaly (Miller-Dieker syndrome), X-linked hydrocephalus
Born too soon, too small	Prematurity	Periventricular leukomalacia
Low Apgar scores, low cord pH, neonatal seizures	Perinatal	Hypoxic-ischemic encephalopathy
Acquired microcephaly, stagnation in developmental gain	Postnatal	Rett syndrome
Postnatal vomiting, failure to thrive, hypoglycemia	Metabolic	Phenylketonuria, urea cycle disorders, organic acidurias, other specific enzyme defects
Cerebral calcifications, congenital or acquired microcephaly	Infectious	Cytomegalovirus encephalopathy, toxoplasmosis, herpes simplex viruses, human immunodeficiency virus, bacterial meningitis
Hemorrhage, infarction, venous thrombosis	Cerebrovascular	Factor V Leiden deficiency, sickle cell disease
Failure to thrive	Nutritional	Prenatal and postnatal protein malnutrition, vitamin and essential element deficiency
Parental drug abuse, neonatal jaundice, acute encephalopathy	Prenatal, perinatal, postnatal toxic exposure	Fetal alcohol syndrome, neonatal hyperbilirubinemia, lead poisoning
Dry skin, hypotonia, hyporeflexia	Endocrine	Hypothyroidism
Extreme poverty, parental drug abuse, low parental educational level, severe plagiocephaly	Sociocultural/environmental	Nonaccidental head trauma, emotional deprivation, lack of infant stimulation
Nonspecific findings	Unknown	Up to one-half of all developmental disabilities

bolic disorders in children with developmental delay is low, ranging from 0% to 5% (8–10). In addition, nonspecific, nondiagnostic, or false-positive abnormalities are common in routine nondirected laboratory testing. This can lead to further laboratory pursuits that do not result in a definitive diagnosis. Most infants and children with true inborn errors of metabolism demonstrate some signs or symptoms of their metabolic disorder such as hepatosplenomegaly, failure to thrive, intolerance of certain food groups, intermittent emesis, recurrent unexplained illnesses, seizures, intermittent somnolence, or fluctuating hypotonia. The various metabolic tests employed under these circumstances are reviewed in Chapter 1. Metabolic screening should be deferred in patients with developmental disor-

ders who lack signs or symptoms of a metabolic disorder (9,11–13).

Many individuals with mental retardation have associated behavioral, emotional, and psychiatric disorders and other congenital anomalies. A composite pattern recognition or cytogenetic testing may lead to a specific diagnosis. In these circumstances the "diagnosis" refers to the most salient aspect of the condition or is noted by an acronym, such as CHARGE association (of congenital anomalies) or eponym (e.g., Angelman syndrome), or by the chromosomal abnormality, such as chromosome 22q11.2. A specific molecular cytogenetic analysis, such as fluorescence *in situ* hybridization (FISH) studies, may be indicated if the child has features of a known mental retardation syndrome (e.g., Williams or fragile X syndromes) or autism (e.g., chromosome 15q11 duplication) (see Chapter 3).

There are no specific neuropathologic correlates in most individuals with mild mental retardation, and neuroimaging has a low diagnostic yield if no suspicious physical findings or localized neurologic deficits exist. The diagnostic yield of neuroimaging studies increases considerably if the child has severe mental retardation, microcephaly or macrocephaly, major motor abnormalities, features of a genetic syndrome, or seizures. Magnetic resonance imaging (MRI) may reveal migrational disorders (e.g., lissencephaly), midline defects (e.g., holoprosencephaly or septo-optic dysplasia), or other brain malformations and disruptions (e.g., schizencephaly) (see Chapter 4). When the history suggests metabolic insult, vascular compromise, infection, or trauma, neuroimaging may reveal evidence of destructive CNS changes.

There is no consensus on which children with developmental delay should be studied by imaging (14,15), and there are considerable technical, methodologic, demographic, and interpretive variations in the few available studies of CT and MRI in children with mental retardation. Thus, the frequency of abnormal neuroimaging findings in persons with mental retardation ranges from 9% to 80% (9,16–20). Developments in functional neuroimaging, using techniques such as positron emission tomography (PET), single photon emission CT (SPECT), functional MRI (fMRI), and volumetric and morphometric MRI provide insights into specific conditions, but have limited overall application in the infant or child with a nonspecific developmental disorder (21,22). A qualified audiologist must rule out hearing loss in all children with language delay, or who have developed some language but may have isolated high-frequency hearing losses. Children with hearing impairment should be followed longitudinally by a developmental speech and hearing center (with a speech pathologist and audiologist) for speech therapy and possible speech amplification.

Electroencephalography (EEG) is indicated if the history suggests seizures or regression or plateau in language acquisition (see Chapter 13). This test can assist in the diagnosis of certain children with developmental disorders (23).

Rehabilitation Model

In the rehabilitation model the physician is less concerned about the specific etiology than the level of function and the implementation of evidence-based, effective, and enabling therapies.

Children considered to have cognitive deficiency may come to attention because of poor academic achievement, abnormal behavior, or both. The physician must determine whether the lack of academic achievement is because of limited cognitive ability or whether it represents underachievement relative to the child's potential because of other (e.g., psychosocial or emotional) reasons. If the child appears to be achieving at his or her maximum level, then special needs are identified, and an individualized educational plan (IEP) is implemented. If the child is underachieving, the causes are sought in the child's school and social setting or emotional well-being. In only a few developmental syndromes, notably attention deficit–hyperactivity disorder (ADHD), can cognitive potential be enhanced by medical means.

Inclusion in Public Education

The Education for All Handicapped Children Act (EHA) was renamed in 1990 to the Individuals with Disabilities Education Act (IDEA). This legislation requires schools to provide an appropriate individualized educational plan to students with disabilities, to be implemented in the "least restrictive environment." The IDEA mandates a nondiscriminatory assessment, active involvement of parents in the educational process with due-process rights and hearing, and access to indicated ancillary services such as physical therapy, counseling, and transportation. The reauthorization of IDEA requires that students with disabilities be educated with their nondisabled peers to the extent possible, that schools actively plan for student transitions (and that traumatic brain injury and autism be considered separate categories). The word *handicapped* in the original version of the law was replaced with the word *disabled*. *Inclusion* refers to the effort to include students with disabilities in general classrooms, while providing special services outside the general classroom as needed. Currently, approximately 70% of all students with disabilities attend mainstream classes during part of the school day.

Quantitative Measurement of Cognition (Standardized Scales)

In infancy and early childhood, receptive and expressive language and play skills are the best indices of cognitive level. The prognostic reliability of cognitive testing improves when children reach an age at which some language competence is expected, and a wider range of test situations is applicable. Language development up to age 3 years can be documented with the Early Language Milestone Scale (24). Essential early cognitive and language developmental milestones in infancy and childhood are summarized in Table 16.1.

The diagnosis of cognitive deficiency relies on the validation of a clinical impression of a "slow learner" by standard psychometric assessment. In infants and children with developmental delays or disabilities, an appropriate assessment depends on the child's age, level of impairment, and the presence of additional sensory deficits. For screening up to age 6 years, the Denver-II (formerly the Denver Developmental Screening Test–Revised) is most commonly used (25). The Denver-II draws on parent history, testing, and observation, and takes approximately one-half hour to administer. The Bayley Scales of Infant Developmental estimate the level of cognitive and motor deficits in infants (26). However, infant cognition is so limited that only sensorimotor functions can be evaluated accurately for normative purposes. These functions are nonspecifically correlated to an infant's later emerging cognitive skills, the lack of which may result in a developmental disability in later years. More specific information about selective deficits in cognitive operations can be gleaned from the results of neuropsycho-

logical testing. A cognitive profile is established, for diagnoses and functional evaluation, the monitoring of further development, and rehabilitation planning. Commonly used measures of cognitive and adaptive behavioral development are summarized in Table 16.3.

A normal IQ test result eliminates mental retardation as the reason for preschool or school achievement below the expected level. It does not eliminate the possibility that specific learning disabilities may compromise the acquisition of some academic skills. Furthermore, no single IQ test measures all cognitive operations and various subtests may involve multiple cognitive processes. Therefore, although a learning disabled child might achieve a low score on a subtest, this may not identify the basic cognitive deficit that prevents the child from learning to read, write, or calculate. The Kaufman Assessment Battery for Children attempts to cover some skills not well measured by other psychometric batteries (32).

Scatter between the levels of subscale subtest scores on an intelligence scale can reflect a disparity in the level of development of different intellectual skills. Verbal performance discrepancy scores are often reported. Children with mild mental retardation tend to score somewhat lower on the Wechsler verbal subscale than on the performance subscale. A much lower verbal than performance IQ accompanies selective language delay; the converse discrepancy is often found in association with developmental difficulties in spatial orientation and visuomotor control.

The Stanford-Binet scale and Wechsler Preschool and Primary Scale of Intelligence (WPPSI) are most commonly used for preschoolers (30). The Wechsler Intelligence Scale for Children (WISC-III) is available for school-aged children (29). These are well-standardized test batteries that call for the use of a range of different cognitive skills. For deaf children, the WISC-III performance scale and the Hiskey-Nebraska Test of Learning Aptitude have been specifically standardized (43). On such tests, deaf children without additional disabilities score close to the population average. For blind children, the Perkins-Binet (44) and the Blind Learning Aptitude Test (45) are

TABLE 16.3. *Common measures of cognitive and adaptive behavioral development in infancy and childhood*

Category of test	Test name/reference	Ages	Description
Screening	Bayley Infant Neuro-development Screen (27)	3–24 mo	Assesses neurodevelopmental skills such as object permanence, imitation, and language
	Denver-II (25)	0–72 mo	Screens for language, fine motor, adaptive personal/social, and gross motor skills
Intelligence measures	Wechsler Preschool and Primary Scale of Intelligence, Revised (28)	Preschoolers	Measures verbal comprehension, perceptual organization, attention/concentration, and visual processing speed
	Wechsler Intelligence Scale for Children-III (29)	School-aged children	Both the Wechsler Preschool and the Wechsler Intelligence Scale give a verbal, performance, and full-scale IQ
	Stanford-Binet Intelligence Scale: Fourth Edition (30)	Variable for each subtest	Measures general intelligence, verbal reasoning, quantitative reasoning, abstract/visual reasoning, and short-term memory
Alternative cognitive measures	Goodenough-Harris Drawing Test (Draw-A-Man) (31)	3–16 yr	Easy to use as a screen of nonverbal intellectual abilities, especially useful for culturally diverse, low-functioning children
	Kaufman Assessment Battery for Children (32)	2.5–12.5 yr	Used to complement Stanford-Binet or Wechsler nonverbal estimates
	McCarthy Scales of Children's Abilities (McCarthy) (33)	2.5–8.5 yr	Provides information on young children with suspected learning disabilities
	Leiter International Performance Scale (34)	2 years to adult	Often used with autistic children as a measure of nonverbal intelligence
Behavior rating scales	Achenbach Child Behavior Checklist (35)	2–3 yr	Allows parents or caregivers to rate a young child's social/emotional development
	Conners' Parent/Teacher Rating Scales (CPRS-48 and CPRS-28) (36)	3–17 yr	The CPRS-48 has 48 items and CPRS-28 items that assess conduct problems, learning problems, impulsivity/hyperactivity, and attention
Adaptive behavioral scales	Battelle Developmental Inventory (37)	Newborn to 8 yr	Assesses personal/social, adaptive, motor, communication, and cognition
	Vineland Adaptive Behavioral Scales (38)	Newborn to 18 yr	Parent questionnaire that assesses communication, daily living skills, socialization, motor skills, adaptive behavior, and maldevelopment; useful in children with cognitive disabilities
Achievement	Wide Range Achievement Test 3 (39)	5 yr to adult	Screening test of basic academic skills, including reading, spelling, and arithmetic
	Woodcock Johnson Psychoeducational Battery–Revised, Part II (40)	3 yr to adult	Psychometric test of academic abilities with subtests in reading, mathematics, and written language
Language	Early Language Milestone Scale (24)	Newborn to 3 yr	Examines listening, speaking, audition, and visual perception
	Peabody Picture Vocabulary Test–Revised (41)	2–6 yr	Vocabulary screening test for children with expressive language difficulties
Nonverbal	Developmental Test of Visual-Motor Integration (42)	4–18 yr	Tests child's abilities to integrate visual perception and motor output by requiring the child to copy increasingly complex geometric forms

available. The most widely used psychometric instruments lack sensitivity in the mental retardation range. Even simple tests that use single words, such as the Peabody Picture Vocabulary Test, cannot be used if the patient is nonverbal (41). The Leiter International Performance Scale is useful for evaluating low functioning individuals (34). The interpretation of psychometric findings in mentally retarded subjects is complicated by uncertainties about the child's test orientation and motivation. Reinforcement schedules can optimize test performance (46). Because IQ values in children younger than 3 years are unstable, the child should be retested for a more definitive evaluation at a later date.

Qualitative Considerations in the Assessment of Learning, Emotion, and Behavior

The developmental history and physical findings in early infancy are unreliable bases for prognosis as to developmental outcome. For example, Apgar scores of 0 to 3 at 15 and 20 minutes are predictive of high mortality and high probability of disability; however, many of these infants score normally in later developmental assessment (see Chapter 5). Intelligence tests in infancy yield a developmental quotient that is necessarily heavily loaded with factors relating to motor development. Within a normal population, the developmental quotient is a poor predictor of individual differences in subsequent cognitive development. It has some success, however, in distinguishing a healthy from a mentally retarded population. Infant testing is highly specialized, but calls for the child's cooperation. If this cannot be enlisted, the mother can be asked standard questions about her child's social development (38).

The IQ scores, taken literally, can underrepresent the child's cognitive potential. Specific adaptive limitations often coexist with strengths in other adaptive skills or other personal capabilities. Limitations in adaptive skills may exist within the context of the child's community. The child's motivation to perform during testing cannot be taken for granted, particularly when the child comes from a cultural or ethnic background that has little understanding of and interest in cognitive testing and its uses. Anxiety can block the child's reasoning processes, alienation and withdrawal can render the child unavailable for the task, thought disorders can intrude, or impulsive behavior can impede performance. Lapses of attention owing to subclinical absence seizures can interrupt concentration, and psychotropic and antiepileptic medication may impair some cognitive processes. The limited attention span of patients with ADHD can impair performance on tasks that demand sustained attention and cognitive effort. In young children, even gross sensory impairment (vision, hearing, tactile) can go unrecognized, and the child's imperfect response to instruction or verbal questioning can be misattributed to defiance or cognitive deficiency. Other factors that affect interpretation of mental status examination performance include extremely low or high parental educational level, poor motivation or failure to expend effort on testing, depression, fatigue, or poor self-esteem. The intelligence test results must be considered in the light of these potential sources of misinterpretation, which cannot be discounted unless they are explicitly ruled out in the psychologist's report.

MENTAL RETARDATION

Terminology and Definitions

The terminology used to characterize persons with cognitive and adaptive behavioral disabilities has evolved, so as to minimize social stigma. Terms such as *cognitive deficiency*, *intellectual disability*, and *learning disability* have been suggested to replace *mental retardation*, a term that misleadingly implies delay and the possibility of catch-up. A similar term is *developmental delay*, which is nonspecific and is more of a chief complaint or a symptom complex than a diagnosis (46). Whereas children with mental retardation may learn new skills as they mature and are taught, most functional neurologic impairments are related to intractable deficits of intellectual capacity. Mental retardation is not a term for a group of diseases, syndromes, or medical disor-

TABLE 16.4. *Classification of mental retardation by measure of IQ and level of adaptive behavior*

Severity (older terminology)	Estimated IQ	Category of support required	Estimate of cognitive/ academic level	Estimate of adaptive behavior as a function of ADL
Borderline	70–85	Intermittent	Adequate language ability, but often develops late	Independent in ADL
			Variable learning disability	Employable
Mild	50/55–70	Intermittent	Adequate language ability, but often develops late	Most are independent in ADL
			Severe learning disability	Employable at simple jobs
			May develop minimal reading ability	
Moderate	35/40–50/55	Limited	Simple language, develops late	Most are trainable in ADL (often need help)
			Most lack even minimal reading ability	May be employable in a sheltered environment
Severe	20/25–35/40	Extensive	May speak some words or be nonverbal	May be trainable in some basic ADL
Profound	<20/25	Complete	May speak a few words; most are nonverbal	Dependent in all ADL

ADL, activities of daily living.

ders. It must be distinguished from disorders resulting from neurodegenerative and progressive neurometabolic diseases, or primary psychiatric disorders.

According to the World Health Organization, mental retardation is "incomplete or insufficient general development of mental capacities." Formal definitions of mental retardation that are currently recognized emphasize a descriptive diagnosis of persons with significant disability because of "subaverage intellectual functioning" and "concurrent deficits or impairments in present adaptive functioning [i.e., the person's effectiveness in meeting the standards expected for his or her age by his or her cultural group]" (47–49). In addition, the manifestation of brain dysfunction must originate during the developmental period of life. The three formal definitions differ slightly in their approach to the diagnosis because of differences in emphasis on adaptive skill symptom menus or underlying etiologic factors.

Because mental abilities are on a continuum, the quantitative definition of mental retardation and its subdivisions based on the IQ is necessarily arbitrary. The operational definition of intellectual functioning is based on performance on standardized intelligence tests. A score is derived by dividing the age at which the child functions

on the test (mental age) by chronologic age to yield an IQ score (mean for the general population is 100). Mild, moderate, severe, and profound mental retardation have been traditionally associated with cutoff points in standard deviations below the mean of -2, -3, -4, and -5, respectively (50) (roughly corresponding to IQs of 70, 50, 35, and 20). But measured intelligence does not reveal the individual's adaptive skills (Table 16.4). There is ongoing controversy on whether to emphasize IQ or adaptive behavioral deficits as the central defining characteristic of mental retardation (51). The level of adaptive skills shape the ultimate life success of persons with mental retardation, but there is no single measure of adaptive behavior. Newer efforts to define mental retardation have emphasized the amount of support needed for an individual to succeed or maintain basic activities of daily living, instead of focusing on the degrees of impairment (52). Support intensities are subdivided into four levels: intermittent, limited, extensive, and pervasive. Support functions are classified into eight categories: teaching, befriending, financial planning, behavioral support, in-home living assistance, community and school access and use, and health assistance. This categorization acknowledges that the diagnosis of mental retardation is useful only

TABLE 16.5. *Examples of genetic syndromes with characteristic behavioral phenotypes*

Syndrome	Behavioral phenotype	References
Fragile X	Poor eye contact, shy, withdrawn, hyperactive, self-injurious	See Chapter 3
Lesch-Nyhan syndrome	Self-injurious, especially compulsive lip and finger biting	72,73
Prader-Willi syndrome	Food seeking, hyperphagic, impulsive, obstinate	74,75
Rett syndrome	Features of autism, stereotypical hand-wringing and hand-flapping, hyperventilation	76
Velocardiofacial syndrome	Ultrarapid cycling bipolar disorder, schizophrenia-like condition	77,78
Williams syndrome	Superficial sociability, musically talented, shy, obsessive	79,80

as a pointer toward providing the individual with additional supports for activities of everyday living, beyond those normative for the child's age.

IQ labeling should not replace repeated educational and achievement assessments (53). The reliability of the IQ score may be affected by the age at which the assessment is done. Visual, spatial, and motor function, as well as expressive language deficits may influence early testing. Over time both the IQ and adaptive behavioral level may be affected by special education and vocational rehabilitation. All assessment techniques must take into account cultural and linguistic diversity, differences in communication ability, behavioral factors, and other limitations in adaptive skills.

Dissociations between Cognitive Domains in Mild Mental Retardation

Although mentally retarded children are by definition impaired in most or all cognitive domains, certain mental retardation syndromes present striking dissociations. Mentally retarded autistic children are disproportionately handicapped in the language and social domain (53), whereas these are relatively strong points for children with Williams syndrome who are especially deficient in spatial and number sense (see Chapter 3) (54). Down syndrome individuals are particularly impaired in language (and motor skills) (55), whereas hydrocephalics are strong in speech production, producing rapid "cocktail chatter." Hydrocephalics are particularly weak in face recognition and social cognition (56). Among X-linked chromosomal aberrations, fragile X syndrome is particularly handicapping in language development (57) as is XXX (58), whereas

Turner syndrome (XO) is associated with visuospatial, arithmetic, and memory deficits (59), and treated phenylketonuric patients are weak in visuospatial and executive functions (60).

Comorbid Psychiatric Disorders in Persons with Mental Retardation (Dual Diagnosis)

Persons with mental retardation are at risk for psychiatric disorders. Mentally retarded children behave deviantly because of one or more of the following: defense against excessive demands, psychopathology, cerebral dysfunction, or environmental deprivation. Compared with the general population, which has an incidence of psychiatric disorders of approximately 7% to 10% (61), approximately one-third of all children with developmental disorders also have psychiatric disorders (61–64). The frequency of psychiatric disorders is much higher in the severely retarded population and approaches two-thirds by adolescence (65). The broad spectrum of psychopathology includes affective disorders (66), anxiety disorders, autistic-like behaviors (67), conduct disorders (68), maladaptive behaviors (repetitive self-stimulating behavior, self-injurious behavior, pica) (69,70), and psychosis. These emotional and behavioral disturbances are caused by multiple factors, including both primary neuropsychological disorders as well as secondary effects of illness, dependency, environmental deprivation, frustration, and low self-esteem (71). Certain recognizable genetic syndromes are associated with typical personality characteristics and reproducible behavioral mannerisms (Table 16.5). Down syndrome children may be irritable and inattentive on account of the frequent association of obstructive sleep apnea.

Epidemiology and Prevalence

The incidence of a disorder is the frequency with which it arises in a population during a stated period of time; the prevalence is its amount within a population at a given time. Thus, the prevalence of the condition is the product of its incidence and its duration. The prevalence of a developmental disorder may change over time because of a variety of factors, including prenatal diagnosis and increased termination of pregnancy, changes in the maternal population, and changes in health care. For example, the prevalence of Down syndrome increased from the 1920s through the 1960s as persons with this condition began to live much longer because of improvements in medical care (81). However, since 1980, further decreases have been slight (82,83).

The prevalence of mental retardation ranges from approximately 6 to 20 per 1,000 (84–87). The prevalence of mental retardation is difficult to assess because of regional differences, ascertainment biases, and variations in diagnostic criteria and study methodology. Mild mental retardation is 10 to 12 times more common than severe retardation. Mental retardation is slightly more common among male subjects because of X-linked syndromes involving mental retardation, especially fragile X syndrome. The male to female ratio ranges from 1.3 to 1.9:1 (88). Medical complications and mortality are increased in persons with severe mental retardation and result in a discrepancy between expected and identified prevalence rates in this subgroup. This is caused not by the mental retardation itself, but by the severe cerebral palsy that is often associated. Total immobility and feeding by tube are the features that are most predictive of curtailed life span (89,90).

Causes of Mental Retardation

Timing

Mental retardation can be caused by genetic, environmental, and ecogenetic factors. The diagnostic process is aided considerably if the timing of a developmental insult can be determined. Prenatal causes of mental retardation, with genetic etiologies as the major subset, account for approximately 60% to 80% of all developmental disorders. Perinatal and postnatal causes are much less common. Perinatal causes include asphyxia and birth trauma. Mental retardation secondary to perinatal causes is almost invariably accompanied by cerebral palsy and probably accounts for 8% to 12% of all cases (91). Postnatal causes, including meningitis, encephalitis, trauma, and malnutrition, may account for up to 10%. Some individuals may have more than one etiologic cause of their developmental disability and the causes may have occurred at different periods of development. For example, a fetus with hypotonia secondary to genetic causes is more likely to sustain perinatal injury (92–94). Moreover, some individuals who were thought to have perinatal causes of their disabilities are later found to have a genetic etiology that is assumed to be primary (95).

Severity

A direct relationship exists between the severity of mental retardation and the likelihood of a specific etiologic diagnosis. Up to 70% to 80% of individuals with severe disabilities have an identifiable cause, as contrasted to barely 50% of individuals with mild mental retardation. At neuroimaging studies or at autopsy, the brains of most severely mentally retarded individuals manifest gross abnormalities. Mild cases of mental retardation for which no specific cause can be uncovered are usually ascribed to polygenic inheritance.

Diagnostic Categories

Chromosomal

Chromosomal aberrations have been reported in 4% to 28% of persons with moderate to severe mental retardation, craniofacial differences, and other congenital anomalies (Table 16.6). The percentage of clinically relevant chromosomal abnormalities varies between studies because of

TABLE 16.6. *Cause of mental retardation by diagnostic category*

	Percent
Chromosome abnormalities	4–28
Recognizable syndromes	3–9
Structural central nervous system malformations	3–17
Complications of prematurity	2–10
Perinatal conditions	8–13
Environmental/teratogenic causes	5–13
Cultural-familial mental retardation	3–12
Metabolic/endocrine causes	1–5
Unknown	30–50

Compiled references 11, 18, and 96–101.

differences in definitions, methodology, ascertainment (population-based versus institutional), and type of cytogenetic study. Down syndrome is by far the most common chromosomal disorder and accounts for 4% to 7% of all cases of mental retardation (101,102). This condition and the various other chromosomal disorders, including the contiguous gene syndromes, are covered in Chapter 3. The fragile X syndrome is also covered in Chapter 3. Primary malformations of the CNS result from multiple genetic and ecogenetic causes. Numerous major and minor developmental malformations may result from disturbances in neuronal proliferation, migration, differentiation, axonal outgrowth, synapse formation, dendritic arborization, and process elimination, depending on the genetic condition or severity and timing of an environmental insult. In the prenatal period it is often impossible to distinguish the degree to which an environmental insult may cause either direct vascular or parenchymal injury or a disruption of gene and signaling molecule expression. The various cerebral dysgeneses are covered in Chapter 4.

Prematurity

Survival rates and morbidity patterns have changed with technological advances in neonatology. There are notable differences in outcome between very-low-birth-weight infants (less than 1,500 g) and extremely low-birth-weight infants (less than 1,000 g). Outcomes in premature infants range from normal to severe disability. In addition, an increased frequency of learning disabilities, sensorineural hearing loss, and ocular and cerebral visual impairment occurs, which complicates later development and learning. The various neurologic complications of prematurity are covered in Chapter 5.

Teratogens and Toxins

The teratogenic and long-term cognitive and behavior effects of exposure to alcohol, marijuana, cigarettes, cocaine, and other street drugs are difficult to determine separately, because polydrug use is the rule. Also, the frequency, quantity, type of substance, and timing of exposure during pregnancy varies greatly. Moreover, drug habits are frequently associated with poor nutrition and lack of prenatal care. However, there are clear associations between maternal alcohol abuse and adverse effects on early brain development. Fetal alcohol syndrome may be the most common cause of mental retardation in North America and Europe. The condition is covered in Chapter 9 as are the complications of prenatal cocaine exposure.

Lead poisoning may cause mental retardation. Chronic subclinical lead poisoning is associated with an increased risk of antisocial and delinquent behavior as well as disorders of cognition and learning, but these outcomes are confounded by the effects of social class and home environment (103,104) (see Chapter 9). Scores on the HOME questionnaire, a measure of the stimulation a child receives at home, are a crucial covariate in any population study of cognitive effects of potential toxins (105). When relevant covariates were held constant in a meta-analysis, the apparent effects of subclinical lead dwindled into insignificance (105). Although mercury is also a potent neurotoxin, it is doubtful that the low-level prenatal exposure to methylmercury from maternal consumption of seafood poses an increased neurodevelopmental risk (106–108).

Nutrition, Poverty, and Other Familial Factors

A complex relationship exists between genetics, nutrition, social environment, and learning (109). The effects of psychosocial deprivation on socialization and motivation may impair performance even in the child with otherwise normal cognitive abilities. Animal experiments have demonstrated a wide range of prenatal deficiency states that can result in congenital anomalies, as well as in stillbirth and prematurity. The various nutritional disorders are covered in Chapter 9.

One American child in five lives in a family with income below the poverty threshold (110). The risk of mental retardation and inferior academic performance increases with decreasing socioeconomic status (111–113). However, on a population basis, the factors that mediate the effects of poverty on child health and development are uncertain (114). Parental nurturing, sociocultural influences, and educational environments are determinants of developmental outcome and ultimate adaptation to society (115). Infants and children who are deprived of maternal attention often become depressed and their cognitive skills decline (116).

Metabolism and Hormones

Thyroid hormone influences brain growth; hypothyroidism is associated with mental retardation presumably by defects in thyroid hormone biosynthesis or through iodine deficiency. Maternal hypothyroidism results in lower IQ of the offspring (117), congenital hypothyroidism only causing mental retardation in children left untreated after birth. Insulin-dependent diabetes mellitus is associated with declining verbal test scores (118). The neurologic complications of thyroid deficiency and diabetes are presented in Chapter 15.

Infection

CNS infection early in life is a major cause of mental retardation, especially in developing countries. Prenatal infections such as toxoplasmosis, syphilis, rubella, cytomegalovirus, herpes, and varicella are associated with microcephaly, intracranial calcifications, cataracts, growth retardation, sensorineural hearing loss, and seizures. Such infections may produce mild, moderate, or severe disabilities. Bacterial, viral, and fungal meningitis and encephalitis, in particular neonatal and childhood herpes simplex encephalitis,

are perinatal and postnatal causes of mental retardation (see Chapter 6).

Radiation

Pelvic nuclear (119) and x-irradiation (120) can lead to mental retardation of offspring, particularly when applied between the seventh and fifteenth weeks of gestation. The degree of retardation is proportional to the amount of irradiation. The incidence of Down syndrome and other chromosomal abnormalities is greater among offspring of women in their late reproductive years who were irradiated during pregnancy (121).

Management

Medical

Stimulant medications, such as methylphenidate, may be beneficial in some mildly mentally retarded children with hyperactivity (122). Numerous other older and newer medications have been used with variable results in an attempt to ameliorate adverse behaviors such as aggression, self-injurious behavior, and severe hyperactivity in persons with mental retardation. Neuroleptics, such as thioridazine in low doses, may have a calming effect in some children, and when given at bedtime may assist sleep. Carbamazepine and propranolol can be beneficial for rage and episodic loss of control. Antidepressants, such as clomipramine and fluvoxamine, are often helpful in decreasing compulsive behaviors and stereotypies. Opioid antagonists, such as naltrexone, are occasionally successful in decreasing self-injurious behaviors (123, 124). Pharmacologic treatment of behavioral disorders should be coordinated with behavior modification programs. On withdrawal, some medications can give rise to tardive dyskinesias, because of dopamine hypersensitivity (125). This tendency can be counteracted by gabergic antiepileptic agents (126).

Nonspecific Nonmedical

Nonmedical management includes family support and education, and the provision of early intervention and special education programs. For most mentally retarded people, specific methods for improving intelligence are not available. The efficacy of early intervention programs in enhancing mental development remains unvalidated (127). The primary goal is to provide for a placement that safeguards the child and at the same time permits the child to function at his or her maximum potential (i.e., the least restricted environment). The child's temperament and level of socialization are important modifying factors that can differ widely among individuals at a given IQ level. For mildly disabled preschool children with adequate comprehension and without behavioral problems, referral to a regular preschool with language therapy may be appropriate. For children with limited attention and concentration, special education teachers use attention-focusing techniques to optimize learning. Best results are obtained in structured rather than flexible settings, because judgment and problem-solving strategies are usually most impaired in individuals with mental retardation. Taught at an appropriate rate in structural settings, a child with mild mental retardation can later become vocationally self-reliant in manual and domestic occupations and in routine industrial tasks such as assembly and production-line operations.

Children with mental retardation who have significant additional language and social dysfunction often do not succeed in the typical classroom settings that are appropriate for students with specific learning disabilities. Self-contained classrooms usually provide a better environment for children with severe mental retardation and severe communication disorders or autistic behaviors. These classrooms ideally have a low teacher-to-student ratio with special education teachers who are familiar with interventions for students with nonverbal learning disabilities and social communication deficits. Some children with severe mental retardation require special education classroom placements that offer behavioral modification programs and school time geared toward life skills such as basic hygiene and self-care (128). Public laws mandate regular reassessments of individual educational programs.

Models of management involve many nonmedical disciplines. Caregivers may need training in the handling, feeding, and toileting of their child, depending on the severity of associated disabilities. Ideally, intervention for children with disabilities is family centered, multidisciplinary or interdisciplinary, and oriented to the severity of the disability and the specific needs of the child. An interdisciplinary approach with effective case management usually results in appropriate health care planning that includes comprehensive diagnostic evaluation, an assessment of disabilities, and an individualized treatment plan for educational, behavioral, pharmacologic, and medical interventions.

AUTISTIC SPECTRUM DISORDERS

Autism is a behaviorally defined developmental disorder that includes a heterogeneous set of symptoms and results from a selection of diverse biological, genetic, and ecogenetic factors (129). Although the broad spectrum of cognitive and behavioral impairments makes a concise definition impossible, in practice, clinicians tend to agree on its predominant features (130,131). Research into the neurobiology of these conditions is complicated by this broad heterogeneity in clinical and biological characteristics (Table 16.7).

Autism was first described by Kanner in 1943 (132). He emphasized a profound withdrawal from contact with people, an obsessive desire to preserve sameness, and a failure to use language for communication. The current criteria for autistic disorder in the *Diagnostic and Statistical Manual of Mental Disorders, Fourth Edition (DSM-IV)*, include qualitative impairment in social interaction, qualitative impairment in communication, and restricted, repetitive, and stereotyped patterns of behavior, interest, and activities (49). Onset is before 3 years of age. Rett syndrome, covered in Chapter 2, and childhood disintegrative disorder are separately classified.

Clinical Characteristics

Autism presents in either of two ways. Approximately one-third of children appear to develop normally until the second year of life, at which time they gradually regress into autism, often in association with emotional or physical trauma (133) and in the context of

TABLE 16.7. *Neurobiological clues to the etiology of idiopathic autism*

Etiologic clue	Description of findings in studies of autism	References
Environmental	Increased complications of pregnancy, labor, and delivery; perinatal problems/illness in some studies but not others	175–179
Genetic	Higher concordance for autism in monozygotic twin pairs	161,163,175, 180–186
	Marked increase in prevalence of autism in siblings of children with autism	
	Increased frequency of cognitive and learning disabilities in siblings of children with autism	
	Increased frequency of mental health disorders in siblings and parents of children with autism	
	Studies of potential susceptibility genes, such as genes within the 15q11-13 region, are ongoing	
Chromosomal/ monogenetic	Numerous case reports and small series of patients with certain single-gene disorders and chromosomal anomalies are reported; these may account for 5% to 14% of all children with features of autism	174,187
Contiguous genes	Features of autism in some children with recognizable conditions such as Williams syndrome or Angelman syndrome; the most common cytogenetic finding in autism to date is the duplication of maternally derived chromosome 15q11-13	188–192
Mitochondrial	Possible effects of abnormal energy metabolism on central nervous system	193–195
DNA expansion	Features of autism in some children with fragile X syndrome	196
Immunology	Abnormal immune function or presence or autoimmune antibodies in some studies of children with autism	197–199
	Reported improvement in some persons to nonspecific immunosup-pressive or immunomodulating therapies	
Infection	Features of autism in some children with congenital rubella and cytomegalovirus infections, among others; inflammatory bowel disease with intracellular measles virus inclusions in some autistic children	156,200,201
Metabolism	Features of autism in some children with phenylketonuria and other metabolic disorders	202–205,240
	Abnormal intestinal permeability	
Neuroanatomy		164
Cerebellum	Selective hypoplasia of the neocerebellar vermis (especially lobules VI and VII) is found in some autopsy and magnetic resonance imaging studies	206–212
	Developmental cellular abnormalities in the posterior inferior cerebellar hemispheres	
Cerebrum	Associated abnormal neuronal migration, cortical cytoarchitecture in septum, hippocampi, amygdala, entorhinal cortex, and mamillary bodies	166,169, 213–219
	Nonspecific differences in positron emission tomography and P nuclear magnetic resonance spectroscopic studies	
	Variable morphologic differences in some magnetic resonance imaging studies	
	Suppressed voluntary oculomotor responses attributed to prefrontal dysfunction	
Electroenceph-alographic findings	Depending on associated brain dysfunction, seizures occur in 6% to 35%, and electroencephalographic abnormalities are reported in 35% to 65% of children with autism	220,221
Brainstem	Associated smaller pons in some studies	222–224
Neurochemistry		
Serotonin	Increased blood concentrations of serotonin in some children with autism	225–228
	Asymmetric serotonin metabolism by positron emission tomographic studies	
Dopamine	Dopamine agonists worsen behavior, and dopamine antagonists improve behavior in some children with autism	229–231
	Increased CSF homovanillic in some studies	
Norepinephrine	Increased plasma norepinephrine in some studies, but in others, normal plasma, urine, and CSF catecholamine metabolites are reported	231–234
Endorphin neuropeptides	Analogy to "insensitivity to pain" in those children with autism who show self-injurious behavior	235–239
	Increased CSF endorphin concentrations in some studies	

seizures (134). The majority of children with autism are clearly different at an early age, moving and crying little, averse to being held, and content to be alone. Scales that promise earlier diagnosis are available and home videos reviewed retrospectively can reveal a previously unsuspected onset during infancy (135,136). Solid foods may be rejected, and toys elicit little interest or are held onto with unusual obstinacy. Motor development is usually normal. During the second year of life, children with autism are typically unusually sensitive to auditory, visual, tactile, and movement stimulation, and repetitive mannerisms or gestures begin to appear. The older child with autism has restricted and stereotyped behaviors and activities and markedly impaired creativity, social relations, language, and perception. Disturbances in social relations are manifested by poor or absent eye contact and a lack of interest in people, whom the child uses instrumentally rather than interactively. Toys are handled bizarrely or are dropped when handed to the child. Mannerisms include repetitive, stereotyped movements, such as hand flapping, ear flicking, or head banging (137). Toe walking, whirling, and rocking are also common. These movements, often complex, increase when the child is anxious or is confronted with a novel situation (138).

Language disturbances can consist of complete lack of speech, failure to communicate by pointing, failure to imitate (139), perseveration, echolalia (repeating words or phrases out of communicative context), and lack of reciprocity in dialogue (140). If speech does develop, its prosody is often monotonal, pronouns are used poorly, and humor is not understood. Speech in children with autism differs qualitatively from the speech of children with mild mental retardation. Within the limits of a decreased vocabulary, children with mild mental retardation typically speak normally, whereas children with autism use abnormal prosody, syntax, semantics, and pragmatics (141). In some cases, termed *hyperlexic*, mechanical language skills, such as reading, are developed out of proportion to spontaneous verbal expression or reading comprehension (142).

Children with autism may be oversensitive to stimuli, notably self-created sounds or spinning objects. This sensitivity can alternate with periods of nonresponsiveness to speech, objects, or pain. Affected children frequently ignore sounds and are "aloof," provoking testing for possible hearing loss. Some have prolonged attention spans during self-initiated activity (143). Observational studies demonstrate hyperselectivity of attention in children with autism, the exclusive focusing on some distinctive aspect of a display, while ignoring its other features (138).

Some children may exhibit transitional or milder degrees of autistic behavior, which after age 5 to 6 years merge with those observed in mental retardation. Others deviate into pervasive developmental disorders, childhood disintegrative disorder, or Asperger syndrome (144,145). The natural history and outcome of autism is variable. Approximately one-third of children with autism do not develop communicative speech. Others develop rudimentary language, although their communication remains literal and concrete and their affect flat. In yet other affected children, characteristics of organic brain disease become apparent over subsequent years, including auditory or visuoperceptual impairment. A small subset of children with autism develop bizarre thoughts and even delusions. Other children with autism make a fairly adequate social adjustment, but retain certain peculiarities of personality, lack of humor, and unawareness of social nuances (146). Neuropsychological testing reveals deficits on problem-solving tasks (147). Approximately one-half of the population with autism has an IQ above 50, and one-fourth to one-third has an IQ above 70. Children who regressed generally are ultimately more impaired cognitively (134,148). Even when enrolled in treatment programs, only some improve significantly. If they do, it is usually during the second half of the first decade of life.

Prevalence

Autism has a prevalence of approximately 5 in 10,000, with a 3 to 4:1 male predominance (149). Epidemiologic evidence is in dispute as to whether the true incidence of classical autism has increased during the past few decades (150,151). However, studies that include the entire autistic spectrum, such as children with social impairments or repetitive behavioral patterns, and Asperger syndrome, report ranges in incidence from 9 to 90 per 10,000 (150, 152–155). Thus, the increase in the number of children diagnosed with autism is so spectacular, that it is unlikely to be merely because health care workers are paying greater attention to this condition (155a). Despite apparent links between measles, mumps, and rubella (MMR) immunizations and autism (156), opposed by energetic disclaimers (157–159), the definitive epidemiologic study that would distinguish causation, a rare inordinate susceptibility, from chance association has not been performed.

Causes of Autism and Its Neurobiological Basis

Autism clearly has genetic factors in its origins. Previous theories that certain family dynamics promote autism have been refuted (160). The importance of genetics in autism is illustrated by the higher incidence of autism in male subjects, a recurrence risk of up to 9% in families with one affected child, a high concordance of autism among monozygotic twins, an increased incidence of developmental and affective disorder in first-degree relatives, and the association of some disorders of known genetic etiology with autism (161–163).

A variety of structural abnormalities has been reported in various brain regions. This neuroanatomic heterogeneity most likely reflects etiologic heterogeneity and there is no consensus on the neural pathophysiology of autism (164). Widespread abnormalities in the frontal and temporal cortices, cerebellar hemispheres, vermis, and brainstem ascending activating systems have been reported (165–168). Increased head and brain size in autism contrasts with the frequent microcephaly of mentally retarded children (169). Rarely, an autistic syndrome arises in the course of an encephalitis (170). Autistic behavior has been documented in numerous genetic syndromes, notably in Rett syndrome and fragile X syndrome (see Chapters 2 and 3) (171). Recurrent seizures and EEG abnormalities are frequent in children with autism. Although perinatal injuries and prematurity are associated with autism with greater than chance frequency (172,173), evidence indicates prenatal maldevelopment in most cases. The relationship of cerebellar pathology to autism remains controversial. Table 16.7 presents genetic, immunologic, metabolic, neuroanatomic, and neurochemical findings associated with autism. Overall, depending on diagnostic criteria and the extent of medical evaluation, a specific etiology for autism remains unknown in approximately 70% to 90% of all cases (174).

External causes of autism subdivide into infectious [e.g., cytomegalovirus (241), herpes simplex (242), rubella embryopathy (243)], toxic [e.g., alcohol (244), cocaine (245), thalidomide (246)], and in utero exposure to valproate (247).

The role of gastrointestinal disorders in the genesis of autism has received considerable attention since the report of Wakefield and coworkers who found that a significant proportion of autistic children had a nonspecific colitis and lymphoid nodular hyperplasia in the ileal region (156). Other workers have observed that autistic children had a high instance (69%) (247a), and have related these gastrointestinal abnormalities to infections with measles, mumps, or other paramyxoviruses (247b).

Differential Diagnosis

Classical autism is one of five subtypes of pervasive developmental disorders described in the *DSM-IV*. The four other subtypes include Rett syndrome (see Chapter 2), Asperger syndrome, childhood disintegrative disorder, and pervasive developmental disorder not otherwise specified. These subgroups may however be better conceived as arranged along a spectrum of autistic disorders (247c).

Asperger Syndrome

Possibly distinct from relatively high functioning autism are the individuals with flat affect, insensitivity to social cues, and obsessively indulged special interests first described by Asperger (145), which some authorities consider to be on a continuum with autism. Their language skills develop normally but the use of language to communicate is aberrant, and they may also have delayed visuomotor development. Like autistic children, children with Asperger syndrome have a need for sameness, but are usually normal and have age-appropriate self-help and adaptive behavioral skills.

Childhood Disintegrative Disorder

First described by Heller (248), this distinct syndrome appears after normal childhood development for 2 to 3 years. The child regresses over weeks and months in language, motor skills, play, and social or adaptive skills, including bowel and bladder control to an autistic endpoint (144).

Pervasive Developmental Disorder Not Otherwise Specified

Pervasive developmental disorder differs from autism in its later age of onset and in the subthreshold or atypical severity of communication, behavioral, and social impairment. Like Asperger syndrome, it may be on a continuum of social and cognitive impairment with autism (249).

Other Conditions

Other conditions that overlap with autism's behavioral characteristics include childhood schizophrenia, elective mutism, developmental language disorders, severe mental retardation, complex motor tics, and obsessive compulsive disorder. Childhood schizophrenia develops in midchildhood and unlike autism, is characterized by thought disorder, delusions, or hallucinations. Children with elective mutism by definition speak normally in some situations and do not show abnormalities in play or nonverbal social interactions. In developmental language disorders, language impairment is not associated with impairment in social interaction and behavior. A small proportion of children with severe language disorders exhibit some aspects of autistic behavior, but relate well, using gestures to communicate (250). Children with congenital ocular or cerebral visual impairment, such as retrolental fibroplasia and septo-optic dysplasia, respectively, may show stereotypic or self-injurious behavior. Autistic behavior patterns are also common in congenital deafness and in mental retardation.

Diagnostic Evaluation

Beyond tests that are applicable to any child with a neurodevelopmental disorder (see previous discussion), further laboratory evaluation may be indicated. High-resolution chromosome analysis leads to a diagnosis in approximately 5% of children with autistic traits. Brain imaging studies are indicated only if there are signs of progressive loss of function, localized neurologic deficits, or persistent focal seizures. An EEG is indicated if a suggestion of seizures exists. Approximately one-third of patients with autism experience one or more epileptic attacks during the first two decades of life. Various seizure types have been described. Of these, the most common are complex partial seizures (221). The question of subclinical seizures is frequently raised in the autistic subtype in which an acquired loss of receptive and communicative abilities occurs, as is observed in Landau-Kleffner syndrome (see Chapter 13). For this reason sleep electroencephalography has been advocated for children whose autistic symptoms develop after 2 to 3 years of age in the hope that anticonvulsant therapy might improve language and social skills (251,252). Lewine and coworkers suggest that magnetoencephalography is more sensitive than electroencephalography in demonstrating the subclinical epileptiform discharges (253).

Metabolic studies, such as serum copper and ceruloplasmin, are indicated if autistic symptoms develop in late childhood or are progressive. Formal cognitive, language, educational, and behavioral assessments establish the level of severity of the child's impairments and serve as a baseline for the individual educational program and additional therapies.

Management Strategies

Medical

Autism may be the most difficult developmental disability to manage. It has no known cure. Impairments in cognition, communication, socialization, and behavior often result in lifelong disability and frustration. Many recent pharmacologic trials report some benefit in controlling problematic behaviors, aggression, and self-injurious behavior. Medications include serotonin reuptake inhibitors such as fluoxetine, dopamine and serotonin receptor antagonists such as risperidone, tricyclics such as clomipramine, antihypertensives such as propranolol and clonidine, anticonvulsants such as valproic acid, and lithium (251,254–258). Some hyperactive autistic children benefit from methylphenidate but others became worse (259). The short- and long-term risks and benefits of various corticosteroid regimens await further investigation. Little evidence exists that children with autism have nutritional deficiencies (260), but various dietary supplements, such as magnesium and pyridoxine, are commonly used. Pharmacotherapy must be coordinated with a comprehensive and individualized treatment program (261).

Nonspecific Nonmedical

The most important role of the physician, teacher, and therapists in the management of a child with autism is to support and advocate for parents and caregivers in their own ability to help their child grow, communicate, and learn. Most families have the best understanding of their child's unique behaviors and developmental needs, and they should be encouraged to be co-therapists in their child's individual education program, and in his or her speech and language, socialization, and behavior modification programs. Families should be informed about publicly funded special education programs, financial aid programs such as social security income (SSI), and developmental disability services that provide funding for respite care. Family support groups, such as the National Society of Autism, offer additional information and family self-help services.

The typical community-based support services, including appropriate educational and voca'communication (e.g., sign language, augmented communication) therapies, and behavioral modification programs, are summarized alphabetically in Table 16.8. Some of the prevalent unconventional and unproved interventions are summarized alphabetically in Table 16.9.

SPEECH AND LANGUAGE DISORDERS

At least 5% to 7% of the school-aged children in the United States (aged 5 to 21 years) have serious deficits of speech or deficits of hearing with which a speech disorder is associated. An additional 5% have relatively minor speech impairments (279,280). Approximately twice as many boys as girls are affected. Speech and language disorders overlap with academic underachievement and behavioral problems in school-aged children (281,282).

Language Development

Precursors

Neonates can perceive virtually all the speech contrasts that are used in natural languages. By the end of the first year, they begin to understand meaningful speech and produce it, and they lose the ability to discriminate contrasts that do not occur in their own language (283).

Even in the first 6 weeks of life, infants vocalize when they orient by head and gaze turning and by hand pointing (tonic neck reflex) in response to a novel stimulus. Babbling begins between 2 and 6 months of age and soon includes all the phonemes in human languages. Babbling is both spontaneous and imitative of the speech of others. Although some severely mentally retarded children are late to begin babbling, the characteristics of babbling, when it occurs, cannot be used to predict the quality of the language that will follow. Additionally, babbling is not causally involved in the child's use of language. For instance, prevention of babbling by long-term tracheotomy does not retard the development of speech once the aperture is closed. Babbling does not initially depend on auditory feedback; even profoundly deaf children babble (284). Toward the end of the first year, however, the deaf child babbles less, and then falls silent.

Early Language

At around 11 to 13 months of age, children begin to utter single words, of which *mama* and *dada* are often, but unreliably, reported first by parents. They look and point with the right hand at the object they are naming (285). Parents report that

TABLE 16.8. *Conventional strategies for children with autism*

Therapy/ intervention	Method	Rationale/benefits	References
Alleviate family distress	Provide diagnostic information Counseling (e.g., social worker)	Helps families deal with guilt and frustration Increases understanding of the cause and possible prognosis	262
Behavioral modification	Modify environmental factors Redirect maladaptive behaviors Engage children with solitary play Deter tantrums, aggression Restrain injurious behavior	Stereotypies, maladaptive and injurious behaviors occur less frequently in structured and stimulating environments	138,263
Communication therapy	Direct speech training Sign language Augmented communication	Increase all forms of communication, not just speech	264,265
Individual education program	Structured teaching to promote communication, cognitive and social learning Limits overstimulation Direct social skills training Self-help, life skills training	Promotes directed cognitive, language, and social learning To help adaptation to new situations	138,266–268
Pharmacologic trials	Individual medication trials should be symptom oriented, time-limited, beginning with low doses and gradual increases until the true benefits of the therapy are determined	May improve attention, impulsivity May decrease agitation, aggression, anxiety May enhance sleep Stop seizures	257

their children produce approximately 4 words at 10 months, 12 words at 1 year, and 80 words at 16 months (286). When children acquire a vocabulary between 50 and 100 words, word combinations begin. There is a burst of vocabulary development toward the end of the second year (approximately 150 to 300 words by age 2 years), and of syntactic development in the third year (287). Simple sentences emerge at around 3 years, and agreement between subject and verb toward the end of the fourth year. At all stages, children can understand more words and phrases than they can utter, and even children who cannot vocalize develop substantial comprehension of spoken speech. Late talkers have a good prognosis if their receptive vocabularies are in the normal range (288).

Ontogenesis of Cerebral Dominance for Language

Lesion and stimulation effects on behavior show that in almost all right-handed individuals, the left hemisphere is primarily concerned with the neural process underlying language, as well as the decoding of symbols and the programming of motor sequences. Some deficits in tasks that are not overtly verbal have been reported in children with language delay, notably discriminating time differentials between rapidly successive stimuli in various modalities (289). With respect to other functions, such as spatial orientation and spatial organization of nonverbal patterns, there is a less striking, but definite, asymmetry in favor of the right hemisphere. This hemisphere specialization emerges progressively during the first decade of life.

The newborn infant shows none of the abilities that derive from hemispheric specialization. Indeed, the infant's cerebrum is barely functional. Yet, most infants more often spontaneously turn their heads and eyes to the right rather than the left, a tendency that subsequently comes under control of the left hemisphere. Congenital left hemispheric maldevelopment

TABLE 16.9. *Unproved intervention programs for children with autistic spectrum disorder*

Therapy/intervention	Method	Rationale/benefits/outcomes	References
Auditory integration training	Use filters to remove frequencies to which the individual is sensitive	Decrease sound sensitivity and hence behavioral disturbances Studies have not shown effectiveness of training	269,270
Cranial osteopathy	Gentle manipulation of cranial bones	No adequate outcome studies exist	
Early intensive interventions	Intensive therapist-parent-teacher behavior therapy during most of the child's waking hours	One-on-one intensive therapy may improve cognition and communication, requires great effort and expense	271
Facilitated communication	An augmented communication technique that requires a facilitator to provide physical assistance for writing or keyboarding	Leads to independent communication in few persons, communication is influenced by the facilitator	272,273
Nutritional restrictions or supplements	Includes numerous restriction diets (e.g., gluten casein) or supplements (e.g., vitamin B_6, magnesium, secretin)	Benefits remain unproven, side effects include sensory neuropathy and photosensitivity	261,274, 275
Patterning exercises	Daily, extensive controlled stimulation of muscle activity	Claims to repair nonfunctional neural networks Little or no benefit from the treatment has been shown, places enormous demands on families	276
Sensory integration therapy	Attempts to improve sensory processing through exposure to auditory, olfactory, visual, and tactile stimuli	Unproven and probably ineffective treatment, but its current use is widespread	277,278

and injury in the first year do not invariably lead to gross language disorder or delay; the right hemisphere assumes language representation (290). Preschoolers show transitory language deficits after left hemisphere injury, but usually only after the first decade does the language disorder assume the characteristic severity and persistence of adult aphasia (291). In very early lateralized lesions of either hemisphere, there is often contralateral compensation, but age and other complex neurologic factors, such as lesion site, lesion size, presence of seizures and use of antiepileptic drugs or hemispherectomy, contribute to variable outcomes (292,293).

In the past, language lateralization was believed to be progressive, from bihemispheric origins toward the end-point of fully established left hemispheric dominance for language, only toward the end of childhood. The weight of evidence is against this theory, however. Instead, it now appears that language processes are lateral-

ized from the beginning, in the same manner as when the individual's brain has fully matured (292,294). This inference has been directly validated by intracranial electrical stimulation in young children, whose language areas were much like those of adults (295).

This invalidates a host of theories that attribute a variety of language disabilities to delay in the "lateralization process." Because no such process exists, therapy programs that purport to accelerate it are irrational.

Left hemispheric control of language involves inhibition of the potential language capability of the right hemisphere. Massive left hemispheric lesions release this inhibition. Disconnection of the hemispheres by section of the corpus callosum reveals that the right hemisphere can decode at least simple speech messages. The same decoding success is observed while the left hemisphere is temporarily anesthetized by intracarotid injection of amobarbital (296). The patient remains responsive to verbal commands, as indicated by left facial and left hand movements. This response perhaps explains why permanent total receptive aphasia is so rare. Right hemisphere compensation for language disorder is more complete for language decoding than encoding (297). When the right hemisphere is involved in language from the start, rather than because the left hemisphere was malfunctioning, as is the case in many non–right-handers, then language develops in the normal manner. There is no basis for attributing language deficits, as in Down syndrome, to right-sided language lateralization. Agenesis of the corpus callosum yields few of the signs of hemispheric disconnection exhibited by patients who have undergone callosal section. Whether compensation involves brainstem commissures, redundant functional specialization in each cerebral hemisphere, or both, is not clear (298). Early right hemisphere damage, in contrast, results in more negative affect, inattentiveness, and impersistence, consonant with early right-sided specialization for emotion (299).

Disorders of Pronunciation and Stuttering

The prevalence of speech disorders is closely related to age. Speech disorders occur most commonly in young children and reach an incidence of 15% in kindergartners (300). Approximately 90% of children younger than 8 years outgrow their speech disorders, but those who still have a speech impairment by 14 years of age can expect improvement only with speech therapy.

The frequency of production of sounds normally increases up to 2.5 years of age, at which time the speech sound pattern closely resembles that of the adult. Children utter phrases averaging 1.5 words at 18 months, 1.8 words at 2 years, 3.1 words at 2.5 years, and 4.1 words at 3 years. Ninety percent of children can correctly articulate all vowel sounds by 3 years of age. For boys, a 90% success rate for consonant sounds comes later: by age 3 years, pronunciation of *p*, *b*, *m*, *h*, *w*, *d*, *n*, *t*, and *k*; by age 4 years, pronunciation of *ng*; by age 5 years, pronunciation of *y*; by age 5 to 6 years, pronuncia-

tion of *j*; by age 6 years, pronunciation of *zh* and *wh*; and by age 7 years, pronunciation of *f*, *l*, *r*, *sh*, *ch*, *s*, *z*, *th*, and *v*. Girls achieve some of these sounds slightly sooner. Sounds are used more accurately in the initial rather than medial position and are used least well terminally. Impaired intelligibility is prognostically less ominous than depressed level of language use, and referral to speech therapy on its account can be delayed until 4 years of age. If speech is also sparse, however, as in the 2-year-old who does not yet utter two-word phrases, earlier referral is justified. Even so, progress is slow, and a special effort by the parents is needed to offer the child experience by talking to him or her more than is usual.

Whereas immaturity in the central control of articulation is by far the most common cause of speech disorders in children, definable neurologic deficits contribute in some cases. Quadriplegia or double hemiplegia associated with suprabulbar palsy causes speech to be slurred, and athetosis renders it jerky, explosive, and indistinct. Congenital suprabulbar palsy can exist as a rare, isolated neurologic deficit. This condition has a major effect on speech. A hyperactive jaw jerk distinguishes congenital suprabulbar palsy from acquired nuclear and infranuclear paralysis of the mechanism of articulation. Some children suffer from buccolingual apraxia, which affects voluntary tongue, lip, and palate movements, but spares automatic movements of these structures (301).

Stuttering develops between the ages of 2 and 4 years, with maximal incidence at age 3 years. Many children stutter only transiently, but in some the stutter persists. The underlying cause of stuttering in childhood is unknown. It rarely appears secondary to organic brain disease, such as focal dystonia. When stuttering forms part of the symptoms of an extrapyramidal disease, it is more likely that an entire word is repeated, rather than a single sound (palilalia). More boys and left-handed persons are affected by stuttering. The notion that stuttering is the result of left hemispheric dysfunction is supported by positron emission tomographic studies (302,303). Cerebral dominance for language may be mixed in children who stutter, with "rivalry" between the hemispheres for control over speech (304,305). Stuttering cannot be a disorder of auditory feedback, because speech, like any highly practiced and automatized process, is not under continual feedback control. However, stutterers do find it difficult to disengage their attention from their own speech, which then cannot be automatic. Stuttering is relieved by noise that is sufficiently loud to mask speech sounds, and it is rare among deaf persons.

The child who stutters has difficulty in passing smoothly from phoneme to phoneme, especially at the beginning of sentences, and with words of more than five letters. The child who stutters explosively reiterates a single sound or blocks speech completely. Moments of self-consciousness and embarrassment yield maximal dysfluency, whereas distraction can result in temporarily normal speech. Singing is spared. Speech therapies include awareness training, regulated breathing, and social support. Treatment outcomes are variable (306).

Distinct from stuttering is cluttering, in which speech is fast, slurred, and dysrhythmic, with omission, reduplication, and transposition of speech sounds and words. Like stuttering, it can rarely result from brain lesions (307).

Secondary Language Disorders

The *DSM-IV* differentiates developmental language disorders from those etiologies such as epilepsy, mental retardation, autism, and severe brain injury that have other prognosis and treatment implications (49). A strong role of genetics in developmental language disorders is implicated in many family studies. However, secondary language disorders may be associated with numerous other risk factors such as socioeconomic status and other family and environmental factors or learning disabilities (308).

Twins who share a secret language, sounding coherent though incomprehensible, rapidly transfer to normal language when they are separated. Blind children of normal intelligence tend to be slow to begin to learn to speak and often pass through an echolalic phase. Subsequently,

vocabulary grows at a normal rate but they lack imitative gestures. Emotionally disturbed children might withhold speech, either totally or only outside the home (so-called elective mutism) (309), but comprehend well. In autism, speech is not only limited, but pervaded by echolalia, stereotypic utterances, and avoidance of the personal pronoun *I*. Children with autism have less difficulty with articulation and more with comprehension than do children with dysphasia who are matched for nonverbal intelligence. When bilingual children have difficulty in acquiring the second language, their ability with the first language is found to be limited also. A bilingual environment may explain some idiosyncratic uses modeled on the first language, but it does not explain delayed language development (310).

The language of culturally deprived children reflects local speaking patterns that are better described as different than impaired. On formal tests, such children score poorly relative to middle-class norms. The healthy child who has been totally deprived of language experience does not speak, but rapidly learns once the opportunity is offered (unless the child is secondarily emotionally disturbed). Extreme instances of children isolated from language, such as "wolf children" (311), have been reported, but even 6 years of total deprivation can supposedly be overcome (312), although a striking counter-example exists (313). The notion of a critical period for first language development remains controversial. Second language learning results in lower ultimate competence the later it is begun, up to age 15 years. Beyond this age, there is no further relationship between age and ultimate level of achievement (314).

Language in the Deaf

Three million American children have hearing deficits; 0.1% of the school population is deaf and 1.5% hard of hearing. Of cases of hearing deficits, 60% are congenital, and most of the rest result from meningitis (see Table 4.18). Children who are born with hearing loss in excess of 70 dB (severe) or even 90 dB (profound) cannot hear conversational speech, and therefore do not learn to talk unassisted. Taught by the oral method, acquisition proceeds through the expected stages, but falls far short of the expected eventual level of proficiency (315). In contrast, young children learn American Sign Language (ASL) spontaneously when exposed to it by their deaf parents. Their ultimate proficiency is a function of the age at which learning began (316). Thus, it is essential to begin as early as possible. Consistent with the status of ASL as a natural language, its use depends on left hemisphere function, even though in execution it is visuospatial (317).

Deafness often goes unnoticed, even by observant parents, when a bright child uses contextual cues to guide his or her behavior. It can be suspected, however, as early as 4.5 to 6 months of age if a child fails to look toward a sound source beyond his or her visual field. In young children, free-field audiometry is used for definitive diagnosis. This study should take place as early as possible so that the child does not go without appropriate language training (after the fitting of a hearing aid, if it is shown to help) and does not acquire the habit of ignoring auditory stimuli. Rarely, the auditory processing disorder is central, calling for tests of auditory attention and discrimination of speech modified in various ways (318). Performance on central auditory processing tests is also impaired in children with ADHD, and improves after stimulant therapy (319). Children with recurrent otitis media also can be at risk for language delays (320).

Congenitally deaf children with the usual high-frequency deafness adopt a harsh "deaf tone." When children become deaf abruptly (usually owing to meningitis), the effect depends on the stage of their language development. Children who become deaf when younger than 5 years gradually lose their ability to control articulation and voice production, sounding increasingly like congenitally deaf persons. Children with as little as 1 year of language experience are substantially easier to train in language skills than the congenitally deaf, whereas children who become deaf before age 2 years become indistinguishable from the congenitally deaf. The early provision of hearing aids and training for all deaf children improves their language progress.

Developmental Language Disorder

In developmental language disorder (alternatively named *specific language impairment*), verbal intelligence develops at a lesser rate than intelligence in other cognitive domains. The selective language delay results in late developing and semantically and syntactically impoverished speech. As indicated previously, the diagnosis of developmental language disorder excludes certain comorbid disorders unless the coexisting condition is unable to account for the severity of the language problem. Thus, an individual with mild mental retardation who is disproportionately impaired in verbal abilities can be considered to have developmental language disorder as well. Approximately 2% to 3% of 3-year-old children have either deficient expression, deficient reception, or both (321). Unlike speech in mental retardation, speech in delayed (dysphasic) language is also characterized by several articulatory disorders. These conditions differ from speech or articulation disorders such as stuttering, cluttering, lisping, and cleft palate nasality in that they are more severe, affect a wider range of phonemes, and involve a far greater difficulty in making the transition from phoneme to phoneme than in pronouncing the phonemes individually. This difficulty results in grossly curtailed word formation. Short binding words ("function" rather than "content" words) are frequently omitted.

In contrast to the relatively fixed deficits of speech disorder, delayed language is sensitive to context, and sound combinations that can be uttered at one time are unavailable at another. Greater mental effort often results in worse rather than better performance. The disorder is not limited to the spoken language; it affects writing, and even lip reading, manual alphabet, sign language, and Braille. Language delay invariably involves expressive speech. Verbal memory is impaired also. In one subtype, speech comprehension can be relatively spared, although affected children have difficulty discriminating speech sounds. In a less common subtype, semantic as well as syntactic comprehension is severely deficient (322). Perhaps the best developed subtyping is that of Rapin (323), who distinguishes five syndromes:

1. Phonologic production and speech planning disorder: These are largely speech problems with other associated motor deficits. Utterances are sparse or fluent, but contaminated by sequencing errors.
2. Lexical-syntactic deficit: Speech is sparse, though intelligible, word finding and paraphasic errors abound, and syntax is immature.
3. Phonologic-syntactic syndrome: Both speech sound formation and syntax are compromised and repetition is difficult. Speech is "telegraphic."
4. Verbal-auditory agnosia: Language expression and reception are generally disordered. The child cannot derive meaning from spoken language.
5. Semantic-pragmatic disorder: The child is fluent and talkative, and syntax is preserved, but comprehension and verbal reasoning are deficient. Utterances are stereotyped and tangential.

When comprehension is severely affected, the problem is often initially mistaken for peripheral deafness. The impression that auditory acuity fluctuates, which leads parents to doubt that the learning disorder is genuine, is borne out by audiometry. Stable hearing thresholds are hard to obtain and repeated testing is apt to lead to radically different audiometric profiles. Recording psychogalvanic skin responses to sound is informative. These instabilities are caused by inconstant focusing of attention on sound, a function normally performed by auditory cortex.

The claim has been made that a defect in auditory perception exists in some developmental language disorders, specifically, a difficulty in discriminating the patterns of transition from speech sound to speech sound (324). This problem is most common in verbal auditory agnosia, and when phonology is permanently impaired. Affected persons may have variable degrees of difficulty in auditory, visual, and linguistic processing. The neuropathology of developmental

language disorder is poorly understood but has been associated with a mild neuronal migrational disorder in left inferior frontal cortex (325).

Acquired Aphasia

Aphasia is considered to be acquired when it results from a condition that occurs after language development has begun, generally after age 2 years (326). Whereas bacterial infections causing encephalopathy used to be the most common causes of acquired aphasia in children, traumatic lesions currently predominate (291). Stroke in childhood is another cause of acquired aphasia, especially when the dominant hemisphere is affected (327).

Acquired aphasia is almost always nonfluent, especially in the youngest children, and loss of spontaneous speech or even mutism occurs more commonly than in adults. Other syndromes analogous to those in adults also have been described in children, and with analogous lesion location. Right hemisphere lesions cause aphasia in children no more frequently than they do in adults (1% to 4%). When they precede the onset of language, lesions of either hemisphere can temporarily retard language and spatial development (328).

Unless the lesion is bilateral, recovery of fluent speech is more likely in children with acquired aphasia than in adults, and disorders of comprehension occur less commonly. The prognosis for recovery from aphasia is also generally better in infants and young children. Residual minor language deficits and consequent school problems are common, however (329,330).

A rare type of acquired aphasia in children, the Landau-Kleffner syndrome, is discussed in Chapter 13, under the section of nonconvulsive status epilepticus. In this clinical entity, there is a severe comprehension deficit, as well as an agnosia for environmental sounds. Oral expression is poorer than written, although both are impaired. Nonverbal intelligence is normal. Seventy percent of children have a correlated severe behavior disorder, featuring hyperactivity, impulsivity, and oppositional behavior. The severity follows fluctuations in the severity of the language disorder (331). Long-term outcome is poor despite anticonvulsant therapy.

Diagnosis of Speech and Language Disorders

An essential diagnostic tool in speech and language disorders is the intelligence test, by use of which the selective nature of the disorder is verified. To verify intact intelligence in nonverbal domains, tests that are verbally based, such as the WISC verbal subscale and the Stanford-Binet, should be avoided in favor of tests that necessitate neither complex verbal instructions nor verbal responses. Examples are the WISC performance subscale, Ravens Colored Progressive Matrices for Children, the Leiter International Performance Scale (34), and the Hiskey-Nebraska Test of Learning Aptitude. A major discrepancy between a child's language and nonverbal developmental levels is integral to the developmental language disorder diagnosis. However, there is no consensus on what differential is critical and how it might vary with age (332). Audiometry excludes cases secondary to high-frequency deafness, and it can reveal the fluctuating impairments of pure tone sensory threshold that are typical of cortical deafness. The language behavior itself is evaluated by one of the standard language test batteries. Physical examination reveals any mechanical or motor deficits of the vocal apparatus. In the rare instances in which receptive aphasia and deafness resist clinical differentiation, the ability to elicit auditory-evoked potentials confirms that the auditory projections to the auditory cortex are intact.

Electroencephalography and neuroimaging are often used to seek structural intracranial abnormalities, but as a rule, yield little information of practical use. Rarely, subclinical seizures thought to disrupt cognitive processes can be detected by EEG (333). In such cases, effective anticonvulsant management, less often excision of circumscribed foci defined by electrocorticography, can sometimes improve cognition. Brain imaging techniques such as PET and functional MRI that index regional metabolic activity yield insights in language dysfunction (334,335). Molecular cytogenetic analysis can explain the cause of developmental language disorders in a small minority of affected children (336–338).

Treatment of Speech and Language Disorders

Language delay with an organic basis resists remediation. Treating the commonly associated impairments of dexterity, attention, and impulse control has little effect on the language problems (339). Speech therapy is at its most effective in improving a child's articulatory skills, although such skills are also apt to improve spontaneously with increasing age. However, the central problem of impoverished vocabulary and syntax and the resulting difficulty in thinking in words, is harder to address, and the so-called enrichment techniques are unrewarding. Syndrome-specific remediation approaches may be more effective (340,341). Parental expectations must be reconciled with the realities of what is often an enduring problem, and the child's education must be organized to enable him or her to learn optimally at an admittedly limited rate. Individual instruction is usually required, as well as family therapy and behavior modification on account of secondary emotional disorder, which involves the whole family.

In cases in which adequate language skills cannot be supplied, augmentation and alternative communication methods (AAC) may succeed. Beyond manual signing as used by the deaf, these methods are applied to children with disordered oral and verbal development caused by cerebral palsy, bulbar palsy, and dysarthria; developmental language disorder; autism; and mental retardation. The need first to verify that intensive speech training does not succeed must be balanced against the advantage of an early onset of AAC training (342), keeping in mind that AAC training may even facilitate verbal production rather than merely replace it. AAC subdivides into unaided (manual signing, finger spelling) and aided (communication board displaying pictures, symbols, or words). Depending on the child's motor capabilities, the child responds with finger, head, or eye indicating, yes and no indicating, or through electronic devices. A frequently used symbol system is Blissymbolics (343). The additional placement of another's hand on the child's hand or arm, combined with an expectation of sophisticated latent communication skills, characterizes the recently propagandized method of facilitated communication (344). This lacks both scientific basis and empirical validity (272,345).

LEARNING DISABILITIES

Definitions

Parents often seek neurologic assessment when their child's performance in school is unexpectedly poor, based on the prevalent but inaccurate assumption that a child who deals intelligently with some topics should also be able to do so with others. Some children, who have ostensibly normal intelligence and are willing to learn, do not benefit as much as expected from conventional methods of education in specific subject areas. The question of a cognitive limitation on certain forms of learning arises.

The term *learning disability* conventionally refers to a developmentally determined impairment in acquisition of certain mental skills that results in a discrepancy between observed performance on an academic achievement test and the expected performance level, as predicted by the child's age and IQ (346,347). The selective failure arises from irregularity of cognitive development, but not from the general failure owing to imperfect control of attention (see the section on ADHD, later in this chapter). An increasingly influential alternative formulation invokes depressed reading level only, regardless of IQ (348). Descriptors variously imply a neurologic basis (minimal cerebral dysfunction), a perceptual deficit (word blindness), or the isolated character of the disorder (selective reading disability or dyslexia). Dyslexia is also often termed *selective*, *specific*, or *pure* and is hypothesized to be organic, congenital, or developmental. However, preoccupation with the brain as the basis of the difficulty can lead to investigations that do not help in planning the child's future. Assumptions about the mechanism of the cognitive deficit preclude a rational search for

exactly what each affected child finds particularly difficult to understand or remember. The diagnostic term *dyslexia* comprises heterogeneous cases that require individualized remedial programs. Terms that characterize the clinical problem are preferable. If only reading and writing are problematic, the condition is called *selective* (or *specific*) *reading disability*. Selective arithmetic and drawing disabilities occur commonly but are much less frequently brought to clinical attention (unless the drawing disability involves the misshaping of letters). This is both because social pressure is concentrated on reading, and because schools use printed texts as vehicles for all forms of learning, especially as the child grows older. Thus, an early reading disability that is left uncorrected will in time broaden out into a general school failure.

In contrast to these initially selective difficulties, which stem from irregularities in cognitive development, more general early school failures occur. Severe hearing impairment is a cause of severe delays in both reading and math achievement, even for those who are skilled users of American Sign Language (349,350). Other school failures reflect differences in brain development and the consequence of the inability to maintain focused attention (see section on ADHD, later in this chapter). Affected children typically are referred for evaluation when they enter school, and their poor attention interferes with school activities.

Prevalence

Approximately 11% of school-aged children (aged 6 to 21 years) in the United States are classified as disabled, and 52% (2.4 million) of these students have learning disabilities (351). Another 10% to 20% of all students have learning or behavior problems that are not severe enough to be classified as disabilities. Other studies estimate that 7% to 8% of early grade-school students have reading disabilities (352).

Selective Reading Disability (Developmental Dyslexia)

There is no consensus on a comprehensive model of reading (353). Beginning reading involves, at the very least, (a) a visual complex of processes: discrimination of form, orientation, and sequence, as well as retention in memory of these three aspects of visual stimuli; (b) an auditory complex, which is the ability to analyze a word sound into its speech sounds, and to synthesize speech sounds into the appropriate spoken word; and (c) an associative complex, which is the ability to relate spoken words to sequences of shapes (whole-word method) and to relate letter sounds to shapes (phonics method). The second component, the ability to analyze the phonologic structure of the word, is the most potent determinant of progress in beginning readers (354). Word decoding ability accounts for much variance in reading skills at all levels (355). Reading difficulties are not confined to any particular orthographic system; they are approximately equally prevalent among readers of English, Japanese, and Chinese (356). Selective reading disability is more frequent in male subjects. In a population study, up to 20% of boys and 5% of girls read significantly less well than the norm (i.e., more than two standard deviations below the mean) (357). This indicates that selective reading disability is not the lower end of a normally distributed continuum of a proficiency in reading, but a distinctive group within the general population.

More advanced reading also requires fluent successive visual fixation and appropriate direction of eye movement, as well as knowledge, explicit or implicit, of the phonologic structure of the language, and the ability to construct meaning from the words in their context. Thus, a deficit that limits beginning readers, once overcome, does not prevent further acquisition of reading skill in a normal manner, whereas a deficit that limits advanced reading might not be foreshadowed in the early stages. Failing readers in early and later stages can show different patterns of cognitive deficit. Perceptual tests discriminate between succeeding and failing readers in the early grades; language tests do so in later grades. Perceptual tests also show different patterns of academic failure. In some cases difficulty is limited to spelling (358).

Numerous component processes, acting together, support reading and writing. Each component process is potentially subject to developmental immaturity. Thus, many different patterns of cognitive immaturity could result in a selective reading disability. No specific pattern of behavioral deficit characterizes dyslexia; slow readers have been reported to have numerous limitations. These implicate visual and auditory memory, the ability to store memories in terms of speech sounds and to integrate visual and auditory information, left and right discrimination, auditory synthesis, analysis of words into speech sounds, rhyming judgments, temporal order judgment, fast sequential processing, and nonword reading (359–363). Reading disability is associated with arithmetic difficulties, immature language, motor incoordination and impersistence, left and right confusion, and difficulty in copying figures, but there are no consistent combinations of these difficulties (364). Although some persons with dyslexia can have above average skills that reflect nondominant hemisphere specialization (365), the long-term outcome for most individuals with reading disabilities indicates persistent global deficits in academics, underemployment, and problems in behavior, social skills, and emotional adjustment (366). The mean IQ of learning disabled samples tends to be below average (355).

Many minor neurologic abnormalities have been uncovered in children with learning disabilities, but these seem haphazard in their occurrence. Soft signs of neuromotor immaturity are frequent in these children, but their presence does not predict problems in any particular cognitive or academic domain (367,368). Soft signs are less prevalent after puberty but remain in excess of those found in normally developed adults. MRI indicates a tendency toward decreased volume of the left posterior perisylvian region in children with learning disabilities. Topographic mapping of EEG activity has demonstrated differences between dyslexic and normal boys. These differences are localized not only to the cortical speech areas, but also in both supplementary motor areas (369). Regional cerebral blood flow is reportedly decreased in both parietal lobes (370). Additionally, multiple foci of microdysgenesis of cortical and thalamic architecture have been documented by anatomic examination of the brains of dyslexic individuals (371,372). These abnormalities are widespread in the left hemisphere, but also extend into the right frontal territory. In contrast, CT scans are rarely revealing, even if there are abnormalities on neurologic examination (373). In short, at none of the three levels of analysis (i.e., behavioral, physiologic, and anatomic) is the notion of a "pure" dyslexia validated. Rather a more widespread abnormality is indicated, particularly in dyslexic adults (374). This is supported by neuropsychological studies of adult dyslexics (375).

Investigation of Failure in School

Because the diagnosis of a learning disability is predicated on the combined presence of normal intelligence and subnormal achievement, the first step is to arrange standard intelligence and achievement tests. Quite often, the results rule out specific learning disability; a child's school failure may be adequately explained by intelligence tests that reveal an unsuspected general mental retardation, or the impression of academic underachievement may be contradicted by the achievement test results. Individual intelligence tests are the best available predictors of academic success. However, the highest correlations that are achieved between IQ and achievement grade equivalents range from 0.5 to 0.6. Thus, the amount of variance in school achievement that is accounted for by measured intelligence, the square of the correlation, is one-fourth, or at best one-third. Most of the remaining variance is accounted for by nonintellectual factors including those discussed in this section. A regression equation has been developed that correlates reading score, age, IQ, and social settings (376). It is necessary to qualify the expected reading level by these factors to avoid overdiagnosing reading disability in low IQ, low socioeconomic status (SES) children, and underdiagnosing it in the reverse type of child.

On educational achievement tests a lag of 2 years behind the norm is accepted as significant, and even a 1-year lag in the early grades. For adults, a quantitative definition of specific reading disability is available (377). But even if the achievement failure is real, and general intellect is adequate, learning disability must not be diagnosed if the child lacks the motivation to learn. If motivation is inadequate, the reason may be a behavior deviancy often involving the whole family, an impulsive or hurried approach to the task, or cultural alienation from middle-class educational aspirations. The lack of motivation can also derive from poor self-image and a sense of hopelessness secondary to cumulative failure.

If the evidence favors learning disability, often the family history features similar problems (378). In a twin study, approximately 29% of the cognitive profile in reading disability was found to be caused by heritable factors (379). In some families with dyslexia, a genetic abnormality with a marker on chromosome 15 has been identified (380). The learning disabled child, twice as often male as female, and more often living in poverty (381), shows soft signs on neurologic examination in perhaps one-half of the cases, when a primary attentional component is also present. At times, the learning difficulty occurs in the context of frank cerebral palsy. Whether family history is positive and whether neurologic abnormalities exist can be used as circumstantial evidence in deciding between a social or cultural and a developmental cause for the learning difficulties. Neither positive family history nor neurologic abnormality, however, helps in identifying the limitation on performance, whether cognitive or attentional, or in assigning a prognosis. For these purposes, it is necessary to scrutinize the psychometric data, to perform further tests, and to find out what kind of mistakes the child makes.

Some authorities favor a unitary hypothesis for the cognitive basis of dyslexia (e.g., verbal coding difficulty) (382). According to Gough and Turner (383), the variances in reading comprehension can be fully accounted for by decoding skill and listening comprehension. "Once the printed matter is decoded, the reader applies to the text exactly the same mechanism which he or she would bring to its spoken equivalent (383)." Listening comprehension relies on storing information in working memory, and slow decoding limits working memory (384). Thus, a wide range of difficulties that the reading disabled person has, with phonologic awareness, speech perception, production, and naming, is amenable to a unitary explanation.

The decoding needs not only to be accurate, it needs to be fluent. The ability to automatize retrieval of names is quantitated by the Rapid Naming Test. Scores in this test have substantial predictive value for poor readers (385).

Others infer multiple causation from the diversity of patterns of test performance. Some children score substantially worse on the verbal than the performance subscale of the WISC. A less common pattern is a lower performance score than verbal score, with a particular deficit appearing on the performance subtests of block design and object assembly, as well as on arithmetic (386). However, specific learning disability or hemisphere dysfunction cannot be inferred from a large verbal performance split alone. Children with verbal deficit have a history of delayed language development, and their mistakes in reading and spelling suggest that they find it difficult to match appropriate letter sounds to a given word. In contrast, children with performance deficit make mistakes of letter sequence rather than letter choice. Their difficulty in remembering sequence is further illustrated in arithmetic, in which they make errors in manipulations (such as subtraction) that involve the relative position of digits. Failure on tests of "finger order sense" is similarly accounted for by difficulty in making use of information about relative position. Typically developing children can distinguish between their right and left sides by 7 years of age.

Another pattern is that of the child, often left-handed, who has a normal psychometric profile, but occasionally reads or writes from right to left. Although these mistakes attract much attention, they are transient and of little consequence. Mirror-image reversal of letters occurs in healthy children who are not yet ready to learn to read and in some older, but selectively immature, children who have difficulty in the initial stages of reading.

Additional attempts to subtype children with reading disability (387) include making distinctions among different language subtypes, for instance a problem in phoneme-grapheme conversion, versus a comprehension problem also implicating heard speech (388). Others distin-

guish a visuospatial subtype (389), even a subtype attributed to right hemisphere dysfunction (390). Yet another typology distinguishes between accuracy-disabled and rate-disabled readers (391). Some studies even raise questions about the more elementary visual functioning of children with dyslexia (392,393). Surprisingly, the dorsal stream of visual information, usually associated with visuospatial rather than with linguistic functioning, may be defective (394,395). However, although it is generally accepted that many reading-disabled children have impaired auditory-phonologic skills, there is no agreement as to whether there are other subtypes of dyslexia, and, if so, how they should be characterized. Further, it has not been demonstrated that instruction is more effective if tailored to subtype. Where specialized facilities are unavailable, the physician can use certain test instruments that do not require special training for administration or interpretation (see Table 16.3). Such measures enable the clinician to determine whether disparities exist between the child's intelligence and achievement, and whether apparent underachievement can be accounted for on the basis of selective language or other cognitive deficit. Such inferences can then be checked against the prevalent error type in reading and spelling (396,397). There appear to be some electrophysiologic correlates of the two main error categories, dysphonetic and dyseidetic dyslexia (398).

Right-handedness almost always reflects left cerebral hemisphere dominance for language. Although some left-handed and mixed-handed individuals have dominant left hemispheres, most have language representation spread across both hemispheres. Pathologic left-handers are genotypic dextrals whose hand preference is shifted on account of left-sided cerebral damage (399). This shift perhaps explains why the incidence of left-handedness among epileptic children, especially those with left-sided EEG foci of early origin, and among mentally retarded children is twice that in the general population. The incidence of sinistrality is proportionate to the severity of the mental retardation (400).

As a group, slow readers have frequently been reported to show an excess of left-handedness, mixed-handedness, and inconsistency of side of preference for hand, foot, and eye. Some large series have shown no such relationship, however. In general, samples that yield a high proportion of left-handed subjects come from clinical sources, whereas samples that do not are drawn from the general school population (401). Samples from clinical sources are more likely to include children who have suffered early brain damage, which leads to pathologic left-handedness, as mentioned previously. The association between left-handedness and dyslexia also can encompass a vulnerability to autoimmune disease (402), and poor readers are more likely to have mothers with immune dysfunction (403). Eye preference, usually inferred from sighting dominance (404), bears no close relationship to hemisphere dominance. It is influenced mostly by minor disparities of visual acuity between the eyes that are not neurologically significant and is not useful in the investigation of learning disabilities. Anomalies of central laterality also have been suggested; for instance, bilateral spatial representation interfering with left-sided verbal processing (405). Anomalous lateral preference is too inconstant to be useful diagnostically, and there is certainly no rationale for trying to correct a learning disability by interfering with a child's established limb preference or by guiding a younger child toward right-handedness. Hiscock and Kinsbourne have reviewed the evidence for the relationship between laterality and learning disability (406).

Investigating reading disability with MRI rarely yields useful information. The EEG is helpful only when absence seizures momentarily interrupt the child's attention with a frequency that is sufficiently great to interfere with the child's ability to follow trains of thought in class. On the average, generalized 3 per second spike-wave discharges lasting 5.5 seconds or more can interfere with mental activity (see Chapter 13) (407). Brain electrical activity mapping (369) reveals interesting group differences and offers prospects for clinical utility for individual diagnosis in learning disability. Neuroimages may reveal reversed hemisphere asymmetry no more fre-

quently than in controls (408), but see reference 409. Gross deficits of hearing and vision must be ruled out as contributing to the problem; however, reading is only impaired when visual acuity is substantially reduced. Orthoptic investigation may reveal poor vergence control and stereoacuity, especially in children who report that the text is subjectively unstable (410). Six months of monocular occlusion reportedly results in better reading (411). Vestibular dysfunction is no more common among children with learning disabilities than in a control population (412). The differentiation of learning and emotional disorder is discussed by Gallico and colleagues (413).

Neurologic Basis and Genetics

More than most disorders of cognition, dyslexia has an extensively documented genetic and neuroimaging substrate. Genetic linkages to reading-related symptoms have been established to chromosomes 6p21 (414,415), 15q21 (415), and chromosome 2p16 (416). This genetic heterogeneity may partly explain range of diverse, bilateral loci that have been implicated in functional neuroimaging studies (417–421, 421a).

Prognosis

By far the best predictors of success in learning are socioeconomic circumstances (422). Holding these constant, the prediction of reading failure in preschool children who are not mentally retarded remains difficult. Reading readiness tests do have a measure of success, but they rely unduly on establishing whether the child entering first grade can already read to some extent. Also, the outcome does not specify the failing child's area of weakness and thus is no guide to how the child should be taught. Selective learning disability, as opposed to learning failures that arise from adverse social and economic circumstances (381), cannot be predicted. Readiness testing is best performed shortly before children enter school, although soon enough to enable decisions based on the outcome to be implemented before the school's openings for the coming year are filled. Longitudinal studies indicate that learning disability persists into adulthood and even broadens into vocational and personal problems, although delinquency is not a common outcome (423).

Treatment

Treatment programs are designed to have an effect at various functional levels hypothesized to relate to reading. In decreasing degree of relevance, they are (a) training with emphasis on concepts fundamental to reading itself, first on visual letter and word recognition and labeling, and then on linguistic and semantic aspects of the reading process. The combination of phonologic awareness training (424) and direct instruction in alphabetic coding is the most effective approach to early reading; (b) behavior modification, with emphasis on maturity, attention, and improved study habits; and (c) training in discriminating sounds, shapes, and directions in various modalities.

Programs that are irrelevant for treating reading disability include optometric exercises (425), improvement of neuromuscular control (e.g., sensory integration therapy) (426,427), labyrinthine stimulation, attempts to change peripheral or central laterality (428), psychoactive drug treatment (429), and antimotion sickness medication (430,431).

Physical training with a view to improving spatial orientation and body image has been claimed to improve mental performance. However, these techniques involve teaching the child accomplishments far removed from the area of the child's difficulty and giving him or her unaccustomed attention. This encouraging experience could improve self-concept and motivation, without specifically improving reading (432,433). Efforts to change hand preference do not address the basic deficits in learning disability and are ineffective. Eye-movement training ignores the fact that, except in rare cases of conjugate gaze palsies, rate of eye movement shift from fixation to fixation is not a limiting factor in reading skill. Visuomotor training is based on the view that early motor ability influences and predicts later intelligence. No evidence supports the claim that either visual training or perceptual training can improve the academic outcome of children with

reading disabilities (434). A motor program based on "patterning" of locomotion (435) is not only ineffective but may be harmful and cause unnecessary expenses, delay in appropriate educational intervention, and give a false sense of security (276). Visuoperceptual training (436) was found to be less effective than specific reading training in helping first-graders to read (437). In general, the notion that cognitive deficits can be remediated by training ontogenetically earlier perceptuomotor skills has been abandoned.

In general, noneducational remedial methods have not been shown to have specific effects on reading readiness, and the time is better used for fundamental instruction in reading or in the language skills on which reading is based. For some children, perceptual training, including "tactile-kinesthetic training," might have some benefits; it focuses attention on stimulus dimensions relevant to reading, such as orientation, that immature children customarily ignore. But the claim that training in activities not directly pertinent to reading generalize to the reading process remains unsubstantiated. Preferable is a systematic, analytic approach to reading itself, in which the information is presented stepwise, while distractions are minimized. Usually, this can only be achieved by individual instruction, to conform to the individual learning requirements of the child. "Language experience" approaches are generally unsuccessful.

To meet these requirements, some educators would "teach to weakness" in the hope of improving the efficiency of the process responsible for reading deficiency; others regard it as more realistic to circumvent the deficiency by teaching to residual strengths. In fact, it is not necessary to adopt an inflexible position. Initial attempts can be made to teach to weakness. If these do not succeed within a reasonable period of time, they should be discontinued before cumulative failure further lowers the child's morale, and teaching to strength should be substituted. It is usually not necessary to remove the child totally from the regular classroom, and doing so is best avoided because it is apt to lead to pessimism and self-denigration by the child, who becomes less willing than ever to try to learn. Instead, the child should be withdrawn from the classroom only during those sessions that would leave him or her floundering, for individual instruction in basics not yet mastered.

Beyond identifying the child who needs individualized reading instruction, many psychoeducational diagnosticians regard it as not only feasible, but also necessary, to determine the child's preferred reading style. Is the child a visual learner, to be taught by the whole-word approach, or an auditory learner, to be taught using phonics? Instruments such as the Illinois Test of Psycholinguistic Abilities (438) and the Wepman Auditory Discrimination Test (439) are deployed for this purpose. Tests such as these have no demonstrated validity for the purpose of choosing a properly individualized reading curriculum, nor are whole-word and phonics approaches mutually exclusive alternatives in a comprehensive tutorial program in reading. Whole-word instruction serves for acquiring a useful but limited initial working sight vocabulary. Phonic-linguistic methods are needed to enable the child to learn the phonologic structure of the language as presented in alphabetic script. Mere ability to learn paired associations suffices for acquiring sight vocabulary, but understanding the phonologic structure calls for specifically linguistic processing skills. By applying phonologic rules, the child is able to read words not yet learned. Popular remedial reading programs include Orton-Gillingham, a multisensory alphabetic method, whereby the child learns letter-sound correspondences, blending of sounds, and syllabication. Computer programs have been used (440).

Finally, lexical knowledge does not guarantee fluency. The child who has mastered phonics may nonetheless emerge as a halting, dysfunctional reader. Fluency training is a necessary sequel. Different children are led through these stages at different rates, encountering different problems on the way. This exacting, long-term effort is not substantially facilitated by any form of diagnostic testing at the time of the original assessment.

NONVERBAL LEARNING DISABILITIES

Attention has focused on children with selective difficulties that impede school performance in spite of satisfactory spoken and written language skills. In the long run, such nonverbal learning disabilities can be more handicapping for employment prospects than selective reading disability (441). These include children with developmental dyscalculia who experience difficulty in mathematics not explained by concurrent verbal difficulties, but instead are associated with visuospatial impairments (442,443). Some children with attention disorders have difficulty in achieving fluency in knowledge of arithmetic facts, such as tables (444). Children with dyscalculia also are described as experiencing difficulty in tactile discrimination, concept formation, fine motor coordination, and dysgraphia (445). Dyscalculia is as prevalent as dyslexia (446) but attracts little attention, perhaps because a fourth-grade arithmetic achievement level suffices for everyday activities (447). Four subtypes of mathematical disability have been suggested, corresponding to weakness in semantic memory, the execution of the procedures, visual and spatial processing, and working memory (448).

One formulation relates such a constellation of symptoms to hypothesized inadequacy of the right hemisphere (449) and invokes impaired social skills as yet another component of such a syndrome (450). Shyness and social isolation are accompanied by lack of eye contact and impaired use of gestures with speech in flat intonation. When soft neurologic signs are present, they tend to be left-sided. An electrophysiologic study reports diminished activity in the 36- to 44-Hz band over the right hemisphere during a face recognition task in dyscalculics (451). A group of children being treated for phenylketonuria was reported as conforming to such a neuropsychological pattern (452). Nonverbal learning disability is common in female carriers of fragile X (453). It is the most common type of learning disability in epilepsy (454).

A high prevalence of nonverbal learning disability exists among children with neurofibromatosis type 1 (455). Affected individuals have visuospatial deficits and reading disabilities; MRI studies that show basal ganglia and cerebellar lesions suggest a role of subcortical structures in the etiology of this condition (456–458).

More generally, children with learning disabilities have low social status among their peers (459). This low status could result both from associated social obliviousness, and from the school failure that children with learning disabilities experience, resulting in low self-concept and negative perception by others.

So-called social learning disability (460) comprises skill deficits, when socially relevant behaviors are not in the child's repertoire, and performance deficits, when they are in the repertoire, but not used (461). They might not be used because the child avoids interactions (self-control skill deficit) or because the child lacks impulse control (self-control performance deficit).

Some children exhibit impaired development of sensorimotor coordination. When impairment cannot be attributed to sensorimotor deficit as elicited during the neurologic examination, it is described as the clumsy child syndrome (462). The difficulty extends beyond motor control to visuoperceptual activities that do not call for hand or eye movement control (463). Information about this unusual, but troublesome and persistent, syndrome has been compiled by Gordon and McKinley (464).

ATTENTION DEFICIT-HYPERACTIVITY DISORDER

The amount of sensory information almost always far exceeds the individual's ability to respond. He or she must prioritize the inputs for their adaptive relevance and selectively attend to whatever is most relevant at the time. Thus, children's adaptive ability depends both on their intelligence and their ability to attend to the relevant aspects of their environment. Children whose cognitive development is otherwise normal may find it abnormally difficult to sustain goal-directed attention.

Characteristics of Attention Deficit-Hyperactivity Disorder

The term *ADHD* refers to the covariation of inattention, hyperactivity, and impulsivity (49). The *DSM-IV* describes three major ADHD subtypes: (a) inattention alone, (b) hyperactivity-impulsivity alone, and (c) a combined type with significant inattention, hyperactivity, and impulsivity. Restlessness may be observed. Children

may be restless during one stage of development but not subsequently. *DSM-IV* does not include developmental qualifiers as a part of the criteria for ADHD but the listed behaviors typically decrease as the child grows older. This does not imply that the disorder grows milder with increasing age, but that its form of presentation changes during development.

The major clinical manifestations of ADHD of developmentally maladaptive attention, activity, and impulse control must be sufficient to cause impairment in social, academic, or occupational functioning (49). Signs of ADHD generally begin before age 7 years and should persist for at least 6 months in two or more settings (e.g., home, school, or play). However, some children may have a later onset of the signs of ADHD (465).

There is consensus on the behavioral characteristics of ADHD that are listed in *DSM-IV* criteria. The most frequently reported primary manifestations of ADHD include cognitive disorganization, distractibility, inattention, impulsivity, and hyperactivity. The most commonly reported secondary manifestations include disruptive behaviors, poor social skills, emotional immaturity, fidgeting, poor academic performance, and excessive talking.

The relationship between the level of motor activity in infants and subsequent hyperactivity is unknown. Mothers often observe in retrospect that their child with hyperactivity was unusually active from birth. Feeding difficulty and sleep disturbances in infancy and the preschool period are commonly reported precursors (466,467). A prospective study found the second year of life the earliest in which ADHD symptoms could be detected, and age 3 to 5 years to be the peak time of onset (468). Children with hyperactivity explore their environment with unusual persistence, which accounts for the increased frequency of accidental poisonings and traumatic brain injury (469,470). In older children, gross motor exuberance can give way to a less flagrant but continual wriggling restlessness. More troublesome is the child's impulsive, distractible, and often antisocial behavior. The hyperactivity becomes less a source of adults' irritation at home and more an occasion for disapproval from teachers at times when school children are expected to sit still and pay attention. This disapproval can be partly responsible for the high stealing and truancy rates among hyperactive children (471). Girls and boys with ADHD are similar in their characteristics of impulsivity, academic performance, social functioning, fine motor skills, parental education, and parental depression (472). Girls tend to show less hyperactivity and externalizing behavior but greater cognitive impairment.

Gross body movements are not always more frequent in children with hyperactivity. In unstructured situations, many children are active, and children with hyperactivity do not stand out. In structured situations, differences appear both in the amount and the relevance of the activity. In a 24-hour study, an ADHD group did exhibit more overall activity than controls night and day (473). Recorded over as much as 1 week, boys with ADHD were significantly more restless than controls at ages 6 to 11 years, but rarely so at older ages. Some children manage to continue to be attentive (e.g., to a television program) while moving around a room. Mostly, however, each movement signals a more comprehensive reorientation of mental set. In infancy, and until the child walks, this continual reorientation appears not to cause concern. Subsequently, complaints gather as the child disrupts the orderly home or classroom, while failing to pay the expected degree of attention to the teacher, the instructional materials, and homework assignments.

Young children with ADHD show no signs of distress initially, but negative reactions from adults and peers gradually engender feelings of inadequacy, and this can lead to withdrawal or aggression. Hyperactive children are seen as quarrelsome, irritable, defiant, untruthful, and destructive by their classmates, as well as by adults (474). The discipline imposed by the school and the need to repeat grades further contribute to learning failure and social maladjustment. Nonhyperactive children with attention deficit are misperceived as undermotivated or lazy, and the diagnosis is often missed.

School work demands increasing effort and organization in fourth grade (475), and the intermittency of attention interferes more with learning and becomes more troublesome to teachers.

Some 10% to 50% of children with ADHD underachieve in reading (476,477). Whether this is caused by the attention deficit, which can impair word attack (478), or to comorbid dyslexia is hard to determine in the individual case (479). Children with ADHD are not, as a group, lower in IQ than attentionally normal children.

Neither restlessness nor inattention is the core of the ADHD syndrome. There are circumstances under which hyperactive children attend as efficiently as normals. This is when they find the task intrinsically interesting or rewarding. It is when the task itself is tedious and the motivation for doing it is remote in the future that their inattention is maximal. The hyperactive child understands consequences and professes the usual concern about them. The consequences make little impression on the child's behavior, however (480). But if the task is attractive or of interest to the child (i.e., if it is intrinsically motivating), then the ADHD child performs as well as a child who is attentionally normal.

Diagnosis of Attention Deficit-Hyperactivity Disorder

There are no definitive dianostic tests for ADHD. Rather, the diagnosis depends on the demonstration of inappropriate behavior for a child's expected level of developmental maturity and subsequent impairment in social and school functioning. Corroborating information can be obtained through child, parental, and teacher interviews; standardized questionnaires; direct observation; and formal psychological and educational evaluations. Behavioral laboratory tests may contribute corroborating evidence. A complete history, physical and neurologic examination should be performed to rule out any identifiable genetic or medical conditions that might simulate ADHD; however, although it may uncover nonspecific soft neurologic signs, the examination rarely contributes to the diagnosis. Neither physiologic nor biochemical measures reliably identify ADHD children (481). Psychiatric consultation is indicated in children with more complex behavioral problems or who have comorbid depression or thought disorders.

Prevalence

ADHD is the most common chronic behavioral disorder in children. It occurs far more frequently in boys (482). The prevalence of ADHD ranges between 2% and 6% and is reported to be highest in inner city populations in the United States (471,483). Through the evolution of the diagnostic criteria and changes in public attitude toward the disorder, the prevalence of ADHD has gradually increased. In a more recent study, primary care providers identified behavioral problems in approximately one in five children and attentional/hyperactivity problems in 9.2% of the entire study sample, but the diagnosis was commonly made solely by parental interview and without the benefit of standardized questionnaires (484).

Although it is most frequently diagnosed in North America, cross-cultural studies have shown comparable levels of prevalence in all countries studied, even in the Third World (482), not only of ADHD, but also of both internalizing and externalizing psychopathology in general (485). In Britain, the diagnostic label is *hyperkinetic disorder* (486). It is reserved for the most severe cases, whereas other children who would have been considered to have ADHD in the United States are termed *conduct disordered* in the United Kingdom (487). This difference in semantic emphasis parallels a difference in prevailing use of management modalities, stimulant therapy being used sparingly in the United Kingdom. Whether ADHD and conduct disorder are truly separable is questionable (488). Those who use *aggressive conduct disorder* as a primary diagnosis find a majority of their patients to be hyperactive also (489). Comorbidities affect both prognosis and treatment (490).

Neurobiological Basis and Genetics

ADHD is not a consistent condition and there is no single underlying cause. It occurs both in the absence of any identifiable risk factors and in association with numerous other childhood conditions such as motor dyspraxia, tics, learning problems, speech and language disorders, sleep disorders, oppositional behavior, enuresis, and encopresis. In addition, overactive and socially disruptive behavior is commonly reported in children who have evidence of injury from infections, head trauma, toxic exposures (491,491a), and extreme prematurity (173,492,493). Minor physical anomalies are frequent (494).

In most cases, hyperactivity is already evident in infancy, and it can persist into adult life as attentional and social problems (495,496). Thus, it has the characteristics of a stable personality trait or temperament, and in most cases is probably genetic in origin. Families of ADHD/conduct-disordered children are notable for the high incidence of sociopathy, alcoholism, and hysteria (497–499).

ADHD is believed to result from an underactivation of some relevant neural system with the dopaminergic mesolimbic-orbital frontal projection having received considerable attention (500). Several linkage studies implicate the dopamine receptor D4 (DRD4) gene, mapped to chromosome 11p (501), and a dompamine transporter, a target of many of the drugs used to treat ADHD, to this condition (502). In addition, there is a marked increase in the density of dopamine transporters in the striatum, as measured by single photon emission computed tomography (SPECT), using labelled altropane, a specific ligand for dopamine transporter (502a). This disorder in dopaminergic function results in a disinhibited sensation-seeking behavioral style (503). The striatum has abnormal morphology in ADHD (504). Regional cerebral blood flow is diminished in striatum and frontal lobes in ADHD, and the deficiency is partly reversible by methylphenidate (505, but see 506). Power spectrum analysis indicates prefrontal underactivation (507), cerebral glucose metabolism is generally diminished, but most notably in prefrontal lobes (508), and some neuropsychologic deficits are seen consistent with prefrontal underactivity. Anatomic imaging reveals modest (approximately 10%) mean reduction in size of the frontal lobes, basal ganglia, and corpus callosum (509–511). The posterior cerebellar vermis is also reduced in size, with the inferior posterior lobe being particularly involved (512). The neurobiological clues to the etiology of ADHD are summarized in Table 16.10.

TABLE 16.10. *Neurobiological clues to the etiology of attention deficit-hyperactivity disorder* (ADHD)

Etiologic clue	Description of findings in studies of ADHD	References
Environmental	Increased incidence of behavioral disorders, sociopathy, and alcoholism in families of children with ADHD.	498,586, 587
Endocrine	Increased frequency of ADHD in patients with resistance to thyroid hormone in some studies.	588,589
Genetic	Increased concordance for hyperactivity/inattentiveness in monozygotic twins (59% to 81%), compared with dizygotic twins (approximately one-third). Increased incidence of ADHD in first-degree (up to 25%) and second-degree relatives of children with ADHD.	590–594
Neuroanatomy		
Cerebrum	Some limited magnetic resonance imaging brain morphology and neuropsychological studies suggest that children with ADHD have a smaller or functionally abnormal right frontal lobe. Other studies show variable asymmetries and volumetric differences in the basal ganglia, corpus callosum, ventricular systems, and subcortical white matter.	595–599
Electroencephalographic findings	Increased anterior absolute theta and decreased posterior relative beta activity in quantified electroencephalographic analysis suggests reduced cortical arousal in adolescents with ADHD.	600
Brainstem	Prolonged latencies of waves III and V, and longer brainstem transmission of waves I–III and I–V in brainstem auditory-evoked potentials of children with ADHD suggest brainstem dysfunction in these children. Activation of reticular midbrain formation and thalamic intralaminar nuclei increases on attention-demanding tasks in a positron emission tomographic study.	601,602
Neurochemistry		
Dopaminergic and noradrenergic systems	Pharmacologic agents that are effective in ADHD (e.g., stimulants and tricyclic antidepressants) increase central nervous system dopamine and norepinephrine transmission. Dopamine deficiency is postulated to account for lack of impulse control in ADHD. Studies that measure catecholamines and their metabolites in blood, urine, and CSF in individuals with ADHD are inconclusive. Regional dopamine inhibitory autoreceptors may play a role in central nervous system catecholamine metabolism. Functional neuroimaging studies support the hypothesis that attention is regulated at multiple levels, especially frontal, parietal, or temporal cortex as well as subcortical structures within the basal ganglia and thalamus.	603–606

Differential Diagnosis

Restlessness and short attention span can be facets of mental retardation, and these abnormal behaviors may be fitting to a patient's developmental quotient. Mental retardation itself can be hard to determine. If the validity of the intelligence tests is uncertain, the educational psychologist may qualify the IQ score with a warning that it could underrepresent the child's cognitive potential, particularly for measures that require sustained attention rather than merely a quick response. Retesting after initiation of stimulant therapy can yield a more realistic estimate. Improvement can be conveniently documented by teachers and parents by means of the Conners rating scales (513). How-

ever, even correction of the attentional problem can leave the educational difficulty unresolved, given the 30% to 40% overlap between ADHD and learning disabilities (514).

When cognitive deficits do not explain the attentional problem, an alternative possibility is overanxious disorder. The anxious child is most restless under emotional stress, as in the classroom and consulting room, and least when unstressed, as on weekends or on vacation. The child is visibly unhappy, either characterologically or because of some maladjustment within the family. The hyperactive child, on the other hand, is typically in good spirits until the child comes up against frustration and adverse attitudes from others. Whereas the time of onset of anxiety can usually be specified, hyperactivity often dates from early infancy. A favorable response to a stimulant supports the diagnosis of ADHD as opposed to anxiety. This can be documented in the laboratory on a time-response and dose-response basis, using a paired-associated learning task (515). The resulting findings contribute to the design of an appropriate drug regimen for the child who responds favorably. Other tasks that can be used in a similar way are the Continuous Performance Test (516) and the Children's Checking Test (517).

Overfocusing is sometimes comorbid with ADHD. This condition represents a difficulty in shifting mental set associated with perseveration and isolating tendencies. It bears some resemblance to high-level autistic behavior, though milder (143). A contrasting temperament of uncertain relation to overfocusing is exhibited by the *behaviorally inhibited* child (518). Irritable in infancy, shy and fearful as a toddler, and cautious, quiet, and introverted in grade school, these children are thought to have increased limbic-sympathetic tone and to be anxiety prone. Disordered sleep, especially caused by obstructive sleep apnea, can render a child inattentive and restless.

Attention deficits are often found among children of schizophrenic parents. These children are themselves at high risk of developing schizophrenia. They perform poorly on vigilance tasks, but are not impulsive (519). Another potentially overlooked differential diagnosis of ADHD is bipolar disorder, particularly when it presents in adolescents with chronic rather than episodic symptomatology. The combination of dysphoric and irritable mood with aggressive conduct, resistant to stimulant therapy, should prompt an examination of the family for bipolar disorder (520). Episodic loss of control is attributed to dysfunction in the limbic cortex (521). Whereas impulsive acts of aggression are common in ADHD, intermittent states of episodic explosive behavior are not. The restless movements of Sydenham chorea are associated with ADHD in one-third of cases and are often accompanied by emotional lability and obsessive-compulsive symptoms (522).

Management Strategies

Medical

Although behavioral modification may be a sufficient first-line therapy in mild cases of ADHD, it is advisable to consider a pharmacologic intervention trial before extensive behavioral management therapies, home interventions, or changes in the educational program or curriculum are instituted (523). The most effective pharmaceutical agents for symptomatic control of hyperactivity are the stimulant medications. Therapy with stimulants leads to significant improvement in at least 70% to 80% of properly diagnosed children with ADHD (524). At the effective dose, stimulants modify the child's activity, improve behavioral control, and permit a more adaptive disposition of attention in relation to the demands of the moment (525,526). A meta-analysis of effect size finds twice as much improvement of behavior as of classroom achievement (527). Stimulants also enhance performance in otherwise normal, healthy individuals, when performance is affected by disinterest, fatigue, or sleep deprivation.

Stimulants are conventionally prescribed for children with hyperactivity according to the child's weight, for instance at a dose of 0.3 mg/kg (528), but there is no empirical justification for prescribing based on body weight. These drugs have a strong affinity for the brain, which approximates its adult size by age 6 years, and the optimal dosage does not increase with increasing age or severity and is not a function of body weight (529).

Stimulant therapy usually remains useful for many years, if not indefinitely. Even after long periods of administration, discontinuing the drug leads to notable relapse within a few hours. Because most stimulants are short-acting, their effectiveness can be evaluated on a daily basis by comparing behavior on and off medication, without the need for drug holidays.

Approximately 20% of children diagnosed with ADHD fail to respond to stimulants or respond adversely (530). In acute overdose, stimulants cause tics, which cease when the medication is stopped. The possibility that stimulant therapy can on rare occasions precipitate Tourette syndrome has been debated (531,532). If tics appear with initiation of stimulant therapy or if an existing tic disorder is aggravated by it, the medication should be discontinued. Approximately 50% of children with Tourette syndrome meet ADHD criteria and one-third feel compulsions to perform risky acts (533). In up to one-half of these children, stimulant therapy exacerbates the tics (534). Desipramine is often an effective alternative treatment of symptoms in children with both ADHD and Tourette syndrome (535). Doses and common adverse effects of medications used in the treatment of ADHD are listed in Table 16.11.

Dexedrine is preferred to the equally effective racemic amphetamine because it produces fewer side effects. The standard tablet is effective for 4 hours but therapeutic effects can be distributed more evenly over time by using the longer-acting dextroamphetamine (Dexedrine Spansules). Any

adverse effects are apparent within 3 days, and if these are worrisome, the dosage should be decreased or discontinued. If no change occurs at the initial dosage, an increase of 2.5 mg is introduced every 3 days until a favorable result occurs or until adverse effects supervene. Usually adverse effects are transient. Insomnia can represent the recurrence of hyperactivity after the stimulant has worn off, or an effect of the stimulant itself. It can be controlled by adjusting dosage and timing. No long-term adverse effects have been substantiated. The claim that high dosages of stimulants retard growth (536) has not been confirmed (537,538). This is the case even though stimulants may interfere with cartilage metabolism by inhibiting somatomedin-stimulated sulfate uptake by tissues (539).

Methylphenidate is far more commonly used than dextroamphetamine. It is effective in about

TABLE 16.11. *Pharmacologic treatment of attention deficit-hyperactivity disorder*

Medication	Dose ranges (mg/kg per day)	Maximum dose (mg per day)	Formulations	Common adverse effects
Stimulants				
D-amphetamine (Dexedrine)	0.1–0.5	40	5-mg tablets; 5-, 10-, 15-mg spansules	Insomnia, poor appetite, stomach ache, tics
D-amphetamine/ L-amphetamine mixture (Adderall)	0.1–0.5	40	5-, 10-, 20-mg tablets	Insomnia, poor appetite, stomach ache, tics
Methylphenidate (Ritalin)	0.5–1.0	60	5-, 10-, 20-mg tablets; 20-mg sustained release	Insomnia, poor appetite, stomach ache, tics
Pemoline (Cylert)	0.5–3.0	112.5	18.75-, 37.5-, 75-mg tablets	Insomnia, tics, stomach ache, movement disorder; rarely: hypersensitivity and hepatic dysfunction
Others				
Clonidine (Catapres)	0.001–0.005	0.3–0.4	0.1-, 0.2-, 0.3-mg tablets 0.1-, 0.2-, 0.3-mg transdermal patch	Somnolence, fatigue, hypotension, bradycardia, headache, dry mouth, constipation
Desipramine (Norpramin)	1–3	100	10-, 75-, 100-mg tablets	Tachycardia, hypertension, arrhythmias; monitor electrocardiogram Rare, unexplained sudden death
Guanfacine (Tenex)	0.5–2 mg/d; 12 yr and older	2	1-, 2-mg tablets	Sedation, fatigue, headaches, insomnia, stomach ache, decreased appetite
Imipramine (Tofranil)	0.5–3	100	10-, 25-, 50-mg tablets	Fatigue, dry mouth, blurred vision Rare, cardiac conduction block

the same proportion of patients (approximately two-thirds) as dextroamphetamine, but not necessarily in the same patients. The regimen is similar, but 5-mg doses are given in increments. Ideally, the drug is administered 30 minutes before meals, because intestinal alkalinity is thought to degrade the product. The side effects are similar to, but less frequent than, those with dextroamphetamine. The long-acting (sustained release) methylphenidate preparation (Ritalin) appears to be effective for approximately 6 hours. Scores on standardized IQ performance subscales may improve in some children who respond to methylphenidate, but it does not treat comorbid learning disabilities. The drug assists performance by helping sustained attention, diminishing impulsiveness, and improving inhibition of hasty incorrect responses (540). In some children the medication improves motor control and handwriting. Methylphenidate can be used in ADHD children with seizure disorders. A double-blind medication and placebo crossover study found that children whose seizure disorders had been well controlled on monotherapy did not relapse on methylphenidate and their EEG tracings remained unchanged (541). This has been confirmed (542,543). The same applies for children with seizures and more severe underlying encephalopathy (544).

The stimulant pemoline has a similar duration of action and the additional advantage of lacking abuse potential. (Children with ADHD have not been reported to abuse their prescribed stimulant medication.) Serum liver enzyme (aspartate aminotransferase/alanine aminotransferase) concentrations can be elevated during pemoline therapy; it is not clear that this is clinically significant but close patient surveillance is recommended (545). A few cases of liver failure attributed to pemoline have been reported.

Clonidine and guanfacine, α_2-adrenergic receptor agonists and antihypertensives, are alternative medications that ameliorate ADHD symptoms, particularly with respect to the frequently associated aggression (546,547). Clonidine has been reported to cause cardiovascular complications, especially when combined with methylphenidate (548). Guanfacine appears to be less sedating and less hypotensive than clonidine and it has a longer half-life (549).

Tricyclic antidepressants or selective serotonin reuptake inhibitors (e.g., fluoxetine, sertraline, and paroxetine) may assist in hyperactivity management, particularly in the presence of depressed affect (550–552). Lithium is an option when aggressive behavior is the outstanding feature of ADHD (258). Barbiturates, used for antiepileptic therapy, have a sedative effect and aggravate hyperactivity (553). When this occurs, nonbarbiturate antiepileptic drugs should gradually be substituted. Methylxanthines such as caffeine and theophylline do not appear to have adverse behavioral effects in children. They may even have a mild positive effect on some externalizing behaviors (554).

Nonspecific Nonmedical

Suggestions abound as to factors that might precipitate hyperactive behavior. These include fluorescent lighting, heavy metals, certain natural foods, notably sugar, and certain food additives, especially dyes. Food additives have been most vigorously propagandized and, therefore, most systematically studied (555).

Additive-free diets show little benefit in open clinical trials and even less in controlled studies. Although there is reliable evidence that an additive challenge in high dosage can impair learning in hyperactive children (556), an overview of available information suggests that restriction of additives is far less effective and less widely applicable than stimulant therapy (557,558). Nevertheless, it is occasionally worth trying. The most vigorous elimination diets appear to be the most successful (559,560). An effect of sugar in rendering children irritable and restless has been reported anecdotally and in open trials, but resists validation in controlled studies (561). A meta-analysis of 16 studies did not show an effect of sugar on children's behavior or cognition (562). The effects of sugar on brain function are complex and interact with whether a protein or carbohydrate meal preceded the challenge (563). A balance between factors promoting and opposing the availability of tryptophan as a serotonin substrate, carbohydrates versus amino acids, should be maintained. In contrast, megavitamin treatment and trace element replacement therapy are not supported by any acceptable evidence (564,565). There is no evidence that artificial sweeteners, such as aspartame, aggravate ADHD (566).

Behavioral Interventions

Short courses of supportive psychotherapy are often necessary for both the child and the child's family and can help to reduce intrafamily tensions that aggravate, or sometimes even precipitate, restless and impulsive behavior. A multimodality regime including intensive psychotherapy reduced the incidence of antisocial behavior in an ADHD cohort (567). For a detailed review of behavioral interventions, see Barkley (568).

Rational management of children who are not relieved of their disability by medication rests on individual attention, frequent and consistent reward of socially acceptable behavior, consistent limit setting, and the gradual phasing in of material to be learned. Although Doubros and Daniels found it possible to extinguish hyperactive behavior by operant conditioning (569), there is no evidence that this effect is lasting, that it generalizes, or that it is practicable to offer this labor-intensive individual management option to many of the large number of affected children. In general, behavior therapy should be an adjunct to effective stimulant therapy rather than the only treatment (570). Cognitive therapy is controversial (571,572), but parent training and school-based interventions may be effective (573–576). Children whose attentional, behavioral, or comorbid needs are not fully met by existing therapies are eligible for benefits under the Americans with Disabilities Act (577).

Prognosis

Whereas the overt restlessness of hyperactive children diminishes in adolescence, their impulsiveness and emotional lability usually persist, with a correspondingly mixed prognosis for long-term adaptive outcome (496). Long-term follow-up of children with ADHD shows an unfavorable outcome in many but not all (578,579). Adults who had ADHD in childhood often continue to

show functional impairment (580). When aggressiveness is a feature, it particularly tends to persist (581) and appears to bear some association with early onset alcoholism (582,583). Impulsive aggressiveness is associated with low concentration of the serotonin metabolite 5-HIAA in cerebrospinal fluid (584). Thus, the ADHD prognosis is intermediate between that of control patients and the more grave outlook for children with frank psychiatric disorder in childhood. Schizophrenia is not a major ADHD outcome. However, children of schizophrenic mothers, at high risk for adult schizophrenia, have been found to be prone to attentional dysfunction and poor social competence (585).

Attempts to relate the prognosis of ADHD to psychoactive drug therapy have been so poorly controlled as to be uninterpretable. In the medium term, stimulant therapy is clearly beneficial for educational progress, and even on a long-term basis, stimulant therapy continues to be effective in most adults in whom clinically diagnosable residual type ADHD persists.

REFERENCES

1. Bouchard TJ, et al. Sources of human psychological differences: the Minnesota study of twins reared apart. *Science* 1990;250:223–228.
2. Denckla MB. Development of motor coordination in normal children. *Dev Med Child Neurol* 1974;16: 729–741.
3. Mickelsen EJ, et al. Neurological status in hyperactive, enuretic, encopretic, and normal boys. *J Am Acad Child Adolesc Psychiatry* 1982;21:75–81.
4. Shafer SQ, et al. Ten-year consistency in neurological test performance of children without focal neurological deficits. *Dev Med Child Neurol* 1986;28:417–427.
5. Woods BT, Eby MD. Excessive mirror movements and aggression. *Biol Psychiatry* 1982;17:23–32.
6. Rutter M. Syndromes attributed to "minimal brain dysfunction" in childhood. *Am J Psychiatry* 1982; 139:21–33.
7. Kinsbourne M. Development of attention and metacognition. In: Rapin I, Segalowitz S, eds. *Handbook of neuropsychology.* Amsterdam: Elsevier Science, 1993;7: 261–278.
8. Wuu KD, et al. Chromosomal and biochemical screening of mentally retarded school children in Taiwan. *Japan J Hum Genet* 1991;36:267–274.
9. Majnemer A, Shevell MI. Diagnostic yield of the neurologic assessment of the developmentally delayed child. *J Pediatr* 1995;127:193–199.
10. Allen WP, Taylor H. Mental retardation in South Carolina. VII. Inborn errors of metabolism. *Proc Greenwood Genet Ctr* 1996;15:76–79.

11. Schaefer GB, Bodensteiner JB. Evaluation of the child with idiopathic mental retardation. *Pediatr Clin North Am* 1992;39:929–943.

12. Levy SE, Hyman SL. Pediatric assessment of the child with developmental delay. *Pediatr Clin North Am* 1993;40:465–477.

13. First LR, Palfrey JS. The infant or young child with developmental delay. *N Engl J Med* 1994;330:478–483.

14. Majnemer A, Shevell M. Neuroimaging studies in children with developmental delay [Letter]. *J Pediatr* 1995;128:302.

15. Cunningham RD. Neuroimaging studies in children with developmental delay [Letter]. *J Pediatr* 1995; 128:302.

16. Moeschler J. The use of the CT scan in the medical evaluation of the mentally retarded child. *J Pediatr* 1981;98:63–65.

17. Lingham S, Kendall BE. Computed tomography in non-specific mental retardation and idiopathic epilepsy. *Arch Dis Child* 1983;58:628–643.

18. Curry CJ, et al. Diagnostic yield of genetic evaluations in developmental delay/mental retardation. *Clin Res* 1996;44:130A.

19. Root S, Carey JC. *Brain dysmorphology and developmental disabilities.* Proceedings of the Annual DW Smith Workshop on Malformation and Morphogenesis, 1996.

20. Kjos BO, Umansky R, Barkovich AJ. Brain MR imaging in children with developmental retardation of unknown cause: results in 76 cases. *Am J Neuroradiol* 1990;11:1035–1040.

21. O'Tuama LA, et al. Functional brain imaging in neuropsychiatric disorders of childhood. *J Child Neurol* 1999;14:207–221.

22. Filipek PA, et al. Volumetric MRI analysis comparing subjects having attention-deficit hyperactivity disorder with normal controls. *Neurology* 1997;48: 589–601.

23. Prensky AL. An approach to the child with paroxysmal phenomena with emphasis on nonepileptic disorders. In: Dodson WE, Pellock JM, eds. *Pediatric epilepsy: diagnosis and therapy.* New York: Demos Publications, 1993.

24. Coplan J, Gleason JR. Quantifying language development from birth to 3 years using the Early Language Milestone scale. *Pediatrics* 1990;86: 963–971.

25. Frankenburg WK, et al. The Denver II: a major revision and restandardization of the Denver Developmental Screening test. *Pediatrics* 1992;89:91–97.

26. Bayley N. *Bayley scales of infant development.* San Antonio, TX: The Psychological Corporation, 1990.

27. Bayley N. *Bayley scales of infant development.* San Antonio, TX: The Psychological Corporation, 1993.

28. Wechsler D. *Wechsler preschool and primary scale of intelligence—revised.* New York: The Psychological Corporation, 1989.

29. Wechsler D. *Wechsler intelligence scale for children—III.* New York:Psychological Corporation, 1991.

30. Thorndike RL, Hagen EP, Samer JM. *Guide for administering and scoring the Stanford-Binet Intelligence Scale,* 4th ed. Chicago: Riverside Publishing, 1986.

31. Goodenough FL, Harris DB. *Manual of the Goodenough-Harris drawing test.* San Antonio: The Psychological Corporation, 1963.

32. Kaufman AS, Kaufman NL. *Kaufman assessment battery for children.* Circle Pines, NM: American Guidance Services, 1983.

33. McCarthy D. *Manual of the McCarthy scales of children's disabilities.* San Antonio: The Psychological Corporation, 1972.

34. Leiter RG. *The Leiter International Performance scale.* California: Western Psychological Services, 1969.

35. Achenbach TM. *Manual for the child behavior checklist/2-3 and 1992 profile.* Burlington, VT: University of Vermont Department of Psychiatry, 1992.

36. Conners CK. *Manual for Conners rating scales.* North Tonawanda, NY: Multi-Health Systems, 1989.

37. Newborg J, Stock JR, Wnek L. *Batelle developmental inventory.* Allen, TX: DLM Teaching Resources, 1984.

38. Sparrow SS, Balla DA, Ciccheui DV. *Vineland adaptive behavior scales.* Circle Pines, MN: American Guidance Services, 1985.

39. Wilkinson GS. *The wide range achievement test—revision 3, administration manual.* Wilmington, DE: Wide Range, 1993.

40. Woodcock RW, Mather N. *Woodcock-Johnson tests of achievement.* Allen, TX: DLM Teaching Resources, 1989.

41. Dunn LM, Dunn LM. *Peabody picture vocabulary test—revised.* Circle Pines, MN: American Guidance Service, 1981.

42. Beery KE. *The developmental test of visual-motor integration,* 3rd revision. Cleveland: Modern Curriculum Press, 1989.

43. McQuaid F, Alovisetti M. School psychological services for hearing-impaired children in New York and the New England area. *Am Ann Deaf* 1981;126: 37–43.

44. Davis CJ. *Perkins-Binet test of intelligence for the blind.* Watertown, MA: Perkins School for the Blind, 1980.

45. Newland TE. The blind learning aptitude test. *J Vis Impair Blind* 1979;73:134–139.

46. Petersen MC, Kube DA, Palmer FB. Classification of developmental delays. *Semin Pediatr Neurol* 1998; 5:2–14.

47. American Association on Mental Retardation. *Mental retardation: definition, classification, and systems of support,* 9th edition. Washington, DC: American Association on Mental Retardation, 1992.

48. World Health Organization. *The ICD-10: classification of mental and behavioural disorders: clinical descriptions and diagnostic guidelines.* Geneva: World Health Organization, 1992.

49. American Psychiatric Association. *Diagnostic criteria from DSM-IV: diagnostic and statistical manual of mental disorders.* Washington, DC: American Psychiatric Association, 1994:63–66.

50. Grossman H. *Manual on terminology and classification in mental retardation.* Washington, DC: American Association of Mental Retardation, 1973.

51. Reschly JD. Mental retardation: conceptual foundations, definitional criteria, and diagnostic operations. In: Hooper SR, Hynd GH, Mattison RE, eds. *Developmental disorders: diagnostic criteria and clinical assessment.* Hillsdale, NJ: Lawrence Erlbaum Associates, 1992:23–67.

52. Luckasson R, et al. *Mental retardation: definition, classification, and systems of support.* Washington,

DC: American Association on Mental Retardation, 1992.

53. Prior M, et al. Autistic children's knowledge of thinking and feeling states in other people. *J Child Psychol Psychiatry* 1990;31:587–602.

54. Udwin O. A survey of adults with Williams syndrome and idiopathic infantile hypercalcemia. *Dev Med Child Neurol* 1990;32:129–136.

55. Dykens EM, et al. Profiles and development of adaptive behavior in children with Down syndrome. *Am J Ment Retard* 1994;98:580–587.

56. Dennis M, et al. The content of narrative discourse in children and adolescents after early-onset hydrocephalus and in normally developing age peers. *Brain Lang* 1994;46:129–165.

57. Wiesniewski KF, et al. Fragile-X syndrome: associated neurological abnormality and developmental disabilities. *Ann Neurol* 1985;18:665–669.

58. Pennington B, et al. Language and cognitive development in 47 XXX females followed since birth. *Behav Genet* 1980;10:31–41.

59. Rovet JF. The psychoeducational characteristics of children with Turner's syndrome. *J Learn Disabil* 1993;26:333–341.

60. Welsh MC, et al. Neuropsychology of early-treated phenylketonuria: specific executive function deficits. *Child Dev* 1990;61:1697–1713.

61. Rutter M, Graham P, Yule W. A neuropsychiatric study in childhood. *Clin Dev Med* 1970;35/36:1–272.

62. Borthwick-Duffy SA. Epidemiology and prevalence of psychopathology in people with mental retardation. *J Consult Clin Psychol* 1994;62:17–27.

63. Bregman JD. Current developments in the understanding of mental retardation: Part II. Psychopathology. *J Am Acad Child Adolesc Psychiatry* 1991;30:861–872.

64. Crews WDJ, Bonaventura S, Rowe F. Dual diagnosis: prevalence of psychiatric disorders in a large state residential facility for individuals with mental retardation. *Am J Ment Retard* 1994;98:724–731.

65. Gillberg C, et al. Psychiatric disorders in mildly and severely mentally retarded urban children and adolescents: epidemiological aspects. *Br J Psychiatry* 1986; 149:68–74.

66. Matson JL, Barrett RP, Helsel WJ. Depression in mentally retarded children. *Res Dev Disabil* 1988; 9:39–46.

67. Dawson JE, Matson JL, Cherry KE. An analysis of maladaptive behaviors in persons with autism, PDD-NOS, and mental retardation. *Res Dev Disabil* 1998;19:439–448.

68. Gath H, Gumley D. Behavior problems in retarded children with special reference to Down syndrome. *Br J Psychiatry* 1986;149:156–161.

69. Matson JL, et al. Characteristics of stereotypic movement disorder and self-injurious behavior assessed with the Diagnostic Assessment for the Severely Handicapped (DASH-II). *Res Dev Disabil* 1997;18:457–469.

70. Buitelaar JK. Self-injurious behavior in retarded children: clinical phenomena and biological mechanisms. *Acta Paedopsychiatrica* 1993;56:105–111.

71. Carr KG, Smith CE. Biological setting events for self-injury. *MRDD Research Reviews* 1995;1.

72. Anderson LT, Ernst M. Self-injury in Lesch-Nyhan syndrome. *J Autism Dev Disord* 1994;24:67–81.

73. Matthews WS, Solan A, Barabas G. Cognitive functioning in Lesch-Nyhan syndrome. *Dev Med Child Neurol* 1995;37:715–722.

74. Whitman BY, Accardo P. Emotional symptoms in Prader-Willi syndrome adolescents. *Am J Med Genet* 1987;28:897–905.

75. Curfs LM, Fryos JP. Prader-Willi syndrome: a review with special attention to the cognitive and behavioral profile. *Birth Defects: Original Article Series* 1992;28: 99–104.

76. Hagberg B. Rett syndrome: clinical peculiarities and biological mysteries. *Acta Paediatrica* 1995;84:971–976.

77. Papolos DF, Faedda GL, Veit S, et al. Bipolar spectrum disorders in patients diagnosed with velo-cardiofacial syndrome: does a hemizygous deletion of chromosome 22q11 result in bipolar affective disorder? *Am J Psychiatry* 1996;153:1541–1547.

78. Motzkin B, et al. Variable phenotypes in velocardiofacial syndrome with chromosomal deletion. *J Pediatr* 1993;123:406–410.

79. Udwin O, Yule W. Expressive language of children with Williams syndrome. *Am J Med Genet* 1990;6:108–114.

80. Rossen ML, Samat HB. Why should neurologists be interested in Williams syndrome? [Editorial] *Neurology* 1998;5:8–9.

81. Kushlik A, Blunden R. The epidemiology of mental subnormality. In: Clarke AM, Clarke AD, eds. *Mental deficiency: the changing outlook.* London: Methuen, 1974;31–81.

82. Down syndrome prevalence at birth: United States 1983–1990. *MMWR Morb Mortal Wkly Rep* 1994; 43:617–622.

83. Steele J, Stratford B. The United Kingdom population with Down syndrome: present and future projections. *Am J Ment Retard* 1995;99:664–682.

84. Strømme P, Valvatne K. Mental retardation in Norway: prevalence and sub-classification in a cohort of 30,037 children born between 1980 and 1985. *Acta Paediatr* 1998;87:291–296.

85. Hagberg B, et al. Mild mental retardation in Swedish school children. II. Etiologic and pathogenetic aspects. *Acta Paediatr Scand* 1981;70:445–452.

86. Murphy CC, et al. The administrative prevalence of mental retardation in 10-year-old children in Atlanta, 1985 through 1987. *Am J Public Health* 1995;85: 319–323.

87. Brett EM, Goodman R. Mental retardation, infantile autism, and related disorders. In: Brett EM, ed. *Paediatric neurology.* London: Churchill Livingstone, 1997:406–423.

88. McLaren J, Bryson SE. Review of recent epidemiological studies of mental retardation: prevalence, associated disorders, and etiology. *Am J Ment Retard* 1987;92:243–254.

89. Eyman RK, et al. The life expectancy of profoundly handicapped people with mental retardation. *N Engl J Med* 1990;323:584–589.

90. Eyman RK, et al. Survival of profoundly disabled people with severe mental retardation. *Am J Dis Child* 1993;147:329–336.

91. Gustavson KH, et al. Severe mental retardation in a Swedish county. II. Etiologic and pathogenetic aspects of children born 1959–1970. *Neuropaediatrie* 1977;8:293–304.

92. Nelson KB. What proportion of cerebral palsy is related to birth asphyxia? *J Pediatr* 1988;112:572–573.

93. Gaffney G, et al. Case-control study of intrapartum care, cerebral palsy, and perinatal death. *BMJ* 1994;308:743–750.

94. Torfs CP, et al. Prenatal and perinatal factors in the etiology of cerebral palsy. *J Pediatr* 1990;116:615–619.

95. Rantakallio P, von Wendt L. Risk factors for mental retardation. *Arch Dis Child* 1985;60:946–952.

96. Laxova R, Ridler MAC. An etiologic survey of the severely retarded Hertfordshire children who were born between January 1, 1965 and December 31, 1967. *Am J Med Genet* 1977;1:75–86.

97. Opitz JM, et al. *The diagnosis and prevention of severe mental retardation*. Cairo: Proceedings, International Conference on Preventable Aspects of Genetic Morbidity, 1982, Vol ll.

98. Fryns JP, et al. A genetic diagnostic survey in an institutionalized population of 173 severely mentally retarded patients. *Clin Genet* 1986;30: 315–323.

99. McQueen PC, et al. Causal origins of major mental handicap in the Canadian mountain provinces. *Dev Med Child Neurol* 1986;28:697–707.

100. Wellesley D, Hockey A, Stenely F. The aetiology of intellectual disability in Westem Australia: a community-based study. *Dev Med Child Neurol* 1991;33: 963–973.

101. Yeargin-Allsopp M, et al. Reported biomedical causes and associated medical conditions for mental retardation among 10-year-old children, metropolitan Atlanta, 1985 to 1987. *Dev Med Child Neurol* 1997;39:142–149.

102. Flint J, Wilkie AO. The genetics of mental retardation. *Br Med Bull* 1996;52:453–464.

103. Schroeder SR, et al. Separating the effects of lead and social factors on IQ. *Environmental Res* 1985;38: 144–154.

104. Needleman HL, et al. Bone lead levels and delinquent behavior. *JAMA* 1996;275:363–369.

105. Pocock SJ, Smith M, Baghurst P. Environmental lead and children's intelligence: a systematic review of the epidemiological literature. *BMJ* 1994;309:1189.

106. Bakir F, et al. Clinical and epidemiological aspects of methylmercury poisoning. *Postgrad Med J* 1980;56: 1–10.

107. Davis LE, et al. Methylmercury poisoning: long-term clinical, radiological, toxicological, and pathological studies of an affected family. *Ann Neurol* 1994;35: 680–688.

108. Myers GJ, Davidson PW. Prenatal methylmercury exposure and children: neurologic, developmental, and behavioral research. *Environ Health Perspect* 1998;3:841–847.

109. Lozoff B. Nutrition and behavior *Am Psychol* 1989; 44:231–236.

110. Bronfenbrenner U, et al. *The state of Americans.* New York: The Free Press, 1996.

111. Kiely M. The prevalence of mental retardation. *Epidemiol Rev* 1987;9:194–228.

112. Roeleveld N, Zielhuis GA, Gabreels F. The prevalence of mental retardation: a critical review of recent literature. *Dev Med Child Neurol* 1997;39: 125–132.

113. Patterson CJ, Kupersmidt JB, Vaden NA. Income level, gender, ethnicity, and household composition as predictors of children's school-based competence. *Child Dev* 1990;61:485–494.

114. Aber JL, et al. The effects of poverty on child health and development. *Annu Rev Public Health* 1997;18: 463–483.

115. Ramer JC, Miller G. Overview of mental retardation. In: Miller G, Ramer JC, eds. *Static encephalopathies of infancy and childhood.* New York: Raven Press, 1992:1–10.

116. Spitz RA. Hospitalism. *Psychoanal Stud Child* 1945;1:53–74.

117. Haddow JE, et al. Maternal thyroid deficiency during pregnancy and subsequent neuropsychological development of the child. *N Engl J Med* 1999;341: 549–555.

118. Kovacs M, Goldston D, Iyengar S. Intellectual development and academic performance of children with insulin-dependent diabetes mellitus: a longitudinal study. *Dev Psychol* 1992;28:676–684.

119. Miller RW. Delayed radiation effects in atomic bomb survivors. *Science* 1969;166:569–574.

120. Dekaban AS. Abnormalities in children exposed to x-radiation and during various stages of gestation: tentative timetable of radiation injury to the human fetus, Part I. *J Nucl Med* 1968;9:471–477.

121. Uchida IA, Holunga R, Lawler C. Maternal radiation and chromosomal aberrations. *Lancet* 1968;2: 1045–1049.

122. Aman MG, et al. Fenfluramine and methylphenidate in children with mental retardation and ADHD: clinical and side effects. *J Am Acad Child Adolesc Psychiatry* 1993;32:851–859.

123. Campbell M, Cueva JE. Psychopharmacology in child and adolescent psychiatry: a review of the past seven years, Part I. *J Am Acad Child Adolesc Psychiatry* 1995;34:1124–1132.

124. Herman BH, et al. Naltrexone decreases self-injurious behavior. *Ann Neurol* 1987;22:550–552.

125. Barnes TR. Tardive dyskinesia. *BMJ* 1988;296: 150–151.

126. Swanson JM, et al. Tardive dyskinesia in a developmentally disabled population: manifestation during the initial stage of a minimal effective-dose program. *Exp Clin Psychopharmacol* 1996;4:1–6.

127. Ottenbacher K, Petersen P. The efficacy of early intervention programs for children with organic handicaps. *Evaluation & Program Planning* 1985;8:135.

128. Lott IT, Touchette P. Neurobehavioral treatment of severe chronic self-mutilation. *Ann Neurol* 1980;8:221.

129. Rapin I, Katzman R. Neurobiology of autism. *Ann Neurol* 1998;43:7–14.

130. Wing L. The autistic spectrum. *Lancet* 1997;350: 1761–1766.

131. American Psychiatric Association. Pervasive developmental disorders, 4th ed. In: *Diagnostic and statistical manual of mental disorders.* Washington, DC: American Psychiatric Association, 1994:65–78.

132. Kanner L. Autistic disturbances of affective contact. *Nervous Child* 1943;2:217–250.

133. Gillberg C. Infantile autism and other childhood psychoses in a Swedish urban region: epidemiological aspects. *J Child Psychol Psychiatry* 1984;25:35–43.

134. Tuchman RF, Rapin I. Regression in pervasive developmental disorders: seizures and epileptiform encephalogram correlates. *Pediatrics* 1997;99:560–566.

135. Baron-Cohen S, et al. Psychological markers in the detection of autism in infancy in a large population. *Br J Psychiatry* 1996;168:158–163.

136. Osterling J, Dawson G. Early recognition of children with autism: a study of first birthday home video tapes. *J Autism Dev Disord* 1994;24:247–257.

137. Bauman ML. Motor dysfunction in autism. In: Joseph AB, Young RR, eds. *Movement disorders in neurology and neuropsychiatry*. Boston: Blackwell Science, 1992:658–661.

138. Lovaas O, Koegel R, Schreibman L. Stimulus overselectivity in autism: a review of research. *Psychol Bull* 1979;86:1236–1254.

139. Smith IM, Bryson SE. Imitation in autism. *Cognitive neuropsychology* 1998;15:747–771.

140. Tuchman RF, Rapin I, Shinnar S. Autistic and dysphasic children: clinical characteristics. *Pediatrics* 1991;88:1211–1218.

141. Rapin I, Dunn M. Language disorders in children with autism. *Semin Pediatr Neurol* 1997;4:86–92.

142. Tirosh E, Canby J. Autism with hyperlexia: a distinct syndrome? *Am J Ment Retard* 1993;98:84–92.

143. Kinsbourne M. Overfocusing an apparent subtype of attention-deficit hyperactivity disorder. In: Amir N, Rapin I, Branski D, eds. *Pediatric neurology: behavior and cognition of the child with brain dysfunction*. Basel: Karger, 1991:18–35.

144. Volkmar FR. The disintegrative disorders: childhood disintegrative disorder and Rett's disorder. In: Volkmar FR, ed. *Psychoses and pervasive developmental disorders in childhood and adolescence*. Washington, DC: American Psychiatric Press, 1996:223–248.

145. Wing L. Asperger's syndrome: a clinical account. *Psych Rev* 1981;11:115–129.

146. Baltaxe CAM, Simmons JQI. A comparison of language issues in high-functioning autism and related disorders with onset in childhood and adolescence. In: Schopler E, Mesibov GB, eds. *High-functioning individuals with autism*. New York: Plenum Publishing, 1991:201–225.

147. Rumsey JM, Hamburger SD. Neuropsychological findings in high-functioning men with infantile autism, residual state. *J Clin Exp Neuropsychol* 1988;10:201–222.

148. Rogers SJ, DiLalla DL. Age of symptom onset in young children with pervasive developmental disorders. *J Am Acad Child Adolesc Psychiatry* 1990;29:863–872.

149. Wing L. The definition and prevalence of autism: a review. *Eur Child Adol Psychiatry* 1993;2:61–74.

150. Wing L. Autistic spectrum disorders: no evidence for or against an increase in prevalence. *BMJ* 1996;312:327–328.

151. Fombonne E. Epidemiological studies of autism. In: Volkmar F, ed. *Autism and developmental disorders*. New York: Cambridge University Press, 1998.

152. Wing L, Gould J. Severe impairments of social interaction and associated abnormalities in children: epidemiology and classification. *J Autism Dev Disord* 1979;9:11–29.

153. Ehlers S, Gillberg C. The epidemiology of Asperger's syndrome: a total population study. *J Child Psychol Psychiatry* 1993;34:1327–1350.

154. Honda H, et al. Cumulative incidence and prevalence of childhood autism in children in Japan. *Br J Psychiatry* 1996;169:228–235.

155. Webb EVJ, et al. The changing prevalence of autistic disorder in a Welsh health district. *Dev Med Child Neurol* 1997;39:150–152.

155a. Department of Developmental Services: Report to the Legislature. Changes in the population of persons with autism and pervasive developmental disorder in California's Developmental Services System: 1987 through 1988. California Health and Human Services Agency, March 1, 1999, 1–19.

156. Wakefield AJ, et al. Ileal-lymphoid-nodular hyperplasia, non-specific colitis, and pervasive developmental disorder in children. *Lancet* 1998;351:637–641.

157. Chen RT, DeStefano F. Vaccine adverse events: causal or coincidental? *Lancet* 1998;351:611–612.

158. Lee JW, et al. Autism, inflammatory bowel disease, and MMR vaccine. *Lancet* 1998;351:905.

159. Taylor B, et al. Autism and measles, mumps, and rubella vaccine: no epidemiological evidence for a causal association. *Lancet* 1999;353:2026–2029.

160. Bettelheim B. *The empty fortress: infantile autism and the birth of the self*. New York: Free Press, 1967.

161. Ritvo ER, et al. The UCLA-University of Utah epidemiologic survey of autism: recurrence risk estimates and genetic counseling. *Am J Psychiatry* 1989;146:1032–1036.

162. Bailey A, et al. Autism as a strongly genetic disorder: evidence from a British twin study. *Psychol Med* 1995;25:63–77.

163. Wolff S, Narayan S, Moyes B. Personality characteristics of parents of autistic children: a controlled study. *J Child Psychol Psychiatry* 1988;29:143–153.

164. Rapin I. Autism in search of a home in the brain. *Neurology* 1999;52:902–904.

165. DeLong GR. Autism: new data suggest a new hypothesis. *Neurology* 1999;52:911–916.

166. Minshew NJ, Luna B, Sweeney JA. Oculomotor evidence for neocortical systems but not cerebellar dysfunction in autism. *Neurology* 1999;52:917–922.

167. Courchesne E, Townsend J, Saitoh O. The brain in infantile autism: posterior fossa structures are abnormal. *Neurology* 1994;44:214–223.

168. Kinsboume M. Cerebral-brain stem relations in infantile autism. In: Schopler E, Mesibov GB, eds. *Neurobiological issues in autism*. New York: Plenum Publishing, 1987:107–125.

169. Bailey A, et al. A clinicopathological study of autism. *Brain* 1998;121:889–905.

170. DeLong GR, Bean SC, Brown FR. Acquired reversible autistic syndrome in acute encephalopathic illness in children. *Arch Neurol* 1981;38:191–194.

171. Hagberg B, et al. A progressive syndrome of autism, dementia, ataxia, and loss of purposeful hand use in girls: Rett syndrome. Report of 35 cases. *Ann Neurol* 1983;14:471–479.

172. Lord C, et al. Pre- and perinatal factors in high-functioning females and males with autism. *J Autism Dev Disord* 1991;21:197–209.

173. Dunn HG, ed. Sequelae of low-birth-weight: The Vancouver Study. *Clin Dev Med* 1986;95/96.

174. Gillberg C, Coleman M. Autism and medical disorders: a review of the literature. *Dev Med Child Neurol* 1996;38:191–202.

175. Folstein SE, Rutter ML. Infantile autism: a genetic study of 21 twin pairs. *J Child Psychol Psychiatry* 1977;18:297–321.

176. Gillberg C, Gillberg IC. Infantile autism: a total population study of reduced optimality in the pre-, peri-, and neonatal period. *J Autism Dev Disord* 1983;13:153–166.

177. Tsai LY, Stewart MA. Etiological implication of maternal age and birth order in infantile autism. *J Autism Dev Disord* 1983;13:57–65.

178. Bryson SE, Smith IM, Eastwood D. Obstetrical suboptimality in autistic children. *J Am Acad Child Adolesc Psychiatry* 1988;27:418–422.

179. Mason-Brothers A, et al. The UCLA-University of Utah epidemiologic survey of autism: prenatal, perinatal, and postnatal factors. *Pediatrics* 1990;86:514–519.

180. Steffenberg S, Gillberg C. Autism and autistic-like conditions in Swedish rural and urban areas: a population study. *Br J Psychiatry* 1986;149:81–87.

181. Bolton P, Macdonald H, Pickles A, et al. A case-control family history study of autism. *J Child Psychol Psychiatry* 1994;35:877–900.

182. Ritvo ER, et al. Concordance for the syndrome of autism in 40 pairs of afflicted twins. *Am J Psychiatry* 1985;142:74–77.

183. Steffenberg S, Gillberg C, Holmgren L. A twin study of autism in Denmark, Finland, Iceland, Norway, and Sweden. *J Child Psychol Psychiatry* 1989;30: 405–416.

184. Piven J, et al. A family history study of neuropsychiatric disorders in the adult siblings of autistic individuals. *J Am Acad Child Adolesc Psychiatry* 1990;29: 177–183.

185. Gillberg C, Gillberg IC, Steffenburg S. Siblings and parents of children with autism: a controlled population-based study. *Dev Med Child Neurol* 1992;34: 389–398.

186. Philippe A, et al. Genome-wide scan for autism susceptibility genes. Paris Autism Research International Sibpair Study. *Hum Mol Genet* 1999;8: 805–812.

187. Ritvo ER, Mason-Brothers A, Freeman BJ, et al. The UCLA-University of Utah epidemiologic survey of autism: the etiologic role of rare diseases. *Am J Psychiatry* 1990;147:1614–1621.

188. Schroer RJ, et al. Autism and maternally derived aberrations of chromosome 15q. *Am J Med Genet* 1998;76:327–333.

189. Reiss AL, et al. Autism associated with Williams syndrome. *J Pediatrics* 1985;106:247–249.

190. Gillberg C, Rasmussen P. Brief report: four case histories and a literature review of Williams syndrome and autistic behavior. *J Autism Dev Disord* 1994;24:381–393.

191. Bundey S, et al. Duplication of the 15q11-13 region in a patient with autism, epilepsy, and ataxia. *Dev Med Child Neurol* 1994;36:736–742.

192. Gurrieri F, et al. Pervasive developmental disorder and epilepsy due to maternally derived duplication of 15q11-q13. *Neurology* 1999;52:1694–1697.

193. Graf WD, et al. Autistic regression associated with a mutation in the mitochondrial tRNAlys gene (G8363A). *Ann Neurol* 1998;44:578.

194. Rogers SJ, Newhart-Larson S. Characteristics of infantile autism in five children with Leber's congenital amaurosis. *Dev Med Child Neurol* 1989;31: 598–608.

195. McKusick VA. *Mendelian inheritance in man: catalogs of autosomal dominant, autosomal recessive, and X-linked phenotypes.* Baltimore: The Johns Hopkins University Press, 1992:1893–1894.

196. Reiss AL, Freund L. The behavioral phenotype of fragile X syndrome: DSM-111-R autistic behavior in males. *Am J Med Genet* 1992;43:35–46.

197. Singh VK, et al. Immunodiagnosis and immunotherapy in autistic children. *Ann N Y Acad Sci* 1988;540: 602–604.

198. Zimmerman A, Frye V, Potter N. Immunological aspects of autism. *Int Pediatr* 1993;8:199–204.

199. Todd RD, et al. Antibrain antibodies in infantile autism. *Biol Psychiatry* 1988;23:644–647.

200. Chess S. Autism in children with congenital rubella. *J Autism Child Schizophr* 1971;1:33–47.

201. Ivarsson SA, et al. Autism as one of several disabilities in two children with congenital cytomegalovirus infection. *Neuropediatrics* 1990;21:102–103.

202. Lowe TL, et al. Detection of phenylketonuria in autistic and psychotic children. *JAMA* 1980;243:126–128.

203. Rutter M, Bartak L. Causes of infantile autism: some considerations from recent research. *J Autism Child Schizophr* 1971;1:20–32.

204. Kotsopoulos S, Kutty KM. Histidinemia and infantile autism. *J Autism Dev Disord* 1979;9:55–60.

205. Gillberg I, Gillberg C, Kopp S. Hypothyroidism and autism spectrum disorders. *J Child Psychol Psychiatry* 1992;33:531–542.

206. Courchesne E, et al. Hypoplasia of cerebellar lobules VI and VII in infantile autism. *N Engl J Med* 1988;318: 1349–1354.

207. Murakami JW, et al. Reduced cerebellar hemisphere size and its relationship to vermal hypoplasia in autism. *Arch Neurol* 1989;46:689–694.

208. Holttum JR, et al. Magnetic resonance imaging of the posterior fossa in autism. *Biol Psychiatry* 1992;32: 1091–1101.

209. Kleiman MD, Neff S, Rosman NP. The brain in infantile autism: are posterior fossa structures abnormal? *Neurology* 1992;42:753–760.

210. Garber HJ, Ritvo ER. Magnetic resonance imaging of the posterior fossa in autistic adults. *Am J Psychiatry* 1992;149:245–247.

211. Piven J, et al. An MRI study of autism: the cerebellum revisited. *Neurology* 1997;49:546–551.

212. Kemper TL, Bauman M. Neuropathology of infantile autism. *J Neuropathol Exp Neurol* 1998;57:645–652.

213. Piven J, et al. Magnetic resonance imaging evidence for a defect of cerebral cortical development in autism. *Am J Psychiatry* 1990;147:734–739.

214. Bauman M, Kemper T. Neuroanatomic observations of the brain in autism. In: Bauman M, Kemper T, eds. *The neurobiology of autism.* Baltimore: The Johns Hopkins University Press,1994:119–145.

215. Horwitz B, et al. Interregional correlations of glucose utilization among brain regions in autistic adults. *Ann Neurol* 1987;22:118.

216. Jacobson R, et al. Selective subcortical abnormalities in autism. *Psychol Med* 1988;18:39–48.

217. Prior MR, et al. Computed tomographic study of children with classic autism. *Arch Neurol* 1984;41.

218. Creasey H, et al. Brain morphometry in autistic men as measured by volumetric computed tomography. *Arch Neurol* 1986;43:669–672.

219. Fombonne E, et al. Microcephaly and macrocephaly in autism. *J Autism Dev Disord* 1999;29:113–119.

220. Minshew NJ. Indices of neural function in autism: clinical and biologic implications. *Pediatrics* 1991;87: 774–780.

221. Tuchman RF, Rapin I, Shinnar S. Autistic and dysphasic children. II. Epilepsy. *Pediatrics* 1991;88: 1219–1225.

222. Bauman ML, Kemper TL. Abnormal cerebellar circuitry in autism? *Neurology* 1989;39:186.

223. Gaffney GR, et al. Morphological evidence of brain stem involvement in infantile autism. *Biol Psychiatry* 1988;24:578–586.

224. Hsu M, et al. Absence of magnetic resonance imaging evidence of pontine abnormalities in infantile autism. *Arch Neurol* 1991;48:1160–1163.

225. Anderson GM, et al. Whole blood serotonin in autistic and normal subjects. *J Child Psychol Psychiatry* 1987;28:885–900.

226. McDougle CJ, et al. Acute tryptophan depletion in autistic disorder: a controlled case study. *Biol Psychiatry* 1993;33:547–550.

227. Cook EH, Leventhal BL. The serotonin system in autism. *Curr Opin Pediatr* 1996;8:348–354.

228. Chugani DC, et al. Altered serotonin synthesis in the dentatothalamocortical pathway in autistic boys. *Ann Neurol* 1997;42:666–669.

229. Gillberg C, Svennerholm L. CSF monoamines in autistic syndromes and other pervasive developmental disorders of early childhood. *Br J Psychiatry* 1987;151:89–94.

230. Ross DL, Klykylo WM, Anderson GM. Cerebrospinal fluid indoleamine and monoamine effects in fenfluramine treatment of autism. *Ann Neurol* 1985;18:394.

231. Narayan M, et al. Cerebrospinal fluid levels of homovanillic acid and 5-hydroxyindoleacetic acid in autism. *Biol Psychiatry* 1993;33:630–6435.

232. Lake CR, Ziegler MG, Murphy DL. Increased norepinephrine levels and decreased dopamine-beta-hydroxylase activity in primary autism. *Arch Gen Psychiatry* 1977;34:553–556.

233. Leventhal BL, et al. Relationships of whole blood serotonin and plasma norepinephrine within families of autistic children. *J Autism Dev Disord* 1990;20: 499–511.

234. Minderaa RB, et al. Noradrenergic and adrenergic functioning in autism. *Biol Psychiatry* 1994;36:237–241.

235. Kalat JW. Speculation on similarities between autism and opiate addiction. *J Autism Child Schizophr* 1978;8:477–479.

236. Ross DL, Klykylo WM, Hitzemann R. Reduction of elevated CSF beta-endorphin by fenfluramine in infantile autism. *Pediatr Neurol* 1987;3:83–86.

237. Coid J, Allolio B, Rees LH. Raised plasma metenkephalin in patients who habitually mutilate themselves. *Lancet* 1983;2:545–546.

238. Herman B. A possible role of proopiomelanocortin peptides in self-injurious behavior. *Prog Neuropsychopharmacol Biol Psychiatry* 1990; 14[Suppl]: S109–139.

239. Gillberg C. Endogenous opioids and opiate antagonists in autism: brief review of empirical findings and implications for clinicians. *Dev Med Child Neurol* 1995;37:239–245.

240. D'Eufemia P, et al. Abnormal intestinal permeability in children with autism. *Acta Pediatr* 1996;85: 1076–1079.

241. Ivarsson SA, et al. Autism as one of several disabilities in two children with congenital cytornegalovirus infection. *Neuropediatrics* 1990;21: 102–103.

242. Ritvo ER, et al. The UCLA-University of Utah epidemiological survey of autism: the etiologic role of rare diseases. *Am J Psychiatry* 1990;147: 1614–1621.

243. Desmond MM, et al. Congenital rubella encephalitis. *J Pediatr* 71;71:311–331.

244. Nanson JL. Autism in fetal alcohol syndrome: a report of six cases. *Alcohol Clin Exp Res* 1992;16:558–565.

245. Davis E, et al. Autism and developmental disabilities in children with perinatal cocaine exposure. *J Natl Med Assoc* 1992;84:315–319.

246. Stromland K, et al. Autism in thalidomide embryopathy: a population study. *Dev Med Child Neurol* 1994;36: 351–356.

247. Christianson AL, Chesler N, Kromberg JGR. Fetal valproate syndrome: clinical and neurodevelopmental features in two sibling pairs. *Dev Med Child Neurol* 1994;36:357–369.

247a. Horvath K, et al. Gastrointestinal abnormalities in children with autistic disorder. *J Pediatr* 1999;135: 559–563.

247b. Montgomery SM, et al. Paramyxovirus infections in childhood and subsequent inflammatory bowel disease. *Gastroenterology* 1999;116:796–803.

247c. Prior M, et al. Are there subgroups within the autistic spectrum? A cluster analysis of a group of children with autistic spectrum disorders. *J Child Psychol Psychiatry* 1998;39:893–902.

248. Heller T. Dementia infantilis. Zeitschrift für die Erforschung und Behandlung des Jugendlichen Schwachsinns 1908;2:141–165.

249. Prior M, et al. Are there subgroups within the autistic spectrum? A cluster analysis of a group of children with autistic spectrum disorders? *J Child Psychol Psychiatry* 1998;39:893–902.

250. Bartak L, Rutter M, Cox A. A comparative study of infantile autism and specific developmental receptive language disorder. I. The children. *Br J Psychiatry* 1975;126:127–145.

251. Plioplys AV. Autism: electroencephalogram abnormalities and clinical improvement with valproic acid. *Arch Pediatr Adolesc Med* 1994;148:220–222.

252. Stefanotos GA, Grover W, Geller E. Case study: corticosteroid treatment of language regression in pervasive developmental disorder. *J Am Acad Child Adolesc Psychiatry* 1995;34:1107–1111.

253. Lewine JD, et al. Magnetoencephalographic patterns of epileptic form activity in children with regressive autism spectrum disorders. *Pediatrics* 1999;104: 405–418.

254. DeLong GR, Teague LA, McSwain-Kamran M. Effects of fluoxetine treatment in young children with idiopathic autism: a case series. *Dev Med Child Neurol* 1998;40:551–562.

255. Nicholson R, Awad G, Sloman L. An open trial of risperidone in young autistic children. *J Am Acad Child Adolesc Psychiatry* 1998;37:372–376.

256. Fankhauser MP, Karumanchi VC, German ML, Yates A, Karumanchi SD. A double-blind, placebo-controlled study of the efficacy of transdermal clonidine in autism. *J Clin Psychiatry* 1992;53:77–82.

257. Cohen DJ, Volkmar FR. *Autism and pervasive developmental disorders: a handbook.* New York: John Wiley, 1997.

258. DeLong GR. Lithium carbonate treatment of select behavior disorders in children suggesting manic-depressive illness. *J Pediatr* 1978;93:689–694.

259. Birmaher B, Quintana H, Greenhill L. Methylphenidate for the treatment of hyperactive autistic children. *J Am Acad Child Adolesc Psychiatry* 1988;27:248–251.

260. Raiten DJ, Massaro T. Perspectives on the nutritional ecology of autistic children. *J Autism Dev Disord* 1986;16:133–144.

261. Pfeffler SI, et al. Efficacy of vitamin B6 and magnesium in the treatment of autism: a methodology review and summary of outcomes. *J Autism Dev Disord* 1995;25:481–494.

262. Howlin P. *Children with autism and Asperger's syndrome: a guide for practitioners and carers.* Chichester: John Wiley & Sons, 1998.

263. Matson JL, et al. Behavioral treatment of autistic persons: a review of research from 1980 to the present. *Res Dev Disabil* 1996;17:433–465.

264. Quill K. *Enhancing children's social-communicative interactions. Teaching children with autism: strategies to enhance communication and socialization.* New York: Delmar, 1995:163–192.

265. Rutter M. Infantile autism. In: Shaffer D, Ehrhardt AA, Greenhill LL, eds. *The clinical guide to child psychiatry.* New York: Free Press, 1985:48–78.

266. Schopler EA. Statewide program for the treatment and education of autistic and related communication handicapped children (TEACCH). In: Volkmar F, ed. *Child and adolescent psychiatric clinics of North America: psychoses and pervasive developmental disorders.* Philadelphia: WB Saunders, 1994: 91–103.

267. Lord C. Facilitating social inclusion. In: Schopler E, Mesibov GB, eds. *Learning and cognition in autism.* New York: Plenum Publishing, 1995:221–239.

268. Mesibov GB. A comprehensive program for serving people with autism and their families: the TEACCH model. In: Matson JL, ed. *Autism in children and adults: etiology, assessment and intervention.* Belmont, CA: Brooks-Cole, 1995:85–97.

269. Gillberg C, et al. Auditory integration training in children with autism: brief report of an open pilot study. *Autism* 1997;1:97–100.

270. Bettison S. The long-term effects of auditory training in children with autism. *J Autism Dev Disord* 1996; 26:361–374.

271. McEachin J, Smith T, Lovaas O. Long-term outcome for children with autism who received early intensive behavioral treatment. *Am J Ment Retard* 1993;4: 359–372.

272. Bebko JM, Perry A, Bryson S. Multiple method validation study of facilitated communication. II. Individual differences and subgroup results. *J Autism Dev Disord* 1996;26:19–42.

273. Howlin P. Prognosis in autism: do specialist treatments affect outcome? *Eur Child Adolesc Psychiatry* 1997;6:55–72.

274. Reichelt KL, Ekrem J, Scott H. Gluten, milk proteins, and autism: dietary intervention effects on behavior and peptide secretion. *J Appl Nutrit* 1990;42:1–11.

275. Horvath K, et al. Improved social skills after secretin administration in patients with autistic spectrum disorders. *J Assoc Acad Minor Phys* 1998; 9–15.

276. American Academy of Pediatrics. The Doman-Delacato treatment of neurologically handicapped children. *Pediatrics* 1982;70:810–812.

277. Mason SM, Iwata BA. Artifactual effects of sensory integrative therapy on self-injurious behaviour. *J Appl Behav Anal* 1990;26:361–370.

278. Hoehn TP, Baumeister M. A critique of the application of sensory integration therapy to children with learning disabilities. *J Learn Disabil* 1994;27:338–350.

279. Burden V, et al. The Cambridge language and speech project (CLASP). I. Detection of language difficulties at 36 to 39 months. *Dev Med Child Neurol* 1996; 38:613–631.

280. Tomblin JB, et al. Prevalence of specific language impairment in kindergarten children. *J Speech Lang Hear Res* 1997;40:1245–1260.

281. Stem LM, et al. The Adelaide preschool language unit: results of follow-up. *J Paediatr Child Health* 1995;31:207–212.

282. Silva PA, Williams S, McGee R. A longitudinal study of children with developmental language delay at age three: later intelligence, reading, and behaviour problems. *Dev Med Child Neurol* 1987;29:630–640.

283. Werker JF. The effects of multilingualism on phonetic perceptual flexibility. *Applied Psycholinguistics* 1986;7:141–156.

284. Lenneberg EH, Rebelsky FG, Nichols IA. The vocalization of infants born to deaf and to hearing parents. *Vita Humana* 1965;8:23–37.

285. Franco F, Butterworth G. Pointing and social awareness: declaring and requesting in the second year. *J Child Lang* 1996;307–336.

286. Bates E, Thal D, Janowsky JS. Early language development and its neural correlates. In: Segalowitz SJ, Rapin I, eds. *Handbook of neuropsychology,* Vol. 7. New York: Elsevier Science, 1992: 69–110.

287. Capute AJ, Accardo PJ. Linguistic and auditory milestones during the first two years of life: a language inventory for the practitioner. *Clin Pediatr* 1978;17: 847–853.

288. Thal D, Tobias S, Morrison D. Language and gestures in late talkers: a one-year follow-up. *J Speech Hear Disord* 1991;34:604–612.

289. Tallal P, Stark RE, Mellits ED. Identification of language-impaired children on the basis of rapid perception and production skills. *Brain Lang* 1985;25: 314–322.

290. Nass R. Language development in children with congenital strokes. *Semin Pediatr Neurol* 1997;4:109–116.

291. Woods BT, Teuber HL. Changing patterns of childhood aphasia. *Ann Neurol* 1978;3:273–280.

292. Vargha-Khadem F, Isaacs EB, Papleloudi H. Development of language in six hemispherectomized patients. *Brain* 1991;114:473–495.

293. Dall'Oglio AM, et al. Early cognition, communication, and language in children with focal brain injury. *Dev Med Child Neurol* 1994;36:1076–1098.

294. Hiscock M, Kinsbourne M. Phylogeny and ontogeny of cerebral lateralization. In: Davidson R and Hugdahl K, eds. *Brain asymmetry.* Cambridge, MA: MIT Press, 535–578.

295. Duchowny M, et al. Language cortex representation: effects of developmental versus acquired pathology. *Ann Neurol* 1996;40:37–38.

296. Wada J, Rasmussen T. Intracarotid injections of sodium amytal for clinical observations. *J Neurosurg* 1960;17:266–282.

297. Kinsbourne M. The minor cerebral hemisphere as a source of aphasic speech. *Arch Neurol* 1971;25: 302–306.

298. Chiarello C. A house divided? Cognitive functioning with callosal agenesis. *Brain Lang* 1980;11:128–158.

299. Nass R, Koch D. Differential effects of early unilateral brain damage on temperament. *Dev Neuropsychol* 1987;3:93–99.

300. Travis LS. *Handbook of speech pathology and audiology.* New York: Appleton-Century-Crofts, 1971.

301. Kools JA, et al. Oral and limb apraxia in mentally retarded children with deviant articulation. *Cortex* 1971; 7:387–400.

302. Braun AR, et al. Altered patterns of cerebral activity during speech and language production in developmental stuttering. An H2(15)O positron emission tomography study. *Brain* 1997;120:761–784.

303. Fox PT, et al. A PET study of the neural systems of stuttering. *Nature* 1996;382:158–161.

304. Geschwind N. Why Orton was right. *Ann Dyslexia* 1982;13–30.

305. Bishop DVM. *Handedness and developmental disorder: clinics in developmental medicine.* Oxford: Blackwell Science, 1990:110.

306. Hancock K, et al. Two- to six-year controlled-trial stuttering outcomes for children and adolescents. *J Speech Lang Hear Res* 1998;41:1242–1252.

307. DeFusio EN, Menken M. Symptomatic cluttering in adults. *Brain Lang* 1979;8:25–33.

308. Mathinos DA. Communication competence of children with learning disabilities. *J Learn Disabil* 1988; 21:437–443.

309. Kolvin I, Fundudis T. Elective mute children: psychological development and background factors. *J Child Psychol Psychiatry* 1981;22:219–232.

310. Kinsbourne M. The neuropsychology of bilingualism. *Ann N Y Acad Sci* 1981;379:50–58.

311. Singh JA, Zingg RM. *Wolf children and feral man.* New York: Harper & Row, 1942.

312. Davis K. Final note on a case of extreme isolation. *Am J Sociol* 1947;52:432.

313. Curtis S. *Genie: a psycholinguistic study of a modern day "Wild Child."* New York: Academic Press, 1977.

314. Johnson J, Newport E. Critical period effects in second language learning: the influence of maturational state on the acquisition of English as a second language. *Cogn Psychol* 1989; 21:60–99.

315. Mogford K. Oral language acquisition in the prelinguistically deaf. In: Bishop D, Mogford K, eds. *Language development in exceptional circumstances.* Edinburgh: Churchill Livingstone,1988:110–131.

316. Mayberry RI, Eichen EB. The long-lasting advantage of learning sign language in childhood: another look at the critical period for language acquisition. *J Mem Lang* 1991;30:486–512.

317. Poizner J, Klima ES, Bellugi U. *What the hands reveal about the brain.* Cambridge, MA: MIT Press, 1987.

318. Dempsey C. Selecting tests of auditory function in children. In: Lasky EZ, Katz J, eds. *Central auditory processing disorders.* Baltimore: University Park Press, 1983:203–222.

319. Gascon GG, Johnson R, Burd L. Central auditory processing and attention deficit disorders. *J Child Neurol* 1986;1:27–33.

320. Klein SK, Rapin I. Intermittent conductive hearing loss and language development. In: Bishop D, Mogford K, eds. *Language development in exceptional circumstances.* London: Churchill Livingstone, 1988:96–109.

321. Silva PA, McGee R, Williams S. Developmental language delay from three to seven years and its signficance for low intelligence and reading difficulties at age seven. *Dev Med Child Neurol* 1983;25: 783–793.

322. Wolfus B, Moscovitch M, Kinsbourne M. Subtypes of developmental language impairment. *Brain Lang* 1980; 10:152–171.

323. Rapin I, Allen DA. Developmental language disorders: nosological considerations. In: Kirk U, ed. *Neuropsychology of language, reading, and spelling.* New York: Academic Press, 1983: 155–184.

324. Tallal P, Stark RE, Mellits D. The relationship between auditory temporal analysis and receptive language development: evidence from studies of developmental language disorder. *Neuropsychologia* 1985; 23:527–534.

325. Cohen M, Campbell R, Yaghmai F. Neuropathological abnormalities in developmental dysphasia. *Ann Neurol* 1989;25:567–570.

326. Van Hout A. Acquired aphasia in children. *Semin Pediatr Neurol* 1997;4:102–108.

327. Cranberg LD, et al. Acquired aphasia in childhood clinical and CT investigations. *Neurology* 1987;37: 1165–1172.

328. Stiles J. The effect of early brain injury on lateralization of cognitive function. *Curr Direct Psychol Science* 1998;7:21–26.

329. Van Dongen HR, Loonen MCB. Factors related to prognosis of acquired aphasia in children. *Cortex* 1977;13:131–136.

330. Cooper JA, Flowers CR. Children with a history of acquired aphasia: residual language and academic impairment. *J Speech Hear Disord* 1987;52:251–262.

331. Appleton RE. The Landau-Kleffner syndrome. *Arch Dis Child* 1995;72:386–387.

332. Lahey M. Who shall be called language disordered? Some reflections and one perspective. *J Speech Hear Disord* 1990;55:612–620.

333. Binnie CD, et al. Interactions of epileptiform EEG discharges and cognition. *Epilepsy Res* 1987;1:239–245.

334. da Silva EA, et al. Landau-Kleffner syndrome: metabolic abnormalities in temporal lobe are a common feature. *J Child Neurol* 1997;12:489–495.

335. Kim KHS, et al. Distinct cortical areas associated with native and second languages. *Nature* 1997;388: 171–174.

336. Friedrich U, et al. Chromosomal studies of children and developmental language retardation. *Dev Med Child Neurol* 1982;24:645–652.

337. Ratcliffe SG. Speech and learning disorders in children with sex chromosome abnormalities. *Dev Med Child Neurol* 1982;24:80–84.

338. Mazzocco MM, Myers GF, Hamner JL, Panoscha R. The prevalence of the FMR1 and FMR2 mutations among preschool children with language delay. *J Pediatr* 1998;132:795–801.

339. Cantwell DP, Baker C. Association between attention-deficit hyperactivity disorder and learning disorders. *J Learn Disabil* 1991;24:88–95.

340. Allen DA, Mendelson L, Rapin I. Syndrome-specific remediation in preschool developmental dysphasia. In: French JH, Havel S, Casser P, eds. *Child neurology and developmental disabilities.* Baltimore: Brooks, 1989: 233–243.

341. Tallal P. Developmental language disorders. In: Kavanagh JF, Truss TJ, eds. *Learning disorders*. Parkton, MD: York Press, 1988:181–272.

342. Owens RE, House LI. Decision-making process in augmentative communication. *J Speech Hearing Disord* 1984;47:18–25.

343. Amir N, Seligman-Wine J, Gross-Tsur V. The role of augmentative communication in impaired language acquisition. In: Amir N, Rapin I, Bianski D, eds. *Pediatric neurology: behavior and cognition of the child with brain dysfunction*, Vol 1. Basel: Karger, 1991:129–145.

344. Bilken D. Communication unbound. *Harv Educ Rev* 1990;60:291–314.

345. Cummus RA, Prior MP. Autism and assisted communication: a response to Bilken. *Harv Educ Rev* 1992; 62:228–241.

346. Kavanagh JF, Truss TJ. *Learning disabilities*. Parkton, MD: York Press, 1988.

347. Lyon GR. Toward a definition of dyslexia. *Ann Dyslexia* 1995;45:3–27.

348. Siegel L. IQ is irrelevant to the definition of learning disabilities. *J Learn Disabil* 1989;22:469–478.

349. Moores DF. *Educating the deaf: psychology, principles, and practices*, 3rd ed. Boston: Houghton-Mifflin, 1987.

350. Ross M. *Hard-of-hearing children in regular schools*. Englewood Cliffs, NJ: Prentice-Hall, 1982.

351. U.S. Department of Education. 17th annual report to Congress on the implementation of IDEA.

352. Shaywitz SE, et al. Prevalence of reading disability in boys and girls. Results of the Connecticut Longitudinal Study. *JAMA* 1990;264:998–1002.

353. Gibson EJ, Levin H. *The psychology of reading*. Cambridge: Harvard University Press, 1975.

354. Kinsbourne M. Looking and listening strategies and beginning reading. In: Guthrie JT, ed. *Aspects of reading acquisition*. Baltimore: The Johns Hopkins University Press,1976:141–161.

355. Stanovitch K. Explaining the variance in reading ability in terms of psychological processes: what have we learned? *Ann Dyslexia* 1986;35:67–96.

356. Stevenson H. Orthography and reading disabilities. *J Learn Disabil* 1984;18:132–135.

357. Rutter M, Yule W. The concept of specific reading retardation. *J Child Psychol Psychiatry* 1975;16: 181–197.

358. Nelson HE, Warrington EK. Developmental spelling retardation. In: Knights RM, Bakker DJ, eds. *The neuropsychology of learning disorders: theoretical approaches*. Baltimore: University Park Press, 1976: 325–332.

359. Lyon GR. Research initiatives in learning disabilities: contributions from scientists supported by the National Institute of Child Health and Human Development. *J Child Neurol* 1995;10:120–S126.

360. Gleitman LR, Rozin P. The structure and acquisition of reading. I. Relations between orthographies and the structure of language. In: Reber AJ, Scarborough DL, eds. *Toward a psychology of reading*. Hillsdale, NJ: Erlbaum, 1977.

361. Bradley L, Bryant P. Categorizing sounds and learning to read—a causal connection. *Nature* 1983;301: 419–421.

362. Tallal P. Auditory temporal perception, phonics, and reading disabilities in children. *Brain Lang* 1980;9: 182–198.

363. Eden GF, et al. Temporal and spatial processing in reading disabled and normal children. *Cortex* 1995;31:451–468.

364. Rutter M. The concept of dyslexia. In: Wolff DH, MacKeith R, eds. *Planning for better learning: clinics for developmental medicine*: 33. London: Heinemann Medical Books, 1969:129–139.

365. Gordon H. Delayed readers are cognitively right. In: Kinsbourne M, ed. *The brain basis of learning disability. Topics in learning and learning disability*, Vol. 3. 1983:29–39.

366. Reynolds AM, Elksnin N, Brown FRI. Specific reading disabilities: early identification and long-term outcome. *MRDD Research Reviews* 1996;2: 21–27.

367. Denckla M. Motor coordination in dyslexic children. In: Duffy F, Geschwind N, eds. *Dyslexia*. Boston: Little, Brown and Company, 1987.

368. Landman GB, et al. Minor neurological indicators and developmental function in preschool children. *J Dev Behav Ped* 1986;7:97–101.

369. Duffy FH, et al. Dyslexia: automated diagnosis by computerized classification of brain electrical activity. *Ann Neurol* 1980;7:421–428.

370. Lou HC, Hendrikson L, Bruhn P. Focal cerebral hypoperfusion in children with dysphasia and/or attention deficit disorder. *Arch Neurol* 1984;41: 825–829.

371. Galaburda AM, et al. Developmental dyslexia: four consecutive patients with cortical anomalies. *Ann Neurol* 1985;18:222–233.

372. Galaburda A, Eidelberg D. Symmetry and asymmetry in the human posterior-thalamus. *Arch Neurol* 1982;39:333–336.

373. Denckla MB, LeMay M, Chapman CT. No CT scan abnormalities found even in neurologically impaired learning disabled children. *J Learn Disabil* 1985;18: 132–135.

374. Johnson D, Balock J. *Adults with learning disabilities*. Orlando: Grune & Stratton, 1987.

375. Kinsbourne M, et al. Neuropsychological deficits in adults with dyslexia. *Dev Med Child Neurol* 1991;33: 763–775.

376. Yule W, Rutter M. Reading and intelligence. In: Knights R, Bakker J, eds. *Neuropsychology of language disorders: theoretical approaches*. Baltimore: University Park Press, 1976.

377. Finucci JM, et al. Derivation and validation of a quantitative definition of specific reading disability for adults. *Dev Med Child Neurol* 1984;26:143–153.

378. Finucci J, Childs B. Are there really more dyslexic boys than girls? In: Ansarer A, Geschwind N, Galaburda A, eds. *Sex differences in dyslexia*. Baltimore, MD: The Orton Society, 1981.

379. LaBuda M, DeFries J. Genetic and environmental etiologies of reading disability: a twin study. *Ann Dyslexia* 1988;38:131–138.

380. Pennington BF. Using genetics to understand dyslexia. *Ann Dyslexia* 1989;39:81–93.

381. Alberman E. The early prediction of learning disorder. *Dev Med Child Neurol* 1973;15:202–204.

382. Vellutino TR. *Dyslexia: theory and research*. Cambridge, MA: MIT Press, 1979.

383. Gough PB, Tunmer WE. Decoding, reading, and reading disability. *Remedial and Special Education* 1986;7:6–10.

384. Shankweiler D, Liberman IY. *Phonology and reading disability*. Ann Arbor: University of Michigan Press, 1989.

385. Meyer MS, et al. Selective predictive value of rapid automatized naming in poor readers. *J Learn Disabil* 1998;31:106–117.

386. Kinsbourne M, Warrington EK. Developmental factors in reading and writing backwardness. *Br J Psychol* 1963;54: 145–156.

387. Satz P, Morris R. Learning disability subtypes: a review. In: Pirozzolo FJ, Wittrock MC, eds. *Neuropsychologic and cognitive processes in reading*. New York: Academic Press, 1981.

388. Doehring DG, Hoschko IM. Classification of reading problems by the Q-technique of factor analysis. *Cortex* 1977;13:281–294.

389. Mattis S, French JH, Rapin I. Dyslexia in children and young adults: three independent neuropsychological syndromes. *Devel Med Child Neurol* 1975;17: 150–163.

390. Bakker DJ. Hemispheric differences and reading strategies. *Bull Orton Soc* 1979;29:84–100.

391. Lovett MW. A developmental perspective on reading dysfunction: accuracy and rate criteria in the subtyping of dyslexic children. *Brain Lang* 1984;22:67–91.

392. Geiger G, Lettvin JY. Peripheral vision in persons with dyslexia. *N Engl J Med* 1987;316:1238–1243.

393. Slaghuis WL, Lovegrove WJ. Spatial-frequency-dependent visible persistence and specific reading disability. *Brain Cogn* 1985;4:219–240.

394. Livingstone MS, Rosen GD, Drislane FW, Galaburda AM. Physiological and anatomical evidence for a magnocellular defect in developmental dyslexia. *Proc Nat Acad Sci U S A* 1991;88:7943–7947.

395. Lehmkuhle S, et al. A defective visual pathway in children with reading disability. *N Engl J Med* 1993;328:989–996.

396. Boder E. Developmental dyslexia: prevailing diagnostic concepts and a new diagnostic approach through patterns of reading and spelling. In: Myklebust HR, ed. *Progress in learning diabilities*. Vol II. New York: Grune & Stratton, 1971.

397. Boder E, Jarrico S. *The Boder Test of Reading-Spelling Patterns*. New York: Grune &Stratton, 1982.

398. Fried I, et al. Developmental dyslexia: electrophysiological evidence of clinical subgroups. *Brain Lang* 1981;12:14–22.

399. Satz P. Pathological left-handedness: an explanatory model. *Cortex* 1972;8:121–135.

400. McAnulty GB, Hicks RE, Kinsbourne M. Personal and familial sinistrality in relation to degree of mental retardation. *Brain Cogn* 1984;3:349–356.

401. Hicks RE, Kinsbourne M. On the genesis of human handedness: a review. *J Motor Behav* 1976;8:257–266.

402. Geschwind N, Behan P. Left-handedness: association with immune disease, migraine, and developmental learning disorder. *Proc Natl Acad Sci U S A* 1982;79: 5097–5100.

403. Crawford SG, Kaplan BJ, Kinsbourne M. The effects of parental immunoreactivity on pregnancy, birth, and cognitive development: maternal immune attack on the fetus? *Cortex* 1992;28:483–491.

404. Porac C, Cohen S. *Lateral preferences and human behavior*. New York: Springer-Verlag, 1981.

405. Witelson SF. Developmental dyslexia: two right hemispheres and none left. *Science* 1977;195: 309–311.

406. Hiscock M, Kinsbourne M. Progress in the measurement of laterality and implications for dyslexia research. *Ann Dyslexia* 1995;45:249–268.

407. Geier S. Minor seizures and behavior. *Electroencephalogr Clin Neurophysiol* 1971;31:499–507.

408. Schultz RT, et al. Brain morphology in normal and dyslexic children: the influences of sex and age. *Ann Neurol* 1994;35:732–742.

409. Leonard CM, et al. Anomalous cerebral structure in dyslexia revealed with magnetic resonance imaging. *Arch Neurol* 1993;50:461–469.

410. Stein JF, Riddell PM, Fowler S. Disordered vergence control in dyslexic children. *Br J Ophthalmol* 1988;72: 162–166.

411. Comelissen P, et al. Covering one eye affects how some children read. *Dev Med Child Neurol* 1992;34: 296–304.

412. Polatajko HJ. A critical look at vestibular dysfunction in learning disabled children. *Dev Med Child Neurol* 1985;27:283–292.

413. Gallico RP, Burns TJ, Grob CS. *Emotional and behavioral problems in children with learning disabilities*. Boston: Little, Brown and Company, 1988.

414. Fisher SE, et al. A quantitative-trait locus on chromosome 6p influences different aspects of developmental dyslexia. *Am J Hum Genet* 1999;64:146–156.

415. Grigorenko EL, et al. Susceptibility loci for distinct components of developmental dyslexia on chromosomes 6 and 15. *Am J Hum Genet* 1997;60:27–39.

416. Fagerheim T, et al. A new gene (DYX3) for dyslexia is located on chromosome 2. *J Med Genet* 1999;36:664–669.

417. Flowers DL, Wood FB, Naylor CE. Regional cerebral blood flow correlates of language processes in reading disability. *Arch Neurol* 1991;48:637–643.

418. Gross-Glenn K, et al. Positron emission tomographic studies during serial word-reading by normal and dyslexic adults. *J Clin Exp Neuropsychol* 1991;13–4: 531–544.

419. Rumsey JM, et al. Right frontotemporal activation by tonal memory in dyslexia, an O15 PET study. *Biol Psychiatry* 1994;36:171–180.

420. Rumsey JM, et al. Normal activation of frontotemporal language cortex in dyslexia as measured with oxygen 15 positron emission tomography. *Arch Neurol* 1994;51:27–38.

421. Rumsey JM, et al. A positron emission tomographic study of impaired word recognition and phonological processing in dyslexic men. *Arch Neurol* 1997;54: 562–573.

421a. Shaywitz SE, et al. Functional disruption in the organization of the brain for reading in dyslexia. *Proc Nat Acad Sci USA* 1998;95:2636–2641.

422. Nichols PL, Chen T-C. *Minimal brain dysfunction: a prospective study*. Hillsdale, NJ: Erlbaum, 1981.

423. Spreen O. Adult outcome of reading disorders. In: Malatesha R, Aaron P, eds. *Reading disorders: varieties and treatments*. New York: Academic Press, 1982:473–498.

424. Ball EW, Blachman BA. Does phoneme awareness training in kindergarten make a difference in early

word recognition and development of spelling? *Read Res Quart* 1991;26:49–66.

425. The 1986/87 Future of Visual Development/Performance Task Force Special Report. The efficacy of optometric vision therapy. *J Am Optom Assoc* 1988;59:95–105.

426. Carte E, et al. Sensory integration therapy: a trial of a specific neurodevelopmental therapy for the remediation of learning disabilities. *J Dev Behav Pediatr* 1984;5:189–194.

427. Cummins RA. Sensory integration and learning disabilities: Ayers' factor analyses reappraised. *J Learn Disabil* 1991;24:160–168.

428. Tomatis A. *Education and dyslexia*. France, Quebec: Les Editions, 1978.

429. Aman MG, Werry JS. Methylphenidate and diazepam in severe mental retardation. *J Am Acad Child Adolesc Psychiatry* 1982;21:31–37.

430. Levinson HN. *A solution to the riddle dyslexia*. New York: Springer-Verlag, 1980.

431. Fagan JE, et al. The failure of antimotion sickness medication to improve reading in developmental dyslexia: results of a randomized trial. *J Dev Behav Pediatr* 1988;9:359–366.

432. McMahon JR, Gross RT. Physical and psychological effects of aerobic exercise in boys with learning disabilities. *J Dev Behav Pediatr* 1987;8:274–277.

433. Kohen-Raz RL. *Learning disabilities and postural control*. London: Freund, 1986.

434. American Academy of Ophthalmology. *Learning disabilities and children: what parents need to know*. San Francisco: American Academy of Ophthalmology, 1984.

435. Delacato CH. *The diagnosis and treatment of speech and reading problems*. Springfield, IL: Charles C Thomas, 1963.

436. Frostig M, Home D. *The Frostig Program for visual perception*. Chicago: Follett, 1964.

437. Rosen CL. An experimental study of visual perceptual training and reading achievement in first grade. *Percept Mot Skills* 1966;22:979–986.

438. Kirk SA, McCarthy JJ, Kirk WD. *Illinois Test of Psycholinguistic Abilities*. Urbana, IL: University of Illinois Press, 1968.

439. Wepman JM. *Auditory Discrimination test*. Western Psychological Services, 1973.

440. Roth SF, Beck IL. Theoretical and instructional implications of the assessment of two microcomputer word recognition programs. *Read Res Quart* 1987;22: 197–218.

441. Semrud-Clikeman M, Hynd GW. Right hemisphere dysfunction in nonverbal learning disabilities: social, academic, and adaptive functioning in adults and children. *Psychol Bull* 1990;107: 196–209.

442. Rourke B, Finlayson M. Neuropsychological significance of variations in patterns of academic performance: verbal and visuospatial abilities. *J Abnorm Child Psychol* 1978;6:121–133.

443. Shalev RS, Wurtmann R, Amir N. Developmental dyscalculia. *Cortex* 1988;24:555–561.

444. Ackerman P, Anhalt J, Dykman R. Arithmetic automatization failure in children with attention and reading disorders: associations and sequela. *J Learn Disabil* 1986;19:222–232.

445. Shalev RS, et al. Persistence of developmental dyscalculia: what counts? Results from a 3-year prospective follow-up study. *J Pediatr* 1998;133:320–321.

446. Badian N. Dyscalculia and nonverbal disorders of learning. In: Myklebust HR, ed. *Progress in learning disabilities*, Vol I. New York: Grune & Stratton, 1983:235–264.

447. Chandler HN. Confusion confounded: a teacher tries to use research results to teach maths. *J Learn Disabil* 1987;11:361–369.

448. Semrud-Clikeman M, Hynd GW. Right hemisphere dysfunction in nonverbal learning disabilities: social, academic, and adaptive functioning in adults and children. *Psychol Bull* 1990;107: 196–209.

449. Geary DC. Mathematical disabilities: cognitive, neuropsychological, and genetic components. *Psychol Bull* 1993;114:335–362.

450. Rourke BP, Fisk JL. Socio-emotional disturbances of learning disabled children: the role of central processing deficits. *Bull Orton Soc* 1981;31:77–88.

451. Mattson AJ, Sheer DE, Fletcher JM. Electrophysiological evidence of lateralized disturbances in children with learning disabilities. *J Clin Exp Neuropsychol* 1992;14:707–716.

452. Pennington BF, van Doorninck WJ. Neuropsychological deficits in early treated phenylketonuric children. *Am J Ment Def* 1985;89:467–474.

453. Pennington BF. Genetics of learning disabilities. *Semin Neurol* 1991;11:28–34.

454. Aldenkamp HP, et al. Neuropsychological aspects of learning disabilities in epilepsy. *Epilepsia* 1990;31 [Suppl 4]:9–20.

455. Eliason MJ. Neuropsychological patterns: neurofibromatosis compared to developmental learning disorders. *Neurofibromatosis* 1987;6:17–25.

456. North K, et al. Specific learning disability in children with neurofibromatosis type 1: significance of MRI abnormalities. *Neurology* 1994;44:878–883.

457. Sevick RJ, et al. Evolution of white-matter lesions in neurofibromatosis type 1: MR findings. *Am J Roentgenol* 1992;159:171–175.

458. Denckla MB. Neurofibromatosis type 1: a model for the pathogenesis of reading disability. *MRDD Research Reviews* 1996;2:48–53.

459. Dudley-Marling C, Edmiaster R. Social status of learning disabled children and adolescents: a review. *Learn Disabil Quart* 1985;8:189.

460. Hazel JS, Schumaker JB. Social skills and learning disabilities: current issues and recommendations for future research. In: Kavanagh F, Truss TJ, eds. *Learning disabilities: proceedings of the national conference*. Parkton, MD: York Press, 1988:293–344.

461. Gresham FM, Reschly DJ. Social skills, deficits and low peer acceptance of mainstreamed learning disabled children. *Learn Disabil Quart* 1986;9:23–32.

462. Gubbay SS. *The clumsy child. A study of developmental apraxic and agnosic ataxia*. Philadelphia: WB Saunders, 1975.

463. Hulme C, Smart A, Moran G. Visual perceptual deficits in clumsy children. *Neuropsychologia* 1982;20: 475–481.

464. Gordon N, McKinley I. *Helping clumsy children*. London: Churchill Livingstone, 1980.

465. Applegate B, et al. Validity of the age-of-onset criterion for ADHD: a report from the DSM-IV field trials. *J Am Acad Child Adolesc Psychiatry* 1997;36: 1211–1221.

466. Kaplan BJ, et al. Sleep disturbances in preschool-aged hyperactive and nonhyperactive children. *Pediatrics* 1987;80:839–844.

467. Cherrin RD, et al. Symptoms of sleep disorders, inattention, and hyperactivity in children. *Sleep* 1997; 20:1185–1192.

468. Palfrey JS, et al. The emergence of attention deficits in early childhood: a prospective study. *J Dev Behav Pediatr* 1985;6:339–348.

469. Stewart MA, Thach BT, Freidin MR. Accidental poisoning and the hyperactive child. *Dis Nerv Syst* 1970; 31:403–407.

470. Gerring JP, et al. Premorbid prevalence of ADHD and development of secondary ADHD after closed head injury. *J Am Acad Child Adolesc Psychiatry* 1998;37: 647–654.

471. Wolraich ML, et al. Comparison of diagnostic criteria for attention-deficit hyperactivity disorder in a countywide sample. *J Am Acad Child Adolesc Psychiatry* 1996;35:319–324.

472. Gaub M, Carlson CL. Gender differences in ADHD: a meta-analysis and critical review. *J Am Acad Child Adolesc Psychiatry* 1997;36:1036–1045.

473. Porrino LJ, et al. A naturalistic assessment of the motor activity of hyperactive boys. I. Comparison with normal controls. *Arch Gen Psychiatry* 1983;40:681–687.

474. Pelham W, Bender NE. Peer relationships in hyperactive children: description and treatment. *Adv Behav Disabil* 1982;1:365–435.

475. Levine MD, Oberklaid F, Meltzer L. Development output failure: a study of low productivity in school-age children. *Pediatrics* 1981;67:18–25.

476. Cantwell DP, Satterfield JH. The prevalence of academic underachievement in hyperactive children. *J Pediatr Psychol* 1978;3:168–197.

477. Lambert NM, Sandoval J. The prevalence of learning disabilities in a sample of children considered hyperactive. *J Abnorm Child Psychol* 1980;8: 33–50.

478. Ackerman PT, Dykman RA, Gardner MY. ADD students with and without dyslexia differ in sensitivity to rhyme and alliteration. *J Learn Disabil* 1990;23: 279–283.

479. Nigg JT, et al. Neuropsychological correlates of childhood attention-deficit/hyperactivity disorder: explainable by comorbid disruptive behavior or reading problems? *J Abnorm Psychol* 1996;107:468–480.

480. Kinsbourne M. Toward a model for the attention deficit disorder. In: Perlmutter M, ed. *Minnesota symposia in child development*. Hillsdale, NJ: Erlbaum, 1983:137–166.

481. Zametkin A, Rapoport JL. The neurobiology of attention deficit disorder with hyperactivity: where have we come in 50 years? *J Am Acad Child Adolesc Psychiatry* 1987;26:676–686.

482. Bhatia MS, et al. Attention deficit disorder with hyperactivity among paediatric outpatients. *J Child Psychol Psychiatry* 1991;32:297–306.

483. Szatmari P. The epidemiology of attention-deficit hyperactivity disorders. *Child Adolesc Psychiatry Clin North Am* 1992;1:361–371.

484. Wasserman RC, et al. Identification of attentional and hyperactivity problems in primary care: a report from pediatric research in office settings and the ambulatory sentinel practice network. *Pediatrics* 1999;103:E38.

485. Lambert MC, et al. Epidemiology of behavioral and emotional problems among children of Jamaica and the United States: parent reports for ages 6 to 11. *J Abnorm Child Psychol* 1994;22:113–128.

486. The ICD-10 classification of mental and behavioral disorders: clinical descriptions and diagnostic guidelines. 1992; World Health Organization.

487. Prendergast M, et al. The diagnosis of childhood hyperactivity: A US-UK cross-national study of DSM-III and ICD-9. *J Child Psychol Psychiatry* 1988;29: 289–300.

488. Hinshaw SP. On the distinction between attentional deficits/hyperactivity and conduct problems/aggression in childhood psychopathology. *Psychol Bull* 1987;101: 443–463.

489. Stewart MA, et al. The overlap between hyperactive and unsocialized aggressive children. *J Child Psychol Psychiatry* 1981;22:35–45.

490. Biederman J, Favarone SV, Laysey K. Comorbidity of diagnosis in attention-deficit hyperactivity disorder. *Child Adolesc Psychiatry Clin North Am* 1992;1: 335–358.

491. Streissguth AP, et al. Association of prenatal alcohol exposure with behavioral and learning problems in early adolescence. *J Am Acad Child Adolesc Psychiatry* 1997;36:1187–1194.

491a. Dennis M, et al. Attention deficits in the longterm after childhood head injury. In: Broma S, Michel ME (eds). *Traumatic head injury om children*. New York: Oxford University Press, 1995.

492. Astbury J, Orgill A, Bajuk B. Relationship between two-year behavior and neurodevelopmental outcome at five years of very low-birth-weight survivors. *Dev Med Child Neurol* 1987;29:370–379.

493. Klebanov PK, Brooks-Gunn J, McCormick MD. Classroom behavior of very low birth weight elementary school children. *Pediatrics* 1994;94:700–708.

494. Krouse JP, Kaufman JM. Morphological anomalies in exceptional children: a review and critique of research. *J Abnorm Child Psychol* 1972;10:247–264.

495. Menkes MM, Rowe JS, Menkes JH. A twenty-five year follow-up on the hyperkinetic child with minimal brain dysfunction. *Pediatrics* 1967;39:393–399.

496. Wender PH, Reimherr FW, Wood DR. Attention deficit disorder ("minimal brain dysfunction") in adults: a replication study of diagnosis and drug treatment. *Arch Gen Psychiatry* 1981;38:449–456.

497. Alberts-Corish J, Firestone P, Goodman JT. Attention and impulsivity characteristics of the biological and adoptive parents of hyperactive and normal control children. *Am J Orthopsychiatry* 1986;53:413–423.

498. Cantwell DP. Psychiatric illness in the families of hyperactive children. *Arch Gen Psychiatry* 1972;27: 414–417.

499. Lahey BB, et al. Psychopathology in the parents of children with conduct disorder and hyperactivity. *J Am Acad Child Adolesc Psychiatry* 1988;27:163–170.

500. Evans RW, Gaultieri CT, Hicks RE. A neuropathic substrate for stimulant drug effects in hyperactive children. *Clin Neuropharmacol* 1986;9:264–281.

501. LaHoste GJ, et al. Dopamine D4 receptor gene polymorphism is associated with attention deficit hyperactivity disorder. *Mol Psychiatry* 1996;1:121–124.

502. Gill M, et al. Confirmation of association between attention-deficit hyperactivity disorder and a

dopamine transporter polymorphism. *Mol Psychiatry* 1997;2:311–313.

502a. Doughety DD, et al. Dopamine transporter density in patients with attention deficit hyperactivity disorder. *Lancet* 1999;354:2132–2133.

503. Zentall SS, Meyer MJ. Self-regulation of stimulation for ADD-H children during reading and vigilance task performance. *J Abnorm Child Psychol* 1987;15: 519–536.

504. Castellanos FX, et al. Quantitative morphology of the caudate nucleus in attention-deficit hyperactivity disorder. *Am J Psychiatry* 1994;151:1791–1796.

505. Lou HC, L, et al. Striatal dysfunction in attention deficit and hyperkinetic disorder. *Arch Neurol* 1990;46:48–52.

506. Matochik JA, et al. Cerebral glucose metabolism in adults with attention-deficit hyperactivity disorder after chronic stimulant treatment. *Am J Psychiatry* 1994; 151:658–664.

507. Satterffield JH, et al. Topographic study of auditory-event related potentials in normal boys and boys with attention deficit disorder with hyperactivity. *Psychophysiology* 1988;25:591–606.

508. Zametkin AJ, et al. Brain metabolism in teenagers with attention-deficit hyperactivity disorder. *Arch Gen Psychiatry* 1993;50:333–340.

509. Hynd GW, et al. Attention-deficit hyperactivity disorder and asymmetry of the caudate nucleus. *J Child Neurol* 1993;8:339 347.

510. Aylward EH, et al. Basal ganglia volumes in children with attention-deficit hyperactivity disorder. *J Child Neurol* 1996;11:112–115.

511. Castellanos FX, et al. Quantitative brain magnetic resonance imaging in attention-deficit hyperactivity disorder. *Arch Gen Psychiatry* 1996;53:607–616.

512. Mostofsky SH, et al. Evaluation of cerebellar size in attention-deficit hyperactivity disorder. *J Child Neurol* 1998;13:434–439.

513. Goyette CH, Conners CK, Ulrich RF. Normative data on revised Conners Teacher and Parent Rating Scales. *J Abnorm Child Psychol* 1978;6:221–236.

514. Aylward EH, Whitehouse D. Learning disability with and without attention deficit disorders. In: Ceci SJ, ed. *Handbook of cognitive, social, and neuropsychological aspects of learning disabilities*. Hillsdale, NJ: Erlbaum Associates,1986–1987:321–342.

515. Swanson J, et al. A time-response analysis of the effect of stimulant medication on the learning ability of children referred for hyperactivity. *Pediatrics* 1978;61: 21–29.

516. Conners CK. The computerized continuous performance test. *Psychopharm Bull* 1985;21:891–892.

517. Keogh BK, Margolis JS. A component analysis of attentional problems of educationally handicapped boys. *J Abnorm Child Psychol* 1976;4:349–359.

518. Kagan J, Reznick JS, Snidman N. Biological bases of childhood shyness. *Science* 1988;40:167–171.

519. Nuechterlein KM. Signal detection in vigilance tasks and behavioral attributes among offspring of schizophrenic mothers and hyperactive children. *J Abnorm Psychol* 1983;92:4–28.

520. Akiskal HS, et al. Affective disorders in referred children and younger siblings of manic depressives. *Arch Gen Psychiatry* 1985;42:996–1003.

521. Rickler KC. Episodic dyscontrol. In: Benson F, Blumer A, eds. *Psychiatric aspects of neurologic disease*, Vol II. New York: Grune & Stratton, 1982.

522. Swedo SE, Leonard HL, Kiessling L. Speculations on antineuronal antibody-mediated neuropsychiatric disorders of childhood. *Pediatrics* 1994;93:323–326.

523. American Academy of Pediatrics Committee on Children with Disabilities and Committee on Drugs. Medication for children with attentional disorders. *Pediatrics* 1996;98:301–304.

524. McDaniel KD. Pharmacologic treatment of psychiatric and neurodevelopmental disorders in children and adolescents, Part 1. *Clin Pediatr (Phila)* 1986;25: 65–71.

525. Barkley RA. Hyperactive boys and girls: stimulant drug effects on mother-child interactions. *J Child Psychol Psychiatry* 1989;30:379–390.

526. Schachar R, et al. Changes in family function and relationships in children who respond to methylphenidate. *J Am Acad Child Adolesc Psychiatry* 1987;26: 728–732.

527. Swanson JM, et al. Effect of stimulant medication on children with attention deficit disorder: a "review of reviews." *Exceptional Children* 1993;60: 154–162.

528. Brown RT, Sleator EK. Methylphenidate in hyperkinetic children: differences in dose effects on impulsive behavior. *Pediatrics* 1979;64:408–411.

529. Rapport MD, duPaul GJ, Kelly KL. Attention-deficit hyperactivity disorder and methylphenidate: the relationship between gross body weight and drug response in children. *Psychopharm Bull* 1989;25:285–290.

530. Greenhill LL, et al. Medication treatment strategies in the MTA study: relevance to clinicians and researchers. *J Am Acad Child Adolesc Psychiatry* 1996;35:1–10.

531. Lowe TL, et al. Stimulant medications precipitate Tourette's syndrome. *JAMA* 1982;247:1729–1731.

532. Comings DE, Comings BG. Tourette's syndrome and attention deficit disorder with hyperactivity. *Arch Gen Psychiatry* 1987;44:1023–1026.

533. Price RA, et al. Gilles de la Tourette's syndrome. Tics and central nervous system stimulants in twins and non-twins. *Neurology* 1986;36:232–237.

534. Cohen AJ, Leckman JF. Sensory phenomena associated with Gilles de La Tourette. *J Clin Psychiatry* 1992;53:519–523.

535. Singer HS, et al. The treatment of attention-deficit hyperactivity disorder in Tourette's syndrome: a double-blind placebo-controlled study with clonidine and desipramine. *Pediatrics* 1995;95:74–81.

536. Roche AF, et al. The effects of stimulant medication on the growth of hyperkinetic children. *Pediatrics* 1979;63:847–850.

537. Gittelman-Klein R, Mannuzza S. Hyperactive boys almost grown up. III. Methylphenidate effects on ultimate height. *Arch Gen Psychiatry* 1988;45:1131–1134.

538. Kalachnik JE, et al. Effect of methylphenidate hydrochloride on stature of hyperactive children. *Dev Med Child Neurol* 1982;24:586–595.

539. Kilgore BS, et al. Alterations in cartilage metabolism by neurostimulant drugs. *J Pediatr* 1979;94:542–545.

540. Campbell SF, Douglas VI, Morgenstern G. Cognitive styles in hyperactive children and the effect of methylphenidate. *J Child Psychol Psychiatry* 1971;12: 55–67.

541. Feldman H, et al. Methylphenidate in children with seizures and attention-deficit disorder. *Am J Dis Child* 1989;143:1081–1086.

542. Gross-Tsur V, et al. Epilepsy and attention deficit disorder: is methylphenidate safe and effective? *J Pediatr* 1997;130:40–44.

543. Pelham WE, et al. Pemoline effects on children with ADHD: a time-response by dose-response analysis on classroom measures. *J Am Acad Child Adolesc Psychiatry* 1995;34:1504–1513.

544. Wroblewski BA, et al. Methylphenidate and seizure frequency in brain injured patients with seizure disorders. *J Clin Psychiatry* 1992;53:86–89.

545. Shevell M, Schreiber R. Pemoline-associated hepatic failure: a critical analysis of the literature. *Pediatr Neurol* 1997;16:141–146.

546. Greenhill LL. Pharmacotherapy: stimulants. *Child Adolesc Psychiatry Clin North Am* 1992;1:411–447.

547. Chappell PB, et al. Guanfacine treatment of comorbid attention-deficit hyperactivity disorder and Tourette's syndrome: preliminary clinical experience. *J Am Acad Child Adolesc Psychiatry* 1995;34:1140–1146.

548. Swanson JM, et al. Clonidine in the treatment of ADHD: questions about safety and efficacy. *J Child Adolesc Psychopharmacol* 1995;5:301–304.

549. Balldin J, et al. Guanfacine as an alpha-2-agonist inducer of growth hormone secretion: a comparison with clonidine. *Psychoneuroendocrinology* 1993;18:45–55.

550. Biederman J, Gastfriend DR, Jellinek MS. Desi-pramine in the treatment of children with attention deficit disorder. *J Clin Psychopharmacol* 1986; 6:359–363.

551. Gammon GD, Brown TE. Fluoxetine and methylphenidate in combination for treatment of attention deficit disorder and comorbid depressive disorder. *J Child Adolesc Psychopharmacol* 1993;3:1–10.

552. Popper CW. Antidepressants in the treatment of attention-deficit hyperactivity disorder. *J Clin Psychiatry* 1997;58:14–29.

553. Wolf SM, Forsythe A. Behavior disturbance, phenobarbital, and febrile seizures. *Pediatrics* 1978;61: 728–731.

554. Stein MA, et al. Behavioral and cognitive effects of methylxanthines. A meta-analysis of theophylline and caffeine. *Arch Pediatr Adolesc Med* 1996;150:284–288.

555. Feingold BF. *Why your child is hyperactive*. New York: Random House, 1975.

556. Swanson JM, Kinsbourne M. Food dyes impair performance of hyperactive children on a laboratory learning test. *Science* 1980;207:1485–1487.

557. Conners CK. *Food additives and hyperactive children*. New York: Plenum Publishing, 1980.

558. Kinsbourne M. Hyperactivity management. The impact of special diets. In: Levine MD, Satz P, eds. *Middle childhood: developmental variation and dysfunction between six and fourteen years*. New York: Appleton-Century-Crofts, 1984:487–499.

559. Egger J, et al. Controlled trial of oligoantigenic treatment in the hyperkinetic syndrome. *Lancet* 1985;1:540–545.

560. Kaplan BJ, et al. Dietary replacement in preschool-aged hyperactive boys. *Pediatrics* 1989;83:7–17.

561. Kinsbourne M. Sugar and the hyperactive child. *N Engl J Med* 1994;330:355–356.

562. Wolraich ML, Wilson DB, White JW. The effect of sugar on behavior or cognition in children. A meta-analysis. *JAMA* 1995;274:1617–1621.

563. Conners CK, Blouin AG. Nutritional effects on behavior of children. *J Psychiatr Res* 1982;17:193–201.

564. American Academy of Pediatrics: Committee on Nutrition. Megavitamin therapy for childhood psychoses and learning disabilities. *Pediatrics* 1971;58:910–911.

565. Haslam RH, Dalby JT, Rademaker AW. Effects of megavitamin therapy on children with attention deficit disorders. *Pediatrics* 1984;74:103–111.

566. Shaywitz BA, et al. Aspartame, behavior, and cognitive function in children with attention deficit disorder. *Pediatrics* 1994;93:70–75.

567. Satterfield JM, Satterfield BT, Schell AM. Therapeutic interventions to prevent delinquency in hyperactive boys. *J Am Acad Child Adolesc Psychiatry* 1987;26: 56–64.

568. Barkley RA. *Attention deficit hyperactivity disorder: a handbook for diagnosis and treatment*. New York: Guilford Press, 1990.

569. Doubros SG, Daniels GJ. An experimental approach to the reduction of overactive behavior. *Behav Res Ther* 1966;4:251–258.

570. Pelham WEJ, et al. Separate and combined effects of methylphenidate and behavior modification on boys with attention-deficit hyperactivity disorder in the classroom. *J Consult Clin Psychol* 1993;61:506–515.

571. Douglas VI, et al. Assessment of a cognitive training program for hyperactive children. *J Abnorm Child Psychol* 1976;4:389–410.

572. Abikoff H. Cognitive training in ADHD children: less to it than meets the eye. *J Learn Disabil* 1991;24:204–209.

573. Patterson GR, Guttman HM. Retraining of aggressive boys by their parents: review of recent literature and follow-up evaluation. *Canad Psychiatry Assoc J* 1974;19:142–161.

574. Gittelman M. *Strategic interventions for hyperactive children*. New York: Armonk, 1981.

575. Braswell L, Bloomquist ML. *Cognitive-behavioral therapy with ADHD children: child, family and school interventions*. New York: Guilford, 1991.

576. Swanson JM. *School-based assessments and interventions for ADD students*. Irvine, CA: KC Publications, 1992.

577. Latham P, Latham P. Who has a disability under the ADA? *Attention* 1999;6:40–42.

578. Mendelson W, Johnson N, Stewart M. Hyperactive children as teenagers: a follow-up study. *J Nerv Ment Dis* 1971;153:273–279.

579. Howell DC, Huessy HR. Hyperkinetic behavior followed from seven to twenty-one years of age. In: Gittelman M, ed. *Strategic interventions for hyperactive children*. New York: Sharpe, 1981:201–215.

580. Roy-Byrne P, et al. Adult attention-deficit hyperactivity disorder: assessment guidelines based on clinical presentation to a specialty clinic. *Compr Psychiatry* 1997;38:133–140.

581. Loney J, Kramer J, Milich R. The hyperactive child grows up: predictors of symptoms, delinquency, and achievement at follow-up. In: Gadow J, Loney J, eds. *Psychosocial aspects of drug treatment for hyperactivity*. Boulder, CO: Westview, 1981:381–415.

582. Kellam SG, Ensminger ME, Simon MB. Mental health in first grade and teenage drug, alcohol, and cigarette use. *Drug Alcohol Depend* 1980;5:273–304.

583. Tarter RE, Alterman AI, Edwards KL. Vulnerability to alcoholism in men: a behavior-genetic perspective. *J Stud Alcohol* 1985;46:329–356.

584. Linnoila VI, Virkkunen M. Aggression, suicidality, and serotonin. *J Clin Psychiatry* 1992;53[Suppl]: 46–51.

585. Marcus J, et al. Review of the NIMH Israeli Kibbutz-City Study and the Jerusalem Infant Development Study. *Schizophr Bull* 1987;13:425–438.

586. Alberts-Corish J, Firestone P, Goodman JT. Attention and impulsivity characteristics of the biological and adoptive parents of hyperactive and normal control children. *Am J Orthopsychiatry* 1986;53:413–423.

587. Lahey BB, et al. Psychopathology in the parents of children with conduct disorder and hyperactivity. *J Am Acad Child Adolesc Psychiatry* 1988;27:163–170.

588. Hauser P, et al. Attention-deficit hyperactivity disorder in people with generalized resistance to thyroid hormone. *N Engl J Med* 1993;328:997–1001.

589. Weiss RE, et al. Low intelligence but not attention-deficit hyperactivity disorder is associated with resistance to thyroid hormone caused by mutation R316H in the thyroid hormone receptor beta gene. *J Clin Endocrinol Metab* 1994;78:1525–1528.

590. Goodman R, Stevenson J. A twin study of hyperactivity. I. An examination of hyperactivity scores and categories derived from Rutter Teacher and Parent Questionnaires. *J Child Psychol Psychiatry* 1989;30:671–689.

591. Hechtman L. Families of children with attention deficit hyperactivity disorder: a review. *Can J Psychiatry* 1996;41:350–360.

592. Faraone SV, Biederman J. Genetics of attention-deficit hyperactivity disorder. *Child Adolesc Psychiatry Clin North Am* 1994;3:285–301.

593. Biederman J, et al. Family genetic and psychosocial risk factors in DSM-III attention deficit disorder. *J Am Acad Child Adolesc Psychiatry* 1990;29:526–533.

594. Faraone SV, Biederman J, Milberger S. An exploratory study of ADHD among second-degree relatives of ADHD children. *Biol Psychiatry* 1994;35:398–402.

595. Hynd GW, et al. Brain morphology in developmental dyslexia and attention-deficit hyperactivity. *Arch Neurol* 1990;47:919–926.

596. Casey BJ, et al. Implication of right frontostriatal circuitry in response inhibition and attention-deficit hyperactivity disorder. *J Am Acad Child Adolesc Psychiatry* 1997;36:374–383.

597. Baumgardner TL, et al. Corpus callosum morphology in children with Tourette's syndrome and attention-deficit hyperactivity disorder. *Neurology* 1996;47:1–5.

598. Semrud-Clikeman M, et al. Attention-deficit hyperactivity disorder: magnetic resonance imaging morphometric analysis of the corpus callosum. *J Am Acad Child Adolesc Psychiatry* 1994;33:875–881.

599. Filipek PA, et al. Volumetric MRI analysis comparing subjects having attention-deficit hyperactivity disorder with normal controls. *Neurology* 1997;48:589–601.

600. Lazzaro I, et al. Quantified EEG activity in adolescent attention-deficit hyperactivity disorder. *Clin Electroencephalogr* 1998;29:37–42.

601. Lahat E, et al. BAEP studies in children with attention-deficit hyperactivity disorder. *Dev Med Child Neurol* 1995;37:119–123.

602. Kinomura S, et al. Activation by attention of the human reticular formation and thalamic intralaminar nuclei. *Science* 1996;271:512–515.

603. Shaywitz BA, Yager RD, Klopper JM. Selective brain dopamine depletion in developing rats: an experimental model of minimal brain dysfunction. *Science* 1976;191:305–308.

604. Cook EHJ, et al. Association of attention-deficit disorder and the dopamine transporter gene. *Am J Hum Genet* 1995;56:993–998.

605. Mercugliano M. Neurotransmitter alterations in attention-deficit hyperactivity disorder. *MRDD Res Rev* 1995;1:220–226.

606. Castellanos FX. Toward a pathophysiology of attention-deficit hyperactivity disorder. *Clin Pediatr* 1997;36:381–393.

Index

Note: Page numbers followed by *f* indicate figures; page numbers followed by *t* indicate tables.

Sternocleidomastoid muscle
    testing in spinal accessory nerve examination, 9
    in torticollis, 454–455
Stevens-Johnson syndrome in anticonvulsant therapy,
        966, 974
Stiff baby syndrome, 189, 1066
Stiff man syndrome, 1066
Stimulant drugs in attention deficit-hyperactivity disorder,
        1193–1195, 1194t, 1196
Stimulation programs in cerebral palsy, 444
Stokes-Adams syndrome, 1003
Storage disorders, lysosomal. *See* Lysosomal
        storage diseases
Strabismus, 7
    in cerebral palsy, 444
Streptococcal infections
    autoimmune neuropsychiatric disorders in, 656, 657
    meningitis in, 468, 490–491
        frequency of, 469t
        and hydrocephalus, 474f
        in neonates, 492, 493
        prognosis in, 485, 486, 490
        treatment of, 482, 483, 483t, 484, 491
    pneumonia in, 491
    rheumatic fever and Sydenham chorea in, 652–657,
        1120, 1193
Streptomycin in tuberculous meningitis, 497
Stroke. *See* Cerebrovascular disorders
Strokelike episodes, in mitochondrial myopathy,
        encephalopathy, and lactic acidosis. *See*
        MELAS
Sturge-Weber syndrome, 872–876, 907
Stuttering, 1177–1178
Subarachnoid space
    cerebrospinal fluid in, 359, 360
        obstruction of, 364–365
    hemorrhage in. *See* Hemorrhage, subarachnoid
Subclavian steal syndrome, 1123
Subcortical laminar heterotopia, 299, 344, 346f
Subiculum, in pontosubicular degeneration, 416–417
Substance abuse
    in pregnancy, 758–759, 1167
        addiction of neonate in, 758–759, 991–992
        of alcohol, 750–752, 1167
        seizures of neonate in, 991–992
    of psychedelic drugs, 757
Substantia nigra
    in Parkinson's disease, juvenile, 186
    in phenylketonuria, 38
Sucrosuria, 66
Sugar and sweeteners in attention deficit-hyperactivity dis-
        order, 1195
Sulfadiazine in congenital toxoplasmosis, 513
Sulfatase deficiency, multiple, 219, 220
Sulfatide accumulation in metachromatic leukodystrophy,
        217–220
Sulfite oxidase deficiency, 131
Sulfur amino acids, metabolic disorders of, 55f, 55–59
Sumatriptan in migraine, 1001

Sunflower cataracts in Wilson disease, 126
Sunstroke, 733–734
Suprabulbar paresis, congenital, 381, 451
Surgery
    in aneurysms, intracranial, 908
    in brachial plexus injury, perinatal, 453
    in brain abscess, 503
    in brain tumors, 802–803
        of brainstem, 826
        of cerebellum, 820, 821, 822
        of cerebral hemispheres, 841
        in craniopharyngioma, 832, 833
        of optic pathway, 834–835
        of pineal region, 837
    cardiac, 1120
        neurologic complications in, 1121–1123
    in cavernous angioma, 906
    in cerebral arteriovenous malformations, 903
    in cerebral palsy, 442–443
    in coarctation of aorta, spinal cord trauma in, 1118
    in craniosynostosis, 354
    in diplomyelia and diastematomyelia, 328
    in facial nerve palsy, 667
    in Galen vein malformations, 905
    in hydrocephalus, 371–376
        in Dandy-Walker syndrome, 364
        fetal (intrauterine), 366
    in moyamoya disease, 892
    in myasthenia gravis, 1045
    in neurodermal sinus, 330
    in pseudotumor cerebri, 373, 848
    in seizures, 976–981
        in chronic focal encephalitis, 590
    shunt procedures in. *See* Shunt procedures
    in spina bifida
        cystica, 320–321
        occulta, 323
        results of, 323–324
    in spinal cord injuries, 729–730
    in spinal cord tumors, 845, 846
    in Sturge-Weber syndrome, 875
    in subdural hematoma, 719–720
    in syringomyelia, 329
    transplantation procedures in. *See* Transplantation
Survival motor neuron *(SMN)* gene, 285t, 295, 1032, 1034
Sutures, cranial, in craniosynostosis, 351–354
Swallowing problems
    in cerebral palsy, 444
    in rabies, 547
Swash-Schwartz disease, 1073
Sydenham chorea, 652–657, 1120
    differential diagnosis of, 1193
    hand positions in, 653, 654f
Sydney line, 268f
Sympathetic dystrophy, reflex, 733
Sympathomimetics, neurotoxicity of, 744t
Synapses, 301
    affecting apoptosis, 295
    excitatory, 928–929